Primary Care for Women

Second Edition

Primary Care for Women

Second Edition

Editors

Phyllis C. Leppert, MD, PhD

Adjunct Professor of Obstetrics and Gynecology
St. Louis University
St. Louis, Missouri

Jeffrey F. Peipert, MD, MPH, MHA

Professor of Obstetrics, Gynecology, and Community Health
Brown University Medical School
Director, Division of Research
Department of Obstetrics and Gynecology
Women and Infants Hospital
Providence, Rhode Island

Lippincott Williams & Wilkins
A **Wolters Kluwer** Company
Philadelphia • Baltimore • New York • London
Buenos Aires • Hong Kong • Sydney • Tokyo

Acquisitions Editor: Lisa McAllister
Developmental Editor: Alyson Forbes
Production Editor: Thomas Boyce
Manufacturing Manager: Benjamin Rivera
Cover Designer: Jeane Norton
Compositor: Lippincott Williams & Wilkins Desktop Division
Printer: Quebecor World–Taunton

530 Walnut Street
Philadelphia, PA 19106 USA
LWW.com

Library of Congress Cataloging-in-Publication Data
Primary care for women / edited by Phyllis C. Leppert, Jeffrey F. Peipert.—2nd ed.
p. ; cm.
Includes bibliographical references and index.
ISBN 0-7817-3790-7
1. Women—Diseases. 2. Women—Health and hygiene. 3. Primary care (Medicine)
I. Leppert, Phyllis Carolyn. II. Peipert, Jeffrey F.
[DNLM: 1. Women's Health. 2. Primary Health Care. 3. Sex Factors. WA 309 P9521 2004]
RC48.6.P75 2004
616′.0082—dc21

2003051686

---

10 9 8 7 6 5 4 3 2 1

To my mother Alice and my brother Mark
for their support and encouragement throughout my career
as a physician-scientist
With love and great respect, PCL

To my wife, Joyce, my children, Ben, Daniel, Allison, and Leah,
my parents, and sister, Julie,
who have been so supportive and understanding
during my life-long education and career
With love, JFP

and

To young investigators everywhere
who will provide the fundamental knowledge for the
next generation of evidence-based primary care for women

Contents

PART 4
Endocrine Problems

PART 5
Cardiovascular Disease

PART 6
Respiratory Problems

PART 7
Gastrointestinal Problems

PART 8
Urinary Tract Problems

Contributing Authors

Roy K. Aaron, MD
100 Butler Drive, Providence, Rhode Island

Saurabh Agarwal, MD
Resident, Department of Urology, Brown University, Rhode Island Hospital, Providence, Rhode Island

Vivian C. Aguilar, MD
Teaching Fellow in Urogynecology, Department of Obstetrics and Gynecology, Division of Urogynecology and Reconstructive Pelvic Surgery, Women and Infants Hospital, Brown University School of Medicine, Providence, Rhode Island

Yousaf Ali, MD, FACR
Assistant Clinical Professor of Medicine, Brown University, Providence, Rhode Island

Scott D. Allen, MD
Clinical Assistant Professor, Department of Medicine, Brown University Medical School, Providence, Rhode Island

Seetharaman Ashok, MD
Resident, Department of Urology, Brown University, Rhode Island Hospital, Providence, Rhode Island

Trimble S. Augur, MD
Department of Internal Medicine, Rhode Island Hospital, Brown University School of Medicine, Providence, Rhode Island

Marie Aydelotte, MD
Clinical Assistant Professor of Medicine, University of Rochester, Rochester, New York

George F. Aziz, MD
Division of Cardiology, The Miriam Hospital, Brown Medical School, Providence, Rhode Island

Gloria Bachmann, MD
Associate Dean of Women's Health, Women's Health Institute, Robert Wood Johnson Medical School; Chief of OB/GYN Service, Department of Obstetrics and Gynecology, Robert Wood Johnson University Hospital, New Brunswick, New Jersey

György Baffy, MD, PhD
Assistant Professor, Liver Research Center, Brown Medical School; Director, Liver Treatment Center, Rhode Island Hospital, Providence, Rhode Island

Jean-Patrice Baillargeon, MD
Division of Endocrinology and Metabolism, Medical College of Virginia, Virginia Commonwealth University, Richmond, Virginia

David A. Baram, MD
Assistant Clinical Professor, Department of Obstetrics and Gynecology, University of Minnesota, Minneapolis, Minnesota

Diane M. Biskobing, MD
Department of Medicine, Medical College of Virginia, Virginia Commonwealth University, Richmond, Virginia

Catherine Blackburn, MD
Division of Obstetric and Consultative Medicine, Women and Infants Hospital, Providence, Rhode Island

Eric M. Bluman, MD, PhD
Department of Orthopaedics, Brown University School of Medicine, Rhode Island Hospital, Providence, Rhode Island

Ann J. Brown, MD
Assistant Professor, Department of Medicine and Obstetrics and Gynecology, Duke University, Durham, North Carolina

Marc D. Brown, MD
Department of Dermatology, University of Rochester School of Medicine and Dentistry; Director, Division of Dermatologic Surgery, Oncology, and MOHS Surgery, Strong Memorial Hospital, Rochester, New York

Gunhilde M. Buchsbaum, MD
Assistant Professor, Department of Obstetrics and Gynecology, University of Rochester; Urogynecologist, Strong Memorial Hospital, Rochester, New York

Douglas M. Burtt, MD
The Miriam Hospital, Providence, Rhode Island

Richard Caesar, MD
Department of Urology, Rhode Island Hospital, Providence, Rhode Island

Joanna M. Cain, MD
Professor, Department of Obstetrics and Gynecology, Oregon Health and Science University, Portland, Oregon

Robert Campbell, MD
Resident, Orthopaedic Surgery, Brown University, Rhode Island Hospital, Providence, Rhode Island

Michelle Carpenter-Bradley, MD
Highland Hospital, University of Rochester, Rochester, New York

Gretchen Champion, MD
Resident Physician, Department of Otolaryngology, Head and Neck Surgery, Washington University School of Medicine, Barnes Jewish Hospital, St. Louis, Missouri

Richard I. Chang, MD
Clinical Instructor of Ophthalmology, University of Rochester, Rochester, New York

Linda Chaudron, MD, MS
Senior Instructor, Department of Psychiatry, University of Rochester School of Medicine; Director, Psychiatric Consultation–Liaison Services, Director, Strong Behavioral Healthcare for Women, Strong Memorial Hospital, Rochester, New York

William T. Chen, MD
Department of Medicine, Division of Gastroenterology, Brown University School of Medicine, Providence, Rhode Island

Steven S. T. Ching, MD
Department of Ophthalmology, Strong Memorial Hospital, Rochester, New York

Maureen A. Chung, MD, PhD
Assistant Professor, Department of Surgery, Brown University, Women and Infants Hospital, Providence, Rhode Island

Jeffrey L. Clemons, MD
Department of Obstetrics and Gynecology, Division of Urogynecology and Pelvic Reconstructive Surgery, Madigan Army Medical Center, Tacoma, Washington

John N. Clore, MD
Professor of Medicine, Department of Internal Medicine, Virginia Commonwealth University School of Medicine, Medical College of Virginia, Richmond, Virginia

Susan E. Cohn, MD, MPH
Associate Professor of Medicine, Department of Medicine, Division of Infectious Diseases, University of Rochester School of Medicine, Rochester, New York

Elise M. Coletta, MD
Clinical Associate Professor, Department of Family Medicine, Brown University School of Medicine, Memorial Hospital of Rhode Island, Pawtucket, Rhode Island

John M. Conte, MD
Assistant Clinical Professor, Department of Medicine, Brown University; Rheumatology Consultant, Department of Medicine, The Miriam Hospital, Rhode Island Hospital, Providence, Rhode Island

Patricia A. Coury-Doniger, RN, FNPC
STD/HIV Program Director, Department of Medicine, Infectious Diseases Unit, School of Medicine and Dentistry, University of Rochester, Rochester, New York

Giuseppe Del Priore, MD
Department of OB/GYN, New York University, New York, New York

Christopher W. DiGiovanni, MD
Assistant Professor, Department of Orthopaedic Surgery, Brown University School of Medicine; Director, Foot and Ankle Service, Department of Orthopaedic Surgery, Rhode Island Hospital, Providence, Rhode Island

Jennifer E. Dominguez, BA
Research Assistant, Department of Obstetrics and Gynecology, Columbia University, New York, New York

Mark Donowitz, MD
Professor of Medicine, Johns Hopkins University, Baltimore, Maryland

Brent DuBeshter, MD
Associate Professor, Department of Obstetrics and Gynecology, University of Rochester School of Medicine and Dentistry; Director of Gynecologic Oncology, Department of Obstetrics and Gynecology, Strong Memorial Hospital, Rochester, New York

Elizabeth deLahunta Edwardsen, MD
Associate Professor, Department of Emergency Medicine, University of Rochester School of Medicine and Dentistry, Rochester, New York

Alison Ehrlich, MD, MHS
Director of Clinical Research, Department of Dermatology, George Washington University Medical Center, Washington, D.C.

Ramy Eid, MD
Assistant Clinical Professor, Department of Gastroenterology, Brown University, Providence, Rhode Island

Boni E. Elewski, MD
Department of Dermatology, University of Alabama at Birmingham, Birmingham, Alabama

Anthony J. Fedullo, MD
Professor, Department of Medicine, University of Rochester; Pulmonary and Critical Care Medicine, Rochester General Hospital, Rochester, New York

David S. Fefferman, MD
Clinical Fellow, Harvard Medical School, Cambridge, Massachusetts

Edward Feller, MD
Clinical Professor, Department of Medicine, Brown Medical School; Director, Division of Gastroenterology, The Miriam Hospital, Providence, Rhode Island

Gary M. Ferguson, MD
Clinical Assistant Professor, Orthopedic Surgery, Brown University; Attending Staff, Orthopedic Surgery, The Miriam and Newport Hospitals, Providence, Rhode Island

Patricia G. Fitzpatrick, MD
Parnell Office Building, Rochester, New York

David C. Foster, MD, MPH
Associate Professor, Department of Obstetrics and Gynecology, University of Rochester School of Medicine and Dentistry, Rochester, New York

Sarah Fox, MD
Assistant Professor, Ambulatory Division, Brown University School of Medicine, Women and Infants Hospital, Providence, Rhode Island

James Frank, MD
Diseases and Surgery of the Retina, Vitreous and Macula, Eye Consultants of Atlanta P.C., Atlanta, Georgia

David F. Gardner, MD
Department of Medicine, Virginia Commonwealth University School of Medicine, Medical College of Virginia Hospitals, Richmond, Virginia

Lynn C. Garfunkel, MD
Department of Pediatrics, University of Rochester; Associate Director, Pediatric and Medicine–Pediatric Training Programs, Department of Pediatrics, Rochester General and Strong Memorial Hospitals, Rochester, New York

Pierre M. Gholam, MD
Department of Medicine, Brown University School of Medicine; Attending Physician, Department of Medicine, Division of Gastroenterology, Rhode Island Hospital and Providence VAMC, Providence, Rhode Island

Paul C. Gordon, MD
Division of Cardiology, The Miriam Hospital, Providence, Rhode Island

Tana A. Grady-Weliky, MD
Associate Professor of Psychiatry and Obstetrics/Gynecology, Department of Psychiatry, Senior Associate Dean for Medical Education, University of Rochester School of Medicine and Dentistry, Rochester, New York

Neil R. Greenspan, MD
Department of Medicine, Division of Gastroenterology, Brown University School of Medicine, Providence, Rhode Island

James A. Hadley, MD, FACS
Clinical Associate Professor, Division of Otolaryngology, University of Rochester Medical Center; Attending Physician, Department of Surgery (Otolaryngology), Strong Memorial Hospital, Rochester, New York

Lucinda Anne Harris, MD
Cornell-New York Hospital, New York, New York

Jane Hitti, MD
Assistant Professor, Department of Obstetrics and Gynecology, University of Washington Medical Center, Seattle, Washington

Kathleen M. Hoeger, MD
Associate Professor, Department of Obstetrics and Gynecology, University of Rochester School of Medicine and Dentistry, Rochester, New York

Joshua Hollander, MD
Associate Professor, Department of Neurology, University of Rochester School of Medicine and Dentistry; Chief, Neurology Unit, Department of Medicine, Rochester General Hospital, Rochester, New York

Gerald W. Honch, MD
Associate Professor, Department of Neurology, University of Rochester School of Medicine and Dentistry; Department of Medicine, Rochester General Hospital, Rochester, New York

Cynthia Howard, MD, MPH
Associate Professor of Pediatrics, Department of Pediatrics, University of Rochester School of Medicine; Director of Mother/Baby Unit, Department of Pediatrics, Rochester General Hospital, Rochester, New York

Fred M. Howard, MD
Department of Obstetrics and Gynecology, University of Rochester, Strong Memorial Hospital, Rochester, New York

Christopher M. Hull, MD
Department of Dermatology, University of Utah School of Medicine, Salt Lake City, Utah

Elizabeth Hyde, MSN, FNP
Family Nurse Practitioner Faculty, Family Practice Residency, Lehigh Valley Hospital, Allentown, Pennsylvania

Maria J. Iuorno, MD
Division of Endocrinology and Metabolism, Medical College of Virginia, Virginia Commonwealth University, Richmond, Virginia

Neil D. Jackson, MD, FACOG
Department of Obstetrics and Gynecology, Brown University School of Medicine; Director, Center for Women's Surgery, Department of Obstetrics and Gynecology, Women and Infants Hospital, Providence, Rhode Island

Wen Jiang, MD
Resident Physician, Department of Otolaryngology, Head and Neck Surgery, Washington University School of Medicine, Barnes Jewish Hospital, St. Louis, Missouri

Brenda L. Johnson, MD
Suburban Medical Group PC, Reading, Massachusetts

Jennifer E. Kacmar, MD
Assistant Professor, Department of Obstetrics and Gynecology, Brown Medical School; Attending Physician, Department of Obstetrics and Gynecology, Division of Ambulatory Care, Women and Infants Hospital of Rhode Island, Providence, Rhode Island

Julia A. Katarincic, MD
Assistant Professor of Orthopaedic Surgery, Brown University Medical School, Providence, Rhode Island

Gary M. Katzman, MD
Assistant Professor, Department of Cardiology, Brown University; Associate Director, Coronary Care Unit, Department of Cardiology, The Miriam Hospital, Providence, Rhode Island

Sripathi R. Kethu, MD
Assistant Professor of Medicine, Division of Gastroenterology, Brown Medical School, Providence, Rhode Island

Michelle Khan, BA
Research Assistant, Women's Health Institute, Robert Wood Johnson Medical School, New Brunswick, New Jersey

Michelle Kang Kim, MD
Weill Medical College, Cornell University, New York, New York

Jonathan D. Klein, MD, MPH
Associate Professor of Pediatrics/Community and Preventitive Medicine, Department of Pediatrics, Division of Adolescent Medicine, University of Rochester, Rochester, New York

Peter A. Kouides, MD
Associate Professor, Department of Medicine, Hematology Unit, University of Rochester School of Medicine; Research Director/Attending Physician, Department of Medicine, Mary M. Gooley Hemophilia Center/ Rochester General Hospital, Rochester, New York

Joseph Kozlowski, MD
Physician's Assistant, Department of OB/GYN, Rochester General Hospital, Rochester, New York

Lucia Larson, MD
Division of Obstetric and Consultative Medicine, Women and Infants Hospital, Providence, Rhode Island

Ruth A. Lawrence, MD
Professor of Obstetrics and Gynecology, Department of Pediatrics, University of Rochester School of Medicine; Director of Newborn Nursery, Department of Pediatrics, University of Rochester School of Medicine, Rochester, New York

Susan H. Lee, MD
Fellow, Breast Diseases, Women and Infants Hospital, Brown University, Providence, Rhode Island

Richard S. Legro, MD
Department of Obstetrics and Gynecology, Penn State University College of Medicine; Staff, Department of Reproductive Endocrinology and Infertility, Milton S. Hershey Medical Center, Hershey, Pennsylvania

Adrian Leibovici, MD
Associate Professor, Department of Psychiatry, University of Rochester School of Medicine and Dentistry; Attending Psychiatrist, Department of Psychiatry, Strong Memorial Hospital, Rochester, New York

Ann M. Lenane, MD
Strong Children's Emergency Department, University of Rochester Medical Center, Rochester, New York

Phyllis C. Leppert, MD, PhD
Adjunct Professor, Department of Obstetrics and Gynecology, St. Louis University, St. Louis, Missouri

Harold Lesser, MD
Clinical Assistant Professor, Department of Neurology, University of Rochester, Rochester General Hospital, Rochester, New York

Vivian Lewis, MD
Department of Obstetrics and Gynecology, University of Rochester School of Medicine and Dentistry; Director, Division of Reproductive Endocrinology, Strong Memorial Hospital, Rochester, New York

Phillip R. Lucas, MD
Clinical Assistant Professor, Chief, Spine Surgery Division, Department of Orthopaedics, Brown University, Rhode Island Hospital, Providence, Rhode Island

H. Trent MacKay, MD
National Institute of Child Health and Human Development, Center for Population Research, Contraceptive and Reproductive Health Branch, Bethesda, Maryland

Donald R. Mattison, MD
National Institute of Child Health and Human Development, Bethesda, Maryland

Sheetal Mehta, MD
Department of Dermatology, University of Illinois at Chicago, Chicago, Illinois

Margaret A. Miller, MD
Director of Division of Ambulatory Internal Medicine, Department of Internal Medicine, Women and Infants Hospital, Providence, Rhode Island

Richard K. Miller, MD
Department of Obstetrics and Gynecology, University of Rochester School of Medicine and Dentistry, Rochester, New York

William L. Miller, MD, MA
Leonard Parker Pool Chair of Family Practice, Department of Family Practice, Lehigh Valley Hospital, Allentown, Pennsylvania

Anne Moss, MD
Department of Neurology, University of Rochester School of Medicine and Dentistry; Attending Neurologist, Department of Medicine, Rochester General Hospital, Rochester, New York

Carl Nath, MD
Department of Obstetrics and Gynecology, General Division, University of Medicine and Dentistry of New Jersey–Robert Wood Johnson Medical School; Instructor, Department of Obstetrics and Gynecology, Robert Wood Johnson University Hospital, Saint Peter's University Hospital, New Brunswick, New Jersey

John E. Nestler, MD
Division of Endocrinology and Metabolism, Medical College of Virginia, Virginia Commonwealth University, Richmond, Virginia

Florian Nickisch, MD
Resident, Department of Orthopaedic Surgery, Brown University Medical School; Resident, Department of Orthopaedic Surgery, Rhode Island Hospital, Providence, Rhode Island

Sarah Nicklin, MD
Family Practice Associate, Department of Family Practice, Lehigh Valley Hospital, Allentown, Pennsylvania

Lynnette K. Nieman, MD
Senior Investigator, Pediatric and Reproductive Endocrinology Branch, National Institute of Child Health and Human Development, National Institutes of Health, Bethesda, Maryland

Angela Novy, MD
Department of Medicine, Medical College of Virginia, Virginia Commonwealth University, Richmond, Virginia

Paul Nyirjesy, MD
Associate Professor, Department of Obstetrics and Gynecology, Department of Medicine (Infectious Diseases), Jefferson Medical College, Philadelphia, Pennsylvania

Martin E. Olsen, MD
Department of Obstetrics and Gynecology, James H. Quillen College of Medicine, East Tennessee State University, Johnson City, Tennessee

Anita S. Pakula, MD
3180 Willow Lane, Westlake Village, California

Mark Palumbo, MD
Assistant Professor, Department of Orthopaedics, Spinal Surgery Division, Brown University, Rhode Island Hospital, Providence, Rhode Island

Jeffrey F. Peipert, MD
Professor of Obstetrics, Gynecology, and Community Health, Brown Medical School, Brown University; Director, Division of Research, Department of Obstetrics and Gynecology, Women and Infants Hospital, Providence, Rhode Island

Edward A. Pensa, MD
Department of Medicine, Division of Gastroenterology, Brown University School of Medicine, Providence, Rhode Island

Pradyumna D. Phatak, MD, FACP
Chief, Hematology/Medical Oncology Unit, Rochester General Hospital, Rochester, New York

William R. Phipps, MD
Department of Obstetrics and Gynecology, University of Rochester School of Medicine and Dentistry; Attending Physician, Strong Fertility and Reproductive Science Center, University of Rochester Medical Center, Rochester, New York

Jay Piccirillo, MD
Associate Professor, Otolaryngology, Head and Neck Surgery, Director, Clinical Outcomes Research Office, Washington University School of Medicine, St. Louis, Missouri

Ronald D. Plotnik, MD
Department of Ophthalmology, University of Rochester Eye Institute, Rochester, New York

Douglas L. Powell, MD
Department of Dermatology, University of Utah School of Medicine, Salt Lake City, Utah

Raymond O. Powrie, MD, FRCP(C), FACP
Obstetric Internist, Women and Infants Hospital, Providence, Rhode Island

Victor E. Pricolo, MD
Professor of Surgery, Brown University, Rhode Island Hospital, Providence, Rhode Island

John T. Queenan, Jr., MD
Associate Professor, Department of Obstetrics and Gynecology, University of Rochester School of Medicine and Dentistry, Rochester, New York

Harlan G. Rich, MD
Department of Medicine, Brown Medical School; Director of Endoscopy, Rhode Island Hospital, Providence, Rhode Island

Christopher T. Ritchlin, MD
Department of Medicine, University of Rochester Medical Center; Director, Clinical Immunology Research, Allergy, Immunology and Rhemumatology Unit, University of Rochester Medical Center, Rochester, New York

Jay K. Roberts, MD
Staff Physician, Department of Otolaryngology, Cleveland Clinic Florida–Naples;
Staff Physician, Department of Otolaryngology, Cleveland Clinic Hospital, Naples, Florida

Steven J. Rose, MD
Clinical Associate Professor, Department of Ophthalmology, University of Rochester School of Medicine; Attending Physician, Department of Ophthalmology, Strong Memorial Hospital, Rochester, New York

Paul J. Russinko, MD
Department of Urology, Brown University, Rhode Island Hospital, Providence, Rhode Island

Ara Sadaniantz, MD
The Miriam Hospital, Providence, Rhode Island

Lawrence M. Samkoff, MD
Associate Professor, Department of Neurology, University of Rochester School of Medicine and Dentistry; Attending Neurologist, Department of Medicine, Rochester General Hospital, Rochester, New York

Nadine Sauvé, MD
Department of Medicine, University of Sherbrooke, Sherbrooke, Québec, Canada

James Segars, MD
Associate Professor, Department of Obstetrics and Gynecology, Uniformed Services University; Unit Chief, Pediatric and Reproductive Endocrinology Branch, National Institute of Child Health and Human Development, National Institutes of Health, Bethesda, Maryland

Jay P. Shah, MD
Instructor, Clinical Acupuncture for Physicians, Harvard Medical School, Beth Israel Deaconess Medical Center, Boston, Massachusetts; Director, Medical Rehabilitation Training Program, Department of Rehabilitation Medicine, Clinical Center, National Institutes of Health, Bethesda, Maryland

Samir A. Shah, MD, FACG
Clinical Assistant Professor of Medicine, Brown University School of Medicine, Gastroenterology Associates, Providence, Rhode Island

Robert Shalvoy, MD
Clinical Assistant Professor, Orthopedic Surgery, Brown University Medical School; Medical Director, New England Center for Athletics, Providence, Rhode Island

Ronald Lewis Sham, MD
Medical Director, Mary M. Gooley Hemophilia Center, Department of Medicine–Hematology, Rochester General Hospital, Rochester, New York

Douglas Shemin, MD
Clinical Associate Professor, Department of Medicine, Brown University School of Medicine; Director, Hemodialysis Program, Division of Renal Diseases, Rhode Island Hospital, Providence, Rhode Island

Bryant Shin, MD
Department of Ophthalmology, Strong Memorial Hospital, Rochester, New York

Cynthia K. Shortell
Rochester General Hospital, Rochester, New York

Winnie W. K. Sia, MD
Royal Alexandra Hospital, Edmonton, Alberta, Canada; Fellow, Department of Medicine, Brown Medical School, Women and Infants Hospital, Providence, Rhode Island

Deborah Martina Smith, MD, MPH
Special Expert, National Institute on Drug Abuse, Center on AIDS and Other Medical Consequences of Drug Abuse, Bethesda, Maryland

Eric Sokol, MD
Fellow, Division of Female Pelvic Medicine and Reconstructive Surgery, Brown University School of Medicine, Women and Infants Hospital, Providence, Rhode Island

Gwen K. Sterns, MD
Chief of Ophthalmology, Rochester General Hospital, Rochester, New York

King To, MD, MMS
Department of Ophthalmology, Brown Medical School, Rhode Island Hospital, Providence, Rhode Island

Gisela Torres, MD
University of Texas Medical Branch, Center for Clinical Studies, Houston, Texas

Eugene Toy, MD
Assistant Professor, Department of Obstetrics and Gynecology, University of Rochester, Rochester, New York

Julie H. Tsai, MD
Department of Ophthalmology, Strong Memorial Hospital, Rochester, New York

Stephen K. Tyring, MD, PhD
University of Texas Medical Branch, Center for Clinical Studies, Houston, Texas

Mauricio A. Valdes, MD
Fellow, Spiral Surgery Division, Brown University, Rhode Island Hospital, Providence, Rhode Island

Charlene B. Varnis, MD
Assistant Professor, Department of Medicine, University of Rochester School of Medicine and Dentistry; Clinical Director, Allergy/Immunology/Rheumatology Unit, University of Rochester Medical Center, Rochester, New York

Madhuri Ventrapragada, MD
Department of Dermatology, University of Illinois at Chicago, Chicago, Illinois

Laura J. von Doenhoff, MD
Clinical Instructor, Department of Medicine/Cardiology, University of Rochester School of Medicine and Dentistry; Attending Physician, Rochester Heart Institute, Rochester General Hospital, Rochester, New York

Matthew Vrees, MD
Rhode Island Hospital, Providence, Rhode Island

Gary W. Wahl, MD
Department of Medicine, University of Rochester; Department of Medicine, Pulmonary and Critical Care Physician, Rochester General Hospital, Rochester, New York

Jean Wang, MD
Clinical Fellow, Johns Hopkins School of Medicine, Baltimore, Maryland

Michelle P. Warren, MD
Department of Obstetrics and Gynecology, Columbia University; Medical Director, Center for Menopause, Hormonal Disorders, and Women's Health, Columbia–Presbyterian Medical Center, New York, New York

David Warshal, MD
Gynecological Oncologist, 124 King Highway West, Haddonfield, New Jersey

Barbara E. Weber, MD, PhD
Rochester General Hospital, General Medicine Unit, Rochester, New York

Arnold-Peter C. Weiss, MD
Professor of Orthopaedics, Department of Orthopaedic Surgery, Brown University School of Medicine, Rhode Island Hospital, Providence, Rhode Island

Roy S. Wiener, MD
Clinical Associate Professor, Department of Medicine, University of Rochester School of Medicine; Cardiologist, Rochester Heart Institute, Rochester General Hospital, Rochester, New York

Sophie M. Worobec, MD
Associate Professor of Dermatology, University of Illinois, Chicago, Illinois

Wen-Chih Wu, MD
Assistant Professor, Department of Medicine, Brown Medical School, Providence Veterans Administration Medical Center, Providence, Rhode Island

Susan M. Yussman, MD
Fellow, Adolescent Medicine, Department of Pediatrics, University of Rochester; Fellow, Adolescent Medicine, Department of Pediatrics, Golisano Children's Hospital at Strong, Rochester, New York

Preface

The second edition of *Primary Care for Women* expands and updates the successful previous edition. As stated in the preface of the first edition, the primary care physician needs a wider range of care knowledge than a subspecialist and a razor-sharp diagnostic ability to truly serve the primary care needs of women. The editors believe that there is a core of knowledge that all providers of primary care for women must acquire and comprehend irrespective of their individual specialty training and education.

Since the first edition was published, there has been widespread recognition of the biological differences between the sexes at all levels, from the basic molecular and cellular levels to that of the whole person. Gender differences, in addition to fundamental genetic differences, are now also widely understood to impact on health.

While the general organization of the text remains, all chapters have been rigorously updated and emphasize evidence-based practice. New chapters, such as those on the topics of pharmacology, chronic pain, and uterine leiomyomas, have been added. New authors have been recruited, and a new editor has contributed to the endeavor of the publication of this second edition.

We are proud of *Primary Care for Women*, second edition, as it presents a text that integrates care for women into a comprehensive whole. We believe that this approach will benefit all women.

Phyllis C. Leppert, M.D., Ph.D.
Jeffrey F. Peipert, M.D., M.P.H., M.H.A.

PART

1

Principles of Primary Care for Women

CHAPTER 1

Uniqueness of Women's Health

Phyllis C. Leppert

The constitution of the World Health Organization defines health as a state of complete physical, mental, and social well-being. Women's health is related to far more than health during the reproductive years and means more than the absence of gynecologic disease. Women's health encompasses the total well-being of each individual woman. Every physiologic system in the female human being is influenced by XX chromosomes and by a lifetime of variations in reproductive hormones. Therefore, women's health incorporates the combined knowledge of all the traditional specialties of medicine, in addition to public health, nursing, midwifery, social work, and other health professions.

At the same time, the perspective of women's health is much broader than that of these traditional health professions. Epidemiology has enabled us to understand that the social and political climate in which a woman finds herself may be the most important determinant of her health. In societies in which women are undervalued, the necessary human, economic, and scientific resources are seldom allocated to women's health. Thus, in such circumstances, the health needs of women are not met. This fact holds true in all countries, and it is true in the United States. The status of women's health, whether it is the shockingly high maternal mortality rate in some parts of Africa, the lack of obstetric resources in Afghanistan, or the unacceptably high prevalence of domestic violence and trauma in the United States, reflects the lack of value placed on women's lives.

In nations that allocate economic resources to maternal and child health, most of the money is all too often used for child health, with the effect that women's health is neglected. Although the health and well-being of children are essential to the survival of the human species and our multitude of cultures, too many nations do not adequately address the compelling health needs of women. Women contribute to the nurture, development, and success of nations and to the world culture, whether or not they are mothers. Nations that value women educate all women to their full intellectual potential. The education of women is a vital element in reducing infant mortality, improving the overall well-being of the family, ensuring optimal health for all women, encouraging women's economic stability, and preparing women for community, national, and world leadership. The fact that women are not valued for their full potential is evidenced by the educational barriers and hurdles that exist for women worldwide.

Women's health is also unique in that the female reproductive system is an anatomically and physiologically complex entity that is subject to a large number of disease processes. The signs and symptoms of disease in the female reproductive tract are more varied and often more subtle than those of disease in the male reproductive tract. Women are subject to disease and dysfunction of the reproductive tract throughout life, not only during their reproductive years; these may occur at any time, from intrauterine life to old age. Such pathologic conditions occur whether or not a woman has borne children; furthermore, having borne children may alter her risk for a particular disease.

The female reproductive tract is a common site for the formation of neoplasms, both benign and malignant. Most of these tumors occur at the end of the reproductive years or in the menopausal period. The multiplicity of the pathologic classification of female reproductive tract neoplasms attests to the wide variety of tumors affecting women at any stage of life. Gynecologic and mammary gland malignancies are so common that all providers of women's primary care must be cognizant of the natural history, signs, symptoms, and methods of diagnosis of these neoplasms. Uterine leiomyomata in females have no equivalent in males. These benign tumors today account for

25% to 30% of the hysterectomies performed in the United States. One study noted that histologic evidence of leiomyomata was found in as many as 77% of specimens obtained during hysterectomies performed for all causes in a community hospital.

Sexually transmitted diseases occur in both men and women, but the consequences of these diseases are more serious in women. For biologic and social reasons, women are more likely to become infected and less likely to seek care, and sexually transmitted disease is often more difficult to diagnose in women. Women with a sexually transmitted disease suffer serious sequelae, including chronic pelvic pain, ectopic pregnancies, and infertility. Women infected with a sexually transmitted disease are more often subject to social discrimination. Prevention is difficult for women because men control the most effective method of prevention, the condom. No method is currently available that a woman can use to protect herself from the sexual transmission of disease without her partner's cooperation. Many women have difficulty in negotiating their sexual partner's cooperation because of concerns of issues of trust and fidelity. The female condom is still not widely accepted by many people.

Women's health care providers must always be cognizant of the fact that a woman's reproductive role means that she faces health risks, including complications and death, related to pregnancy. Too many and too closely spaced pregnancies are a health risk for women. A woman's ability to control fertility so that all pregnancies are wanted and occur at the appropriate time is fundamental to her health and well-being.

Pregnancy can be prevented by methods controlled by an individual woman. Many of these methods, however, pose potential health risks. Abstinence is the only certain and sure way to prevent both unwanted pregnancy and sexually transmitted disease. However, abstinence as the only strategy to prevent both pregnancy and sexually transmitted disease in the age of AIDS is unrealistic. Furthermore, health care providers must consider that most women worldwide live in social situations in which they are compelled by custom or physical force to have sexual intercourse when they do not want it. In these circumstances, women bear a heavy health and social burden of pregnancy and sexually transmitted disease.

It is being increasingly recognized that the results of research conducted in men do not necessarily apply to women, another area in which women's health care is unique. In response to this recognition, the National Institutes of Health has initiated many studies of women's health and gender differences in health and disease and various programs to train young physicians and scientists in women's health research.

IMPACT OF EDUCATIONAL STATUS ON WOMEN'S HEALTH

The educational attainment of women in any society correlates with their health because education increases the ability of women to be partners in their own health care. If they understand what constitutes good health and know the risk factors that lead to disease and disability, women can choose lifestyles that decrease the risks for disease and thus prevent or mitigate disease. It is assumed that an educated woman will make wise lifestyle choices based on knowledge within the context of her individual culture.

Recently, science has demonstrated that both behavior and susceptibility to disease are linked to biologic and genetic factors. Therefore, it has become more important than previously for women and their health care providers to share knowledge regarding health and disease prevention. It is well established that health care providers can influence a woman's lifestyle through education. For example, alcohol dependence has a biologic basis. An individual predisposed to alcoholism needs to understand her risk and adopt a lifestyle that provides for avoidance of alcohol. In this situation, the primary physician is obligated to educate the patient about ways to avoid alcohol and support her efforts at avoidance. Obesity, another serious health problem, is a risk factor for heart disease and diabetes. Health care providers must use effective ways to educate all women about healthful lifestyles to mitigate these health problems. These two examples demonstrate that a woman's health reflects her individual biologic and genetic inheritance, the attitudes of the society in which she resides, the resources allocated to women's health, her social values, and her lifestyle choices. The truly educated woman is able to understand all these influences and make wise choices regarding her health.

In the final analysis, all women, no matter how poor or uneducated, respond positively to compassionate, competent care. Compassion and competence should pervade the complete care of a woman that leads to her physical, mental, and social well-being.

CULTURE AND HEALTH

The world is made up of numerous groups of people, each with different ways of living that have developed during centuries and been transmitted through many generations. The sum of the language, ideas, customs, skills, and arts of a given people makes up their culture and traditions. Culture and tradition influence the way people look at and respond to health and illness in both spoken and unspoken ways. Physicians and other health care professionals have a culture with traditional codes of conduct and behavior that are unique to the health care professions. This culture is pervasive. When people are initiated into the culture of medicine, they become socialized by it and adopt it. Thus, they may not necessarily accept all the values of the culture of their birth and may have as much difficulty in relating to persons of their own culture as to those of a different culture. The North American continent, and the United States in particular, are becoming more multiracial and more multicultural than in the past. The primary physician must acquire the necessary competency to relate to persons from many cultures and appreciate that a physician's own cultural values may influence the understanding and acceptance of those from different cultural backgrounds.

Many aspects of a woman's life, especially those of her reproductive life, are intertwined with culturally derived ideas of what is considered necessary for health. Tradition and culture affect in broad ways a person's behavior and attitudes toward illness. Reproductive health is an extremely important component of women's health, both individually and globally. In many cultures, traditional beliefs and practices come into conflict with modern medical and scientific knowledge and practice. Cultural competency reduces sociocultural barriers to health care by improving patient-physician relationships. The modern, future-thinking health care provider accepts cultural diversity and educates patients for autonomy, personal decision making, and self-care. Modern physicians do not simply accept patients' unhealthful practices but rather work within their cultural values and present to them the evidence for sound medical practice so as to arrive at an appropriate management plan.

Sometimes, particular cultural practices are very harmful to women, and it becomes difficult for physicians to accept them.

One example is female circumcision. The health consequences of this practice are severe; it can lead to pelvic infections and difficult childbearing. Many professional organizations, such as the International Federation of Obstetrics and Gynecology and the American College of Obstetricians and Gynecologists, have made extensive efforts to educate the medical profession and the public regarding this practice. Female circumcision is practiced predominantly in Africa. However, it is also practiced in some form in other countries, including Yemen, the United Arab Emirates, Malaysia, Indonesia, Pakistan, and India. Jews, Christians, Muslims, and followers of many other religions practice female circumcision. About 130 million women in the world have been circumcised. Immigration patterns are such that it is estimated that approximately 168,000 girls and women in the United States in 1990 had either undergone circumcision or were at risk for the procedure. Most of these women and young girls live in the states of California, Florida, Georgia, Illinois, Maryland, Massachusetts, New Jersey, New York, Ohio, Pennsylvania, Texas, and Virginia. Almost half reside in large cities. Thus, primary care physicians need to understand this practice and how to provide health care to women and young girls who have been circumcised.

First, female circumcision is defined as any type of genital alteration performed in young girls and young women for nontherapeutic purposes. The persons performing female circumcision vary from culture to culture. In some, the procedure is performed by nonmedical persons; in others, physicians, midwives, and nurses are involved.

Female circumcision is classified by the World Health Organization into four types. Type I is clitoridectomy, type II is excision (clitoridectomy and partial or total excision of the labia minora), type III is infibulation (clitoridectomy, excision of the labia minora and labia majora, and infibulation or reapproximation of the remnant labia majora and creation of a new introitus), and type IV is any other form (e.g., introcision, stretching, nicking, cauterization, manipulation, and application of corrosive substances).

Immediate complications include hemorrhage, infection, urinary retention, hypotension, shock, and death. Complications that develop over time include keloids, sebaceous cysts, vesicovaginal fistulae, dyspareunia, dysmenorrhea, hematocolpos, infertility, vaginitis, urinary tract problems, and HIV infection/AIDS. Women who have undergone type I or II circumcision are at less risk for obstetric complications than women who have been subjected to type III, in whom obstetric examinations are difficult and in some cases impossible. It is also difficult to manage labor in these women. Thus, the best solution is to discuss deinfibulation, a procedure in which the scar tissue is incised surgically. Although obstetric care presents a difficult challenge, women with type III circumcision should be allowed a trial of labor. Cesarean sections should be performed only for maternal or fetal indications. Increased rates of perineal wound infections, separation of episiotomy, postpartum hemorrhage, and sepsis have also been documented. In developing nations, obstructed labor has caused fetal compromise and intrauterine fetal demise. In countries such as the United States and Canada, these complications are uncommon because of the availability of fetal monitoring and operative deliveries.

It is essential in caring for circumcised women that physicians conduct themselves in a culturally competent manner. Counseling must be done in a sensitive manner and psychosocial issues considered. Individual beliefs and attitudes must be accepted. By considering the total health, emotional, and cultural needs of circumcised women, the primary provider will optimize their care.

SOME TRENDS IN WOMEN'S HEALTH TODAY IN THE UNITED STATES

Birth and death rates and life expectancy are the parameters usually evaluated in comparing the nation's health with that of other countries. These rates are also used as indicators of the overall status of women's health. Both biologic and lifestyle factors influence the rates, which are also used as the basis for observing trends.

Birth Rates

In 2001, there were 4,025,933 births in the United States, a rate 1% lower than the rate in 2000, which was the highest in 30 years. The year 2000 was the first since 1993 that the number of births exceeded 4 million. In 2000, women in the United States averaged 2.1 births during their lifetime. This fertility level maintains a steady-state population. In 2000, Hispanic women had a fertility rate of 3.1, the highest of any ethnic group. In 2001, 33.5% of all births were to unmarried women. The birth rate for teenagers fell for the 10th consecutive year. During the past decade, births to young women ages 15 to 17 years fell by more than a third. The birth rate for African-Americans in this age group declined by almost a half.

A significant trend during the past decade has been an increase in the birth rate for women older than 30 years (Fig. 1.1).

The birth rate for married women has decreased. This decrease has resulted in a noticeable increase in the proportion of births to unmarried women. Some of these changes are a consequence of women's ability to control their own fertility because of the general availability of contraception. Data from

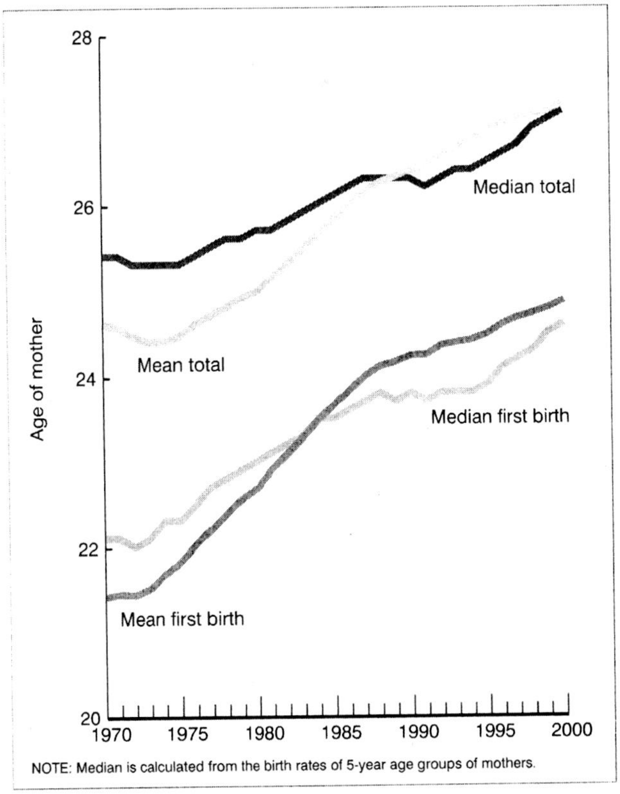

FIG. 1.1. Mean and median ages of mother by order of live births, 1970–2000. (From Mathews TJ, Hamilton BE. Mean age of mother, 1970–2000. *National vital statistics reports,* vol 51, no 1. Hyattsville, MD: National Center for Health Statistics, 2002.)

studies of unwanted births suggest that unmarried women accept single motherhood and plan for it.

The treatment of infertility with assisted reproductive technology (ART) has increased significantly. In 2000, 383 fertility clinics reported outcome data to the Centers for Disease Control and Prevention. In that year, 99,639 ART cycles (a cycle begins when a woman starts taking drugs to stimulate ovulation) resulted in 25,228 live births and 35,025 babies. Of these reported live births, 35% were births of more than one infant, 30.7% were births of twins, and 4.3% were births of triplets or a greater number of babies. The number of ART cycles has increased from the 64,724 reported in 1996. Of the ART cycles in which fresh, nondonor eggs or embryos were used, 70% were in women ages 30 to 39 years. Very few women younger than 22 years of age used ART, and very few women older than 46 years used ART with their own eggs. This increase in the use of ART is attributed to the increasing numbers of women entering the work force and thus delaying childbearing. The definition of delayed childbearing is not standard. Some argue that delayed childbearing should be defined as birth to women older than 40 years.

The third National Health and Nutrition Examination Survey (NHANES III) showed that highly educated women are more likely to postpone childbearing. The rates of births to women older than 30 years have been increasing since 1985, as noted previously. However, an initial pregnancy and birth after the age of 35 years remains uncommon despite the increased number of births to women in this age group.

Careful analysis of the NHANES III data for women at age 50 who delivered a child when they were older than 35 demonstrates that delayed childbirth increases the risks for acute myocardial infarction and congestive heart disease, but not stroke. The increased risks are related to increases in blood pressure and glucose abnormalities. Therefore, delayed childbearing may have long-term consequences for women, especially those with a familial risk for cardiovascular disease and the associated risk factors of diabetes and hypertension.

In 2001, the percentage of preterm births (before 37 weeks) increased to 11.9%, the highest in two decades. The rate of low birth weight was 7.7% in 2001, an increase of 13% since the mid-1980s. Some of this increase was a consequence of the increase in multiple births during the past decade. The infant mortality rate for 2000 (the latest year available) was 6.9 infant deaths per 1,000 live births, compared with 7.1 in 1999. Black infant mortality decreased from 14.6 to 14.0. Congenital malformations and chromosomal abnormalities were the leading cause of infant death. These accounted for 20.7% of all infant deaths. Preterm birth with a low birth weight was the second leading cause of death, accounting for 15.4% of all deaths. The third leading cause of infant death was sudden infant death syndrome.

Trends in Heath Related to Lifestyle

OBESITY

During the past few decades, the prevalence of overweight and obesity has increased significantly. Obesity, defined as a body mass index (BMI) of 30 or more, and overweight, defined as a BMI of 25 to 29, have increased more among women of childbearing age than among older women or men. In women ages 20 to 29 years, the rate of obesity has increased from 7% in 1960–1962 to 17% in 1988–1997. The percentage of those who are overweight has increased to 19% from 11% in that same period. The weight of women ages 30 to 44 years changed little or not at all.

The risk for premature death from all causes is increased in obese and overweight persons. Obesity during pregnancy is associated with a risk for maternal death. The incidence of heart diseases, including myocardial infarction, congestive heart failure, sudden cardiac death, angina, chest pain, and arrhythmias, is increased in overweight persons. Overweight and obesity are associated with an increased risk for endometrial cancer. The rates of colon, gallbladder, kidney, and postmenopausal breast cancer are increased in persons who are overweight as well as in those who are obese.

Overweight appears to be a serious problem in women immediately before pregnancy. One third of all women gain more weight during pregnancy than is recommended. This weight gain is not lost after pregnancy in many cases. In addition, the 10-year risk for obesity of a woman with one live birth is twice that of a woman without a live birth.

CIGARETTE SMOKING

Almost 3 million women in the United Stated have died prematurely since 1980 as a consequence of smoking. Of all smoking-related deaths, 39% are in women, more than double the number reported in 1965. The Centers for Disease Control and Prevention, the National Institutes of Health, and other federal agencies are committed to curbing the epidemic of tobacco-related disease in young people and women. Smokers who quit derive immediate health benefits secondary to improved respiration. The excess risk for coronary heart disease is substantially reduced 1 or 2 years after smoking cessation.

In addition, smoking during pregnancy is associated with serious risks, especially for the delivery of a low-birth-weight infant. The percentage of women smoking during pregnancy in 2000 was 12.2%, representing a decline of more than one third since 1989. This trend is very encouraging because it clearly shows that women are responding to the important health education message that smoking has serious consequences for both mothers and infants.

Chronic Conditions

Data from three national health surveys and vital statistics collected in the United States demonstrate the effects of seven chronic conditions by age and sex: arthritis, visual impairment, hearing impairment, ischemic heart disease, chronic obstructive pulmonary disease, diabetes mellitus, and malignant neoplasms. The effects are divided into three categories: limitation of activity, visits to physicians, and hospital stays.

Data indicate that the effects of all conditions in limiting activity, or reducing daily functioning, increase in both sexes from young adulthood (ages 18–44 years) to middle adulthood (ages 45–64 years). The effects of all conditions in limiting activity increase only slightly more in women after the age of 65, except for visual impairment, which limits the activity of both sexes. The effect of heart disease in limiting activity is greatest in both sexes at ages 45 to 64; in persons 18 to 44 years of age, heart disease has the effect of limiting activity predominantly in men. The effect of chronic obstructive pulmonary disease is somewhat less and the effect of visual impairment is greater in women than in men at all ages. For instance, cataracts are ranked fourth in prevalence for women but tenth for men.

The likelihood that a person with a given condition will visit a physician is similar for both men and women for all conditions, except that more care is sought by young men with heart disease, and more care is sought by women with visual impairment at all ages. Cancer and diabetes increase the number of physician visits more among middle-aged women than among middle-aged men.

The likelihood that a person with a given condition will be hospitalized is similar for both men and women for all conditions, except that young men with ischemic heart disease are hospitalized more frequently than young women with ischemic heart disease. It has been suggested that young men are more likely than young women to receive aggressive treatment rather than that their illness is more severe. In middle-aged and older people, the rates of hospitalization for ischemic heart disease do not differ by sex.

The leading causes (principal diagnoses) of hospital stays are also revealed by analyzing survey data. Among women ages 18 to 44 years, the leading causes of hospitalization are complications of pregnancy, other genital tract problems, diseases of the pelvic organs, and complications of HIV infection/AIDS. In other words, the major causes of hospitalization are related to reproductive health. Among men in this age range, the major causes of hospitalization are fractures, alcohol dependence syndrome, and lacerations and open wounds.

In people ages 45 to 79 years, the primary cause of hospitalization in both women and men is malignant neoplasm, with the rate for women slightly higher than that for men. Among women, the next-ranked conditions are diseases of the urinary system and benign neoplasms, whereas in men, they are ischemic heart disease and acute myocardial infarction. Among people ages 65 years and older, malignant neoplasms and cerebrovascular disease are the leading causes of hospitalization in both men and women. The third-ranked conditions leading to hospitalization differ in this age group: fractures for women and prostate and other genital disorders for men. Only in this age group is a condition related to reproductive health one of the three main causes of hospital stays for men. However, among women, conditions related to reproductive health are major causes of hospitalization in the three age groups.

The principal diagnoses for visits to a physician's office differ between the sexes in persons 18 to 44 years of age. For example, diseases of the reproductive system ranked prominently in women ages 18 to 44 years, including diseases of the pelvic organs (ranked second), other female genital tract problems (ranked fourth), diseases of the urinary system (ranked fifth), complications of pregnancy (ranked sixth), and menstrual disorders (ranked ninth). In contrast, fewer reproductive system conditions were noted among men; prostate and other genital problems ranked eighth in the 18- to 44-year-old age group.

The diagnoses are more similar in patients ages 45 to 64 years. The three leading reasons for visits to a physician's office in both men and women are essential hypertension, ischemic heart disease, and diabetes. In persons ages 65 years and older, the diagnoses in men and women are again similar, with office visits made for essential hypertension and chronic eye conditions. However, the third-ranked condition differs between men and women: diabetes for women and malignant neoplasms for men.

Death Rates

The total number of people who died in the United States in 2000 was 2,403,351. The crude death rate was 873.6 per 100,000 population, which is a decrease from 877.0 per 100,000 in 1999. The age-adjusted death rate, which accounts for the age distribution in the population as a whole, reached a low of 872.4 per 100,000 U.S. standard population. The number of women of all ages who died in 2000 was 122,773. Heart disease and cancer remain the leading causes of death in women of all races (Table 1.1).

Cardiovascular disease is the leading cause of death and includes heart disease and stroke. In 2000, 365,953 women died of heart disease and 102,892 women died of stroke. The risk factors for heart disease are older age, hypertension, high level of cholesterol, diabetes, lack of physical activity, and cigarette smoking. A high level of cholesterol significantly increases the risk for cardiovascular disease. These levels begin to rise at age 20 and decrease rapidly at menopause. The number of women with a high cholesterol level (>240 mg/dL) has been declining in the past four decades. However, it has been reported that approximately 41% of women older than 55 years should lower their cholesterol level. Physical activity reduces the risk for heart disease by helping to control cholesterol, weight, and blood pressure.

The symptoms of heart disease tend to develop 10 years later in women than in men. The rate of coronary heart disease is 10-fold higher among women older than 55 years of age than it is among younger women. The risk for coronary heart disease in younger women is less than that in men, but as women age, the mortality associated with heart disease increases. By age 75, the incidence of heart disease is essentially the same in both sexes.

TABLE 1.1. Deaths and Percentage of Total Deaths for the 10 Leading Causes of Death by Sex: United States, 2000

Cause of death (based on the 10th revision of the International Classification of Diseases, 1992)	Males			Females		
	Rank[a]	Deaths	Percentage of total deaths	Rank[a]	Deaths	Percentage of total deaths
All causes.	...	1,177,578	100.0	...	1,225,773	100.0
Diseases of heart. . . . . (I00–I09,I11,I13,I20–I51)	1	344,807	29.3	1	365,953	29.9
Malignant neoplasms . . . . (C00–C97)	2	286,082	24.3	2	267,009	21.8
Cerebrovascular diseases . . . . (I60–I69)	3	64,769	5.5	3	102,892	8.4
Accidents (unintentional injuries). . (V01–X59,Y85–Y86)	4	63,817	5.4	8	34,083	2.8
Chronic lower respiratory diseases . . . . (J40–J47)	5	60,004	5.1	4	62,005	5.1
Diabetes mellitus . . . . (E10–E14)	6	31,602	2.7	5	37,699	3.1
Influenza and pneumonia . . . . (J10–J18)	7	28,658	2.4	6	36,655	3.0
Intentional self-harm (suicide). . . . . . . (X60–X84,Y87.0)	8	23,618	2.0	...	5,732	0.5
Nephritis, nephrotic syndrome . . (N00–N07,N17–N19, and nephrosis . . . . N25–N27)	9	17,811	1.5	9	19,440	1.6
Chronic liver disease and cirrhosis . . . . (K70,K73–K74)	10	17,214	1.5	...	9,338	0.8
Alzheimer disease . . . . (G30)	...	14,438	1.2	7	35,120	2.9
Septicemia . . . . (A40–A41)	...	13,537	1.1	10	17,687	1.4

[a]Rank based on number of deaths.
... Category not applicable.
Source: *National Vital Statistics Report* 2002;50:8, with permission.

Because women ages 55 and older are at a higher risk for coronary artery disease, it is hypothesized that the increased risk is associated with the changes of menopause.

Research efforts aimed at understanding heart disease have included predominantly men because the symptoms of heart disease typically develop in women at later stages of life. Therefore, because they are older at the onset of cardiovascular disease and have other medical conditions and diseases thought to be confounding factors in study design, women are not included in the studies. Furthermore, treatment studies tend to include middle-aged men at high risk for the simple reason that conclusions can be reached fairly quickly with a smaller sample size.

Cancer is the second leading cause of death among white, black, and Native American women in the United States. A 5-year survival in a patient with cancer is considered a potential cure. The 5-year survival rate, which includes a calculation of the normal, age-adjusted life expectancy, is used as a measure for the detection and treatment of early-stage cancer. Although some cancers, such as breast cancer, may recur 5 years after diagnosis of the primary cancer, a 5-year survivor is usually considered cured.

Except for lung cancer deaths, cancer deaths have declined in women during the past decade. In women ages 85 years and older, cancer ranks as the third leading cause of death. However, in Native Americans and Native Alaskans, lung, colorectal, and breast cancer rates have not declined. Lung cancer remains a leading cause of death in women. Approximately 90% of these deaths are related to smoking.

Because symptoms of lung cancer appear at advanced stages of the disease, it is difficult to detect in its earliest stages. Lung cancer is a preventable disease; if cigarette smoking were stopped, most lung cancer cases would be eliminated.

In 1998, the rates of breast cancer among women were highest in blacks, but the rate decreased in white women. Although the incidence is higher for white women, the mortality rates are higher for blacks. Breast cancer mortality rates are related to how early the disease is diagnosed, the availability of treatment, and lifestyle. Women who have never had children and women who delay having a first birth until age 30 are at increased risk for breast cancer. Obesity increases the risk for postmenopausal breast cancer, as noted previously.

The risk for breast cancer increases as women age, and the disease occurs more frequently among white women 45 years of age and older than among black women of the same age. Screening for breast cancer through mammography, self-examination, and clinical examination is an essential element in health care for women. To date, not all women are obtaining the screening examinations and mammograms necessary to detect breast cancer early. During the past decades, breast cancer has been treated successfully with less aggressive surgical intervention, so that the quality of life and self-image of women with this disease have improved.

Cervical cancer is related to sexual activity. Sexually transmitted infection with certain subtypes of human papillomavirus (HPV) is a strong risk factor for cervical cancer. Early intercourse, having multiple sexual partners, and having a partner with multiple sexual partners all increase the chances of HPV infection and cervical cancer. Therefore, the primary measure to prevent cervical cancer is the promotion of healthy sexual behaviors, such as having fewer sexual partners, using condoms, and abstaining in appropriate situations. The clinical trial of a vaccine against HPV-16, one of the subtypes of HPV linked to cervical cancer, has recently been published. Smoking may increase the risk for cervical cancer by exposing the cervical tissues to carcinogens. The risk for cervical cancer is increased among women who use oral contraceptives. This is not a direct effect; rather, it is most likely a consequence of the fact that these women do not use barrier methods of contraception.

Cervical cancer is prevented by the Papanicolaou smear, which identifies very early cancer and its precursors. Nevertheless, an estimated 13,000 new cases of invasive cervical cancer were diagnosed in 1991. The incidence of cervical cancer is twice as high in black women than in white women. The incidence is also higher in Hispanic and Native American women. Sexual behavior plays a part in the risk for cervical cancer; multiple sexual partners and first intercourse at an early age increase the risk for the development of cervical cancer.

Endometrial cancer is more common among white women than among black women, and it is more common in older women than in younger women, both black and white. The incidence increased quickly during the decade when unopposed estrogen was given to postmenopausal women to prevent the complications of menopause. Estrogen replacement therapy was more often given to white women, which may explain the fact that endometrial cancer is more common among white women. Endometrial cancer is related to nulliparity, infertility, obesity, and hormone replacement therapy with estrogen only. Certainly, many of these risk factors are related to lifestyle.

Ovarian cancer is rare. However, it is particularly worrisome because it often does not cause symptoms until the disease is in a late stage. Furthermore, the risk for ovarian cancer increases with age. The use of oral contraceptives and increased parity decrease the risk for this disease. The 5-year survival rate for patients with ovarian cancer is a low 38%. Ovarian cancer is the fifth leading cause of death among women. The risk for the development of ovarian cancer increases with age and with the number of ovulation cycles a woman has during her lifetime. Mutations in the epithelial surface and exposure to ovulation-inducing drugs are thought to be a partial cause of this observation; however, more research into this risk factor is indicated.

The primary prevention of cancer in women includes the reduction and cessation of smoking, the reduction of promiscuous sexual behavior, and screening with Papanicolaou smears, mammography, and regular gynecologic and general examinations. Basic, clinical, and epidemiologic research must focus on the multiple unanswered questions involving the etiology, prevention, and treatment of cancers in women.

Deaths in women caused by AIDS have increased since the beginning of the epidemic in the United States. Half of the women with AIDS were exposed to HIV by injecting drugs. Of those exposed through heterosexual contact, almost two thirds indicated that their sexual partners were intravenous drug users.

AIDS continues to be a serious epidemic in women. In 1999, the women in whom AIDS was diagnosed represented 23% of new cases, although the overall incidence of AIDS has been declining. In the United States, women with HIV infection are economically poor and often lack access to competent medical care. The most common means of HIV acquisition is heterosexual contact, followed by injection drug use. However, these two methods overlap in many cases.

Major depressive disorders are more common in women than in men. The consensus among health care professionals is that the observed differences between women and men are real. Depression occurs most frequently in women younger than 24 years. Suicide and attempted suicide indicate depression, and many in our society who attempt suicide are depressed. Again, further research is needed to determine the biologic and psychosocial factors leading to depression.

Life Expectancy

Women are living longer than in previous generations, which is a major reason why they now require more than reproductive health care. Menopausal and postmenopausal health care has become an essential component of health care. During the past century, women's life expectancy has increased. Although the life expectancy of black women lags behind that of white women, the gap seen in previous years has narrowed. In 2000, the life expectancy of white women was 80.0 years, and that of black women was 75.0 years. The life expectancy for women of all races was 79.5 years.

Women are more likely than men to have many debilitating diseases, such as osteoporosis, lupus, and rheumatoid arthritis, that restrict independent living. Women are also more likely than men to be the objects of violence and rape, with attendant psychosocial difficulties. It has been estimated that violence against women accounts for about 5% of the disease and incapacitation in women worldwide.

During the last 20 years, women have become more articulate in stating their health needs. All women require universal access to quality health care, including reproductive health care, and must be made aware of their individual rights—goals that all health care providers must strive to achieve.

These trends in women's health are not exhaustive. They illustrate the totality of a woman's health care environment based on physical, social, cultural, educational, and political factors, all of which potentially contribute to her well-being.

BIBLIOGRAPHY

Alonzo A. Long-term health consequences of delayed childbirth: NHANES III. *Women's Health Issues* 2002;12:37–45.

American College of Obstetricians and Gynecologists. *Female circumcision/female genital mutilation.* Washington, DC: American College of Obstetricians and Gynecologists, 1999.

Cogswell ME, Perry GS, Schieve LA, et al. Obesity in women of childbearing age: risks, prevention, and treatment. *Primary Care Update for Obstetricians/Gynecologists* 2001;8:3:89–105.

Department of Heath and Human Services, Agency for Health Care Research and Quality. *Care of women in U.S. hospitals, 2000.* Available at www.ahrq.gov/data/hcup/factbk3/factbk3.htm. Accessed February 27, 2002.

Department of Health and Human Services, Centers for Disease Control and Prevention. *Assisted reproductive technology success rates. National summary and fertility clinic reports.* Atlanta, GA: Centers for Disease Control and Prevention, 2002. 502 pp.

Department of Health and Human Services, Centers for Disease Control and Prevention. National Center for Health Statistics National Vital Statistics System. Available at www.cdc.gov. Accessed February 26, 2003.

Fathalla M, ed. World report on women's health. Special issue. *Int J Gynaecol Obstet* 1994;1:258.

Fletcher SW. Commentary: Summing up epidemiology's effect on women's health and vice versa. *Ann Epidemiol* 1994;4:174.

Haseltine FP, Jacobson BG. *Women's health research: a medical primer.* Washington, DC: Health Press International, 1997. 364 pp.

Leibman-Smith J. Social consequences of delayed childbirth: NHANES III. *Women's Health Issues* 2002;12:37–45.

Leigh WA. *The health status of women of color.* Washington, DC: Women's Research and Educational Institute, 1994.

Leppert PC. Overview of women's health. *Clin Obstet Gynecol* 2002;45:1073–1079.

Misra D, ed. *The women's health data book,* 3rd ed. *A profile of women's health in the United States, 2001.* Washington, DC: Jacobs Institute of Women's Health and the Henry J. Kaiser Family Foundation, 2001.

Verbrugge LM, Patrick DL. Seven chronic conditions: their impact on U.S. adults' activity levels and use of medical services. *Am J Public Health* 1995;85:173.

Volker R. A new agenda for women's health. *JAMA* 1994;272:7.

World Health Organization. Female genital mutilation: a joint WHO/UNICEF/UNFPA statement. Geneva: World Health Organization, 1997.

CHAPTER 2
The Well Woman Visit: Prevention and Screening

Barbara E. Weber

Preventive health care services are increasingly being incorporated into patient care. Clinical preventive services include screening tests, counseling, immunizations, and chemoprophylaxis. Several organizations, including the American College of Physicians (ACP), the Canadian Task Force on Preventive Health Care (CTFPHC), and the U.S. Preventive Services Task Force (USPSTF), have developed practice guidelines that emphasize critical appraisal of the evidence rather sole reliance on expert opinion to recommend specific interventions. This chapter reviews the theory behind these guidelines, discusses several approaches to disease prevention, and provides summary tables of preventive services.

THEORY

Screening is defined as the detection of disease at an asymptomatic or preclinical stage. The purpose of screening is to improve patient outcomes, often evaluated as decreased morbidity or mortality. Screening should be assessed according to the following major principles:

- Burden of suffering caused by the target condition. For screening to be appropriate, the target condition or disease should be prevalent and a significant cause of mortality, and it must have a preclinical phase that can be detected.
- Efficacy of the screening test. The screening test should be inexpensive, harmless, accurate, and reliable. The test should make it possible to detect the target condition earlier than without screening, and it should be sufficiently accurate that large numbers of false-positive and false-negative results are avoided.
- Effectiveness of early detection. Effective intervention should be available for patients with a positive screening test result, and the intervention should favorably influence outcome. Patients with disease that is detected early should have a better clinical outcome than those whose disease is detected without screening. Early detection should also be cost-effective.
- Population benefit. The total number of deaths prevented by the screening test should be considered, not simply the relative reduction in risk. The costs, both direct (the screening test) and indirect (false-positive and false-negative results), should be considered.

Screening always advances the diagnosis (lead time bias) and thereby improves survival from the time of diagnosis, but not necessarily from the time when the patient would have presented clinically. This difference is crucial in assessing the effectiveness of a screening intervention (Fig. 2.1).

Although a test may be accurate (good sensitivity and specificity), the true usefulness of the test is best determined by the positive predictive value (PPV = true positives/[true positives + false positives]) or the likelihood ratio positive (LR+ = sensitivity/[1 – specificity]). The predictive value of a positive screening test result increases as the prevalence of the target condition

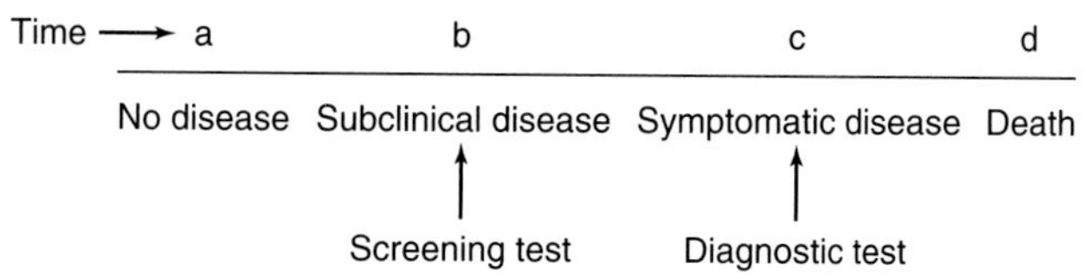

FIG. 2.1. If *d* occurs at the same time whether the disease is detected at time *b* or time *c*, the screening test is not effective. If the time until *d* occurs is extended, if the disease is detected at time *b* rather than time *c*, the screening test is effective.

increases. Screening for some target conditions is best performed for an entire population (blood pressure determination for hypertension), whereas other screening tests should be performed only for selected high-risk populations (thyroid palpation for thyroid cancer in patients exposed to upper body radiation).

OTHER CONSIDERATIONS

The need for evidence of effectiveness is especially important when cost is considered. Ensuring that benefits outweigh risks is critical, especially when interventions are recommended to healthy, asymptomatic patients.

Recommendations for preventive care occasionally conflict. Conflicts may be related to differences in the intended target population, in the objectives of the intervention, or in the interpretation of evidence of the effectiveness of the intervention.

The periodic health assessment should be thought of as more than a traditional history (current symptoms, past medical history, past surgical history, medications, allergies, family history, and review of systems) and physical examination. It should focus on evaluating risk factors, screening for disease, immunization, and health education. Acquiring a complete database (e.g., tobacco use, family history of cancer) allows the clinician to determine whether a patient is at average or high risk for the development of certain diseases. Equally important is the establishment of the clinician-patient relationship.

BARRIERS

Both patient and clinician barriers must be overcome to ensure compliance with preventive care guidelines. Patient barriers include lack of knowledge about the role of preventive health care, fear of screening tests (e.g., discomfort, anxiety generated by a false-positive test result in a healthy patient), and cost. Clinician barriers include concern about conflicting recommendations, cost, uncertainty that outcomes will be improved, and inadequate tracking systems to identify patients eligible for screening. Methods for surmounting these barriers include educating both patients and clinicians, cautiously selecting highly accurate screening tests, minimizing costs to patients, improving the identification of patients due for preventive services, and improving access for patients, especially those who are elderly, members of minority groups, or of low socioeconomic status.

DISEASE-FOCUSED APPROACH

Prevention can be thought of in terms of the target condition (cervical cancer, accidental injury, influenza) or the intervention (Papanicolaou smear, counseling about the use of seat belts, immunization). The next two sections and Tables 2.1 and 2.2 summarize the epidemiology of the leading causes of death (burden of suffering) and provide an overview of the effectiveness of interventions used to decrease the morbidity and mortality associated with these diseases. Subsequent chapters address each specific disease.

Mortality

The most common cause of death for women of all ages is heart disease, followed by cancer, cerebrovascular disease, unintentional injury (accidents), chronic lower respiratory disease, diabetes mellitus, pneumonia and influenza, and intentional self-harm (suicide). The number of deaths caused by each of these diseases varies with age (Table 2.1). Risk factor modification and disease prevention are key to decreasing the mortality associated with these conditions.

TABLE 2.1. Reported Deaths for the Ten Leading Causes of Death in Women by Age, United States, 1999

Age (y)	20–39	40–59	60–79	80+
All causes	30,157	117,773	415,988	630,276
	Unintentional injuries (accidents) 6,300	Cancer 46,757	Cancer 131,972	Heart diseases 238,579
	Cancer 5,747	Heart diseases 20,249	Heart diseases 111,350	Cancer 78,550
	Heart diseases 2,768	Unintentional injuries (accidents) 6,256	Chronic lower respiratory diseases 30,453	Cerebrovascular diseases 68,709
	Intentional self-harm (suicide) 1,915	Cerebrovascular diseases 5,262	Cerebrovascular diseases 27,981	Chronic lower respiratory diseases 26,912
	Assault (homicide) 1,841	Diabetes mellitus 4,199	Diabetes mellitus 17,204	Pneumonia and influenza 26,531
	HIV disease 1,659	Chronic lower respiratory diseases 3,889	Pneumonia and influenza 7,400	Alzheimer disease 25,679
	Cerebrovascular diseases 804	Chronic liver disease and cirrhosis 2,892	Unintentional injuries (accidents) 6,971	Diabetes mellitus 15,192
	Diabetes mellitus 605	Intentional self-harm (suicide) 2,372	Nephritis, nephrotic syndrome, and nephrosis 6,843	Unintentional injuries (accidents) 10,483
	Chronic liver disease and cirrhosis 546	HIV disease 1,673	Septicemia 6,002	Nephritis, nephrotic syndrome, and nephrosis 9,917
	Congenital anomalies 439	Septicemia 1,539	Alzheimer disease 5,373	Septicemia 9,230

Source: Adapted from Jemal A, Thomas A, Murray T, et al. Cancer statistics, 2002. *CA Cancer J Clin* 2002;52:23–47, with permission.

TABLE 2.2. Reported Deaths for the Five Leading Cancer Sites in Women by Age, United States, 1999

Age (y)	20–39	40–59	60–79	≥80
All sites 264,006	All sites 5,747 Breast 1,426 Uterine cervix 519 Leukemia 494 Lung and bronchus 432 Brain and other nervous system 384	All sites 46,757 Breast 11,525 Lung and bronchus 10,182 Colon and rectum 3,571 Ovary 2,964 Pancreas 1,860	All sites 131,972 Lung and bronchus 38,260 Breast 17,773 Colon and rectum 12,940 Pancreas 7,747 Ovary 7,100	All sites 78,550 Lung and bronchus 13,786 Colon and rectum 12,044 Breast 10,415 Pancreas 5,202 Non-Hodgkin lymphoma 3,983

Source: Adapted from Jemal A, Thomas A, Murray T, et al. Cancer statistics, 2002. *CA Cancer J Clin* 2002;52:23–47, with permission.

Heart Disease

Risk factors for coronary heart disease include tobacco smoking, hypercholesterolemia, hypertension, diabetes mellitus, obesity, a sedentary lifestyle, and deprivation of estrogen after menopause. Most research to date on the primary prevention of coronary heart disease has been performed in men. Although the risk factors for disease and the strategies for preventing disease in women may be similar to those in men, the magnitude of the effects may be different. Table 2.3 provides an overview of the interventions used for the primary prevention of coronary heart disease in women. The American Heart Association recommends comprehensive risk assessment and risk reduction for the primary prevention of cardiovascular disease and stroke.

Treatment for a risk factor may be recommended, but the clinician must also consider the efficacy of screening for that risk factor. Screening for hypertension is recommended for all women, yet screening for hypercholesterolemia is controversial, especially in women younger than 45 years with no known risk fac-

TABLE 2.3. Reductions in the Risk for Coronary Heart Disease Among Women According to Type of Intervention

Intervention	Source of data	Estimated mean reduction in risk for coronary heart disease[a]
Smoking cessation	Prospective observational studies in women	Lower risk (50%–80%) in former than in current smokers within 5 years after cessation
Reduction in serum cholesterol level	Randomized trials with >15% women Observational studies Randomized trials in men	No statistically significant reduction in risk in women Positive association between total cholesterol levels and coronary heart disease in women Decline in risk of 2% to 3% for every 1% reduction in serum cholesterol
Treatment of hypertension	Metaanalysis of randomized trials	Relative risk reduction of 15% after 2–5 years of treatment (not statistically significant), similar to the risk reduction found for men
Treatment of isolated systolic hypertension	One randomized trial with 57% women	Relative risk reduction of 25%
Maintenance of normoglycemia in type 2 diabetics	Randomized trial (40% women)	Relative risk reduction of 36%; 6.4% absolute risk reduction (diet plus metformin vs. diet alone); no separate analysis for women
Avoidance of obesity	Prospective observational studies in women	Lower risk (35%–60%) for those at ideal weight than for obese (≥20% above desirable weight) women
Physical activity	Small prospective and retrospective observational studies in women	Lower risk (50%–60%) for physically active women than for sedentary women
Small-to-moderate alcohol consumption	Prospective observational studies in women	Relative risk reduction of 40% in women who consume 3–9 drinks per week compared with nondrinkers
Prophylactic low-dose aspirin	Metaanalysis of randomized trials Subgroup analysis for two trials including women	Relative risk reduction of 42% in male aspirin users compared with nonusers Relative risk reduction of 19% (not statistically significant) in female aspirin users compared with nonusers
Antioxidant vitamin supplementation	Prospective observational studies in women	Insufficient data

[a]Estimated risk reductions refer to the independent contribution of each risk factor to the risk for myocardial infarction and do not account for the many known and hypothesized interactions among factors.

Source: Rich-Edwards JW, Manson JE, Hennekens CH, et al. The primary prevention of coronary heart disease in women. *N Engl J Med* 1995;332:1758–1766, with permission.

Additional data from the following: Walsh JM, Grady D. Treatment of hyperlipidemia in women. *JAMA* 1995;274:1152–1158; Gueyffier F, Boutitie F, Boissel JP, et al. Effect of antihypertensive drug treatment on cardiovascular outcomes in women and men: a meta-analysis of individual patient data from randomized, controlled trials. *Ann Intern Med* 1997;126:761–767; UK Prospective Diabetes Study (UKPDS) Group. Effect of intensive blood-glucose control with metformin on complications in overweight patients with type 2 diabetes (UKPDS 34). *Lancet* 1998;352:854–865; Mosca L, Manson JE, Sutherland SE, et al. Cardiovascular disease in women: a statement for healthcare professionals from the American Heart Association. *Circulation* 1997;96:2468–2482; Stampfer MJ, Colditz GA, Willett WC, et al. A prospective study of moderate alcohol consumption and the risk of coronary disease and stroke in women. *N Engl J Med* 1988;319:267–273; Hayden M, Pignone M, Phillips C, et al. Aspirin for the primary prevention of cardiovascular events: a summary of the evidence for the U.S. Preventive Services Task Force. *Ann Intern Med* 2002;136:161–172.

tors for coronary heart disease. Mathematical models suggest a mortality benefit from blood pressure and cholesterol reduction and smoking cessation in women at high risk for ischemic heart disease. Women must be educated about their risk for coronary heart disease and counseled to avoid smoking, maintain a diet low in saturated fat, and engage in a moderate level of physical activity to help control weight. If these behaviors do not also control hypertension or diabetes, pharmacologic intervention is often necessary. An estimation of the future risk for cardiovascular events assists in determining how aggressively risk factors should be modified; various risk calculators are available, such as the one from the National Cholesterol Education Program (http://nhlbi.nih.gov/guidelines/cholesterol/index.htm).

Cerebrovascular Disease

Risk factors for stroke (cerebrovascular accident, or CVA) include age, non-Caucasian race, hypertension, diabetes, tobacco use, hyperlipidemia, heart disease, transient ischemic attack (TIA), and atrial fibrillation. Rare risk factors, but unique to women, include fibromuscular dysplasia, choriocarcinoma, mitral annular calcification, current pregnancy, migraine, mitral valve prolapse, antiphospholipid antibody syndrome, Takayasu arteritis, and systemic lupus erythematosus. Modifiable risk factors include hypertension, smoking, and hyperlipidemia. Hypertension is the most prevalent risk factor and has the strongest association with stroke. Treating hypertension, including isolated systolic hypertension, reduces the risk for stroke by as much as 36%. The information on the best treatment for women is still limited, given the preponderance of men in antihypertensive trials. Smoking cessation decreases the risk for stroke by 50% within 1 year, and the risk returns to baseline after 5 years. Treating hyperlipidemia in patients with coronary artery disease can decrease the risk for stroke by 30%. The primary prevention of stroke with aspirin is not recommended for all women; however, certain patients at high risk for coronary heart disease (multiple risk factors) or cerebrovascular disease (prior TIA or CVA) may benefit from aspirin. Concerns about the efficacy of aspirin in women are not supported by the data; therefore, women should be considered for secondary stroke prevention.

Diabetes Mellitus

The risk for the development of type 2 diabetes increases with age, obesity, and lack of physical activity. Type 2 diabetes is more common in persons with a family history of the disease and in members of certain racial/ethnic groups. It occurs more frequently in women with prior gestational diabetes mellitus or polycystic ovary syndrome and in persons with hypertension, dyslipidemia, impaired glucose tolerance, or impaired fasting glucose. The decision to screen for type 2 diabetes should ultimately be based on clinical judgment and patient preference because of the lack of data from prospective studies on the benefits of screening and the relatively low cost-effectiveness of screening. The American Diabetes Association recommends screening the general population at 3-year intervals beginning at age 45. The rationale for this interval is that false-negative results will be repeated before substantial time elapses, and it is unlikely that any of the complications of diabetes will develop to a significant degree within 3 years after a negative screening test result. Testing should be considered at a younger age or be carried out more frequently in persons with one or more of the risk factors previously mentioned.

Strong evidence indicates that comprehensive lifestyle interventions, including sustained weight reduction and moderately intense physical activity, reduce the incidence of type 2 diabetes. The risk for diabetes was reduced by 58% in obese, glucose-intolerant patients who received individualized counseling aimed at reducing weight, total intake of fat, and intake of saturated fat and increasing intake of fiber and physical activity in comparison with similar control patients.

The aggressive treatment of diabetes can decrease the morbidity and mortality of the disease by decreasing its chronic complications (42% risk reduction for diabetes-related death and 36% for all-cause mortality). Lowering blood glucose reduces the incidence of microvascular complications in type 2 diabetes by 25%.

Pneumonia and Influenza

Immunization with pneumococcal and influenza vaccines has been shown to be safe and cost-effective in preventing pneumococcal pneumonia and influenza and reducing serious complications of these diseases.

Chronic Lower Respiratory Disease

Cigarette smoking accounts for 82% of deaths from chronic obstructive lung disease. With smoking cessation, the rate of loss of ventilatory function declines, but lost function cannot be regained.

Unintentional Injury (Accidents) and Intentional Self-Harm (Suicide)

For women 18 to 85 years of age, the most common causes of unintentional injury are related to motor vehicles and falls (Web site: Office of Statistics and Programming, National Center for Injury Prevention and Control, Centers for Disease Control and Prevention data source for numbers of deaths in 1999: National Center for Health Statistics Vital Statistics System) (http://webapp.cdc.gov/sasweb/ncipc/leadcaus10.html). All patients should be counseled regarding the use of seat belts and proper protective gear during exercise (e.g., bicycle helmets). Guns in the home should be kept unloaded and locked. Elderly patients should be assessed for their risk for falling (see Chapter 14).

According to the National Center for Injury Prevention and Control (www.cdc.gov/ncipc), males are four times more likely than females to die by suicide; however, females are more likely than males to attempt suicide. Suicide rates increase with age; risk factors for suicide among older persons differ from those among the young. In older persons, the prevalence of depression, the use of highly lethal methods, and social isolation are greater. They make fewer attempts per completed suicide, and the male-to-female ratio is higher than in other groups. Older persons often visit a health care provider before committing suicide and have more physical illnesses. Screening for depression can be accomplished with simple instruments such as the Primary Care Evaluation of Mental Disorders (PRIME-MD); however, because of a lack of data from randomized trials, the USPSTF does not recommend the routine use of case-finding instruments. Clinicians should remain alert for symptoms of depression, particularly in high-risk patients. The diagnosis and treatment of depression are addressed in Chapter 145.

Cancer

The most common sites of cancer causing death in women of all ages are the lung and bronchus, followed by the breast, colon and rectum, pancreas, and ovary. The number of deaths caused by cancer at each of these sites varies with age (Table 2.2).

Subsequent chapters in this book address specific details regarding screening for some of the more common cancers. This section discusses the recommendations for women at average risk for each of the cancers mentioned.

Despite advances in the treatment for lung cancer, long-term survival has improved little. Screening for lung cancer with chest radiography or sputum cytology has not proved to be effective. Although the results of studies of the detection of early-stage lung cancers with spiral computed tomography are promising, no data suggest reduced mortality. Primary prevention may be more effective than screening because cigarette smoking is responsible for more than 90% of all lung cancers.

Screening for breast cancer can be accomplished by clinical breast examination (physical examination), mammography (test), or self-performed breast examination (counseling). Tables 2.4 (clinical examination), 2.5 (mammography), and 2.6 (self-examination) provide recommendations for each of these interventions. Breast palpation accounts for 50% to 67% of the value

TABLE 2.4. History and Physical Examination Recommendations

Area	ACP	USPSTF	Others
Height and weight			
General	Measure to determine BMI in all patients	[B] 18+ every 1–3 y[a]	IOM: 18+ every 5 y AHA: 18+ every 2 y
Selective			CTF: [B] 18+ if one or more: woman of low socioeconomic status, food faddist, adolescent woman, Native American or Inuit.
Blood pressure measurement			
General	[B] 18+ y every 1–2 y and at every visit for other reasons	[A] 21+ every 2 y	IOM: 18+ every 5 y JNC, AHA: 18+ every 2 y
Selective	18+ every 1 y if diastolic BP is 85–89 mm Hg 18+ at least every 1 y if one or more: previous HTN, DM, known cardiovascular disease, moderate or extreme obesity, black race, history of HTN in parents or siblings	[A] 21+ every 1 y if diastolic BP is 85–89 mm Hg	JNC, AHA: 18+ every 1 y if diastolic BP is 80–89 mm Hg; measure BP more frequently if diastolic BP >89 mm Hg.
Assessment of cognitive impairment			
General	"Elderly" functional assessment screening, including measures of cognitive status	[I] No recommendation[b] [I] No recommendation [2003]	NIH: Clinical evaluation CTF 1994: [C] No recommendation for or against Mini-Mental Status Exam; clinician should remain alert for symptoms of cognitive impairment.
Selective	No recommendation		
Assessment of depression and suicidal intent[c]			
General	"Elderly," functional assessment screening, including measures of emotional status	[B] 2002 Screen adults in clinical practices that have systems in place to ensure accurate diagnosis, effective treatment, and follow-up.	ACOG: Stay alert to symptoms of depression; question patients about psychosocial stressors and family history of depression.
Selective	No recommendation	[C] 2002 Keep a high index of suspicion for depressive symptoms in adolescents and young adults, persons with a family or personal history of depression, with chronic illnesses, who perceive or have experienced a recent loss, and those with sleep disorders, chronic pain, or multiple unexplained somatic complaints.	
Assessment for problem drinking			
General	Screen all patients for hazardous drinking of alcoholic beverages or alcohol dependence using a rapid screening test such as the CAGE or AUDIT questionnaire.	[B] Screen to detect problem drinking and hazardous drinking for all adult and adolescent patients. Screening should involve assessment of quantity and frequency; use the CAGE or AUDIT for further assessment.	CTF 1994: [B] Screen routinely using a standardized questionnaire (MAST, CAGE, or AUDIT). NIAAA: Screen for quantity and frequency.
Selective		[B] All pregnant women should be screened for evidence of problem or hazardous drinking (2 drinks per day or binge drinking)	NIAAA: Screen drinkers with CAGE.

(continued)

TABLE 2.4. (*continued*)

Area	ACP	USPSTF	Others
Assessment for drug abuse			
General	Not considered	[C] No recommendation for or against routine screening for drug abuse with standardized questionnaires or biologic assays.	
Selective		Including questions about drug use when taking a history from adolescent and adult patients may be recommended on other grounds, including the prevalence of drug use and the serious consequences of drug abuse and dependence.	
Assessment for violence			
General	Routinely ask about domestic violence of all patients at each initial visit and at periodic intervals (when a woman's relationship status changes, when a woman is pregnant)	[C] 1996: No recommendation for or against the use of specific screening instruments to detect family violence; recommendations to include questions about physical abuse when taking a history from adult patients may be made on other grounds.	ACOG: Screen all patients for intimate partner violence.
Selective	Look for symptoms or behaviors that may be associated with abuse.	Clinicians should be alert to the various presentations of child abuse, spouse and partner abuse, and elder abuse.	ACOG: Screen pregnant women at various times during a pregnancy. CTF 1994: [C] No recommendation to search for elder abuse in the periodic health examination; be alert for indicators of elder abuse and institute measures to prevent further abuse.
Assessment of visual impairment			
General	Not considered	[C] No recommendation	AAO: 20–39 once; 40–64 every 2–4 y; 65+ every 1–2 y
Selective	Not considered	[B] 65+ routine Snellen acuity testing	AAO: More frequent screening if personal or family history of eye disease; African-American; previous serious eye injury; on certain medications or have systemic diseases that affect the eye (e.g., diabetes).
Assessment of hearing impairment			
General	[C] <50 y do not screen	[B] 65+ by history	IOM: Once each during ages 40–59, 60–74, 75+
Selective	[B] Perform pure-tone audiometry testing at regular intervals in at-risk populations, such as persons exposed to excessive noise and those with a family history of hearing loss before age 50	[C] 18–64 if regularly exposed to excessive noise	
Examination of oral cavity to detect oral cancer			
General	Not considered	[C] No recommendation	NCI: Recommend against ACS: 20+ every 3 y; 40+ every 1 y
Selective	Not considered	18+ if one or more: tobacco use, excessive alcohol exposure, suspect lesions detected through self-examination	
Carotid auscultation for cervical bruit			
General	Not considered	[C] No recommendation	CTF: [D] Do not auscultate if asymptomatic
Selective	No recommendation	Discuss with high-risk patients	CTF: 40+ if one or more TIA symptoms, previous stroke, HTN, smoking, CAD, atrial fibrillation, DM

(continued)

TABLE 2.4. (*continued*)

Area	ACP	USPSTF	Others
Thyroid palpation for cancer			
General	No recommendation	[D] No recommendation	
Selective	[B] Perform periodic screening for thyroid nodules in persons who have received radiation to the thyroid region.	[C] 18+ if personal history of upper body radiation in infancy or childhood	
Complete skin examination			
General	[C] Annual skin examination by an experienced clinician	[I] 2001 No recommendation[d]	ACS: 20–39 every 3 y, 40+ every 1 y
Selective	[B] High-risk persons, such as those with dysplastic nevi or family history of melanoma, should have a thorough skin examination to include the scalp, ears, and feet every 6–12 months.	18+ if one or more: increased sun exposure, personal or family history of skin cancer, dysplastic nevi, or congenital nevi (by skin cancer specialist)	
Breast examination by clinician (CBE)			
General	No active recommendations since 1989	[I] 2002 No recommendation (CBE alone)	ACS: 40+ every 1 y ACOG: 18+ every 1 y CTF: Because the relative contributions of mammography and clinical examination have not yet been fully ascertained, recommend CBE every 1 y ages 50–69.
Selective		Not considered	ACS: "more frequently"
Pelvic examination by bimanual palpation			
General	Recommend against	[D] Recommendation against[e]	ACS, NCI: 20–40 every 1 to 3 y; 40+ every 1 y ACOG: 18+ every 1 y NIH: recommend against CTF: [D] recommend against
Selective	Recommend against[a]	[C] No recommendation	NIH: if 1 or more 1st degree relatives with ovarian cancer, consult MD; if hereditary ovarian cancer syndrome, every 1 y[f] CTF: [C] no recommendation

[a]The USPSTF recommends routine evaluation of height and weight using a table of desirable weights or a BMI of more than 27.3 in women as a basis for further intervention.
[b]Clinicians should periodically inquire about the functional status of elderly patients at home and at work and remain alert to changes in performance with age. When possible, information about daily activities should be solicited from family members or other persons.
[c]Refers to use of formal instruments to screen for depression.
[d]Although routine screening for skin cancer by complete skin examination is not recommended, clinicians should be alert to skin lesions with malignant features when examining patients for other reasons.
[e]Although the USPSTF states that screening of asymptomatic women for ovarian cancer is not recommended, they advise examination of the adnexa when performing gynecologic examinations for other reasons.
[f]ACP and NIH recommend against screening asymptomatic women for ovarian cancer with CA-125 or pelvic ultrasound. For women at increased risk for ovarian cancer (more than one first-degree relative with ovarian cancer), the decision to screen should be individualized after discussing the lack of evidence that screening decreases mortality from ovarian cancer. For women from a family with the rare hereditary ovarian cancer syndrome, referral for specialist care is recommended.
Note (Tables 2.4–2.8): The recommended intervention is listed in the first column. "General" screening refers to routine testing of asymptomatic persons who have no risk factors, other than age or gender, associated with the target condition. "Selective" screening refers to testing of asymptomatic persons who are at increased risk for the target condition.
ACP, American College of Physicians; USPSTF, U.S. Preventive Services Task Force.
Square brackets enclose a one-letter "strength of recommendation" code, if available. Indicated next is the age range to which the recommendation applies and how often the test should be done (in years) if specified by the health organization. For selective screening strategies, risk factors are listed. The original articles describing the recommendations are available in the tables provided by Hayward et al. and Sox; citations in this chapter refer to articles that have appeared since 1994, when the article by Sox was published. Not all panels graded recommendations for all topics.
[A] denotes a strong recommendation based on good evidence.
[B] denotes a favorable recommendation based on at least fair evidence.
[C] denotes an intermediate recommendation in which the evidence is too weak to support a positive or a negative recommendation despite grade C evidence ("Yes [C]" or "No [C]"), but the usual recommendation with grade C evidence is "no recommendation."
[D] denotes an unfavorable recommendation (exclude the intervention) based on fair evidence.
[E] denotes an unfavorable recommendation based on good evidence.
"Not considered" indicates that the health organization has not published a practice guideline about the preventive care intervention.
"Recommend against" means that the intervention should be excluded from routine preventive care for the age, sex, and risk status indicated.

(continued)

TABLE 2.4. (*continued*)

"No recommendation" indicates that an authority considered the intervention but, for lack of convincing evidence, refrained from making a specific recommendation either for or against it.
The 2002 USPSTF Web site offers an update to their grading system:
[A] The USPSTF strongly recommends that clinicians routinely provide [the service] to eligible patients. (The USPSTF found good evidence that [the service] improves important health outcomes and concludes that benefits substantially outweigh harms.)
[B] The USPSTF recommends that clinicians routinely provide [the service] to eligible patients. (The USPSTF found at least fair evidence that [the service] improves important health outcomes and concludes that benefits outweigh harms.)
[C] The USPSTF makes no recommendation for or against routine provision of [the service]. (The USPSTF found at least fair evidence that [the service] can improve health outcomes but concludes that the balance of the benefits and harms is too close to justify a general recommendation.)
[D] The USPSTF recommends against routinely providing [the service] to asymptomatic patients. (The USPSTF found at least fair evidence that [the service] is ineffective or that harms outweigh benefits.)
[I] The USPSTF concludes that the evidence is insufficient to recommend for or against routinely providing [the service]. (Evidence that [the service] is effective is lacking, of poor quality, or conflicting and the balance of benefits and harms cannot be determined.)
Other sources of preventive care guidelines are indicated by organization abbreviation:
AAFP, American Academy of Family Physicians; ACC, American College of Cardiology; ACIP, Advisory Committee on Immunization Practices; ACOG, American College of Obstetrics and Gynecology; ACS, American Cancer Society; ADA, American Diabetes Association; AGS, American Geriatrics Society; AHA, American Heart Association; ATA, American Thyroid Association; CDC, Centers for Disease Control and Prevention; CTF, Canadian Task Force (on Preventive Health Care); ICSI, Institute for Clinical Systems Improvement; IOM, Institute of Medicine; JNC, Joint National Committee; NIAAA, National Institute on Alcohol Abuse and Alcoholism; NCEP, National Cholesterol Education Program; NCI, National Cancer Institute; NIH, National Institutes of Health.
Other abbreviations used in the tables: BMI, body mass index; BP, blood pressure; BSE, breast self-examination; CAD, coronary artery disease; CHD, coronary heart disease; CSF, cerebral spinal fluid; CVA, stroke; DM, diabetes mellitus; first-degree relative—parent, sibling, or child; HDL, high-density lipoprotein; HIV, human immunodeficiency virus; HTN, hypertension; IVDU, intravenous drug user; LDL, low-density lipoprotein; PVD, peripheral vascular disease; STD, sexually transmitted disease; TB, tuberculosis; TIA, transient ischemic attack; VZV, varicella-zoster virus.
Source: From Hayward RSA, Steinberg EP, Ford DE, et al. Preventive care guidelines: 1991. *Ann Intern Med* 1991;114:758–783 [Erratum, *Ann Intern Med* 1991;115:332]; Sox NC. Preventive health services in adults. *N Engl J Med* 1994;330:1589–1595, with permission.

TABLE 2.5. Laboratory Test Recommendations

Test	ACP	USPSTF	Others
Hemoglobin measurement for iron deficiency anemia			
General	Recommendation against	[C] Recommendation against	
Selective	18+ if one or more: recent immigrant from underdeveloped country, institutionalized elderly	[B] Pregnant women at first prenatal visit	IOM: 40+ every 20 y
Urinalysis			
General	Recommendation against screening for asymptomatic bacteriuria	[D] Recommendation against	CTF: [C] No recommendation to screen for bacteriuria CTF: [D] Recommendation against dipstick screening for proteinuria IOM: 40+
Selective	Screen for asymptomatic bacteriuria if pregnant, are about to undergo an invasive urologic procedure, have recently had a urinary catheter removed, or are recent renal transplant recipients.	[A] Pregnant women 12–16 weeks of gestation (screen for bacteriuria with culture, not dipstick [D]) [C] Diabetic or elderly (screen for bacteriuria with dipstick)	
Fasting plasma glucose			
General	Consider if <55 years old	[I] No recommendation [2003]	IOM: 40+ every 5 y ADA: 45+ every 3 y CTF: [D] Recommend against AHA: 20+ every 5 y
Selective	18+ if one or more: family history of type 2 DM; obesity; HTN; personal history of gestational DM; membership in ethnic group with high prevalence of DM; atherosclerotic disease	[B] If HTN or hyperlipidemia [2003] [I] No recommendation if pregnant [2003]	ADA: 18+ every 2 y if one or more: family history of DM in first-degree relative; >20% over ideal body weight; Native American, Hispanic, or black race; previously identified impaired glucose tolerance; conditions associated with insulin resistance (acanthosis nigricans, HTN, dyslipidemia, polycystic ovary syndrome); personal history of gestational DM or birth weight of babies >9 lb

(*continued*)

TABLE 2.5. (*continued*)

Test	ACP	USPSTF	Others
Fasting cholesterol[a]			
General	20+ fasting lipid profile every 5 y	[A] 45+ every 5 y	AHA, NCEP: 20+ every 5 y
Selective	65+ continue to screen if in generally good health	[B] 20–45 if one or more: DM; family history of cardiovascular disease before age 50 y in male relatives or age 60 y in female relatives; family history suggestive of familial hyperlipidemia; multiple coronary heart disease risk factors (e.g., tobacco use, hypertension).[b]	AHA: 20+ every 2 y if risk factors present
Thyroid function testing[c]			
General	No recommendation	[D] Recommendation against	ATA: 35+ every 5 y
Selective	Screen every 5 y if one or more: 50+; pre-conception; early pregnancy	[C] No recommendation, but it may be clinically prudent to screen elderly and postpartum women, and persons with Down syndrome.	ATA: "More frequent" serum TSH testing if one or more risk factors: personal history of previous thyroid dysfunction, goiter, surgery, or radiotherapy affecting the thyroid gland; DM; vitiligo; pernicious anemia; leukotrichia (prematurely gray hair); medications and other compounds (e.g., lithium carbonate, amiodarone hydrochloride, radiocontrast agents, expectorants containing potassium iodide, and kelp); or family history of thyroid disease, pernicious anemia, DM, or primary adrenal insufficiency.
Hepatitis B virus surface antigen			
General	Not considered	[D] Recommendation against	CDC 2002: Prevaccination testing is not cost-effective in adolescents.
Selective		[A] Recommended for all pregnant women at their first prenatal visit; may be repeated in the third trimester in women who are initially HbSAg-negative and who are at increased risk for HBV infection during pregnancy. [C] Certain persons who are at high risk may be screened to assess eligibility for vaccination.	
Human immunodeficiency virus (HIV) serology			
General	Recommendation against	[C] No recommendation	
Selective	Screen if currently or previously (any time since the late 1970s) exposed to unprotected sexual activity or blood, blood products, tissues, and organs (specifically patients who have shared needles, received blood, blood products, or tissues in the United States, before effective screening of the blood supply in approximately 1986), have received blood products more recently outside of the U.S. or Western Europe, or have received medical care other than transfusions in developing countries.	[A] Screen if one or more: recent STD, past or present injection drug users; persons who exchange sex for money or drugs, and their sex partners; women and men whose past or present sex partners were HIV-infected, bisexual, or injection drug users; and persons with a history of transfusion between 1978 and 1985. Screen pregnant women in these categories, and those from communities where the prevalence of seropositive newborns is increased.	ACOG: Every pregnant woman in the U.S. regardless of her apparent risk, should be tested for HIV as a routine part of prenatal care.

(*continued*)

TABLE 2.5. (*continued*)

Test	ACP	USPSTF	Others
Syphilis serology			
General	No recommendation	No recommendation	
Selective	Use a nontreponemal serologic test (RPR or VDRL) to screen for latent syphilis in patients with any of the following: history of or current STD, multiple sexual partners, sexual partner with a STD (including HIV), history of substance abuse.	[A] Screen: all pregnant women (at their first prenatal visit), commercial sex workers, persons who exchange sex for money or drugs, persons with other STDs (including HIV), . and sexual contacts of persons with active syphilis. For women at high risk of acquiring syphilis during pregnancy (e.g., women in the high-risk groups listed above), repeated serologic testing is recommended in the third trimester and at delivery	CDC 2002: Screen all pregnant women at the first prenatal visit. Screen in the third trimester if at high risk for syphilis, living in areas of excess syphilis morbidity, . previously untested, or have positive serology in the first trimester
Resting electrocardiogram			
General	No recommendation	[C] No recommendation [D] Recommend against routine ECG screening as part of the periodic health visit or preparticipation sports physical for asymptomatic adolescents and young adults.	IOM: 40–45 once
Selective	As part of disease management (e.g., diagnosis of end-organ damage in patients with HTN)	Screening those with multiple cardiac risk factors is indicated only when results would influence treatment decisions (e.g., use of lipid-lowering drugs in asymptomatic persons). Screening individuals in certain occupations (e.g., pilots, truck drivers) can be recommended on other grounds, including possible benefits to public safety.	AHA: As part of disease management
Exercise stress test			
General	No recommendation	[C] No recommendation	
Selective	Consider screening the following groups with exercise stress testing: asymptomatic patients who have physically strenuous jobs (e.g., firefighters), asymptomatic patients who could jeopardize public safety (e.g., airline pilots), women over 50 who are planning to embark on a vigorous exercise program, women with significant cardiac risk factors who plan to or have become pregnant, especially patients with type 1 DM for >10 y.	Screening those with multiple cardiac risk factors is indicated only when results would influence treatment decisions (e.g., use of lipid-lowering drugs in asymptomatic persons). Screening individuals in certain occupations (e.g., pilots, truck drivers) can be recommended on other grounds, including possible benefits to public safety.	ACC, AHA: No recommendations for women
Assessment of intraocular pressure			
General	Not considered	[C] No recommendation	AAO: 40+ every 3–5 y; 65+ every 1–2 y
Selective	Not considered	An eye specialist should screen populations with >1% prevalence of glaucoma: blacks >40, whites >65, family history of glaucoma, diabetes, severe myopia.	AAO: 20–39 every 3–5 y if black race

(continued)

TABLE 2.5. (*continued*)

Test	ACP	USPSTF	Others
Tuberculin skin testing (PPD)			
General	No recommendation	Recommendation against	
Selective	Screen those at higher risk of exposure to or of contracting TB, including close contact to a person known or suspected to have TB; foreign-born persons from areas where TB is common; residents and employees of high-risk congregate settings; health care workers who serve high-risk clients; medically underserved, low-income populations; high-risk racial or ethnic minority populations, defined locally as having an increased prevalence of TB (e.g., Asian and Pacific Islanders, Hispanics, African-Americans, Native Americans, migrant farm workers, or homeless persons); IVDU; children exposed to adults in high-risk categories.	[A] Screen if one or more: HIV, close contacts of persons with known or suspected TB, medical risk factors associated with TB, immigrants from countries with high TB prevalence, medically underserved low-income populations (including high-risk racial or ethnic minority populations), alcoholics, IVDU, and residents of long-term care facilities (e.g., correctional institutions, mental institutions, nursing homes). 1996	CDC 2000: Screen those at higher risk for exposure to or infection with *M. tuberculosis:* close contacts of persons known or suspected to have TB; foreign-born persons, including children, from areas that have a high TB incidence or prevalence; residents and employees of high-risk congregate settings (e.g., correctional institutions, nursing homes, mental institutions, other long-term residential facilities, and shelters for the homeless); health care workers who serve high-risk clients; some medically underserved, low-income populations as defined locally; high-risk racial or ethnic minority populations, defined locally as having an increased prevalence of TB (e.g., Asians and Pacific Islanders, Hispanics, African-Americans, Native Americans, migrant farm workers, or homeless persons); infants, children, and adolescents exposed to adults in high-. risk categories; and IVDU Screen those at higher risk for developing TB disease once infected with *M. tuberculosis:* HIV; recently infected with *M. tuberculosis* (within the past 2 y); medical conditions known to increase the risk for disease if infection occurs, (e.g., DM, end-stage renal disease); IVDU; and those with a history of inadequately treated TB.
Chest radiograph to detect lung cancer			
General	Recommendation against	[D] Recommendation against	ACS: Recommendation against
Selective	Recommendation against if smoker	[D] Recommendation against if smoker	
Bone mineral content testing[d]			
General	Recommendation against	[C] No recommendation <60 [C] No recommendation 60–64 who are not at increased risk for osteoporotic fractures	NIH 2000: No recommendation. Bone density measurement should be considered when it would help the patient decide whether to institute treatment to prevent osteoporotic fracture. CTF: [D] Recommendation against
Selective	Screen postmenopausal women who have at least one additional risk factor for osteoporosis (history of fracture as an adult, history of fragility fracture in first-degree relative, current smoker, low body weight, frailty, white or Asian race, low calcium intake, alcoholism, inadequate physical activity/impaired mobility, cognitive impairment, recurrent falls, impaired eyesight, residence in a nursing home, use of long-acting benzodiazepines or anticonvulsants); postmenopausal women in whom the discovery of low bone density, and therefore an increased risk for fracture, would result in an accepted therapeutic recommendation; any woman concerned about her bone health; any person in whom routine radiography detects low bone mass or bone deformity that suggests osteoporosis.	[B] 2002: Screen all women >65 y Screen high-risk women (Caucasian, surgical or early natural menopause, slender build) if it would help the patient decide whether to institute treatment to prevent osteoporotic fracture.	NIH 2000: Recommendation for bone density measurement in patients receiving glucocorticoid therapy for 2 months or more and patients with other conditions that place them at high risk for osteoporotic fracture.

(continued)

TABLE 2.5. (*continued*)

Test	ACP	USPSTF	Others
Mammography			
General	Screen 40+ every 1 y Individualize this decision for each woman; there is no consensus on an upper age limit for discontinuing screening mammography.	[B] 2002 Recommend screening with or without CBE every 1–2 y for women 40+ Evidence is strongest for women 50–69 and generalizable to women 70+.	ACOG: 40–49 every 1–2 y; 50+ every 1 y ACS: 40+ every 1 y; stop based on comorbidity, not age CTF 2001: [C] no recommendation 40–49 CTF 1998: [A] 50–69 every 1–2 y AAFP: 50+ every 1–2 y; counsel about risks and benefits of screening before making decisions if 40–49. NIH 1997: Counsel about potential benefits and harms before making decisions about screening if 40–49. AGS 1999: 65–75 every 1–2 y; 75+ every 2–3 y with no upper age limit if estimated life expectancy ≥4 y.
Selective	Screen 5–10 y earlier than the age when breast cancer occurred in a first- or second-degree relative (especially if there is a strong family history for breast cancer at a young age, particularly if it is associated with ovarian cancer at any age).	40+ Recommend screening . women at increased risk (e.g., those with a family history of breast cancer in a mother or sister, a previous breast biopsy revealing atypical hyperplasia, or first childbirth after age 30)	AAFP: 40+ See text for discussion of controversy.
Papanicolaou smear (cervical cytology)[e]			
General	Last revised 1990 20–65 every 3 y	1996 [A] 18+ (or at the onset of sexual activity) if a cervix is present. [B] Repeat at least every 3 y. [D] 65+ discontinue regular testing in women who have had regular previous screenings in which the smears have been consistently normal. [I] Do not screen routinely for human papilloma virus infection.	ACS, ACOG: Screen every 1 year if 18+ or younger if sexually active. After three consecutive normal Pap smears, screen less frequently. AGS: Screen every 1 to 3 y at least until age 70. Any older woman who has never had a Pap smear may be screened with at least two negative Pap smears 1 year apart.
Selective	20–65 every 2 y if at increased risk after consideration of main risk factors (multiple sexual partners, early onset of sexual activity, smoking) and additional risk factors (Black, Hispanic, Native American ethnic origins; certain partner characteristics, history of STD, oral contraceptive use) 66–75 every 3 y if not screened in the 10 y before age 66	18+ more frequently if one or more: early onset of sexual activity, multiple sexual partners, low socioeconomic status, HIV. 65+ every 1–3 y if no documentation of consistently normal cervical cytology in the previous 10 y. [D] Do not screen if s/p total hysterectomy for benign disease.	CDC 2002: During the evaluation of an STD, if a woman has not had a Pap test during the previous 12–36 months, a Pap smear may be obtained as part of the routine pelvic examination. ICSI: Women with one or more risk factor (e.g., HIV, moderate dysplasia on Pap smear <5 y, intercourse within 1 y of menarche, no prior screening, human papillomavirus, six or more lifetime sexual partners, low socioeconomic class, black, smoker, oral contraceptive user) have a greater need to be screened, but do not need to be screened more frequently as long as their prior Pap smears have been normal.
Gonorrhea culture[f]			
General	Not considered	1996 [D] Recommend against screening low-risk adults.	

(continued)

TABLE 2.5. (*continued*)

Test	ACP	USPSTF	Others
Selective	Screen those with new or multiple sexual partners, history of STDs or unprotected intercourse.	[B] Recommend routine screening of asymptomatic women at high risk of infection (e.g., prostitutes, persons with a history of repeated episodes of gonorrhea, and women under age 25 with two or more sex partners in the last year). In communities with high prevalence of gonorrhea, broader screening of sexually active young women may be warranted. [B] Recommend screening at the first prenatal visit for pregnant women who fall into one of the high-risk categories; an additional test in the third trimester is recommended for those at continued risk of acquiring gonorrhea. [C] No recommendation for universal screening of pregnant women.	CDC 2002: Screen at the first prenatal visit for women at risk or for women living in an area in which the prevalence of *N. gonorrhoeae* is high. A test should be repeated during the third trimester for those at continued risk.
Chlamydia testing[g]			
General	Screen sexually active women age <24 years every 1 y	2001 [A] Recommend routine screening for all sexually active women ages 25 and younger. [C] No recommendation for routine screening for asymptomatic women ages 26 and older at low risk for infection.	
Selective	Screen those with new or multiple sexual partners, history of STDs or unprotected intercourse. Screen pregnant patients by the third trimester. Screen high-risk pregnant patients during the first trimester.	[A] Recommend routine screening for asymptomatic women at increased risk for infection (e.g., more than one sexual partner, history of STD, not using condoms consistently and correctly). [B] Recommend routine screening for asymptomatic pregnant women ages 25 and younger and other pregnant women at increased risk for infection. [C] No recommendation for routine screening of asymptomatic, low-risk pregnant women age 26 and older.	CDC 2002: Screen at the first prenatal visit. If <25 y or at increased risk for chlamydia (i.e., women who have a new or more than one sex partner), also test during the third trimester.
Endometrial aspirate or biopsy, or transvaginal ultrasound[h]			
General	Not considered	Not considered	NCI 2002: There is insufficient evidence to establish whether a decrease in mortality from endometrial cancer occurs with screening by endometrial sampling or transvaginal ultrasound
Selective	Not considered	Not considered	ACOG 2000: Recommend against screening. ACS: At menopause, if one or more: history of infertility, obesity, anovulation, uterine bleeding, estrogen therapy Memorial Sloan-Kettering Cancer Center 2000: Recommend against screening women with breast cancer who are taking tamoxifen.

(continued)

TABLE 2.5. (*continued*)

Test	ACP	USPSTF	Others
Testing for fecal occult blood			
General	(Colorectal cancer screening guidelines not recently updated) 50+ every 1 y	2002 [A] Recommend screening 50–80 every 1 y	ACS: 50+ every 1 y CTF 2001: [A] 50+ every 1–2 y NCI 2002: 50–80 every 1–2 y ACOG 2000: 50+ every 1 y plus flexible sigmoidoscopy every 5 y or colonoscopy every 10 y or double contrast barium enema every 5–10 y.
Selective	40+ every 1 y if one or more: personal history of inflammatory bowel disease, familial polyposis coli, family history of colon cancer in first-degree relative	1996 Recommend screening before age 50 if family history of colorectal cancer at younger age.	See text for discussion of controversy
Sigmoidoscopy			
General	50+ every 5 y[i]	[A] 50+ every 5 y (optimal interval unknown) 2002 [C] 40+ no recommendation 1996 [D] 18–39 recommendation against 1996	ACS, NCI, ACOG: 50+ every 3–5 y (optimal interval unknown) CTF 2001: [B] 50+ (optimal interval unknown)
Selective	40+ every 5 y if family history of colon cancer in first-degree relative, especially if cancer was before age 60.	1996 [C] 50+ every 3–5 y if one or more: personal history of adenomatous polyps or colorectal cancer or inflammatory bowel disease, first-degree relative with colorectal cancer after age 40 [C] 50+ every 3–5 y if personal history of one or more: endometrial, ovarian, breast cancer	CTF 2001: [B] Periodically if history of familial adenomatous polyposis See text for discussion of controversy.
Colonoscopy			
General	50+ every 10 y	2002 50+ every 10 y (there is no direct evidence that colonoscopy is effective in reducing colorectal cancer mortality)	ACS, ACOG: 50+ every 10 y CTF 2001: [C] 50+
Selective	40+ (or 10 y younger than the earliest diagnosis in the family, whichever comes first) every 5 y if personal history of inflammatory bowel disease, familial polyposis coli, family history of colon cancer in first-degree relative	1996 [A] 18+ if family history of hereditary polyposis syndromes [B] 18+ if personal history of 10 or more years of ulcerative colitis [B] 18+ if personal history of colorectal cancer or adenomatous polyps [B] 40+ if two or more first-degree relatives with colorectal cancer, particularly if age of onset is before 40 y	CTF 2001: [B] periodically if history of hereditary nonpolyposis colon cancer. CTF 2001 [C]: No recommendation if family history of colorectal polyps or cancer but do not meet criteria for hereditary nonpolyposis colon cancer. See text for discussion of controversy.

[a]If the testing opportunity is nonfasting, only the values for total and HDL cholesterol will be usable. If the total cholesterol is ≥200 mg/dL or the HDL is <40 mg/dL, a fasting lipoprotein profile is needed for appropriate management based on LDL.
[b]The optimal interval for screening is uncertain. On the basis of other guidelines and expert opinion, reasonable options include every 5 years, shorter intervals for people who have lipid levels close to those warranting therapy, and longer intervals for low-risk people who have had low or repeatedly normal lipid levels. An age to stop screening is not established. Screening may be appropriate in older people who have never been screened, but repeated screening is less important in older people because lipid levels are less likely to increase after age 65 years.
[c]Sensitive thyrotropin (TSH) immunoradiometric assay.
[d]Methods for assessing the risk for osteoporosis-related fractures with bone mineral content testing include single-photon absorptiometry, dual-photon absorptiometry (DEXA), and quantitative computed tomography. DEXA has the highest accuracy and precision of any densitometry technique.
[e]The ACP, the ACS, the CTF, and the USPSTF suggest initiating screening with 2 to 3 annual smears at the onset of sexual activity. Recommendations pertain to women who are sexually active. After three normal annual examination results, the Papanicolaou test may be done less frequently at the discretion of the physician.
[f]Culture from urethral, rectal, throat, or endocervical swabs.
[g]Culture or immunofluorescent assay of endocervical or urethral swabs.
[h]All women should be taught to report postmenopausal bleeding.
[i]Air-contrast barium enema every 5 years may be substituted for sigmoidoscopy.

TABLE 2.6. Counseling Recommendations

Topic	ACP	USPSTF	Others
Dietary assessment and nutritional counseling			
Caloric balance and type	18+ Identify individuals who are at risk for obesity and complications by noting one or more: body weight increasing at a rate above 1 to 2 per year, strong family history of being overweight, waist circumference >88 cm (35 in), low level of physical activity. Counsel at-risk individuals about the importance of controlling calorie intake, lowering fat intake for weight loss or weight maintenance, increasing dietary fiber. Explain the importance of understanding the increased risk for weight gain in smokers who stop smoking, increasing weight with age, diabetes, heart disease, sleep apnea.	Both diet and exercise should be designed to achieve and maintain a desirable weight by keeping caloric intake balanced with energy expenditures. [A] 18+ limit dietary intake of fat to <30% of total calories (saturated fat to <10% of total calories). [B] 18+ limit dietary intake of cholesterol to <300 mg/d. [B] 18+ maintain caloric balance in diet; emphasize fruits, vegetables, and grain products containing fiber. [C] No recommendation to reduce dietary sodium intake or increase dietary intake of iron, β-carotene, or other antioxidants. Recommendation to reduce sodium intake may be made on other grounds, including the potential beneficial effects on blood pressure in salt-sensitive persons.	NAS/IOM: 18+ advise to balance food intake and physical activity to maintain appropriate body weight. Carbohydrates: 45%–65% of total calories Fat: 20%–35% of total calories Protein: 10%–35% of total calories Fiber: 25 g if ≤50 y; 21 g if >50 y AHA: Do not recommend widespread use of folic acid and B vitamin supplements to reduce the risk of heart disease and stroke. Advise a healthy, balanced diet that includes five servings of fruits and vegetables a day. AHA 2000: Balance the number of calories eaten with the number used each day. General recommendations (daily): Eat 5+ servings of a variety of fruits and vegetables; 6+ servings of a variety of grain products, including whole grains; include fat-free and low-fat milk products, fish, legumes (beans), skinless poultry, and lean meats; choose fats with 2 g or less saturated fat per serving, such as liquid and tub margarines, canola oil, and olive oil. Limit intake of foods high in calories or low in nutrition, high in saturated fat, *trans* fat, and cholesterol.
Sodium	Counsel patients at risk for HTN about the importance of dietary sodium reduction.	1996: Reduce intake of dietary sodium in people with sodium-dependent hypertension or who are likely to develop it in the future.	AHA 2000: Advise to limit total daily intake of salt to <6 g (sodium chloride = 2.4 g sodium) NAS: 18+ advise to limit total intake of salt to 6 g/d or less by avoiding salty foods and limiting salt added to foods.
Calcium	Recommend daily intake at least: 1,000 mg/d in adults <50 y 1,200–1,500 mg/d in adults >50 y	[B] 18+ counsel to consume recommended quantities of calcium: Adolescents and young adults: 1,200–1,500 mg/d Adults 25–50 y: 1,000 mg/d Postmenopausal: 1,000–1,500 mg/d Pregnant or nursing: 1,200–1,500 mg/d	NAS/IOM 2001: <18 y 1,300 mg/d; 18–50 y 1,000 mg/d; >50 y 1,200 mg/d ACOG: Premenopausal 1,200 mg/d; postmenopausal 1,500 mg/d
Vitamin D	Recommend daily intake: <50 y: 200 to 400 IU 51–70 y: 400 IU >70 y: 600 IU	Not considered	IOM 1997: Recommend daily intake: 18–50 y, pregnant, lactating: 200 IU 50–70 y: 400 IU >70 y: 600 IU ACOG: >65 y: 400 IU/d
Iron	Not considered	[C] No recommendation for or against the routine use of iron supplements for pregnant women who are not anemic. Adequate dietary iron intake may be important for menstruating women and for young children to maintain iron stores and prevent iron deficiency anemia.	IOM/NAS 2001: Recommend daily intake: 18–50 y: 18 mg Lactating or >50 y: 8 mg Pregnant: 27 mg ACOG: >65 y: 5 mg/d; pregnant: 30 mg/d; nonpregnant: 15 mg/d
Physical activity and exercise	[C] 2002: No recommendation to counsel adults in the primary care setting to increase physical activity. Counsel individuals at risk for obesity about the importance of exercising for 30 minutes, five times per week.	[I] 2002: No recommendation for or against behavioral counseling in primary care settings to promote physical activity.[a]	AHA 2000: Walk or do other activities for at least 30 minutes on most days. NAS/IOM: Recommend ≥1 hour of moderately intense physical activity per day. CTF 1994 [B]: Recommend ≥30 minutes moderate activity most days of the week.

(continued)

TABLE 2.6. (*continued*)

Topic	ACP	USPSTF	Others
Cancer surveillance and risk reduction			
Melanoma	Counsel to reduce risk: wear protective clothing, avoid peak hours of the sun, wear sunscreen with at least SPF 15; limit sun exposure; strictly avoid sun burning.	[C] 1996 No recommendation for or against counseling patients to perform periodic self-examination of the skin. Clinicians may wish to educate patients with established risk factors for skin cancer concerning signs and symptoms suggesting cutaneous malignancy and the possible benefits of periodic self-examination.	ACS: Advise monthly skin self-exam and prevention (sunscreen use and avoid sun exposure).
Breast cancer	20+ Counsel monthly BSE	[I] 2002 No recommendation for or against teaching or performing routine BSE	ACS: Advise monthly BSE. ACOG: Advise monthly BSE.
Cervical cancer	Not considered	[C] 1996 No recommendation for or against routine counseling. Include information about the potential reduced risk of cervical cancer in barrier contraception users when counseling women about contraceptive options.	
Sexual practices			
STD	Advise patients to limit the number of sexual partners and to use barrier methods of contraception to decrease the risk of acquiring gonorrhea, *Chlamydia,* and trichomoniasis.	[B] 1996: 18+ recommend advising about risk factors for STDs and counseling about effective measures to reduce risk of infection.	CDC 2002: Recommending interactive counseling approaches directed at a patient's personal risk, the situations in which risk occurs, and use of goal-setting strategies is effective in STD prevention. Prevention counseling is believed to be more effective if provided in a nonjudgmental manner appropriate to the patient's culture, language, sex, sexual orientation, age, and developmental level.
HIV	Counsel at-risk individuals (sexually active individuals, those contemplating the potential for sexual encounters) about the routes of HIV transmission (any mucosal exposure to genital secretions) and risk reduction strategies (sexual abstinence, decreased numbers of sexual partners, consistent use of barrier protection for all sexual intercourse). Counsel pregnant women, as well as couples contemplating pregnancy, about the risks of maternal-fetal transmission and include the option of HIV testing as a routine part of prenatal care. Counsel IVDU or individuals who use percutaneous needles for any reason about the risks of HIV transmission and encourage risk reduction behaviors (sharps disposal, avoid needle sharing).	Patients who have sex with multiple partners, casual partners, or other persons who may be HIV-infected should be advised to use a latex condom at each encounter and to avoid anal intercourse.	
Unintended pregnancy	Not considered	[B] 1996: 18+ recommend periodic counseling about effective contraceptive methods.	

(continued)

TABLE 2.6. (*continued*)

Topic	ACP	USPSTF	Others
Substance abuse			
Tobacco	18+ Encourage smoking cessation in all patients who smoke.	[A] Recommend tobacco cessation counseling on a regular basis for all patients who use tobacco products. [A] Counsel pregnant women and parents with children living at home on the potentially harmful effects of smoking on fetal and child health. [A] Include antitobacco messages in health promotion counseling of non-smoking adolescents and young adults.	AHA: Advise tobacco cessation and avoidance of exposure to second-hand smoke.
Alcohol	18+ Counsel patients about ways to stop alcohol and drug use and give information about existing rehabilitation programs; encourage patients with prior use of alcohol and drugs to continue abstinence.	18+ Counsel to limit alcohol consumption, stop alcohol consumption during pregnancy, not to drive after drinking.	AHA 2000: Advise no more than 1 alcoholic drink per day (1 drink = ½ oz pure alcohol, 12 oz beer, 4 oz wine, 1.5 oz 80-proof spirits or 1 oz 100-proof spirits). NIAAA: Advise ≤1 drink per day; none when pregnant or considering pregnancy.
IV street drugs	See above	Inform patients who report potentially harmful use of drugs of the risks associated with their drug use and advised to cut down or stop. Advise IVDU of measures that may reduce the risk of infections due to drug use (e.g., use a new sterile syringe with each use, never share or reuse injection equipment, use clean [sterile, if possible] water to prepare drugs, clean the injection site with alcohol prior to injection, and safely dispose of syringes after use). Advise pregnant women about the potential risks to the fetus of drug use during pregnancy and the potential to transmit drugs to infants through breast-feeding.	
Injury prevention			
Motor vehicle accidents	Not considered	[A] Counsel patients to use seat belts. [A] Urge operators of vehicles carrying infants and toddlers to use child safety seats. [A] Counsel those who operate or ride on motorcycles to wear safety helmets. [A] Counsel patients regarding the dangers of operating a motor vehicle while under the influence of alcohol or other drugs, as well as the risks of riding in a vehicle operated by someone who is under the influence of these substances. [B, C] Counseling to avoid accidents has not been uniformly proved to be effective.	CDC: Counsel all bicycle riders to wear a helmet when bicycling.
Back injuries	Recommend exercise and fitness awareness to patients, despite the lack of data to support a specific intervention for the primary prevention of low back pain. Advise patients that it is helpful to engage in regular aerobic physical activity and that this might decrease the likelihood of back pain.	[C] No recommendation for or against counseling patients to exercise to prevent low back pain; recommendations for regular physical activity can be made based on other proven benefits. [C] No recommendation for or against the routine use of educational interventions, mechanical supports, or risk factor modification to prevent low back pain; although there is some evidence that exercise protects against the development of low back pain, the effect is modest.	

(continued)

TABLE 2.6. (*continued*)

Topic	ACP	USPSTF	Others
Falls among the elderly	Counsel to reduce environmental hazards in the home (e.g., ensure adequate lighting, install handrails in the bathroom and on the stairs, remove loose cords and rugs, store the most frequently used items in the kitchen within easy reach). Explain that poor vision, muscular weakness, and certain medications are modifiable risk factors for falls.	[B] Counsel elderly patients on measures to reduce the risk of falling, including exercise (particularly training to improve balance), safety-related skills and behaviors, and environmental hazard reduction, along with monitoring and adjusting medications [B] Recommend intensive individualized home-based multifactorial intervention to reduce the risk of falls for high-risk elderly patients (ages ≥75 years or ages 70–74 with one or more additional risk factors, including use of certain psychoactive and cardiac medications, use of ≥4 prescription medications, impaired cognition, strength, balance, or gait) in settings where adequate resources are available to deliver such services. [C] No recommendation for or against the routine use of external hip protectors to prevent fall injuries.	CDC: Counsel elderly to maintain a regular exercise program to improve strength, balance, and coordination. Counsel to make living areas safer (remove tripping hazards, use non-slip mats in the bathtub and on shower floors, have grab bars put in next to the toilet and in the tub or shower, and have handrails put in on both sides of all stairs). Counsel patients to have an annual vision test.
Fire injuries	Not considered	Counsel to install and maintain smoke detector; discuss danger of smoking near bed or upholstery.	
Domestic violence/ firearm injuries	Provide information about domestic violence; obtain patient information materials from national and local domestic violence programs or medical societies, display information in both public and private areas, educate staff to answer questions about domestic violence, discuss safety and respect in relationships as part of safe sex counseling. Emphasize that danger and entrapment will increase, and that extra safety precautions will be necessary if the victim decides to leave the perpetrator.	[C] Counsel to remove firearms from the home or keep them unloaded in a locked compartment. [B] Counsel to avoid engaging in potentially dangerous activities (e.g., swimming, boating, handling of firearms, smoking in bed, hunting, bicycling) while intoxicated.	
Promoting dental health			
Dental hygiene teaching	Not considered	[C] Counsel patients to visit a dental care provider on a regular basis [B] Counsel patients to brush their teeth daily with a fluoride-containing toothpaste and to clean thoroughly between their teeth with dental floss daily. [C] The effectiveness of clinician counseling to encourage these behaviors has not been adequately evaluated.	

[a]The USPSTF found insufficient evidence to determine whether counseling patients in primary care settings to promote physical activity leads to sustained increases in physical activity among adult patients. It did not review the evidence for the effectiveness of physical activity to reduce chronic disease morbidity and mortality, which has been well documented in other recent reviews, or review evidence of counseling in other settings.

of breast examination and mammography. Significant controversy exists about the value and role of each of the screening interventions, particularly for women younger than 50 years. Although many experts recommend an annual clinical breast examination (CBE) for women older than 40 years, no screening trials have examined the benefit of CBE alone (without an accompanying mammogram) in comparison with no screening. Mammography has been the best-studied intervention. Eight randomized controlled trials have been conducted since the 1963 Health Insurance Plan trial. A metaanalysis of the efficacy of screening mammography showed a relative risk for breast cancer mortality of 0.74 (95% confidence interval [CI], 0.66–0.83) in women ages 50 to 74 and of 0.93 (95% CI, 0.73–1.13) in women ages 40 to 49. The results for women younger than 50 years are controversial. Two other metaanalyses performed by the USPSTF and the Cochrane Collaboration came to different conclusions. In 2002, the USPSTF revised its recommendations to suggest screening mammography, with or without a clinical breast examination, every 1 to 2 years for women ages 40 years and older, stating that there is

> ... fair evidence that mammography screening every 12–33 months significantly reduces mortality from breast cancer. Evidence is strongest for women aged 50–69, the age group generally included in screening trials. For women aged 40–49, the evidence that screening mammography reduces mortality from breast cancer is weaker, and the absolute benefit of mammography is smaller, than it is for older women. Most, but not all, studies indicate a mortality benefit for women undergoing mammography at ages 40–49, but the delay in observed benefit in women younger than 50 makes it difficult to determine the incremental benefit of beginning screening at age 40 rather than at age 50. The absolute benefit is smaller because the incidence of breast cancer is lower among women in their 40s than it is among older women.

The Cochrane Collaboration reviewed the topic in 2001. When the data from all eligible randomized trials (excluding flawed studies) were considered, their metaanalysis found no benefit for overall mortality (relative risk after 13 years, 1.01; 95% CI, 0.99–1.03) and a modest benefit for breast cancer mortality (relative risk after 13 years, 0.80; 95% CI, 0.71–0.89). Breast cancer mortality is considered to be an unreliable outcome and biased in favor of screening. The controversy emanates from differences in study design, quality and type of mammography, length of follow-up, and performance of mammography in the control arm. The evidence also suggests that mammography is less effective in women older than 70 years. Experts agree on the need for annual mammography beginning at age 50, recognizing that 75% of all breast cancers occur in women older than 50 years. Some organizations recommend mammography for women ages 40 to 49. Self-examination of the breasts is not recommended by any of the three panels because of a low rate of accuracy.

Screening for colorectal cancer can be performed with a digital rectal examination, fecal occult blood testing, barium enema, sigmoidoscopy, or colonoscopy. The effectiveness and optimal frequency of use of each of these interventions are controversial. Screening with the detection and removal of adenomatous polyps can be considered preventive given the known progression of adenomas to carcinomas. Published reports show a decrease in mortality from colon cancer after screening with fecal occult blood testing (33%) or sigmoidoscopy (70%). Fecal occult blood testing assumes that tumors bleed, relies on a second test with visualization of the colon in a patient with a positive test result, has poor sensitivity, and is associated with poor patient compliance, factors that limit its usefulness. Because there are barriers to the use of sigmoidoscopy (e.g., cost, patient discomfort and fear), the quality of evidence is inferior, and prospective data are unlikely to be available for years, some experts advise cautiously proceeding with the ACP guidelines of regular (every 3–10 years) sigmoidoscopy after the age of 50 years.

Screening for ovarian cancer with a bimanual rectovaginal pelvic examination, testing for cancer antigen-125, or transvaginal ultrasonography has not proved effective in women with one or no first-degree relative with ovarian cancer. Because the prevalence of ovarian cancer is low, even if a screening test had a specificity of 99% and a sensitivity of 100%, the positive predictive value would still be less than 5%. Thus, the National Institutes of Health (NIH) consensus panel concluded that women at average risk should not be screened for ovarian cancer. The NIH and the ACP concur that screening should be individualized for women at increased risk, although the evidence does not support a mortality benefit.

Screening for pancreatic cancer with abdominal palpation, serologic markers, or ultrasonography has not proved to be an effective intervention. The screening tests are not accurate, and early intervention has not been found to decrease mortality.

Morbidity

Although the principles of effective screening emphasize a mortality benefit, the prevention of acute illness and symptoms should not be neglected. Significant morbidity is associated with alcohol and substance abuse (Chapter 148), sexually transmitted disease (Chapters 22, 25, 86), low back pain (Chapter 98), sexual abuse (Chapters 150–152), upper respiratory tract infection (Chapter 54), urinary tract infection (Chapter 75), incontinence (Chapter 81), osteoporotic fractures (Chapters 97, 100), obesity, and impaired vision and hearing. Counseling to prevent such morbidity is addressed in Table 2.6.

In the elderly, health should be defined by the absence of disease, the maintenance of optimal function, and the presence of an adequate support system. The USPSTF major principles of screening are less applicable to the elderly, for whom the concept of compression of morbidity is especially important. Evidence is inadequate to support the effects of many preventive services on morbidity or mortality in the elderly.

INTERVENTION-FOCUSED APPROACH

Expert panels such as the ACP, CTFPHC, and USPSTF have evaluated the evidence for the effectiveness of a broad range of preventive services. Each recommendation is linked to the strength of the evidence. Tables 2.4 through 2.8 review each preventive service and the recommended policy for its implementation in general and selected populations. The tables are organized by intervention: history and physical examination, testing, counseling, immunization, and chemoprophylaxis. Evidence-based recommendations and expert opinion are represented. The tables were adapted from preventive care guidelines published in 1991, 1994, and 1996 and updated with current data:

History and physical examination: A history and physical examination should be performed to assess risk factors and document baseline abnormalities. Emphasis should be placed on maneuvers that will assess risk and influence recommendations for further testing, counseling, immunization, and

TABLE 2.7. Adult Immunization Recommendations

Vaccine	ACP	USPSTF	Others
Hepatitis B inactivated virus vaccine			
General	Recommend vaccinating all newborn infants and unvaccinated children.	[A] All young adults not previously immunized.	
Selective	Recommend vaccinating adolescents who use injection drugs or have multiple sex partners, health care workers, public safety workers, institutionalized clients and workers, hemodialysis patients and staff, household and sexual contacts of HBV carriers, international travelers, IVDU, women with other STDs or high-risk sexual behaviors, patients with chronic hepatitis C and other chronic liver disease.	[A] 18+ initial series if one or more: IVDU and their sex partners; history of sex with multiple partners in the previous 6 months or recent STD; blood product recipients (e.g., hemodialysis patients); health care worker with blood product exposure.	CDC: 18+ initial series if one or more: health care worker with blood product exposure, client or staff of institution for the developmentally disabled, staff of nonresidential day care programs, hemodialysis patient, person with multiple sexual partners or recent STD, prostitute, IVDU in household, sexual contact with HBV carriers, inmate of long-term correctional facilities, recipient of certain blood products.
Hepatitis A inactivated virus vaccine			
General	Not considered	No recommendation	
Selective		[B] 18+ initial series if one or more: persons living in, traveling to, or working in areas where the disease is endemic and periodic hepatitis A outbreaks occur (e.g., Alaska Native, Pacific Islander); IVDU; military personnel; certain hospital and laboratory workers; institutionalized persons (e.g., in prisons and institutions for the developmentally disabled) and workers in these institutions and in day care centers.	CDC: Initial series if one or more: travel to endemic area; IVDU; persons with clotting factor disorders; persons with chronic liver disease.
Inactivated influenza vaccine			
General		[A] 65+ every 1 y (1996)	ACIP/CDC 2002: Every 1 y if desired by low-risk patient.
Selective	Vaccinate every 1 y if increased risk of influenza-related complications (e.g., >50; residents of nursing homes and other long-term care facilities that house persons with chronic medical conditions; 18+ with chronic disorders of the pulmonary or cardiovascular systems (including asthma); 18+ who have required regular medical care or hospitalization during the preceding year because of chronic metabolic diseases (including DM), renal dysfunction, hemoglobinopathies, or immunosuppression (including HIV); women who will be in the second or third trimester of pregnancy during the influenza season. Vaccinate every 1 y if person can transmit influenza to persons at increased risk for complications (e.g., health care workers, employees of nursing homes and other long-term care facilities, home caregivers for high-risk persons, household members of high-risk persons).	[A] 18+ every 1 y if one or more: resident of chronic care facility, chronic cardiopulmonary disease, hemoglobinopathy, metabolic disease (e.g., DM), renal dysfunction, immunosuppression; health care provider for high-risk patients.	ACIP/CDC 2002: Every 1 y if one or more: at increased risk for influenza-related complications (e.g., ≥65 y; any age with certain chronic medical conditions); increased prevalence of certain chronic medical conditions (50–64 y); persons who live with or care for persons at high risk (e.g., health care workers and household members who have frequent contact with persons at high risk and can transmit influenza to persons at high risk); residents of nursing homes and other long-term care facilities. Chronic medical conditions: chronic disorders of the cardiovascular or pulmonary systems including asthma; chronic metabolic diseases including DM; renal dysfunction; hemoglobinopathies; immunosuppression; requiring regular medical follow-up or hospitalization during the preceding year; women who will be in the second or third trimester of pregnancy during the influenza season.

(continued)

TABLE 2.7. (*continued*)

Vaccine	ACP	USPSTF	Others
Measles live virus vaccine[a]			
General	No recommendation	No recommendation	
Selective	18+ two doses if born after 1956 and without proof of immunity or documentation of receipt of live vaccine; revaccinate if college student or health care worker and previously given only one dose of vaccine or killed measles vaccine	[A] 18+ once if born after 1956 and lack proof of immunity, documentation of receipt of live vaccine or physician-documented measles. [B] Give a second measles vaccination to adolescents and young adults in settings where such individuals congregate (e.g., high schools, technical schools, and colleges) if they have not previously received a second dose. Administration of the MMR or measles vaccine during pregnancy is not recommended.	CDC: 18+ if health care worker or student born after 1956 and lacking evidence of two live measles vaccinations, physician-diagnosed measles disease, or laboratory evidence of measles immunity.
Meningococcal quadrivalent polysaccharide serogroups A, C, Y, and W-135 vaccine			
General	Not considered	Not considered	No recommendation
Selective			CDC 2000: 18+ of one or more: terminal complement component deficiencies; anatomic or functional asplenia; travelers to countries in which disease is hyperendemic or epidemic. Counsel college freshmen, especially those who live in dormitories, regarding meningococcal disease and the vaccine so that they can make an educated decision about receiving the vaccination. AAFP: Colleges should take the lead on providing education on meningococcal infection and vaccination and offer it to those who are interested. Physicians need not initiate discussion of the meningococcal vaccine as part of routine medical care.
Pneumococcal polysaccharide 23-valent vaccine			
General	65+ once	[B] Immunocompetent 65+; . consider revaccination at 75 if vaccinated more than 5 years previously	CDC 1997: [A] 65+ [C] Revaccinate if patient received vaccine ≥5 y previously and were age <65 y at time of vaccination.
Selective	Vaccinate <64 y if on or more: residence in special environments (e.g., long-term care facilities); chronic illnesses (e.g., cardiovascular disease, chronic obstructive pulmonary disease [not asthma], DM, alcoholism, chronic liver disease [cirrhosis], cerebrospinal fluid leaks, functional or anatomic asplenia); Alaskan natives and American Indians; immunocompromised persons (e.g., HIV, leukemia, lymphoma, multiple myeloma, malignancy, chronic renal disease, nephrotic syndrome) immunosuppressive therapy (e.g., long-term corticosteroids). Revaccinate once anyone 65 y or older who initially was vaccinated more than 5 y earlier at an age younger than 65 y; immunocompromised patient 5 y after vaccination.	[B] Vaccinate high-risk groups: institutionalized persons 50+; 18+ with certain medical conditions, including chronic cardiac or pulmonary disease, DM, and anatomic asplenia (excluding sickle cell disease), and certain Native American and Alaska Native persons who live in social settings with an identified increased risk of pneumococcal disease; consider revaccination at 65 if vaccinated more than 5 y previously. [C] No recommendation in <65 y immunocompromised patients (e.g., alcoholism, . cirrhosis, chronic renal failure, nephrotic syndrome, sickle cell disease, multiple myeloma, malignancy) immunodeficiency (e.g., HIV, organ transplant)	[A] 18–64 if one or more: chronic cardiovascular disease, chronic pulmonary disease or DM; revaccination not recommended [B] 18–64 if one or more: alcoholism, chronic liver disease, or CSF leak; revaccination not recommended. [A] 18–64 if functional or anatomic asplenia; revaccinate ≥5 y after first dose. [C] 18+ if one or more: HIV, leukemia, lymphoma, myeloma, malignancy, chronic renal failure, nephrotic syndrome, transplant recipient, chemotherapy or steroid use; revaccinate once if ≥5 y have elapsed since first dose.

(continued)

TABLE 2.7. (*continued*)

Vaccine	ACP	USPSTF	Others
Rubella live virus vaccine [a]			
General	Recommendation against	Recommendation against	
Selective	18+ once if lacking documentation of receipt of live vaccine or after first birthday, particularly women of childbearing age and young adults studying or working in educational, health care, or military institutions.	[A] 18 to menopause once if lacking proof of vaccination or serologic evidence of immunity and agreeing not to become pregnant for 3 months.	CDC 1998: 18+ once if nonpregnant and lacking adequate documentation of immunity, serologic laboratory evidence, or record of immunization on or after first birthday. Do not vaccinate pregnant women or those planning to become pregnant in the next 4 weeks. If pregnant and susceptible, vaccinate as early in postpartum period as possible.
Tetanus-diphtheria toxoid (Td booster)			
General	18+ every 10 y or 1 booster at age 50 for persons who have completed the full pediatric series, including the teenage/young adult booster (1994).	[A] 18+ at least once every 10 y; in the U.S. intervals of 15–30 y between boosters are likely to be adequate in persons who received a complete five-dose series in childhood; every 10 y for international travelers.	CDC 1991: Primary series and booster every 10 y.
Selective		No recommendation	
Varicella live attenuated virus vaccine			
General	Vaccinate children, adolescents, and adults who have never had varicella (chickenpox).	[B] Vaccinate healthy adults with no history of varicella infection or previous vaccination.	CDC 1999: 18+ if no reliable clinical history of varicella infection or no serologic evidence of VZV infection *and* one or more: health care workers and family contacts of immunocompromised persons; live or work in environments where transmission is likely (e.g., teachers of young children, day care employees, and residents and staff members in institutional settings); persons who live or work in environments where VZV transmission can occur (e.g., college students, inmates and staff members of correctional institutions, and military personnel); adolescents and adults living in households with children; women who are not pregnant but who may become pregnant in the future; international travelers.
Selective	Vaccinate susceptible if one or more: persons who have close contact with other individuals who are at high risk for serious varicella complications (e.g., health care workers and family contacts of immunocompromised persons); persons in environments in which VZV transmission is likely (e.g., teachers of young children, day care employees, and residents and staff in institutional settings); persons in other environments in which varicella transmission can occur (e.g., college students, inmates, and military personnel); nonpregnant women of childbearing age; nternational travelers; patients who are receiving inhaled corticosteroids for the treatment of pulmonary disease; after VZV exposure to prevent or modify the disease. Recommend against vaccinating pregnant women or individuals with diminished cell-mediated immunity caused by either disease or drug therapy.	Vaccinate if one or more: susceptible health care workers; family contacts of immunocompromised individuals; susceptible adults who live or work in environments with a high likelihood of varicella transmission (e.g., day care centers, residential institutions, colleges, military bases).	Do not vaccinate pregnant women or those planning to become pregnant in the next 4 weeks. If pregnant and susceptible, vaccinate as early in postpartum period as possible.

[a]Most authorities advise using a combined mumps, measles, and rubella vaccine.

TABLE 2.8. Adult Chemoprophylaxis Recommendations

Drug	ACP	USPSTF	Others
Aspirin			
General	Not considered	No recommendation	
Selective	[A] Nonvalvular atrial fibrillation: first choice warfarin, second choice ASA 325 mg/d [C] ASA may not be useful >75 y [A] Prior TIA, CVA; [C] Any dose	[A] Those at increased risk for CHD	
Tamoxifen or raloxifene			
General	Not considered	[D] Recommend against	
Selective		[B] Recommend for women at high risk for breast cancer and at low risk for adverse effects of chemoprevention	
Folate			
General	Not considered	[A] All women planning pregnancy: daily multivitamin or multivitamin-multimineral supplement containing folic acid 0.4–0.8 mg beginning at least 1 month prior to conception and continuing through the first trimester. [B] All women capable of becoming pregnant: daily multivitamin containing folic acid 0.4 mg. Offering counseling to increase dietary folate intake to women who do not wish to take folic acid supplements may be recommended on other grounds, including low risk, low cost, and likely benefit.	IOM 1998: Childbearing age: folic acid 0.4 mg from food and/or supplements AHA: Supplements only when diet provides <0.4 mg daily
Selective		[A] Women planning pregnancy who have previously had a pregnancy affected by a neural tube defect: folic acid 4 mg/d beginning 1–3 months prior to conception and continuing through the first trimester. [C] Women taking drugs that interfere with folate metabolism (e.g., methotrexate, pyrimethamine, trimethoprim, phenytoin), women at increased risk of vitamin B_{12} deficiency (e.g., vegans or persons with AIDS), and those with epilepsy whose seizures are controlled by anticonvulsant therapy should consult with their clinician regarding potential risks and benefits prior to considering folic acid supplementation.	

chemoprophylaxis. The database should include information on the family and social history, personal habits (e.g., diet, exercise, substance abuse), and past medical and surgical history and a pertinent review of symptoms. The history and physical examination can be the most cost-effective aspect of preventive care.

Laboratory testing: Performance should be based on explicit goals and documented efficacy of the test.

Counseling: Although "talk is cheap," clinicians should consider the cost and inconvenience of recommendations for behavior modification. Tobacco cessation must be emphasized because it is responsible for more than one of every six deaths in the United States and is the most important single preventable cause of death and disease in our society. Cigarette smoking accounts for 21% of coronary heart disease deaths, 87% of lung cancer deaths, and 30% of all cancer deaths. Tobacco use is a major risk factor for chronic bronchitis and obstructive lung disease; cancer of the lung, larynx, pharynx, oral cavity, esophagus, pancreas, and bladder; respiratory infections; and peptic ulcers. Because coronary heart disease is the number one cause of death in women, it is practical for clinicians to focus counseling efforts on modifying the risk factors for cardiovascular disease (Table 2.3). This paradigm addresses many features of a healthy lifestyle.

Immunization: True primary prevention can be accomplished, but the efficacy of vaccines in the groups most at risk for disease is controversial.

Chemoprophylaxis: This section is limited to advice about the prevention of coronary heart disease with aspirin and the prevention of breast cancer with tamoxifen or raloxifene. The use of calcium and vitamin D for the prevention of osteoporosis is addressed under counseling.

The arm of the Women's Health Initiative Study comparing combination hormone replacement therapy with placebo was discontinued in 2002 after 5.2 years of follow-up; although the risks for colorectal cancer (hazard ratio [HR], 0.63) and hip fractures (HR, 0.66) were decreased, the risks for invasive breast cancer (HR, 1.26), heart attacks (HR, 1.29), strokes (HR, 1.41), and thromboembolic events (HR, 2.11) were increased in the treatment group. Combination hormone replacement therapy can no longer be recommended solely for the prevention of cardiovascular events.

A recent comprehensive review of the use of vitamins for long-term disease prevention concluded that all adults should take one multivitamin daily.

CONCLUSION

This chapter has emphasized disease prevention and screening (testing in asymptomatic women). Interventions should be considered for general implementation after the four major principles of screening have been considered. Women at average risk for disease differ considerably from those at high risk. Care must always be individualized, and patient preferences should be considered.

BIBLIOGRAPHY

Ahlquist DA, Weiand HS, Moertel CG, et al. Accuracy of fecal occult blood screening for colorectal neoplasia. *JAMA* 1993;269:1262–1267.

American College of Physicians. *Guide for adult immunization,* 3rd ed. Philadelphia: American College of Physicians, 1994.

American College of Physicians. Guidelines for medical treatment for stroke prevention. *Ann Intern Med* 1994;121:54–55.

American College of Physicians. Periodic health examination: a guide for designing individualized preventive health care in the asymptomatic patient. Medical Practice Committee, American College of Physicians. *Ann Intern Med* 1981;95:729–732.

American College of Physicians. Screening for ovarian cancer: recommendations and rationale. *Ann Intern Med* 1994;121:141–142.

American Diabetes Association. Screening for diabetes. *Diabetes Care* 2002;25: S21–S24.

Anastos K, Charney P, Charon RA, et al. Hypertension in women: what is really known? *Ann Intern Med* 1991;115:287–293.

Canadian Task Force on the Periodic Health Examination. *The Canadian guide to clinical preventive health care*. Ottawa: Canada Communications Group, 1994.

Carlson KJ, Skates SJ, Singer DE. Screening for ovarian cancer. *Ann Intern Med* 1994;121:124–132.

Carney DN. Lung cancer—time to move on from chemotherapy. *N Engl J Med* 2002;346:126–127.

Chemoprevention of breast cancer. Recommendations and rationale. Rockville, MD: Agency for Healthcare Research and Quality, 2002. Available at www.ahrq.gov/clinic/3rduspstf/breastchemo/breastchemorr.htm.

Colditz GA, Bonita R, Stampfer MJ, et al. Cigarette smoking and the risk of stroke in middle-aged women. *N Engl J Med* 1988;318:937–941.

Eddy DM. Clinical decision making: from theory to practice—resolving conflicts in practice policies. *JAMA* 1990;264:389–391.

Eddy DM. *Common screening tests*. Philadelphia: American College of Physicians, 1991.

Expert Panel on the Detection, Evaluation, and Treatment of High Blood Cholesterol in Adults. Executive summary of the third report of the National Cholesterol Education Program (NCEP) Expert Panel on the Detection, Evaluation, and Treatment of High Blood Cholesterol in Adults (Adult Treatment Panel III). *JAMA* 2001;285:2486–2497.

Fiebach N, Beckett W. Prevention of respiratory infections in adults: influenza and pneumococcal vaccines. *Arch Intern Med* 1994;154:2545–2557.

Fletcher RH, Fairfield KM. Vitamins for chronic disease prevention in adults: clinical applications. *JAMA* 2002;287:3127–3129.

Franz MJ, Bantle JP, Beebe CA, et al. Evidence-based nutrition: principles and recommendations for the treatment and prevention of diabetes and related complications. *Diabetes Care* 2002;25:148–198.

Goldstein LB, Adams R, Becker, et al. Primary prevention of ischemic stroke. *Stroke* 2001;32:280–299.

Gueyffier F, Boutitie F, Boissel JP, et al. Effect of antihypertensive drug treatment on cardiovascular outcomes in women and men: a meta-analysis of individual patient data from randomized, controlled trials. *Ann Intern Med* 1997;126: 761–767.

Hayden M, Pignone M, Phillips C, et al. Aspirin for the primary prevention of cardiovascular events: a summary of the evidence for the U.S. Preventive Services Task Force. *Ann Intern Med* 2002;136:161–172.

Hayward RSA, Steinberg EP, Ford DE, et al. Preventive care guidelines: 1991. *Ann Intern Med* 1991;114:758–783. [Erratum, *Ann Intern Med* 1991;115:332.]

Jemal A, Thomas A, Murray T, et al. Cancer statistics, 2002. *CA Cancer J Clin* 2002; 52:23–47.

Kawachi I, Colditz GA, Stampfer MJ, et al. Smoking cessation and decreased risk of stroke in women. *JAMA* 1993;269:232–236.

Kerlikowske K, Grady D, Rubin SM, et al. Efficacy of screening mammography: a meta-analysis. *JAMA* 1995;273:149–154.

Klinkman MS, Zazove P, Mehr DR, et al. A criterion-based review of preventive health care in the elderly. Part 1. Theoretical framework and development of criteria. *J Fam Pract* 1992;34:205–224.

Littenberg B, Garber AM, Sox HC. Screening for hypertension. *Ann Intern Med* 990;112:192–202.

Mandel JS, Bond JH, Church TR, et al. Reducing mortality from colorectal cancer by screening for fecal occult blood. *N Engl J Med* 1993;328:1365–1371. [Erratum, *N Engl J Med* 1993;329:672.]

Matchar DB, McCrory DC, Barnett HJM, et al. Medical treatment for stroke prevention. *Ann Intern Med* 1994;121:41–53.

Mosca L, Manson JE, Sutherland SE, et al. Cardiovascular disease in women: a statement for healthcare professionals from the American Heart Association. *Circulation* 1997;96:2468–2482.

Mulrow CD, Williams JW, Gerety MB, et al. Case-finding instruments for depression in primary care settings. *Ann Intern Med* 1995;122:913–921.

National Institutes of Health Consensus Development Panel on Ovarian Cancer. Ovarian cancer: screening, treatment, and follow-up. *JAMA* 1995;273:491–497.

Nystrom L, Rutqvist LE, Wall S, et al. Breast cancer screening with mammography: overview of Swedish randomised trials. *Lancet* 1993;341:973–978.

Olsen O, Gøtzsche PC. Screening for breast cancer with mammography [Cochrane Review]. In: *The Cochrane Library*, Issue 2, 2002. Oxford: Update Software.

Pearson TA, Blair SN, Daniels SR. AHA guidelines for the primary prevention of cardiovascular disease and stroke: 2002. Update: Consensus panel guide to comprehensive risk reduction for adult patients without coronary or other atherosclerotic vascular diseases. *Circulation* 2002;106:388–391

Ransohoff DF, Lang CA. Sigmoidoscopic screening in the 1990s. *JAMA* 1993;269: 1278–1281.

Rich-Edwards JW, Manson JE, Hennekens CH, et al. The primary prevention of coronary heart disease in women. *N Engl J Med* 1995;332:1758–1766.

Screening for breast cancer: recommendations and rationale. Rockville, MD: Agency for Healthcare Research and Quality, 2002. Available at www.ahrq.gov/clinic/3rduspstf/breastcancer/brcanrr.htm.

Screening for lipid disorders: recommendations and rationale. Article originally in *Am J Prev Med* 2001;20:73–76. Rockville, MD: Agency for Healthcare Research and Quality. Available at www.ahrq.gov/clinic/ajpmsuppl/lipidrr.htm.

Selby JV, Friedman GD, Quesenberry CP Jr, et al. A case-control study of screening sigmoidoscopy and mortality from colorectal cancer. *N Engl J Med* 1992; 326:653–657.

Selby JV, Friedman GD, Quesenberry CP Jr, et al. Effect of fecal occult blood testing on mortality from colorectal cancer: a case control study. *Ann Intern Med* 1993;118:1–6.

Shapiro S. Periodic screening for breast cancer: the health insurance plan project and its sequelae, 1963–1986. Baltimore: Johns Hopkins University Press, 1988.

SHEP Cooperative Research Group. Prevention of stoke by antihypertensive treatment in older persons with isolated systolic hypertension: final results of the Systolic Hypertension in the Elderly Program. *JAMA* 1991;265:3255–3264.

Sox HC. Preventive health services in adults. *N Engl J Med* 1994;330:1589–1595.

Stampfer MJ, Colditz GA, Willett WC, et al. A prospective study of moderate alcohol consumption and the risk of coronary disease and stroke in women. *N Engl J Med* 1988;319:267–273.

Taylor WC, Pass TM, Shepard DS, et al. Cholesterol reduction and life expectancy: a model incorporating multiple risk factors. *Ann Intern Med* 1987;106:605–614.

Tuomilehto J, Lindstrom J, Eriksson JG, et al. Prevention of type 2 diabetes mellitus by changes in lifestyle among subjects with impaired glucose tolerance. *N Engl J Med* 2001;344:1343–1350.

U.K. Prospective Diabetes Study (UKPDS) Group. Effect of intensive blood-glucose control with metformin on complications in overweight patients with type 2 diabetes (UKPDS 34). *Lancet* 1998;352:854–865.

U.S. Department of Health and Human Services, Public Health Service. *Healthy people 2000. National health promotion and disease prevention objectives*. Washington, DC: Department of Health and Human Services, 1990.

U.S. Preventive Services Task Force. *Guide to clinical preventive services*, 2nd ed. Alexandria, VA: International Medical Publishing, 1996.

Walsh JM, Grady D. Treatment of hyperlipidemia in women. *JAMA* 1995;274: 1152–1158.

Wolf PA, D'Agostino RB, Kannel WB, et al. Cigarette smoking as a risk factor for stroke: the Framingham study. *JAMA* 1988;259:1025–1029.

Women's Health Initiative Writing Group. Risks and benefits of estrogen plus progestin in healthy postmenopausal women. Principal results form the Women's Health Initiative Randomized Controlled Trial. *JAMA* 2002;288:321–333.

Zazove P, Mehr DR, Ruffin MT, et al. A criterion-based review of preventive health care in the elderly. Part 2. A geriatric health maintenance program. *J Fam Pract* 1992;34:320–347.

CHAPTER 3

The Importance of the Gynecologic Examination

Phyllis C. Leppert and Jay P. Shah

Because a woman's reproductive tract health from birth to death is essential for her total health, the gynecologic examination is especially important. Unfortunately, this examination often is not performed as part of the complete physical examination, or if it is, it may not be carried out adequately. The gynecologic history is distressing for many women because the physician must ask very personal questions to understand the woman's problem or prevent disease. A history and examination include an assessment of the total woman and her physical, psychological, and cultural well-being. Many women avoid a gynecologic examination for fear of discomfort or embarrassment; many more avoid it because they fear an abnormality will be found.

ATTITUDES TOWARD HEALTH PROVIDERS

A physician or provider of either sex is an authority figure; thus, women will relate to individual providers based on their own experience with authority. Women with less money or less education than the physician may view the physician in an unfavorable light because of past negative experiences with persons in authority. Although health care providers who are not physicians, such as midwives and physician assistants, are perceived as having less power than physicians, the same dynamics may apply, especially among medically underserved women in poor communities. When women in focus groups in a medically underserved neighborhood were asked why they did not keep regular appointments for gynecologic examinations, they stated that they thought the doctor might report them for legal transgressions (e.g., to the county government about welfare issues). In this case, the women's image of the physician was one of a person who had power over them. People who are sick are in a dependent situation, especially if they are seriously ill. This extreme dependency further distances them from the physician. A woman may then subconsciously see the physician as a father or mother figure. This subconscious thought is especially apt to interfere with an adequate pelvic examination unless physicians conducting pelvic examinations understand how to accept and deal with the feelings of the women they treat.

Both male and female physicians must understand that a totally professional, caring attitude is essential to ease any psychological distress connected with the pelvic examination that is a consequence of cultural attitudes toward sexuality and the reproductive tract. The United States includes many diverse cultural groups. Some of these groups believe that the only man to whom a woman should reveal her genital organs is her mate. Other women may be uncomfortable with a woman physician because of culturally derived attitudes toward sexuality.

GYNECOLOGIC TEACHING ASSOCIATES

In the mid-1970s, departments of obstetrics and gynecology (or in some instances departments of medicine) in U.S. medical schools began to use gynecologic teaching associates to educate students in the art of the gynecologic examination. However, gynecologic teaching associates are more than surrogate patients; in well-organized departments, these well-versed women are teachers too, and they instruct students in teams without the presence of a physician. Instruction by gynecologic teaching associates, more than any other recent innovation in medical education, has greatly encouraged the sensitive performance of a thorough gynecologic examination.

Medical students are taught that the problem-solving skills essential to making an accurate diagnosis require a completely open and nonjudgmental attitude. A woman must have confidence in her health care provider.

WHEN A GYNECOLOGIC EXAMINATION SHOULD BE PERFORMED

A gynecologic examination is mandatory in any of the following circumstances:

- A general physical examination
- A prenatal examination
- A premarital examination, or an examination before any method of contraception is prescribed
- Examination of a women taking hormones or exposed to hormones, such as diethylstilbestrol
- Examination of a woman with any abdominal or genital complaint.

The four essential parts of a complete gynecologic examination are (a) the initial contact, (b) a detailed history, (c) the physical examination, and (d) the post-examination interview.

INITIAL CONTACT

As in all physician-patient relationships, the initial contact begins well before the woman seeking care actually meets the doctor. An impression of the sort of caring or uncaring provider the physician is begins with the first phone call to the office. The receptionist is a key part of the establishment of trust. He or she must be kind, courteous, and well-mannered. The receptionist must be skilled in distinguishing acute or emergency problems from chronic situations and must be able to ask enough questions to delineate the problem at hand. After the physician-patient relationship has been established, the receptionist is vital in maintaining this professional alliance. A woman with vaginal bleeding should be scheduled in a more urgent manner than a woman requesting an annual examination. Routine examinations are not usually scheduled when a patient is menstruating. It is helpful for the receptionist to ask a patient to bring valuable medical records and a carefully written menstrual calendar. The patient should be advised about routine laboratory procedures included in the examination, such as a Papanicolaou smear. Women should know that they should not use a douche for at least 2 days before a gynecologic examination. A woman who has pain at a particular point in her menstrual cycle should be scheduled at approximately that time in her cycle.

The first meeting between the physician and a woman patient should occur in a consultation room or other suitable place. The patient should be dressed and sitting face to face with the physician. It is inappropriate and leads to discomfort to have the patient lying on an examination table the first time she meets a provider. On the surface, this may appear to be the most efficient way to initiate contact and proceed with the examination, but it is not. It is impossible to perform an adequate examination on an uncomfortable, tense patient, so important history and physical findings are missed. This scenario is inefficiency at its worst.

TAKING A DETAILED HISTORY

A gynecologic examination cannot be performed without a careful history. Although a nurse or another person may obtain a preliminary screening history, the physician should personally obtain the medical history from the patient. It is only by obtaining a careful history that a differential diagnosis can be made and then narrowed. Thus, a physician who takes an unhurried, accurate history in a relaxed setting ultimately is a more efficient health care provider than one who is hurried; in the latter case, inadequate care and misdiagnosis result.

All health care providers must appreciate and respect the patient's temperament. Initially, some personal conversation develops the physician-patient relationship. A good beginning is, "What brings you to the office?" Open-ended questions can be asked regarding the history of the presenting problem. In this type of questioning, no particular response is suggested. At times, some questions need to be directed to avoid irrelevancies. These questions should be used only as necessary. The historical interview is one of the most important skills a health care provider must master. The physician should have the attitude that the physical findings confirm a careful history.

After the precise history of the problem at hand has been elicited, a review of systems should be carried out. The purpose of the systematic review is to uncover problems or diseases that may have been missed in obtaining the history of the present problem. Questions are asked in a logical sequence regarding anatomic areas, beginning with the head and neck and proceeding down to the feet. Clues to gynecologic illness may be obtained in this fashion. Information may point to a systemic problem as a cause of the gynecologic problem. At an initial visit to a physician administering primary care to a woman, a complete history includes a past history, family history, and social history. Information pertinent to the gynecologic examination is asked in an interested but matter-of-fact professional manner. Information to be elicited includes the patient's age at menarche, the type of menstrual cycle normal for her, her last menstrual period, and the previous menstrual period. An inexperienced practitioner may believe that a woman's periods are heavy when in fact the menstrual flow is normal for her. Therefore, the number of perineal pads or tampons usually worn, how often they are generally changed, and any use of double pads should be ascertained. A history of menstrual changes that interfere with work or other activities is significant. If a woman describes pelvic pain, this must be related to the timing of the menstrual period. Without such information, ovulatory pain, a ruptured corpus luteal cyst, ectopic pregnancy, or endometriosis cannot be diagnosed with accuracy. Equally important are the number of pregnancies and the amount and type of sexual activity and experience. Careful, gentle questioning regarding contraception use and any history of sexually transmitted disease is mandatory.

The physician who explains to the woman the reasons for these very personal questions will obtain a more accurate and useful history than the one who is rushed and judgmental. Exceptional skill in framing questions yields the most accurate diagnosis. This area of expanded diagnosis separates the professional approach from the nonprofessional "cookbook" approach to the history. A woman's personal and social history offers a portrait of her lifestyle and gives the physician an idea of how her environment may be contributing to her presenting problem. Information on smoking, consumption of alcoholic beverages, and use of illicit drugs is essential. It is necessary to inquire about a history of sexual assault or possible domestic violence. Questions of this nature may well be asked during the physical examination, especially if the findings suggest possible abuse. A sensitive provider is attuned to the possibility that a woman may initially deny sexual abuse by a partner.

The actual symptoms elicited, placed in sequence in the course of a gynecologic history, usually identify a problem; the physical examination provides the correct diagnosis. The three most common symptoms described by women are abnormal vaginal bleeding, vaginal discharge, and pelvic pain. Abnormal bleeding suggests pregnancy or malignancy, but other conditions can also cause abnormal bleeding. A good history determines the quality and quantity of the blood loss and whether hormones or other medications are being taken. Abnormal bleeding may indicate malignant disease, leiomyomata, pelvic inflammatory disease, or endometriosis. In young women of childbearing age, bleeding or spotting at the time of a normal period may indicate an unruptured ectopic pregnancy or an early intrauterine pregnancy. A history of spotting or bleeding after several missed menstrual periods suggests a threatened abortion. Irregular bleeding suggests carcinoma of the cervix, endometrial or cervical polyps, dysfunctional uterine bleeding secondary to hormonal abnormalities, or endometrial cancer.

When evaluating vaginal discharge, the physician must appreciate that not all discharge is pathologic. Some women may have excessive vaginal discharge without a single symptom, but others with a slight discharge may have many symptoms. A heavy discharge associated with normal vaginal flora often makes the proper diagnosis difficult. A cheesy white discharge is a classic symptom of moniliasis and must be confirmed by a wet smear. A chronic, irritating moniliasis is difficult to eradicate and is often associated with diabetes or HIV infection. An irritating, foul-smelling, frothy, yellow-green discharge of trichomoniasis may be worse after a menstrual period. The diagnosis is made by a hanging drop smear. The discharge of bacterial vaginosis is also irritating and often has a fishy smell. A discharge may mean a gonococcal infection. The physician must ask when the discharge began, the amount of discharge, the nature of the odor, and if blood is seen in the discharge. Knowledge of whether the patient has been taking antibiotics is helpful. Finally, questions determining the relation of the discharge to sexual intercourse and the menstrual cycle are essential.

Pain is probably the most difficult symptom to deal with, from the point of view of both the women and the practitioner. In the case of dysmenorrhea, it is important to ascertain whether the problem is primary or secondary. The type of pain needs to be elicited. Is it sharp? Aching? Dragging? Burning? Cramping? Colicky? Is it bearing-down, pressure-type pain? Is it steady or intermittent? Is it present before, during, or after menses? At what point in the cycle is the pain most intense? What is its location, and does it radiate? Does position change the pain?

Ovarian and fallopian tube pain may be referred to the lower abdomen just above the groin. It may radiate down the medial aspect of the thigh. Pain in the lower rectum may radiate to one or both legs. The physician should ask if the pain interferes with work or sleep. A backache of pelvic origin is never higher than S1. Uterine pain can be diffuse; it may be hypogastric in location or transmitted to the inner aspect of the thigh, but it is never below the knee.

PHYSICAL EXAMINATION

A gynecologic examination is not merely an examination of the genitalia and pelvic organs. A general physical examination should be completed first to look for signs that may explain the presenting symptomatology. For instance, the condition and texture of the patient's hair and its pattern of growth should be observed and noted because these features can reflect her hormonal status. Careful attention should be paid to the thyroid because abnormal thyroid function often causes disturbances in the menstrual cycle.

Breast Examination

The breast examination must include inspection, palpation, and the examination of any secretions. When examining the breasts, a careful physician instructs the patient how to carry out a breast self-examination. This is also an opportune moment to educate the patient about the appropriate timing of mammography.

Both breasts should be carefully palpated as a part of every complete physical examination. Palpation should be performed as a routine measure, and not only in women who have particular signs and symptoms. The early detection of breast cancer depends on an accurate physical examination and the appropriate use of mammography.

A systematic approach to the examination is most important. The patient should disrobe so that adequate observation can be made. A towel or gown can cover her breasts except for the time of the actual examination. The patient should first be sitting up when her breasts are examined and then asked to lie flat with the opposite arm elevated above her head.

The first part of the examination is inspection. This cannot be overlooked or rushed because important information is acquired. The physician must remember that the breasts look and feel different early in the menstrual cycle from the way they do later in the same cycle. All women have a degree of asymmetry of the breasts. However, an increase in the size of one breast over the other may indicate the development of a tumor, cyst, or inflammation. The size and symmetry of the breasts are noted with the patient in a sitting position. The skin overlying the breasts is carefully observed. Edema may be associated with certain carcinomas. An ulceration of the nipple is seen in Paget disease. Skin retraction usually indicates carcinoma. For the physician to see this sign best, the patient should sit erect and raise her arms overhead. This position exerts a pull on the suspensory ligaments of the breasts, and any lesion that is shortening these ligaments will cause skin retraction and deviation of the nipple. Alternative methods of eliciting this information are asking the patient to put both palms of her hands together and push them against each other, or asking her to place her hands on her hips and push against them. Another way is to ask the patient to lean forward at the waist with her hands on the back of a chair. These procedures are helpful in detecting early lesions. Lastly, the nipples should be inspected carefully for evidence of bleeding, discharge, retraction, or ulceration, and the axillary and supraclavicular regions must be observed for evidence of bulging, edema, and retraction.

Next, palpation is performed. The consistency of normal breast tissue varies widely from one woman to another, and it also varies according to age, weight, stage of the menstrual cycle, and pregnancy. Palpation of the breast should be carried out systematically so that all areas of the breasts and their lymphatic drainage can be evaluated. Most providers usually begin with the left breast. Palpation is done with the fingertips, lightly at first. It is carried out in a clockwise fashion until the entire breast has been examined. The nipple is palpated and the presence of discharge determined; this can be accomplished by a gentle stripping motion of the nipple. The right breast is then examined in a similar fashion. Palpation is performed with the patient sitting, then lying down, then with her arms at her sides, and finally with her arms overhead. The axillary and supraclavicular areas are also palpated.

After the examination has been completed, any abnormalities found should be reported accurately. The location should be described by quadrant, and it should be noted whether the lesion is multiple or solitary. The consistency and extent of the mass should be described, in addition to any tenderness. The examiner should record whether the mass is movable or fixed to the wall, whether the nipple is displaced or retracted, and whether the regional lymph nodes are palpable.

The breast examination must be conducted in a complete manner. Mammograms have an important place in the screening of women for breast cancer, but they do not replace a thorough manual and visual examination and an indicated biopsy.

Pelvic Examination

The pelvic examination is an essential part of any complete physical examination of a woman and is considered a basic skill for all providers, just as an examination of the heart and lungs is a basic skill for all. For the nonspecialist, the examination is carried out to ascertain that the reproductive organs are normal and to identify women who require referral to a specialist.

Because women feel differently about the pelvic examination than about the examination of other parts of the body, many are embarrassed. They may be less embarrassed with a female provider, but this is not always the case.

The patient must be comfortable. She should be helped into the lithotomy position and draped adequately for the examination. Gentleness is essential; it is not only reassuring but also essential for the accurate completion of the examination, and it prevents involuntary contraction of the anal sphincter, which makes the examination uncomfortable. Roughness interferes with the accuracy of the examination. Thus, the movements of the examiner's hands must be light at first and deliberate. Quick, darting, or jabbing motions hurt the patient and make the examination impossible. A careful beginning of the examination is essential to the rest of the examination.

First, the external genitalia are inspected. This inspection usually takes 2 minutes. Abnormalities to be noted are erythema, skin lesions of the perineum, and evidence of vaginal discharge. Palpation is conducted to determine the presence of Bartholin cysts or abscesses, and whether the Skene glands are enlarged or inflamed. The areas are gently stripped upward and observed for purulent discharge from the urethral meatus. The strength of the perineal support is ascertained by asking the patient to bear down. Cystoceles and rectoceles may be detected by this method.

The cervix and upper vagina are next inspected by using a vaginal speculum. One of the most important considerations in this examination is choosing a speculum of the right size. This minimizes patient discomfort and allows adequate observation. Vaginal specula are nondisposable metal or disposable plastic. If a disposable speculum is used, great care must be taken not to pinch the skin as the bills are being opened. A disadvantage of disposable specula is that they tend to be all one size and thus are not tailored to the patient. Metal specula are either the Graves (duckbill) type or the Pedersen type. The bills of the Graves speculum are wide and spoon-shaped; those of the Pedersen speculum are narrowed. Both speculum types come in various sizes, from large to small. Except for very obese women, a medium-sized Pedersen speculum is adequate and more comfortable. The vaginal speculum has a movable anterior blade and a fixed posterior blade. A metal speculum can be warmed beforehand, and most modern examination tables have a warming tray at the foot in which the speculum can be kept. If lubrication is needed, warm water can be used.

The technique of inserting the speculum is most important. The speculum is held firmly by the blades between the index and middle fingers. When the speculum is inserted, the blades should be held obliquely and pressure placed against the posterior fourchette. The angle of insertion should be downward toward the sacrum. The blades should not be inserted in a horizontal manner because doing so stretches the introitus and causes pain. When the blades are vertical, the suburethral area is touched and pain is felt. When the blades are almost past the introitus, they should be rotated to a horizontal position and the handle elevated. When the speculum is fully inserted, the blades should be separated. The examiner's thumb presses the thumb piece on the side to elevate the top blade and the hand lifts the handle to lower the fixed posterior blade.

The cervix can then be inspected. The Papanicolaou smear is performed. The most important part of this examination is to obtain an adequate endocervical sample. A cytobrush is inserted into the endocervical canal and turned several times. The material obtained is spread immediately on a slide. (A cytobrush is not used for pregnant patients.) The cervical face and vaginal pool samples are next obtained by using the hand of the wooden Ayres spatula. The traditional method of collection includes spreading the sample on a slide. Because the cellular specimen must be fixed immediately, the slide and the bottle of fixative or spray should be prepared and labeled in advance to ensure prompt fixing of the cells. Alternative methods of cytologic specimen collection and preparation use liquid-based technology. Data regarding the improved sensitivity of these methods in comparison with the traditional collection method are not conclusive, although some studies indicate a small increase in test sensitivity. In addition, the Food and Drug Administration has approved the use of a computer-based system to read Papanicolaou smears. The role of human papillomavirus testing as a screening tool is under investigation.

Cervical cytology does not replace a biopsy. If an apparent lesion or a suspect area is noted, it should be sampled. In fact, any lesion noted by the naked eye should be sampled. Tissue with abnormal cytology should be evaluated by colposcopy, and abnormal areas of the cervix noted in this examination should be sampled. If an abnormality is noted, a negative cytologic report does not obviate the need for a biopsy.

As the speculum is removed, the walls of the vagina should be inspected for lesions. After the speculum has been removed, a bimanual examination is conducted. The abdominal hand brings the pelvic structures to the intravaginal fingers for palpation. The abdominal hand must be positioned to hold the pelvic organs between it and the intravaginal hand. If the abdominal hand is placed too low on the abdomen, the pelvic organs will be missed. This hand should be placed at least three fourths of the way to the umbilicus. The fingers examining intravaginally must be well lubricated and gently inserted into the vagina over the posterior fourchette. The elbow of the intrapelvic hand can rest on the examiner's knee if the physician places a foot on a stool or footrest.

The cervix is easily palpated. It usually points away from the fundus—in other words, if the cervix points posteriorly, the fundus is found anteriorly. Movement of the cervix should be painless. Pain resulting from pathologic conditions such as an ectopic pregnancy or pelvic inflammatory disease is indicated by the patient without questioning.

The uterus should be held between the examining hands and its size, contour, and mobility noted. The cul-de-sac should be examined for masses, tenderness, and irregularities. The broad ligament and fallopian tubes are usually not palpable. The intravaginal fingers should go posteriorly under the broad ligament while the abdominal fingers on the sides of the uterus can approach the broad ligament. Next, the intravaginal fingers should move down and toward the lateral wall on one side, and the abdominal hand should move to just inside the anterior-superior spine of the ilium. This process should be repeated on the opposite side. In this manner, the size, shape, and mobility of the ovaries are noted. In postmenopausal women, the ovaries should not be palpable.

In place of the vaginal fingers, a vaginal ultrasonic probe can accurately detect abnormalities of the reproductive tract. To ease discomfort, the patient is instructed to insert the probe herself under guidance. After the probe has been inserted, the provider manipulates it to facilitate examination of the reproductive organs. Used in this manner, vaginal probe ultrasonography is considered an essential part of the examination, just as sphygmomanometry is essential to determine blood pressure. With ultrasonographic examination, ectopic pregnancies can be diagnosed before rupture and ovarian masses can be discovered at an earlier stage, with great benefit to the health and well-being of patients.

The bimanual pelvic examination is completed by rectovaginal abdominal palpation. The middle finger should be inserted into the rectum and the index finger into the vagina. The examiner palpates the adnexal areas, the posterior surface of the broad ligament, and the rectum.

The health care provider must explain to the woman the steps of the physical examination as it is conducted. The possibility of discomfort must be expressed honestly and in an open manner.

Approaches to the Patient with Chronic Pelvic Pain

A thorough examination of the patient with chronic pelvic pain should include a neuromusculoskeletal evaluation to acquire an understanding of the likely pain mechanisms occurring in a given patient (see Chapter 6). This examination should be included if the cause of the pain is unclear and traditional pharmacologic and surgical treatments have not been helpful. A neuromusculoskeletal evaluation should definitely be conducted if further invasive procedures are being contemplated, especially when the rationale for further procedures is unclear.

According to Weiss, "the additive effect of tense pelvic floor holding patterns, trauma, inflammation, or pelvic organ disease can overload the muscles, stimulating the development of myofascial trigger points (MTrPs) and pelvic floor hypertonus. The increased tenderness and tension in these muscles may refer pain into the lower back, abdomen, or perineum, or it may cause urethral, vaginal, or anal symptoms by compression." This self-sustaining process leads to a constant barrage of noxious stimuli at the dorsal horn of the spinal cord which can lead to *central sensitization*. Clinically, one observes allodynia, hyperalgesia and the spread of symptoms.

An MTrP is a hyperirritable spot, usually located within a taut band of skeletal muscle or its fascia, that is painful on compression and can give rise to characteristic referred pain, tenderness, and autonomic phenomena. The MTrP is the end result of muscle injury at the motor endplate by acute, sustained, or repetitive overloading. The MTrP can then refer pain along a muscle or to surrounding muscles. According to Weiss, it can "set off autonomic nervous system symptoms in the reference zone, weaken the muscles, and increase their sensitivity. The affected muscle and fascia contract, establishing a shortened position and causing surrounding muscle groups to compensate." As a result, MTrPs may also develop in the surrounding muscles, causing the symptoms to spread.

Pelvic floor muscles are uniquely vulnerable to the development of MTrPs because of their anatomically central location, where forces are transmitted between the upper and lower body. Weiss notes "their constant functional activity (supportive, sphincteric and sexual), and their eccentric or elongating contractions contribute to making these muscles a major target of stress."

An MTrP can be asymptomatic (latent) or symptomatic (active), depending on the severity of muscle injury and the predisposition to injury. The evaluation for MTrPs can be carried out only through a history and physical examination because no imaging or blood tests can diagnose myofascial pain. This is a clinical diagnosis that depends solely on the clinical suspicion and acumen of the provider. Unfortunately, it is often undiagnosed or misdiagnosed. Myofascial pain often leads to diagnostic confusion because it frequently co-exists with other pain generators (see Chapter 6). Fortunately, it is very treatable with pharmacologic and non-pharmacologic methods.

In patients with chronic pelvic pain, the benefits of using a broad neuromusculoskeletal approach to find and eradicate all incoming noxious stimuli that maintain the nerve sensitization cannot be overstated. This will help to prevent continued or recurrent pain.

POST-EXAMINATION INTERVIEW

On completion of the physical examination, brief comments should be offered regarding the findings of the examination so that the patient is not left to imagine them. Either reassurance or a brief discussion of abnormal findings is in order. The woman is then asked to get dressed. Afterward, a post-examination discussion of the physical findings is held in a separate consultation room or in the examination room. Good health habits and preventive measures should be stressed. If necessary, specific procedures or tests indicated for diagnostic purposes should be described and the reasons for them explained. Time must be allotted to answer the patient's questions. Therapeutic measures, prescriptions, and side effects should also be explained.

Communication between the health care provider and patient is best when the patient's anxiety is lessened—hence the need for a brief summation of the findings before the more detailed post-examination conference. The post-examination conference is conducted after the patient is fully clothed because the discussion then takes place on a more equal footing. The patient is more comfortable and thus is more likely to pay attention to recommendations and comply with a health care program or specific therapeutic measures.

It is fashionable in the name of efficiency to "move female patients through a system." The woman sees the physician quickly and then meets with a nurse or other worker for the post-examination conference. Although a nursing or dietitian conference has a role in teaching about health or a specific illness, it is false economy to leave all teaching to other professionals. First, it interferes with the trust necessary to the relationship between the primary provider and patient. Second, compliance is improved if the provider and other health care professionals spend time with the patient. Third, it is an opportunity for the provider to obtain important feedback.

Surveys have demonstrated that patients want and need advice and information regarding prescription drugs from the person prescribing the medication, not from the pharmacist. Patients want and need time from their primary care provider, not from a nurse, to review laboratory and diagnostic tests. Taking time to educate a female patient saves time in the long run.

CONCLUSION

In summary, a careful examination of the reproductive system is an essential part of a complete physical examination for women. Skill in performing this examination should be part of the armamentarium of every primary care practitioner.

BIBLIOGRAPHY

American College of Obstetrics and Gynecology. *Technology assessment in obstetrics and gynecology. Cervical cytology screening*. Washington, DC: American College of Obstetrics and Gynecology, 2003:689–693.

Bishop FM, Forelich RE. Interviewing techniques. In: Rakel RE, ed. *Essentials of family practice*. Philadelphia: WB Saunders, 1992:103.

Female genitalia. In: Barkauskas VH, Stoltenberg-Allen K, Baumann LC, et al., eds. *Health and physical assessment*. St. Louis: Mosby, 1994:661.

Female genitalia. In: Bates B, ed. *A guide to physical examination and history taking*, 5th ed. Philadelphia: JB Lippincott, 1991:385.

Gerwin RD, Dommerholt J. Treatment of myofascial pain syndromes. In: Weiner R, ed. *Pain management: a practical guide for clinicians*. Boca Raton, FL: St. Lucie Press, 1997:217–229.

Giamberardino MA, Berkley KJ, et al. Pain threshold variations in somatic wall tissues as a function of menstrual cycle, segmental site, and tissue depth in non-dysmenorrheic women, dysmenorrheic women, and men. *Pain* 1997;71:187–197.

King GD. Female pelvic examination. In: Judge RD, Zuidema GD, eds. *Clinical diagnosis: a physiologic approach*. Boston: Little, Brown, 1989:389.

Timor-Tritsch I, Greenidge S, Admon D, et al. Emergency room use of transvaginal ultrasonography by obstetrics and gynecology residents. *Am J Obstet Gynecol* 1992;166:866.

Timor-Tritsch IE, Monteagudo A. Transvaginal sonography. In: Nichols DH, Sweeney PJ, eds. *Ambulatory gynecology*, 2nd ed. Philadelphia: JB Lippincott, 1995:350.

Travell JG, Simons DG. *Travell and Simons' myofascial pain and dysfunction: the trigger point manual*, vol 2. *Lower half of the body*. Baltimore: Williams & Wilkins, 1983.

Weiss JM. Chronic pelvic pain and myofascial trigger points. *The Pain Clinic* 2001:13–18.

Zuidema GD. Breast. In: Judge RD, Zuidema GD, eds. *Clinical diagnosis: a physiologic approach*, 5th ed. Boston: Little, Brown, 1989:311.

CHAPTER 4

Exercise, Nutrition, and Women's Health

Ann J. Brown

The conveniences of living in a highly industrialized society have greatly altered the physical activity and nutrition habits of the people who enjoy them. The by-product of fast food and suburban living is a U.S. population that is more sedentary and overweight than ever before. In this environment, the prevalence of diseases associated with inactivity and excess body fat has increased dramatically, so that the term *epidemic* has been invoked to describe the alarming rise in some diseases, such as type 2 diabetes. Some groups are experiencing a disproportionate increase, including children, adolescents, Hispanics, African-Americans, and Native Americans. In addition, gender differences in physical activity and overweight have been noted. Although the poor health that results from these social changes must be addressed by public health measures, providers nonetheless must find effective ways to help individual patients make therapeutic lifestyle changes to prevent and treat disease.

BACKGROUND

In its 2002 Annual Report, the World Health Organization (WHO) calls the trend toward inactivity and overweight a result of "living dangerously." In recognition of their enormous health consequences, the WHO places inactivity and overweight among the top 10 health threats in the world today. In the United States, *Healthy People 2010* identifies these lifestyle elements as important targets of efforts to improve the nation's health.

One source of data fueling national concern is the National Health and Nutrition Examination Survey (NHANES). The 1999–2000 survey found that obesity, defined as a body mass index (BMI) of 30 or higher, now affects 31% of adults, up from 23% in the prior survey conducted a decade earlier. Rates of obesity are higher among black women (50%) and Mexican-American (40%) women, but not among men in these ethnic groups. Sixty-five percent of adults are now overweight (BMI, 25–29.9) or obese (BMI ≥30), compared with 56% just 10 years ago. Among children and adolescents, the prevalence of overweight has also increased. The 1999–2000 NHANES found that about 15% of children and adolescents are overweight, defined as a BMI at or above the 95th percentile for age. A decade ago, the rate was about 11%, and in 1960 it was just 4% to 5% (Fig. 4.1). This group reflects the same ethnic trends seen in adults, with African-American and Mexican-American children and adolescents showing rates almost twice that of white children.

CHRONIC DISEASES

Obesity and inactivity contribute to many chronic diseases, including coronary heart disease, stroke, colon cancer, anxiety and depression, arthritis, hyperlipidemia, and type 2 diabetes. Now considered an epidemic, type 2 diabetes affects 7% of the population, up from 4.5% in 1960. Among adolescents, the increase in type 2 diabetes has been most disturbing; prevalence rates reached 7.5 per 100,000 in 1994, up from 0.7 per 100,000 in 1982. Although most diabetic children and adolescents have type 1 diabetes, the proportion in whom type 2 diabetes is diagnosed has increased from just 5% in the early 1980s to approximately 33% now. The young age at diagnosis raises concerns for the development of long-term complications at a correspondingly early age. One report has shown the appearance of renal failure by the age of 30 years in patients given a diagnosis of type 2 diabetes while in their teens.

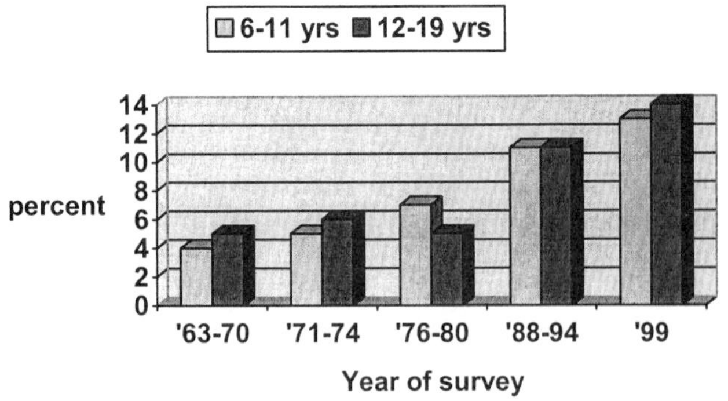

FIG. 4.1. Prevalence of overweight in children and adolescents ages 6 through 19 according to the National Health and Nutrition Examination Survey (NHANES). (From *Physical activity fundamental to preventing disease*. Washington, DC: U.S. Department of Health and Human Services, 2002.)

METABOLIC SYNDROME

The National Cholesterol Education Program (NCEP), WHO, and other organizations have recognized the existence of a preclinical state that is fueled by inactivity and overweight and identifies persons at high risk for cardiovascular disease and diabetes. Called *metabolic syndrome, syndrome X,* or *insulin resistance syndrome,* this state has been defined clinically in various ways. In its most recent guidelines from the spring of 2001, the NCEP Adult Treatment Panel III defines the metabolic syndrome as the presence of three or more of the following: waist circumference of more than 35 inches (women) or more than 40 inches (men); a fasting triglyceride level of 150 mg/dL or higher; a high-density lipoprotein cholesterol level below 50 mg/dL (women) or below 40 mg/dL (men); blood pressure of 130/85 mm Hg or higher; and a fasting blood glucose level of 110 mg/dL or higher (Table 4.1). According to this definition, the NHANES III (1988–1994) survey estimated that one in four (approximately 24%) U.S. adults, or 47 million persons, have this syndrome. The rates for African-American and Mexican-American women are much higher, 26% and 36%, respectively, than those for men in these ethnic groups. Among African-American women, the rates were 62% higher (16% for African-American men vs. 26% for African-American women), and for Mexican-American women, the rates were 78% higher (28% for Mexican-American men vs. 36% for Mexican-American women).

The NCEP Adult Treatment Panel III recommends that persons with the metabolic syndrome receive aggressive counseling about therapeutic lifestyle changes as an initial step in their management. The Association for Clinical Endocrinologists in a recent conference added that it is important to recognize two other disorders strongly linked with the metabolic syndrome and insulin resistance: polycystic ovary syndrome and nonalcoholic fatty liver disease. This conference also suggested that the 2-hour post-glucose challenge test be used to improve detection of the insulin resistance syndrome.

PHYSICAL ACTIVITY: OVERVIEW OF THE PROBLEM

Therapeutic lifestyle changes consist primarily of physical activity and healthful nutrition. Physical activity improves muscle strength and agility and decreases the risk for osteoporotic fracture. It improves cardiovascular health, joint health, and mood and decreases the risk for diabetes. Metabolic benefits of activity are noted even with minimal or no weight loss, and they are realized even when exercise is only moderate, not vigorous. Regular physical activity can benefit all persons, regardless of their baseline level of activity, weight, burden of chronic disease, disability, age, or gender. Based on these observations, the Centers for Disease Control and Prevention and the American College of Sports Medicine recommend a goal of at least 30 minutes of moderate-intensity activity, such as brisk

TABLE 4.1. National Cholesterol Education Program Adult Treatment Panel III Definition of the Metabolic Syndrome

Metabolic syndrome—three or more of the following:	
Waist circumference	>35 inches (women) or >40 inches (men)
Fasting triglycerides	≥150 mg/dL
High-density lipoprotein cholesterol	<50 mg/dL (women) or <40 mg/dL (men)
Blood pressure	≥130/≥85 mm Hg
Fasting blood glucose	≥110 mg/dL

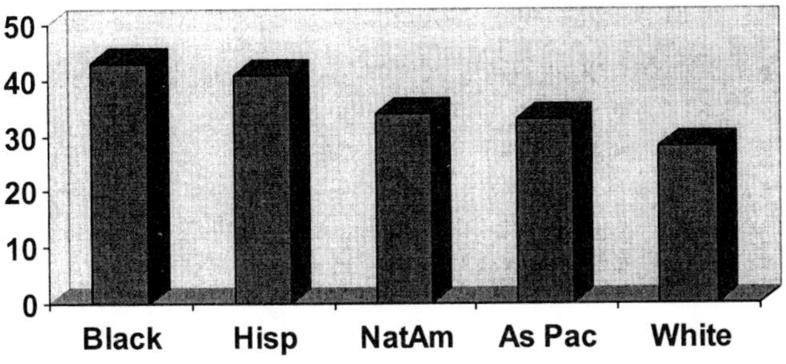

FIG. 4.2. Percentage of women with no leisure time physical activity. (From *Behavior risk factor surveillance survey 1992–1994.*)

walking, on at least 5 days, and preferably on most days, of the week (150 min/wk). By definition, only one fourth of U.S. adults meet this goal, and 38.3% of adult respondents to the 1997–1998 NHANES reported no leisure time physical activity at all. African-American and Hispanic women reported the least activity, with about 40% reporting no leisure time activity, in comparison with 28% of white women (Fig. 4.2). About two thirds of high school students engage in vigorous physical activity, and about one fourth in moderate activity. Girls engage in vigorous activity less frequently than boys (57% vs. 72%). These data support the common sense observation that important habits in regard to activity are set early in life, and that the carryover to adulthood has important implications for chronic disease.

NUTRITION: OVERVIEW OF THE PROBLEM

The Third Report on Nutrition Monitoring provides an overview of the composition of the U.S. diet. According to this report, fewer than one third of Americans include at least five fruits and vegetables in their diet daily. For women, iron intake (12.8 mg) and calcium intake (774 mg) are below the recommended daily allowances. Sodium intake is higher than recommended, with men consuming 4 g daily and women consuming 2.8 g daily. Total fat intake and saturated fat intake remain above the recommended limits of 30% and 10%, respectively, despite vigorous public health campaigns to limit fat intake. The report finds that many pregnant women are not getting the recommended daily amounts of folate, calcium, vitamin B_6, iron, zinc, and magnesium. And finally, as further testament to the influence of social changes on health, one third of family food expenses go toward food prepared outside the home.

Because a high-fat diet has been linked to hyperlipidemia, coronary artery disease, and insulin resistance, it is apparent that poor diet, in addition to sedentary lifestyle and overweight, is contributing to the burden of chronic disease.

PHYSICAL ACTIVITY: OBSERVATIONAL DATA

Epidemiologic studies have reported lower mortality and lower rates of several important diseases in women who engage in regular physical activity. Documented benefits of activity include a decreased risk for coronary heart disease, stroke, type 2 diabetes, colon cancer, breast cancer, and anxiety/depression. The reduction in the risk for diabetes in persons who exercise regularly is substantial, with several studies estimating a reduction of 25% to 40%.

NUTRITION: OBSERVATIONAL DATA

The Dietary Guidelines for Americans published by the U.S. Department of Agriculture illustrates dietary recommendations with its Food Pyramid. The Pyramid advocates a daily intake of 6 to 11 servings of grains, 2 to 4 servings of fruit, 3 to 5 servings of vegetables, 2 to 3 servings of meat/beans/nuts, 2 to 3 servings of dairy, and the sparing use of fats, oils, and sweets. Data from a variety of sources suggest important refinements to the Food Pyramid. For instance, the Nurses' Health Study and the Iowa Women's Health Study showed that the consumption of whole grains instead of refined grains (bran removed) decreases the risk for type 2 diabetes, heart disease, and stroke. The fiber in whole grains delays the absorption of carbohydrates and slows the postprandial rise in glucose and insulin. This effect may help delay progression of the metabolic syndrome to diabetes and perhaps contributes to the observed decrease in the risk for diabetes in women consuming a high-fiber diet.

Another analysis of the Nurses' Health Study showed that the consumption of ω-6 and ω-3 fatty acids reduces the risk for diabetes, whereas the consumption of *trans* fatty acids appears to increase the risk. This observation illustrates the concept that some fats are actually good for health and that not all fats should be assigned uncritically to the "use sparingly" category. In fact, substituting monounsaturated fats for carbohydrates, provided the difference in their caloric density is kept in mind, can result in a decrease in triglycerides. And ω-3 fatty acids (fish oil capsules) are frequently used as a lipid-lowering therapy in patients with hypertriglyceridemia. On the other hand, a diet high in carbohydrate can exacerbate hypertriglyceridemia, a component of the metabolic syndrome and a common finding in persons with diabetes. Thus, adjusting the balance of carbohydrates and certain fats can be therapeutic in some cases.

The U.S. Department of Agriculture Food Pyramid categorizes red meat with poultry, fish, nuts, and beans. Because red meat typically contains more fat, and more saturated fat, than the other choices in this category, the authors of the Nurses' Health Study suggest that it might better be categorized as a "use sparingly" food. They also raise questions about the "dairy" category. They point out that although dairy products such as milk are an excellent source of calcium, they are not the only source. Other sources, such as calcium-fortified orange juice and breakfast cereals, tofu, and broccoli, are low in fat, particularly in comparison with dairy products made from whole milk. These, and milk products that are reduced in fat, are better choices and should be emphasized in this category.

The Food Pyramid guidelines offer a diet with a caloric distribution that emphasizes carbohydrates (~60%), with 25% to 30% calories coming from fat and 10% to 15% from protein. The dramatic rise in obesity at a time when low-fat diets were advocated, combined with popular interest in low-carbohydrate diets, has spurred research on diets with a lower carbohydrate intake. At present, however, no scientific evidence indicates that low-carbohydrate diets are more effective at promoting weight loss than diets based on the Food Pyramid. For patients who prefer to reduce their intake of carbohydrate, it is prudent to encourage more healthful choices of proteins and fats, such as lean meats, beans, or nuts instead of red meat, foods containing monounsaturated and polyunsaturated fats rather than saturated fats, and whole grains rather than refined carbohydrates.

RANDOMIZED CLINICAL TRIALS

Randomized controlled clinical trials that evaluate the influence of a specific dietary pattern on disease are difficult to perform and rare in the literature. However, two key trials with metabolic outcomes have been published. The Dietary Approaches to Stop Hypertension (DASH) and the DASH-Sodium studies both recruited an ethnically diverse, gender-balanced group of people with higher than normal blood pressure or stage 1 hypertension (120–159/80–95 mm Hg). During the study, participants received all meals from the study kitchen. The DASH diet emphasized fruits, vegetables, and low-fat dairy foods and included whole grains, poultry, fish, and nuts. It minimized fats, red meats, sweets, and sugar-containing beverages. At the end of 8 weeks, during which weight and sodium intake remained constant, the DASH diet had lowered blood pressure by 5.5/3.0 mm Hg overall. Reductions in blood pressure were even greater in African-Americans and persons with hypertension. In the subsequent DASH-Sodium trial, sodium restriction in addition to the DASH diet further reduced blood pressure. The PREMIER trial demonstrated that the DASH diet can be successfully implemented outside of a feeding study, by patients making their own food choices. The DASH diet is now recommended for the treatment of hypertension by the Joint National Committee on the Prevention, Detection, Evaluation and Treatment of HTN (JNC VII) report.

Several trials have investigated the use of weight loss and activity interventions to prevent or treat chronic disease. The largest of these is the Diabetes Prevention Program, completed in 2001. The Diabetes Prevention Program studied 3,224 persons with impaired glucose tolerance, defined as a fasting glucose level of 95 to 125 mg/dL or a 2-hour glucose level of 141 to 199 mg/dL during a 75-g oral glucose tolerance test. The group was diverse, with 20% African-Americans, 16% Hispanics, and 5% Native Americans. Women made up 68% of the participants. Individuals were randomized to one of three arms: intensive lifestyle, 850 mg of metformin twice daily plus standard lifestyle, and placebo plus standard lifestyle. Participants receiving the standard lifestyle intervention were advised to lose 7% of their initial body weight and engage in moderate physical activity, such as brisk walking, 150 minutes each week. The intensive lifestyle group received the same advice but with more intensive support, such as one-on-one counseling with a case manager. The people in the intensive lifestyle group lost 5.6 kg and increased their physical activity, whereas those in the standard lifestyle group lost only 0.1 kg and did not increase their physical activity. Persons in the metformin group lost 2.1 kg and did not change their level of activity. In the intensive lifestyle group, the 3-year conversion rate from impaired glucose tolerance to diabetes decreased by 58%. In the metformin group, the conversion rate decreased by 31%. This study demonstrates that moderate physical activity and modest weight loss can prevent or delay the progression of impaired glucose tolerance to diabetes and justifies vigorous efforts to support lifestyle changes to prevent disease.

IMPLEMENTATION TRIALS

The studies previously described, both observational and mechanistic, provide a basis for recommending therapeutic lifestyle interventions for the treatment and prevention of chronic disease. One large question that remains is how providers can help individuals and populations implement healthy changes. Several trials have addressed this issue, basing their interventions on the recommendation to achieve 30 minutes of moderate exercise on at least 5 days, and preferably on most days, of the week.

The Activity Counseling Trial evaluated the effectiveness of two different strategies implemented in primary care practices in increasing activity among adults. A control group received advice from their physician about physical activity and also written educational materials. The "assistance" group received the same, plus interactive mail and behavioral counseling at physician visits. This intervention was augmented in the "counseling" group by the addition of regular telephone counseling and behavioral classes. At the end of 24 months, women in the "assistance" and "counseling" groups had modestly increased their cardiorespiratory fitness, measured by the maximum oxygen consumption ($V_{O_2}max$), by approximately 5%. Neither of the interventions resulted in improved fitness in men.

Project Active compared a structured exercise program with a strategy in which participants increased moderate activity in their daily routine. At the end of 24 months, both interventions resulted in increased energy expenditure and improved cardiorespiratory fitness. Both groups also experienced significant reductions (3–5 mm Hg) in blood pressure. Neither group lost weight, but the percentage of body fat decreased significantly for both.

Both of these studies provide evidence that counseling women to increase their physical activity, either in a structured way or by increasing the activity in their daily routine, is effective in improving fitness.

CONCLUSION

Physical activity and nutrition interventions should be standard tools used in clinical practice to prevent and manage disease. This is especially important as diseases associated with a low level of activity and poor nutrition become increasingly prevalent, particularly in younger persons. Clinical studies, both observational and randomized trials, have provided data about the magnitude of the lifestyle changes needed to bring about a clinical result and about how interventions can be structured to promote adherence. However, much more research is needed to characterize important interventions fully. In addition, we must explore other means of reaching the goals established in documents such as *Healthy People 2010*. These include making low-cost recreational facilities widely available to persons of various ages, people with chronic disease, and those with disabilities, and providing more healthful fast food. Changing the health practices of a population, and thus the disease burden to individuals and society, will require both medical interventions and cultural change.

BIBLIOGRAPHY

Dunn AL, Marcus BH, Kampert JB, et al. Comparison of lifestyle and structured interventions to increase physical activity and cardiorespiratory fitness: a randomized trial. *JAMA* 1999;281:327–334.

Fagot-Campagna A. Emergence of type 2 diabetes mellitus in children: epidemiological evidence. *J Pediatr Endocrinol* 2000;13[Suppl 6]:1395–1402.

Ford ES, Giles WH, Dietz WH. Prevalence of the metabolic syndrome among U.S. adults: findings from the third National Health and Nutrition Examination Survey. *JAMA* 2002;287:356–359.

Jakicic JM, Clark K, Coleman E, et al. Appropriate intervention strategies for weight loss and prevention of weight regain in adults. *Med Sci Sports Exerc* 2001;33:2145–2156.

Knowler WC, Barrett-Connor E, Fowler SE, et al. Reduction in the incidence of type 2 diabetes with lifestyle intervention or metformin. *N Engl J Med* 2002;346:393–403.

Mokdad AH, Bowman BA, Ford ES, et al. The continuing epidemics of obesity and diabetes in the United States. *JAMA* 2001;286:1195–1200.

Stewart KJ. Exercise training and the cardiovascular consequences of type 2 diabetes and hypertension: plausible mechanisms for improving cardiovascular health. *JAMA* 2002;288:1622–1631.

Writing Group for the Activity Counseling Trial Research Group. Effects of physical activity counseling in primary care. The Activity Counseling Trial: a randomized controlled trial. *JAMA* 2002;286:677–687.

CHAPTER 5

Acute Abdominal Pain

Fred M. Howard

The woman with acute abdominal pain represents a challenging dilemma to the primary care physician. Although some patients require urgent operative intervention, most benefit from a methodic approach to evaluation and treatment. It is important to develop the clinical acumen and judgment that enable one to identify a patient who must be rushed to the operating room immediately, such as a woman with exsanguinating hemorrhage from a ruptured ectopic pregnancy. In such instances, only a few minutes may be available to assess the critical nature of the problem, and all obstacles must be swept aside to get the patient to surgery immediately. Fortunately, such circumstances are relatively uncommon.

DIAGNOSIS AND ETIOLOGY

Many disorders present with acute abdominal pain. Often, it is helpful to organize and conceptualize them according to the mechanisms by which they cause pain (Table 5.1). Pain may be of somatic or visceral origin, or both. Visceral sources include the reproductive organs, vascular system, gastrointestinal tract, and urinary tract. Somatic sources include the abdominal and pelvic muscles, fascia, parietal peritoneum, subcutaneous tissue, and skeletal system. An example of pain of both somatic and visceral origin is the pain of parietal peritoneal inflammation resulting from appendicitis.

Visceral pain has characteristics that contribute notably to the complexity of the diagnosis. The viscera contain relatively few nociceptive nerve endings, so that visceral pain is difficult to localize. Furthermore, the pathways within the same spinal segments of pelvic and abdominal viscera overlap significantly (viscerovisceral convergence), as do pathways within the same spinal segments of visceral and somatic structures (viscerosomatic convergence).

Visceral pain may be classified as true visceral pain, referred pain without hyperalgesia, or referred pain with hyperalgesia. Understanding the differences between these classes of visceral pain is clinically useful. *True visceral pain* is a deep, dull, vague, poorly defined sensation. True visceral pain originating in the pelvic organs is usually perceived in the periumbilical area. It is accompanied by a sense of malaise, discomfort, and oppression and by autonomic phenomena, such as pallor, sweating, nausea and vomiting, blood pressure changes, diarrhea, and changes in body temperature. Additional stimulation of the perceived painful area does not increase the pain. Diseases of the viscera tend to manifest true visceral pain in their early stages, when they pose especially difficult diagnostic dilemmas.

Referral is a fundamental and common characteristic of visceral pain. Referred pain is a consequence of viscerosomatic convergence and is felt at a location distant from the diseased organ. *Referred visceral pain without hyperalgesia* is felt in areas of the somatic metameres that relate to the viscus of origin, but the pain is not increased by stimulation of the areas of referred pain. *Referred visceral pain with hyperalgesia* is also felt in somatic areas that are metamerically connected to the affected viscus, but it is accompanied by allodynia, in which non-noxious stimulation of the somatic area of referred pain increases pain, and by secondary hyperalgesia, in which the threshold of pain is decreased in the somatic areas of pain referral. A state of sustained contraction of the muscles in the area also develops in many cases. Visceral diseases with referred pain and hyperalgesia are somewhat less problematic diagnostic dilemmas.

Visceral pain tends to result from the distention of a viscus or organ capsule, spasm of intestinal muscular fibers, infection and inflammation, ischemia secondary to vascular disturbances, hemorrhage, or neoplasm. Obstruction of the small or large intestine, gallbladder, or a ureter may cause distention or spasm and visceral pain. Similarly, vascular disturbances that result in ischemia or hemorrhage of the intestines, kidneys, or spleen may lead to visceral pain. Inflammation of the appendix, gallbladder, liver, stomach, intestine, mesenteric lymph nodes, pancreas, fallopian tubes, uterus, or kidneys is a common cause of abdominal pain. Generally, such inflammation extends to the peritoneum and also causes somatic pain.

Somatic mechanisms causing acute abdominal pain are often related to inflammation of the parietal peritoneum.

TABLE 5.1. Classification of Causes of Abdominal Pain

Visceral
Mechanical obstruction of hollow viscera
Obstruction of the small or large intestine
Obstruction of the biliary tree
Obstruction of the ureter
Distention of visceral surfaces (e.g., hepatic or renal capsules)
Vascular disturbances
Embolism or thrombosis
Vascular rupture
Pressure or torsional occlusion
Sickle cell anemia
Referred from nonabdominal viscera
Thorax (e.g., pneumonia, referred pain from coronary occlusion)
Metabolic causes
Black widow spider bite
Lead poisoning and others
Uremia
Diabetic ketoacidosis
Porphyria
Allergic factors (C1 esterase inhibitor deficiency)
Somatic
Parietal peritoneal inflammation
Bacterial contamination (e.g., perforated appendix, pelvic inflammatory disease)
Chemical irritation (e.g., perforated ulcer, pancreatitis, mittelschmerz)
Abdominal wall
Distortion or traction of mesentery
Trauma or infection of muscles
Spine (e.g., radiculitis from arthritis)
Neurogenic causes
Tabes dorsalis
Herpes zoster
Causalgia and others
Functional

Because somatic nerves innervate the parietal peritoneum, the pain is located directly over the inflamed area. Pain receptors in the peritoneum are stimulated in many diseases and disorders, whether by leakage of purulent matter into the peritoneal cavity, intraperitoneal bleeding, necrosis of an intraabdominal structure, or inflammation secondary to infection. The pain caused by inflammation of the parietal peritoneum is usually steady and aching. However, tension on the peritoneum during palpation or movement, as in coughing or sneezing, invariably increases the pain. Thus, the patient with peritonitis lies quietly in bed in an effort to avoid any movement. These characteristics lead to the clinically useful finding of constant pain with occasional sharp exacerbations. The pain is well localized. Abdominal tenderness, involuntary guarding, and rebound tenderness and guarding are also noted. The intensity of pain and inflammation varies depending on the nature of the inciting factor and how long the peritoneum has been exposed to the factor. For example, a given quantity of gastric or pancreatic fluid causes much more pain than the same quantity of feces, sterile bile, blood, or urine. Intraperitoneal blood and urine may actually go undetected if the peritoneal exposure has not been sudden and massive. In bacterial infection, as in pelvic inflammatory disease, the pain is usually of gradual onset and does not become intense until bacterial multiplication is sufficient to cause the production and release of inflammatory, irritating substances.

Abdominal pain may be of metabolic origin. When the cause of abdominal pain is obscure, a metabolic origin should be considered. Familial Mediterranean fever, porphyria, lead colic, uremia, diabetes, hyperlipidemia, and angioneurotic edema may be causes of abdominal pain. Porphyria and lead colic cause severe hyperperistalsis and abdominal pain that is difficult to distinguish from that of intestinal obstruction. In certain instances, such as hyperlipidemia, the metabolic disease itself may be accompanied by an intraabdominal process such as pancreatitis, and the patient may be subjected to an unnecessary laparotomy unless this is recognized.

Occasionally, abdominal pain has a neurogenic cause. Certain diseases and conditions may injure sensory nerves; these include herpes zoster, arthritis, tumors, a herniated nucleus pulposus, diabetes, multiple sclerosis, and syphilis.

Psychogenic disorders may cause abdominal pain, but the mechanism is hard to define. Ovulation or some other natural event that causes brief, mild abdominal discomfort may be experienced as an abdominal catastrophe by a person with a psychological disorder.

Somatic abdominal pain is not infrequently associated with conditions of the anterior abdominal wall. These include myofascial trigger points, hernias, hematomas, muscle strain or injury, myositis, and trauma.

In addition, pain referred from an intrathoracic site of disease must be considered in patients with abdominal pain. For example, pneumonia, esophagitis, and myocardial infarction occasionally present with abdominal pain.

The disorders that must be considered in the differential diagnosis of abdominal pain are listed in Table 5.2. Most of these are discussed in detail in other chapters of this textbook. Only a few that are not discussed elsewhere are reviewed in this chapter.

TABLE 5.2. Differential Diagnosis of Acute Abdominopelvic Pain

Gastrointestinal
Appendicitis
Bowel obstruction
Cholecystitis
Constipation
Diverticulitis
Esophagitis
Fecal impaction
Gastroenteritis
Hepatitis
Hirschsprung disease
Incarcerated hernia
Intussusception
Irritable bowel syndrome
Meckel diverticulitis
Neoplasm
Pancreatitis
Peptic ulcer disease
Perforated viscus
Regional ileitis (Crohn disease)
Ulcerative colitis
Volvulus
Urologic
Cystitis
Neoplasm
Urethritis
Pyelonephritis
Calculi
Musculoskeletal
Abdominal wall hematoma or infection
Trauma
Herniated disc
Arthritis
Strain or sprain
Hernia
Neoplasm
Gynecologic
Pregnancy complications
Abortion
Dysmenorrhea
Ectopic pregnancy
Fitz-Hugh and Curtis syndrome
Pelvic inflammatory disease
Endometritis
Neoplasm
Ovarian cyst
Salpingitis
Torsion of adnexa
Rupture of ovarian cyst
Endometriosis
Vascular
Abdominal aortic aneurysm
Ischemic bowel
Myocardial infarction
Neoplasm
Sickle cell crisis
Splenic infarction
Splenic rupture
Metabolic
Adrenal crisis
Black widow spider bite
Diabetic ketoacidosis
Lactose intolerance
Lead poisoning
Neurologic
Abdominal epilepsy
Abdominal migraine
Depression
Herpes zoster
Neoplasm
Other
Pneumonia

Abdominal Aneurysm

An aneurysm is a focal dilation of a blood vessel. An abdominal aortic aneurysm is defined as having a diameter at least one and one-half times the diameter measured at the level of the renal arteries. Abdominal aneurysms are much less common in women than in men. Most patients with an abdominal aneurysm have few symptoms, if any, unless the aneurysm is rapidly dilating or a rupture is impending or has been contained. The pain associated with impending rupture may be throbbing or aching in quality and may be more severe in the back or lumbar region than in the abdomen. The pulsatile abdominal mass of a small aneurysm can be difficult to palpate, particularly in an obese patient. Tenderness of a palpable aneurysm or significant pain in a patient with a known aneurysm should prompt an immediate referral for surgical evaluation and intervention because leakage or impending rupture must be presumed. Plain films can demonstrate aortic calcifications; computed tomography (CT), arteriography, and ultrasonography often define the anatomy and size of an aneurysm. Aneurysms with a diameter of 6 cm or more are highly likely to rupture and should be repaired promptly, even if the patient has no symptoms. Free rupture of an aneurysm into the abdominal cavity can result in sudden shock and death.

Acute Appendicitis

Appendicitis is infection of the vermiform appendix. Acute appendicitis is the most common disorder requiring emergent operation in the nongravid patient and the most common nonobstetric emergency of pregnancy. The correct diagnosis is made in only 40% of menstruating young women. The classic sequence of signs and symptoms in appendicitis is the following: epigastric pain; the development of anorexia, nausea, and emesis (emesis usually occurs only once or twice); right lower quadrant tenderness; right lower quadrant peritoneal signs; and the later development of generalized peritonitis. This sequence of development is so consistent that any deviation should lead one to question the diagnosis.

Acute Intermittent Porphyria

Acute intermittent porphyria, although rare, can present with attacks of abdominal pain that may be quite severe. This is an inherited deficiency of the hepatic enzyme porphobilinogen deaminase, which causes a buildup of the heme precursors δ-aminolevulinic acid and porphobilinogen. Abnormally high levels of these compounds are responsible for pain and metabolic disturbances. Patients may give an antecedent history in which the ingestion of alcohol, barbiturates, or sulfonamides precipitates the pain and not be aware of a familial trait. The symptoms typically include severe and colicky abdominal pain, vomiting, and constipation. The pain is often central but may radiate widely. The patient may have noticed prior episodes of rash or intolerance to sun exposure and a reddish brown discoloration of the urine on exposure to sunlight. Fever and leukocytosis may be present.

Adnexal Torsion

Adnexal torsion is usually torsion of an ovarian cyst. The mechanism of pain is most likely ischemia. Adnexal torsion presents with the acute development of hypogastric pain and a tender pelvic mass. Vomiting occurs with the onset of pain but is not always present. A sitting position may relieve the symptoms, whereas a supine position may accentuate the pain. Ultrasonography and laparoscopy are diagnostic. The presentation of fallopian tube torsion, usually secondary to a hydrosalpinx, is similar but usually less severe.

Drug Withdrawal

Acute withdrawal from narcotics, opiates, and other drugs can result in severe, cramping abdominal pain. Other signs may be present, such as tachycardia, diaphoresis, pupillary dilation or constriction, and evidence of drug use (e.g., pockmarked skin, needle tracks, absence of patent vessels in the upper extremity). Oral or inhaled drugs may be used, however. The clinician should remember that drug abuse occurs in all social strata.

Endometriosis

Endometriosis is defined as the presence of endometrial glands and stroma outside the endometrial cavity and uterine musculature. The mechanism of pain production is not known but is probably related to inflammatory mediators. Endometriosis most often involves the ovaries, anterior and posterior cul-de-sac, posterior broad ligaments, uterosacral ligaments, uterus, fallopian tubes, sigmoid colon and appendix, and round ligaments. It is most often asymptomatic. When pain symptoms are present, they are most often chronic pelvic pain, dysmenorrhea, and dyspareunia. At times, acute flares of pain may present clinically as acute abdominal pain. A past history of similar pain should raise the possibility of endometriosis. The diagnosis can be confirmed only by operative visualization and biopsy.

Hemolytic Disorders

Various hemolytic disorders can result in acute abdominal pain and tenderness. The frequency of episodes tends to be in proportion to the degree of anemia or developing jaundice. Sickle cell crisis is a classic example. Pigmented gallstones may also develop in these patients and give rise to symptomatic cholecystitis.

Meckel Diverticulum

A Meckel diverticulum is a congenital outpouching of the intestine 2 to 5 ft from the ileocecal valve and is found in about 2% of the population. It is a remnant of the vitelline duct and may contain aberrant gastric or pancreatic tissue. Meckel diverticulum is less common in women than in men (male-to-female ratio of 2:1). Most cases are asymptomatic, but a Meckel diverticulum can cause an acute abdomen as a result of infection, bleeding, perforation, or bowel obstruction secondary to intussusception, torsion, or volvulus about a bandlike remnant of the vitelline duct. The pain is usually periumbilical, but at times it may be difficult to distinguish from the pain of acute appendicitis. A Meckel diverticulum may bleed if an ulcer forms in the adjacent distal ileum. A suspected Meckel diverticulum can be localized by radionuclide scanning with technetium.

Mesenteric Adenitis

Mesenteric adenitis may present with acute lower abdominal pain and tenderness. The patient may have a febrile course. The pain may be colicky but should not progress to signs of localized peritonitis. Both viral and bacterial causes have been implicated. *Yersinia* infection accounts for many cases in adults.

Mesenteric Ischemia

Mesenteric ischemia can result from several conditions. The index of suspicion should be increased in an elderly patient, anyone with a known cardiovascular disease or arrhythmia or a coagulopathy, or a patient who has sustained a hypotensive insult secondary to sepsis or trauma. The pain is often sudden in onset, severe, and unrelenting. The patient may writhe in bed, and the physical examination findings are generally much less impressive than the severity of the symptoms. Prompt diagnosis and surgery are necessary. The classic symptoms and signs of bloody diarrhea, metabolic acidosis, elevated creatine phosphokinase or amylase values, pneumatosis intestinalis, and "thumbprinting" of the bowel on x-ray films are variable and nonspecific or absent in many cases. Many of these signs appear late and may herald an irreversible course. Vigorous fluid resuscitation, prompt arteriography, and surgery are key to survival. Irreversible necrosis of the bowel is invariable after 6 hours of warm ischemia. Segmental ischemia can be treated successfully with judicious resection and "second look" procedures. The survival of patients with short gut syndrome after massive small bowel resection has been greatly improved by the use of total parenteral nutrition and elemental diets.

Ovarian Cysts

An ovarian cyst, such as an endometrioma, most often causes acute abdominal pain by rupture. Torsion, as previously noted, may also be a cause of acute pain. Cyst rupture causes iliac fossa, hypogastric, or diffuse lower abdominal pain, vomiting, and low-grade fever. Overt peritoneal signs are rare. A bimanual pelvic examination may demonstrate fullness of the cul-de-sac and ovarian tenderness with or without slight ovarian enlargement. A history of endometriosis or prior cysts is helpful but may not be noted. Ultrasonography may show excessive pelvic fluid and an ovarian cyst. Laparoscopy is diagnostic. Observation and the use of analgesics can be helpful; the symptoms are often self-limiting.

Pyelonephritis

Pyelonephritis is infection of the kidney. It may present with severe abdominal pain and associated nausea. Urinary frequency, dysuria, and urgency often precede an episode of pyelonephritis. Acute pyelonephritis presents with fever and often with rigors secondary to bacteremia. Flank pain is present, and percussion elicits tenderness over the costovertebral angle. Pyuria is noted on microscopic urinalysis. Ultrasonography may reveal hydronephrosis.

Splenic Artery Aneurysm

Rupture of a splenic artery aneurysm tends to occur in women who are pregnant or taking oral contraceptives. Splenic artery aneurysm may present as a pulsatile or expanding mass in the upper abdomen. A rupture can cause sudden collapse as a consequence of massive intraabdominal hemorrhage. A calcified lesion may be noted on abdominal x-ray films or CT scans. Prompt surgical intervention is required for expanding, leaking, or ruptured aneurysms. Arteriography may be helpful in establishing the diagnosis.

Splenic Rupture

Rupture of the spleen is almost always caused by trauma; the spleen is the organ most commonly injured in blunt abdominal trauma. Patients with splenic injuries may present with diffuse abdominal tenderness, left upper quadrant pain, or left shoulder pain secondary to diaphragmatic irritation from subphrenic blood. If the patient is hemodynamically unstable, immediate surgery is mandatory. Nonoperative management is appropriate if the patient is hemodynamically stable and shows steady improvement.

Tuberculosis

Tuberculosis can cause tuberculous peritonitis, which is relevant given the increase in the number of HIV-positive and immunocompromised patients. This disease is called "the great mimicker" because it is associated with a wide variety of symptoms and signs. The patient may present with vague abdominal pain, abdominal distention, and ascites. Evidence of pulmonary tuberculosis can be helpful in establishing the diagnosis. Tuberculosis can also result in intestinal perforation or obstruction that requires surgical intervention in addition to treatment with antituberculous drugs. The emergence of resistant strains is of great concern.

CLINICAL HISTORY

Taking a systematic, painstakingly detailed history is essential. This can be laborious and time-consuming but often leads to a reasonably accurate diagnosis. Keeping the most frequent diagnoses in mind during evaluation of the patient is essential to formulating a differential diagnosis (Table 5.2), yet the clinician must remain sufficiently open-minded and unhurried to avoid missing important information.

When a woman has an acute abdominal crisis, it is crucial that the history be obtained expeditiously so as not to jeopardize survival. An acute abdominal crisis usually presents with a combination of symptoms and signs that may include pain, vomiting, muscular rigidity, abdominal distention, and shock. However, pain may be the sole symptom, so the ability to home in on potentially life-threatening conditions is crucial. In taking the history of pain symptoms, it is helpful to use the acronym *PQRST*—provocation-palliation (What causes the pain? What makes it worse? What makes it better?); quality (characteristics and nature of the pain); region-radiation-referral (Where does it hurt? Where does the pain move or radiate?); severity (How much does it hurt?); and temporality (duration, frequency, and pattern of pain). These historical characteristics define the type of pain and often suggest the underlying cause or causes.

Provocation-Palliation

Epigastric or right upper quadrant pain that is frequently accentuated by recumbency and relieved by an upright position is consistent with gradual dilation of the pancreatic ducts, as in carcinoma of the head of the pancreas.

Acute abdominal pain that is exacerbated by movement and coughing is generally consistent with peritoneal inflammation or irritation. Most often, it indicates an infectious process, but the pain of visceral rupture, including rupture of an ovarian cyst, is also aggravated by motion, cough, or the Valsalva maneuver. Pain referred from the spine may also be exacerbated in this way. Usually, compression or irritation of the nerve roots is involved in association with hyperesthesia over the involved dermatomes, and the pain is characteristically intensified by coughing, sneezing, or straining.

Causalgia, which is pain caused by diseases that injure the sensory nerves, is characteristically burning in quality and is intensified by normal stimuli such as touch or change in temperature.

Acute intermittent porphyria, although uncommon, can present with attacks of abdominal pain that may be quite severe. Patients may give an antecedent history in which the ingestion of alcohol, barbiturates, or sulfonamides precipitates the pain.

Quality

Colicky pain is wavelike; spasms develop and abate in a somewhat rhythmic pattern. It is characteristic of intestinal disorders, especially obstruction. In small bowel obstruction, colicky pain is severe, but as the intestine becomes progressively dilated and loses muscular tone, the colicky nature of the pain may diminish. Colicky pain in colonic obstruction is generally less intense than in small intestinal obstruction. Colicky pain is also characteristic of acute intermittent porphyria.

Steady or constant pain is characteristic of a distended gallbladder or kidney. Sudden distention of the biliary tree causes steady rather than colicky pain, so that the term *biliary colic* is misleading.

Sharp, well-localized pain is characteristic of peritoneal inflammation. As previously noted, causalgia tends to be burning in quality.

Pain that is lancinating or burning often suggests an origin in the spinal nerves or roots, as in herpes zoster, arthritis, tumors, herniated nucleus pulposus, diabetes, or syphilis.

Abdominal wall pain is constant and aching when it is caused by trauma or myofascial trigger points.

Region-Radiation-Referral

The location of pain often provides a significant clue to the diagnosis. It is important to inquire about the initial location in addition to the location at the time of the clinical presentation. Table 5.3 summarizes the location of pain in some common disorders that cause acute abdominal pain.

Radiation of pain occurs in many disorders that cause abdominal pain. For example, abdominal pain with radiation to the sacral region, flank, or genitalia should always suggest possible rupture of an abdominal aortic aneurysm. In acute obstruction of the intravesical portion of the ureter, severe suprapubic and flank pain radiates to the labia or inner aspect of the upper thigh. Acute distention of the gallbladder usually causes pain in the right upper quadrant with radiation to the right posterior region of the thorax or tip of the right scapula. With a distended common bile duct, pain in the epigastrium often radiates to the upper part of the lumbar region. Referral of pain to the shoulder is common when the diaphragm is involved, as in perihepatitis secondary to pelvic inflammatory disease or hemoperitoneum secondary to a ruptured ectopic pregnancy.

Pain caused by myofascial trigger points is poorly localized and regional, with referral to the entire muscle in addition to subcutaneous tissues and joints.

Pain referred to the abdomen from the thorax can be a difficult diagnostic problem. Diseases of the upper part of the abdomen, such as acute cholecystitis and perforated ulcer, often cause intrathoracic complications. It is important to consider the possibility of intrathoracic disease in every patient with abdominal pain, especially in the upper part of the abdomen. Systematic questioning directed toward detecting myocardial

TABLE 5.3. Location of Pain in Some Common Diseases That Cause Acute Abdominopelvic Pain

Right upper quadrant	
	Dilation of the biliary tree (carcinoma of the head of the pancreas)
	Acute distention of the gallbladder
	Diaphragmatic pleuritis
	Amebic abscess or hydatid disease of the liver
Epigastric	
	Intestinal colic
	Gastroenteritis
	Early acute appendicitis
	Early small bowel obstruction
	Mesenteric thrombosis or ischemia
	Acute pancreatitis
	Carcinoma of the head of the pancreas
	Distention of the common bile duct
Left upper quadrant	
	Myocardial infarction
	Pulmonary infarction
	Pneumonia
	Pericarditis
	Esophageal disease
	Localized gastric perforation
	Rupture of a splenic artery aneurysm
	Splenic rupture
	Inflamed jejunal diverticulum
	Acute pancreatitis
Periumbilical	
	All visceral diseases in their early stages
	Abdominal trauma
	Abdominal wall hernias
	Bowel obstruction
Diffuse or generalized	
	All visceral diseases late in their course
	Pelvic inflammatory disease
	Endometriosis
	Muscular strain or sprain
	Bowel obstruction
Left lower quadrant	
	Adnexal torsion
	Constipation
	Crohn disease
	Diverticulitis
	Ectopic pregnancy
	Endometriosis
	Inflammation or perforation of colonic carcinoma
	Irritable bowel syndrome
	Ovarian cyst or ruptured ovarian cyst
	Pyelonephritis
	Salpingitis
	Urinary calculi
Right lower quadrant	
	Appendicitis
	Ectopic pregnancy
	Adnexal torsion
	Ovarian cyst or ruptured ovarian cyst
	Urinary calculi
	Endometriosis
	Pyelonephritis
	Meckel diverticulitis
	Regional enteritis (Crohn disease)
	Salpingitis
Suprapubic	
	Obstruction of the urinary bladder
	Cystitis
	Urinary calculi
Lumbar radiation	
	Colonic obstruction
	Pyelonephritis
	Urinary calculi
Flank	
	Urinary calculi
Costovertebral angle	
	Obstruction of the ureteropelvic junction (urinary calculi)
	Pyelonephritis

or pulmonary infarction, pneumonia, pericarditis, or esophageal disease often elicits sufficient clues to establish the correct diagnosis. Furthermore, thoracic and abdominal diseases frequently coexist and may be difficult to differentiate. For example, a patient with known biliary tract disease often experiences epigastric pain during a myocardial infarction, and in a patient with known angina pectoris, pain is referred to the precordium or left shoulder during an episode of biliary colic.

Severity

The severity of pain does not necessarily correlate with the severity of disease and is not always helpful diagnostically. In bowel ischemia, for example, the degree of pain is generally disproportionate to the abdominal examination findings. In many cases, when pain is especially severe, it may be difficult for the clinician to arrive at an accurate diagnosis. Nevertheless, an initial assessment of the severity of pain is important in planning treatment and in monitoring the response to treatment.

Temporality

The chronology of events is important, especially in cases of pain of visceral origin. The nature of the pain at onset, the timing of the onset, and the duration of pain are crucial diagnostic elements. For example, onset after trauma must be ascertained. The timing of the onset and the severity of associated symptoms, such as fever, diarrhea, constipation, and urinary or vaginal symptoms, must also be determined.

In general, a sudden onset is consistent with perforation, hemorrhage, torsion, or rupture, whereas a gradual onset is consistent with inflammation, infection, or obstruction. It is often assumed that the pain of intraabdominal ischemia is always sudden and catastrophic. Although the pain of embolism or thrombosis of the superior mesenteric artery may be severe and diffuse, this condition just as frequently presents with only mild, continuous, diffuse pain that lasts for 2 or 3 days before vascular collapse or peritonitis develops. The early, seemingly insignificant pain is caused by hyperperistalsis rather than peritoneal inflammation.

The timing of pain in relation to the menstrual cycle may be important. For example, a ruptured graafian follicle causes pain at or near the middle of the cycle (mittelschmerz), whereas a ruptured corpus luteal cyst causes pain at or near the onset of menses.

Associated Symptoms

The symptoms associated with pain may be significant. An accurate menstrual history is essential. Vaginal bleeding may suggest an origin in the reproductive system, especially pregnancy-related disease. Fever and chills may suggest an infectious process.

Anorexia, nausea, vomiting, and diarrhea often indicate a gastrointestinal origin, such as appendicitis or bowel obstruction. A condition requiring surgical intervention is less likely when emesis precedes the onset of abdominal pain. For example, viral and bacterial enteritis present with prominent episodes of nausea, vomiting, and diarrhea before the onset of pain, whereas in appendicitis, pain appears first. The character of the vomitus (e.g., bilious, green, feculent) may help differentiate gastroenteritis from early or late obstruction of the small bowel. The patient with an incompetent ileocecal valve and large bowel obstruction exhibits feculent emesis. Changes in bowel function may also be important, such as constipation, melena, hematochezia, and changes of stool caliber or color.

Syncopal symptoms may indicate significant intraabdominal, rectal, or vaginal hemorrhage, or hematemesis. Dysuria and urinary frequency often imply cystourethritis. Inflammation of the peritoneum covering the bladder may cause bladder pain. For example, it is not unusual for a patient to note an episode of urinary urgency at the time of initial rupture of an ectopic pregnancy or ovarian cyst. Hematuria suggests urinary calculi or infection.

CLINICAL EXAMINATION

Like a careful history, an unhurried examination is invaluable. How much information is obtained depends greatly on the clinician's ability to perform a gentle and thorough examination. Once a patient with peritoneal inflammation has been examined brusquely, accurate further assessment becomes almost impossible. Examination of the abdomen, pelvis, and rectum is critical. The need for other components of the general physical examination is indicated by the history and findings. For example, palpation of the peripheral pulses to detect a pulse deficit or unequal femoral pulses may be important if vascular disease is suspected.

An examination of the patient with acute abdominal pain begins with an observation of her appearance, particularly a global assessment of how ill she appears. Simple critical inspection of the patient's facial expression, position in bed, and respiratory activity may provide valuable clues. For example, a patient with pelvic peritonitis is frequently most comfortable with one or both hips flexed, depending on the site and extent of the peritonitis, and tries to minimize movement. A determination of the vital signs, including temperature, blood pressure, and pulse, and possibly orthostatic measurement of the blood pressure and pulse are essential. Tachycardia and hypotension obviously suggest significant hypovolemia secondary to blood loss or dehydration. Fever suggests an infectious cause. Noting the respirations may be helpful because referred pain of thoracic origin is often accompanied by splinting of the involved hemithorax, marked respiratory lag, and excursion decreased more than is usual with acute abdominal pain.

Abdominal Examination

Inspection is important. During the progression of peritoneal inflammation, the abdomen becomes distended as peristalsis is inhibited and loops of bowel fill with gas and fluid. Increasing distention without rigidity, in association with pain and multiple episodes of emesis, usually signifies intestinal obstruction. Increasing distention without rigidity, accompanied by constipation but little or no emesis, indicates large bowel obstruction. Distention and abdominal rigidity, with pain and persistent vomiting, occur in spreading peritonitis. In cases of suspected obstruction, the patient must be examined carefully for inguinal, femoral, or incisional hernias. Uremia may also present with abdominal distention and vomiting. Ureteral obstruction secondary to tumor encasement (e.g., ovarian carcinoma) should be considered.

The skin changes of jaundice, herpes zoster, and cellulitis should be noted. Some masses can be seen at the time of inspection, especially in thin women. A pulsatile abdominal mass confirmed by palpation suggests an aortic aneurysm.

Auscultation for abnormal bowel sounds is a critical part of the abdominal examination. As peristalsis is decreased by ileus or peritonitis, the bowel sounds may diminish or disappear. High-pitched bowel sounds and rushes may be heard if obstruction is present. These findings are often unreliable, however. Not infrequently, the bowel sounds seem normal in catastrophic diseases such as strangulating small intestinal obstruction and perforated appendicitis. Conversely, absent or diminished bowel sounds suggestive of peritonitis or ileus may occur in small bowel obstruction if the part of the intestine proximal to the obstruction becomes markedly distended and edematous.

Next, palpation is performed. The abdomen is assessed especially for tenderness, rebound tenderness, and masses. Gentleness, as previously pointed out, is particularly pertinent to this part of the examination. A brusque, overly vigorous palpation will induce spasm and anxiety and make it impossible for the clinician to obtain reliable findings during the rest of the examination. A palpable gallbladder will be missed if the palpation is so brusque that voluntary muscle spasm becomes superimposed on involuntary muscular rigidity. Eliciting rebound tenderness in a patient with suspected peritonitis by suddenly releasing a deeply palpating hand is cruel and unnecessary. Asking the patient to cough will elicit true rebound tenderness and obviates the need for placing a hand on the abdomen. Gentle percussion of the abdomen can also be used to identify rebound tenderness. A forceful attempt to identify rebound tenderness will startle and induce protective spasm in almost any patient with abdominal pain, especially if she is nervous or worried, even when true rebound tenderness is not present. Abdominal tenderness, involuntary guarding, and rebound tenderness are characteristic of peritoneal inflammation of any cause.

Severe abdominal pain, collapse, and generalized rigidity of the abdominal wall often indicate perforation of a viscus, such as the stomach or duodenum, as a consequence of peptic ulcer disease. This represents a true surgical emergency.

Several findings have names or eponyms worth pointing out. The Rovsing sign, in which palpation of the left lower quadrant causes pain in the right lower quadrant, suggests appendicitis. In McBurney point tenderness, which is associated with appendicitis, palpation of the right lower quadrant at a point two-thirds the distance between the umbilicus and right anterior superior iliac crest causes pain. The Murphy sign is a pause in inspiration during palpation under the liver and suggests cholecystitis. The psoas sign is pain on flexion of the thigh and suggests inflammation around the psoas muscle. The obturator sign is pain on rotation of the flexed thigh, especially internal rotation, and occurs when inflammation surrounds the internal obturator muscle.

A tender or discolored hernia site may suggest current or recent bowel incarceration.

Black widow spider bites cause intense pain and rigidity in the abdominal muscles and back, an area infrequently involved in intraabdominal disease.

Causalgia is distinct from other types of abdominal pain in that it is usually limited to the distribution of a single peripheral nerve. The demonstration of irregularly spaced areas of cutaneous pain may be the only indication of an old nerve lesion underlying causalgia. Because allodynia is commonly present, tenderness may be precipitated by gentle palpation, but rigidity of the abdominal muscles is absent, and the respirations are not disturbed. Distention of the abdomen is uncommon.

When abdominal pain is referred pain of thoracic origin, the abdominal area of referred pain usually is not tender, and palpation does not accentuate the pain; in many instances, palpation actually seems to relieve pain in this setting.

Palpation should be directed at detecting possible abdominal masses in addition to tenderness. In hematoma of the rectus sheath, now most frequently encountered in association with anticoagulant therapy, a mass may be present in the lower quadrants of the abdomen. A pulsatile abdominal mass may be palpable in a patient with an abdominal aneurysm.

Patients whose findings are consistent with generalized peritonitis (guarding and rebound tenderness in all four quadrants of the abdomen), are commonly said to have a "surgical abdomen" because it is often not possible to arrive at a clear diagnosis without operative evaluation. It should be noted, though, that the diagnosis of acute surgical abdomen is based on signs and symptoms of peritonitis, which can be caused by a tremendous array of disease processes—not all of which require surgical treatment. An immediate surgical or medical decision is crucial in such cases, but some patients have disorders that do not absolutely require surgical evaluation and treatment. An example is the woman with acute gastrointestinal bleeding who clearly requires emergency care but possibly not surgery. A clinical decision is often difficult in cases of acute surgical abdomen. Thus, reevaluation every 2 to 3 hours may be necessary to note the development of other clinical signs and symptoms.

Pelvic Examination

Like the abdominal examination, the pelvic examination of a woman with acute abdominal pain must be gentle. Abdominal signs are occasionally virtually or totally absent in cases of pelvic peritonitis, so a careful pelvic and rectal examination is mandatory in all patients with abdominal pain. Tenderness noted during the pelvic or rectal examination in the absence of other abdominal signs can be caused by a perforated appendicitis, diverticulitis, or torsion of an ovarian cyst, all of which are operative indications. With peritoneal irritation of any cause, diffuse tenderness is noted during examination of the uterus and adnexa, including cervical motion tenderness. Although cervical motion tenderness is often thought to be specific for pelvic inflammatory disease, this notion is incorrect.

Adnexal masses may be palpable in cases of ovarian cyst, cancer, leiomyoma, tuboovarian abscess, or ectopic pregnancy. Bimanual pelvic examination may demonstrate fullness of the cul-de-sac in a patient with a ruptured ovarian cyst.

Rectal Examination

A rectal mass or tenderness may be noted in cases of ovarian cyst, cancer, leiomyoma, tuboovarian abscess, or ectopic pregnancy. A rectal examination in patients with pelvic appendicitis reveals right iliac tenderness.

LABORATORY AND OTHER DIAGNOSTIC STUDIES

Laboratory and imaging studies should be performed based on the differential diagnosis as determined by the history and physical examination. Laboratory data may be of great value but rarely establish a definitive diagnosis. Studies usually indicated include a complete blood cell count, urinalysis, urine culture, pregnancy test, and measurement of electrolytes.

The complete blood cell count is used to assess for leukocytosis, a shift of white blood cells, and anemia. Leukocytosis should never be the single factor in deciding whether surgery is indicated because it is unreliable in distinguishing surgical from nonsurgical disease. A white blood cell count above 20,000/μL may be noted in many disorders, such as perforation of a viscus, pancreatitis, acute cholecystitis, pelvic inflammatory disease, and intestinal infarction. Conversely, a normal white blood cell count is not unusual in cases of perforated abdominal viscus and of abdominal or pelvic infection or inflammation.

Urinalysis is used to assess particularly for pyuria, hematuria, glucosuria, and ketones. Pyuria is most often secondary to urinary tract infection, but it may also be caused by an abscess adjacent to the ureter, as in ruptured retrocecal appendicitis. Gross or microscopic hematuria can reflect the passage of a stone or perhaps exacerbation of an underlying pathologic process, such as neoplasia or interstitial or lupus cystitis. Urinalysis may reveal the state of hydration or rule out severe renal disease or diabetes.

Reliable pregnancy testing, with the detection of β-human chorionic gonadotropin in serum or urine, should be performed in all women of reproductive age who have acute abdominal pain. It is the fastest way to rule out ectopic pregnancy or abortion. In addition, pregnancy in a patient with a pathologic process unrelated to the pregnancy may affect the presentation of the disease and influence management.

The measurement of serum electrolytes, glucose, blood urea nitrogen, and bilirubin levels may be helpful. Patients with diabetic ketoacidosis may present with severe acute abdominal pain; therefore, testing the blood and urine for glucose and ketones is essential. The serum lipase level should be measured if pancreatic disease is possible. This is more accurate parameter than the serum amylase level in diagnosing pancreatic disorders. Serum amylase levels may be increased by many diseases, such as perforated ulcer, strangulating intestinal obstruction, and acute cholecystitis.

Cultures for gonococci and chlamydial organisms should be obtained at the time of the pelvic examination. Although not useful for immediate management decisions, they may aid in guiding therapy if the patient is thought to have a pelvic infection.

Plain x-ray films of the abdomen may be helpful. Dilated loops of bowel with air-fluid levels are seen in cases of bowel obstruction or paralytic ileus. The presence of free air under the diaphragm on an upright film indicates perforation of a viscus and requires immediate intervention. An upright film that does not show the diaphragm is inadequate for evaluating a woman with acute abdominal pain. Occasionally, loss of the psoas shadow is noted on the right side, supporting a diagnosis of appendicitis. An appendicolith in association with right lower quadrant pain should be considered diagnostic of appendicitis. In addition, renal calculi may be seen on plain films, which may also show an intraabdominal mass or aortic aneurysm. Plain films are less helpful in diagnosing gynecologic causes of acute abdomen.

Occasionally, barium or water-soluble contrast studies are indicated. Upper gastrointestinal tract studies with contrast may demonstrate partial intestinal obstruction that eludes diagnosis by other means. It is important to remember that if there is any question of obstruction of the colon, the oral administration of barium sulfate should be avoided. In cases of suspected colonic obstruction, a contrast enema may be diagnostic. The barium enema examination may be useful in difficult cases of suspected appendicitis. The findings of cecal spasm, edema, extrinsic compression of the cecum by a mass, partial visualization or nonvisualization of the appendix, and irregular filling of the appendiceal lumen suggest appendicitis. However, the absence of appendiceal filling as the sole abnormality on a full-column barium enema is a nonspecific finding; in 20% of normal adults, the appendiceal lumen is obliterated. The barium enema is helpful in differentiating appendicitis from regional enteritis involving the terminal ileum and from colon carcinoma affecting the cecum or ascending colon.

Chest roentgenography is sometimes appropriate, especially in a patient with upper abdominal pain referred from a thoracic problem, such as pneumonia or a pleural effusion. Additionally, chest roentgenography may show a pneumoperitoneum caused by a perforated stomach, duodenum, or colon.

Abdominal ultrasonography, pelvic ultrasonography, and CT are often helpful. Ultrasonography has proved useful in detecting enlargement of the gallbladder or pancreas, gallstones, hydronephrosis, an enlarged ovary or cyst, pelvic abscess, uterine masses, intrauterine pregnancy, excessive free fluid or hemorrhage in the cul-de-sac, and tubal pregnancy. Ultrasonography may also be helpful in diagnosing appendicitis; a distended appendiceal lumen, thickened appendiceal or cecal walls, and localized fluid collections are often considered diagnostic findings.

Radioisotope scans (hepatic 2,6-dimethyliminodiacetic acid, or HIDA) may help differentiate acute cholecystitis from acute pancreatitis.

CT may demonstrate an enlarged pancreas, ruptured spleen, a thickened colonic or appendiceal wall, and streaking of the mesocolon or mesoappendix, which is characteristic of diverticulitis or appendicitis. Spiral CT without contrast can often determine the location and size of stones in patients with renal colic. Traditional intravenous pyelography is a slower alternative in such cases. CT with intravenous contrast is helpful only in patients with suspected vascular rupture who are stable. CT with intravenous and oral contrast is indicated when a condition involving bowel that warrants surgery or an intraperitoneal hemorrhage is suspected. CT with rectal contrast is highly accurate only in detecting appendicitis.

Electrocardiography should be considered part of the evaluation in women with upper abdominal pain who are older than 40 years or who have risk factors for coronary artery disease.

Peritoneal lavage and culdocentesis are diagnostic procedures that have been almost entirely supplanted by ultrasonography, CT, and laparoscopy. In the absence of trauma, peritoneal lavage is rarely performed. Similarly, culdocentesis, an easily performed but painful diagnostic procedure that examines the contents of the peritoneal cavity, is rarely necessary in an evaluation of gynecologic causes of pelvic pain.

Laparoscopy is especially helpful in diagnosing pelvic conditions such as ovarian cysts, tubal pregnancies, salpingitis, and acute appendicitis.

TREATMENT

Sometimes, a definitive diagnosis cannot be established at the time of the initial examination, yet it is clear to an experienced and thoughtful physician that surgery is indicated. Quite often, however, it is not clear whether surgery is indicated. If the decision is questionable, watchful waiting with repeated questioning and examination will often elucidate the true nature of the illness and indicate the proper course of action. It is important to note that although many perceive the acute surgical abdomen as a problem that always requires surgical intervention, in many instances medical management is more appropriate. An acute abdomen does not dictate the type of management, only the need to come to a decision rapidly and implement appropriate therapy as expeditiously as possible.

It is imperative that an ill patient with acute abdominal pain be stabilized initially. When emergent laparotomy or laparoscopy is appropriate, such as in a woman who is hemodynamically unstable with suspected rupture of an ectopic pregnancy, large-bore intravenous access and fluid resuscitation are crucial. Supplemental oxygen and intensive monitoring are also indicated. In such cases, surgery should never be delayed. The operating room should be notified, and blood work, including a complete blood cell count and cross-matching, should be sent as the patient is being moved to the operating room. Such expeditious management is not always required. Most cases of localized peritonitis can be diagnosed outside the operating room, so that more time is available to consider therapeutic options and fully correct the patient's fluid, glucose, electrolyte, and acidotic status. In this type of case, narcotics or analgesics should not be withheld pending a definitive diagnosis or formulation of a plan; obfuscation of the diagnosis by adequate analgesia is unlikely. Antiemetics increase the patient's comfort and can usually be administered when appropriate. Antibiotics should be initiated as soon as possible when an infectious process is suspected, especially one with the potential to cause perforation or peritonitis.

The specific treatments for the most common diseases that cause acute abdominal pain are covered in other chapters of this text. Only the treatment of appendicitis, which is not addressed elsewhere, is discussed in this chapter.

Treatment of Appendicitis

The appropriate management of acute or suspected appendicitis is prompt surgery. Traditionally, this is performed through a muscle-splitting incision in the right lower quadrant. The vermiform appendix is removed whether or not the patient has appendicitis. In cases of appendiceal abscess, the appendix cannot always be removed safely, and sometimes only irrigation and drainage are performed. If appendicitis is not present at the time of surgical evaluation, the surgeon must rule out other surgically relevant processes. The traditional right lower quadrant incision is not optimal for a full evaluation of the abdomen and pelvis. Laparoscopy is particularly useful in such cases, and recent surgical literature supports the usefulness of laparoscopy in patients with right lower quadrant abdominal pain in whom appendicitis cannot be ruled out. In addition, in most cases, it is possible to perform the appendectomy laparoscopically.

ABDOMINAL PAIN IN PREGNANCY

The pregnant patient with acute abdominal pain is a difficult diagnostic challenge. The clinical evaluation is generally confounded because symptoms typical of illnesses that cause abdominal pain are common in pregnancy itself, and physical examination of the abdomen is hampered by the pregnant state.

The primary care provider must be familiar with the anatomic and physiologic changes of pregnancy. By 12 weeks' gestation, the uterine fundus rises from the pelvis and becomes an abdominal organ. The adnexal structures also become abdominal organs. As the uterus enlarges, it displaces the intestines and omentum superiorly and laterally. By late pregnancy, the appendix is likely to be closer to the gallbladder than to the McBurney point. The anterior abdominal wall is also elevated, so that any underlying inflammation is less likely to cause the usual symptoms of direct parietal peritoneal irritation. The leukocyte count varies considerably during normal pregnancy. The white cell count during pregnancy is normally elevated to 12,000 to 16,000/μL, a level that overlaps those expected in intraabdominal inflammatory conditions.

The causes of acute abdominal pain in pregnancy can be categorized as obstetric or nonobstetric. The most common nonobstetric causes of acute abdominal pain in the pregnant patient are appendicitis, cholecystitis, pyelonephritis, hepatitis, pancreatitis, and degenerating uterine myomata.

Nonobstetric Causes

ACUTE APPENDICITIS

Acute appendicitis occurs in 1 in 1,600 pregnancies and is the most common nontraumatic, nonobstetric surgical condition that complicates pregnancy. The diagnosis during pregnancy is often challenging because the typical symptoms (anorexia, nausea, and vomiting) mimic those of normal pregnancy; furthermore, the location of the appendix during pregnancy differs from that in the nonpregnant state (Fig. 5.1). Appendicitis should always be considered when a pregnant woman presents with abdominal pain, nausea, vomiting, fever, and leukocytosis. Surgical evaluation and treatment should not be delayed when appendicitis is strongly suspected on clinical grounds. The differential diagnosis includes preterm labor, abruptio placentae,

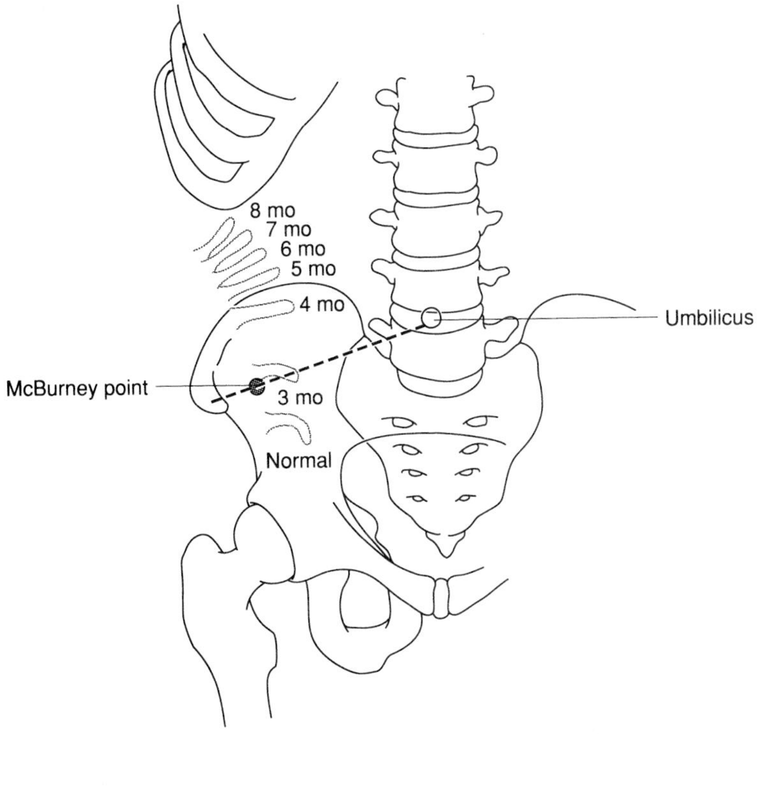

FIG. 5.1. Location and orientation of the appendix in pregnancy.

degenerating myoma, and adnexal torsion. Postoperative antimicrobial agents are recommended for perforation, peritonitis, and periappendiceal abscess. The administration of tocolytic agents is indicated during the postoperative period in a patient with evidence of preterm labor and no clinical infection.

CHOLECYSTITIS/CHOLELITHIASIS

Cholelithiasis occurs in 3% to 4% of pregnant women and is the cause of more than 90% of cases of cholecystitis in pregnancy. Pregnancy does not notably change the clinical presentation of acute cholecystitis. Medical management, consisting of intravenous hydration, nasogastric suction, and analgesics, is usually preferred during pregnancy. Surgical therapy is reserved for patients with recurrent attacks of biliary colic, suspected perforation, sepsis, or peritonitis. Prophylactic antibiotics in the preoperative period are recommended.

HEPATITIS

Viral hepatitis is the most common serious liver disease in pregnant women. Although pregnancy has little effect on the presentation and course of hepatitis, hepatitis significantly affects the pregnancy, fetus, and neonate, depending on the type of hepatitis and how far the pregnancy is advanced at the onset of infection. Consultation with a perinatologist is advisable in most cases.

PANCREATITIS

Acute pancreatitis complicates 1 in 1,000 to 1 in 10,000 pregnancies. Gallbladder disease is the most common cause; medications, infection, and hyperlipidemia are less frequent causes. The signs and symptoms are similar to those in women who are not pregnant. Medical management includes bowel rest with nasogastric suction, relief of pain, and correction of fluid and electrolyte imbalances. Patients with pancreatic abscess, ruptured pseudocyst, or hemorrhagic pancreatitis may require surgery while they are still pregnant.

PYELONEPHRITIS

Pyelonephritis is identified in 1% to 2% of all pregnancies. Untreated pyuria during pregnancy increases the risk for pyelonephritis. The treatment includes parenteral antibiotics and intravenous hydration. Close monitoring for complications, such as renal impairment, hematologic abnormalities, septic shock, and pulmonary dysfunction, is critical in the pregnant patient. Ampicillin is not recommended as single-agent therapy because of the high degree of bacterial resistance. Extended-spectrum penicillins or cephalosporins are safe, and cure rates of 85% to 90% are typical.

UTERINE LEIOMYOMATA

The most common cause of acute pain associated with myomata during pregnancy is red or carneous degeneration. This is a hemorrhagic infarction that usually results from an acutely inadequate blood supply to the myoma. The pain and tenderness are usually localized but can be severe. Low-grade fever and leukocytosis may develop. Preterm labor may be initiated as a consequence of irritation of the adjacent myometrium. Ultrasonography is helpful in making the diagnosis. The management is nonsurgical, with analgesics and hydration if necessary. The patient should be observed for preterm labor. Surgical management during pregnancy is rarely, if ever, indicated.

Obstetric Causes

PRETERM LABOR

In preterm labor, cyclic or rhythmic episodes of acute abdominal pain that increases and decreases alternate with intervals of complete resolution. Palpation reveals uterine contractions at the time of the episodes of pain. True preterm labor is defined as regular uterine contractions with cervical dilation or effacement. Treatment includes the administration of tocolytic agents between 20 and 34 weeks of gestation and antenatal steroids (dexamethasone or betamethasone) between 24 and 34 weeks of gestation.

ABRUPTIO PLACENTAE

Acute abdominal pain develops during premature separation of the placenta (abruptio placentae). This condition occurs about once in every 150 deliveries. The cause is unknown. Risk factors include older age of the mother, multiparity, pregnancy-induced or chronic hypertension, prematurely ruptured membranes, external trauma, cigarette smoking, cocaine abuse, and uterine leiomyomata. The signs and symptoms include vaginal bleeding, uterine tenderness, back pain, high-frequency contractions, hypertonus, and idiopathic preterm labor. Abruptio placentae can cause profound blood loss, anemia, coagulopathy, and fetal death, which usually occurs when the degree of separation exceeds 50%. The treatment varies depending on the status of the mother and fetus. In general, in cases of massive external bleeding, intense therapy with blood and an electrolyte solution and prompt delivery to control the hemorrhage can be lifesaving for mother and fetus. In cases of slower blood loss, provided the fetus is alive without evidence of compromise and the maternal hemorrhage is not causing serious hypovolemia or anemia, close observation with facilities for immediate intervention may be adequate management.

PREECLAMPSIA

Preeclampsia typically develops in the mid to late part of the third trimester of pregnancy. Hepatic involvement occurs in 10% of women with severe preeclampsia and can cause severe right upper quadrant and epigastric pain. Associated nausea and vomiting, hypertension, and proteinuria suggest the diagnosis. Tender hepatomegaly is found on physical examination. The alkaline phosphatase and transaminase levels are elevated. The serum bilirubin is elevated in 10% of cases. Thrombocytopenia and disseminated intravascular coagulation with microangiopathic hemolytic anemia may be present. In patients who present in hypovolemic shock, hepatic hematoma and ruptured liver should be considered immediately. Hepatic rupture has a maternal mortality rate of 70%. Delivery is the recommended management for severe preeclampsia and should be carried out once the patient has been medically stabilized. In a patient with suspected hepatic rupture, surgical intervention is mandatory. Hepatic artery ligation, partial hepatic resection, laceration repair, and packing are the suggested intraoperative treatments.

ACUTE FATTY LIVER OF PREGNANCY

This complication of 1 in 10,000 to 15,000 pregnancies usually occurs in the third trimester. Patients typically present with an abrupt onset of nausea, persistent vomiting, abdominal pain, and jaundice. Laboratory findings include hyperbilirubinemia, elevated alkaline phosphatase and serum transaminase levels, thrombocytopenia, hypoglycemia, elevated serum ammonia levels, and a prolonged coagulation time. The initial management is medical, with correction of fluid, electrolyte, and coagulation abnormalities. Prompt delivery is the only known cure. Recurrences in subsequent pregnancies are unusual.

CONCLUSION

The decision of whether an acute process requires surgical intervention or referral to a specialist is based on the clinical skill of the provider. A complete history and careful physical examination (including a rectal and pelvic examination), the judicious use of laboratory and radiologic studies, and frequent reevaluation are required to reach a firm diagnosis. The primary care physician should not hesitate to seek advice from a surgeon, gynecologist, or other specialist.

The difficulties of diagnosing abdominal pain in pregnancy are well-known. A prompt clinical diagnosis and surgical intervention when indicated are necessary to minimize maternal and fetal mortality. When the diagnosis is uncertain, the advice of surgical and obstetric consultants should be sought.

BIBLIOGRAPHY

Ankum WM, Wieringa-De Waard M, Bindels PJ. Management of spontaneous miscarriage in the first trimester: an example of putting informed shared decision making into practice. *BMJ* 2001;322:1343.

Attard AR, et al. Safety of early pain relief for acute abdominal pain. *BMJ* 1992; 305:554.

Cervero F, Laird JM. Visceral pain. *Lancet* 1999;353:2145.

Cook IJ, Van Eeden A, Collins SM. Patients with irritable bowel syndrome have greater pain tolerance than normal subjects. *Gastroenterology* 1987;93:727.

Drossman DA, Zhiming L, Andruzzi E, et al. U.S. householders survey of functional gastrointestinal disorders: prevalence, sociodemography, and health impact. *Dig Dis Sci* 1993;38:1569.

Fischer MG, Farkas AM. Diverticulitis of the cecum and ascending colon. *Dis Colon Rectum* 1984;27:454.

Kaminski DL. Arachidonic acid metabolites in hepatobiliary physiology and disease. *Gastroenterology* 1989;97:781.

Ragan L, Rai R. Epidemiology and the medical causes of miscarriage. Best practice and research. *Clin Obstet Gynecol* 2000;14:839.

Scott HJ, Rosin RD. The influence of diagnostic and therapeutic laparoscopy on patients presenting with an acute abdomen. *J R Soc Med* 1993;86:699.

CHAPTER 6

Management of Chronic Pain in Women

Jay P. Shah

Chronic pain is a vast and rapidly evolving topic about which entire textbooks have been written. To attempt to condense this information into a single chapter would allow only a superficial discussion and shed little light on recent significant advances. The reader is advised to consult other textbooks for comprehensive information on the evaluation and treatment of specific pain syndromes.

The author's intent is to introduce five emerging, underappreciated, and clinically relevant areas for consideration:

1. The elucidation and integration of pain mechanisms into a clinical reasoning model
2. The association between gender and pain
3. The differences between chronic pain and chronic pain syndrome
4. The problems with the fibromyalgia construct (see Chapter 88)
5. The importance of accurately diagnosing and treating myofascial pain.

The International Association for the Study of Pain defines pain as "an unpleasant sensory and emotional experience associated with actual or potential tissue damage or described in terms of such damage." Pain is a *subjective* experience. In other words, pain is what the patient says it is. It has also been called the "fifth vital sign," along with blood pressure, temperature, respiratory rate, and pulse. As such, it is an indication of possible illness or pathology.

One's personality, mood, ethnic background, and past experiences of pain influence the perception and reaction to pain. Furthermore, *gender* is emerging as an important factor and is discussed later in this chapter. Pain is indeed unpleasant and therefore frequently an emotional experience. Thus, pain has three components—sensory, emotional, and as it is defined by the patient.

No laboratory or imaging study can show pain. Therefore, it is important that clinicians *believe* their patients. Chronic pain is often a multidimensional experience. Melzack and Casey describe three distinct dimensions:

1. Sensory-discriminative dimension is the physical, sensory component of pain and is described in terms of time (e.g., intermittent vs. constant, acute vs. chronic) and space (anatomical location).
2. Cognitive-evaluative dimension represents the ongoing perception and assessment of the meaning of the sensation for which there is great variation among individuals. It can be described in terms of time (present, past, or future). It represents the coping dimension of pain, i.e., the "Why is this happening to me?" dimension of pain.
3. Affective-motivational dimension is the mood dimension of pain and like the cognitive-evaluative dimension, there is great variation among individuals.

All three dimensions are often seen to varying degrees in most pain experiences especially in chronic pain states. Treatment strategies are more effective if they address these distinct dimensions.

Traditional categorizations of pain states, such as duration (acute vs. chronic), causative factors (e.g., runner's knee, cumulative trauma disorder), and affected body parts (e.g., knee pain, wrist pain), are inadequate for several reasons. They *do not* predict outcome, guide treatment, allow a search for risk factors, or identify subcategories that may respond to certain therapies.

MECHANISMS OF PAIN

A new model for understanding pain states is emerging thanks to advances in basic science research and the integration of pain mechanisms into clinical evaluation. Butler recommends the following:

- Pain should be categorized in terms of its *mechanisms* or processes, thus essentially its neurobiology and biochemistry.
- *A comprehensive model* of all pain states must include peripheral and central factors.
- Pain mechanisms are *not diseases* or specific injuries—they simply represent a process or biologic state categorized according to (a) input to the central nervous system, (b) central processing, and (c) output.

Input-related mechanisms

Nociceptive: pain secondary to tissue damage at the end of a neuron. It is usually associated with ischemia and inflammation in the tissue.

Peripheral neurogenic: pain originating in neural tissue distal to the dorsal horn of the spinal cord. Peripheral nerve entrapments such as carpal tunnel syndrome and radiculopathy are common examples.

Processing-related mechanisms

Centrally evoked symptoms: pain originating from within the spinal cord and/or central nervous system neurons. For example, an afferent barrage of impulses may be generated within the dorsal horn itself. This is a form of central sensitization.

Affective or emotional influences: the meaning of the situation, which depends on past experiences of pain, cultural factors, etc., affects the perception of pain.

Output-related mechanisms

Autonomic and motor signs and symptoms: autonomic effects may cause changes in skin temperature and color, abnormal sweating patterns, edema, or trophic changes in the hair, skin or nails (complex regional pain syndrome is the classic example). There may be associated motor dysfunction such as weakness, tremor, and reduced movement.

Various combinations of all the aforementioned categories may be operational at any one time. These pathobiologic mechanisms may be adaptive and protective (in response to a noxious stimulus) or maladaptive (with sensation of pain long after the noxious stimulus has been removed).

Pain and nociception are different, although the terms are often used interchangeably. Nociception is activity in a neural structure considered capable of causing or contributing to a sensation of pain. Unlike pain, nociception can be measured in the laboratory in individual nociceptors of what could be painful stimuli. It is essentially a laboratory measure of the number of action potentials in a nociceptor in response to a potentially noxious stimulus. A nociceptor is defined as a receptor preferentially sensitive to a noxious stimulus or a stimulus that would become noxious if prolonged. Nociceptors serve two critical functions: to encode noxious stimuli and maintain tissue health by initiating and maintaining reaction to injury.

New research in animals and humans indicates that men and women differ greatly in nociceptive processing. Young et al. cogently observe:

- Estrogen alters the receptive properties of important nerves, and evidence clearly indicates that pregnancy and the hormone progesterone affect nerve conduction.
- Sex hormones affect many central nervous system pathways involved in pain transmission.
- Electrophysiologic and brain imaging studies have revealed gender-based differences at many stages of pain processing.
- Hormones affect levels of serotonin, other neurotransmitters, and various biochemicals involved in processing pain.
- Hormones can affect nociceptor receptivity; for example, nociceptors may be sensitized (which lowers their threshold for activation) by ovarian hormones. Furthermore, central nervous system pain processing may vary with the stage of the menstrual cycle.

Basic science and clinical studies indicate that multiple mechanisms, operating at different sites and at different times, produce the sensation of pain. Pain is not a homogeneous sensation but is, rather, a collection of different sensitivities in normal and diseased states. The same symptom may be produced by different mechanisms (e.g., nociceptive, peripheral neurogenic, central sensitization), and a single mechanism may elicit different symptoms. Woolf et al. emphasize that it is essential to differentiate etiologic factors or diseases from mechanisms of pain.

Etiologic factors, such as cancer pain, postoperative pain and osteoarthritic pain, are important in initiating pain mechanisms, but it is the pain mechanisms that produce the pain symptoms. Because the same disease, such as cancer, may activate different mechanisms, a disease-based classification is of use primarily for disease-modifying therapy, not for treating pain. One can appreciate that the term cancer pain does not explain the mechanism(s) responsible for the experience of pain. For example, the pain may be caused by neuropathic, visceral, bony, or soft tissue mechanisms, secondary to tumor infiltration, or a combination of these.

Butler developed a reasoning model as an ongoing, dynamic process in which relevant knowledge and clinical skills are applied to the management of individual patients. The cornerstone is a thorough history and physical examination.

History

Woolf et al. developed the following questionnaire and cogently argued that it accompany the standard medical history in order to determine the likely pain mechanisms operant in a given individual:

Is the pain spontaneous or evoked?

What is the nature and intensity of the stimulus?

For evoked pain,

- Is there static mechanical hypersensitivity (i.e., punctate, blunt, or distributed)?
- Is there dynamic mechanical hypersensitivity (i.e., brush or distributed touch or movements)?
- Is there sensitivity to heat or cold?
- Is such sensitivity associated with body movements?
- Is there chemical sensitivity?

What is the quality of the spontaneous/evoked pain?

Is it:

- Burning
- Sharp
- Pulsing
- Cramping
- Shooting
- Crushing
- Pricking
- Tingling
- Stabbing
- Stinging?

What is the localization/distribution of pain?

Is it:

- At the sites of injury
- Beyond the sites of injury
- Dermatomal/nondermatomal
- Beyond the nerve territory
- Asymmetric?

What is the timing of the pain?

Is the pain continuous or intermittent?

Finally, what is the intensity of the pain on a visual analogue scale of 1 to 10?

Physical Examination

A thorough neuromusculoskeletal examination includes an evaluation of posture, body mechanics, range of motion, strength, palpation of tissue texture, and myofascial trigger points; a standard neurologic examination; selective tension diagnosis; and arthrokinematic assessment. Using the aforementioned historical and physical findings, the clinician makes a *hypothesis* of the specific pain mechanisms (e.g., nociceptive, peripheral neurogenic, central sensitization) operant in a particular patient. According to Foley, individual pain mechanisms then are *prioritized* so that *strategies* for a comprehensive treatment program, including pharmacologic treatments and standard and complementary nonpharmacologic interventions (joint and soft tissue techniques, electric modalities, effective self-management), are targeted at the mechanisms likely responsible for the pain and dysfunction.

Butler notes that organizing information in this manner logically guides diagnostic decision making and suggests the optimal treatment based on available data. Further evaluation and patient response to treatment either confirms one's prioritization of the treatment focus or indicates a need for reassessment.

GENDER AND PAIN

Gender differences have become an important issue on the national research agenda. The National Institutes of Health (NIH) Pain Research Consortium organized and sponsored a conference titled "Gender and Pain: A Focus on How Pain Impacts Women Differently than Men," held at the NIH in 1998. The conference was the first of its kind to be completely devoted to this topic, bringing together 30 top clinicians and researchers from a variety of disciplines. Studies presented at the conference underscored the following facts; to wit:

- Women experience more pain than men.
- Women discuss pain more than men.
- Women cope with pain better than men.
- Society's attitudes toward men and women in pain may influence physicians' treatments.
- The open expression of pain sometimes helps people control pain better, but being perceived as "too emotional" may work against a woman and lead to inadequate care.
- Pain treatment that works for one sex may not work as well, or at all, for the other.

Riley et al. found that women show lower pain thresholds and tolerances for a variety of experimental pain stimuli compared to men, and the effect sizes for these sex differences are moderate. Riley et al. also conducted a metaanalysis and found that pain sensitivity was greater in the premenstrual vs. postmenstrual phase for most pain stimuli. Furthermore, gender differences have also been reported for physiologic indices including pain-related muscle reflexes, and brain responses.

Women are more likely than men to seek medical attention for pain. They are better able, or more willing, to describe their pain experience fully and talk about their feelings. It is also more socially acceptable for women to express emotional distress. Unfortunately, women's descriptions of pain are often viewed with skepticism, or their complaints are dismissed as "hysterical." Young et al. note that depression or histrionic and somatization disorders are much more likely to be diagnosed in women with chronic pain than in men with chronic pain.

Unruh found that women seek more pain-related health care than men. Unfortunately, women are more often treated with psychotropic drugs than men. In the National Ambulatory Medical Care Survey, researchers found that women with an identical complaint, diagnosis, and visit history were 37% more likely than men to receive medication for anxiety and were 82% more likely to be given an antidepressant. These results were replicated in a later study published in 1998. As previously mentioned, a knowledge of pain mechanisms and the ability to conduct a thorough neuromusculoskeletal examination will enable the primary care physician to prioritize pain mechanisms and understand the anxiety and suffering of women with chronic pain.

Zubieta et al. found greater mu-opioid receptor activation among males in the nucleus accumbens, amygdala, ventral pallidum/substantia innominata and thalamus. Furthermore, in women circulating estrogen has been found to be inversely correlated with mu opioid receptor binding on the amygdala and the hypothalamus. Miaskowski et al. reviewed 18 studies of postoperative opioid analgesic use and reported greater opioid consumption among males in 10 (56%) and no gender difference in 8 (44%) of the studies. However, pain was assessed in only three of the studies; therefore, it is unknown whether the sex differences in opioid use are due to enhanced analgesia in women. There are also gender differences in the effects of morphine on electrical pain. As reported by Sarton et al., morphine-induced increases in electrical pain threshold and tolerance were greater for women than men. Interestingly, onset of analgesia was earlier in men but lasted longer in women.

There also appear to be gender differences in the effectiveness of non-opioid analgesics and non-pharmacologic treatments. Shafer et al. found that cholinergic agonists produce greater analgesia in women than in men. Males showed a significant increase in electrical pain tolerance after taking ibuprofen, but women did not. In patients with spinal pain, women showed improved health-related quality of life following behavioral medicine rehabilitation intervention, while men did not. Krogstad et al. found in patients with temporomandibular joint disorder, women reported significant reductions in pain following multidisciplinary interventions, while men reported no change.

Other studies show that commonly used pain relievers are less effective for women than for men. For example, in a study of experimentally induced pain, ibuprofen was less effective at relieving pain in women than in men. Young et al. suggest that perhaps gender should be considered when doses of nonsteroidal antiinflammatory drugs are prescribed. Women are more likely than men to use analgesics even after controlling for differences in pain, other medical conditions and economic factors.

Unfortunately, studies indicate that women do get less pain medication. In one study of 180 adults who had undergone appendectomy, the men received significantly more narcotic pain relievers than the women for the initial postoperative dose, although the total dose during the recovery period was about the same. Furthermore, in a study of people who had undergone coronary artery bypass graft surgery, the men received morphine significantly more often than the women. Interestingly, the women received more sedative drugs for anxiety or agitation. Young et al. suggest this difference may have reflected the nurses' belief that women are more emotional and more likely to complain of pain than men. Unfortunately, other research has shown that even among patients with metastatic cancer, being a woman is a significant predictor of inadequate pain management.

Studies presented at the 1998 NIH conference on gender and pain emphasized that some common diseases affect women more frequently or more severely than men. These include osteoarthritis (OA), rheumatoid arthritis (RA), migraine headaches, heart disease, temporomandibular disorder (TMD) and fibromyalgia syndrome (FMS).

- Osteoarthritis: Keefe et al. found that women reported 40% more OA pain and more severe pain than men. However, the women had better coping strategies than the men. For example, they spoke more about their pain with others, sought spiritual support and distractions, and asked for help more often than the men in the study. Furthermore, the day after experiencing severe OA pain, the women were less likely to report negative moods than the men were.
- Rheumatoid arthritis: women are two and one-half times more likely to develop RA than men and it may also affect them

more severely. Women also report that their joints are more painful and more swollen and report worse function than men.

- Migraine headaches: these occur more frequently in women (approximately 3:1) and are more severe and longer lasting in women than in men. Women are frequently afflicted at the time of ovulation, near menstruation and during pregnancy which suggests a hormonal contribution.
- Heart disease: prior to age 50 (pre-menopausal), women have more chest pain but less heart disease then men do. However, after age 50, women have more silent heart disease than men do. Studies have shown that both premenopausal women with high estrogen levels and postmenopausal women on estrogen replacement therapy had more frequent and more severe chest pain that was not caused by heart disease.
- TMD: the prevalence of TMD is seven times greater in women than men and affects one in four young women. Evidence suggests that TMD is not just a regional pain syndrome. TMD sufferers have greater sensitivity to a variety of noxious stimuli in other parts of the face and arm than non TMD sufferers. This suggests that people with TMD have central sensitization, whose hallmarks are allodynia and hyperalgesia.
- FMS: this is a disorder of chronic widespread pain with tenderness, fatigue, sleep disturbance and psychological distress. It is nine times more common in women than men, and affects 3.4% of women in North America. Recently, a physiologic term for FMS was coined, *chronic, widespread allodynia*, that more accurately describes this syndrome of chronic central sensitization and neurochemical pain amplification.

Finally, presenters and attendees at the NIH conference on gender and pain agreed on several key issues for future practice and research. To wit:

- Physicians need to consider gender when they diagnose illness and prescribe treatment.
- Women need to pay attention to variations in illness and pain tied to their menstrual cycle and to bring their observations to the attention of their physicians.
- Men need to develop a broader repertoire of active coping strategies.
- Parents need to give children age-appropriate information about medical procedures, telling them, for example, that an injection will sting. They need to help children receiving medical care understand what is happening, take charge of their bodies, and learn active pain-reducing coping strategies.
- Researchers studying pain at every level, from the molecular and genetic to the clinical, must assess the possible impact of gender. Use of males, whether animal or human, as the norm for research studies is outmoded.

CHRONIC PAIN VERSUS CHRONIC PAIN SYNDROME

Acute pain can persist, eventually becoming subacute and, with time, chronic (if pain has been present for 3-6 months) in nature. The hallmark of chronic pain is pain that persists long after the expected healing time. Most people with chronic pain gradually adapt physiologically, functionally and behaviorally. They learn to adapt to and cope with pain in different ways. On the other hand, persons with the chronic pain syndrome exhibit maladaptive patterns of behavior for dealing with persistent pain. The term chronic pain syndrome refers to a constellation of biological, neurophysiological and psychological changes that develop, often insidiously, over time.

The five *D*s of chronic pain syndrome are the following:

- Drug abuse or misuse
- Dysfunction or decreased function in life
- Disuse resulting in loss of flexibility and endurance
- Depression or depressed mood
- Disability resulting in an inability to perform the activities of daily living or pursue gainful employment.

Patil et al. added a sixth *D*—disturbed sleep pattern, in which stage 4 sleep is adversely affected.

According to Patil et al., the following factors may be associated with a predisposition to the development of chronic pain syndrome in a person with chronic pain:

- A past history of anxiety, depression, panic attacks, or child abuse
- Poor working conditons or no job to return to
- Substance abuse
- Multiple medical problems
- Limited education with poor command of the local language
- Tendency to miss medical appointments
- Inconsistent physical findings
- Preexisting medical conditions
- Failure to respond to different modalities of treatment
- Previous injury claims with difficult rehabilitation

The challenge to primary care physicians is to identify early warning signs of chronic pain syndrome or predisposing factors in their patients so that appropriate interventions can be made to prevent this devastating condition from developing. However, if the diagnosis of chronic pain syndrome is established, Patil et al. recommend the following 10 steps:

1. Accept that a patient's pain is real and try to determine to what degree the various dimensions of pain are contributing to the total pain experience.
2. Avoid excessive, unnecessary invasive procedures that do not facilitate the management of pain and merely perpetuate the chronic pain process.
3. Set realistic goals by making it clear that you are trying to manage pain rather than cure it.
4. Evaluate patients' level of function and enlist their aid in setting realistic goals of increasing function gradually (e.g., increase their tolerance for sitting, standing, walking) so that they learn to work around their pain rather than allowing it to restrict their daily activities and quality of life.
5. Prescribe pain medication on a time-contingency basis rather than as needed because the latter may reenforce pain behavior.
6. Prescribe an exercise program to improve flexibility, strength, and endurance. Many patients with chronic pain become deconditioned as a consequence of inactivity brought about by the fear of pain.
7. Educate patients and their families about the chronic pain process. A better understanding of the problem improves their compliance with the program.
8. Encourage patients to become involved in recreational and pleasurable activities. This will keep them physically and mentally occupied, less focused on their pain and facilitate their compliance with an exercise program.
9. Take action to help restore a normal sleep pattern in patients not getting enough hours of stage 4 sleep. 44%–88% of chronic pain patients are poor sleepers. Poor sleep may exacerbate pain the following day.
10. Identify and treat depression.

THE FIBROMYALGIA CONSTRUCT

As mentioned, fibromyalgia (see Chapter 88) is a common medical condition of chronic widespread pain that is accompanied by tenderness to palpation at multiple anatomically defined areas, fatigue, sleep disturbance, and psychological distress.

Although much of the pain and many of these defined areas are located in muscle, the allodynia is believed to be due to central sensitization and neurochemical pain amplification. Not only do sufferers experience allodynia (pain to normally non-noxious stimulus) but they also experience hyperalgesia (increased pain to a noxious stimulus). This may occur all over the body, not just in the clinically mapped and measured "tender points."

Although fibromyalgia is often reported to be a disorder primarily of young women, it is most common in women ages 50 years and older.

The 1990 American College of Rheumatology (ACR) criteria for the classification of fibromyalgia suggest that fibromyalgia can be diagnosed if a combination of the following criteria are met:

- A history of widespread pain (defined as pain in the left side of the body, pain in the right side of the body, pain above the waist, and pain below the waist, plus axial pain) for at least 3 months
- Pain in 11 of 18 anatomically defined tender points during palpation with approximately 4 kg of force. The tender points include the following nine paired locations: occiput, low cervical, trapezius, supraspinatus, second rib, lateral epicondyle, gluteal, greater trochanter, and knee.

Dommerholt has cogently argued that when one symptom (tenderness) is used to define an entire syndrome, circular reasoning is inevitable. For example, in an all too common scenario, a patient with chronic widespread pain and dysfunction is evaluated by a physician in a 15 minute office visit. The clinician is familiar with the criteria, has little time and does not really know what to do with this unfortunate patient. The clinician performs the tender point count and concludes that the patient has FMS. The patient is looking for a diagnosis and wants to know why she has pain. A common reply by the clinician is "because you have FMS." In other words, the message to the patient is "you have pain, because you have pain."

Dommerholt notes that the ACR criteria do not include the typical symptoms of sleep disturbance, fatigue, stiffness, and psychological distress. While sleep disturbance, fatigue, and stiffness were noted in more than 75% of patients with fibromyalgia, a combination of the three symptoms was noted in only 56% of patients and lacked the "high sensitivity, specificity, and accuracy of the tender point count." Though the report did suggest that these typical symptoms be considered, they are not essential for categorization purposes. Dommerholt notes that unfortunately, in clinical practice, it appears that many clinicians diagnose FMS based primarily on the tender point count together with the patient's history.

The criteria for FMS are classification criteria, designed for entry of subjects into research or epidemiological studies. Dommerholt notes that there is no validity anywhere in the literature that supports using these classification criteria for clinical diagnostic purposes. Furthermore, according to the criteria, the diagnosis is inclusive and should be made "irrespective of other diagnoses," meaning that in a patient with widespread pain that can be attributed to other treatable diagnoses, fibromyalgia syndrome must also be diagnosed if the criteria are met.

Of course, there are many entities that cause widespread pain, such as widespread burns, myofascial pain syndrome, parasitic diseases, hypothyroidism and other metabolic diseases (e.g., myoadenylate deaminase deficiency), whiplash, side effects of medications (especially the statin drugs), psychological or emotional stress, hypermobility syndrome, other rheumatic diseases, etc. Dommerholt concludes that patients diagnosed with FMS are at great risk for not getting the proper diagnosis and therefore not the proper treatment, which would make FMS an iatrogenic syndrome, created by physicians who do not perform an adequate differential diagnosis.

Like Dommerholt and his colleagues, the author has evaluated and successfully treated many patients who carried a diagnosis of fibromyalgia (some for many years) and, in fact, had a treatable condition that is also characterized by widespread pain.

As mentioned above, the ACR criteria were not developed for diagnostic purposes, so that they do not consider the potentially devastating psychological and emotional consequences of "a diagnosis of inclusion" for patients and their families. The current treatment modalities for fibromyalgia are unable to resolve the symptoms adequately, so that people in whom this condition is diagnosed may actually exhibit iatrogenic illness behavior. According to Dommerholt, "Specific patient beliefs, including a sense of hopelessness or the idea that one is disabled, are predictive of patient physical and psychological dysfunction and pain behaviors. It is likely that patients with fibromyalgia adjust to living with a chronic pain syndrome, frequent pain, loss of hope, and poor expectations rather than focusing on a positive treatment outcome." Unfortunately, this attitude unnecessarily complicates the rehabilitation process.

In conclusion, it is incumbent upon primary care physicians who evaluate patients with widespread chronic pain (even if they carry a diagnosis of fibromyalgia) to do a thorough workup to determine the underlying cause of the pain and then offer the appropriate intervention. Therefore, the diagnosis of FMS should not be made until all other possible causes have been investigated, treated and ruled out-in other words, fibromyalgia should be a diagnosis of exclusion.

MYOFASCIAL PAIN, THE "GREAT MIMICKER"

Myofascial pain has been called the "great mimicker" because it is often mistaken for other musculoskeletal conditions or even internal medicine-related diagnoses (Table 6.1). Therefore, the primary care physician who understands the nature, diagnosis, and treatment of myofascial pain will be able to identify the soft tissues and probable pain mechanism(s) involved, and institute the appropriate treatment for the patient with pain. According to the most commonly accepted concept (as described by Simons et al.), the myofascial pain syndrome is characterized by myofascial trigger points (MTrPs) in a taut band of muscle fibers. An MTrP is a hyperirritable spot in skeletal muscle that is associated with a hypersensitive palpable nodule in a taut band. Myofascial pain can go undetected if the physician is not prepared to identify MTrPs and does not actively search for them. It is often mistakenly diagnosed as fibromyalgia (Table 6.2).

An "active" myofascial trigger point causes pain or other abnormal sensory symptoms and often motor dysfunction (stiffness and restricted range of motion). A "latent" myofascial trigger point often causes motor dysfunction without pain. Otherwise, latent MTrPs exhibit all the characteristics of active MTrPs, although usually to a lesser degree. An active MTrP usually produces a referred pain pattern typical of the muscle in which it is located, restricted range of motion, and a visible local twitch response during mechanical stimulation.

The primary peripheral sensing apparatus in muscle involves group III (thinly myelinated and low threshold, identical to A-δ fibers in the skin) and group IV (unmyelinated and high threshold, identical to C fibers in the skin) afferent nerve fibers. These fibers cause cramping pain when stimulated.

There are several important characteristics of the central projections of these fibers: (a) reduced spatial resolution due to a lower innervation density of muscle tissue compared to the skin, thus making it more difficult to localize muscle pain; (b) convergence of sensory input into the same area of the dorsal horn from skin, muscle, periosteum, bone and viscera, making

TABLE 6.1. Common Referral Diagnoses When Overlooked Trigger Points are Actually the Cause of Symptoms

Initial diagnosis	Some likely trigger point sources
Angina pectoris (atypical)	Pectoralis major
Appendicitis	Lower rectus abdominis
Atypical angina	Pectoralis major
Atypical facial neuralgia	Masseter Temporalis Sternal division of sternocleidomastoid Upper trapezius
Atypical migraine	Sternocleidomastoid Temporalis Posterior cervical
Back pain, middle	Upper rectus abdominis Thoracic paraspinals
Back pain, low	Lower rectus abdominis Thoracolumbar paraspinals
(Bicipital) tendinitis	Long head of biceps brachii
Chronic abdominal wall pain	Abdominal muscles
Dysmenorrhea	Lower rectus abdominis
Earache (enigmatic)	Deep masseter
Epicondylitis	Wrist extensors Supinator Triceps brachii
Frozen shoulder	Subscapularis
Myofascial pain dysfunction	Masticatory muscles
Occipital headache	Posterior cervicals
Postherpetic neuralgia	Serratus anterior Intercostals
Radiculopathy, C8	Pectoralis minor Scalenes
Scapulocostal syndrome	Scalenes Middle trapezius Levator scapulae
Subacromial bursitis	Middle deltoid
Temporomandibular joint disorder	Masseter Lateral pterygoid
Tennis elbow	Finger extensors Supinator
Tension headache	Sternocleidomastoid Masticatory muscles Posterior cervicals Suboccipital muscles Upper trapezius
Thoracic outlet syndrome	Scalenes Subscapularis Pectoralis minor and pectoralis major Latissimus dorsi Teres major
Tietze syndrome	Pectoralis major enthesopathy Internal intercostals

Adapted from Simons et al. with permission.

TABLE 6.2. Clinical Features Distinguishing Myofascial Pain Caused by Trigger Points from Fibromyalgia

Myofascial pain (trigger points)	Fibromyalgia
Female-male ratio 1:1	Female-male ratio 4:1–9:1
Local or regional pain	Widespread, general pain
Focal tenderness	Widespread tenderness
Muscle feels tense (taut bands)	Muscle feels soft and doughy
Restricted range of motion	Hypermobile
Examine for trigger points	Examine for tender points
Immediate response to injection of TrPs	Delayed and poor reaction to injection of TrPs
Twenty percent also have fibromyalgia	Seventy-two percent also have active TrPs

TrP, trigger point.
Adapted from Simons et al. with permission.

it difficult to distinguish the origin of the pain compared to the skin; and (c) divergence of sensory input into the dorsal horn with sustained noxious input leads to the opening of previously ineffective connections; this is especially true of group IV fibers in animal models. These group IV fibers then begin to respond at lower levels of stimulation (mechanical allodynia).

Compared to normal muscle and muscle with latent MTrPs, muscle with active MTrPs is more tender and mechanically sensitive, suggesting that peripheral nociceptors are already sensitized. If already sensitized, the group IV afferents are likely firing, even though they are normally high-threshold nociceptors. For example, Mense et al. found that an increase in sympathetic stimulation or injection of bradykinin or prostaglandins in the muscle near the active MTrP will cause the group IV afferents to begin responding at much lower levels of stimulation. This phenomenon is believed to contribute to the unusual referral patterns that are seen in myofascial pain syndrome. For example, active MTrPs in the suboccipital muscles may refer pain to the frontal region, or active MTrPs in the piriformis may refer pain in a sciatic nerve distribution.

Therefore, the opening up of previously ineffective connections can have a profound effect on the one's pain experience and can lead to neuroplastic changes in the dorsal horn (central sensitization). These experimentally induced changes are well documented in animal models. They occur exclusively only after stimulation of the group IV afferents in skeletal muscle and tendon and are believed to be mediated by N-methyl-d-aspartate (NMDA) receptors. The astute clinician who is aware of this phenomenon should undertake a systematic examination of the soft tissue to identify the nociceptive foci of MTrPs that may be a generator of the patient's pain experience.

MTrPs can be accurately diagnosed only by systematic palpation by a trained and experienced clinician; there are no imaging or laboratory tests diagnostic for MTrPs or myofascial pain. Most commonly, the patient gives a history of acute, sustained, or repeated overload of the muscle. Examination of the affected muscle reveals painfully restricted full range of motion and exquisite localized tenderness of a nodule in a palpable taut band. Pressure applied directly on such a tender spot evokes pain that patients recognize as familiar (i.e., localization of an MTrP).

Clinically, an MTrP is a hyperirritable spot in skeletal muscle that is associated with a hypersensitive palpable nodule in a taut band. According to Simons et al., "the spot is painful on compression and can give rise to characteristic referred pain, referred tenderness, motor dysfunction, and autonomic phenomena (vasoconstriction, pilomotor response, ptosis, and hypersecretion)." Electromyographic (EMG) studies of MTrPs reveal a group of electrically active loci, each of which is associated with a contraction knot and a dysfunctional motor endplate in skeletal muscle.

MTrP nociceptors become activated in response to noxious stimulation. Muscle trauma and muscle ischemia are two factors commonly responsible for this. MTrP nociceptors are activated when the muscle containing them is exposed to sudden direct injury or when the muscle becomes actively, chronically, or recurrently overloaded. Furthermore, repeated episodes of microtrauma (e.g., repetitive strain injury, cumulative trauma disorder, etc.) can activate MTrP nociceptors.

Sola and colleagues, in a study of 200 fit U.S. Air Force personnel, found latent MTrPs in the shoulder girdle muscles in 54% of the women and 45% of the men. As mentioned, a latent MTrP may become active in response to any noxious lesion, usually trauma to the muscle. Some suggest that this is a phenomenon of central sensitization in the spinal cord. However, the central sensitization may be a response to peripheral activation and sensitization of MTrP nociceptors. Newborns demonstrate a pain reaction in response to noxious stimuli at all sites in a muscle. However, as they grow, they exhibit a stronger reaction to noxious stimuli in an MTrP than at other sites in the same muscle. Therefore, latent trigger points appear to develop gradually as a child gets older.

The prevalence of the myofascial pain syndrome in the community is not known, but myofascial trigger point pain is commonly diagnosed by experienced clinicians. For example, MTrPs were the primary source of pain in 74% of 96 patients with musculoskeletal pain evaluated by a well-trained and experienced neurologist in a community pain medical center and in 85% of 283 patients consecutively admitted to a comprehensive pain center. These and other epidemiologic studies suggest that MTrP pain is a significant, albeit overlooked source of morbidity in the community.

The diagnosis of myofascial pain syndrome is made exclusively by the systematic palpation of the muscle for taut bands and MTrPs after a review of the patient's history (including perpetuating factors) and an assessment of the posture and functional movement patterns. The patient's pain description and restriction of range of motion usually guides the clinician to the most likely involved muscles. According to Gerwin and colleagues, the minimum criteria that must be satisfied to distinguish an MTrP from any other tender area in muscle are a taut band and the presence of a tender point within the taut band. The presence of a local twitch response or referred pain or the ability to reproduce the patient's symptomatic pain increases the certainty and specificity of the diagnosis of myofascial pain syndrome. Systematic palpation differentiates between myofascial taut bands and general muscle spasms. Spasm can be defined as electromyographic activity caused by an increase in the neuromuscular tone of an entire muscle.

There are a variety of pharmacologic treatments used for myofascial pain though there are no controlled trials studying drug efficacy. Agents commonly used include nonsteroidal anti-inflammatory drugs, tramadol (a weak opioid agonist and inhibitor of the reuptake of serotonin and norepinephrine in the dorsal horn), tricyclic antidepressants, alpha 2 adrenergic agonists, and anticonvulsants (Borg-Stein and Simons). Inactivation of the MTrPs is the main short-term goal. It is essential to improve the circulation at the site of the MTrP, to decrease pathologic nociceptive activity, and to eliminate the abnormal biomechanical force patterns generated by the taut bands. To that end, there are a variety of minimally invasive physical medicine and nonpharmacologic approaches commonly used including postural, mechanical and ergonomic modifications, manual therapy, relaxation training, therapeutic exercise, the use of electrotherapy modalities (e.g., transcutaneous electrical nerve stimulation), and trigger point injections (e.g., with short- or long-acting anesthetics and botulinum toxin type A).

Hong found that dry needling (using a hypodermic without any solution) into an MTrP as effective as lidocaine injection in inactivating a trigger point and providing symptomatic relief. The author's preference is to use a 32-gauge acupuncture needle for dry needling MTrPs. An acupuncture needle has a rounded tip compared to the beveled edge of a hypodermic needle and is therefore less painful and less traumatic to tissue. Furthermore, it affords the clinician superior proprioceptive feedback that is very helpful in guiding the needle toward the active MTrPs, which are often firm and initially resistant to needle passage. Many authors also recommend investigation and treatment of possible underlying medical disorders that predispose to the development or maintenance of MTrPs.

CONCLUSION

Pain is merely a symptom. Fortunately, advances in the neuroscience of pain now make it possible to understand pain mechanisms based on a thorough history and neuromusculoskeletal examination. Integrating this information into a treatment plan can greatly assist the clinician in selecting effective therapeutic strategies (pharmacologic, nonpharmacologic, complementary) and fosters interdisciplinary intervention.

Women with chronic pain pose unique challenges to the medical community. It is hoped that this chapter will enable primary care physicians to make an accurate diagnosis and select appropriate interventions, and also reassure their female patients that their pain is real and manageable.

BIBLIOGRAPHY

Borg-Stein J, et al. Focused review: myofascial pain. *Arch Phys Med Rehabil* 2002;83(3 Suppl 1):S40–S47, S48–S49.

Butler DS. *The sensitive nervous system*. Adelaide, Australia: NOI Group Publications, 2000.

Derbyshire et al. Cerebral responses to noxious thermal stimulation in chronic low back pain patients and normal controls. *Neuroimage* 2002;16:158–168.

Dommerholt J. Muscle pain syndromes. In: Cantu RI, Grodin AJ, eds. *Myofascial manipulation: theory and clinical application*. Gaithersburg, MD: Aspen Publishers, 2001:93–125.

Fillingim R. *Sex-related differences in the experience of pain*. Glenview, IL: American Pain Society, 2001.

Fishbain DA, et al. Male and female chronic pain patients characterized by DSM-III psychiatric diagnostic criteria. *Pain* 1986;26:181–197.

Foley R. Complex regional pain syndromes: focus on the autonomic nervous system. Adelaide, Australia: NOI Group Publications, 2000.

Gerwin RD. A study of 96 subjects examined both for fibromyalgia and myofascial pain. *J Musculoskeletal Pain* 1995;3[Suppl 1]:121(abst.).

Hong C-Z. Lidocaine injection versus dry needling to myofascial trigger point: the importance of the local twitch response. *Am J Phys Med Rehabil* 1994;73:256–263.

Isaacson D, et al. Attitudes towards drugs: a survey in the general population. *Pharm World Sci* 2002;24(3):104–110.

Keefe FJ, et al. The relationship of gender to pain, pain behavior, and disability in osteoarthritis patients: the role of catastrophizing pain. *Pain* 2000;87:325–334.

Krogstad BS, et al. The reporting of pain, somatic complaints, and anxiety in a group of patients with TMD before and 2 years after treatment: sex differences. *J Orofac Pain* 1996;10(3):263–269.

Mense S, Simons DG. *Muscle pain: understanding its nature, diagnosis, and treatment*. Philadelphia: Lippincott Williams & Wilkins, 2001.

Miaskowski C, et al. Sex-related differences in analgesic responses. In: Fillingim RB, ed. *Sex, gender and pain*. Seattle: IASP Press, 2000:209–230.

NIH Pain Research Consortium. *Gender and pain: a focus on how pain impacts women differently than men*. Future Directions, 1998.

Patil JJ, et al. Pain management. In: O'Young BJ, et al., eds. *Physical medicine and rehabilitation secrets*, 2nd ed. Philadelphia: Hanley & Belfus, 2002:363–369.

Paulson PE, et al. Gender differences in pain perception and patterns of cerebral activation during noxious heat stimulation in humans. *Pain* 1998;76:223–229.

Riley JL, et al. Sex differences in the perception of noxious stimuli: a meta-analysis. *Pain* 1998;74:181–187.

Sarton E, et al. Sex differences in morphine analgesia: an experimental study in healthy volunteers. *Anesthesiology* 2000;93(5):1245–1254; discussion 6A.

Shafer S, et al. Cerebrospinal fluid pharmacokinetics and pharmacodynamics of intrathecal neostigmine methylsulfate in humans. *Anesthesiology* 1998;(Nov)89 (5):1074–1088.

Simons DG, et al. *Travell and Simons' myofascial pain and dysfunction: the trigger point manual*, vol 1. *Upper half of body*. Baltimore: Williams & Wilkins, 1999.

Sola, et al. Incidence of hypersensitive areas in posterior shoulder muscles. *Am J Phys Med* 1955;34:585–590.

Unruh AM. Gender variations in clinical pain experience. *Pain* 1996;65:123–167.

Woolf CJ, et al. Implications of recent advances in the understanding of pain pathophysiology for the assessment of pain in patients. *Pain* 1999;(Suppl 6): S141–S147.

Young M, et al. *Women and pain: why it hurts and what you can do*. New York: Hyperion, 2002.

Zubieta JK, et al. Mu-opioid receptor-mediated antinociceptive responses differ in men and women. *J Neuroscience* 2002;22:5100–5107.

CHAPTER 7

Care of the Cancer Patient

Joanna M. Cain

A woman with cancer enters a complex world of specialists and a bewildering array of possible treatments, and the entire basis of her life view is challenged. In the midst of this maelstrom, the primary care provider may be called on to provide complex supportive therapy, such as treatment of neutropenic sepsis, or guidance and psychological support during this confusing process. To be an adequate guide, the primary care provider must have a current understanding of the genetic nature of cancer and the implications for future therapy, a basic understanding of the terminology of cancer staging and therapy, a clear view of the psychosocial sequelae of the diagnosis and treatment of cancer, and an awareness of the particular complications or side effects of cancer therapy that may arise during the primary care of such patients.

THE NATURE OF CANCER

A complex interaction of inherited factors, environmental influences, and chance ultimately results in a genetic alteration that leads to cancer. Our understanding of oncogenes and how they function is rapidly expanding, along with the potential for treatments based on this knowledge. Such advances also may allow the presymptomatic testing of individuals for genetic tendencies toward cancer, which in turn raises several issues in primary care. All these discoveries have been based on laboratory tools developed along with the genome project and sequencing initiative. Most changes are too small to be seen by cytogenetic analysis, which, for example, reveals relatively gross triploidy and polymorphisms. Instead, restriction enzymes are used that generate sequences or clipped bits of DNA sized differently from normal sequences. Southern blot analysis detects these restriction fragment length polymorphisms; however, the process takes several days and detects only 1% to 5% of altered DNA. Furthermore, fresh tissue is required. More recently, polymerase chain reaction with primers and short sequences of DNA that stick to certain areas but are too far apart to yield a product in normal tissue has been used to fingerprint cancers. Polymerase chain reaction is 10 times more sensitive than Southern blot analysis and can be performed on fixed tissues. These techniques are merely ways of identifying commonalities among cancers; the actual sequencing of defects and identification of the genetic sequence of interest, such as in breast cancer, are far more elegant and far from complete.

The underlying biology of cancer is being understood at a much more complex level than before. Most somatic cell mutations are phenotypically silent, especially those in nonessential or redundant genes. If they are in essential genes, they more often result in death of the affected cells, but they sometimes cause changes in the growth patterns of the cells, either by directly stimulating growth or by attracting growth factors to stimulate growth and prevent normal cell death (apoptosis). This abnormal growth is propelled by oncogenes, which are altered genes that lead to cancer. Their normal counterparts are known as *protooncogenes* (sometimes termed *wild-type genes*); these have a normal gene sequence and produce the proteins that control cellular growth and function.

Oncogenes are uncovered in three ways. The number of copies of a gene (e.g., the HER-2/*neu* or c-*erb*-B2 protooncogene) can be increased in a process called *amplification*. This gene determines the number of receptors for epidermal growth factor (EGF) and is of particular interest in ovarian and breast cancers. When the number of copies in each cancer cell is amplified, the upstream decrease or modulation in the number of receptors is lost, and the cell is stimulated by EGF to grow inappropriately.

The second way an oncogene is uncovered is by a change in the sequence of the DNA (e.g., the *ras* oncogene). A change in a single three-base codon is enough to create an oncogene.

The third type of event requires the loss of a matching gene (loss of heterozygosity), which destroys function. Most oncogenes are heterozygous and are affected by the loss of matching normal alleles and also by transpositions that change the upstream control of the gene. The best example is the Philadelphia chromosome of chronic myelocytic leukemia, in which the ABL gene transfers from chromosome 9 to chromosome 22 and forms BCR-ABL, which is oncogenic. This is also how Burkitt lymphoma works, with transpositions from chromosome 8 to chromosome 14.

Loss of heterozygosity is particularly important in tumor suppressor genes. The absence of these genes causes cancer, as in retinoblastoma, in which Knudson's two-hit (or loss) theory has been proved. One allele is missing in the germ cell line, so only the loss of the second tumor suppressor gene in the somatic cell lines is needed for the cancer to occur. Other important tumor suppressor genes code for proteins p53 and p16 and for multiple tumor suppressor I, a cell cycle regulator.

The p53 protein is a nuclear phosphoprotein that arrests cells in G_1. For progression to synthesis, the gene that encodes p53 must be inactivated. This gene should be at p13 on the short arm of chromosome 17. Often, the remaining p53 allele harbors point mutations, and the mutant allele remains after the normal p53 allele is lost. Normal functioning of p53 is closely tied to programmed cell death (apoptosis); this area may provide new therapeutic opportunities.

Extension of Genetic Findings to New Directions in Cancer Therapy

An area of active interest is the identification of genes that code for recognizable antigens or cytokines that might be placed into cells to attract the attention of the immune system. As an example, genes that code for antibiotic sensitivity, tumor necrosis factor, or interleukin-2 could be placed specifically into tumor cells. Treatment would then be targeted accordingly. For example, ganciclovir would be administered to tumor cells with a gene conferring sensitivity to ganciclovir, and the cells would be differentially destroyed.

The new genetic information will also be used in immunotherapy. Trials performed in the past relied on passive or adoptive immunotherapy. T cells can recognize single amino acid substitutions that differentiate a tumor antigen from a self-antigen. They then secrete inflammatory cytokines, such as interleukin-2, to attract other cells, so that leukocytes (tumor-infiltrating leukocytes and activated killer cells) and macrophages can infiltrate and potentially eradicate solid tumors. In early attempts, the entire immune system was stimulated, but results were not as successful as had been hoped. These therapies, often administered as intraperitoneal infusions, have been evaluated in trials of patients with ovarian cancer, but probably because of a lack of specificity, they have not been particularly successful. Tumor cells have a remarkable ability to use growth factors and other antigenic markers to evade the immune system.

Presymptomatic Testing

Presymptomatic testing for oncogenes will require the identification of genes associated with different cancers and a far better understanding of their variable expression. Major areas of difficulty are the sensitivity and specificity of these tests and the fact that environmental factors continue to play a major role in the ultimate development of cancer. Presymptomatic testing is fraught with ethical, psychological, and economic pitfalls. Even when no current presymptomatic test is available, genetic counseling can be offered to patients, but this too is beset with issues such as unwarranted life changes, depression, and suicide if it is not undertaken by persons adequately trained in the field. Furthermore, the inclusion in a medical record of a "family history of" may be used to deny a patient insurance coverage for all ovarian or colon cancer therapy, even when the risk is only minimally increased over baseline.

When presymptomatic testing is available, the effect of such information on the patient is only one of the factors that must be considered. The current concept of informed consent and autonomy is challenged by this genetic diagnostic technique, which inherently requires the consent and involvement of other genetically related family members. The potential for insurance and job discrimination based on an inherited tendency to acquire a particular cancer or a susceptibility to certain environmental toxins is real. The physician who includes such testing in the primary care of patients must carefully consider the medical and societal consequences, making sure that appropriate safeguards and education have been provided.

STAGING

Once a cancer has been diagnosed, the therapy chosen is closely tied to the stage of the malignancy. Staging is carried out by various measures, depending on the tumor site and type. A stage is assigned at the time of the original diagnosis and never changes after that, even if disease recurs. A patient with a recurrent cancer is described as having a cancer of the original stage, with recurrent disease. An erroneous description can lead a consultant to an incorrect conclusion regarding the need for referral, further evaluation, or therapy. For example, the therapeutic options and evaluation requirements of a patient a stage I carcinoma of the cervix with a central recurrence are entirely different from those of a patient with stage III cancer of the cervix. Clear communication between providers is essential to optimize therapy and advance knowledge about cancer, and staging is one means of communication.

Most cancers are staged by the TNM system according to tumor size (T), the presence or absence of suspect or positive nodes (N), and the presence or absence of metastatic disease (M). For some cancers unique to women, staging follows guidelines set by the International Federation of Gynecologists and Obstetricians. Staging systems for common cancers in women and cancers unique to women are outlined in Table 7.1.

PSYCHOSOCIAL CONTEXT OF CANCER

Women undergoing surgery, radiation, and chemotherapy for malignancy present particular challenges to primary care providers. A primary care provider who is familiar with the psy-

TABLE 7.1. Staging of Common Cancers

Site	Most common site of metastasis	T definition	Methods for staging
Lung	Depends on cell type	**AJC** T1, <3 cm T2, >3 cm or pleural atelectasis, pneumonitis, or hilar involvement T3, direct extension beyond T2	Bronchoscopy Chest roentgenography Biopsy, radionuclide scan, or computed tomography as appropriate
Colon	Liver	Dukes by extension from mucosa T1, mucosa T2, serosa or peritoneal fat T3, adjacent structures	Resection required for staging
Breast	Regional lymph nodes	**AJC/UICC** T1, <2 cm T2, >2 cm, <5 cm T3, >5 cm T4, direct extension	Physical examination Biopsy Bone scan
Cervix	Regional lymph nodes	**FIGO** I, confined to cervix II, in parametrium III, to side wall IV, direct extension or distant	Physical examination Biopsy Other radiographic tests as appropriate
Ovary	Abdominal cavity	**FIGO** I, ovaries only II, ovaries plus pelvis III, abdomen IV, outside abdominal cavity	Surgically staged Chest roentgenography
Uterus	Regional nodes	**FIGO** I, uterine cavity II, uterine cavity plus cervix III, plus pelvic area IV, distant	Surgically staged Chest roentgenography

AJC, American Joint Commission; UICC, International Union Against Cancer; FIGO, International Federation of Gynecologists and Obstetricians.

chological and physical side effects of cancer treatment can clarify the appropriateness of therapy and support the patient while she undergoes treatment. The process of helping a patient live with a diagnosis of cancer often begins with informing her of the results of a biopsy and the diagnosis. This is the start of a period of intense personal challenge for the patient, and gentle truthfulness on the part of caregivers enables her to make choices and trust her caregivers. Withholding information from a patient rarely serves her best interests and does not respect her right to make choices on matters ranging from whether referral is appropriate to whether a particular proposed therapy is acceptable.

Identifying problems of social and psychological adjustment, closely monitoring the availability of support systems and encouraging the patient to use them, and clearly communicating that the primary care provider is available for consultation for any reason can help assuage the terrible feelings of isolation and loneliness raised by a diagnosis of cancer.

Psychologic Effects

A diagnosis of cancer profoundly affects the fundamental assumptions of daily life, particularly the notion that we control our destiny, and raises the specter of death. In addition, a woman's ability to carry out her various roles, particularly that of caregiver in her relationships, is altered, which adds to her distress. Finally, many aspects of cancer treatment affect a woman's self-image, from the loss of hair to the loss of body parts integral to her identity as a woman. Thus, the psychological context of cancer care should be the first consideration in the primary care of women with cancer.

Adjustment to the Diagnosis

A woman's reaction to a diagnosis of cancer depends on three major factors: her prior psychological adjustment, her societal or cultural context, and the medical factors of the particular diagnosis. The morbidity and mortality rates of women with cancer clearly differ between racial, ethnic, and socioeconomic groups. The legacy of poverty for women includes unemployment with a lack of health coverage, malnutrition, higher rates of smoking, lack of basic health education, and a cognitive fatalism; all these affect choices in seeking health care. Improving the social and economic status of women, particularly minority women, will improve the medical and psychological outcomes of women with cancer and is a proper concern for the primary caregiver.

The coping abilities a woman has had before the diagnosis of cancer are brought into the spotlight after the diagnosis. If her coping was poor, it will still be poor in response to this challenge. Her emotional maturity, her ability to modify plans, and the availability of emotional support are also the same as before the diagnosis. A major role of the primary care provider can be to identify support systems and coping patterns to sustain the patient through this turbulent time. However, it is unreasonable to assume that her ability to deal with stress will be improved miraculously by a diagnosis of cancer. Patients who are stoic remain so, and those who lose all ability to function in crises tend to do so. The two axioms of support for primary caregivers are these:

Do not expect the patient to change her coping mechanisms. Accept her approach and suggest more successful strategies.

If the woman is well-known to the primary caregiver and pretest (e.g., before biopsy) counseling can be arranged before the diagnosis, this should be offered if possible.

Sexual Dysfunction

One of the factors affecting a woman's response to certain types of cancer is the inextricable cultural link between the breasts, ovaries, and uterus and womanhood. Although much has been made of the connection and the ultimate effect of those cancers on a woman's sexuality and body image, her previous sexual satisfaction and psychological health are actually more important factors in her response. According to Schover's 1991 article, which included a review of the work of multiple authors, breast-conserving strategies for the treatment of breast cancer clearly resulted in a better body image but had little or no effect on marital satisfaction, psychological adjustment, frequency of sex, and sexual dysfunction. In patients with gynecologic cancers, the extent of sexual disruption is overshadowed by their overall coping skills, so that it is difficult to assess the sequelae independently. The available data strongly suggest, however, that the number of sexually active women drops during and after treatment, that the frequency of intercourse declines, and that arousal deficits emerge. As Anderson noted in 1989, "The cancer-related sexual difficulties for couples may provide a sufficient, added vulnerability if sexual intercourse is already problematic for other reasons." Also, pelvic surgery may affect sensation or exacerbate dyspareunia.

Chemotherapy and hormonal therapies can have significant effects on the vaginal mucosa, in addition to other side effects, with resultant dyspareunia and sexual dysfunction. Schover and colleagues in 1995 found chemotherapy to be a major predictor of greater psychosocial distress and sexual dysfunction.

Of particular concern to primary caregivers should be the 1994 finding by Thranov and Klee that although 74% of patients with gynecologic cancers expressed little or no desire for sexual relations, 54% had had sexual relations within the past month, primarily those younger than 55 years. This observation suggests that such women are trying to fulfill their normal roles and retain normal sexual function without concomitant support, and their sexual problems are being neglected.

Given the general lack of attention paid to this area of life in medicine overall, it is important to initiate such inquiries and provide support to all patients. Caregivers must not assume that older women are less concerned about sexual dysfunction after cancer has been diagnosed and treated. The discrepancy between sexual desire and actual sexual relations reported for younger women does not seem to be as great in women older than 55 years, but this seems to be the consequence of a concomitant finding that many of the elderly patients' partners also have no desire for a sexual relationship. Thus, although sexual function appears to be less discordant and problematic for older women than for the younger ones, individual patients may still desire a better evaluation and greater support in dealing with these issues, regardless of age. Sexual functioning is another area in which the primary caregiver can be of particular assistance.

Quality of Life

Much has been said about quality-of-life issues in cancer therapy, but the measurement of such factors and our ability to affect the various domains of the psychological and functional adaptation to cancer remain in the early stages. It is important for medical caregivers to note that estimates of a patient's quality of life by others, including medical caregivers, correlate poorly with the patient's own assessment. Listening to a patient talk about whatever part of her quality of life is most troublesome during the diagnosis and treatment of cancer is the approach most likely to allow primary caregivers the opportunity to address these issues adequately. For some patients, spirituality or sexuality rather than physical function is the biggest concern, and failure to pay attention to their concerns will result in a poorer outcome.

The entire family's experience is often important to women with cancer. The partner's or family's quality of life affects the perceived quality of life of a woman with cancer, so it may be appropriate to assess more than just the patient. Some suggest that because spouses have different coping styles, quality-of-life assessments should be carried out separately.

PHYSICAL CHANGES RELATED TO CANCER THERAPY

Surgical changes related to cancer care encompass many organ systems and have varying sequelae. It is important for the caregiver to understand the complications that may develop during the general care of women with cancer. A few selected problems are outlined here.

Venous Access Devices

A subcutaneous port (arm or chest wall) or a transcutaneous catheter is often placed in a patient undergoing chemotherapy. These devices are used for the frequent blood draws required during chemotherapy, and maintenance of skin integrity and avoidance of infection are critical. A Dacron cuff portion may stabilize a transcutaneous catheter in the subcutaneous tissue. If the transcutaneous catheter does not have such a cuff, fixation to the skin with sutures must be maintained, and a lost stabilizing suture must be replaced. The primary caregiver should be able to draw blood through the various catheter systems and evaluate these devices for infection. Breakdown of the skin over a port or extension of erythema and purulent drainage above the Dacron cuff of a transcutaneous catheter (or down the catheter channel in those without a cuff) warrants expert evaluation. Deep venous thrombosis in an upper extremity, evidenced by arm or neck edema, also requires immediate attention because of the risk for pulmonary embolism.

Limb Edema Associated with Cancer Surgery

The removal of regional lymph nodes, particularly axillary and groin dissection, can cause lymphedema of a limb. Multiple systems for diminishing lymphedema are available; passive compression and sequential compression are the major functional elements in these strategies. The use of sleeves or socks with varied pressure (Jobst) often prevents the accumulation of fluid in a limb. The major complication of lymphedema is lymphangitis or local skin cellulitis as a consequence of poor drainage of the tissues. Often, the only change noted is slight redness or a sensation of heat in the affected extremity. The usual agents are skin flora, and antibiotic therapy should be instituted as soon as lymphangitis or cellulitis is suspected. Avoidance of blood draws, establishment of intravenous sites, and trauma to the arms after axillary dissection is based on this risk for infection.

Radical Pelvic Surgery

Radical pelvic surgery for malignancies in women is never undertaken lightly. The physical changes that follow such surgery affect self-image and sexual function and create a new set of problems.

URINARY RECONSTRUCTION

Techniques of urinary reconstruction range from bladder augmentation to the placement of ileal urinary conduits. Health-related quality of life appears to be better after bladder substitution (continent) than after placement of an ileal conduit because of the decreased risk for leaks and the avoidance of ostomy appliances. However, all reconstructive surgery of the urinary tract increases the risk for pyelonephritis and stone formation with entrapment at anastomotic strictures, and for the development of partial or complete ureteral obstruction with strictures. Infections can be particularly difficult to assess because reconstructions with ostomies are chronically colonized. Fever, back pain, or ureteral symptoms should alert the practitioner to the need for careful evaluation for one of the sequelae of such surgery.

PELVIC EXENTERATION AND RECONSTRUCTION

New surgical techniques have made it possible to preserve bowel and bladder function and to reconstruct the pelvis and vagina after exenterative surgery for recurrent cervical or colon cancers. A major advance has been the development of multiple graft techniques to restore normal anatomy.

SKIN AND MUSCLE GRAFTS

When an area has been subjected to significant radiation therapy, the microvascular blood supply is often inadequate for normal healing. The use of myocutaneous and other flaps makes it possible to reconstruct a new vagina after such surgery. These flaps may be plumper than the original vaginal and surrounding tissue and can cause discomfort from compression. In addition, the cutaneous sensation continues to be transmitted to the brain, at least initially, as if originating from the donor site. For instance, if a gracilis myocutaneous graft is used, sensation is referred to the medial thigh. This is normal for such grafts. Anesthesia of a graft site can also develop if the graft nerves are significantly damaged or, with the use of free flaps, if the original neural bundle is not maintained. Because grafts are placed in the original tumor bed, it is important to examine these areas for abnormalities to detect recurrent disease.

SIDE EFFECTS OF CANCER TREATMENT AND THEIR MANAGEMENT

Hair Loss

Hair loss during chemotherapy is common. It is also a visible sign of cancer therapy to the patient and others, and it notably changes the patient's appearance. A proactive approach to hair loss (e.g., teaching about alternative head wraps, selection of wigs or hairpieces made with the patient's own hair) should be undertaken before or shortly after the first chemotherapy session. Women must be reminded that they are likely to lose more heat and be more susceptible to sunburn with thinner hair or a bald scalp. The hair follicles can also become quite sensitive early in hair loss, and the use of loosely fitted, 100% cotton scarves or turbans can help manage this sensitivity.

Pain

The pain associated with cancer treatment, whether the anticipated outcome is death or cure, is woefully undertreated. The causes of pain may be multiple. The cancer itself with surrounding nerve pressure and inflammation can cause pain. Procedures (even diagnostic) and therapies can also cause various types of pain and anxiety. It is important to differentiate neuropathic pain from the pain of tissue damage because the therapy for each differs markedly. Anticonvulsants and antidepressants are appropriate for neuropathic pain, whereas the more traditional pain medications, from nonsteroidal antiinflammatory drugs through the opiates, are appropriate for tissue damage pain. Corticosteroids and local radiation therapy may be required for osseous pain.

The routine assessment of pain on a scale with which the practitioner is comfortable substantially improves pain control. The most important aspect of cancer pain management, however, is believing the patient's perspective and reassuring her regarding the "addictive" properties of opioids. The difference between addiction or drug-seeking behavior and the habituation that occurs when patients take substantial doses of narcotics for a long time is commonly misunderstood. Although habituation means that patients cannot stop their pain medicine abruptly without experiencing withdrawal symptoms, appropriate withdrawal from narcotics when they are no longer needed is successful. Patient and family education regarding pain therapy with narcotic medications is usually required, and the health care team must encourage the patient to report pain. No patient with cancer should have to suffer untreated pain.

Futile Care

The concept of quality of life is also used to address ethical issues in cancer therapy. For example, when is further curative therapy of no further benefit to the patient? What constitutes a "life not worth living" to an individual patient? These are often difficult decisions for patients and their caregivers. The need to treat and offer assistance is integral to the practice of medicine, but treatment can be given with palliative as well as curative intent. It is important for the caregiver to make an honest assessment of the likelihood of cure with additional treatment (and the probable side effects), to determine when further curative therapy is unlikely to meet this goal, and to transmit this information in a supportive setting. Such actions respect the patient's right to make choices about what the benefits and harms of a particular treatment mean to her quality of life.

Of course, the information given must be correct. Some patients with metastatic disease are told that no further therapy will be of benefit. It may be quite true that although no therapy is curative, therapies with relatively tolerable side effects are available that can both prolong life and delay or attenuate pain, bowel obstruction, and other difficult terminal symptoms. To ignore this information is clearly not in the best interests of the patient. The choice should be hers, based on her evaluation of how the side effects will affect her life. Telling the truth and eliciting the patient's goals and wishes in a respectful way allow the patient and caregiver to make the best decision about terminal therapy.

INTRODUCTION TO CHEMOTHERAPY

Chemotherapy in the treatment of malignancy is always directed at a potential site of metastasis or a verified disease process. Localized cancers are generally treated with radiation, surgical extirpation, or both. Chemotherapy is combined with radiation and surgery to treat localized tumors when either the potential for metastases (as in breast cancer) is great or the local response is enhanced by its radiation-sensitizing effects. The principles guiding the use of chemotherapy have been outlined by Skipper and colleagues. In short, chemotherapeutic drugs in general kill a constant fraction of cancer cells regardless of the tumor size (first-order kinetics); therefore, smaller tumors are more curable than large tumors. Second, resistance may be present de novo or emerge during treatment, so that chemotherapy with multiple agents is preferred as a means of overcoming resistance in different populations of cancer cells. The drugs included in combination chemotherapy must each be at least partially effective when used alone for the cancer being treated. It also is theoretically important to combine drugs that act during different phases of the cell cycle or cell division, in the hope that the mechanism of resistance to one agent is different from that to the others. Given the theoretic advantage of combining drugs that have different mechanisms and targets of action (with the presumed avoidance of cross-resistance), the major chemotherapeutic drugs are reviewed according to mechanism of action. The largest group damages the nucleic acids of cancer cells by alkylation, strand scission, and intercalation.

Chemotherapeutic Drugs

ALKYLATING AGENTS

Alkylating agents were the first class of chemotherapeutic drugs developed. Nitrogen mustard was introduced in the 1940s—the forerunner of this group—and is still used for lymphoma therapy. The most commonly administered agents are cisplatin and carboplatin, both of which work by cross-linking DNA strands. The platinum-containing alkylating agents are unique in that they are the only heavy metal compounds commonly used for chemotherapy. The drugs in this class, with their likely toxicities and therapeutic targets, are outlined in Table 7.2.

ANTITUMOR ANTIBIOTICS

Antitumor antibiotics are a subset of the drugs that attack nucleic acids. They work either by intercalation or by strand scission (bleomycin). The anthracyclines (doxorubicin and daunomycin) are the agents in this class most commonly used to treat solid tumors, particularly of the breast and lung, and leukemias. The anthracyclines have the unique side effect of cardiotoxicity; this can develop both as an acute syndrome that is not dose-dependent and as a cumulative cardiomyopathy that is directly related to the overall dose.

ENZYME INHIBITORS

The point of interfering with various enzymatic processes of the cell is to have fewer building blocks available for DNA synthesis and eventual division. Different agents specifically block different pathways. 5-Fluorouracil, widely used for gastrointestinal malignancies, specifically inhibits thymidylate synthetase. Methotrexate, used for gestational trophoblastic disease and now for some ectopic pregnancies, inhibits dihydrofolate reductase. Cytosine arabinoside, used for hematologic malignancies, inhibits DNA polymerase. Often, the normal product of a blocked metabolic path, such as leucovorin (5-formyl tetrahydrofolate), is combined with these agents, either to "rescue" normal cells when large doses are given or to propel the cell systems toward a blocked path, as when leucovorin is combined with 5-fluorouracil.

Whereas these enzyme inhibitors are focused on general cellular function, new classes of enzyme inhibitors are specifically directed against known molecular targets; for example, ST571, a tyrosine kinase inhibitor, has been developed against a specific target in chronic myelogenous leukemia. As the genetic analysis of tumor abnormalities continues, this class of designer inhibitors will likely grow.

MITOTIC SPINDLE AGENTS

The mitotic spindle agents affect the function of the mitotic spindle in various ways to inhibiting division. Vincristine, vinblastine, and the taxanes are the agents of this group in widest use.

Hormonal Therapies

Hormonal therapies are generally considered cytostatic rather than cytotoxic because they do not directly cause the death of cells. The most commonly used agents are the selective estrogen receptor modulators (SERMs), which selectively block estrogen receptors, and the progestational agents. Two SERMs, tamoxifen and raloxifene, are widely used to treat hormonally associated tumors, such as breast cancers. Aromatase inhibitors are being used increasingly often in breast cancer and potentially other cancers to inhibit the intracellular enzymes that metabolize substrates into estrogenic substances. Even estrogen itself, usually diethylstilbestrol, has been used to treat advanced metastatic breast cancer in the past (and prostate cancer) with some success.

Side Effects of Chemotherapy Agents

Primary care providers may be called on to identify and treat the side effects of chemotherapy, some of which can present management dilemmas. These side effects are not specifically associated with classes of drugs; rather, they are part of the individual profile of each drug. Therapy for the common side effects and the consequences for further chemotherapy are outlined in the next sections.

HYPERSENSITIVITY REACTIONS

With some drugs, such as paclitaxel, the potential for hypersensitivity is great enough that all patients receive prophylaxis before therapy. With others, hypersensitivity is idiosyncratic and related to the mode of delivery. Major drugs associated with hypersensitivity include L-asparaginase, the platinum-based drugs, etoposide, and the anthracycline antibiotics. Treatment of the reaction is usually acute and includes the management of hypotension in addition to the administration of histamine H_1 and H_2 receptor blockers. Re-treatment with a drug is generally contraindicated when severe hypotension develops. However, milder reactions may be alleviated by substituting analogues, if possible, or pretreating with corticosteroids and H_1 and H_2 blockers when a particular agent is important to the success of cancer therapy.

SKIN REACTIONS

The extravasation of a drug can have direct and dramatic effects on the skin, tendons, and subcutaneous tissues. The major treatment is avoidance by careful administration technique, particularly with doxorubicin, and a demonstration of blood return and free flow of fluids before injection. The management of an area after a recognized extravasation varies; removal of fluid from the area, if possible, is the first option. Injecting substances into the skin to lessen toxicity has also been proposed, but the substance to be used is different for each agent. Most pharmacies mixing chemotherapy drugs maintain a list of such substances. Ultimately, some cases of extravasation are severe enough that skin debridement and grafting are eventually required.

Skin burns can be caused by a radiation-association effect, regardless of the relative timing of the administration of radiation and drug (called *after-radiation recall*), and by sunlight. The most significant reactions occur in patients given actinomycin D, although doxorubicin, 5-fluorouracil, and hydroxyurea can also initiate reactions. Major sunburns can develop in patients receiving methotrexate, 5-fluorouracil, and the vinca alkaloids who do not protect themselves from exposure to the sun. This side effect is more important than ever as the use of methotrexate to treat ectopic pregnancies in young women increases.

Finally, other cutaneous side effects, such as pigmentation, tanning in areas of trauma (such as in areas that are scratched), and nail changes are associated with various agents. Some of the skin changes are permanent; therefore, care should be taken at all times to maintain the integrity of the skin.

ORAL LESIONS

Mucositis with subsequent poor nutrition can be caused by many chemotherapeutic agents. The management of oral lesions is critical to maintaining comfort and nutrition. Unfortunately, the natural course of the lesions associated with chemotherapy is not shortened by any specific treatment. Differentiation from a herpetic outbreak is critical, as is monitoring

TABLE 7.2. Chemotherapeutic Drugs

Class	Selected drug	Most frequent side effects	Used commonly for
Alkylating (nucleic acid)	Cisplatin	Nausea, vomiting, nephrotoxicity (Mg, Ca wasting), ototoxicity, neurotoxicity	Ovarian, lung, endometrial
	Carboplatin	Milder symptoms than cisplatin	Ovarian, lung, endometrial
	Cyclophosphamide	Hemorrhagic cystitis, myelosuppression	Ovarian, breast, others
	Etoposide	Nausea, myelosuppression, neuropathy (especially when combined with vincristine)	Lung, ovarian, lymphoma, testicular
Antibiotics (nucleic acid)	Bleomycin	Pulmonary fibrosis, fever, skin pigmentation, hypersensitivity	Cervix, germ cell malignancies
	Actinomycin D	Mucositis, stomatitis, diarrhea, myelosuppression, "radiation recall"	Germ cell, gestational trophoblastic disease
	Doxorubicin	Cardiac toxicity, skin necrosis with extravasation, myelosuppression	Breast cancer, sarcoma
Enzymes	Cytosine arabinoside	Nausea, myelosuppression, stomatitis, hepatotoxicity	Leukemia
	5-Fluorouracil	Nausea, myelosuppression, hand and foot syndrome when combined with leucovorin	Colon, breast, ovarian
	Hydroxyurea	Myelotoxicity	Leukemia
	Methotrexate	Mucositis, myelosuppression, nephrotoxicity at high doses	Gestational trophoblastic disease
	Tyrosine kinase inhibitors (imatinib mesylate)	Occasional nausea, periorbital edema, muscle cramps, skin rash, diarrhea *(Mild)*, myelosuppression	CML, others
Mitotic spindle	Vincristine and vinblastine	Neuropathy (vincristine), myelosuppression (vinblastine)	Leukemia, lymphoma, pediatrics
	Paclitaxel	Hypersensitivity, neutropenia	Ovarian, breast, others?

CML, chronic myelogenous leukemia.

for secondary infections, both of which can be treated directly. Maintaining oral hygiene by rinsing the mouth with saline solution and cleaning the teeth gently (with a foam brush) are key. Spicy, acidic, rough, very hot, and very cold foods should be avoided. For pain, local anesthetic agents such as Viscous Xylocaine or various mixtures of antacids and anesthetic agents can be used before eating and between meals. The use of nutritional liquid supplements is often critical to maintaining nutrition at this time.

NAUSEA AND VOMITING

Many chemotherapeutic regimens are highly emetic, and a wide variety of therapies have been developed to control nausea and vomiting. In many cases, nausea has two components: anticipatory and chemical. Anticipatory nausea (and, frequently, vomiting) occurs before any drug is given and is fairly frequent when prior antiemetic therapy has been inadequate. Anticipatory nausea is best treated by adding anxiolytic agents such as lorazepam to the planned regimen. For example, if nausea generally develops before the patient leaves home for treatment, then therapy should begin 30 minutes before that time.

Treatment for chemotherapy-induced nausea and vomiting has progressed significantly through the years, and major new classes of drugs, particularly the serotonin antagonists, have been developed to manage this problem. Most antiemetic chemotherapy regimens include metoclopramide, ondansetron, or granisetron. Both metoclopramide and ondansetron can be given orally. For sustained nausea after chemotherapy, the oral medication should be continued and is very effective. An evaluation of the electrolyte status and nutritional indices is indicated for a patient with anorexia and nausea related to chemotherapy. Intervention with dietary supplementation or even total parenteral nutrition is occasionally required.

NEPHROTOXICITY

An awareness of the nephrotoxicity of different agents is important in the long-term care of patients who have received chemotherapeutic agents. Some complications, such as the rapid release of uric acid during the treatment of rapidly proliferating tumors (e.g., lymphomas and leukemias) with subsequent hyperuricemic nephropathy, are immediate effects of chemotherapy; other sequelae are permanent. Most patients receiving directly nephrotoxic drugs (e.g., streptozotocin or cisplatin) are routinely followed with evaluation of the calculated or direct creatinine clearance to decrease the risk for renal compromise at re-treatment. However, some nephrotoxicity, such as that related to the nitrosoureas (carmustine [BCNU], semustine [meCCNU]) may not appear for several months to years after chemotherapy, particularly when doses of BCNU and meCCNU are higher than 1,500 mg/m^2.

A true nephropathy can be induced by inorganic platinum coordination complexes, particularly cisplatin, and can usually be prevented by maintaining high-volume renal flow with fluid management during therapy. Unfortunately, the dehydration associated with emesis and poor intake for several days after treatment can also contribute to nephropathy, so dehydration in any patient on platinum-based therapy must be taken seriously. The nephropathy is related to tubular necrosis, and hypomagnesemia and hypocalcemia often develop secondary to urinary magnesium wasting. Even without significant increases in the creatinine level, such wasting can occur. The obvious outcome of unmonitored loss is seizures and tetany. Monitoring with replacement of electrolytes is an important preventive strategy in the long-term primary care of these patients.

NEUTROPENIA AND ANEMIA

In most cases, the neutropenia and anemia associated with chemotherapy develop 7 to 21 days after a dose of chemotherapy. Much of this is anticipated, and the development of various cytokines to stimulate the production of white and red cells has significantly decreased the number of admissions for neutropenia. A few guiding principles of granulocyte colony-stimulating factor (G-CSF) therapy are appropriate, however. First, during the 3 days immediately following the administration of G-CSF, the white cell counts climb rapidly, sometimes in multiples of 10,000. This increase does not mean that the G-CSF should be discontinued because it represents the demargination of white cells. Second, in combination chemotherapy, the expected nadir of the white blood cell count may be different for each drug, so the treatment should cover the expected nadir of all drugs.

Summary of Chemotherapy

In chemotherapy, a wide variety of injectable agents are administered that modify the growth of cancer cells. Because new agents become available all the time, it is prudent to keep track of their major acute and chronic toxic effects. Neutropenia and bone marrow suppression are the most constant of the acute side effects. However, the long-term sequelae of chemotherapeutic agents can affect everything from the dermis to the kidneys, so that the attention and vigilance of the primary care provider are essential.

PRINCIPLES OF RADIATION THERAPY

Simply stated, the benefit of radiation therapy for cancer is based on the tissue damage inflicted when radiation energy is absorbed by tissue. The extent of the damage depends on the energy of the photons emitted from linear accelerators and betatrons. Higher energy, in general, penetrates more deeply into tissue, whereas lower energy (such as electron beam) penetrates only superficially. The intensity of the dose delivered from a source to adjacent tissue or personnel is governed by the inverse square law; the intensity of the radiation varies inversely as the square of the distance from the source. Therefore, the best way to avoid exposure to radiation or lessen its toxicity is to increase the distance from the source (and also limit the duration of exposure to the source). This phenomenon explains why the intensity of an implanted source of radiation rapidly decreases as the distance from the source increases. The amounts of radiation at different points beyond a source are often described in isodose curves.

In general, radiation therapy is administered in average fractionated doses of 200 cGy/d to achieve the final dose. This dosing allows for the differential killing of cancers and repair of normal tissues in the field. The complications of radiation therapy are caused primarily by the exposure of normal tissue within the radiated field. Multiple treatment adaptations have been developed to decrease side effects, including using computers to target tumors, rotation, shrinking the field to be treated later, shielding normal tissue, and brachytherapy, in which interstitial implants direct higher doses only to the tissue of interest (e.g., breast or cervix). Most interstitial and brachytherapy implants have a removable source that can be loaded afterward (afterloaded) to decrease exposure of the staff to radiation. If any problem arises in the care of a patient, the source can be removed rapidly.

Occasionally, patients are irradiated with isotopes in suspension (^{32}P); this technique has been used for the intraperitoneal treatment of ovarian carcinoma and mesothelioma. This form of radiation has a short half-life (14 days) and an effective penetration of only millimeters, so that exposure is not a major concern for caregivers. However, the surface dose is high and predisposes women patients to bowel complications, including obstruction and fistula. Other isotopes (e.g., ^{125}I) are occasionally implanted in internal tissues but also provide very little exposure beyond several centimeters. Again, the risk for exposure to caregivers is minimal, but if a patient dies during the decay period of the isotope, removal at autopsy is required for radiation safety. Clearly, the presence of either of these isotopes precludes close and extended personal contact (e.g., a child should not be held on the patient's lap), at least until the half-life of the isotope has elapsed.

Complications of Radiation

Side effects during radiation therapy include skin burning or tanning, local mucositis with concurrent nausea, and bowel mucositis with diarrhea. Most of these side effects are easily controlled with local skin care (e.g., Silvadene or antibiotic ointment) and oral therapy for nausea and diarrhea (e.g., Lomotil). Pelvic radiation may be associated with a mild cystitis and vaginal mucositis, which are also treated conservatively. Vulvar radiation is often the most painful, and the use of local therapies such as sitz baths and air-drying the area with a hair dryer rather than toilet tissue may be helpful. The pain resolves after the therapy has been completed.

In children and young women, pelvic radiation is associated with the significant problem of loss of fertility. Numerous efforts to prevent such loss have included surgically moving the ovaries above the irradiated field and behind the uterus in some cases of targeted lymphatic radiation. More recently, preservation by transposing the ovaries outside the abdomen (arm), freezing fertilized ova, or even freezing ova and ovaries has been an area of active research. It is clear that one or several of these options will be feasible in the future.

Late Complications

During longer follow-up, radiation induces intense fibrosis in many tissues. Only 20% to 30% of patients experience some of the major long-term complications mentioned here, but it is worthwhile to identify their association with the radiation a woman has previously received and the unique treatment problems they represent. A woman who underwent radiation treatment as a child (generally before the age of 2 years) is at risk for multiple late effects. These include bone deformity, endocrine deficiency (depending on the site of radiation), and atrophic skin changes; second malignancies develop in 7%.

Subcutaneous tissue that has been exposure to a high local dose (head, neck, or groin radiation) often has a woody, indurated feeling that can be permanent. In the lung, variable fibrosis develops with secondary restrictive lung disease. In the liver, if hepatic radiation is used in place of total-body irradiation or whole-abdomen radiation, the result can be a radiation hepatitis that initially behaves like veno-occlusive disease, with the development of anicteric ascites 2 to 4 months after the administration of radiation.

The bowel syndromes associated with radiation vary. In 30% of patients, increases in gastrointestinal motility require medication and dietary adjustment. Lactase deficiency often develops in patients with significant mucosal damage from radiation, and avoiding milk products may significantly relieve diarrhea. Also, avoiding cruciferous vegetables and other foods that increase gut motility can be beneficial. In all patients, local microvascular function in the areas exposed to radiation is diminished, with a concurrent decline in reparative function. The risk for gastrointestinal complications is cumulative over time.

Late effects in the entire gastrointestinal tract, depending on which portions were within the irradiated field, include dysmotility, benign stricture formation, gastric ulceration, bleeding, frequency, fistula formation, and obstruction. A long-term sequela of pelvic radiation is proctitis that is associated with the formation of telangiectases in the mucosal lumen and uncontrolled bleeding. Alternatives for management include local corticosteroid therapy, diversion, argon plasma coagulation, and embolization in cases of uncontrolled bleeding. Unfortunately, the same pathophysiology that causes these lesions predisposes to failure of healing after surgical intervention, so the risk for complications of surgery in an irradiated field is quite high. Attempts to control bleeding locally or manage side effects medically should always be made first.

Similar side effects develop in the urinary tract; hemorrhagic cystitis and ureteral and urethral strictures are the more serious late complications. Also, fibrosis and edema can lead to significant contracture of the bladder. Surgical repair can be especially challenging in such cases, and replacement of function with a conduit or the use of a patch of intestine not involved in the radiated field is sometimes required. Hyperbaric oxygen therapy has been proposed for many of these abnormalities of repair in radiated fields because the adequate delivery of oxygen is essential to normal reparative function. However, no long-term or large studies have evaluated the efficacy of this approach. Hyperbaric oxygen can promote the healing of hemorrhagic cystitis and of nonhealing ulcers and surgical wounds within a radiated field.

Radiation is curative therapy for a number of cancers, but it is not without side effects. The unique feature of the side effects of radiation is that they are long-lasting; late risks are significant. Second surgeries and diagnostic procedures within the radiation field are associated with an increased risk for poor wound healing and, depending on the organ involved, fistula formation.

BIBLIOGRAPHY

Anderson B. Yes, there are sexual problems: now what can we do about them? *Gynecol Oncol* 1994;52:10.

Bonica JJ. Cancer pain. In: Bonica JJ, ed. *The management of pain,* 2nd ed, vol 1. Philadelphia: Lea & Febiger, 1990:400.

Cain J, Stacey L, Jusenius K, et al. The quality of dying: financial, psychological, and ethical dilemmas. *Obstet Gynecol* 1990;76:149.

Cascinu S. Drug therapy in diarrheal diseases in oncology/hematology patients. *Crit Rev Oncol Hematol* 1995;18:37.

Cleeland CS. Barriers to the management of cancer pain. *Oncology* 1987;1:19.

Coia LR, Myerson RJ, Tepper JE. Late effects of radiation therapy on the gastrointestinal tract. *Int J Radiat Oncol Biol Phys* 1995;31:1213.

Farncombe M, Daniels G, Cross L. Lymphedema: the seemingly forgotten complication. *J Pain Symptom Manage* 1994;9:269.

Green D. Preserving fertility in children treated for cancer: preventing the effects of radiation and chemotherapy on gonadal function. *BMJ* 2001;323:1201–1203.

Gross PE, Strasser K. Aromatase inhibitors in the treatment and prevention of breast cancer. *J Clin Oncol* 2001;19:881–894.

Holland JC. Fears and abnormal reactions to cancer in physically healthy individuals. In: Holland JC, Rowland JH, eds. *Handbook of psychooncology: psychological care of the patient with cancer*. New York: Oxford University Press, 1989:13.

Ignoffo RJ, Friedman MA. Therapy of local toxicities caused by extravasation of cancer chemotherapeutic drugs. *Cancer Treat Rev* 1980;7:17.

Korf B. Molecular medicine: molecular diagnosis. *N Engl J Med* 1995;332:1218.

Lawrence TS, Robertson JM, Anscher MS, et al. Hepatic toxicity resulting from cancer treatment. *Int J Radiat Oncol Biol Phys* 1995;31:1237.

Lerman C, Rimer BK, Engstrom PF. Cancer risk notification: psychosocial and ethical implications. *J Clin Oncol* 1991;9:1275.

Letschert JG, Lebesque JV, Aleman BM, et al. The volume effect in radiation-related late small bowel complications: results of a clinical study of the EORTC in patients treated for rectal carcinoma. *Radiother Oncol* 1994;32:116.

Management of cancer pain: clinical practice guidelines. Rockville, MD: Agency for Health Care Policy and Research, 1994: publication no 94-0592.

Munro M, O'Dwyer M, Heinrich M, et al. STI571: a paradigm of new agents for cancer therapeutics. *J Clin Oncol* 2002;20:325–334.

Quaid KA. Psychological and ethical considerations in screening for disease. *Am J Cardiol* 1993;72:64D.
Rosenthal N. Regulation of gene expression. *N Engl J Med* 1994;331:931.
Sachs BP, Korf B. The Human Genome Project: implications for the practicing obstetrician. *Obstet Gynecol* 1993;81:458.
Schneiderman LJ, Jecker NS, Jonsen AR. Medical futility: its meaning and ethical implications. *Ann Intern Med* 1990;112:949.
Schover LR, Yetman RJ, Tuason LJ, et al. Partial mastectomy and breast reconstruction: a comparison of their effects on psychosocial adjustment, body image, and sexuality. *Cancer* 1995;75:54.
Stewart A, McQuade B, Cronje JD, et al. Ondansetron compared with granisetron in the prophylaxis of cyclophosphamide-induced emesis in outpatients: a multicenter, double-blind, double-dummy, randomized, parallel-group study. Emesis Study Group for Ondansetron and Granisetron in Breast Cancer Patients. *Oncology* 1995;52:202.
Taieb S, Rolachon A, Cenni JC, et al. Effective use of argon plasma coagulation in the treatment of severe radiation proctitis. *Dis Colon Rectum* 2001;44: 1766–1771.
Williams LT, O'Dwyer JL. Guidelines for oral hygiene, denture care, and nutrition in patients with oral complications. In: Peterson DE, Sonis ST, eds. *Oral complications of cancer chemotherapy.* Baltimore: Kluwer Academic, 1983.

CHAPTER 8
Sexuality

David A. Baram

IMPORTANCE OF SEXUALITY

Sexuality is an important and integral part of every woman's life. Questions and concerns about sexuality span a woman's entire lifetime, from adolescence to menopause and aging. The primary health care provider for women should include a sexual history as a routine part of a woman's periodic health assessment.

In recent surveys, almost two thirds of the women questioned had concerns about their sexuality. One third of them lacked interest in sex, 20% said sex was not always pleasurable, 15% experienced pain during intercourse, up to 50% experienced difficulty becoming aroused, 50% noted difficulty reaching orgasm, and up to 25% were unable to experience orgasm.

The primary provider should routinely inquire about a history of childhood sexual abuse or adult sexual assault because these experiences are common and often have a lasting and profound effect on a woman's mental and sexual function in addition to her general health and well-being. One of eight American women will be forcibly raped during her lifetime, and nearly one third of women in the United States report some type of contact sexual victimization. Fifty percent of American women report uninvited sexual attention in the workplace.

Despite the importance of these issues to their health care, many women find it difficult to talk to their physicians about sexual concerns, and many physicians are uncomfortable discussing sexual issues with their patients. In a recent survey, 71% of adults said they thought their doctor would dismiss any concerns about sexual problems, and 68% said they were afraid that a discussion of sexuality would embarrass their physician. Surveys of primary care physicians reveal that fewer than one half ask their new patients about sexual practices and concerns and that many physicians make incorrect assumptions about their patients' sexual activity based on marital status, profession, age, race, and socioeconomic status.

Physicians may worry that patients will be offended by questions about their sexual practices, or they may believe that little useful information will be gained by asking about sexual concerns or a history of sexual assault. In addition, some physicians may believe they have too little time to obtain a sexual history; they may also be anxious about their perceived inability to treat sexual concerns, distressed by a patient's history of sexually related violence, or personally uncomfortable when discussing sexual matters with their patients. However, surveys of patients reveal that they expect their physician to be able to address sex-related concerns and believe it is appropriate for questions about sexuality to be included as a routine part of the gynecologic history. Indeed, not asking about sexuality or sexual abuse suggests to the patient that sexuality is not important and not to be discussed, and that sexual assault has no long-term consequences.

Physicians will feel more comfortable talking to their patients about sex if they have an understanding of the normal sexual response and know how to approach the evaluation and treatment of common forms of sexual dysfunction. Asking about sexual concerns gives physicians an opportunity to educate patients about the risk for sexually transmitted infections, counsel them about safe sex practices, evaluate their needs for contraception, and dispel sexual myths and misconceptions. Furthermore, patients are given permission to address sexual issues in a professional, confidential, and nonjudgmental setting. Even if patients are initially uncomfortable discussing these sensitive and private issues, they know that their physician will be receptive in the future if they have sexual concerns to discuss.

It is important to allow the patient to feel comfortable and safe when a sexual history is taken. The physician's personal values and potential biases should be left out of the discussion. Use straightforward language that the patient can understand and acknowledge that many people find it difficult to discuss sensitive and intimate issues. Remember that most sexual concerns can be managed successfully by providing factual information, reassurance, and appropriate medical intervention. Only a few open-ended questions are all that is necessary to elicit a basic sexual history from patients. These questions should be a part of the medical history during a routine examination:

1. Are you currently sexually active? With men, women, or both?
2. Are you or your partner having any sexual difficulties at this time? Has there been any change in your sexual activity?
3. Have you ever experienced any unwanted or harmful touching or sexual activity?

If any of these questions elicits a positive response, further evaluation of the patient may be warranted. Follow-up questions might include the following: Are you having difficulty initiating a sexual encounter or becoming aroused when you want to be sexual? Do you experience as much arousal as you would like? Do you experience vaginal dryness during intercourse? Do you have orgasms when you want to? Are you satisfied with your sexual relationship? Do you have pain during intercourse? Has this difficulty always been present or is it new to you? Have you had this difficulty with all of your partners or just with the current one? Is the difficulty always there or just some of the time? Does anything make it better or worse? How much of a concern is this for you and your partner? Do you have any idea what may have caused your sexual difficulty? Have you received any treatment for this difficulty? What are your expectations and goals of treatment?

Further inquiries about specific sexual dysfunction or the sequelae of sexual abuse can be addressed when appropriate, and the patient can be referred for psychological counseling or sex therapy when necessary.

Two recent comprehensive surveys provide an interesting and useful description of the sexual behavior of Americans. Sexual activity among adolescents in the U.S. has increased significantly during the past 20 years. The average age at first intercourse in both men and women is 16 years. By 19 years of age, 66% to 75% of women and 79% to 86% of men will have had intercourse. Most young men and women have multiple, serial sexual partners. They use condoms infrequently and inconsistently, thus exposing themselves to sexually transmitted infections and unintended pregnancy. A survey of American men and women between the ages of 18 and 59 years revealed that most men and women are satisfied with their sex life, even those who rarely have sex. Among married men and women, 87% reported that they were satisfied with their sexual relationship.

Sexual dysfunction was reported in 43% of women and was more likely among women in poor physical and emotional health, unmarried women, younger women, uneducated women, women who had experienced sexual victimization, women who were sexually inexperienced, and women who had had negative experiences in prior sexual relationships.

Women have sex with a partner from a few times per month (47%) to two or three times per week (32%) to four or more times a week (7%). Twelve percent of women have sex a few times per year, and 3% have never been sexually active.

The most appealing sexual activity for both men and women is vaginal intercourse. Watching their partner undress and receiving and giving oral sex were also considered very pleasurable. Most Americans are monogamous. Seventy-five percent of married men and 85% of married women said they had never been unfaithful.

The number of homosexuals may be smaller than previously believed—2.7% of men and 1.3% of women had a homosexual partner in the past year. Since puberty, 7.1% of men and 3.8% of women had partners of the same gender.

Twenty-two percent of women said they had been forced to do something sexual, usually by someone they loved, but only 3% of men admitted to forcing themselves on a woman. Perhaps men and women have different ideas about what constitutes sexual coercion.

SEXUAL RESPONSE CYCLE

The sexual response cycle in women is mediated by a complex interplay of psychological, environmental, and physiologic (hormonal, vascular, muscular, and neurologic) factors. The initial phase of the sexual response cycle is interest and desire, followed by arousal, orgasm, and resolution. The way in which women respond sexually varies widely, and each phase can be affected by aging, illness, medication, alcohol, illicit drugs, and relationship factors.

Sexual desire is the motivation and inclination to be sexual. It is a "state of subjective feeling" that may be triggered by both internal (fantasy) and external (an interested partner) sexual cues and depends on adequate neuroendocrine functioning. Desire is under the influence of dopamine-sensitive excitatory centers located in the limbic system. Testosterone is responsible for desire and arousal in both men and women. Drive is the biologic component of desire and is characterized by sexual thoughts, erotic interest in others, genital tingling, and the seeking of sexual activity. Desire is influenced by a person's sexual orientation, preferences, psychological mind-set, beliefs and values, expectations, willingness to behave sexually, and environmental setting.

The arousal (excitement) phase is mediated by the parasympathetic nervous system and is characterized by erotic feelings and the appearance of vaginal lubrication. Sexual arousal increases the blood flow to the vagina, and the resulting vascular congestion and changes in capillary permeability create a condition that increases the capillary filtration fraction. The filtered capillary fluid transudes between the intercellular spaces of the vaginal epithelium, causing droplets of fluid to form on the walls of the vagina. In addition to feelings of sexual tension, sexually excited women experience tachycardia, rapid breathing, an elevation in blood pressure, a generalized feeling of warmth, breast engorgement, generalized muscle tension (myotonia), nipple erection, mottling of the skin, and a maculopapular erythematous rash (sex flush) over the chest and breasts. During this phase, the clitoris and labia become swollen; the vagina lengthens, distends, and dilates; and the uterus elevates out of the pelvis. During the latter stages of arousal, sexual tension and erotic feelings intensify, and vascular congestion reaches maximum intensity. The skin becomes more mottled, the breasts become more engorged, and the nipples become more erect. The labia become more swollen and turn dark red, and the lower third of the vagina swells and thickens to form the "orgasmic platform." The clitoris becomes more swollen and elevates to lie nearer the symphysis pubis. The uterus elevates fully out of the pelvis. With adequate sexual stimulation, women reach the point of orgasmic inevitability (threshold point).

Orgasm is a myotonic response mediated by the sympathetic nervous system. It is experienced as a sudden release of the tension that has built up during arousal. Orgasm is the most intensely pleasurable of the sexual sensations. It consists of multiple (3–15) 0.8-second reflex rhythmic contractions of the muscles (pubococcygeal) surrounding the vagina, perineum, anus, and orgasmic platform. Many women also experience uterine contractions during orgasm. Thus, some women report that the sensation of orgasm is different after hysterectomy. Many women who are orgasmic prefer to have orgasms before intercourse, during the time when clitoral stimulation is most intense. Unlike men, who are relatively unresponsive to sexual stimulation after orgasm (refractory period), women are potentially multiorgasmic and capable of experiencing more than one orgasm during a single sexual cycle. Thus, they can experience orgasms both before and during intercourse if adequate clitoral stimulation is provided.

Following the sudden release of sexual tension brought about by orgasm, women experience a feeling of relaxation and well-being. The physiologic changes that took place during arousal are reversed, and the body returns to a resting state. Complete uterine descent, detumescence of the clitoris and orgasmic platform, and decongestion of the vagina and labia take about 5 to 10 minutes.

AGING AND SEXUALITY

Aging and the cessation of ovarian function accompanying menopause have a significant effect on the sexual response cycle of women. Sexual desire and the frequency of intercourse decrease gradually as women age, although women retain an interest in sex and continue to have the potential for sexual pleasure for their entire lives. The need for closeness, love, and intimacy does not change with age. The way women function sexually as they grow older largely depends on health status, partner availability, and how frequently they had sex and how much they enjoyed sex when they were younger.

The anatomic changes that accompany aging (reduced vaginal size and thinning of the vaginal walls, shrinkage of the labia minora and majora, decreased clitoral size and sensitivity, and loss of perineal muscle tone) predispose women to more frequent episodes of vulvovaginitis and urinary tract infections. These anatomic changes, along with a decrease in vaginal lubrication, may cause dyspareunia. The effects of aging on sexual physiology include a decrease in sexual desire, a decrease in vaginal lubrication, an increase in the amount of stimulation needed to become orgasmic, and a decreased intensity of orgasms. Women who remain coitally active after menopause experience less vulvar and vaginal atrophy than abstinent women.

Several psychosocial factors may influence an older woman's sexual activity. Older women may lack a sexual partner. Their partner may develop erectile dysfunction. The couple may have had an unsatisfactory sexual relationship earlier in life and may not be able to negotiate successfully the changes and possible sexual dysfunction that occur with aging. Couples may find that they can no longer function sexually as they did in the past and are unable to make the transition or adapt to a new (noncoital) way of lovemaking. Other factors include privacy issues (such as living in a nursing home), reluctance to masturbate, and the negative attitudes of society toward sexuality in older women. Aging men and women may experience performance anxiety as they enter into new relationships. As women age, many become less fit. Recent studies indicate that improved physical fitness is positively related to the frequency of sexual intimacy, which in turn is related to longevity.

The management of sexual difficulties in older women should include supplementation of estrogen or testosterone, or both. Local or systemic estrogen supplementation can alleviate vaginal dryness, urinary tract symptoms, and dyspareunia. Estrogen replacement restores cells, decreases pH, and increases blood flow in the vagina, thereby alleviating vaginal dryness, urinary tract symptoms, and dyspareunia. Estrogen replacement appears to increase sexual desire, fantasy, arousal, and enjoyment and the frequency of orgasms in postmenopausal women. In addition, estrogen supplementation relieves insomnia, hot flushes, and other menopausal symptoms that may interfere with sexual function. The addition of progesterone to the hormone replacement therapy regimen partially opposes the beneficial effects of estrogen by decreasing vaginal blood flow. Estrogen supplementation also decreases the levels of free testosterone by nearly 50% because it increases the levels of sex hormone-binding globulin.

Testosterone levels decrease gradually as women age. Testosterone supplementation, either alone or in combination with estrogen, has been shown to increase libido, arousal, sexual responsiveness, frequency of sexual fantasies and dreams, clitoral sensitivity, and frequency of orgasm in women who are deficient in testosterone (<30 ng/mL) as a consequence of surgical or natural menopause. In addition, the restoration of normal testosterone levels can have beneficial effects on muscle tone, physical energy, mood, and sense of well-being, and it can relieve genital atrophy not responsive to estrogen supplementation. Side effects of testosterone include acne, hirsutism, deepening of the voice, clitoromegaly, hepatotoxicity, alopecia, and undesirable changes in lipoprotein levels. The lowest effective dose of androgens should be prescribed, and patients should be carefully monitored for side effects.

Sildenafil, an effective treatment for erectile dysfunction in men, has been investigated for the treatment of sexual dysfunction in women. One study demonstrated the effectiveness of sildenafil in reversing female sexual dysfunction induced by selective serotonin reuptake inhibitors (SSRIs). Another study failed to demonstrate any improvement in sexual function in postmenopausal women but did note an increase in vaginal lubrication and clitoral sensitivity. The effectiveness of sildenafil and other recently developed pharmacologic agents in the treatment of sexual dysfunction in women awaits further investigation.

Other suggestions for aging patients might include taking a warm bath before lovemaking to loosen joints, making love in the morning when the couple is less fatigued, and experimenting with oral or manual sexual stimulation to orgasm without having intercourse.

A variety of prescription and nonprescription medications, including alcohol and illicit drugs, can alter the normal sexual response. These agents include antihypertensives, antidepressants, anxiolytics, antipsychotics, narcotics, and oral contraceptives. The patient's use of such drugs should be assessed as part of the medical history and adjustments in dosage or formulation suggested, if appropriate. For patients taking certain medications, such as the SSRIs, it may be appropriate to suggest a short holiday from the drug to allow a temporary return of sexual function.

Both acute (e.g., myocardial infarction) and chronic (e.g., chronic renal disease, arthritis) illnesses can cause depression, a distorted body image, physical discomfort, and disturbances in the hormonal, vascular, and neurologic integrity required for sexual functioning. Neurologic disorders that impair sexual functioning include multiple sclerosis, alcoholic neuropathy, and spinal cord injury. Endocrine and metabolic disorders, such as diabetes mellitus, hyperprolactinemia, testosterone deficiency, estrogen deficiency states, and hypothyroidism, can affect the sexual response.

The diagnosis and treatment of breast cancer can affect sexuality. However, most women cope well with the stress of treatment, without the development of major psychiatric disorders or significant sexual dysfunction. A number of studies have compared women undergoing mastectomy and women undergoing lumpectomy with breast conservation; these studies have revealed little difference between the two groups in regard to postoperative marital satisfaction, psychological adjustment, frequency of sex, or incidence of sexual dysfunction. The frequency of breast stimulation during sexual activity does decrease after mastectomy. Many men and women avoid looking at the surgical scar after mastectomy. Women who undergo lumpectomy have more positive feelings about their bodies, especially their appearance in the nude, than women who undergo mastectomy. The strongest predictor of sexual satisfaction after cancer is not the extent of surgery but rather the woman's overall psychological health, satisfaction with her relationship, and level of sexual functioning before cancer. Interestingly, many women report that their physician did not discuss the effect of breast surgery on sexuality before they underwent surgery.

A number of studies have demonstrated that abdominal hysterectomy does not adversely affect sexual functioning if the vagina is not shortened excessively and the ovaries are preserved. However, concern about sexual functioning after hysterectomy is often the most common anxiety patients experience before this procedure. Many women report a decrease in dyspareunia, an increase in the frequency and strength of orgasms, and an increase in libido and frequency of intercourse after hysterectomy for benign disease. Some gynecologists prefer to perform supracervical hysterectomies in an effort to preserve full sexual function.

Women who undergo surgery for gynecologic cancer experience more sexual dysfunction (inhibited sexual desire, decreased arousal, dyspareunia, anorgasmia) and are less sexually active than healthy women of the same age. Dyspareunia may be related to a decrease in vaginal lubrication caused by surgical menopause or to vaginal shortening and scarring resulting from radiation therapy. Some patients, especially those with cervical cancer, may worry that the resumption of sexual activity will cause their disease to recur. Among patients with gynecologic cancer, sexual activity after treatment does not appear to be related to the type of cancer or stage of the disease.

Physicians should discuss sexual concerns with patients and their partners before surgery, attempt to dispel myths and misconceptions, and continue to offer counseling after treatment. Specific technical advice (water-based lubricating jelly, noncoital sexual activity for patients with severe dyspareunia, vaginal dilators, Kegel exercises) should also be provided. Women who functioned well sexually before surgery and had a positive self-image are better able to cope with the sexual difficulties resulting from gynecologic cancer treatment than women whose sexual adjustment was poor before their illness.

PREGNANCY

The physical, emotional, and economic stresses of pregnancy often significantly affect a couple's sexual and marital relationship. Sexual attitudes and behavior during pregnancy are influenced by sexual value systems, folklore (taboos), religious beliefs, physical changes, and arbitrary medical restrictions. In a pregnancy uncomplicated by preterm labor, antepartum bleeding, or an incompetent cervix, no evidence has been found to indicate that intercourse increases the risk for complications of pregnancy.

Most women and men experience a longitudinal decrease in sexual desire, frequency of orgasm, sexual satisfaction, and frequency of intercourse as pregnancy progresses. Sexual satisfaction in pregnancy is closely correlated with being happy about the pregnancy, feeling attractive, and experiencing orgasm during lovemaking. Toward the end of the third trimester, physical discomfort and concerns about labor and delivery and the health of the child increase significantly. At this time, many couples decrease their sexual activity or become abstinent. However, the need for closeness, emotional support, and nurturing during late pregnancy can still be met by engaging in touching, caressing, holding, and noncoital lovemaking.

SEXUAL DYSFUNCTION

Forms of sexual dysfunction include the following:

1. Disorders of sexual desire (hypoactive or inhibited sexual desire and sexual aversion)
2. Disorders of sexual arousal
3. Orgasmic disorders
4. Sexual pain disorders (vaginismus, dyspareunia, and noncoital sexual pain)
5. Sexual disorders resulting from general medical conditions and substance abuse.

Each disorder can be further classified as either:

1. Lifelong or acquired (after a period of normal sexual functioning)
2. Generalized (i.e., not limited to a specific partner or situation) or situational
3. Caused by psychological or medical factors.

During an evaluation of a patient with sexual dysfunction, it is important to obtain the following information:

1. A specific description of the dysfunction and an analysis of current sexual functioning
2. When the dysfunction began and how it progressed over time
3. Any precipitating factors
4. The patient's theory about what caused the dysfunction
5. What effect the dysfunction has had on her relationship
6. Past treatment and outcomes
7. The patient's expectations and goals of treatment
8. The patient's understanding of sexual physiology and sexual behavior
9. Any myths or misinformation the patient may believe.

Although many physicians have some feelings of anxiety about discussing sexual issues with their patients and believe that they lack the basic skills to provide sexual counseling, most sexual concerns can be treated by the general gynecologist. The PLISSIT model is a useful method of sexual counseling and therapy that consists of four levels of therapeutic intervention. With use of the first three levels of this model, approximately 80% to 90% of sexual concerns can be addressed. The PLISSIT model follows:

1. *Permission* validates the patient's feelings and gives her permission to address her sexual concerns.
2. *Limited information* provides the patient with information about sexual physiology and behavior.
3. *Specific suggestions* involve specific reeducation regarding the patient's sexual attitudes and practices.
4. *Referral for intensive therapy* is reserved for those patients who do not respond to the first three levels of intervention and who may require intensive individual or couple therapy.

Hypoactive Sexual Desire Disorder

DEFINITION AND ETIOLOGY

Hypoactive sexual desire disorder (HSDD) is a recurrent deficiency or absence of sexual fantasies/thoughts and desire for sexual activity that causes marked distress and interpersonal difficulty. Patients with HSDD have little interest in seeking sexual stimuli but often retain the ability to become sexually aroused and experience orgasm if they are approached sexually by their partner. This disorder usually develops in adulthood, often after a period of adequate sexual interest and functioning. HSDD is the most common sexual dysfunction in both women and men and the most difficult to treat. It is often accompanied by another sexual disorder, such as dyspareunia or anorgasmia. Some persons may experience sexual aversion—a complete avoidance of all sexual activity with a partner.

The physiologic causes of HSDD include medications, chronic medical illness, depression, stress, substance abuse, aging, and hormonal alterations. The serum testosterone and prolactin levels should be evaluated in any patient presenting with the recent onset of HSDD because elevated prolactin levels (from a pituitary adenoma) or low testosterone levels (sometimes following natural or surgical menopause) can be responsible. Some postmenopausal women who experience dyspareunia secondary to vaginal atrophy may avoid intercourse. This condition will resolve with systemic or vaginal estrogen replacement therapy. Some women with HSDD benefit from testosterone supplementation.

Individual causes of HSDD include religious orthodoxy, anhedonic or obsessive-compulsive personality (these patients may lack the capacity for play and find it difficult to display emotion and let themselves go), masked sexual deviation (e.g., transvestism), fear of pregnancy or sexually transmitted infections, and object choice issues (i.e., the patient may be a homosexual trying to function sexually in a heterosexual relationship). Some individuals unconsciously and involuntarily suppress sexual desire and actively avoid sexual situations. They may suppress desire by evoking negative thoughts or by allowing spontaneously emerging negative thoughts to intrude when a sexual opportunity arises (anti-fantasies).

Sexual desire can also be inhibited by performance anxiety, a negative body image, chronic stress, a low level of self-esteem, depression, the anticipation of an unpleasant sexual experience, fear of intimacy, or residual guilt about sex and pleasure. Women who have been sexually abused as children or sexually assaulted as adults may exhibit sexual avoidance or aversion. Some patients may fear loss of control over their sexual feelings and therefore suppress them completely. If a patient experiences another form of sexual dysfunction, such as dyspareunia or anorgasmia, she may also experience HSDD.

The way a couple functions sexually is often a good barometer of other aspects of the relationship. Therefore, whenever a woman presents with sexual concerns or sexual dysfunction, it is important to inquire about the relationship in general. If a couple is experiencing significant problems in their relationship in addition to sexual concerns, they should be referred for counseling.

Relationship causes of HSDD include a lack of sexual attraction to the partner (because of factors such as poor hygiene), the poor lovemaking skills or sexual inexperience of one or both partners, marital conflict, lack of commitment, or discomfort with physical closeness because of distrust of the partner or a sense of vulnerability. Some couples experience sexual difficulties because the two partners do not want the same degree of closeness in the relationship. One partner may want to be very close, whereas the other wants more distance. Couples may be sexually incompatible, with one partner making sexual demands the other is unable or unwilling to accommodate. Couples may have difficulty with the timing or manner of initiation of sexual activity, or the partners may have incompatible or very different levels of sexual desire. Spouse abuse, financial problems, concerns about children, and marital issues of power and control can significantly affect the way a couple functions sexually. It is difficult for people to feel sexual if they feel unloved or are depressed, overwhelmed by career and household responsibilities, unhappy about their relationship, or afraid of or angry with their partner.

TREATMENT

The treatment of patients with HSDD may require both individual therapy and relationship counseling. Insight-oriented psychotherapy may allow a patient to identify the negative feelings that inhibit her erotic impulses and gain insight into the underlying causes of her low level of sexual desire. Individual "homework" assignments include identifying erotic feelings, body awareness exercises, reading about human sexuality and sexual techniques, and fantasy training. In addition, the couple may benefit from learning how to perform structured sexual exercises known as *sensate focus exercises*. These behavior modification exercises are designed to reduce sexual anxiety and provide a nondemanding, nonthreatening, and reassuring environment in which a couple can address performance anxiety, issues of sexual communication, and lack of sexual experience and knowledge.

Meeting with a couple for a few sessions to assess their sexual knowledge, attitudes, and practices is often beneficial. Many of the sexual problems couples encounter are caused by a deficit of knowledge or experience, sexual misconceptions, or an inability to communicate about what they would like to give and receive in the sexual part of their relationship. Brief counseling and education by the obstetrician-gynecologist regarding the sexual response cycle and the encouragement of open and honest communication are often all that is needed to help couples achieve a fulfilling sexual relationship.

Arousal Phase Disorders

Arousal phase disorders, in which women experience sexual desire and orgasm but lack vaginal lubrication and other signs of sexual stimulation, are relatively rare. A lack of lubrication may lead to dyspareunia and eventually impair a woman's subjective sense of arousal and pleasure. Women with arousal phase disorders may benefit from the use of intravaginal lubricants or estrogen replacement therapy.

Orgasmic Dysfunction

Orgasmic dysfunction in women is characterized by a persistent or recurrent delay in or absence of orgasm following a normal sexual excitement phase that results in distress or interpersonal difficulty. Orgasmic dysfunction is more prevalent in younger and less sexually experienced women. Primary (lifelong) anorgasmia is found in approximately 5% to 10% of women and is more common than secondary (acquired) anorgasmia. Secondary anorgasmia develops in some women because of relationship problems, depression, substance abuse, prescription medications (e.g., SSRIs), chronic medical illness (e.g., diabetes), estrogen deficiency, or neurologic disorders (e.g., multiple sclerosis). Many women who are orgasmic during masturbation or noncoital sex may be distressed because they are not orgasmic during intercourse, do not have multiple orgasms or an orgasm during every sexual encounter, or do not have an orgasm at the same time as their partner. Surveys of sexual behavior demonstrate, however, that most couples do not experience orgasm simultaneously and that many women are more likely to be orgasmic during foreplay, when they receive more direct and intense clitoral stimulation, than during intercourse. The most common psychological cause of anorgasmia is obsessive self-observation and monitoring during the arousal phase, which is often accompanied by anxiety and distracting, negative, and self-defeating thoughts. Inhibited orgasm may be related to a history of sexual abuse, negative feelings about sexuality, relationship problems, an inattentive partner, ineffective sexual technique, a low level of self-esteem, a poor body image, or fear of losing control.

Numerous programs have been proposed to treat orgasmic dysfunction. Approaches include the evaluation and treatment of medical and psychiatric disorders (including substance abuse), sex education, communication and sexual skills training, marital therapy, group therapy, erotic fantasy, and counseling to reduce sexual anxiety and performance anxiety. The most effective treatment for primary anorgasmia is a program of directed masturbation during erotic fantasy. Success rates of 80% to 90% have been reported with the use of this technique. Several excellent books are available to help women learn how to become orgasmic through masturbation, including Heiman and LoPiccolo's *Becoming Orgasmic* and Barbach's *For Yourself*. These self-help books instruct women how to increase their self-awareness by exploring their genital area in a nondemanding way. Once a woman has identified the most sensitive and pleasure-producing parts of her body, she can manually stimulate her clitoris and other erogenous areas while engaging in erotic fantasy until she reaches orgasm.

Vaginismus

Vaginismus is the recurrent or persistent involuntary contraction of the perineal muscles surrounding the outer third of the vagina whenever vaginal penetration is attempted with a penis, finger, tampon, or speculum. Vaginismus is an involuntary reflex precipitated by real or imagined attempts at vaginal penetration. It can be global (the woman is unable to place anything inside her vagina) or situational (she is able to use a tampon and can tolerate a pelvic examination but cannot have intercourse). Many women with vaginismus have normal sexual desire, experience vaginal lubrication, and are orgasmic but are unable to have intercourse. Vaginismus can be primary (the woman has never been able to have intercourse) or secondary, often to acquired dyspareunia. Some couples may cope with this difficulty for years before asking for help. They usually seek treatment because they want to have children or decide they would like to consummate their relationship. Vaginismus is relatively rare, affecting approximately 1% of women.

Vaginismus can be a conditioned response to an unpleasant experience, such as past sexual trauma or abuse, a painful first pelvic examination, or a painful first attempt at intercourse. It may be secondary to religious orthodoxy, a negative sexual upbringing, or concerns about sexual orientation. Many women with vaginismus have an extreme fear of penetration and misconceptions about their anatomy and the size of their vagina. They may believe that their vagina is too small to accommodate a tampon or penis and that great physical harm will result if anything is placed inside their vagina.

Although medical conditions are rarely the cause of vaginismus, conditions such as endometriosis, chronic pelvic inflammatory disease, partially imperforate hymen, and vaginal stenosis must be ruled out by a careful pelvic examination, which should be performed, if possible, in the presence of the woman's partner. The pelvic examination allows the physician to educate the couple about normal female anatomy and dispel misconceptions about the size of the introitus and vagina. Allowing the patient to observe the examination in a mirror is helpful. Because vaginismus is usually psychophysiologic in origin, patients with this condition should not undergo surgery to "enlarge" their introitus unless they have a partially imperforate hymen or other valid indication for surgery.

The treatment of vaginismus is directed at extinguishing the conditioned involuntary vaginal spasm. This can be accomplished by helping the woman become more familiar with her anatomy and more comfortable with her sexuality, teaching her techniques to help her relax when she anticipates vaginal penetration, and instructing her in the use of Kegel exercises and graduated vaginal dilators.

The protocol for dilator use is discussed with the patient while she is in the office, but the dilators are actually placed by the patient when she is at home. It is important for the patient to maintain total control over application of the dilators and use them in an environment that is comfortable and safe. The dilators should be covered with a warm, water-soluble lubricant. She should initially try to place the dilators (or her finger) in her vagina when she is alone and relaxed. If she is unable to relax enough to place to smallest dilator in her vagina, she may be able to reduce her anxiety by learning relaxation or self-hypnosis techniques. Medications such as propranolol and alprazolam may also reduce anxiety. Once the patient has been able to place the smallest dilator in her vagina, she can progressively insert the larger dilators, practicing Kegel exercises while the dilators are in place. Once she is comfortable inserting the larger dilators, she can teach her partner how to place the dilators in her vagina while she maintains control over how quickly and deeply they are placed. She may then be ready to proceed to intercourse. Again, this must be under her control, with her sitting or kneeling over her partner and inserting his penis herself. Most couples that follow this protocol are successful and able to have intercourse.

Dyspareunia

Dyspareunia ("difficult mating") is genital pain that occurs before, during, or after intercourse in the absence of vaginismus. The repeated experience of pain during intercourse can cause marked distress, anxiety, and interpersonal difficulties, leading to anticipation of a negative sexual experience and eventually sexual avoidance. Like other forms of sexual dysfunction, dyspareunia can be generalized or situational, lifelong or acquired. Secondary dyspareunia occurs, on average, about 10 years after the onset of sexual activity.

Dyspareunia is one of the most common forms of sexual dysfunction and is estimated to affect about two thirds of women during their lifetime. Women with dyspareunia usually discuss the pain with their sexual partner, but fewer than half of them consult a physician. Because dyspareunia is a psychophysiologic condition, both psychological and physical factors must be considered in the assessment. In many cases, no exact cause of dyspareunia can be found. Even when a source of dyspareunia is identified and successfully treated, fear of pain and the presence of anxiety before and during intercourse can inhibit arousal, interfering with vaginal lubrication and causing further discomfort. Many women who have dyspareunia report more physical symptoms, difficulty with pelvic examinations and tampon insertion, a history of sexual abuse or assault, psychological distress, and relationship issues than women who do not have pain during intercourse.

ETIOLOGY

Causes of pain during stimulation of the external genitalia include chronic vulvitis and clitoral irritation and hypersensitivity. Pain at the introitus during penile entry can be caused by a rigid hymenal ring, scar tissue in an episiotomy repair, a müllerian abnormality, vaginitis resulting from infection with one of the many common vaginal pathogens (e.g., *Candida, Trichomonas, Gardnerella*), or irritation resulting from the use of over-the-counter vaginal sprays, douches, or contraceptive devices. Other causes include Bartholin gland inflammation, radiation vaginitis, infection with human papillomavirus, urethral syndrome, cystitis, vaginal trauma, chronic constipation, and proctitis. Vaginal infection is a very frequent cause of successfully treated dyspareunia. Dyspareunia is common in women after childbirth, affecting 45% for as long as 1 year postpartum. Another common cause of dyspareunia is friction secondary to inadequate sexual arousal. This situation can be resolved by counseling the couple to spend more time in foreplay, which ensures that the woman's vagina is adequately lubricated before intercourse. The use of a water-soluble lubricant is often helpful. Vaginal atrophy resulting from hypoestrogenic states (menopause and lactation) can be treated with systemic or vaginal estrogen replacement.

Vulvar vestibulitis syndrome is a constellation of symptoms that include severe pain or burning when the vestibule is touched and vaginal entry is attempted. Women with vulvar vestibulitis report difficulty with sexual arousal, decreased lubrication, dyspareunia, and negative emotions during sexual encounters. On examination, diffuse or focal vulvar erythema is noted around the orifices of Bartholin or the Skene, periurethral, or vestibular glands. This syndrome may be caused by an infection (subclinical human papillomavirus infection, bacterial vaginosis, chronic candidiasis), irritants (soaps, detergents, douches, vaginal sprays), or an altered vaginal pH secondary to a decrease in lactobacilli. Vulvar vestibulitis may also be secondary to the treatment of human papillomavirus infection with podophyllin, trichloracetic acid, or laser.

Causes of midvaginal pain include a congenitally shortened vagina, interstitial cystitis, and urethritis. Pain during orgasm may be associated with uterine contractions. Dyspareunia during deep vaginal penetration may be associated with inadequate vaginal lengthening and lubrication secondary to inadequate sexual arousal, chronic pelvic inflammatory disease, endometriosis, a fixed retroverted uterus, a pelvic mass, a uterus enlarged by myomata or adenomyosis, inflammatory bowel disease, irritable bowel syndrome, or pelvic relaxation.

A careful history should be directed toward a complete chronology of the discomfort and an assessment of the effect of the dyspareunia on the patient and her partner. Any prior attempts to treat the condition should be noted. The patient should be asked about the specific location of the pain, when during the course of lovemaking the pain occurs, how long it lasts, its nature and quality, what relieves or aggravates the discomfort, and the severity of the pain. It is useful to ask the patient about her theory of how the pain began and to assess her expectations and goals of treatment. Patients should be carefully asked about a history of childhood sexual or physical abuse or adult sexual assault because these may be associated with dyspareunia. Patients who are anxious about their sexuality because of sexual misconceptions, guilt, fear of pregnancy or sexually transmitted disease, or prior unpleasant sexual experiences may be unable to relax during lovemaking, so that arousal and lubrication are impaired. Some women note an exacerbation of their symptoms when they are anxious, depressed, or stressed or when their coping resources are limited.

Significant problems in a couple's relationship or communication may also contribute to dyspareunia. It is often useful to approach dyspareunia as a couple issue. It can be helpful to interview the partners together because they can frequently provide useful information about the cause of the pain. Conflicts about family size, contraception, frequency of intercourse, and sexual technique may lead to anger, distrust, misunderstanding, depression, and ultimately pain. The patient's partner may pick an inconvenient time or may not spend enough time for her to become adequately aroused and lubricated.

PHYSICAL EXAMINATION

During the physical examination, attempts should be made to identify any subtle organic factors contributing to the discomfort. Physiologic changes that take place during sexual arousal may account for pain that is present during intercourse but absent at other times, such as during a routine pelvic examination. Examples are Bartholin gland cysts, which swell during intercourse, and adhesive bands that form between portions of the hymenal ring only during arousal.

The physical examination should both evaluate and educate the patient. She should be examined, if possible, with her partner present and be given a hand mirror to help her indicate where her pain is coming from. The physician should watch the patient's face while performing the pelvic examination to see if pain is elicited and if dyspareunia is re-created when specific anatomic sites are palpated. Careful inspection of the external genitalia can identify ulcerations, erythema, or pigment changes. Palpation with a moist cotton-tipped swab can identify sites of vulvar vestibulitis.

The vagina should be gently and carefully examined with one finger; any scars from previous surgery or episiotomy should be noted, and involuntary spasm of the muscles of the introitus or levator sling should be sought. Having the patient contract her pelvic floor muscles while the examiner's finger is placed inside her vagina helps to assess the tone of the pelvic floor and identify these muscles as a possible source of dyspareunia. Stroking the base of the bladder and the urethra may reproduce pain caused by trigonitis, interstitial cystitis, chronic urethritis, or a urethral diverticulum. A speculum should be used to obtain cervical cultures and vaginal secretions for a wet mount examination and to assess the vagina for atrophy.

The bimanual and rectovaginal examination should be carried out in a systematic manner. Pain during manipulation of the cervix may identify it as a source of dyspareunia. Pain during uterine palpation may be caused by adenomyosis or uterine myomata. A fixed, tender, and retroverted uterus may indicate endometriosis. Tenderness of the adnexa, possibly secondary to endometriosis or an ovarian cyst, may be the cause of deep thrust dyspareunia. A rectovaginal examination may help identify endometriosis, retroperitoneal lesions, inflammatory bowel disease, and rectal masses.

In patients who are difficult to examine because of obesity, tenderness, or anxiety, pelvic ultrasonography may further evaluate the pelvic organs and provide possible clues to the cause of pain. Many patients who cannot tolerate a pelvic examination are survivors of childhood sexual abuse or adult sexual assault or may have experienced a traumatic and uncomfortable first pelvic examination. These patients must be approached in a gentle, sensitive, and reassuring way and allowed as much control as possible over the examination.

TREATMENT

When vulvovaginitis is treated, attempts should be made to diagnose a specific pathogen with vaginal cultures, wet preparations, and a determination of the vaginal pH. In many cases, a specific organism is not found. Patients often become less symptomatic when some hygiene habits and potentially harmful self-treatment practices are changed. Patients should use unperfumed soap, not apply soap to the vaginal area, dry the vulva after bathing with a hair dryer, and avoid douches, vaginal sprays, and scented tampons. Wearing cotton underwear and loose-fitting clothing often helps. Many detergents contain enzymes and should be avoided. Patients should wash their underwear in Dreft or Woolite.

The treatment of vulvar vestibulitis syndrome is empiric because the cause is unknown. Some patients respond favorably to cognitive-behavioral therapy and biofeedback rehabilitation of the pelvic floor muscles. Symptomatic treatments include the application of topical steroid ointments or anesthetic creams, the injection of a long-acting local anesthetic, and the administration of antidepressants or antihistamines. Associated infections should be treated, and vulvovaginal irritants should be eliminated. Surgery (vestibulectomy with vaginal advancement) should be reserved for patients with severe dyspareunia who have not responded to conservative management.

Patients who experience urinary urgency and frequency or dysuria without an identifiable infection may respond to urinary antispasmodics, low-dose antibiotics, or antidepressants. Vaginal strictures or vaginal shortening following surgery or radiation therapy can be treated with estrogen vaginal cream and progressive vaginal dilation with dilators.

Deep thrust dyspareunia can be caused by endometriosis, pelvic adhesions, pelvic relaxation, symptomatic uterine retroversion, myomata, or adnexal pathology. The treatment of endometriosis is described elsewhere, but mitigation or worsening of dyspareunia can be a guide to the success or failure of treatment. Many patients note relief of chronic pelvic pain after the laparoscopic lysis of pelvic adhesions. Laparoscopy can also be used to diagnose and treat adnexal masses and to suspend a fixed retroverted uterus.

In addition to treating specific physical problems, the physician can assign the patient and her partner behavioral therapy exercises they can practice at home. These can desensitize the patient to the discomfort she may anticipate during vaginal penetration and help her extinguish the learned pain response to intercourse. Suggested exercises may include assigned reading, progressive sexual fantasies, masturbation, instruction in deep muscle relaxation, and couple-pleasuring exercises. As in the treatment of vaginismus, Kegel exercises and the use of graduated vaginal dilators can help the patient overcome her discomfort. Once the patient has gained voluntary control over her levator muscles, she may want to proceed to intercourse, eventually incorporating sexual responsiveness and a variety of coital positions into lovemaking.

BIBLIOGRAPHY

American College of Obstetricians and Gynecologists. *Androgen treatment of decreased libido. Technical bulletin.* Washington, DC: American College of Obstetricians and Gynecologists, 2000:244.

American Psychiatric Association. *Diagnostic and statistical manual of mental disorders,* 4th ed. Washington, DC: American Psychiatric Association, 1994.

Barrett G, Pendry E, Peacock J, et al. Sexual function after childbirth: women's experiences, persistent morbidity, and lack of professional recognition. *Br J Obstet Gynaecol* 1997;104:330–335.

Bergeron S, Binik YMJ, Khalife S, et al. Vulvar vestibulitis syndrome: reliability of diagnosis and evaluation of current diagnostic criteria. *Am J Obstet Gynecol* 2001;98:45–51.

Crenshaw TL, Goldberg JP. *Sexual pharmacology: drugs that affect sexual functioning.* New York: Norton, 1996.

DeCherney AH. Hormone receptors and sexuality in the human female. *J Womens Health Gender-Based Med* 2000;9[Suppl 1]:s9–s13.

Francoeur RT, Kock PT, Weis DL. *Sexuality in America: understanding our sexual values and behavior.* New York: Continuum, 1998.

Heiman J, Meston CM. Evaluating sexual dysfunction in women. *Clin Obstet Gynecol* 1997;40:616–629.

Heiman JR, LoPiccolo J. *Becoming orgasmic: a sexual and personal growth program for women,* 2nd ed. New York: Simon & Schuster, 1988.

Kilpatrick DG, Edmunds CN, Seymour AK. *Rape in America.* New York: National Victim Center, 1992.

Kohn II, Kaplan SA. Female sexual dysfunction: what is known and what can be done. *Contemp Obstet Gynecol* 2000;45:25–46.

Laumann EO, Paik A, Rosen RC. Sexual dysfunction in the United States. *JAMA* 1999;281:537–544.

Leiblum SR. Redefining female sexual response. *Contemp Obstet Gynecol* 2000;45:120–126.

Leiblum SR, Rosen RC. *Sexual desire disorders.* New York: Guilford Press, 1988.

Michael RT, Gagnon JH, Laumann EO, et al. *Sex in America.* Boston: Little, Brown, 1994.

Rhodes JC, Kjerulff KH, Langenberg PW, et al. Hysterectomy and sexual functioning. *JAMA* 1999;282:1934–1941.

Risen CB. A guide to taking a sexual history. *Psychiatr Clin North Am* 1995;150:1033–1038.

Schover LR, Jensen SB. *Sexuality and chronic illness: a comprehensive approach.* New York: Guilford Press, 1988.

Shifren JL, Braunstein GD, Simon JA, et al. Transdermal testosterone treatment in women with impaired sexual function after oophorectomy. *N Engl J Med* 2000;343:682–688.

Spector IP, Carey MP. Incidence and prevalence of the sexual dysfunctions: a critical review of the empirical literature. *Arch Sex Behav* 1990;19:389–408.

PART 2

Age Specific Issues in Women's Health Care

CHAPTER 9
Newborns and Children

Lynn C. Garfunkel

Although the needs of all healthy infants are similar, the routines of newborn care—feeding, diaper changing, comforting, bathing, and dressing—vary based on the parents, their previous experience, the child's temperament and, to some extent, gender. Many textbooks of pediatrics are available that address the health care, growth and development, and illnesses of infants and children. Several of the ways in which girls differ physically from boys warrant specific attention. This chapter focuses on health issues unique to female infants and toddlers and girls of preschool and school age.

FEMALE EMBRYOLOGY

The differentiation of the male and female internal genitalia is illustrated in Fig. 9.1. In the early embryo, the male and female gonads are indistinguishable; the external genitalia are female-like and similarly undifferentiated. Remnants of the nonfunctional renal system develop into both the müllerian (paramesonephric) and wolffian (mesonephric) ducts, which exist side by side in the sixth to seventh week of embryonic development. At 6 to 7 weeks gestation, the gonads differentiate according to the presence or absence of the Y chromosome. The sex-determining region of the Y chromosome (SRY) is responsible for testicular differentiation. The Sertoli cells produce müllerian inhibiting substance (also known as *müllerian inhibiting factor* or *antimüllerian hormone*). The Leydig cells produce androgens, specifically testosterone. In the absence of a Y chromosome and SRY, the undifferentiated gonads develop into ovaries, which produce 20 million oocytes by 20 weeks gestation. This number declines to 1 to 2 million by birth. Müllerian inhibiting substance inhibits the müllerian system and enhances differentiation of the wolffian ducts into the epididymis, vas deferens, and seminal vesicles. In the absence of müllerian inhibiting substance, the wolffian ducts do not develop, and the müllerian ducts differentiate into the fallopian tubes, uterus, and upper two thirds of the vagina. In the presence of testosterone, the external genitalia become the penis, penile urethra, and scrotum. Ovaries do not produce androgens; in the absence of testosterone, the external genitalia becomes the labia majora and minora, female urethra, and clitoris. The lower one third of the vagina develops from the urogenital sinus.

NORMAL GROWTH AND DEVELOPMENT IN NEWBORNS AND CHILDREN

The genitalia of normal newborns respond to maternal estrogen, which passively crosses the placenta. In girls, the effects of estrogen include swollen labia majora, prominent and pink labia minora, a redundant and thickened pink hymen with a barely perceptible vaginal orifice, and a physiologic vaginal discharge with a low pH. Some female newborns exhibit estrogen withdrawal bleeding, generally within 1 week after birth. The effects of estrogen on the genitalia recede during the first few months such that by 6 to 24 months, girls have flat labia majora, a red and thinned hymen and labia minora, a neutral vaginal pH, and no discharge. The vaginal orifice becomes less covered (as the labia minora and hymen involute) and so is more easily irritated. The labia minora have a large number of nerve endings and are thus very sensitive. The normal shape of the orifice in young girls can vary from annular to crescentic, and the orifice may be septate or fimbriated. The clitoral size appears relatively large in preterm female infants. The infant uterus, stimulated by maternal estrogens before birth, decreases in size during the first 2 years of life and does not begin to enlarge again until puberty.

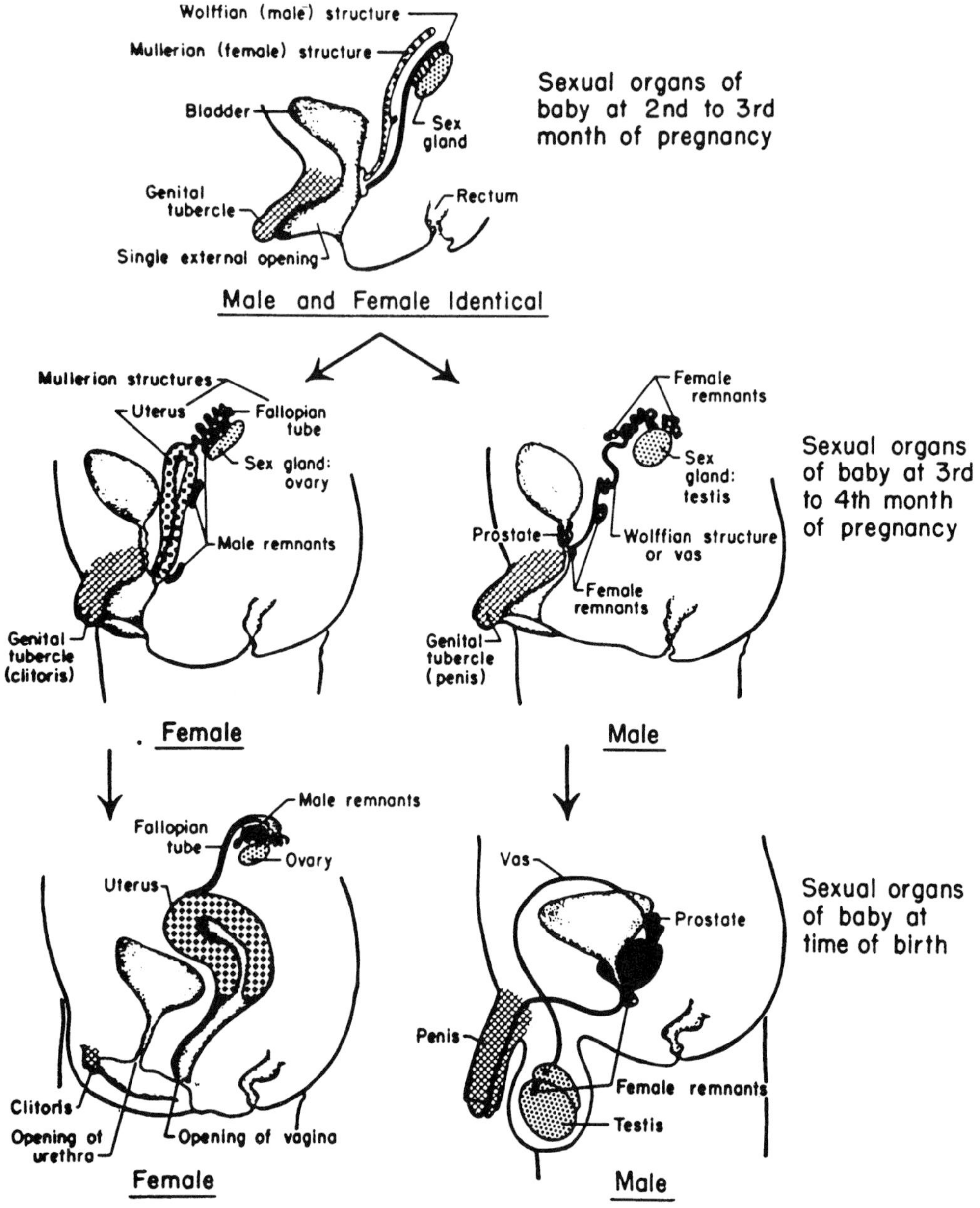

FIG. 9.1. Teaching diagram: differentiation of the internal genitalia. (From Money J. Psychological aspects of disorders of sexual differentiation. In: Carpenter SE, Rock JA, eds. *Pediatric and adolescent gynecology.* New York: Raven Press, 1992:109, with permission.)

Fetal breast tissue enlarges in both sexes after a gestational age of 28 weeks because of its responsiveness to maternal estrogen. The breast bud size of a newborn is a component of the assessment of its gestational age. An infant breast maturity rating of 4 indicates a 5- to 10-mm breast bud and full areola. Occasionally, glandular secretions ("witch's milk") are noted. The enlarged breast buds are at increased risk for infection and inflammation (mastitis), especially after local manipulation or trauma. The breast buds usually resolve during the first several months of life as estrogen levels fall, but they may not recede for up to 12 to 13 months.

Premature thelarche, the isolated development of breast buds in early childhood (typically in 1- to 3-year-old girls) without other signs of puberty, represents a slight increase in function of the hypothalamic-pituitary-ovarian axis. The estrogen level, not estrogen sensitivity, as previously thought, is mildly increased. These toddlers and preschoolers maintain Tanner stage 2 breast buds until the onset of true puberty, which occurs at the usual time and with a normal cadence.

Intelligence, defined in Western societies as a series of traits, includes the use of language and numbers, discrimination of objects in space, separation of an element from its background, problem solving, reasoning, and mastery of concepts. Not all these skills are present at birth, nor are they all learned in childhood; they are acquired throughout childhood, adolescence, and young adulthood. Gender differences in some areas begin in adolescence. Girls score higher in verbal ability, and boys generally score higher in spatial and mathematical ability. However, these abilities are reversed in boys raised in father-absent families, and girls in mother-absent families exhibit more "male" abilities, findings that indicate that environmental factors may modify what were previously considered hereditary traits.

A girl's family, school, and peers greatly influence her social, psychological, physical, and intellectual development. Proposed reasons for lower achievement in science by girls in grade school and high school include low expectations by families, educators, and peers. The National Assessment of Educational Progress shows gaps in science achievement scores between girls and boys as early as the age of 9 years. Studies show that self-confidence in mathematics is an important determinant of success in science. Therefore, with family encouragement, a supportive learning environment, and qualified, caring teachers and mentors, girls achieve equally. Practitioners must encourage parents to help develop their daughters' intelligence and their athletic and creative abilities.

PHYSICAL EXAMINATION OF NEWBORNS AND CHILDREN

The most important aspect of conducting a physical examination in a young girl is gentleness and patience on the part of the physician. These qualities are essential for all aspects of the pediatric examination, but examination of the genitalia of a prepubescent female demands particular sensitivity. Any lack of rapport with the child may prevent an adequate examination or pose a risk for inadvertent or perceived sexual abuse. Especially when the patient is a school-age girl, the history should be obtained with the child fully dressed. Before examining the child, the physician should explain the process to the mother and child in terms they understand. Any instruments that will be used to examine the genitals and collect specimens should also be explained. For some parents, the idea that the "hymen will be broken" is threatening. The examiner must take time to point out that the introitus will continue to be "virginal" and that it is unusual for the hymen to be imperforate, even at birth.

An initial evaluation of hormonally sensitive tissue provides information about the endocrine status. The production of female sex steroids can be determined by breast development and the vaginal mucosal maturation index. (The prepubertal mucosa is red, thin, and very tender; during estrogenization in early puberty, the mucosa becomes thicker and pinker.) Inferences about androgen production can be made based on the pattern of hair growth and apocrine and sebaceous gland activity. Careful examination of the abdomen may allow palpation of enlarged ovaries. An inguinal hernia may represent an undescended testis in a child with undiagnosed male pseudohermaphroditism (genetic XY with either gonadal dysgenesis or androgen insensitivity). The external genitalia, including the clitoris, labia, hymen, and introitus, should be inspected carefully. In newborns, this is easily accomplished with the infant supine and the thighs abducted and externally rotated—the frog leg or lithotomy position. Older infants, toddlers, and preschool girls may be more comfortable in their mother's lap in the lithotomy position. The knee-chest position (Fig. 9.2) may be ideal for the examination of preschool or school-age prepubescent girls because the cervix can potentially be visualized during deep (relaxed) breathing. However, this position can be quite threatening because the patient is unable to see the examiner, and it should be used only with consent of the patient and parent.

The ovaries and uterus can be palpated during a gentle rectal examination. A digital vaginal examination is rarely, if ever, indicated in a prepubescent girl. The ovaries are not completely quiescent in the prepubertal period, so functional cysts may be present. Ovarian cysts larger than 9 mm in diameter are considered abnormal in girls younger than 12 years. Torsion of ovarian cysts is more common in young girls than in adult women,

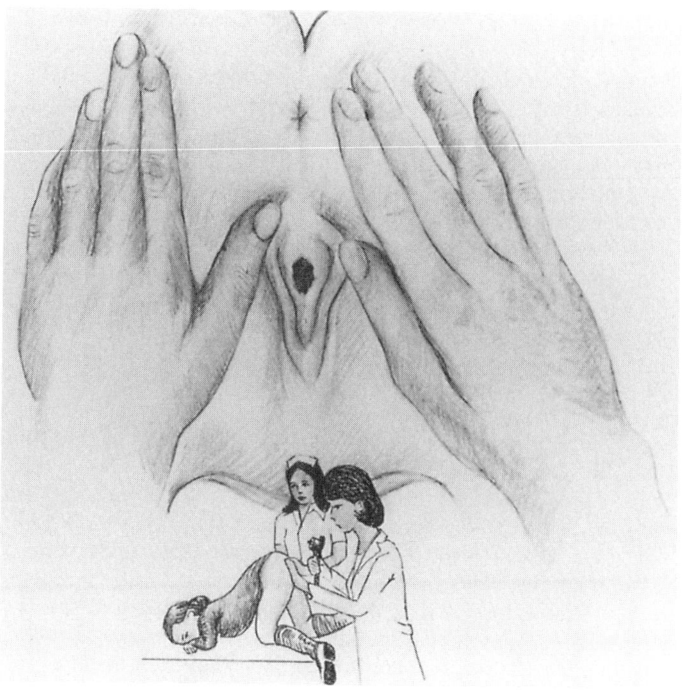

FIG. 9.2. Examination of the prepubertal child in the knee-chest position. (From Emans SJ, Goldstein DP, eds. *Pediatric and adolescent gynecology.* Boston: Little, Brown, 1982, with permission.)

especially around puberty. Any ovarian cyst that does not resolve in 6 to 8 weeks, or any cyst in which the ultrasonographic findings suggest malignancy, must be evaluated by surgical exploration.

Occasionally, a young girl must be examined under anesthesia if an adequate evaluation is to be completed. An examination under anesthesia is mandatory in cases of undiagnosed vaginal bleeding, especially in a patient with a history of trauma or a suspected vaginal foreign body.

CHILDHOOD VULVAR DISEASE

Labial adhesions, which are likely a consequence of the hypoestrogenic state of prepubescent girls, are often asymptomatic, do not require therapy, and usually resolve spontaneously at puberty. Parents may mistake labial adhesions for vaginal agenesis; reassurance is important. If labial adhesions must be treated because of obstruction (urine or vaginal secretions), an estrogen cream is applied to the adhesion while gentle traction is administered twice a day for 2 weeks, then once a day for 1 to 2 weeks. Continued application of Vaseline or another barrier ointment for a few weeks to a few months after the completion of estrogen therapy may help prevent re-formation of the adhesions. Rarely is surgical separation needed.

Sexually transmitted diseases are not uncommon in prepubescent girls. They may be acquired during sexual abuse or, less commonly, transmitted from the mother. Gonococci infect the thin vaginal epithelium and produce a vaginal discharge that can irritate the vulva. The infection is treated with antibiotics and appropriate referral to child protective services. One dose of 125 mg of ceftriaxone is given intramuscularly for children who weight less than 40 kg; those with a weight of more than 40 kg are given 250 mg. Alternatively, 8 mg of cefixime per kilogram (maximum, 400 mg) can be given orally. A child older than 8 years should also receive 100 mg of doxycycline every 12 hours for 7 days, or 10 mg of azithromycin per kilogram (maximum, 1 g) orally. In children, the gonococcus does not usually cause cystitis. Soothing lotions or cool sitz baths can be used to relieve perineal irritation or dysuria, both of which may accompany the vaginitis.

Not limited to girls, congenital syphilis can result in stillbirth, hydrops fetalis, or prematurity. The disease can present with hepatosplenomegaly, snuffles, lymphadenopathy, mucocutaneous lesions, rashes, osteochondritis, and blood dyscrasias; it may even be asymptomatic. Syphilis is transmitted (vertically) to an infant by an infected mother. It is diagnosed by antibody tests of the blood and must be treated with adequate doses of penicillin to prevent systemic sequelae. It is customary to test the mother's blood or cord blood obtained at delivery, or both, to screen for congenital syphilis. Syphilis acquired in childhood is divided into stages. (a) Primary syphilis is the chancre(s)—painless indurated ulceration(s) at the inoculation site. (b) The secondary stage is characterized by a maculopapular, generalized rash of the palms and soles, fever, lymphadenopathy, and constitutional symptoms. (c) Tertiary syphilis develops years to decades after the primary infection and is characterized by gummatous changes of the skin, bones, or internal organs and cardiovascular disease. It is rare or nonexistent in childhood. (d) In latent syphilis, the patient is seroreactive but without clinical evidence of disease. The diagnosis is made by dark-field examination or direct fluorescent antibody testing of lesion or tissue exudate. The presumptive diagnosis is made with the rapid plasma reagent (RPR) and Venereal Disease Research Laboratory (VDRL) tests (nontreponemal) and confirmed with the fluorescent treponemal antibody absorption (FTA-ABS) test (treponemal). However, both types of tests can yield false-positive results, and false-negative results of nontreponemal tests are possible in early and late syphilis. Quantitative nontreponemal tests are used to assess the adequacy of treatment. Syphilis is treated with parenteral penicillin G or with erythromycin in case of penicillin allergy. The evaluation criteria for newborn infants with congenital infection is outlined in the 25th edition of *Redbook 2000* (American Academy of Pediatrics), as is the treatment regimen. Retreatment is necessary if a sustained increase in the titer occurs or if clinical signs and symptoms recur. After adequate treatment, the original titers should decrease fourfold.

Herpes simplex can be transmitted to an infant from an infected mother at birth. Most pregnant women are therefore followed carefully for evidence of herpes simplex, and if they are infected, a cesarean section is planned. However, maternal herpetic lesions are not always apparent. Therefore, herpes in the first month of life strongly suggests maternal infection and transmission to the infant. In the newborn period, vertically acquired herpes presents in one of three forms: (a) localized central nervous system disease (meningitis, encephalitis) (35%); (b) disseminated disease involving multiple organs, especially the liver and lungs (25%); or (c) localized skin and mucous membrane infection (40%). Infants are treated with intravenous acyclovir, but the prognosis in both disseminated herpes and central nervous system herpes is poor. Patients with ocular involvement also require topical antiviral therapy. Herpes simplex can be acquired in childhood by sexual contact. The lesions have a classic appearance, and the diagnosis is usually made easily; herpes culture, an immunofluorescence test, or the Tzank preparation are diagnostic. Acyclovir given orally four times a day for 3 to 5 days is a consideration, although it does not alter the rate or severity of recurrences. Other sexually transmitted diseases may also be present, and therefore if an infant has any sexually transmitted disease, cultures should be performed for all agents of sexually transmitted disease, including HIV.

Condyloma acuminatum can be transmitted to an infant at the time of birth or during sexual contact. The incubation period for human papillomavirus (HPV) infection is long, and lesions acquired at birth may not become apparent until months or even years later. HPV may infect the larynx, causing hoarseness or upper airway obstruction with respiratory distress. Condylomata have been seen in the vagina, urethra, and perineal and perianal regions. The ideal treatment for anogenital HPV infection has not been identified, but treatments include topical podophyllum or podophyllum resin, cryotherapy, trichloracetic or bichloracetic acid, topical imiquimod, intralesional injections of interferon, electrocautery, laser surgery, and surgical excision. Recurrences are common.

Molluscum contagiosum caused by the poxvirus may affect the vulva of young girls. The definitive diagnosis is made under local anesthesia by biopsy with a small key punch. Spontaneous remission usually occurs in 3 months, although molluscum may cause widespread infection in immunocompromised infants.

Candidiasis of the vulva is common in infants and diapered toddlers, especially during or after antibiotic use or if the perineum has been irritated (i.e., after a diarrheal illness). A topical antifungal ointment, cream, or lotion, such as nystatin or clotrimazole, is effective when applied for 5 to 10 days. Pruritus or irritation and excoriation can be intense. In these cases, low-dose (1%) hydrocortisone cream can be applied gingerly 1 to 2 times per day for a very short period (1–3 days) in addition to the antifungal agent. The antiinflammatory effects of glucocorticoids disrupt effective fungal treatment, and therefore topical steroids should be used to treat fungal skin infections only briefly, if at all. Lotions, ointments, and creams that contain both antifungal and antiinflammatory ingredients should be avoided.

In infants, irritant diaper rash can be treated with zinc oxide or other similar barrier or lubricating ointments; in serious cases, 1% hydrocortisone cream can be added. If the diaper rash does not respond to frequent changing and barrier medications, a monilial infection should be suspected and treated.

Eczema can present in the perineum; however, this is rare because the area tends to be well hydrated. Vitiligo and lichen sclerosis of the perineum in girls may look similar. Lichen sclerosis is a depigmented area of the perineum with sensitive, thinned skin caused by androgen receptor insensitivity. The area of involvement ends abruptly in the mid labia majora. The patient may remain asymptomatic but frequently presents with pruritus, hypopigmentation, or hemorrhage. Secondary infection and bleeding are common in this easily traumatized tissue. The diagnosis is usually clinical, but in suspected cases of child abuse (prominent in the differential diagnosis of lichen sclerosis), the diagnosis can be made histologically. Treatment with topical testosterone may quell the symptoms in a prepubertal child; during puberty, the symptoms resolve.

Some young girls are especially sensitive to bubble baths, perfumes, or soaps, which can act as irritants and cause both vulvitis and vaginitis. The chemical irritant should be discontinued and the girl should be taught to practice good perineal hygiene.

Pinworm infestation may also lead to vulvitis. The classic symptom of pinworm infestation is perianal and vulvar itching at night. The diagnosis is often made by the parents. The perineal and perianal area is checked at night (when child is sleeping) because that is when the parasites are visible. Alternatively, the pinworm eggs can be recovered on cellophane tape applied to the rectum overnight. The treatment is one 100-mg dose of oral mebendazole given to the child and all members of the household older than 2 years and repeated after 2 weeks.

Irritant dermatitis of the vulva can also be caused by vaginal discharge. Efforts should be made in these cases to identify the cause of the discharge (see later discussion). With appropriate treatment of the vaginal discharge, the dermatitis should resolve.

Group A β-hemolytic streptococcal infection can present as a vaginal discharge (vaginitis) or as a perianal or perineal cellulitis in toddlers and young children. The nonspecific discharge or reddened perineal or perianal skin is key to the diagnosis. The diagnosis is based on a positive culture and a high degree of suspicion. The infection is treated with penicillin or amoxicillin (or erythromycin in children allergic to penicillin) for 10 days.

Tumors of the vulva include hemangioma, for which the initial treatment is observation and reassurance. If the urethra or other structures are obstructed, either intralesional steroid injections to reduce the size of the hemangioma or laser or surgical excision is required. Most hemangiomas do not continue to enlarge after 9 to 12 months and then begin to regress, usually completely by the time the child is 5 years old. Malignant tumors, such as carcinoma and embryonal rhabdomyosarcoma, are extremely rare.

VAGINITIS AND VAGINAL BLEEDING IN YOUNG GIRLS

Because the vagina at birth has been stimulated by maternal estrogen, the epithelium is thickened; however, after a few weeks, the epithelium becomes smooth, thin, and atrophic. The vagina of a young girl is made susceptible to colonic bacterial overgrowth by a neutral pH and a lack of lactobacilli. The prepubertal girl has no labial fat pads, no pubic hair, small labia minora, and a rectum in close proximity to the vagina, all of which contribute to a tendency to acquire vulvovaginitis. Poor perineal hygiene, including incorrect cleaning practices by young girls, also contributes to the problem. Girls may present with vaginal discharge, itching, perineal irritation, or cellulitis. Proper perineal hygiene, which includes wiping from front to back after voiding, frequent changes of underpants, adequately drying the perineum after bathing and voiding, and avoiding bubble baths, usually leads to resolution of the discharge and irritation. Rarely are broad-spectrum antibiotics necessary.

Besides mixed bacterial overgrowth resulting from poor perineal hygiene, foreign body insertion (usually toilet tissue) with secondary infection is another cause of vaginal discharge in prepubertal girls. The discharge may be mucoid, white, green, yellow, or bloody. If the foreign body is not obvious or cannot be easily removed, the cultures are negative, or empiric antibiotic treatment has been unsuccessful, examination under anesthesia with removal of the object(s) is necessary.

A vaginal discharge in a young girl with otherwise normal examination findings, even if she has no history of sexual abuse or foreign body insertion, must be properly diagnosed. Vaginal cultures (they need not be cervical) for *Chlamydia,* gonococci, *Trichomonas,* bacterial vaginosis (BV), *Candida,* and streptococci in addition to routine bacterial cultures should all be obtained. An appropriate collection technique includes the use of swabs moistened with nonbacteriostatic sterile saline solution to avoid trauma to the delicate vaginal mucosa. Test results positive for sexually transmitted disease must be reported to child protective services so that an investigation to ensure the child's continued safety can be initiated. The child must be treated with appropriate antibiotics, and an interdisciplinary team should provide long-term support and counseling.

Any girl in whom vaginal bleeding develops before puberty must be examined carefully. Withdrawal bleeding is not uncommon in the first few days to week of life, but vaginal bleeding beyond this period is abnormal. Causes include urethral prolapse, hemangioma, neoplasms, precocious puberty, vaginal foreign body, and genital trauma resulting from sexual abuse or a straddle injury. It is rare for a blood dyscrasia (i.e., von Willebrand disease) to present as vaginal bleeding in prepubescent girls, although it is a common cause of menorrhagia after menarche.

TRAUMA TO THE VULVA AND VAGINA AND SEXUAL ABUSE OF FEMALE CHILDREN

Trauma to the vulva and vagina may occur accidentally or as the result of sexual abuse. Up to 90% of perineal injuries to girls are caused by sexual abuse. A seemingly minor vulvar or vaginal injury in a young girl can be extensive. Therefore, vaginal bleeding in a child with a traumatic injury must be investigated with the patient under anesthesia for possible extension of the laceration into the peritoneum, broad ligament, bladder, or rectum. Vulvar and perineal trauma followed by microscopic hematuria should be evaluated by computed tomography (CT). If gross hematuria is present, both CT and voiding cystourethrography may be necessary.

The examination of a young girl with trauma begins with a primary survey. First, the airway must be evaluated and maintained. Breathing, circulation, and neurologic status are quickly and accurately assessed, followed by a search for gross bleeding. Only if these parameters are stable can a further examination be carried out. Sedation may be needed before the perineum is examined. The labia are gently retracted, and the examiner looks closely for hematomas, blood, and feces. A rectal and abdominal examination should be performed in a prepubertal girl. A small hematoma of the vulva may be treated conservatively, but any hematoma of the vulva that appears to be extensive or expanding must be opened under general anesthesia and points of bleeding ligated appropriately. A vaginal inspection with small vaginoscopes or small nasal specula must be conducted. Accurate and complete written documentation is necessary. If a bladder injury is suspected, a cystoscopic examination should be carried out. A rectoscopic examination should be conducted in cases of suspected anorectal trauma. If the wound penetrates the peritoneum, an exploratory laparotomy is required.

The vulva and vagina of a young girl may be accidentally injured in several ways. Straddle injuries, thought to account for 75% of all accidental genital injuries, occur commonly as the result of straddling playground or gym equipment or the center bar of a boy's bicycle. These injuries usually involve the anterior perineum, including the mons pubis, clitoris, and anterior labia majora, and less frequently the urethra. They are often not symmetric around the midline. External injuries rarely extend vaginally. The lesions may be treated conservatively with cold, gentle compression, careful observation for extension, and adequate analgesia.

Accidental penetration by a foreign body can also injure the vulva or vagina. Girls of preschool age (2 to 4 years old) can fall on a sharp object, such as a pen or pencil, or other foreign bodies may be placed in the vagina as a result of curiosity, pruritus, or self-manipulation. Sometimes, ecchymosis or an obvious puncture wound is observed, but it is not unusual for a child to present with hematuria, vaginal discharge, or bleeding. Small pieces of toilet tissue and rarely buttons, coins, or toys can lodge in the vagina and cause bleeding or secondary infection with discharge. Any young girl or toddler with persistent vaginal discharge requires a vaginal examination to detect a foreign body. Before a foreign body that has been in the vaginal vault for a prolonged time is removed, antibiotic therapy should be initiated. The vagina can also be injured when a young girl is held directly over a swimming pool fountain by the high-pressure force of the water. Lacerations of the perineum and vagina can occur during sudden abduction of the lower extremities, as in water skiing or motor vehicle accidents.

The incidence of sexual abuse in children is difficult to estimate. It has been said to occur in 5% to 10% of reported cases of maltreatment of children. However, many authorities believe that the true incidence is higher than that reported. Victims often repress sexual abuse. Surveys indicate that as many as 20% to 30% of women have had unwanted sexual experiences during childhood. Childhood sexual abuse is often overlooked, underreported, and ineffectually treated by medical personnel.

Sexually abused children are exposed to, or engage in, sexual activities that are inappropriate for their developmental level or chronologic age with an older or more mature person. The sexual abuse of children includes fondling of their genitalia or breasts, orogenital contact, and vaginal or anal penetration. It also includes exhibitionism, voyeurism, involvement in child pornography, and the deliberate exposure of children to sexually explicit photographs or materials.

More than 90% of perpetrators are male, and up to 90% are known to the victim (one third are relatives). Sexual abuse is most common in school-age children, but children of all ages and socioeconomic groups are subjected to sexual abuse. The usual course when the perpetrator is known to the victim is a steady increase in the establishment of sexual contact. The perpetrator encourages secrecy by threatening or rewarding the victim. Disclosure may be late and unfortunately is possible only with a receptive caretaker; suppression of abuse is common, the victim often blaming herself.

The physical examination of a child suspected of being abused must be carried out in as nonthreatening and gentle a fashion as possible. Care must be taken that the examiner does not reinforce the child's sense of victimization. A thorough physical examination is conducted and any signs of trauma noted. An anal examination without digital evaluation is included. The genital examination is performed with the patient in either the supine (lithotomy or frog leg) or knee-chest position. The hymen can be visualized by applying gentle outward traction to the labia majora. The hymen is carefully examined (to note whether it is annular, crescentic, fimbriated, septate, or imperforate—all normal findings) for tears and scars, and its transverse diameter should be documented. Lesions in the 3- to 9-o'clock position (posterior half of the hymen and introitus) are more suspect than anterior clefts or notches, although all may be normal. In most cases of proven sexual abuse, the findings are normal or nonspecific. The primary care clinician should refer the child and the family to the appropriate local or regional facility for multidisciplinary care in cases of suspected abuse. Vaginal specimens should be collected with moistened swabs (nonbacteriostatic saline solution) to decrease the chance of further injury to the sensitive vaginal mucosa.

FEMALE CIRCUMCISION

Female circumcision is practiced in 28 African countries and among many immigrants to the United States and Canada. Girls may be circumcised at any age. Female circumcision is classified into four types. In type I, or Sunna circumcision, part or all of the clitoris is removed. In type II, the clitoris and part of the labia minora are excised. Bleeding from the clitoral artery and raw surfaces is stemmed by sutures of catgut or thorn, or by the application of poultices. Type III is a modified or intermediate infibulation. The clitoris and labia minora are removed, and the labia majora are incised. The anterior two thirds of the labia majora are then stretched and sutured together. Type IV is total infibulation. The clitoris and labia minora are removed, and the labia majora are incised and stretched together to cover the entrance of the vagina with a hood of skin; only a very small posterior opening is left for the passage of urine and menstrual blood. Complications of these procedures include hemorrhage, severe pain, and shock and death in some cases. Severe anemia and local and systemic infections also develop. Long-term complications include chronic infections of the pelvis and urinary tract and renal damage. Dermoid cysts may form along the scar, and the victim may experience severe dyspareunia. Childbirth is a risk because of the potential for large perineal tears; fetal death and vesicovaginal fistula formation have also been reported. The children of women who have undergone infibulation need not be delivered by cesarean section; however, a deinfibulation procedure should be performed to allow a vaginal birth.

These abhorrent practices were thought to ensure a good marriage in certain cultures in which marriage was essential for a woman. In 1992, the International Federation of Gynecology and Obstetrics and the World Health Organization published a joint statement condemning female circumcision, and in 1993, the World Health Assembly issued a similar statement. As Toubia has stated, no ethical defense can be made for preserving a cultural practice that damages a woman's health.

AMBIGUOUS GENITALIA AND OTHER CONGENITAL DEFECTS

Usually, a rapid glance at the external genitalia is sufficient to determine the sex of a newborn. The birth of an infant with ambiguous genitalia is difficult for all present and is considered a medical emergency. The midwife or obstetrician must explain immediately that the baby looks well (if this is indeed true) but that its sex cannot be determined by a simple examination. The parents must be told that specialists will be consulted and that several laboratory tests are needed to determine the sex of the child. The team examining the infant will consist of the pediatrician or family physician, a pediatric endocrinologist, and a urologist; a psychologist experienced in the diagnosis of sex differentiation can also be consulted. The family is told that it will take several days before the results are known. The members of the health care team treating the infant and family must keep a neutral opinion regarding the sex, using words such as *baby*, *gonads*, and *phallus* (rather than penis or clitoris). Surgical and medical therapy depends on an accurate diagnosis.

It is important to establish the preferred sex for rearing the child. This decision is best made during the first days of life. It is extremely difficult to make a sex change after a year. Assignment of sex in these cases is complex and best handled by an expert medical team; therefore, prompt referral to a tertiary care facility is mandatory. A scheme for determining the pathology related to ambiguous genitalia based on the karyotype is presented in Fig. 9.3.

The genetic mutation that causes the most common form of 46,XX ambiguous genitalia (21-hydroxylase deficiency) may have other life-threatening effects. The salt-losing forms of congenital adrenal hyperplasia associated with ambiguous genitalia (21-hydroxylase deficiency and 3β-hydroxysteroid dehydrogenase deficiency) may present with acute adrenal crisis—hyponatremia, hyperkalemia, hypoglycemia, metabolic acidosis, dehydration (weight loss), or frank shock—between days 2 and 21 of life. Without glucocorticoids, death occurs.

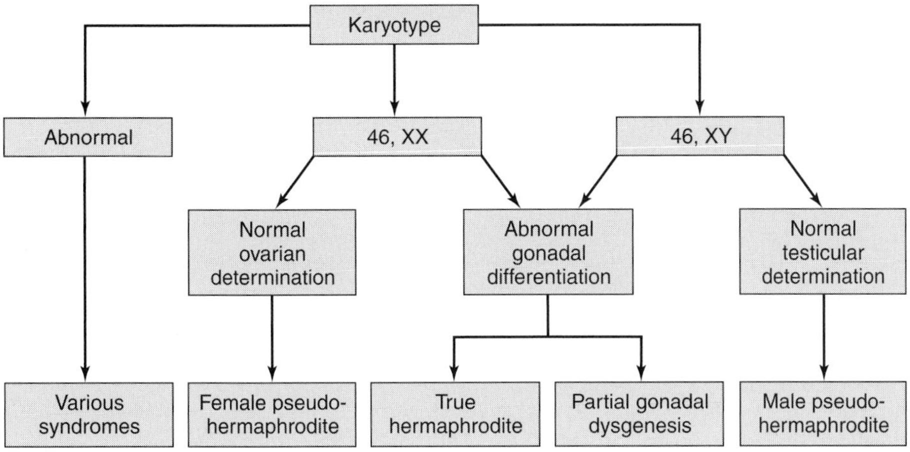

FIG. 9.3. Scheme determining the pathology related to ambiguous genitalia based on the karyotype. In 46,XY infants with normal testicular formation, the condition is termed *male pseudohermaphroditism.* In 46,XX infants with normal ovarian formation, the condition is termed *female pseudohermaphroditism.* In 46,XX or 46,XY infants with abnormal gonadal differentiation, the condition may be true hermaphroditism or partial gonadal dysgenesis. (From Carpenter SE, Rock JA, eds. *Pediatric and adolescent gynecology.* New York: Raven Press, 1992, with permission.)

Imperforate hymen can present in the neonatal period as a bulge in the vagina caused by pooled secretions. The imperforation may go unnoticed, and the secretions, if present, are generally resorbed within the first few days of life. Girls with an imperforate hymen usually present at puberty with abdominal pain or symptoms of urinary retention or constipation. Examination reveals a vaginal bulge or abdominal mass resulting from the retention of vaginal secretions (including blood). Blood may be localized to the vagina (hematocolpos), and the vaginal bulge will have a blue hue. Blood can also be found in the uterus (hematometra). Treatment to drain occluded fluids is generally not necessary until puberty and includes a hymenectomy.

Other congenital anomalies of the uterus also may not present until puberty, the initiation of sexual activity, or pregnancy. Symptoms include difficulty in inserting a tampon, dysmenorrhea, menorrhagia, and difficult intercourse. A palpable mass may be noted. The congenital uterine anomaly may first be noted on an intravenous pyelogram, during a dilatation and curettage procedure, or on a pelvic ultrasonogram. Fetal malpresentation or an abnormal uterine contour during pregnancy, or a pregnancy that occurs despite the presence of an intrauterine device, suggests the possibility of a uterine anomaly.

PRECOCIOUS PUBERTY

The accepted age at which puberty normally begins is decreasing. Previously, the lower age limit for normal breast development was 7.5 years, and for menarche, it was 9.5 years. A large pediatric office-based study reported in 1997 defined the development of breasts or pubic hair at age 7 in white girls and at age 6 in African-American girls as the lower limit of normal. Precocious puberty is either central hypothalamic-pituitary (true) puberty or puberty that occurs independently of pituitary gonadotropin (peripheral precocious puberty or autonomous gonadal function). In girls, "idiopathic" central precocious puberty is the most common form, and although it occurs early, a specific organic lesion is found only rarely. Central nervous system tumors, such as hypothalamic hamartomas, gliomas, and neurofibromas, and hydrocephalus are associated with central precocious puberty. Other causes of central precocious puberty include head trauma and infections or irradiation of the central nervous system.

Central precocious puberty is associated with advanced linear growth, an advanced skeletal age, and levels of luteinizing hormone (LH) and follicle-stimulating hormone (FSH) in the pubertal range. Samples to measure LH and FSH levels should (ideally) be drawn late at night or in the very early hours of the morning (between 2 and 3 a.m.) because this is when levels of these hormones typically rise in early central puberty. A gonadotropin-releasing hormone (GnRH) stimulation test that shows an increase in both LH and FSH but LH more than FSH indicates central puberty. True central precocious puberty is treated with GnRH agonists, such as leuprolide acetate (Lupron Depot).

One form of primary hypothyroidism is associated with pituitary enlargement, galactorrhea, and precocious puberty (Van Wyck-Grumbach syndrome). Low levels of LH and FSH in a pubertal girl may indicate autonomously functioning gonads. Ovarian or adrenal estrogen-producing tumors and severe, prolonged hypothyroidism (associated with the formation of multicystic ovaries) may cause the onset of puberty without central mediation.

The McCune-Albright syndrome is the triad of café au lait spots, polyostotic fibrous dysplasia, and ovarian cysts. The autonomously functioning cysts produce estradiol that causes breast development and vaginal bleeding—that is, precocious puberty. Autonomous ovarian function is treated with aromatase inhibitors (i.e., ketoconazole, testolactone), but they are not always effective and have not been approved.

Estrogen from exogenous sources can cause precocious puberty. A young girl may ingest oral contraceptives or use skin creams containing estrogen. One authority cites eating meat from an estrogen-treated animal as a cause of precocious puberty.

Isolated premature breast development (premature thelarche) in early childhood (typically between 6 months and 2 years of age) appears to be caused by a mild increase in the pituitary-ovarian axis with mildly elevated estrogen levels. Although no treatment is given if *no* other signs of puberty are present, close follow-up is indicated.

Premature pubarche (the early appearance of pubic hair) is caused by adrenal androgen secretion (adrenarche). This condition is more common in overweight, African-American, and Latino girls. These girls may also have hyperinsulinism secondary to insulin resistance that stimulates adrenal androgen production. Nonclassical adrenal hyperplasia (partial or late-onset 21-hydroxylase deficiency) may present as premature adrenarche without congenital genital ambiguity and is treated with oral cortisone. A young girl with premature sexual development should be referred to a pediatric endocrinologist.

HIRSUTISM

Virilization is caused by excessive androgen from adrenal gland tumors, congenital adrenal hyperplasia, ovarian tumors, other androgen-producing tumors, or exogenous androgen exposure or ingestion (danazol, methyltestosterone, stanozolol). Masculinization occurs in girls with extremely elevated levels of androgen. It is characterized by upper body obesity, temporal and frontal baldness, clitoromegaly, hirsutism, absence of breast development, and an increase in muscle mass.

However, hirsutism may also occur without androgen excess, as in acromegaly and chronic skin irritation. Phenytoin causes hypertrichosis, not hirsutism. Hypertrichosis is an increase in vellus hair that creates a "fuzzy" look. Hirsutism and clitoromegaly may develop in the peripubertal period in young girls with incomplete testicular feminization (46,XY partial androgen insensitivity) or XY gonadal dysgenesis.

The syndrome of congenital adrenal hyperplasia, discussed previously, is caused by a deficiency of one of several different enzymes involved in the adrenocortical synthesis of cortisol, most commonly 21-hydroxylase. Because of a block in the synthesis of cortisol and mineralocorticoids, the steroid precursors are shunted to the androgen pathway. This leads to masculinization and hirsutism. Late-onset adrenal hyperplasia occurs in up to 6% of girls and women with hirsutism. The treatment is corticosteroid replacement.

Hirsutism is seen in hyperandrogenism and may be associated with insulin resistance, acanthosis nigricans, and obesity. Cushing syndrome, androgenic tumors, and hyperthecosis (persistent estrogen secretion by islands of hyperplastic, luteinized theca cells, as in polycystic ovarian syndrome) may also lead to hirsutism. Occasionally, a girl with hirsutism has normal levels of free and total androgen; in this case, the hirsutism is labeled idiopathic.

The workup includes a careful history of the onset and progression of the hirsutism, pubertal development, vaginal bleeding, and drug use. A physical examination should be conducted to detect signs of androgen excess, clitoromegaly, and cushingoid features and to determine the Tanner stage. Acne is frequently present. The size of the thyroid gland and any hypothyroid or hyperthyroid symptoms should be noted. Appropriate laboratory evaluations should be carried out to determine the total and free serum testosterone, sex hormone-binding globulin, dehydroepiandrosterone sulfate (DHEAS), and 17-hydroxyprogesterone levels (see Chapter 40).

TUMORS OF THE VULVA, VAGINA, CERVIX, UTERINE CORPUS, AND OVARY

Tumors of the reproductive tract in newborn and young girls are very uncommon. Because of their rarity, neoplasms may be confused with other conditions, so that diagnosis and treatment are seriously delayed.

Vulvar lesions must be carefully evaluated. The most common neoplasm of the lower genital tract in infants and young girls is embryonal rhabdomyosarcoma of the botryoid type. Endodermal sinus tumors may be seen in the infant vagina. Clear cell adenocarcinoma has been seen in the vagina and cervix of infants and young girls exposed to diethylstilbestrol in utero. The use of diethylstilbestrol decreased in the mid-1950s, so that these tumors are now rare. In children, the most common clinical symptom of a uterine tumor is vaginal bleeding. Only 5% of all ovarian malignancies occur in children and adolescents. Almost two thirds of these tumors are germ cell tumors.

BIBLIOGRAPHY

Altchek A. Finding the cause of genital bleeding in prepubertal girls. *Contemp Pediatr* 1996;13:80–92.
Baldwin DD, Landa HM. Pediatric gynecology: evaluation and treatment. *Contemp Pediatr* 1995;Nov:35–58.
Ballard, et al. Gestational age assessment. *J Pediatr* 1979;95:769–774.
Carpenter SE, Rock JA, eds. *Pediatric and adolescent gynecology.* New York: Raven Press, 1992.
Craighill MC. Pediatric and adolescent gynecology for the primary care pediatrician. *Pediatr Clin North Am* 1998;45:1659–1673.
Emans SJH, Goldstein DP, eds. *Pediatric and adolescent gynecology.* Boston: Little, Brown, 1982.
Herman-Giddens ME, Slora EJ, Wasserman RC, et al. Secondary sexual characteristics and menses in young girls seen in office practice: a study from the Pediatric Research in Office Setting Network. *Pediatrics* 1997;99:505–512.
Hoekelman R, Friedman SB, Nelson NM, et al. *Primary pediatric care,* 2nd ed. St. Louis: Mosby–Year Book, 1992.
Money J, Lamacz M. Genital examination and exposure experience as nosocomial sexual abuse in childhood. *J Nerv Ment Dis* 1987;175:713.
Mroueh J, Muram D. Common problems in pediatric gynecology: new developments. *Curr Opin Obstet Gynecol* 1999;11:463–466.
Preminger MK, Pokorny SF. Vaginal discharge—a common pediatric complaint. *Contemp Pediatr* 1998;April:115–122.
Toubia N. Female circumcision as a public health issue. *N Engl J Med* 1994;331:11.

CHAPTER 10
Adolescent Health Care

Susan M. Yussman and Jonathan D. Klein

In this chapter, we review the biologic, psychological, and social developmental issues of adolescents. We explore communication between adolescents and their families, and the effect of such communication on the major health problems affecting young women today. We review the major causes of morbidity and mortality, most of which are preventable health problems amenable to primary care interventions. We examine the special health care needs and issues of greatest concern to practitioners. Finally, we discuss special issues affecting the accessibility and availability of primary care services to adolescents.

BIOPSYCHOSOCIAL MODEL APPLIED TO ADOLESCENT DEVELOPMENT

The biopsychosocial model is an appropriate paradigm for the primary care of female adolescents because it recognizes the complex interaction of the biologic, psychological, and social phenomena influencing them during this stage of development. In many situations related to the primary health care of adolescent women, a biopsychosocial approach, although time-consuming, is essential. For instance, a biologic problem such as diabetes mellitus in a 14-year-old girl will affect, and be influenced by, her psychological development and social interactions with her family and peers. A psychological problem such as depression in a 15-year-old girl may result in, or begin with, a loss of friends and social isolation, but it may also be associated with a biologic deficiency of central nervous system neurotransmitters, such as serotonin; depression from either cause can lead to attempted suicide. A social problem such as recurrent runaway behavior in a 16-year-old may be associated with numerous other high-risk behaviors, including substance abuse, exposure to sexually transmitted diseases, unintended pregnancy, and violence. Yet, such behavior may represent an attempt to escape sexual abuse at home.

Thus, the "psychosocial" aspects of primary care adolescent medicine are best incorporated into the overall preventive care of the adolescent and not evaluated only after specific behavioral problems arise. The physician must be observant and become acquainted with both the adolescent and her family, peers, and school. The provider must interview in a style that resembles conversation more than interrogation and adopt a developmentally oriented approach to the patient and a systems-oriented approach to the family.

Physical Growth and Development

Growth and development during puberty are the consequence of biologic changes that occur during this phase. The most visible changes of puberty, which begins in girls between the ages of 8 and 14 years, result from the effects of gonadal hormones on the maturation of the musculoskeletal and reproductive systems. Equally significant but less obvious changes occur in the adolescent's cognitive abilities, as a young woman acquires the ability to engage in formal operational thought. Additionally, adolescents undergo a predictable process of psychosocial development. Each of these developmental processes may affect a young woman's health.

Clinicians may find it useful to consider four tasks of adolescence related to these pubertal, cognitive, and psychosocial developmental processes. To enter adulthood, the following tasks must be completed: (a) acceptance of physical changes resulting in an adult body and reproductive capability, (b) attainment of independence and autonomy from the family of origin, (c) emergence of a stable identity, and (d) development of adult thinking patterns.

Key concepts with respect to female adolescent pubertal growth and development include secular trend, sequencing, tempo, and variability. *Secular trend* is the reduction in the age of pubertal development from the middle of the 19th to the middle of the 20th century in industrialized countries. Although this was thought to have plateaued during the last few decades, recent evidence indicates that many girls are demonstrating pubertal changes by the age of 8 years; thus, the standards for normal growth and pubertal development used in primary care have recently been reconsidered. *Sequencing* is the progression of secondary sex characteristics, which follows a predictable order. *Tempo* refers to the timing of the onset and the velocity of changes in secondary sex characteristics. The *interindividual variability* of sequencing is small, but that for tempo is great.

Pubertal maturation occurs as a result of activation of the hypothalamic-pituitary-gonadal system. The exact triggering mechanism for puberty is unknown. Puberty in girls begins when a progressive decrease in the sensitivity of the hypothalamus to the negative feedback of estrogen results in the cyclic release of gonadotropins during sleep. Hypothalamic gonadotropin-releasing hormone (GnRH) acts on the anterior pituitary gland to produce follicle-stimulating hormone (FSH) and luteinizing hormone (LH). FSH stimulates the production of estrogen and growth of the ovarian follicle. LH stimulates and initiates ovulation, the corpus luteum, and the production of progesterone.

The physical changes associated with puberty and the average time course for these events are shown in Fig. 10.1. As noted, the events of puberty progress in a relatively fixed and predictable sequence, but the timing of the events is quite variable. Thus, chronologic age differs widely within any given maturational stage. A determination of sexual maturation based on the development of breast and pubic hair, with the use of Tanner's maturational stages as a reference standard, is an important part of the routine care of young women. Plotting and monitoring growth and development are critical to helping young women and their families understand the normal nature of the changes taking place. Staging pubertal changes is of substantial value in predicting the likely course of developmental events because pubertal growth is completed in most girls within 4 years after onset. Additionally, a sexual maturity rating (SMR) has implications in the assessment of pubertal delay, short stature or other growth failure, and amenorrhea.

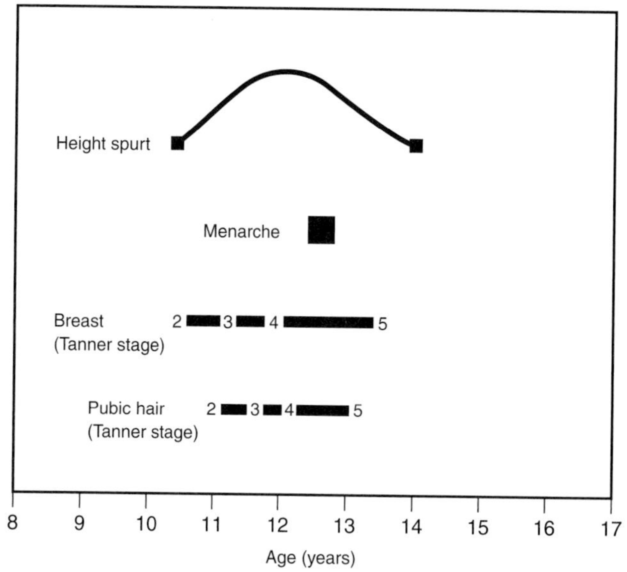

FIG. 10.1. Pubertal events in girls. (From Copeland KC, Brookman RR, Rauth JL. *Assessment of pubertal development.* Ross Laboratories PREP Series. Columbus, OH: Ross Laboratories, 1986:6, with permission.)

The earliest visible change resulting from increasing estrogen levels following activation of the hypothalamic-pituitary-gonadal axis is breast budding (thelarche), which occurs at a mean age of 10.0 years in white girls and 8.9 years in African-American girls. The appearance of dark, straight pubic hair over the mons veneris (adrenarche or pubarche) indicates activation of the hypothalamic-pituitary-adrenal axis and takes place at a mean age of 10.5 years in white girls and 8.8 years in African-American girls. Thelarche and adrenarche mark the onset of SMR (Tanner stage) 2. Breast development proceeds to SMR 5 (adult) during the next 4 years; the completion of breast development may take as little as 18 months or as long as 9 years (Fig. 10.2). The development of pubic hair is completed in about 18 to 40 months (Fig. 10.3). About 1 year after the initiation of breast development, during SMR 3, a very rapid increase in height takes place in girls. The peak of this growth spurt (peak height velocity) precedes the onset of menstruation (menarche) by about 6 months (Figs. 10.4, 10.5). Menarche is regularly preceded by the peak growth spurt, but it may occur as early as age 10 or as late as age 16, with a mean age of 12.9 years in white girls and 12.2 years in African-American girls. Thus, menarche is a relatively late pubertal event, occurring during or just before the SMR 4 stage of breast development.

Pubertal girls gain lean body mass and body fat. The average fat-to-lean ratio changes from 1:5 at the start of the growth spurt to 1:3 at the time of menarche. Weight gain and weight velocity standards are shown in Figs. 10.6 and 10.7. As the external appearance changes, the internal organs also develop. For

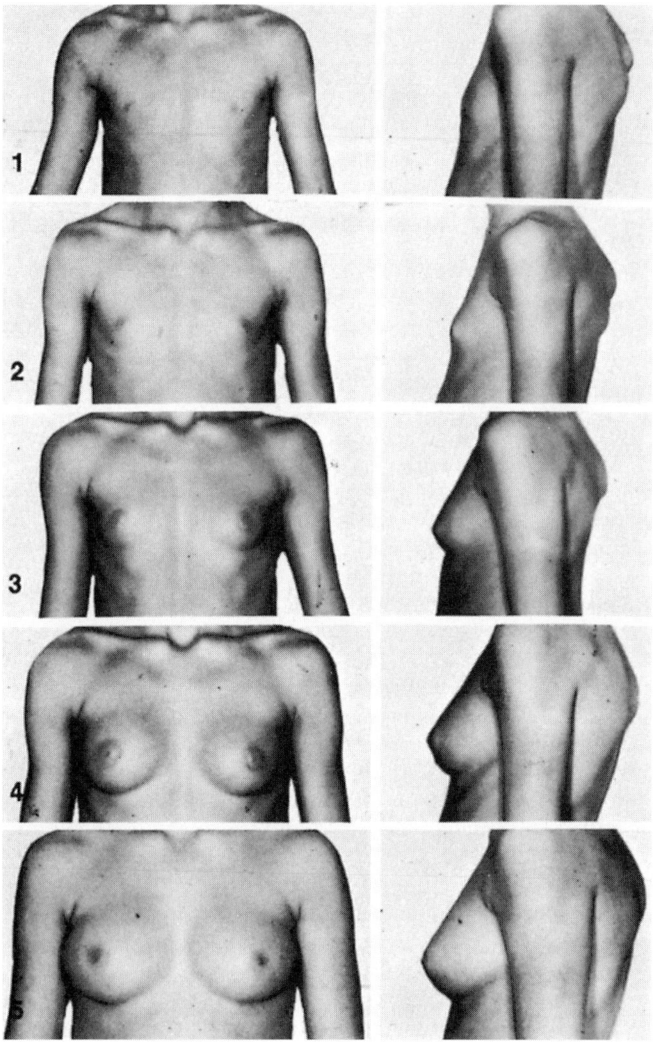

FIG. 10.2. Sexual maturity ratings—pubertal development of the female breast. Stage 1: Preadolescent—elevation of the papillae only. Stage 2: Breast bud—the elevated breast and papilla form a small mound. Stage 3: Continuing enlargement of the breast and areola without separation of their contours. Stage 4: The areola and papilla project to form a secondary mound above the level of the breast. Stage 5: Mature adult—the areola has recessed to the contour of the breast. (From Tanner JM. *Growth at adolescence,* 2nd ed. Oxford: Blackwell Science, 1962, with permission.)

example, the mucus-secreting cells lining the uterus may produce a scant, thin, acidic, odorless vaginal discharge before menarche, called *physiologic leukorrhea.*

Psychological and Cognitive Development during Adolescence

Piaget first described the transition from concrete to formal operational thought as occurring in the early and middle teen years. Although the variations in development are considerable, most young people acquire the ability to think abstractly between the ages of 12 and 16 years. Before such ability is acquired, young people have difficulty in applying general principles to different situations and realistically appraising and planning for the future. In contrast, formal operational thought includes the capacity to think about abstractions, such as ideas and thoughts. This developmental task is a gradual transition from primarily egocentric or concrete thinking to formal operational thought. Mature cognitive ability facilitates adolescents' thinking about independence, interdependence, careers, and personal moral choices. However, some people successfully function as independent adults without ever becoming capable of formal operational thinking.

The development of formal operational thought is also a crucial milestone with regard to planning the care of adolescents. For example, youths whose thought is concrete operational are probably not capable of true emancipation or informed consent. Adolescents capable of formal operational thought can consider the consequences and the risks and benefits of immediate decisions with a realistic orientation to the future. However, this ability may be inconsistently applied in emotionally charged situations, such as arise within family and sexual relationships.

Finally, the psychosocial tasks of adolescence should be considered. The traditional Eriksonian task of adolescence is identity formation, which allows the development of independence from parents and intimacy with other individuals as adults. In contrast, Baumrind and other recent developmental theorists have defined the goals of adolescent social development as

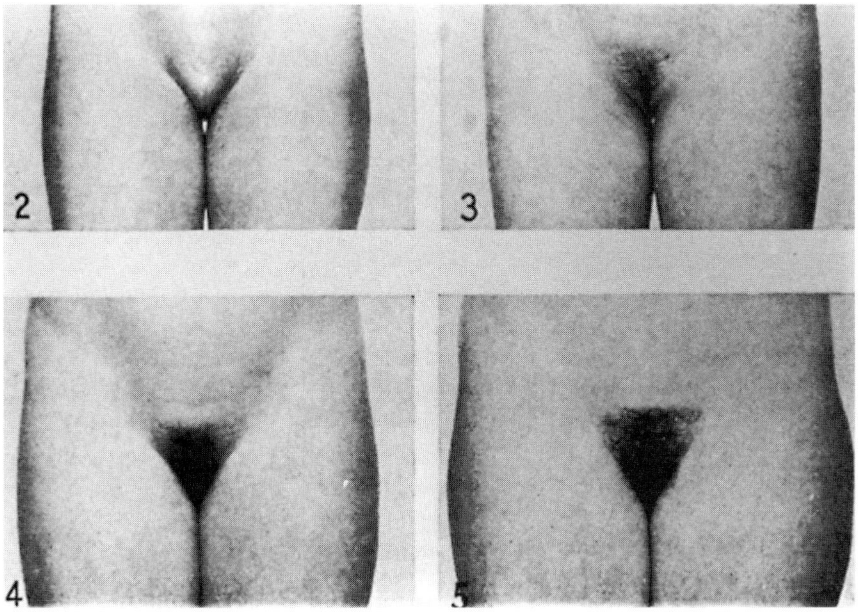

FIG. 10.3. Sexual maturity ratings—pubertal development of pubic hair. Stage 1: Preadolescent—no pubic hair. Stage 2: Sparse growth of long, slightly pigmented, straight or slightly curly pubic hair along the labia only. Stage 3: Darker, coarser, and more curled hair spreading upward over the pubic area. Stage 4: Adult type and pattern of hair, without extension onto the thighs. Stage 5: Adult type, quantity, and pattern of hair, with extension onto the thighs. (From Tanner JM. *Growth at adolescence,* 2nd ed. Oxford: Blackwell Scientific, 1962, with permission.)

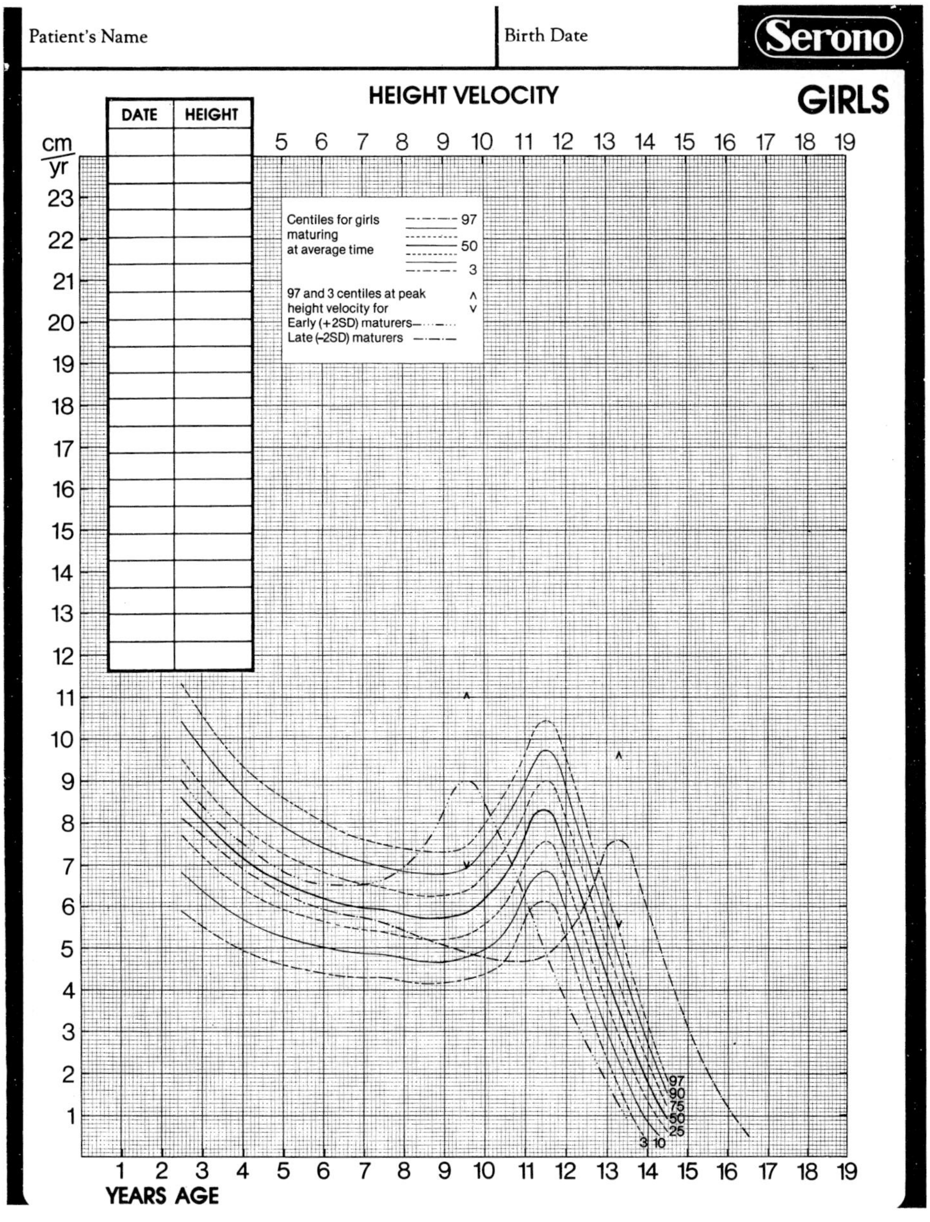

FIG. 10.4. Height attained for adolescent girls. (Modified from Tanner JM, Davies PW. Clinical longitudinal standards for height and height velocity for North American children. *J Pediatr* 1985;107;317, with permission.)

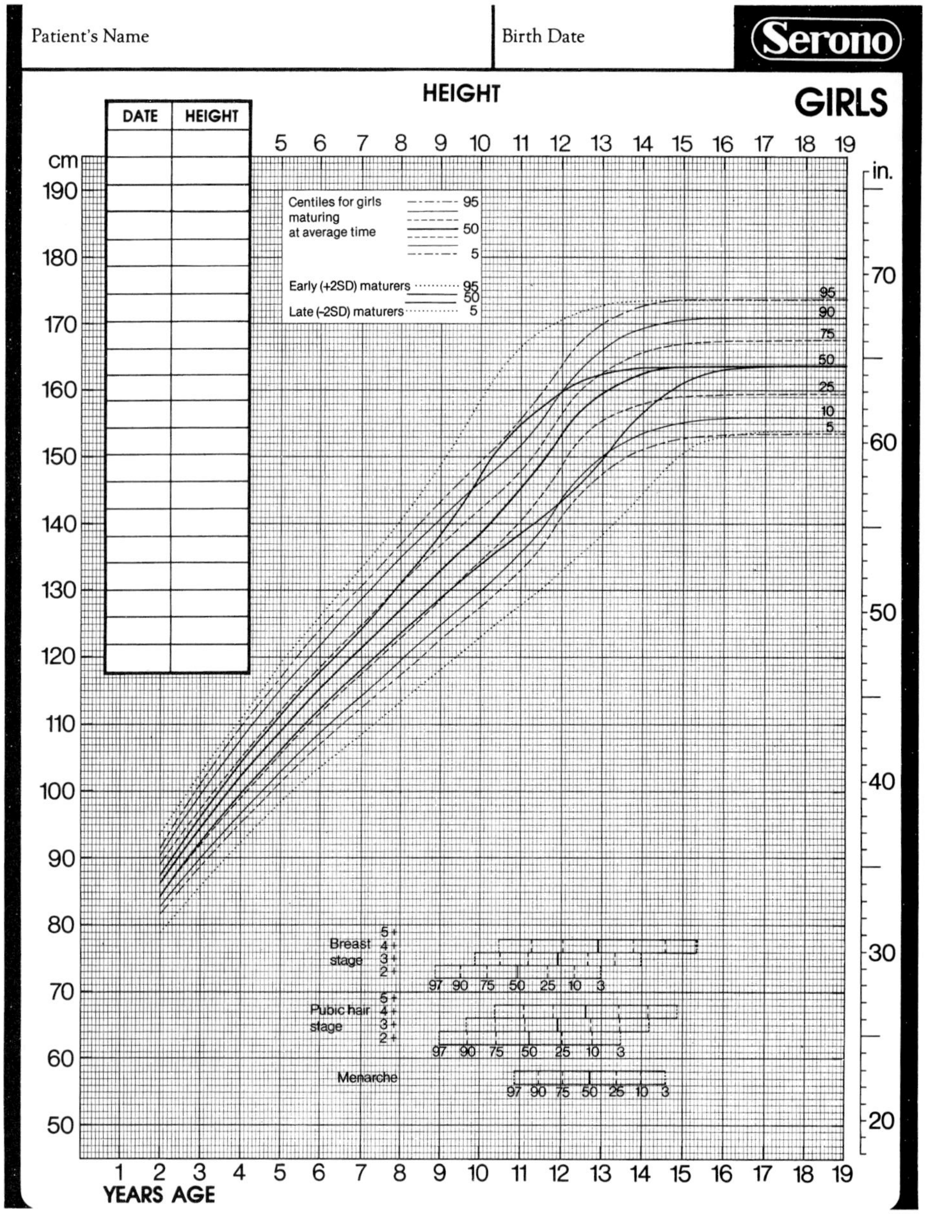

FIG. 10.5. Height velocity for adolescent girls. (Modified from Tanner JM, Davies PW. Clinical longitudinal standards for height and height velocity for North American children. *J Pediatr* 1985;107:317, with permission.)

interdependence, reflecting the continuing relationships and importance of the connections between adult children and their families.

It is useful to divide adolescence into three stages: early (10–14 years), middle (15–16 years), and late (17–21 years). Each stage can be understood in regard to adolescents' changing relationships with family, school, and peers. The developmental changes of adolescents also affect their risks, evaluation, management, and outcome. The early onset of puberty in girls (and also the later onset of puberty in boys) is associated with increased levels of risky behavior. Under stress, the ability to think and solve problems in formal operational ways may regress. Because the thought processes of early adolescents are concrete, the motivation for behavioral change depends on short-range goals (e.g., don't smoke because it may make you smell bad, keep you from running fast, or stain your teeth, rather than because it increases your risk for lung cancer or heart disease).

EARLY ADOLESCENCE (10–14 YEARS OLD)

The early adolescent years are marked by rapid physical growth, both somatically and sexually. Increases in sex hormones are partly responsible for these changes, preparing the girl for womanhood and reproduction. Physical and sexual changes lead the girl in early adolescence to question her identity in terms of "Am I normal?" As she begins to identify more with her peer group, she gradually seeks autonomy or independence. Insecurity and self-consciousness characterize this stage. Although some 13-year-old girls are sexually active, it is usually for nonsexual reasons, such as seeking peer approval or

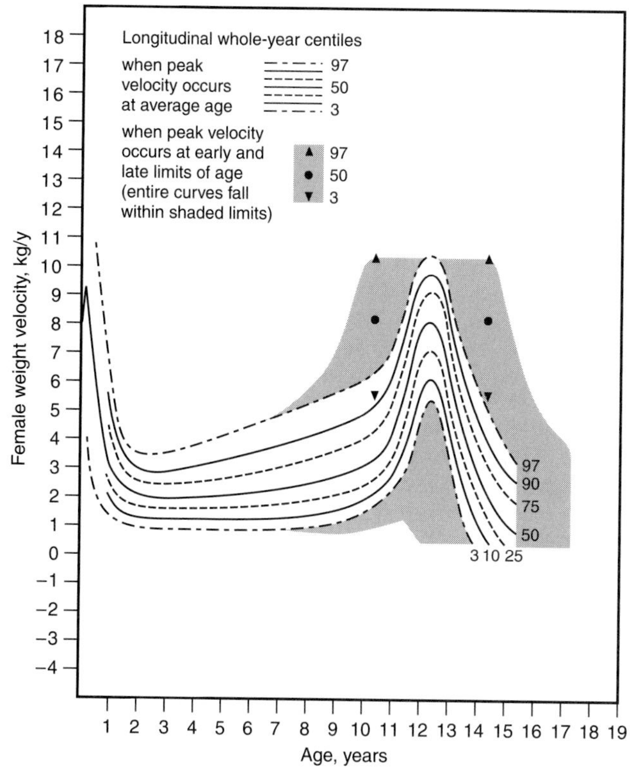

FIG. 10.6. Weight attained for adolescent girls. (Modified from Tanner JM, Whitehouse RH. Clinical longitudinal standards for height, weight, height velocity, weight velocity, and stages of puberty. *Arch Dis Child* 1976;51:170, with permission.)

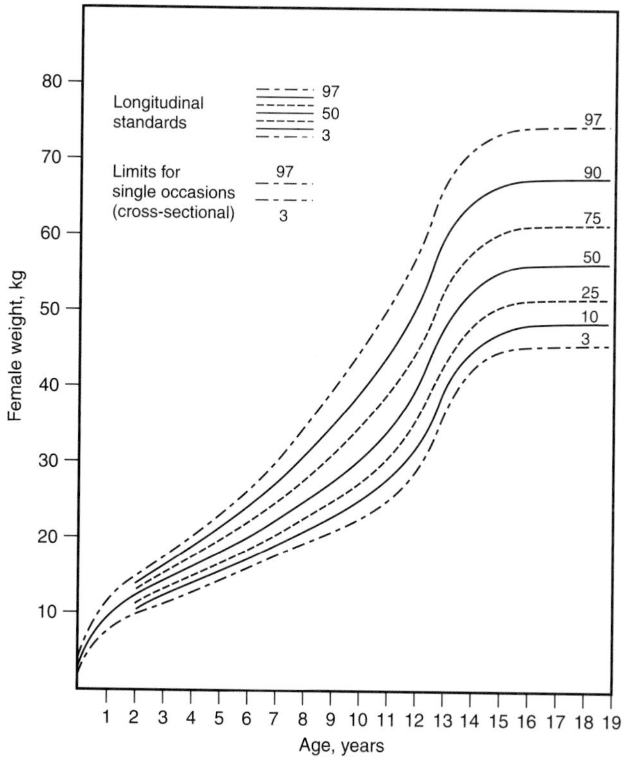

FIG. 10.7. Weight velocity for adolescent girls. (Modified from Tanner JM, Whitehouse RH. Clinical longitudinal standards for height, weight, height velocity, weight velocity, and stages of puberty. *Arch Dis Child* 1976;51:170, with permission.)

independence, rather than sexual reasons, such as a true desire for intimacy, which is developmentally impossible to achieve until late adolescence or young adulthood. Furthermore, even though a girl may strive for independence from her family, when challenged by a crisis she will most often retreat to them. For girls, relationships generally are of greater value than the achievement and domination implied in the term *independence*. Thus, dependency in childhood tends to give way to interdependence in adolescence and young adulthood for girls. Even the cognitive structure of the early adolescent is fluctuating and highly variable, primarily limited to the present (concrete operational) and occasionally expanding to a consideration of abstractions, things as they might be, or the future (formal operational).

MIDDLE ADOLESCENCE (15–16 YEARS OLD)

The middle adolescent has already experienced most of her physical growth and development. Most middle adolescents accept their adult body and reproductive capacity, but the growth and development of adolescents with chronic illness may be delayed. A desire for autonomy, conflict with authority, testing of limits, and experimentation characterize middle adolescent behavior. "Who am I?" is the critical question of the emerging identity during middle adolescence. Sexuality usually is directed toward partners of the opposite sex, and individual dating is often initiated, even in women who will be lesbians as adults. Formal operational cognition also allows consideration of the feelings of others and the development of insight and a future orientation.

Although middle adolescents do not bring the same egocentricity to concrete objects that younger children do, they remain quite narcissistic and egocentric, and they often believe that others share their thoughts. This gives rise to what has been called the "imaginary audience," through which an adolescent believes everyone is concerned about and attentive to her unique, special actions. It also results in the "personal fable," in which adolescents see themselves as invulnerable to harm.

LATE ADOLESCENCE (17–21 YEARS OLD)

The late adolescent is even more concerned about the future than the middle adolescent. Adult habitus has usually been achieved. Issues concerning future education, vocation, individuation, and sexuality assume primacy in her developmental scheme. Her emerging identity question at this stage is, "Who am I in relation to other people and to the future?" Late adolescents and young adults often physically or emotionally move away from their families and face the responsibilities of economic and physical independence, marriage, and working and the reality of an uncertain future. Experimental behaviors may lessen as adult sexual identity is acknowledged. Thus, although the patient may appear as an adult physically, it is important for the primary care provider to recognize that she is developmentally vulnerable because of a lack of adult experiences and skills. The female late adolescent may have the thinking skills and body of a woman but still be vulnerable and unready for adulthood because of unresolved issues relating to her experiences, skills, autonomy, and identity.

HEALTH RISK BEHAVIOR AND PREVENTIVE CARE OF YOUNG WOMEN

Many adolescents engage in risky behaviors that affect their health. The leading cause of death among all adolescents is unintentional injury, mostly caused by motor vehicle accidents. In teen driver fatalities, alcohol is involved about 35% of the

TABLE 10.1. Death Rates per 100,000 for the Leading Causes of Death in Adolescents and Young Adults by Age and Gender, 1999

	Males			Females		
Cause	**10–14 y**	**15–19 y**	**20–24 y**	**10–14 y**	**15–19 y**	**20–24 y**
All causes	25.3	96.3	137.6	16.7	41.7	48.0
Unintentional injuries (including MVAs)	10.8	45.1	59.0	5.8	21.5	17.6
Homicide	1.5	17.2	26.6	1.0	3.6	5.2
Suicide	1.9	13.3	21.6	0.5	2.8	3.5
Malignant neoplasms	2.8	4.4	6.3	2.4	3.1	4.6
Cardiovascular disease	0.9	2.9	4.0	0.7	1.7	2.7
Congenital anomalies	1.1	1.4	1.3	1.1	0.9	1.0
Infectious disease (including HIV)	0.3	0.3	1.5	0.2	0.4	1.6
Chronic lower respiratory disease	0.6	0.6	0.7	0.3	0.5	—

MVA, motor vehicle accident.
Source: Adapted from National Center for Health Statistics. *National vital statistics report,* vol 49, no 11, October 12, 2001. Available at www.cdc.gov/nchs/fastats/pdf/nvsr49_11tbl.pdf. Accessed January 4, 2002.

time. Homicide and suicide are the second and third leading causes of death for all adolescents, followed by neoplasms, cardiovascular diseases, and congenital anomalies. Many of these causes of death are associated with preventable behavioral choices that place young people at risk for adverse outcomes. As many as one in four adolescents are also at high risk for substance abuse, sexually transmitted diseases, unintended pregnancy, interpersonal violence, and school failure. These choices, along with choices about diet, exercise, and other issues (e.g., safety, use of seat belts), have profound implications for the prevention of adult chronic disease. The lifestyles and behaviors adopted by teens often persist, resulting in excess adult morbidity and mortality.

The use of tobacco, alcohol, and marijuana remains epidemic among adolescents, with as many as one in three adolescents smoking cigarettes. Nearly 80% of high school students have drunk alcohol; of greater concern, 28% of female students and 35% of male students have reported engaging in binge drinking (more than five drinks at one sitting) in the past month.

Violence has emerged as a significant issue during the past decade. In 1999, 27% of female students and 44% of male students were involved in one or more physical fights. Seventeen percent of high school students reported carrying a gun or other weapon in the past 30 days, and 7% brought a weapon onto school property. Although carrying a weapon does not always lead to injury, it is associated with intimidation, threats, fear, and vulnerability.

Sexual intercourse is reported by half of high school students, just under half of whom describe using a contraceptive during their last intercourse. Although it is estimated that 10% of 15- to 19-year-olds became pregnant in 1998, the teen birth rate dropped almost 20% in the 1990s. The proportion of teens reporting regular condom use continues to increase each year. Yet, nearly half of all young people who are sexually active do not take adequate precautions against HIV infection, other sexually transmitted diseases, and pregnancy.

Much of the morbidity and mortality among our nation's adolescents is preventable; thus, effective health promotion and disease prevention for adolescents is a critical part of their primary care (Tables 10.1, 10.2). In addition to school- and community-based strategies, clinical preventive services delivered by primary care providers play an important role in efforts to

TABLE 10.2. Death Rates per 100,000 for the Leading Causes of Death in Adolescents and Young Adults by Age and Race, 1999

	Black			White			Native American		
Cause	**10–14 y**	**15–19 y**	**20–24 y**	**10–14 y**	**15–19 y**	**20–24 y**	**10–14 y**	**15–19 y**	**20–24 y**
All causes	29.4	93.6	156.4	19.8	66.2	83.5	22.9	104.4	151.8
Unintentional injuries (including MVAs)	10.1	25.4	35.0	8.2	36.1	39.8	10.5	55.4	81.8
Homicide	2.6	37.2	61.2	1.0	5.6	8.2	—	11.5	17.0
Suicide	0.9	5.9	10.8	1.3	8.6	13.1	—	22.2	22.1
Malignant neoplasms	3.2	4.6	6.6	2.5	3.6	5.3	—	—	—
Cardiovascular disease	1.5	4.3	7.8	0.7	2.1	2.6	—	—	—
Congenital anomalies	1.8	1.4	1.5	1.0	1.1	1.1	—	—	—
Infectious disease (including HIV)	—	0.7	5.5	0.2	0.3	0.5	—	—	—
Chronic lower respiratory disease	1.6	1.2	1.6	0.3	0.4	0.4	—	—	—
Anemias	—	0.8	2.3	—	—	—	—	—	—

Note: Hispanics may be of any race.
MVA, motor vehicle accident.
Source: Adapted from National Center for Health Statistics. *National vital statistics report,* vol 49, no 11, October 12, 2001. Available at www.cdc.gov/nchs/fastats/pdf/nvsr49_11tbl1.pdf. Accessed January 4, 2002.

promote health and prevent disease. Most adolescents see a physician or other provider each year, but only 15% of all visits are for preventive care. Additionally, most providers offer recommended preventive services at a relatively low rate.

Various guidelines for adolescent preventive services summarize the comprehensive screening and counseling that should be provided to teenagers. These include the American Medical Association *Guidelines for Adolescent Preventive Services* (GAPS) and the guidelines in the Maternal and Child Health Bureau *Bright Futures*, in addition to recommendations made by primary care specialty organizations. Although some vary in specific content, the major guidelines are in agreement regarding the content of care. Adolescent care guidelines help primary care providers organize and deliver comprehensive preventive services to adolescents. For example, the GAPS recommendations address the organization of services, the promotion of healthy lifestyles, screening for physical, emotional, and behavioral problems, and immunizations. Additionally, the goals of the GAPS and other materials available from the American Medical Association are to make the entire clinical visit part of a health-promoting experience. One way to facilitate this is to use a trigger (screening) questionnaire during health visits. A trigger questionnaire helps identify the range of topics to be addressed. It allows for both extensive screening and prioritization and efficiency during the clinical encounter. Additionally, the use of trigger questionnaires improves the likelihood that health risks or problems will be detected and can improve the documentation of care delivery. The GAPS trigger questionnaires are available on line at www.ama-assn.org/ama/pub/category/2280.html.

MEDICAL CONDITIONS AFFECTING ADOLESCENTS

The medical conditions affecting adolescents can be the residual effects of childhood illness, the start of an adult disease process, or a condition unique to adolescence. Additionally, a few conditions manifest differently in adolescence than in adulthood or childhood. In the following sections, we briefly review conditions characteristically found in adolescents, with attention focused on diagnosis and management in primary care settings.

Acne

Acne occurs in more than 85% of adolescents and is identified as a major health concern by nearly all teenagers. Acne pimples, or comedones, are formed by the thickening, occlusion, and inflammation of hair follicles on the face, forehead, back, and chest. Androgens stimulate and estrogens inhibit the secretion of the pilosebaceous glands. Thus, most adolescent girls report acne flares, often just before menarche. The increased growth of *Propionibacterium acnes* during puberty contributes to the number of comedones and the increase in symptomatic acne during adolescence. Although most adolescents outgrow acne, 5% to 10% of young adults continue to report acne lesions into their 20s.

To evaluate acne, the type, number, and severity of lesions should be documented. Unless an androgen or corticosteroid excess is suspected, laboratory studies are not indicated. Oral contraceptives may relieve or exacerbate acne; the use of progestational contraceptive agents is usually associated with an exacerbation of acne. Several other drugs, including corticosteroids, anabolic steroids, isoniazid, lithium, and phenytoin, can cause papular and pustular acneiform lesions. Similarly, cosmetics and hair care products can cause or exacerbate acne, although fatty foods and chocolate do not aggravate acne.

The recognition and treatment of acne are an important part of adolescent practice. The goals of therapy are to prevent scarring, improve self-esteem, and reduce the number and severity of comedones. Picking and squeezing lesions should be avoided because scarring is more likely to occur. Routine skin care should be limited to washing with a mild soap twice a day, and the use of cosmetics or cover-ups should be discouraged; if used, they should be noncomedogenic.

Topical treatment is usually the first line of therapy. The application of over-the-counter 2.5% to 5% topical benzoyl peroxide cream once or twice daily is recommended as initial therapy. Tretinoin cream at an initial concentration of 0.025% may also be used, both to prevent new lesions and to treat existing ones. The use of gel preparations, as well as stronger concentrations, of either of these medications may dry and irritate the skin. Topical erythromycin or clindamycin is often added to benzoyl peroxide or tretinoin. Systemic erythromycin or tetracyclines are also used effectively, especially in cases of moderate to severe inflammatory acne. If oral tetracyclines are given, the patient's pregnancy status must be carefully monitored because these drugs are teratogenic. It is controversial whether oral antibiotics alter the metabolism of estrogens in oral contraceptives; thus, barrier contraceptives should be considered in sexually active women whose acne is being treated with systemic antibiotics. Additionally, both topical and systemic acne treatments can increase sensitivity to ultraviolet radiation, so that use of an adequate sunscreen should be recommended.

A period of 4 to 6 weeks is generally required to assess the efficacy of any particular treatment, and sufficient time should be allowed before additional therapies are added or the current regimen is abandoned. Combination regimens often result in increasingly effective treatment. Many adolescents with severe, resistant, and cystic acne also benefit from systemic isotretinoin. Adolescents with severe acne or significant scarring and candidates for isotretinoin therapy should be referred to a dermatologist. The initial course is generally 16 to 20 weeks long and may be associated with significant side effects. Because retinoic acid is highly teratogenic, intensive counseling, serial pregnancy testing, and the use of two effective methods of birth control are recommended (see Chapter 134).

Vision and Hearing Disorders

The onset of myopia most frequently occurs between the ages of 11 and 13 years. Adolescence is also often a time when preexisting nearsightedness undergoes rapid change. Additionally, adolescents are at relatively high risk for traumatic eye injuries sustained during sports or motor vehicle accidents. Hyphema, or hemorrhage into the anterior chamber of the eye, is a common form of injury; baseball, tennis, and soccer are the leading causes. Corneal abrasion is also a frequent result of trauma to the eye.

Protective eye guards should be used by adolescents who have only one functioning eye and by those who engage in sports involving projectiles (e.g., baseball). Patients with significant eye trauma should be referred for ophthalmologic evaluation without delay.

During adolescence, the differential diagnosis of bacterial conjunctivitis must be broadened to include infections with gonococci, *Chlamydia*, and herpes simplex virus in addition to other bacteria and viruses. Mechanical and allergic causes must also be considered. These conditions, which are easily treated by the primary care provider, must be differentiated from acute glaucoma, corneal abrasion or inflammation, acute iritis, and acute scleritis, all of which present with varying degrees of pain in the affected eye and require prompt referral to an ophthalmologist.

Hearing loss is a common chronic health disorder in adolescents. Of 12- to 19-year-olds, 13.0% have a high-frequency hearing loss of at least 16 decibels, and 6.6% have a low-frequency hearing loss of at least 16 decibels. Although the most common cause of hearing loss in adolescents used to be meningitis secondary to *Haemophilus influenzae* infection, hearing loss is now more likely to be caused by exposure to environmental noise. More than 15% of teens have noise-induced shifts in their hearing threshold, a progressive hearing problem caused by continued exposure to loud noise, which can lead to difficulty in discriminating among high-frequency sounds. Irreversible acoustic trauma may result from single and recurrent exposures to noise louder than 80 decibels, either loud music or occupational noise. In general, adolescents should be counseled to limit such noise exposures, allow recovery time between episodes, and use protective earplugs. Those with a significant history of exposure should be screened for hearing loss on a regular basis and counseled accordingly.

Pharyngitis and Oral Conditions

Pharyngitis, one of the most common presenting complaints in children, remains common among adolescents. Viral infections and streptococcal pharyngitis are still the leading causes of disease in adolescents; however, the spectrum of viral and bacterial agents differs from that in younger children. For example, in 1% to 4% of adolescents with *Neisseria gonorrhoeae* infection, the pharynx is the only site of infection. Other sexually transmitted pathogens can also cause pharyngitis; however, oropharyngeal involvement in sexually transmitted disease is usually seen together with genitourinary symptoms rather than alone. Additionally, infectious mononucleosis may present with pharyngitis in adolescents, although the incidence of concurrent infection with Epstein-Barr virus and streptococcal disease is at least 30%. Streptococcal pharyngitis, in particular, requires accurate diagnosis and treatment with antimicrobials because post-streptococcal systemic disease remains a significant and preventable cause of morbidity. Rheumatic heart disease accounts for 25% to 45% of cases of cardiovascular disease in all age groups (see Chapter 126).

Sexually transmitted diseases are also a major cause of oral ulcerative disease in adolescents. Primary herpes simplex viral infection may cause extensive and painful oral lesions. Treatment with oral acyclovir, if initiated early in the course of herpes infection (whether oral or genital), shortens the duration and decreases the severity of symptoms. Acyclovir may also be effective in the suppression of frequently recurring lesions, although persistence or spread of herpes simplex lesions should prompt an investigation of the patient's ability to mount an immune response.

In addition to herpes, syphilis must also be considered in the differential diagnosis of ulcerative lesions. Aphthous oral ulcers may be a sign of extraintestinal inflammatory bowel disease or rheumatologic diseases, such as Behçet or Reiter syndrome. Adolescence is a time when systemic manifestations of these chronic conditions often become apparent. Because such signs may be the first manifestations of chronic disease, clinicians must remain keep these diagnoses in mind, especially in the face of atypical or persistent (>2 weeks in duration) ulcerative disease (see Chapter 86).

Issues in the dental and oral care of adolescents include traumatic injury to the teeth, adequate dental hygiene and prophylaxis, the use of smokeless tobacco products, and the onset of periodontal disease. Thus, the primary care provider has an important role to play in promoting appropriate dental hygiene, including brushing and the use of preventive dental services. Like the counseling regarding other preventive health behaviors, the recommendations for dental care are important in that health habits adopted during the teenage years are likely to persist throughout adulthood. Screening for injury and tobacco exposure, counseling about the use of protective helmets and mouth guards during sports, and recommendations about smoking cessation are essential in primary care practice. Adolescents with bulimia nervosa and some patients with anorexia nervosa who vomit are at risk for dental erosion; regurgitated gastric acid may dissolve tooth enamel and dentin on the lingual surface of the teeth.

During adolescence, the third molars ("wisdom teeth") erupt, and these may require extraction. Additionally, gingivitis and gum hypertrophy occasionally develop in female adolescents, similar to the gingivitis seen during pregnancy. This inflammation, which may occur in response to oral contraceptives, is believed to be caused by a combination of local and hormonal influences. Although a condition that arises spontaneously may persist for years, cases caused by oral contraceptive use generally resolve when the additional hormone is withdrawn. Therapy consists of frequent oral hygiene and removal of plaque.

Respiratory and Environmental Conditions

The lung volume and alveoli grow throughout adolescence, corresponding to increases in the height and other dimensions of the thorax. Asthma remains a highly prevalent disease, affecting more than 5% of children and adolescents; nearly half of these patients have some functional impairment in their ability to perform normal daily activities. Although many school-age children with asthma become symptom-free during adolescence, 60% to 70% of these adolescents exhibit airway hyperreactivity when challenged, and many adults with reactive airway disease first became symptomatic during adolescence. The incidence of asthma and the rate of subsequent death from asthma have risen in recent decades. Exercise-induced asthma, which also often starts in adolescence, may present with cough or shortness of breath in addition to wheezing. The condition of girls is less likely to improve during adolescence, and the female-to-male ratio for asthma changes from 1:3 to 1:1 between childhood and adulthood (see Chapter 55).

Exposure to particulate and chemical toxins, including cigarette and marijuana smoke, pollution, and occupational dust and chemical fumes, may increase during adolescence. All these exposures irritate the lungs and may destroy lung tissue. Passive exposure to environmental smoke and sniffing glue or other inhalants may also exacerbate reactive airway disease. Thus, appropriate screening and history taking and counseling regarding protective measures should be part of routine primary care. Similar consideration should also be given to the dermatologic and systemic manifestations of occupationally or environmentally mediated diseases. Some chemical exposures (e.g., petrochemicals, solvents) can cause pneumonia, aspiration, pulmonary edema, and death. Occupational medicine and toxicology consultations, available in many centers, may be appropriately used by primary care providers to evaluate harmful vocational or recreational exposures and take action to reduce them.

Once a patient reaches the stage of mild persistent reactive airway disease (symptoms 3–6 days per week or 3 to 4 nights per month), a daily inhaled corticosteroid becomes the long-term therapy of choice. Long-acting bronchodilators, such as salmeterol, and leukotriene modifiers, such as monteleukast or zafirlukast, are newer long-term oral therapies that may be used in addition to inhaled steroid medication. Exercise-induced asthma is treated with a short-acting β-agonist or inhalation of a mast cell stabilizer (e.g., cromolyn sodium) 15 minutes before exercise or a long-acting β-agonist the morning of exercise. The mainstays of acute asthma management still consist of inhaled short-acting β-agonists, inhaled anticholinergics, and oral steroids.

Current therapeutic interventions for asthma should include explicit algorithms for home medication use so that patients do not overestimate their margin of safety with regard to respiratory failure. Understanding how adolescents comply with the long-term use of medication and adapt to chronic illness is also key in the successful management of asthma during adolescence.

In patients with cystic fibrosis, several issues are affected by puberty. First, pubertal development and menarche are often delayed by several years. Second, their appearance (clubbed fingers, barrel-shaped chest, cachexia) and behaviors (coughing, sputum production, foul-smelling stools, frequent hospitalizations) may make social integration with peers difficult. Third, up to 20% of girls with cystic fibrosis are fertile, and their average life expectancy is now well into the third decade. Contraception must be addressed in sexually active girls with cystic fibrosis because pregnancy is likely to worsen pulmonary function. Information about the effects of other risky health behaviors on the adolescent's pulmonary status should also be provided, along with routine preventive health counseling.

Cardiovascular Diseases

The growth and sexual maturation of puberty result in a variety of changes in the cardiovascular system. The heart rate slows and the stroke volume, cardiac output, and blood pressure gradually increase to adult levels. Because physical size is important to these physiologic measurements, it is necessary to use age- and gender-referenced norms (Fig. 10.8).

The risk for coronary artery disease is well established by adolescence, and the first visible lesions of atherosclerosis often appear during the second decade of life. High-fat diets, inactivity, and smoking are the major causes of preventable cardiovascular mortality in the United States. Other risk factors include obesity, hyperlipidemia, hypertension, and diabetes mellitus. Even though these risk factors may be genetically determined, modifications of diet and activity clearly benefit adolescents in regard to both immediate health effects (e.g., smoking cessation, weight reduction) and long-term cardiovascular risk reduction. Many providers manage adolescents with high cholesterol and triglyceride levels; nutritional consultation is often helpful in promoting healthful dietary and exercise habits.

Sudden cardiac death, although rare, is of concern to families and schools, in part because it tends to occur during vigorous exercise. Most of these deaths are caused by hypertrophic cardiomyopathy. Less commonly, they are caused by a congenital coronary artery anomaly, an arrhythmia (most often prolonged

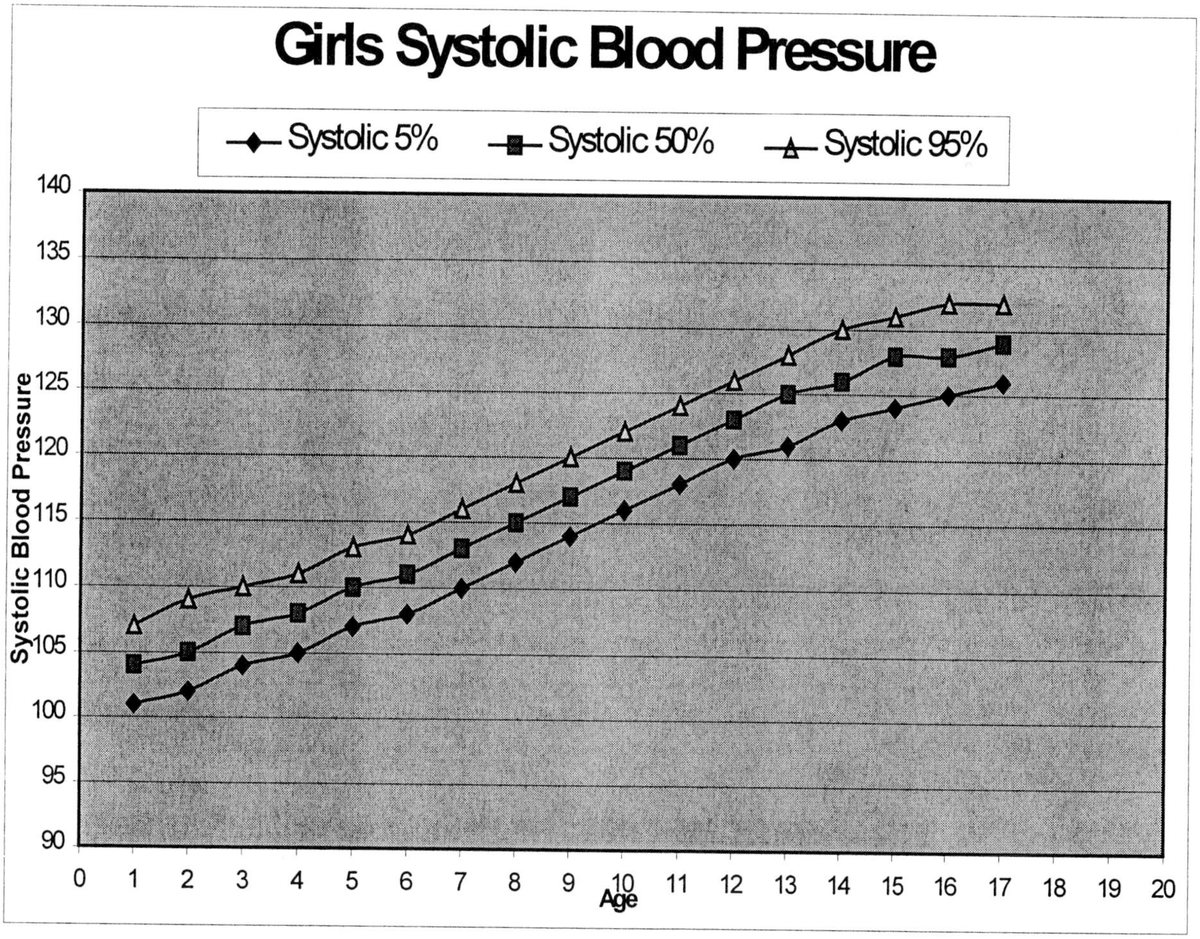

FIG. 10.8. Systolic blood pressure in girls. (Adapted from Bickley LS. *Bates' guide to physical examination and history taking,* 8th ed. Philadelphia: Lippincott Williams & Wilkins, 2002.)

QT syndrome), or preexisting structural cardiac disease. Screening by history and physical examination is recommended. Adolescents with a prior history of cardiovascular disease or syncope, a family history of cardiac or unexplained sudden death, or a potentially pathologic murmur should be referred to a pediatric cardiologist for a comprehensive evaluation.

Relatively few congenital or acquired cardiac defects are first detected during puberty. However, primary care providers increasingly share in caring for adolescents and young adults who have undergone repair of a congenital cardiac lesion. The management of endocarditis prophylaxis, exercise restriction, family planning, and psychosocial adjustment should be coordinated with the patient's cardiologist.

Heart murmurs are caused by turbulent blood flow. The timing, location, and other characteristics of heart murmurs are determined by their anatomy. Most heart murmurs in female adolescents arise from turbulent flow in an anatomically normal heart. However, no diastolic murmurs are normal. Normal systolic murmurs include pulmonary ejection murmurs (heard best during midsystole at the second left intracostal space with radiation to the axilla); pulmonary souffle murmurs (also heard best at the second left intracostal space, especially in states of high cardiac output, as a soft, midsystolic murmur without radiation); venous hums (heard above the clavicle only with the patient in an upright position); and Still murmurs, which are soft, short, musical or vibratory ejection murmurs heard over the precordium. Adolescents with murmurs that do not fall into one of these categories should be evaluated by a cardiologist.

Mitral valve prolapse is one of the cardiac conditions often detected during adolescence. The mid-late systolic click of mitral valve prolapse is common in normal adolescents and young adults, noted in fewer than 2% of children and in about 20% of persons by the third decade of life. The high-pitched or honking murmur of mitral valve regurgitation is also relatively common. Mitral valve prolapse is three times more common in women than in men and is most often diagnosed in tall, slender women. It is associated with Marfan syndrome and connective tissue disorders. Thus, adolescents who have murmurs consistent with mitral valve prolapse must be evaluated for these conditions. The major differential diagnosis of a midsystolic click is normal splitting of the first heart sound.

A cardiology referral is indicated, as is echocardiography, to assess the extent of mitral regurgitation. The electrocardiographic findings are normal in more than 80% of patients and are significant only for nonspecific T-wave changes in those with positive results. Because the risk for bacterial endocarditis is increased 10 times in persons with mitral regurgitation, endocarditis prophylaxis is indicated for adolescents with mitral valve prolapse. Additionally, arrhythmias are somewhat more common in adolescents with mitral valve prolapse, although they remain relatively rare overall. In controlled studies, chest pain and panic and anxiety attacks were not found to be more frequent in persons with mitral valve prolapse than in controls.

Hematologic Conditions

Puberty causes an increase in hemoglobin and red cell volume, especially in boys (testosterone directly stimulates erythropoiesis). Boys ages 12 to 14 years have an average hemoglobin concentration of 14 g/dL, with an increase of 1 g/dL through age 18 and another 1 g/dL after age 18. Although the hemoglobin concentration does not increase dramatically in girls, the mean corpuscular volume increases in both boys and girls from 84 fL to the adult value of 90 fL. During puberty, because of menstrual blood loss, the dietary iron requirements for girls increase.

Some mild disorders of bleeding escape detection until adolescence. As many as 20% of adolescent girls with severe menorrhagia presenting at menarche have a primary coagulation disorder (most often von Willebrand disease; see Chapter 90).

Iron deficiency anemia is not uncommon among adolescents, especially menstruating girls. The total body iron represents a balance between dietary intake and gastrointestinal absorption and excretion. Iron is lost through the skin and stool at a rate of approximately 0.75 mg/d. Girls also lose an average of 0.6 mg/d in menstrual blood. In contrast, the average intake of dietary iron is 10 to 12 mg/d, of which approximately 10% is absorbed. Because many adolescent girls do not consume a diet rich in heme iron (e.g., meat), iron deficiency anemia may develop. Athletes are at particular risk because losses are increased during sweating and by physical red cell damage and hematuria during exercise.

As many as 20% to 30% of adolescent girls are thought to have an iron deficiency without frank anemia. Fewer have symptoms of lethargy and decreased exercise tolerance. Mild iron deficiency generally presents as a normocytic anemia and reduced serum ferritin level. Later, a more typical microcytic anemia develops, with elevated free erythrocyte protoporphyrin, increased iron-binding capacity, and decreased serum iron. The differential diagnosis of iron deficiency anemia includes the hemoglobinopathies and the anemia of chronic disease.

The treatment of iron deficiency anemia includes replacing the body iron stores and treating any abnormal source or rate of ongoing blood loss. Ferrous sulfate in a dose that provides 6 mg of elemental iron per kilogram per day is generally recommended for symptomatic iron deficiency. Absorption is facilitated by taking the iron with orange juice. Although the reticulocyte count rises within days and the hemoglobin level rises by 0.5 to 1.0 g/dL per week, therapeutic doses are recommended for 2 to 3 months to replenish the body iron stores. Doses of 2 mg/kg per day are recommended for prevention in patients with known blood loss or low intake of iron.

Megaloblastic anemias are uncommon among adolescents, although they occasionally take medications (e.g., oral contraceptives, anticonvulsants) that can interfere with folate absorption. However, because folate deficiency has been associated with congenital anomalies (including neural tube defects), folate supplementation is recommended before conception and during early pregnancy for adolescents and young adults. Because many pregnancies during adolescence are unplanned, some authorities recommend routine multivitamin use by women. Vitamin B_{12} deficiency is rare except among people maintaining a strict vegetarian diet (see Chapter 89).

Endocrine Conditions

Graves disease and autoimmune (chronic lymphocytic or Hashimoto) thyroiditis are the most common causes of hyperthyroidism and hypothyroidism, respectively, during adolescence. Behavioral changes may be part of the initial manifestation of thyroid disease. Similarly, growth failure, weight loss or gain, and amenorrhea or menorrhagia may be part of the presentation of thyroid dysfunction in young women. Hypothyroidism may also present as depression in adolescents and as precocious puberty or precocious thelarche in younger girls. Providers should consider thyroid hormone abnormalities when approaching patients with generalized problems, examine patients for thyroid bruits or goiter, and determine the thyroid hormone and thyroid-stimulating hormone levels as indicated in the evaluation of adolescents with most systemic illnesses (see Chapter 34).

TABLE 10.3. Causes of Delayed Adolescence in the Phenotypic Male and Female

Hypergonadotropic conditions
Variants of ovarian and testicular dysgenesis
Gonadal toxins (antimetabolite and radiation treatment)
Enzyme defects (17α-hydroxylase deficiency in the genetic male or female and 17-ketosteroid reductase deficiency in the genetic male)
Androgen insensitivity (testicular feminization)
Other miscellaneous disorders
Hypogonadotropic conditions
Multiple tropic hormone deficiency
Isolated growth hormone deficiency
Isolated gonadotropin deficiency
Miscellaneous syndrome complexes (e.g., Prader-Willi syndrome)
Systemic conditions, nutritional and psychogenic disorders, increased energy expenditure
Other endocrine causes: hypothyroidism, glucocorticoid excess, hyperprolactinemia
Constitutional delay in growth and development
Eugonadotropic conditions: delayed menarche
Gonadal dysgenesis variants with residually functioning ovarian tissue
Abnormalities of müllerian duct development
Polycystic ovary disease
Hyperprolactinemia

Source: Updated from McAnarney ER, Kreipe RE, Orr D, et al. *Textbook of adolescent medicine.* Philadelphia: WB Saunders, 1992, with permission.

Most cases of complete congenital adrenal hyperplasia are diagnosed in early childhood. However, the diagnosis of partial enzyme deficiencies causing milder endocrine disturbances is often delayed until adolescence. The most common of these disorders is 21-hydroxylase deficiency, which results in excess levels of 17-hydroxyprogesterone. Some patients are asymptomatic; more typically, signs of androgen excess are seen, including hirsutism, premature growth of pubic hair, advanced bone age, and accelerated growth. These symptoms may be difficult to differentiate from those of polycystic ovarian syndrome, or Stein-Leventhal syndrome (see Chapters 35 and 37).

Delayed puberty in women is generally defined as the absence of breast development by age 13 or the absence of menstrual periods by age 16 (Table 10.3). However, these statistical norms mean that maturation begins in about 2.5% of girls outside this age range. In constitutional delay, puberty is delayed but the woman is otherwise normal. The most common cause of hypergonadotropic hypogonadism is gonadal dysgenesis. Thus, determination of the karyotype, in addition to the FSH and LH levels (and in younger girls the bone age), should be part of an initial evaluation for pubertal delay. Carefully reviewing the growth history, plotting and assessing the height and weight and growth velocity, and examining the anatomic structures are also important. The workup should include a sedimentation rate to help rule out a chronic illness such as Crohn disease; 30% to 40% of cases of Crohn disease present during adolescence. Nutritional compromise, chronic illness, malignancies and their treatment, and infectious disease are also relatively common causes of pubertal delay.

Diabetes

Although diabetes is not unique to adolescents, several challenges arise during adolescence that can make diabetes control difficult. (Many of these issues apply to all young persons with chronic disease.) For example, dietary compliance may become more difficult when medical regimens conflict with peer group behaviors, especially as young people begin to take responsibility for their own management, independently of their parents' or family's role. Thus, adolescents must learn to think ahead and adjust their insulin appropriately for dietary and exercise changes. Additionally, as young people become capable of formal operational thought and assume direct control of the management of their diabetes, they may realize in a new way that their condition is permanent. This realization may result in denial, anger, and other stages of mourning for a loss of normalcy. Although such adjustments to chronic disease are normal, adolescents, their families, and their health care providers should anticipate conflicts and may need help in managing the adjustment period.

In addition to the adjustment of a developing adult to a chronic disease, pregnancy and alcohol use pose special risks for diabetics. Nephropathy and retinopathy are more likely to develop during pregnancy in women whose diabetes is poorly controlled. Additionally, congenital anomalies are much more common in the infants of diabetic mothers whose sugar is poorly controlled. Alcohol use can affect glucose metabolism, causing an initial rise in blood glucose levels, followed by a drop. Alcohol also enhances the glucose-lowering effects of insulin and prolongs its effect for up to 8 to 36 hours after consumption, thereby increasing the risk for hypoglycemia. Because of these serious potential effects, adolescents should be counseled about the effects of alcohol on their blood sugar. The American Diabetes Association recommends that alcohol should be consumed only if diabetes is well controlled, that drinking should be in moderation (no more than two drinks once or twice a week), and that insulin doses need not be changed.

Others recommend that adolescents avoid high-carbohydrate beverages (i.e., beer) and consume foods with complex carbohydrates, protein, and fat while drinking to provide excess glucose during the period when their glucose-regulatory mechanisms may be impaired (see Chapter 39).

Eating Disorders

Eating disorders (see Chapter 149) affect up to 5% of female adolescents and young adults, resulting in medical, psychological, and social dysfunction. Because the symptoms of an eating disorder may cause a young woman to visit (or cause her parents to bring her to) a primary care provider, practitioners must be able to recognize, evaluate, and initiate appropriate treatment and, when necessary, make a referral for more intensive treatment.

Anorexia nervosa is a syndrome in which caloric intake insufficient to maintain weight is associated with a delusion of being overweight and an obsession to be thinner, neither of which diminishes with weight loss. Patients with anorexia nervosa truly believe they are fat, even when emaciated (delusion). Likewise, they are driven to lose weight (obsession) through a variety of means (compulsions), including dieting and enhancing caloric output. The primary method of increasing caloric output is exercise, used by more than 75% of patients; vomiting and cathartics are less common means. A feature that differentiates simple dieting from anorexia nervosa is the difficulty that an anorexic person has in identifying, or being satisfied with, a healthful weight goal. Affected persons relentlessly pursue thinness; thus, they repeatedly lower their goal weight as they continue to lose weight. Anorexia may result in severe malnutrition.

The key clinical feature of bulimia nervosa is binge eating (not, as is often assumed, vomiting). Awareness that the pattern of binge eating (ingesting large amounts of food within a short interval) is abnormal leads to depressed moods and self-deprecating thoughts. Temporary relief of the distress precipitated by a binge is sought through means intended to rid the body of the effects of calories; more than 80% of patients with bulimia nervosa engage in self-induced vomiting or laxative or diuretic abuse for this purpose. Fasting or exercise also may be used to avoid weight gain, but many patients with bulimia nervosa remain at normal to slightly above normal weight. Patients with bulimia are more likely than those with anorexia nervosa to be impulsive in regard not only to eating behavior but also to the use of drugs and alcohol, self-mutilation or self-harm, sexual promiscuity, lying, stealing, and other manifestations of personality disturbance.

Anorexia nervosa and bulimia nervosa are not mutually exclusive diagnoses. Approximately 40% of patients with anorexia nervosa exhibit a bulimic phase during the course of their illness or recovery. Binge-eating disorder is also common in young adult women and is not associated with significant medical morbidity other than weight gain, but it is associated with emotional distress.

Regardless of how well a patient may appear, a detailed physical examination is indicated whenever eating problems are a concern. For example, because of the recent availability of low-fat or nonfat foods and new food-labeling laws, some adolescents limit their intake of fat to unhealthful levels, often to less than 10 g/d. Signs noted during the physical examination can be used as evidence that the patient is unhealthy. The presence of an organic condition, such as inflammatory bowel disease, thyroid disease, or a central nervous system lesion, must also be ruled out.

In patients with eating disorders, the serum protein and albumin levels are generally normal. The serum liver enzymes may be mildly elevated (up to two times normal values). The cholesterol levels are often elevated, sometimes dramatically, in states of starvation. Some practitioners also routinely perform thyroid screening; when the results are abnormal, the triiodothyronine level is usually low, a means of reducing the metabolic rate when the caloric intake is small. In these patients, the clinical picture typically suggests both hypothyroidism (fatigue, constipation, bradycardia, hypothermia) and hyperthyroidism (weight loss, excessive activity, anxiety), but the treatment for the symptoms is healthful nutrition and weight gain. The other endocrinopathy suggested by a constellation of weight loss, fatigue, and a small heart is Addison disease; the serum cortisol level tends to be high in anorexia nervosa, however. An electrocardiogram may be useful to determine the nature of profound bradycardia.

Overweight

An increasing proportion of adolescents in the United States are physically unfit and overweight. Up to 14% of adolescents were considered overweight in 1999. The term *overweight* is preferred to *obesity* because of the potential negative social connotations of the latter. Based on the 2000 growth charts of the Centers for Disease Control and Prevention, being "at risk" for overweight is defined as having a body mass index (BMI)-for-age between the 85th and 95th percentiles. Overweight is defined as a BMI-for-age at or above the 95th percentile. The BMI is the weight in kilograms divided by the height in square meters (kg/m^2). Standard growth charts for plotting the BMI from height and weight are available from the Centers for Disease Control and Prevention, Maternal and Child Health Bureau (MCHB), and other sources.

Normal puberty in girls is associated with at least a doubling of the percentage of body weight that is fat. Thus, increases in weight in female adolescents must be interpreted in the light of pubertal development, exercise patterns, and body composition. However, overweight during childhood and adolescence occurs at least three times more often in girls than in boys, especially those of low socioeconomic status, and is more likely to persist into adulthood. Medical consequences of overweight include hyperlipidemia, glucose intolerance, hepatic steatosis, cholelithiasis, hypertension, and early maturation. Overweight children and adolescents are at increased risk for adverse health consequences later in life, including cardiovascular disease and premature death.

The primary cause of most female adolescent obesity is a combination of excessive caloric intake and inadequate expenditure of energy in exercise. Ready access to high-fat, calorically dense fast foods and snacks, together with an increasingly sedentary lifestyle, accounts for numerous cases of adolescent obesity. Furthermore, pregnancy among some adolescents is associated with weight gain that is not lost postpartum. Depressed moods, low self-esteem, and feelings of inadequacy are also common in obese female adolescents, although the cause-and-effect relationship is unclear.

In an evaluation of weight gain in early adolescence, it is important also to chart changes in height. Exogenous obesity, in which excessive calories account for the increase in weight, is characterized by an increase in height; endocrine causes of obesity are marked by growth retardation rather than acceleration. Recent evidence underscores the importance of genetic influences; however, environmental influences also play a major role in obesity. Thus, even if the patient has a family history of obesity, it is still prudent to institute effective weight management practices.

An adolescent identified as being overweight requires an in-depth medical evaluation and weight management program. When an adolescent is identified as being at risk for overweight, the physician should obtain a thorough family history and determine the blood pressure and total cholesterol level. If any of these are abnormal, the patient requires a complete medical evaluation, with weight management initiated right away. Otherwise, the patient can be screened again 1 year later. An in-depth medical evaluation consists of a medical, family, and dietary history, an assessment of physical activity, a psychological assessment, a physical examination, and laboratory studies.

A weight loss program is indicated for adolescents who are overweight or at risk for overweight with medical complications. For those who are markedly overweight (BMI >35) or have health consequences such as hypertension or hyperlipidemia, weekly weight loss of up to 1 to 2 lb is recommended.

It is difficult to treat obese female adolescents successfully (Table 10.4). Early adolescents may be especially difficult to treat because they lack motivation. Food is often used as a source of comfort or as a reward; its ready availability ensures immediate gratification. Diets may be seen as restrictive, punitive, or controlling. If a parent institutes limitations in caloric intake without the active participation of the adolescent, she may interpret this as rejection by the parent. Such circumstances often lead to surreptitious eating and acting out. On the other hand, permissive parents often find it onerous to restrict their daughter's intake, perceiving such behavior as uncaring, even when the adolescent herself wants to lose weight. Thus, even though a primary care provider may recognize the value of weight loss for medical or psychosocial reasons (Table 10.5), it is best not to institute definitive therapy until the younger adolescent and at least one of her parents are interested in change. For older adolescents, individual motivation may be sufficient. Regardless, it is best to provide information about ways to control weight in a nonthreatening and nonjudgmental manner.

TABLE 10.4. Evaluation of the Overweight Adolescent Patient

History
Family history: obesity and stature, endocrine problems, psychiatric problems
Past medical history: serious illnesses, surgery, menarche, sexual developmental history
History of obesity: abrupt onset versus chronic history, physical or developmental problems at time of rapid weight gain
Dietary history: 24-hour diet recall; review of eating habits, including timing and circumstances of meals and snacks, history of previous weight loss attempts
Physical activity history: exercise, television, video games, Internet, transportation to and from school
Social history: family, school, and individual stressors, especially at times of rapid weight gain
Psychological assessment: self-esteem, depression, anxiety
Physical examination
Anthropometrics: height, weight, body mass index
Sexual maturity rating
Vital signs, including blood pressure taken with cuff of appropriate size
Complete physical examination for causes of secondary obesity and complications of obesity
Laboratory tests
Routine screening with cholesterol and triglyceride levels
Endocrine studies only if suggested by history or physical examination findings
Estimate of basal metabolic rate sometimes helpful

Source: Updated from McAnarney ER, Kreipe RE, Orr D, et al. *Textbook of adolescent medicine.* Philadelphia: WB Saunders, 1992, with permission.

Treatment for obesity is often viewed as futile, but primary care providers can use many effective strategies to help overweight adolescents adopt healthful lifestyles. "Dieting: the best way to gain weight" is a popular aphorism that underscores the importance of changing eating habits and patterns rather than dieting, which may be viewed as restraining and limiting. Unfortunately, adolescents and young adults are bombarded by advertisements that promise quick, effortless weight loss through dieting programs of dubious value. No scientific evidence has substantiated most of the claims of these diets or formulas. Diets alone rarely lead to healthful, sustained weight loss.

Rather than prescribing a diet, the primary care provider should help the adolescent learn to make nutritional choices that are balanced, healthful, sustainable, and enjoyable (Table 10.6). Thus, preprinted diets are of less value than an exchange system of meal planning, in which the patient can choose from a wide variety of foods that will meet her daily preferences and requirements while also allowing her to control her weight in a healthful manner.

Weight reduction programs that do not include an increase in physical activity are doomed to failure. School buses, escalators, elevators, and remote control devices are all conveniences that reduce physical activity. Adolescents trying to lose weight should be encouraged to seek ways to burn calories in their activities of daily living. In addition, they should be involved in a regular exercise program for at least 20 minutes a day, 3 to 5 days a week.

Although intensive, multicomponent interventions are effective in some populations, little evidence is available to indicate that group weight loss programs or drugs that induce anorexia are useful in adolescents. Ephedra, a compound found in many over-the-counter diet pills, should especially be discouraged

TABLE 10.5. Complications of Overweight

During adolescence
Psychosocial
Disturbed body image
Poor self-image/self-esteem
Poor family relations: scapegoat and source of embarrassment
Poor peer relations and social isolation
Exclusion from activities, especially dating
Acting out and depression
Medical
Potentially lethal
Obstructive sleep apnea, pickwickian syndrome
Pancreatitis
Heart failure from cardiomyopathy
Less severe
Cardiovascular: hypertension
Endocrine: early maturation, pseudogynecomastia
Gastrointestinal: hepatic steatosis, cholelithiasis
Orthopedic: slipped capital femoral epiphysis, coxa vara, Perthes disease, ankle fracture, genu valgum
Metabolic: hyperlipidemia, glucose intolerance
Skin problems: candidal infections, breakdown
Neurologic: pseudotumor cerebri
Increased risk for adult obesity
During adulthood
Psychosocial
Job discrimination
Others as during adolescence
Medical
Cardiovascular disease: hypertension, hypercholesterolemia, diabetes mellitus, coronary artery disease, cerebrovascular disease (increased with "android" fat distribution), premature death
Cancer: endometrial, breast, prostate, colon
Orthopedic: gouty and degenerative arthritis
Genitourinary incontinence, male sexual dysfunction
Surgical: increased operative morbidity and mortality

Source: Updated from McAnarney ER, Kreipe RE, Orr D, et al. *Textbook of adolescent medicine.* Philadelphia: WB Saunders, 1992, with permission.

because of its association with cardiac toxicity. Current efforts to decrease the weight of adolescents concentrate on prevention at the community level, such as changes in school lunch options, removal of soda machines from schools, and increased opportunities to join local physical fitness clubs (see Chapter 4).

TABLE 10.6. Principles of Healthful Eating

Use the Food Pyramid (6–11 servings of bread, cereal, rice, or pasta; 3–5 servings of vegetables; 2–4 servings of fruit; 2–3 servings of milk, yogurt, or cheese; 2–3 servings of meat, dry beans, eggs, or nuts as sources of protein; sparse use of oils, fats, and sweets) to plan the daily intake.
Avoid "good food"/"bad food" dichotomies that can lead to unhealthful, monotonous choices and feelings of guilt when a "bad" food is ingested.
Spread daily intake evenly over three well-balanced meals plus one or two snacks.
Recognize breakfast as the most important meal of the day.
Reduce intake of calories gradually and not excessively.
Consider how foods are prepared, in addition to their intrinsic caloric content and density.
Combine reduction of caloric intake with increase in caloric expenditure through regular, moderate exercise.
Accept small weight losses.
A number of these goals can be more easily achieved within a behavior modification system that increases motivation and rewards appropriate actions.

Menstrual Cycle Disorders

Menstrual periods begin relatively late in puberty, usually during Tanner stage 4 (Figs. 10.2, 10.3). The normal menstrual cycle averages 28 days, with a range of 21 to 35 days. Adolescents often have even longer cycles, especially during the first 2 years of menstruation (see Chapter 11). A negative effect of estradiol on the hypothalamus and pituitary is present throughout infancy and childhood. However, a positive effect of estrogens on the pituitary, with a resultant surge in LH, develops in middle to late puberty. Positive feedback increases as the hypothalamus becomes decreasingly sensitive to negative feedback during early puberty. However, without positive feedback, ovulation does not occur. Thus, ovulation is often irregular for several years after menarche, and most young women have a mixture of ovulatory and anovulatory cycles. Many early adolescent cycles are a consequence of negative feedback and the cyclic production of gonadotropin and estrogen, and many of them are anovulatory. In fact, 28- to 42-day cycles of FSH and LH hormone levels occur in pubertal girls even before menarche. During these anovulatory periods, the stimulation of ovarian hormonal activity may result in physiologically normal ovarian enlargement and multiple cyst formation. Dysmenorrhea may become significantly worse after a few years of menstrual cycles as predominantly ovulatory cycles develop in a young woman.

The spectrum of menstrual irregularity in young women ranges from frequent, prolonged bleeding to complete amenorrhea. Although the most common cause of amenorrhea or abnormal uterine bleeding is pregnancy, this can be diagnosed easily. Primary care providers should be aware of the high likelihood of anovulatory cycles during puberty and should be familiar with the diagnosis and management of menstrual disorders.

Persistent stimulation of the endometrium by estrogen, in the face of inadequate LH to induce ovulation, may present as short cycles, excessive bleeding, oligomenorrhea, or amenorrhea. In contrast, a low-estrogen state, secondary to a lack of gonadotropin stimulation or end-organ unresponsiveness (ovarian failure), results in an atretic uterine lining and amenorrhea. Amenorrhea in young women may also be a consequence of severe underweight or abnormal body composition resulting from chronic illness, poor nutrition, or excessive exercise. These conditions probably suppress the release of GnRH from the hypothalamus; thus, amenorrhea may also develop during high levels of stress or in response to drugs. Amenorrhea presenting with galactorrhea is likely caused by a prolactinoma, elevated prolactin levels secondary to drugs (including phenothiazines, cocaine, and marijuana), or pregnancy.

Another common pattern of menstrual irregularity is associated with androgen excess. Generally, estrogen levels are normal or high, but the gonadotropin levels do not fluctuate normally, LH levels are quite high, and the ratios of LH to FSH exceed 3:1. These patients appear hirsute and obese. Some present with premature pubic hair and acne, occasionally a consequence of mild 21-hydroxlase deficiency or another adrenal cause of androgen excess. However, most present with hirsutism, acne, and accelerated weight gain during puberty without any enzymatic deficiency. When associated with oligomenorrhea, these symptoms characterize Stein-Leventhal syndrome, or polycystic ovarian syndrome. The differential diagnosis of amenorrhea and obesity in adolescents also includes adrenocorticoid excess (both endogenous and exogenous) and hypothyroidism. However, hypothyroidism may also present as excessive menstrual bleeding, especially later in puberty (see Chapters 34 and 36).

The management of irregular menses in adolescents requires an accurate history and a careful physical examination. Menstrual calendars may help with regard to bleeding, hormonally related cyclic changes, and other symptoms. For example, anovulatory bleeding is usually painless and not accompanied by the breast soreness or cramps often associated with ovulatory cycles. A review of the patient's developmental and sexual history should be obtained. The history should include sexual activity, chronic illness, congenital anomalies, herniorrhaphy (which suggests an XY karyotype), radiation, central nervous system insult, and drug exposure.

The examination should include a careful evaluation for the developmental stage, hirsutism, galactorrhea, and the genital anatomy. Estrogenization of the vaginal introitus should be assessed; this can be quantified by Papanicolaou fixation of a vaginal smear. Enlargement of the clitoris suggests androgen excess. The vagina should be examined either digitally or with a cotton-tipped applicator, and a bimanual vaginal or rectal examination should be performed to assess the uterine size and adnexa. Laboratory studies should include measurement of the urinary β-human chorionic gonadotropin level to rule out pregnancy, thyroid function tests, and measurement of the serum LH, FSH, and prolactin levels. Often, a progestin challenge with 10 mg of medroxyprogesterone (Provera) per day for 10 days or 20 mg/d for 5 days is sufficient to induce menses and diagnose anovulatory cycles in a nonpregnant amenorrheic patient. If an LH-to-FSH ratio greater than 3:1, hirsutism, or other signs of androgen excess are present, the androgen levels should also be measured. In patients with polycystic ovaries, low-progestin oral contraceptives allow regular cycles and lower the androgen levels. The results of studies of metformin in adolescents with polycystic ovarian syndrome also appear promising. Weight control is an important component of therapy. Oral contraceptives are often the treatment of choice for excessive dysfunctional uterine bleeding (see Chapter 15), dysmenorrhea (as a first-line therapy for sexually active teens, and as a second choice after nonsteroidal antiinflammatory drugs for women who are not sexually active; see Chapter 17), and premenstrual syndrome.

Orthopedic Conditions and Sports-Related Injuries

Scoliosis, or lateral curvature of the spine, is a common problem during adolescence. Because it is not specific, the screening examination for scoliosis in school settings generates many unnecessary referrals. However, regular screening in primary care practice is indicated.

A screening examination for scoliosis is performed by first observing the young woman from behind to look for asymmetric shoulder height, a prominent scapula, unequal arm-to-trunk length, asymmetric hip height, or palpable lateral curves of the spine. The patient should next be asked to bend forward from the waist with her palms opposed and her elbows straight. Elevation of one scapula is characteristic of scoliosis; the right scapula is elevated in 95% of cases. Patients should also be observed closely for asymmetry of the chest wall or lumbar area.

Scoliosis is usually idiopathic, or it may be caused by neuromuscular disease, a congenital anomaly, a congenital injury, or an intraspinous process. The significance of scoliosis depends on the location and degree of the curvature. The severity of scoliosis is determined by radiologic evaluation. In general, nonprogressive and painless curves of less than 25 degrees do not require active treatment. Curves of more than 25 degrees, in addition to all curves accompanied by pain or neurologic symptoms, should be referred to an orthopedic surgeon for further evaluation. Scoliosis tends to progress most rapidly during the growth spurt, or SMR 2 and 3 in girls. Thus, adolescents should be monitored as frequently as every 3 months during this period of rapid growth. Bracing prevents curves of more than 30 degrees from progressing but does not eliminate a preexisting curve. Curves of more than 40 degrees generally progress into adulthood, and surgery is often required to halt progression.

Although relatively rare, slipped capital femoral epiphysis almost always occurs during the adolescent growth spurt. Rapid growth, obesity, trauma, inflammatory diseases, and genetic factors all play a role in this condition. Most cases are subacute, with limping and mild intermittent pain the most common presenting symptoms. The physical examination findings include pain on motion and limited internal rotation and abduction of the affected hip; the leg preferentially is held flexed and externally rotated. The limp is typically a Trendelenburg gait caused by weak hip abductors on the affected side. A high index of suspicion, an accurate radiographic diagnosis (anteroposterior and frog leg lateral views), and rapid fixation to prevent further slipping and, if needed, realign the trochanter and the femoral head are indicated to minimize the risk for avascular necrosis and degenerative joint disease.

The greatest risk factor for a sports injury in an adolescent is a prior significant sports injury. Several organizational guidelines have addressed sports participation examinations, and a model form is shown in Fig. 10.9. The goals of these examinations are to detect potentially life-threatening conditions and previous or incompletely rehabilitated injuries and to direct developing athletes into activities that maximize their opportunity for performance while minimizing their risk for injury. This evaluation should not take the place of regular routine well care, and the sports physical can be combined with regular preventive service visits without jeopardizing the importance of the pre-participation safety assessment.

Primary care physicians often are called on to assess sports injuries. Most injuries are sprains, strains, or contusions and can be managed initially with rest, ice, compression, and elevation (RICE). Injuries that should be evaluated by an orthopedist include those associated with rapid or obvious swelling, a popping or snapping noise at the time of occurrence, anatomic deformity, limited range of motion, neurovascular compromise, or joint instability.

Rheumatologic Conditions

The most common rheumatologic conditions affecting adolescents are rheumatoid arthritis, systemic lupus erythematosus, and dermatomyositis. Caring for patients with these conditions should involve consultation with experts in pediatric rheumatology (see Chapters 83 and 94).

The most common form of chronic arthritis in adolescent girls is pauciarticular rheumatoid arthritis. This condition, which affects fewer than five joints, usually begins between the ages of 12 and 16 years. Patients are generally well except for asymmetric inflammation of the larger joints of the lower extremity, most often the knee. If only one joint is inflamed, septic arthritis, particularly with *Neisseria gonorrhoeae,* must be considered in the differential diagnosis. Antinuclear antibody (ANA) is used as a marker of an increased risk for uveitis and iridocyclitis, unrelated to the extent of pauciarticular joint involvement. Thus, female adolescents with pauciarticular arthritis who are ANA-positive should have an eye examination annually, regardless of the activity of joint inflammation. HLA-B27 is associated with this form of arthritis in fewer than 10% of girls.

Polyarticular arthritis is characterized by symmetric inflammation in at least five joints, usually the smaller ones of the hands and feet, wrists, and elbows. Positivity for rheumatoid factor is found in only 10% to 15% of cases of juvenile polyarticular arthritis; it is more common in girls and is associated with the onset of progressive joint destruction at a median age of 12 years. Rheumatoid factor-negative disease, on the other hand, is usually marked by exacerbations and remissions, and patients have a good long-term prognosis.

The management of adolescents with juvenile arthritis consists of medications (systemic, intraarticular, or both), physical therapy, and supportive therapy; surgery may be required for destructive forms. Nonsteroidal antiinflammatory drugs are the primary medications used, although low-dose systemic corticosteroids can be a very effective short-term adjunctive. Cytotoxic medications and cyclosporine also have a place in the treatment of juvenile arthritis but should be prescribed only by those familiar with their use.

Systemic lupus erythematosus is a multisystem disease with protean manifestations, sparing no organ. Females are affected five times more often than males, with the onset commonly at puberty. A familial predisposition to lupus has been noted, and HLA loci associated with the disease include Al, B8, and DR3. ANA positivity, the presence of various antinuclear subunit antibodies (particularly anti-Ro and anti-La), and an elevated erythrocyte sedimentation rate are highly sensitive but not specific for the diagnosis. Up to half of adolescents with lupus present with primarily behavioral or psychiatric manifestations. Long-term management can be difficult because of the chronic nature of the illness and the prominence of mental health problems.

Juvenile dermatomyositis is an inflammatory myopathy characterized by vasculitis of the skin and skeletal muscles. A female predominance is noted during adolescence. HLA loci DR3 and B8 are associated with dermatomyositis. A light, violaceous, scaling, mildly edematous "heliotrope" rash usually affects the eyelids. Scaling, erythematous to violaceous papular lesions are generally found over the interphalangeal joints, elbows, knees, and malleoli and may progress to become thickened, smooth, and shiny (Gottron patches). Muscle involvement is primarily proximal, and the heart is involved rarely. In about 25% of affected female adolescents, complications develop in the gastrointestinal tract, joints, or skin (calcinosis cutis). Treatment involves aggressive physical therapy to preserve range of motion and strength, together with systemic corticosteroids and, in resistant cases, immunosuppressive therapy.

Neurologic Conditions

Seizures, nonepileptic paroxysmal disorders, multiple sclerosis, myasthenia gravis, and Wilson disease are among the neurologic conditions that may present in adolescence. All these conditions require close coordination of care by the primary care provider and neurologist (see Chapters 105, 111, and 115).

Epilepsy is a symptom complex defined as recurrent, episodic paroxysms (seizures) that develop when the cerebral cortex and gray matter are activated. Seizures may be caused by tumors, metabolic disturbances, or infection, but they are often idiopathic. The location and the pattern of spread of activity determine the clinical expression. Few forms of epilepsy begin in adolescence, but epileptic seizures may worsen during adolescence because of hormonal changes (especially in relation to the menstrual cycle), changes in the metabolism of anticonvulsant medication during puberty, or failure to comply with treatment because of psychosocial conflicts. These may include hav-

Part C – PHYSICAL EXAMINATION RECORD

NAME ____________ DATE ________ AGE ________ BIRTHDATE ____________

Height ________ Vision: R ______/______, corrected ______, uncorrected ______

Weight ________ L ______/______, corrected ______, uncorrected ______

Pulse ________ Blood Pressure ____________ Percent Body Fat (optional) ____________

	Normal	Abnormal Findings					Initials
1. Eyes							
2. Ears, Nose, Throat							
3. Mouth & Teeth							
4. Neck							
5. Cardiovascular							
6. Chest and Lungs							
7. Abdomen							
8. Skin							
9. Genitalia - Hernia (male)							
10. Musculoskeletal: ROM, strength, etc.							
a. neck							
b. spine							
c. shoulders							
d. arms/hands							
e. hips							
f. thighs							
g. knees							
h. ankles							
i. feet							
11. Neuromuscular							
12. Physical Maturity (Tanner Stage)		1.	2.	3.	4.	5.	

Comments re: Abnormal Findings: ____________

PARTICIPATION RECOMMENDATIONS:

1. No participation in: ____________
2. Limited participation in: ____________
3. Requires: ____________
4. Full participation in: ____________

Physician Signature ____________

Telephone Number ____________ Address ____________

American Academy of Pediatrics

A

FIG. 10.9. Pre-participation sports screening examination form, 1990. Parts **A** and **B** show both sides of form. (Courtesy of the American Academy of Pediatrics.)

SPORTS PARTICIPATION HEALTH RECORD

This evaluation is only to determine readiness for sports participation. It should not be used as a substitute for regular health maintenance examinations.

NAME ______________________ AGE ________(YRS) GRADE ________ DATE ________

ADDRESS ______________________ PHONE ________

SPORTS ______________________

The Health History (Part A) and Physical Examination (Part C) sections must both be completed, at least every 24 months, before sports participation. The Interim Health History section (Part B) needs to be completed at least annually.

PART A — HEALTH HISTORY:
To be completed by athlete and parent

	YES	NO
1. Have you ever had an illness that:		
a. required you to stay in the hospital?	____	____
b. lasted longer than a week?	____	____
c. caused you to miss 3 days of practice or a competition?	____	____
d. is related to allergies? (ie, hay fever, hives, asthma, insect stings)	____	____
e. required an operation?	____	____
f. is chronic? (ie, asthma, diabetes, etc)	____	____
2. Have you ever had an injury that:		
a. required you to go to an emergency room or see a doctor?	____	____
b. required you to stay in the hospital?	____	____
c. required x-rays?	____	____
d. caused you to miss 3 days of practice or a competition?	____	____
e. required an operation?	____	____
3. Do you take any medication or pills?	____	____
4. Have any members of your family under age 50 had a heart attack, heart problem, or died unexpectedly?	____	____
5. Have you ever:		
a. been dizzy or passed out during or after exercise?	____	____
b. been unconscious or had a concussion?	____	____
6. Are you unable to run 1/2 mile (2 times around the track) without stopping?	____	____
7. Do you:		
a. wear glasses or contacts?	____	____
b. wear dental bridges, plates, or braces?	____	____
8. Have you ever had a heart murmur, high blood pressure, or a heart abnormality?	____	____
9. Do you have any allergies to any medicine?	____	____
10. Are you missing a kidney?	____	____

11. When was your last tetanus booster? ________

12. **For Women**
   a. At what age did you experience your first menstrual period? ________
   b. In the last year, what is the longest time you have gone between periods? ________

EXPLAIN ANY "YES" ANSWERS ________

____

____

____

I hereby state that, to the best of my knowledge, my answers to the above questions are correct.

Date ________

Signature of athlete ________

Signature of parent ________

PART B — INTERIM HEALTH HISTORY:
This form should be used during the interval between preparticipation evaluations. Positive responses should prompt a medical evaluation.

1. Over the next 12 months, I wish to participate in the following sports:
   a. ________
   b. ________
   c. ________
   d. ________

2. Have you missed more than 3 consecutive days of participation in usual activities because of an injury this past year?
   Yes ________ No ________
   If yes, please indicate:
   a. Site of injury ________
   b. Type of injury ________

3. Have you missed more than 5 consecutive days of participation in usual activities because of an illness, or have you had a medical illness diagnosed that has not been resolved in this past year?
   Yes ________ No ________
   If yes, please indicate:
   a. Type of illness ________

4. Have you had a seizure, concussion or been unconscious for any reason in the last year?
   Yes ________ No ________

5. Have you had surgery or been hospitalized in this past year?
   Yes ________ No ________
   If yes, please indicate:
   a. Reason for hospitalization ________
   b. Type of surgery ________

6. List all medications you are presently taking and what condition the medication is for.
   a. ________
   b. ________
   c. ________

7. Are you worried about any problem or condition at this time?
   Yes ________ No ________
   If yes, please explain: ________

____

____

____

I hereby state that, to the best of my knowledge, my answers to the above questions are correct.

Date ________

Signature of athlete ________

Signature of parent ________

B

FIG. 10.9. *(continued).*

ing a chronic illness with few visible manifestations, undesirable side effects of medications, limit testing of persons in authority, fear of losing control during a seizure, and being unable to participate in activities, especially driving.

Syncope and hyperventilation are two common nonictal paroxysmal disorders in female adolescents. A prodrome is associated with each, which may be followed by secondary epileptic phenomena. Therefore, the history of events immediately before the attacks must be sought. Syncope is characterized by malaise, vertigo, lightheadedness, and blurring or fading of vision, followed by a loss of postural tone and passing out; pallor and limpness are often noted by witnesses. Hyperventilation causes similar lightheadedness and blurring of vision, but patients also characteristically report perioral paresthesias and a tingling sensation in the fingertips (see Chapter 48).

Multiple sclerosis, the most common demyelinating disease in adolescent girls, is an immune-mediated disorder characterized by the gradual development of demyelination and scarring in the white matter in multiple central nervous system sites. The differential diagnosis includes idiopathic optic neuritis, acute disseminated encephalomyelitis, the inherited leukodystrophies, and the collagen-vascular diseases. Most adolescents with multiple sclerosis experience well-delineated exacerbations and remissions, with complete or nearly complete recovery, but a few have a severe, rapidly progressive form of the disease. Although no definitive cure is available, treatment consists of symptomatic management in combination with various immunomodulators.

Myasthenia gravis is an immunologically mediated disorder of the neuromuscular junction that results in episodic or progressive skeletal muscle weakness. Juvenile myasthenia is more common in girls than in boys and is associated with acetylcholine receptor antibodies. The insidious onset of weakness of the ocular, facial, and oropharyngeal muscles is characteristic; patients often report ptosis or diplopia, and symptoms tend to worsen late in the day or during stress or fatigue. Generalized muscle weakness, if it occurs, progresses slowly. The intravenous administration of edrophonium chloride (Tensilon) generally results in an abrupt improvement in strength and provides a presumptive diagnosis. Almost all adolescents respond, at least initially, to treatment with cholinesterase inhibitors.

Wilson disease, an autosomal-dominant condition resulting from an inborn error of copper metabolism, often presents in adolescents with tremor, chorea, dystonia, and dysarthria. Because of behavioral abnormalities, it may initially be mistaken for a primary psychiatric condition. The deposition of copper in the cornea produces the pathognomonic Kayser-Fleischer ring, which is always present when neurologic symptoms are evident. The diagnosis is confirmed by the findings of an excessive copper concentration and a decreased ceruloplasmin level in the blood.

Psychological Conditions

Among the many mental health issues important in the care of women, two are particularly relevant to primary care practice: depression and somatoform disorders.

Depression in older adolescents presents much as it does in adults, with sadness, depressed mood, sleep disturbances, anhedonia, and other vegetative (or agitated) symptoms. However, during early and middle adolescence, depression may present in a masked form and be hard to differentiate from oppositional or behavioral problems. In young adolescents in particular, depression often does not present as sadness but as boredom, irritability, aggression, or acting-out behavior. As adolescents mature, their increasing cognitive ability makes it possible to think about thinking, and thus to express sadness and manifest more adult-like depressive symptoms (see Chapter 145).

Many adolescents experience transient depression. As many as 25% to 66% of adolescents report feeling sad or depressed. However, younger adolescents with depression may report boredom as their only symptom. In 1999, 20% of high school students reported having seriously considered suicide, and 8% actually attempted suicide. Many of these youths never received medical or mental health care after their attempts. Major depression is defined by either a depressed mood or a loss of interest or pleasure in nearly all activities for at least 2 weeks. The prevalence of major affective disorders in adolescents has been estimated at 4% to 6%. Although bipolar disease is much rarer that depressive illness, the peak period for the onset of bipolar disease is between ages 15 and 25. The differential diagnosis of depression includes depressed mood resulting from a social condition, such as bereavement, or a medical condition, such as hypothyroidism or substance abuse.

Adolescents who attempt or complete suicide present to primary care providers in the 2- to 4-week period before their attempt, often with vague or nonspecific complaints. Thus, systematic and careful screening for depressed mood and suicidality is an important part of adolescent primary care practice. A mildly depressed mood or occasional suicidal thoughts without specific intent are normal, and adolescents can be reassured and informed of the availability of resources should they require more intensive counseling. Most primary care providers should be comfortable in diagnosing and treating depressive illness and in managing first-line pharmacologic therapy with selective serotonin reuptake inhibitors (fluoxetine, sertraline, paroxetine, citalopram). The use of these medications is reviewed in Chapter 145. Tricyclic antidepressants are given less often as first-line agents because of the risk for overdose and subsequent cardiotoxicity. Primary care providers should have crisis services available so that adolescents at high risk for self-destructive behaviors can be assessed by mental health professionals without delay.

The somatoform disorders include a variety of conditions in which the physical symptoms are attributed to emotional or psychological factors. These disorders are often considered when an adolescent's symptoms suggest a medical problem but her history, physical examination findings, and laboratory studies do not support an organic cause, so that a psychological basis is presumed. The somatoform disorders are often classified as conditions in which the symptoms are under voluntary control (malingering and factitious disorders) and those in which the symptoms are involuntary (somatization disorder, conversion disorder, hypochondriasis). The professional providing primary care to female adolescents must avoid common pitfalls in approaching the diagnosis and management of these disorders.

In clinical practice, it is usually countertherapeutic to label the cause of symptoms as organic or psychological and the symptoms as voluntary or involuntary. The rare patient with malingering or factitious disorder generally seeks care from other sources after her diagnosis is discovered. The vast majority of female adolescents in primary care with somatoform disorders first have symptoms as part of an organic process (e.g., a viral illness or trauma), but then the symptoms persist or gradually change as the organic process subsides. They seek care because their symptoms are not under their control and interfere with their daily activities. Thus, attempts to determine whether the symptoms are voluntary are met, understandably, with resistance and frustration. Making the diagnosis by exclusion ("I can't find anything wrong. Your symptoms must be caused by psychological problems") rarely is accepted because it implies that the symptoms are imaginary or being feigned. Referral to a mental health provider, although possibly worthwhile, is usually rejected because the symptoms are experienced somatically and are not "all in her head."

Perhaps the best example of the futility of diagnosing a somatoform disorder by exclusion is adolescent dysmenorrhea. In the early 1970s, a reputable pediatric publication described the cause of adolescent dysmenorrhea as "psychogenic." A decade later, that same publication reported that dysmenorrhea was caused by increased and irregular myometrial pressure related to prostaglandin levels. In the intervening decade, the knowledge of menstrual physiology had increased; in the absence of knowledge, psychogenic causes had been presumed. The absence of proof of organic causation does not rule out organic pathology. Thus, symptoms should be assumed to be involuntary unless proven otherwise. Finally, if psychological conflict is discovered while a patient is being evaluated, it should be acknowledged and addressed, whether or not it is causally related to the presenting symptoms.

When an adolescent girl with a somatoform disorder is approached, communication during the evaluation is part of the intervention; active listening is essential on the part of the primary care provider. A dichotomous, "rule out" approach is counterproductive. When the patient seems disappointed to learn that "all the tests are normal," this does not necessarily mean she wants to play the sick role (factitious disorder). More likely, she may interpret negative test results as evidence that her symptoms either are not being taken seriously or cannot be relieved.

A functional pathophysiologic explanation is needed and should be based on data obtained during the evaluation. For example, tension headaches in the temporal region are best attributed to sustained contraction of the temporalis and masseter muscles. To emphasize this, it is often helpful to have the patient bite down hard while placing her fingers on the temporal region. The palpable movement of the painful area as her affected jaw and scalp muscles contract demonstrates the biologic substrate of her pain.

The examiner should identify any concomitant developmental or psychological problems during the evaluation rather than attempt to identify psychological "causes" of the symptom. Often, a family member has a similar problem, so it is essential to include the family in the treatment program.

Finally, primary care providers can institute face-saving therapies in an attempt to relieve the symptoms. These can include physical therapy, biofeedback, and attention to adequate sleep, nutrition, and exercise. The use of a symptom journal can be effective in documenting the conflicts that may be related to the symptoms. Additionally, seeing these patients regularly (regardless of symptoms), examining them at each visit, and performing only those laboratory tests indicated by the physical findings help to limit unnecessary testing and often allow for recovery over time.

BIBLIOGRAPHY

American Medical Association. *Guidelines for adolescent preventive services*. Chicago: American Medical Association, 1992.

Emans SJ, Goldstein DP. *Pediatric and adolescent gynecology*, 4th ed. Boston: Little, Brown, 1998.

McAnarney ER, Kreipe RE, Orr DP, et al. *Textbook of adolescent medicine*. Philadelphia: WB Saunders, 1992.

Neinstein LS. *Adolescent health care: a practical guide*, 4th ed. Philadelphia: Lippincott Williams & Wilkins, 2002.

U.S. Congressional Office of Technology Assessment. *Adolescent health*. Washington, DC: U.S. Congressional Office of Technology Assessment, 1991: OTA-H-468.

WEB SITE RESOURCES

For Health Care Providers

American Medical Association Adolescent Health On-Line: www.ama-assn.org/ama/pub/category/1947.html.

Centers for Disease Control and Prevention Adolescent Health State of the Nation: www.cdc.gov/nccdphp/dash/ahson/ahson.htm.

Konopka Institute for Best Practices in Adolescent Health, University of Minnesota: http://allaboutkids.umn.edu/konopka.

National Eating Disorders Association: www.nationaleatingdisorders.org.

For Patients and Families

American Social Health Association Teen Health Information: www.iwannaknow.org.

Children's Hospital Boston, The Center for Young Women's Health: www.youngwomenshealth.org.

Children's Medical Center of Atlantic Health System Teen Health Information: www.teenhealthFX.com.

Girls Incorporated (national nonprofit organization that provides education to young women): www.girlsinc.org.

CHAPTER 11

The Reproductive-Age Woman

Phyllis C. Leppert

For more than half her life, a woman is physiologically capable of bearing children. In North America, the physiologic reproductive age extends, in general, from ages 12 to 55 years. However, this entire period is not optimal for childbearing. The best time for reproduction is between the ages of 20 and 29 years; the outcomes of pregnancy in women younger than 20 years and in their 30s or older are not as successful. A U-shaped curve describes pregnancy outcome by age, with the least desirable and more complicated pregnancies occurring in young teens and in women ages 35 and older.

In addition to the physiologic readiness to conceive and bear healthy children, women of reproductive age face the social and psychological aspects of pregnancy, birth, and child rearing. Human infants are extremely dependent at birth, and human childhood is long compared with that of other species. At a fundamental level, a woman needs a partner in the process of child rearing. All human societies have understood this fact and have stressed within their cultures the importance of the family unit. The family unit often comprised not only biologic parents and children but also grandparents, aunts, uncles, and other kin. This basic unit reinforced the importance of the social and economic support of women in their reproductive role. In modern society, the need for social and economic support continues.

Modern society has presented challenges to women and families. More than anything else in the lifetime of women living in the last half of the 20th century, modern methods of contraception have contributed to their ability to develop roles in the world beyond motherhood. This change has come about as a consequence of the scientific understanding of reproductive biology. All forms of contraception, including and especially natural family planning, are based on the tremendous scientific advances in reproductive biology that have been made during the past 50 years or so. Without a fundamental scientific understanding of the complexities of the menstrual cycle and ovulation, modern contraception would not be possible. In this essential way, modern women owe a great deal to the basic sciences, which have advanced reproductive health and thus the general health of women. Since 1900, the number of pregnancies each woman has in a lifetime has declined. Also, the number of children born to each woman has decreased. Therefore, reproductive-age women have been freed from the stress of endless pregnancies and childbearing without rest between children. These changes have enhanced women's health overall and allowed them to pursue education and careers in addition to motherhood.

Pregnancy and lactation cause numerous physiologic and psychological alterations, but they also protect women from certain diseases, such as breast cancer. Lifestyle issues, including the more sedentary behavior of our times, contribute to some of the diseases women acquire. The environmental pollution of industrial societies is also associated with the development of disease.

Despite changes in societal roles and lifestyle, women still link their general health and well-being with their reproductive health. Given the centrality of reproductive hormones in female physiology, this attitude is inevitable. As long as a woman is actively menstruating, pregnancy is possible, and this physiologic fact creates a sense of psychological vulnerability in many women. Modern women need to assimilate the facts of reproductive physiology into their lives and accept them. Unfortunately, some women tend to embrace pregnancy and motherhood for its own sake, often at an inappropriate point in their lives. Conversely, some modern women assume an unbalanced view toward motherhood and ignore their reproductive potential. Others tend to delay childbearing and do not realize that such delay has health consequences for them and their children. Thus, physicians who provide primary care to women must guide each patient toward an integrated and "appropriate for her" approach to reproduction and reproductive health. Such an integrated approach does not negate the role of a woman's reproductive health in her total health and well-being, nor does it mean that all women should be mothers. It means simply that all women ought to be encouraged to discern the right decision for them regarding pregnancy and birth in a responsible manner.

THE MENSTRUAL CYCLE

For a reproductive-age woman, menstruation is a central reality, and the primary care provider must be knowledgeable about menstrual physiology.

Changes in the Endometrium

During the menstrual cycle, the endometrium undergoes distinct changes. Throughout the cycle, a dynamic paracrine-juxtacrine interaction takes place between the endometrial epithe-

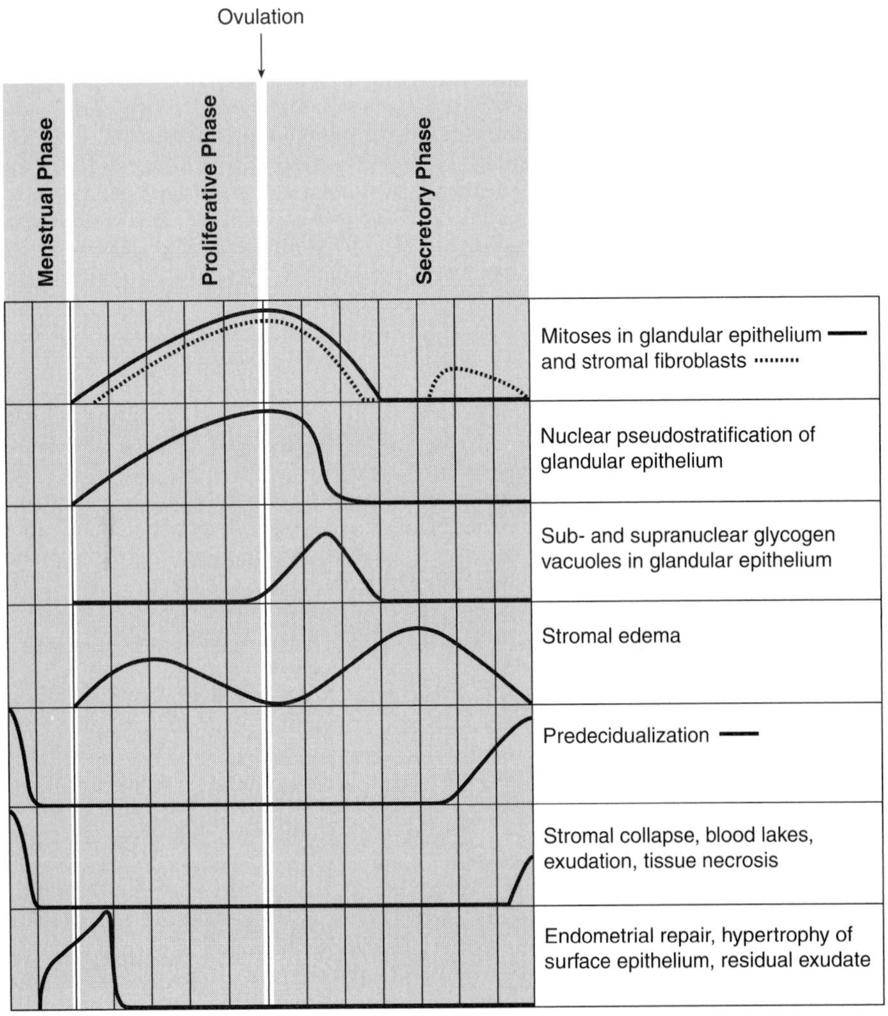

FIG. 11.1. Dating the endometrium. (Redrawn from Speroff L, Glass RH, Kase NG. *Clinical gynecologic endocrinology and infertility,* 5th ed. Baltimore: Williams & Wilkins, 1994:120, with permission.)

lium and the stroma. The first day of bleeding is customarily considered the first day of the menstrual cycle, a convention important in prescribing contraceptive pills.

The endometrial lining of the uterus consists of two layers. The upper, or functional, layer makes up two thirds of the lining, and the lower basalis layer comprises one third. The endometrium regenerates from the basalis layer after menstruation. A sequence of specific histologic and functional changes occurs within the glandular, vascular, and stromal parts of the endometrium. Five phases occur in concert with changes in the ovaries, pituitary gland, and hypothalamus. The menstrual endometrial phase occurs between days 1 and 4 of the cycle, the proliferative phase begins at day 4 or 5, and the secretory phase occurs after ovulation, followed by the implantation preparation and endometrial breakdown phases. The endometrial changes throughout the 28-day cycle are shown in Fig. 11.1.

MENSTRUAL PHASE

During the menstrual phase, the endometrial tissue contains fragmented blood vessels and disarrayed and broken glands. Stromal necrosis, white cell infiltration, and interstitial diapedesis of red cells are evident throughout the tissue, and the supporting matrix is collapsed. As much as two thirds of the functioning endometrium is lost during menstruation. A short menstrual flow is associated with rapid tissue loss, whereas flow is heavier and blood loss greater when shedding is delayed or incomplete. During endometrial shedding in a normal menstrual cycle, tissue repair takes place along with loss of the functional endometrium. The rapid growth of new epithelium is noted beginning on days 2 to 3 of the cycle. By days 5 to 6, the entire endometrium has acquired new epithelium.

PROLIFERATIVE PHASE

The proliferative phase occurs in conjunction with growth of the ovarian follicle and an increase in estrogen secretion. The endometrial glands are lined by low columnar epithelial cells and are narrow and tubular. Mitosis develops and becomes predominant in these cells, which are pseudostratified. The glandular epithelium extends, and the glands become linked with adjacent glands. The endometrial stroma is densely cellular during the menstrual phase. For a brief time, it is edematous, and at the end it becomes a loose, syncytium-like tissue. Blood vessels course through the stroma. The spiral arteries extend in an unbranched manner to just below the epithelial binding membrane, where they form a loosely organized capillary network. The proliferative phase peaks at day 8 to 10; a marked increase in mitotic cytoplasmic RNA synthesis is followed by maximal intranuclear concentrations of estrogen and progesterone receptors at midcycle, just before ovulation.

SECRETORY PHASE

An early sign of ovulation is the appearance of glycogen vacuoles in the glandular epithelium. These are seen in the subnuclear intracytoplasmic compartment of the glandular cells. The nuclear membranes unfold under the influence of progesterone into a nucleolar channel system.

The tissue continues to grow, but because it is confined to a fixed area, the glands become increasing tortuous, with progressively intense curling of the spiral cells. Glycoproteins and peptides are secreted into the endometrial cavity. The secretions also contain a plasma transudate. Circulating immunoglobulins are secreted into the endometrial cavity by an epithelial binding protein. Seven days after the midcycle surge in gonadotropin, secretory activity peaks. If conception occurs, the peak secretory activity coincides with implantation of the blastocyst.

IMPLANTATION PHASE

Implantation is thought to occur on days 20 to 24. Marked changes take place in the endometrium. At the beginning of this phase, the secretory glands appear tortuous, with very little stromal tissue between them. Three separate zones develop in the endometrium. One fourth of the endometrial tissue is basalis, which contains straight blood vessels and spindle-shaped stroma. The middle zone, which makes up half of the endometrium, is the stratum spongiosum, a lacelike layer composed of loose, edematous stroma and tightly coiled, densely packed spiral vessels and ribbons of exhausted glands. Pinopods replace the microvilli of the luminal epithelium. These domelike structures exist for less than 48 hours. They develop between days 20 and 22, with variations seen in individual women. Over the spongiosum is the stratum compactum, which comprises the remaining fourth of the endometrial tissue. In this layer, the stromal cells are large and polyhedral and compress one another. The glands in this area are compressed, and the subepithelial capillaries and spiral vessels are prominent and engorged. Receptors for estrogen and progesterone during this phase are located in the walls of the endometrial blood vessels. The enzymes necessary for prostaglandin synthesis are within the muscle walls and endothelium of the endometrial arterioles.

If a pregnancy occurs, the stromal cells are transformed into decidua, producing a multitude of hormones and growth factors. They secrete prolactin, relaxin, renin, insulin-like growth factor, and insulin-like growth factor binding proteins. Decidual cells are derived from primitive uterine mesenchymal stem cells. The process of deciduation begins in the late luteal or implantation phase under the influence of progesterone. Eighty-four percent of successful implantations occur on days 22 to 24 of the cycle.

ENDOMETRIAL BREAKDOWN PHASE

If conception, implantation, and secretion of human chorionic gonadotropin (hCG) from the trophoblast do not ensue, the corpus luteum dies, and the estrogen and progesterone levels fall. By day 25, the upper compactum layer is transformed. The stroma secretes proteases (matrix metalloproteases) that help degrade the endometrium. Tissue necrosis, vascular thrombosis, and extravasation of red blood cells take place. The matrix metalloproteases degrade the extracellular matrix and basement membrane.

As the estrogen and progesterone levels begin to fall, the height of the tissue shrinks, blood flow within the spiral vessels decreases, venous drainage decreases, and vasodilation occurs. The spiral arterioles rhythmically constrict and relax. The spasms become progressively longer, leading finally to endometrial blanching, ischemia, and stasis. Red blood cells escape into the interstitial space 24 hours before the onset of menstruation. White cells migrate into the tissue, and the prostaglandin content in the secretory endometrium peaks. Thrombin platelet plugs appear in the vessels. Finally, breaks develop in the superficial arterioles and capillaries. New thrombin platelet plugs are formed. Tissue breakdown continues. The endometrium shrinks further, and the coiled spiral arteries are compressed and buckled. Thus, ischemic breakdown progresses. A cleavage plane between the basalis and spongiosum is breached, and the spongiosum desquamates and collapses. Menstrual flow then ceases as the consequence of a combination of vasoconstriction, tissue collapse, vascular stasis, and estrogen-stimulated repair and clot formation over the stumps of the endometrial spiral arterioles. The basalis endometrium remains, and repair originates from this layer.

Menstrual flow consists of red blood cells, inflammatory exudate, proteolytic enzymes, and functionalis that has undergone autolysis.

Ovarian Changes

The menstrual cycle is divided into a follicular and a luteal phase. The average or typical cycle is said to be 28 days, although the cycle length varies considerably both between women and within the same woman. The follicular phase is more variable; the luteal phase is more constant in duration, lasting 13 to 15 days.

FOLLICULAR PHASE

During the follicular phase, a new group of primordial follicles begins to grow and develop. These follicles have been "recruited" during the luteal phase of the preceding menstrual cycle, when a number of antral follicles (2 to 4 mm in diameter) are active. An aromatase activity develops in the antral follicles that is stimulated by follicle-stimulating hormone (FSH). The follicles, usually three to five in number, form the cohort of follicles that develop during the next follicular phase. FSH stimulates growth of the follicular granulosa cells and the conversion of androgens in the granulosa cells into estrogen. Thus, concentrations of 17β-estradiol increase during the follicular phase.

During the first 5 days of the menstrual cycle, a selection process occurs. Only one of the three to five FSH-stimulated follicles from the previous luteal phase grows to become the preovulatory graafian follicle. Vascularization and blood flow increase in this follicle. The rising concentration of estradiol in the follicle increases the sensitivity of the follicular granulosa cells to FSH as the number of FSH receptors increases. Over time, the dominant follicle secretes sufficient estradiol to elevate peripheral estradiol concentrations. When this happens, FSH secretion is suppressed, and the nondominant follicles stop growing. As the follicular phase continues, the dominant follicle grows to a diameter of 10 to 20 mm, its final size. As a result, the secretion of estradiol increases exponentially. The sharp increase in estrogen (Fig. 11.2), causes the glandular endometrium to proliferate. The rise in estrogen also causes an increase in the secretion of cervical mucus in which viscosity is decreased and the pH increased. Cornification of the vaginal smear occurs at this time. These changes are the basis of a simple, indirect test of normal ovulation.

Peak estradiol secretion is associated with follicular maturation and signals the readiness of the reproductive tract for ovulation to the brain and the pituitary gland. Estrogen stimulates a surge in the gonadotropins luteinizing hormone (LH) and FSH. The surge persists for 1 to 2 days and leads to the final stage of follicular maturation. The high concentrations of gonadotropins arrest granulosa cell growth and secretory activity. As the granulosa cells stop growing, estradiol secretion abruptly ceases. LH induces theca luteinization, with a small preovulatory rise in progesterone. Follicle rupture and ovulation occur 24 to 36 hours after the beginning of the LH and FSH surge (Fig. 11.2). At the time of ovulation, the first meiotic division is completed, and a secondary oocyte has formed.

LUTEAL PHASE

The luteal phase is characterized by major changes in the dominant follicle. Shortly after the LH and FSH surge, secretory activity in the granulosa cell stops. The basal lamina is invaded by capillaries of the theca interna. A new structure, the corpus luteum, forms. The corpus luteum secretes both progesterone and 17β-estradiol. Progesterone dominates the luteal phase. Changes in the reproductive tract occur in preparation for the potential implantation of a fertilized ovum. Secretory activity increases in the endometrial glands, and the cervical mucus becomes thick and viscous. Progesterone affects the hypothalamic thermoregulatory center, and the basal body temperature rises (Fig. 11.2).

The corpus luteum matures 8 to 9 days after ovulation. Midway through the luteal phase, the levels of estradiol and pro-

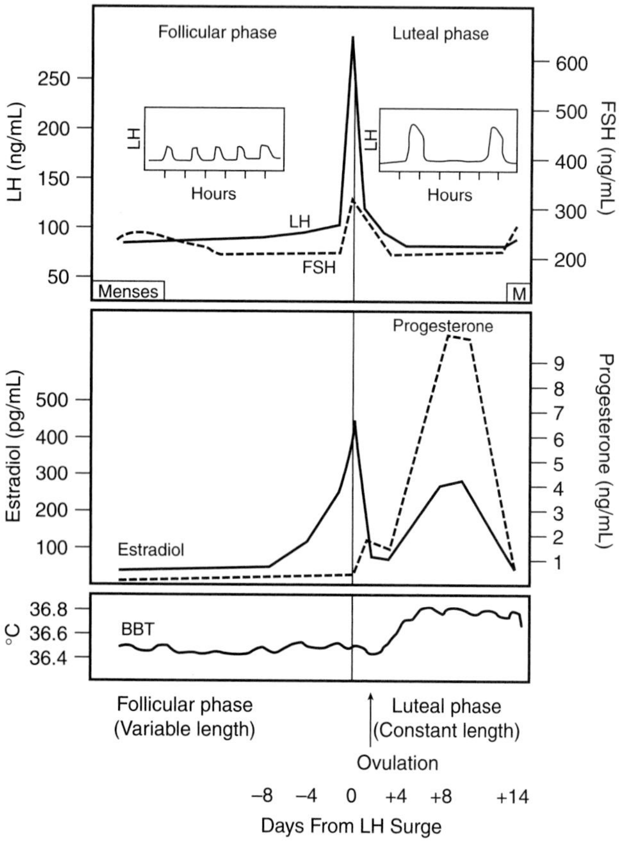

FIG. 11.2. The human menstrual cycle. (Redrawn from Speroff L, Glass RH, Kase NG. *Clinical gynecologic endocrinology and infertility,* 5th ed. Baltimore: Williams & Wilkins, 1994, with permission.)

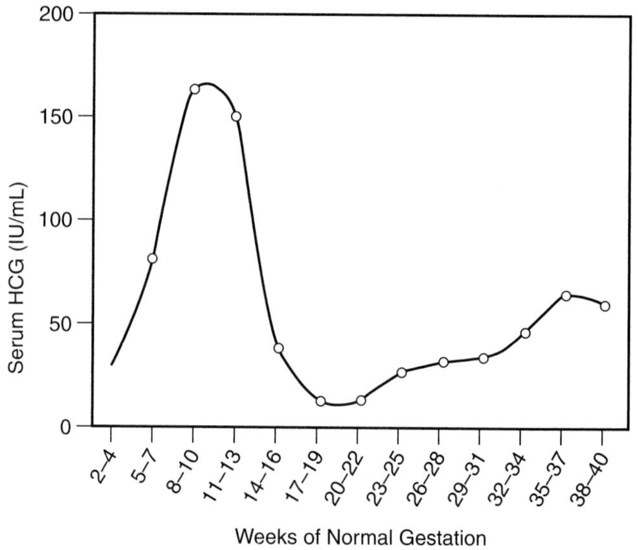

FIG. 11.3. Fluctuation of serum levels of human chorionic gonadotropin during normal intrauterine gestation. (Redrawn from Speroff L, Glass RH, Kase NG. *Clinical gynecologic endocrinology and infertility,* 5th ed. Baltimore: Williams & Wilkins, 1994, with permission.)

gesterone decrease. Thus, menstruation follows ovulation by 13 to 15 days. When and if a pregnancy occurs, hCG extends the life of the corpus luteum and maintains the secretion of estrogen and progesterone (Fig. 11.3). In nonfertile cycles, luteolysis occurs. A decrease in luteal hormonal secretion is followed by an increase in FSH.

Hormonal Changes

The endometrial and ovarian changes are under the control of positive and negative feedback from the reproductive hormones. As in other endocrine systems, the major form of feedback is inhibitory. Estradiol and progesterone secreted by the target organ, the ovary, inhibit the secretion of gonadotropin-releasing hormone (GnRH) in the hypothalamus and the secretion of gonadotropins in the pituitary gland. This is the negative or inhibitory feedback loop. In the positive or stimulatory feedback loop, the increase in ovarian steroids increases gonadotropin secretion. In the first, negative feedback system, 17β-estradiol inhibits the secretion of gonadotropins in the anterior pituitary. Small increases in estradiol cause a decrease in gonadotropins. In the follicular phase of the menstrual cycle, the LH and FSH levels are determined by the circulating estradiol concentration (Fig. 11.2). At menopause, or after surgical removal of the ovaries, LH and FSH secretion is increased continuously.

In the second, positive feedback loop during the late follicular phase, large increases in estradiol initiate the midcycle surge in gonadotropins (LH and FSH). Experimental studies indicate that a preovulatory rise in progesterone plays an important role in the midcycle gonadotropin surge. However, large amounts of circulating progesterone inhibit the estrogen-induced LH surge.

LH and FSH are released from the anterior pituitary in a pulsatile manner (Fig. 11.2). Estradiol and progesterone affect the pulsatile release of the gonadotropins. Estradiol affects the pulse amplitude, and progesterone affects the frequency. However, over time, the estradiol negative feedback loop selectively suppresses FSH more than LH.

The secretion of LH and FSH in the anterior pituitary is regulated by the hypothalamus. Neurohormones are secreted and transported through the portal blood vessels to the anterior pituitary sinusoids. GnRH is a small protein comprising 10 amino acids. The prohormone contains 92 amino acids and is degraded before release to the decapeptide. GnRH-secreting cells are located in the arcuate nucleus of the hypothalamus. The cells extend to the portion of the hypothalamus known as the *median eminence*. Although some GnRH cells originate in the preoptic area of the hypothalamus, it appears that in women the GnRH neurons in the arcuate nucleus are the most important cells. During embryogenesis, GnRH cells originate in the olfactory placodes outside the brain and then migrate into the central nervous system. This is of interest because Kallmann syndrome (hypogonadotropic hypogonadism, delayed puberty, and anosmia) reflects a defect in the migration of GnRH cells during embryogenesis.

GnRH is secreted in a pulsatile fashion that is related to the pulsatile secretion of LH and FSH. The pulsatile mechanism of GnRH release is present at birth but is suppressed. During the prepubertal period, the pulsatile pattern of gonadotropin release begins, stimulated by the GnRH pulse-generator region of the hypothalamus. At first, the phenomenon occurs at night during sleep; in adulthood, LH secretion takes place during 24 hours. The hormone inhibin, a glycoprotein with α- and β-subunits, is present in follicular fluid and is secreted into the circulation. This hormone inhibits FSH secretion.

Declining levels of inhibin in the peripheral circulation and the type of GnRH pulse frequency that occurs at the end of the luteal phase stimulate the early rise of FSH in a new follicular phase. Thus, the menstrual cycle begins again.

Common Abnormalities of the Menstrual Cycle

Small disturbances of the feedback systems that regulate the ovary and anterior pituitary affect the menstrual cycle.

If the amount of FSH released at the end of a cycle is less than normal, follicular growth becomes difficult. As a result, the estrogen concentration is subnormal and the luteal phase short. Progesterone levels are then also low. Sometimes, a premature surge in LH halts follicular maturation. In obese women, the conversion of androstenedione to estrone in adipose and other tissue, such as skin, causes anovulation. Polycystic ovarian syndrome is characterized by irregular menses, infertility, insulin resistance, and increased androgen production (see Chapters 36 and 37). Abnormalities of the hypothalamus or pituitary gland may also cause anovulatory cycles.

The menstrual cycle can be suppressed by pituitary tumors, especially prolactin-secreting adenomas and craniopharyngiomas. Severe postpartum hemorrhage and ischemic shock are associated with Sheehan syndrome. Amenorrhea can be caused by hypothalamic tumors and by head trauma.

Hypothalamic amenorrhea is associated with poor nutrition and is associated with anorexia nervosa, stress, and strenuous exercise. Psychological stress can cause chronic amenorrhea. Anorexia nervosa is discussed in Chapter 149, amenorrhea in Chapter 16, and dysmenorrhea in Chapter 17.

Because of the complex interaction of the hypothalamic-pituitary unit, the pituitary-ovarian unit, and the positive and negative feedback regulatory systems, the diagnosis of menstrual irregularities can be challenging. Therefore, if amenorrhea persists despite treatment for 6 months, or if symptoms of headache, visual disturbances, or galactorrhea occur, referral to a specialist is necessary.

PREGNANCY

In women of reproductive age, the single most common cause of amenorrhea is pregnancy. Because pregnancy is a time of major physiologic change for women, every woman ideally should plan for pregnancy and childbearing to occur at the optimal time in her life. A woman should be as physically and psychologically healthy as possible and in a stable economic and social environment with a supportive family and friends.

Preconceptual Counseling

Because women have fewer pregnancies than in previous generations, it is essential that each child born be wanted, loved, and treasured by parents who love and support each other. This is the ideal, but of course, not all situations are ideal. The goal of preconceptual counseling, then, is to maximize the chances of a successful pregnancy outcome for each woman.

Preconceptual counseling should include the woman's family and especially her spouse or significant other. By including the others, the primary care provider emphasizes the fact that childbearing is a shared endeavor. To be a parent is a joyful privilege, but it is also a responsibility. When this responsibility is a shared one, the woman, her partner, and the child all benefit.

Preconceptual counseling includes a careful medical history that focuses on familial medical problems and the woman's past medical and reproductive history. While obtaining this information, the provider can note areas of concern and begin to educate the couple regarding health matters. One short but to-the-point remark of a physician made at the appropriate time can be a powerful agent of behavioral change toward a more healthful lifestyle. Health care providers who take care of women of childbearing age find that pregnancy and childbirth are a crucial time in a woman's life when changes to a more healthful lifestyle can be encouraged and effected.

Women contemplating pregnancy must be counseled to reach an appropriate weight, so that nutritional education is essential. Pregnancy is not a time to lose weight. Conversely, if a woman is underweight before pregnancy or does not gain enough weight during pregnancy, the outcome is usually suboptimal. Women who take 0.4 mg of folic acid per day around the time of conception significantly reduce the risk for having an infant with spina bifida.

Exercise is important and must be carried out routinely and in moderation. Many women now work outside the home, so counseling and education about diet and exercise must include strategies for the workplace. Women need to know how to select healthful foods at restaurants and workplace cafeterias. Working women should be encouraged to walk and climb stairs during their working hours. Some helpful strategies are to climb stairs rather than take elevators, and to walk outdoors at lunchtime in fair weather. Exercise and nutrition are discussed in Chapter 4.

In many health care settings, preconceptual classes are held for women contemplating a pregnancy, and many women benefit from a referral to such classes for additional information.

Before a pregnancy, a woman should stop smoking cigarettes. Cigarette smoke is responsible for more low-birth-weight infants than any drug. Because binge consumption of alcoholic beverages and the use of illicit drugs are harmful, a complete preconceptual counseling session covers these areas. It is easiest to address these aspects of education during counseling sessions. By asking questions about smoking, alcohol consumption, and recreational drug use, the health care provider can ascertain which women will benefit from referrals to other resources.

A history of genetic and congenital diseases in the families of the woman and her partner is ascertained. Genetic diseases now encompass many problems, such as colon cancer and some breast and ovarian cancers. The primary care provider must understand basic genetic concepts, but definitive counseling should be carried out by genetic centers.

As the human genome becomes better understood and the area of genetic disease more complex, large regional referral centers that serve numerous academic medical centers will be the rule. They will house vast databases, and genetic counseling based on this information will be available to persons contemplating a pregnancy. Genetic testing must be voluntary. Women older than 35 years must fully appreciate the genetic risks of pregnancy. Amniocentesis and chorionic villus sampling should be explained. Some couples with a family history of significant genetic disease elect to undergo a preimplantation diagnosis in the context of in vitro fertilization. People interpret relative risks for disease in ways that are acceptable to them in their individual circumstances, and the right of a woman and her partner to make their own choices is an important ethical consideration. The age of the potential mother should be explored. If she is a teenager, it should be pointed out that it would be advisable to wait several years. On the other hand, a woman nearing her mid-30s should be encouraged to have a child as soon as possible.

A thorough history of infectious diseases that can affect a pregnancy is obtained. Rubella vaccine is given to any woman who has not already had the disease. Past exposure to sexually transmitted disease, including HIV infection and herpes simplex, should be discussed in a matter-of-fact and nonjudgmental manner. Most women are extremely honest with their care provider regarding this history when they appreciate how important the information is to a successful outcome of childbearing. If a woman is in a profession, such as health care, in which she may acquire hepatitis B, she should be immunized rather than risk becoming infected during pregnancy.

The workplace environment should be discussed in some detail. The possibility of exposure to environmental toxic chemicals should be explored. Cigarette smoking still continues in some workplaces, so the need to avoid passive smoke should be indicated. The possibility of acquiring infectious diseases potentially harmful to an embryo or fetus during the first months of pregnancy should be mentioned. For instance, nurses working in a neonatal intensive care unit have acquired cytomegalovirus infections that have damaged a fetus. Workers in child day care centers are also exposed to infectious diseases. The aim is to help each woman determine her own particular risks, and the actual plan for dealing with these risks must be individualized. Primary care providers must be aware that for many women, work is an economic necessity.

Women in professional careers, such as medicine, law, business, and the clergy, must understand the demands their careers will place on their role as a mother. Often, these women are extremely goal-oriented and high achievers. Realistic plans for parenthood need to be part of their lives. At a preconceptual counseling session, a woman has to look at these issues and find the right solutions. She must be aware of the availability of day care facilities for infants and toddlers. Professional women do not have the option, as do women in other careers, of dropping out for several years to raise children because they lose too much career momentum. Professional musicians and others in the entertainment field face the same dilemma. Each woman makes her own choice, but these issues must be addressed.

The potential father must be a part of these discussions. His role is to maintain a caring and loving partnership throughout the pregnancy, provide emotional support and company during labor, and be a caring and dependable member of the extended family. Childbirth is a time when families can be strengthened. At a time when society seems to weaken families, it is a privilege and responsibility of health care providers, especially primary care physicians, to use childbearing as a way to strengthen the family. The patient's family may not be a traditional one, but there is always a family that can be strengthened.

It is worthwhile to recommend childbirth classes and preparation for parenthood classes as important experiences during pregnancy. Some mention of health care providers—pediatrician, family physician, pediatric nurse practitioner—for the planned-for infant is also helpful in preconceptual counseling.

Any special needs of the mother must be addressed. A diabetic should be instructed that she must have good glucose control before conception. Her eyes should be examined for retinopathy and her renal status determined. Women with chronic hypertension should be in good normotensive control. Women with this disease should not stop taking their antihypertensive medication when they conceive, nor should women with thyroid disease discontinue their thyroid medication. The goal for women with medical disease is to prevent as many complications as possible. If the primary care physician does not understand the specific risks, a referral should be made to the appropriate specialist, or a computer search can be undertaken. No physician, especially a primary care physician, can know everything and rely on memory, or even textbooks, and large data banks can be of help. Primary physicians are excellent persons to perform the initial preconceptual counseling because they know the woman and her partner best and have established some trust in an ongoing relationship.

TABLE 11.1. Planning for Pregnancy

Reproduction
Fetal growth and development
Nutrition
Exercise
Substance use or abuse (illegal drugs, alcohol, cigarettes)
Medication use (prescription, over-the-counter)
Infectious diseases (e.g., sexually transmitted diseases, HIV, rubella, toxoplasmosis)
Medical history (e.g., diabetes, hypertension)
Genetics
Environmental issues
Specific issues and concerns of men
Parenting issues
Childbirth options
Community resources

The concept of a maternity care team should be explained to the woman and her partner during preconceptual counseling. The woman's primary care provider is one member of the team, and other physicians, midwives, nurses, health educators, and nutritionists on the team are available to provide the best care for an optimal pregnancy outcome. The team approach provides an appropriate, caring, and scientifically up-to-date pregnancy experience. Each member of the team brings his or her own special expertise to the care of the childbearing woman, and the advantages of a team approach should be conveyed during the preconceptual counseling session.

Childbearing has been a central part of women's lives in the past. Although most modern women have only two or three children on average, pregnancy and birth remain an extremely important part of the total health of individual women. First, the physiologic changes of pregnancy affect all organ systems, and some of the effects are long-term. Second, if women are to maintain their modern roles and careers, the goal should be for every pregnancy to be healthy. Table 11.1 summarizes the topics that should be addressed during planning for pregnancy.

Conception and Diagnosis of Pregnancy

Classically, amenorrhea is the most significant sign of pregnancy in a healthy woman. Slight bleeding at the time of implantation can be mistaken for a menstrual period. Therefore, the woman should be carefully questioned regarding the duration and characteristics of the last episode of vaginal bleeding. This is especially important because abnormal vaginal bleeding is often associated with an ectopic pregnancy.

Other subtle signs of pregnancy are a slight tingling in the breasts, noticed especially by primigravid women. Morning sickness occurs at any time in the day, usually from weeks 4 to 14 of gestation, but only in about 50% of pregnant women. Many pregnant women describe bladder irritability in the first 12 weeks of pregnancy, usually noted as an increased frequency of urination that is not accompanied by pain or burning. Some women note skin changes of chloasma or linea nigra and a darkening of the primary areola and formation of a secondary areola of the breasts. It is not uncommon for a woman to tell her health care provider, "I just know I am pregnant. I feel pregnant." Many women feel tremendous fatigue. A careful and thorough physician does not ignore such a comment but takes it seriously and follows up with the appropriate diagnostic evaluation.

During the physical examination, classic probable signs of pregnancy can be noted (Table 11.2). In our era of accurate ultrasonography and immunologic testing for pregnancy, it is tempting to ignore these signs, but they are helpful adjunct findings and should not be overlooked.

Physical signs are important clues to the need for further diagnostic tests. Primary care providers for women must appreciate these signs, especially in a managed care environment; if they are overlooked or not appreciated, a pregnancy will not be diagnosed as soon as possible. Especially in the early weeks, not all pregnancies are normal. Ectopic pregnancies and incomplete spontaneous abortions are associated with life-threatening hemorrhage (see Chapter 20). Without immunologic tests and vaginal probe ultrasonography, these two abnormalities of pregnancy cannot be diagnosed until late in their course. When a pregnancy is suspected, an immunologic test for pregnancy should be performed. If the results are abnormal, vaginal probe ultrasonography can then usually confirm the diagnosis.

IMMUNOLOGIC TESTS FOR PREGNANCY

Immunologic tests measure hCG, which is produced by the syncytiotrophoblast of the placenta. The level of placental hCG corresponds to the level in the urine, and a characteristic pattern of hCG is seen in normal pregnancy (Fig. 11.3). The tests reliably determine pregnancy if they are performed on urine collected 14 days or more after a missed, expected menstrual period. However, hCG appears in the urine about 9 days after conception. When the hCG level is between 1,000 to 2,000 mIU/mL (first and second International Reference Preparation), a gestational sac is usually noted on vaginal probe ultrasonography. A positive test result does not confirm a viable embryo or fetus; results are also positive in women with a hydatidiform mole, invasive mole, choriocarcinoma, or blighted ovum. In women in whom ovulation has been induced, the fail-

TABLE 11.2. Signs of Pregnancy

Sign	Time of occurrence	Description
Hegar sign	6th to 12th weeks	Because of the softness of the isthmus at this stage, the two fingers of the examiner's vaginal hand almost meet the abdominal hand. The sign helps to establish the gestational age.
Jacquemier sign[a]	8th week	The vaginal mucous membrane has a blue to violet discoloration.
Osiander sign[a]	8th week onward	Increased pulsation is palpated in the lateral fornices.
Uterine signs	8th week onward	The uterus is enlarged, soft, and globular in shape.
Cervical softening	10th week	The cervix has the consistency of the lips. In nonpregnant women, it has the consistency of the tip of the nose.
Uterine souffle[a]	16th week onward	A blowing sound is heard on auscultation that is synchronous with the mother's pulse.

[a]Can also be present in other clinical circumstances.

ure to detect a gestational sac 24 days or longer after conception is evidence of an abnormal pregnancy.

The definitive diagnosis is made when fetal heart activity is noted. The most reliable method for detecting fetal heart pulsation in early gestation is real-time ultrasonography, especially when performed with a vaginal probe. Fetal movement felt by the mother is not a positive sign of pregnancy; she may be imagining movement.

Prenatal Care

The concept of antenatal care was initiated in the early decades of the 20th century as a means to prevent severe preeclampsia, eclampsia, and maternal mortality. Before the universal acceptance of prenatal care, pregnant women were urged to stay at home. Being "in the family way" was not a time to be in society. Pregnant women would see a midwife or physician infrequently, if at all. It is a tremendous achievement that prenatal care has achieved its goals, although other factors, such as the availability of blood products, good anesthesia, and improved delivery practices, have also contributed. The maternal mortality rate in 1940 was 376 deaths per 100,000 births. The pregnancy-related death rate was 10.3 per 100,000 in 1991 and 12.9 per 100,000 in 1997. Black women, older women, and women with no prenatal care are at increased risk for pregnancy-related death. The risk for pregnancy-related death is almost four times higher in black than in white women. The number of women receiving prenatal care increased in 2001. Only 1% of pregnant women during that year did not receive prenatal care.

Prenatal care was not developed specifically to prevent the poor pregnancy outcomes of low-birth-weight infants and premature delivery. This has become a modern expectation of prenatal care, with conflicting evidence regarding success. Prenatal care currently encompasses many activities. The traditional practices of weighing women, taking their blood pressure, and checking their urine for albumin or protein all are aimed at the early diagnosis and treatment of preeclampsia and other maternal complications. Until science understands totally what role molecular, biochemical, and physiologic events play in the initiation of labor and preterm labor, prenatal care cannot be expected to eradicate the problem of low birth weight. About a third of cases of preterm labor are associated with infection. Therefore, activities to eradicate and prevent infection should be included in prenatal care. It is also necessary to continue to fund basic research into the physiology of parturition.

The most important aspect of prenatal care may be educating childbearing women and their families. Another goal is to motivate each woman to become responsible for her own health. This can become complicated. Physicians are not taught the principles of education, and until recently, medical schools did not traditionally teach the principles of communication and interviewing very well. Primary care providers must learn to be effective teachers and communicators. Nurses, midwives, social workers, dietitians, and genetic counselors often learn the principles of teaching as part of their basic professional education.

Most hospitals and health care facilities offer prenatal education. These programs prepare prospective parents for labor and delivery and emphasize methods for coping with labor. They also present all the information necessary for a healthy pregnancy, emphasizing diet, rest, recreation, exercise, and avoidance of cigarette smoke, alcohol, and illicit drugs. Education about sexually transmitted diseases is essential. These important programs complement but do not replace the ongoing prenatal education and emphasis on lifestyle change that should take place at each prenatal visit to the primary care provider.

The three components of prenatal care are education about pregnancy and infant care, along with advice on how to reduce risks; screening and risk assessment; and treatment of medical conditions throughout pregnancy.

Education includes advice to eliminate or reduce alcohol intake, stop smoking, and avoid illegal drugs. Patients should be instructed about proper diet, appropriate weight gain, and the use of vitamin and mineral supplements. Women should also be encouraged to prepare for childbirth and breast-feeding.

Screening should include blood pressure monitoring, cervical cytology, urinalysis, documentation of weight gain, a physical examination that includes a pelvic examination, and a medical history. Screening for genetic disease or congenital anomalies should be performed with ultrasonography and measurements of α-fetoprotein, estradiol, and β-hCG. Screening for infectious disease, especially group B streptococcal infections, is also conducted. Vaginal and rectal cultures are obtained at 36 to 37 weeks of gestation from all pregnant women to prevent group B streptococcal infection in their infants. Amniocentesis or chorionic villus sampling is performed in women with a family history of genetic disorders, women older than 35 years, and those with other appropriate indications. Women who take care of cats should avoid their litter to prevent toxoplasmosis.

The first prenatal visit is extremely important because trust and communication between patient and provider are established then. The primary care provider must allow enough time so that the visit is not hurried and the pregnant woman's questions can be answered to her satisfaction. Adequate time must be allowed to listen to the woman and her partner. Their concerns, fears, and anxieties can be discerned and then addressed. It is also essential to understand and accept the patient's dreams and expectations. The goal of this visit is to establish a mutual partnership that will work toward a successful outcome of the pregnancy and birth.

A thorough medical history should be obtained and documented, and a complete medical examination should be conducted. A careful pelvic examination should ensue, including an assessment of the adequacy of the pelvis for childbirth. The blood type, Rh blood group, and hematocrit are determined, a urinalysis is performed, and ultrasonography is performed as appropriate. The individual pregnancy risk should be determined and documented. Educational material and counseling about a healthful lifestyle should be provided at this first visit. It is essential to obtain some idea of the family's traditions regarding pregnancy and birth and begin the process of developing a safe but culturally appropriate plan for the birth experience. The expectations of both mother and physician should be clearly stated. The importance of good nutrition for the mother and of breast-feeding for the infant should be stressed. Table 11.3 lists the screening tests that should be performed.

Subsequent visits should be planned to monitor the growth and well-being of the fetus and the health of the pregnant woman. Table 11.4 lists the tests to be performed at subsequent visits. The blood pressure, weight, and urine protein are monitored to diagnose and treat preeclampsia during its earliest stages. Current studies indicate that weight gain in pregnancy should not be limited to 20 or 25 lb. However, excessive weight gain is inappropriate and ultimately harmful; many women first become obese during pregnancy. Obesity is a serious health problem for women in the United States, and providers of primary care to women must educate them about the need for appropriate weight gain to enhance their welfare and that of their unborn children.

The traditional pattern of prenatal care visits is once a month until the 28th week, every other week from the 28th to 36th

TABLE 11.3. Screening Tests

Hematocrit
Blood type and Rh and antibody screening
Venereal Disease Research Laboratory test
Rubella titer
Hepatitis B screening
Urine culture
Cervical cytology
Cervical cultures for gonococci (and β-streptococci and *Chlamydia*, as indicated)
Sickle cell screening in women at risk
HIV counseling and testing
Genetic counseling and amniocentesis for women older than 35 years or with a family history of genetic disease
Tuberculin testing

week, then once a week from the 36th week until delivery; however, this schedule should be modified depending on the circumstances. Women with greater educational needs, serious social difficulties, such as the use of illicit drugs, or medical complications, such as diabetes, should be seen more frequently.

A postdate pregnancy should be followed carefully, with biweekly antenatal testing for fetal well-being. The accepted management is to induce labor in patients with a softened cervix at 40 weeks' gestational age. If the cervix is not favorable, it is prepared for induction pharmacologically.

The aims of prenatal care are to keep the mother in good health, prepare her for labor and childbirth, and ensure the birth of a viable, healthy baby no earlier than 36 weeks.

Common Problems of Pregnancy and Danger Signs

Nausea and vomiting, or "morning sickness," is common and may occur at any time of the day. Pregnant women should eat frequent light meals. It is useful to have dry foods such as toast or crackers available during periods of nausea. Pregnant women with constant vomiting or diarrhea require urgent evaluation by a primary care physician, and if dehydration is severe, referral to a specialist is indicated.

During the first trimester, the enlarging uterus compresses the bladder, causing more frequent urination. The patient should be reassured.

Backaches may occur during the second and third trimesters. Excellent posture, wearing low-heeled, comfortable shoes, sleeping on a firm mattress, and instruction in pelvic rocking as an exercise are helpful strategies to alleviate this problem.

Leg muscle cramps are usually caused by increased pressure on veins, but they may also be caused by low levels of calcium and high levels of phosphorus. Pregnant women should drink milk and consume other dairy products; they should also take a vitamin and mineral supplement. Leg cramps may be relieved by lying on the back with the affected leg extended. The knee should be kept straight and the foot flexed up and down.

TABLE 11.4. Prenatal Studies at Subsequent Visits

Screen for neural tube defects and trisomy 21	(14–16 wk)
α-Fetoprotein, estradiol, and β-human chorionic gonadotropin	
Complete obstetric ultrasonography encouraged	(18–20 wk)
One-hour 50-g glucose screen	(26 wk)
Herpes culture in symptomatic patients or in patients with history of herpes	
Cultures for β-streptococcal infection) (vaginal and rectal	(36–37 wk)

Heartburn may develop, especially after a large meal. It is relieved by antacids and reduced by eating frequent small meals throughout the day.

When a pregnant woman stands or moves quickly, tension in the round ligament causes a pulling pain in the right or lower left abdomen. A pregnant woman should rise slowly from a sitting or lying position. Lying on the same side as the round ligament pain provides relief.

Most pregnant women notice some swelling of the ankles and feet, especially during hot weather. Elevating the feet and walking rather than standing improve the circulation. Edema of the face and hands should be reported to the physician.

Braxton-Hicks contractions of the uterus typically become more noticeable near the time of delivery. They are usually irregular and last about 30 seconds. They are self-limited.

Varicosities are common during pregnancy and are treated with support stockings. Pregnant women should be encouraged to take "walk breaks" at least twice a day and should drink plenty of fluids. The legs may be raised against a wall above the heart for 15 to 20 minutes a day.

Constipation and hemorrhoids are common. Fluids and a mild laxative may help. Because progesterone can cause some decrease in intestinal motility, walking and exercise are important. Sitz baths and analgesic ointments are helpful for hemorrhoids. The pregnant woman should be able to reduce hemorrhoids easily by herself; if they become thrombosed, they must be evaluated.

A "pregnancy mask" of dark blotches around the eyes, mouth, and forehead may occur, but it disappears after delivery. Many women worry about stretch marks. The skin discoloration of these marks also disappears after delivery. They are caused by hormonal changes, not the growing fetus.

Pregnant women should call their obstetrician immediately if vaginal bleeding or spotting occurs. During the first trimester, this can indicate a threatened abortion. Late in pregnancy, it can indicate abruptio placentae or placenta previa. Headache and blurred vision can be a sign of preeclampsia. Severe abdominal pain may be a sign of abortion, ectopic pregnancy, or infection. Chills and a fever of 38.3°C (101°F) without symptoms of upper respiratory infection indicate pyelonephritis, especially if the woman has a history of urinary tract infections. Fluid escaping from the vagina can indicate rupture of membranes.

NORMAL BIRTH

Physicians must learn the mechanisms and physiology of normal birth as part of their fundamental medical knowledge. Just as physicians who are not cardiologists must have a fundamental appreciation of normal cardiac and circulatory physiology, all physicians must understand the process of childbirth because it deeply affects women at many levels—physiologically, emotionally, and spiritually.

Every woman has a profound need to share her own experience of childbirth. One woman will tell another her story, even a stranger. Childbirth is a major life event, and women talk about it to each other as a way of coming to terms with the experience. It is not unusual for a health care provider taking a history from a postmenopausal woman to hear a detailed and complete account of her childbirth history. Such storytelling helps the woman understand exactly what happened to her and puts the experience, whether it was a normal birth or an operative delivery, into context in her life. Birth to women is not just a medical or physiologic event; it is a social, psychological, and spiritual event.

Both positive and negative feelings need to be expressed. Expressing through storytelling her disappointment with any aspect of birth allows these feelings to be resolved.

Retelling a birth experience allows a new mother to accept her baby as a separate human being, not just the fetus she carried for 9 months. The baby is often different from what the new mother expected. Retelling her story lets each woman acknowledge her strength. Labor and birth are among the most incredible and physically and emotionally challenging of life events. After childbirth, women discover what they are capable of, and it is not unusual for women to use this strength as a basis for renewing their lives. Women see themselves in a new light. Birth is a physical triumph. All physicians need to understand this very fundamental aspect of the birth experience.

Retelling the story of childbirth aids a woman in assuming her new role of mother and also helps her relate to her own mother. Finally, in telling her birth story, every woman shares with others the miracle of life. All physicians need to respect and revere this sense of the miracle of birth as part of life and to encourage it in their patients.

No primary care text can present in great detail all aspects of labor and delivery, so the student is encouraged to read and study further. What follows is a description of the essential events of normal birth.

Stages of Labor

Before the onset of parturition, the cervix softens, and the presenting part of the fetus descends into the pelvis. In normal pregnancy, the cervix becomes soft and effaced or thin, and it easily admits one examining finger. Its length is usually less than 1.3 cm. This process can be evaluated by a Bishop score (Table 11.5); a score of 9 or higher indicates that the cervix is ready for parturition because it can easily be dilated with the onset of contractions. The mucus that has plugged the cervix throughout pregnancy is passed and usually appears dark and bloody.

Women often describe irregular contractions of the uterus that increase in intensity and frequency as the pregnancy advances toward term (36–41 weeks). Other signs of impending labor include the development of a spurt of energy, usually 24 hours before the onset of contractions that dilate the cervix. Because of a decrease in progesterone levels, women tend to lose 1 to 1.5 lb about 1 to 2 days before the onset of labor.

Labor begins as a series of mild but regular uterine contractions that at first are usually 20 or 30 minutes apart. They are experienced as pressure, cramps, or sometimes a backache. With time, the contractions become stronger, more noticeable, and closer together. At some point, they cause pain, and the pregnant woman involuntarily stops what she is doing and must rest and breathe deeply to cope with the pain of the contractions. In early labor, the woman feels the need to be active and to eat and drink. However, as labor progresses to a more active phase, the digestive process slows, and most are not hungry. The woman begins to focus her energy on labor, and her concentration turns inward.

Labor is divided into three stages. The *first stage* is further subdivided into a latent phase and an active phase. The latent phase varies in length and starts with the onset of contractions and cervical change. During this phase, the contractions become stronger, efficient, and polarized and are accompanied by cervical softening. The cervix becomes thinner and is easily stretched. In nulliparas, the average length of the latent phase is 8.6 hours; in multiparas, it is 5.3 hours. The Friedman curve in Fig. 11.4 demonstrates this. The normal limit of the latent phase is 20 hours in nulliparas and 14 hours in multiparas. The length of this phase is correlated with the degree of cervical softness at the onset of labor.

The active phase starts when the cervix is 3 to 4 cm dilated. The extracellular matrix of the cervix has been altered to allow more rapid dilation; thus, the active phase of labor is 5.8 hours in nulliparas and 2.5 hours in multiparas (Fig. 11.5). This phase normally should not exceed 12 hours in nulliparas and 6 hours in multiparas.

A transition phase of variable but short duration occurs between the first and second stages. The transition phase corresponds to the time between 8 and 10 cm of dilation, or full dilation. At this phase, it is normal for women to experience a full gamut of emotions that range from wonderful, happy, powerful, and elated to angry, sad, overwhelmed, and scared.

The *second stage* of labor begins with full dilation of the cervix and ends with the birth of the baby. Once the transition phase has been completed and the cervix is fully dilated, the second or expulsive stage commences. The laboring woman instinctively feels an urge to push. Pushing, accomplished by a Valsalva maneuver, increases the force of the contractions by 20% to 30% to allow the fetus to pass through the pelvis. Pushing may be more effective if done between contractions. Progress of the second stage of labor is measured by the station of the presenting part (Fig. 11.6). The membranes, if not ruptured artificially, usually rupture spontaneously during the active phase. In some cases, the membranes rupture before the onset of labor, and in most such cases, the contractions begin spontaneously within 12 hours. The time between spontaneous rupture of the membranes and the onset of labor normally does not exceed 24 hours.

TABLE 11.5. Bishop Score

Factor	Points: 0	1	2	3
Dilation of cervix (cm)	0	1–2	3–4	5–6
Effacement of cervix (%)	0–30	40–50	60–70	80
Consistency of cervix	Firm	Medium	Soft	
Position of cervix in the vagina	Posterior	Middle	Anterior	
Station	−3	−2	−1.0	+1, +2

Source: From Oxorn H. *Oxorn-Foote human labor and birth,* 5th ed. Norwalk, CT: Appleton & Lange, 1986:918, with permission.

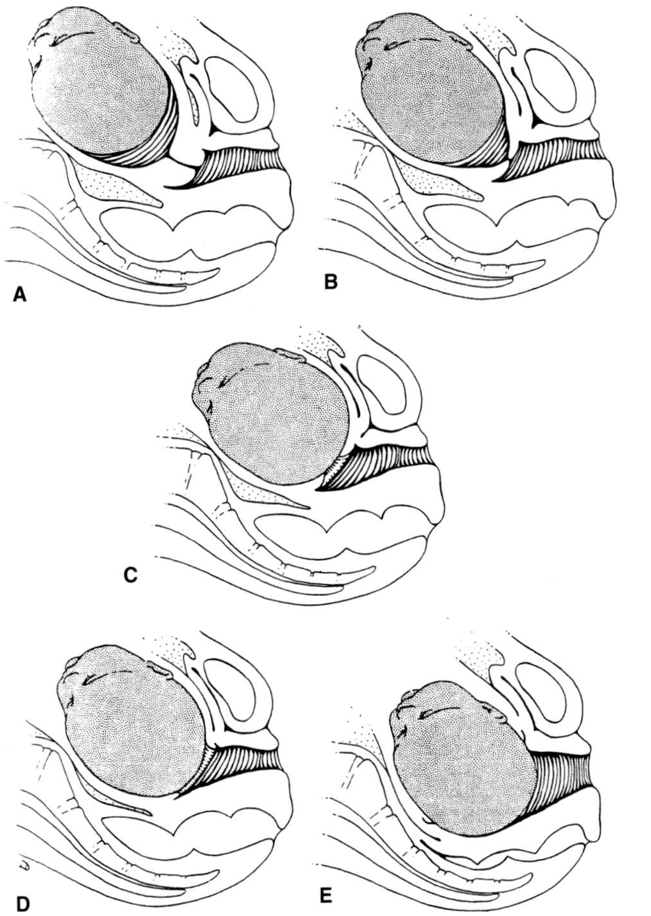

FIG. 11.4. Dilation of the cervix. A: Cervix thick and closed. B: Cervix effaced. C: Cervix effaced and dilated 2 to 3 cm. D: Cervix half open. E: Cervix fully dilated and retracted.

The normal mechanisms of labor that allow the fetus to pass through the pelvic bones are descent and flexion, internal rotation, extension, restitution, and external rotation, followed by delivery. These classic mechanisms occur as the force of the mother's expulsive efforts and the force of the contractions cause the fetal presenting part to meet the resistance of the pelvis. Thus, the fetal presenting part turns passively as it makes its way through the pelvic canal. The mechanisms of labor are illustrated in Figs. 11.4, 11.7, and 11.8.

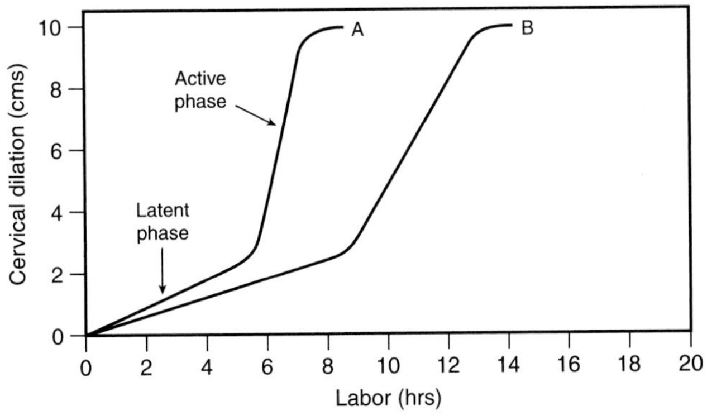

FIG. 11.5. First stage of labor: Friedman curves. *A*, multipara; *B*, nullipara.

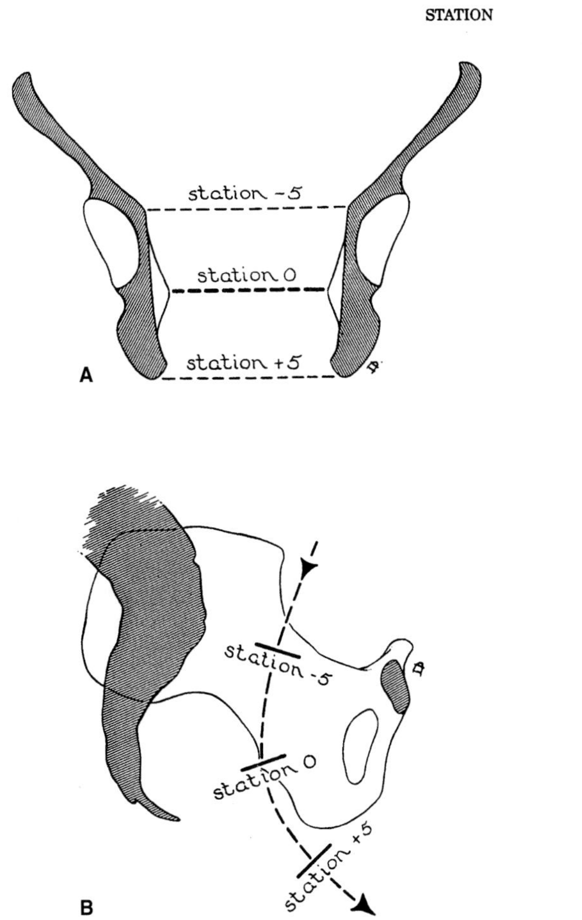

FIG. 11.6. Station of presenting part. A: Anteroposterior view. B: Lateral view.

The *third stage* of labor is delivery of the placenta. In a normal birth, this stage is accomplished easily, with spontaneous separation and expulsion of the placenta. The third stage should not exceed 30 minutes; the placenta should be removed manually under anesthesia after 30 minutes. Care must be taken to ensure that the entire placenta is delivered because even small portions of retained membranes can cause postpartum hemorrhage. Normal blood loss is 200 to 250 mL.

After the infant is born, the physician or midwife must ensure that the mother's uterus is well contracted to prevent hemorrhage. This is accomplished by giving the mother 20 U of oxytocin (Pitocin) intravenously. Putting the infant to breast immediately causes the uterus to contract and therefore helps to prevent hemorrhage.

Care of the Fetus/Infant

During labor, the well-being of the fetus is monitored carefully by electronic techniques. The primary care provider must know what is accepted as a normal fetal heart rate tracing and, when deviations occur, what constitutes appropriate care. A consultation with a specialist may be required. At birth, the physician or midwife suctions the infant's nasopharynx of secretions and mucus and helps the infant adjust to extrauterine life. The infant must be kept warm.

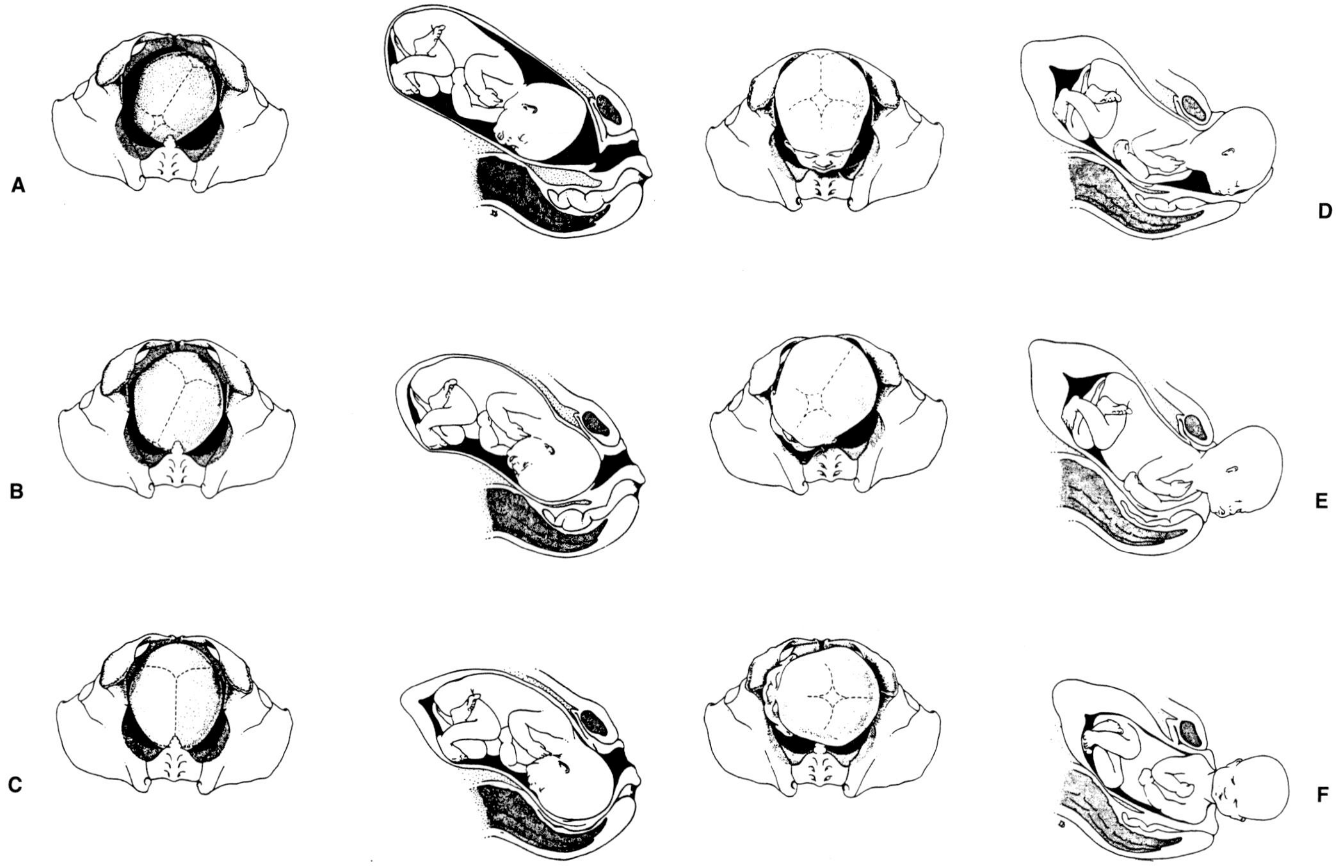

FIG. 11.7. Summary of mechanism of labor. **A–C:** Anterior positions of the occiput. **A:** Onset of labor. **B:** Descent and flexion. **C:** Internal rotation: left occiput anterior to occiput anterior. **D–F:** Left occiput anterior. **D:** Extension. **E:** Restitution: occiput anterior to left occiput anterior. **F:** External rotation: left occiput anterior to left occiput transverse.

Complications of Parturition

When a women is at risk for preterm birth, she should be referred to a specialist immediately.

The antenatal administration of glucocorticoids to the mother is one of the most important means of preventing respiratory complications in the newborn. In 2001, more than 20% of births were induced; the rate of induced labor doubled from 1989 to 2001. In 2001, cesarean births increased to the highest level since 1989. In 2002, the rate was 22.9%. The subjects of abnormal labor and delivery, including malpresentations such as breech and occiput posterior and multifetal pregnancies, the induction of labor, and cesarean section are beyond the scope of this book, and the reader is referred to a textbook of obstetrics.

This summary of normal birth is not meant to be a presentation of obstetric management and the conduct of labor, including methods of pain management and appropriate anesthesia; these topics belong to the realm of specialists in the field. However, all physicians should have an understanding of the birth process.

OTHER ISSUES OF REPRODUCTIVE HEALTH

Family planning and contraceptive care, essential to women of reproductive age, are discussed in Chapter 19. Abnormalities of pregnancy, such as ectopic pregnancy and spontaneous abortion, are discussed in Chapter 20.

A discussion of the reproductive health of women must always address the issue of termination of pregnancy. Unfortunately, abortion has become a polarizing topic in our society. Most women take a position somewhere in the middle; they are aware of a woman's needs and the fact that in some cases a pregnancy is detrimental to a woman physically or psychologically, but at the same time they understand that using abortion as a means of birth control undermines a woman's health. This position acknowledges the fact that the decision to terminate a pregnancy is a difficult one and not made lightly. Counseling is an indispensable part of all abortion services. In an open society with diverse opinions, respect for an individual's choice and beliefs must be paramount, and part of this respect is providing access to safe clinical services for abortion. All cultures have practiced termination of pregnancy. Even when abortion was illegal, women sought abortion providers, at great risk to their health. The American College of Obstetricians and Gynecologists has stated that their residents must be exposed to and educated about the proper management of termination of pregnancy. Residents with religious or moral objections to the procedure are not obligated to perform abortions but must state their reasons in writing.

CHRONIC MEDICAL CONDITIONS AND REASONS FOR HOSPITALIZING WOMEN OF REPRODUCTIVE AGE

The most common reasons for hospitalizing women ages 18 to 44 years are complications of pregnancy, followed by other gen-

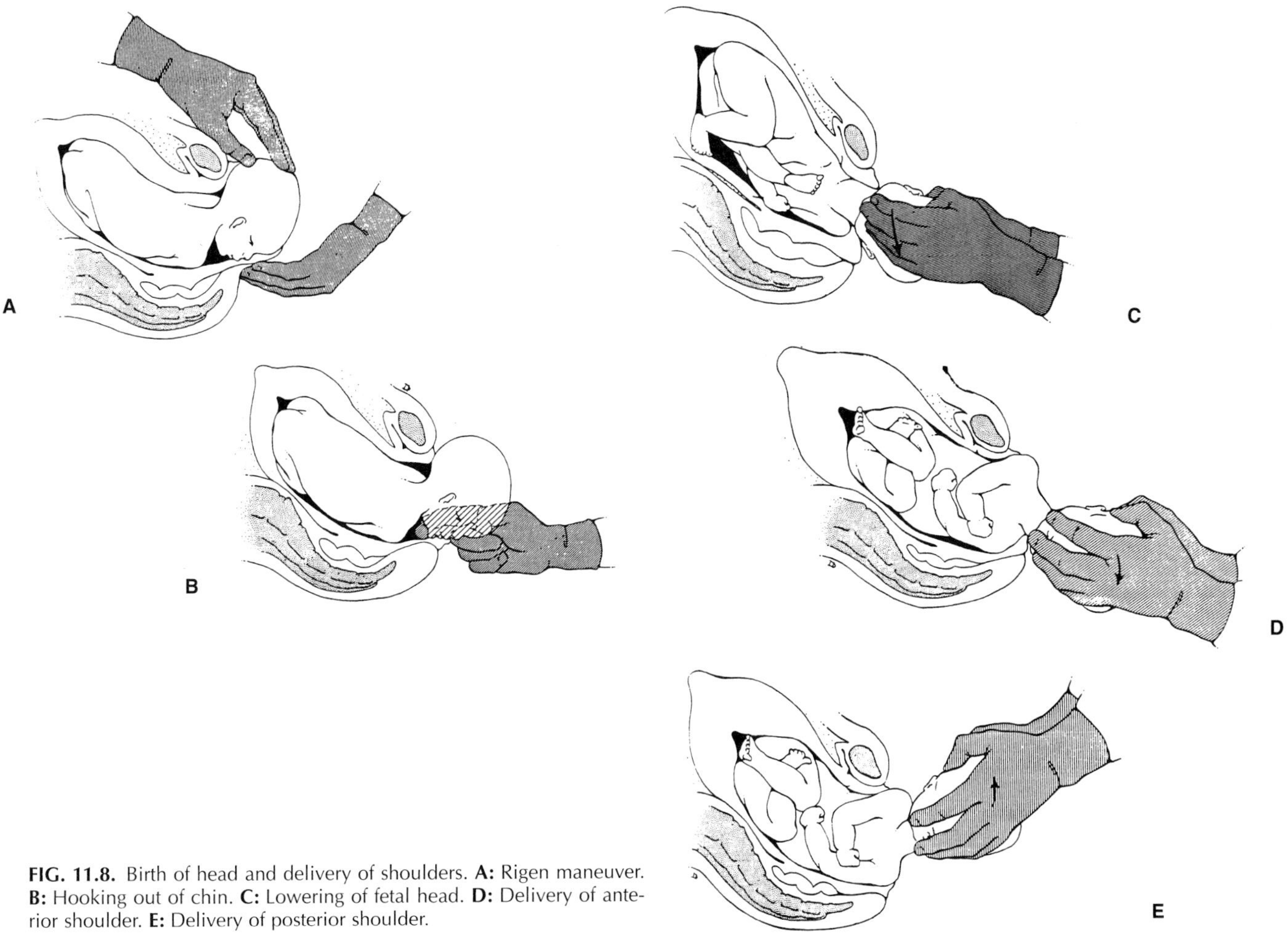

FIG. 11.8. Birth of head and delivery of shoulders. **A:** Rigen maneuver. **B:** Hooking out of chin. **C:** Lowering of fetal head. **D:** Delivery of anterior shoulder. **E:** Delivery of posterior shoulder.

ital tract problems and diseases of the female pelvic organs. The fourth most common reason is spontaneous abortion and termination of pregnancy. This list underscores the importance of reproductive health in women 18 to 44 years of age.

The reasons for hospitalization are completely different from the most common chronic conditions in women of reproductive age. These are most often treated on an ambulatory basis. The most common chronic conditions are the following: chronic sinusitis; hay fever without asthma; chronic obstructive pulmonary disease, which includes chronic bronchitis, asthma, and emphysema; HIV infection; orthopedic deformities, especially of the back; migraine headaches; arthritis; diseases of the female genital tract; hemorrhoids; high blood pressure; and dermatitis. When chronic medical conditions that impair activity are considered, the most common conditions of women ages 18 to 44 are the following: back deformity; deformity of the lower extremities; chronic obstructive pulmonary disease; arthritis; intervertebral disc disorders; high blood pressure; visual impairment; deformity of the upper extremities; heart disease, including congestive heart disease but not ischemic disease; diabetes; and hearing impairment.

The variations in the lists show that ambulatory care and hospital care facilities treat and manage different problems in this age group. It is therefore tempting to think that health care providers for women may easily and rationally be divided into two groups—primary providers of ambulatory care and specialized providers of hospital care. The problem with this analysis is that it is incomplete; prenatal care is recorded as complete care, including delivery, so that prenatal care is not included in ambulatory care statistics. Because pregnancy-related problems are the most common reasons for hospitalization, it follows that prenatal care is a common reason for women to seek ambulatory care.

BIBLIOGRAPHY

American College of Obstetricians and Gynecologists. *Compendium of selected publications.* Washington, DC: American College of Obstetricians and Gynecologists, 2003:733.

Berg CJ, Chang J, Callagahan WM, et al. Pregnancy-related mortality in the United States, 1991–1997. *Obstet Gynecol* 2003;101:289–297.

Cooper RL, Goldenberg RL, DuBard MB, et al., and the Collaborative Group on Preterm Birth Prevention. Risk factors for fetal death in white, black, and Hispanic women. *Obstet Gynecol* 1994;84:490.

Cunningham FG, Gant NF, Leveno KJ, et al. *Williams' obstetrics,* 21st ed. Columbus, OH: McGraw-Hill, 2003:1488.

Farook AA. *Colour atlas of childbirth and obstetric techniques.* Aylesbury, UK: Wolfe Publishing, 1990.

Herschel M, Hsieh H, Mittendorf R, et al. Risk factors for fetal death in white, black, and Hispanic women [Letter]. *Obstet Gynecol* 1995;85:318.

Lessey BA. Adhesion molecules and implantation. *J Reprod Immunol* 2002;55: 101–112.

Myles ME. *Textbook for midwives with modern concepts of obstetric and neonatal care,* 10th ed. Edinburgh: Churchill Livingstone, 1985.

Oxorn H. *Oxorn-Foote human labor and birth,* 5th ed. Norwalk, CT: Appleton & Lange, 1986:918.

Robert Wood Johnson Foundation. *Special report: Medicaid expansions for pregnant women and children.* Princeton, NJ: Robert Wood Johnson Foundation, 1995.

Speroff L, Glass RH, Kase NG. *Clinical gynecologic endocrinology and infertility,* 6th ed. Philadelphia: Lippincott Williams & Wilkins, 1999:201–246.

Sullivan LE. The birth experience. *Working Mothers,* June 1995.

CHAPTER 12

Sex Matters in Pharmacology: Principles of Pharmacology for Women

Donald R. Mattison

Men and women differ in how they respond to drug treatment. Anatomic, physiologic, and molecular differences between the sexes account for diversity in clinical therapeutics. In this review, sex is defined as biologic differences, and gender as the socially constructed and individual created characterization of a man or a woman.

To design safe and effective drug treatments, it is essential to understand how men and women differ in the way they dispose of drugs and respond to drugs. Clinical therapeutics focuses on what the body does to a drug (pharmacokinetics) and what the drug does to the body (pharmacodynamics). This chapter summarizes how pharmacokinetics and pharmacodynamics differ between men and women and between pregnant and nonpregnant women. This area is evolving rapidly, and it is essential for the practitioner to review the information on drug labels and the recent literature to understand sex-related differences in therapeutics.

SEX DIFFERENCES IN THE ADVERSE EFFECTS OF DRUGS

The adverse events data of the U.S. Food and Drug Administration (FDA) suggest that women experience more frequent and more serious adverse events (Table 12.1). For example, the General Accounting Office reviewed the 10 drugs withdrawn from the market from January 1997 through December 2000 and noted that eight of them had been withdrawn because of a greater risk for adverse effects in women. Given the pharmacokinetic differences between men and women, it is possible that women are more frequently overdosed, with drugs reaching a higher free concentration or being eliminated more slowly. Women may be more sensitive; the concentration of free drug and length of time it is in the body are similar for the two sexes, but the response of women is greater. Another explanation, given that women take more medications (including oral contraceptives) than men, is that adverse events result from drug interactions.

In another FDA study, which explored the influence of sex on bioequivalence, differences in pharmacokinetic parameters of more than 20% were observed between the sexes in approximately 40% of the drugs studied. Unfortunately, the inclusion of women in clinical studies still lags considerably. As a consequence, physicians who care for women frequently have to estimate the appropriate dose, dosing schedule, and treatment interval with only a modest knowledge of the appropriate use of the drug.

PRINCIPLES OF CLINICAL PHARMACOLOGY

Clinical pharmacology is the study of uptake, distribution, elimination, and effects of drugs in humans (Fig. 12.1). The goals of clinical therapeutics are to minimize therapeutic misadventures and enhance therapeutic efficacy, thereby optimizing the effects of drugs. Both goals can be achieved by understanding how a drug is absorbed into the body, distributed throughout, metabolized, and ultimately eliminated (pharmacokinetics), and how the body responds to the drug when it reaches its sites of action (pharmacodynamics).

Pharmacokinetics

Pharmacokinetics can be described from two perspectives: (a) absorption, distribution, metabolism, and elimination (Fig. 12.1) and (b) volume of distribution (V_d), clearance, and half-life ($t_{1/2}$).

CLEARANCE, VOLUME OF DISTRIBUTION, AND HALF-LIFE

The concept of clearance was developed to characterize renal function by describing the volume of blood cleared of urea or creatinine by the kidneys during some fixed interval of time. This concept is applied similarly to drugs. For example, the clearance of intravenous diazepam is 0.038 L/h per kilogram of body weight in women and 0.029 L/h per kilogram of body weight in men. After the intravenous administration of a dose of diazepam, 38 mL of plasma is cleared of diazepam per hour per kilogram of body weight in a woman, and 29 mL in a man. Understanding clearance is important because both renal and nonrenal pathways of drug elimination may be affected by age, sex, and disease, so that the drug dose and frequency of administration must be altered.

The volume of distribution is an important theoretic volume. It is defined as the amount of drug administered divided by the initial plasma concentration, *with the assumption of instantaneous absorption and distribution throughout the body*. Values for the volume of distribution depend on molecular weight, lipid and water solubility, and protein binding. Water-soluble drugs (not highly protein-bound, molecular weights <400) typically have a volume of distribution close to total body water (~700 mL/kg).

TABLE 12.1. Sex Differences in Adverse Events

Possible clinical factors	Pharmacologic factors	Physiologic and molecular factors
Women are overdosed.	Pharmacokinetics	Volume of distribution smaller Free fraction of drug larger Clearance from the body slower
Women take more medications.	Drug interactions	Alteration in pharmacokinetics (see preceding row) Alteration in pharmacodynamics (see next row)
Women are more sensitive.	Pharmacodynamics	Alteration in receptor number Alteration in receptor binding Alteration in signal transduction pathway following receptor binding

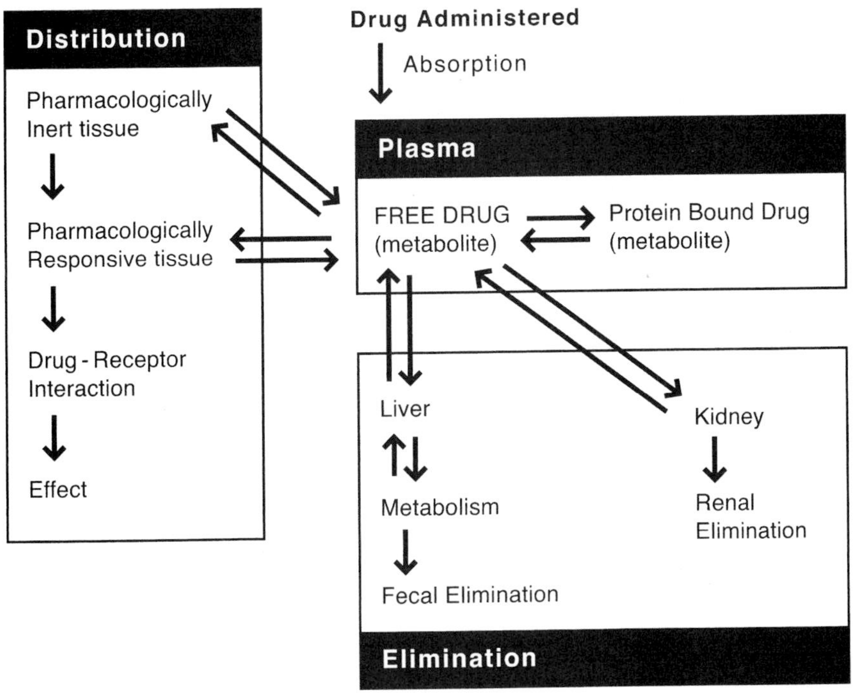

FIG. 12.1. Schematic representation of pharmacokinetic and pharmacodynamic processes. Differences in these processes between men and women are the result of sex-related differences in anatomy, physiology, and cellular and molecular biology.

Examples include acetaminophen (950 mL/kg) and ethanol (540 mL/kg, with a smaller volume of distribution in women than in men). Drugs that are highly tissue-bound may have a volume of distribution of thousands of milliliters per kilogram, including azithromycin (31,000 mL/kg) and fluoxetine (35,000 mL/kg). Some drugs have a small volume of distribution, including dicloxacillin (86 mL/kg) and heparin (58 mL/kg).

Understanding clearance and volume of distribution makes it possible to predict the concentration of drug, amount in the body, and length of time in the body, information critical for effective therapy and the prevention of toxicity. The half-life ($t_{1/2}$), determined by the clearance and volume of distribution, is the time during which half of the drug is removed from the blood.

ABSORPTION, DISTRIBUTION, METABOLISM, AND ELIMINATION

Although the concepts of clearance, elimination half-life, and volume of distribution provide much of the information needed to use a drug, the concepts of absorption, distribution, metabolism, and elimination allow a richer anatomic, physiologic, and molecular description of drug disposition and action (Fig. 12.1).

Absorption. Absorption is the process by which a drug administered by various routes reaches the blood. Examples of sex differences in absorption include rifampicin, which women absorb more efficiently, and benzylamine, which is absorbed transdermally more completely in women than in men. Absorption occurs at different sites along the gastrointestinal tract and is influenced by multiple factors, including gut transit times, lipid solubility of the agent, pH at the site of absorption, and ionization and molecular weight of the agent. Gut transit times are shorter in men (44.8 hours) than in women (91.7 hours). Gastric juice is more acidic in men (pH 1.92) than in women (pH 2.59), and the rates of basal and maximal flow of gastric juice and acid secretion are higher in men. Gastric acid secretion is reduced by 30% during pregnancy. The gastrointestinal absorption of iron and ethanol differs between men and women. In preadolescent girls, 45% of ingested iron is incorporated into erythrocytes, versus 35% in boys. Ethanol is metabolized more rapidly in the gut in men; as a result, less is available for absorption.

Distribution. Distribution is the process by which a drug is moved throughout the body from the site of absorption. Body composition, which differs between the sexes and between pregnant and nonpregnant women, influences the concentration of a drug at the target site, and variations in body composition result in varying responses. On average, total body water, extracellular water, intracellular water, total blood volume, plasma volume, red blood cell volume, and muscle mass are greater in men than in women. Therefore, if average men and women are exposed to the same dose of a water-soluble drug that is not highly tissue-bound, the volume of distribution is larger in men and the concentration of the drug is lower. For example, the volume of distribution of ethanol and the fluoroquinolones is smaller in women, so that peak concentrations are higher; the volume of distribution of vancomycin is larger in women.

The total concentrations of protein and serum albumin do not differ significantly between men and nonpregnant women; however, the total protein concentration decreases during pregnancy. Pregnancy-related changes in body weight, plasma proteins, plasma volume, extracellular fluid volume, total body water, and body fat alter drug distribution. Decreases in plasma binding proteins increase the free fraction of drug, but the concentrations of free drug are unaltered in the case of drugs such as phenytoin, which are restrictively eliminated. Oral contraceptives, frequently used by women of reproductive age, alter the plasma proteins and free fractions of some drugs.

The percentage of total body weight that is fat is higher in women than in men and increases with age. The total body fat for a male adult is 13.5 kg. Body fat increases by about 25% during pregnancy, from 16.5 kg in a nonpregnant woman to 19.8 kg in a pregnant woman at 40 weeks' gestation. The larger proportion of body fat in women and the increase in body fat during pregnancy may increase the burden of lipid-soluble, slowly metabolized drugs.

Metabolism. Two processes are typically responsible for stopping the action of a drug—metabolism and elimination. (Distribution is responsible for stopping the action of drugs such as lidocaine and thiopental when they are administered by bolus injection.) Although drugs can be eliminated from the body in sweat, tears, breast milk, and expired air, the most common routes of elimination are in feces and urine.

Most drug metabolism occurs in the liver. The consequence of drug metabolism is usually that a drug becomes more soluble in water and is more easily eliminated from the body. Metabolic processes are divided into phase I reactions (addition of an oxygen or other similar atom) and phase II reactions (conjugation with a large polar molecule to enhance elimination in urine or bile).

Phase I Reactions. Most differences in phase I reactions between the sexes relate to oxygenation by cytochrome P-450 (CYP) monooxygenases. The CYP enzymes are a superfamily of isoenzymes responsible for most drug metabolism. Depending on which CYP enzyme metabolizes a drug, the drug may be metabolized more rapidly in men or in women, or metabolism may take place at the same rate in both sexes.

Research indicates that drug transporters removing a drug from cells influence the amount of drug available for metabolism, and that the role of the various CYPs is more complicated than previously thought. Differences in both CYPs and drug transporters between the sexes may explain the more rapid metabolism of methylprednisolone, nifedipine, and cyclosporine in women. Drugs more rapidly metabolized in women because of the effects of CYPs include sparteine, codeine, dextromethorphan, amitriptyline, imipramine, and propranolol. Drugs metabolized more rapidly in men include caffeine, theophylline, and clozapine. Drugs that are metabolized similarly in both sexes include warfarin, phenytoin, tolbutamide, and naproxen.

Phase II Reactions. Phase II reactions include glucuronidation, sulfation, acetylation, and methylation. Rates of phase II metabolism are generally more rapid in men.

Drug Transporters. Drug transporters are plasma membrane–bound proteins that transport drugs out of cells. They play a role in the absorption, metabolism, and elimination of drugs in various organs. Drug transporters are responsible for the drug resistance observed in cancer patients. Adding to the complexity of the situation is the overlap of substrates transported by drug transporters and metabolized by CYPs. Metabolism is a major factor in pharmacokinetics, and sex-dependent differences in biotransformation have been observed for a few specific drugs, such as nicotine, chlordiazepoxide, flurazepam, acetylsalicylic acid, and heparin.

Elimination. Drugs are generally eliminated from the body by renal or hepatic routes. Drugs can be excreted in the urine by glomerular filtration, passive diffusion, or active secretion. Increases in renal blood flow and the glomerular filtration rate increase the rate at which a drug is cleared by the kidneys. When standardized for body surface area, the rates of renal blood flow, glomerular filtration, tubular secretion, and tubular reabsorption are all higher in men than in nonpregnant women. During pregnancy, changes in renal blood flow, the glomerular filtration rate, hepatic blood flow, bile flow, and pulmonary function affect maternal drug elimination. The maternal renal plasma flow is increased to 1.4-fold the value for nonpregnant women and 1.1-fold the value for men. The glomerular filtration rate also increases during pregnancy. By mid gestation, the glomerular filtration rate has increased to approximately 1.5-fold the value for nonpregnant women and 1.2-fold the value for men.

Pharmacodynamics

Pharmacodynamics describes the effects of a drug on the body, which are a consequence of receptor interactions (Fig. 12.1). Given the complex effects of drugs at various sites of action, it is not surprising that research on the differences in pharmacodynamics between the sexes is scarce.

Although the beneficial or adverse effect of a drug depends on its concentration at the target site, the plasma concentration is a good surrogate. Keeping the plasma concentration in mind is a challenge for the practitioner, who typically thinks of dose and frequency of administration rather than concentration in developing a therapeutic strategy. However, it is essential to focus on concentration because the dose-effect relationship is much more variable than the concentration-effect relationship. Additionally, adverse effects are more easily prevented by considering plasma concentration than dose and frequency of administration.

Differences between the sexes in the risk for and treatment of cardiovascular disease are interesting, especially in that the cardiovascular effects (predominantly torsade de pointes with prolonged repolarization) of many drugs withdrawn by the FDA between 1997 and 2000 were different for men and women. Different responses to risk factors include the greater effects of smoking, diabetes, low-density lipoproteins, and triglycerides in women. Because differences between the sexes in risk for cardiovascular disease have been thought to be related to estrogen, it is useful to comment briefly on the differences observed between men and women in the pharmacodynamic response to steroid hormones (through sex hormone receptors).

Estrogen, like many hormones, is bound to a protein in the circulation, steroid hormone–binding globulin; about 2% of estrogen is free, or unbound. Metabolism occurs in the liver via hydroxylation or sulfation (phase I) and glucuronidation (phase II); the metabolites are eliminated in bile. Free estrogen has access to several types of estrogen receptors (α- and β-subtypes) within cells; the receptors bind estrogen, are modified, and enter the nucleus, where they bind DNA and modify gene expression. Because the two subtypes of estrogen receptor respond differently to estrogen and are distributed differently in various tissues throughout the body, the responses of the tissues to estrogen differ (i.e., the effect of estrogen in the body differs according to the receptor types and signal transduction pathways present).

Cardiac function is clearly influenced by sex, including the effects of steroid hormones on cardiac electrophysiology and repolarization, reflected in the QT interval. Because the QT interval is longer in women, fatalities are more likely to occur in women after the administration of drugs that delay repolarization. Other observations include menstrual cycle–dependent differences in the risk for torsade de pointes, which is increased during the follicular and ovulatory phases of the cycle. During adolescence, the major hormonal effect appears to be that of testosterone; shortening of the QT interval is noted in men, rather than prolongation of the QT interval by estrogen or progesterone in women. Four of the drugs withdrawn by the FDA from January 1997 through December 2000 were associated with a risk for torsade de pointes. Despite these differences, women remain underrepresented in published cardiovascular clinical trials. This is especially troublesome in clinical therapeutics because the effect of a lack of clinical studies is to deny women access to safe, effective, evidence-based therapy.

Differences in pulmonary development and function have also been observed between the sexes, with associated effects on pharmacodynamics. At birth, the lungs of female infants are smaller and more mature than those of male infants, so that the production of surfactant and response to prenatal steroid treatment are greater. Airway hyperresponsiveness to a range of challenges differs between the sexes, with less hyperresponsiveness noted in women than in men. Sex differences in asthma vary across the life span; in children up to the age of 14 years, the incidence of asthma is twice as high in boys; during the reproductive years, the incidence of asthma is greater in women, but around the time of menopause, the incidence rates equalize. These observations are consistent with the greater risk for lung cancer and chronic obstructive lung disease in women smokers than in men smokers after dose adjustment by pack-years or cumulative tar delivered.

Use of Pharmacokinetic and Pharmacodynamic Data

In this section, selected data are reviewed to illustrate differences between the sexes in pharmacodynamics and pharmacokinetics (Table 12.2). Theophylline is cleared more rapidly by women. Smoking induces CYP IA1 and CYP IA2, increasing clearance in both men and women. Interestingly, although smoking increases the clearance of theophylline in both men and women, urinary metabolites are increased only in women. Cimetidine, which inhibits CYP metabolism, decreases the clearance of theophylline and the appearance of urinary metabolites.

Methylprednisolone is eliminated more rapidly by women than by men, whereas the volume of distribution and protein binding are similar, so that the area under the concentration

TABLE 12.2. Sex Differences in Pharmacokinetics

Drug	Pharmacokinetic parameter	Comments
Acebutolol	Area under the concentration-time curve	The concentration-time profile is larger in women than in men, suggesting greater therapeutic and potential side effects.
Acetaminophen	Clearance, half-life	Clearance is increased and the half-life decreased during pregnancy.
Aspirin	Clearance, half-life	Aspirin is cleared more rapidly from women than from men.
β-Blockers	Clearance, volume of distribution	Lower oral clearance and lower volume of distribution in women result in higher systemic exposure. The greater reduction in blood pressure in women is a consequence of pharmacokinetic, not pharmacodynamic, differences.
Cefazolin	Clearance, volume of distribution, half-life	Clearance increases during pregnancy as a consequence half-life decreases. There is no change in volume of distribution during pregnancy.
Cefotaxime	Clearance	Clearance is slower in women.
Clorazepate	Volume of distribution, half-life	Both volume of distribution and half-life are increased during pregnancy; initial concentration will be lower but drug will persist longer in the body during pregnancy.
Diazepam	Plasma binding	Plasma binding decreases during pregnancy; as a result, the free fraction increases.
Digoxin	Clearance	Clearance increases during pregnancy; as a result, more frequent administration may be needed.
Erythromycin	Oral availability	Oral availability decreases during pregnancy; as result, circulating concentrations are decreased.
Ethanol	Volume of distribution, clearance, first-pass metabolism	First-pass metabolism is greater in men; volume of distribution is smaller in women.
Gemcitabine	Clearance	Clearance is slower in women than in men.
Heparin	Clearance	Clearance is slower in women than in men.
Iron	Absorption measured as percentage of dose incorporated into red blood cells	More ingested iron is absorbed by women than by men.
Lithium	Clearance	Clearance is increased during pregnancy.
Mefloquine	Clearance, half-life	Clearance is increased during pregnancy.
Methylprednisolone	Plasma binding, clearance, volume of distribution, half-life	Plasma binding and volume of distribution are similar in men and women. Clearance is faster in women, and as a consequence, half-life is shorter.
Metoprolol	Plasma binding, clearance, volume of distribution, half-life	Oral availability decreases during pregnancy. Plasma binding is unaffected by gender or pregnancy. Clearance increases during pregnancy but is slower in women than in men. Volume of distribution is smaller in women than in men but increases during pregnancy.
Midazolam	Considered to be probe for CYP 3A4, not substrate for PGP, the drug transport proteins	No sex difference in clearance following either oral or intramuscular administration. Interpretation complicated by differences in intestinal and hepatic CYP 3A4 levels.
Naratriptan	Oral availability, peak concentration	Oral availability is greater in women than in men; therefore, the peak concentration is higher in women.

(continued)

TABLE 12.2. ***(continued)***

Drug	Pharmacokinetic parameter	Comments
Ondansetron	Oral availability, clearance	Oral availability is increased in women.
Phenobarbital	Plasma binding, clearance	Plasma binding is unchanged, clearance is increased during pregnancy.
Phenytoin	Plasma binding	Plasma binding decreases during pregnancy. However, the intrinsic clearance is unchanged, so the free concentration is unchanged.
Prazosin	Clearance, half-life	Clearance decreases during pregnancy.
Propranolol	Plasma binding, clearance, volume of distribution, half-life	Plasma binding is similar in men and women; however, plasma binding increases during pregnancy. Propranolol is cleared more rapidly in men, as are its metabolites. Volume of distribution is similar in men and women and does not appear to be altered during pregnancy. Half-life is shorter in women in comparison with men but does not appear to be altered during pregnancy. Potential for therapeutic and adverse effects is greater in women.
Quinidine	Plasma binding	Plasma binding decreases during pregnancy.
Quinine	Plasma binding, clearance, volume of distribution, half-life	Plasma binding is unaltered during pregnancy, as is clearance. Volume of distribution decreases during pregnancy, as does half-life.
Rizatriptan	Urinary excretion, clearance, volume of distribution, half-life	Urinary excretion is similar in men and women. Clearance is greater in men.
Selective serotonin reuptake inhibitors	Volume of distribution	Plasma concentrations are higher in women than in men. Decreased metabolism by hepatic CYP.
Sulfisoxazole	Plasma binding	Plasma binding decreases during pregnancy.
Theophylline	Plasma binding, clearance, volume of distribution	Plasma binding decreases during pregnancy. Distribution volume is increased as expected from protein binding and changes in physiologic spaces. Decreased hepatic clearance is offset by increased renal clearance.
Valproic acid	Plasma binding	Plasma binding decreases during pregnancy.
Verapamil, calcium channel blockers	Clearance	Clearance following intravenous administration is more rapid in women, but oral clearance is greater in men than in women. Substrate for both CYP 3A4 and PGP. Sex differences in hepatic and gut CYP 3A4 and PGP lead to complex differences in clearance between men and women. Bioavailability from the gut is greater in women than in men. The . greater bioavailability leads to increased systemic exposure in women, which results in larger decreases in heart rate

CYP, cytochrome P-450; PGP-p-glycoprotein, the drug transport protein.

curve is larger in men. Women, however, appear to be more sensitive to cortisol suppression, and they may also be more sensitive to the effects on basophils and T helper lymphocytes. Overall, the data indicate that the differences in pharmacokinetics and pharmacodynamics between the sexes are balanced; as a result, men and women should receive the same dose and treatment schedule.

Propranolol is cleared more rapidly by men than by women a consequence of a higher rate of metabolism; interestingly, the volume of distribution is not different. The difference in clearance appears to be related to responses to sex hormones. Side chain oxidation and glucuronidation are increased by testosterone in men (and perhaps women), whereas ring oxidation is not. The effects of circulating endogenous hormone levels on the disposition of propranolol in women appears to be minimal, although synthetic hormones (oral contraceptives) appear to alter the disposition. Little difference is noted between the sexes nor variation during the menstrual cycle on the plasma binding of propranolol. In contrast, a significant decrease in binding is observed in women treated with oral contraceptives.

Caffeine is a frequently consumed drug; because high concentrations cause toxicity (restlessness, anxiety, palpitations), the dose ingested may be titrated according to the physical or mental status. For example, during pregnancy, both the volume of distribution (increasing from 25 to 33 L) and the half-life (increasing from 3.5 to 10.5 hours) are altered. As a consequence of the increase in half-life during pregnancy, the dose required to reach the same blood concentration falls by more than half. Caffeine metabolism, which occurs along several pathways, is generally slower in women than in men, although cigarette smoking can stimulate it.

Ethanol is distributed throughout the body water. Given that the volume of body water is smaller in women, higher peak concentrations would be expected; however, other pharmacokinetic processes must also be considered. For example, both the stomach and liver participate in ethanol metabolism, but at what appears to be a lower rate in women. Following absorption, alcohol is cleared from the blood more rapidly in women than in men. It has been suggested that the slower clearance in men is a consequence of higher testosterone levels; testosterone inhibits alcohol dehydrogenase. Interestingly, the pharmacodynamics of ethanol appear to differ between men and women, with women more sensitive to sedation than men.

SUMMARY

To minimize therapeutic misadventures, the physician responsible for treating women must pay attention to the following:

Clear therapeutic goals must be established for the drug of choice before treatment is started.

- Will the results of treatment be judged by clinical signs and symptoms or by laboratory test values?
- Will drug toxicity be evaluated by clinical or laboratory parameters?
- What determines the appropriate duration of treatment?

The principles of clinical pharmacology must be understood as they apply to the drug of choice.

- Absorption—what influences the rate at which the drug reaches the blood?
- Distribution—how is the drug distributed throughout the body?
- Metabolism—what happens to the drug in the liver or kidneys?
- Elimination—how is the drug removed from the body?

The principles of clinical pharmacodynamics must be understood as they apply to the drug of choice.

- What is the relationship between the drug concentration and the desired biologic effect at the site of action?
- What is the mechanism of action of the drug?
- What is the effect of the chosen drug on the patient's signs, symptoms, and laboratory test results?

ACKNOWLEDGMENT

Whereas all the errors in this review are mine, I appreciate the comments of Drs. Arthur J. Atkinson, Jr., Charlotte Catz, and Mary J. Berg, which have improved the accuracy of this brief chapter and made it more understandable.

BIBLIOGRAPHY

Atkinson AJ, Daniels CE, Dedrick RL, et al., eds. *Principles of clinical pharmacology.* New York: Academic Press, 2001.

Becklake MR, Kauffmann F. Gender differences in airway behavior over the human life span. *Thorax* 1999;54;1119–1138.

Berg MJ. Pharmacokinetic differences between men and women. In: Atkinson AJ, Daniels CE, Dedrick RL, et al., eds. *Principles of clinical pharmacology.* New York: Academic Press, 2001:265–275.

Chen ML, Lee SC, Ng MJ, et al. Pharmacokinetic analysis of bioequivalence trials: implications for sex-related issues in clinical pharmacology and biopharmaceutics. *Clinical pharmacology and therapeutics* 2000;68:510–521.

Collins P, Stevenson JC, Mosca L. Spotlight on gender. *Cardiovasc Res* 2002;53: 535–537.

Cummins CL, Wu CY, Benet LZ. Sex-related differences in the clearance of cytochrome p450 3a4 substrates may be caused by p-glycoprotein. *Clin Pharmacol Ther* 2002;72:474–489.

Heinrich J. Letter to Senators Harkin, Snowe, and Mikulski and Congressman Waxman. Drug safety: most drugs withdrawn in recent years had greater health risks for women. Washington, DC: General Accounting Office, 2001: GAO-01-286R.

Mattison DR. Gender differences in response to drugs and environmental toxicants. In: Ness RB, Kuller LH, eds. *Health and disease among women: biological and environmental influences.* New York: Oxford University Press, 1999:33–57.

Meibohm B, Beierle I, Derendorf H. How important are gender differences in pharmacokinetics? *Clin Pharmacokinet* 2002;41:329–342.

Schwartz JB. The influence of sex on pharmacokinetics. *Clin Pharmacokinet* 2003;42:107–121.

Wizemann TM, Pardu ML, eds. *Exploring the biological contributions to human health: does sex matter?* Washington, DC: Institute of Medicine, National Academy Press, 2001.

CHAPTER 13

The Menopausal Woman

Carl Nath, Michelle Khan, and Gloria Bachmann

Menopause, the permanent cessation of ovarian endocrine function and menstruation, occurs among women in the United States at a median age of 51 years. Women today can expect to spend more than one third of their life past the age of menopause (Fig. 13.1). Because the average life expectancy for female Americans is 79.5 years, women who reach the menopause are expected to live another 30 years. Clinicians who interact with perimenopausal and postmenopausal women therefore have a wonderful opportunity to affect their future health and should be deeply committed to providing preventive health care.

The term *menopause* has been defined as the period of time following a woman's last menstrual cycle, and retrospectively, it is said to have occurred when a woman has been amenorrheic for 9 months. More accurately, menopause is the cessation of menstruation that results from the diminution of ovarian steroid levels secondary to follicle attrition. The *perimenopause* is the 3- to 5-year period before menopause during which estrogen levels begin to drop. This period is usually characterized by menstrual irregularity and can be evidenced clinically through rising serum levels of follicle-stimulating hormone and a menopausal symptom complex including vasomotor, urogenital, and psychological symptoms. The *climacteric* encompasses the period of endocrine, somatic, and transitory psychological changes occurring during the transition to menopause.

The loss of estrogen at menopause is associated with significant increases in the incidence of sexual dysfunction, cardiovascular disease, and osteoporotic fractures. Statistics show coronary artery disease to be the major cause of death in women after menopause, with almost twice as many women dying of heart disease than of all forms of cancer combined. The risk for fractures of the hip, spine, or distal forearm in women after the age of 50 is approximately 40%. Postmenopausal women are therefore at risk for potentially debilitating or life-threatening events that are related to ovarian failure and estrogen deprivation.

PHYSIOLOGY OF MENOPAUSE

Most women in the perimenopausal period experience variations in cycle length beginning 2 to 8 years before menopause. The major determinant of cycle length is the variation of the follicular phase. A change in the length of a woman's menstrual cycle is accompanied by elevated levels of follicle-stimulating hormone (FSH) and luteinizing hormone (LH) and decreased levels of inhibin and estradiol (Fig. 13.2). As the ovary ages, fewer follicles develop until the follicular supply is completely depleted and cessation of menses occurs. However, until the cessation of menses, ovulation may take place, leading to the possibility of an unexpected pregnancy. Because of this variability in ovarian function, the use of contraception should be recommended until the postmenopausal state is confirmed.

Nongravid women synthesize two biologically active estrogens, estradiol (E_2) and estrone (E_1). During the reproductive years, the ovaries are the main source of estrogen, whereas postmenopausally the periphery, including adipose tissue, muscle,

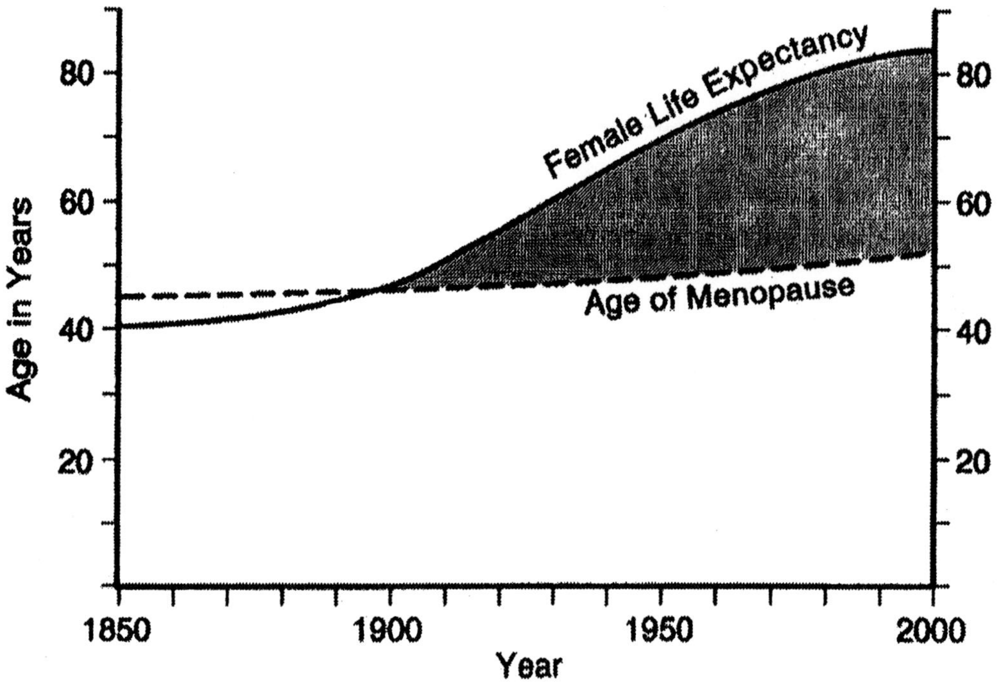

FIG. 13.1. Changes in the life expectancy and age of women at the menopause during the past 150 years. (From Nachtigall LE. The aging woman. In: Sciarra JJ, ed. *Gynecology and obstetrics.* Philadelphia: JB Lippincott, 1995: Chapter 28, with permission.)

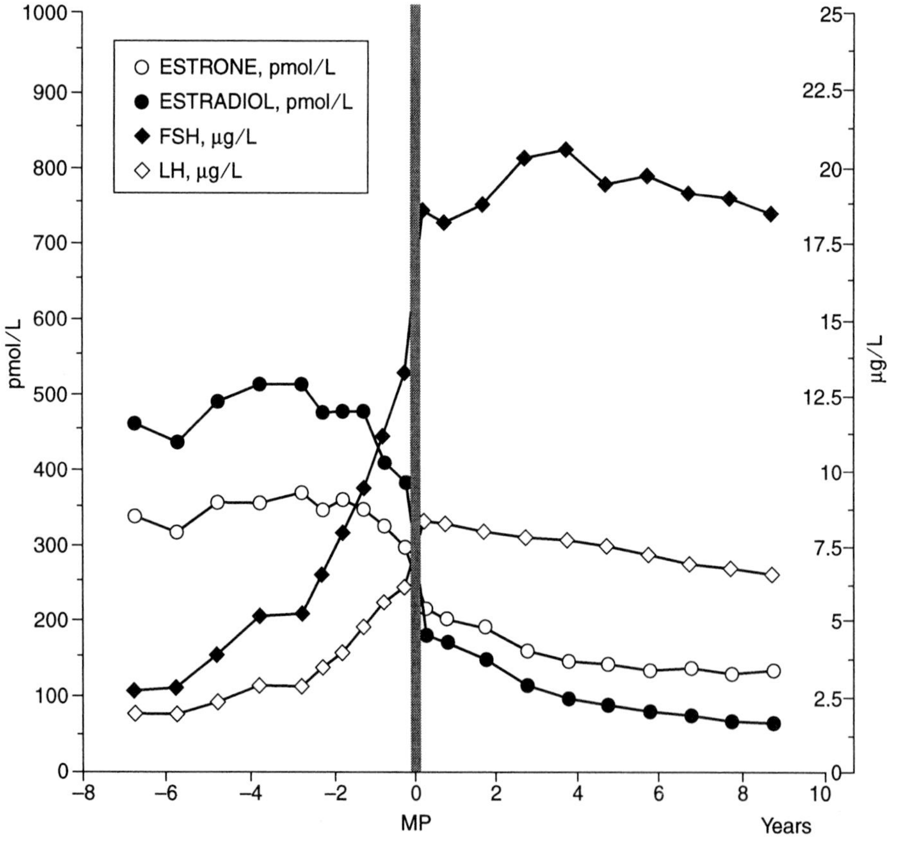

FIG. 13.2. Mean serum levels of follicle-stimulating hormone, luteinizing hormone, estradiol, and estrone during the perimenopausal transition. (From Rannevik G, Jeppsson S, Johnell O, et al. A longitudinal study of the perimenopausal transition: altered profiles of steroid and pituitary hormones, SHBG, and bone mineral density. *Maturitas* 1995;21:103–113, with permission.)

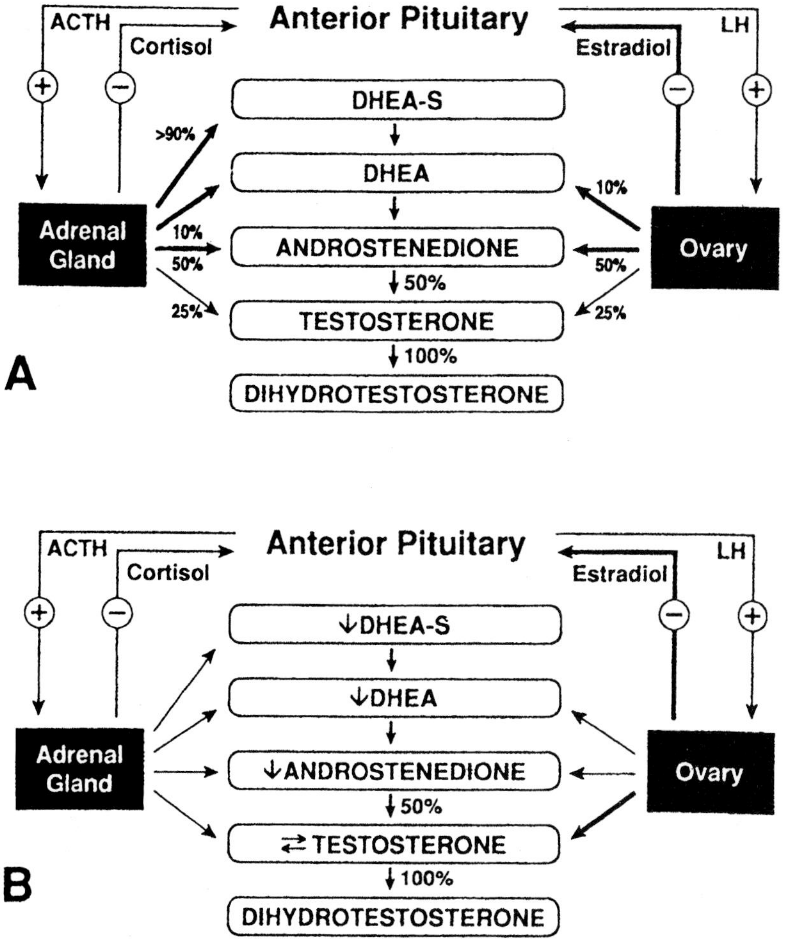

FIG. 13.3. Androgen dynamics in **(A)** premenopausal and **(B)** postmenopausal women. Menopausal levels of luteinizing hormone drive the ovarian stroma to produce more testosterone, compensating in part for the age-related loss of adrenal androgens and androgen precursors. (From Buster JE, Casson PR. DHEA: biology and use in therapeutic intervention. In: Lobo RA, Kelsey J, Marcus R, eds. *Menopause: biology and pathobiology.* New York: Academic Press, 2000:625–638, with permission.)

and the adrenal glands, plays a larger role in supplying a woman's body with estrogen. It should be noted that circulating levels of androgens (androstenedione, testosterone, dehydroepiandrosterone [DHEA], and dehydroepiandrosterone sulfate [DHEAS]), which are precursors of the estrogens, are also present in both premenopausal and postmenopausal women (Fig. 13.3).

Estrogen, a steroid hormone, diffuses through the cell membrane and interacts with a nuclear receptor. The activated ligand-and-receptor complex then enters the nucleus and induces biologic change by acting on DNA-response elements within target genes. Steroid receptors are widespread in the body. The two major subtypes of estrogen receptors, the alpha (ER-α) and beta (ER-β) forms, are distributed differently in tissues; ER-α is dominant in the breasts, kidneys, endometrium, ovaries, and vagina, whereas ER-β is concentrated in the brain, ovaries, bladder, and lungs. Each activated ER-ligand complex displays unique properties, depending on the tissue involved and the structural relationship between the particular ligand and estrogen receptor. For example, the tamoxifen–ER-α complex acts as an estrogen antagonist in breast tissue but as an estrogen mimetic in the endometrium. On the other hand, the raloxifene–ER-α complex functions as a pure anti-estrogen in endometrium. The distinctive properties of ligand-receptor complexes have important pharmacologic implications because they result in selective actions of pharmacologically administered estrogens in different tissues.

Many of the symptoms of menopause can be explained by the effect of estrogen deprivation on different target organs. The response of each organ to decreased estrogen levels may or may not produce clinically apparent symptoms in the postmenopausal woman. For example, estrogen deprivation in the reproductive tract leads to atrophy of the endometrium and vagina, which often causes dryness, irritation, and dyspareunia in menopausal women. On the other hand, estrogen deprivation in bone leads to an increase in the overall remodeling process of bone and a concomitant decrease in bone mineral density in the first few years after menopause. This organic response, in contrast to reproductive tract symptoms, may not be clinically apparent until many years later or until a fracture occurs.

SYMPTOMS DURING MENOPAUSE

Estrogen deprivation is primarily responsible for the classic symptoms of menopause: abnormalities in vasomotor reactivity, urogenital atrophy, and psychological alterations such as mood disorder, depression, irritability, insomnia, and decreased libido. Although many changes that women go through during the menopause are related to a drop in estrogen levels, some are merely a result of the aging process.

Vasomotor Symptoms

The prevalence and intensity of vasomotor symptoms among menopausal women are variable. The symptoms include hot flushes, perspiration, and palpitations. The vasomotor flush, or "hot flush," viewed as the hallmark of the climacteric, is the most common symptom of perimenopause. A hot flush is a sudden feeling of heat that rushes the body and face. The skin may redden to a blush, and profuse perspiration may occur. The duration of hot flushes varies from a few seconds to several minutes, and the frequency from rarely occurring to recurrent every few minutes. Hot flushes are more frequent and severe at night, sometimes leading to sleep disruption and insomnia.

Urogenital Atrophy

Estrogen depletion leads to atrophy of the urogenital tissue, which in turn causes vulvar, vaginal, and urinary symptoms; these include pruritus, dyspareunia, urinary urgency, incontinence, urethritis, and cystitis. Estrogen maintains a moist and healthy vaginal environment through the transudation of secretions secondary to increased blood flow and through glycogenation of the vaginal mucosa. The resulting *Lactobacillus*-dominant environment maintains a normal acidic pH below 4.5, which discourages the growth of *Escherichia coli* and promotes a healthy vaginal ecosystem. Because women on systemic hormone replacement therapy (HRT) may have atrophic vaginitis, supplemental local vaginal estrogen can be therapeutic.

Psychological Variables

The menopause is a time of great physiologic change for a woman, and changes in both body function and individual life circumstances can greatly affect her psyche. Many women experience mood changes throughout the climacteric, with one half of perimenopausal women reporting feeling irritated or depressed and about one third experiencing a decrease in libido. Although a drop in hormone levels is an important factor in the urogenital atrophy and decreased sexual functioning that women experience during menopause, evidence is lacking to demonstrate that the depressive symptoms and mood changes of the perimenopausal and postmenopausal period are associated with hormonal changes.

Abnormal Uterine Bleeding

Fluctuating hormone levels can cause erratic changes in the menstrual cycle. The perimenopause may be associated with anovulatory cycles that lead to irregularity in the menses, such as decreased flow, prolonged flow, or spotting between periods. Women should be counseled by their physicians before the climacteric, so that they know what to expect during the perimenopause and do not become unduly alarmed at the onset of menstrual irregularity.

MENOPAUSE AND CARDIOVASCULAR DISEASE

Heart disease is the number one killer of women in the United States, and the incidence of cardiovascular disease-related morbidity and mortality increases dramatically following the menopause. Long-term estrogen replacement therapy (ERT), alone or in combination with progesterone, has long been viewed as an effective means of reducing the risk for postmenopausal cardiovascular morbidity and mortality. Evidence supporting the use of HRT to prevent cardiovascular disease has been derived mainly from cohort, case control, and descriptive studies. Two short-term, randomized, placebo-controlled trials have addressed cardiovascular outcomes with HRT use. The Postmenopausal Estrogen/Progestin Interventions (PEPI) Trial looked at the development of cardiovascular risk factors in healthy postmenopausal women as measures of outcome. The Heart and Estrogen/Progestin Replacement Study (HERS) studied the effect of HRT on cardiovascular event and death rates in women with known coronary artery disease.

The PEPI Trial compared the effects of placebo, unopposed estrogen, and each of three estrogen/progestin combination therapies on risk factors for cardiovascular disease, including lipoproteins, fibrinogen, insulin, and blood pressure. This 3-year multicenter, randomized, double-blinded trial demonstrated that 0.625 mg of conjugated equine estrogen (CEE), given either alone (ERT) or with cyclic medroxyprogesterone acetate (MPA) or cyclic micronized progesterone, improves the lipoprotein profile by decreasing levels of low-density lipoprotein (LDL) cholesterol and increasing levels of high-density lipoprotein (HDL) cholesterol. In addition, the placebo group was found to have a significantly higher increase in mean fibrinogen levels than any of the treatment groups. As had been documented previously, the use of unopposed estrogen in the CEE group was associated with a significantly increased risk for endometrial hyperplasia. The PEPI Trial Investigators therefore recommended unopposed estrogen for women with a prior hysterectomy and combination estrogen/progestin for women with a uterus as the most favorable treatment options for lowering selected risk factors for cardiovascular disease in postmenopausal women.

The HERS was a secondary prevention trial evaluating the recurrence of coronary heart disease events and the use of HRT in women with established coronary artery disease. Subjects were randomized to receive either CEE-MPA (0.625 mg of CEE per day and 2.5 mg of MPA per day) or placebo. Although no significant differences were observed in any cardiovascular outcomes between the treatment and placebo groups at the end of the 4-year study, the treatment did increase the risk for venous thromboembolic events and gallbladder disease. In addition, a time trend was noted, with significantly more cardiovascular events occurring in the treatment group in the first year after the initiation of therapy. This increased risk for coronary heart disease disappeared after 2 or more years of active HRT therapy, at which time women in the treatment group actually exhibited fewer adverse outcomes. The HERS Research Group concluded in 1998 that starting HRT for the secondary prevention of CHD could not be recommended, whereas women already receiving the treatment could continue, given the favorable effects demonstrated after several years of therapy. However, after an additional 2.7 years of follow-up, the investigators found that the favorable cardiovascular effects did not persist in the treatment group. The new recommendation is that HRT should not be used for the secondary prevention of cardiovascular disease.

The Women's Health Initiative (WHI), one of the most important ongoing women's health studies, is being sponsored by the National Heart, Lung, and Blood Institute in collaboration with other units of the National Institutes of Health. This randomized controlled trial, like the PEPI Trial, is assessing the effects of HRT in healthy postmenopausal women. However, unlike the PEPI Trial, which looked at risk factors for cardiovascular disease, the WHI is the first randomized primary prevention trial designed to answer numerous questions about the role of HRT and the outcomes of chronic disease (cardiovascular disease, cancer, osteoporosis) in postmenopausal women. A total of 161,809 healthy postmenopausal women between the ages of 50 and 79 years were enrolled in the WHI between 1993 and 1998. The initiative is examining several issues, including a low-fat dietary pattern, calcium and vitamin D supplementation, estrogen-only HRT, and estrogen plus progestin HRT.

Originally planned to continue for 8.5 years, the estrogen plus progestin trial of the WHI was stopped prematurely and the results were released in July 2002 because of a noted increased risk for invasive breast cancer and overall health risks that exceeded benefits during an average follow-up of 5.2 years in 16,608 women with an intact uterus. The objective of the estrogen plus progestin trial was to examine the effect of combined HRT in preventing fractures and heart disease and to observe the associated risks for breast and colon cancer. The treatment was found to have a hazard ratio (HR) of 1.26 (95% confidence interval [CI], 1.00–1.59) for invasive breast cancer, which tipped the scales in terms of benefits versus risks and caused the study to be stopped. Other results included an HR of 1.22 (95% CI, 1.09–1.36) for total heart disease, including an HR of 1.41 (95% CI, 1.07–1.85) for stroke and 2.13 (95% CI, 1.39–3.25) for pulmonary embolism. The benefits found in the study were an HR of 0.63 (95% CI, 0.43–0.92) for colorectal cancer, 0.76 (95% CI, 0.69–0.85) for total fractures, and 0.66 (95% CI, 0.45–0.98) for hip fractures alone.

The results of the estrogen plus progestin trial of the WHI have far-reaching implications for the estimated 6 million postmenopausal American women currently taking the therapy. Many women have stopped their medication because of fears of heart disease, breast cancer, or stroke. However, it must be emphasized that the results of the WHI show a statistically significant increase in disease risk for the overall population, which does not translate directly to individual patients. In addition, the mean age of the women participating in the WHI was older than that of most women who begin HRT for vasomotor symptoms. The risk for the development of breast cancer in an individual postmenopausal woman on an estrogen/progestin regimen is less than 0.1% per year. The bottom line for clinicians is that the initiation or continuation of HRT in postmenopausal women should be approached in an individualized manner, with the benefits of HRT weighed against each woman's personal risks for cardiovascular disease, stroke, thromboembolism, and cancer.

The estrogen-only trial of the WHI is continuing, and the final results are expected in March 2005, along with the results of the low-fat dietary and calcium/vitamin D supplementation studies.

NEUROLOGIC FUNCTION DURING MENOPAUSE

Perimenopausal women may report cognitive changes, including difficulty recalling words or numbers, forgetting events and actions, and difficulty concentrating. This decline in cognitive function has been associated with a loss of estrogen. Estrogen has been shown to improve verbal memory in postmenopausal women, both endogenously and as part of HRT, and may be a key factor in synapse formation in specific types of neurons (Table 13.1). Studies also show that estrogen increases cerebral blood flow in postmenopausal women, and the increased blood flow can improve cognitive abilities. More research needs to be done to validate the role of estrogen in cognition because the evidence is contradictory.

TABLE 13.1. Effects of Estrogen on Brain Function

Organizational actions
Neurotrophic actions
Neuroprotective actions
Effects on neurotransmitters
Effects on glial cells
Effects on proteins involved in Alzheimer disease

Source: Modified from Henderson VW. Estrogen, cognition, and a woman's risk of Alzheimer's disease. *Ann J Med* 1997;130[Suppl 3A]:11–18, with permission.

The use of estrogen to prevent Alzheimer disease awaits the results of long-term, prospective, randomized controlled trials. Studies to date have suggested a promising role for estrogen in delaying the onset of Alzheimer disease or the reducing risk for this disease in postmenopausal women. However, estrogen intervention is effective only when administered early, before significant neuronal degeneration has taken place. Women at high risk for Alzheimer disease may be promising candidates for ERT. Most studies have not demonstrated any improvement in cognitive function in women who already have Alzheimer disease.

In addition to its beneficial effects on cognition, HRT improves mood and sleep and reduces stress levels. In one randomized study, postmenopausal women using ERT reported that they slept better, found it easier to fall asleep, and experienced less nocturnal restlessness and awakening after 3 months of ERT. The improvement in sleep was associated with an alleviation of menopausal symptoms, including vasomotor symptoms, mood changes, palpitations, and muscular pain. A decrease in stress-induced cortisol production and an attenuation of total-body responses to stress have been demonstrated after estrogen supplementation. Furthermore, estrogen may improve the mood of postmenopausal women without clinical depression.

SEXUALITY DURING MENOPAUSE

A reduction in sexual intimacy and satisfaction is extremely common during the menopause. Changes that postmenopausal women frequently experience include a decrease in libido and sexual responsiveness and an increase in dyspareunia. These alterations in postmenopausal female sexual functioning may arise from a host of causes. A drop in sex hormone levels with subsequent urogenital atrophy and mood changes are often at the root of the problem, but factors that are not physically related, such as religious beliefs, fear of abandonment, shamefulness, and loss of touch with inner self, may also contribute to sexual dysfunction and be overlooked by women and their health care practitioners.

During menopause, circulating levels of E_2 drop to approximately 5% of premenopausal levels and are mainly derived from the peripheral conversion of E_1, which in turn is derived from the peripheral conversion of androstenedione. The ratio of androgen to estrogen changes dramatically during menopause, heralded in some women by the onset of mild hirsutism and hair loss. Interestingly, some women who do not receive HRT may experience an increase in libido as a consequence of the higher circulating level of androgen in proportion to estrogen.

The withdrawal of estradiol during menopause results in a reduction of mitotic activity in the vaginal and urethral mucosa, which in turn leads to a thinning and decrease in the elasticity of this layer. Furthermore, collagen and adipose tissue are lost in the vulva, and the clitoral glans loses its protective covering. Clinically, the vaginal and urethral mucosal layer appears thin, dry, pale, and flattened. These hypoestrogenic changes are associated with vaginal dryness, burning, and dyspareunia, and an increased incidence of urethritis and urinary incontinence. Clinicians commonly prescribe HRT to alleviate these symptoms. The vaginal epithelium of postmenopausal women who do not receive HRT is often thin and dry, so that they are more susceptible to trauma and abrasion during sexual activity.

In addition to systemic HRT, estrogen creams and tablets and an estradiol-impregnated vaginal ring are available that can effectively treat and reverse local vaginal atrophy. However, the ready absorption of locally administered vaginal estrogen preparations through the mucosa leads to significant increases in circulating levels if the vaginal dose of estrogen is standard or high.

Other characteristics of menopause, such as hot flushes, sleep disorders, fatigue, and mood changes, may combine to affect sexuality and sexual behavior adversely.

An additional issue concerning the sexuality of women during menopause is their willingness, or lack thereof, to discuss their symptoms with their health care providers and actively seek answers to their questions. Often, menopausal women may not express their difficulties because they are embarrassed to discuss their sexual needs with their health care provider, who may not directly question patients about this subject. Many patients feel that no medical treatment for their problem is available or that their physician would be uncomfortable or dismissive of their concerns. Clinicians should be cognizant of the changes in sexuality that occur during menopause and should approach this topic with their patients in the form of a simple, forthright question about sexual function. Initiation by the clinician may be helpful in discussing a topic that women might otherwise be embarrassed or hesitant to bring up.

BREAST CANCER

The incidence of breast cancer increases as women age (Fig. 13.4). This age-associated increase may be explained in part by an extended duration of estrogen exposure, such as occurs in patients with early menarche, late menopause, or obesity. For a woman between the ages of 50 and 59 years, the lifetime risk of having breast cancer diagnosed is 1 in 36, whereas for a woman between the ages of 70 and 79 years, the risk increases to 1 in 24.

Two retrospective observational studies examined the association of breast cancer and the use of estrogen/progestin HRT regimens. In one study, researchers reviewed data on 46,355 postmenopausal women who were monitored for 15 years in the Breast Cancer Detection Demonstration Project. In 2,082 incident cases of breast cancer, the investigators found that among women with current or recent HRT use (within the past 4 years), the risk was increased 1.2-fold in those taking estrogen alone and 1.4-fold in those taking estrogen plus a progestin. The other study matched 1,897 breast cancer cases with a control group and also found a statistically higher risk for breast cancer in patients using estrogen/progestin HRT.

The American College of Obstetrics and Gynecology has calculated that the projected absolute lifetime risk for nonusers of estrogen is about 10 cases of breast cancer per 100 women. This baseline risk increases to approximately 12 cases per 100 women with unopposed estrogen use and to 14 cases per 100 women with combined HRT use. Therefore, combination HRT seems to have a more deleterious effect with respect to breast cancer than estrogen alone. A deleterious effect of the combined estrogen/progestin regimen on the incidence of breast cancer was confirmed by the trial of the WHI, which was ended prematurely when an HR of 1.26 (95% CI, 1.00–1.59) was found for the use of estrogen plus progestin for an average of 5.2 years.

The most important preventive measure for improving breast cancer outcome is early detection. All menopausal women should be encouraged to perform monthly breast self-examinations, have regular physical examinations, and receive screening mammograms.

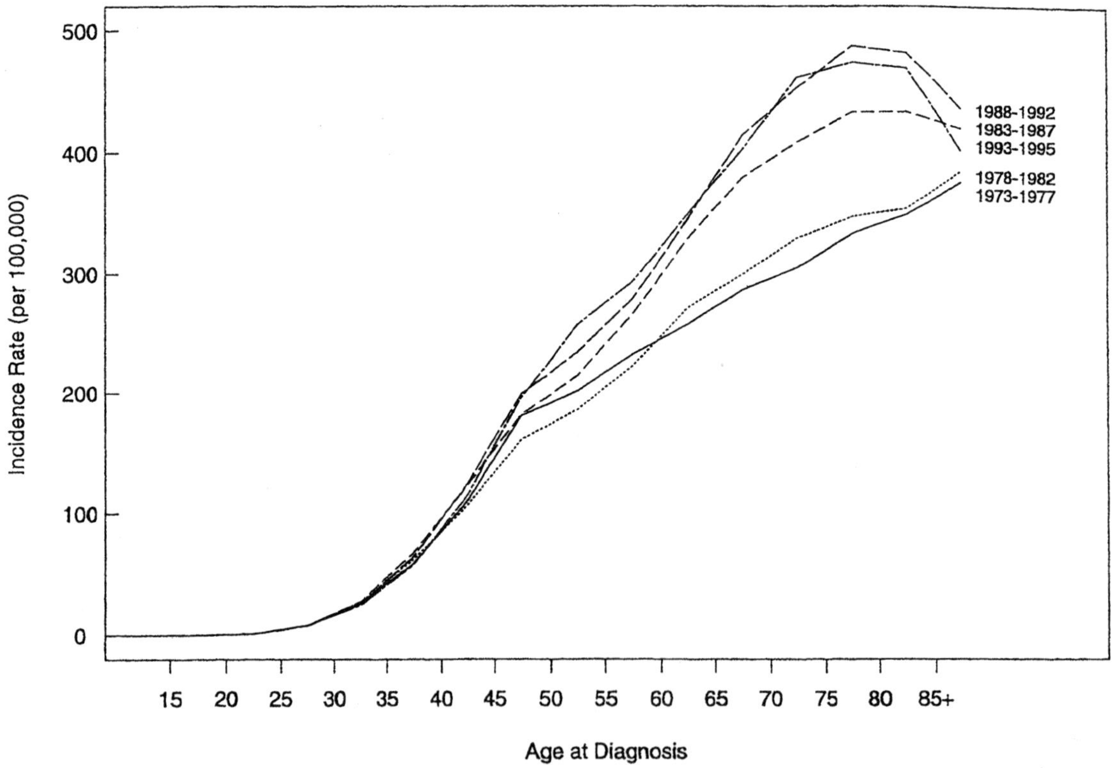

FIG. 13.4. Incidence rates of invasive breast cancer by age and time period. (From Karagas MR, Kelsey J, McGuire V. Cancers of the female reproductive system. In: Lobo RA, Kelsey J, Marcus R, eds. *Menopause: biology and pathobiology*. New York: Academic Press, 2000:359–381, with permission.)

Mammography screening has been shown to decrease breast cancer deaths. The initial age at screening and the optimal screening interval to maximize the detection of breast cancer are controversial. The American Cancer Society recommends a baseline mammogram from ages 35 to 39, mammography at 1- to 2-year intervals from ages 40 to 49, and an annual mammogram for women ages 50 and older. For women at high risk, a baseline mammogram is recommended at age 30. A negative screening mammogram should not exclude a cancer diagnosis when a palpable breast mass is present. Rather, for preventive measures, a biopsy specimen or aspirate should be obtained in a timely fashion.

Even though patients with breast cancers detected at an early stage have a favorable prognosis, many menopausal women do not undergo screening mammography at the recommended intervals. The health care professional should review the increase in risk with age, recommended screening intervals, and performance of the breast self-examination with their patients. Mammography and appropriate follow-up should be recommended for women in the perimenopausal and postmenopausal age range.

OVARIAN CANCER

Nearly 8 million women in the United States take some form of ERT. The association between ERT and ovarian cancer was reported to be significant in an observational study. In a follow-up of the women in the Breast Cancer Detection Demonstration Project, ever-use of estrogen and use for 10 to 19 years and 20 or more years were significantly associated with ovarian cancer, with relative risks of 1.6 (95% CI, 1.2–2.0), 1.8 (95% CI, 1.1–3.0), and 3.2 (95% CI, 1.7–5.7), respectively. The association between ovarian cancer and estrogen/progestin HRT was not significant; however, randomized controlled trials to study the risk for ovarian cancer with both ERT and combined regimens are warranted. The WHI is continuing the trial with ERT alone, and the results expected in 2005 may clarify the role of estrogen in the development of ovarian cancer.

OSTEOPOROSIS

Aging is associated with a gradual loss of bone mineral density in both men and women. In women, the bone mineral density decreases by approximately 1% per year between the ages of 35 and 45 years; the rate of decrease then accelerates at the onset of menopause to approximately 3% per year for the first 5 years, returning to 1% per year thereafter. Bone loss enhances fragility and increases the risk for fractures. Osteopenia or osteoporosis is diagnosed in many women soon after they go through menopause. *Osteopenia,* or decreased bone mass, is defined by the World Health Organization as a bone mineral density between 1 and 2.5 standard deviations below the mean value for young adults. *Osteoporosis* is diagnosed when the bone mineral density is 2.5 standard deviations or more below the mean for young adults. The National Osteoporosis Foundation estimates that in 2002, between 17 and 23 million postmenopausal women had osteopenia or osteoporosis. Factors related to the development of osteoporosis include genetic background, nutritional state, level of activity, and level of estrogen.

Bone is a dynamic tissue that undergoes constant loss and replacement in a remodeling cycle. The remodeling process consists of two simultaneous and opposing forces. Bone resorption occurs when osteoclasts secrete acid hydrolases, collagenases, and other proteolytic enzymes that degrade the matrix and minerals of bone; bone replacement occurs when osteoblasts secrete osteoid, which then undergoes calcification and vascularization. A loss of bone mineral density is the result of a shift in the bone remodeling process so that bone resorption exceeds bone replacement.

Osteoporosis is usually asymptomatic until fractures occur. Eighty percent of total bone mass is cortical bone, with trabecular bone comprising the rest. Trabecular bone is more vulnerable to alterations in the bone remodeling process because remodeling occurs eight times faster in trabecular bone than in cortical bone. The vertebral bodies are composed mainly of trabecular bone, and compression fractures of the vertebrae are the most common type of fracture in menopausal women. Hip fractures occur frequently 15 to 25 years after menopause. Women in this age range are at high risk because of the combination of reduced bone mass and an increased number of falls. In addition to the considerable morbidity associated with fractures, hip fractures are associated with an excess mortality of 10% to 20%, so that osteoporosis is a cause of great concern.

An effective approach for the early detection of osteopenia and osteoporosis is bone mineral density testing. Several techniques are available; however, dual-energy x-ray absorptiometry (DEXA) remains the "gold standard." DEXA offers the advantages of rapid results, a high level of precision, and minimal radiation exposure, approximately 10% that of standard chest roentgenography. Limitations of DEXA include the cost of equipment, the need for a certified x-ray technician, and a lack of portability. Other methods frequently used for bone mineral density testing are ultrasonographic densitometry for screening peripheral bone and quantitative computed tomography.

The National Osteoporosis Foundation has established guidelines for the prevention and treatment of osteoporosis. Specific recommendations include bone mineral density testing for all postmenopausal women age 65 years or older, postmenopausal women younger than 65 years who have one or more risk factors for osteoporosis or who present with fractures, and women who have been on HRT for a prolonged period (Fig. 13.5).

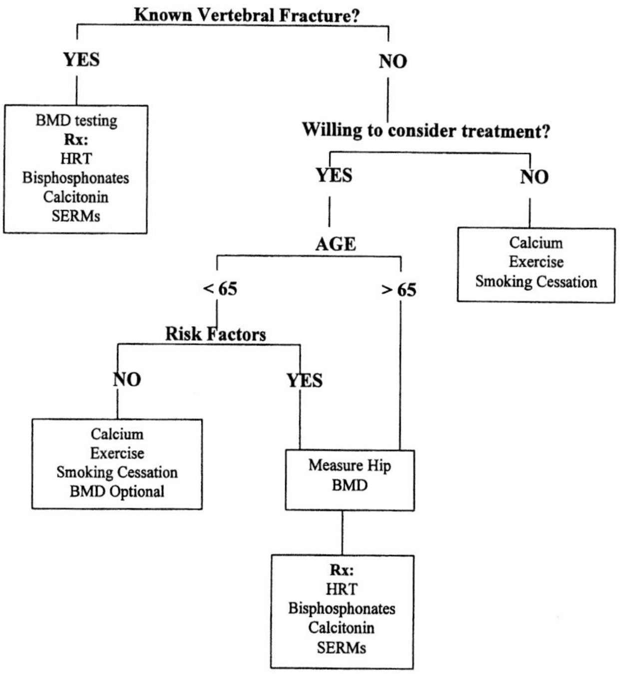

FIG. 13.5. Guidelines for the prevention and treatment of postmenopausal osteoporosis. (Modified from the National Osteoporosis Foundation, Washington, DC, with permission.)

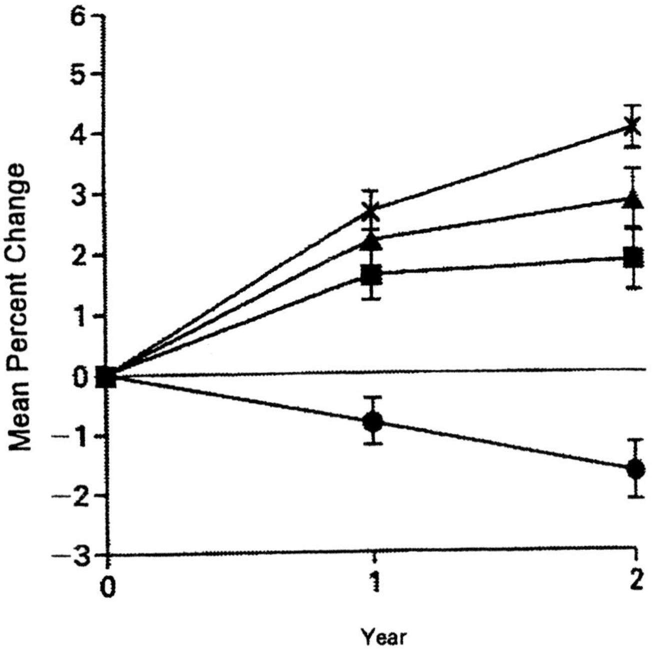

FIG. 13.6. Mean percentage change from baseline in bone mineral density of the hip in postmenopausal women given estrogen/progestin (x), 5 mg of alendronate (▲), 2.5 mg of alendronate (■), or placebo (●). (From Hosking D, Chilvers CED, Christiansen C, et al. Prevention of bone loss with alendronate in postmenopausal women under 60 years of age. *N Engl J Med* 1998;338:485–492, with permission.)

HRT has been the conventional therapy for the treatment and prevention of postmenopausal osteoporosis. Standard doses of estrogen that are currently used include 0.625 mg of conjugated estrogen or 0.5 mg of micronized estradiol. Other pharmacologic therapies that are effective in preventing bone loss include the bisphosphonates, selective estrogen receptor modulators (SERMs), and calcitonin (Fig. 13.6). Alternative therapies, particularly soy and magnesium, may also be of benefit in increasing bone mineral density, but no randomized controlled trials have been performed to evaluate their effect on osteoporotic fractures.

The prevention of osteoporosis should incorporate a lifelong strategy, beginning in early adolescence and continuing during the reproductive years and through to menopause. With the onset of menopause, the practitioner should readdress the dietary needs for calcium and vitamin D with patients and emphasize the benefits of exercise, lifestyle modification, preventive surveillance, and available treatments.

SUMMARY

The menopause and postmenopausal years encompass a substantial proportion of a woman's life. Managing the spectrum of conditions and risk factors that accompany this period poses a challenge to women and their physicians. The approach to each woman's menopause should take into account her symptoms, such as vasomotor and urogenital problems, in addition to her personal risk factors for cancer, osteoporosis, and heart disease. Other life circumstances that may affect her overall health should also be considered, such as smoking, obesity, lack of exercise, and personal relationships. With appropriate preventive and interventional care, most women will be able to live through their postmenopausal years sound in body and mind.

BIBLIOGRAPHY

Brinton LA, Hoover RN. Estrogen replacement therapy and endometrial cancer risk: unresolved issues. The Endometrial Cancer Collaborative Group. *Obstet Gynecol* 1993;81:265–271.

Centers for Disease Control and Prevention, National Center for Health Statistics. Fast stats A to Z: life expectancy. June 13, 2002. Available at www.cdc.gov/nchs/fastats/lifexpec.htm. Accessed July 18, 2002.

Dennerstein L, Dudley EC, Hopper JL, et al. A prospective population-based study of menopausal symptoms *Obstet Gynecol* 2000;96:351–358.

Ettinger B. Optimal use of postmenopausal hormone replacement. *Obstet Gynecol* 1988;72[Suppl]:31S–36S.

Grady D, Herrington D, Bittner V, et al. Cardiovascular outcomes during 6.8 years of hormone therapy: Heart and Estrogen/Progestin Replacement Study Follow-up (HERS II). *JAMA* 2002;288:49–57.

Hulley S, Grady D, Bush T, et al., for the Heart and Estrogen/Progestin Replacement Study (HERS) Research Group. Randomized trial of estrogen plus progestin for secondary prevention of coronary heart disease in postmenopausal women. *JAMA* 1998;280:605–613.

Komesaroff PA, Esler MD, Krishnankutty S. Estrogen supplementation attenuates glucocorticoid and catecholamine responses to mental stress in perimenopausal women. *J Clin Endocrinol Metab* 1999;84:606–610.

Kuiper GG, Carlsson B, Grandian K, et al. Comparison of the ligand-binding specificity and transcript tissue distribution of estrogen receptors alpha and beta. *Endocrinology* 1997;138:863–870.

Lacey JV Jr, Mink PJ, Lubin JH, et al. Menopausal hormone replacement therapy and risk of ovarian cancer. *JAMA* 2002;288:334–341.

Maki PM, Resnick SM. Longitudinal effects of estrogen replacement therapy on PET cerebral blood flow and cognition. *Neurobiol Aging* 2000;21:373–383.

McEwen B. Estrogen actions throughout the brain. *Recent Prog Horm Res* 2002;57:357–384.

Mitchell ES, Woods NF. Midlife women's attributions about perceived memory changes: observations from the Seattle Midlife Women's Health Study. *J Womens Health Gender-Based Med* 2001;10:351–362.

Mulnard RA, Cotman CW, Kawas C, et al. Estrogen replacement therapy for treatment of mild to moderate Alzheimer's disease: a randomized controlled trial. Alzheimer's Disease Cooperative Study. *JAMA* 2000;283:1007–1015.

National Cancer Institute. Lifetime probability of breast cancer in American women. July 5, 2001. Available at http://cis.nci.nih.gov/fact/5_6.htm. Accessed July 17, 2002.

National Osteoporosis Foundation. *Physician's guide to prevention and treatment of osteoporosis*. Washington, DC: National Osteoporosis Foundation, 2000.

Obermeyer CM. Menopause across cultures: a review of the evidence. *Menopause* 2000;7:184–192.

Polo-Kantola P, Erkkola R, Helenius H, et al. When does estrogen replacement therapy improve sleep quality? *Am J Obstet Gynecol* 1998;178:1002–1009.

Portin R, Polo-Kantola P, Polo O, et al. Serum estrogen level, attention, memory, and other cognitive functions in middle-aged women. *Climacteric* 1999;2:115–123.

Ross RK, Paganini-Hill A, Wan PC, et al. Effect of hormone replacement therapy on breast cancer risk: estrogen versus estrogen plus progestin. *J Natl Cancer Inst* 2000;92:328–332.

Schairer C, Lubin J, Troisi R, et al. Menopausal estrogen and estrogen-progestin replacement therapy and breast cancer risk. *JAMA* 2000;283:485–491.

Sherwin BB. Affective changes with estrogen and androgen replacement therapy in surgically menopausal women. *J Affect Disord* 1988;14:177–187.

Tang M-X, Jacobs D, Stern Y, et al. Effect of oestrogen during menopause on risk and age at onset of Alzheimer's disease. *Lancet* 1996;348:429–432.

Wolf OT, Kirschbaum C. Endogenous estradiol and testosterone levels are associated with cognitive performance in older women and men. *Horm Behav* 2002;41:259–266.

Writing Group for the PEPI Trial. Effects of estrogen or estrogen/progestin regimens on heart disease risk factors in postmenopausal women. The Postmenopausal Estrogen/Progestin Intervention (PEPI) Trial. *JAMA* 1995;273:199–208.

Writing Group for the Women's Health Initiative Investigators. Risks and benefits of estrogen plus progestin in healthy postmenopausal women: principal results from the Women's Health Initiative randomized controlled trial. *JAMA* 2002;288:321–333.

CHAPTER 14

The Elderly Woman

Michelle Carpenter-Bradley, Marie Aydelotte, Brenda L. Johnson, and Phyllis C. Leppert

The field of geriatrics is not limited to the practice of the geriatrician or internist. With the exception of the pediatrician, all medical specialists care for elderly patients. Before the 20th century, few people lived beyond the age of 75 years, whereas more than 50% of the U.S. population now reaches age 75. In the years between 1960 and 2000, the population of persons older than 65 years almost doubled in the United States. It is estimated that by 2030, persons past that age will number 70.3 million, accounting for 20% of the projected population. By virtue of their increased longevity, the majority of these people will be women. In the United States, the number of persons ages 85 or older will increase from 4.3 million in 2000 to an estimated 19.4 million in 2050, or from 1.6% to 4.8% of the total population by 2050.

It is currently accepted that 22 million adults are the informal caregivers for ill or fragile persons older than 50 years of age. They provide most of the long-term care in the United States today. Usually, these informal caregivers are middle-aged women, many of whom are married with children. It is estimated that the economic value of their work was $196 million in 1997. This figure is not included in the official cost-of-illness figures. Great demands are placed on informal caregivers, and in many instances, they have to cope with confused behavior, wandering, sleep-wake disturbances, and sometimes aggression. Thus, many adult caregivers experience chronic distress. The other side of this coin is that many adult caregivers feel isolated when the elderly person in their care is hospitalized or placed in a long-term care facility.

The scope of geriatrics is much too large to include here in its entirety. Virtually every organ system is affected by both the normal and pathologic changes of aging. We have attempted to cover a few specific conditions that, because of their frequency and severity, greatly affect elderly women. By no means, however, are these the only important issues concerning the elderly woman. Pelvic organ prolapse occurs in 21% of women older than 70 years of age and is discussed in Chapter 32. Urinary incontinence, a common problem for elderly women, is discussed in Chapter 81.

SCREENING AND PREVENTIVE CARE

During the last century, the periodic health examination, cancer screening, and preventive care have been studied, and guidelines have been developed by several organizations based on the efficacy of tests and interventions (see Chapter 2). Most of these guidelines apply to adults up to the age of 65, and some to the age of 75, but few recommendations are made for persons beyond this age. As the population ages, these types of data and assessment take on greater importance. For example, when should a healthy elderly woman be counseled to stop having mammograms?

Healthy—that is, disease-free—old age is not uncommon. Only 30% of people older than 85 years are impaired in one of the activities of daily living, and only 20% reside in nursing homes. Dysfunction may become more common with age, but age alone is not an explanation for dysfunction.

The *assessment of functional status* has gained acceptance as an important reflection of an elderly person's overall health. The goal of including this type of assessment in the periodic health examination of patients older than 65 years is to diagnose problems early, target appropriate areas of intervention, and reduce morbidity and mortality. The questions and observations deal with areas commonly affecting the elderly population: vision, hearing, use of arms and legs, continence of urine, nutrition, mental status, depression, activities of daily living, home environment, and social support (Table 14.1).

Advance directives and the identification of a *health care proxy* should be addressed in one or several discussions and documented in the chart; any legal documents that have been completed should be included. The patient, physician, and proxy should discuss specific issues, and the physician and proxy should attempt to acquire an optimal understanding of the patient's wishes in various circumstances, such as cardiac or respiratory arrest or a vegetative state.

In making decisions regarding screening tests for elderly patients, as for persons of all ages, it is wise to inform them of the significance of a positive test result and the likely recommended follow-up, such as colonoscopy, breast biopsy, or chemotherapy. Some patients may not agree to these invasive tests in the absence of an established problem, so that it becomes unnecessary to perform the initial screening test. The elderly population is heterogeneous, and care must be taken to individualize treatment based on multiple factors, such as functional status, comorbidity, and the patient's goals for successful aging, rather than on age alone.

HYPOTHERMIA

Elderly persons are very susceptible to accidental hypothermia resulting from environmental circumstance. Symptoms of hypothermia are an irregular heat beat, slurred speech, slowed breathing, confusion, and sluggishness. The body temperature is 96°F. In this situation, blankets should be placed around the person to keep him or her warm and dry. The victim should be hospitalized because this in a medical emergency. Precautions that should be taken to prevent hypothermia in an elderly person include dressing in layers of clothing both indoors and outside, wearing a hat and gloves in cold weather, wearing enough warm clothing and having enough blankets in bed, eating a balanced diet, keeping active, and having someone responsible check on him or her daily during cold weather. The home temperature of 68°F should be adequate unless the elderly person is sick. Other preventive measures include refraining from drinking alcoholic beverages because they can cause the body core temperature to fall. The elderly often are taking numerous medications, and these also contribute to a fall in the core temperature when the environment is cold. Elderly persons living alone are particularly at risk because they may have been confused about paying heating bills, although most states have laws that provide safeguards against disconnecting utilities in such cases.

OSTEOPOROSIS AND HIP FRACTURE

Progressive loss of bone mass begins in all women after the third decade of life, and it accelerates rapidly in the years after menopause. Clinically significant osteoporosis resulting in fracture occurs in about one in four women older than 65 years. The morbidity, mortality, and costs associated with this disease are tremendous. These topics are discussed in greater detail in Chapter 97.

TABLE 14.1. Procedure for Functional Assessment Screening in the Elderly

Target area	Assessment procedure	Abnormal result	Suggested intervention
Vision	Test each eye with Jasger card while patient wears corrective lenses (if applicable).	Inability to read greater than 20/40.	Refer to ophthalmologist.
Hearing	Whisper a short, easily answered question such as "What is your name?" in each ear while the examiner's face is out of direct view.	Inability to answer question.	Examine auditory canals for cerumen and clean if necessary. Repeat task; if still abnormal in either ear, refer for audiometry and possible prosthesis.
Arm	Proximal: "Touch the back of your head with both hands." Distal: "Pick up the spoon."	Inability to perform task.	Examine the arm fully (muscle, joint, and nerve), paying attention to pain, weakness, limited range of motion. Consider referral for physical therapy
Leg	Observe the patient after instructing as follows: "Rise from your chair, walk 10 feet, return, and sit down."	Inability to walk or transfer out of chair.	Do full neurologic and musculoskeletal evaluation, paying attention to strength, pain, range of motion, balance, and traditional assessment of gait. Consider referral for physical therapy.
Continence of urine	Ask, "Do you ever lose your urine and get wet?"	"Yes."	Ascertain frequency and amount. Search for remarkable causes, including local irritations, polyuric states, and medications. Consider referral.
Nutrition	Ask "Without trying, have you lost 10 pounds or more in the last 8 months?" Weigh the patient. Measure height.	"Yes" or weight is below acceptable range for height.	Perform appropriate medical evaluation.
Mental status	Instruct as follows: "I am going to name three objects (pencil, truck, book). I will ask you to repeat their names, now and then again a few minutes from now." (See text for discussion.)	Inability to recall all three objects after 1 minute.	Administer Folstein Mini-Mental Status Examination. If score is less than 34, search for causes of cognitive impairment. Ascertain onset, duration, and fluctuation of overt symptoms. Review medications. Assess consciousness and effect. Perform appropriate laboratory tasks.
Depression	Ask, "Do you often feel sad or depressed?" or "How are your spirits?"	"Yes" or "Not very good, I guess."	Administer Geriatric Depression Scale. If positive (score above 5), check for antihypersensitive, psychotropic, or other pertinent medications. Consider appropriate pharmacologic or psychiatric treatment.
ADL-IADL	Ask, "Can you get out of bed yourself?" "Can you dress yourself?" "Can you make your own meals?" "Can you do your own shopping?"	"No" to any question.	Corroborate responses with patient's appearance; question family members if accuracy is uncertain. Determine reasons for the inability (motivation compared with physical limitation). Institute appropriate medical, social, or environmental interventions.
Home environment	Ask, "Do you have trouble with stairs inside or outside your home?" Ask about potential hazards inside the home with bathtubs, rugs, or lighting.	"Yes."	Evaluate home safety and institute appropriate countermeasures.
Social support	Ask, "Who would be able to help you in case of illness or emergency?"		List identified persons in the medical record. Become familiar with available resources for the elderly in the community.

ADL-IADL, activities of daily living-instrumental activities of daily living.
Source: Modified from Lache MG, et al. A simple procedure for general screening for functional disability in elderly patients. *Ann Intern Med* 1990;112:899, with permission.

Multiple factors affect the development of osteoporosis, including hormones, nutrition, genetics, and lifestyle. In postmenopausal women, a lack of estrogen causes bone resorption and a net loss of calcium. Malabsorption of calcium and vitamin D commonly develops during aging, which may increase the likelihood of osteoporosis. Lifestyle factors such as alcohol and tobacco use are associated with an increased incidence of the disease. Weight-bearing exercise may be protective. Causes of secondary osteoporosis include medications (e.g., corticosteroids, phenytoin, excess thyroid hormone, heparin) and medical conditions (e.g., hyperparathyroidism, Cushing disease, hyperthyroidism, athletic amenorrhea). Genetic inheritance primarily affects the attainment of peak bone mass during the third decade of life. Osteoporosis is more likely to develop in women of slight stature or with a positive family history.

Hip fracture is the most dreaded complication of osteoporosis for many elderly women. One in seven women who reach the age of 80 sustain a hip fracture. Disability after hip fracture is common. Up to 50% of patients with a hip fracture require short- or long-term nursing home care, and 35% are able to ambulate only with a cane or walker. Mortality is also increased in the months after fracture and may be as high as 15% to 30%. The risk for death is highest in persons of advanced age or with severe medical comorbidity.

The etiology of hip fracture is multifactorial. The major contributors to the risk for hip fracture are osteoporosis and falls, with lesser factors including orientation during a fall and body habitus. Preventing falls may be of major benefit in avoiding hip fracture. Some particularly important ways to decrease the risk for falls include correcting visual impairment and minimizing the use of medications (especially of benzodiazepines, narcotics, and drugs that cause orthostatic hypotension). Correcting environmental hazards, such as poor lighting or throw rugs, may be beneficial.

Types of hip fracture and management techniques are discussed in Chapter 97. A preoperative medical evaluation and the prevention of postoperative complications are helpful in ensuring a good outcome. Delirium, infection, congestive heart failure, and depression are common after fracture repair and should be recognized and treated. Deep venous thrombosis prophylaxis is routine during the postoperative period. Early weight bearing is usually permitted. Intensive rehabilitation therapies begun immediately after surgery are crucial in helping patients achieve the best functional outcome.

FALLS

Falls are a common and serious problem in the elderly. At least 30% of elderly persons living in the community fall one or more times each year. This percentage rises to 50% in the nursing home population. The National Safety Council lists accidents as the sixth leading cause of death in the elderly. The vast majority of these accidents are the result of falls.

Although falls are not a problem only in elderly women, osteoporosis increases the chances of a serious injury in elderly women in comparison with men of the same age. Elderly women are also at greater risk for falling than men, probably because of a number of factors to be discussed later (see section "The Female Faller").

The economic cost of falls is huge. In a study performed in the state of Washington by Alexander and colleagues, $53 million in hospital charges in 1989 were attributable to fall-related trauma in patients older than 65 years of age. This cost did not take into account the long-term sequelae of falls. Falls may result in nursing home placement. The cost of a fall does not end with the hospital discharge.

Fall Injuries

Only about 5% of falls result in a fracture. Conversely, the vast majority of hip fractures are the result of falls.

Even without a fracture, significant soft tissue injuries can cause serious disability. Other consequences include dehydration or rhabdomyolysis as a result of lying on the floor for a prolonged time. Extended contact with a hard surface may also cause serious pressure ulcers.

A fall often triggers a cascade of disability. Bed rest or limited activity following an injury leads to deconditioning. This, in turn, can worsen a person's gait and increase the risk for further falls. An elderly person's ability to take care of herself deteriorates. The loss of independence can be devastating.

The most serious consequence of a fall is death. This can be caused directly by the fall (e.g., serious head injury) or indirectly (e.g., hip fracture leading to deep venous thrombosis that causes pulmonary embolism and death). Mortality is higher in fallers than in near-fallers, partly as a consequence of the fall itself but partly also as a consequence of the overall increased frailty of those who fall.

Psychological Sequelae

Studies have reported that as many as 48% of persons who have fallen fear falling again. Their fear may be disproportionately large in comparison with the degree of injury sustained in the preceding fall. Those who have not personally fallen but express a fear of falling are probably influenced by the fall of a family member or acquaintance.

To varying degrees, a fear of falling limits people's lives and affects their quality of life. It limits their ability to perform the activities of daily living, their physical functioning, and even the activities in which they engage. When severe, fear of falling also prevent people from participating in social activities.

Types of Falls

Falls are generally classified as extrinsic or intrinsic based on etiology. *Extrinsic falls* are caused by environmental hazards, both indoors (objects on the floor, loose throw rugs, telephone and electric cords) and outdoors (slippery sidewalks, loose stones, automobiles). *Intrinsic falls* are caused by personal factors. Many falls are caused by a combination of extrinsic and intrinsic factors. For example, an elderly person with limited vision and slow reflexes is not able to see and avoid an obstacle in her path.

Risk Factors for Falling

A number of risk factors are intrinsic to the elderly patient. Disability and frailty contribute greatly to falls. An elderly person may be getting by without falling until a new problem, such as an acute illness, develops and precipitates a fall.

Neurologic factors are important in falling. Poor vision is a powerful risk factor. Weakness of the lower extremities and disturbances of gait also predispose the elderly to falling. A previous stroke increases the risk for falling by adversely affecting lower extremity strength, balance, vision, and judgment. A fall can often be the presenting symptom of an acute stroke. The neurologic changes of normal aging, such as an increased reaction time and a less organized response to a presented obstacle, can cause falls. Parkinson disease, associated with abnormalities of gait, predisposes to falls. Cerebellar atrophy causes falls through abnormalities of gait and balance. Any vestibular disturbances, including labyrinthitis, Méenière disease, drugs, and benign positional vertigo, affect balance and so increase the risk for falling.

A very strong risk factor for falling is dementia, which acts through a number of mechanisms, including impaired judgment and decreased attention span. The demented patient is unable to devise and carry out an effective movement strategy.

Depression is a risk factor, probably secondary to the decreased attention span associated with this condition.

Joint disease in the elderly contributes to falls. Reduced flexibility and increased stiffness of the joints and muscles lead to lower extremity disability and falls.

Medications are implicated in falls. Both the number and types of medications are factors. Taking more than four prescription drugs and sedatives concurrently has been associated with an increased risk. Cardiac drugs as a class may not be a risk factor, but the orthostatic blood pressure changes associated with many of these medications are a problem. Heavy alcohol use also causes falls.

Decreased hearing is common in the elderly and contributes to falls by decreasing the sensory input that can warn the potential faller of hazards.

Cardiovascular disease can predispose to falls. Syncope can result from arrhythmias, aortic stenosis, or hypotension and precipitate sudden falls. Falls can also occur in the setting of an acute myocardial infarction. Carotid atherosclerosis is a risk factor through its consequences of cerebral hypoperfusion and stroke.

Some metabolic conditions contribute to falls. Hypoglycemia with a decrease in mental status is one of these.

Hyponatremia results in unsteadiness. Dehydration and subsequent hypotension cause falling. Malnutrition indirectly causes falls by contributing to muscle weakness and fatigue.

All these facts would imply that the greater the burden of disease or frailty, the greater the risk for falling. This is true, but research has shown that the vigorous elderly are more likely to be seriously injured when they do fall. The vigorous elderly are more likely to encounter hazardous extrinsic factors and to fall while on the stairs or away from home. Thus, concern and education about falling must to be extended to all elderly patients.

The Female Faller

Elderly women are at greater relative risk for falling than elderly men because of a number of intrinsic and extrinsic factors.

The important risk factors for falling are different in elderly women and elderly men. In women, they are increased age, use of psychotropic medications, inability to rise from a chair without using the arms, polypharmacy, and living alone. In men, they are arthritis of the knees, a past history of stroke, and weak grip strength.

Elderly women living alone are probably at increased risk for falling for several reasons. An elderly woman who lives alone is more likely to undertake physical tasks that put her in danger of falling, such as taking out the garbage or standing on a stool. She may also become fatigued from these physical efforts and be more likely to fall as a result. Or, she may limit her activities outside the home because she is reluctant to do things on her own and thus becomes deconditioned and falls more often. An elderly woman living alone does not have the benefit of an arm to support her or steady her during a walk or to catch her if she trips.

Assessment

It is important to assess the elderly person who has fallen. As in all illnesses, a good history and physical examination are critical. In most cases, these reveal the cause of the fall.

Particular attention should be given to the circumstances of the fall. It should be determined where the fall occurred and what, if any, extrinsic factors played a role. Information about whether a person's shoes fit, the apartment is cluttered, or the person was outside shoveling is helpful.

What symptoms were experienced just before the fall? Dizziness, palpitations, and chest pain can all help point to the cause. The patient's baseline features are important—how is her vision and hearing?

A medication history is necessary. One or several medications may be the culprit. The faller should be questioned about alcohol use. Light to moderate intake may be of no significance, but heavy use probably is.

The symptomatology of acute illness should be sought. Respiratory illness and urinary tract infections are common causes of falls. Questions about unilateral weakness, slurred speech, or new gait disturbances are helpful in determining whether a neurologic event has occurred.

Once a careful history has been obtained, an examination should be performed. The orthostatic vital signs should be noted. If orthostatic changes are present, the underlying cause should be sought. Is there evidence of bleeding, dehydration, or diabetes with an autonomic neuropathy, or are medications causing the changes? The patient's temperature must be taken to check for infectious illnesses.

A meticulous cardiopulmonary examination is important. The lung examination reveals acute respiratory illness or congestive heart failure. The cardiac examination detects valvular disease or arrhythmias. Listening for carotid bruits helps to uncover carotid disease.

The abdominal examination may reveal a source of infection. Suprapubic tenderness and costovertebral angle tenderness suggest that a urinary tract infection may have led to the fall. The symptom of urinary incontinence points to this diagnosis. Incontinence may also indicate that the person has had a seizure and fallen as a result.

The musculoskeletal examination, particularly of the lower extremities, is very important. Muscle strength must be tested. The feet should be checked for deformities, evidence of ill-fitting shoes, corns, calluses, erythema, and pressure ulcers. The knees must be examined for range of motion, deformities, and inflammation. The hips should be checked for the same. Upper body strength should also be evaluated, particularly in those who use assistive devices for ambulation, because good arm and shoulder strength are needed in this situation.

The neurologic examination should start with an evaluation of the special senses. It is important to check the vision because decreased vision is such a strong risk factor for falls. The hearing should be evaluated. Otitis media or impacted cerumen may be causing vertigo.

Testing the muscles and reflexes may reveal a recent or past stroke. Cogwheeling, rigidity, and tremor may help diagnose Parkinson disease. Cerebellar testing may indicate balance problems. During the assessment of balance, see how the patient stands alone and nudge her a bit, with and without her eyes closed, to see if she is able to recover her balance. Nystagmus may be the clue to vestibular disease.

Sensation to pain and vibration should be examined to determine the presence of neuropathy. Proprioception is an essential sensory input in preventing falls and should be tested.

A functional examination includes an evaluation of gait and body sway. The patient should be observed as she rises from a chair to see whether she can get up with or without using the arms, or whether she needs assistance. She should be observed to see whether her feet slide out from under her when she tries to stand. Once she is up, it is important to see whether she stands firmly over her feet or leans backward or forward. A patient's gait is critical. Simple observation of the patient ambulating, with or without an assistive device, can give the examiner a good idea of whether she has a gait disorder.

Although a number of other maneuvers have been devised by researchers, a good, careful examination reveals the cause or causes of many falls. Sometimes, further evaluation with laboratory testing, electrocardiography, and roentgenography is indicated. Anemia may be detected. A chemistry profile may aid in the diagnosis of dehydration, malnutrition, or other metabolic derangements. An electrocardiogram is helpful in detecting an arrhythmia. Radiologic procedures can delineate orthopedic deformities. Computed tomography (CT) or magnetic resonance imaging of the head may be necessary to diagnose central nervous system disorders.

Treatment

Any acute illnesses precipitating the fall should be treated first. Because falls are often the result of the cumulative effect of a number of factors, treating the acute event can be of benefit in preventing further falls.

Efforts should be made to decrease the total number of medications the patient is taking. Individual medications should be evaluated for adverse effects. If orthostatic hypotension is a problem, decreasing or discontinuing diuretics or antihypertensive medications should be considered. Antidepressants should be chosen from or changed to those with the least effect on orthostasis. Anticholinergic medications should be avoided because they cause or exacerbate confusion in the elderly. Sedatives should be discontinued if possible. Psychotropic medications, with their side effects of increased rigidity and sedation, make falls more likely and should be stopped if possible.

Improving vision is very helpful in preventing further falls. An eye examination should be performed and new glasses prescribed if needed. It may also be necessary to increase the lighting in the patient's home.

It is important to educate the faller. She should be advised to change from a lying to a standing position slowly and pause for a few minutes between each change of posture. In this way, the vascular system can adjust, and falls secondary to orthostasis are prevented. The patient should also be advised to avoid hazardous activities, such as climbing a ladder.

Attempts should be made to modify the patient's environment if possible. Hazards such as clutter on stairs and in rooms and hallways can be removed. Loose throw rugs should be taped down or removed. Bathroom safety can be improved with a raised toilet seat, shower, tub seat, and grab bars as needed. A bedside commode can be provided. Enhancing visual contrast with tape on the stairs or patterned flooring may help.

Physical therapy can strengthen the lower extremities and improve gait. The physical therapist evaluates whether a mobility aid, such as a cane or walker, will facilitate ambulation.

Plans must be individually tailored to each patient. It should be realized, however, that many causes of falls are not reversible or treatable, and that the patient will remain at risk for falling.

Research reinforces that efforts must be made to evaluate persons who fall fully and help prevent further falls. Evidence suggests that all people older than 65 years are at risk. They should be educated about risk factors and means to reduce them.

DEMENTIA

Dementia has a huge impact on the elderly woman. She is not only at risk for acquiring dementia herself but also more likely to be the primary caregiver for a spouse with dementia. Although the risk for dementia increases with age, dementia is not a characteristic of normal aging.

Dementia is a clinical syndrome in which an acquired deterioration of cognitive function is manifested as a decline in memory and other deficits of higher cortical function, including language and visuospatial skills.

The incidence of dementia is higher in elderly women, but this is a consequence of advancing age rather than a true increase in risk associated with the female sex. Dementia, including Alzheimer disease, is also discussed in Chapter 108.

Differential Diagnosis and Types of Dementia

Dementia must be differentiated from other disorders that cause cognitive decline. Delirium is commonly mistaken for dementia, particularly in hospitalized patients; delirium may occur in as many as 33% of elderly people admitted. Delirium can present in persons with or without an underlying dementia. It is critical to diagnose delirium because the associated mortality is approximately 25%. Delirium is characterized by the acute or subacute presentation of a confusional state; inattentiveness and a reduced level of consciousness are the hallmarks. Agitation or lethargy may be present, and the patient is likely to be easily distracted. Visual hallucinations are common. Tremors and myoclonus may be seen. Delirium is caused by medications, worsening of the underlying medical condition, or both.

Depression also may mimic dementia in the elderly. Depressed elderly patients may demonstrate bradykinesia and lack of motivation. Agitation often accompanies depression in the elderly. However, a depressed person has few or no memory deficits and no abnormalities of other cortical functions on testing.

Structural defects of the central nervous system can both cause and mimic dementia. These include normal-pressure hydrocephalus, meningiomas, and subdural hematomas. Although such disorders are considered "reversible" causes of dementia, cognitive dysfunction often persists after they have been corrected surgically.

Alzheimer disease is the most common dementing illness. It is associated with a 5-year mortality rate of 95%. The absolute diagnosis of Alzheimer disease depends on the histologic identification of neuropathologic changes of neurofibrillary tangles and plaques on biopsy specimens or brain tissue examined postmortem. The term *Alzheimer disease* is something of a misnomer because the condition likely represents a group of diseases that result in these pathologic features. Alzheimer disease is discussed in detail later in this chapter.

The incidence of multi-infarct dementia may be increasing as the survival of persons who have had strokes increases. Multi-infarct dementia is characterized by an abrupt onset with or without a history of a cerebrovascular accident. The course is usually fluctuating, with stepwise deterioration noted. Multi-infarct dementia is associated with hypertension and coronary artery disease. The examination reveals focal neurologic signs, including dysarthria, increased tone or spasticity, an abnormal small-stepped gait, a Babinski reflex, hemiparesis, and often a labile affect. Laboratory tests may indicate end-organ damage, such as renal disease with elevated blood urea nitrogen and creatinine levels. Treatment focuses on the underlying disorders: control of hypertension, smoking cessation, administration of antiplatelet agents, control of arrhythmias, and administration of anticoagulants for atrial fibrillation. It is important to diagnose and treat multi-infarct dementia because most of these people die of their cardiac disease.

Parkinson disease is often associated with dementia. A patient with Parkinson dementia demonstrates slow mentation on examination, but with preservation of language function. The speech may be difficult to understand because the articulation is affected. Bradykinesia, increased rigidity, pill-rolling tremor, a masklike facies, and cogwheeling are other findings that suggest the diagnosis of Parkinson disease. Treating the Parkinson disease does not cure the dementia.

Conditions that are generally considered to be reversible causes of dementia are thyroid disease, vitamin B_{12} deficiency, neurosyphilis, thiamine deficiency, and hypercalcemia. The incidence of some conditions, such as vitamin B_{12} deficiency, increases with age, and these may simply coexist with Alzheimer disease. Thus, treating reversible causes may improve a person's cognitive abilities but not restore them fully.

Infections such as Jakob-Creutzfeldt disease and herpes encephalitis can cause dementia. Jakob-Creutzfeldt disease is very rare and passed by human-to-human transmission. The onset is sudden, with rapid progression over weeks to months. Bizarre behavior, clumsiness, spasticity, myoclonus, and cortical blindness are characteristic. The results of laboratory tests, cerebrospinal fluid examination, and CT of the head may all be normal, but electroencephalography shows a characteristic burst-suppression pattern. Herpes encephalitis has a subacute presentation of fever, headache, and seizures associated with deterioration of memory or language. Examination of the cerebrospinal fluid demonstrates an elevated red blood cell count and protein level. Head CT may show rarefication of the temporal lobes. If herpes encephalitis is strongly suspected clinically, acyclovir should be started immediately.

Clinical Presentation of Alzheimer Disease

The presentation of Alzheimer disease is often subtle; memory deficits make it difficult for the patient to balance the checkbook, pay bills, or find her way home along a familiar route. The family may bring her in for an evaluation but often attribute her behavior to "getting old." Radical behavioral changes, such as agitation, sleep-wake cycle disturbances, and hallucinations, are more likely to prompt an evaluation.

In Alzheimer dementia, the primary motor and sensory modalities are maintained until late in the disease. The dementia is characterized in the early phase by memory loss and personality and psychiatric changes, such as anxiety, depression, apathy, and withdrawal. In this phase, social skills are relatively well preserved.

Memory is affected in virtually all people with Alzheimer disease. If the memory is not impaired, the diagnosis should be doubted. Patients with early Alzheimer disease usually exhibit mild anomia (i.e., difficulty naming objects).

As the disease progresses to the middle phase, intellectual function deteriorates further. Apraxia, which is the inability to perform complex motor tasks such as manipulating forks and toothbrushes, develops. Agnosia, the inability to recognize or interpret what is seen, felt, or heard, also worsens. Language disorders develop or worsen and can progress to complete aphasia. Visuospatial problems become more severe, impairing the patient's ability to recognize or navigate through familiar environments. The ability to recognize close family members may be lost. Urinary incontinence develops secondary to a loss of inhibitory fibers from the cerebral cortex. Hallucinations, delusions, and paranoia may escalate. Disruptive behaviors, including agitation, wandering, and sleep-wake cycle disturbances, are frequent.

In the late stages of Alzheimer disease, double incontinence (bowel and bladder) develops. Awareness of self and the environment is lost. Patients can become bedridden in a fetal position. They may stop eating. Aspiration becomes a problem. Death often results as a consequence of sepsis and malnutrition.

Evaluation of Dementia in the Elderly

The first step in the evaluation is a complete history and physical examination. The history should include information from the family about the person's acuity and progression of symptoms. This can indicate whether the patient may have more acute and potentially reversible dementia. Attention should be paid to all medications, including over-the-counter medications. A history of caffeine, alcohol, tobacco use, and any other substance abuse should be elicited. A nutritional history is valuable. A previous history of head trauma may be pertinent.

A functional history is necessary. It is important to understand a person's previous cognitive function. An education and employment history and the patient's age at and reason for retirement aid in establishing this. Details about a person's ability to perform the activities of daily living (ADLs), such as bathing and dressing, are important. Instrumental activities of daily living include using the phone and operating a stove. These also should also be determined. A driving history must be taken.

The psychosocial history is important. The support system of a patient with Alzheimer disease is critical and determines how the person will be cared for.

The physical examination must be thorough. The patient should be weighed and the orthostatic blood pressure and pulse changes evaluated. Close attention should be paid to the cardiovascular examination.

The neurologic examination is of paramount importance. Focal neurologic signs may provide clues that the patient's dementia is multi-infarct dementia rather than Alzheimer dementia. Alzheimer disease occasionally presents atypically with focal neurologic deficits, dominant hemispheric signs including aphasia, or nondominant signs including visual agnosia, dressing apraxia, and constructing apraxia. Although rigidity, cogwheeling, postural instability, and loss of facial expression may indicate Parkinson disease, approximately 30% of patients with Alzheimer disease exhibit these parkinsonian features.

Formal mental status testing must be performed. A tool such as the Folstein Mini-Mental State Examination (MMSE) (Fig. 14.1) is useful because it is standardized and the results can be duplicated by other examiners. The MMSE provides the most information in the greatest number of domains, although it does not specifically assess goal-setting behavior. The domains to be evaluated are attention, recent memory, cortical functioning (including language and visuospatial skills), and goal setting or executive function. Executive function is responsible for motivation, intention, and organizational skills. The total score on the MMSE is not necessarily of value, but the specific areas of deficits provide clues to the diagnosis. For example, the performance of serial sevens may be poor because of a lack of education rather than dementia.

The MMSE can be supplemented by additional questions. A forward digit span test asking for the immediate recall and repetition of at least five digits can be helpful in circumventing the educational influence. The inability to repeat five numbers implies significant inattention. The naming section of the MMSE is insensitive to early language problems. This can be expanded by asking the patient to name the parts of a watch (e.g., face, hands, wrist band). Executive function can be tested by asking the patient to list for 1 minute items to buy in the supermarket. This test is invalidated if the examiner prompts the patient with "What else?"

Ideally, a functional assessment should be performed in the home. This is most helpful in determining the requirements for home care or need for alternate living arrangements. The assessment of a person's ability to use a stove safely can be lifesaving. Often, physicians are unable to perform this assessment, but they can be assisted by a home care nurse or occupational therapist.

Further evaluation is recommended with various routine laboratory tests: complete blood cell count with platelet count, electrolyte measurement, metabolic panel, thyroid function test, vitamin B_{12} and folate level measurement, syphilis serology, and urinalysis. Other tests, including measurement of drug and cortisol levels, a toxin screen, and HIV testing, can be performed depending on diagnostic suspicion. A lumbar puncture is indicated if neurosyphilis or an infectious process is suspected. The National Institutes of Health also recommends electrocardiography and chest roentgenography. Head CT is often performed to evaluate for structural lesions and multi-infarct dementia. Positron emission tomography and single photon emission computed tomography provide functional information about central nervous system metabolism, which has been shown to be impaired in Alzheimer disease. These tests are very expensive and experimental.

MINI-MENTAL STATE EXAM

ADAPTED FROM FOLSTEIN 1975

SCORE=one point for each correct response unless otherwise specified. — MAXIMUM SCORE — ACTUAL SCORE

ORIENTATION

1. Ask for the date. Then specifically ask for parts omitted.
   "What is the (year) (season) (date) (month) (day) ?" (5) ____

2. "Can you tell me the name of the (state) (country) (town) (hospital) (floor) ?" (5) ____

REGISTRATION

SCORE=number of words correct on first attempt (0–3) Allow up to 6 trials.
Ask the patient if you may test his/her memory. Then say the words clearly and slowly.

3. "Remember these 3 words: cup, pencil, airplane."
   After you have said all 3, ask him/her to repeat them.
   (NUMBER OF REPETITIONS REQUIRED____) (3) ____

ATTENTION and CALCULATION

SCORE both tasks, but count only the best one toward the total score

4. "I want you to count backwards from 100 by 7's." Stop after 5 subtractions.
   (93,86,79,72,65)
   (SCORE=one point for each correct subtraction of 7 from the previous number ____)
   "Now spell 'WORLD' backwards."
   (SCORE=number of letters in correct order. ie. DLROW=5, DLORW=3 ____) (5) ____

RECALL

5. "Do you remember the words I gave you earlier? What were they?" (3) ____

LANGUAGE

6. NAMING: Point to a wrist watch and ask him/her what it is. Repeat for pencil. (2) ____

7. REPETITION: Ask the patient to repeat "No ifs, ands, or buts." (1) ____

8. COMPREHENSION: Place a piece of paper in front of the patient and say, "Take the paper in your right hand, fold it in half, and put it on the floor." (3) ____

9. READING: CLOSE YOUR EYES.
   Ask the patient to read it and to do what it says. (1) ____

10. WRITING: Ask the patient to write a sentence on the back of the page.
    Do not dictate a sentence. It should contain a subject and a verb and make sense. Correct grammar and punctuation are not necessary. (1) ____

VISUO-SPATIAL

11. Ask the patient to copy the design. All 10 angles must be present and they must intersect in order to get credit. Tremor and rotation are ignored.
    Allow 1 minute to start and 1 minute to complete task (1) ____

TOTAL SCORE (30) ____

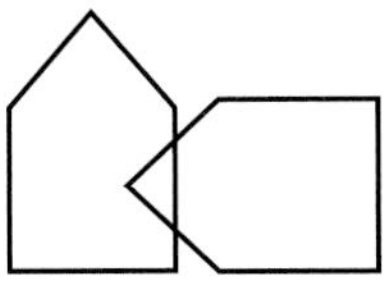

FIG. 14.1. Mini-Mental State Examination. (Adapted from Folstein MF, Folstein SE, McHugh PR. "Mini-mental state." A practical method for grading the cognitive states of patients for the clinician. *Psychiatr Res* 1975;12:189, with permission.)

Treatment

No restorative or curative treatments are available for Alzheimer disease. Most therapies are aimed at alleviating symptoms. Therapy should be tailored for specific symptoms or behaviors. Not all behaviors are amenable to pharmacologic therapy.

Wandering, inappropriate sexual behavior, disrobing, hoarding and hiding objects, and repetitive questioning are examples of behaviors poorly responsive to drug treatment. Behavioral approaches can be successful at managing some of these problems. A safe path for wandering can be established, or a walking group to provide safe exercise.

Behavioral approaches should be attempted before pharmacologic treatment. Searching for the precipitant of agitation can be productive. Pain, for example, can cause agitation in a person who is not able to tell anyone about it. Environmental factors, such as being too hot or too cold, can also cause agitation. Agitation is the only expression left in a severely demented person's repertoire. Relieving the discomforts can calm the agitation.

To avoid agitation, a person with Alzheimer disease should be approached with a quiet, friendly, soothing manner. Although she may no longer understand the content of language, she is still responsive to tone.

A structured environment with limited changes of routine and people is often helpful. Catastrophic deterioration often occurs when a person is placed in a new environment, such as a hospital or nursing home. Meals should be offered in a setting as devoid of distractions as possible (i.e., few people, no television, quiet room).

Agitation and hyperactivity sometimes respond to pharmacologic treatment. Appropriate pharmacologic therapy is discussed in detail in other textbooks of internal medicine, neurology, and pharmacology.

The treatment of intercurrent illnesses is important. Often, an acute medical illness worsens the behavior of a person with Alzheimer disease. Treating chronic medical illnesses may improve mentation—for example, by increasing the oxygenation and thus improving the mental status of a person with emphysema or congestive heart failure. Attention must be paid to the medication regimen. Medications that can affect the mental status should be eliminated; those with anticholinergic properties, such as antihistamines, are particular offenders.

Psychosocial Issues

The person with Alzheimer disease should be informed of the diagnosis and involved in as much decision making as possible. Guidelines for resuscitation and artificial intubation should be addressed while the person is still able to comprehend. Even with significant mental impairment, a person is still often able to make decisions regarding these issues. Legal matters also must be dealt with early, before the patient is no longer able to make decisions concerning finances or appoint a power of attorney.

Finally, the primary caregivers of these patients should be considered at all times and given as much support as possible. They need to be kept informed of all services and options available to them. They require financial guidance through the federal regulations concerning Medicaid if placement issues arise. A number of support groups and agencies are available to help. Social workers are vital in providing support and assisting with obtaining services. The emotional needs of caregivers should not be ignored. Alzheimer disease is as devastating, if not more so, to the family as it is to the patient. The primary care provider should be as helpful as possible in guiding both patients and caregivers through this difficult disease process.

CORONARY HEART DISEASE

For many years, coronary heart disease has been viewed primarily as a disease of men. Women have been perceived as unlikely to die of a heart attack, even if they have known coronary disease. This perception is wrong.

Coronary heart disease accounts for 250,000 to 500,000 deaths per year in women in the United States. These amount to one third to one half of all deaths in women.

Until menopause, the incidence of coronary disease in women lags well behind that in men. By the age of 75 years, the incidence is about equal, but because there are more women than men of that age, more women die of coronary disease. Coronary heart disease in women is mostly a disease of elderly women.

Risk Factors

The incidence of coronary disease in women increases with aging because their risk factors change. Estrogen is the major protective influence in women. That protection is altered by menopause. The influence of estrogen lingers, however, delaying the presentation of disease until an older age.

Estrogen favorably affects the lipid profile. Among persons of the age range that precedes menopause in women, the incidence of hypercholesterolemia is higher in men. After menopause, hypercholesterolemia becomes more prevalent in women. Women do continue to have higher levels of high-density lipoprotein (HDL) cholesterol than men, but their levels of HDL cholesterol decline after menopause.

Estrogen may have a direct effect on the vasculature. It may alter thrombotic mediators, thereby decreasing the risk for thrombosis and infarction. A decrease or loss of this effect is associated with the estrogen deficiency state of postmenopausal women.

The incidence of hypertension increases as women age. The use of antihypertensive medication is a predictor of coronary disease in elderly women, probably reflecting the risk associated with the long-term effects of hypertension, even if current blood pressures are controlled. A number of studies have demonstrated that hypertension is not a benign norm in the elderly and that treatment is important.

Smoking is another risk factor that shows a crossover effect with age. Higher numbers of young men and older women die. Smoking contributes to the increased incidence of coronary disease in elderly women. Even women who have not smoked but who have lived with smokers are at increased risk.

Hyperglycemia is a very strong risk factor for coronary disease. It, too, is more common in older women. Direct effects on the vasculature, in addition to associated lipid abnormalities, make diabetes a major contributor to coronary disease.

Obesity is another major risk factor, probably because it is associated with or causes most of the previously listed risk factors—hypertension, hypercholesterolemia, and diabetes. Weight increases with age in women, at least until extreme old age, when it tends to decrease. The incidence of coronary disease is highest in women 65 to 74 years old who have the highest Quetelet index (weight in kilograms divided by height in square meters). Interestingly, the incidence is second highest in those with the lowest weight who also report the greatest previous weight loss, suggesting that fluctuation in weight is also a risk.

The factors that affect mortality from coronary disease are different in women and men. The strongest predictors of mortality in women are diabetes and current smoking. Other influences, although less strong, are hypertension and known cardiac disease. In men, only the use of hypertensive medications is significantly associated with cardiac mortality.

Research demonstrates that the association between risk factors and myocardial infarction or coronary artery disease mortality is stronger in women. It may be that the risk factors have stronger biologic effects in postmenopausal women or that the men susceptible to the risk factors have already died at an earlier age.

Clinical Presentation

Silent ischemia occurs more frequently in the elderly, particularly diabetics. Thus, the elderly woman who has the significant risk factor of diabetes is somewhat more likely to present atypically without prominent chest pain.

Dementia in the elderly also plays a role in the atypical presentation. This is less the result of a lack of symptoms than a problem of interpreting nonverbal signs and symptoms. Agitation may be the only clue to a problem.

In elderly women, the only indication of angina is often exertional shortness of breath. In other women, congestive heart failure, resulting from ischemia and subsequent diastolic dysfunction, is the presenting symptom. Other atypical presentations include palpitations, syncope, and sweating during exertion.

Most elderly women do have typical anginal symptoms as the first indication of coronary disease (i.e., chest pain, radiation to the left arm). Men are more likely to present with myocardial infarction or sudden death. Anginal symptoms cause more disability in elderly women than in men. Their symptom complex also tends to be more aggressive.

Some evidence indicates that women have a poorer prognosis than men after acute myocardial infarction. This increased mortality is probably related to the older age of women with coronary disease and to their concurrent illnesses.

Diagnosis

Because the presentation is often less straightforward in elderly women, the diagnosis of coronary disease may be more difficult. It is much easier to diagnose coronary disease in the setting of an acute myocardial infarction than in atypical angina. The history is still important and helpful in women with typical anginal symptoms.

The physical examination may not be particularly helpful. Often, the findings are nonspecific. The resting electrocardiogram also may not be helpful, with only nonspecific changes in the ST-T wave, often in association with left ventricular hypertrophy.

Women tend to more chest pain with causes other than coronary artery disease. These include mitral valve prolapse and angina secondary to vasospasm of a nonstenotic coronary artery. For this reason, the results of the initial and most frequently used test for coronary artery disease, the exercise tolerance test, are often unreliable.

The positive predictive value of the exercise tolerance test result is lower in women than in men. The incidence of false-positive results is higher in women because of the noncoronary causes of chest pain mentioned previously. Elderly women are less likely to be able to perform adequately to achieve a sufficiently high work load. They are limited not only by coronary disease but also by other factors, such as deconditioning and degenerative joint disease. The electrocardiographic criteria for a positive exercise tolerance test result may be different for women. Rather than ST-segment depression, a change in R-wave height may be used more reliably to define a positive test result.

A thallium exercise tolerance test may be more reliable diagnostically. However, shadowing of the breast can decrease its accuracy.

In general, noninvasive tests are less accurate in women, particularly elderly women. Clinicians must consider invasive testing earlier in elderly women with possible coronary disease.

The decision to undertake angiography is complicated by the greater difficulty of performing the procedure in the elderly and the increase in associated risks. Technically, the procedure can be made more difficult by the presence of generalized arteriosclerosis with plaques in the iliac and aortic arteries. Renal function decreases during the normal aging process and often is worsened by concurrent illnesses and medications. The elderly patient is at higher risk for renal compromise after the administration of contrast dye required for angiography.

Provided these factors are taken into consideration, coronary angiography is the most informative test. Before angiography is performed, it should be determined whether the patient is a candidate for surgery. If concurrent medical illness contraindicates surgery or the patient is unwilling to undergo surgery, then angiography is probably not indicated.

Many times in the frail elderly, empiric treatment and the subsequent response are the only, and best, diagnostic tools available.

Sex Bias

A number of studies performed in recent years suggest a sex bias against women in the diagnosis and treatment of coronary artery disease. Much of the bias stems from the misconception that coronary disease is less frequent and less severe in women. According to another school of thought, coronary disease in women is actually being diagnosed and treated appropriately, and men are being overtreated. Some earlier studies reported a higher mortality of coronary artery bypass grafting in women, and this may have played a role in dissuading physicians from referring women to angiography and subsequent surgery.

The answer probably lies somewhere in the middle. Women are initially referred less often for noninvasive testing. Even when they are referred and the results of exercise tolerance testing are positive, fewer are referred for angiography. This holds true after adjustments for age differences between men and women.

After myocardial infarction, women are less likely to receive thrombolytic therapy than men. Elderly women, in particular, are less likely to receive thrombolytic therapy because the trials have been performed in populations younger than 70 years and have included few women. The effect of sex bias on angioplasty in persons with prior myocardial infarction is less evident but still present.

Angiography after myocardial infarction is one area in which the sex bias is less operational. Once age has been controlled for, women are equally likely to be referred for angiography after myocardial infarction. The implication of this finding is that age limits referral to angiography.

After angiography, women are almost as likely as men to be referred to surgery. Results of studies of whether women are referred at a later stage and are sicker at the time of bypass surgery are conflicting. This may be appropriate because the sickest patients have the most to gain from surgery.

The greatest effect of referral bias is probably on the early diagnosis of coronary artery disease. The question then arises of how much morbidity and mortality might be avoided by the earlier diagnosis of coronary disease in elderly women.

Older women are also less likely to be referred for cardiac rehabilitation after myocardial infarction despite evidence that older women benefit as much as men in terms of increasing their maximal exercise capacity.

Treatment

Risk reduction as primary prevention of coronary disease in elderly women is important. This includes treating hypertension and hyperlipidemia and avoiding weight gain and, thus, hyperglycemia. Discontinuing smoking is also of paramount importance. It is not clear that aggressive treatment of elevated cholesterol levels in the general elderly population is warranted, but it is indicated in elderly patients with established coronary disease. Reducing hyperlipidemia before old age is most useful in reducing risk.

Exercise also probably continues to be valuable in reducing risk in elderly women. Some evidence suggests that exercise slows age-related increases in coronary disease. This benefit is probably derived from the effects of exercise in lowering blood pressure and increasing HDL cholesterol. Exercise is important in elderly women who have had a myocardial infarction because it prevents deconditioning and improves exercise tolerance. This is why a cardiac rehabilitation referral is helpful. A better-conditioned elderly woman is more likely to be able to continue functioning independently.

Once coronary disease has developed in a woman, medical management is usually the first line of therapy (see Chapters 42 and 43). However, polypharmacy with subsequent drug interactions and increased side effects in general is more problematic in the elderly. Also, the clearance of drugs is decreased in the elderly secondary to decreased renal function and decreased hepatic perfusion, which increase drug levels and the risk for toxicity.

The procedural morbidity of angioplasty is greater in women than in men. The incidence of internal tears and coronary dissections is increased, perhaps because of smaller arterial size and the use of oversized balloons. Concurrent illnesses also increase risk.

Several studies have addressed the question of whether mortality after coronary artery bypass grafting is increased in women, with conflicting results. Earlier reports indicated that the smaller body size of women influenced mortality, but this finding has not been supported in more recent studies. Improvements in surgical technique since the original studies were performed may explain the discrepancy.

Mortality after coronary artery bypass grafting may be increased in women because of the less frequent use of internal mammary grafts. Women tend to be referred when they are in a worse functional class, and they are older when cardiac disease develops, factors that increase operative mortality. The effect of age may be the most important factor.

However, the benefits of surgery are greatest in those with the most severe disease, so older women may have the most to gain. Possibly, women with less severe disease who are not referred miss an opportunity for a better quality of life that could be achieved with earlier surgery.

Coronary artery disease is far from a benign and rather rare disease in elderly women. It is a leading cause of death and significant morbidity. Treatment options and decisions are made more complex by advancing age.

BIBLIOGRAPHY

Alexander BH, Rivara FP, Wolf ME. The cost and frequency of hospitalization for fall-related injuries in older adults. *Am J Public Health* 1992;82:1020.

Arfken CL, Lach HW, Birge SJ, et al. The prevalence and correlates of fear of falling in elderly persons living in the community. *Am J Public Health* 1994;84:565.

Bennett DA, Knopman DS. Alzheimer's disease: a comprehensive approach to patient management. *Geriatrics* 1994;49:20.

Bickell NA, Pieper S, Lee KL, et al. Referral patterns for coronary artery disease treatment: gender bias or good clinical judgment? *Ann Intern Med* 1992;116:791.

Campell AJ, Spears GF, Borrie MJ. Examination by logistic regression modelling of the variables which increase the relative risk of elderly women falling compared to elderly men. *J Clin Epidemiol* 1990;43:1415.

Department of Health and Human Services, National Institutes of Health, National Institute on Aging. Available at www.nia.nih./gov. Accessed February 24, 2003

Department of Health and Human Services, National Institutes of Health, National Institute of Nursing Research. Available at www.nih.gov/ninr. Accessed February 24, 2003.

Eisdorfer C, Olson EJ, eds. Management of patients with Alzheimer's and related dementias. *Med Clin North Am* 1994;78:4.

Eysmann SB, Douglas PS. Reperfusion and revascularization strategies for coronary artery disease in women. *JAMA* 1992;268:1903.

Harrell LE. Alzheimer's disease. *South Med J* 1991;84:S32.

Gorelick PB, Bozzola FG. Alzheimer's disease: clues to the cause. *Postgrad Med* 1991;89:231.

Krumholz HM, Douglas PS, Lauer MS, et al. Selection of patients for coronary angiography and coronary revascularization early after myocardial infarction: is there evidence for a gender bias? *Ann Intern Med* 1992;116:785.

Mandelblatt JS, et al. Breast cancer screening for elderly women with and without comorbid conditions: a decision analysis model. *Ann Intern Med* 1992; 116:722.

O'Loughlin JL, Robitaille Y, Boivin JF, et al. Incidence of and risk factors for falls and injurious falls among the community-dwelling elderly. *Am J Epidemiol* 1993;137:342.

Oettgen P, Douglas PS. Coronary artery disease in women: diagnosis and prevention. *Adv Intern Med* 1994;39:467

Seeman T, Mendes de Leon C, Berkman L, et al. Risk factors for coronary heart disease among older men and women: a prospective study of community-dwelling elderly. *Am J Epidemiol* 1993;138:1037.

Steingart RM, Packer M, Hamm P, et al. Sex differences in the management of coronary artery disease: survival and ventricular enlargement investigators. *N Engl J Med* 1991;325:226.

Tinetti ME, Baker DL, McAvay G, et al. A multifactorial intervention to reduce the risk of falling among elderly people living in the community. *N Engl J Med* 1994;331:821.

Williams EL, Winkleby MA, Fortman SP Changes in coronary heart disease risk factors in the 1980s: evidence of a male-female crossover effect with age. *Am J Epidemiol* 1993;137:1056.

PART

3

Reproductive Tract Problems

CHAPTER 15
Abnormal Vaginal Bleeding

William R. Phipps

Between menarche and the menopause, any vaginal bleeding not occurring on the basis of regular ovulatory menstrual cycles can be considered abnormal. Such bleeding may be secondary to a wide array of specific underlying problems. Although the characteristics of normal menses (Table 15.1) are pertinent, the menstrual patterns of many women without clinically significant abnormalities fall outside these norms, and a patient is actually most likely to consult a physician when she detects a pattern that she considers abnormal for her. Along these same lines, the decision to intervene should be governed by the individual circumstances, not the presence or absence of a specific pattern.

The terminology used to describe abnormal bleeding can be confusing. Traditionally, the term *oligomenorrhea* has been used to designate a pattern in which the intervals between episodes of bleeding are longer than 35 days, and *polymenorrhea* to describe a pattern in which the intervals are shorter than 24 days. *Menorrhagia* refers to episodes of excessive flow or prolonged duration occurring at regular normal intervals, and *metrorrhagia* describes such episodes occurring at irregular intervals. The term *dysfunctional uterine bleeding (DUB)* refers to abnormal uterine bleeding that is not a consequence of structural or systemic disease. Usually, DUB is related to anovulatory menstrual cycles, referred to here as *anovulatory DUB*. Women with ovulatory cycles may also have DUB, specifically referred to here as *ovulatory DUB*.

TABLE 15.1. Characteristics of Normal Menses

	Mean	Normal range
Menarche	12–13 y	8–16 y
Interval	28–30 d	24–35 d
Duration	4–5 d	2–8 d
Amount of flow	30–40 mL	20–80 mL
Menopause	50–52 y	40–60 y

ETIOLOGY AND DIFFERENTIAL DIAGNOSIS

As shown in Table 15.2, a very large number of entities may present with abnormal vaginal bleeding. Although DUB, the main focus of this chapter, is ultimately diagnosed in many, if not most, patients with abnormal bleeding, it is important that the other entities listed be excluded with reasonable certainty before treatment is initiated; in fact, the diagnosis of either anovulatory or ovulatory DUB is one of exclusion.

The pathophysiology and optimal treatment of anovulatory DUB are best understood by comparing anovulatory DUB with the bleeding that occurs as part of the normal menstrual cycle. In the proliferative phase of the normal cycle, estradiol produced by the dominant follicle causes the endometrial glands and stroma to proliferate. Following ovulation, the corpus luteum produces large amounts of progesterone in addition to estrogen, causing secretory changes in the endometrium. In the absence of pregnancy, regression of the corpus luteum is associated with the withdrawal of progesterone and estrogen, which leads to a normal menses, an orderly and self-limited event that involves desquamation of the entire endometrium.

Anovulatory DUB differs from normal menstrual bleeding in that the endometrium is exposed to estrogen unopposed by progesterone for a relatively long time. Prolonged exposure to estrogen results in an abnormally high and structurally unstable endometrium. The tissue is delicate and undergoes essentially spontaneous breakdown with associated bleeding. The

TABLE 15.2. Causes of Abnormal Vaginal Bleeding

Group	Specific entities
Dysfunctional uterine bleeding	Anovulatory Ovulatory
Pregnancy-related bleeding	Threatened, missed, or incomplete abortion Ectopic pregnancy Molar pregnancy Third-trimester or puerperal bleeding
Bleeding diatheses	Coagulopathies (especially platelet disorders) Anticoagulation therapy Severe hepatic disease
Benign anatomic lesions	Endometrial hyperplasia Uterine myoma(ta) or adenomyosis Endometrial or endocervical polyp(s) Cervical or vaginal endometriosis Vaginal adenosis Müllerian anomalies associated with partial outflow obstruction
Pelvic malignancies	Endometrial adenocarcinoma Uterine sarcoma Cervical or vaginal carcinoma Gestational trophoblastic neoplasia
Inflammatory processes	Endometritis, cervicitis Infectious or atrophic vaginitis
Miscellaneous	Pelvic lacerations/trauma Intrauterine device Intravaginal foreign body Drug-related (including oral contraceptives and hormone replacement therapy) Hypothyroidism Uterine sarcoidosis

process is not an orderly one, may continue more or less indefinitely, and involves different portions of the endometrium at different times.

Ovulatory DUB differs from anovulatory DUB in that for the most part ovulation occurs on a regular basis. The heavy bleeding of ovulatory DUB is thought to be at least in part a consequence of the effects of abnormal arachidonic acid metabolism on endometrial function, with excess production of vasodilator as opposed to vasoconstrictor prostaglandins.

Pregnancy-related bleeding may occur in both abnormal and essentially normal pregnancies, and the possibility of pregnancy must always be considered before intervention. In particular, it is important to diagnose an ectopic pregnancy as early as possible to allow the option of medical rather than surgical treatment. The abnormal bleeding that occurs vaginally in a tubal pregnancy is nearly always a consequence of endometrial shedding, which is in turn secondary to abnormal corpus luteum function, and it usually precedes the development of pelvic pain, which is generally caused by tubal rupture or intrapelvic bleeding.

The possibilities of a bleeding diathesis or either a benign or malignant anatomic lesion should also be considered in all patients presenting with abnormal vaginal bleeding. In particular, platelet disorders often present as menorrhagia, especially in adolescents. In older patients, malignancies are relatively more common, and it is especially important to rule out endometrial hyperplasia and adenocarcinoma. In this same vein, cancer must always be ruled out in the case of bleeding in a postmenopausal woman not taking hormone replacement therapy.

HISTORY

A careful history is of course essential to the management of any patient presenting with abnormal bleeding. The date of onset of the presenting episode and the prior menstrual history must be ascertained, along with concurrent symptoms of any kind. Information about the general obstetric and gynecologic history, including pregnancies, infertility, prior pelvic surgery, abnormalities noted on earlier examinations, Papanicolaou smear results, and methods of contraception, must also be obtained. A history of any significant medical problems should be noted, and it is also particularly important to inquire about symptoms suggestive of endocrine and bleeding disorders, and whether or not any family members have had similar problems.

The typical history in cases of anovulatory DUB is one of irregular episodes of often painless bleeding occurring in an unpredictable fashion, ranging from a day of spotting to several weeks of continuous, heavy bleeding. Long periods of amenorrhea may or may not alternate with episodes of bleeding. The cyclic symptoms of mittelschmerz and molimina are absent. Patients particularly at risk include postmenarchal teenagers, perimenopausal women, and women with polycystic ovarian syndrome (PCOS) or obesity-related anovulation.

Women with ovulatory DUB in general present with menorrhagia. A monthly loss of more than 80 mL of blood is considered abnormal and often associated with iron deficiency anemia. As a practical matter, it is difficult to quantify blood loss precisely, and thus decisions about both investigating and treating a patient for menorrhagia largely hinge on her subjective complaints.

A history of mucocutaneous bleeding, such as epistaxis, gingival bleeding, or easy bruising, may suggest von Willebrand disease, idiopathic thrombocytopenia purpura, or another bleeding diathesis. Von Willebrand disease, the most common inherited bleeding diathesis, is an autosomal-dominant condition with considerable molecular and clinical heterogeneity. The overall prevalence is about 1%, and it should particularly be considered when an adolescent patient presents with abnormal uterine bleeding. The family history may not always be helpful because of the variable penetrance associated with mild to moderate von Willebrand disease (type I), and in particular male subjects may not be symptomatic.

The history will also often provide diagnostic clues when a benign or malignant anatomic lesion is the cause of abnormal bleeding. A patient with regular menstrual cycles who has an enlarging submucosal myoma often presents with a gradually increasing amount or duration of bleeding and perhaps increasing dysmenorrhea. An ovulatory woman with a bleeding endometrial or endocervical polyp may present with erratic episodes of bleeding essentially superimposed on a normal menstrual cycle. Women with endometrial hyperplasia or adenocarcinoma often have a long history of obvious anovulation and symptoms consistent with PCOS.

It is also important to note that some women who have conditions usually associated with menorrhagia, such as ovulatory DUB, a submucosal myoma, or a bleeding diathesis, may ovulate infrequently. Accordingly, such women would be expected to present with irregular and heavy menses, mimicking the usual pattern of anovulatory DUB.

PHYSICAL EXAMINATION

A careful physical examination may reveal findings suggestive of a specific diagnosis. Obviously, the patient's vital signs are important, especially in the presence of acute or substantial bleeding, when immediate medical or surgical intervention may be in order. A goiter may suggest hypothyroidism. Acne and hirsutism may suggest PCOS, often associated with anovulatory DUB. The pelvic examination is particularly important. The vagina and cervix should be thoroughly inspected for lesions, and the amount of ongoing bleeding noted. A bimanual examination may reveal evidence of an intrauterine or ectopic pregnancy, uterine myomata or adenomyosis, a müllerian anomaly with partial outflow obstruction, or an ongoing pelvic infection.

LABORATORY AND IMAGING STUDIES

Decisions about what diagnostic studies should be performed must be individualized, although in most cases, at least a complete blood (CBC) count cell should be performed. In general, it is mandatory to rule out pregnancy with a serum or sensitive urine pregnancy test in any patient who could be pregnant, regardless of the contraceptive method used or the specific bleeding pattern noted. If the patient is not pregnant, in most cases her ovulatory status should be established. Basal body temperature charting, serum progesterone determinations, or endometrial sampling may be required. Given the high prevalence of autoimmune thyroid disease in women, the concentration of thyroid-stimulating hormone should also be routinely assessed, even in the absence of other evidence for thyroid disease.

Younger patients especially should usually be assessed for a bleeding diathesis. In less striking cases, determinations of the CBC, platelet count, prothrombin time, activated partial thromboplastin time (aPTT), and bleeding time are in order. Although the bleeding time and aPTT are usually at least somewhat abnormal in cases of von Willebrand disease, they may be normal. Thus, depending on the level of suspicion, additional testing more specific for von Willebrand disease may be appropriate, including the ristocetin cofactor assay of von Willebrand factor, quantification of von Willebrand factor antigen, and factor VIII assay.

A variety of imaging studies may also be useful in establishing the diagnosis, but again the specific studies warranted depend on the individual circumstances. Transvaginal ultrasonography may be very useful if an anatomic lesion is suspected, such as a submucosal or intramural myoma, adenomyosis, or polyp. In obviously anovulatory patients, a thicker endometrial lining as assessed by ultrasonography may lower the threshold for performing an endometrial biopsy. Especially when endometrial polyp(s) or submucosal myoma(ta) are suspected, the instillation of saline solution into the uterus coupled with transvaginal ultrasonography (sonohysterography) is warranted because this technique better delineates intracavitary lesions. In selected cases, such as when an unusual müllerian anomaly is suspected, a traditional hysterosalpingogram can be useful. Diagnostic hysteroscopy may also be invaluable in certain cases.

When a tentative diagnosis of anovulatory DUB has been made, the decision about whether or not to perform endometrial sampling depends primarily on the risk for endometrial hyperplasia or adenocarcinoma, two conditions that also may occur as a consequence of chronic anovulation. Most women older than 35 years and virtually all women older than 40 years who present with apparent anovulatory bleeding should undergo endometrial sampling, as should many younger women with a long history of anovulation, particularly if they are obese or hyperinsulinemic. Such sampling can usually be accomplished easily in the office setting with the use of a Pipelle endometrial suction curette or similar device. From a diagnostic standpoint, traditional dilation and curettage have minimal role, if any, except in conjunction with hysteroscopy.

TREATMENT

Treatment is tailored to the individual circumstances, which include not only the underlying cause but also a host of other factors, including the degree of ongoing bleeding and the patient's hemodynamic status.

In the case of a patient with a positive pregnancy test result, treatment is dictated by the nature of the pregnancy and is not discussed here further. Similarly, most patients with benign or malignant anatomic lesions require surgical intervention of some sort, depending on the nature of the lesion.

For women with apparent anovulatory DUB, after the initial diagnostic measures have been completed, attention is directed to therapeutic intervention. The first goal of therapy is to stop the acute bleeding, which can nearly always be accomplished without surgical intervention. If uterine curettage is performed, this by itself does provide a substantial acute therapeutic effect, although in general there is no reason not to start medical therapy immediately after endometrial sampling of any kind. In most cases of anovulatory DUB, the bleeding can be stopped with the administration of a progestin. A typical progestin regimen is 10 to 20 mg of medroxyprogesterone acetate (Provera) given orally once daily for 10 days. The bleeding usually stops while the Provera is being administered; more or less orderly withdrawal bleeding then starts immediately after the Provera has been discontinued. This sequence of events is similar to what occurs during the secretory phase of the normal cycle. It is important to advise the patient at risk for pregnancy that occasionally ovulation will occur as a result of progestin administration.

Another therapeutic option useful in stopping acute anovulatory DUB is to administer oral contraceptive pills (OCPs), each containing 30 to 35 µg of ethinyl estradiol and a progestin. A variety of regimens may be used—for example, having the patient take two to four pills daily for 5 days, which often stops the bleeding within 1 or 2 days, then one pill daily for another 21 days; withdrawal bleeding can be expected within a few days after the last pill. For the patient who has been bleeding heavily for a prolonged period of time and has little residual endometrial tissue, it may be best to give high-dose estrogen therapy initially—for example, two or three 25-mg doses of conjugated estrogens (Premarin) by intravenous bolus every 4 hours. The immediate improvement with such therapy is more a consequence of the pharmacologic effect of estrogen on small vessel hemostasis than of the ability of estrogen to induce proliferation and healing of endometrial tissue. Once the bleeding has stopped in response to the Premarin, in general an OCP regimen should be started immediately.

Patients in whom anovulatory DUB has been diagnosed but who do not respond to the regimens previously outlined require additional evaluation. This may include endometrial sampling if not already performed, transvaginal ultrasonography, or hysteroscopy.

Once the acute episode of anovulatory DUB has been treated, attention is directed toward the possible need for long-term treatment. If the patient usually ovulates and it is thought that bleeding is unlikely to recur, a period of observation may be all that is necessary. On the other hand, some form of long-term therapy is indicated for a patient whose anovulatory state, responsible for the DUB, is unlikely to abate spontaneously. The goals of long-term therapy, which must include a progestin component, are to prevent recurrent unpredictable episodes of bleeding and endometrial hyperplasia and to lower the risk for endometrial cancer. An iron supplement may also be started at this time if needed.

Long-term treatment with OCPs administered in the usual cyclic fashion is the best option for most patients with anovulatory DUB. Such therapy is particularly useful for women who occasionally ovulate spontaneously and require birth control, and for those with PCOS because OCPs mitigate the associated hyperandrogenism. Patients who are not candidates for OCP therapy may be treated with cyclic progestin—for example, 10 mg of Provera taken orally once daily the first 10 to 14 days of each month, or even every second or third month. Anovulatory patients with DUB who desire pregnancy should undergo an appropriate hormonal evaluation followed by ovulation induction therapy.

Patients in whom ovulatory DUB is diagnosed can be treated successfully with either OCPs or a nonsteroidal antiinflammatory drug (NSAID) regimen, such as 400 mg of ibuprofen taken orally every 6 hours; this is started on cycle day 1 and continued through the cessation of menses. Both of these treatments not only decrease the amount of bleeding but also address the often associated problem of dysmenorrhea. The mechanism by which NSAIDs work is not entirely clear but appears to involve a disproportionate reduction in the uterine concentrations of vasodilator prostaglandins relative to that of prostaglandin $F_{2\alpha}$, a potent vasoconstrictor.

Another option for patients with ovulatory DUB is danazol—for example, 200 mg taken orally daily. Most patients on such a dose continue to have regular menses, although androgenic side effects may be a problem. Furthermore, barrier contraception is needed for patients who are sexually active. Still another possible treatment modality is an antifibrinolytic agent, such as ε-aminocaproic acid. Strong evidence indicates that the antifibrinolytic agent tranexamic acid is a very effective treatment for ovulatory DUB, but unfortunately it is not generally available in the United States. Finally, another option is a progestin-releasing intrauterine device, such as the Mirena levonorgestrel-releasing intrauterine system.

At times, patients with either anovulatory or ovulatory DUB show a consistently poor response to the long-term medical options described or experience unacceptable side effects. In that situation, treatment with a long-acting gonadotropin-releasing hormone (GnRH) agonist, such as leuprolide acetate, may be considered to induce a menopause-like state. Long-term treatment with a GnRH agonist is problematic for most patients, however, largely because of the adverse effects on bone density. In general, patients with DUB failing to respond to the regimens described are best treated surgically, either by endometrial ablation, which is usually performed hysteroscopically, or hysterectomy.

For women with a diagnosed bleeding diathesis, consultation with a hematologist may be in order. Patients with less severe forms of von Willebrand disease can often be successfully treated with OCPs because estrogens increase the concentration of von Willebrand factor. Another option for these patents is a concentrated desmopressin acetate intranasal spray (Stimate Nasal Spray).

BIBLIOGRAPHY

American College of Obstetricians and Gynecologists. Management of anovulatory bleeding. ACOG Practice Bulletin Number 14, 2000.

American College of Obstetricians and Gynecologists. Von Willebrand's disease in gynecologic practice. ACOG Committee Opinion Number 263, 2001.

Bevan JA, Maloney KW, Hillery CA, et al. Bleeding disorders: a common cause of menorrhagia in adolescents. *J Pediatr* 2001;138:856–861.

Brenner PF. Differential diagnosis of abnormal uterine bleeding. *Am J Obstet Gynecol* 1996;175:766–769.

Ewenstein BM. The pathophysiology of bleeding disorders presenting as abnormal uterine bleeding. *Am J Obstet Gynecol* 1996;175:770–777.

Farquhar CM, Lethaby A, Sowter M, et al. An evaluation of risk factors for endometrial hyperplasia in premenopausal women with abnormal menstrual bleeding. *Am J Obstet Gynecol* 1999;181:525–529.

Kadir RA, Economides DL, Sabin CA, et al. Frequency of inherited bleeding disorders in women with menorrhagia. *Lancet* 1998;351:485–489.

Lusher JM. Screening and diagnosis of coagulation disorders. *Am J Obstet Gynecol* 1996;175:778–783.

Munro MG. Medical management of abnormal uterine bleeding. *Obstet Gynecol Clin North Am* 2000;27:287–304.

Munro MG. Dysfunctional uterine bleeding: advances in diagnosis and treatment. *Curr Opin Obstet Gynecol* 2001;13:475–489.

Speroff L, Glass RH, Kase NG. Regulation of the menstrual cycle. *Clinical gynecologic endocrinology and infertility,* 6th ed. Philadelphia: Lippincott Williams & Wilkins, 1999:201–246.

Speroff L, Glass RH, Kase NG. Dysfunctional uterine bleeding. *Clinical gynecologic endocrinology and infertility,* 6th ed. Philadelphia: Lippincott Williams & Wilkins, 1999:575–593.

CHAPTER 16
Amenorrhea

Kathleen M. Hoeger

Amenorrhea is the absence of menstruation. If menstruation has not begun by the age of 16 years, the amenorrhea is primary. If menstruation has begun but subsequently ceases for a period of 6 months or longer, the amenorrhea is secondary. Although some conditions always present as primary amenorrhea, this distinction is arbitrary for many diagnoses, and the same evaluation applies to both situations.

The pathophysiology of amenorrhea can be defined by dysfunction at one of the levels of the hypothalamic-pituitary-ovarian-uterine axis. A thorough history and physical examination can elucidate most causes of amenorrhea. A carefully planned laboratory assessment based on the initial clinical impression can further substantiate the diagnosis.

NORMAL FEMALE REPRODUCTIVE CYCLE

The normal female reproductive cycle depends on the cyclic interaction of hypothalamic, pituitary, and ovarian hormones. The pulsatile release of gonadotropin-releasing hormone (GnRH) from the hypothalamus stimulates the release of the pituitary gonadotropins, follicle-stimulating hormone (FSH) and luteinizing hormone (LH). These in turn stimulate the ovary to produce estradiol and progesterone in sequence, resulting in timed uterine bleeding. The system is controlled by strict negative feedback in childhood until activation of the hypothalamic-pituitary axis by an unknown mechanism at puberty initiates the pulsatile release of GnRH and subsequently FSH and LH. The axis matures predictably during approximately 2 to 3 years; initially, nocturnal pulses are followed by a carefully orchestrated release of FSH every 90 minutes. In the mature system, controlled ovarian follicular development and subsequent ovulation result in regular and predictable menstrual cycles. If the axis is disrupted in any way, cycles are abnormal or absent (see Chapter 11). Hypothalamic-pituitary dysfunction can be caused by both organic and functional conditions. In many common syndromes, such as polycystic ovary syndrome (PCOS), the disruption of normal hormonal production on several levels of the axis leads to chronic anovulation and amenorrhea.

CAUSES OF AMENORRHEA

Hypothalamic Dysfunction

FUNCTIONAL HYPOTHALAMIC AMENORRHEA

The normal secretion of GnRH from the hypothalamus can be disrupted by either structural or functional problems. Stress, either physical or emotional, is one of the most common causes of amenorrhea. Under conditions of extreme stress, GnRH secretion is suppressed, so that the pulsatile secretion of FSH and LH is diminished. All forms of hypothalamic suppression with amenorrhea can lead to estrogen deficiency. In the absence of normal gonadotropin secretion, the ovaries no longer produce sex steroids. Treatment of this condition is directed at determining and eliminating the sources of stress.

EATING DISORDERS

A loss of body fat and extremes of body weight can lead to hypothalamic-pituitary dysfunction and amenorrhea. Anorexia nervosa is an eating disorder characterized by significant weight loss, amenorrhea, and a distorted body image with the constant impression that one remains fat despite often skeletal proportions. However, loss of weight even to 10% to 15% below ideal weight can result in amenorrhea. Treatment is directed at weight gain. A psychiatric referral is often necessary for patients with anorexia nervosa (see Chapter 149).

TUMORS

Suprasellar tumors, such as craniopharyngiomas and hamartomas, and inflammatory disorders, such as sarcoidosis, interrupt the normal hypothalamic-pituitary connections via the portal system, so that the GnRH-induced secretion of FSH and LH is disrupted. Suprasellar tumors often develop before puberty and present as primary amenorrhea; however, they may occur anytime. They can be diagnosed with central nervous system (CNS) imaging studies. Tumors can cause abnormally elevated prolactin levels by interfering with the normal dopamine suppression of prolactin secretion. Other symptoms, such as headache and various CNS changes may be noted, but hypothalamic suppression with amenorrhea may be the only symptom of a CNS tumor.

KALLMANN SYNDROME

A rare cause of primary amenorrhea is Kallmann syndrome, in which an absence of GnRH neurons in the hypothalamus is associated with anosmia. The diagnosis is suspected when a patient with primary amenorrhea and a failure of sex steroid production is challenged with a strong odor, such as that of coffee, and is unable to identify an odor. GnRH neurons have been found in the olfactory placode of these patients and do not migrate to the arcuate nucleus of the hypothalamus in utero. Treatment is directed at hormone replacement therapy (HRT). The ovaries are capable of oocyte production, and fertility is possible with the administration of exogenous gonadotropins.

DRUGS

Chronic illicit drug use has been associated with hypothalamic suppression. Inquiries into drug use should be made at the first assessment.

Pituitary Dysfunction

ADENOMAS

A prolactin-secreting adenoma with subsequent hyperprolactinemia is the most common pituitary-related cause of amenorrhea. The diagnosis should be suspected in a patient who has amenorrhea with galactorrhea and elevated prolactin levels. No absolute level of prolactin has been found to be associated with adenomas, and no lower cutoff of elevated prolactin levels rules out the possibility of an adenoma. If all other sources of hyperprolactinemia have been eliminated, CNS imaging of the pituitary gland is recommended. Dopamine agonist therapy, with either bromocriptine or cabergoline, has been used successfully to suppress prolactin secretion and reduces the size of adenomas. Surgical therapy is not usually needed.

SHEEHAN SYNDROME

Sheehan syndrome is characterized by postpartum hemorrhage and resultant anterior pituitary necrosis. Generalized pituitary failure is often heralded by a failure of lactation in the postpartum period. Other pituitary hormones may be deficient to various degrees. Estrogen replacement is necessary to manage the amenorrhea, but pregnancy is possible if exogenous gonadotropins are administered.

Polycystic Ovary Syndrome

PCOS is a common clinical syndrome affecting approximately 5% of women of reproductive age. It is characterized by chronic anovulation and hyperandrogenism in the absence of other causes of hyperandrogenism. PCOS may present as either primary or secondary amenorrhea. Most patients with PCOS have irregular menstrual cycles and features of androgen excess at puberty. Although PCOS occurs in patients of normal weight, most (~70%) are overweight. In general, weight gain and obesity exacerbate the symptoms of PCOS. Insulin resistance is found in most patients with PCOS in comparison with weight-matched control subjects. The cause of the insulin resistance is not known, but it is suspected to result from a post-receptor mechanism. Insulin has been shown to have a direct effect on testosterone secretion in the ovary. Reducing insulin secretion, either through weight reduction or the use of insulin sensitizers, improves the ovulatory status. Currently, it is not known whether the use of insulin sensitizers such as metformin will diminish the long-term sequelae of PCOS, such as an increased risk for type 2 diabetes and possibly an increased cardiovascular risk. The administration of oral contraceptives or cyclic progestins is indicated to induce regular menstrual cycles because estrogen production continues in these patients, and unopposed estrogen can increase the risk for endometrial cancer (see Chapters 36 and 37).

Gonadal Abnormalities

OVARIAN FAILURE

Turner Syndrome

Turner syndrome is characterized by an abnormal X-chromosome count in a phenotypic female. The classic karyotype is 45,X, but other karyotypes (e.g., 46,XX/45,X) may be seen. Notable features of the syndrome are short stature, amenorrhea, webbed neck, increased carrying angle, and shield chest. Micrognathia, a high-arched palate, low-set hairline, and abnormal angulation of the eustachian tube resulting in repeated childhood ear infections may also be seen. Abnormalities of the heart (particularly coarctation of the aorta) and kidneys are frequent, as is hypothyroidism. Ovarian failure is a uniform finding. Most often, secondary sex characteristics fail to develop, but spontaneous puberty occurs in a small percentage of subjects. The diagnosis is suspected by the physical findings and confirmed by an elevated FSH level and a karyotype revealing the deleted X chromosome.

Treatment is directed at hormone replacement to induce secondary sexual characteristics and menstruation. If the condition is detected in childhood, growth hormone replacement therapy can be initiated to maximize height. HRT can be delayed to accommodate the treatment for short stature. Once estrogen replacement is initiated and continued, the epiphyseal plates eventually close, and no further growth takes place. Evaluation of the heart (particularly to detect aortic root dilation) and kidneys should be performed regularly, in addition to yearly monitoring for hypothyroidism.

Patients who present with secondary amenorrhea after spontaneous puberty should also be offered HRT to allow appropriate bone deposition. Patients with Turner syndrome are at risk for osteoporosis secondary to estrogen deficiency. After ovarian failure is noted, fertility is usually not possible without the use of donor oocyte technology. Careful physical assessment and consultation are appropriate before pregnancy is attempted, given the increased risk for adverse outcomes.

Other X-chromosome Abnormalities

Because genetic information determining the rate of follicular atresia is carried on the long arm of the X chromosome, any loss of the long arm results in premature ovarian failure. The extent of long arm loss determines the chronologic age at which ovarian failure occurs. For example, if the loss is substantial, ovarian failure may develop before puberty. If the loss is slight, ovarian failure may occur after several pregnancies. Karyotyping is indicated in patients with premature ovarian failure to assess for the possibility of sex chromosome abnormality.

Alkylating Chemotherapy

Alkylating chemotherapy alters the follicular membrane surrounding the oocyte so that it becomes resistant to gonadotropins. As a result, temporary signs and symptoms of ovarian failure may develop in women who have been treated with alkylating agents for Hodgkin lymphoma, leukemia, breast cancer, and other neoplastic disease. Destruction of the ovarian follicles may also occur and lead to permanent ovarian failure. It is often difficult to determine immediately after therapy whether spontaneous resumption of ovulation is possible. A 6-month evaluation for return of menses is generally indicated. If the FSH level remains elevated, HRT should be started. With HRT, spontaneous ovulation and pregnancy have been reported in patients with presumed ovarian failure secondary to chemotherapy. Ovarian failure may also occur years after the primary insult.

Other Causes of Premature Ovarian Failure

If a women presenting with evidence of ovarian failure has a normal karyotype and no history of antecedent chemotherapy or radiation, other causes of premature ovarian failure should be sought. Ovarian failure develops in patients with galactosemia, an autosomal-recessive trait resulting in a deficiency of galactose-1-phosphate uridyltransferase. Autoimmune disease and lymphocytic oophoritis can result in ovarian failure. Autoimmune failure can be seen in multiple endocrine glands, such as the thyroid, parathyroid, and adrenal glands, and these hormonal axes should be carefully evaluated if autoimmune ovarian failure is diagnosed (see Chapter 36).

MALE PSEUDOHERMAPHRODITISM

Swyer Syndrome

An XY karyotype may be found in patients who present with sexual infantilism and an elevated FSH level. If they have a müllerian system, Swyer syndrome or gonadal dysgenesis of the primordial gonad is diagnosed. The testes do not form, and therefore no müllerian inhibiting factor is secreted. No testosterone is secreted in utero, so no wolffian ducts develop. The abdominal streak gonads must be removed because of a significant risk for neoplastic transformation. HRT should be initiated at the time of anticipated puberty.

Androgen Insensitivity Syndrome

Women with androgen insensitivity syndrome have a 46,XY karyotype but abnormal cytosol androgen receptors. Because testosterone cannot bind to the receptors and its androgenic influence on the external or internal genitalia is lost, the patients have female characteristics. The testes are often intra-abdominal and secrete testosterone, which is converted to estradiol in the periphery. Therefore, breasts develop at puberty. Because müllerian inhibiting factor is produced by the fetal testes, no uterus, fallopian tubes, or vagina forms, and the patient presents with primary amenorrhea. Very little pubic or axillary hair is noted because these are androgen-dependent. Intra-abdominal or inguinal testes must be removed because of the risk for neoplasia. HRT should then be initiated.

Anatomic Abnormalities

MÜLLERIAN AGENESIS

Müllerian agenesis is a birth defect resulting from failure of fusion and canalization of the müllerian ducts. Unless the defect is recognized at birth, the presenting sign is primary amenorrhea. In most cases, no functioning müllerian tissue is present, although remnant structures may be seen. Because ovarian function is normal, secondary sex traits develop normally at the expected time. It is possible to have a functioning uterus with outflow obstruction. In these cases, pelvic pain is often associated with primary amenorrhea and a pelvic mass. Vaginoplasty with dilators or the surgical creation of a new vagina is indicated in müllerian agenesis.

IMPERFORATE HYMEN

In imperforate hymen, menstrual fluid is obstructed at the vaginal introitus. A large amount of menstrual effluent can accumulate in the vaginal vault before symptoms develop. A bluish, bulging imperforate hymen is the characteristic feature. Incising the hymen evacuates the accumulated effluent and provides immediate and long-term resolution of the problem.

ASHERMAN SYNDROME

Asherman syndrome usually develops after dilation and curettage of a postpartum uterus for retained products of conception. It presents as secondary amenorrhea. Curettage of a uterus several days after delivery can denude the endometrium so that it cannot regenerate; without endometrial regeneration, menstruation cannot occur. The diagnosis is made by hysterosalpingography or hysteroscopic visualization of the endometrial cavity. On the hysterosalpingogram, the endometrial cavity shows signs of scarring. Lysis of adhesions by hysteroscopy can sometimes restore menstruation and fertility. If the scarring is very extensive, the likelihood of restoring menstruation and fertility is poor. Ovarian function is normal in this syndrome.

EVALUATION

History

An evaluation for pubertal abnormalities should be initiated if no secondary sexual characteristics have appeared by the age of 13 years. If the breasts have begun to develop but menses do not begin within 2 years after the start of breast development, or if menses do not begin by the age of 16 years, the patient should be evaluated for primary amenorrhea. After the initiation of menses, if no further menstrual cycles occur for 6 months, an evaluation should be undertaken. One should carefully record the rate of childhood growth and whether the patient had any unusual childhood illnesses. The dates of onset of pubertal change should be noted. The patient should be questioned about evidence of hormonal changes, such as cyclic breast tenderness, mood changes, acne, or bloating. Eating habits and exercise patterns should be carefully elicited. Changes in body weight should be noted and inquiries made about illicit drug use. The patient's lifestyle, including work, school, and family stressors, should be carefully evaluated. Any changes in the patient's energy level, hair or skin, frequency of headaches, or bowel habits should be noted.

Physical Examination

A careful physical examination often uncovers findings that suggest the cause of amenorrhea. The body habitus, particularly truncal obesity or extreme slenderness, can frequently be linked to amenorrhea. Skin changes, such as acanthosis nigricans, acne, or hirsutism, suggest PCOS. Hair loss may be seen in thyroid disorders or anorexia nervosa. Abdominal striae may be seen in cases of cortisol excess, either endogenous or exogenous.

The Tanner stage of the breasts is determined in cases of primary amenorrhea. Any galactorrhea should be noted. The pelvic examination often provides clues to the estrogen status. In estrogen-deficient patients, the vaginal mucosa is thin, pale or red, and dry. Cervical mucus is lacking. Clues to anatomic causes of primary amenorrhea are also often found during the pelvic examination. If only a vaginal pouch is present without growth of pubic hair, then androgen insensitivity should be considered. The same findings with normal development of pubic hair should raise the possibility of müllerian agenesis. Pelvic masses may indicate obstructed menstrual flow.

Laboratory Evaluation

Hormonal studies can be very useful in distinguishing the cause of amenorrhea (Fig. 16.1). If evidence of an anatomic abnormality has been noted, the serum testosterone and FSH levels should be

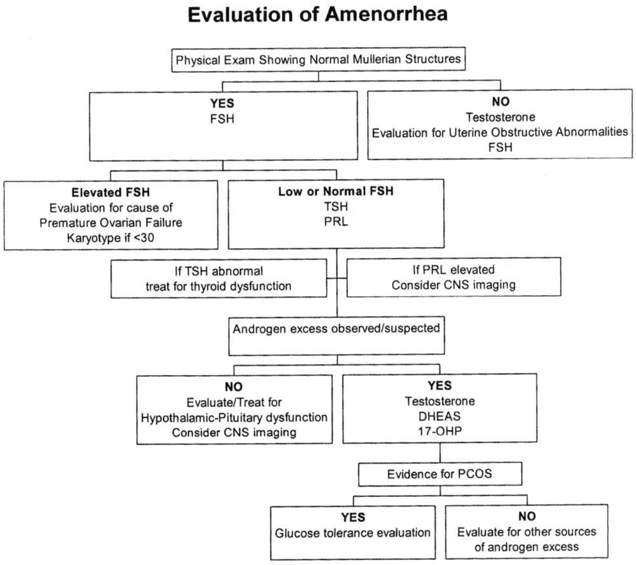

FIG. 16.1. Flow chart for the evaluation of amenorrhea.

determined initially to assess for male pseudohermaphroditism, such as androgen insensitivity. If normal müllerian structures are present, then the FSH level is helpful to categorize the amenorrhea as a primary ovarian or a hypothalamic-pituitary disorder. If the FSH level is high, the karyotype should be determined to evaluate for sex chromosomal abnormalities. If the FSH level is low or normal, the causes of hypothalamic-pituitary dysfunction should be sought. If evidence of androgen excess is found, the serum levels of testosterone, dehydroepiandrosterone sulfate (DHEAS), and 17-hydroxyprogesterone, a marker for the late onset of 21-hydroxylase deficiency, should be measured. Androgen excess with amenorrhea, in the absence of other causes of increased testosterone, should be considered evidence of PCOS, and the glucose metabolism should be assessed, especially if the patient is overweight.

TREATMENT

Once the cause of amenorrhea is established, treatment is directed according to the needs of the patient. Patients who wish to conceive are managed differently from those who require reestablishment of the menstrual cycle, estrogen replacement, or control of symptoms of androgen excess.

For a patient with PCOS, one of the most common causes of amenorrhea, many different needs may have to be addressed: protecting the endometrium from hyperplasia, decreasing androgenic symptoms, establishing regular menstruation, and possibly inducing ovulation so that she can conceive. The endometrium can be protected by administering cyclic progestin to establish monthly withdrawal bleeding or an oral contraceptive. The oral contraceptive provides the additional benefits of decreasing both testosterone production and the amount of free testosterone, thereby lessening the symptoms of androgen excess. If the patient is significantly overweight or obese, weight reduction has been shown to restore normal ovulatory cycles and menstrual bleeding. Weight reduction strategies should be discussed with these patients as a first line of therapy. Recently, insulin-sensitizing therapies, such as metformin, have been shown to restore ovulation in patients with PCOS. At present, it is unclear whether the long-term use of metformin alone is appropriate care for the patient with PCOS who does not wish to become pregnant, but it should be considered for the patient desiring pregnancy (see Chapters 36 and 37).

Patients with premature ovarian failure are deficient in estrogen. They must be informed of the long-term consequences of estrogen deprivation, such as osteoporosis and possibly cardiovascular disease, especially those who are still young. HRT can be given as low-dose estrogen with cyclic medroxyprogesterone acetate or as an oral contraceptive. Patients with Turner syndrome should also undergo a cardiac and renal evaluation because anomalies in these areas are common, as is thyroid dysfunction.

Hypothalamic-pituitary abnormalities should be addressed to restore normal ovulatory cycles. Hyperprolactinemia can be treated with a dopamine agonist, such as bromocriptine or cabergoline. Once the prolactin level is suppressed to within a normal range, the menses will return. Weight gain in patients with anorexia restores the normal axis in most cases. Severe eating disorders may require the intervention of a clinical psychologist or psychiatrist who is knowledgeable in the management of these conditions because anorexia nervosa can be life-threatening (see Chapter 149). Patients with functional hypothalamic-pituitary dysfunction should be encouraged to identify and moderate the sources of stress that led to suppression of the hormonal axis. Often, doing so restores menstrual function. For those with permanent disruption of the axis secondary to tumor or a congenital abnormality, hormone replacement in the form of estrogen-progestin should be encouraged.

The surgical correction of amenorrhea is indicated for patients with obstructive abnormalities of the outflow tract. In a patient without müllerian structures, a new vagina must be created. Remnant uterine structures must be removed only if they contain active endometrial tissue. A patient with gonadal dysgenesis and evidence of a Y chromosome or androgen insensitivity syndrome should undergo gonadectomy because of the possibility of malignancy in such gonads. HRT should be initiated subsequently.

SUMMARY

Amenorrhea is a symptom of disease in the reproductive axis. Disorders of the hypothalamic-pituitary axis, ovaries, or uterus can all cause amenorrhea. The evaluation and treatment of a patient presenting with amenorrhea should be comprehensive and thoughtful, based on the history and physical examination findings. The long-term consequences of amenorrhea should be addressed so that the patient can receive appropriate counseling and treatment.

BIBLIOGRAPHY

Aiman J, Smentek L. Premature ovarian failure. *Obstet Gynecol* 1985;66:9.
Berga SL. Functional hypothalamic chronic anovulation. In: Adashi E, Rock J, Rosenwaks Z, eds. *Reproductive endocrinology, surgery and technology*. Philadelphia: Lippincott-Raven, 1996:1061.
Dunaif A, Segal K, Futterweit W, et al. Profound peripheral insulin resistance independent of obesity in polycystic ovary syndrome. *Diabetes* 1989;38:1165.
Filicori M, Santoro N, Merriam GR, et al. Characterization of the physiological pattern of episodic gonadotropin secretion throughout the menstrual cycle. *J Clin Endocrinol Metab* 1986;62:1136.
Griffen JE. Androgen resistance—the clinical and molecular spectrum. *N Engl J Med* 1992;326:611.
Griffen JE, Edwards C, Ladden JD, et al. Congenital absence of the vagina. *Ann Intern Med* 1988;85:224.
Hoeger K. Obesity and weight loss in polycystic ovary syndrome. *Obstet Gynecol Clin North Am* 2001;28:85.
Manuel M, Katayama KP, Jones Jr HW. The age of occurrence of gonadal tumors in intersex patients with a Y chromosome. *Am J Obstet Gynecol* 1976;124:293.
Reindollar RH, Novak M, Tho SPT, et al. Adult-onset amenorrhea: a study of 262 patients. *Am J Obstet Gynecol* 1986;155:531.
Saenger P. The current status of diagnosis and therapeutic intervention in Turner's syndrome. *J Clin Endocrinol Metab* 1993;77:297.
Schlechte J, Sherman B, Halm N, et al. Prolactin-secreting pituitary tumors. *Endocr Rev* 1980;1:295.
Warren MP. Effect of exercise and physical training on menarche. *Semin Reprod Endocrinol* 1985;3:17.
Warren MP, Vandewiele RL. Clinical and metabolic features of anorexia nervosa. *Am J Obstet Gynecol* 1973;117:435.

CHAPTER 17
Dysmenorrhea

Fred M. Howard

Dysmenorrhea is defined as severe, cramping pain in the pelvis, lower abdomen, lower back, and upper thighs that occurs just before or during menses. The prevalence of dysmenorrhea seems to be as high as 75%, with about 15% of women having symptoms sufficiently severe to limit their daily activities. In the United States, absenteeism from work because of dysmenorrhea is estimated at 600 million work hours, and the economic consequences are estimated to be $2 billion per year.

Dysmenorrhea is usually classified as primary or secondary. *Primary dysmenorrhea* is painful menses with no pelvic pathology found to account for the pain and is a diagnosis of exclusion. It is particularly a problem of young women, with an onset before age 20. Although the condition becomes less severe in some women after age 25, many have undiagnosed disorders, such as endometriosis. Pregnancy and vaginal delivery, per se, do not necessarily cure primary dysmenorrhea. *Secondary dysmenorrhea* is diagnosed in women with pelvic pathology that causes pain with menses, such as leiomyomata, adenomyosis, or endometriosis. It is more common in women older than 20 years.

ETIOLOGY

Tissue hypoxia and ischemia are thought to cause the pain of primary dysmenorrhea. An elevation in the basal tone of the uterus, combined with an increase in the strength and frequency of contractions, leads to vasospasm and a reduction in uterine blood flow. Primary dysmenorrhea appears to be caused principally by prostaglandins, in particular prostaglandin $F_{2\alpha}$ (PGF_2) and PGE_2, released from the endometrium at menses. Prostaglandins are unsaturated fatty acids with a cyclopentane ring and two side chains that are synthesized from arachidonic acid. Polyunsaturated fatty acids, including arachidonic acid, are constituents of all cell membranes and are converted to prostaglandins or leukotrienes via two major pathways, the cyclooxygenase (COX) and lipoxygenase pathways (Fig. 17.1). In the COX (prostaglandin synthetase) pathway, free arachidonic acid, released by phospholipase, is converted into cyclic endoperoxides, then into PGE_2, $PGF_{2\alpha}$, prostacyclin, or thromboxane A_2. $PGF_{2\alpha}$ is especially important in dysmenorrhea, and it has been shown that both estradiol and progesterone levels influence the synthesis and levels of endometrial $PGF_{2\alpha}$.

In 1989, it was determined that the COX enzyme exists in at least two isoforms. Although they are 60% homologous in the amino acid sequences considered important for the catalysis of arachidonic acid, they are the products of two different genes and differ in regulation and expression. Nonsteroidal antiinflammatory drugs (NSAIDs) specifically inhibit COX and thereby reduce the conversion of arachidonic acid to $PGF_{2\alpha}$. COX-l is a "housekeeping enzyme" that regulates normal cellular processes and is stimulated by hormones or growth factors. It is constitutively expressed in most tissues and is inhibited by

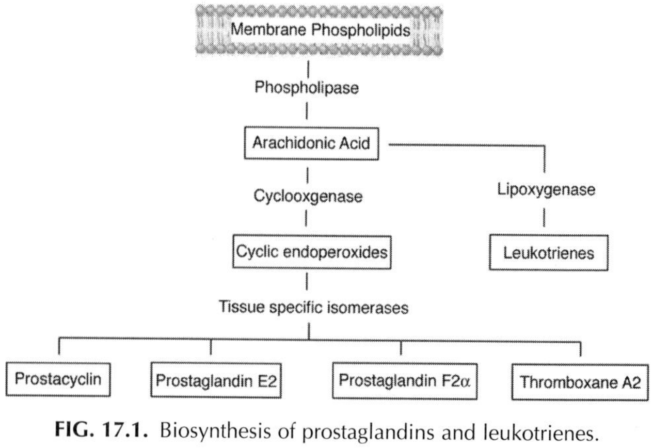

FIG. 17.1. Biosynthesis of prostaglandins and leukotrienes.

all NSAIDs to varying degrees. COX-1 is important in maintaining the integrity of the gastric and duodenal mucosa. Many of the toxic effects of NSAIDs on the gastrointestinal tract are attributed to inhibition of COX-1. The other isoform, COX-2, is an inducible enzyme. Levels of COX-2 are usually very low or undetectable in most tissues, but expression is increased during states of inflammation. COX-2 is also constitutively expressed in the brain, in the female reproductive tract, in the male vas deferens, in bone associated with osteoblast activity, and perhaps in human kidney. Traditional NSAIDs are effective antiinflammatory drugs because they inhibit COX-2, whereas many of their potential toxic effects can be attributed to inhibition of COX-l.

The other metabolic pathway for arachidonic acid metabolism, the lipoxygenase pathway, leads to the formation of leukotrienes. Leukotrienes cause uterine muscle contractions and are potent vasoconstrictors and bronchoconstrictors. Many NSAIDs block the COX pathway, but they do not block the lipoxygenase pathway.

The association between increased uterine $PGF_{2\alpha}$, increased myometrial activity, and dysmenorrhea is now well established. Higher concentrations of $PGF_{2\alpha}$ have been noted in the menstrual fluid of dysmenorrheic women. In anovulatory cycles without dysmenorrhea, progesterone levels are low and endometrial prostaglandin levels are not increased. The intravenous injection of $PGF_{2\alpha}$ reproduces uterine cramps and pain. $PGF_{2\alpha}$ can also cause diarrhea, vomiting, headache, and syncope, symptoms frequently associated with primary dysmenorrhea. Also, prostaglandin synthetase inhibitors relieve dysmenorrhea and decrease menstrual flow and uterine contractility. The observation that prostaglandin synthetase inhibitors block the COX pathway, but not the lipoxygenase pathway, may explain why these drugs do not relieve primary dysmenorrhea in all patients.

In addition to prostaglandins, several other factors may play a role in the development of dysmenorrhea. One is vasopressin, a powerful stimulant of the uterus, particularly at the onset of menstruation. The circulating levels of vasopressin during menstruation are fourfold higher in women with dysmenorrhea than in asymptomatic women. The effect of vasopressin is not thought to be mediated by prostaglandins because vasopressin levels are not decreased when dysmenorrhea is relieved by prostaglandin synthetase inhibitors.

Purely psychological factors are rarely if ever the cause of dysmenorrhea. However, psychological factors may significantly intensify or diminish the pain of dysmenorrhea. The clinical observation that primary dysmenorrhea is relieved in some women after childbirth may be explained by the fact that short adrenergic neurons in the myometrium tend to be destroyed during pregnancy and do not regenerate afterward.

By definition, secondary dysmenorrhea is caused by a pathologic condition within the pelvis. A variety of conditions may lead to secondary dysmenorrhea (Table 17.1).

Endometriosis, the presence of endometrial glands and stroma outside the uterine epithelium, is a major cause of secondary dysmenorrhea. Approximately 7% of women in the United States have endometriosis, and at least half of these women experience dysmenorrhea. A definitive diagnosis requires direct visualization during laparoscopy or laparotomy and a tissue biopsy for histologic confirmation. Prostaglandins are believed to cause the increased pain of endometriosis. Investigators have shown that the levels of prostaglandins are significantly higher in endometriotic implants than in other pelvic structures. Endometriotic implants in severely dysmenorrheic patients have also been shown to produce larger amounts of 6-keto-PGF.

TABLE 17.1. Common Causes of Secondary Dysmenorrhea

Uterine
Adenomyosis
Leiomyomata
Endometrial polyps
Congenital malformation (e.g., redundant uterine horn)
Cervical stenosis
Extrauterine
Endometriosis
Pelvic inflammatory disease
Pelvic congestion syndrome
Allen-Masters syndrome
Iatrogenic
Intrauterine contraception device
Psychogenic
Uncommon (learned behavior?)

Cervical stenosis can increase both the intrauterine pressure and retrograde menstrual flow, thereby causing lower abdominal discomfort, dysmenorrhea, and even endometriosis. A narrow or stenotic os may be a congenital abnormality or the result of trauma, infection, or surgery such as conization or cryocautery.

Imperforate hymen is a cause of obstructive dysmenorrhea associated with failure of canalization of the urogenital sinus. This also can lead to retrograde menstruation and the development of endometriosis. Similarly, blind rudimentary horns may present with dysmenorrhea and cause endometriosis.

Pelvic infections, including tuberculosis, also cause secondary dysmenorrhea, possibly through tissue destruction.

Adenomyosis is the presence of ectopic endometrial glands and stroma in the myometrium of the uterus. Symptoms of adenomyosis classically include dysmenorrhea and menorrhagia. On physical examination, the uterus generally is soft, globular, and uniformly enlarged. Typically, the uterus is tender just before and during menstruation. Diagnostic aids include pelvic ultrasonography, magnetic resonance imaging, and hysterosalpingography.

Other reported causes of secondary dysmenorrhea include small intracavitary leiomyomata or polyps that can become engorged and painful at time of menstruation. Investigators have found a significant relation between functional bowel disorder and dysmenorrhea. Pelvic congestion syndrome may also be a cause of secondary dysmenorrhea.

CLINICAL SYMPTOMS AND FINDINGS

Primary Dysmenorrhea

Primary dysmenorrhea usually begins 6 to 12 months after menarche, at the onset of ovulatory cycles. Some patients, however, experience pain with the first cycle. A survey by Andersch and Milsom reported that in 38% of girls, dysmenorrhea developed in the first year after menarche, whereas in 21%, it developed 4 years later. The pain is significantly correlated with ovulatory cycles because only endometrial tissue exposed to both estrogen and progesterone produces abnormal levels of prostaglandins. Patients experience spasmodic, colicky, or cramping lower abdominal pain that may radiate suprapubically, to the inner aspect of the thighs, or the lower back. The pain may also be of a continuous, dull, aching character. Other symptoms may accompany the pain, such as headache, nausea, vomiting, diarrhea, and fatigue. In most cases, the pain starts a few hours before menstruation or at the onset of menstruation. The symptoms typically last 48 hours or less, but sometimes up to 72 hours. The severity of pain is variable. About 15% of women with primary dysmenorrhea have severe pain. Occasionally, the accompanying vasoconstriction in the acute phase may be so marked that the patient appears to be in shock.

The family history is important because dysmenorrhea has been found to run in families. The overall demeanor of the patient is sometimes helpful in assessing whether the pain has a psychiatric component. The psychosocial history should be ascertained. The sexual history should be elicited; often, this requires that the parents be absent during questioning. It should be noted that the history of a prior pregnancy does not negate the possibility of primary dysmenorrhea. In a study by Chan and Dawood, the pain of primary dysmenorrhea returned in almost 20% of patients following vaginal delivery.

A careful history and detailed examination are of key importance in diagnosing primary dysmenorrhea. In a young woman with suspected primary dysmenorrhea, the pelvic examination may be difficult because of her anxiety and discomfort. The clinician must be sensitive to this. If a vaginal examination is not feasible, sometimes a rectal examination can be performed and will suffice in many cases.

Primary dysmenorrhea is a diagnosis of exclusion. The general physical examination and pelvic examination reveal no abnormality. Laparoscopy may be required rule out pelvic pathology, particularly endometriosis. Endometriosis is relatively common in adolescents and may be the cause of more cases of "primary" dysmenorrhea than is generally recognized.

Secondary Dysmenorrhea

The symptoms of secondary dysmenorrhea, caused by identifiable pathologic conditions (Table 17.1), are similar to those of primary dysmenorrhea, but secondary dysmenorrhea tends to start at a later age. Patients may have a history of menorrhagia, pelvic inflammatory disease, infertility, dyspareunia, or use of an intrauterine contraceptive device.

The timing of pain relative to the menses can be helpful. Pain starting before menstruation is often caused by pelvic inflammatory disease, pelvic congestion syndrome, endometriosis, or premenstrual syndrome. On the other hand, pain starting at menstruation is sometimes associated with uterine pathology, such as submucous leiomyomata or endometrial polyps.

A history of surgical procedures involving the cervix may suggest cervical stenosis. The diagnosis of cervical stenosis should be considered in a patient who has a history of hypomenorrhea and severe pelvic pain during menses, or whose external cervical os is less than 5 mm in diameter. During the physical examination, the physician should attempt to pass a uterine sound into the endometrial cavity. If a clear passage through the cervical canal cannot be documented, further investigation is warranted.

Intrauterine contraceptive devices are another cause of secondary dysmenorrhea; therefore, the contraceptive history should be discussed.

The physical examination may reveal findings consistent with anemia secondary to heavy menstrual bleeding. A careful pelvic examination should be performed to look for uterine enlargement or irregularity, pelvic masses, or pelvic tenderness. A rectal examination should be performed to detect nodularity and tenderness along the uterosacral ligaments and cul-de-sac, findings suggestive of endometriosis. The presence of an intrauterine device may be confirmed by finding its string at the cervix.

LABORATORY AND IMAGING FINDINGS

No laboratory test results are diagnostic or specific in primary or secondary dysmenorrhea. The levels of cancer antigen-125 (CA-125) may be elevated in patients with endometriosis or leiomyomata, but the CA-125 levels are elevated in several other conditions not related to dysmenorrhea. The results of cervical cultures for gonorrhea and tests for *Chlamydia* may be positive and helpful if pelvic inflammatory disease is suspected. Although prostaglandin levels have been measured experimentally in menstrual fluid, this test is not useful clinically.

Ultrasonography, especially when performed transvaginally, may be useful to look for uterine leiomyomata, uterine enlargement, adnexal masses, endometrial polyps, or an unsuspected intrauterine device. It may also be useful for the nonoperative diagnosis of adenomyosis, but further investigation is needed.

Hysterosalpingography often detects uterine anomalies, endometrial polyps, or Asherman syndrome. In cases of cervical stenosis, hysterosalpingography may reveal a narrow cervical canal.

Laparoscopy remains an important diagnostic procedure to assess the pelvis for endometriosis or other pathologic conditions. Simultaneous hysteroscopy to evaluate the uterine cavity for submucosal leiomyomata or endometrial polyps may also be useful.

TREATMENT

Many women seek medical help for dysmenorrhea. The primary care physician should be sensitive to the concerns of each patient and provide treatment that is specific to her needs. The usual goal of therapy is to decrease pain sufficiently so that the patient can resume her daily life without being disabled by dysmenorrhea. Successful management can be challenging. In selecting the appropriate treatment, it is usually helpful to determine whether the dysmenorrhea is primary or secondary.

Primary Dysmenorrhea

For many women, oral contraceptives provide significant relief from primary dysmenorrhea. They suppress ovulation, markedly reduce spontaneous uterine activity, and prevent fluctuations of endogenous progesterone levels, thereby reducing pain and other symptoms associated with primary dysmenorrhea. Oral contraceptives are a good first-line therapy for many young women, especially if contraception is also needed. Continuous oral contraceptives may be more effective, but many patients consider the amenorrhea induced by continuous oral contraceptives unnatural. However, sometimes they are willing to compromise by taking long-cycle contraceptives in a pattern so that they have only three or four menses a year.

The NSAIDs that inhibit prostaglandin synthetase have been pivotal in the treatment of primary dysmenorrhea for the last 20 years (Table 17.2). Unlike oral contraceptives, these agents must be taken only 2 or 3 days per month and do not suppress the hypothalamic-pituitary-ovarian axis. Their primary therapeutic benefit is inhibition of prostaglandin formation. They provide relief in up to 75% of patients. It is hypothesized that in patients whose pain is not relieved by NSAIDs, the activity of the alternate lipoxygenase pathway of prostaglandin production is increased. The choice of a particular NSAID depends on clinical efficacy, side effects, patient acceptance, and individual clinical experience. NSAIDs should be started at or just before the his-

TABLE 17.2. Nonsteroidal Antiinflammatory Drugs and Cyclooxygenase-2 Inhibitors Commonly Used for Dysmenorrhea

Drug	Trade name	Recommended dosage
Ibuprofen	Motrin, Advil, Rufen	40 mg q6–8h
Naproxen	Naprosyn	250–500 mg q6–8h
Mefenamic acid	Ponstel	250–500 mg q6h
Diclofenac	Voltaren, Cataflam	50 mg q8h
Naproxen sodium	Anaprox	275–500 q6–8h
Celecoxib	Celebrex	200 mg q12h
Rofecoxib	Vioxx	50 mg qd
Valdecoxib	Bextra	20 mg q12h

torical time of onset of pain and continued regularly during the symptomatic period on an "as-needed" basis. If pain control with an as-needed regimen is insufficient, a trial of regularly scheduled dosing is sometimes worthwhile. If the pain is still inadequately controlled, the loading dose may be increased by up to 50% during the next cycle, but the maintenance dose should be kept the same. A trial of several months may be needed to demonstrate effective relief of symptoms. If a particular NSAID is ineffective, a different one should be tried because individual responsiveness to the NSAIDs varies significantly. The side effects of NSAIDs include gastric irritation, heartburn, abdominal pain, nausea, vomiting, headache, occasional visual disturbances, allergic reactions, and blood disorders. These are unusual when NSAIDs are used on an intermittent basis for dysmenorrhea, but therapy with NSAIDs should be discontinued if adverse side effects develop. COX-2 inhibitors are also effective and may cause fewer gastrointestinal side effects than NSAIDs.

If neither NSAIDs nor oral contraceptives alone alleviate primary dysmenorrhea, the two can be used together. If combination therapy also fails, the patient should be reevaluated and a diagnostic workup initiated for secondary dysmenorrhea.

Calcium antagonists such as verapamil and nifedipine reduce uterine activity and contractility and have relieved pain in some resistant cases of dysmenorrhea. The mechanism may be different—decreasing the severity of myometrial contractions decreases intrauterine pressure and the resultant pain. They have no effect on other symptoms, such as vomiting or diarrhea.

Nonpharmacologic treatments include transcutaneous electric nerve stimulation (TENS), acupuncture, application of a lower abdominal heating pad, supplemental vitamin B_1 (100 mg daily) or magnesium (400 mg daily), and a low-fat vegetarian diet.

The neural pathways from the uterus may be surgically interrupted to decrease the pain of dysmenorrhea. The efficacy of presacral neurectomy in relieving midline dysmenorrhea is more than 80%. Uterine nerve ablation achieved by transecting the uterosacral ligaments may be more easily performed than a presacral neurectomy, but its efficacy is less reliable. Cervical dilation has historically been used to relieve dysmenorrhea thought to be secondary to cervical stenosis, but its value is debatable.

Secondary Dysmenorrhea

In addition to the treatments described for primary dysmenorrhea, therapy for secondary dysmenorrhea should be directed at the underlying condition.

The treatment of endometriosis may be medical, surgical, or both. Oral contraceptives, gonadotropin-releasing hormone agonists (e.g., leuprolide depot), danazol, or high-dose progestins are all beneficial in relieving pain. Surgical treatment may be conservative, with ablation and resection of lesions and adhesions, or extirpative, with hysterectomy and oophorectomy.

Adenomyosis may be treated with medical suppression of ovarian function or may respond to conservative treatment with NSAIDs. However, most cases go undiagnosed until a histologic evaluation is performed at the time of a hysterectomy. Endomyometrial ablative or resection procedures may be effective treatment in some cases.

Cervical stenosis may be treated by dilating the cervical canal with laminaria tents or by formal dilation under anesthesia. These procedures are usually of limited therapeutic benefit and must be repeated frequently. Symptoms typically resolve completely with pregnancy and vaginal delivery.

Women using intrauterine devices can be treated with NSAIDs or COX-2 inhibitors, or the device can be removed. NSAIDs may offer an added benefit of reduced menstrual flow. Naproxen, mefenamic acid, and ibuprofen are frequently used (Table 17.2). It is important to rule out pelvic inflammatory disease in women with an intrauterine device.

Leiomyomata uteri may be treated surgically with myomectomy or hysterectomy, depending on the patient's age, parity, and severity of symptoms.

Endometrial polyps may be removed via hysteroscopy or dilation and curettage.

BIBLIOGRAPHY

Akin MD, Welngand KW, Hengehold DA, et al. Continuous low-level topical heat in the treatment of dysmenorrhea. *Obstet Gynecol* 2001;97:343.

Andersch B, Milsom I. An epidemiological study of young women with dysmenorrhea. *Am J Obstet Gynecol* 1982;144:655–657.

Anderson KE, Ulmsten U. Effects of nifedipine on myometrial activity and lower abdominal pain in women with primary dysmenorrhea. *Br J Obstet Gynaecol* 1978;85:142–144.

Barbieri RL. Stenosis of the external cervical os: an association with endometriosis in women with chronic pelvic pain. *Fertil Steril* 1998;70:571–573.

Chan WY, Dawood MY. Prostaglandin levels in menstrual fluid of nondysmenorrheic and dysmenorrheic subjects with and without oral contraceptive or ibuprofen therapy. *Adv Prostaglandin Thromboxane Res* 1980;8:1443–1446.

Chan WY, Dawood MY, Fuchs F. Relief of dysmenorrhea with the prostaglandin synthetase inhibitor Ibuprofen: effect on prostaglandin levels in menstrual fluid. *Am J Obstet Gynecol* 1979;135:102–104.

Chatman DL, Ward AB. Endometriosis in adolescents. *J Reprod Med* 1982;27:156.

Crowell MD, Dubin NH, Robinson JC, et al. Functional bowel disorders in women with dysmenorrhea. *Am J Gastroenterol* 1994;89:1973–1977.

Fedele L, Blanchi S, Boccioione L, et al. Pain symptoms associated with endometriosis. *Obstet Gynecol* 1992;79:767.

Helms JM. Acupuncture in the management of primary dysmenorrhea. *Obstet Gynecol* 1987;69:51–56.

Jordan VC, Pokoly TB. Steroid and prostaglandin relations during the menstrual cycle. *Obstet Gynecol* 1971;49:449–451.

Kaplan B, Rablnerson D, Pardo J, et al. Transcutaneous electrical nerve stimulation (TENS) as a pain-relief device in obstetrics and gynecology. *Clin Exp Obstet Gynecol* 1997;24:123.

Milsom I, Hedner N, Mannheimer C. A comparative study of the effect of high-intensity transcutaneous nerve stimulation and oral naproxen on intrauterine pressure and menstrual pain in patients with primary dysmenorrhea. *Am J Obstet Gynecol* 1994;170:123–126.

Morrison BW, Daniels SE, Kotey P. Rofecoxib, a specific cyclooxygenase-2 inhibitor, in primary dysmenorrhea: a randomized controlled trial. *Obstet Gynecol* 1999;94:504–508.

Owen PR. Prostaglandin synthetase inhibitors in the treatment of primary dysmenorrhea: outcome trials reviewed. *Am J Obstet Gynecol* 1984;148:96–99.

Pickles VR, Hall WJ, Best FA, et al. Prostaglandin in endometrium and menstrual fluid from normal and dysmenorrheic subjects. *Br J Obstet Gynaecol* 1965;72: 185–187.

Proctor ML, Roberts H, Farquhar CM. Combined oral contraceptive pill (OCP) as treatment for primary dysmenorrhoea [Cochrane Review]. In: *Cochrane Library*, issue 4. Oxford, UK: Update Software, 2001.

Sundell G, Milson I, Andersch B. Factors influencing the prevalence and severity of dysmenorrhea in young women. *Br J Obstet Gynaecol* 1990;97:588.

Widholm OM, Kantero RA. A statistical analysis of the menstrual patterns of Finnish girls and their mothers. *Acta Obstet Gynecol Scand Suppl* 1971;14:1–2.

Wilson L, Cendella RJ, Butcher RL, et al. Levels of prostaglandins in the uterine endometrium during the ovine estrous cycle. *J Anim Sci* 1972;34:93–96.

Wilson ML, Murphy PA. Herbal and dietary therapies for primary and secondary dysmenorrhea. *Cochrane Database Syst Rev* 2001;3:CD002124.

CHAPTER 18
Infertility

John T. Queenan, Jr.

The primary care provider is frequently the first clinician to be consulted by the infertile couple. The workup is ideally suited to the ambulatory, primary care setting. Primary care practitioners will find that the evaluation and treatment of infertility can be very satisfying.

The scope of the problem is huge. Approximately 15% to 20% of couples of reproductive age have difficulty in initiating a pregnancy or maintaining one that has been established. The desire for childbearing has compelled millions of couples to seek competent care from physicians.

Infertility is classically defined as a failure to conceive within 1 year of unprotected intercourse. This chapter discusses the basic concepts involved in the diagnosis and treatment of the infertile couple. Practitioners will learn how to recognize those patients who merit evaluation and which couples should be referred for further evaluation or treatment.

ETIOLOGY

During the past two decades, fertility has declined consistently. Our society has witnessed many trends that contribute to this pattern. Contraceptive methods have become plentiful and accessible. The arrival of family planning has enabled women to develop careers on a par with those of their male counterparts. The changing role of women in society has brought about greater access to the workplace and higher education. All these factors have led to a delay of marriage and a postponement of childbearing. Today, one in five women gives birth to her first child when she is older than 35 years. Maternal age is significant, but it is far from the only explanation for the rise in infertility.

The failure to establish an ongoing gestation is a complex condition with many possible causes. Infertility can result from an anatomic abnormality, endocrine dysfunction, a genetic abnormality, an immune system problem, or a prior infection. Any of these conditions can arise in the male partner, the female partner, or both. The cause may be an external factor. Fertility is compromised in persons who engage in substance abuse, have an eating disorder, or are environmentally exposed to toxic substances. The basis for infertility may be very simple, such as infrequent intercourse, poor timing, or a lack of motivation on the part of one of the partners.

Frequently, a thorough evaluation does not identify any etiologic factor. Unexplained infertility is a source of considerable frustration for both patients and physicians. At the other end of the spectrum, infertility may be multifactorial. The wide variety in clinical presentation highlights the need for a complete and systematic evaluation of the couple.

A formal evaluation is warranted for those who fail to conceive after 1 year of unprotected intercourse. Earlier intervention is indicated for the patient who is older than 35 years or who has oligomenorrhea/amenorrhea, moderate to severe endometriosis, known or suspected uterine/tubal pathology, or a partner with a history of subfertility.

CLINICAL SYMPTOMS/HISTORY

Historical information regarding fertility issues may help the clinician to formulate a diagnosis and direct the evaluation and treatment. It makes sense to begin with age, parity, and outcomes of prior pregnancies. The duration of infertility should be determined. A history of adequate coital exposure should confirm that at least two acts of intercourse per cycle in the ovulatory period took place during repeated monthly attempts in the course of a year. Lubricants known to be spermicidal, such as K-Y jelly, should not have been used.

Forty percent of infertile women have ovulatory dysfunction and 40% have tubal/pelvic pathology, which can often be identified by the history alone. The age at menarche and the menstrual interval should be documented. Evidence of ovulation includes mittelschmerz, an increase in midcycle cervical mucus, and symptoms of molimina (premenstrual breast tenderness, abdominal bloating). Questioning regarding tubal or pelvic pathology is intended to elicit risk factors for pelvic adhesions or endometriosis. Patients should be asked about a history of in utero exposure to diethylstilbestrol (DES), intrauterine device use, pelvic inflammatory disease, genital infection or sexually transmitted disease, prior pelvic surgery, a family history of endometriosis, pelvic pain, dysmenorrhea, and dyspareunia.

The male factor history involves inquiring about age, prior paternity, impotence or other sexual dysfunction, exposure to drugs, heat, or toxins, congenital abnormality, and prior infection, injury, or surgery involving the reproductive organs. The man and woman should both be questioned about current medications, substance abuse, and any family history of mental retardation, congenital anomalies, or reproductive failure. A history of prior fertility testing and treatment should be obtained.

CLINICAL SYMPTOMS/PHYSICAL EXAMINATION

A careful examination can detect signs that suggest a specific cause for infertility. The examination should begin with a measurement of weight and body mass index. The thyroid should be evaluated, particularly for goiter, nodularity, and tenderness. Thyroid dysfunction is associated with ovulatory abnormalities and recurrent miscarriage. The breasts should be examined for galactorrhea. Hyperprolactinemia and galactorrhea are associated with ovulatory dysfunction. A detailed skin examination will reveal signs of androgen excess, such as acne, oily skin, hirsutism, and possibly acanthosis nigricans. Hirsutism commonly presents as facial hair and a male pattern escutcheon. This finding is usually a manifestation of elevated circulating androgen levels. When performing a pelvic examination, the clinician should inspect for genital malformations, vaginal and cervical abnormalities characteristic of in utero DES exposure, vaginal or cervical discharge, and other pathology, such as cervical polyps. A bimanual examination evaluates the size, mobility, positioning, and tenderness of the uterus and adnexa. Pertinent findings include nodularity of the uterosacral ligaments suggestive of endometriosis, fixation of the uterus or adnexa, uterine masses suggestive of fibroids, and adnexal masses that require evaluation for ovarian pathology.

The physical examination of the male partner includes an evaluation for anatomic abnormalities such as varicocele, hypospadias, and congenital absence of the vas deferens. Male hypogonadism is characterized by a testicular volume of less than 10 cc as measured with the orchidometer and receding secondary sex characteristics. In the evaluation for infection, the genitourinary tract is checked for potential sources, including urethritis, epididymitis, prostatitis, and pyelonephritis.

LABORATORY AND IMAGING STUDIES

The number of tests and the rate at which the problem is addressed vary from patient to patient. It is entirely appropriate to tailor the workup to suit individual patient circumstances, such as advancing age. The basic evaluation for infertility includes an assessment of ovulation and the uterine/tubal anatomy and a semen analysis. Secondary tests include the postcoital test for cervical factor, endometrial biopsy to diagnose inadequate luteal phase progesterone production, and laparoscopy to diagnose peritoneal factor. The endometrial biopsy should not be used as a screening test.

Male Factor

Forty percent of cases of infertility are attributed solely to a male factor. It makes sense to perform a semen analysis early in the workup. Unwillingness of the male partner to produce a specimen for evaluation may be an early sign of his lack of support in the process. The man should be evaluated by semen analysis before the woman undergoes invasive tests and treatments. The man is instructed to collect a masturbated semen specimen in a sterile container. For men who cannot do this, nonspermicidal condoms are available to collect a sample during intercourse.

The World Health Organization has provided guidelines for interpreting the semen analysis. "Normal" values are the following: volume, more than 2 mL; sperm concentration, more than 20 million per milliliter; motility, more than 50% with forward progression; morphology, more than 30% normal forms; and white blood cells, fewer than 1 million per milliliter. Considerable overlap is seen between fertile and subfertile men with regard to the above semen parameters. Recent research suggests that subfertility should be suspected when the sperm concentration is less than 13.5 million per milliliter, motility is less than 30%, and normal morphology is less than 9% with the use of strict criteria.

Men with semen parameters outside the World Health Organization guidelines are asked to undergo a second test because each ejaculate is different. Large fluctuations between samples may be caused by individual variation or other factors, such as a febrile illness or exposure to medication. The semen should be collected close to the laboratory to prevent thermal artifact. A persistent abnormality in the semen analysis should prompt a recommendation for urologic evaluation. Urologists may be helpful in defining congenital, acquired, hormonal, or infectious abnormalities. Severe oligospermia (concentration < 5 million per milliliter) is associated with genetic abnormalities such as Klinefelter syndrome or microdeletions of the Y chromosome. A karyotype should be obtained in this setting.

Evaluation of Ovulation

The ovulatory function of all infertile patients should be assessed because a history of monthly menses is inadequate to conclude that ovulation is occurring and optimal for conception. About 5% of women with apparent menstrual cycles are anovulatory. An elevated follicle-stimulating hormone level on day 3 may reflect a perimenopausal state as the underlying cause of ovulatory dysfunction. The prolactin and thyroid-stimulating hormone levels should be checked when an ovulatory abnormality is suspected. Basal body temperature charts are also used to evaluate ovulation. These show a biphasic pattern—a rise in temperature at ovulation that is maintained for 12 days or more. This pattern indicates ovulation with an adequate luteal phase. Ovulation predictor kits that detect the surge in luteinizing hormone in a urine sample or luteinizing hormone assays that detect the surge in serum also help to predict ovulation accurately.

Ultrasonography in the late follicular phase should show a mature follicle with a diameter of more than 18 mm. Ultrasonography after ovulation often reveals the disappearance of a lead follicle or a shrunken, collapsed, or absent follicle. Echolucency of the follicle may be replaced by echodensity, indicative of organizing hemorrhage or luteinizing tissue. Fluid may be observed around the ovary or in the cul-de-sac.

An evaluation of the luteal phase includes measurement of the progesterone levels and endometrial biopsy. The progesterone levels peak in the mid luteal phase on day 21 of an idealized 28-day cycle. Progesterone levels above 3 ng/dL are consistent with ovulation, yet levels above 10 to 15 ng/dL are needed to maintain a normal pregnancy. Progesterone is secreted in a pulsatile manner, so that the value of a single reading representing only one point in time is limited. Multiple visits for venipuncture are inconvenient for patients, and many clinicians prefer the endometrial biopsy.

An endometrial biopsy allows a histologic evaluation of the endometrium. It is performed with a plastic endometrial suction curette. This is a brief procedure but may cause cramping. The histology is judged by the criteria of Noyes and associates. The biopsy is performed 2 to 3 days before the expected menses, when the cumulative hormonal effects of the preceding menstrual cycle are evident in the endometrium. Some argue that dating is more sensitive in the midluteal phase, when the state of the endometrium at the time of implantation can be observed. There is a small risk that an existing pregnancy may be interrupted. It is wise to obtain a pregnancy test and informed consent before the test is performed. Current studies indicate that endometrial biopsy should not be used as a test screening.

A pathology report of the biopsy may identify proliferative endometrium, which indicates anovulation or endometritis that precludes dating. Patients with endometritis should be treated with 100 mg of doxycycline twice each day for 14 days and undergo biopsy again to confirm resolution. An adequate report indicates a secretory endometrium characteristic of a postovulatory day. The patient is instructed to call to report the day of onset of menses after the biopsy. For purposes of interpreting the endometrial biopsy, the first day of bleeding is called day 28; the clinician must count backward from the day of onset of menses to the day the biopsy was performed. For example, if the biopsy was performed 3 days before the onset of menses, the specimen should be dated as secretory day 25 endometrium. Alternatively, the specimen can be dated by counting forward from the time of ovulation if a urine or serum surge in luteinizing hormone was detected, with day 14 counted as the day of ovulation.

A histologic lag of more than 2 days on two endometrial biopsy specimens indicates a luteal phase defect. The ambiguity of this diagnosis stems from the large number of isolated cycles fitting these criteria in normally fertile women, in addition to the high rate of interobserver discrepancies in dating the endometrium. The diagnosis is more substantial when the histologic lag increases to 5 days or more, as evidenced by a higher conception rate in response to treatment.

Hysterosalpingography

The uterine and tubal status is best assessed by hysterosalpingography. Other diagnostic modalities include saline sonohysterogram, hysteroscopy, and laparoscopy.

Hysterosalpingography is performed in a radiology suite under fluoroscopic guidance. One or more x-ray films are made for a permanent record. The patient may be instructed to take a dose of a nonsteroidal antiinflammatory drug 30 to 60 minutes before the examination to act as an antispasmodic because some cramping is commonly associated with the procedure. A paracervical block or the application of a topical anesthetic helps to alleviate discomfort and decrease the false-positive result of cornual obstruction secondary to tubal spasm.

Important uterine findings include congenital abnormalities, such as a unicornuate or septate uterus, and acquired abnormalities, which are seen as filling defects that represent polyps, fibroids, or synechiae (intrauterine scarring). The tubes are assessed for patency, site of any obstruction, degree of dilation, presence of ampullar rugae and other abnormalities (e.g., cornual polyps, salpingitis isthmica nodosa, atypical position), and pattern of contrast dispersion. Loculated contrast dispersion suggests adnexal adhesions; free dispersion suggests that these are absent.

Abnormalities of the cavity usually must be verified by saline sonohysterogram or endoscopic examination. Hysteroscopy allows a direct visual diagnosis of the causes of filling defects. Most uterine polyps, adhesions, and septa and many submucosal fibroids can be resected by operative hysteroscopy at the time of diagnosis. Tubal occlusion may necessitate laparoscopy. Chromotubation can confirm tubal obstruction and allow a visual assessment of the fimbriae and rest of the pelvis. Tubal occlusion can be treated surgically in some cases. Many couples choose in vitro fertilization instead of surgery to overcome tubal infertility.

Postcoital Testing (Sims-Huhner Test)

Postcoital testing is performed in vivo to evaluate the interaction between the sperm and the cervical mucus. Patients should be instructed to have intercourse the day before or on the day of expected ovulation. Optimally, the man should abstain from ejaculating 2 to 3 days before the postcoital test. The woman should be examined about 2 to 12 hours after intercourse. Showering before postcoital testing does not affect the results, but douches and vaginal lubricants should not be used.

Either a tuberculin syringe without a needle or a nasal speculum is used to collect mucus from the cervical canal. The mucus is placed on a glass slide, covered with a cover slip, and examined under 200× magnification. The cervical mucus at midcycle should appear clear, acellular, and thin; it should be stretchable to 8 to 10 cm (*spinnbarkeit*) and display a fern pattern on drying, which reflects a high salt content. Sperm should be present and exhibit linear motion. The finding of one or more motile sperm per high-power field is within the normal range; the presence of more than 20 motile sperm per high-power field indicates an increased likelihood of conception. A clearly abnormal postcoital test result shows no sperm, no motile sperm, or no sperm with forward progression (shakers). Shakers can be further evaluated with sperm antibody testing. A normal postcoital test result confirms appropriate coital technique, correct timing at midcycle, good-quality cervical mucus without hostile factors, and the ability of sperm to survive in the cervical mucus. An abnormal postcoital test result may indicate incorrect timing of the test, poor-quality mucus or semen, the presence of sperm antibody, or improper coital exposure, such as nonvaginal ejaculation. The most common reason for an abnormal postcoital test result is incorrect timing of the test.

LAPAROSCOPY

Laparoscopy is an endoscopic evaluation of the pelvis. The procedure is invasive and usually requires general anesthesia. Because it test involves surgical risks and disability from work for 2 to 4 days, this test is usually the last diagnostic procedure undertaken. Historical, physical examination, hysterosalpingographic, or ultrasonographic findings that suggest tubal or peritoneal factors may indicate that laparoscopy is appropriate earlier in the evaluation.

Diagnostic laparoscopy identifies pelvic abnormalities in about 50% of cases. The most common findings are pelvic adhesions and endometriosis. Most of these can be treated at the time of the diagnostic laparoscopy. In a few cases, diagnostic laparoscopy leads to laparotomy because of the location or extent of pathology.

TREATMENT

Cervical Factor

If a cervical factor, defined by an abnormal postcoital test result, is the sole reason for infertility, it can be effectively treated by intrauterine insemination, for which the cumulative pregnancy rate is 35% in three or four cycles. A less reliable alternative treatment is the addition of estrogen during the follicular phase, such as 0.625 to 1.25 mg of conjugated estrogen daily. Guaifenesin is a mucolytic agent used to treat thick cervical mucus. It is popular with patients as a home remedy, but no data show that such treatment increases pregnancy rates.

If cervical cultures are positive for *Chlamydia trachomatis* or *Ureaplasma urealyticum*, the patient and her partner are treated with 100 mg of doxycycline orally twice a day for 7 days. If external lubricants are needed for intercourse at midcycle, vegetable oil can be used without detrimental effects on sperm.

Ovulatory Dysfunction

Anovulation is treated by administering clomiphene citrate or human menopausal gonadotropins to induce ovulation. Ovulatory abnormalities, such as oligo-ovulation or luteal phase defect, are treated by enhancing ovulation with the same agents. Metformin has been shown to restore ovulation in patients with polycystic ovary syndrome. Hyperprolactinemia is treated with bromocriptine. Thyroid dysfunction is treated to produce a euthyroid state. Empiric treatment with bromocriptine or thyroid hormone replacement in the face of normal thyroid function and normal prolactin levels is not helpful.

Uterine Factor

Corrective surgery for uterine septa, leiomyomata, polyps, or synechiae may optimize the endometrium for implantation. Surgery may involve hysteroscopy, laparoscopy, or laparotomy. Bicornuate, unicornuate, or hypoplastic uteri secondary to DES exposure usually do not benefit from surgical intervention.

Peritoneal Factor

Lysis of adnexal adhesions by laparoscopy or laparotomy is advocated to optimize pickup of the ovum by the fallopian tube. Endometriosis is treated with laser vaporization, cauterization, or sharp excision to restore functional adnexal anatomy, prevent disease progression, and minimize toxic peritoneal factors.

Tubal Factor

The likelihood of a pregnancy after tubal surgery depends on the degree of tubal damage. Multiple sites of internal obstruction in a fallopian tube preclude surgical repair. Proximal tubal obstruction may be managed by tubal cannulization, resection, and reanastomosis, or by reimplantation. Isthmic and ampullar obstructions require resection and reanastomosis. Distal tubal surgery may involve fimbrioplasty or neosalpingostomy. If surgical repair is impossible, if an attempt at repair fails, or if the tubes are patent after repair but conception does not occur, in vitro fertilization is indicated. In vitro fertilization involves ovarian hyperstimulation, ovum retrieval, fertilization, and embryo transfer into the uterus, so that the function of the fallopian tubes in gamete and embryo transport and placement for fertilization is bypassed.

Male Factor

Reproductive tract infections require antibiotic treatment. Varicocelectomy should be considered when a varicocele is associated with infertility and compromised semen and no other cause can be found. Hypogonadotropic hypogonadism may respond to hormonal treatment with clomiphene citrate or human chorionic gonadotropin.

The most common abnormality of semen is asthenospermia (low motility), followed by oligoasthenospermia (low count and low motility). Identifiable exacerbating factors should be relieved, including excess heat in the environment (from sources such as hot tubs, saunas, spas, and heated water beds), medications, recreational drugs, alcohol, and tobacco. Pregnancy rates are improved by a combination of superovulation and intrauterine insemination. If this treatment is unsuccessful, assisted reproductive technologies may be required.

Cervical insemination or intrauterine insemination in a natural cycle has not proved more beneficial than intercourse alone in cases of asthenospermia or oligoasthenospermia. Aspermia, severe compromise of the semen, failed in vitro fertilization, and in vitro fertilization with intracytoplasmic sperm injection are indications for the use of donor sperm.

Unexplained Infertility

When factors contributing to infertility cannot be identified, it is reasonable to offer empiric treatment. This may involve measures with multiple effects intended to enhance a couple's chance of conceiving. Enhancement of ovulation with clomiphene citrate or human menopausal gonadotropins, with or without intrauterine insemination, or an assisted reproductive technology such as in vitro fertilization or gamete intrafallopian transfer may be tried.

REFERRAL

A patient who has tried to conceive unsuccessfully for a year or who has a known impediment to conception, such as amenorrhea, and desires a pregnancy requires an evaluation. The evaluation and treatment may be undertaken by any physician with appropriate training. Patients should be referred for the evaluation and treatment of infertility when they request a referral or when the physician feels that a referral is appropriate, based on the available facilities and the physician's training and level of comfort in caring for infertile patients and willingness to provide such care. The time at which a referral to a gynecologist or reproductive endocrinologist should be made varies widely.

It is reasonable to inform patients that 15% of couples do not conceive after 1 year and only 7% do not conceive after 2 years. Therefore, about half of couples conceive without active intervention between the first and second year of attempts at conception. However, it is inappropriate to tell couples that if they could just relax and forget about trying, they would be able to have a baby. Timely evaluation, treatment, and referral must be instituted for all patients requesting care. Advancing age is one of the more pressing issues.

BIBLIOGRAPHY

American Society for Reproductive Medicine. *Optimal evaluation of the infertile couple: a Practice Committee opinion.* Birmingham, AL: American Society for Reproductive Medicine, 2000:1–6.

Guzick DS, Overstreet JW, Factor-Litvak P, et al. Sperm morphology, motility, and concentration in fertile and infertile men. *N Engl J Med* 2001;345:1388–1393.

Rowe PJ, Comhaire FH, Hargreave TB, et al. *World Health Organization manual for standardized investigation and diagnosis of the infertile couple.* Cambridge, UK: Cambridge University Press, 1993.

Seibel MM. *Infertility: a comprehensive text,* 2nd ed. East Norwalk, CT: Appleton & Lange, 1997.

Speroff L, Glass RH, Kase NG. *Clinical gynecologic endocrinology and infertility,* 6th ed. Philadelphia: Lippincott Williams & Wilkins, 1999.

Whitman-Elia GF, Baxley EG. A primary care approach to the infertile couple. *J Am Board Fam Pract* 2001;14:33–45.

CHAPTER 19
Contraception and Sterilization

H. Trent MacKay

Despite the availability of numerous effective methods of contraception, the United States has one of the highest rates of unintended pregnancy among developed nations. Primary care physicians are in a key position to prevent these unintended pregnancies because they frequently provide contraceptive services. However, they must be knowledgeable about all the methods; they must also be prepared to help their patients choose a method and counsel them to ensure compliance.

The choice of contraception often depends on whether a couple plans to have additional children. Hormonal contraceptives are the most popular choice among women planning future pregnancies, whereas sterilization is the most popular method among women who have completed childbearing. Education and counseling by the primary care physician play a major role in lowering the failure rate and increasing compliance. With proper guidance and accurate information, every couple can make an informed decision and rationally choose the method most appropriate for them.

ORAL CONTRACEPTIVE PILLS

Oral contraceptive pills (OCPs) are the most widely chosen form of reversible contraception and are used by 27% of women ages 15 to 44 years who are practicing contraception. Three major types of OCP formulations are available: fixed-dose combination, multiphasic combination, and daily progestin-only. OCPs contain synthetic steroids. The only estrogen used is ethinyl estradiol. In contrast, five older progestins (norethindrone, norethindrone acetate, ethynodiol diacetate, norethynodrel, and levonorgestrel) and three newer progestins (desogestrel, norgestimate, and drosperinone) are included in current formulations. The combination formulations are the most widely used. Tablets containing both an estrogen and a progestin are taken continuously for 3 weeks, followed by a 1-week steroid-free interval that allows withdrawal bleeding to occur. The multiphasic combination OCPs were developed to lower the total dose of steroid, primarily the progestin, without increasing the incidence of breakthrough bleeding. These formulations contain two or three different amounts of the same estrogen and progestin.

The progestin-only formulations consist of tablets containing a progestin without any estrogen. They must be taken daily without a steroid-free interval. They are used by women who cannot tolerate estrogen or for whom estrogen intake is contraindicated. The incidence of breakthrough bleeding and the pregnancy rate are slightly higher.

Many of the most common symptoms experienced by women taking combination OCPs are caused by the estrogen component. These include nausea, breast tenderness, and fluid retention. However, the incidence of these side effects is low because the current formulations contain less estrogen than the earlier ones; nonetheless, the efficacy of the current OCPs, which contain a threefold to fourfold lower dose of estrogen and 10-fold lower dose of progestin, is not decreased in comparison with that of the earlier OCPs.

The effectiveness of OCPs is based primarily on consistent inhibition of the midcycle gonadotropin surge, which prevents ovulation. Other effects include alteration of the cervical mucus to make it viscid and scanty, so that sperm penetration is retarded. They also alter the motility of the uterus and fallopian tubes, impairing transport of both ova and sperm. The endometrium is altered so that the glandular production of glycogen is diminished and less energy is available for the blastocyst to survive in the uterine cavity.

OCPs also have substantial metabolic effects; the estrogen component and progestin component have different, and sometimes opposite, effects. The symptoms most commonly caused by the estrogen component include nausea, breast tenderness, and fluid retention (a consequence of decreased sodium excretion). The progestins, because they are structurally related to testosterone, may cause weight gain, acne, and nervousness.

OCPs also offer many health benefits unrelated to contraception. Because of the antiestrogenic action of progesterone, the endometrium is thinner than that seen in a normal cycle, so that less blood is lost and the risk for iron deficiency anemia is reduced 50%. Menorrhagia or irregular menstruation is less likely to develop in OCP users, and endometrial cancer is half as likely to develop. By inhibiting ovulation, OCPs decrease dysmenorrhea and premenstrual tension and may protect against functional ovarian cysts. The risk for ovarian cancer is reduced 40% in OCP users. The incidence of clinical salpingitis among OCP users was 50% less than that in a control group using no method.

OCPs have not been shown to interfere with the action of other drugs despite being metabolized in the liver. However, some drugs can interfere clinically with the action of OCPs, decreasing their effectiveness. These include barbiturates, phenytoin, primidone, carbamazepine, and rifampin. Women should be instructed to use some form of barrier contraception while taking these drugs.

OCPs can be prescribed to most healthy women of reproductive age. The few absolute contraindications are current or previous vascular disease, including thromboembolism, deep venous thrombophlebitis, atherosclerosis, and cerebrovascular accident; a known or suspected estrogen-dependent tumor; a history of a benign or malignant tumor of the liver; active liver disease (however, women with a history of liver disease whose liver function test results are normal may use OCPs); migraine headaches with focal neurologic signs; diabetes with vascular or other complications; and age older than 35 years with heavy cigarette smoking (>15 cigarettes per day).

Relative contraindications to OCP use include treated hypertension, hyperlipidemias, migraine headaches without focal neurologic signs, diabetes without complications, existing gallbladder disease, systemic lupus erythematosus, and sickle cell disease. Women in whom frequent or severe migraine headaches associated with neurologic signs develop should stop taking OCPs immediately. In addition, women in whom mild hypertension develops while they are using OCPs should be advised to stop.

Women who have disorders that may lead to hyperkalemia, such as renal or adrenal insufficiency, or who are daily taking drugs on a long-term basis that may increase serum potassium levels, such as angiotensin-converting enzyme inhibitors, potassium-sparing diuretics, or nonsteroidal antiinflammatory drugs, should not use the OCP that contains drosperinone.

The prescribing guidelines for OCPs are relatively simple. The Planned Parenthood Federation of America and the World Health Organization have now approved the initiation of OCPs without a physical examination, although a thorough history should be taken and the blood pressure measured. However, ideally, at the initial office visit, a history should be obtained and a physical examination should be performed. The physical examination should include a breast and pelvic examination with a Papanicolaou smear. The blood pressure and weight should be recorded. If the patient has no medical contraindication to the use of OCPs, she should be informed of the benefits, risks, and alternatives. She should be seen at least once a year, at which time a history should be taken, the blood pressure and weight measured, and a physical examination performed.

In determining which formulation to use, it is best initially to prescribe one with 35 μg of ethinyl estradiol or less. The formulation with the lowest dose of a particular progestin should be chosen to mitigate the progestational metabolic and clinical adverse effects. Many women cease using OCPs because of these progestational effects, which often include androgenic side effects. Thus, the OCP formulations that contain the newer progestins (including desogestrel, norgestimate, and drosperinone, as previously noted) may increase compliance rates.

Primary care physicians must improve patient compliance with OCPs. Discontinuation falls into the category of noncompliance and contributes to the alarming number of unintended pregnancies seen each year. About 25% of OCP users in the United States discontinue this method during the first year, many without adopting an alternative means of birth control. Among women who stop using OCPs, side effects or the fear of potential side effects are most frequently cited as the reason. Careful education and anticipatory guidance regarding the nuisance side effects are a necessity. Women must be made aware of the fact that breakthrough bleeding, amenorrhea, actual or perceived weight gain, nausea, headaches, and mood changes are often transient.

A woman should take the pill at night (to lessen the possibility of nausea) and should use a given OCP for at least three cycles to evaluate its effects. During the first month of use, up to 30% of women may experience breakthrough bleeding; the proportion drops to less than 10% during the third month. Other clinical recommendations for improving oral contraceptive compliance are listed in Table 19.1. The efficacy during the first year of use of combination OCPs is 99.9% with perfect use and 92.4% with typical use.

TABLE 19.1. Clinical Recommendations for Improving Oral Contraceptive Compliance

1. All oral contraceptive users should know three things before they start taking their pills:
   a. How to take the oral contraceptive prescribed.
   b. What to do if they miss a pill or pills.
   c. Which side effects are common and usually transient (breakthrough bleeding and nausea), and which are potentially serious and should be brought immediately to their clinician's attention.
2. Simple instructions should be provided to all patients both verbally and in writing; a copy of written instructions should be discussed with the patient point by point during the visit. Another copy of written instructions should be offered at each follow-up visit.
3. Show each patient who is starting a new brand of pill (and especially first-time oral contraceptive users) how to use the specific package being prescribed. Use of the 28-day package enhances compliance.
4. Help women select a specific time of day to take their pills; a brief discussion of their daily schedules may help identify an optimal time of day. Taking the pill after dinner or with a bedtime snack lessens the possibility of nausea. Patients who skip breakfast may find that taking the pill in the morning leads to nausea and sometimes vomiting.
5. The refill prescription should include an additional cycle to accommodate missed pills or lost packets.
6. The use of a back-up method and the availability of emergency contraception should be discussed.
7. Discuss prevention of sexually transmitted diseases. Provide the oral contraceptive user with a condom and discuss its proper use.
8. On follow-up visits, ask patients if they have had any problems taking their pills; ask what they did when they missed pills. A nonjudgmental approach encourages honesty and can help uncover and solve potential problems.
9. Oral contraceptive users who continually have difficulty remembering to take their pills or who have other serious compliance problems should be counseled about other available methods.

Source: From Grimes DA. Oral contraceptive compliance: strategies for ensuring correct and continued use of the pill. *Contraception Rep* 1994;5:3, with permission.

OTHER COMBINATION HORMONAL CONTRACEPTIVES

Several other combination hormonal contraceptives have been introduced, including an injectable, a patch, and a vaginal ring. The injectable contains depot medroxyprogesterone acetate (DMPA) and estradiol cypionate and is administered monthly. The transdermal patch contains norelgestromin and ethinyl estradiol; it is applied to the lower abdomen, upper torso, or buttock once a week for 3 weeks and then is not applied for 1 week. In a small number of women, irritation may develop at the site of the patch. The vaginal ring has a diameter of approximately 2 inches and contains etonogestrel and ethinyl estradiol. The ring is inserted for 3 weeks, removed for 1 week, and replaced. Users may experience an increased incidence of vaginal discharge. The systemic side effects, efficacy, and mechanism of action of these methods are very similar to those of OCPs.

LONG-ACTING CONTRACEPTIVE STEROIDS

Two long-acting, progestin-only methods of contraception have been available in the United States—an injectable, Depo-Provera, and a six-rod subdermal implant, Norplant. They provide a highly effective, long-acting, estrogen-free, reversible method of contraception. However, Norplant has been removed from the market in the United States, although many women continue to use the method. A single-rod implant, Implanon, is currently under evaluation by the Food and Drug Administration.

Of the injectable steroid formulations, three types are available, but only one, DMPA (Depo-Provera), has been approved for use in the United States. It is used by approximately 3% of women practicing contraception. DMPA is an aqueous suspension of microcrystals that is administered by intramuscular injection every 12 weeks. Contraceptive protection is immediate. DMPA acts by inhibiting the midcycle surge of luteinizing hormone. The first injection is preferably given within the first 5 days after menses. Side effects include amenorrhea, mild weight gain, and headache. Less common untoward reactions include abdominal discomfort, nervousness, dizziness, depression, and acne. In addition, the return of fertility is delayed in comparison with other contraceptive methods. A reduction in bone mineral density in long-term DMPA users has been reported, but it appears to be reversible after discontinuation.

Candidates for DMPA include women in whom exogenous estrogen is contraindicated, who cannot tolerate estrogens, who dislike taking a pill daily or simply cannot remember to do so (therefore, this is often an ideal method for adolescents), or who want a long-acting, coitus-independent, convenient method of birth control. DMPA can be used immediately after delivery whether or not the mother is nursing. The injection should be given before the mother is discharged from the hospital.

The second method of contraception in this category is a subdermal implant system, Norplant, which is no longer on the market in the United States. In this form of birth control, six Silastic capsules containing levonorgestrel are placed subdermally. It too is a highly effective, estrogen-free, long-term method of contraception. The six capsules are implanted just under the skin of the upper, inner area of the arm in an outpatient procedure. They are effective for 5 years. The primary mechanism of action is inhibition of the midcycle surge of luteinizing hormone, which prevents ovulation. Other actions include effects on the cervical mucus and sperm penetration, endometrial lining, and implantation. The major side effect is similar to that of DMPA—menstrual irregularity. Other untoward effects include headache, weight gain, acne, depression, anxiety, abdominal discomfort, and hirsutism. Removal may be difficult, given the need to locate six capsules. The efficacy rates, with both perfect and typical use, of these two long-acting contraceptive steroids are similar, more than 99%.

BARRIER CONTRACEPTION

Barrier contraception includes the diaphragm, cervical cap, and male and female condoms. The vaginal sponge is available in Canada and may return to the market in the United States.

Diaphragm and Cervical Cap

The diaphragm and cervical cap are used by 2% of U.S. women. The diaphragm comes in a large range of sizes and types and must be carefully fitted by the practitioner. The largest size that does not cause discomfort or undue pressure on the vaginal mucosa or urethra should be used. The cervical cap comes in only four sizes. It is smaller than the diaphragm, fits closely over the cervix, and is kept in place by suction. Advantages include comfort and that it can be left in place for up to 48 hours. A spermicide should be used and applied inside each device. Both devices should be left in place for at least 6 hours after the last coital act, but the diaphragm for no longer than 24 hours and the cervical cap for no longer than 48 hours. If intercourse is repeated or if coitus is performed more than 6 hours after insertion, additional contraceptive cream or jelly should be applied. The risk for clinical gonococcal infection is lower in diaphragm users than in nonusers, but the rate of cystitis is higher. Effectiveness requires motivation, and failure rates decline with increasing age and increasing use. Overall, efficacy is 94% with perfect use and 88% with typical use.

Male Condom

Male condom use has increased during the past two decades from 12% of couples practicing contraception in 1982 to 20% in 1995. The male condom is made of latex rubber or animal intestine. It should not be applied too tightly. The tip should extend beyond the end of the penis by about half an inch to collect the ejaculate. Latex condoms can reduce the transmission rate of sexually transmitted diseases, including HIV infection. The incidence of cervical neoplasia is also reduced. For men or women with an allergy to latex or men who desire greater sensitivity, condoms made of lamb's intestine are available, but they do not protect against HIV infection.

Candidates for use of the condom as the primary form of birth control include highly motivated couples inasmuch as it is coitus-dependent. Any man or woman with multiple sexual partners should be encouraged to use a condom, regardless of whether another form of birth control is also being used. Efficacy is 97% with perfect use and 86% with typical use.

Female Condom

The female condom is made of polyurethane that resists tearing during use. It too reduces the transmission rate of sexually transmitted diseases, including HIV infection. It is disposable and designed for a single coital act. It can be inserted several hours before sexual intercourse. Again, the ideal candidates are highly motivated couples. Efficacy is 95% with perfect use and 79% with typical use.

SPERMICIDES

Vaginal spermicides include foams, creams, suppositories, and jellies and are used by approximately 1% of women. All spermicides marketed in the United States contain a surfactant, nonoxynol-9, that immobilizes or kills sperm on contact. Because they also provide a chemical barrier, spermicides must be placed into the vagina before each coital act. They are most effective when used with a device to hold them in place. Spermicides may prevent certain sexually transmitted diseases and the development of cervical cancer. However, with very frequent use, vaginal irritation may actually enhance HIV transmission, and nonoxynol-9 spermicides are not recommended for the prevention of HIV transmission.

Vaginal spermicides require a moderate degree of motivation, so that effectiveness increases with age. The ideal candidates are older women who are unable or unwilling to use other forms of birth control. They should be instructed to use this method in combination with a barrier contraceptive. Efficacy is 94% with perfect use and 74% with typical use.

NATURAL FAMILY PLANNING OR PERIODIC ABSTINENCE

These methods involve no drugs, devices, or surgery and are currently used by approximately 2% of couples practicing contraception. If they are to be effective, the couple must be highly motivated and able to predict their most fertile interval accurately. Most women with regular menstrual cycles must abstain for almost one third of the days of each cycle; thus, the rate of failure and discontinuation is high.

Four methods are used to determine the fertile interval: calendar rhythm, basal body temperature, cervical mucus, and symptothermal. The latter is the most effective, although a new variation of the rhythm method, the standard days method, also appears to be effective. In the symptothermal method, several indices, rather than a single physiologic index, are used to determine the fertile period. Calendar calculations and changes in the cervical mucus are used to estimate the onset of the fertile period, and changes in the mucus and basal temperature to estimate its end. Although more effective than the other methods, the symptothermal method is more difficult to learn. In the standard days method, a string of beads is used to remind women to avoid intercourse from days 8 through 19 of the cycle. This method is effective for women with 26- to 32-day cycles.

With the need to abstain from sexual intercourse for many days during the menstrual cycle, many women choose to use barrier methods or spermicides during the fertile period. In addition, home ovulation predictor kits may help define the fertile interval more accurately. Because such assays make it possible to reduce the number of days of abstinence, they may improve the effectiveness and acceptance of this method.

Candidates for natural family planning must be highly motivated and sufficiently intelligent to comprehend the subtleties of this method. This may be the only method available to strict Roman Catholics and other religious couples. The efficacy of perfect use varies from 91% to 99%, depending on the method. Overall, efficacy with typical use is approximately 80%.

INTRAUTERINE DEVICE

The intrauterine device (IUD) is a highly effective method of birth control in which interest has been renewed. Advantages include a lack of systemic metabolic effects and the lack of a need for coitus-related responsibility; furthermore, long-term use is possible after only a single act of motivation. For these reasons, in addition to the need to visit a health care professional to have the device removed, the continuation rate for IUDs is one of the highest of those for reversible methods of birth control. However, because of concerns related to infections associated with the Dalkon Shield in the 1980s, fewer than 1% of U.S. women were using IUDs in 1995. Classic contraindications to the IUD include nulliparity, a history of pelvic infection, current involvement in a nonmonogamous relationship, and uterine malformation, although more recent studies have challenged these long-held concepts. For example, many believe that placing an IUD in a properly selected nulliparous woman is no longer contraindicated.

Two IUDs are currently marketed in the United States: the levonorgestrel-releasing IUD (Mirena), which is approved for 5 years of use, and the T 380A intrauterine copper contraceptive (ParaGard), which is approved for 10 years of use. The main mechanism of action of an IUD is spermicidal, in which the presence of a foreign body in the uterus causes a local sterile inflammatory reaction. The levonorgestrel-releasing IUD also thickens the cervical mucus. Adverse effects include uterine bleeding, perforation of the uterus at the time of insertion, infection-related complications, pregnancy-related complications, and expulsion. The rate of intrauterine infection is increased slightly during the first 3 weeks of use, but subsequently, the risk for infection is related primarily to sexual transmission of disease. During the first year of IUD use, the expulsion rate is about 5%, but in up to 20% of cases, expulsion is unnoticed by the user. Thus, clinicians must stress the importance of periodically palpating the string. Women using the levonorgestrel-releasing IUD experience irregular bleeding during the first 3 to 6 months of use. However, the menstrual flow subsequently decreases markedly, with oligomenorrhea or amenorrhea developing in many cases after 3 to 6 months. Dysmenorrhea is also markedly decreased with use of this IUD. The incidence of all major adverse events, including unintended pregnancy, steadily diminishes in subsequent years and with increasing age.

Several epidemiologic studies have shown that if pregnancy occurs with an IUD in place, it is more likely to be an ectopic pregnancy. Thus, if a pregnancy does occur, the patient must be followed diligently with quantitative measurement of serum levels of β-human chorionic gonadotropin and early transvaginal ultrasonography to confirm the location of the pregnancy.

Resumption of fertility after IUD removal is not delayed. It returns at the same rate as after discontinuation of mechanical methods of contraception, such as the condom or diaphragm.

To avoid the risk for pelvic infection with sexually transmitted organisms, the best candidates for IUD use are parous women with stable, monogamous sexual relationships. For women who have completed their families but do not opt for sterilization, or women who cannot take OCPs, this may be the method of choice. The first-year failure rate ranges from less than 1% to 3.7%, but as previously noted, this declines steadily in subsequent years.

EMERGENCY CONTRACEPTION

Emergency contraception is used to prevent pregnancy after unprotected intercourse, failure of a barrier method, or rape. Although the magnitude of the protective effect is debatable, few people question the important role that emergency contraception can play in preventing unwanted pregnancy and thus maternal mortality and morbidity resulting from unsafe abortion. Every primary care practitioner concerned with improving women's reproductive health should be familiar with postcoital contraception and provide it when appropriate.

The development of hormonal methods of postcoital contraception dates back to the 1960s, when the first human trials of postcoitally administered high-dose estrogens were undertaken. The most popular current regimens include the administration of two combined high-dose estrogen-progesterone pills twice 12 hours apart (Preven), or the administration of 0.75 mg of levonorgestrel twice 12 hours apart (plan B). The administration of 1.5 mg of levonorgestrel in a single dose is also effective. Treatment should begin as soon as possible after coitus. If initiated within 72 hours after an isolated midcycle act of intercourse, efficacy is very good: approximately 75% for the combination regimen and 85% for the levonorgestrel regimens. If more than one episode of coitus has occurred or if treatment is initiated 72 hours after intercourse, the method is less effective. However, even at 120 hours after intercourse, efficacy exceeds 60% for the single or two-dose levonorgestrel regimen. The placement of a copper IUD within 5 days after unprotected intercourse is at least as effective as the hormonal regimens.

SURGICAL STERILIZATION

Sterilization is the most frequently used method of contraception in the United States. In 1995, among persons ages 15 to 44 years practicing contraception, 38.6% used sterilization (female sterilization rate, 27.7%; male sterilization rate, 11.9%). Female sterilization is generally an effective method for preventing future pregnancies. However, the overall cumulative failure rate at 10 years is 1.85% and may be as high as 3.65%, depending on the specific procedure. Female sterilization is also relatively simple and safe, with major complications occurring in fewer than 1% of cases.

Different surgical techniques are of comparable safety but may vary somewhat in efficacy. In the selection process, the surgeon's preference and expertise combined with the patient's needs determine the technique of choice in each case. It is important that primary care providers be able to explain to patients the different options and modalities available when permanent surgical contraception is being considered.

Female Sterilization

Female sterilization, which is chosen by about 28% of couples, can be performed on an outpatient basis, usually by the laparoscopic two-puncture technique, or on an inpatient basis after a vaginal delivery. It can also be performed at the time of cesarean section. Female sterilization, regardless of technique, is more complicated than male sterilization. The laparoscopic technique requires general anesthesia, with its inherent risks. In addition, although rare, bowel or bladder injury is a risk. In a relatively new method, an intratubal device that causes scarring and occlusion of the proximal fallopian tube is placed hysteroscopically on an outpatient basis. The efficacy of female sterilization methods after 10 years varies from 99.25% for unipolar coagulation and postpartum tubal ligation to 97.5% for bipolar coagulation and 96.35% for the Hulka clip.

Male Sterilization

Male sterilization, or vasectomy, is chosen by about 11% of couples. This is an outpatient procedure that takes about 20 minutes and requires only local anesthesia. Complications include hematoma, sperm granulomas, infection, and spontaneous reanastomosis (if this is to occur, it does so within a short time after the procedure). Unlike female sterilization, effective male sterilization is not immediate. The man is not considered sterile until two sperm-free ejaculates have been produced. Semen analyses should be performed 1 and 2 months after the procedure. Usually, about 15 to 20 ejaculations are required after the operation before the man is sterile. The efficacy rate is about 99.9%.

The ideal candidate for sterilization, male or female, has completed reproduction and is certain that no additional children will be wanted, regardless of the possibility of remarriage.

Preoperative Evaluation

A complete history and physical examination are mandatory. Furthermore, considerable care must be taken to identify anesthesia, surgical, and psychosocial risk factors. Gynecologic pathology, such as abnormal cervical cytologic findings, menstrual disorders, symptomatic pelvic relaxation, and neoplasia, must be excluded or, if identified, treated appropriately.

Risk factors for regret after sterilization should be considered during preoperative counseling (Table 19.2). It has been well documented that age at the time of surgery is inversely related to the likelihood of regretting a surgical sterilization.

A discussion of the long-term effects of tubal sterilization should be part of the counseling. The existence of a syndrome of menstrual abnormalities after tubal ligation has been debated for decades. Data from the U.S. Collaborative Review of Sterilization were used to determine whether persistent menstrual abnormalities were more likely to occur in women who had undergone tubal sterilization than in women who had not. The investigators found that women who had undergone sterilization were no more likely than those who had not undergone the procedure to report persistent changes in intermenstrual bleeding or length of the menstrual cycle. Although women with gynecologic disorders before tubal sterilization were more likely to undergo hys-

TABLE 19.2. Regret after Tubal Sterilization by Selected Baseline Characteristics[a]

Characteristic	Rate	Odds ratio	Confidence interval
Age (y)			
<20	6.5	2.9	1.2–7.0
20–24	4.3	1.9	1.4–2.5
25–29	3.1	1.3	1.0–1.7
30–34	2.4	1	Referent
>34	1.2	0.5	0.4–0.7
Timing of sterilization			
Interval	2.1	1	Referent
Postvaginal delivery	3.0	1.4	1.0–2.0
Postcesarean section	4.4	2.1	1.5–2.9
Postabortion	2.6	1.2	0.7–2.1
History of abortion			
Yes	3.0	1.3	1.1–1.7
No	2.3	1	Referent
Method of payment			
Private insurance	2.1	1	Referent
Medicaid	3.7	1.8	1.4–2.3
Time after sterilization (y)			
1	1.8	1	Referent
2	2.8	1.5	1.3–1.8
3	2.5	1.4	1.2–1.7
4	2.2	1.2	0.9–1.6
5	3.1	1.7	1.4–2.1
Marital status			
Married	2.3	1	Referent
Not married	2.7	1.2	0.9–1.5
Education (y)			
<13	2.4	1	Referent
13–16	2.3	0.9	0.7–1.2
>16	3.4	1.4	0.9–2.4
Employed			
Yes	2.7	1	Referent
No	2.1	0.8	0.6–1.0
No. of living children			
0	1.9	0.8	0.5–1.4
1	2.7	1.2	0.9–1.6
2	2.2	1	Referent
>2	2.5	1.1	0.9–1.4
Race			
White	2.4	1.0	Referent
Black	2.4	1.0	0.8–1.3
Other	2.2	0.9	0.5–1.8

[a]Adjusted rate per 100 women, adjusted odds ratios, and 95% confidence interval rates and odds ratios adjusted for all other characteristics listed in table and for institution.

Source: From Wilcox LS, Chu SY, Eaker ED, et al. Risk factors for regret after tubal sterilization: 5 years of follow-up in a prospective study. *Fertil Steril* 1991;55:930, with permission.

terectomy during the 14 years after sterilization than women without these disorders, the majority of sterilized women in both categories did not subsequently undergo hysterectomy.

An evaluation of preexisting medical conditions influences the choice of anesthesia. The most commonly used surgical techniques have been performed successfully with the patient under sedation and local anesthesia, but general anesthesia is preferred. Tubal sterilization should be presented as a permanent procedure. Rates of failure (intrauterine or ectopic pregnancy) and complications related to the surgical technique must be adequately discussed and documented. In the case of a patient who is mentally retarded or has a psychiatric disorder, consultation is warranted to determine the capability of the patient to understand and consent to the procedure.

Surgical Techniques

The pelvis can be accessed through the vaginal or abdominal route. Minilaparotomy and laparoscopy are the choices for interval abdominal surgery, infraumbilical incision for postpartum tubal sterilization, and posterior colpotomy if the procedure is performed vaginally. A newer method is the transcervical hysteroscopic placement of a tubal occlusive device on an outpatient basis.

In the laparoscopic approach, either a closed or an open technique can be used. The closed method is preferred by most gynecologic laparoscopic surgeons. The patient is placed in a low dorsal lithotomy position, the abdomen and vagina are cleaned, the bladder is emptied, and a uterine manipulator is inserted. In the closed technique, a small periumbilical incision is created and the abdominal wall is elevated, after which a 10- or 11-mm trocar is inserted. Under direct visualization, a pneumoperitoneum is developed by insufflating with carbon dioxide. The pneumoperitoneum can be developed with a Veress needle before the trocar is inserted if the surgeon prefers. In the open technique, a similar periumbilical incision is used, but the incision is continued in layers until the peritoneal cavity is entered, the fascia is sutured with 0 synthetic absorbable suture in each corner, and a special trocar designed for the open method is inserted and secured. The main advantage of open laparoscopy is that major vascular injury is prevented. Although rare, such injury is a very serious complication, requiring immediate laparotomy. For patients with documented abdominopelvic adhesive disease or with risk factors for such disease, a left upper quadrant entrance is an excellent option. Once the laparoscope is inserted, the operator decides on the number of punctures and the size of the extra trocars required for the type of surgical procedure selected, with a single puncture or double puncture being the most popular.

If the selected incision is a minilaparotomy, a 3-cm transverse incision is created 2 to 3 cm above the superior aspect of the symphysis pubis in layers. A transverse incision of the fascia of the rectus abdominis exposes the muscles, which are then separated in the midline, after which the peritoneum is opened and the abdominopelvic cavity entered. The use of a uterine manipulator greatly facilitates minilaparotomy sterilization procedures.

In vaginal tubal sterilization procedures, the cervix is grasped at the posterior lip with a tenaculum or sutured temporarily with any 0 suture material (the author prefers modern synthetic absorbable). This allows the operator to retrovert the uterus, exposing the fallopian tubes through a posterior colpotomy incision of 3 to 4 cm made transversely between the uterosacral ligaments 1 to 2 cm under the cervicovaginal junction. After hemostasis has been secured, vaginal retractors are inserted and the tubes are exposed with the further help of ring forceps.

With the significant advances in laparoscopic instrumentation, almost any technique developed for minilaparotomy (e.g., Pomeroy) can be performed laparoscopically with only minor modifications. Also, a significant number of techniques designed for minilaparotomy or laparoscopic sterilization procedures can be performed safely and successfully through the vaginal route.

Regardless of the incision or method selected for the tubal sterilization, appropriate identification of the relevant anatomic structures and the fimbriated end of each fallopian tube is mandatory. Although tubal sterilization is considered permanent, it is inappropriate to select surgical techniques that involve excessive and unnecessary destruction of the fallopian tube, thereby precluding tubal reversal. It is important to be sensitive to the fact that when a woman decides on a tubal reversal, her decision may be surrounded by a personal tragedy, such as the loss of a child or a change in marital status.

The remainder of this chapter discusses the most commonly used surgical techniques and the preferred incisions.

SILASTIC BAND (FALOPE RING)

The preferred incision for the Silastic band technique is laparoscopy. The Falope ring applicator is loaded with two Silastic bands and inserted through the operative laparoscope with a single-puncture technique, or through a 7- or 8-mm trocar placed 3 cm above the symphysis pubis in the midline with a two-puncture technique. A midportion of the fallopian tube is grasped with the tongs of the applicator, and a Silastic band is applied. The same procedure is carried out contralaterally (Fig. 19.1). Tubal engorge-

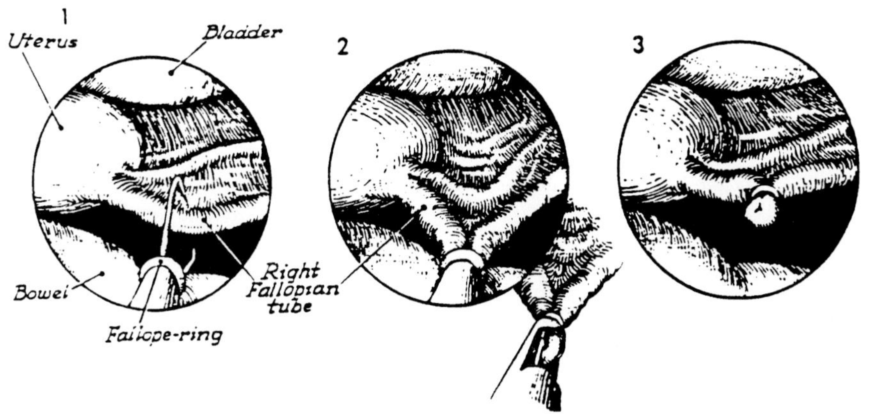

FIG. 19.1. Silastic band technique (Falope ring). (From Wheeless CR. *Atlas of pelvic surgery,* 2nd ed. Philadelphia: Lea & Febiger, 1988:258, with permission.)

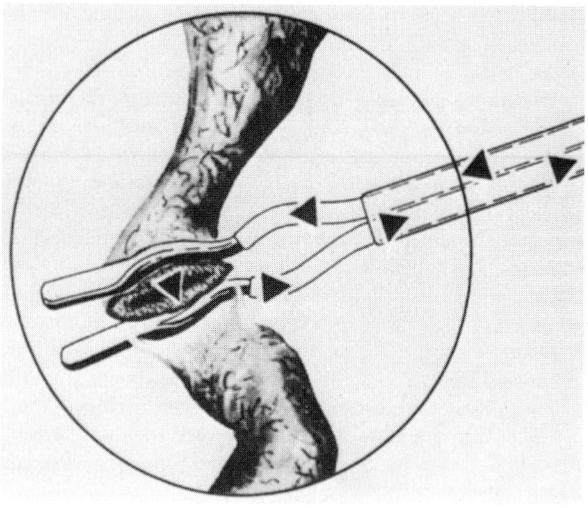

FIG. 19.2. Bipolar electrocoagulation (Kleppinger forceps). (From Thompson JD, Rock JA. *TeLinde's operative gynecology,* 7th ed. Philadelphia: JB Lippincott, 1992:343, with permission.)

ment (e.g., in postabortal sterilization) makes this technique difficult because of the limitation of the diameter of the applicator. Also, the fallopian tube must be adequately mobile to prevent transection of the tube. Severe tubal ischemic pain is one of the most common problems associated with this method. The preoperative use of nonsteroidal antiinflammatory medications and spraying the tubes or injecting the mesosalpinx with local anesthetics help to reduce immediate postoperative pain. The cumulative failure rate at 10 years is 1.77%.

BIPOLAR ELECTROCOAGULATION (KLEPPINGER FORCEPS)

Coagulation of a mid segment of the fallopian tube with the bipolar cautery is one of the preferred methods of laparoscopic sterilization (Fig. 19.2). This technique has also been successfully used during vaginal sterilization. The current flows from the active tong to the ground tong of the forceps, so that spread to other structures is eliminated. The advantages of bipolar electrocoagulation are the following: (a) It is fast and easy to master; (b) the size or mobility of the tube is not an issue; (c) it minimizes the possibility of bowel injury and excessive destruction of the tube associated with the use of unipolar current; (d) it is probably the least painful technique; and (e) only 6 to 8 mm of tissue is destroyed, so that the probability of reversal is as good as with Falope ring or Hulka clip sterilization. The cumulative failure rate at 10 years is 2.48%.

UNIPOLAR ELECTROCOAGULATION

The unipolar technique is very similar to bipolar electrocoagulation (Fig. 19.3). The main difference is that with unipolar technique, the current flows from the tip of the forceps through the body to a grounding pad or return electrode placed on the patient's thigh. The disadvantages in comparison with bipolar coagulation have been mentioned. The cumulative failure rate at 10 years is 0.75%.

HULKA AND FILSHIE CLIPS

The Hulka clip technique was introduced in 1972 as a method of laparoscopic sterilization. The greatest advantage of this procedure is that less than 1 cm of tissue is destroyed in the area of the isthmus; therefore, the potential for reversal is excellent.

In this technique, a plastic Hulka clip with interlocking teeth is loaded into a special applicator. The spring-loaded clip is then applied perpendicular to the fallopian tube in the isthmus (Fig. 19.4). The Filshie clip, which is made of titanium lined with silicone rubber, has now been introduced in the United States. It is applied with a special applicator in a manner similar to that used for the Hulka clip. The cumulative failure rate of the Hulka clip at 10 years is 3.65%. Comparable data are not available for the Filshie clip.

POMEROY METHOD

The Pomeroy method is one of the most popular and simple techniques for tubal sterilization. After the fallopian tubes with their respective fimbriated ends have been adequately identified, the midportion of one tube is grasped with a Babcock clamp, the tube is elevated, and a loop is formed. A single strand of absorbable suture material is placed around the 1.5-cm knuckle and tied firmly, after which the loop is excised with scissors (Fig. 19.5). The same procedure is carried out contralaterally. In the initial description of this method, 0 plain catgut was the suture of choice. Currently, we have the option of using high-quality, rapidly absorbed synthetic suture material with a smaller diameter, which has the advantage of causing less tissue reaction. This technique can easily be carried out through a minilaparotomy or vaginal incision during interval sterilization, or through a small infraumbilical incision during the early puerperium. With the availability of endoloop sutures, it is also possible to apply this method laparoscopically. The cumulative failure rate at 10 years for postpartum tubal excision procedures such as the Pomeroy method is 0.75%.

PARKLAND PROCEDURE

Although most commonly used for postpartum sterilization, the Parkland procedure is an easy and effective method for performing interval sterilizations by minilaparotomy. The fallopian tube is identified, grasped, and elevated as described for the Pomeroy method. The mesosalpinx is entered through an avascular space with a small Kelly clamp. The isolated portion of the tube is excised after being ligated proximally and distally with absorbable suture material (Fig. 19.6).

KROENER FIMBRIECTOMY

In Kroener fimbriectomy, the distal portion of the ampulla with its fimbriated end is excised. This is a simple procedure that can easily be carried out through a minilaparotomy or the vaginal route. The distal end of the fallopian tube is grasped with a Babcock clamp, double-sutured or clamped and double-ligated, then excised with scissors (Fig. 19.7). This technique has lost popularity in view of an almost nonexistent potential for reversal.

Other Techniques

The Irving procedure is shown in Fig. 19.8, and the Uchida technique in Fig. 19.9. These are highly effective methods for sterilization with low failure rates. Nevertheless, because they are more complex, they are less popular.

A new method of transcervical sterilization, Essure, has been approved by the Food and Drug Administration. An expanding microcoil of titanium is placed into the proximal fallopian tube under hysteroscopic guidance. Short-term efficacy rates are similar to those of other methods.

Although an ideal method of contraception will probably never be devised, current methods are such that with proper education, counseling, and support, every patient should have the opportunity to prevent an unintended pregnancy. Because of their unique relationship with patients, primary care physicians can obtain a proper and thorough sexual history and help prevent the 3 million unintended pregnancies that occur in the United States each year.

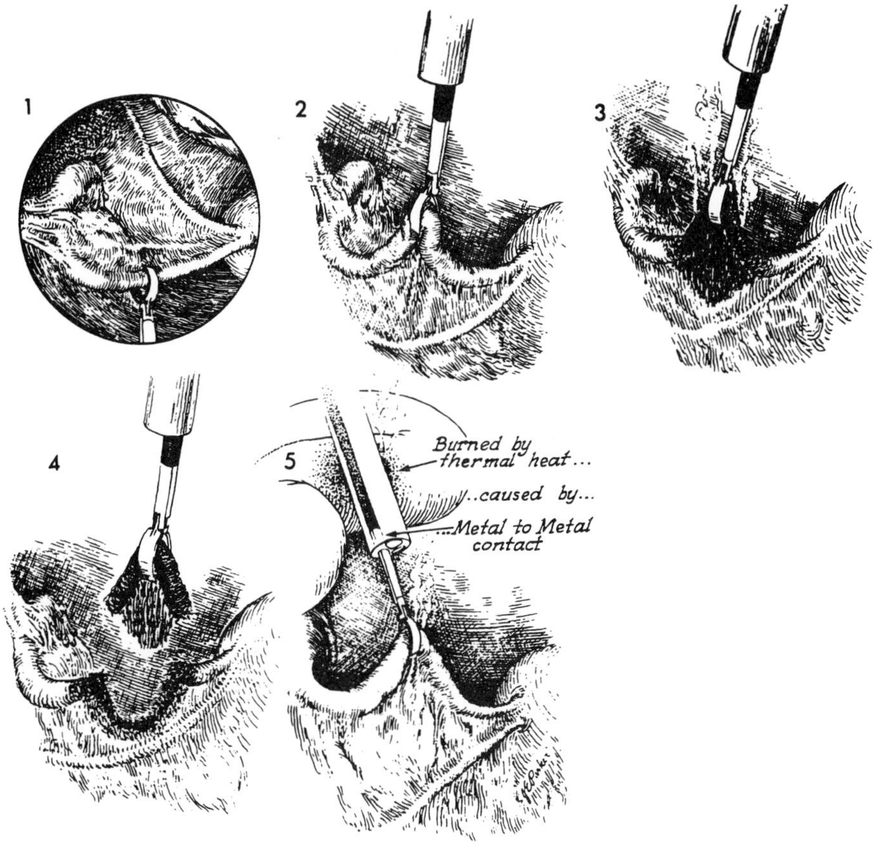

FIG. 19.3. Unipolar electrocoagulation. (From Wheeless CR. *Atlas of pelvic surgery,* 2nd ed. Philadelphia: Lea & Febiger, 1988:258, with permission.)

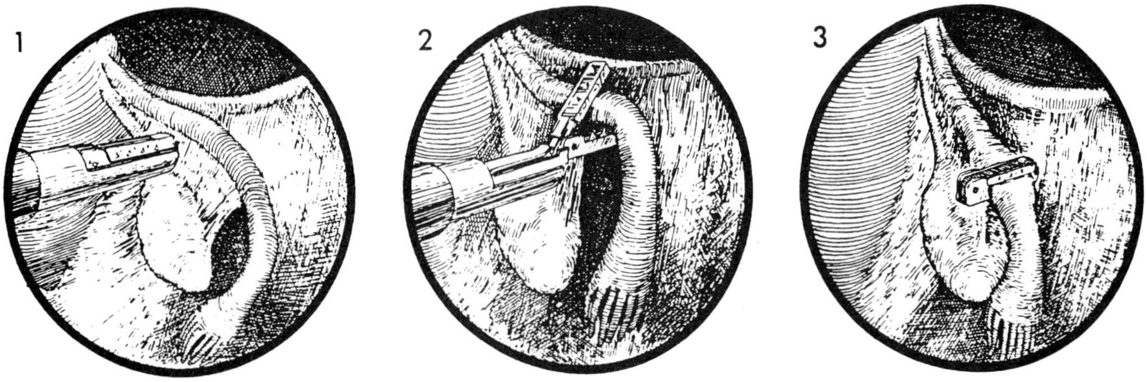

FIG. 19.4. Hulka clips technique. (From Wheeless CR. *Atlas of pelvic surgery,* 2nd ed. Philadelphia: Lea & Febiger, 1988:258, with permission.)

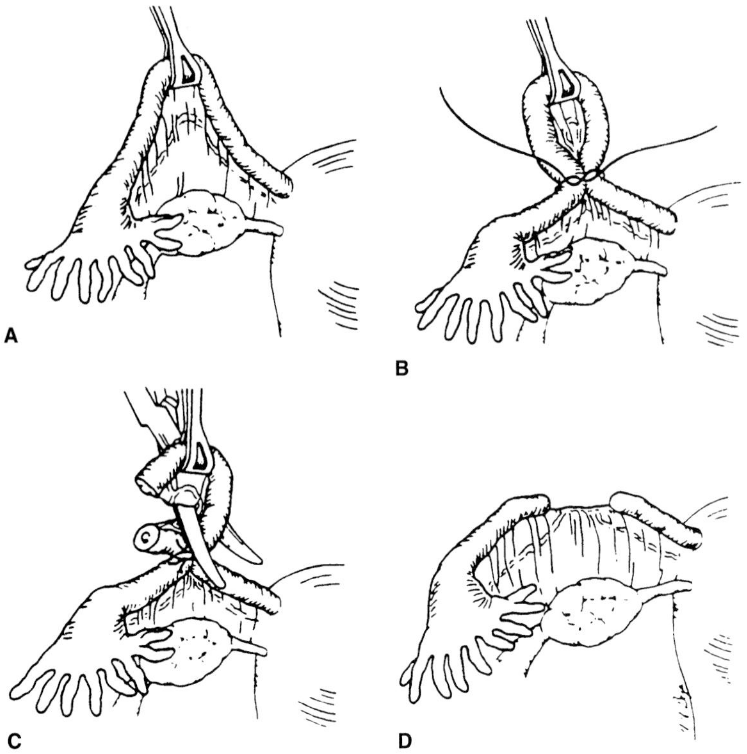

FIG. 19.5. Pomeroy technique. (From Sciarra JJ. Surgical procedures for tubal sterilization. In: Sciarra JJ, Steege JF, eds. *Gynecology and obstetrics,* vol 6. Philadelphia: Lippincott-Raven, 1996:3, with permission.)

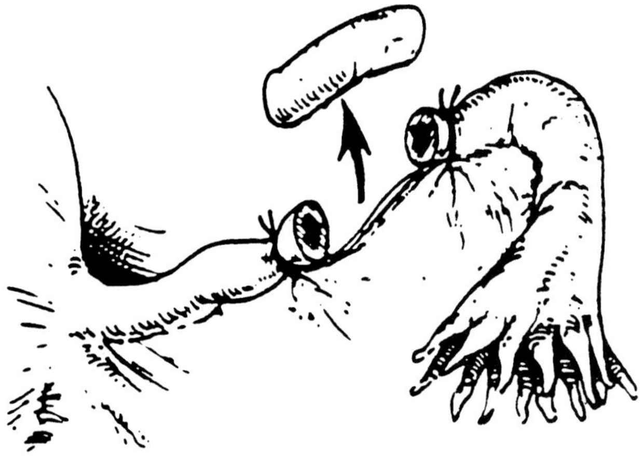

FIG. 19.6. Parkland procedure. (From Cunningham FG, MacDonald PC, Gant NF. *Williams obstetrics,* 19th ed. Norwalk, CT: Appleton & Lange, 1993:1354, with permission.)

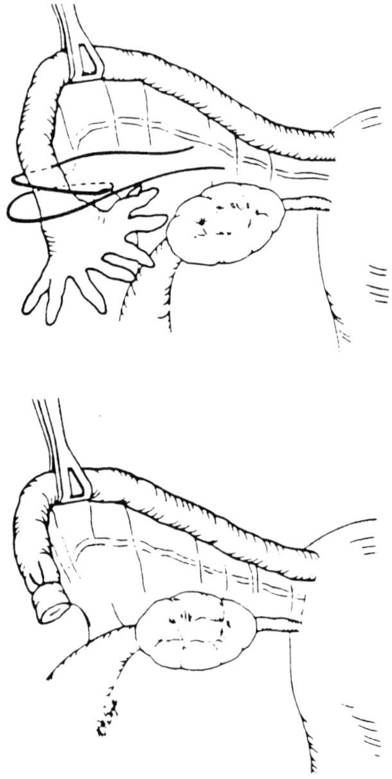

FIG. 19.7. Kroener fimbriectomy. (From Sciarra JJ. Surgical procedures for tubal sterilization. In: Sciarra JJ, Steege JF, eds. *Gynecology and obstetrics,* vol 6. Philadelphia: Lippincott-Raven, 1996:3, with permission.)

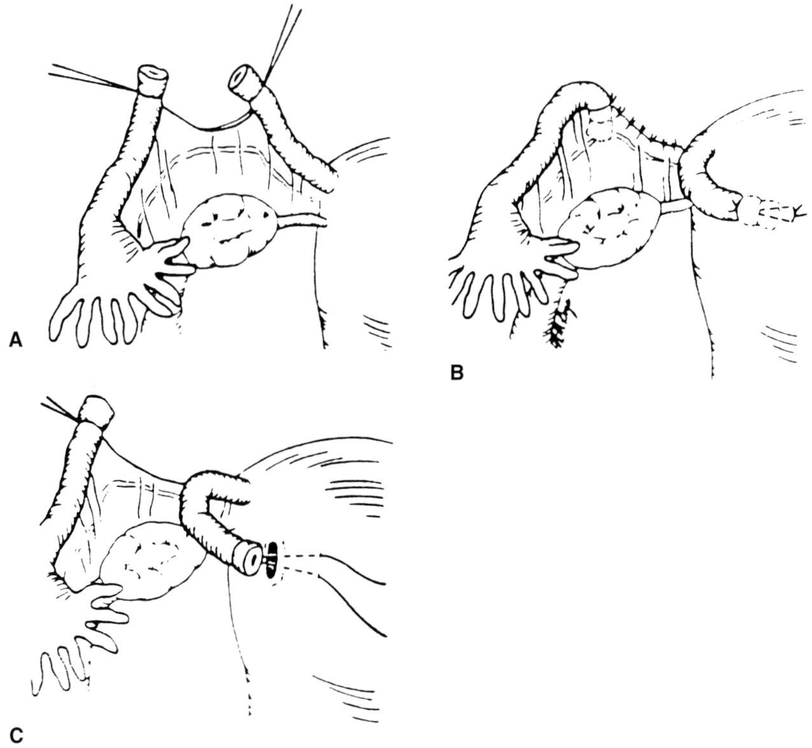

FIG. 19.8. Irving procedure. (From Sciarra JJ. Surgical procedures for tubal sterilization. In: Sciarra JJ, Steege JF, eds. *Gynecology and obstetrics,* vol 6. Philadelphia: Lippincott-Raven, 1996:3, with permission.)

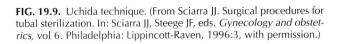

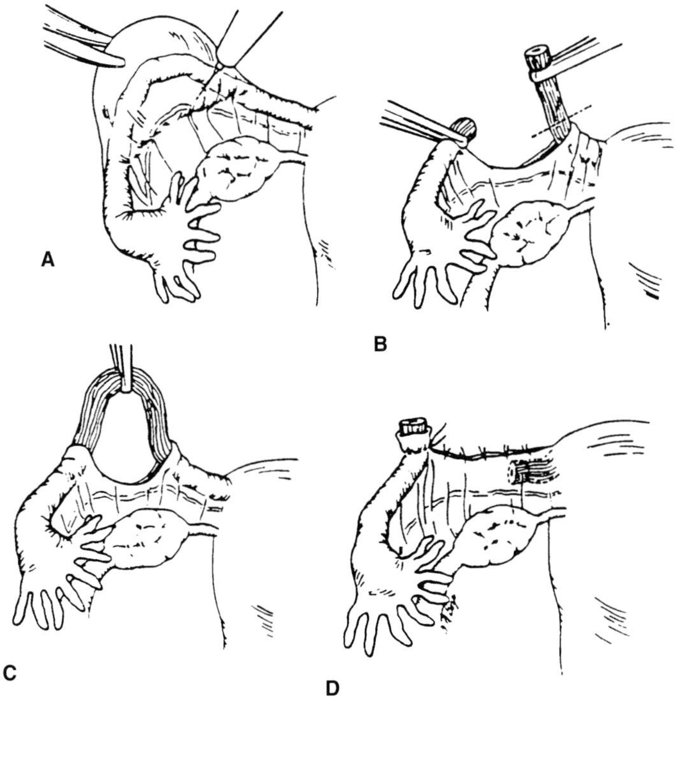

FIG. 19.9. Uchida technique. (From Sciarra JJ. Surgical procedures for tubal sterilization. In: Sciarra JJ, Steege JF, eds. *Gynecology and obstetrics,* vol 6. Philadelphia: Lippincott-Raven, 1996:3, with permission.)

BIBLIOGRAPHY

Cunningham FG, Gant NE, Leveno KJ, et al. *Williams obstetrics,* 21st ed. New York: McGraw-Hill, 2001:1555.

Grimes DA. Oral contraceptive compliance: strategies for ensuring correct and continued use of the pill. *Contraception Rep* 1994;5:3.

Grimes DA. Intrauterine device and upper-genital-tract infection. *Lancet* 2000;356:1013.

Hartfield JV. Female sterilization by the vaginal route: a positive reassessment and comparison of four tubal occlusion methods. *Aust N Z J Obstet Gynaecol* 1993;33:408.

Hatcher RA, Nelson AL, Zieman M, et al. *A pocket guide to managing contraception 2002–2003.* Tiger, GA: Bridging the Gap Foundation.

Hillis SD, Marchbanks PA, Tylor LR, et al. Tubal sterilization and long-term risk of hysterectomy: findings from the U.S. Collaborative Review of Sterilization. *Obstet Gynecol* 1997;89:609.

Kaunitz AM. Injectable long-acting contraceptives. *Clin Obstet Gynecol* 2001;44:73.

Kerin JF, Carignan CS, Cher D. The safety and effectiveness of a new hysteroscopic method for permanent birth control: results of the first Essure PBC clinical study. *Aust N Z J Obstet Gynaecol* 2001;41:364.

Mishell DR Jr. Noncontraceptive benefits of oral contraceptives. *J Reprod Med* 1993;38:1021.

Peterson HB, Jeng G, Folger SG, et al. The risk of menstrual abnormalities after tubal sterilization. U.S. Collaborative Review of Sterilization Working Group. *N Engl J Med* 2000;343:1681.

Peterson HB, et al. The risk of pregnancy after tubal sterilization: findings from the U.S. Collaborative Review of Sterilization. *Am J Obstet Gynecol* 1996;174:1161.

Piccinino LJ, Moser WD. Trends in contraceptive use in the United States: 1982–1995. *Fam Plann Perspect* 1998;30:4.

World Health Organization, Reproductive Health and Research. *Improving access to quality care in family planning: medical eligibility criteria for contraceptive use.* Geneva: World Health Organization, Reproductive Health and Research, 2000.

World Health Organization, Reproductive Health and Research. *Selected practice recommendations for contraceptive use.* Geneva: World Health Organization, Reproductive Health and Research, 2002.

Thompson JD, Rock JA. *TeLinde's operative gynecology,* 7th ed. Philadelphia: JB Lippincott, 1992:343.

Van Damme L, Ramjee G, Alary M, et al. Effectiveness of COL-1492, a nonoxynol-9 vaginal gel, on HIV-1 transmission in female sex workers: a randomised controlled trial. *Lancet* 2002;360:971–977.

Von Hertzen H, Piaggio G, Ding J, et al. Low dose mifepristone and two regimens of levonorgestrel for emergency contraception: a WHO multicentre randomised trial. *Lancet* 2002;360:1803.

Westhoff C, et al. Tubal sterilization: focus on the U.S. experience. *Fertil Steril* 2000;73:913.

Wheatley SA, Millar JM, Jadad AR. Reduction of pain after laparoscopic sterilisation with local bupivacaine: a randomised, parallel, double-blind trial. *Br J Obstet Gynaecol* 1994;101:443.

Wheeless CR. *Atlas of pelvic surgery,* 2nd ed. Philadelphia: Lea & Febiger, 1988:258.

Wilcox LS, Chu SY, Eaker ED, et al. Risk factors for regret after tubal sterilization: 5 years of follow-up in a prospective study. *Fertil Steril* 1991;55:927.

CHAPTER 20
Abortion and Ectopic Pregnancy

Fred M. Howard and H. Trent MacKay

ABORTION

Abortion is the termination of pregnancy before 20 gestational weeks. Another definition is the loss of a fetus weighing less than 500 g. Although the true rate of embryonic or fetal wastage is much higher, clinically recognized spontaneous abortion occurs in about 15% to 20% of known human pregnancies. (Elective or therapeutic abortion is discussed in Chapter 21.) Most abortions (80%) are early abortions, occurring in the first trimester. Abortions between 12 and 20 weeks of gestation, or late abortions, are less common. The abortion rate is relatively constant from 5 to 12 weeks of gestation, but it drops steadily and rapidly after 12 weeks.

Several stages of abortion may be clinically defined. Threatened abortion is uterine bleeding at less than 20 weeks of gestation without cervical dilation or effacement. This occurs in about 30% of pregnancies; about half of patients with threatened abortion miscarry. Missed abortion is the presence of a nonviable pregnancy documented by ultrasonography, with or without bleeding, but without cervical dilation. Inevitable abortion is uterine bleeding at less than 20 weeks of gestation with cervical dilation but without the passage of placental or fetal tissue. Incomplete abortion is uterine bleeding with expulsion through the cervix of some but not all placental and fetal tissue at less than 20 weeks of gestation. Complete abortion is the expulsion through the cervix of all placental and fetal tissue at less than 20 weeks of gestation. Septic abortion is an abortion associated with uterine infection.

Ultrasonography, especially when performed transvaginally, provides significantly more information than the clinical history and examination. It shows that in a first-trimester abortion, most fetuses die before 8 weeks and are retained in the uterus for several weeks before clinical symptoms develop. This situation, termed *intrauterine fetal death,* may be diagnosed ultrasonographically when cardiac activity is lacking in a fetus with a crown-rump length of 15 mm or more. Ultrasonography also detects a blighted ovum (anembryonic gestation), a pregnancy of more than about 7 weeks with a gestational sac but no fetus. If the fetus is shown by ultrasonography to be viable at less than 12 weeks, the risk for subsequent abortion is only 2% to 3%.

The risk for abortion is increased by both maternal and paternal age. In regard to maternal age, the risk of a woman older than 40 years (25%–30%) is twice that of a woman younger than 25 years (10%–15%). In regard to paternal age, the risk for abortion when the father is 45 years of age or older (23%) is about double the risk when the father is younger than 25 years (12%).

The reproductive history is the best predictor of risk for miscarriage. The risk for abortion is increased by a history of prior abortion, particularly in a woman with no prior pregnancy past 20 weeks of gestation. The risk for abortion is only slightly increased by a history of one prior abortion. However, with a history of two prior abortions, the risk is about 35%; with three, it is about 50% (in women with no parity). At least one live birth decreases the statistical risk for recurrent abortion after three prior abortions to 30%. The occurrence of three or more abortions is sometimes diagnosed as recurrent or habitual abortion. In clinical practice, however, couples with two consecutive abortions warrant an evaluation for treatable causes of abortion (Fig. 20.1).

Etiology

Numerous diseases and abnormalities, both congenital and acquired, can result in abortion (Table 20.1). Abortions are most commonly caused by genetic abnormalities. Cytogenetic studies show that chromosomal anomalies account for about 50% of all abortions. Most of these are aneuploidies—numeric abnormalities in which the number of chromosomes is more or less than the normal 46. Table 20.2 summarizes the chromosomal abnormalities most often associated with spontaneous abortion. Autosomal trisomies are the most common abnormality; about one third of the trisomies are trisomy 16. Monosomy 45,X is the most common single-chromosomal abnormality associated with abortion. About 1 in 300 concepti with a 45,X karyotype survives (Turner syndrome). Only about 5% of chromosomal anomalies are structural, with a euploid 46-chromosome karyotype. This finding is of clinical relevance because in such cases, a chromosomal carrier state may be detectable in one of the

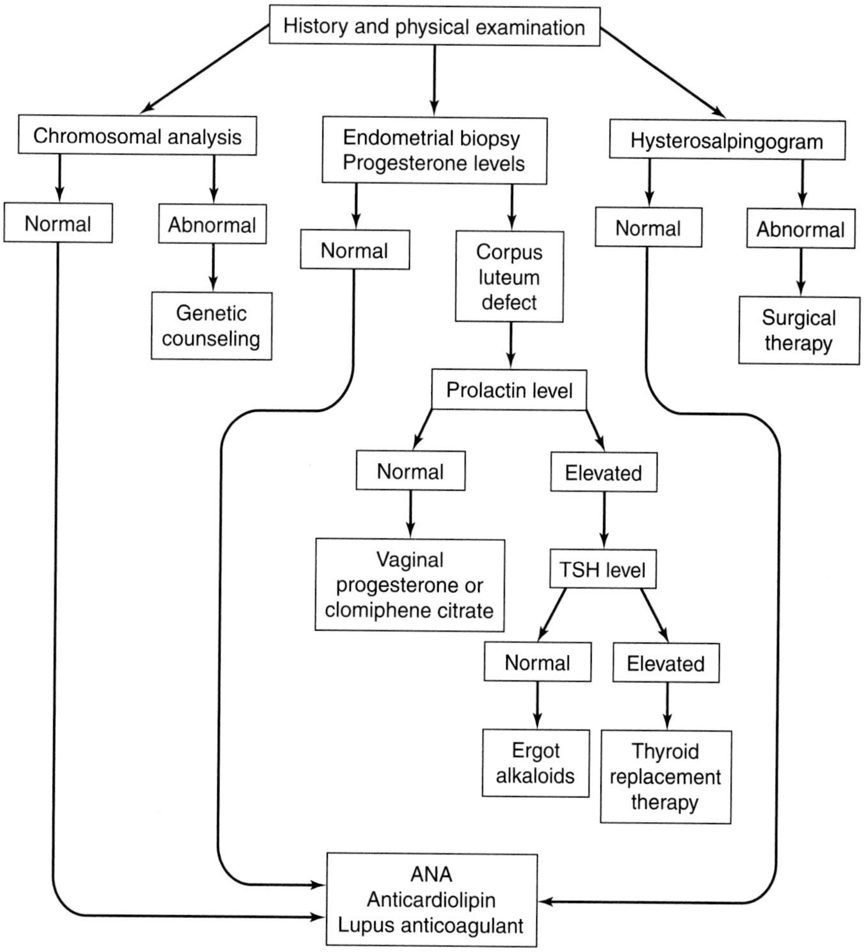

FIG. 20.1. One possible evaluation scheme for recurrent abortions.

TABLE 20.1. Classification of Causes of Spontaneous Abortion

Chromosomal
- Autosomal trisomy
- Monosomy 45,X
- Triploidy
- Tetraploidy
- Chromosomal structural abnormality

Uterine abnormalities
- Congenital
  - Unicornuate
  - Bicornuate
  - Septate
  - Diethylstilbestrol exposure
- Acquired
  - Leiomyomata
  - Incompetent cervix
  - Intrauterine adhesions (Asherman syndrome)

Hormonal
- Progesterone deficiency (corpus luteum defect)
- Thyroid disease
- Diabetes mellitus
- Polycystic ovarian syndrome

Thrombophilias

Immunologic
- Lupus anticoagulant activity
- Anticardiolipin antibodies

Infections

Smoking, alcohol, drugs

partners of a couple experiencing recurrent spontaneous abortion.

Advancing maternal and paternal age both independently increase the risk for spontaneous abortion. However, paternal age does not correlate with an increase in chromosomal anomalies as a cause of abortion. Maternal age correlates only with an increase in trisomies, particularly of groups D and G chromosomes, as a cause of miscarriage. The relation of age to the incidence of chromosomally abnormal abortion is not intuitive.

Most abortions caused by chromosomal abnormalities occur in the first trimester. Generally, chromosomally normal fetuses abort later in gestation than those with abnormal chromosomes; the peak incidence is at 12 to 13 weeks for chromosomally normal fetuses and at 11 weeks for chromosomally abnormal fetuses.

TABLE 20.2. Abnormal Karyotypes Observed in Spontaneous Abortions

Karyotype	Frequency (%)
Autosomal trisomy	50
Monosomy 45,X	20
Triploidy	15
Tetraploidy	10
Structural abnormality	5

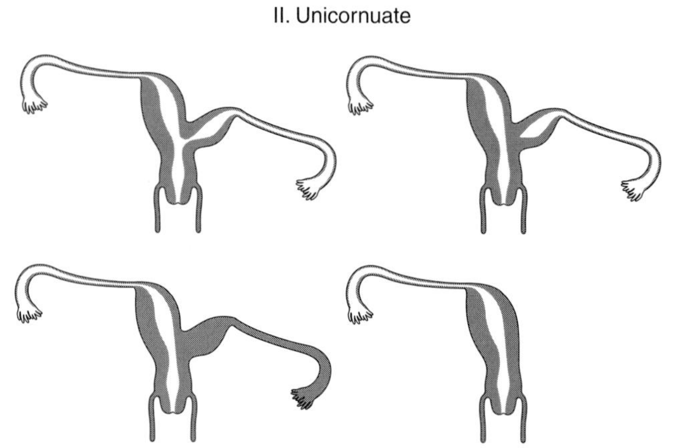

FIG. 20.2. Variations of possible types of unicornuate uteri. (*Roman numerals* indicate the AFS classification of the anomalies.)

The other general category of conditions that cause abortion may be said to be environmental, or maternal (Table 20.1). These are less common causes of abortion, although they are often causes of recurrent abortion. Anomalies of uterine development result from abnormal fusion of the müllerian system and probably occur in 1 in 200 to 600 women. About 25% of women with müllerian anomalies have reproductive problems. Most such anomalies may cause reproductive problems, but unicornuate uterus (Fig. 20.2) carries the greatest risk for abortion (~50%). Bicornuate and septate uteri (Fig. 20.3) are the anomalies most amenable to surgical correction but carry only about a 25% risk for abortion. Uterine septa can usually be resected hysteroscopically, after which the rates of abortion are normal. Bicornuate uteri usually require a transabdominal Strassman reunification procedure. Abortion rates are subsequently decreased to 12% to 25%. Uterine anomalies usually cause second-trimester abortions.

Leiomyomata are present in about 25% of women of reproductive age and are not a frequent cause of abortion. However, they may occasionally be a cause of miscarriage, particularly when located submucosally. Myomectomy may improve pregnancy outcomes.

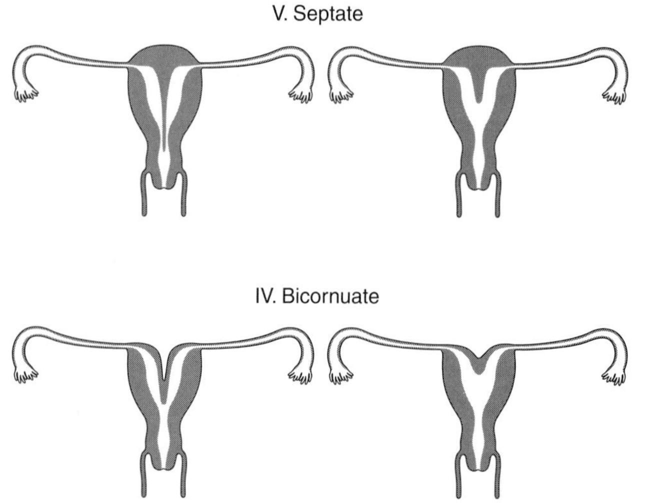

FIG. 20.3. Variations of types of septate and bicornuate uteri. (*Roman numerals* indicate the American Fertility Society [AFS] classification of the anomalies.)

Incompetent cervix is a syndrome in which asymptomatic cervical dilation leads to pregnancy loss in the second trimester. It may be congenital, sometimes associated with congenital uterine anomalies, or acquired during traumatic cervical dilation. Placement of a cervical cerclage is often an effective treatment (Fig. 20.4).

Intrauterine adhesions may cause infertility or recurrent abortion. These most often develop after vigorous postpartum uterine curettage but have also been reported after curettage for incomplete abortion, missed abortion, or diagnostic evaluation. To prevent this problem, vigorous, sharp endometrial curettage is best avoided. Genital tuberculosis may also be a cause.

In utero exposure to diethylstilbestrol (DES) may cause subsequent müllerian abnormalities, but this should now be a rare clinical occurrence. The risks for anomalies and vaginal adenocarcinoma are well known, and therefore DES should not be used during pregnancy. In utero exposure to DES results in a small endometrial cavity and possibly a TIQ2-shaped uterus, and it increases the likelihood of cervical incompetence.

Endocrine dysfunction may also cause abortion, especially recurrent abortion. Viability during the first 7 weeks of gestation depends on the production of progesterone by the corpus luteum. If production is insufficient (luteal insufficiency), then abortion may result. Midluteal progesterone levels are normally above 9 ng/mL. Consistently lower mid luteal levels suggest a diagnosis of luteal insufficiency as a cause of recurrent abortion.

Uncontrolled diabetes mellitus increases the rate of abortion and fetal anomalies. However, when blood glucose levels are well controlled, the risk for abortion is not increased in women with diabetes. A risk for abortion is directly correlated with elevated levels of glycosylated hemoglobin (HbA_1). Hypothyroidism is another endocrine dysfunction often cited as a cause of abortion, although little objective evidence has been found of such a relation. Some evidence suggests that women with thyroid dysfunction and thyroid autoantibodies are at increased risk for abortion.

Lupus anticoagulant activity or anticardiolipin antibodies have been associated with an increased risk for abortion and intrauterine fetal death. The mechanism by which these factors cause abortion is unclear, but evidence supports testing women with recurrent abortion for lupus anticoagulant activity and anticardiolipin antibodies.

Endometritis secondary to infection with certain bacteria, viruses, and parasites may cause spontaneous abortion, although probably not frequently. *Toxoplasma gondii,* herpes simplex virus,

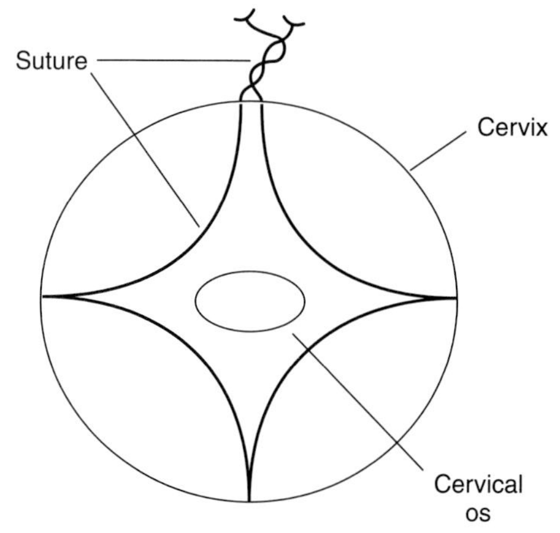

FIG. 20.4. McDonald cerclage placement for incompetent cervix.

and *Ureaplasma urealyticum* appear to be proven causes of abortion. *U. urealyticum* and possibly *Mycoplasma hominis* may occasionally cause recurrent abortion.

Cigarette smoking, alcohol consumption, and possibly exposure to radiation or environmental toxins increase the risk for abortion.

Differential Diagnosis

Ectopic pregnancy is the major diagnosis that the clinician may easily confuse with a possible abortion (Table 20.3). Both may present with a positive pregnancy test result, abdominopelvic pain, and irregular bleeding. Often, the two cannot be differentiated clinically by the history and physical examination findings, but current methodologies with transvaginal ultrasonography and quantitative measurement of human chorionic gonadotropin (β-hCG) levels usually allow an accurate diagnosis.

Molar pregnancy may also present similarly to abortion. Again, ultrasonography and quantitative β-hCG levels generally allow an accurate diagnosis to be made preoperatively. Also, the routine histologic evaluation of aborted products of conception makes it possible to identify hydatidiform molar pregnancies, including partial and incomplete molar pregnancies, in most cases.

The most common causes of bleeding in the first 20 weeks of gestation are summarized in Table 20.3.

History

Patients with abortion have a history of amenorrhea or irregular bleeding. Their chief symptoms at presentation are usually vaginal bleeding and cramping pain in the lower abdomen and pelvis. Women with threatened abortion who do not subsequently miscarry usually do not experience cramping pain.

Although 15% to 20% of pregnant women abort, twice this number bleed during the first half of pregnancy. Thus, bleeding by itself is a symptom of abortion only half the time; a pregnant woman with bleeding during the first 20 weeks of pregnancy has about a 50% chance of miscarrying. Bleeding for 3 days or more is associated with a greater risk for abortion than bleeding that lasts only 1 or 2 days.

Associated fever and foul vaginal discharge, especially in a patient with a history of uterine instrumentation, should raise a concern of possible septic abortion, as should any symptoms suggestive of infection without a clear origin outside the genital tract.

TABLE 20.3. Causes of Vaginal Bleeding before the 20th Week of Gestation in 1,549 Patients

Diagnosis	Number	Percentage (%)
Threatened abortion	211	13.6
Inevitable and incomplete abortion	951	61.4
Complete abortion	203	13.1
Septic abortion	67	4.3
Missed abortion	27	1.7
Hydatidiform mole	12	0.8
Tubal ectopic pregnancy	78	5.1

Source: From Cavanagh D, Fleisher A, Ferguson JH. *Am J Obstet Gynecol* 1964;90:216, with permission.

Physical Examination and Clinical Findings

The status of the cervix at the time of the examination may allow a definitive diagnosis. If the cervix is dilated without a history of passage of tissue, the diagnosis is inevitable abortion. If tissue has passed or is within the cervical os and the cervix is dilated, the diagnosis is incomplete abortion. If all fetal and placental tissue has passed and the cervix is closed, usually with a decrease to minimal bleeding and cessation of cramping, the diagnosis is complete abortion.

Abortions before 6 weeks or after 14 weeks of gestation are more likely to be complete. Those between 6 and 14 weeks are often incomplete. If cervical motion tenderness, foul cervical discharge, and marked abdominopelvic tenderness are present, then septic abortion is likely. Pelvic inflammatory disease can occur during pregnancy but is uncommon. If pelvic inflammatory disease is thought to be the explanation for these findings, the patient should be treated in the hospital with intensive observation. Gram-negative endotoxins can cause septic shock can develop rapidly in a patient with a septic abortion.

Laboratory and Imaging Studies

With ultrasonography, particularly transvaginal ultrasonography, it is almost always possible to identify a gestational sac by 5 weeks of gestation (34 days) and a fetal pole by 6 weeks (40–42 days) in a normal pregnancy. Generally, this correlates with a β-hCG level of 1,500 to 2,000 mIU/mL. Fetal cardiac activity can usually be detected by 7 weeks (47–49 days). Thus, ultrasonography can diagnose intrauterine death or anembryonic gestation and clearly differentiate between threatened abortion and incomplete or missed abortion. Although the usual abortion rate is about 15%, once fetal viability is ultrasonographically established at 8 weeks or more of gestation, the abortion rate is only 3% to 4%.

Although parental chromosomal abnormalities are an uncommon cause of abortion, if a couple has had two or more consecutive abortions, the prevalence of major chromosomal anomalies is 3%. About half of these are balanced translocations and about a fourth are robertsonian translocations. Thus, with such a history, parental karyotyping is indicated. If a translocation is found, 80% of pregnancies will abort, and in 3% to 5% of those that do not abort, the fetal chromosomes will be unbalanced. For this reason, amniocentesis for fetal karyotyping is indicated in the second trimester for a couple with a parental translocation.

For couples with two or more consecutive abortions, hysterosalpingography and hysteroscopy may be indicated to evaluate for intrauterine adhesions, especially if the woman has previously undergone curettage. Hysterosalpingography may also demonstrate uterine anomalies as a cause of abortion. A complete blood cell count, measurement of thyroid-stimulating hormone (TSH) levels, lupus anticoagulant activity, anticardiolipin antibody levels, and midluteal progesterone levels, or endometrial biopsy may also be indicated for patients with multiple miscarriages (Fig. 20.1).

Treatment

THREATENED ABORTION

No specific treatment has been shown to alter the course of threatened abortion, but most clinicians nonetheless recommend bed rest, abstaining from coitus, and restriction of activities. Increasing pain or bleeding necessitates reevaluation.

Progesterone supplementation is indicated only for patients in whom luteal insufficiency has been diagnosed before pregnancy. Initiating progesterone in a patient who is already pregnant, whether for bleeding, low progesterone levels, or a history of recurrent abortion, is of no proven benefit. If luteal insufficiency has been diagnosed before pregnancy, progesterone vaginal suppositories (25 mg twice daily) or intramuscular progesterone (12.5 mg/d) may be effective if started about 3 days after ovulation and continued through the first 8 to 12 weeks of gestation.

MISSED ABORTION

Missed abortion may be managed either expectantly or with uterine evacuation. Typically, the patient who desires termination undergoes curettage. However, some evidence suggests that medical treatment with the prostaglandin misoprostol may be a useful alternative. In one study of patients with missed abortion, 800 μg of misoprostol was placed in the posterior vaginal fornix. Patients were seen 24 and 48 hours after the initial dose, and misoprostol was readministered only if ultrasonography revealed evidence of persistent pregnancy tissue. By 72 hours after initiation of the study, if either a gestational sac or placental tissue was present, the medical treatment was considered a failure, and uterine curettage was performed. In 15 of 25 patients, the termination of pregnancy was successful, and they did not require curettage.

INEVITABLE ABORTION

Outpatient suction curettage is probably the best treatment for inevitable abortion, particularly during the first trimester. Because the cervix is open, it can be performed comfortably and safely with conscious sedation or local anesthesia. Although an intravenous line and intravenous fluids are ideal, they may sometimes be omitted if bleeding is not profuse. In addition to conscious sedation, a paracervical block with 20 mL of 1% lidocaine can be used. Care must be taken to avoid intravascular injection of the local anesthetic. Various methods of paracervical block have been shown to be efficacious. The injection of 1 mL into the anterior cervical lip allows painless grasping of the cervix with a Jacobs or single-tooth tenaculum; the remaining anesthetic can then be injected at the 3- and 9-o'clock positions at the cervicovaginal junction. A suction curet is introduced just through the internal cervical os, suction is initiated to a pressure of about 60 cm H_2O, and the curet is gently rotated 360 degrees several times. When tissue and blood stop passing through the curet and frothy bubbles start to appear, the procedure is usually finished. A gentle curettage with a sharp curet may be performed to ensure that all the products of conception have been evacuated, but this must not be vigorous or deep. Manual vacuum aspiration with a prepackaged syringe and suction cannula may also be used. Ergonovine (0.2 mg intramuscularly) or oxytocin (10–20 units intravenously or intramuscularly) is usually given during or at the end of the procedure.

The patient should be observed for bleeding and her vital signs measured for 2 to 8 hours, depending on her preoperative and intraoperative blood loss and level of consciousness. At discharge, the patient is given 0.2 mg of ergonovine every 4 hours for six doses, and 100 mg of doxycycline twice daily for 2 or 3 days. Prophylactic antibiotic treatment may decrease the risk for postoperative infection after elective abortion. Discharge instructions include rest for 24 to 72 hours and nothing per vagina for 2 weeks.

INCOMPLETE ABORTION

Between 6 and 14 weeks of gestation, most clinicians recommend curettage for incomplete abortion. However, in the absence of demonstrable residual tissue on ultrasonography, evidence suggests that expectant management without curettage may decrease the risk for infection, with only 1.5 days more of bleeding on average than after traditional treatment with curettage. The duration of pain, time required for convalescence, and need for transfusion are similar with either expectant or surgical management in this setting.

SEPTIC ABORTION

If the history, physical examination, and laboratory findings suggest septic abortion, the patient and physician must recognize that this is a potentially fatal condition. Hospital admission is mandatory. Cultures of the cervix and blood should be obtained. A complete blood cell count, electrolyte measurements, chemistries, and coagulation studies are advisable. Broad-spectrum antibiotics should be initiated immediately. A preferred regimen is triple antibiotic coverage with ampicillin, gentamicin, and clindamycin. After antibiotics have been started, dilation and suction curettage or evacuation are performed. Rarely, the infection is severe enough to necessitate hysterectomy. If septic shock or disseminated intravascular coagulation develops, intensive care is required, possibly including Swan-Ganz catheterization, vasopressors, and blood products.

RECURRENT ABORTION

A couple with two consecutive abortions, especially if they have had no live births, should be evaluated and treated for recurrent abortion. Most of the known causes and the evaluation of recurrent abortion have been discussed previously. Treatment is based on the results of the diagnostic evaluation (Fig. 20.1).

A history and physical examination specifically directed toward incompetent cervix, cigarette smoking, illicit drug use, alcohol abuse, and exposure to environmental toxins should be completed. A complete blood cell count is obtained, and the TSH level, lupus anticoagulant activity, anticardiolipin antibody level, and several midluteal progesterone levels determined. A hysterosalpingogram should be performed to look for intrauterine adhesions, leiomyomata, or uterine anomalies. If the results of all these studies are normal, then chromosomal abnormalities in either the man or woman should be sought by karyotyping both.

If luteal insufficiency is diagnosed based on mid luteal progesterone levels of less than 9 ng/mL, progesterone vaginal suppositories (25 mg twice daily) or intramuscular progesterone (12.5 mg/d) may be effective if started 3 days after ovulation and continued through the first 8 to 12 weeks of gestation.

If the TSH levels are high, then thyroid replacement should be initiated and studies to evaluate possible autoimmune thyroid disease performed.

If intrauterine adhesions are diagnosed, surgical treatment is indicated. Hysteroscopic adhesiolysis, followed by endometrial distention with a Foley catheter and then high-dose estrogen (e.g., 2.5 mg of conjugated estrogen) for 30 to 60 days, results in a normal abortion rate postoperatively.

Lupus anticoagulant activity or anticardiolipin antibodies have been associated with recurrent abortion. If either of these is present in a woman with abortion, treatment is probably indicated, although no general agreement has been reached regarding the best therapy. Corticosteroids, aspirin, and heparin have all been used.

RHESUS FACTOR IMMUNE GLOBULIN

With any of the categories of abortion, the patient's blood type should be known. Prophylaxis against Rhesus factor (Rh) sensitization with Rh immune globulin should be administered to a patient with Rh-negative blood. The need for Rh immune globulin in cases of threatened abortion is debated, but prophylaxis is clearly indicated in all other cases. In the first trimester, a decreased dose (50 mg) may be adequate rather than the usual 300-mg dose.

Postabortion Counseling

It has been reported that conception within the first 3 months after a live birth is associated with an increased rate of abortion. Extrapolation of this information has led to a clinical recommendation that women not attempt conception for at least 3 months after a spontaneous abortion, although the recommendation is not based on any clear evidence.

If the abortion is the woman's first, she can be counseled that the risk for abortion is not increased in the next pregnancy. However, after two or more abortions, the subsequent risk is 30% to 50%.

The clinician must be aware of the loss that a woman suffers with an abortion. Most women have bonded with their baby, even in the first trimester, and grieve for their lost child. Physicians and other providers involved in a woman's care should be sensitive to this suffering and offer her appropriate psychosocial support and counseling. In many locales, active support groups are available that are helpful to many women. Well-intentioned comments are often painful to the woman and are best avoided, such as, "At least this happened before it was a real baby" and "Don't worry, you can always get pregnant again." Every effort should be made to make the woman's medical experience during an abortion as supportive as possible.

ECTOPIC PREGNANCY

An ectopic pregnancy is one that develops after implantation of the blastocyst at any site other than the endometrium of the uterine cavity. The most common ectopic site of implantation is the fallopian tube, in which 97% to 98% of all ectopic pregnancies occur. The remaining 2% to 3% are abdominal, ovarian, cornual (interstitial), or cervical implantations (Fig. 20.5).

Ectopic pregnancy is a life-threatening condition. With the availability of early diagnosis, blood transfusions, and effective surgical and medical therapies, the death rate has decreased more than sevenfold during the past three decades and is now less than 5 per 10,000 cases. However, ectopic pregnancies still cause 40 to 50 deaths per year in the United States, and ectopic pregnancy is the leading cause of maternal mortality in black women. Because this is a disease of young women who have a life expectancy of 50 to 70 years or more, any deaths are particularly tragic. Early diagnosis and treatment are essential if serious or fatal complications are to be avoided. Primary care physicians must always consider the possibility of ectopic pregnancy in a woman of reproductive age with irregular vaginal bleeding or abdominopelvic pain.

During the past three decades, the rate of ectopic pregnancy appears to have increased threefold to fourfold and is currently 16 to 20 per 1,000 pregnancies in the United States. The rate is higher in nonwhite than in white women and higher in parous women than in nulligravidas.

Etiology

Normally, the fertilized ovum passes through the fallopian tube to implant in the decidual endometrium at about 7 days of age.

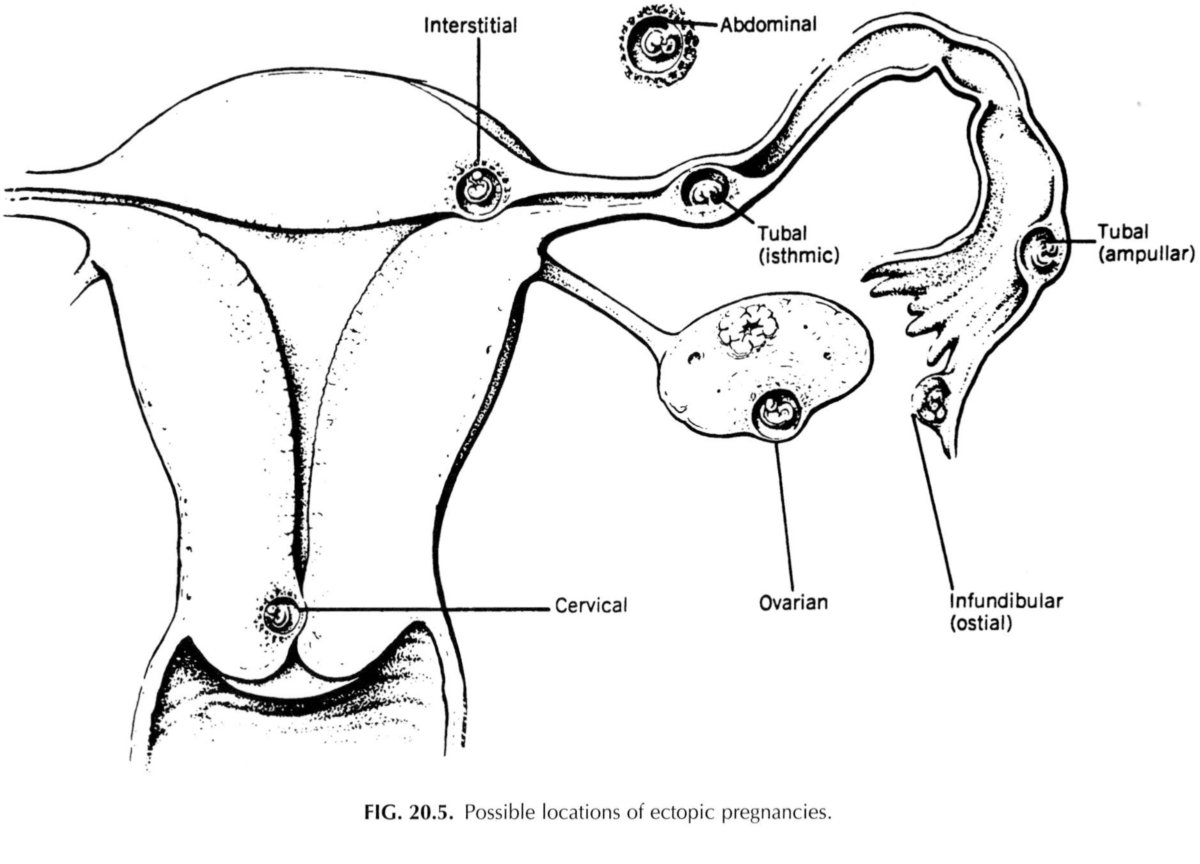

FIG. 20.5. Possible locations of ectopic pregnancies.

It appears that any factor impeding this migration may cause a tubal implantation (Table 20.4). The most common factor seems to be tubal damage secondary to acute salpingitis. In about half of all women with a first ectopic pregnancy, morphologic changes are found that can be attributed to previous acute salpingitis. Further evidence contributing to the hypothesis that acute salpingitis is a major cause of ectopic pregnancy comes from a 1981 study by Westrom and colleagues, who followed 900 women with laparoscopically confirmed salpingitis and observed a rate of ectopic pregnancy of 68.8 per 1,000 conceptions, sixfold higher than the rate in a control population without prior salpingitis. Scarring and agglutination of the endosalpinx are probably the mechanisms by which salpingitis causes tubal implantation. Adhesions of the tubal serosa to the bowel or peritoneum often develop after salpingitis and may impede normal tubal motility and play a role. Adhesions may also develop after pelvic surgery, which appears to be another risk factor for ectopic pregnancy.

Any surgery performed on the fallopian tube increases the risk for a tubal ectopic pregnancy. Often, surgery is undertaken to treat infertility secondary to salpingitis; however, the surgery does not correct the salpingian damage resulting from salpingitis, so that if conception occurs, the same factors discussed previously lead to a tubal implantation. When surgery is performed on a relatively normal tube (e.g., for tubal reanastomosis after sterilization), the risk for an ectopic pregnancy is less than when surgery is performed on an abnormal tube. However, the risk is still higher than in women who have not undergone surgery because tubal surgery, even when carried out with the most meticulous technique, inevitably causes some damage.

Tubal sterilization is a particularly important risk factor for ectopic pregnancy. Although tubal sterilization is an effective method of permanent contraception, when it fails, tubal implantation is a particular risk. Tubal coagulation and Falope ring techniques may carry a higher risk for ectopic pregnancy when they fail than other methods of tubal sterilization. As tubal sterilization has become a more popular method of family planning, it has also become a more frequent cause of ectopic pregnancy.

Another suspected factor in the etiology of tubal ectopic pregnancy is a hormonal imbalance in which levels of estrogen, progesterone, or both are excessive. Elevated levels are thought to impede normal tubal motility and contractility, slowing the transit of the fertilized ovum through the tube. This mechanism probably accounts for the increase in ectopic pregnancies among women who conceive while taking progestin-only oral contraceptives, ovulation-inducing drugs such as clomiphene and human menopausal gonadotropin, and progesterone-releasing intrauterine devices (IUDs). The risk associated with these factors is less than that associated with salpingitis; the increase in the rate of ectopic pregnancy ranges from 50% to 300%. These contraceptive methods do not put a woman at risk for ectopic pregnancy; they decrease her chance of conceiving and thus the chance of an ectopic pregnancy. However, when they fail, the progestin-only pill and the IUD carry a higher risk for tubal implantation. Failure of diaphragms, condoms, and combination oral contraceptives does not increase the rate of ectopic pregnancy above that in women not practicing contraception.

The etiologic mechanisms underlying other types of ectopic pregnancy—cervical, ovarian, interstitial, and abdominal—are less well understood. Abdominal pregnancies are thought to occur often after abortion of a tubal pregnancy, with reimplantation and development (secondary abdominal ectopic pregnancy). However, abdominal and ovarian pregnancies also appear to arise primarily after direct implantation of the blastocyst on the peritoneum or ovary.

Differential Diagnosis

Abdominopelvic pain or bleeding in a young woman may have numerous other causes, the most frequent of which are listed in Table 20.5. It is worth dividing the differential diagnosis into conditions directly related to pregnancy and those that may also occur in women who are not pregnant. (We assume that the pregnancy test result is positive; the results of modern, sensitive pregnancy tests are almost never negative in a woman with an ectopic pregnancy.) These conditions are extensively covered in Chapters 5 and 23, so only those specific to pregnancy are reviewed here.

Abortion is a common cause of bleeding and pain during the first half of pregnancy. The pain is usually cramping, located in the midline, and accompanied by vaginal bleeding, which is often heavy with clots. An open cervical os with obvious products of conception often allows a clinical diagnosis without further laboratory or imaging tests. However, a decidual cast, passed in about 10% of women with an ectopic pregnancy, may lead to an incorrect diagnosis of abortion. Histologic evaluation of any passed or curetted tissue is a safeguard against such a misdiagnosis. A frozen section evaluation can be performed if the diagnosis is uncertain and reveals chorionic villi in most cases of abortion. Floating the tissue on saline solution is a useful clinical technique to identify chorionic villi, but a histologic evaluation must still be performed. Permanent sections may show an Arias-Stella reaction (hyper-

TABLE 20.4. Risk Factors for Ectopic Pregnancy

History of salpingitis
Prior ectopic pregnancy
Progesterone-releasing intrauterine device
Progestin-only birth control pill failure
Pharmacologic ovulation induction
Pelvic adhesions
Prior pelvic surgery
Prior tubal surgery (tubal sterilizations or tuboplasties)
Two or more induced abortions

TABLE 20.5. Differential Diagnosis of Ectopic Pregnancy

Abortion
Heterotopic pregnancy
Acute salpingitis
Functional ovarian cyst
Ovarian tumor
Appendicitis
Adnexal torsion
Endometriosis
Pelvic adhesions
Leiomyomata
Cystitis
Polycystic ovarian disease
Urinary calculus
Gastroenteritis

secretory endometrial glands with hyperchromatism, pleomorphism, increased mitotic activity, and hypertrophy), which in the absence of obvious chorionic villi should make the clinician highly suspicious of an ectopic pregnancy rather than an abortion.

A heterotopic pregnancy is one in which an intrauterine pregnancy and an ectopic pregnancy are combined. Although rare (1 in 4,000–30,000 pregnancies), it may be more frequent after induced ovulation. The correct diagnosis can be made only when a high index of suspicion leads the clinician to obtain further laboratory and imaging studies.

Appendicitis during the first trimester of pregnancy may be confused with ectopic pregnancy. As in ectopic pregnancy, the pain is usually unilateral early in the disease (right lower quadrant). Bleeding is not a characteristic symptom of appendicitis. The temperature is usually higher in appendicitis than in ectopic pregnancy; temperature elevation in ectopic pregnancy is usually minimal. White blood cell counts in appendicitis are usually elevated above the normal pregnancy range of up to 14,000/mL. Both diseases may present with anorexia, nausea, and vomiting.

History

The classic symptoms of ectopic pregnancy are abdominopelvic pain, absence of menses, and irregular vaginal bleeding (Table 20.6). Pain is almost always present. Usually, it is unilateral at first; then, as the course progresses, it becomes bilateral or generalized. The quality of the pain is not characteristic. At first, it may be colicky or vague; at times, it is sharp or stabbing. The pain characteristically becomes intense with tubal rupture. Right shoulder pain may develop secondary to diaphragmatic irritation by a hemoperitoneum. Occasionally, patients experience rectal pain or an urge to defecate.

More than 75% of patients have amenorrhea, but this may be difficult to elicit because about 75% of them also have a history of irregular bleeding. On careful inquiry, most women at the time of clinical presentation are found to be 6 weeks or more past their last normal menstrual period. The irregular bleeding is characteristically spotting but occasionally heavy enough to resemble menstrual flow. It is not usually as heavy as the bleeding of a miscarriage. As previously noted, in up to 10% of cases, a decidual cast is passed that resembles the tissue passed in a spontaneous abortion.

Before the diagnosis is made, about 25% of women experience dizziness or syncope. Ideally, the diagnosis should be made before this symptom develops because most young, healthy women can compensate for significant blood loss before true syncope occurs. Pregnancy molimina is common, and breast tenderness, nausea, and constipation are not unusual.

TABLE 20.6. Symptoms and Signs of Ectopic Pregnancy

>75% of Cases
Abdominopelvic pain
Abnormal uterine bleeding
Normal-sized uterus
Adnexal tenderness
50%–75% of Cases
Generalized abdominopelvic pain
Amenorrhea
25%–50% of Cases
Unilateral abdominopelvic pain
Syncopal symptoms
Unilateral adnexal mass
Cervical motion tenderness
<25% of Cases
Shoulder pain
Passage of uterine cast
Fever
Tachycardia
Orthostatic changes

Physical Examination and Clinical Findings

An assessment of the vital signs reveals tachycardia or low-grade fever (≤38°C) in up to 20% of patients. Orthostatic changes in pulse and blood pressure are also found in up to 20% of patients.

Most patients have abdominal tenderness that may be unilateral, bilateral, or generalized. Rebound tenderness may also be present but does not necessarily indicate a hemoperitoneum; conversely, the patient may have a hemoperitoneum without rebound tenderness. Pelvic tenderness is usually present and may be unilateral, bilateral, or diffuse. Cervical motion tenderness is not unusual. An adnexal mass is palpable in about half of patients but usually represents a corpus luteum cyst, not the ectopic pregnancy; in fact, in up to 20% of patients, the mass is on the contralateral side. The uterus is usually enlarged, but almost never to the size of more than 8 weeks of gestation. Uterine bleeding may be noted but is usually not heavy. The cervical os is almost always closed, except with passage of a decidual cast.

Laboratory and Imaging Studies

In all women with an ectopic pregnancy, the serum pregnancy test result is positive if a sensitive radioimmunoassay type of test is performed. A negative serum assay for β-hCG makes the diagnosis quite unlikely. In addition to a pregnancy test, a complete blood cell count, blood typing, and Rh determination should be performed when an ectopic pregnancy is suspected. About 25% of women have a hematocrit of 30% or less at presentation. Consistent with the changes of pregnancy, up to a third have a white cell count of 10,000 to 15,000/mm^3. Fewer than 20% have a significant leukocytosis above 15,000/mm^3.

If the diagnosis is not apparent and the patient is clinically deemed not to be in imminent danger, the diagnosis may be established in a rational, judicious approach by means of a combination of serial quantitative β-hCG measurements and transvaginal ultrasonography. A baseline β-hCG level is always obtained if an ectopic pregnancy is suspected and the patient is stable, but this value is rarely diagnostic. Although the β-hCG levels are usually lower than normal in an ectopic pregnancy, the variation of levels at a given gestational age and the usual uncertainty about the date of conception do not allow a diagnosis with one level. If the turnaround time for the β-hCG level is short, then the clinician may wish to wait for the value before ordering ultrasonography. When the β-hCG level is 1,500 to 2,000 mIU/mL, transvaginal ultrasonography can detect almost 100% of cases of normal intrauterine pregnancy. If no intrauterine pregnancy is apparent, then the diagnosis is almost certainly abortion or ectopic pregnancy. If transvaginal ultrasonography is unavailable, then abdominal ultrasonography may be used, but it does not reliably detect an intrauterine pregnancy until the β-hCG level is 6,500 mIU/mL or higher. In most patients

TABLE 20.7. Lower Limits of Percentage Increase in β-Human Chorionic Gonadotropin Levels Early in Pregnancy[a]

Sampling interval (d)	Percentage increase (%)
1	29
2	66
3	114
4	175
5	255

[a] In 85% of normal pregnancies, the increase is greater than these lower limits.
Source: Adapted from Kadar N, Caldwell BV, Romero R. A method of screening for ectopic pregnancy and its indications. *Obstet Gynecol* 1981;58:162, with permission.

with an ectopic pregnancy, the β-hCG level does not become this high.

If the initial β-hCG level is less than 1,500 mIU/mL, the fact that the β-hCG levels double about every 48 hours may be used to aid in the diagnosis (Table 20.7). In a classic study, the levels failed to increase 66% or more within 2 days in only 15% of normal pregnancies, and the normal increase in β-hCG was noted in only 13% of ectopic pregnancies. Following the doubling times allows continued observation so long as the patient is stable until a β-hCG level of 2,000 mIU/mL is reached and ultrasonography can confirm an intrauterine pregnancy. Prolongation of the normal doubling time indicates an abnormal pregnancy, and intervention with dilation and curettage or laparoscopy, if clinically indicated, can be undertaken to allow a definitive diagnosis and treatment.

It has been suggested that the progesterone levels may also be useful in the evaluation of patients with a suspected ectopic pregnancy. A single measurement that is pathologically low suggests an inevitable abortion or an ectopic pregnancy. Published pathologically low values are 5 to 9 mg/mL, but each institution should establish its own levels. A normal progesterone level is not diagnostic because it may be consistent with normal pregnancy, inevitable abortion, or ectopic pregnancy. Following the progesterone levels to observe a pathologic decline does not seem to offer any additional benefit over following the β-hCG levels alone.

Ultrasonography is probably most useful when combined with measurement of the β-hCG levels. However, in some cases, it reveals an adnexal gestational sac and leads to a direct diagnosis of ectopic pregnancy, as was reported in up to 65% of cases in one series, although a direct diagnosis by ultrasonography is usually made much less often. Ultrasonography may also show free blood in the pelvis, suggesting an ectopic pregnancy and indicating surgical exploration.

Laparoscopy as a diagnostic technique is accurate but has been reported to miss 2% to 5% of ectopic pregnancies. It has the advantage of allowing treatment via laparoscopy if an ectopic pregnancy is diagnosed.

Many algorithms have been proposed for the diagnosis of ectopic pregnancy (Fig. 20.6) and may assist the clinician in organizing the diagnostic evaluation. The clinician caring for a woman whose differential diagnosis includes ectopic pregnancy should fully understand the utility and pitfalls of the available diagnostic tests, particularly the β-hCG levels and ultrasonography, and should tailor the evaluation to the clinical situation.

Treatment

Surgical removal remains the mainstay of current therapy, but medical management has assumed a greater role. Radical surgical therapy consists of removal of the involved fallopian tube, sometimes with the ipsilateral ovary, or hysterectomy and salpingo-oophorectomy. Radical therapy is not usually indicated, but if the fallopian tube has ruptured or if no further pregnancies are desired, then complete or partial salpingectomy may be appropriate. If the ovary is intimately involved in the adnexal pathology, oophorectomy is occasionally necessary. No evidence suggests that removing the ipsilateral ovary decreases the risk for a subsequent ectopic pregnancy, so prophylactic oophorectomy is not indicated. Occasionally, significant uterine pathology coincident with an ectopic pregnancy may justify a hysterectomy, but in general, the additional morbidity of a hysterectomy is not justified, particularly in an unstable patient with hemorrhage from an ectopic pregnancy.

Conservative surgical therapy is treatment with preservation of the fallopian tube. Either salpingostomy (incision into the tube without subsequent closure of the incision) or salpingotomy (incision into the tube with subsequent closure of the incision) may be performed. Because the outcomes and sequelae appear to be the same with either procedure, salpingostomy is usually preferred because it is simpler and faster. Hemostasis is sometimes difficult to obtain with either procedure, so that a segmental salpingectomy is required; this may also be necessary in cases of tubal rupture. If preservation of fertility is desired, segmental resection is preferred to complete salpingectomy because reanastomosis is then possible.

Laparoscopy is usually preferable to laparotomy because less blood is lost and the hospital stay is shorter. Salpingostomy, salpingotomy, segmental salpingectomy, and total salpingectomy may all be performed laparoscopically. If the patient is hemodynamically unstable or if a skilled laparoscopic surgical team is unavailable, laparotomy is still appropriate. Regardless of the incisional approach, if fertility is to be preserved, then the microsurgical principles of using a fine, nonreactive suture material, obtaining complete hemostasis, and causing minimal tissue trauma, destruction, and drying should be followed.

In cases of interstitial or cornual implantation, wedge or cornual resection is usually necessary. Preoperative and intraoperative bleeding may be massive because the myometrium and large uterine vessels are involved. These cases have been managed laparoscopically but are more difficult and should be treated via laparotomy except by a very skilled laparoscopic team. Attempts to reimplant the tube at the time of the primary operation are discouraged; this may be done later if indicated.

Medical therapy of unruptured ectopic pregnancy with methotrexate was introduced in 1982 and has become popular. Its major advantage is the avoidance of surgery and anesthesia. Subsequent rates of conception and intrauterine pregnancy are comparable with those after surgical therapy. Numerous protocols have been used, but two appear to be the most practical clinically: a high dose of methotrexate with citrovorum rescue and a single low dose of methotrexate. Tables 20.8 and 20.9 provide two examples of such protocols. Treatment with methotrexate fails in up to 10% of cases, and hemorrhage sometimes requires transfusion and emergency surgery. These complications can be avoided by careful patient selection and follow-up. It is probably wisest not to give methotrexate if an adnexal mass is larger than 3.5 cm, a fetal heart-

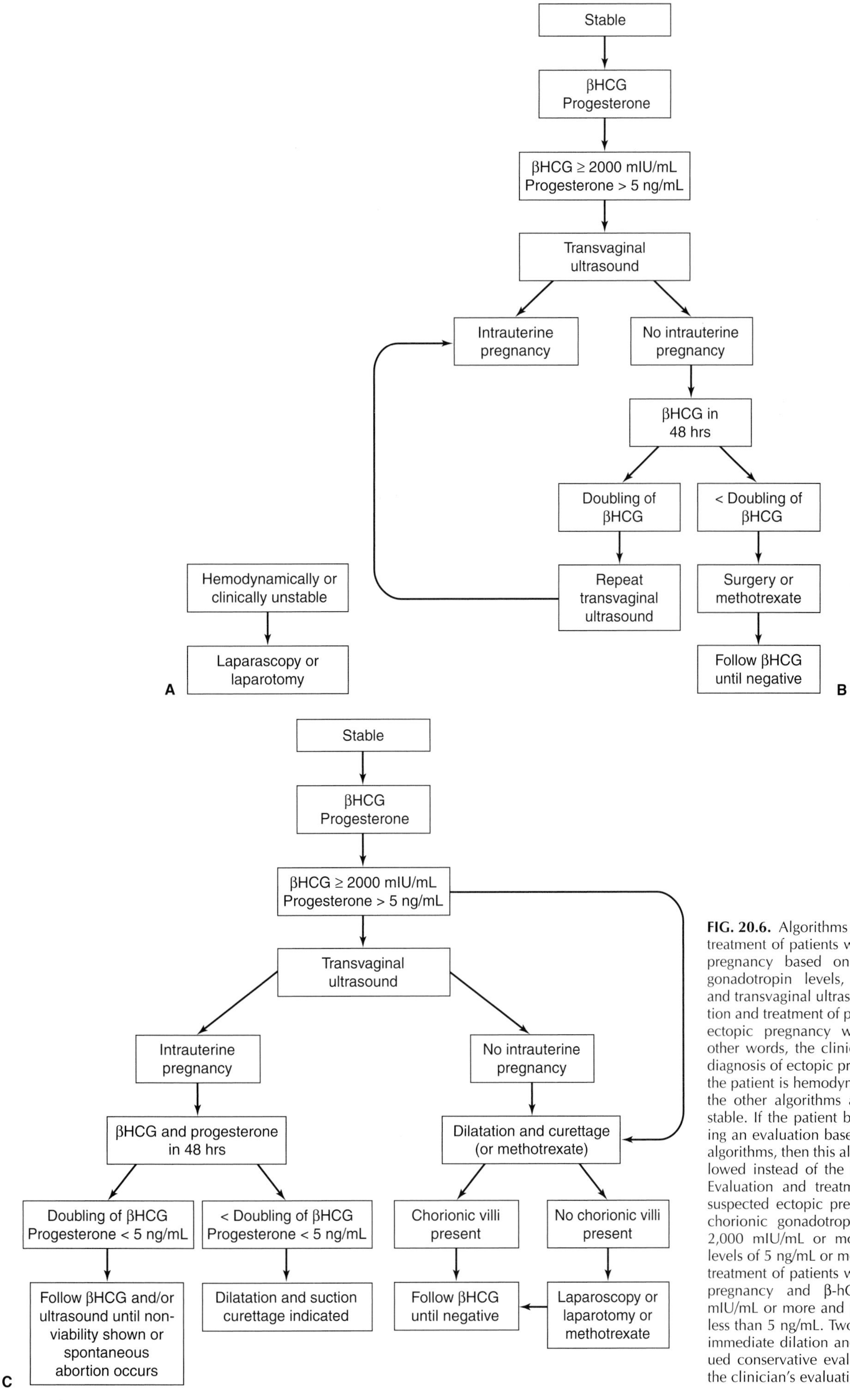

FIG. 20.6. Algorithms for the evaluation and treatment of patients with suspected ectopic pregnancy based on β-human chorionic gonadotropin levels, progesterone levels, and transvaginal ultrasonography. **A:** Evaluation and treatment of patients with suspected ectopic pregnancy who are unstable—in other words, the clinical findings make the diagnosis of ectopic pregnancy very likely or the patient is hemodynamically unstable. All the other algorithms assume the patient is stable. If the patient becomes unstable during an evaluation based on any of the other algorithms, then this algorithm should be followed instead of the original algorithm. **B:** Evaluation and treatment of patients with suspected ectopic pregnancy and β-human chorionic gonadotropin (β-hCG) levels of 2,000 mIU/mL or more and progesterone levels of 5 ng/mL or more. **C:** Evaluation and treatment of patients with suspected ectopic pregnancy and β-hCG levels of 2,000 mIU/mL or more and progesterone levels of less than 5 ng/mL. Two options are possible: immediate dilation and curettage or continued conservative evaluation, depending on the clinician's evaluation.

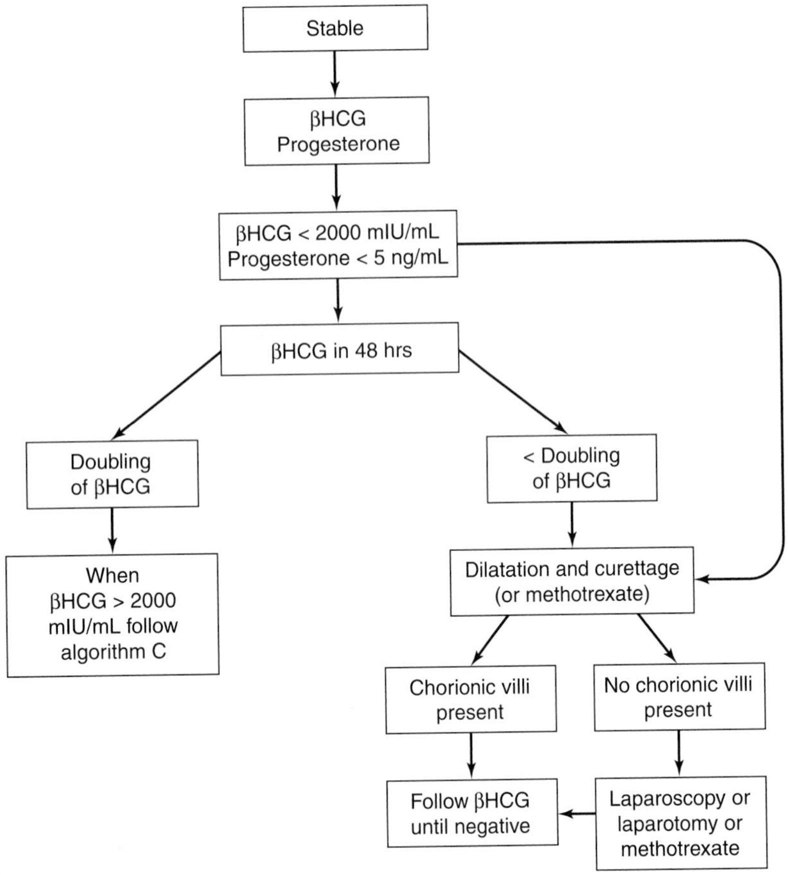

D

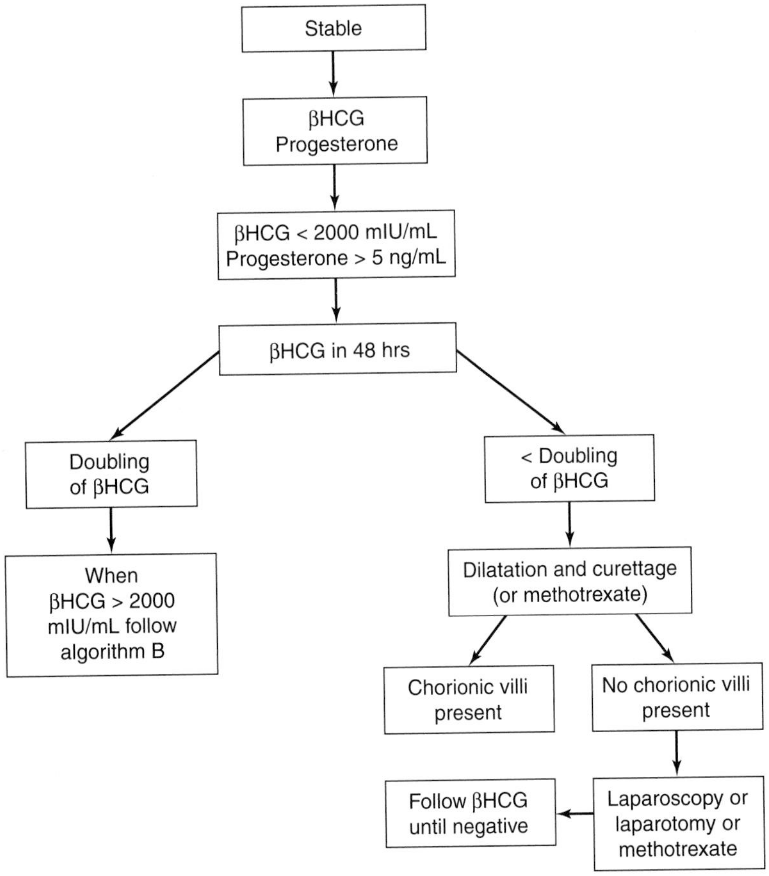

E

FIG. 20.6. ***(continued)*** **D:** Evaluation and treatment of patients with suspected ectopic pregnancy and β-hCG levels of less than 2,000 mIU/mL and progesterone levels of less than 5 ng/mL. Two options are possible: immediate dilation and curettage or continued conservative evaluation, depending on the clinician's evaluation. **E:** Evaluation and treatment of patients with suspected ectopic pregnancy and β-hCG levels of less than 2,000 mIU/mL and progesterone levels of 5 ng/mL or more.

TABLE 20.8. Multiple-Dose Methotrexate Regimen with Citrovorum Rescue for Treatment of Ectopic Pregnancy

Day	Time	Therapy, laboratory tests
1	0800	Methotrexate IM, 1.0 mg/kg CBC, SGOT, type and Rh, creatinine, BUN, β-hCG
2	0800	Citrovorum IM, 0.1 mg/kg β-hCG
3	0800	Methotrexate IM, 1.0 mg/kg β-hCG
4	0800	Citrovorum IM, 0.1 mg/kg β-hCG
5	0800	Methotrexate IM, 1.0 mg/kg β-hCG
6	0800	Citrovorum IM, 0.1 mg/kg β-hCG
7	0800	Methotrexate IM, 1.0 mg/kg β-hCG
8	0800	Citrovorum IM, 0.1 mg/kg β-hCG, CBC, SGOT, type and Rh, creatinine, BUN

BUN, blood urea nitrogen; CBC, complete blood cell (count); β-hCG, β-human chorionic gonadotropin; Rh, Rhesus factor; SGOT, serum glutamic-oxaloacetic transaminase.

beat is sonographically visible in the adnexa, evidence of hemoperitoneum is noted on ultrasonography, or the pretreatment β-hCG level is above 10,000 mIU/mL. Measuring the β-hCG levels daily or every other day is important. Levels that fail to decline by 15% to 20% every 2 to 3 days, or levels that plateau or rise, may indicate the need for repeated treatment or surgical intervention. Side effects of methotrexate therapy develop in about 20% of patients, but with the regimens used, these are minor and transient. Bone marrow suppression does not occur, and the reported side effects have not altered or stopped the treatment.

After conservative therapy for ectopic pregnancy, whether surgical or medical, the β-hCG levels must be followed until they are negative. Because of the persistence of trophoblastic tissue, subsequent surgical or medical re-treatment is necessary in up to 7% of cases managed conservatively. A rising or persistent β-hCG level or acute abdominal signs and symptoms may indicate persistent trophoblastic tissue. Even in cases of persistent ectopic pregnancy, the β-hCG levels may initially decline rapidly. However, if the β-hCG level exceeds 10% of the pretreatment level 12 days after conservative therapy, persistent ectopic gestation should be considered likely.

TABLE 20.9. Single-Dose Methotrexate Regimen for Treatment of Ectopic Pregnancy

Day	Therapy, laboratory tests
1	Methotrexate IM, 50 mg/m^2 β-hCG, CBC, SGOT, BUN, creatinine
2	β-hCG
4	β-hCG
7	β-hCG
8	Repeat protocol if <15% drop in β-hCG between days 4 and 7

BUN, blood urea nitrogen; CBC, complete blood cell (count); β-hCG, β-human chorionic gonadotropin; Rh, Rhesus factor; SGOT, serum glutamic-oxaloacetic transaminase.

Similarly, increasing levels after 6 days are very suggestive of persistence. The choice of surgical or medical treatment of persistent trophoblastic tissue depends on the patient's condition and preference.

Observation may be appropriate in selected cases of ectopic pregnancy; up to 60% of cases resolve without surgical or medical therapy. However, the potential for life-threatening hemorrhage is significant, so hospitalization seems prudent if this approach is chosen. A major drawback is that the average time of hospitalization to document resolution exceeds 1 month.

Many treatment algorithms have been proposed, but again, a fundamental understanding of the disease and treatment options and the physician's experience are most important. The algorithm proposed by Vermesh and Presser in 1992 is useful for the clinician who is planning treatment for a woman with an ectopic pregnancy (Fig. 20.7).

All women with an ectopic pregnancy should undergo Rh screening. Rh sensitization may develop secondary to ectopic pregnancy, although the magnitude of this risk is unknown. However, because the risk associated with the administration of Rh immune globulin is nil, any patient with an ectopic pregnancy should be given Rh immune globulin if she is Rh-negative. Before 12 weeks of gestation, a 50-mg dose may be used, but the full 300-mg dose is advised after 12 weeks of gestation.

It is difficult to counsel a woman who has had an ectopic pregnancy about her future fertility because many factors (e.g., age, prior infertility, tubal disease, adhesions, ruptured or unruptured tube) influence the statistics. Rates of repeated ectopic pregnancy are 8% to 20%, with a mean of about 15%. Rates of subsequent intrauterine pregnancy range from 45% to 70%. If the ectopic pregnancy was associated with an IUD, the risk for a subsequent ectopic pregnancy does not appear to be increased. If the woman is parous, the subsequent fertility rate is higher than if her first pregnancy is ectopic. Gross evidence of salpingitis also predicts a lower fertility rate and higher recurrence rate. Diagnosis and treatment before rupture of the fallopian tube improve the prognosis, so every effort should be made to diagnose the situation early and provide immediate treatment.

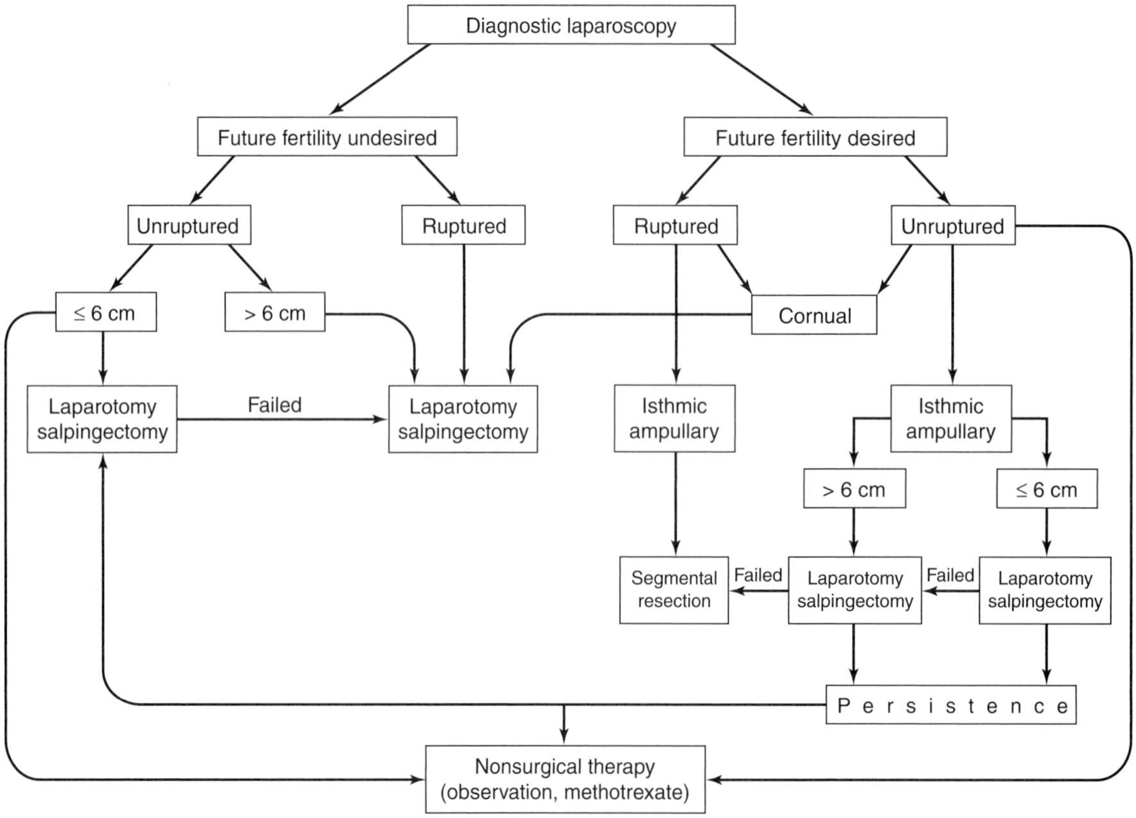

FIG. 20.7. Algorithm for the operative management of tubal ectopic pregnancy. (Adapted from Vermesh M. Conservative management of ectopic pregnancy. *Fertil Steril* 1992;51:559, with permission.)

BIBLIOGRAPHY

Barnhart K, Mennuti MT, Benjamin I, et al. Prompt diagnosis of ectopic pregnancy in an emergency department setting. *Obstet Gynecol* 1994;84:1010.

Ben-Baruch G, Schiff E, Moran O, et al. Curettage vs. nonsurgical management in women with early spontaneous abortions. *J Reprod Med* 1991;36:644.

Buster JE, Heard MJ. Current issues in medical management of ectopic pregnancy. *Curr Opin Obstet Gynecol* 2000;12:525–527.

Coumans AB, Huijgens PC, Jakobs C, et al. Haemostatic and metabolic abnormalities in women with unexplained recurrent abortion. *Hum Reprod* 1999;14:211.

Luciano AA, Roy G, Solima E. Ectopic pregnancy from surgical emergency to medical management. *Ann N Y Acad Sci* 2001;943:235–254.

Muffley PE, Stitely ML, Gherman RB. Early intrauterine pregnancy failure: a randomized trial of medical versus surgical treatment. *Am J Obstet Gynecol* 2002;187:321.

Ness RB, Grisso JA, Hirschinger N, et al. Cocaine and tobacco use and the risk of spontaneous abortion. *N Engl J Med* 1999;340:333.

Ohno M, Maeda T, Matsunobu A. A cytogenetic study of spontaneous abortion with direct analysis of chorionic villi. *Obstet Gynecol* 1991;77:394.

Shalev E, Romano S, Peleg C, et al. Spontaneous resolution of ectopic tubal pregnancy: natural history. *Fertil Steril* 1995;63:15.

Shepherd RW, Patton PE, Novy MJ, et al. Serial β-HCG measurements in the early detection of ectopic pregnancy. *Obstet Gynecol* 1990;75:417.

Stovall TG, Ling FW. Ectopic pregnancy: diagnostic and therapeutic algorithms minimizing surgical intervention. *J Reprod Med* 1993;38:807.

Tay JI, Moore J, Walker JJ. Ectopic pregnancy. *West J Med* 2000;173:131–134.

Vermesh M, Presser SC. Reproductive outcome after linear salpingostomy for ectopic gestation: a prospective 3-year follow-up. *Fertil Steril* 1992;57:682.

Washington AE, Katz P. Ectopic pregnancy in the United States: economic consequences and payment source trends. *Obstet Gynecol* 1993;81:287.

Westrom L, Bengtsson LPH, Mardh P-A. Incidence, trends, and risks of ectopic pregnancy in a population of women. *Br Med J* 1981;282:15.

CHAPTER 21

Elective Termination of Pregnancy

H. Trent MacKay

Elective termination of an unwanted pregnancy is one of the oldest surgical procedures known, but even today, the ethical, moral, and religious debates surrounding this issue continue to rage. In recent years, the worldwide trend has been toward liberalizing abortion laws. According to the Alan Guttmacher Institute, 40% of the world's population live in countries where induced abortion is permitted on request (the "least restrictive" category), and 25% live in countries where abortion is allowed only if the woman's life is in danger (the "most restrictive" category). Countries in the least restrictive category include China, Russia, the United States, Turkey, Greece, Singapore, France, Germany, Austria, Denmark, Sweden, and Canada. The countries with the most restrictive abortion laws include Angola, Botswana, Chad, Libya, Mali, Mozambique, Nigeria, Somalia, Sudan, Zaire, Iran, Iraq, Laos, Lebanon, Pakistan, Syria, Guatemala, Haiti, Mexico, Brazil, Colombia, and Venezuela.

In 1973, the U.S. Supreme Court legalized abortion in this country. That year, 744,000 abortions were performed. Since 1980, the reported termination of more than 1.5 million pregnancies per year has made abortion the most frequently performed surgical procedure in the United States. Despite this fact, and largely because of the stigma associated with the procedure, scientific literature on the subject of the elective termination of pregnancy is scant. Scarcer still are textbooks, review articles, and organized meetings for those who wish to perform this service in a medically safe manner.

HISTORICAL ASPECTS

Abortion was practiced legally from colonial times under the common law of England. Abortion continued to be practiced legally after the birth of the United States and well into the 19th century, at which time numerous states began passing restrictive abortion laws. In 1830, the state of New York enacted the nation's first statute making it illegal to terminate a pregnancy after "quickening." The person performing the abortion was criminally liable, not the woman. Early abortion remained legal. By 1850, 17 states had enacted similar laws, and by the end of the 19th century, every state except Kentucky had passed antiabortion legislation. Abortion had effectively been forced into the medical underground, in both the United States and England.

All this began to unravel in the famous *Rex v Bourne* decision in England, handed down in 1939. The defendant, a prominent London obstetrician, performed an abortion on a 14-year-old girl who had become pregnant after a gang rape by three British soldiers. The trial judge, in an unusual move, instructed the jury to consider a definition of "preserving the life of the woman" broader than simply preventing her imminent death. The jury was asked, for the first time, to consider that preserving the woman's life also meant preventing her from becoming a "physical or mental wreck." The defendant was acquitted, and a new concept of "preservation of life" emerged.

The effect of *Rex v Bourne* was eventually felt in the United States, but 28 years passed before Colorado became the first state to pass a liberalized abortion statute. For the first time, consideration of preserving the mother's mental health was added to consideration of preserving her life. By 1971, 17 states had followed Colorado's lead. A patchwork quilt of state laws varied widely in how they restricted abortion. Even among the states that allowed abortion, the requirements varied with respect to gestational limits, the need for hospitalization, parental consent, and residency. When the U.S. Supreme Court rendered its historic *Roe v Wade* (Texas) and *Doe v Bolton* (Georgia) decisions on January 22, 1973, it effectively stripped the states of their power to prohibit abortion, except after the onset of fetal viability. The powers of the states were limited to ensuring the availability of adequate facilities and duly licensed physicians.

PREOPERATIVE COUNSELING

Preoperative counseling must be individualized. Counseling should be tailored to the patient's needs, education, and emotional state. Some patients are resolute in their choice to terminate a pregnancy; others are ambivalent and require considerable guidance. The counselor must maintain complete neutrality about the patient's decision. The counselor's role is not to advocate a particular outcome but to facilitate the patient's decision-making process. Counseling should always include some inquiry into the circumstances surrounding the pregnancy: Was it the result of contraceptive failure, unwillingness to use contraception, forcible sex, or the sudden departure of a sexual partner? In other cases, counseling requires some assessment of the risk of roentgenographic, chemical, or alcohol exposure. Counseling may provide information that seriously affects a patient's decision to terminate a pregnancy. Perhaps the most important role of the counselor is to help the patient separate the medical from the emotional realities of this difficult decision.

INFORMED CONSENT

Physicians often misunderstand the meaning of informed consent, generally mistaking it for a signed document. Informed consent is a conversation that a health care provider has with a woman who has elected to terminate a pregnancy. Physicians have the obligation to explain, in terms the patient understands, the substantive risks, benefits, and alternatives associated with elective abortion. The informed consent document, which the patient signs, is merely supportive evidence that such a conversation has taken place.

In most states, a minor may give informed consent to terminate a pregnancy electively. Other states may require some form of notification of a parent or legal guardian. If any doubt arises as to whether a minor, or an adult, is competent (based on her mental or emotional ability) to give informed consent for an abortion, the court has indicated that parental or judicial consent may be required.

FACILITIES FOR TERMINATION OF PREGNANCY

Pregnancies can be terminated in various facilities, ranging from a private practice setting to a hospital inpatient unit. With careful selection of patients and proper staffing, most pregnancies can safely be terminated electively in an office or outpatient setting up to the 18th week of gestation.

Wherever abortions are carried out, the following are of critical importance:

- Properly trained counselors
- A practice-specific protocol
- Well-trained, compassionate, and experienced staff
- Proximity to a hospital with blood-banking facilities
- Parenteral sedation, narcotic analgesics, uterotonic agents, and crystalloid solution and antibiotics
- Emergency equipment (including oxygen, resuscitation equipment, narcotic antagonists, intravenous catheters, and atropine)
- Pulse oximetry
- Immediate access to ultrasonographic equipment
- An adequate sterilizer
- Means to transfer the patient to the hospital in an emergency
- Access to contraception and information regarding contraceptive use.

In many communities, practitioners hesitate to terminate a pregnancy electively in an office environment beyond the 12th week. Often, patients are treated in a hospital outpatient or inpatient department where the necessary "hardware" is available but the trained and compassionate staff critical to their well-being is lacking. The physical and emotional needs of patients must be entrusted to professionals with the proper credentials. Abortion providers must be dedicated to the physical and emotional safety of their patients.

ANALGESIA AND ANESTHESIA

A choice of analgesia and anesthesia should be offered to a patient terminating a pregnancy. It makes little sense to offer a service that can be provided only under paracervical block anesthesia; it is equally punitive to insist that all patients undergo general anesthesia. A variety of methods should be available, ranging from simple paracervical block, to intravenous conscious sedation (with or without narcotics), to full general anesthesia provided by a board-certified anesthesiologist. This approach applies to patients in both the first and second trimesters.

Occasionally, a patient arrives at a facility in a state of terror brought on by innumerable issues, including fear of surgery, anesthesia, and loss of control. Such fear may be compounded by feelings of guilt arising from political, moral, and religious concerns about abortion. In these cases, the patient must be reassured immediately on arrival that

- Every precaution will be taken to minimize the risk for complications.
- The patient can choose from a variety of analgesics and anesthetics.
- The patient will be treated with dignity and respect in a confidential, nonjudgmental manner.
- All possible precautions will be taken to safeguard the patient's future reproductive choices.
- All possible precautions will be taken to safeguard the patient's privacy and keep her medical record confidential.

Some women have difficulty deciding, in advance, whether they wish to undergo a pregnancy termination procedure under paracervical block, intravenous sedation, or general anesthesia. The author's recommendation is that for a patient who has been pregnant for less than 10 weeks, the procedure be initiated under paracervical block, with the understanding that intravenous conscious sedation can be added at any time. The patient is therefore asked to avoid food or liquids for at least 4 hours before the procedure. She must have someone drive her home.

IMPORTANCE OF ACCURATE DETERMINATION OF FETAL GESTATIONAL AGE

Safe abortion services require accurate preoperative information regarding the gestational age of the fetus. The need for accurate information must be balanced, however, against the cost of expensive technology. For example, the use of routine ultrasonographic examinations is not recommended in the first trimester, when a simple urine pregnancy test, combined with the hands of an experienced examiner, often suffices. However, the selective use of transvaginal ultrasonography in the first trimester is highly recommended in the assessment of a pregnancy complicated by bleeding, pelvic pain, syncope, hyperemesis gravidarum, or uncertain dates. Additionally, teenagers, poor historians, and obese and difficult-to-examine patients are best served with a careful sonographic examination.

Because of the potential risks associated with second-trimester abortions, routine ultrasonographic dating is required. The importance of a routine ultrasonographic examination for these patients cannot be overstated. A miscalculation or an inaccurate bimanual examination may result in the performance of an illegal abortion, beyond the limits established by a state or municipality.

TERMINATION OF PREGNANCY IN THE FIRST TRIMESTER

First-trimester abortions are those performed before the 14th week of gestation, measured from the first day of the last menstrual period. These can be subdivided into those performed before 10 weeks and those performed between 10 and 14 weeks (ending at the onset of the 14th week).

Before 10 Weeks

During the first 9 weeks (63 days), pregnancy can be safely terminated by either medical or surgical intervention. For medical intervention, two drug regimens are available. Mifepristone (RU-486) in combination with the prostaglandin misoprostol, although approved by the Food and Drug Administration for pregnancy termination through 49 days of gestation, is highly effective up to 63 days of gestation. The second regimen consists of a combination of methotrexate, an antifolate used in gestational trophoblastic disease, and misoprostol. This regimen is effective up to 49 days of gestation.

Medical abortifacients are important because they offer an alternative to surgical intervention before the eighth week of gestation and may reduce complications and the fear of an invasive alternative. However, more than one medical visit is required, and the side effects, including possible prolonged cramping and bleeding, are not acceptable to all women.

Dilation and suction curettage is used to perform most abortions before 10 weeks of gestation. The safety of suction curettage during the first 10 weeks has been well established; during this period, it is associated with a mortality rate of 0.5 per 100,000—less than the mortality associated with a single oral dose of penicillin.

Up to the 10th week of gestation, surgical abortion can be performed at a single visit without the insertion of laminaria tents. With some exceptions, most abortions can be performed safely with the careful use of a paracervical block anesthetic, with or without conscious sedation (usually intravenous midazolam). Because of its excellent safety record, 1% lidocaine is recommended. The procedure is begun as 1 to 2 mL is injected just under the anterior cervical mucosa to facilitate placement of the tenaculum. The rest of the lidocaine (9–14 mL) is slowly injected in the area of the uterosacral ligaments and the accompanying nerve plexus. The patient is allowed to rest for a few minutes, and then dilation, if necessary, is accomplished with the gentle use of Hank or Denniston dilators (Fig. 21.1). This is normally followed by suctioning with an appropriate disposable plastic suction curet. The procedure can be performed with either electric vacuum curettage or manual vacuum aspiration. Before 10 weeks, it is often possible to perform the procedure with a 5- to 7-mm soft suction curet without cervical dilation.

Uterine perforation is rare provided that the tissues are handled delicately and the position of the uterus has been assessed correctly. Occasionally, ultrasonography is necessary to gain this information in an obese patient or one who is difficult to examine.

From 10 to 14 Weeks

Terminating a pregnancy during the interval from 10 to 14 weeks requires two visits to the physician's office: one for laminaria insertion and a second for the suction procedure. The visits are scheduled 24 hours apart so that cervical dilation can be safely accomplished beginning the day before the suction procedure. Some physicians prefer to use hygroscopic dilators;

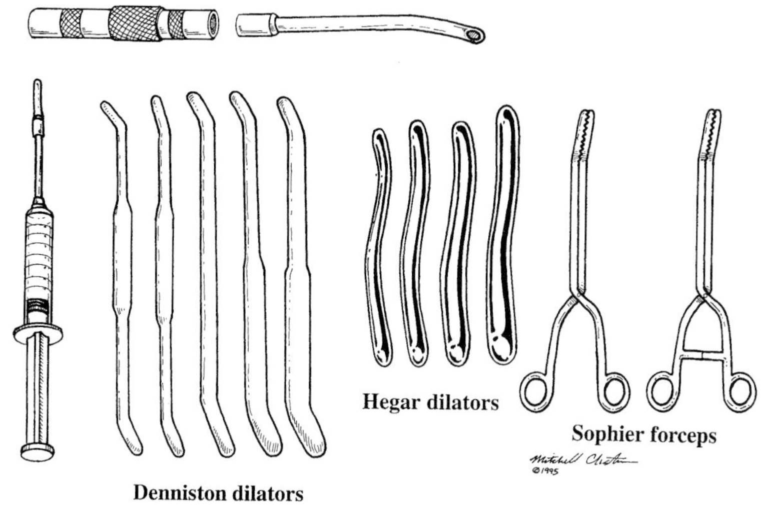

FIG. 21.1. Commonly used instruments for first- and second-trimester abortions.

these accomplish dilation within 3 to 4 hours, and the procedure can then be performed in a single day, which is a consideration if the patient must travel a long distance. Both of these methods safely dilate the cervix and minimize the risk for tears and subsequent stenosis.

Although laminaria tents are occasionally inconvenient and time-consuming to use, and not absolutely necessary before 12 weeks, they obviate many of the complications of aggressive and overzealous dilation of the cervix. Among these are rupture of the cervix, lacerations of the anterior cervical lip, uterine perforation, and incomplete removal of the products of conception. The use of laminaria, therefore, provides an important margin of safety that should not be overlooked. Often, women who have recently delivered vaginally or who have a soft, patulous cervix can undergo a procedure without undue concern for cervical tears. Patients who have demonstrated poor compliance in keeping appointments may be better served by not using laminaria because prolonged retention of these devices can result in life-threatening sepsis. The administration of 600 to 800 μg of misoprostol vaginally 2 to 4 hours before the procedure also promotes cervical softening and dilation.

After an appropriate anesthetic or sedative-hypnotic has been selected, the laminaria is removed. Occasionally, some mechanical dilation is necessary after the cervix has been secured with a tenaculum. A thorough curettage is then performed with an appropriate suction catheter. A good rule for choosing a suction catheter of the right size is to select one with a diameter 1 to 2 mm less than the gestational age in weeks. For example, at 12 weeks of gestation, a suction catheter with a diameter of 10 mm is used. In most instances, performing an abortion during this interval does not require intrauterine manipulation with forceps.

TERMINATION OF PREGNANCY IN THE SECOND TRIMESTER

The safety principles for abortions performed in the middle trimester are identical to those for abortions performed in the first trimester. Most abortions up to the 18th week of gestation or beyond can be performed safely in an office setting so long as appropriate equipment is available, including a pulse oximeter for conscious sedation, and the personnel are well trained. However, physicians who are poorly equipped would better serve their patients by using an appropriate hospital or clinic facility. Although the maternal risks and consequences of middle-trimester abortions increase with gestational age, they do not exceed those associated with a pregnancy continued to term. Most large studies in the United States and Canada demonstrate an increase in maternal mortality from less than 1 per 100,000 in the first trimester to between 2 and 5 per 100,000 in the middle trimester. The lower end of the range for maternal mortality applies to abortions performed before 18 weeks. Morbidity, in contrast, does not vary widely between the first and second trimesters.

Abortions performed in the middle trimester are said to confront the provider with the destructive nature of the procedure, which may explain the paucity of providers who perform this service. Most studies support the notion that middle-trimester abortion by dilation and evacuation is safer than other methods of terminating pregnancy. During the procedure, the cervix is dilated with one or more laminaria tents, after which limited suction curettage is applied. The use of destructive instruments such as Sopher forceps (Fig. 21.1) is necessary to assist in the evacuation of all fetal and placental tissue. The uterus must be completely emptied of all products of conception. This is accomplished by several methods, including examination of all fetal parts and ultrasonographic examination of the uterus.

It is safest to perform middle-trimester abortions under ultrasonographic guidance (Fig. 21.2). This generally reduces the length of the procedure and may play an important role in reducing uterine perforations.

Middle-trimester abortions require meticulous attention to the patient's well-being. The use of sedative-hypnotics, narcotic analgesics, and parenteral nonsteroidal antiinflammatory agents must be strongly considered. Many physicians prefer general anesthesia for abortions performed in this interval. However, except in the most difficult cases, such as those complicated by massive obesity or vaginismus, conscious sedation is preferable because the uterine atony and associated blood loss that may occur with general anesthesia are avoided.

PROPHYLACTIC ANTIBIOTICS

The incidence of infections associated with termination of pregnancy varies with such factors as socioeconomic class, race, marital status, and geographic location. Several authors advo-

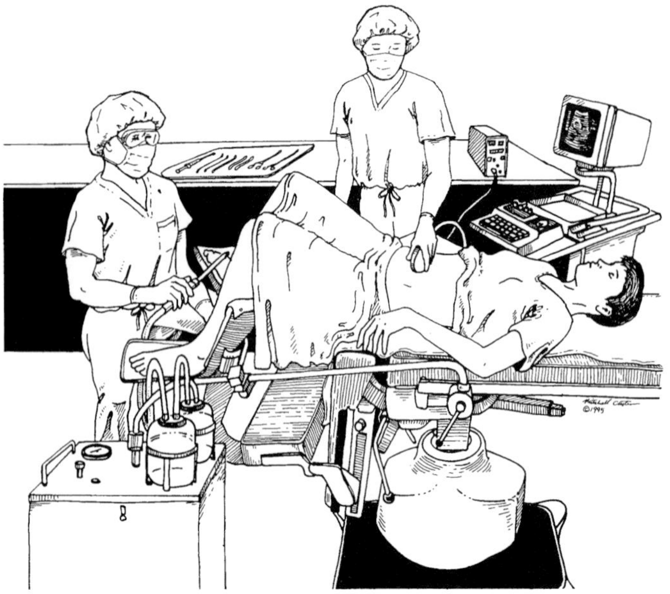

FIG. 21.2. Office operating room setup for termination of pregnancy under ultrasonographic guidance.

cate the routine use of prophylactic antibiotics as a way to reduce the incidence of subsequent endometritis/salpingitis. A variety of antibiotic regimens have been used. A popular one includes either 200 mg of doxycycline or 500 mg of metronidazole given preoperatively. If metronidazole is used, an additional two or three 500-mg doses may be given every 4–6 hours.

COMPLICATIONS

Because of the political debate that surrounds the abortion issue and also because abortion is the most frequently performed surgical procedure in the United States, few if any surgical procedures have been studied as extensively. Among the organizations that regularly track abortions and their complications are the Alan Guttmacher Institute, the National Abortion Federation, and the Centers for Disease Control and Prevention. Most state health departments collect and analyze data on the demographics of abortion facilities in addition to the complications of abortion.

The morbidity and mortality of abortion vary with the gestational age. The mortality associated with first-trimester abortion is about 1 per 100,000. This increases to 1.2 per 100,000 at 13 to 15 weeks of gestation and to 5.8 per 100,000 beyond 16 weeks.

The morbidities most often associated with first-trimester abortion are upper genital tract infections and excessive blood loss. The latter may require repeated suctioning, blood transfusions, or both. Perforation injuries are uncommon, and the rate varies inversely with operator experience. Rarely, perforation injuries lead to subsequent hysterectomy. Other complications of first-trimester abortion include failure to terminate the pregnancy, failure to diagnose an ectopic pregnancy, and severe vasovagal reactions.

Second-trimester abortions carry equivalent complications. However, because gestation is more advanced, uterine perforation injuries and incomplete abortion take on much greater significance. Some physicians use prostaglandin gels or suppositories to perform middle-trimester abortions. These have been associated with hypertonic uterine contractions and lower segment ruptures. On rare occasions, prostaglandins have been associated with the unplanned birth of a live fetus.

Middle-trimester abortions are best handled by highly experienced physicians in an optimal clinical environment. The proper credentialing of a physician learning to perform this demanding procedure requires training supervised by an experienced gynecologist.

Many women who present for middle-trimester abortion are ambivalent about their choice, so that gentle psychological support is extremely important. Other patients require additional education about the need to avoid, when possible, abortion in the middle trimester. For some patients, middle-trimester abortion is a difficult choice that they have made after learning of a significant congenital malformation or even fetal demise. Care must be individualized, and the abortion provider must often coordinate consultations from genetic counselors and perinatal experts.

CONTRACEPTION

Abortion providers must dispense information about various contraceptive methods. Many women accept contraceptive counseling readily when faced with the difficult decisions that the termination of a pregnancy entails. For others, the fear that may accompany the process of terminating a pregnancy does not allow them to absorb and weigh additional medical information for the while. Instead, they may be better served with some written information and a follow-up appointment to discuss various contraceptive choices. For a more complete discussion of contraceptive choices, the reader is referred to Chapter 19.

BIBLIOGRAPHY

Atrash HK, MacKay HT, Binkin NJ, et al. Legal abortion mortality in the United States: 1972–1982. *Am J Obstet Gynecol* 1987;156:605.

Crenin MD, Vittinghoff E, Keder L, et al. Methotrexate and misoprostol for early abortion: a multicenter trial. *Contraception* 1996;53:321.

Grimes DA, Cates W. Complications from legally induced abortion: a review. *Obstet Gynecol Surv* 1979;34:177.

Paul M, Lichtenberg ES, Borgatta L, et al. *A clinician's guide to medical and surgical abortion*. New York: Churchill Livingstone, 1999.

Schaff EA, Fielding SL, Eisinger SH, et al. Low-dose mifepristone followed by vaginal misoprostol at 48 hours for abortion up to 63 days. *Contraception* 2000; 61:41.

Sawaya GF, Grady D, Kerlikowske K, et al. Antibiotics at the time of induced abortion: the case for universal prophylaxis based on a meta-analysis. *Obstet Gynecol* 1996;87:884.

CHAPTER 22

Pelvic Inflammatory Disease

Jennifer E. Kacmar and Jeffrey F. Peipert

Pelvic inflammatory disease (PID) is an infectious process of the upper genital tract and may include any or all of the following: endometritis, salpingitis, oophoritis, parametritis, pelvic peritonitis, and tubo-ovarian abscess. As the most common serious infection in young women, PID is a costly and important public health problem. An accurate diagnosis and prompt treatment are extremely important in managing acute disease and preventing serious long-term sequelae, such as infertility, ectopic pregnancy, and chronic pelvic pain.

ETIOLOGY

PID is polymicrobial in nature. Infection with *Neisseria gonorrhoeae* or *Chlamydia trachomatis* is highly associated with PID. In fact, upper genital tract infection eventually develops in 10% to 20% of women with cervical *N. gonorrhea* or *C. trachomatis* infection. In addition, one or both of these sexually transmitted organisms is identified in the majority of proven cases of PID (up to 75%). Investigators have isolated many other aerobic and anaerobic organisms from the endometrium, fallopian tubes, ovaries, and pelves of women with acute PID (Table 22.1). The type and number of species identified vary depending on the geographic location and patient population studied, the prevalence of lower genital tract disease, and stage of disease at the time of culture.

Most cases of acute PID develop when organisms spread along mucosal lines from the vagina and cervix to the upper genital tract. Chlamydial or gonococcal organisms likely begin the destructive process within the fallopian tubes, which is followed by an invasion of bacteria from the lower tract. Concurrent bacterial vaginosis has been associated with PID, suggesting that an alteration of the vaginal environment with an overgrowth of endogenous organisms increases the risk for upper tract infection. In addition, more than 50% of cases occur within 7 days after the last menstrual period, which indicates an increased risk associated with a break in the protective cervical mucus.

Causes other than ascending sexually transmitted infection are much less common. Hematogenous spread likely accounts for tuberculous infection of the pelvis, an extremely uncommon event in the United States. Direct transperitoneal extension of appendicitis or diverticulitis is possible, but such spread is estimated to occur in fewer than 1% of cases of PID.

Although the exact incidence is unknown, endometritis, salpingitis, or abscess formation can occur after instrumentation of the cervix or uterus that exposes the upper genital tract to colonization by vaginal flora. For this reason, patients should be screened for chlamydial or gonococcal cervicitis in addition to bacterial vaginosis and treated as indicated before such procedures are undertaken. Some experts suggest empiric treatment or prophylaxis for high-risk or unscreened patients at the time of instrumentation.

EPIDEMIOLOGY

Many of the risk factors for PID are the same as those for any sexually transmitted infection (STI). Early age at first intercourse, multiple recent sexual partners, frequent sexual activity, numerous past partners, unsafe sexual practices, and living in an area with a high prevalence of STIs are associated with an increased risk for PID. The incidence of PID decreases with increasing age; 75% of cases occur in women younger than 25 years. The risk for the development of PID in sexually active adolescents is 1 in 8, compared with 1 in 80 for women older than 25 years. Table 22.2 lists identified risk factors for PID.

Barrier contraceptive methods decrease the risk for PID. The consistent correct use of barrier contraceptives and spermicides protects against STI and PID. In addition, some observational studies report that oral contraceptives decrease the risk for upper genital tract infection despite an increased risk for cervical chlamydial infection. More recent data have questioned this finding and suggest that oral contraceptives may modify the clinical presentation of PID. Tubal ligation also reduces the risk for PID.

Reports from the 1970s and 1980s suggested that intrauterine devices (IUDs) were associated with higher rates of PID. Further investigation revealed a correlation with a specific type of IUD (i.e., the Dalkon Shield) that was subsequently withdrawn

TABLE 22.1. Microorganisms Frequently Isolated from the Fallopian Tubes of Women with Pelvic Inflammatory Disease

Sexually transmitted
Chlamydia trachomatis
Neisseria gonorrhoeae
Mycoplasma hominis
Aerobic or facultative
Streptococcus species
Staphylococcus species
Haemophilus species
Escherichia coli
Anaerobic
Bacteroides species
Peptococcus species
Peptostreptococcus species
Clostridium species
Actinomyces species

TABLE 22.2. Risk Factors for Pelvic Inflammatory Disease

Young age (younger than 25 years)
New or multiple sexual partners
Young age at first intercourse
Frequent episodes of intercourse
Single or divorced marital status
African-American race
Inconsistent or non-use of contraception
Previous sexually transmitted infection or pelvic inflammatory disease
Recent insertion of intrauterine device
Recent invasive gynecologic procedure
Cervical ectopy
Current cervical infection
Bacterial vaginosis
Symptoms within 7 days after menses
Frequent vaginal douching
Cigarette smoking and substance abuse
Geographic area with high prevalence of sexually transmitted infection

from the market. More recent data suggest that patients using IUDs are at no greater risk for PID than women who do not use contraceptives when screened carefully for sexual history and other risk factors for PID. Because IUD insertion disrupts the cervical mucous barrier, patients may be at slightly higher risk immediately after insertion.

DIFFERENTIAL DIAGNOSIS

An accurate diagnosis of PID is difficult because the presenting signs and symptoms vary widely. Many other entities must be considered in the differential diagnosis (Table 22.3). Misdiagnoses are quite common (Table 22.4). It is imperative to rule out other possible conditions (e.g., appendicitis, ovarian torsion) as early as possible during the evaluation of a patient for PID. However, because of the potential for severe long-term sequelae if the treatment of PID is delayed or omitted, health care providers should maintain a low threshold for treating suspected cases of PID.

CLINICAL SIGNS/HISTORY

Patients with PID exhibit a wide range of nonspecific presenting symptoms. Some are completely asymptomatic, whereas others present with evidence of sepsis and diffuse peritonitis. Laparoscopic studies have shown no correlation between the number and severity of symptoms and the severity of the inflammatory process.

Most patients with PID present with diffuse lower abdominal pain. This is usually characterized as constant and dull, with occasional cramping, and is exacerbated by movement, coitus, or physical activity. Fewer than 10% of patients report localized or unilateral pain. Typically, they have had pain for 7 days or less before seeking medical attention. About 5% to 10% of women with PID report right upper quadrant pain, often with a pleuritic quality.

Increased vaginal discharge is reported by about half of patients. Examination usually reveals a yellow or greenish tinge, consistent with purulence. Irregular vaginal bleeding—spotting or menorrhagia—is reported in about 40% of cases.

Fever or chills are noted by 30% to 40% of women with PID. Urinary symptoms, such as urgency or frequency, are reported by 20% to 30%. Nausea and vomiting may be present but usually develop in the later stages of PID, when peritoneal inflammation is more extensive.

A careful sexual and gynecologic history should be obtained to evaluate the patient for risk factors. Reports of frequent douching or a history of previous STI or PID should lead the examiner to suspect a current infection. A recent surgical or invasive procedure, such as pregnancy termination, IUD insertion, endometrial biopsy, or hysterosalpingogram, should also raise suspicion.

TABLE 22.3. Differential Diagnosis of Pelvic Inflammatory Disease

Appendicitis
Ectopic pregnancy
Pyelonephritis/urinary tract infection
Gastroenteritis
Endometriosis
Ovarian cyst or tumor
Adnexal torsion
Pelvic adhesions[a]
Chronic salpingitis[a]
Uterine leiomyoma[a]
Intra-abdominal hemorrhage[a]
Ruptured or perforated viscus[a]
Peritonitis from other causes[a]
Diverticulitis[a]
Mesenteric lymphadenitis[a]

[a]Less common causes.

TABLE 22.4A. Misdiagnosis: Women in Whom Pelvic Inflammatory Disease Was Incorrectly Diagnosed Clinically

Laparoscopic diagnosis	Percentage (%)
Acute appendicitis	24
Endometriosis	16
Corpus luteum bleeding	12
Ectopic pregnancy	11
Pelvic adhesions only	7
Benign ovarian tumor	7
Chronic salpingitis	6
Miscellaneous	15

TABLE 22.4B. Incorrect Preoperative Clinical Diagnoses in Women in Whom Pelvic Inflammatory Disease Was Diagnosed at the Time of Surgery

Clinical diagnosis	Percentage (%)
Ovarian tumor	22
Acute appendicitis	20
Ectopic pregnancy	18
Chronic salpingitis	11
Acute peritonitis	7
Endometriosis	5
Uterine myoma	5
Uncharacteristic pelvic pain	5
Miscellaneous	7

CLINICAL FINDINGS/PHYSICAL EXAMINATION

The clinical findings in patients with suspected PID also vary. However, some frequent ones have been identified. The abdominal examination usually reveals direct abdominal tenderness, primarily in the lower quadrants. Rebound tenderness may be present but is not a consistent finding. The bowel sounds are typically normal but may be decreased or absent in severe peritonitis. The pelvic examination typically demonstrates cervical and uterine tenderness with movement and adnexal tenderness on palpation. According to the 2002 guidelines of the Centers for Disease Control and Prevention for the treatment of sexually transmitted diseases, empiric treatment of PID should be initiated in women at risk if the following minimal criteria are present and no other cause(s) of the illness can be identified:

- Uterine/adnexal tenderness
- Cervical motion tenderness.

In any patient at high risk for infection, PID should be considered if pelvic tenderness and signs of lower genital tract inflammation (white blood cells in saline microscopic examination) are noted. In cases complicated by tubo-ovarian abscess, a mass may be palpated, but this is a relatively insensitive test for

TABLE 22.5. Criteria for the Diagnosis of Pelvic Inflammatory Disease

Minimal clinical criteria
Uterine/adnexal tenderness
Cervical motion tenderness
Supportive criteria
Oral temperature >101°F (38°C)
Abnormal cervical or vaginal mucopurulent discharge
Presence of white blood cells on saline microscopy of vaginal secretions
Elevated erythrocyte sedimentation rate
Elevated C-reactive protein level
Laboratory documentation of cervical infection with *Neisseria gonorrhoeae* or *Chlamydia trachomatis*
Elaborate/most specific criteria
Endometrial biopsy specimen showing histopathologic evidence of endometritis
Transvaginal sonography showing thickened, fluid-filled tubes with or without free pelvic fluid or complex tubo-ovarian structure
Laparoscopic abnormalities consistent with pelvic inflammatory disease

PID. Many patients are too uncomfortable for an adequate bimanual examination to be performed.

About one third of patients with acute PID present with a temperature higher than 38°C. In 5% to 10% of women, right upper quadrant tenderness consistent with the perihepatic inflammation of Fitz-Hugh and Curtis syndrome is noted.

Because most women with classic PID exhibit abdominal, cervical/uterine, and adnexal tenderness on examination, these are considered minimal clinical criteria for the diagnosis of PID. Minimal, supportive, and elaborate (most specific) clinical criteria for PID are listed in Table 22.5.

Some reports have emphasized that a substantial number of patients with upper genital tract infection present with atypical or nonclassic signs and symptoms. For example, a young woman with previously normal, regular menstrual cycles who begins to experience irregular cycles or spotting may have chlamydial endometritis. Other patients may present with adnexal tenderness but no cervical motion or uterine tenderness, or with complaints of vaginal discharge and discomfort but no appreciable tenderness. Patients with chlamydial or gonococcal cervicitis or bacterial vaginosis may have silent PID (PID without symptoms), which may explain why a substantial number of patients with tubal factor infertility have no clinical history of PID. Thus, clinicians must maintain a low threshold for the diagnosis of upper genital tract infection.

LABORATORY AND IMAGING STUDIES

Recognizing that the clinical criteria used to diagnose PID are neither sensitive nor specific, the Centers for Disease Control and Prevention and the Infectious Disease Society for Obstetrics and Gynecology have specified laboratory criteria to assist in the diagnosis (Table 22.5). An elevated erythrocyte sedimentation rate, elevated C-reactive protein level, or increased white blood cell count supports a diagnosis of PID.

Cervical secretions should be obtained for *N. gonorrhoeae* and *C. trachomatis* testing and microscopic evaluation for inflammatory cells. A saline preparation and pH determination of vaginal discharge should be obtained to evaluate for leukorrhea (more white blood cells than epithelial cells) and bacterial vaginosis.

Because ectopic pregnancy is a potentially life-threatening process and is still occasionally misdiagnosed as PID, a sensitive pregnancy test should be performed for all women suspected of having a pelvic infection.

Additional laboratory tests may be necessary to differentiate PID from other disease processes. For example, urinalysis and urine culture may be useful to rule out a urinary tract infection or pyelonephritis. In addition, measurement of electrolytes and liver function tests may be useful in patients with upper abdominal symptoms or emesis. Chest roentgenography and right upper quadrant ultrasonography may occasionally be required.

Ultrasonography is of limited value in the diagnosis of PID. However, in patients with a palpable mass or exquisite tenderness precluding an adequate bimanual examination, pelvic ultrasonography may be helpful. In addition, the positive predictive value of ultrasonographic findings of a dilated, fluid-filled tube with thickened walls is high for PID. However, the sensitivity of these findings is very limited. Abdominal computed tomography may help to distinguish appendicitis from PID but should be used selectively.

Endometrial biopsy revealing acute endometritis has been shown to be highly sensitive and specific in the diagnosis of PID. However, clinicians are often reluctant to have a patient with pain and possible infection undergo a biopsy. A finding of acute or chronic endometritis on biopsy can provide valuable information. If the endometrium is sampled, the clinician should begin treatment pending the final histologic results.

Laparoscopy is considered the gold standard in the diagnosis of PID. However, because it is invasive and costly, a laparoscopic evaluation is not often performed. It may be indicated in cases of severe illness when appendicitis, adnexal torsion, or another acute intraperitoneal process cannot otherwise be ruled out, when the diagnosis is uncertain, or when the patient does not respond appropriately to therapy.

Patients with suspected PID should be treated appropriately (see next section) and without delay. Expectant management and observation have no role in cases of suspected infection because delay in diagnosis and treatment is associated with adverse reproductive outcomes. In the study of Hillis and colleagues, patients whose therapy was delayed longer than 3 days were more likely to be infertile.

TREATMENT

Treatment for PID should be instituted as soon as a presumptive diagnosis is made and must provide empiric, broad-spectrum coverage. The Centers for Disease Control and Prevention has established guidelines for parenteral and oral treatment (Table 22.6) and indications for hospitalization (Table 22.7).

Until recently, no data were available to compare the efficacy of oral and parenteral therapies or inpatient and outpatient regimens. The Pelvic Inflammatory Disease Evaluation and Clinical Health (PEACH) Study is a randomized trial of inpatient versus outpatient therapy. Data from this study demonstrate that outpatient or ambulatory therapy of uncomplicated PID is as efficacious as inpatient (intravenous) therapy in terms of fertility and other important long-term health outcomes. However, the study did not include patients with tubo-ovarian abscess or patients who could not tolerate ambulatory (outpatient) oral antibiotics. Thus, hospitalization is recommended for cases complicated by tubo-ovarian abscess, severe symptoms, intolerance of outpatient therapy, pregnancy, an uncertain diagnosis, possible surgical emergencies, or failed outpatient therapy. In general, patients who are unable or unlikely to comply with oral treatment or with complicating medical conditions (e.g., HIV infection) should be hospitalized.

TABLE 22.6A. Parenteral Antibiotic Regimens Recommended by the Centers for Disease Control for the Treatment of Pelvic Inflammatory Disease

Regimen A
Cefotetan 2 g IV every 12 hours
OR
Cefoxitin 2 g IV every 6 hours
PLUS
Doxycycline 100 mg orally or IV twice daily
Discontinue after 24 hours of improvement.
THEN
Doxycycline 100 mg orally for 14 days
Regimen B
Clindamycin 900 mg IV every 8 hours
PLUS
Gentamicin loading dose IV or IM (2 mg/kg body weight) followed by maintenance dose (1.5 mg/kg body weight) every 8 hours OR single daily dosing
THEN
Doxycycline 100 mg orally twice daily for 14 days
OR
Clindamycin 450 mg orally four times daily for 14 days
Alternative regimens
Ofloxacin 400 mg IV every 12 hours
OR
Levofloxacin 500 mg IV once daily
WITH OR WITHOUT
Metronidazole 500 mg IV every 8 hours
OR
Ampicillin/sulbactam 3 g IV every 6 hours
PLUS
Doxycycline 100 mg orally or IV every 12 hours
THEN
Oral antibiotics for 14 days as above

TABLE 22.6B. Oral Antibiotic Regimens Recommended by the Centers for Disease Control for the Treatment of Pelvic Inflammatory Disease

Regimen A
Ofloxacin 400 mg orally twice daily for 14 days
OR
Levofloxacin 500 mg orally once daily for 14 days
WITH OR WITHOUT
Metronidazole 500 mg orally twice daily for 14 days
Regimen B
Ceftriaxone 250 mg IM in a single dose
OR
Cefoxitin 2 g IM in a single dose and probenecid 1 g orally administered concurrently as a single dose
OR
Other parenteral third-generation cephalosporin
PLUS
Doxycycline 100 mg orally twice daily for 14 days
WITH OR WITHOUT
Metronidazole 500 mg orally twice daily for 14 days

Table 22.6 outlines the current recommendations for parenteral and oral therapy. All parenteral regimens should be continued for at least 24 to 48 hours after clinical improvement is noted. A 14-day course of therapy with oral antibiotics should then be completed.

Whether oral or parenteral therapy is used, clinical improvement should be noted within 3 to 5 days after treatment is initiated. An objective decrease in fever, reduced abdominal tenderness, or reduced uterine, adnexal, or cervical motion tenderness suggests clinical improvement. Women treated as outpatients should be followed closely by their provider and reassessed within 72 hours after the initiation of treatment. If they show no signs of improvement, the diagnosis should be reevaluated and parenteral treatment considered.

TABLE 22.7. Indications for Hospitalization of Patients with Pelvic Inflammatory Disease

Surgical emergency (e.g., appendicitis) cannot be ruled out
Pregnancy
Inadequate response to outpatient treatment
Tubo-ovarian abscess or complex
Inability to comply with or tolerate an outpatient regimen
Severe illness, nausea and vomiting, or high fever
Complicating medical disease (e.g., HIV infection)

Failure to respond to appropriate antibiotic therapy may indicate a misdiagnosis or more severe disease (e.g., tubo-ovarian abscess). Surgical evaluation with laparoscopy or exploratory laparotomy may be indicated in these cases. Extirpative therapy is rarely necessary with current antibiotic regimens. Pelvic abscesses may require drainage. This can often be achieved percutaneously with ultrasonographic or computed tomographic guidance or by laparoscopy. Generally, more conservative interventions are preferred.

From a public health standpoint, it is important to evaluate and treat the male sexual partners of women in whom PID is diagnosed. Empiric treatment for *N. gonorrhea* and *C. trachomatis* infection should be offered regardless of the pathogen isolated from the patient.

LONG-TERM SEQUELAE

Major medical sequelae of PID include recurrent PID and tubo-ovarian abscess. PID recurs in 20% to 25% of cases, and the risk for recurrence increases dramatically with each subsequent infection. In addition, in some reported series, up to one third of women hospitalized for the treatment of PID require surgery, usually because of abscess formation. Tubal factor infertility occurs in 20% of women with at least one episode of laparoscopically proven PID. This risk doubles with each episode. The rate of ectopic pregnancy increases sixfold to 10-fold after acute PID. Chronic pelvic pain with an alteration in the daily functional status develops in 20% to 25% of women with a history of PID.

PREGNANCY CONSIDERATIONS

PID is uncommon in pregnancy. In any pregnant woman with a suspected diagnosis of PID, septic abortion and ectopic pregnancy must be ruled out.

When PID does occur in pregnancy, it tends to be a first-trimester infection, although some cases have been reported later in pregnancy. The presenting signs and symptoms are similar to those in women who are not pregnant. The causative organisms are the same and the etiologic factors are probably similar—ascending infections from the lower genital tract that develop before 12 weeks of gestation. Fetal wastage approaches 50% in pregnancies complicated by PID. Aggressive early medical treatment may improve this poor prognosis.

Because pregnant women with PID are at higher risk for maternal morbidity, fetal wastage, and preterm delivery, hospitalization and parenteral treatment are preferred. Of the inpatient regimens described previously, parenteral regimen B (gentamicin and clindamycin) is preferred because doxycycline is contraindicated during pregnancy. In clinical practice, erythromycin is substituted for doxycycline during ongoing outpatient treatment after hospital discharge, but little evidence is available to support its effectiveness in treating PID.

BIBLIOGRAPHY

Blanchard AC, Pastorek JG, Weeks T. Pelvic inflammatory disease during pregnancy. *South Med J* 1987;80:1363.

Centers for Disease Control and Prevention. Sexually transmitted diseases treatment guidelines 2002. *MMWR Morb Mortal Wkly Rep* 2002;51(RR-6):48–52.

Droegemueller W. Infections of the upper genital tract: endometritis, acute and chronic salpingitis. In: Mishell DR, Stenchever MA, Droegemueller W, et al., eds. *Comprehensive gynecology,* 3rd ed. St. Louis: Mosby–Year Book, 1997:661.

Hagdu A, Westrom L, Brooks CA, et al. Predicting acute pelvic inflammatory disease: a multivariate analysis. *Am J Obstet Gynecol* 1986;155:954.

Hillis SD, Joesoef R, Marchbanks PA, et al. Delayed care of pelvic inflammatory disease as a risk factor for impaired fertility. *Am J Obstet Gynecol* 1993;168: 1503–1509.

Jacobsen JL. Differential diagnosis of acute pelvic inflammatory disease. *Am J Obstet Gynecol* 1980;130:1006.

Kahn JG, Walker CK, Washington AE, et al. Diagnosing pelvic inflammatory disease. *JAMA* 1991;266:2594.

Korn AP, Bolan G, Padian N, et al. Plasma cell endometritis in women with symptomatic bacterial vaginosis. *Obstet Gynecol* 1995;85:387–390.

Livengood CH, Hill GB, Addison WA. Pelvic inflammatory disease: findings during inpatient treatment of clinically severe, laparoscopy-documented disease. *Am J Obstet Gynecol* 1992;166:519.

Ness RB, Soper DE, Holley RL, et al. Effectiveness of inpatient and outpatient treatment strategies for women with pelvic inflammatory disease: results from the Pelvic Inflammatory Disease Evaluation and Clinical Health (PEACH) randomized trial. *Am J Obstet Gynecol* 2002;186:929–937.

Peipert JF, Boardman L, Hogan JW, et al. Laboratory evaluation of acute upper genital tract infection. *Obstet Gynecol* 1996;87(5 Pt 1):730–736.

Peipert JF, Montagno A, Cooper A, et al. Bacterial vaginosis as a risk factor for upper genital tract infection. *Am J Obstet Gynecol* 1997;177:1184.

Peipert JF, Soper DE. Diagnostic evaluation of pelvic inflammatory disease. *Infect Dis Obstet Gynecol* 1994;2:38.

Safrin S, Schacter J, Dahrouge D, et al. Long-term sequelae of acute pelvic inflammatory disease. *Obstet Gynecol* 1992;166:1300.

Sweet RL. Pelvic inflammatory disease and infertility in women. *Infect Dis Clin North Am* 1987;1:199.

Washington AE, Aral SO, Wolner-Hanssen P, et al. Assessing risk for pelvic inflammatory disease and its sequelae. *JAMA* 1991;266:2581.

Wiesenfeld HC, Hillier SL, Krohn MA, et al. Lower genital tract infection and endometritis: insight into subclinical pelvic inflammatory disease. *Obstet Gynecol* 2002;100:456–463.

Wolner-Hanssen P, Eschenbach DA, Paavonen J, et al. Association between vaginal douching and acute pelvic inflammatory disease. *JAMA* 1990;263:1936.

Wolner-Hanssen P, Eshenbach DA, Paavonen J, et al. Decreased risk of symptomatic chlamydial inflammatory disease associated with oral contraceptive use. *JAMA* 1990;263:54.

CHAPTER 23
Chronic Pelvic Pain

Fred M. Howard

When pelvic pain persists for longer than 6 months, it is considered to be chronic. For the purposes of this discussion, solely dysmenorrhea (painful menses) and dyspareunia (painful coitus) lasting for more than 6 months are not considered to be chronic pelvic pain (CPP). One or both of these symptoms are often part of the symptom complex of CPP, however. CPP is a common and significant affliction of women. In the United Kingdom, the prevalence of CPP was found to be greater than that of migraine and similar to that of asthma and back pain. In a Gallup poll in the United States, 16% of women reported pelvic pain. CPP is the indication for 12% of all hysterectomies and more than 40% of gynecologic diagnostic laparoscopies. It often leads to years of disability and suffering, with loss of employment, marital discord and divorce, and numerous untoward and unsuccessful medical interventions. Clearly, pelvic pain is an important part of the practice of any clinician who provides health care for women.

CPP is a frustrating problem for most physicians because they tend to think of pain within the context of the classic cartesian model, which postulates that pain is the direct result of tissue trauma that activates specific neuroreceptors and neural pain fibers. It also postulates that the severity of pain is directly proportional to the severity of the traumatic insult. As a corollary, pain that is not associated with identifiable tissue injury is regarded as spurious or psychogenic. This model is not applicable to chronic pain. Attempts to find sufficient organic pathology to explain chronic pain have routinely been frustrating, and the relationship of somatic conditions such as endometriosis, adhesions, and leiomyomata to CPP is at best uncertain. Considering chronic pain solely a psychiatric disorder is also frustrating and not supported by the available scientific evidence. The most useful model for chronic pain is a biopsychosocial one that takes into account the influences of nociceptive stimulation, individual psychological characteristics, and social and cultural determinants of pain.

Observations of psychological changes in women with CPP have led to a search for identifiable psychosocial characteristics. Psychological interviews suggest they are anxious, depressed, and highly dependent, with a low level of self-esteem and a high level of somatization. Psychometric testing shows a characteristic personality profile of patients with CPP, who score high on scales of hysteria, hypochondriasis, and depression. These personality profiles are noted whether or not organic pathology can be found. Such psychological changes tend to maintain or increase the level of pain, regardless of the degree of physical disease. Additionally, when the pain is treated successfully, the hysteria, hypochondriasis, and depression scores revert to normal values.

The diagnosis and treatment of CPP must integrate many influences: the patient's personality and affect, cultural influences, level of stress, organic changes that may trigger nociceptive signals, sensory thresholds or gates, and cognition about pain. Clearly, in cases of chronic pain, no clear distinction can be made between psychological and physical causes, nor are attempts to make such a distinction useful. Rather than try to establish organic versus functional causes, it is more useful to ask in each case whether the patient has any physical disease or abnormality that requires medical or surgical treatment, and whether she has any emotional or psychological distress that requires treatment.

ETIOLOGIC DIAGNOSIS

Occasionally, the primary care physician is the first to evaluate the patient, and a single diagnosis can be made and curative treatment provided. More often, the pain is long-standing, and the patient has previously been given numerous diagnoses and treatments. Such patients often either lack a demonstrable organic injury or disease that accounts for their pain or have organic pathologies with an uncertain relationship to the pain. Therefore, a continued search for one cause is frequently futile. It is generally more useful to evaluate the pain itself as a diagnosis and consider the possibility that several psychological, somatic, or visceral disorders may be contributing to the pain. Many disorders can cause or contribute to CPP (Table 23.1), and a multidisciplinary approach to diagnosis and treatment is usually needed. The primary care physician may have to serve as

TABLE 23.1. Diseases That May Cause or Contribute to Chronic Pelvic Pain in Women

Gynecologic: extrauterine
Adhesions
Adnexal cysts
Chronic ectopic pregnancy
Chlamydial endometritis or salpingitis
Endometriosis
Ovarian retention syndrome (residual ovary syndrome)
Ovarian remnant syndrome
Ovarian dystrophy or ovulatory pain
Pelvic congestion syndrome
Postoperative peritoneal cysts
Residual accessory ovary
Subacute salpingo-oophoritis
Tuberculous salpingitis
Gynecologic: uterine
Adenomyosis
Atypical dysmenorrhea or ovulatory pain
Cervical stenosis
Chronic endometritis
Endometrial or cervical polyps
Intrauterine contraceptive device
Leiomyomata
Symptomatic pelvic relaxation (genital prolapse)
Urologic
Bladder neoplasm
Chronic urinary tract infection
Interstitial cystitis
Radiation cystitis
Recurrent acute cystitis
Recurrent acute urethritis
Stone/urolithiasis
Uninhibited bladder contractions (detrusor dyssynergia)
Urethral diverticulum
Urethral syndrome
Urethral caruncle
Gastrointestinal
Carcinoma of the colon
Chronic intermittent bowel obstruction
Colitis
Constipation
Diverticular disease
Hernias
Inflammatory bowel disease
Irritable bowel syndrome
Musculoskeletal
Abdominal wall myofascial pain (trigger points)
Chronic coccygeal pain
Compression of lumbar vertebrae
Degenerative joint disease
Disc disease
Faulty or poor posture
Fibromyositis
Hernias: ventral, inguinal, femoral, spigelian
Low back pain
Muscular strains and sprains
Neoplasia of spinal cord or sacral nerve
Neuralgia of iliohypogastric, ilioinguinal, or genitofemoral nerve
Pelvic floor myalgia (levator ani spasm)
Piriformis syndrome
Rectus tendon strain
Spondylosis
Other
Abdominal cutaneous nerve entrapment in surgical scar
Abdominal epilepsy
Abdominal migraine
Bipolar personality disorders
Depression
Familial Mediterranean fever
Neurologic dysfunction
Porphyria
Shingles
Sleep disturbances
Somatization

the organizer of a multidisciplinary team. For example, interstitial cystitis, irritable bowel syndrome, poor posture, and emotional stresses may all be contributing factors in a single patient, who requires simultaneous urologic, gastroenterologic, and psychological treatments and physical therapy.

It must also be remembered that acute and serious illnesses, such as appendicitis and cystitis, are no less likely to develop in women with CPP than in the rest of the population. Thus, if the patient experiences an acute exacerbation of pain, it is important to remember to review the symptoms and reevaluate her appropriately to rule out acute medical or surgical conditions.

Adhesions

Adhesions may be caused by pelvic inflammatory disease, endometriosis, perforated appendix, prior surgery, or inflammatory bowel disease. Whether adhesions cause CPP is controversial. Evidence from conscious laparoscopic pain mapping suggests that adhesions may be painful.

Depression

At least 50% of patients with CPP are clinically depressed, and about 70% report sleep disorders. Depression is often overlooked and, when untreated, can worsen or prolong CPP. With somatization, depression may sometimes be an underlying cause of CPP. It may not be a coincidence that sleep, pain perception, and depression are all at least partially mediated by serotoninergic neurons, which may be a unifying factor.

Endometriosis

Endometriosis is the ectopic occurrence of endometrial glands and stroma. Currently, only evaluation by laparoscopy or laparotomy can diagnose endometriosis in the pelvis, the most common location. Biopsy with histologic confirmation is advisable because of the potential error of 10% to 90% associated with solely visual diagnosis at laparoscopy. Not all women with endometriosis experience dysmenorrhea, dyspareunia, or CPP, and it is not known why some but not all women with endometriosis experience pelvic pain. Although published research on endometriosis is extensive, most of it does not specifically address CPP.

Hernias

Hernias may be an underrecognized cause of chronic abdominopelvic pain. Incisional hernias may develop after any abdominal surgery. Spigelian hernias are small, spontaneous ventral hernias that protrude through the transversus abdominis aponeurosis lateral to the edge of the rectus abdominis muscle but medial to the spigelian line. The spigelian line is the point of transition of the transverse abdominal muscle to its aponeurotic tendon. Spigelian hernias are often difficult to palpate and diagnose. Inguinal hernias, either direct or indirect, may also be a source of abdominopelvic pain. Obturator and sciatic hernias may also cause pelvic pain, and both are quite difficult to diagnose. Spigelian, inguinal, obturator, and sciatic hernias may all be diagnosed via laparoscopy.

Irritable Bowel Syndrome

Irritable bowel syndrome is a common functional bowel disorder of uncertain cause. It is characterized by a chronic, relapsing pattern of abdominopelvic pain and bowel dysfunction with constipation, diarrhea, or both. Irritable bowel syndrome affects 50% to 80% of women who have CPP and is one of the disorders most frequently associated with CPP in women.

Interstitial Cystitis

Interstitial cystitis is a chronic inflammatory condition of the bladder characterized by urinary frequency, urgency, and nocturia. Often, CPP and dyspareunia are also symptoms. The cause is unknown. The diagnostic criteria are controversial, but most often, interstitial cystitis is diagnosed when objective evidence of another disease that could be causing the symptoms is lacking and characteristic cystoscopic glomerulations or Hunner ulcer of the bladder is found. It has been suggested that hypersensitivity to potassium chloride instilled into the bladder is a diagnostic finding. Interstitial cystitis may be a relatively frequent diagnosis in women with CPP.

Musculoskeletal Pain

Many disorders and dysfunctions of the musculoskeletal system may cause CPP (Table 23.1). Most of the evidence linking these with CPP is anecdotal. The muscles most often involved in CPP are the iliopsoas, piriformis, obturator internus, levator ani, abdominal muscles, and quadratus lumborum. Frequent periods of prolonged sitting, unilateral standing patterns, inactive lifestyles, and sleeping on the side or stomach are physical habits frequently observed in patients with CPP. These may lead to poor posture, particularly "typical pelvic pain posture," which is a persistent lordosis or kyphosis-lordosis with an anterior pelvic tilt.

Other musculoskeletal abnormalities may be important in some patients. For example, asymmetric pelvic posture resulting from an anatomically short leg may exert traction forces on the abdominal, paravertebral, and gluteal muscles and cause muscular strain and pain presenting as CPP.

In pelvic floor myalgia, tension or spasm of the musculature of the pelvic floor causes pain in these muscles or their areas of attachment to the sacrum, coccyx, ischial tuberosities, and pubic rami. Several factors are believed to cause habitual contraction or chronic spasm of the pelvic floor muscles: inflammatory processes, such as urethritis, anal fissures, and hemorrhoids; general muscular deconditioning and poor posture, as previously described; and prior orthopedic or gynecologic surgery. This syndrome is more common in women than in men (ratio of 5:1) and occurs most frequently in persons between 40 and 50 years of age. Symptoms are often vague, but patients generally describe aching, throbbing, or heavy discomfort in the pelvis, rectum, or lower back. The pain is most consistently exacerbated by sitting for more than a half-hour. Numerous treatments have been recommended with varying success, including rectal diathermy, Thiele massage (rectal massage of the levators), relaxation exercises, immersion in a hot tub twice a day, and pelvic floor training with biofeedback.

Trigger point pain is a not uncommon finding, occurring in up to 75% of patients with CPP. Myofascial trigger points associated with CPP may involve the iliopsoas, piriformis, coccygeus, obturator internus, levator ani, abdominal muscles, or quadratus lumborum. Additionally, trigger points may be found in the subcutaneous tissue on the anterior abdomen within the T11, T12, and L1 dermatomes, posteriorly over the same dermatomes on the mid back, or in the S2, S3, and S4 dermatomes over the sacrum in patients with CPP.

The pain of musculoskeletal problems may mimic that of gynecologic disease in many ways. It may be altered by hormonal influences and therefore be cyclic. It may be dull, aching, stabbing, or cramping in character. It may vary with posture, position, or specific activity, particularly decreasing with rest.

Ovarian Remnant Syndrome

After hysterectomy and bilateral oophorectomy, CPP may be caused by ovarian remnant syndrome. The diagnosis is sometimes confirmed by the finding of premenopausal levels of follicle-stimulating hormone or estradiol in a patient not taking hormone replacement therapy. The diagnosis may also be confirmed by a significant rise in estradiol levels 7 to 10 days after dosing with a gonadotropin-releasing hormone (GnRH) agonist. This syndrome has also been reported after unilateral oophorectomy without hysterectomy, with persistence of ovarian tissue and pelvic pain on the ipsilateral side.

Ovarian Retention Syndrome (Residual Ovary Syndrome)

Ovarian retention syndrome is the development of persistent pelvic pain, dyspareunia, or a pelvic mass after a hysterectomy in which one or both ovaries have been conserved. Ovarian retention syndrome is also called *residual ovary syndrome*. Unfortunately, both these terms are easily confused with *ovarian remnant syndrome*.

Pelvic Congestion Syndrome

Pelvic congestion syndrome is characterized by pelvic varicosities and delayed or slow venous return in the ovarian veins. It may be diagnosed by transfemoral, transjugular, or transcervical pelvic venography. The symptoms of pelvic congestion syndrome are vague and nonspecific, including dull aching pelvic pain, congestive dysmenorrhea, postcoital pain, backache, excessive vaginal discharge, pelvic pressure, deep dyspareunia, and urinary symptoms. Almost all patients either experience postcoital aching pain in the lateral lower abdomen or exhibit ovarian tenderness on palpation.

Pelvic Inflammatory Disease

The chance for the development of CPP after an episode of pelvic inflammatory disease is as high as 30%. The risk increases with the number of infections. Although chronic or recurrent pelvic inflammatory disease is not infrequently diagnosed in women with CPP, the evidence is clear that the pain is not caused by a chronic or recurrent infectious process.

Peritoneal Cysts

Peritoneal mesothelial cysts are rare. At least two distinct types of multicystic masses are associated with CPP. One is related to surgical adhesive disease and is called *postoperative peritoneal cyst* or *peritoneal inclusion cyst*. The formation of peritoneal cysts is an infrequent postoperative complication and has been reported only in women. The other, *benign cystic mesothelioma* or *multicystic peritoneal mesothelioma*, is a reactive mesothelial proliferation and may or may not be related to surgery and adhesive disease. Although relatively rare, benign cystic mesotheliomas have been reported more frequently than postoperative peritoneal cysts. Benign mesothelial cysts have been reported in men but are much more common in women.

Tuberculous Salpingitis

This insidious infection may cause CPP, abnormal uterine bleeding, and infertility. The diagnosis is difficult in some cases but may be confirmed by a positive tuberculin skin test result, an endometrial biopsy showing tuberculous granulomas and acid-fast bacilli, and possibly a positive culture of menstrual blood. Findings at laparoscopy of miliary pelvic visceral and peritoneal disease are characteristic of tuberculous salpingitis. Although tuberculous pelvic infections are now rare, with the recent increase in the number of cases of pulmonary tuberculosis, they may become more common.

CLINICAL HISTORY

The diversity of potential etiologic or contributing conditions requires a multidisciplinary diagnostic approach. The primary care physician may not have the expertise to diagnose or manage all the possible causes but can obtain a thorough, exploratory history that will direct further evaluation and requisite referrals. Although the history is directed to the patient's pain, a thorough review of systems must not be neglected. Because pain may be of visceral or somatic origin, or both, attention should be given to a review of symptoms in the gastrointestinal, reproductive, urologic, and musculoskeletal systems.

The location of pain is a crucial part of the history. Any radiation of the pain may also be important. A useful technique at the initial interview and at intervals during care is to have the patient create a "pain map" on a diagram of the human anatomy (Fig. 23.1). Other locations of pain are often revealed in this manner. For example, up to 60% of women with CPP also have headaches, and up to 90% have backaches. The location of chronic pain is sometimes, although not always, useful in the

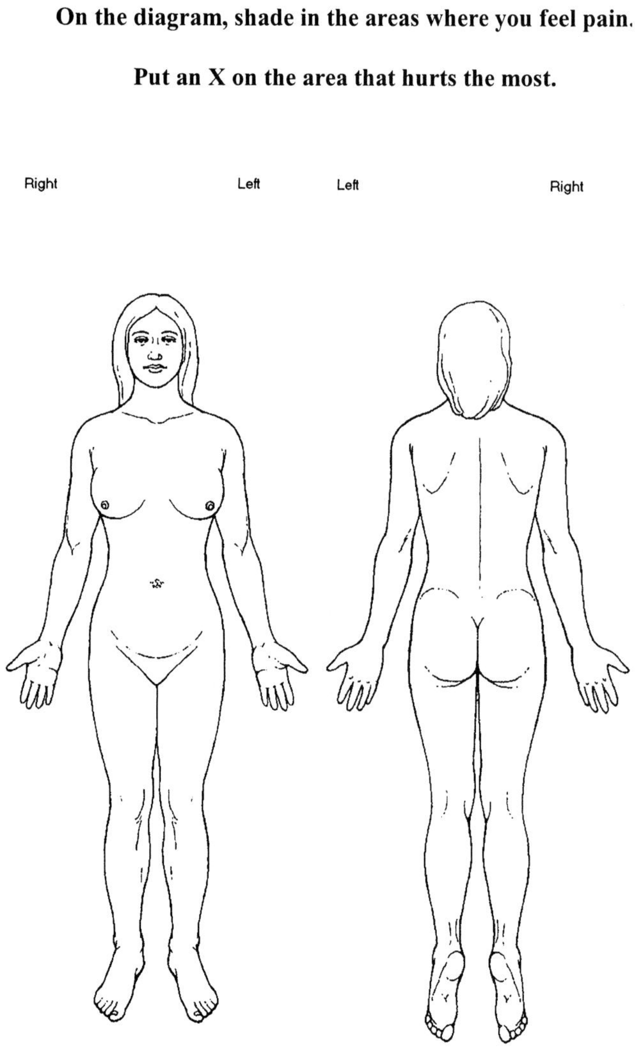
On the diagram, shade in the areas where you feel pain.
Put an X on the area that hurts the most.
Right
Left
Left
Right

FIG. 23.1. Example of an instrument used to document the location of chronic pelvic pain.

differential diagnosis. Visceral pain is not as well localized as somatic pain, so patients with chronic pain and visceral pathology may have trouble localizing their pain. Lateral pelvic pain is often of adnexal or sigmoid colonic origin. Midline infraumbilical pain is often caused by disease of the uterus and cervix. Pain from the bladder or vagina may localize over the mons pubis, pubic bone, or groin. Lower sacral and midline pain may be from the uterosacral ligaments and posterior cul-de-sac. Descriptions of pain that is both ventral and dorsal often suggest intrapelvic pathology, whereas low back pain alone suggests a musculoskeletal origin.

The severity, frequency, and timing of pain should be investigated. Determining whether the pain is constant or cyclic is useful; for example, the examiner asks if the symptoms are the same 24 hours a day, 7 days a week, every week. Stress-related and musculoskeletal pain may vary with the day of the week and the corresponding level of work or activity. The patient should use some type of rating system for her pain and other symptoms. Either a visual or verbal analogue scale, with ratings from 0 to 10, is most often used for pain, with a rating of 0 representing no pain, 4 to 5 moderate pain, and 10 the worst pain possible. A simple "no pain, mild pain, moderate pain, severe pain" rating system may also suffice. In the McGill Pain Questionnaire, the patient uses "mild," "discomforting," "distressing," "horrible," and "excruciating" as descriptors or ratings of the degree of pain.

The quality or nature of pain should be sought. For example, the pain of cutaneous nerve entrapment is often described as sharp, piercing, or burning. The patient should be asked about factors that provoke, intensify, and palliate the pain. For example, rest often relieves pain of musculoskeletal or adnexal origin but has no effect on pain of mostly psychological origin. Questions about the amount, type, and effectiveness of pain medications should be included in this part of the history.

The primary care physician should explore aspects of the psychosocial history. Sexuality, abuse (physical or sexual), health habits, sleep habits, depression, and anxiety are some of the areas that may be evaluated. It is important to assess the consequences of the patient's pain on her functional ability. The degree of incapacity caused by the pain, especially as it affects work and family roles, appears to be a significant indicator of success of traditional treatment. It is particularly important to seek symptoms of depression, not only because of the association of depression and chronic pain but also because a large percentage of depressed patients consult their primary care physician 1 to 2 months before they commit suicide.

During the history and discussion, nothing should be dismissed as ridiculous, impossible, or unimportant. Communicating such an attitude to the patient is counterproductive and only creates distrust. It is important that the examiner be tolerant while listening to the patient relate and interpret her history. A major goal in caring for women with CPP is to establish rapport. For this reason, even though a questionnaire may be very helpful for a busy primary care practitioner, it must not replace a conversation with the patient in which she is allowed to tell her story directly to the physician.

CLINICAL FINDINGS

A major goal of the examination of a patient with pain is to detect the exact location or locations of pain and tenderness. This requires a systematic and methodic attempt to duplicate the pain by movement and palpation.

Ideally, the examination should start as the patient enters the office or examination room. Gait and posture are observed, especially any limp, altered or asymmetric gait, lordosis, kyphosis-lordosis, scoliosis, or standing on one leg. It may be helpful to evaluate forward bending. Normally, this reverses the concave lumbar lordotic curve, but in patients with the typical posture of pelvic pain, the reversal does not occur and the curvature remains convex during forward bending. The primary care physician can also evaluate unequal iliac crest heights by placing flattened palms on the superior aspects of the iliac crests and noting asymmetry; a difference of more than one fourth of an inch is significant and may be associated with a short leg or a habit of unilateral standing. Also with the patient standing, an evaluation for femoral and inguinal hernias is performed by palpating both with and without a Valsalva maneuver. Palpation for tenderness of the upper and lower back and sacrum should be performed, including single-digit palpation for trigger points.

After the patient lies down, inspection and palpation for lordosis or pelvic tilt are repeated. Surgical scars should be noted. The leg can be flexed, knee to chest, to elicit low back dysfunction, low back pain, and abdominal muscle weakness. Head raise and leg raise can be used similarly. The abdominal palpation should initially be superficial, with allodynia noted. Next, single-digit palpation for trigger points is carried out carefully and systematically and includes the inguinal areas. This technique is also used to localize cutaneous nerve entrapment. The point of maximal tenderness is localized with one finger, and the patient confirms that palpation here duplicates her pain. The abdominal wall tenderness test may be useful in distinguishing abdominal wall (myofascial) tenderness from visceral tenderness. In this test, while the area of abdominal tenderness is palpated, the patient tenses her abdominal muscles voluntarily or by raising her head or legs. A lack of change or increase in the pain suggests that the patient has no intra-abdominal disease and that the pain is of myofascial origin. A decrease in the pain suggests the presence of intra-abdominal disease. Any myofascial pain suggested by the abdominal wall tenderness test may be caused by muscular strain, nerve entrapment, viral myositis, trauma, rupture of the epigastric artery, or an abdominal wall hernia in addition to myofascial trigger points. Palpation to detect hernial defects should be performed, including careful palpation of any surgical scars.

The usual components of the abdominal examination should not be neglected. Examination for distention, bowel sounds, shifting dullness, and vascular bruits and palpation for deep tenderness, guarding, and rigidity are essential. A palpable, tender sigmoid colon may suggest irritable bowel syndrome.

The external genitalia should be visually inspected, and any redness, discharge, abscess formation, excoriation, atrophic changes (thinning, paleness, loss of vaginal rugae, protruding urethral mucosa), or signs of trauma particularly noted. Any fistulae and fissures should also be noted and may rarely be the first objective evidence of inflammatory bowel disease. A cotton applicator may be used to evaluate the vestibule for the localized tenderness of vulvar vestibulitis (Fig. 23.2).

The traditional speculum examination is performed to allow a full visual inspection and obtain the requisite cytologic and bacteriologic specimens. Cervical deviation may suggest endometriosis. Examination with a single speculum blade or Sims-type retractor may reveal evidence of pelvic relaxation.

The digital pelvic examination should always be initiated with a single index finger and any introital tenderness or spasm noted. Next, the levator ani muscles are directly palpated for tone, tenderness, and trigger points. The insertion of the levators should also be palpated if possible, both laterally at the arcus tendineus and anteriorly at the pubic rami. The urethral and trigonal areas should be gently palpated to elicit any areas of tenderness, induration, or thickening. The urethra should also be massaged to elicit any secretions. The "gutter" on either side of the urethra should then be evaluated for any fullness, fluctuance,

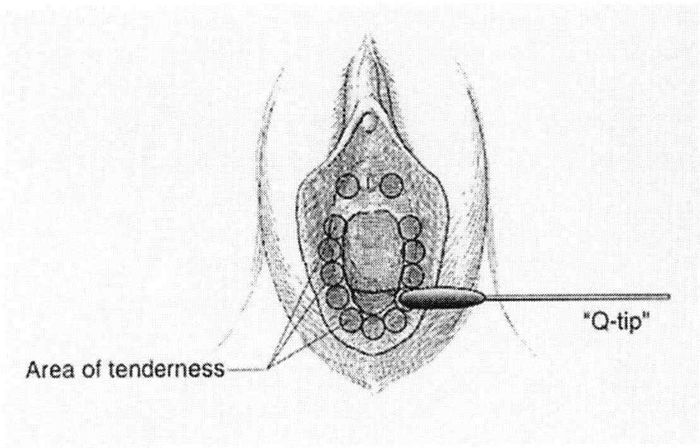

FIG. 23.2. Q-tip test of the minor vestibule to detect the vestibular tenderness of vulvar vestibulitis.

or discomfort that might suggest a urethral diverticulum or vaginal wall cyst. The base of the bladder is evaluated for tenderness. With deeper palpation, tenderness of the cervix or vaginal fornix is sought. The piriformis, coccygeus, and obturator internus should be palpated for tenderness that reproduces pelvic pain.

The traditional bimanual and rectovaginal examinations are the last components of the pelvic examination in the patient with pelvic pain. A fixed, retroverted uterus may suggest endometriosis or cul-de-sac adhesions. Endometriosis is also suggested by tenderness of the posterior uterus, nodularity of the uterosacral ligaments and cul-de-sac, and narrowing of the posterior vaginal fornix. Pelvic nodularity, however, is not diagnostic of endometriosis and may occur in other conditions, particularly ovarian carcinoma. Asymmetric, enlarged ovaries, particularly if fixed to the broad ligament or pelvic side wall, may indicate endometriosis. Bilateral or unilateral ovarian tenderness almost always accompanies pelvic congestion syndrome. Marked discomfort during the digital rectal examination is often noted in patients with irritable bowel syndrome or chronic constipation, in addition to hard feces in the rectum. The rectal examination should also include an evaluation for rectal masses because many colorectal carcinomas can be palpated in this way.

Basic sensory testing to sharpness, dullness, and light touch may be indicated, in addition to testing of muscle strength and the deep tendon reflexes of the trunk and lower extremities. Further neurologic, musculoskeletal, gastrointestinal, gynecologic, and urologic aspects of the physical examination may be indicated by the clinical history. Consultation outside the primary care physician's areas of expertise should be liberally obtained.

LABORATORY AND DIAGNOSTIC FINDINGS

In most women with CPP, cervical cultures or smears for gonococci and chlamydiae, a complete blood cell count, measurement of the sedimentation rate, stool guaiac testing, urinalysis, and urine culture should all be performed. Other tests depend on the history and physical findings.

Imaging studies are useful mostly to rule out specific diagnoses suggested by the clinical findings. For example, intravenous pyelography, cystography, skeletal or pelvic roentgenography, ultrasonography, or computed tomography may each be useful in certain patients but certainly should not be performed routinely.

TREATMENT

Not infrequently, the primary care physician must help the patient with CPP to set clear goals of treatment that are short of a "cure." Examples of such goals are the following: (a) relieve suffering by treating identifiable symptoms and concurrent psychological morbidity; (b) restore normal function without specific goals regarding level of pain; (c) improve quality of life and minimize disability by managing pain and other symptoms with analgesics, physical therapy, acupuncture, nerve blocks, and other modalities; and (d) prevent recurrence of chronic symptoms and disability by means of ongoing compliance and treatment.

Also, as previously mentioned, the primary care physician may have to assemble a multidisciplinary team to treat the patient with CPP. Special multidisciplinary clinics that treat chronic pain are not available to all patients because of geographic, time, and financial constraints. The physician may be able to provide similar, although not identical, care by using appropriate referral and consultation. In such a setting, the primary care physician serves as the ongoing care provider and resource person for the patient.

Surgery

Various surgical procedures, including neurolysis, extirpation of nerves or organs, and selective removal of abnormal tissue, continue to be an important component of the management of CPP, but both the surgeon and the patient must recognize the limitations of surgery.

ADHESIOLYSIS

Uncontrolled observational studies suggest that 50% to 70% of patients with CPP and abdominopelvic adhesions obtain significant relief from symptoms of pain for more than 6 months after laparoscopic adhesiolysis. However, the only randomized study of adhesiolysis (performed by laparotomy after diagnostic laparoscopy) failed to show any effectiveness of adhesiolysis except in cases of dense intestinal adhesions.

APPENDECTOMY

Chronic appendicitis and periappendiceal adhesions as causes of CPP are controversial. Up to 15% of patients with endometriosis have endometriosis of the appendix, but this is rarely an isolated finding. Laparoscopic appendectomy has been reported to relieve pain in up to 80% of patients with persistent right lower quadrant abdominopelvic pain and either appendiceal endometriosis, adhesions, or a history suggestive of chronic appendicitis.

EXCISION OR DESTRUCTION OF ENDOMETRIOSIS

In a randomized clinical trial of laparoscopic laser treatment of endometriosis versus no treatment, 62% of patients who underwent surgical treatment experienced relief of pain at 6 months, versus 20% of the group who underwent diagnostic laparoscopy only. The recurrence rate of endometriosis after conservative surgical treatment is variously reported as 15% to 100%. The average time to recurrence after initial surgery by laparotomy is 40 to 50 months, but this may depend on the thoroughness of the original surgery or effectiveness of subsequent medical treatment.

LAPAROSCOPY

As a diagnostic procedure, laparoscopy serves at least three useful functions: diagnostic confirmation, histologic documentation, and patient reassurance. It also may prevent unnecessary laparotomy and allow simultaneous surgical treatment via operative laparoscopy. Abnormalities are found at laparoscopy in more than 50% of women with CPP who have normal physical examination findings. However, the routine use of laparoscopy for all women with CPP may be unnecessary.

HYSTERECTOMY

According to discharge diagnosis data, about 12% of all hysterectomies in the United States are performed for pelvic pain. In the Maine Women's Health Study, 74 (18%) of 418 women underwent hysterectomy for a primary indication of CPP. Furthermore, 45% of the women who underwent hysterectomy for leiomyomata had experienced pain for more than 8 days per month, and 66% of those with bleeding as the preoperative indication had experienced similar pain, suggesting that in many cases, pelvic pain is a primary or secondary diagnosis for women undergoing hysterectomy. Hysterectomy has a useful role in the treatment of women with CPP attributable to reproductive tract disease. Among women who undergo hysterectomy for CPP, 75% to 90% are relieved of pain at follow-up 1 year later.

OOPHORECTOMY

Bilateral oophorectomy must be undertaken with great caution in young women because of the long-term risks for osteoporosis if they do not comply with estrogen replacement therapy. However, oophorectomy may at times be necessary—for example, if endometriosis involves the adnexa or in cases of pelvic congestion syndrome.

OVARIAN CYSTECTOMY

Benign ovarian cysts other than those secondary to endometriosis are rarely a cause of CPP. Adnexal surgery results in significant adhesive disease, so caution must be exercised in deciding to perform ovarian cystectomies for CPP in young women of reproductive age.

PRESACRAL NEURECTOMY

Resection of the superior hypogastric plexus (presacral nerve) partially interrupts afferent nociception from the cervix, uterus, and proximal fallopian tubes. Presacral neurectomy is particularly useful for central dysmenorrhea but does not effectively relieve pain that is not menstrual or pain that is localized in the lateral pelvic area. The indications for presacral neurectomy are limited and include dysmenorrhea secondary to endometriosis or adenomyosis and primary dysmenorrhea that does not respond to nonsurgical treatments.

UTERINE SUSPENSION

Uterine suspension is usually performed to establish and maintain anteversion of a fixed, retroverted uterus as part of overall surgery for pathology outside the uterus, such as endometriosis or adhesions. It has been suggested that women in whom penile collision with a retroverted uterus causes dyspareunia may also benefit from uterine suspension. The procedure may be carried out via laparotomy or laparoscopy.

Trigger Point Therapies

Injections at trigger points should not be considered curative. They are a means of diagnostically evaluating and then temporizing or modulating the pain response. Reports of effectiveness vary, but Slocumb has reported that 80% to 90% of patients with trigger points obtain partial or complete relief after injection of a local anesthetic. However, if repeated injections are needed, the rate of response declines. Most patients experience recurrences related to stress or specific activities within a few months after successful treatment.

Hormonal Therapies

Induction of a hypoestrogenic state with GnRH agonists, medroxyprogesterone acetate, or danazol has been shown to relieve pain in patients with endometriosis. GnRH agonists may be similarly effective in women with irritable bowel syndrome or bladder pain syndromes. However, in most cases, symptoms of pelvic pain recur within 3 years after the completion of danazol or GnRH agonist treatment. GnRH agonists and danazol are contraindicated in patients who have undiagnosed abnormal uterine bleeding or who are pregnant or breast-feeding. Danazol is also contraindicated in patients with impaired renal, cardiac, or hepatic function. During treatment with GnRH agonists, bone density is lost, but loss can be prevented by add-back treatment with norethindrone.

Suppression of the normal hormonal changes of the menstrual cycle may be useful in women who have functional menstrual pain, such as atypical dysmenorrhea or pelvic congestion syndrome, or who have pain in association with premenstrual syndrome. This may be accomplished with oral contraceptives, GnRH analogues, danazol, or high-dose medroxyprogesterone acetate.

Antidepressants

Antidepressants, particularly tricyclics, have been shown in placebo-controlled studies to reduce levels of pain and increase tolerance of pain in some chronic pain syndromes. The most frequently used are imipramine, amitriptyline, nortriptyline, and doxepin. Doses lower than those used to treat depression seem to be effective for chronic pain. Like the antidepressant effect, the analgesic effect of antidepressants is not noted before 2 to 3 weeks of therapy.

The use of antidepressants specifically for CPP has been little studied. In one uncontrolled evaluation of nortriptyline for CPP, a decrease in the intensity and duration of pain, in addition to change in the character of pain, was noted. However, half of the enrolled patients discontinued nortriptyline before the study was completed because of drug side effects at doses of 100 mg or less. A small trial of sertraline failed to show any effect on the severity of pain in women with CPP.

Analgesics

The optimization of analgesic therapy is sometimes overlooked during the initial treatment of CPP. Often, this is best accomplished with a scheduled regimen rather than an "as-needed" regimen. In a scheduled regimen, effectiveness is improved because the patient takes the analgesic before severe pain develops and does not focus on symptoms of pain (which may actually exacerbate pain), as occurs during as-needed dosing. However, a scheduled regimen also presents some hazards. For example, scheduled dosing of nonsteroidal antiinflammatory medications may cause gastric irritation or renal damage, and scheduled dosing of opioids may lead to constipation, sedation, habituation, addiction, or diminished analgesic potency.

Although the role of opioid analgesics in the management of acute pain is well recognized, their use in the treatment of chronic pain is controversial. Concerns about long-term opioid use for pain that is not associated with cancer include the following: tolerance that results in increasing doses; potent smooth muscle–relaxing effects that exacerbate dysmotility diseases (especially constipation); sedation that limits the restoration of normal function because of debilitating side effects such as apathy, lethargy, and depression; and possible iatrogenic addiction and substance abuse. However, it appears that long-term opioid therapy may allow a return of normal function without significant adverse side effects in patients in whom other treatments for pain have failed. Estimates are that 3% to 16% of patients with chronic pain become addicted to opioids, and surveys show that 50% to 75% of patients referred to chronic pain centers take opioids regularly.

Opioid maintenance therapy for chronic pain should be considered only after all reasonable attempts at pain control have failed and persistent pain is the major impediment to improved function. Also, it appears important that "the committed involvement of a single physician who will evaluate ongoing medical and psychological problems, as well as pain-related issues, should be available before institution of opioid maintenance therapy is considered." A formal written consent or a detailed notation in the chart documenting that the patient has failed nonnarcotic treatment and has knowingly undertaken a trial of opioid maintenance may be advisable. The risks for alcohol or other drug interactions and possible psychological dependence and any pregnancy issues should be explained to the patient before opioid maintenance is initiated. A written or documented verbal contract or agreement with the patient should be prepared that includes at least the following:

1. The treating doctor is the sole provider of opioids.
2. The patient is seen by this physician before her opioid prescription is refilled.
3. Lost medications or prescriptions will not be refilled.
4. The patient agrees she will actively participate in strategies to develop alternative pain therapies.

Some physicians have advocated inclusion of random urine drug testing as a condition of opioid maintenance therapy.

Antibiotics

Antibiotic therapy should be used only when upper genital tract infection is suspected, cervical cultures are positive, or urinary tract symptoms and bacteriuria are noted. Some effectiveness of prolonged antibiotic treatment for urethral syndrome has been suggested. Empiric antibiotic treatment for "chronic pelvic inflammatory disease" is ill advised because it is ineffective. Furthermore, the diagnosis is controversial and greatly overused; the evidence indicates that no chronic infectious process is present in women with CPP after acute salpingitis.

Placebo Treatment

Although many of the therapies for CPP may have a placebo effect, the deliberate use of placebo medication has no role in the diagnosis or treatment of CPP. It is not true that if a patient responds to placebo, the pain must be of psychological origin.

Psychological Treatments

Psychogenic CPP is uncommon, but psychological factors are always important in patients with CPP. Unfortunately, referral for psychological evaluation is difficult. Many of these women have been told, "The pain is in your head," a statement that only angers them because they tend to focus continually on a physical diagnosis and medical cure. For this reason, when a physician fails to deduce a specific physical diagnosis and suggests a psychiatric diagnosis, the patient continues to fear she has an occult disease that is continuously missed by physicians and seeks a new physician who will pay attention anew to her perceived occult physical problem. Even when sufficient rapport has been established that psychological evaluation and therapy can be suggested as an adjunct to pain treatment, ambivalence often makes this difficult to accomplish. Unfortunately, the cost of such care, which is usually inadequately covered by health insurance, may also be an impediment. If possible, it is generally helpful if a psychologist or psychiatrist trained in pain therapy can participate in the treatment plan.

Multidisciplinary Clinics

In planning the treatment of a patient with CPP, it is useful to stress the differentiation between acute pain and chronic pain, both psychologically and physiologically, and to consider chronic pain as a diagnosis rather than as a symptom. With our currently incomplete understanding of chronic pain, it is necessary to acknowledge that CPP must often be managed rather than cured. As previously articulated, management is best provided through a multifaceted, biopsychosocial approach that involves a multidisciplinary team of health care providers. To meet this need, pain centers have been developed where the expertise of psychologists, anesthesiologists, neurologists, and physical therapists is available. In clinics dedicated specifically to CPP, gynecologists, urologists, and gastroenterologists are also often members of the staff. Many women have neither access to nor the means to pay for care at a multidisciplinary pain center. In such cases, the primary care physician may have to try to emulate the multidisciplinary pain clinic approach by enlisting the aid of a select pool of consultants and formulating a multidisciplinary plan of treatment.

CONCLUSION

CPP is a serious problem. It is a much more common affliction than is generally recognized, affecting women more often than migraine or asthma. The estimated direct and indirect costs of CPP in the United States are more than 2 billion dollars per year. CPP is often a devastating disorder for those afflicted, leading to years of disability and suffering, loss of employment, and marital discord and divorce. It is the indication for 12% of all hysterectomies and more than 40% of gynecologic diagnostic laparoscopies.

Many different diseases of the reproductive, gastrointestinal, urologic, and musculoskeletal systems are associated with CPP in women. Primary care physicians especially must be familiar with endometriosis, adhesions, irritable bowel syndrome, interstitial cystitis, myofascial pain, and depression because these are the diseases most commonly diagnosed in women with CPP. Often, the pain is associated with several conditions, so that an interdisciplinary approach is likely to be most effective in diagnosis and treatment. Standardized protocols or algorithms do not appear to facilitate the care of women with CPP and often lead to costly and unnecessary diagnostic studies.

The diagnosis and treatment of CPP can be complex, and the goals of treatment must be realistic. Sometimes, one or more specific diseases can be treated, such as endometriosis and irritable bowel syndrome, but often, the pain itself must be considered as a diagnosis and treated accordingly. Although it may be difficult for both clinician and patient to accept chronic pain as a diagnosis, this is an important concept in the management of CPP. It allows the use of pain-directed therapies that, albeit not curative, permit the patient to progress toward a more normal life that is not dominated by pain. It also breaks the traditional hold of the cartesian model of pain, so that if no organic lesion is found that can be cured, the patient is not led to believe that her pain is not real. Finally, it offers hope that with future research, the psychologic and neurologic dysfunctions responsible for CPP may be identified and definitive, curative treatments developed.

BIBLIOGRAPHY

Al Salilli M, Vilos GA. Prospective evaluation of laparoscopic appendectomy in women with chronic right lower quadrant pain. *J Am Assoc Gynecol Laparosc* 1995;2:139–142.

Beard RW, Kennedy RG, Gangar KF, et al. Bilateral oophorectomy and hysterectomy in the treatment of intractable pelvic pain associated with pelvic congestion. *Br J Obstet Gynaecol* 1991;98:988–992.

Beard RW, Reginald PW, Wadsworth J. Clinical features of women with chronic lower abdominal pain and pelvic congestion. *Br J Obstet Gynaecol* 1988;95:153–165.

Candiani GB, Fidele L, Vercellini P, et al. Repetitive conservative surgery for recurrence of endometriosis. *Obstet Gynecol* 1991;77:421.

Carlson KJ, Miller BA, Fowler FJ Jr. The Maine Women's Health Study: I. Outcomes of hysterectomy. *Obstet Gynecol* 1994;83:556–565.

Engel CC Jr, Walker EA, Engel AL, et al. A randomized, double-blind crossover trial of sertraline in women with chronic pelvic pain. *J Psychosom Res* 1998;44:203–207.

Hornstein MD, Surrey ES, Weisberg GW, et al. Leuprolide acetate depot and hormonal add-back in endometriosis: a 12-month study. Lupron Add-Back Study Group. *Obstet Gynecol* 1998;91:16–24.

Howard FM, Sanchez R, El-Minawi A. Conscious pain mapping by laparoscopy in women with chronic pelvic pain. *Obstet Gynecol* 2000;96:934–939.

Howard FM. The role of laparoscopy in chronic pelvic pain: promise and pitfalls. *Obstet Gynecol Surv* 1993;48:357–387.

Jamieson DJ, Steege JF. The prevalence of dysmenorrhea, dyspareunia, pelvic pain, and irritable bowel syndrome in primary care practices. *Obstet Gynecol* 1996;87:55–58.

Ling FW. Randomized controlled trial of depot leuprolide in patients with chronic pelvic pain and clinically suspected endometriosis. Pelvic Pain Study Group. *Obstet Gynecol* 1999;93:51–58.

Mathias SD, Kuppermann M, Liberman RF, et al. Chronic pelvic pain: prevalence, health-related quality of life, and economic correlates. *Obstet Gynecol* 1996;87:321–327.

Miotto K, Compton, Ling W, et al. Diagnosing addictive disease in chronic pain patients. *Psychosomatics* 1996;37:223–235.

Peters AAW, Trimbos-Kemper GCM, Admiraal C, et al. A randomized clinical trial on the benefit of adhesiolysis in patients with intraperitoneal adhesions and chronic pelvic pain. *Br J Obstet Gynaecol* 1992;99:59–62.

Peters AAW, Van Dorst E, Jellis B, et al. A randomized clinical trial to compare two different approaches in women with chronic pelvic pain. *Obstet Gynecol* 1991;77:740–746.

Portenoy RK, Foley KM. Chronic use of opioid analgesics in non-malignant pain: report of 38 cases. *Pain* 1986;25:171–186.

Sidall-Allum J, Rae T, Rogers V, et al. Chronic pelvic pain caused by residual ovaries and ovarian remnants. *Br J Obstet Gynaecol* 1994;101:979–985.

Slocumb JC. Neurological factors in chronic pelvic pain: trigger points and the abdominal pelvic pain syndrome. *Am J Obstet Gynecol* 1984;149:536–543.

Steege JF, Stout AL. Resolution of chronic pelvic pain after laparoscopic lysis of adhesions. *Am J Obstet Gynecol* 1991;165:278.

Stovall TG, Ling FW, Crawford DA. Hysterectomy for chronic pelvic pain of presumed uterine etiology. *Obstet Gynecol* 1990;75:676.

Sutton CJ, Ewen SP, Whitelaw N, et al. Prospective, randomized, double-blind, controlled trial of laser laparoscopy in the treatment of pelvic pain associated with minimal, mild, and moderate endometriosis. *Fertil Steril* 1994;62:696–700.

Telimaa S, Puolakka J, Ronnberg L, et al. Placebo-controlled comparison of danazol and high-dose medroxyprogesterone acetate in the treatment of endometriosis. *Gynecol Endocrinol* 1987;1:13–23.

Tjaden B, Schlaff WD, Kimball A, et al. The efficacy of presacral neurectomy for the relief of midline dysmenorrhea. *Obstet Gynecol* 1990;76:89–94.

Walker EA, Roy-Byrne PP, Katon WJ, et al. An open trial of nortriptyline in women with chronic pelvic pain. *Int J Psychiatry Med* 1991;21:245–252.

Zondervan KT, Yudkin PL, Vessey MP, et al. Prevalence and incidence in primary care of chronic pelvic pain in women: evidence from a national general practice database. *Br J Obstet Gynaecol* 1999;106:1149–1155.

CHAPTER 24
Vaginitis

Paul Nyirjesy

For any clinician involved in women's health care, vaginitis remains an unavoidable problem. It is estimated that vaginitis accounts for more than 10 million office visits each year, and it is the most common reason why a patient visits her obstetrician-gynecologist. Over-the-counter antifungal therapies rank

TABLE 24.1. Effect of Estrogen on the Vaginal Environment

Age	Estrogen source	Dominant flora	Vaginal pH
Newborn	Maternal	Lactobacilli	<4.5
Prepubertal	Peripheral fat	Skin organisms Fecal flora	>4.5
Reproductive	Ovaries	Lactobacilli	<4.5
Menopausal	Peripheral fat	Variable	Variable
	Hormone therapy	Lactobacilli	<4.5

among the top 10 best-selling over-the-counter products, with about $500 million dollars yearly in sales. Despite these numbers, vaginitis is trivialized by many within the medical community. This lack of interest results in misdiagnosis and mistreatment, which in turn complicate efforts at further evaluation and the treatment of vaginal symptomatology.

Most studies confirm that the three most common vaginal infections are bacterial vaginosis (30%–35%), vulvovaginal candidiasis (20%–25%), and trichomoniasis (15%–20%). The remaining causes of vaginitis include a host of miscellaneous conditions, the most common of which are a heavy but physiologic discharge, atrophic vaginitis, and vulvar disorders.

Estrogen plays a crucial role in determining the vaginal microbial flora (Table 24.1). Lactobacilli, the dominant vaginal microorganisms in healthy women, and their role in regulating the vaginal environment have been extensively scrutinized. Colonization of the vagina by lactobacilli has been thought to be a consequence of the relatively high levels of glycogen in vaginal epithelial cells, which are in turn caused by estrogen. Although previous theories focused on lactic acid produced by lactobacilli and its effects, it is now felt that hydrogen peroxide produced by lactobacilli inhibits the growth of other organisms in vitro and in vivo and is crucial to the regulation of a healthy vaginal microflora.

However, even during the reproductive years, a woman's flora contains a wide variety of organisms. For example, the skin and fecal organisms present during the prepubertal years, such as *Staphylococcus epidermidis* and *Escherichia coli,* remain as part of the normal flora and can be isolated from vaginal cultures with relative ease. Indeed, pathogenic organisms such as *Streptococcus agalactiae* (group B streptococci), *Mycoplasma hominis, Ureaplasma urealyticum, Gardnerella vaginalis,* and *Candida albicans* are each present in about 20% of healthy, asymptomatic women, with wide variations noted depending on the patient population.

EVALUATION

All too often when seeing women with vaginal symptoms, physicians avoid obtaining a complete history, perhaps out of fear of embarrassing the patient or themselves. However, as with any disorder, a complete history is essential to obtaining an accurate diagnosis. The symptoms related to vaginitis include a broad spectrum of manifestations, not just vaginal discharge, irritation, itching, and burning. A thorough historian asks about the nature, quantity, and color of discharge but then focuses on symptoms other than discharge, which are often those causing the patient's distress. Pertinent areas of inquiry include the location of the symptoms (vulvar, introital, or vaginal), their duration, any variations with the menstrual cycle, any association with sexual relations, and their response to past therapy. With the widespread use of over-the-counter antifungal agents, a particularly important question is when the patient last used any treatment, so that it can be determined whether she is partially treated. These nuances within the history often allow a better evaluation.

The physical examination should begin with a careful assessment of the vulva and vestibule, particularly if they are the focus of symptoms. Palpation with a cotton-tipped applicator helps discern areas of tenderness. After the speculum has been inserted, the vagina and cervix are inspected thoroughly. If secretions are present, an effort is made to determine if they are cervical or vaginal in origin.

The laboratory evaluation of vaginal symptoms is summarized in Table 24.2. Each part of this workup is an essential component of the office visit. The experienced clinician can perform all these tests in at most 5 minutes, and they yield an accurate diagnosis in the vast majority of cases.

When the vagina is sampled, it is important to swab its middle third, not the pooled vaginal secretions in the posterior fornix. Because the latter consist of cervical and vaginal secretions, they may hinder a determination of the vaginal pH and an examination of the saline smear. When the swab touches pH paper with a range of 3.5 to 5.5, not nitrazine paper, the characteristic color change of a high pH is unmistakable. A whiff test for the presence of amines is most easily performed by obtaining an additional swab and placing a drop of 10% potassium hydroxide on it, then checking for the characteristic fishy odor. Like the vaginal pH test, this simple test is easy, unequivocal, and underused.

In a few complicated cases, adjunctive studies may be indicated. These include a culture for herpes simplex virus in a patient with ulceration or mucopurulent cervicitis, in addition to cultures for *Trichomonas vaginalis* and yeast. Given the wide

TABLE 24.2. Evaluation of Acute Vaginal Symptoms

Test	Potential diagnostic use
History	Extent, nature, location, and duration of symptoms
Physical examination	Localization of symptoms, abnormal physical findings
Cervical samples for *Chlamydia* and *N. gonorrhoeae* DNA testing or culture	Cervicitis
Vaginal pH	Hormonal status, bacterial vaginosis, trichomoniasis
Whiff test	Bacterial vaginosis, trichomoniasis
Saline smear	White blood cell–epithelial cell ratio Vaginal cytology Bacterial floral pattern Trichomonads Clue cells
10% Potassium hydroxide smear	Hyphae, blastospores

range of organisms that can be part of the normal flora and their potential for misleading the clinician, vaginal bacterial cultures play little role in the evaluation of vaginal symptoms.

A physiologic discharge, the result of secretions from the uterus, including the cervix and fallopian tubes, the glands that line the vagina, and the vestibular glands, can sometimes be quite heavy. Any alteration in these organs can cause a change in the physiologic discharge; the classic example is the heavy discharge associated with fallopian tube carcinoma. More common factors affecting the normal vaginal discharge are age, the menstrual cycle, the use of oral contraceptives, and pregnancy. In general, a physiologic discharge is described as odorless; clear or white; viscous, flocculent, or homogeneous; having little or no odor; and associated with little vaginal pooling. However, normal discharge varies widely, even in the same person at different times. Because American society is often unwilling to acknowledge the existence of normal discharge, women who have no infection may present for an evaluation. Only with a thorough evaluation can potential infections be excluded and the patient be reassured that her discharge is normal. Although it might appear to be easier to take a quick look and write a prescription, the lack of response to inappropriate and unnecessary therapy frustrates patient and physician alike in the longer term.

TRICHOMONIASIS

Trichomoniasis is the one of the most common protozoan infections in the United States, with an estimated 3 million cases annually. Although occasional nonsexual transmission (e.g., fomites) has been suggested, the primary mode of transmission is sexual. Therefore, the prevalence of the disease depends in large part on the overall level of sexual activity of the group of women being studied, with a range of 5% in family planning clinics to 75% in prostitutes. Asymptomatic men serve as a large reservoir for reinfection.

Even in women, trichomoniasis is often harbored asymptomatically. When symptomatic, it can cause an abnormal purulent, frothy, or bloody discharge. Vaginal malodor, pruritus, and dyspareunia are other relatively frequent complaints. *T. vaginalis* can invade the bladder and urethra, so some women also experience dysuria or urinary frequency.

Findings on examination include varying degrees of erythema and excoriation of the vulva, erythema and edema of the vagina, an abnormal discharge, and punctate hemorrhage of the cervix ("strawberry cervix"). This latter feature, considered pathognomonic for trichomoniasis, is noted in about 2% of cases. In most offices, the diagnosis ultimately rests the detection of live motile trichomonads on a wet smear examined under the microscope. Additional microscopic findings include an increase in white blood cells and a shift away from the normal bacillary flora. Unfortunately, the sensitivity of the wet smear is relatively poor (22%–76%). Although a positive whiff test and an elevated pH are helpful clues if the smear is negative, they do not distinguish between trichomoniasis and bacterial vaginosis. The sensitivity of the Papanicolaou smear is higher, but its false-positive rate is about 20%. The gap between these two methods of detection can be bridged by culture systems, a sensitive method of detection. They are affordable and easy to use, but unfortunately they are not always readily available. Newer tests for *T. vaginalis* are currently under development.

The only medication available in the United States that is effective against *T. vaginalis* is metronidazole. The most commonly prescribed regimen, a single oral 2-g dose, achieves a cure in more than 90% of cases if sexual partners are treated simultaneously. Common side effects of metronidazole, especially at higher doses, include nausea, a disulfiram-like effect if alcohol is ingested, and a metallic taste. Patients who are allergic to metronidazole can frequently be managed with either oral or intravenous desensitization protocols. For patients who fail this treatment, the standard therapy consists of 500 mg twice a day for 7 days, after reinfection from the partner has been excluded as the cause of failure. For patients with metronidazole-resistant infections, increased doses may be required. If higher doses fail to effect a cure, therapy with tinidazole, a nitroimidazole agent not currently marketed in the United States, is frequently effective.

Although case control studies have failed to reveal an association between birth defects and metronidazole, this drug is generally avoided in the first trimester of pregnancy because it has shown mutagenic activity in in vitro assay systems. In a severely symptomatic patient in early pregnancy, topical clotrimazole or douches with pH-lowering solutions such as vinegar may inhibit growth sufficiently to alleviate symptoms. In large studies evaluating infection, pregnancy, and outcome of pregnancy, trichomoniasis has been associated with preterm delivery, preterm premature rupture of membranes, and low-birth-weight infants. However, the only prospective randomized study to evaluate the effect of metronidazole treatment on asymptomatic trichomoniasis in pregnancy demonstrated a potential increase in adverse outcomes.

BACTERIAL VAGINOSIS

Bacterial vaginosis (BV), formerly known as *nonspecific vaginitis* or *Gardnerella vaginitis,* is a polymicrobial infection of the vagina. As its name suggests, this is an abnormal condition of the vagina marked by a paucity or absence of hydrogen peroxide-producing lactobacilli and a subsequent overgrowth of facultative anaerobic organisms. Gardner and Dukes initially implicated *Gardnerella vaginalis* (then known as *Haemophilus vaginalis*) as the causative organism, but subsequent studies and the realization that *G. vaginalis* did not actually fulfill Koch's postulates demonstrated that the organism is not the cause of this syndrome. Rather, a multitude of organisms, including *G. vaginalis,* genital mycoplasmata, *Mobiluncus* species, *Bacteroides* species, and other anaerobes, appear to act synergistically to produce this syndrome.

The prevalence of this infection is highly variable. As in patients with trichomoniasis, the prevalence is related to the general level of sexual activity, with 5% noted in college populations and up to 60% in clinics treating patients with sexually transmitted disease. However, whether BV is sexually transmitted remains controversial. It is rare in women who have never been sexually active, and it is associated with multiple sexual partners. Furthermore, studies have shown that relatively frequent intercourse and intercourse with a new partner are associated with a loss of hydrogen peroxide–producing lactobacilli, and such loss may represent the first step toward the development of BV. BV is found in virginal women, and treatment of the male partner has not prevented recurrences.

Up to 50% of women with BV are asymptomatic. Women with symptoms have a profuse, malodorous discharge. The fishy odor may be more noticeable during menses or after intercourse, when the high pH of blood or semen increases the volatility of the amines that cause the odor. Although it is not part of the classic description, itching is reported in up to 67% of cases.

The diagnosis of BV is based on the clinical findings, not on a positive culture for *Mycoplasma* or *Gardnerella.* Three of the four following conditions should be met: presence of a homogeneous gray or white discharge, a vaginal pH above 4.5, a positive whiff test, and more than 20% clue cells on a wet preparation. In addition, a shift from the normal bacillary flora to a coccobacillary pattern is noted, along with an increase in flora on the smear. If performed as an ancillary test or as part of a research protocol, a Gram stain will demonstrate this shift in flora more clearly than saline microscopy.

Acceptable treatment regimens include the following: 500 mg of metronidazole twice a day for 7 days, one 5-g applicator of 0.75% metronidazole gel daily for 5 days, one 5-g applicator of 2% clindamycin cream for 7 days, 100-mg clindamycin ovules intravaginally for 3 days, and 300 mg of clindamycin twice a day for 7 days. The current treatment guidelines from the Centers for Disease Control and Prevention prefer the metronidazole-containing regimens. Vulvovaginal candidiasis as a sequela of therapy develops in up to 10% of treated patients. *Clostridium difficile* colitis has occurred rarely after therapy with clindamycin cream.

In the past decade, the awareness of BV has been increasing because of its consistent association with many of the infectious morbid conditions of the female genitourinary system. In women who are not pregnant, it is associated with a greater risk for urinary tract infections, cuff cellulitis after hysterectomy, and pelvic inflammatory disease. It is also associated with a greater risk for acquiring HIV infection. In pregnant women, BV is a risk factor for some of the most common causes of perinatal morbidity and mortality: premature labor, premature rupture of membranes, preterm delivery, and postpartum endometritis. Antepartum treatment with metronidazole significantly decreases these problems in patients with a previous preterm birth. However, in a low-risk population of pregnant women with asymptomatic BV, treatment did not benefit the pregnancy. Less clear is whether to treat the asymptomatic gynecologic patient who is not undergoing any type of surgery. Because of the association of BV with other infectious morbid conditions of the female reproductive tract, the trend has been for clinicians to treat asymptomatic BV.

VULVOVAGINAL CANDIDIASIS

Vulvovaginal candidiasis (VVC) is one of the most common infections of the female genital tract. About 75% of women at some time in their lives experience the discomfort of a vaginal yeast infection. For most, these infections are rare and respond to a multitude of therapies. However, an estimated 5% suffer chronic or recurrent episodes of VVC, despite the absence of underlying medical illnesses or predisposing factors. Theories to explain these repeated infections have focused on vaginal reinfection, either from a gastrointestinal source or from sexual transmission, or on vaginal relapse, which hypothesizes that recurrent infections are due to the same infecting organism, suppressed only temporarily by antifungal therapy. The bulk of controlled data supports the vaginal relapse theory. Although a precipitating factor such as pregnancy, the use of oral contraceptives, diabetes mellitus, systemic diseases requiring the use of antibiotics or corticosteroids, or HIV infection is sometimes found, most of these women have no underlying medical disorders.

C. albicans is the cause of about 95% of cases of VVC, but other yeast species have been implicated in selected cases. In certain centers that treat chronic vaginitis, non-albicans species such as *Candida (Torulopsis) glabrata*, *C. parapsilosis*, *C. tropicalis*, and *Saccharomyces cerevisiae* (baker's or brewer's yeast) may account for up to a third of infections. Although competing claims of clinical efficacy against these non-*C. albicans* organisms are being made, no adequate clinical studies have been done to show that any of the drugs on the market are effective against anything other than *C. albicans*. Anecdotal evidence from a variety of case series suggests that non-*C. albicans* cases are more resistant to imidazole and triazole therapy.

Patients with candidiasis complain primarily of vulvar or vaginal pruritus, irritation, or burning. In chronic cases, dyspareunia may become a more prominent symptom. Although a white discharge resembling oral thrush is sometimes found, many patients with VVC notice no change in their discharge.

Vulvar or vaginal erythema should prompt a search for candidiasis, as should the presence of vaginal thrush. The vaginal pH is normal with VVC. Diagnosis is made on the basis of hyphae or blastospores, visualized either on wet mount or KOH prep. Although *C. albicans* can produce either blastospores (budding yeast) or hyphae on clinical samples, smears positive for *C. glabrata* and *S. cerevisiae* contain only blastospores. In these cases, as well as those in which the history is strongly suggestive for VVC but the smears are unrevealing, fungal cultures may help confirm the diagnosis as well as identify the species of the pathogen. However, because yeast can be present as part of the normal vaginal flora, asymptomatic patients with yeast on either a vaginal culture or a Pap smear should not be treated.

Prior to selecting therapy, a clinician should determine whether a patient has uncomplicated versus complicated candidiasis. Women with uncomplicated candidiasis have sporadic infections, exhibit mild-to-moderate symptoms and findings, are thought to have a *C. albicans* infection, and have no significant illnesses predisposing them to VVC. These women will respond to any of the various therapies available for the treatment of VVC (Table 24.3). Topical regimens are generally well tolerated, but 5% of patients note itching and burning from the therapy. A single

TABLE 24.3. Therapy for Vulvovaginal Candidiasis

Drug	Formulation	Dose
Nystatin	100,000-U vaginal tablet	100,000 U × 14 d
Butoconazole	2% cream	5 g × 3 d
	2% sustained-release cream	5 g × 1 d
Clotrimazole	1% cream	5 g × 7 d
	100-mg vaginal inserts	100 mg × 7 d
		100 mg bid × 3 d
	500-mg vaginal tablet	500 mg × 1 d
Miconazole	2% cream	5 g × 7 d
	100-mg vaginal suppository	100 mg × 7 d
	200-mg vaginal suppository	200 mg × 3 d
Terconazole	0.4% cream	5 g × 7 d
	0.8% cream	5 g × 3 d
	80-mg vaginal suppository	80 mg × 3 d
Tioconazole	6.5% cream	5 g × 1 d
Fluconazole	150-mg oral tablet	150 mg × 1 d

oral dose of fluconazole has been shown to be as effective as a week of miconazole, clotrimazole, and terconazole in uncomplicated cases of VVC. Side effects such as headaches, nausea, and diarrhea tend to be self-limited. There are insufficient data to support its use in pregnancy. There are also interactions with other drugs, particularly rifampin, theophylline, phenytoin, warfarin, cyclosporine, and oral hypoglycemic agents.

Patients with complicated VVC complain of recurrent (four or more per year) episodes, exhibit severe symptoms or findings, are thought to have a non-albicans infection, or have factors predisposing them to VVC. These women require more aggressive therapy. For women with severe VVC, a more prolonged course of therapy, such as giving a second dose of fluconazole three days after the first, significantly increases cure rates. Women with recurrent infections caused by *C. albicans* may require a long-term maintenance regimen, either topical (clotrimazole 500-mg vaginally once a week) or oral (ketoconazole 100-mg daily; fluconazole 100, 150 or 200 mg once or twice a week). Treating the partners of women with recurrent VVC does not seem to decrease the risk of recurrent disease. In non-albicans infection, therapy with boric acid suppositories seems to be of use. In pregnant women, one of the 7-day topical azole therapy regimens is recommended.

ATROPHIC VAGINITIS

As noted earlier, estrogen plays a central role in maintaining the homeostasis of the vaginal environment. Therefore, any woman who no longer produces estrogen is theoretically at risk for developing atrophic vaginitis. With the recent trend away from systemic hormone replacement therapy in menopausal women, there will probably be an increase in the incidence of this condition.

Atrophic vaginitis should be suspected in any post-menopausal woman who complains of abnormal vaginal discharge, dryness, itching, or burning. Examination may reveal atrophy of the labia minora or majora, vaginal pallor, or loss of rugal folds. However, the genitalia often appear normal. The diagnosis is relatively easy to make by routinely checking the vaginal pH and looking at vaginal cytology when examining saline smears. With estrogen deficiency, the pH rises above 4.5. On the microscopic wet mount, many of the vaginal epithelial cells are parabasal or intermediate cells. The vaginal flora is scant and often is composed of bacilli and cocci, as opposed to the normal predominantly bacillary flora. A whiff test is negative.

The only therapy that truly reverses atrophic changes is estrogen therapy, either topical or oral. It may take several weeks before the patient begins to notice an improvement in symptoms, and once she stops therapy, her symptoms are likely to recur.

CHRONIC VAGINITIS

With the treatment approaches discussed here, most women should achieve a satisfactory resolution of their symptoms. However, when the patient fails to respond to seemingly appropriate therapy, the clinician must reassess the initial evaluation and diagnosis (Table 24.4) before proceeding with further therapy. Of these pitfalls, self-diagnosis and telephone diagnosis may represent the greatest traps that have been validated in prospective studies. One small prospective study demonstrated that 60% of women about to self-treat for a yeast infection had a vaginal problem for which antifungal therapy is not indicated. Meanwhile, diagnosis over the telephone seems to be comparable to random chance. In patients with short-lived symptoms, these two pitfalls may not lead to much morbidity, although they probably contribute to an overuse of over-the-counter antifungal therapy. However, in women with more chronic problems, treatment without an accurate diagnosis can prolong the time it takes to accurately diagnose and treat the cause of a woman's symptoms. In certain cases, it may be helpful to discontinue all therapy to see whether the remaining symptoms are due to the treatment itself. Other causes of "chronic vaginitis" encompass a wide spectrum of dermatologic conditions. For the woman with refractory symptoms, referral to a center that specializes in vulvovaginal disorders may be helpful.

TABLE 24.4. Pitfalls in the Treatment of Vaginitis

Patient self-diagnosis and treatment
Failure to see the patient (telephone diagnosis)
Patient seen but not examined
Failure to examine vulva and vestibule
Failure to perform laboratory tests
Treating *Escherichia coli, Enterococcus, Gardnerella vaginalis,* and other normal flora as pathogens
Use of shotgun therapy
Guessing at therapy
Overuse of topical steroids
Relying on Papanicolaou smear to make diagnosis
Failure to recognize that topical therapy may exacerbate symptoms

Source: Adapted from Sobel JD. Vaginal infection in adult women. *Med Clin North Am* 1990;74:1573, with permission.

BIBLIOGRAPHY

Allen-Davis JT, Beck A, Parker R, et al. Assesment of vulvovaginal complaints: accuracy of telephone triage and in-office diagnosis. *Obstet Gynecol* 2002; 99:18–22.

Carey JC, Klebanoff MA, Hauth JC, et al. Metronidazole to prevent preterm delivery in pregnant women with asymptomatic bacterial vaginosis. *N Engl J Med* 2000;342:534–540.

Centers for Disease Control and Prevention. Sexually transmitted diseases treatment guidelines 2002. *MMWR Morb Mortal Wkly Rep* 2002;51(RR-6):1.

Ferris DG, Nyirjesy P, Sobel JD, et al. Over-the-counter antifungal drug misuse associated with patient-diagnosed vulvovaginal candidiasis. *Obstet Gynecol* 2002;99:419–425.

Gardner HL, Dukes CD. *Haemophilus vaginalis* vaginitis: a newly defined specific infection previously classified as "nonspecific" vaginitis. *Am J Obstet Gynecol* 1955;69:962.

Hillier SL, Krohn MA, Klebanoff SJ, et al. The relationship of hydrogen peroxide-producing lactobacilli to bacterial vaginosis and genital microflora in pregnant women. *Obstet Gynecol* 1992;79:369.

Kent HL. Epidemiology of vaginitis. *Am J Obstet Gynecol* 1991;165:1168.

Klebanoff SJ, Hillier SL, Eschenbach DA, et al. Control of the microbial flora of the vagina by H_2O_2-generating lactobacilli. *J Infect Dis* 1991;164:94.

Klebanoff MA, Carey JC, Hauth JC, et al. Failure of metronidazole to prevent preterm delivery among pregnant women with asymptomatic *Trichomonas vaginalis* infection. *N Engl J Med* 2001;345:487–493.

Morales WJ, Schorr S, Albritton J. Effect of metronidazole in patients with preterm birth in preceding pregnancy and bacterial vaginosis: a placebo-controlled, double-blind study. *Am J Obstet Gynecol* 1994;171:345.

Nyirjesy P. Managing resistant *Trichomonas* vaginitis. *Curr Infect Dis Rep* 1999;1: 389–392.

Nyirjesy P, Seeney SM, Grody MHT, et al. Chronic fungal vaginitis: the value of cultures. *Am J Obstet Gynecol* 1995;173:820.

Piper JM, Mitchel EF, Ray WA. Prenatal use of metronidazole and birth defects: no association. *Obstet Gynecol* 1993;82:348.

Schaaf VM, Perez-Stable EJ, Borchardt K. The limited value of symptoms and signs in the diagnosis of vaginal infections. *Arch Intern Med* 1990;150:1929.

Sobel JD. Vaginal infections in adult women. *Med Clin North Am* 1990;74:1573.

Sobel JD. Candidal vulvovaginitis. *Clin Obstet Gynecol* 1993;36:153.

Sobel JD, Faro S, Force RW, et al. Vulvovaginal candidiasis: epidemiologic, diagnostic, and therapeutic considerations. *Am J Obstet Gynecol* 1998;178:203–211.

Sobel JD, Nyirjesy P, Brown W. Tinidazole therapy for metronidazole-resistant vaginal trichomoniasis. *Clin Infect Dis* 2001;33:1341–1346.

CHAPTER 25
Breast-Feeding

Cynthia Howard and Ruth A. Lawrence

Nourishing a child to provide for its proper growth and development is an essential task of parenthood. Parents judge their competency by how well or poorly their infant grows, and physicians use growth as an overall indicator of an infant's health. Issues surrounding the choice of an infant feeding method are thus of great concern to expectant and new parents. Although many mothers make their decision regarding infant feeding before pregnancy, a substantial proportion seek the advice of their physician. Women in the United States are increasingly choosing to breast-feed, so that lactation management is becoming a significant part of clinical practice for primary care physicians. This chapter discusses the management of breast-feeding mothers and infants and the treatment of common lactation problems.

Breast milk is the ideal food for infants. Breast-feeding is acknowledged by the American College of Obstetricians and Gynecologists, the American Academy of Pediatrics, and the World Health Organization as the optimal way to nourish an infant. The Institute of Medicine of the National Academy of Sciences recommends breast-feeding for all infants in the United States under ordinary circumstances and believes that exclusive breast-feeding is the preferred method for feeding most infants from birth to the age of 6 months.

Breast-feeding is considered to be so important to the health of mothers and infants that national health goals for the year 2010 include the objectives that 75% of women initially breast-feed their infants, that 50% continue to breast-feed them until they are 6 months of age, and that 25% breast-feed them through 12 months. Despite strong medical support for breast-feeding, only about 64% of women in the United States choose to breast-feed their infants, and as few as 29% continue to 6 months and 16% to 12 months. Although U.S. breast-feeding rates are on the increase, the promotion of breast-feeding as optimal infant nutrition must remain a priority for physicians, public health officials, and organizations with an interest in maternal and child health.

BENEFITS TO MOTHER AND INFANT

Human milk is species-specific and thus the ideal source of nourishment for human infants. Various features of breast milk, such as the concentrations of cholesterol and taurine and the specific amino acid profile, are believed to be essential for optimal central nervous system development, nerve myelinization, and retinal development. Also, active enzymes in human milk facilitate the digestion and absorption of nutrients in breast-fed infants while enhancing gut maturation and repair.

Women who breast-feed derive health benefits, including a concurrent reduction in fertility, a lowered risk for breast cancer, and probable protection against osteoporosis and adult-onset obesity. In the United States, the body weight of a woman who has given birth tends to be heavier than ideal, and breast-feeding may promote postpartum weight loss. It is normal for lactating women to lose an average of 0.5 to 1.0 kg (1–2 lb) per month during the first 6 months of breast-feeding.

Breast-feeding is beneficial for infants. Among the most important benefits is increased protection against many common infectious diseases. Human milk reduces exposure to contaminated food sources, enhances the nutritional status of at-risk infants, and prevents infection via several antiinflammatory, immune system–stimulating, and antimicrobial factors. The preventive effects of breast-feeding are especially evident in the third world, where infant mortality rates are many times higher in artificially fed than in breast-fed infants.

Although the protective effects of breast-feeding are more difficult to document in industrialized nations, epidemiologic evidence suggests a decreased risk for gastrointestinal and lower respiratory tract disease, otitis media, and bacteremia and sepsis in breast-fed infants living in developed nations. Additionally, breast-feeding may protect children from the development of food allergies and some chronic diseases, including childhood-onset diabetes mellitus, lymphoma, and Crohn disease. In a landmark randomized clinical trial conducted in the Republic of Belarus, breast-feeding protected children from gastrointestinal disease and atopic skin disease during the first year of life. The continued follow-up of the more than 16,000 children who participated in this study will be vital in evaluating the effects of breast-feeding on a variety of short- and long-term health outcomes, including intelligence and the development of cardiovascular disease.

ANATOMY AND PHYSIOLOGY OF THE LACTATING BREAST

Breast development, under the influence of estrogen, progesterone, and lactogenic hormones, begins in early fetal life and extends into puberty and adult life. Only during pregnancy does the breast become fully mature, with a rapid growth of ducts and alveoli in response to prolactin and placental lactogen. Small amounts of milk synthesis and secretion begin during the second trimester of pregnancy. Lactogenesis, the onset of the copious secretion of milk around the time of parturition, is triggered by the decrease in progesterone after delivery (Fig. 25.1).

Once the production of milk begins, prolactin and oxytocin provide the hormonal environment for maintaining it. Prolactin is released in response to the amount and frequency of suckling and controls milk synthesis and secretion. Suckling also promotes the release of pituitary oxytocin. Oxytocin causes the myoepithelial cells in the breast to contract, so that the ejection of milk, or "letdown," occurs. During ejection, milk moves from the alveoli into the lacteal sinuses of the breast, where it is easily removed by the infant (Fig. 25.2).

Milk production also responds to local negative feedback in the breast. Local distention and increases in pressure in the breast, such as occur during engorgement, may decrease milk production. The major negative effect of engorgement is to decrease vascular flow in the breast and thus to slow the transport of prolactin and oxytocin to target cells in the breast.

Most women can successfully breast-feed, but a few experience primary failure of lactation as a consequence of inadequate glandular tissue, neurohormonal disruption, or prolactin deficiency. Normal changes during pregnancy include an increase in breast size, increased pigmentation of the nipple and areola, and hypertrophy of the Montgomery tubercles. A lack of normal changes during pregnancy should alert the clinician to possible lactation problems. These women and their infants benefit from close postpartum follow-up to ensure adequate milk production.

Women who have undergone surgical procedures that interrupt ducts and sever or damage nipple nerves may also produce inadequate supplies of milk. Those who have undergone augmentation procedures usually have few problems in breast-

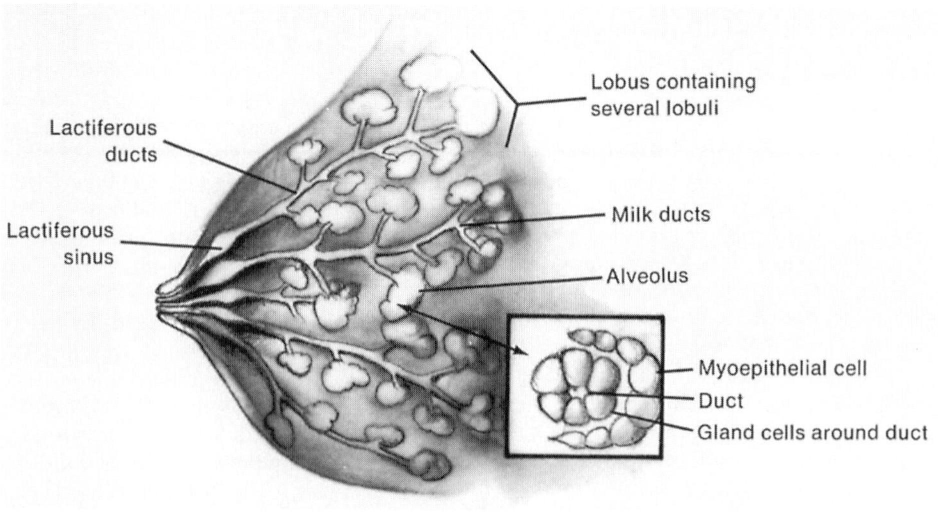

FIG. 25.1. Anatomy of the breast. (From Lawrence RA. *Breast-feeding: a guide for the medical profession*, 5th ed. St. Louis: Mosby, 1999, with permission.)

feeding. The physician, however, must be aware that some women who undergo augmentation for an improved cosmesis do so because of breast features associated with inadequate glandular tissue. Many articles can be found in the literature about illness associated with silicone gel implants, including reports of esophageal motility problems in the breast-fed infants of mothers with implants. Currently, it is not known whether breast-feeding by a woman who has breast implants affects the nursing infant. Silicone, however, is present in many substances, including some antacid preparations.

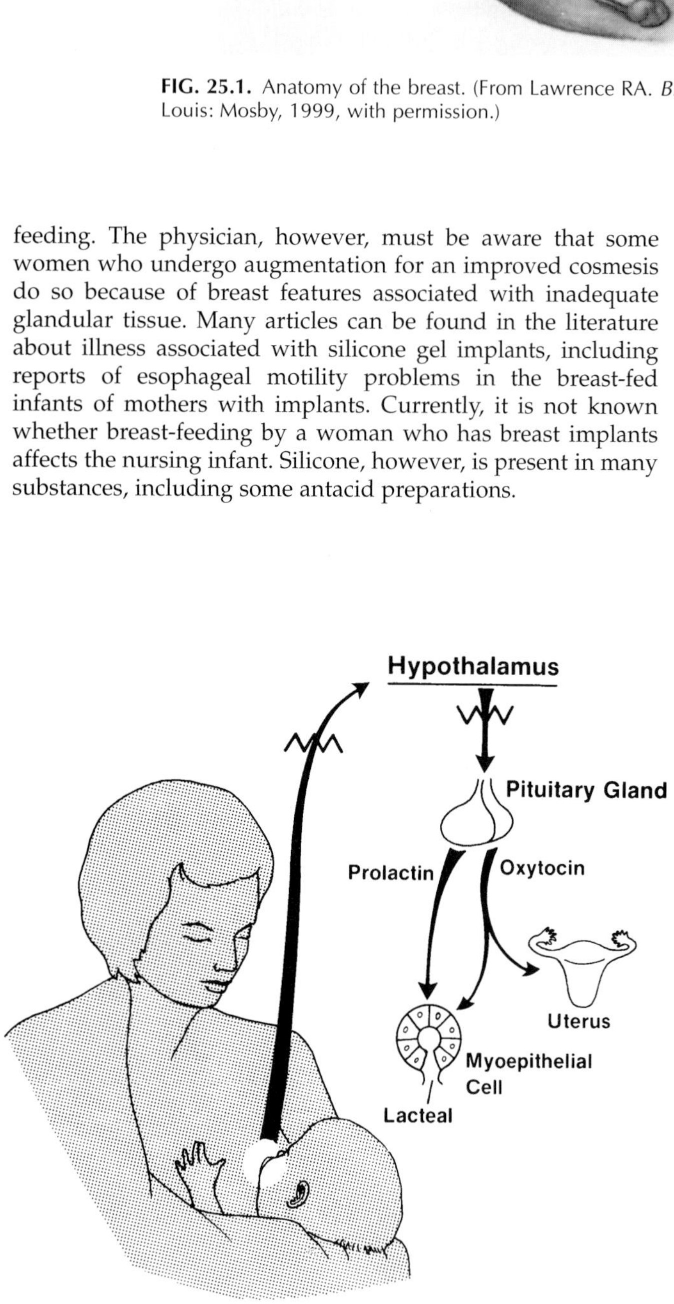

FIG. 25.2. Ejection reflex arc. (From Lawrence RA. *Breast-feeding: a guide for the medical profession*, 5th ed. St. Louis: Mosby, 1999, with permission.)

MANAGEMENT

Maternal Nutritional Needs and the Production and Composition of Milk

The amount of milk produced on the first postpartum day ranges from about 50 to 150 mL. Production rapidly increases after about 36 hours postpartum. The volume of milk produced does not appear to be affected by maternal nutrition, body composition (adiposity), and energy or nutrient intake. Average milk production is about 750 to 800 mL/d in women with wide variations in dietary intake and nutritional status. If a lactating woman is overweight, a weight loss of up to 2 kg (4.5 lb) per month is unlikely to affect milk volume; however, women should be alert to signs that the infant's appetite is not being satisfied. In general, women can produce much more breast milk than an infant is likely to require.

Characteristics of the infant, such as ineffective or infrequent suckling by a low-birth-weight or preterm infant, can affect the amount of milk produced. In the early postpartum period, frequent suckling (10 ± 3 sessions per day) is important to the establishment of an adequate supply of milk. Mothers whose infants are hospitalized can develop an adequate supply by pumping their breasts (using an electric breast pump) at least five times a day (at least 100 minutes of total pumping time per day) in the first postpartum month.

Maternal factors that may contribute to inadequate milk production include pain, stress, fatigue, and the use of alcohol, cigarettes, and some oral contraceptives. Pain, stress, and fatigue inhibit the release of oxytocin and thus milk ejection. The use of barrier contraceptives, spermicides, and progestin-only and combination oral contraceptives with less than 2.5 mg of 19-norprogestogen and 50 μg of ethinyl estradiol or 100 μg of mestranol is compatible with breast-feeding. Milk yield may be decreased with larger doses of combination oral contraceptives. Smoking may also decrease milk volume by decreasing the response to prolactin and oxytocin. Although sipping small amounts of alcohol has traditionally been recommended to enhance letdown, ethanol in sufficient amounts inhibits the release of oxytocin. The Institute of Medicine states, "There is no scientific evidence that consumption of alcoholic beverages has a beneficial impact on any aspect of lactation performance.

If alcohol is used, advise the lactating woman to limit her intake to no more than 0.5 g of alcohol per kg of maternal body weight per day. Intake over this level may impair the milk ejection reflex." For the average 60-kg (132-lb) woman, 0.5 g of alcohol per kilogram of body weight corresponds to approximately 2 to 2.5 oz of liquor, 8 oz of wine, or two cans of beer. Although nursing mothers should maintain adequate fluid intake, fluids consumed in excess of thirst do not appear to increase milk volume, and forcing fluids may decrease production.

The composition of milk varies among women and with the stages of lactation, although individual differences in well-nourished women are insignificant. More than 200 different constituents make up human milk, providing both nutritive and nonnutritive benefits for the infant. These are synthesized in the mammary secretory cells from precursors in the plasma, produced by other cells in the mammary gland, or transferred directly from the plasma to milk. The composition of milk is thus influenced by physiologic and biochemical processes that affect the plasma and by hormonal and biosynthetic processes in the mammary gland. Table 25.1 lists the components of human milk.

The composition of milk changes most rapidly during the first few weeks of lactation. Colostrum is the fluid secreted by the mammary gland immediately after delivery. It is produced in smaller quantities than mature milk and is higher in protein, minerals, and immunoglobulin. Beginning on about day 7, the composition of milk begins a slow transition during about 2 weeks to that of mature milk.

By using their body stores, women can produce milk with adequate amounts of protein, fat, carbohydrate, and most minerals, even if their own supply of nutrients is limited. Maternal diet strongly affects the fatty acid content of human milk, but the total fat and cholesterol content is independent of diet. The content of human milk is most likely to be affected by a low maternal intake of vitamins, especially vitamins B_6, B_{12}, A, and D. Breast-feeding women should consume good sources of all essential nutrients for their own health and to replenish their body stores.

The total amounts of nutrients that a lactating mother secretes are directly related to the amount and duration of breast-feeding. If nutrient intake is inadequate, maternal body stores of macronutrients, many minerals, and folate may be sacrificed to maintain the composition of milk. Because of the substantial margin of safety included in the Recommended Daily Allowances (RDAs) for lactating women, women's needs are easily met by an average American diet containing 2,700 kcal/d. At energy intakes of less than 2,700 kcal/d, the nutrients most likely to be deficient are calcium, magnesium, zinc, vitamin B_6, and folate. Table 25.2 lists food sources rich in these nutrients, and women should be encouraged to consume these foods. Iron-rich foods are important once the mother's menstrual cycle returns. Adolescents, women who are complete vegetarians (vegans), and those who avoid dairy products, diet to lose weight during lactation, or are impoverished may be at risk for nutritional deficiencies during lactation. Table 25.3 contains suggestions for increasing nutrient intake in women at risk for nutritional deficiencies during lactation. Current evidence does not indicate that routine vitamin-mineral supplementation for lactating women is warranted.

Prenatal Preparation

A knowledgeable, supportive physician is an essential part of any effort to promote breast-feeding. Because most women make decisions about infant feeding before the third trimester, physicians caring for women are in an ideal situation to influence the choice to breast-feed. Although physicians must support the mother's decision either way, they also must educate her so that her decisions are based on facts. Except for some sophisticated families, most discussions about infant feeding are initiated by the physician. Given the overwhelming evidence in support of breast-feeding, physicians should sensitively but openly encourage women to choose breast-feeding.

The physical examination early in pregnancy provides a good opportunity to discuss breast-feeding and any breast abnormalities. Any questions about lactation or the mother's ability to produce sufficient milk should be addressed at this time. The size of the mammary gland does not predict a mother's ability to nourish her infant, although failure of the

TABLE 25.1. Constituents of Human Milk

Nitrogen compounds	**Water-soluble vitamins**	**Lipids**
Proteins	Thiamin	Triglycerides
Caseins	Riboflavin	Fatty acids
α-Lactalbumin	Niacin	Phospholipids
Lactoferrin	Pantothenic acid	Sterols and hydrocarbons
Surface IgA, other immunoglobulins	Biotin	Fat-soluble vitamins A, D, E, K
β-Lactoglobulin	Folate	**Minerals**
Lysozyme	Vitamin B_6	Calcium
Enzymes	Vitamin B_{12}	Phosphorus
Hormones	Vitamin C	Magnesium
Growth factors	Inositol	Potassium
Nonprotein nitrogen	Choline	Sodium
Urea	*Cells*	Chlorine
Creatine	Leukocytes	Sulfur
Creatinine	Epithelial cells	Iodine
Uric acid	**Carbohydrates**	Iron
Glucosamine	Lactose	Copper
α-Amino nitrogen	Oligosaccharides	Zinc
Nucleic acids	Bifidus factors	Manganese
Nucleotides	Glycopeptides	Selenium
Polyamines		Chromium
		Cobalt

Source: National Academy of Sciences. *Nutrition during lactation.* Washington, DC: National Academy Press, 1991, with permission.

TABLE 25.2. Food Sources for Nutrients Most Likely to be Deficient in the Diet of the Lactating Woman

Calcium	Zinc	Magnesium	Vitamin B_6[a]	Thiamin[a]	Folate
Milk	Meat	Nuts	Bananas	Pork	Leafy vegetables
Cheese	Poultry	Seeds	Poultry	Fish	Fruit
Yogurt	Seafood	Legumes	Meat	Whole grains	Liver
Fish with edible bones	Eggs	Whole grains	Fish	Organ meats	Green beans
Tofu made with calcium sulfate	Seeds	Green vegetables	Potatoes	Legumes	Fortified cereals
Bok choy	Legumes	Scallops	Sweet potatoes	Corn	Legumes
Broccoli	Yogurt	Oysters	Spinach	Peas	Whole-grain cereals
Kale	Whole grains		Prunes	Seeds	
Collard greens			Watermelon	Nuts	
Mustard greens			Some legumes	Fortified cereal grain	
Turnip greens			Fortified cereals		
Breads made with milk			Nuts		
Seeds and nuts					

[a]In general, this nutrient is widely distributed in food rather than concentrated in a small number of foods.
Source: National Academy of Sciences. *Nutrition during lactation.* Washington, DC: National Academy Press, 1991, with permission.

gland to enlarge during pregnancy may be associated with inadequate production. If the mother has any anatomic abnormalities or has previously undergone breast surgery, however, potential problems should be discussed. Particular attention should be paid to the nipple and areola. Nipples should be tested for protrusion. Inverted nipples are caused by the persistence of fibers involved in invagination of the mammary dimple in the embryo and become evident when the areola is squeezed or compressed (Fig. 25.3).

A prenatal visit with a pediatric care provider may provide expectant mothers with useful information about infant feeding. Many hospitals also conduct prenatal education classes that are excellent sources of information about breast-feeding. Additionally, Lamaze classes and La Leche League representatives may serve as educational resources. The American Academy of Pediatrics, the American College of Obstetricians and Gynecologists, and the La Leche League publish patient education materials about breast-feeding. Patient education materials published by formula companies are inappropriate sources of breast-feeding information.

The Academy of Breast-feeding Medicine is a multidisciplinary physician organization that is a good resource for physician education regarding breast-feeding. It produces clinical protocols on a variety of breast-feeding management issues (www.bfmed.org). The American Academy of Pediatrics section on breast-feeding produces educational resources for pediatricians and patient information. Additionally, the Lactation Study Center at the University of Rochester School of Medicine and Dentistry (585-275-0088) provides information on medications, lactation, and lactation management issues and maintains a computer data bank of lactation literature.

Preparation of the Breasts

In general, no special preparation of the breasts is necessary in anticipation of breast-feeding. Women should avoid applying soap, alcohol, or other drying agents to the nipples. Secretions from the Montgomery glands clean and lubricate the areola and nipple. Studies have not shown ointments or creams to be effective in preventing sore nipples; in fact, they may cause the nip-

TABLE 25.3. Suggested Measures for Improving Nutrient Intake of Women with Restrictive Eating Patterns

Eating pattern	Corrective measures
Excessive restriction of food intake (i.e., ingestion of <1,800 kcal of energy per day, which ordinarily leads to unsatisfactory intake of nutrients compared with the amounts needed by lactating women)	Encourage increased intake of nutrient-rich foods to achieve an energy intake of at least 1,800 kcal/d; if the mother insists on curbing food intake sharply, promote substitution of foods rich in vitamins, minerals and protein for those lower in nutritive value. In individual cases, it may be advisable to recommend a balanced multivitamin-mineral supplement. Discourage the use of liquid weight loss diets and appetite suppressants.
Complete vegetarianism (avoidance of all animal food, including meat, fish, dairy products, and eggs)	Advise intake of a regular source of vitamin B_{12}, such as special vitamin B_{12}-containing plant food products or a 2.6-μg vitamin B_{12} supplement daily.
Avoidance of milk, cheese, or other calcium-rich dairy products	Encourage increased intake of other culturally appropriate dietary calcium sources, such as collard greens for blacks from the southeastern United States. Provide information on the appropriate use of low-lactose dairy products if milk is being avoided because of lactose intolerance; if correction by diet cannot be achieved, it may be advisable to recommend 600 mg of elemental calcium per day taken with meals.
Avoidance of vitamin D-fortified food, such as fortified milk or cereal, combined with limited exposure to ultraviolet light	Recommend 10 μg of supplemental vitamin D per day.

Source: National Academy of Sciences. *Nutrition during lactation.* Washington, DC: National Academy Press, 1991, with permission.

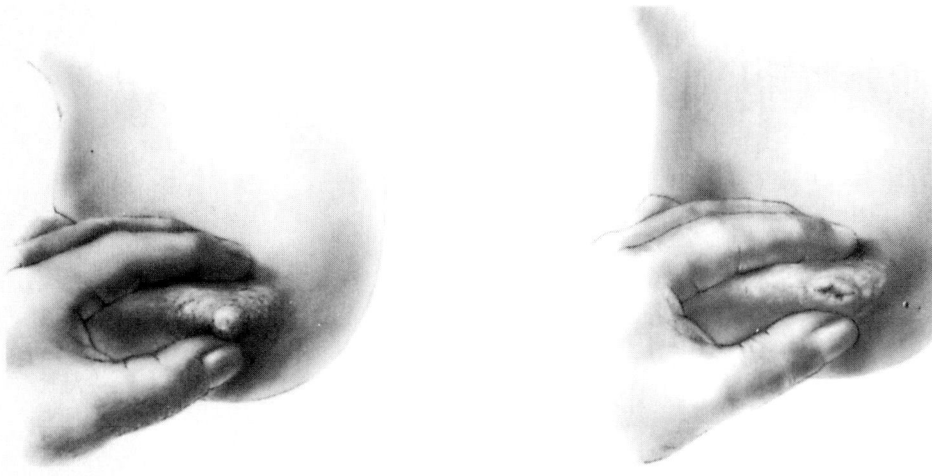

FIG. 25.3. A: Normal nipple everts with gentle pressure. **B:** Inverted or tied nipple inverts with gentle pressure. (From Lawrence RA. *Breast-feeding: a guide for the medical profession*, 5th ed. St. Louis: Mosby, 1999, with permission.)

ples to macerate and become more susceptible to irritation. In extremely dry climates where lubricating ointments are necessary for skin integrity, however, such an ointment may be indicated. Nipple rolling and other manipulations are also ineffective in preventing sore nipples and should be avoided because of the risk for inducing uterine contractions and premature labor.

As many as 10% of pregnant women have inverted (nonprotractile) nipples that may make it difficult for an infant to obtain a proper grasp on the breast. Although Hoffman exercises (stretching and pulling the nipple and areola) and breast shells have been recommended for the treatment of inverted nipples, an effective prenatal treatment of this condition has never been identified. Hoffman exercises are contraindicated because they may induce uterine contractions.

Ideally, prenatal preparation for breast-feeding includes an early breast examination with a discussion encouraging breast-feeding as the optimal method of infant feeding, early treatment of any breast problems, a prenatal visit later in pregnancy with a pediatric care provider, and referrals to helpful community resources (e.g., breast-feeding classes, La Leche League).

Care in the Hospital

The success of breast-feeding depends to a large part on hospital policies and routines. An experienced nursing staff is critical to the management of the nursing mother and infant in the first few days after birth. All labor and delivery, newborn nursery, neonatal intensive care, and postpartum nurses should be adequately trained to assist the nursing mother. Care should be taken to ensure that advice given in the hospital is consistent between providers. A written breast-feeding policy with input from physicians and nurses ensures that advice given to mothers is consistent and accurate. Policies that promote successful breast-feeding include early (preferably within an hour after delivery) and frequent opportunities to breast-feed, rooming-in, "demand" feeding schedules, and the avoidance of routine water or formula supplements. These policies are part of the baby-friendly hospital initiative supported by the United Nations Children's Fund (UNICEF)/World Health Organization (WHO) and administered in the United States by Baby Friendly USA.

Mothers who become ill postpartum, have a difficult delivery, or deliver multiple infants, may find it difficult to breast-feed because of such problems as a sleepy infant, late initiation of breast-feeding, an increased need for supplementation, infrequent night feedings, and a delayed increase in milk supply. Excellent supportive care is essential for these mothers. Key factors in early management include the following:

- *Proper positioning at the breast*: Mothers must be taught to position the infant properly at the breast. The infant's abdomen should be against the mother's abdomen, and the infant's head should be well supported and kept in line with his or her body. After eliciting a rooting response by stimulating the infant's lower lip with the nipple, the mother should bring the infant's head toward her breast by moving her arm or hand. The head should not be pushed toward the breast; doing so may cause the infant to arch back. If the infant's arms are not swaddled, they should be around the mother's thorax.
- *Supporting the breast*: The mother should be taught to support her breast by using a palmar or scissors grasp (whichever works best for her). The mother's grasp must not interfere with the infant's position on the breast. The infant's lips should be positioned on the areola about 1 or 1.5 inches from the base of the nipple. The infant's lower lip should not be folded in so that he or she sucks on the lip.
- *Detaching the infant from the breast:* The mother should be taught to break the suction at the breast by inserting her finger in the infant's mouth when removing the infant from the breast.
- *Waking a sleepy baby:* Mothers should be taught ways to awaken a sleepy infant for feedings, such as unwrapping, diapering, and gentle stimulation. Rooming-in and skin-to-skin contact between mother and baby will enhance opportunities to breast-feed and hasten lactogenesis.
- *Frequency of feedings:* Feedings should be frequent, every 2 to 2.5 hours from the start of one feeding to the start of the next. To equalize stimulation of the breasts, mothers should alternate the breast that is offered first at each feeding.
- *Length of feedings:* Some mothers benefit from general guidelines to nurse about 10 to 15 minutes per side in the first few days. Generally, infants need to suckle about 2 or 3 minutes before milk letdown occurs, especially during the first week or two. Frequent small feedings provide good breast stimulation and prevent undue tiredness in the mother. If rooming-in is impossible, infants should be taken to their mothers to nurse at night.

TABLE 25.4. Factors that Promote Breast-Feeding

Prenatally	Immediately postpartum	Immediately during infancy
General health information Breast-feeding education	Early maternal-infant contact Rooming in	Counseling and support Avoidance of exposure to formula samples and advertising
Encouragement by health professional	"Demand" feeding schedules Avoidance of supplementation Supportive atmosphere for breast-feeding women	Information about breast pumping, counseling regarding return to work

Source: Adapted from Kramer MS. Poverty, WIC, and promotion of breast-feeding. *Pediatrics* 1991;87:399, with permission.

Breast-fed infants should not be given supplementation that is not medically indicated because early supplementation is consistently associated with a shortened duration and increased rates of early cessation of breast-feeding. Supplementation interferes with the supply-and-demand nature of breast-feeding by lessening demand and reducing the production of milk. Also, mechanical differences between breast-feeding and bottle feeding may cause an infant to refuse the breast or learn to suckle ineffectively. Commercial formula discharge packs should not be given to breast-feeding mothers. The distribution of advertising and formula samples to breast-feeding women in the hospital lessens the duration of exclusive and overall breast-feeding. Factors that promote successful breast-feeding are listed in Table 25.4.

Supplements for the Breast-Feeding Infant

Vitamin K prophylaxis should be administered to all infants regardless of feeding method to prevent hemorrhagic disease of the newborn.

A growing number of cases of nutritional rickets have been reported in breast-fed infants, largely those with darkly pigmented skin. "The development of rickets in breast-fed infants is not due to deficiency of vitamin D in breast milk but to failure of the infant to receive adequate sunlight exposure. Because of concerns about sun exposure in young infants and a lack of information about the necessary dose of sunlight needed to prevent rickets in infants with darkly pigmented skin, adequate sunlight exposure cannot be adequately defined." Increased skin pigmentation, avoidance of the sun, the use of sun block, and cultural shrouding may all affect maternal and infant vitamin D status. The American Academy of Pediatrics currently recommends that all breast-fed infants receive supplemental vitamin D while exclusively or predominantly breast-feeding.

Neonatal iron stores meet the needs of a term infant for the first 6 months of life. Iron in human milk is highly bioavailable, so that the depletion of these stores is delayed until after 6 months of life. At that time, other sources of iron, such as iron-fortified infant cereal, should be added to the diet.

Fluoride supplements are no longer recommended for infants younger than 6 months of age. Infants and children 6 months to 3 years old living in areas where the fluoride content of the water is less than 0.3 parts per million should receive a supplement of 0.25 mg/d.

Postpartum Follow-Up

The nursing mother and infant should be assessed frequently throughout their hospital stay for the successful establishment of lactation. With the increasing frequency of early hospital discharge, however, many mothers and infants go home before the mother's milk supply increases. These women and infants require close outpatient monitoring. Ideally, breast-fed infants discharged 48 to 72 hours after delivery should be seen in follow-up within 2 to 3 days. Infants discharged from the hospital earlier require follow-up within 48 hours and again at 1 week of age. La Leche League representatives, peer support groups, hospital hotlines, and lactation consultants may all be useful to mothers in the early postpartum period. Issues related to breast-feeding should also be a regular part of obstetric postpartum care.

Some useful clinical criteria that signal the successful establishment of breast-feeding at 5 to 7 days include the following:

- The quantity of the mother's milk has increased. Mothers generally note their milk "coming in" between postpartum days 2 and 4, when their breasts become firm and full.
- The mother and infant have established an appropriate feeding schedule of every 2 to 3 hours, with one longer sleep interval of about 5 hours. The infant should not be receiving any supplemental feedings (water or formula).
- Any nipple tenderness the mother experienced during the first postpartum days should be mild and resolving.
- The infant should be having at least three or four breast milk stools (mustard-colored seedy stools) and six to eight clear voids per day (at least one diaper per day should be soaked). Urate crystals (the color of brick dust) in the urine are a clue to inadequate hydration.
- The infant's weight loss since birth should be no more than 7%. After the quantity of the mother's milk increases, the infant should gain about 30 g/d. The birth weight should be regained by 2 weeks of age.

CONTRAINDICATIONS TO BREAST-FEEDING

Contraindications to breast-feeding are rare. However, some medications, infectious agents, and toxic substances may appear in breast milk and pose a risk to the nursing infant. In the assessment of any exposure, potential risks must be weighed against the many benefits of breast-feeding. Mothers with life-threatening illnesses, however, must give their own medical treatment priority.

Most medications are safe for use during breast-feeding. The risk that a mother's medication poses to her infant depends on its route of administration and pharmacokinetics (absorption, metabolism, and excretion) and on the infant's physiologic maturity (ability to absorb, metabolize, and excrete the drug).

Drugs contraindicated during breast-feeding include therapeutic radioactive pharmaceuticals, lithium, lactation-suppressing drugs, some antithyroid drugs, illicit or street drugs, and synthetic anticoagulants. During short courses of medications such as radioactive pharmaceuticals, antiprotozoal compounds, and a few antibiotics (e.g., chloramphenicol), mothers may have to pump their breasts temporarily and discard the milk. Other drugs may be contraindicated depending on the infant's age (e.g., sulfa-containing medications should be avoided when an infant is younger than 1 month of age).

If the mother has been exposed to high levels of insecticides, heavy metals, or other contaminants that appear in breast milk, breast-feeding is not recommended without an evaluation of levels. Pesticides such as chlorophenothane (DDT), polychlorinated biphenyls (PCBs), and hexachlorobenzene have been identified in the milk of women with heavy exposures. Although a matter of concern, the levels of heavy metals such as lead, mercury, arsenic, and cadmium are generally lower in breast milk than in water. If a mother has been exposed to a heavy metal, the levels in her breast milk and the infant's serum should be measured.

Mothers in whom mastitis develops may with rare exceptions continue to breast-feed. Women should be counseled to seek early medical care at the first signs of infection (mastitis is discussed later in this chapter). The mothers of infants in whom galactosemia is diagnosed should not breast-feed; a milk substitute with a nonlactose sugar source should be chosen.

Infectious diseases are rarely a contraindication to breast-feeding. Neither cytomegalovirus infection nor hepatitis B or C is a contraindication. To breast-feed safely, infants whose mothers are positive for hepatitis B antigen should be vaccinated and protected against infection with 0.5 mL of hepatitis B immunoglobulin as soon as possible after birth. If a mother requires rubella immunization after delivery, she may still breast-feed.

Of greater concern is the possible transmission of HIV infection through breast milk. The Public Health Service and the Centers for Disease Control and Prevention recommend that women who test seropositive for HIV antibody in the United States not breast-feed to prevent postnatal transmission to infants who may not be infected. In developing countries, the situation is complex, and studies designed to clarify the relative risks and benefits of HIV-infected women breast-feeding their infants are ongoing. Issues including the availability of antiretroviral medications, the safety of water supplies, and the availability and safe storage of breast milk substitutes affect the situation in individual settings. Recommendations from the World Health Organization include the following:

- Exclusive breast-feeding should be protected, promoted, and supported for 6 months in women who are known not to be infected with HIV or whose infection status is unknown.
- When replacement feeding is acceptable, feasible, affordable, sustainable and safe, avoidance of all breast-feeding by HIV-infected mothers is recommended; otherwise, exclusive breast-feeding is recommended during the first months of life.
- To minimize the risk for HIV transmission, breast-feeding should be discontinued as soon as feasible, depending on local circumstances, the individual woman's situation, and the risks associated with replacement feeding (including infections other than HIV infection and malnutrition).
- HIV-infected women should have access to information, follow-up clinical care, and support, including family planning services and nutritional support.

COMMON PROBLEMS

Sore Nipples

Mothers commonly experience some discomfort in the early days of breast-feeding during the initial grasp and suckling of the breast. This is caused by negative pressure on empty ductules and typically resolves as the milk supply increases. Any nipple pain that persists throughout a breast-feeding or fails to resolve within the first week may indicate more serious problems and requires evaluation.

Early in breast-feeding, the most common cause of nipple trauma and subsequent pain is poor positioning of the infant at the breast. Poor positioning results in nipple pain when the infant attaches only to the nipple during suckling, the infant sucks his or her lower lip in and irritates the underside of the nipple, or the mother does not break the suction before removing the infant from her breast.

Sometimes, the infant's nursing style causes pain. The suckling of a very vigorous infant may result in temporary discomfort for the mother. Especially delicate tissues may benefit from air-drying after nursing. Because human milk has many antiinfectious and healing properties, expressing a few drops of milk and allowing them to dry on the areola may also help.

Candidal infection is associated with stabbing pain that radiates throughout the breast. This type of infection often develops after antibiotic treatment has been administered (to mother or infant) or when the infant has a candidal infection (e.g., thrush, diaper rash).

Addressing an underlying cause such as poor positioning is the first step in the treatment of soreness, but a careful assessment of any other contributing factors is also important. Soaps or self-prescribed treatments may lead to drying of the area and subsequent contact dermatitis. If the skin is particularly dry, lubrication may be beneficial, but the routine use of ointments is not recommended because the sebaceous glands and Montgomery glands are easily plugged. Vitamin A & D Ointment is not harmful to the infant, but vitamin E and local anesthetic creams should not be used. Purified lanolin ointments that are free of alcohol and allergens are safe if an ointment is indicated. Some dermatologists recommend moist healing of sore and cracked nipples, citing insufficient moisture coupled with poor positioning of the infant as the cause. Certainly, surface moisture from milk or occlusive plastic in nursing pads aggravates the problem and should be avoided. After gentle drying, however, the area may benefit from the application of a nonirritating ointment to restore moisture in the tissues.

Nipple shields are devices made of rubber or synthetic material designed to be worn over the areola while the infant is nursing. They reduce the amount of milk the infant receives and may cause the infant to learn to suckle improperly. Subsequent weaning back to the bare breast may be difficult. In general, the use of these devices should be avoided.

Flat or inverted nipples may make it difficult for an infant to grasp the breast properly. Compressing the areola between two fingers to cause the nipple to protrude as much as possible helps the infant grasp the breast. Expressing a small amount of milk before a feeding to soften the areola and entice the infant is also helpful. Additionally, breast shells may be worn between feedings to promote nipple protrusion. If these techniques fail, the nipple can be drawn out before breast-feeding with a pump. Inverted nipples often respond to these measures within the first 1 or 2 days postpartum.

If the mother's nipples are cracked, bleeding, or blistered, she may also benefit from shorter, more frequent feedings and the use of a short-acting analgesic before nursing. She should begin the feeding with the breast that is less sore and limit the amount of nonnutritive sucking (that is not associated with swallowing) by the infant. If cracking has not yet developed, dry heat followed by lubrication with cream or ointment between feedings is most effective. Cracks are often caused by poor positioning combined with excessive dryness. Pain is eased by proper positioning and by the application of a therapeutic ointment, such as Vitamin A & D Ointment, purified lanolin, or a synthetic corticoid (available by prescription). If nursing is stopped on the affected side, engorgement, reduced flow, and plugged ducts are likely to develop.

It is not uncommon to isolate *Staphylococcus aureus* or *Candida* species from severely cracked nipples. Local treatment with mupirocin or nystatin cream as indicated by the results of culture aids healing. Studies show that mastitis develops in as many as 20% of women in whom *S. aureus* isolates are detected. When the nipple is severely affected and fungal and bacterial infections have been ruled out, the physician may wish to prescribe 1% cortisone ointment to be rubbed into the nipple and areola after each feeding. Usually, only a short course of treatment (2 days) is needed. The infant receives an insignificant amount of medication from such treatment. The underlying cause of the problem, such as poor positioning, should always be addressed.

Engorgement

Engorgement is characterized by congestion, increased vascularity, and the accumulation of milk in the breast. Either primarily the areola or the entire breast may be affected. Some degree of fullness and swelling, however, is normal as the quantity of milk increases in the early postpartum period. A woman who does not experience such changes in her breasts may be at risk for lactation failure. The best treatment for engorgement is prevention, with early and frequent nursing to enhance the quantity of milk and empty the breast adequately. Engorgement often becomes evident when the infant has been left in the nursery overnight so that the mother can rest.

In areolar engorgement, swelling flattens the nipple, so that attachment is difficult for the infant. If the infant attaches improperly, sucking only on the nipple, breast-feeding is painful and the nipple may be traumatized. Improper attachment to the nipple also makes milk withdrawal inefficient, and the infant receives little nourishment.

The treatment of engorgement is directed at emptying the breast. Often, the manual expression of a small amount of milk allows the infant to grasp the breast properly and nurse efficiently. The application of warm compresses to the breast before expression facilitates blood flow and letdown. Mothers may also find it easier to express milk manually while in a warm shower. During manual expression, the mother compresses the breast just behind the areola back into the chest and then brings her fingers gently together to express milk. When an engorged breast is presented to the infant, the areola should be softened by expression and compressed between two fingers to make the nipple protrude.

Engorgement involving the entire breast usually occurs on the second postpartum day and is largely a consequence of increased vascularity. The mother experiences throbbing pain in breasts that are full, hard, and tender. Breast swelling may extend from the clavicle to the lower rib cage and into the axilla. Treatment, as before, involves emptying the breast adequately. In addition to expressing milk, wearing a well-fitting bra is important to support the breast and provide comfort. Analgesics, including acetaminophen, aspirin, or codeine, may provide further relief; if they are taken a half-hour before nursing, the infant will receive little medication in the milk. It is important to empty the breast adequately to prevent a subsequent decrease in the production of milk. Frequent feeding around the clock to empty the breast is essential in the treatment of engorgement. Milk production and vascularity stabilize after a few days of treatment. Between feedings, cool compresses may provide additional relief.

Plugged Ducts

The lactating breast is lumpy, but the lumps appear in different places and are not tender. Mildly tender lumps in the breasts of a lactating women who shows no other signs of systemic illness are probably caused by a plugged collecting duct. She should continue to nurse to ensure adequate emptying of the breast. Applying warm compresses and massaging the affected area before nursing may further aid in emptying the breast. Women may also be counseled to alternate nursing positions because different areas of the breast empty better depending on the infant's position at the breast (Madonna, cross cradle, or football hold). A good nursing bra is helpful because regular bras with wire stays or constricting straps may contribute to milk stasis in a compressed area.

Mastitis

Mastitis is a common condition in lactating women, with an estimated prevalence of 20% in the 6 months postpartum. Most cases occur in the first 6 weeks, but mastitis can develop at any time during lactation. Certain conditions may predispose to mastitis, including milk stasis (engorgement or plugged ducts) and lowered maternal defenses secondary to fatigue and stress. Cracked or sore nipples may lead to milk stasis when a woman avoids nursing on a painful breast. Engorgement, plugged ducts, and sore nipples should be treated vigorously to prevent the development of mastitis.

Few research trials have been conducted in this area. The usual clinical definition of mastitis is a tender, hot, swollen, wedge-shaped area of breast associated with a temperature of 38.5°C or higher, chills, flulike aching, and systemic illness. The term *mastitis,* however, means "inflammation of the breast," and this may or may not involve a bacterial infection. Redness, pain, and heat may all be present when an area of the breast is engorged, "blocked," or "plugged," but an infection is not necessarily present. If the symptoms of mastitis are mild and have been present for less than 24 hours, conservative management (effective milk removal and supportive measures) may be sufficient. If the symptoms do not abate within 12 to 24 hours, or if the woman is acutely ill, antibiotics should be started.

The most common pathogen in infective mastitis is penicillin-resistant *S. aureus*. Less often, the organism is a streptococcus or *Escherichia coli*. Bacteria infect a secreting lobule in the breast by way of the lactiferous ducts, through a traumatized nipple to the periductal lymphatics, or by hematogenous spread. Early diagnosis and treatment are essential to prevent progression of the disease to abscess formation or chronic mastitis. Cultures of milk and cell counts (bacteria, $>10^3$/ml; leukocytes, $>10^6$/ml) may be helpful in the diagnosis, but antibiotic therapy should not await culture results. Uninfected human milk normally contains 1,000 to 4,000 cells per cubic milliliter. Adverse outcomes such as recurrent mastitis and abscess formation are clearly associated with delays between the onset of symptoms and treatment.

The affected breast should be regularly emptied by nursing or pumping. The woman may continue to nurse, beginning with the unaffected breast, to enhance letdown on the affected side and lessen discomfort when the infant latches on. The breast-fed infant generally remains well during episodes of acute mastitis, and the choice of antibiotics should be compatible with continued breast-feeding. Sulfa drugs should be avoided if the infant is younger than 1 month of age. The antibiotic therapy chosen should account for likely organisms, local sensitivities, and exposure to resistant organisms. Staphylococcal disease responds readily to dicloxacillin or nafcillin, and streptococcal disease to penicillin. Cephalexin is usually safe in women with suspected penicillin allergy, but clindamycin is suggested for cases of severe penicillin hypersensitivity. Antibiotics should be given for at least 10 to 14 days. Adequate rest and stress reduction are essential. Warm compresses often hasten drainage of the involved area and provide additional pain relief. Analgesics such as aspirin or acetaminophen and a supportive bra are also helpful.

CHRONIC MASTITIS

Chronic mastitis can result from inadequate or delayed treatment of acute mastitis. The clinician must stress the importance of a full 10 to 14 days of treatment for acute mastitis. A culture of breast milk, best obtained as a midstream sample, should guide antibiotic therapy. The woman should manually express her milk after carefully washing her hands and cleaning the breast with water. The first 3 mL of expressed milk is discarded and a midstream sample obtained for culture.

Recurrent mastitis should be aggressively treated with antibiotics for at least 2 weeks. Treatment should also include the measures described for acute mastitis. If treatment fails, chronic bacterial infection, fungal infection, or underlying breast disease such as a tumor or cyst must be considered. Cysts or tumors present as unchanging masses in the lactating breast.

Monilial Infection

Monilial infection of the breast typically presents as stinging, burning pain radiating throughout the breast during and after nursing. The infection is a common complication of recent antibiotic treatment, maternal candidal vaginitis, or fungal infection in the infant (thrush or candidal diaper rash). The nipple may be normal or appear pink and shiny with typical satellite lesions. A 2-week course of treatment with a topical antifungal agent rubbed into the nipple and areola after breast-feeding is usually effective. Other sources of infection in the mother, such as vaginitis, should also be treated. The infant should always be treated simultaneously with oral nystatin to prevent recurrences. Such therapy is indicated even if the infant shows no signs of concurrent thrush or candidal diaper rash.

Colic and Breast Rejection

Some breast-fed infants exhibit colicky symptoms that are believed to be associated with specific foods in the mother's diet, such as garlic, onions, cabbage, turnips, broccoli, and beans. Other often-cited foods are apricots, rhubarb, prunes, melons, peaches, and other fresh fruits. Strong spices in foods or teas may also cause symptoms. If a mother has questions regarding foods in her diet, she should carefully document any effects in the 24 hours after ingestion of the suspected irritant. Caffeine, which appears in breast milk, is slowly metabolized by infants and may cause irritability and wakefulness. Most infants, however, tolerate a maternal intake of one or two cups of a caffeinated beverage without problems. Smoking decreases the production of milk and may also cause irritability; cotinine (a metabolite of nicotine) appears in breast milk.

Colic in breast-fed infants has also been attributed to cow's milk in the mother's diet. Numerous components of cow's milk appear in breast milk. A positive family history of allergies, especially to cow's milk, suggests this diagnosis, and the infant may benefit if the mother eliminates cow's milk from her diet; a week-long trial of elimination is usually diagnostic. Alternative sources of calcium and vitamin D may be necessary for the mother who eliminates all dairy products.

Infants 3 to 4 months old sometimes temporarily refuse to breast-feed for several days. The rejection is often associated with spicy foods in the mother's diet, illness in the infant, or the return of menstruation in the mother. Breast rejection is usually temporary. Addressing dietary causes and underlying disease and increasing cuddling and soothing during breast-feeding usually remedy the situation. Breast rejection secondary to menses usually lasts only for the first 1 or 2 days of the cycle. Rarely, one breast is permanently rejected; the milk supply in that breast declines, and the supply in the opposite breast increases to meet the infant's demands.

BIBLIOGRAPHY

American Academy of Pediatrics and American College of Obstetricians and Gynecologists. Maternal and newborn nutrition. In: American Academy of Pediatrics and American College of Obstetricians and Gynecologists. *Guidelines for perinatal care*. Elk Grove Village, IL: American Academy of Pediatrics, 1997:284.

American Academy of Pediatrics, Working Group on Breast-feeding. Breast-feeding and the use of human milk. *Pediatrics* 1997;100:1035–1039.

American College of Obstetricians and Gynecologists, Committees on Health Care for Underserved Women and Obstetric Practice. *Breast-feeding: maternal and infant aspects*. Washington, DC: American College of Obstetricians and Gynecologists, 2000:1–15.

Gartner LM, Greer FR. Prevention of rickets and vitamin D deficiency: new guidelines for vitamin D intake. *Pediatrics* 2003;111:908–910.

Centers for Disease Control and Prevention. *Final report: vitamin D expert panel meeting, October 11–12, 2001*. Atlanta, GA: Centers for Disease Control and Prevention, 2002.

Committee on Drugs, American Academy of Pediatrics. The transfer of drugs and other chemicals into human milk. *Pediatrics* 2001;108:776–789.

Hopkinson JM, Schanler RJ, Garza C. Milk production by mothers of premature infants. *Pediatrics* 1988;81:815–820.

Innocenti declaration on the protection, promotion, and support of breast-feeding. New York: United Nations Children's Fund (UNICEF), 1990.

Institute of Medicine. *Nutrition during lactation: report of the subcommittee on nutrition during lactation of the committee on nutritional status during pregnancy and lactation*. Washington, DC: National Academy Press, 1991.

Institute of Medicine. *Safety of silicon implants*. Washington, DC: National Academy Press, 2000:248–263..

Kinlay JR, O'Connell DL, Kinlay S. Incidence of mastitis in breast-feeding women during the six months after delivery: a prospective cohort study. *Med J Aust* 1998;169:310–312.

Kramer MS, Chalmers B, Hodnett ED, et al. Promotion of Breast-feeding Intervention Trial (PROBIT): a cluster-randomized trial in the republic of Belarus. *JAMA* 2001;285:1–15.

Kreiter SR, Schwartz RP, Kirkman HN Jr, et al. Nutritional rickets in African American breast-fed infants. *J Pediatr* 2000;137:153–157.

Lawrence RA, Lawrence RM. *Breast-feeding: a guide for the medical profession*, 5th ed. St. Louis: Mosby, 1999.

Lawrence RM, Lawrence RA. Given the benefits of breast-feeding, what contraindications exist? *Pediatr Clin North Am* 2001;48:235–251.

Livingstone VH, Willis CE, Berkowitz J. *Staphylococcus aureus* and sore nipples. *Can Fam Physician* 1996;42:654–659.

Neifert M, DeMarzo S, Seacat J, et al. The influence of breast surgery, breast appearance, and pregnancy-induced breast changes on lactation sufficiency as measured by infant weight gain [see Comments]. *Birth* 1990;17:31–38.

Neifert MR. Prevention of breast-feeding tragedies. *Pediatr Clin North Am* 2001;48:273–297.

Neville MC. Anatomy and physiology of lactation. *Pediatr Clin North Am* 2001;48: 13–34.

Protocol Committee of the Academy of Breast-feeding Medicine. Clinical protocol no 4: mastitis. Available at *www.bfmed.org*. Rochester, NY: Academy of Breast-feeding Medicine, 2002.

U.S. Department of Health and Human Services, Office on Women's Health. *HHS blueprint for action on breast-feeding*. Washington, DC: U.S. Department of Health and Human Services, 2000:1–31.

U.S. Department of Health and Human Services, Public Health Service. *Healthy people 2010: national health promotion and disease prevention objectives*. Washington, DC: U.S. Department of Health and Human Services, 1999.

World Health Organization, Department of Child and Adolescent Health and Development. *Mastitis: causes and management*. Geneva: World Health Organization, 2000:1–45.

World Health Organization, United Nations Children's Fund. Protecting, promoting and supporting breast-feeding: the special role of maternity services (a joint WHO/UNICEF statement). *Int J Gynecol Obstet* 1990;31[Suppl 1]:171–183.

CHAPTER 26

Breast Cancer: Approach to Diagnosis and Management

Susan H. Lee and Maureen A. Chung

Breast carcinoma is a common disease in women, and its prevalence will increase as the baby boomer population enters menopause and more women survive this malignancy. The presentation and diagnosis of breast cancer have changed with the implementation of widespread screening mammography, the introduction of minimally invasive techniques, and the increased proportion of women in whom early-stage disease is diagnosed. It is imperative that primary care providers know the risk factors for breast cancer, the screening guidelines, and the appropriate diagnostic tests for evaluating women who present with breast abnormalities. This chapter provides the rationale for screening mammography, a guideline for the use of diagnostic tests, and an overview of breast cancer management.

RISK FACTORS

The etiology of breast cancer is still unknown. Two major risk factors for breast cancer are female gender and advancing age. Of all breast cancers, 99.5% are diagnosed in women. The diagnosis is infrequent in women younger than 40 years and increases in those past the age of 50. Other risk factors are late age at menopause, early onset of menarche, nulliparity, and delayed first parity (first birth after 35 years of age). Environmental risk factors include alcohol use, a diet high in saturated fat, obesity, and exposure to ionizing radiation.

The role of exogenous hormones in the subsequent development of breast cancer is controversial. Much of the debate on hormone replacement has centered on the use of exogenous hormones in postmenopausal women and has increased since the results of the Women's Health Initiative Study were reported. The Women's Health Initiative Study was the first randomized controlled trial to evaluate the risks and benefits of continuous hormone replacement therapy (HRT) in postmenopausal women. A 26% increase in the risk for breast cancer (95% confidence interval, 1.00–1.59) was noted in women taking continuous combination hormone replacement. More importantly, no reduction in the risk for coronary artery disease, the major cause of death in postmenopausal women, was demonstrated. The results of the Women's Health Initiative Study did not include cyclic combined replacement or estrogen-only replacement. Furthermore, the duration of risk after cessation of HRT is unclear.

Atypical ductal hyperplasia (ADH) and lobular carcinoma in situ (LCIS) increase a woman's risk for breast cancer; either breast may be affected. Invasive breast carcinoma develops during the next 10 to 15 years in 10% of women in whom ADH is diagnosed on a breast biopsy specimen. In the Nurses Health Study, women with atypical hyperplasia on breast biopsy specimens had a relative risk for cancer in either breast of 3.7. In women with a positive family history for breast cancer, this risk increased to 7.3. Women with ADH are candidates for chemoprevention (tamoxifen).

LCIS is a risk factor for breast cancer but not a precursor lesion. The incidence of LCIS ranges from 0.8% to 3.6%. LCIS usually occurs in premenopausal women, is asymptomatic, involves multiple lobules (multifocal), and is found incidentally during biopsies for mammographic or palpable abnormalities. The risk for cancer in either breast regardless of the side affected by LCIS is 1% to 1.5% per year, or a 20% to 30% lifetime risk. The treatment for LCIS is observation or chemoprevention (i.e., tamoxifen). If a patient has additional strong risk factors or desires surgical management, bilateral simple mastectomies with immediate reconstruction is the operation of choice. Chemotherapy or radiation therapy has no role in treatment.

A positive family history is an important risk factor for breast cancer. Approximately 15% to 20% of all breast cancer patients have a positive family history; however, a germ-line mutation can be identified in only 5% to 10%. The number of affected relatives, the degree of kinship, and the age at which the disease presented in the relatives all affect breast cancer risk.

The most prevalent germ-line mutations identified in breast cancer are *BRCA1* and *BRCA2*. Both are associated with ovarian cancer, and *BRCA2* is associated with an increased risk for male breast cancer. Less frequent germ-line mutations associated with breast cancer include Li-Fraumeni syndrome, Cowden disease, Muir-Torre syndrome, Peutz-Jeghers syndrome, ataxia-telangiectasia, and Lynch type I syndrome. Patients who appear to be at an increased risk for carrying one of these germ-line mutations should be offered genetic counseling and testing. Genetic testing is most efficacious if the family member affected with breast cancer is tested initially. Genetic susceptibility testing has important ethical, social, and legal implications, and these factors must be taken into consideration before any genetic workup is undertaken. Proper counseling is necessary if genetic testing is to be implemented.

SCREENING

Screening for breast cancer has been shown to be an effective modality for decreasing mortality. Screening modalities range from monthly breast self-examination and annual mammography to tests such as ultrasonography. The effect of breast self-examination on breast cancer mortality has been studied in few trials. The results of one randomized trial indicated that breast self-examination, when used alone, does not affect cancer mortality. A woman may perform monthly breast self examinations if she is comfortable with doing them, however, she should have a clinical breast examination performed annually by a health care provider.

Mammography for breast cancer screening has been studied in eight randomized trials. A metaanalysis of these studies indicates that mammography decreases breast cancer mortality. Overall, in women older than 50 years, a 22% decrease in breast cancer mortality was noted after 14 years of observation in women offered mammography versus controls. A 20% decrease in breast cancer mortality was also noted in women between the ages of 40 and 49 years, but these results were not apparent until 11 years after the start of the program. Breast density in young women tends to limit mammographic sensitivity. The benefits of screening mammography identified in populations with a high level of screening included a decrease in tumor size, an increase in the number of cases of in situ disease diagnosed, and a decrease in breast cancer mortality. The current recommendation of the American Cancer Society, National Cancer Institute, American College of Radiology, and American Medical Association is that all women older than 40 years be offered an annual screening mammography, which should be combined with breast self-examination. Women with a significant family history of breast cancer should be screened starting at an age 10 years younger than that of the affected relative when the disease was diagnosed. An annual physical examination by a primary care provider is part of breast cancer screening.

Other tests for breast cancer screening that are currently being evaluated in clinical trials are ultrasonography, magnetic resonance imaging (MRI), positron emission tomography (PET), and ductal lavage. No substantial data are available to support their use for screening the general population. Ultrasonography remains an important diagnostic test. It has been shown to be effective in identifying lesions missed on mammograms in women with dense breasts. However, it has not been evaluated as a screening tool in the general population because of a lack of standardization, its inability to identify microcalcifications, and its unknown sensitivity and specificity. The expertise and commitment of time necessary for the successful use of ultrasonography in population screening may not be available.

CLINICAL EXAMINATION

Although many patients present with abnormal mammographic findings, a substantial number present with problems such as nipple discharge, skin and nipple changes, and a palpable breast lump. All patients who present to their primary care physicians with a breast problem should undergo a complete breast examination. A history should be obtained of any previous problems related to the breast, the duration of symptoms, and precipitating factors. The physical examination includes a visual inspection and palpation of the breasts to detect asymmetry, retraction or dimpling of the skin or nipple, scars from previous surgeries, and skin lesions. Each breast should be palpated in a systematic (linear or circular motion) fashion and evaluated for masses, nodules, point tenderness, and nipple discharge. It is important to include the retroareolar area because this portion of the breast is often missed during the examination. Axillary and supraclavicular adenopathy must be noted and evaluated.

If the patient presents with abnormal findings on the screening mammogram and normal physical findings, the diagnostic workup must include an evaluation of the mammographic abnormality. Patients who present with a palpable lump should undergo the appropriate imaging. Although mammography should be the initial test in women older than 40 years and ultrasonography the primary test in women younger than 40 years, in many cases, both tests are used. Nipple discharge should be evaluated for occult blood, after which mammography, retroareolar ultrasonography, or both are performed. Ductograms are no longer encouraged for women with nipple discharge because of the high false-positive and false-negative rates. Patients presenting with skin changes should undergo the appropriate imaging test coupled with a punch biopsy of the involved skin. All patients who present with abnormal findings should receive a histologic or cytologic diagnosis. The only exceptions are women who present with palpable lumps where aspiration proves them to be simple cysts. Cytology of the cyst fluid is not necessary if the cyst completely resolves after aspiration, the fluid is not bloody, and the cyst does not recur. If the previously mentioned criteria are not met, these women should be appropriately evaluated with ultrasonography and biopsy.

LABORATORY TESTING

As previously indicated, mammography and to a lesser extent ultrasonography remain the most important imaging modalities used to diagnose breast cancer. All mammograms are standardized according to the breast imaging reporting and data system (BIRADS). A BIRADS rating of 0 indicates an inconclusive result, and additional imaging is required. For BIRADS rating of 1 (normal findings) or a rating of 2 (benign findings), annual screening mammography is recommended. A BIRADS rating of 3 indicates that the abnormality is probably benign but short-term follow-up is recommended, usually a 6-month follow-up mammogram. The risk for malignancy in a patient with a BIRADS 3 mammogram is less than 2.5%. Patients with BIRADS 4 and 5 ratings have indeterminate or suspect findings, and biopsy is recommended. In a patient with a BIRADS rating of 4, the chance of malignancy is greater than 20%, and in a patient with a BIRADS rating of 5, it is more than 50%. A patient with a BIRADS rating of 4 should undergo a core needle biopsy guided by mammography (stereotactic biopsy) or ultrasonography. If the core needle biopsy reveals histologic findings of benign disease that are concordant with the mammographic findings, the patient can be followed with 6-monthly mammography. If malignant or atypical cells are identified or the pathology results are inconclusive or discordant with the radiologic presentation, surgical excision should be performed. BIRADS 5 may suggest carcinoma or a radial scar, and excisional biopsy is recommended; core needle biopsy of radial scars should not be performed because the pathologic interpretation is difficult.

Ultrasonography is a useful adjunct to mammography and should be the initial imaging test in women younger than 40 years. With ultrasonography, it is possible to differentiate a simple cyst from a complex cyst or solid lesion and to characterize the likelihood of malignancy. All solid or complex cystic lesions identified by ultrasonography should be sampled. If the histologic findings are benign and concordant with the ultrasonographic characteristics, the patient can be followed without surgical excision.

MANAGEMENT

The management of breast cancer can be divided into treatment of the breast, axilla, and systemic disease. The breast and axilla are managed with surgery and radiotherapy. Systemic treatment usually consists of cytotoxic chemotherapy or hormonal agents.

Breast cancer can be treated surgically with either breast conservation surgery or removal of the breast (mastectomy). Surgical excision of the tumor with a margin of noncancerous tissue is performed if a woman wants to keep her breasts. The nomenclature for this procedure includes *lumpectomy, wide local excision, excisional breast biopsy,* and *partial mastectomy*. If the tumor cannot be palpated, wire localization is required before removal. Approximately 80% of patients are candidates for breast conservation surgery. Patients who have tumors in different parts of a breast or a large tumor in a small breast, who are not candidates for radiotherapy or have previously received radiation, or who have extensive disease beyond one quadrant of the breast should be treated with mastectomy. If a lumpectomy is performed for primary breast cancer, adjuvant radiotherapy of the breast may be required to decrease total recurrence. Radiotherapy can be delivered either externally or from indwelling catheters (brachytherapy). If external beam radiotherapy is used, 50 Gy is delivered to the breast within a 5- to 6-week period. Brachytherapy, a newer technique, is currently being evaluated to deliver radiation directly to the breast cancer site. It offers the advantage of providing the maximum therapeutic dose within a short period of time. In mastectomy, the entire breast along with the nipple-areolar complex is removed.

Most patients who undergo mastectomy do not require radiotherapy. Plastic surgery may be offered to patients who desire breast reconstruction.

Evaluation of the axilla is an essential part of breast cancer therapy because nodal metastasis is the most important prognostic indicator of outcome. The results of clinical examination and imaging of the axilla are often inaccurate. An axillary evaluation may include axillary node dissection or a sentinel node biopsy. In axillary node dissection, level 1 and level 2 lymph nodes are removed. This is a safe procedure, and the axillary recurrence rate is less than 2%. However, the morbidity associated with axillary node dissection can be substantial, including decreased range of motion, paresthesias, and lymphedema. In sentinel node biopsy, tracers are injected that are picked up by the lymphatic channels and concentrated in the lymph node (sentinel node) draining the breast cancer. The sentinel lymph node can then be removed through a small incision. Occasionally, more than one sentinel lymph node is removed. Many studies have shown that if the sentinel lymph node is negative for cancer, the chance of metastases being found in any axillary lymph node is less than 5%. Moreover, the clinical axillary recurrence rate after a negative result of a sentinel lymph node biopsy is reported to be 1.5%. An axillary node dissection may be required if the patient has a positive sentinel lymph node. It is currently recommended that patients who present with a clinically negative axilla initially undergo a sentinel lymph node biopsy. If the sentinel lymph node is negative, then they require no further axillary surgery. If the sentinel lymph node is positive, axillary node dissection should be performed. Patients who present with a clinically positive axilla should undergo an axillary node dissection as the primary surgical procedure. Axillary radiation is reserved for those patients who present with multiple positive lymph nodes or extensive extracapsular disease.

Systemic Therapy

The nodal status is the most important prognostic factor in breast cancer because it guides therapeutic decisions regarding adjuvant systemic treatment. The systemic treatment of breast cancer includes cytotoxic chemotherapy and hormonal manipulation. In 2000, a consensus conference was convened to consider adjuvant therapy for breast cancer. Prognostic factors felt to indicate a need for systemic therapy include the presence of one or more positive axillary lymph nodes, a tumor larger than 1 cm, young age of the patient, and a lack of hormone receptor expression in the primary tumor. Important secondary prognostic factors include a high nuclear grade; expression of molecular markers such as HER-2/*neu*, p53, and Ki-67; S-phase; and ploidy. These factors should not be used alone to determine the need for adjuvant treatment. It is recommended that all women with positive lymph nodes and premenopausal women without nodal metastases but with tumors larger than 1 cm be evaluated for cytotoxic chemotherapy. The major regimens for cytotoxic chemotherapy consist of multiple agents that include an anthracycline or methotrexate. Metaanalyses have shown, particularly in premenopausal women, that anthracycline-based chemotherapy is the treatment of choice. Side effects of anthracycline-based therapy include bone marrow suppression, alopecia, gastrointestinal irritability, and cardiotoxicity. In older women who may not be able to tolerate the morbidity of anthracycline-based therapy, combination therapy including methotrexate may be used. Women with a substantial risk for systemic relapse, manifested by the presence of metastatic disease in more than three lymph nodes, may receive a taxane in addition to anthracycline-based therapy. Overall, cytotoxic chemotherapy has been shown to reduce the risk for systemic occurrence by approximately one-third. Multiple-institutional and single-institutional trials have shown no significant survival benefit obtained with high-dose chemotherapy followed by bone marrow rescue.

Hormonal therapy remains an important part of the systemic treatment of breast cancer. Approximately 80% of all breast cancers express hormone receptors and are amenable to hormonal manipulation. Currently, the primary agent for hormone treatment is tamoxifen. Studies have shown a reduction of almost 50% in the recurrence of local breast cancer and a 30% decrease in mortality with the use of tamoxifen. Tamoxifen also prevents the development of new breast cancers. Although it is recommended that tamoxifen be taken for 5 years, its survival benefit may persist for 10 years after the initiation of treatment. The major side effects of tamoxifen are an increased risk for endometrial cancer and thromboembolic events secondary to hypercoagulability. A potential benefit of tamoxifen is a reduced incidence of osteoporosis.

The supply of estrogen in postmenopausal women is derived from the peripheral conversion of androstenedione to estrone in adipose tissue. This process requires an enzyme called *aromatase,* and pharmaceutical agents have been developed that interfere with aromatase activity. The most popular of these agents is anastrazole (Arimidex). In early trials, the agents decreased the risk for systemic relapse in postmenopausal women with estrogen receptor–positive tumors. Unlike tamoxifen, anastrazole is not associated with hypercoagulability or an increased risk for endometrial cancer. It can be used only by postmenopausal women. In premenopausal women, surgical or medical ovarian ablation is a viable option. The benefit of oophorectomy in premenopausal women with estrogen receptor–positive tumors is similar to that of tamoxifen.

OUTCOME

The most important predictors of outcome in breast cancer are tumor size and nodal status. Disease can be staged by tumor size, nodal status, and the presence or absence of metastases (TNM system). Survival rates, which decrease as the clinical stage advances, have been increasing annually since 1989. Overall, patients with stage I cancer have a 10-year survival of 75%. The long-term survival of patients with stage I cancer and tumors smaller than 1 cm (T1a, T1b) is greater than 90%. The 5-year survival rate of patients with stage IV disease is less than 20%.

EFFECTS OF PREGNANCY

Approximately 3% of breast cancers are diagnosed in pregnant women, complicating 1 in 3,000 pregnancies. If breast cancer is suspected in a pregnant woman, the pregnancy itself should not impede the diagnosis. Ultrasonography is the preferred diagnostic imaging modality. If required, mammograms may be used because the risk associated with mammography is negligible but appropriate shielding should be used. Fine needle aspiration and core biopsies are not contraindicated in pregnancy. Once breast cancer has been diagnosed, termination of the pregnancy does not affect the prognosis.

The treatment of breast cancer during pregnancy depends on the gestational age, and in the absence of systemic disease, a modified radical mastectomy is usually recommended. Breast conservation surgery is not recommended unless the disease is diagnosed in the late third trimester because adjuvant radiation therapy is required. If disease is detected in the third trimester, radiotherapy can be delayed until the postpartum period. Systemic chemotherapy can be administered after the first trimester. The chemotherapeutic agents most often used are cyclophosphamide and doxorubicin. Methotrexate, an antimetabolite, should not be used in the first trimester because of its toxicity to trophoblastic tissue. 5-Fluorouracil is also an antimetabolite and should be used with caution. Neoadjuvant chemotherapy after the first trimester may be considered for patients with tumors larger than 3 cm or axillary nodal metastases confirmed by fine needle aspiration or biopsy.

The effect of radiation on the fetus depends on the gestational age. In early embryonic development, from before implantation to 2 weeks of gestation, radiation results in an "all or none" phenomenon—either death or no obvious effect. The fetus is most susceptible to teratogenic effects during organogenesis between 2 and 10 weeks of gestation. After 10 weeks of gestation and until birth, fetal exposure to radiation may result in microcephaly, mental retardation, ocular lesions, and developmental delays. Despite adequate shielding, the amount of radiation to which the fetus is exposed during breast radiotherapy is beyond the safety limit because of abdominal scatter.

Patients with pregnancy-associated breast cancer have larger tumors and a higher incidence of axillary metastases than age-matched controls with breast cancer who are not pregnant. This finding may be explained by various factors associated with pregnancy. Hormonally induced changes in the breast during pregnancy make it more difficult to palpate a breast lump. Women do not undergo screening mammography during pregnancy or lactation, and they are reluctant to undergo invasive procedures. However, stage for stage, the prognosis for patients with pregnancy-associated breast cancer is the same as for their counterparts who are not pregnant.

Subsequent pregnancies do not appear to affect recurrence or survival in women who have been treated for breast cancer. No data are available to support a defined waiting period for pregnancy after successful treatment for breast cancer. However, a 2- to 3-year delay is usually recommended because most recurrences develop during this critical observational period.

BIBLIOGRAPHY

Abrams JS. Adjuvant therapy for breast cancer—results from the USA consensus conference. *Breast Cancer* 2001;8:298–304.

American College of Radiology. *Breast imaging reporting and data system (BI-RADS)*, 2nd ed. Reston, VA: American College of Radiology, 1995.

Chung MA, Fulton J, Cady B. Trends in breast cancer incidence and presentation in a population screened for breast cancer. *Semin Breast Dis* 1999;2:55–63.

Chung MA, Steinhoff MM, Cady B. Clinical axillary recurrence in breast cancer patients after a negative sentinel node biopsy. *Am J Surg* 2002;184:310–314.

Dawes LG, Bowen C, Venta LA, et al. Ductography for nipple discharge: no replacement for ductal excision. *Surgery* 1998;124:685–691.

Dekaban A. Abnormalities of children exposed to x-irradiation during various stages of gestation: tentative timetable of radiation injury to the human fetus. Part 1. *J Nucl Med* 1988;2058.

Dicato M. High-dose chemotherapy in breast cancer: where are we now? *Semin Oncol* 2002;29:16–20.

Donegan W. Breast cancer and pregnancy. *Obstet Gynecol* 1977;50:244.

Early Breast Cancer Trialists' Collaborative Group. Polychemotherapy for early breast cancer: an overview of the randomised trials. *Lancet* 1998;352:930–942.

Early Breast Cancer Trialists' Collaborative Group. Tamoxifen for early breast cancer: an overview of the randomized trials. *Lancet* 1998;351:1451–1467.

Giuliano AE, Kirgen DM, Guenther JM, et al. Lymphatic mapping and sentinel lymphadenectomy for breast cancer. *Ann Surg* 1994;222:391–401.

Haagensen CD, Lane N, Lattes R, et al. Lobular neoplasia (so-called lobular carcinoma in situ) of the breast. *Cancer* 1978;42:737–769.

Humphrey LL, Helfand M, Chan BKS, et al. Breast screening: a summary of the evidence for the U.S. preventative services task force. *Ann Intern Med* 2002;137: 347–360.

King R, Welch J, Manton J, et al. Carcinoma of the breast associated with pregnancy. *Surg Gynecol Obstet* 1985;160:228.

Kolb TM, Lichy J, Newhouse JH. Comparison of the performance of screening mammography, physical examination, and breast US and evaluation of factors that influence them: an analysis of 27,825 patient evaluations. *Radiology* 2002; 225:165–175.

London SJ, Connolly JL, Schnitt SJ, et al. A prospective study of benign breast disease and the risk of breast cancer. *JAMA* 1992;267:941.

Nielsen M, Jensen J, Andersen J. Precancerous and cancerous breast lesions during lifetime and at autopsy: a study based on 225 postmortem examination. *Cancer* 1951;54:612–615.

Orel SG, Kay N, Reynolds C, et al. BI-RADS categorization as a predictor of malignancy. *Radiology* 1999;211:845–850.

Page DL, Dupont WD, Rogers LW, et al. Atypical hyperplastic lesions of the female breast: a long-term follow-up study. *Cancer* 1985;55:2698–2708.

Petrek J. Pregnancy safety after breast cancer. *Cancer* 1994;74:528.

Sorosky JI, Scott-Conner CEH. Breast disease complicating pregnancy. *Obstet Gynecol Clin North Am* 1998;25:353.

Swain SM. Noninvasive breast cancer: part 2. Lobular carcinoma in situ—incidence, presentation, guidelines to treatment. *Oncology* 1989;3:30–40.

The Arimidex, Tamoxifen Alone or in Combination (ATAC) Trialists' Group. Anastrazole alone or in combination with tamoxifen versus tamoxifen alone for the adjuvant treatment of postmenopausal women with early breast cancer: first results of the ATAC randomized trial. *Lancet* 2002;359:2131–2139.

Thomas DB, Gao DL, Ray RM, et al. Randomized trial of breast self-examination in Shanghai: final results. *J Natl Cancer Inst* 2002;94:1445–1457.

Wingo P, Tong T, Bolden S. Cancer statistics, 1995. *CA Cancer J Clin* 1995;45:8.

CHAPTER 27

Premalignant Lesions in the Cervix, Vagina, and Vulva

David C. Foster

A vast majority of cases of intraepithelial neoplasia of the anogenital tract, although not all, are associated with genital human papillomavirus (HPV) infection, the most common sexually transmitted disease in the United States. Certain types of HPV cause abnormalities on Papanicolaou (Pap) smears and are etiologically related to cervical, vaginal, vulvar, and anal neoplasia. Other types of HPV cause genital warts and "atypical" or low-grade abnormalities on Pap smears. This chapter reviews the evaluation and management of intraepithelial neoplasia in various regions of the female lower genital tract. Selected topics relevant to non–HPV-related neoplasia are also discussed.

CERVICAL INTRAEPITHELIAL NEOPLASIA

Approximately 12,900 cases of invasive cervical cancer occur annually, with 4,400 women expected to die of disease. The major risk factor for cervical cancer, and also for many vaginal and vulvar malignancies, is HPV infection. Other risk factors for cervical malignancy include cigarette smoking, multiple sexual partners, early age at first intercourse, and lower socioeconomic status.

Early detection through the Pap smear has clearly been the prime example of a successful screening method. Pap smear screening has decreased the incidence of invasive cervical cancer by 70%. Each year, approximately 50 million women undergo Pap smear screening in the United States, and a Pap smear abnormality is detected in 7% of them. Evidence-based guidelines have now been published. These recommendations are based on several events, including the following: (a) a National Cancer Institute–initiated revision and clarification of the Bethesda system, which is a standardized classification of Pap terminology; (b) the publication of several major studies, including the ASC-US/LSIL Triage Study of the National Cancer Institute; and (c) the development of new technologies, including liquid-based cytology and sensitive molecular methods for the detection of HPV. The recommendations based on the evidence-based analysis are summarized in Table 27.1.

Atypical Squamous Cells on Papanicolaou Smear

The Bethesda system divides the Pap classification of atypical squamous cells into two subtypes: (a) atypical squamous cells of undetermined significance (ASC-US) and (b) atypical cells—cannot exclude a high-grade squamous intraepithelial lesion (ASC-H). The chance that a woman with ASC-US has cervical intraepithelial neoplasia (CIN) 2 or 3 is 5% to 17%, and the chance of a woman with ASC-H is 24% to 94%. For this reason, women with ASC-H require additional surveillance and management (Table 27.1).

Atypical Glandular Cells on Papanicolaou Smear

In contrast to the ASC category, atypical glandular cells are associated with a greater risk for cervical neoplasia. The Bethesda system divides atypical glandular cells into three subtypes: (a) atypical glandular cells—endocervical, endometrial, or not otherwise specified (AGC, NOS); (b) atypical glandular cells, favor neoplasia (AGC, favor neoplasia); and (c) adenocarcinoma in situ (AIS). Although all atypical glandular cells carry a risk for malignancy, "AGC, favor neoplasia" carries a greater risk for high-grade lesions (27%–96%) than AGC, NOS (9%–41%). AIS carries an even higher risk for in situ carcinoma (48%–69%) or invasive adenocarcinoma (38%). The recommended management of each type of AGC (Table 27.1) reflects these differences in risk.

Low-Grade Squamous Intraepithelial Lesion on Papanicolaou Smear

In the majority of women with a low-grade squamous intraepithelial lesion (LSIL) on the Pap smear, biopsy reveals either CIN 1 or no pathology, whereas 15% to 30% have CIN 2 or 3. In most women with CIN 1, the lesion regresses spontaneously or is completely removed by the biopsy. Because of the tendency of LSIL to regress, expensive HPV testing or immediate large-loop excision of the transformation zone (LLETZ) does not appear to be justified. According to the ASC-US/LSIL Triage Study, 83% of women with LSIL are infected with a high-risk type of HPV, yet limited specificity of the test in predicting who may progress to CIN 2 to 3 is evident. LLETZ procedures for LSIL often yield no evidence of neoplasia on pathology. For these reasons, the recommendations in Table 27.1 advise a less invasive approach for patients with this category of disease.

High-Grade Squamous Intraepithelial Lesion on Papanicolaou Smear

A high-grade squamous intraepithelial lesion (HSIL) on the Pap smear identifies a woman at significant risk for CIN 2 or 3 or worse. In women with HSIL, the chance of having CIN 2 or 3 is 70% to 75%, and the chance of having invasive carcinoma is 1% to 2%. Colposcopy and endocervical sampling are considered the best approach for evaluating this group of women.

Special Circumstances

HSIL in a pregnant woman: Colposcopy without endocervical sampling is recommended. Biopsy is appropriate during pregnancy when the colposcopic findings suggest invasive disease.

ASC-US in a postmenopausal woman: Atypical cells may arise from estrogen deficiency. If atrophy is evident, a course of topical estrogen is recommended, with a Pap smear follow-up after several months of therapy.

ASC-US or worse in an immunosuppressed woman: Colposcopy is recommended for any woman infected with HIV in whom a Pap smear abnormality is detected irrespective of her $CD4^+$ cell count or viral load.

History of diethylstilbestrol (DES) exposure in utero: DES was administered to several million women in the United States and Europe to prevent spontaneous abortion and premature delivery. Herbst and colleagues reported a clear association between DES exposure and clear cell carcinoma of the vagina in 1971. The largest proportion of the DES cohort in the United States (68%) comprises women born between 1950 and 1959, who are therefore in the fifth or sixth decade of life. No new cases of clear cell carcinoma have been documented in members of the

TABLE 27.1. Papanicolaou Management Guidelines

Papanicolaou smear report	Recommended management	Special circumstances or additional comments
Atypical squamous cells of undetermined significance (ASC-US)	Repeat cytology 4 to 6 months OR immediate colposcopy OR HPV DNA testing	Immunosuppressed women with ASC should be managed with colposcopy and increased surveillance because of increased risk for CIN 2,3 and high risk for HPV infection.
Atypical squamous cells cannot exclude high-grade squamous intraepithelial lesion (ASC-H)	Colposcopy	If colposcopy is negative or unsatisfactory with negative endocervical sampling, follow up in 6 to 12 months with Pap and colposcopy for ASC-US.
Atypical glandular cells (AGC)	Colposcopy with endocervical sampling (and endometrial sampling)	If colposcopy negative, repeat Pap every 4 to 6 months until four consecutive negative studies.
Atypical glandular cells "favor neoplasia" or adenocarcinoma in situ (AIS)	Colposcopy with endocervical sampling (and endometrial sampling)	If colposcopy is negative, diagnostic excisional procedure (cone or LLETZ).
Low-grade squamous intraepithelial lesion (LSIL)	Colposcopy	If colposcopy is negative or unsatisfactory with negative endocervical sampling, follow up in 6 to 12 months with Pap and colposcopy for ASC-US.
High-grade squamous intraepithelial lesion (HSIL)	Colposcopy	In presence of negative colposcopy or unsatisfactory colposcopy with negative endocervical sampling, excisional diagnostic procedure should be performed.

CIN, cervical epithelial neoplasia; HPV, human papillomavirus; LLETZ, large-loop excision of transformation zone.

DES cohort older than 30 years. No overall increase in the incidence of any cancer other than clear cell carcinoma of the vagina has been found in more than 4,500 women followed for an average of 16 years. An earlier report suggested a twofold increased risk for CIN after DES exposure. However, the increased risk may be associated with surveillance bias and requires further confirmation. No increased risk for invasive squamous cell cancer of the cervix has been noted.

VAGINAL INTRAEPITHELIAL NEOPLASIA

The vagina is the rarest site of intraepithelial neoplasia in the lower genital tract. Like CIN, vaginal intraepithelial neoplasia (VAIN) is usually detected by Pap smear, followed by a confirmatory colposcope-directed biopsy. A history or the concurrent presence of neoplasia elsewhere in the anogenital tract is noted in up to 68% of cases. Well-designed clinical trials of the treatment of VAIN are lacking. Much of the management is individualized and may consist of disappearance after biopsy, topical application of 5-fluorouracil, laser surgery, combined 5-flourouracil and surgery, or partial or total vaginectomy. Conceptually, the reader may consider vaginectomy to be more "definitive," but recurrences at the surgical margin or within graft sites after vaginectomy have been reported. In general, less mutilating procedures are recommended, with close surveillance. Despite surveillance, invasive disease occurs in up to 5% of women followed for VAIN.

VULVAR INTRAEPITHELIAL NEOPLASIA

Because the appearance of vulvar intraepithelial neoplasia (VIN) is variable, the practitioner should perform diagnostic biopsies liberally, particularly for recurrent lesions and those that change color, ulcerate, or are hyperpigmented. VIN can present as red, white, dark, raised, or eroded lesions on the vulva. Cigarette smoking has been shown to be a risk factor for both in situ and invasive vulvar carcinoma. The risk for VIN and squamous cell carcinoma of the vulva is higher in "current" smokers, so that a smoking cessation program may theoretically improve the long-term prognosis. Wide local excision and meticulous surveillance for recurrences are likely to reduce the chance of the development of invasive vulvar cancer. In a 15-year follow-up of VIN, disease recurrence or persistence was noted in 48% of the patients who were surgically managed, and the disease progressed to frankly invasive carcinoma in 7%. The risk for the development or recurrence of VIN in women infected with the HIV virus may be more than threefold higher. Nonsurgical immunotherapy of VIN remains an option not yet proven by clinical trial. In a small case series, immunotherapy with the topical application of 5% imiquimod three times per week was found to clear VIN 3.

Vulvar Dermatoses as Premalignant Lesions

Despite the strong evidence that HPV may be the primary etiologic agent in CIN and a risk factor for the development of cervical cancer, the evidence that HPV is the primary etiologic agent in vulvar cancer is not quite as clear. Both epidemiologic and pathologic research suggests that at least two major groups are at risk for the development of vulvar cancer in association with different etiologic agents. Undoubtedly, HPV infections significantly increase the risk for VIN, as noted in the work of Brinton and colleagues. An analysis of vulvar carcinoma, on the other hand, finds only 58% of patients positive for HPV. Vulvar dermatoses such as lichen sclerosus and lichen planus have been implicated in the development of non–HPV-associated vulvar cancer. A small but clear association of lichen sclerosus with vulvar carcinoma is best managed by examining the patient frequently, at least every 6 months, and performing a biopsy when mucocutaneous ulceration or thickening is identified. Like lichen sclerosus, lichen planus may be associated with an increased risk for malignancy and therefore also requires frequent monitoring and biopsy of visibly suspect regions.

Vulvar Paget Disease

Vulvar Paget disease (extramammary Paget disease) is an infrequent neoplastic condition that is symptomatically associated with itching, burning, and bleeding. Presenting findings include a brick red, scaly, eczematoid plaque with a sharply demarcated border and sometimes a verrucous surface. One should consider the diagnosis if presumed vulvar eczema does not respond to topical steroids. The rate of concurrent noncontiguous adenocarcinoma has been reported to be as high as 26%, and that of contiguous vulvar adenocarcinoma to be 4%. Therefore, after vulvar Paget disease has been diagnosed, the workup should include colonoscopy, cystoscopy, mammography, and colposcopy. The cutaneous margin of Paget cell infiltration usually extends beyond the visibly demarcated margin, so that adequate surgical margins are difficult to attain. Therapy for vulvar Paget disease is excision with a border of at least a 2 to 3 cm from the visible margin and is best performed in consultation with a gynecologic oncologist. The local recurrence rates are 31% for radical vulvectomy and 43% for wide local excision. Unlike excision, laser ablation is not appropriate because of the need for deep tissue destruction. The overall prognosis is determined by the nature of the coexisting adenocarcinoma, if present.

TOOLS FOR THE DIAGNOSIS AND MANAGEMENT OF CERVICAL INTRAEPITHELIAL NEOPLASIA, VAGINAL INTRAEPITHELIAL NEOPLASIA, AND VULVAR INTRAEPITHELIAL NEOPLASIA

Colposcopy and Biopsy of the Cervix and Vagina

The colposcope is a microscope designed to visualize the cervix under sixfold to 40-fold magnification. High-intensity illumination and a green filter make it possible to visualize the vascular changes characteristic of squamous cervical intraepithelial lesions. The use of colposcopy has been expanded to evaluate the entire lower genital tract, including the vagina and vulva. The basic equipment, besides the colposcope, consists of Graves specula of different sizes, cotton swabs, sponges, ring forceps, an endocervical speculum, endobrushes, an endocervical curet, punch biopsy forceps (e.g., Burke, Tischler, Kevorkian), 3% acetic acid solution, Lugol iodine solution, and Monsel solution or silver nitrate sticks for hemostasis.

The patient is placed in the dorsal lithotomy position and the speculum inserted. The acetic acid is applied by spraying the cervix with a 5-mL syringe or with a cotton swab. The acetic acid solution makes it easy to remove the cervical mucus and accentuates the difference between the squamous and columnar epithelium, making the latter turn white, so that the squamocolumnar junction is easily identified. Also, abnormal tissue in the transformation zone appears as aceto-white epithelium, in contrast with the pink color of normal squamous epithelium. Vascular patterns contrast with the white background, so that it is easy to identify areas of punctation, mosaicism, or atypical vessels. All such lesions must be sampled. An endocervical specimen is obtained either with the endobrush or by endocervical curettage. The iodine test is helpful when no lesion is apparent during the initial part of the procedure. Iodine darkly stains cells with a high content of glycogen, such as normal squamous epithelium, leaving abnormal cells and columnar cells basically unstained. If a lesion extends inside the endocervical canal, an effort should be made to visualize it fully; this can be achieved by using the endocervical speculum. If visible lesions extend down the vaginal canal, vaginal colposcopy can be performed to identify the extent and degree of atypicality of vaginal lesions.

The procedure is considered "satisfactory" if the squamocolumnar junction and transformation zone are entirely identified and the full extent of any lesion is seen. If the colposcopy is "unsatisfactory," punch biopsies may be deferred and replaced with a more advanced diagnostic procedure, such as a "top hat" LLETZ or a cone biopsy (laser or cold knife cone). If invasive disease is suspected, a punch biopsy should be performed even if the lesion is not completely visualized. Other indications for conization include a positive endocervical specimen, findings on colposcopy suggestive of occult invasive disease regardless of the results of the punch biopsy, a discrepancy of two grades between cytology and histology, and the presence of microinvasive disease on the punch biopsy specimen. If microinvasive disease is suspected, cold knife cone biopsy is the diagnostic procedure of choice to avoid any thermal damage that could impair an accurate histologic diagnosis. After the colposcopy and biopsy, the patient is instructed to avoid vaginal intercourse or the use of tampons for 2 weeks, and a follow-up appointment is scheduled for 2 to 4 weeks later to discuss the results.

Vulvar Colposcopy

Colposcope-directed biopsies have replaced older techniques, such as 2% toluidine blue–directed biopsies, which have a lower specificity. It is important to allow adequate time (up to 5–10 minutes) between the application of 3% to 5% acetic acid and the beginning of the colposcopic examination so that areas of hyperkeratosis and hyperplasia will be accentuated. In a patient who has known VIN with perianal involvement, colposcopy of the anal canal should be performed. The anal examination is particularly important in immunocompromised patients, in whom an increased rate of anal carcinoma has been documented.

Vulvar Biopsy

As a general rule, vulvar biopsies should be performed liberally in a patient with atypical mucocutaneous findings of the lower genital tract. A significant delay in the diagnosis of vulvar cancer has been found to result from the lack of a timely confirmatory biopsy. In a review of 102 women with vulvar cancer, the biopsy diagnosis was delayed longer than 6 months in 88%, and longer than 5 years in 28%. Previous biopsy specimens from unfamiliar outside facilities should be reviewed microscopically before management is offered based on a prior diagnosis. This rule also applies to biopsies of the cervix and vagina performed elsewhere.

SURGICAL MANAGEMENT OF PRENEOPLASTIC LESIONS OF THE LOWER GENITAL TRACT

The regimens for the surgical treatment of preneoplastic lesions comprise two major types: (a) destructive/ablative techniques and (b) excisional techniques. The destructive/ablative procedures include cryosurgery and laser vaporization. Treatment destroys the presumed diseased tissue and a confirmatory pathology specimen cannot be obtained, a major disadvantage of the destructive/ablative techniques. Undiagnosed adenocarcinoma or microinvasive lesions may be present in 2% to 3% of specimens, and for this reason, treatment failure or recurrence is a risk. An advantage of the destructive/ablative techniques is that less tissue is removed and postoperative morbidity is less than with excisional techniques. Excisional techniques include "cold knife" excision, LLETZ, and laser excision. A pathology specimen can be obtained with all three excisional techniques, but LLETZ and laser excision may cause various degrees of burn artifact at the surgical margin, potentially limiting pathologic interpretation. A randomized clinical trial of cryotherapy, laser vaporization, and the loop electrosurgical excision procedure (LEEP) found no statistically significant differences in complications and persistence or recurrence of disease.

Destructive/Ablative Techniques

CRYOTHERAPY

Cryosurgery is a commonly implemented treatment for CIN and, to a lesser degree, VAIN and VIN. It is an office procedure that usually does not require anesthesia. The equipment consists of a gas tank containing nitrous oxide connected to a pistol. The pistol delivers gas to the cryotip, producing temperatures below −70°C. The cervix is inspected and the extension of the lesion defined. A cryotip that will cover the entire lesion is selected and applied to the affected area. The addition of water-based lubricant to the cryotip helps to create an evenly applied ice ball, particularly in the case of an irregularly shaped cervix. Freezing is continued until the ice ball extends 5 mm away from the edges of the cryotip, which correlates with tissue destruction to a depth of 4 to 5 mm. The other option is the 3-minute freeze, 5-minute thaw, and 3-minute freeze.

During and immediately after the procedure, the patient may experience mild uterine cramping that usually responds to nonsteroidal antiinflammatory agents. It is important to explain to the patient that a profuse watery vaginal discharge with an odor is to be expected for 4 weeks. Tampons and intercourse should be avoided for 3 to 4 weeks. If fever or pelvic pain beyond mild cramps develops, immediate evaluation is warranted because infection is the most common complication of cryotherapy. A Pap smear is performed 3 to 4 months after the procedure, and at 6-month intervals thereafter. After two or three negative results of cytology, annual screening can be resumed. Although the procedure is highly successful, one disadvantage of cryosurgery is the potential development of cervical stenosis, which may preclude visualization of the newly healed squamocolumnar junction.

CARBON DIOXIDE LASER ABLATION

The carbon dioxide laser machine has an output of up to 100 watts and can be adjusted to deliver a continuous or pulsatile flow of energy, depending on the procedure. The wattage chosen depends on whether the laser is being used as an ablative instrument or a cutting device—low wattage (10–30 W) is preferred for ablation. The laser is ideal for the treatment of genital warts or extensive cervical, vaginal, or vulvar disease limited to glabrous (non–hair-bearing) skin.

All personnel in the room, including the patient, must wear glasses designed to protect the eyes from the carbon dioxide laser. The patient is prepared for a vaginal procedure, and a nonreflective speculum is placed. The cervix is reevaluated, either by another colposcopy or by staining with Lugol iodine solution. A cervical block is created by using 10 mL of 1% lidocaine with epinephrine or any other equivalent solution of local anesthetic with vasoconstrictive medication. This is not a paracervical block; the goal is to infiltrate the cervical stroma, and a waiting period until complete blanching is seen is recommended. The laser joystick can be attached to the colposcope or used freely. The transformation zone is identified and marked with 3 mm of clearance of normal tissue. It is divided into quadrants, and each quadrant is treated independently until complete vaporization is achieved to a depth of 7 mm. If bleeding occurs, hemostasis can be obtained by defocusing the laser beam or by using electrocautery.

The role of laser therapy in the management of benign genital warts on the vulva is limited, given the availability of other economical and effective modalities, such as electrocautery and surgical excision. The use of laser vaporization to treat VIN has been found to result in a higher recurrence rate. In a comparison of laser vaporization and laser excision, the cure rate was better for laser excision (33 [87%] of 38 cases) than for laser vaporization (11 [79%] of 14 cases). An advantage of standard surgical excision or laser excision over laser vaporization is the ability to submit a specimen for pathologic interpretation. Recurrence of VIN after laser vaporization may be particularly problematic in hair-bearing parts of the vulva, and standard surgical excision is preferable. In hair-bearing regions of the vulva, dysplastic cells may be found in the deeper epithelial surfaces of the hair follicles (mean depth, 1.90 ± 0.84 mm), whereas dysplastic cells in the glabrous skin of the vestibular mucosa are not as deeply situated (mean depth, 0.52 ± 0.23 mm). If laser treatment is carried to adequate levels to destroy VIN in the hair-bearing areas, excessive scarring and deformity may result.

Excisional Techniques

LARGE-LOOP EXCISION OF THE TRANSFORMATION ZONE (LOOP ELECTROSURGICAL EXCISION PROCEDURE)

LLETZ, or LEEP, is performed in the office under local anesthesia, and it may be undertaken in the same session as colposcopy, an important strategy for clinics with a significant number of noncompliant patients. The success rate is 90% to 98% for the treatment of squamous intraepithelial lesions. It is well accepted by patients; mild discomfort is reported by a minority of patients. A diathermy ground plate is attached to the patient. A nonconductive speculum is applied, and a suction tube is attached to aspirate fumes and allow adequate visualization. The cervix is inspected with the colposcope or Lugol solution and the extent of the lesion assessed. A loop of appropriate size is selected. Whether the lesion is taken totally or in parts depends on its extent. For lesions extending into the canal, a follow-up excision of the canal with a smaller square loop (1 × 1 cm) in a "top hat" fashion is recommended after the initial excision. The power setting is selected according to the size of the loop. A stromal infiltration of 1% lidocaine with epinephrine is used, and after complete blanching of the cervix is seen, the procedure is performed. Hemostasis is secured by using the ball cautery.

LASER WIDE LOCAL EXCISION AND LASER CONE

Conization of the cervix and wide local excision of vaginal or vulvar lesions can be performed with the laser. The power is increased to a higher wattage (30 W), and the spot diameter is decreased to make the laser beam function as a knife. This procedure can be performed under local anesthesia in the same approach described previously. The patient is positioned, and a nonreflective speculum is inserted with the suction tube attached. The lesion and the transformation zone are identified and then marked; 3-mm margins are left around the lesion. A small hook device is used to mobilize the specimen until it is completely excised.

SURGICAL "COLD KNIFE" EXCISION: COLD KNIFE CONE

Conization or wide local excision has been considered the "gold standard" for the definitive treatment of carcinoma in situ and HSIL. Nevertheless, for many intraepithelial neoplastic conditions, it has been replaced by office-based techniques, such as electrosurgery (LLETZ). Although usually performed under general anesthesia, "cold knife" cone or wide local excision can also be performed with a combination of conscious sedation and a local anesthetic block, as described previously. It remains a useful technique for patients with lesions extending up the endocervical canal that cannot be visualized with an endocervical speculum. The cervical branches of the uterine artery are bilaterally ligated with a hemostatic figure-of-eight suture of 1-0 absorbable synthetic material. This initial ligation helps minimize bleeding and aids in traction and exposure of the cervix. The stroma of the cervix is infiltrated with a local anesthetic and a vasopressor solution of epinephrine. With a scalpel, the cone is completed; careful attention is given to attaining clear endocervical and ectocervical margins. Hemostasis is secured by using a suction cautery device or by placing individual figure-of-eight sutures of synthetic absorbable material.

WIDE EXCISION OF VAGINAL OR VULVAR LESIONS

Standard excisional techniques are used, with particular attention paid to maintaining a surgical margin that is free of disease in the submitted specimen. A 1-cm disease-free margin is generally recommended. Exceptions to this rule may be necessary in specific anatomic regions, such as the clitoris or urethral orifice. A valuable aid in ascertaining the visible margin is intraoperative colposcopy; visible lesions can be outlined with a cutaneous marking pen.

HYSTERECTOMY FOR CERVICAL INTRAEPITHELIAL NEOPLASIA

Although widely used in the past to treat premalignant conditions of the cervix, hysterectomy is not as popular today in view of the highly successful, less invasive therapeutic options available. Hysterectomy can be considered when the margins of the cone (cold knife) are diseased, or when several more conservative therapies have failed. The type or route of the hysterectomy (abdominal, vaginal, laparoscopically assisted vaginal) depends mostly on the surgeon's preferences and skills. If the abdominal route is selected, particular care must be taken to ensure that the diseased portion of the cervix is adequately removed because the ectocervix is not visible at the time of uterine removal. After the hysterectomy, it is important to continue Pap smear surveillance in these cases because vaginal dysplasia, although rare, has been reported. Furthermore, the same etiologic factors that induced the cervical changes are still present in the lower genital tract.

MEDICAL AND MEDICAL/SURGICAL OPTIONS FOR THE MANAGEMENT OF INTRAEPITHELIAL NEOPLASIA

Immune Augmentation with Imiquimod

Imiquimod (5%) cream has been shown to be highly effective in clearing genital warts (>80% cleared); the recurrence rate is 20%. The cream is applied manually by the patient on wart tissue three times per week for up to 16 weeks. The side effects are primarily skin irritation and erythema in as many as 60% of patients. Clinical follow-up may be considered every 2 to 4 weeks to evaluate lesion status and patient tolerance.

5-Fluorouracil with and without Associated Surgery

Although topical 5-fluorouracil cream alone has a limited effect on intraepithelial neoplasia, it is often given as an adjunct to surgery. Topical 5-fluorouracil is used in several treatment schedules: preoperatively to facilitate superficial excision (chemosurgery) and postoperatively to prevent recurrence. The widely available 5% preparation may cause a marked reaction, particularly when applied vaginally. Close initial monitoring of the response and less frequent use or a reduction of the concentration to 2.5% may be necessary. A once-a-week application of 1 to 2 g of a 2.5% to 5% cream may be a reasonable initial dosage.

SUMMARY

HPV is a "common denominator" in many neoplasms of the lower genital tract. Once intraepithelial neoplasia is diagnosed in one region of the lower genital tract, careful evaluation of the remaining regions is mandatory. Excisional or ablative therapeutic options vary according to the specific region involved. The clinician should also bear in mind the small number of non-HPV causes of neoplasia, such as vulvar dermatoses.

BIBLIOGRAPHY

Benedet JL, Wilson PS, Matisic JP. Epidermal thickness measurements in vaginal intraepithelial neoplasia: a basis for optimal CO_2 laser vaporization. *J Reprod Med* 1992;37:809–812.

Brinton LA, Nasca PC, Mallin K, et al. Case-control study of cancer of the vulva. *Obstet Gynecol* 1990;75:859–866.

Buscema J, Naghashfar Z, Sawada E, et al. The predominance of human papillomavirus type 16 in vulvar neoplasia. *Obstet Gynecol* 1988;71:601–606.

Carlson JA, Ambros R, Malfetano J, et al. Vulvar lichen sclerosus and squamous cell carcinoma: a cohort, case control, and investigational study with historical perspective—implications for chronic inflammation and sclerosis in the development of neoplasia [Review]. *Hum Pathol* 1998;29:932–948.

Davis G, Wentworth J, Richard J. Self-administered topical imiquimod treatment of vulvar intraepithelial neoplasia: a report of four cases. *J Reprod Med* 2000; 45:619–623.

Fanning J, Lambert HC, Hale TM, et al. Paget's disease of the vulva: prevalence of associated vulvar adenocarcinoma, invasive Paget's disease, and recurrence after surgical excision [Review]. *Am J Obstet Gynecol* 1999;180:24–27.

Felix JC, Muderspach LI, Duggan BD, et al. The significance of positive margins in loop electrosurgical cone biopsies. *Obstet Gynecol* 1994;84:996–1000.

Feuer GA, Shevchuk M, Calanog A. Vulvar Paget's disease: the need to exclude an invasive lesion. *Gynecol Oncol* 1990;38:81–89.

Franck JM, Young AWJ. Squamous cell carcinoma in situ arising within lichen planus of the vulva. *Dermatol Surg* 1995;21:890–894.

Hatch EE, Palmer JR, Titus-Ernstoff L, et al. Cancer risk in women exposed to diethylstilbestrol in utero. *JAMA* 1998;280:630–634.

Herbst AL, Ulfelder H, Poskanzer DC. Adenocarcinoma of the vagina: association of maternal stilbestrol therapy with tumor appearance in young women. *N Engl J Med* 1971;284:878–881.

Herod JJ, Shafi MI, Rollason TP, et al. Vulvar intraepithelial neoplasia: long-term follow-up of treated and untreated women [see Comments]. *Br J Obstet Gynaecol* 1996;103:446–452.

Jones BA, Davey DD. Quality management in gynecologic cytology using interlaboratory comparison. *Arch Pathol Lab Med* 2000;124:672–681.

Jones RW, Joura EA. Analyzing prior clinical events at presentation in 102 women with vulvar carcinoma: evidence of diagnostic delays. *J Reprod Med* 1999;44: 766–768.

Jones RW, Rowan DM, Kirker J, et al. Vulval lichen planus: progression of pseudoepitheliomatous hyperplasia to invasive vulval carcinomas. *Br J Obstet Gynaecol* 2001;108:665–666.

Kobak WH, Roman LD, Felix JC, et al. The role of endocervical curettage at cervical conization for high-grade dysplasia. *Obstet Gynecol* 1995;85:197–201.

Korn AP, Abercrombie PD, Foster A. Vulvar intraepithelial neoplasia in women infected with human immunodeficiency virus-1. *Gynecol Oncol* 1996;61:384–386.

Krebs HB. Treatment of vaginal intraepithelial neoplasia with laser and topical 5-fluorouracil. *Obstet Gynecol* 1989;73:657–660.

Larsen J, Petersen CS, Weismann K. Prolonged application of acetic acid for detection of flat vulval warts. *Dan Med Bull* 1990;37:286–287.

Lin WM, Ashfaq R, Michalopulos EA, et al. Molecular Papanicolaou tests in the twenty-first century: molecular analyses with fluid-based Papanicolaou technology. *Am J Obstet Gynecol* 2000;183:39–45.

Mitchell MF, Tortolero-Luna G, Cook E, et al. A randomized clinical trial of cryotherapy, laser vaporization, and loop electrosurgical excision for treatment of squamous intraepithelial lesions of the cervix. *Obstet Gynecol* 1998;92: 737–744.

Robboy SJ, Noller KL, O'Brien P, et al. Increased incidence of cervical and vaginal dysplasia in 3,980 diethylstilbestrol-exposed young women: experience of the National Collaborative Diethylstilbestrol Adenosis Project. *JAMA* 1984;252: 2979–2983.

Sillman FH, Fruchter RG, Chen YS, et al. Vaginal intraepithelial neoplasia: risk factors for persistence, recurrence, and invasion and its management. *Am J Obstet Gynecol* 1997;176:93–99.

Smith RA, Mettlin CJ, Davis KJ, et al. American Cancer Society guidelines for the early detection of cancer. *CA Cancer J Clin* 2000;50:34–49.

Solomon D, Schiffman M, Tarone R, et al. Comparison of three management strategies for patients with atypical squamous cells of undetermined significance: baseline results from a randomized trial [see Comments]. *J Natl Cancer Inst* 2001;93:293–299.

Unger ER, Vernon SD, Lee DR, et al. Human papillomavirus type in anal epithelial lesions is influenced by human immunodeficiency virus. *Arch Pathol Lab Med* 1997;121:820–824.

Wright TCJ, Cox JT, Massad LS, et al. 2001 Consensus guidelines for the management of women with cervical cytological abnormalities [Review] [see Comments]. *JAMA* 2002;287:2120–2129.

CHAPTER 28

Gynecologic Cancers

Brent DuBeshter, Giuseppe Del Priore, David Warshal, and Eugene Toy

UTERINE CARCINOMA

Uterine cancer is the most common malignancy of the female genital tract in the United States, with 38,000 cases diagnosed annually and 1 in 100 women acquiring it during their lifetime. Although it is generally detected in early (curable) stages, more than 6,000 women die of this disease each year in the United States. The peak incidence of nearly 200 cases per 100,000 women per year occurs at about the age of 65 years. Although uterine cancer is a disease of older women, up to 15% of cases develop in women younger than 40 years. The prevalence and incidence data vary at least fourfold among nationalities and ethnic groups and correlate highly with socioeconomic factors and race. For instance, the rate of endometrial cancer in whites may be twice that of minorities in the United States.

The mainstay of the therapy of endometrial cancer is surgery, including hysterectomy, removal of the ovaries, and lymph node biopsy to determine the extent of tumor. However, radiation treatment, chemotherapy, and hormonal therapy are used in selected instances based on the patient's age, extent of the tumor, and histology of the cancer. The most common histologic subtype is endometrioid adenocarcinoma, which accounts for 80% to 90% of cases. Papillary serous and clear cell carcinomas are less common subtypes known for their virulent behavior.

Etiology

Risk factors for adenocarcinoma of the endometrium include obesity, early menarche, late menopause, ovarian granulosa cell tumors, polycystic ovarian syndrome, and nulliparity. Of these factors, obesity is the most important; the risk of patients more than 50 lb overweight is increased 10-fold. Most risk factors for endometrial cancer are related to unopposed estrogen stimulation of the endometrium. In obese women, endogenous estrogen is produced via the peripheral conversion of androstenedione to estrone in adipose cells. In polycystic ovarian syndrome, estrogen is produced without normal progesterone secretion, and granulosa cell tumor of the ovary may be associated with the abnormal production of endogenous estrogen.

Whereas unopposed estrogen, whether exogenous or endogenous, has been unequivocally linked to the development of endometrial cancer, progestin treatment is protective. If estrogen is prescribed to a woman with an intact uterus, progestin treatment should always be included. The risk for endometrial cancer is reduced 50% in women who have used oral contraceptives with a progestin component. Progestin treatment is unnecessary in a woman whose uterus has been removed. Estrogen replacement therapy in postmenopausal women offers some benefits, including the alleviation of hot flashes and the prevention of osteoporosis, but studies have shown an increased risk for heart attack and strokes, which has dampened many practitioners' enthusiasm for recommending this type of treatment.

Tamoxifen is a synthetic steroid with weak estrogenic activity in the endometrium. It is also associated with endometrial hyperplasia and adenocarcinoma, although the causal relation is controversial. The epidemiologic association between tamoxifen use and uterine neoplasms may be genetic, in that women with breast cancer receiving tamoxifen may be genetically predisposed to uterine cancer. Until more information is available, women receiving tamoxifen who experience uterine bleeding should undergo endometrial biopsy. The routine surveillance of asymptomatic patients with ultrasonography or biopsy is not warranted.

The most significant risk factor for development of uterine adenocarcinoma is the presence of complex endometrial hyperplasia with atypia on histologic examination. Hyperplasia results from excessive estrogen stimulation, as occurs in many of the conditions previously mentioned. Hyperplasia can be simple or complex, with or without atypia. Cancer develops in up to 30% of patients with untreated atypical hyperplasia; consequently, hysterectomy is usually recommended. Simple hyperplasia without atypia progresses to a malignancy in fewer than 2% of cases.

Numerous genetic abnormalities have been described in all histologic types of uterine cancer. These include abnormal expression of p53 and the retinoblastoma genes. A syndrome associated with an inherited predisposition to certain cancers, the Lynch type II syndrome, has been described and includes endometrial cancer in addition to mammary, colonic, and ovarian neoplasms. No guidelines are available for recommending prophylactic hysterectomy to women at increased risk for endometrial cancer by virtue of their family history.

History

The most common presenting symptom of uterine cancer is postmenopausal bleeding, but in some patients, the only symptom is discharge or odor. Rarely, endometrial cancer is discovered in asymptomatic patients when abnormal endometrial cells are noted on the Papanicolaou (Pap) smear.

Most postmenopausal women with vaginal bleeding do not have endometrial cancer. The risk is age-related and ranges from 10% in women ages 50 to 59 years to more than 50% in women older than 80 years. Overall, about 30% of women with postmenopausal bleeding have a malignancy. Postmenopausal bleeding is always an indication for endometrial biopsy or dilation and curettage. A biopsy should also be performed when any women older than 35 years has abnormal bleeding, once pregnancy has been excluded.

Physical Examination

In most patients with endometrial cancer, the physical examination reveals no abnormalities. An enlarged uterus is the most common abnormality, but this is not specific. Adnexal masses are unusual but may occur in cases of simultaneous ovarian cancer. Cervical or vaginal involvement may be noted and is associated with a more advanced stage. Manifestations of distant metastases, such as dyspnea from pulmonary involvement, seizures from brain metastases, or pain from bone metastases, are rare. Other physical findings are nonspecific and usually related to coexistent obesity, hypertension, or diabetes.

Laboratory and Imaging Studies

A speculum examination with biopsy of any suspect lesion, a Pap smear, and a pelvic examination should be performed in any patient with postmenopausal bleeding. In addition, an office endometrial biopsy is mandatory; the specimen should be obtained with small flexible catheters. If the results of office endometrial sampling are unsatisfactory, further evaluation with dilation and curettage is warranted.

Transvaginal ultrasonography may be helpful when the results of biopsies are not definitive; in patients with a thin (<5 mm) endometrial stripe, the risk for malignancy is low. The endometrial stripe is frequently thickened in patients receiving hormone replacement therapy or tamoxifen.

Although a Pap smear is not a screening test for endometrial carcinoma, abnormal findings occasionally lead to the diagnosis of endometrial cancer in an asymptomatic patient. The presence of endometrial cells on the Pap smear of a postmenopausal patient is abnormal and requires endometrial evaluation. In addition, the presence of malignant endometrial cells on cervical cytology in patients with endometrial cancer indicates a more advanced lesion with a higher risk for extrauterine spread.

The only metastatic survey routinely indicated for patients with uterine cancer is chest roentgenography. If the pelvic examination is difficult or a mass is suspected, pelvic ultrasonography may be helpful. Screening for other malignancies with mammography, a stool guaiac test, and flexible sigmoidoscopy may be warranted and is usually performed according to age-appropriate guidelines.

Treatment

Endometrial hyperplasias without atypia are usually treated with cyclic progestins. A daily dose of 10 to 20 mg of medroxyprogesterone acetate (Provera) is taken for 14 days each month. A biopsy should be repeated after 3 months of treatment to exclude persistent hyperplasia. Because simple hyperplasia without atypia is sometimes seen in younger women with infertility secondary to anovulation, induction of ovulation may be the therapy of choice in these patients. For older patients in whom the induction of ovulation is not an objective, the recommended treatment consists of continuous progestin therapy with 40 to 160 mg of megestrol acetate (Megace) per day for 12 weeks, followed by repeated endometrial sampling.

Endometrial hyperplasia with atypia requires more thorough evaluation and treatment. If this diagnosis is made by office endometrial biopsy, dilation and curettage is warranted to exclude a coexistent cancer, which is found in about 25% of patients. In a premenopausal woman who desires fertility, management by ovulation induction or the long-term administration of megestrol acetate may still be appropriate. If progestin treatment is chosen, it must be continued indefinitely because hyperplasia or carcinoma recurs in up to 50% of patients who discontinue treatment. Postmenopausal patients or those who do not desire childbearing are better treated by hysterectomy.

The mainstay of the treatment of endometrial cancer is total abdominal hysterectomy and bilateral salpingo-oophorectomy with lymph node dissection. Selected patients who are not operative candidates may be treated solely with pelvic radiation, but the chance of cure is compromised. During hysterectomy, lymph node specimens should be obtained from the pelvis and aortic areas to define those who may benefit from postoperative adjuvant therapy. Omental biopsy or removal may be indicated if an advanced stage is suspected (Table 28.1).

After surgery, patients at high risk for recurrence and those with extrauterine disease should receive adjuvant radiation treatment. Patients with evidence of cancer in the upper abdomen may be treated with progestins or systemic chemotherapy. Whole-abdominal radiation has also been used in those in whom tumor has been completely removed. Chemotherapy is preferred for large, unresectable lesions.

Most patients with uterine cancer are cured, but recurrence in the pelvis is associated with 50% mortality. Because most recurrences develop within the first 2 years after treatment, close surveillance is usually continued during this interval. A physical examination including a pelvic examination and Pap smear three or four times a year for 2 years and every 6 months thereafter is appropriate. Routine metastatic surveillance is not indicated because systemic disease is usually not curable. For disseminated disease, either chemotherapy or progestins may be useful. Patients with an isolated recurrence of disease, usually at the vaginal apex, may be treated with radiation if this has not been given previously, or rarely with pelvic exenteration if the recurrence is isolated and within a previously irradiated field.

Considerations in Pregnancy

Pregnancy is associated with a lifetime reduction in risk for the development of endometrial adenocarcinoma. Vaginal bleeding is common during pregnancy but is rarely the manifestation of a neoplastic process. When it is, a cervical neoplasm is almost always the cause. Therefore, uterine cancer is not usually included in the differential diagnosis of bleeding during pregnancy.

TABLE 28.1. Surgical Staging of Uterine Cancer

Stage	Characteristics
IA	Confined to the endometrium.
IB	Myometrial invasion <50%.
IC	Myometrial invasion >50%.
IIA	Tumor involves endocervical glands.
IIB	Tumor involves endocervical stroma.
IIIA	Tumor involves uterine serosa or adnexa. Cytology positive for malignant cells.
IIIB	Vaginal metastases.
IIIC	Pelvic or aortic node metastases.
IVA	Tumor metastases to bowel or bladder mucosa.
IVB	Other distant metastases or positive inguinal nodes.

OVARIAN CARCINOMA

In the United States, ovarian carcinoma remains the leading cause of death from gynecologic malignancy, with 14,300 deaths expected in 2003. The number of deaths has not changed during the past decade despite the introduction of many new chemotherapeutic agents. Ovarian cancer is the second most frequent gynecologic cancer, with an estimated 25,400 new cases diagnosed in 2003, and the sixth most common malignancy among women. It is estimated that a woman's risk for the development of ovarian carcinoma during the course of her lifetime is 1 in 70.

The neoplastic potential of the ovary is diverse. The classification system adopted by the World Health Organization has been a useful framework for clinicians and pathologists (Table 28.2). Neoplasms intrinsic to the ovary have been divided into three broad categories based on their cellular origin.

Epithelial tumors arise primarily from the coelomic epithelium of the ovary and are the most frequent and important type of ovarian cancer. Ninety-five percent of epithelial tumors are of serous or mucinous histology. On a stage-for-stage basis, the histologic subtype of ovarian cancer has little bearing on treatment decisions, with the exception of clear cell carcinoma, which is known to behave in a virulent fashion.

Sex cord-stromal tumors, such as granulosa cell tumors and thecomas, develop from the sex cords and specialized stroma, or mesenchyme, of the ovary. Although uncommon, they are important because they are frequently hormonally functional, producing estrogen, progesterone, or various androgens. Most of these malignancies are indolent.

Germ cell tumors, derived from the primitive germ cells of the ovary, can replicate embryonic, extraembryonic, or adult-type tissue. The dermoid cyst is the most common benign ovarian neoplasm of childhood and accounts for up to half of all benign ovarian tumors in women of reproductive age. Primitive germ cell malignancies, such as endodermal sinus tumor, dysgerminoma, and immature teratoma, occur predominantly in young women.

TABLE 28.2. Modified World Health Organization Classification of Ovarian Tumors

- Epithelial tumors
  - Serous
  - Mucinous
  - Endometrioid
  - Clear cell
  - Brenner
  - Mixed
  - Undifferentiated
- Sex cord-stromal tumors
  - Granulosa stromal cell
    - Granulosa cell
    - Thecoma-fibroma
  - Sertoli-Leydig cell
  - Lipid cell
  - Gynandroblastomas
- Germ cell tumors
  - Dysgerminomas
  - Endodermal sinus tumors
  - Embryonal carcinomas
  - Polyembryomas
  - Choriocarcinomas
- Teratomas
  - Immature
  - Mature
  - Monodermal (struma ovarii, carcinoid)

They are important because they affect young patients, and the management usually includes preservation of reproductive function in addition to chemotherapy. Advances in the use of chemotherapy have significantly reduced the mortality associated with these tumors, particularly endodermal sinus tumor.

Etiology

The etiology of ovarian carcinoma is not known. Most empiric evidence suggests that the risk for ovarian cancer is related to incessant ovulation because oral contraceptives and pregnancy have a protective effect. Genetic factors, with mutations in the tumor suppressor genes *BRCA1* and *BRCA2*, have been the focus of intense research. However, only 5% to 10% of cases of ovarian cancer are familial; most occur sporadically in women with no family history or demonstrable genetic abnormality.

The major reproductive risk factor for epithelial ovarian carcinoma is nulliparity. Multiple studies have reported that a single full-term pregnancy reduces the risk by approximately 40%. Subsequent pregnancies each appear to reduce the risk by an additional 14%. Oral contraceptive use has also been shown to reduce the risk for ovarian carcinoma. The risk decreases 10% for each year of use and reaches a maximum of 50% with 5 years of use. Infertility has been associated with increased risk, and some studies have shown an increased risk with the long-term use (>1 year) of clomiphene.

History

The development of epithelial ovarian carcinoma is insidious; only 25% of patients present with disease confined to the ovaries. The presenting symptoms are nonspecific and frequently attributed to gastrointestinal ailments. Gastrointestinal problems of early satiety, dyspepsia, and nausea are common and affect most women for months before the diagnosis is made. Abdominal discomfort and distention caused by a large pelvic mass or ascites are frequently signs of advanced disease. Constipation, urinary frequency, and dyspareunia may develop as the mass enlarges. Rapidly enlarging masses occasionally present as surgical emergencies caused by torsion, intracystic hemorrhage, or rupture. Shortness of breath and fatigue are occasionally noticed and may be related to massive ascites or pleural effusions. Paraneoplastic syndromes such as cerebellar degeneration and hypercalcemia occur rarely at presentation.

Sex cord-stromal tumors, which are often hormonally active, may present as precocious puberty in a premenarchal patient. Menstrual cycle irregularity is the most common presentation in women of reproductive age. In postmenopausal women, symptoms and signs of estrogen production, including vaginal bleeding, often develop. Occasionally, virilization is present.

Germ cell tumors occur primarily in young women. They present with abdominal pain and a pelvic mass. Occasionally, symptoms and signs of abnormal endocrine activity, including precocious puberty or hyperthyroidism, occur.

Physical Examination

An annual pelvic examination is recommended for all women as part of their routine health care. Although ovarian carcinoma is sometimes first detected during a pelvic examination, it is not of proven value as a screening method for ovarian cancer. Adnexal masses in women of reproductive age are malignant in fewer than 5% of cases. In women older than 50 years of age, the risk for malignancy increases to approximately 50%.

A rectovaginal examination is an essential component of the pelvic examination in any women with a pelvic mass. A stool guaiac test should be performed routinely. An increased risk for malignancy is associated with adnexal masses that are bilateral, solid, fixed, or nodular. Ascites is also suggestive of malignancy and can be detected during the physical examination as shifting dullness during abdominal percussion. Relevant aspects of the general physical examination include palpation of the inguinal and supraclavicular lymph nodes and evaluation for pleural effusion. A breast examination is necessary because this is a common site of primary disease metastatic to the ovary.

Laboratory and Imaging Studies

The primary modality used to evaluate an adnexal mass is ultrasonography. Basic ultrasonographic features that are essential in decisions regarding the management of any adnexal mass are the size and nature of the mass (solid or cystic; if cystic, either multilocular or unilocular). The patient's age, size of the mass, and ultrasonographic characteristics are the basic factors affecting treatment decisions.

Although cancer antigen-125 (CA-125) is commonly used in the evaluation of adnexal masses, its value is unproven. The CA-125 level is elevated in more than 80% of patients with an advanced ovarian epithelial carcinoma, but it is normal in 50% of cases of early-stage disease. In addition to its generally poor sensitivity, its specificity is also poor, particularly in premenopausal patients, in whom a wide variety of benign conditions can result in elevated levels. The most valuable use of the CA-125 level is in monitoring patients with ovarian carcinoma for response to therapy and for recurrence of disease.

Computed tomography is frequently performed in patients with an adnexal mass but is unnecessary when ultrasonography has already confirmed the presence of an adnexal mass or ascites. Other tests, such as colonoscopy or barium enema, are performed if the symptoms suggest a gastrointestinal primary tumor or if the result of a stool guaiac test is positive.

Routine preoperative studies should include chest roentgenography to rule out pleural effusions and metastatic disease. Liver function tests are used to evaluate metastatic disease and ascites. Elevated serum levels of hepatic enzymes necessitate imaging of the liver. A cervical cytologic examination should be performed if the patient has not had one recently. Mammography should be performed in women older than 40 to 50 years of age.

Treatment

Surgical intervention is warranted for any multilocular mass more than 5 cm in diameter. Asymptomatic unilocular cysts less than 5 to 8 cm in diameter, particularly in premenopausal patients, may be observed because the risk for malignancy is low. Multilocular or solid masses in postmenopausal patients always require surgical intervention.

The initial management of any medically fit patient with an adnexal mass suspected of being ovarian carcinoma is surgical exploration. The aims of operative management are confirmation of the diagnosis, accurate staging, and maximal tumor resection if advanced disease is discovered. Consultation with a gynecologic oncologist is often beneficial. Mechanical bowel preparation with preoperative antibiotics and deep venous thrombosis prophylaxis are indicated.

The International Federation of Gynecology and Obstetrics (FIGO) has adopted a surgical-pathologic staging system for ovarian carcinoma (Table 28.3). Accurate staging, especially in cases of apparently early disease, requires a systematic approach based on an understanding of the patterns of dissemination.

TABLE 28.3. International Federation of Gynecology and Obstetrics (FIGO) Staging of Ovarian Cancer (1988)

Stage I	Growth limited to the ovaries
Stage IA	Limited to one ovary; no malignant ascites, no tumor on external capsule, capsule intact
Stage IB	Limited to ovaries; no malignant ascites, no tumor on external capsule, capsule intact
Stage IC	Limited to ovaries; malignant ascites or washing, tumor on external capsule, or capsule ruptured
Stage II	Growth involving one or both ovaries with pelvic extension
Stage IIA	Extension to uterus, tubes, or both
Stage IIB	Extension to other pelvic tissues
Stage IIC	Stage IIA or IIB with malignant ascites or washings; or tumor on capsule; or capsule ruptured
Stage III	Extrapelvic peritoneal implants or positive retroperitoneal or inguinal nodes; extension to small bowel omentum
Stage IIIA	Tumor grossly limited to true pelvis with negative nodes but microscopic seeding of abdominal peritoneal surfaces
Stage IIIB	Nodes negative, implants on abdominal peritoneal surfaces or omentum ≤2 cm in diameter
Stage IIIC	Nodes positive or implants on abdominal peritoneal surfaces or omentum >2 cm in diameter
Stage IV	Growth involving one or both ovaries with distant metastases, malignant pleural effusion or parenchymal liver metastases

Direct spread along the peritoneal surfaces is the most common mechanism of tumor dissemination. Lymphatic metastasis occurs primarily via the infundibulopelvic ligaments to the periaortic nodes and along the broad ligament and parametria to the pelvic nodes. Hematogenous spread, most frequently to the liver or lung, is less common. Surgical exploration should be performed through a midline vertical incision, which allows maximum exposure of the pelvis and upper abdomen. If gross upper abdominal disease is not apparent, ascites or peritoneal washings from the pelvis and upper abdomen should be collected for cytologic evaluation. After verification of malignancy, total abdominal hysterectomy and bilateral salpingo-oophorectomy are usually performed. Young patients with early-stage ovarian cancer may be treated with preservation of fertility. Meticulous examination of all peritoneal surfaces, the bowel and its mesentery, the liver, and the omentum is necessary. Adhesions and roughened surfaces often are indicative of metastatic disease and should be sampled. The staging of early disease is completed with pelvic and periaortic lymph node sampling, infracolonic omentectomy, and random sampling of the pelvis, pericolic gutters, and diaphragm.

Operative efforts in advanced-stage epithelial disease are directed toward removal of as much tumor as possible. Optimal cytoreduction has been demonstrated in multiple studies to improve the prognosis. Cytoreduction to residual tumor nodules with a maximal diameter of 1 cm is generally considered optimal. In patients with a large volume of residual disease, the resection of large tumor masses may be of palliative benefit, reducing the production of ascitic fluid or delaying impending bowel obstruction.

Conservative surgical management of early-stage ovarian carcinoma is acceptable in younger women who wish to preserve their reproductive potential. Unilateral oophorectomy with complete surgical staging, including ipsilateral pelvic and bilateral periaortic lymph node sampling, is adequate for well-differentiated stage IA disease. Cystectomy has been shown to be effective therapy for similar patients with borderline malignancies. Biopsy of a normal-appearing contralateral ovary is not needed. Close follow-up with removal of the retained ovary is recommended once childbearing is completed.

Ovarian germ cell malignancies affect young women and are usually stage I. They are generally unilateral with the exception of dysgerminomas, which are grossly bilateral in 10% of cases and covertly bilateral in an additional 10% of cases. After unilateral oophorectomy and staging, preservation of the contralateral ovary and uterus is indicated.

In a well-selected patient population, laparoscopic evaluation of an adnexal mass is appropriate. When cancer is suspected, effort is made to remove the ovary intact and avoid tumor spill. Patients must be prepared for a laparotomy if cancer is discovered. Although studies have failed to confirm that intraoperative tumor rupture is a poor prognostic factor in early-stage disease, numerous cases have been reported of port site seeding of cancer in patients who did not undergo immediate laparotomy after a laparoscopic diagnosis of ovarian malignancy.

Patients with well-differentiated stage IA or IB epithelial carcinoma with no poor prognostic factors are at low risk for recurrence and do not require adjuvant therapy. Factors increasing the risk for recurrence include high-grade disease, capsular excrescences or adhesions, a clear cell histologic type, and malignant peritoneal cytologic findings. The management of patients with early-stage disease who are at high risk for recurrence usually includes adjuvant chemotherapy. The most frequently used regimen is the combination of paclitaxel (Taxol) and carboplatin.

The mainstay of postoperative therapy for advanced-stage disease has been platinum-based combination chemotherapy. An outpatient regimen with Taxol and carboplatin is used in most centers. More recently, docetaxel (Taxotere) and carboplatin have been used to avoid some of the neurotoxicity associated with Taxol. Whole-abdominal radiation therapy has a limited role in advanced-stage disease.

Monitoring for the response to chemotherapy is generally by means of physical examination and serial determinations of the serum CA-125 level. An elevated CA-125 level more than 3 months beyond the start of chemotherapy is a strong predictor of persistent disease at the completion of chemotherapy. Computed tomography and other imaging examinations are not used routinely but occasionally may be useful in evaluating symptoms in patients with normal physical examination findings and a normal CA-125 level.

Patients with a complete response to therapy should be examined every 3 months for 2 years. Examinations every 6 months for the subsequent 3 years are recommended, with yearly follow-up thereafter. CA-125 levels should be obtained at each visit. A rising CA-125 level is a strong indicator of recurrent disease and is often noted 3 months or more before disease is detected by other clinical means.

Salvage chemotherapy for recurrent disease is individualized according to the agents used previously and the length of the disease-free interval. Extended survival for patients with recurrent disease is rare.

Postoperative therapy is usually not recommended for patients with ovarian epithelial tumors of low malignant potential or with sex cord-stromal tumors. Malignant germ cell tumors, with the exception of early-stage dysgerminomas and immature teratomas, require aggressive chemotherapy with multiple agents.

Considerations in Pregnancy

Most ovarian masses discovered during pregnancy are benign. In the past, surgical exploration at 16 to 18 weeks of gestation was recommended for patients with adnexal masses larger than 6 cm in diameter. Of the patients who underwent exploration, fewer than 5% had malignancies. More recently, unless malignancy is strongly suspected, most asymptomatic cases have been managed expectantly. If the mass persists postpartum, then surgical intervention is necessary.

The malignancies most frequently presenting during pregnancy are germ cell tumors and epithelial tumors of low malignant potential. Conservation of the pregnancy is usually possible. Postoperative therapy is similar to that for patients who are not pregnant. Chemotherapy may be administered in the last two trimesters because no teratogenic or long-term effects have been well documented.

CERVICAL CARCINOMA

Invasive cervical carcinoma is arguably the most preventable malignancy in women. Although more widespread screening has reduced the incidence in the United States, cervical cancer remains the fourth most common female malignancy. Despite a long and treatable preinvasive phase (cervical intraepithelial neoplasia), 12,200 new cases and 4,100 deaths were expected in 2003. Early detection of cervical intraepithelial neoplasia is critical, and fortunately Pap smear screening is widely available.

Risk factors strongly associated with the development of cervical carcinoma, such as early age at first coitus and multiple partners, support the view that a sexually transmitted agent is an important causative factor. The human papillomavirus (HPV) is extremely prevalent in sexually active women and is considered an important cofactor in the development of cervical cancer. HPV types 16, 18, 31, 33, 35, and 39 have been associated with high-grade dysplasia and carcinoma, but the role of HPV subtyping in the management of dysplasia and carcinoma remains uncertain.

Etiology

The cause of cervical cancer is unknown. However, it would appear that women are particularly susceptible to some inciting event associated with coitus for several years after menarche, a time during which the transformation zone of the cervix is undergoing active squamous metaplasia. Epidemiologic studies strongly support a sexually transmitted agent, probably HPV, as an important cofactor. The risk of cervical cancer for women beginning intercourse before the age of 15 years is double the risk of those first engaging in coitus after age 20. Squamous cell carcinoma of the cervix is virtually unknown among nuns. A "male factor" also may be important; the risk is three times higher for the current wife of a man whose previous wife had cervical cancer. These facts are all consistent with the theory that a sexually transmittable agent, probably HPV, has a role in cervical carcinogenesis.

Screening

No consensus has been reached regarding the optimal, most cost-effective program of cervical cytologic screening. The American College of Obstetricians and Gynecologists recommends that Pap smears be performed in women when they reach the age of 18 years or become sexually active, and annually thereafter. For patients who have had normal findings on three or more annual smears, the interval of testing may be increased at the discretion of the physician. However, the false-negative rate of cervical cytology is 20% to 30% for squamous lesions and up to 40% for adenocarcinomas. In most patients, therefore, an annual pelvic examination including a Pap smear is the most prudent recommendation.

In the past, cervical cytologic findings were reported as class I to V (Table 28.4). The 1988 Bethesda system of reporting cervical/vaginal cytology was introduced in an attempt to standardize cervical cytology. In this system, smears with HPV atypia and mild dysplasia are reported as low-grade squamous intraepithelial lesions (LSIL). The updated 2001 Bethesda system now further qualifies atypical squamous cells as "of undetermined significance" (ASC-US) or "cannot exclude high-grade squamous intraepithelial lesions" (ASC-H). High-grade squamous intraepithelial lesions (HSIL) include moderate and severe dysplasia and carcinoma in situ. Cases with ASC-H, LSIL, or HSIL require further evaluation by colposcopy and biopsy.

Precursors of Cervical Cancer

The site where the columnar epithelium of the endocervix meets the squamous epithelium of the portio of the cervix is the squamocolumnar junction. During female life, this junction progressively migrates from the cervical portio in newborns to well within the endocervical canal in postmenopausal women. The transformation zone where this occurs, through a process called *squamous metaplasia,* is the part of the cervix most prone to the development of malignancy. The metaplastic squamous epithelium in this zone is abundant early in the postmenarchal period and is undoubtedly susceptible to oncogenic triggers such as exposure to HPV.

Cervical intraepithelial neoplasia (CIN), or cervical dysplasia, is a precursor of cervical cancer that may antedate invasive cervical cancer by 10 or more years. Although at one time it was thought that malignant change progressed from mild dysplasia (CIN 1) to severe dysplasia and carcinoma in situ (CIN 3), it is impossible to correlate the degree of dysplasia with the eventual risk for malignancy or the timing of progression to a cancer. Therefore, for most patients, the appropriate management is to treat any dysplasia confirmed by biopsy. However, up to two thirds of cases with mild dysplasia regress spontaneously. Consequently, selected patients with mild dysplasia may be monitored with periodic Pap smears and colposcopy if reliable follow-up is ensured.

The initial evaluation of all patients with LSIL or HSIL should consist of a colposcopic examination of the cervix and vagina (after the application of 3% acetic acid) and directed biopsies, including endocervical curettage. Therapy should be undertaken only for biopsy-proven dysplasia and depends on the results of biopsies and the colposcopic findings.

TABLE 28.4. Bethesda Classification of Papanicolaou Smears

Class	Dysplasia	Bethesda
I	Normal	Normal
II	Atypical	ASC-US (undetermined significance)
		ASC-H (cannot rule out high-grade SIL)
III	Mild dysplasia	Low-grade SIL
	Moderate dysplasia	High-grade SIL
	Severe dysplasia	High-grade SIL
IV	Carcinoma in situ	High-grade SIL
V	Invasive cancer	Invasive cancer

ASC, atypical squamous cells; SIL, squamous intraepithelial lesion.

In cases in which colposcopy is adequate (the entire transformation zone and lesion are fully visualized) and the results of endocervical curettage are negative, various ablative methods can be used with success. Cryocautery of the cervix is acceptable, but the transformation zone is usually located well within the endocervical canal after healing, so that recurrent dysplasia may be more difficult to evaluate. Laser ablation of the cervix is particularly well suited to patients whose lesions extend onto the vaginal fornices. The most widely used treatment of CIN is the loop electrosurgical excision procedure (LEEP), in which a loop cautery is used to excise the entire lesion and transformation zone. This method has become popular because it is simple, can be performed in an office setting, and is applicable whether or not colposcopy is adequate.

An invasive cancer must be excluded in cases with a positive result of endocervical curettage, an inadequate colposcopy, or cytologic evidence of an invasive process. A cone biopsy is mandatory in these instances. In the past, this was performed in the operating room with a scalpel, but currently LEEP is used in most instances.

History

CIN and early cervical cancer are usually asymptomatic, so early detection depends on routine cytologic screening.

Abnormal vaginal bleeding is the most common symptom associated with cervical cancer. All patients with abnormal bleeding should undergo a pelvic examination, and often a Pap smear, cervical biopsy, and endometrial biopsy are indicated. Vaginal discharge and odor frequently accompany the bleeding but may be the primary complaint. The classic symptom of postcoital spotting seldom occurs alone, although an early cervical carcinoma occasionally presents in this fashion.

Weight loss, pelvic pain, fatigue, and weakness are not uncommon in patients with more advanced cancers. Flank pain may accompany obstructive uropathy.

Physical Examination/Clinical Findings

In many patients with early cervical cancer and most with CIN, no abnormalities are detected during a routine physical examination. Occasionally, an area of cervical leukoplakia may be seen on the speculum examination, but usually, early cases are detectable only by colposcopy, with the application of acetic acid to the cervix.

More advanced cervical cancers are virtually always accompanied by an abnormal appearance or consistency of the cervix. Although exophytic lesions are usually easily detected, endophytic growth patterns may be concealed by normal overlying mucosa, so that the diagnosis is more difficult. In most of these cases, the cervix is abnormally enlarged and firm. Biopsy is mandatory whenever a cervical lesion is detected, and the clinician should not be reassured by a normal Pap smear. Even in the presence of invasive cervical cancer, only inflammatory changes may be noted on the Pap smear, particularly in cases with an endophytic growth pattern.

The size of the tumor and any vaginal or parametrial involvement should be noted. Parametrial involvement, manifested by thickening of the tissue adjacent to the cervix, is accompanied by fixation of the cervix and is best detected on rectovaginal examination.

Systemic disease may be manifested by an enlarged supraclavicular lymph node. When this is detected, aspiration or biopsy is warranted.

Laboratory and Imaging Studies

Patients with preinvasive disease (CIN) or very early cancers without metastatic potential require no special laboratory or radiologic assessment. In the presence of an invasive cancer, a complete blood cell count and SMA-12 (sequential multiple analysis—12-channel biochemical profile) are routinely performed.

Although various radiologic procedures have been used in patients with invasive cervical carcinoma, most are of limited usefulness and should be performed only in specific circumstances (Table 28.5). Chest roentgenography and urography (intravenous pyelography [IVP] or computed tomography [CT]) are routine. Other tests, such as magnetic resonance imaging, ultrasonography, and radionuclide bone scans, should be used only for specific indications.

A tumor marker, squamous cell carcinoma antigen, has been found to correlate with tumor status in patients with invasive cervical carcinoma. However, it is unclear whether this test is of value in the management of patients with cervical cancer, and its routine use is discouraged.

Staging

The staging of cervical carcinoma is clinical and depends primarily on the results of the pelvic examination and routine radiologic tests (e.g., chest roentgenography, IVP) allowed by the FIGO staging system (Table 28.6). In most cases, an examination under anesthesia with cystoscopy and proctoscopy is performed to assess the extent of local disease. Chest roentgenog-

TABLE 28.5. Radiologic Assessment in Cervical Carcinoma

Method	Use	Recommended
Chest roentgenography	Exclude metastases	Routine
IVP	Exclude hydronephrosis	Routine
CT	Detect lymphadenopathy, hydronephrosis, liver metastases	Routine for advanced-stage or large tumors
MRI	Define tumor extent	Optional
Ultrasonography	Define tumor extent	Optional
Skeletal roentgenography	Confirm suspicious bone scan	With equivocal result of bone scan
Bone scan	Detect bony metastases	Increased alkaline phosphatase or bone pain

CT, computed tomography; IVP, intravenous pyelography; MRI, magnetic resonance imaging.

TABLE 28.6. International Federation of Gynecology and Obstetrics (FIGO) Staging of Cervical Carcinoma

FIGO Stage	Description
IA_1	Microinvasive with minimal stromal invasion
IA_2	Invasion < 5 mm
IB_1	Tumor confined to cervix ≤ 4 cm
IB_2	Tumor confined to cervix > 4 cm
IIA	Vaginal involvement confined to upper two thirds
IIB	Parametrial involvement
IIIA	Lower-third vaginal involvement
IIIB	Hydronephrosis or parametrial involvement to side wall
IV	Bladder or rectal mucosal involvement, metastatic beyond pelvis

raphy and CT are the only tests routinely used to detect metastatic disease. Although CT has supplanted IVP in most centers, abnormal findings are uncommon in patients with early-stage cancers.

Treatment

The treatment of cervical cancer depends on the stage, with surgical excision the predominant mode in patients with early cancer and radiation therapy in those with more advanced disease. Various other factors, such as the patient's age, histology, desire for childbearing, and medical condition, are considered in formulating an individualized treatment plan.

CERVICAL INTRAEPITHELIAL NEOPLASIA

Local methods (cryotherapy, laser ablation, sharp knife conization, and more recently LEEP) are used predominantly to treat CIN 1 to CIN 3. The type of local method chosen depends on the results of colposcopy with biopsy and endocervical curettage. Ablative methods such as cryotherapy and laser ablation, which preclude a comprehensive pathologic assessment, are appropriate only if an invasive cancer has been excluded. Routine hysterectomy is not indicated for patients with CIN but may be appropriate in postmenopausal women with persistent disease or in patients with recurrent disease when prior treatment has compromised the ability to use a local method.

Stage IA

Stage IA is meant to encompass so-called microinvasive cervical carcinoma, in which the potential for metastatic spread is limited. However, the subgroups IA_1 and IA_2 do not adequately distinguish between cases with a negligible risk for lymph node spread. In 1974, the Society of Gynecologic Oncologists adopted a more useful definition of microinvasive carcinoma: "A microinvasive lesion is one in which the neoplastic epithelium invades the stroma in one or more places to a depth of 3 mm or less below the base of the epithelium, and in which lymphatic or blood vessel involvement is not demonstrated."

Substage IA fits this definition of microinvasive carcinoma, and cervical cancer at this early stage is associated with a very limited (<1%) risk for lymph node spread. In patients who desire childbearing, cervical conization is adequate treatment if the margins of resection are uninvolved. In older patients or those who do not want more children, hysterectomy may be considered.

In substage IA_2, up to 5 mm of stromal invasion is allowed. With 1 to 3 mm of stromal invasion, treatment is similar to that for stage IA_1. However, with 4 to 5 mm of stromal invasion, the risk for lymph node spread is about 5%, so more radical treatment methods are usually used; radical hysterectomy with pelvic lymphadenectomy or pelvic radiation may be appropriate.

Stage IB or IIA

Tumors clinically confined to the cervix are stage IB. This stage is subdivided according to whether the lesion is 4 cm or smaller (stage IB_1) or larger than 4 cm (stage IB_2). Treatment depends on the patient's age and medical condition and the tumor size. In general, young patients who are good surgical candidates are treated with radical hysterectomy. Selected patients with stage IIA disease and minimal vaginal involvement are also candidates for radical surgical treatment. In other cases, pelvic radiation is used. In patients with a bulky cervical lesion, combined radiation and surgery may be appropriate.

Stages IIB through IV

For tumors that extend beyond the cervix, pelvic radiation in conjunction with radiosensitizing chemotherapy is usually used. Cisplatin, alone or in combination with an infusion of 5-fluorouracil, is administered during external beam treatment. One or two brachytherapy implants are routinely inserted after external beam treatment.

Considerations in Pregnancy

The diagnosis of CIN during pregnancy is uncommon, and invasive cancer complicates only 1 in 2,200 pregnancies. The treatment of cervical cancer in pregnant patients depends entirely on the extent of tumor and the stage of gestation. Although normal delivery can be anticipated for patients with preinvasive lesions, cesarean section may be appropriate in more advanced cases.

The pregnant patient with a Pap smear showing either a low- or high-grade squamous intraepithelial lesion should be referred to an experienced colposcopist for evaluation. If an invasive lesion is excluded, periodic reevaluation during pregnancy with anticipation of a normal delivery is appropriate. When a suspect lesion is found colposcopically, biopsy is necessary, and management depends on whether invasion is identified.

Microinvasive carcinoma of the cervix can be managed expectantly during pregnancy. This diagnosis can be made only by cervical conization. Conization should be performed during pregnancy only when a biopsy has shown an early invasive lesion or when invasive cancer is strongly suspected.

The treatment of more advanced invasive cancers during pregnancy depends on the stage of gestation. If the cancer is discovered in the third or late in the second trimester, treatment may be delayed until fetal viability. In these cases, cesarean section is usually used to avoid hemorrhage from the tumor. If cancer is discovered during the first trimester, treatment is initiated without regard to the fetus.

BIBLIOGRAPHY

Burke TW, Eifel PJ, Muggia FM. Cancer of the uterine body. In: DeVita VT Jr, Hellman S, Rosenberg SA, eds. *Cancer principles and practice of oncology*, 5th ed. Philadelphia: Lippincott-Raven, 1997:1478–1499.

Disaia PJ, Creasman WT. *Clinical gynecologic oncology*, 6th ed. St. Louis: Mosby, 2002.

Berek JS, Hacker NF, eds. *Practical gynecologic oncology*, 3rd ed. Philadelphia: Lippincott Williams & Wilkins, 2000.

DuBeshter B, Lin JY, Angel C. Tumors of female reproductive organs. In: Rubin P, ed. *Clinical oncology: a multidisciplinary approach for physicians and students*, 7th ed. Philadelphia: WB Saunders, 1993.

Morrow CP, Curtin JP, Townsend DE. *Synopsis of gynecologic oncology*, 4th ed. New York: Churchill Livingstone, 1987.

Stenchever MA, Droegemuller W, Herbst AL, et al. *Comprehensive gynecology*, 4th ed. St. Louis: Mosby, 2001.

CHAPTER 29
Vulvar Disease

David C. Foster

Unique embryologic and immunologic aspects of the vulva contribute to the diagnostic and therapeutic challenges of managing vulvar problems. Individual variations in the care of the genital region, defined by personal and societal "norms," may exacerbate vulvar problems and should be reviewed with the patient with the intent of *preventing* vulvar disease.

GENERAL DIAGNOSTIC APPROACH (DEVELOPMENT OF THREE-DIMENSIONAL MATRIX)

In systematically approaching the evaluation and management of vulvar disease, three dimensions should be emphasized: (a) lesion type, (b) lesion location, and (c) associated systemic and laboratory findings. Once a list of differential diagnoses has been developed, the practitioner should assign a likelihood to each diagnosis based on factors such as the patient's age, hormonal status, and sexual activity.

Dimension 1: type of lesion

- Macule (color)
- Plaque
- Ulcer
- Papule, nodule, cyst
- Pustule, abscess, cellulitis, and infestations
- Other conditions: pain syndromes and traumatic conditions.

Dimension 2: location of lesion

- Where in the lower genital tract (external vulva, vestibule, vagina, or urethra) is the lesion located?
- Is it bilateral or unilateral?
- Is a single or more than one site affected?

Dimension 3: associated findings

- Other skin areas
- Mouth mucosa and gingiva
- Nails
- Vaginal discharge (wet preparation findings)
- Vaginal pH
- Maturation index
- Urinary/fecal incontinence
- Wood lamp
- Specific vaginal cultures.

RASHES, MACULES, AND PLAQUES

In the "normal" female lower genital tract, a color change is apparent at the junction of the stratified squamous epithelium of the vulva (ectodermal origin) and the stratified squamous epithelium of the vestibule (endodermal origin). At the Hart line, as the junction is called, the skin of the external vulva joins the mucosa of the vulvar vestibule, each with a characteristic texture and color. In the presence of a rash or macule, additional colors and textures may be superimposed on the normal ones of the vulva. Variables to be considered in the evaluation of a rash or macule include location, symmetry, color, texture, duration, and associated pain or pruritus. The common rashes and macules (Table 29.1) include eczema (endogenous and exogenous), vulvovaginal infections (candidiasis, trichomoniasis, bacterial vaginosis, dermatophytoses), and chronic dermatoses (the "three lichens" and other generalized dermatoses, such as psoriasis).

Eczema

The two major types of eczema are exogenous and endogenous. Exogenous eczema can be either "irritant" or "allergic" contact dermatitis. Eczematous lesions are symmetric and found on areas of the vulva that may come in contact with environmental irritants or antigens. Endogenous eczema, also known as *atopic dermatitis,* may affect multiple sites, including the vulva, umbilicus, retroauricular areas, and scalp. Atopic dermatitis may coexist with asthma or allergic rhinitis. Regardless of the type of eczema, the first line of therapy for the primary skin eruption is the same: topical corticosteroids, discussed later. In the case of exogenous eczema, a careful documentation of potential irritants or allergens may be help prevent recurrences. Patch testing is of limited value given the nearly unlimited number of potential irritants and allergens.

Recurrent Vulvovaginal Candidiasis

When vulvovaginal candidiasis becomes chronic or recurrent, management becomes more problematic. Symptomatic, culture-proven candidiasis has been associated with repetitive receptive oral sex and spermicide use. When adjustments were made for these variables, other hypothesized factors, such as antibiotic use, menstrual hygiene products, and fre-

TABLE 29.1. Common Vulvar Rashes, Macules, and Plaques

Condition	Location/characteristics	Condition	Location/characteristics
Irritant (contact) vulvar dermatitis	Symmetric and extending into areas of "irritant" contact	*Lichen simplex chronicus*	Symmetric, variable pigmentation, leathery or coarse texture
Allergic (contact) vulvar dermatitis	Symmetric and extending into areas of "allergic" contact	*Lichen sclerosus*	"Keyhole" distribution, depigmentation, submucosal hemorrhage, loss of elasticity
Vulvar eczema	Search other crural folds, scalp, umbilicus, extremities	*Lichen planus*	Erosive type involves vaginal mucosa, demarcated edge; classic type with cutaneous violaceous plaques
Infectious vulvitis	Commonly *Candida* etiology, culture for resistant strains, also consider dermatophytes (tinea cruris and tinea rubra)	*Psoriasis*	Pink vulvar plaques, elbows and knees often affected, greater scaling in extragenital regions

quent vaginal intercourse, had little effect on recurrence of infection. Obtaining fungal cultures during symptomatic episodes helps to confirm the presence of a fungal organism and determine the species. Both oral and topical antifungal agents are available; however, oral agents may be preferable because they are easily administered, and messy, possibly skin-sensitizing creams can be avoided. A 2- to 3-month course of 200 mg of fluconazole weekly may effectively clear long-standing fungal infections. Resistant species of yeast may require higher doses of fluconazole. The adjunctive use of boric acid vaginal suppositories (400 mg three times weekly) may provide additional long-term suppressive therapy. Caution should be exercised in administering fluconazole together with other drugs, such as the "statins."

Vulvar Dermatoses ("Three Lichens")

LICHEN SIMPLEX CHRONICUS

Lichen simplex chronicus, a common vulvar dermatosis, is characterized by leathery skin with accentuated cutaneous markings. Symptoms of itching and burning predominate. A number of acute disorders may evolve into lichen simplex chronicus, including recurrent vaginal infections and long-standing eczema. Additionally, lichen simplex chronicus may coexist with other chronic dermatoses, such as lichen sclerosus and lichen planus. Essentially, lichen simplex chronicus is an end-stage disorder caused by a wide array of irritative or infectious factors. Treatment includes removal of the irritants or allergens, if discovered, and the topical application of mid- to high-potency corticosteroids, as discussed later.

LICHEN SCLEROSUS

Lichen sclerosus is visually characterized by depigmentation, a loss of mucocutaneous markings, and submucosal hemorrhage. Reduced elasticity of the skin surface may result in fissuring at the perineal body. Lichen sclerosus may involve the labia minora, clitoris, interlabial sulcus, inner portion of the labia majora, and perianal areas. The descriptive term "keyhole distribution" has been used to characterize involvement of the vaginal introitus and perianal region with lichen sclerosus. The etiology of lichen sclerosus remains unknown. Clinical trials comparing clobetasol and testosterone found the long-term response (1 year) to be significantly better with clobetasol. In another clinical trial, patients were treated for 3 months with one of four topical drugs: testosterone (2%), progesterone (2%), clobetasol propionate (0.05%), or a cream placebo. The response was best in the patients treated with clobetasol. Only the clobetasol group displayed gross and histologic improvement after treatment. Excisional surgery with skin grafting has not been effective because of recurrence of disease in the grafted tissue. Perineoplasty, which superimposes vaginal rather than cutaneous tissue, effectively corrects perineal fissuring and the accompanying dyspareunia. A low but clear risk for vulvar carcinoma in afflicted patients is best managed with frequent examinations and biopsy when mucocutaneous ulceration or thickening is identified.

LICHEN PLANUS

Lichen planus may present as either of two types: (a) "classic," consisting of sharply demarcated, flat-topped plaques on oral and genital membranes, or (b) "erosive," in which an erosive, erythematous lesion originating in the vestibule variably extends up the vaginal canal. Opinion varies as to whether desquamative vaginitis is a type of erosive lichen planus. In addition, a significant diagnostic overlap exists between lichen planus and lichen sclerosus. Lichen sclerosus does not affect the vagina, so that erosive vaginal inflammation is more indicative of lichen planus. The mouth lesions in "classic" lichen planus are lacy, white, and weblike. The gingivitis of "erosive" lichen planus appears as a demarcated erythema at the gingival-dentate junction. If a biopsy specimen of the mucosal lesion is taken, the histologic findings include irregular acanthosis of the epithelium, a bandlike infiltrate of lymphocytes and colloid bodies (degenerated keratinocytes) seen in the basal layers of the epidermis. The "erosive" version of lichen planus may be quite nonspecific histologically because of the complete loss of vaginal epithelium. In regard to the treatment of both oral and vulvar lichen planus, no strong evidence supports the effectiveness of any single therapy. Therapeutic options tested in small studies have included cyclosporine, corticosteroids, PUVA (psoralen plus ultraviolet light of A wavelength), tacrolimus, and topical/systemic retinoids. Without question, lichen planus is the most difficult of the "three lichens" to treat, and a supportive, encouraging approach by the clinician is pivotal for effective management. Like lichen sclerosus, lichen planus may be associated with an increased risk for malignancy.

Psoriasis

In psoriasis, cutaneous plaques with a silver scale develop diffusely over the body and generally make the diagnosis obvious. However, the plaques of the vulva may be more intensely pink or red and lack the silver scale. In the event of psoriasis limited to the vulva, local treatment with mid- to high-potency topical corticosteroids, injectable corticosteroids, or topical tacrolimus may be effective. Following standard treatments such as PUVA phototherapy for extensive psoriasis, recalcitrant psoriatic plaques may be found on the vulva as a consequence of the inability to apply phototherapy adequately to this region.

ULCERS

The causes of vulvar ulcers include neoplastic, infectious, and other "systemic" conditions (Table 29.2). Three important components of the physical examination should be the following: (a) a careful evaluation of the appearance and consistency of the ulcer and the degree ulcer tenderness when palpated with a gloved hand; (b) an evaluation of the lymph node status, particularly local or general lymphadenopathy, nodal tenderness, and suppuration; and (c) a general physical examination with particular focus on the skin, mouth, and eyes. Laboratory testing should include the following: (a) biopsy of the ulcer; (b) cultures and smears of the ulcer base; and (c) serum tests, including specific antibody testing for syphilis, HIV, Epstein-Barr virus (EBV), and herpes simplex virus (HSV).

Herpes Simplex Virus and Epstein-Barr Virus Infections

Primary infection with HSV-1 or HSV-2 presents with multiple, superficial, painful ulcerations on the lower genital tract. In the primary infection, tender inguinal lymphadenopathy, fever, and malaise may coexist with ulceration. Although exceptions have been documented, recurrent lesions are usually less severe and less often associated with lymphadenopathy and systemic symptoms. The diagnosis is confirmed by culture, which usually requires several days. Newer immunofluorescent or enzyme tests may provide same-day results with reasonably good sensitivity and specificity. Blood antibody testing for HSV-1 and HSV-2 is of limited utility. Given a negative antibody

TABLE 29.2. Common Vulvar Ulcers

Condition	Location/characteristics	Condition	Location/characteristics
Vulvar neoplasia: squamous cell, basal cell, or melanoma	Commonly solitary, nontender, with raised or indurated edge and clean base	*Pyoderma gangrenosum, anorectal Crohn disease*	Elongated "knife cut" ulcer in skin fold (Crohn disease), necrotic center with rolled edge (pyoderma gangrenosum)
Herpes simplex, Epstein-Barr virus infection	Commonly multiple, painful; herpes simplex may be recurrent	*Syphilis, lymphogranuloma venereum, chancroid, donovanosis*	Ulcer appearance variable; may be single or multiple, hard or soft, deep or superficial
Behçet disease, cicatricial pemphigoid, aphthous	Commonly multiple, painful, recurrent, scarred edge (pemphigoid)	*Decubitus, traumatic*	Ulcers located in areas of direct pressure or trauma

result, HSV-1 and HSV-2 infection can be excluded as the cause of recurrent vulvar ulceration. On the other hand, a positive antibody titer indicates only a history of infection. The treatment regimens with antiviral medications may used episodically or continuously, depending on the frequency of recurrence. No long-term side effects have been found with suppressive therapy.

Particularly in the adolescent, combined symptoms of fever, sore throat, cervical lymphadenopathy, and genital ulcerations may develop during an acute episode of infectious mononucleosis, which is an EBV infection. The diagnosis of EBV infection is likely in an adolescent with multiple painful genital ulcerations, associated lymphadenopathy, splenomegaly, and a negative herpesvirus culture. The diagnosis is confirmed by the demonstration of atypical lymphocytes on the blood smear and a positive result of a heterophile antibody test, such as Monospot. Treatment is limited to relieving pain and managing bacterial superinfection of the genital ulcers. Sitz baths in dilute povidone iodine followed by the application of topical lidocaine cream or gel can be soothing.

Behçet Syndrome, Aphthous Ulcers, and Cicatricial Pemphigoid

Behçet syndrome is a vasculitis of unknown cause, although it is genetically associated with histocompatibility antigens HLA-B51 and HLA-DR4. The syndrome is characterized by a waxing and waning pattern; oral and genital mucosal ulcers are found concurrently or individually. Ulcers develop in areas of potential mucosal trauma, demonstrating the phenomenon of pathergy. In addition to oral ulceration, at least two of the following must be present to confirm the diagnosis of Behçet syndrome: (a) genital ulceration or scarring; (b) an acne-like eruption or erythema nodosum involving the arms, legs, and trunk; (c) retinal vasculitis or uveitis; (d) a positive pathergy test result. The therapeutic efficacy of various drugs has been difficult to ascertain because of the natural waxing and waning pattern of the disease.

In a patient with both oral and genital ulcers who lacks the other criteria of Behçet syndrome, the default diagnosis is *oral-genital aphthosis*. The common condition of recurrent aphthous ulcers presents with superficial, painful mucosal ulcers of the vulva and oral cavity. Unfortunately, no confirmatory histologic, culture, or blood testing is available, and therefore aphthosis remains a diagnosis of exclusion. Diagnostic tests for other causes of ulcers may have to be performed depending on the level of suspicion. The initial treatment is to relieve pain and eliminate bacterial superinfection. In the event of prolonged aphthosis, further treatments are available.

Cicatricial pemphigoid is an autoimmune blistering disease most often affecting the mucosal surfaces in older, postmenopausal patients, who may present with superficial vulvovaginal ulcerations, desquamative vaginitis, and conjunctivitis. Progressive scarification of the conjunctivae often causes severe disability and should be treated aggressively. The intact blister, a hallmark of the acantholytic group of conditions, is rarely identified in cicatricial pemphigoid. The confirmatory diagnosis of the vulvovaginal lesion is by biopsy. Direct immunofluorescence reveals autoantibodies directed against the basement membrane in most cases. Other blistering diseases, such as pemphigus vulgaris and bullous pemphigoid, may also present on the vulva, but these bullous conditions are usually diagnosed on the basis of preexisting generalized cutaneous findings.

Pyoderma Gangrenosum

Pyoderma gangrenosum manifests a characteristic ulcer with a well-defined violaceous border, necrotic base, and overhanging edge. The ulcers may be single or multiple and are routinely painful, so that the patient often requires narcotic relief. They generally develop in regions of the vulva that sustain minor injury, a response known as *pathergy*. The disease coexists with systemic illnesses half of the time, such as inflammatory bowel disease, symmetric polyarthritis, and hematologic malignancies. Biopsy is nondiagnostic but helpful in distinguishing pyoderma gangrenosum from other conditions, such as Behçet syndrome. As a first line of therapy, oral prednisone can be effective.

Anorectal Crohn Disease

Extraintestinal Crohn disease may present with recurrent serpiginous ulcers located in the interlabial sulcus, perineum, or intercrural folds; it may also present with spontaneous rectovaginal, anocutaneous, or rectal-Bartholin gland fistulae. Anorectal Crohn disease remains a difficult diagnosis because vulvar fistulae and abscess formation may precede active intestinal disease by years. Repeated studies of the colon over time may be necessary to rule out the presence of Crohn disease entirely. Because anorectal Crohn disease sometimes precedes the onset of inflammatory bowel symptoms, any spontaneously developing fistulae, recurrent fistulae, or recurrent perineal abscesses should raise the possibility of Crohn disease. Histology confirms the diagnosis by demonstrating noncaseating granulomas and multinucleated giant cells. A trial of therapy for Crohn disease with oral metronidazole may be administered before additional surgery is considered. In the face of confirmed Crohn disease, fistula repair carries a notoriously high failure rate and should be attempted only after other treatment options have failed.

Syphilis

Treponema pallidum often enters the body through an abrasion or injury and causes a chancre to develop close to the entry site (see Chapter 86). The ulcer is painless and raised with a clean base and is associated with painless lymphadenopathy. A dark-field examination or direct fluorescent antibody test confirms the diagnosis of primary syphilis. The results of specific and nonspecific treponemal tests may be negative during a significant portion of the period when the ulcer is present. Following spontaneous clearing of the chancre ulcer, within 3 to 6 weeks, the results of specific and nonspecific treponemal tests become positive. In addition to the generalized maculopapular rash found predominantly on the hands and bottoms of the feet, secondary syphilis may manifest with condyloma latum, which is a flat, smooth, raised vulvar papule.

Chancroid

Haemophilus ducreyi initially enters genital mucocutaneous abrasions or traumatized areas to form a tender papule (see Chapter 86). The papule ulcerates in several days, and a superficial ulcer with a ragged edge and an inflamed surrounding region develops. In contrast to the lesion of syphilis, the ulcer and regional lymph nodes are tender and may suppurate. Multiple ulcers are common in women, so that distinguishing chancroid from the multiple painful ulcers of HSV infection requires a negative HSV culture. A presumptive diagnosis can be made if a Gram stain of the exudate from the ulcer shows Gram-negative rods in a "school of fish" pattern (50% sensitivity). The diagnosis of chancroid by culture is problematic because a special culture medium is required for *H. ducreyi* that is not readily available, and the sensitivity of the culture is 80% or less. The Centers for Disease Control and Prevention therefore does not recommend that chancroid be diagnosed based on culture. A probable diagnosis, for both clinical and surveillance purposes, can be made if the following criteria are met: (a) The patient has one or more painful genital ulcers; (b) the patient has no evidence of *T. pallidum* infection by dark-field examination of the ulcer exudate or by a serologic test for syphilis performed at least 7 days after the appearance of the ulcers; and (c) the clinical features are typical of chancroid in respect to the appearance of the genital ulcers and the presence of regional lymphadenopathy. Polymerase chain reaction testing for *H. ducreyi* may become available soon.

Lymphogranuloma Venereum

The *Clamydia trachomatis* strain associated with lymphogranuloma venereum differs in serotype from the organism associated with chlamydial salpingitis (see Chapter 86). Infection begins with a painless papule that ulcerates and finally heals spontaneously without scarring. Within 1 to 4 weeks after the appearance of the initial lesion, inguinal lymphadenopathy and buboes may develop. The classic "groove sign" is a consequence of infection of nodes on both sides of the inguinal ligament. Needle aspiration of enlarged inguinal nodes can help to differentiate chancroid-associated lymphadenopathy (purulent aspirate) from lymphogranuloma venereum-associated lymphadenopathy (nonpurulent aspirate). Late-stage disease presents months to years after the primary infection with massive scarring, the formation of rectal strictures, deformity, and an increased risk for rectal adenocarcinoma. The confirmatory diagnosis is made with the complement fixation test for *C. trachomatis* antibodies, with a titer of more than 1:64 being diagnostic.

Donovanosis (Granuloma Inguinale)

A highly fastidious Gram-negative organism, *Calymmatobacterium granulomatis*, causes a low-grade infection of the lower genital tract (see Chapter 86). A painless papule or nodule frequently develops on the labia or vaginal introitus. Within several days, the papule or nodule ulcerates into a soft, beefy, "granulomatous" ulcer. Regional lymphadenopathy usually accompanies the ulcer, but the lymph nodes are characteristically not tender. Because of the fastidious nature of the organism, culture confirmation is generally not possible. The disease is confirmed by identifying the "Donovan body" by Giemsa or Wright stain of a crushed tissue fragment from the ulcer.

Decubitus Ulcer

Decubitus ulcers develop in frail, elderly, or disabled individuals who require prolonged bed or chair rest. Decubiti of the vulva are characteristically located over the ischial tuberosities or sacrococcygeal region, or adjacent to the urethra in cases of prolonged catheterization. A digital examination of deep decubiti may detect tissue destruction extending to the underlying bone and indicating a possibility of osteomyelitis.

NODULES AND TUMORS

A myriad of nodules and tumors may arise from glandular elements of the vulvar skin or vestibule, embryologic remnants, an infection, or a hernia. Clinical variables include location of the lesion, size, consistency, whether it is single or multiple, and surface color. In most cases, the excision of solid vulvar lesions is both diagnostic and therapeutic. "Cystic" lesions must be approached cautiously from a surgical standpoint, particularly in regions where hernias develop, such as the upper half of the labia majora and the inguinal canal. Less than careful surgical technique may increase the risk for inadvertent visceral injury. Painless, firm, Bartholin masses, especially following menopause, should be excised to rule out Bartholin gland malignancy. Table 29.3 lists common vulvar nodules, cysts, and tumors.

Genital Warts (Condylomata Acuminata)

Exophytic genital warts are most often found on the labia minora, fourchette, perineum, and perianal areas (see Chapter 141). The exophytic wart is one manifestation of "low-risk" HPV infection, but a greater proportion of HPV infections are believed to exist in a latent or subclinical form. Most genital warts have a classic appearance, and confirmatory biopsy is not necessary. Biopsy should be performed to "rule out" vulvar intraepithelial neoplasia or squamous carcinoma when rapid growth, increased pigmentation, coexisting ulceration, or fixation to underlying connective tissue is noted. One should also be careful not to misdiagnose condyloma latum as a genital

TABLE 29.3. Common Vulvar Nodules, Cysts, and Tumors

Condition	Location/characteristics	Condition	Location/characteristics
Infectious: condyloma acuminatum, molluscum contagiosum	"Warty" surface; variable size, shape, and location; molluscum—umbilicated center, 2 to 4 mm in diameter, commonly multiple	*Mesenchymal cell origin: lipoma, leiomyoma, fibroma, granular cell myoblastoma*	Variable size and consistency, excision diagnostic and therapeutic in most instances
Apocrine and eccrine gland: hidradenoma, Fox-Fordyce disease, syringoma	Note cutaneous location; hidradenoma with umbilicated center, 1–1.5 cm; Fox-Fordyce and syringomata—1 to 2 mm in diameter; Fox-Fordyce—pruritic	*Embryologic remnants: mucocele, mesonephric duct cyst*	Simple thin-walled cyst, soft consistency, commonly unifocal, located in upper vestibule (mucocele)
Keratinocyte: epidermal inclusion cyst, angiokeratoma, seborrheic keratosis	Coloration characteristic: epidermal inclusion cyst—yellow, angiokeratoma—red/purple/brown, seborrheic keratosis—brown to black; location—labia majora and outer labia minora	*Bartholin cyst, cyst of canal of Nuck, minor vestibular adenoma*	Location and consistency to palpation important, large "cysts" in upper labia may contain viscera, excision of indurated Bartholin gland mass to rule out carcinoma
Vulvo-edema and posttraumatic hematoma	With edema consider hypoalbuminemia, cardiac failure, chronic liver disease, or prior lymphadenectomy; variable location	*Hemangioma and vulvar varicosities*	Purple to red in color, varicosities characteristic bluish wormlike appearance, associated pain aggravated by prolonged standing

wart and not to overdiagnose "micropapillomatosis" of the vestibule as evidence of HPV infection. Treatment may be applied by either the physician or the patient.

Molluscum Contagiosum

A viral skin infection caused by a double-stranded DNA virus of the poxvirus family, molluscum contagiosum is transmitted though direct contact or by fomites. The infection is usually asymptomatic and produces multiple 2- to 3-mm papules with umbilicated centers. Confirmatory diagnosis and treatment follow excisional biopsy or dermal curettage. No long-term sequelae of this infection are known.

Hidradenoma, Fox-Fordyce Disease, and Syringoma

Hidradenoma is a 0.5- to 2-cm tumor of apocrine origin found most often in the interlabial sulcus. The nodule is usually solitary, may have an umbilicated center, and is generally not tender to palpation. The lesion shells out easily with excision, and the initial impression on histopathology may suggest an adenocarcinoma. However, close inspection of the glandular structure and individual cells confirms the benign nature of this nodule. Excision is curative.

In Fox-Fordyce disease, pruritic papules of apocrine gland origin are found on the mons, labia majora, and axillae. They are more common in darkly pigmented patients, may cause cyclic pruritus, and sometimes resolve after the menopause. Proposed treatments include oral contraceptives, retinoic acid, and surgical excision, although none have been studied in clinical trials.

Syringomata are benign papules of eccrine gland origin found most often on the eyelids and malar area and occasionally on the labia majora. They are of the same color as the skin. The papules tend to be asymptomatic or sometimes cause mild pruritus.

Edema and Hematoma

Vulvar edema may present spontaneously or at the time of delivery. Some helpful laboratory tests include measurement of the levels of serum albumin, serum electrolytes, blood urea nitrogen, creatinine, and C4 complement for angioedema. Acute infections may also cause edema, including herpes simplex, filariasis, and lymphogranuloma venereum, and appropriate cultures and serologic tests should be considered. Vulvar hematomas may occur in either obstetric or nonobstetric settings. A progressively expanding hematoma may require surgical exploration. However, conservative management with the application of ice and compression is preferable in most cases because of the inherent difficulty of locating a source of bleeding during surgical exploration.

PUSTULES, ABSCESSES, CELLULITIS, AND INFESTATIONS

Abscesses and cellulitis present with classic features of inflammation: redness, swelling, and pain. Specific regions of the vulva commonly affected include the hair follicles, Bartholin glands, Skene glands, and apocrine sweat glands. Some vulvar infections may be associated with various degrees of cellulitis.

Bartholin Gland Abscess

A unilateral swollen, tender, posterior labial mass is most commonly a Bartholin gland abscess. Because of the relatively high prevalence of Bartholin gland abscesses, one must be careful not to misdiagnose an unrelated swelling or abscess. The Bartholin abscess should occur in the anatomically appropriate spot, which is the lower third of the introitus between the vestibule and the labia majora. Because of the natural desire to treat an abscess expeditiously to relieve pain, a frequent management error is premature incision and drainage. It is generally best to allow the abscess to form a defined, walled-off structure, which may take several days after the initial presentation. Until the abscess "matures," the patient should receive adequate analgesics and oral antibiotics and be instructed to take frequent warm sitz baths. The bacteria found in a Bartholin gland abscess are commonly mixed flora arising from the vaginal milieu. However, other pathogens, such as gonococci, may also infect the gland. Once the abscess has matured, an incision should be created on the mucosal (vestibular) side at a point where the abscess cavity is closest to the mucosal surface. The surgical options include simple incision and drainage, insertion of a Word catheter, or marsupialization.

Hidradenitis Suppurativa

Hidradenitis suppurativa may involve apocrine glands anywhere within the "milk line" running from the labia majora to the axilla. It occurs more often in darkly skinned persons, begins after menarche, and abates after the menopause. Long-standing hidradenitis results in multiple skin abscesses, draining subcutaneous sinus tracts, scarring, and deformity. Medical treatments, discussed later, may resolve mild cases of hidradenitis or temporarily relieve severe cases. Invariably, severe hidradenitis suppurativa is managed surgically to provide long-term relief. Because apocrine glands are not found on the inner aspects of the labia minora and vestibule, an abscess in these areas should raise suspicion of another condition, such as anorectal Crohn disease.

Necrotizing Fasciitis

The combination of cellulitis, deteriorating vital signs, and a deep, spreading, painful erythema should raise concern for necrotizing fasciitis. This rapidly progressive infection is often caused by mixed aerobic and anaerobic bacteria. Unfortunately, antibiotic treatment usually proves ineffective. Necrotizing fasciitis is a surgical emergency requiring extensive debridement of the necrotic fascia to prevent septic shock and fatal complications. Magnetic resonance imaging of the fascial layer in question can effectively diagnose the condition. Risk factors for necrotizing fasciitis include diabetes mellitus, arteriosclerosis, obesity, hypertension, and prior irradiation.

Infestations and Parasitic Infections

In *scabies,* which is caused by the itch mite, *Sarcoptes scabiei,* a characteristic darkened cutaneous burrow is associated with an erythematous papule. The burrows can be found on the vulva, axillae, buttocks, and particularly the webs of the fingers and toes. The main symptom is pruritus. The diagnosis can be confirmed by microscopic identification of the itch mite in skin scrapings of the burrow.

Pediculosis pubis is a vulvar infestation with the crab louse, *Phthirus pubis*. In addition to the pubic regions, other hair-bearing areas may be involved, including the axillae, eyelashes, eyebrows, and scalp. The infestation is usually associated with pruritus but may be asymptomatic. It is spread by close physical or fomite contact. The diagnosis is confirmed by seeing the crab louse and its eggs deposited on pubic hair (nits).

Endemic in some populations, pinworm infection is caused by *Enterobius vermicularis*. The condition causes perianal pruritus, especially at night. The diagnosis is made with the cellophane tape test.

VULVAR PAIN SYNDROMES

Vulvar Dysthesia (Vulvodynia)

The 1999 World Congress of the International Society for the Study of Vulvovaginal Disease updated the classification of chronic vulval pain. A discussion group was formed to focus on the ill-defined category of chronic vulval pain *without a visible dermatosis* and proposed the term *vulvar dysesthesia (vulvodynia)* for this category. Vulvar dysesthesia was further divided into "generalized" and "localized" types. *Generalized vulvar dysesthesia* is synonymous with the formerly named *dysesthetic vulvodynia. Localized vulvar dysesthesia* is synonymous with the term *vulvar vestibulitis syndrome* and includes vestibulodynia and clitorodynia.

Vulvar Vestibulitis

Vulvar vestibulitis (localized vulvar dysesthesia or vestibulodynia) is characterized by dyspareunia or pain in response to light touch, one or more painful foci in the vulvar vestibule, and no identifiable cause of pain, such as herpes simplex, candidiasis, or pemphigoid. The Friedrich criteria remain the accepted standard for diagnosis and include the following: (a) severe pain when the vestibule is touched or vaginal entry is attempted, (b) tenderness localized within the vestibule, and (c) physical findings of erythema of various degrees. Reliability between raters and test-retest reliability have been found to be good in the assessment of localized tenderness but not in the assessment of erythema.

Pudendal, Ilioinguinal, and Genitofemoral Neuralgia

Pudendal nerve injury may follow obstetric or mechanical trauma, an outbreak of shingles, or the surgical management of prolapse. It presents with unilateral burning or lancinating pain in a pudendal nerve pattern. Ilioinguinal neuropathy may result from surgery performed close to the external inguinal ring and presents with unilateral burning or lancinating pain that radiates to the ipsilateral labium majus and inner thigh.

TRAUMATIC/ANATOMIC CONDITIONS

Perineal Trauma after Delivery

"Routine" episiotomy at childbirth has been the subject of randomized trials. It does not lower the risk for third- and fourth-degree extensions, does not reduce the duration and severity of postpartum perineal pain, and fails to improve postpartum sexual functioning. A purported "benefit" of episiotomy is a reduced risk for pelvic relaxation and urinary tract disorders. No such benefit has been demonstrated. For patients with prolonged pain and sexual dysfunction after episiotomy in whom conservative measures have failed, the perineoplasty may be an effective treatment option.

Female Genital Mutilation

An estimated 80 million women have been subjected to female genital mutilation. The condition may be found in émigrées from North Africa, the Middle East, and Southeast Asia. The spectrum of crudely performed operations can be categorized into three types: sunna, in which the hood of the clitoris is cut; excision, in which all or part of the clitoris is removed; and infibulation, in which the clitoris, labia minora, and all or part of the labia majora are amputated. Female genital mutilation can lead directly to sexual dysfunction, urinary tract infection, and long-term emotional suffering. At the time of delivery, it is usually necessary to cut the infibulation scar. General gynecologic care requires a gentle, understanding approach, and in accordance with Islamic practices, female practitioners are often requested. See Chapters 1 and 9.

Body Piercing

In genital piercing, objects such as metal rings, loops, and studs are attached to various anatomic areas of the vulva, including the labia minora and clitoris. Piercing may be associated with cellulitis, metal-induced dermatitis ("nickel itch"), and additional trauma to skin if the metal object becomes dislodged. A number of medical problems may result from genital piercing, including local inflammation, skin thickening in the vicinity of the piercing object, and further skin trauma following sexual activity.

DIAGNOSTIC AIDS

Analysis of Vaginal Secretions

Problems of the vulva and vagina may coexist. Therefore, both anatomic areas should be evaluated to acquire a full understanding of many lower genital tract problems. A determination of the vaginal pH and vaginal maturation index adds important diagnostic clues to the routine assessment. Standard nitrazine paper easily differentiates normal pH (yellow nitrazine strip) from abnormal pH (green to blue nitrazine strip). An office-based estimate of maturation index is useful in evaluating the hormonal milieu and monitoring the response to therapy for vaginal atrophy, desquamative vaginitis, or erosive lichen planus. In a patient with regular menstrual cycles, evidence of parabasal cells, which are rounded vaginal cells with large nuclei, should be considered abnormal. Careful microscopic inspection of bacterial and fungal morphology in the vaginal secretions will help to identify specific pathogens, such as *Mobiluncus* and *Candida glabrata*.

Cultures

Routine bacterial cultures of the vaginal flora are of limited diagnostic value because a large number of the bacteria found on routine culture are considered a normal part of the vaginal flora. On the other hand, fungal cultures are generally underused by most practitioners. Fungal cultures are important adjuncts to potassium hydroxide smears because the sensitivity of vaginal smears for identifying fungi is low, approximately 60%. The fungal culture also makes it possible to identify species, such as *C. glabrata,* that may be resistant to standard therapies. With the problem of recurrent candidal vulvovaginitis, self-culture by the patient may provide a timely and simplified documentation of the presence of a fungus during symptomatic episodes.

Biopsy

As a general rule, vulvar biopsies should be performed liberally when atypical mucocutaneous findings of the lower genital tract are present. The diagnosis of vulvar cancer has been found to be delayed significantly by the lack of a timely confirmatory biopsy. Direct immunofluorescence may prove helpful in a number of problems associated with immunoglobulin deposition, such as cicatricial pemphigoid, linear immunoglobulin A disease, and lichen planus. Previous biopsy specimens from unfamiliar outside facilities should be microscopically reviewed before management is offered based on a prior diagnosis.

Colposcopy

Colposcope-directed biopsies have replaced older techniques, such as 2% toluidine blue-directed biopsies, which have a lower specificity. Before the colposcopic examination is begun, it is important to allow adequate time for the application of 3% to 5% acetic acid (up to 5–10 minutes) so that areas of hyperkeratosis and hyperplasia are accentuated.

Photography

Digital photography helps to monitor changes in the vulvar appearance over time. In the selection of a digital camera, slight differences in digital quality may be less important than the capability to record rapidly and store digital files in individual records.

Blood Tests

Certain blood tests may provide diagnostic assistance. Selective testing is generally preferable to extensive screening, and the choice of tests should be based on the history, presenting symptoms, and signs.

- SS-A/SS-B for Sjögren syndrome presenting with vulvovaginal dryness
- HSV antibody for recurrent focal ulcers or focal irritation
- EBV-heterophile antibody (Monospot) for EBV-associated acute ulcers
- HIV screening.

Sensory Testing for Allodynia and Hypesthesia

In mucocutaneous allodynia, light touch with a cotton-tipped applicator evokes a painful response. The use of a numeric analogue scale ranging from 0 ("no pain") to 10 ("worst possible pain") may help the practitioner to quantify a patient's level of pain and map the pain to specific vulvovaginal areas. Localized vulvar dysesthesia (also known as *vulvar vestibulitis, vestibulodynia,* or *clitorodynia*) often presents with chronic burning pain and highly localized allodynia. In contrast, generalized vulvar dysesthesia is characterized by a wider distribution of allodynia on testing with a cotton-tipped applicator and may also demonstrate regions of reduced sensation (hypesthesia). Allodynia or hypesthesia in response to touch with a cotton-tipped applicator may also map unilaterally to a pudendal or ilioinguinal nerve pattern, suggesting pudendal or ilioinguinal neuralgia.

Wood Lamp

Ultraviolet light diagnoses erythrasma. This is a cutaneous mycotic infection that glows coral red under illumination with a Wood lamp.

MEDICAL THERAPEUTIC OPTIONS

Corticosteroids (Oral, Topical, or Injectable)

For patients with allergic or chemical dermatitis that fails to respond to conservative behavioral changes and for those with the chronic vulvar dermatoses, topical corticosteroids are the mainstay of treatment. Severe cases may require brief pulses of ultra–high-potency corticosteroids, such as 0.05% clobetasol, for 7 to 10 days monthly. Ointment preparations are preferred to creams or lotions, which can be drying and irritating. Once symptoms are controlled, the frequency of application and potency of the steroid can be reduced. Caution must be exercised to prevent secondary atrophy and rebound inflammation, which result from the long-term use of ultra–high-potency steroids. Consider the use of mid- to high-potency steroids, such as triamcinolone, betamethasone, and fluocinolone, for short periods of time and dispense in small tubes with no refills. Safer yet are low-potency steroids when the dermatitis is mild. Give low-potency topical steroids, such as 2.5% hydrocortisone, to patients who have thinner skin or prefer to apply a topical preparation regularly. Consider the use of an Aquaphor base in patients who are sensitive to compounded preparations. Concurrent infection may require the addition of topical or oral antifungals to the therapeutic regimen. Oral steroids are less familiar to the gynecologist but should remain an option. An adequate dose (40–60 mg) and an adequate length of taper (2–4 weeks) are important. A number of chronic vulvar conditions associated with pruritus, including lichen sclerosus and lichen simplex chronicus, have shown a favorable long-term response to injectable steroids.

Other Immune Response Modifiers

Steroid-sparing treatments may be considered for patients who respond partially to corticosteroids or who require extended therapy. Steroid-sparing agents may carry a risk for significant side effects, so that the therapeutic response must be monitored carefully, and the benefits must outweigh the risks. Difficult dermatoses, such as lichen planus, may respond only to steroid-sparing agents. Newer agents, such as topical tacrolimus, have been developed, and older products, such as thalidomide, brought back into use based on an increased understanding of the role of proinflammatory factors in chronic vulvar conditions.

SURGICAL OPTIONS

In the presence of a unitary nodule or tumor, surgical therapy may be both diagnostic and therapeutic. Particular care must be taken in certain conditions, such as an unrecognized hernia, in which viscera may be injured, and procedures, such as Bartholin gland *excision,* in which excessive blood loss from the vestibular venous plexus may surprise a less experienced surgeon.

BEHAVIORAL PRECAUTIONS FOR TREATMENT AND PREVENTION

Personal practices leading to irritant contact dermatitis of the vulva contribute substantially to chronic vulvar symptoms. The vulva is one of the most persistently covered regions of the body, usually with layers of fabric that are minimally pervious to moisture. Continued contact of the vulvar skin with excessive moisture can result in maceration and predispose to trauma, itching, and burning. The vulva may be injured by societal practices of questionable benefit (e.g., shaving, piercing, washing with caustic agents, infibulation) or occasionally iatrogenically. According to one study, nearly all women with chronic vulvar problems first treat themselves empirically with over-the-counter antifungal drugs, nearly half of them acting against practitioner recommendations. Self-treatment is associated with a prolongation of symptoms. The physician should particularly

- Modify activities of daily living
- Minimize telephone diagnoses
- Be cognizant of iatrogenic vulvar trauma or inflammation
- Be careful in prescribing potent topical steroids, such as clobetasol.

BIBLIOGRAPHY

1998 Guidelines for treatment of sexually transmitted diseases. *MMWR Morb Mortal Wkly Rep* 1998;47(RR-1):1–118.

Adelson MD, Joret DM, Gordon LP, et al. Recurrent necrotizing fasciitis of the vulva: a case report. *J Reprod Med* 1991;36:818–822.

Alevizon SJ, Finan MA. Sacrospinous colpopexy: management of postoperative pudendal nerve entrapment. *Obstet Gynecol* 1996;88:713–715.

Argentine Episiotomy Trial Collaborative Group. Routine vs. selective episiotomy: a randomised controlled trial. *Lancet* 1993;342:1517–1518.

Ashley RL. Sorting out the new HSV type-specific antibody tests [Review]. *Sex Transm Infect* 2001;77:232–237.

Bergeron S, Binik YM, Khalife S, et al. A randomized comparison of group cognitive-behavioral therapy, surface electromyographic biofeedback, and vestibulectomy in the treatment of dyspareunia resulting from vulvar vestibulitis. *Pain* 2001;91:297–306.

Bergeron S, Binik YM, Khalife S, et al. Vulvar vestibulitis syndrome: reliability of diagnosis and evaluation of current diagnostic criteria. *Obstet Gynecol* 2001;98:45–51.

Bornstein J, Heifetz S, Kellner Y, et al. Clobetasol dipropionate 0.05% versus testosterone propionate 2% topical application for severe vulvar lichen sclerosus. *Am J Obstet Gynecol* 1998;178:80–84.

Bracco GL, Carli P, Sonni L, et al. Clinical and histologic effects of topical treatments of vulval lichen sclerosus: a critical evaluation. *J Reprod Med* 1993;38:37–40.

Brothers TE, Tagge DU, Stutley JE, et al. Magnetic resonance imaging differentiates between necrotizing and non-necrotizing fasciitis of the lower extremity. *J Am Coll Surg* 1998;187:416–421.

Cardosi RJ, Speights A, Fiorica JV, et al. Bartholin's gland carcinoma: a 15-year experience. *Gynecol Oncol* 2001;82:247–251.

Carlson JA, Ambros R, Malfetano J, et al. Vulvar lichen sclerosus and squamous cell carcinoma: a cohort, case control, and investigational study with historical perspective—implications for chronic inflammation and sclerosis in the development of neoplasia [Review]. *Hum Pathol* 1998;29:932–948.

Chopda NM, Desai DC, Sawant PD, et al. Rectal lymphogranuloma venereum in association with rectal adenocarcinoma. *Indian J Gastroenterol* 1994;13:103–104.

Edwards L, Hays S. Vulvar cicatricial pemphigoid as a lichen sclerosus imitator: a case report. *J Reprod Med* 1992;37:561–564.

Ehrlich GE. Diagnostic criteria for Behçet's disease. *J Rheumatol* 2000;27:2049–2050.

Friedrich EG. Vulvar vestibulitis syndrome. *J Reprod Med* 1987;32:110–114.

Geiger AM, Foxman B. Risk factors for vulvovaginal candidiasis: a case-control study among university students. *Epidemiology* 1996;7:182–187.

Guaschino S, De S, Sartore A, et al. Efficacy of maintenance therapy with topical boric acid in comparison with oral itraconazole in the treatment of recurrent vulvovaginal candidiasis. *Am J Obstet Gynecol* 2001;184:598–602.

Handa VL, Stice CW. Fungal culture findings in cyclic vulvitis. *Obstet Gynecol* 2000;96:301–303.

Hillier SL, Krohn MA, Rabe LK, et al. The normal vaginal flora, H_2O_2-producing lactobacilli, and bacterial vaginosis in pregnant women. *Clin Infect Dis* 1993;16 [Suppl 4]:S273–S281.

International Study Group for Behçet's Disease. Criteria for diagnosis of Behçet's disease [Review]. *Lancet* 1990;335:1078–1080.

Jones RW, Joura EA. Analyzing prior clinical events at presentation in 102 women with vulvar carcinoma: evidence of diagnostic delays. *J Reprod Med* 1999;44:766–768.

Jones RW, Rowan DM, Kirker J, et al. Vulval lichen planus: progression of pseudoepitheliomatous hyperplasia to invasive vulval carcinomas. *Br J Obstet Gynaecol* 2001;108:665–666.

Kelly RA, Foster DC, Woodruff JD. Subcutaneous injection of triamcinolone acetonide in the treatment of chronic vulvar pruritus. *Am J Obstet Gynecol* 1993;169:568–570.

Klein MC, Gauthier RJ, Robbins JM, et al. Relationship of episiotomy to perineal trauma and morbidity, sexual dysfunction, and pelvic floor relaxation. *Am J Obstet Gynecol* 1994;171:591–598.

Klein MC, Janssen PA, MacWilliam L, et al. Determinants of vaginal-perineal integrity and pelvic floor functioning in childbirth. *Am J Obstet Gynecol* 1997;176:403–410.

Kopera D, Soyer HP, Cerroni L. Vulvar syringoma causing pruritus and carcinophobia: treatment by argon laser. *J Cutan Laser Ther* 1999;1:181–183.

Lewis FM. Vulval lichen planus [Review]. *Br J Dermatol* 1998;138:569–575.

Marin MG, King R, Sfameni S, et al. Adverse behavioral and sexual factors in chronic vulvar disease. *Am J Obstet Gynecol* 2000;183:34–38.

Moscicki AB, Hills N, Shiboski S, et al. Risks for incident human papillomavirus infection and low-grade squamous intraepithelial lesion development in young females. *JAMA* 2001;285:2995–3002.

Nwokolo NC, Boag FC. Chronic vaginal candidiasis. Management in the postmenopausal patient [Review]. *Drugs Aging* 2000;16:335–339.

O'Hare PM, Sherertz EF. Vulvodynia: a dermatologist's perspective with emphasis on an irritant contact dermatitis component. *J Womens Health Gender-Based Med* 2000;9:565–569.

Patton LW, Elgart ML, Williams CM. Vulvar erythema and induration: extraintestinal Crohn's disease of the vulva. *Arch Dermatol* 1990;126:1351–1352.

Propst AM, Thorp JMJ. Traumatic vulvar hematomas: conservative versus surgical management. *South Med J* 1998;91:144–146.

Rouzier R, Haddad B, Deyrolle C, et al. Perineoplasty for the treatment of introital stenosis related to lichen sclerosus. *Am J Obstet Gynecol* 2002;186:49–52.

Sangwan YP, Coller JA, Barrett MS, et al. Unilateral pudendal neuropathy: significance and implications. *Dis Colon Rectum* 1996;39:249–251.

Schaaf VM, Perez-Stable EJ, Borchardt K. The limited value of symptoms and signs in the diagnosis of vaginal infections. *Arch Intern Med* 1990;150:1929–1933.

Sihvo S, Ahonen R, Mikander H, et al. Self-medication with vaginal antifungal drugs: physicians' experiences and women's utilization patterns. *Fam Pract* 2000;17:145–149.

Sisson BA, Glick L. Genital ulceration as a presenting manifestation of infectious mononucleosis. *J Pediatr Adolesc Gynecol* 1998;11:185–187.
Sobel JD. Vulvovaginitis due to *Candida glabrata*: an emerging problem [Review]. *Mycoses* 1998;41[Suppl 2]:18–22.
Tay YK, Tham SN, Teo R. Localized vulvar syringomas—an unusual cause of pruritus vulvae. *Dermatology* 1996;192:62–63.
Tucker P. Female genital mutilation presents array of medical and cultural challenges. Washington, DC: American College of Obstetricians and Gynecologists, 1995:1–10 (ACOG Newsletter 1-1-0095).
Unger ER, Vernon SD, Lee DR, et al. Human papillomavirus type in anal epithelial lesions is influenced by human immunodeficiency virus. *Arch Pathol Lab Med* 1997;121:820–824.
Vettraino IM, Merritt DF. Crohn's disease of the vulva [Review]. *Am J Dermatopathol* 1995;17:410–413.
Viravan C, Dance DA, Ariyarit C, et al. A prospective clinical and bacteriologic study of inguinal buboes in Thai men. *Clin Infect Dis* 1996;22:233–239.
Virgili A, Bacilieri S, Corazza M. Managing vulvar lichen simplex chronicus. *J Reprod Med* 2001;46:343–346.

CHAPTER 30
Premenstrual Syndrome

Tana A. Grady-Weliky and Vivian Lewis

Premenstrual syndrome (PMS) is a complex of mild to moderate emotional and physical symptoms. Up to 75% of reproductive-age women experience premenstrual symptoms. A severe form of PMS, premenstrual dysphoric disorder (PMDD), affects 3% to 8% of reproductive-age women and typically interferes with the patient's functioning. Premenstrual symptoms occur exclusively during the luteal phase of the menstrual cycle and remit within 3 days after the onset of menses. The etiology of PMS is multifactorial. A role of fluctuating hormones across the menstrual cycle is presumed because PMS does not affect prepubertal girls or menopausal women. Studies have also suggested a role of serotonin and other neurotransmitters in the etiology of PMS.

ETIOLOGY

Although many theories have been advanced, none provides a unified explanation of the complex of PMS symptoms. Because of its relationship to corpus luteum function, the most obvious explanation of PMS would be that it is a consequence of the systemic and psychological effects of sex steroids produced by the corpus luteum. However, multiple studies have shown no difference between women with PMS and controls in respect to circulating levels of progesterone and estrogen. Investigators have examined daily steroid levels, peak steroid levels, and ratios of progesterone to estradiol, generally with the same conclusion—that no significant difference can be found between women with PMS and controls.

Nonetheless, adequate evidence suggests that intrinsic differences in sensitivity to physiologic levels of estrogen and progesterone may be a factor. Administering a gonadotropin-releasing hormone (GnRH) agonist, which suppresses the output of estrogen and progesterone, to women with PMS can relieve their psychological symptoms, whereas the mood of women without PMS does not change consistently. In some cases, reintroducing estrogen and progesterone to the women with PMS reproduces the syndrome. A progesterone metabolite, allopregnenolone, which is produced in the ovary and brain, has been thought to play an important role because it can influence γ-aminobutyric acid (GABA) receptors. However, the results of studies comparing allopregnenolone levels in women who have PMS with those in controls have been conflicting. Recent efforts have focused mainly on neurotransmitter sensitivity to steroid hormones.

The serotoninergic pathway has received the most attention, in part because of the therapeutic implications. Animal studies suggest that estradiol and progesterone can influence central serotoninergic activity. Administering the serotonin agonist *m*-chlorophenylpiperazine in women with PMS acutely relieves depression and anxiety. Furthermore, in placebo-controlled trials, serotonin reuptake inhibitors (SRIs) have clearly shown efficacy in the treatment of PMS.

Other neurotransmitter factors of potential importance include the GABA system, opiate system, and adrenergic receptor functioning. In some studies, decreases in plasma GABA levels have been observed in women with PMS during the luteal phase. Peripheral levels of β-endorphins have been shown to be lower in women with PMS during the luteal phase, but not cerebrospinal fluid levels. Despite the known role of α-adrenergic receptor function in depression, inconsistent results have been obtained in studies of these receptors in women with PMS. A role for β-adrenergic receptor function in both disorders is under study.

The physical symptoms of PMS are largely unexplained. Many women with PMS experience mastalgia, fluid retention, and bloating. No consistent differences in prolactin, cortisol, or thyroid hormone levels have been shown in women with PMS. Progesterone is a substrate for deoxycorticosterone—a potent mineralocorticoid. Renal 21-hydroxylase converts progesterone to deoxycorticosterone in the kidney. This extraglandular deoxycorticosterone is thought by some to mediate the bloating and fluid retention of PMS. However, one study of deoxycorticosterone levels showed similar variations during the menstrual cycle in controls and women with PMS.

In summary, the etiology of PMS is not understood. Current knowledge suggests that many of the psychological symptoms occur because of an increased central sensitivity to physiologic levels of estrogen and progesterone. Sensitivity appears to be enhanced through serotonin-mediated pathways. Other mediators are under study. The physical manifestations of PMS are not understood but may ultimately prove to be another manifestation of increased sensitivity to normal cyclic hormonal variation.

DIFFERENTIAL DIAGNOSIS

Confirming the diagnosis of PMS requires a comprehensive assessment to rule out other causes of the emotional and physical symptoms. The differential diagnosis includes molimina, hypothyroidism, perimenopause, and major mood or anxiety disorders. Most ovulatory women experience some physical changes (e.g., breast tenderness, bloating, food cravings) during the luteal phase. By definition, if these symptoms do not interfere with normal life functions, the term *molimina* can be applied. Hypothyroidism may share many of the symptoms of PMS; however, no cyclic variation should occur. A thyroid-stimulating hormone level is a sufficient screen if warranted by clinical suspicion. The symptoms of perimenopause and those of PMS also overlap considerably. Many women experience symptoms of emotional irritability, cyclic mastalgia, bloating, and hot flashes as part of the symptom complex associated with perimenopause. It is likely that similar pathophysiologic factors mediate the symptoms in both disorders. In a practical sense, to document PMS, women should maintain a calendar of symptoms that can be correlated with the reproductive cycle. For PMDD, women must meet the specific diagnostic criteria outlined in the *Diagnostic and Statistical Manual of Mental Disorders*, 4th edition—text revision.

Distinguishing the emotional symptoms of PMS from those of other major mood or anxiety disorders (e.g., major depressive disorder, dysthymia, panic disorder) is important because the treatment strategies differ. Women with PMS respond to unique therapeutic interventions, such as calcium carbonate, GnRH agonists, and intermittent dosing with SRIs. If patients present with mood or anxiety symptoms that continue across the menstrual cycle, PMS cannot be diagnosed. If patients exhibit mood or anxiety symptoms across the menstrual cycle that become more severe during the luteal phase, the appropriate diagnosis is premenstrual exacerbation of the underlying condition, not PMS. The diagnostic verification of PMS is best accomplished through the prospective daily recording of symptoms ("charting") for at least two menstrual cycles.

A number of valid and reliable diagnostic instruments (e.g., Calendar of Premenstrual Experiences, PMS Diary, Daily Record of Severity of Problems) are available to document emotional and physical symptoms across the menstrual cycle. These forms list emotional, physical, and functional symptoms that patients rate or "chart" daily with a Likert-type scale to document the presence, timing, and severity of symptoms. The diagnosis of PMS/PMDD is verified by the following: (a) demonstrated evidence of a relative absence of symptoms during the follicular phase of the menstrual cycle; (b) a significant increase in emotional and physical symptoms during the luteal phase of the menstrual cycle; and (c) functional impairment during the luteal phase of the menstrual cycle.

CLINICAL SYMPTOMS AND HISTORY

PMS is characterized by mood swings, depressed mood, irritability, or anxiety, which may be accompanied by physical symptoms. The symptoms occur exclusively during the luteal phase of the menstrual cycle. Physical symptoms frequently observed in PMS are breast tenderness, abdominal bloating, headache, and joint and muscle aches. In women with PMDD, social or occupational functioning is also significantly reduced. The functional impairment tends to be in social rather than occupational domains.

TREATMENT

In the initial phase of treatment, the patient charts her symptoms for two menstrual cycles, during which limited interventions are started. If the patient remains symptomatic after the charting period, phase 2 treatment strategies should be initiated.

Phase 1: Diagnostic Interventions

While patients are charting, clinicians may recommend health-promoting lifestyle behaviors, including dietary modifications. Patients with mild to moderate premenstrual symptoms report that reducing the intake of caffeine, refined sugars, or sodium is helpful. Vitamin and mineral supplementation may also be beneficial. Vitamin B_6 in daily doses of 50 to 100 mg was found to relieve premenstrual mood and physical symptoms. In another study, the daily administration of 1,200 mg of calcium carbonate significantly reduced physical and emotional premenstrual symptoms.

Spironolactone, a diuretic and steroid antagonist, may reduce premenstrual bloating, weight gain, and negative emotions. Moreover, limited data suggest that the combination of an oral contraceptive and drosperinone, an analogue of spironolactone, is useful for the treatment of premenstrual emotional and physical symptoms.

Phase 2: Treatment Interventions

SRIs are first-line agents for the treatment of PMS/PMDD. Numerous controlled clinical trials have shown that almost all SRIs are superior to placebo for the management of premenstrual emotional and physical symptoms. Most of these trials have shown symptom relief within three cycles of active treatment.

Fluoxetine has been shown to be more effective than placebo in all studies performed to date. Steiner and colleagues compared 20 and 60 mg of fluoxetine with placebo in 277 patients who had severe PMS. In this study, both doses of fluoxetine were superior to placebo in reducing premenstrual emotional and physical symptoms. The 60-mg daily dose caused more side effects and higher dropout rates without better efficacy than the 20-mg daily dose. Sertraline has also been found to be more effective than placebo for PMDD in multiple randomized controlled trials. In a placebo-controlled study of 243 women with PMDD, 50 to 100 mg of sertraline daily relieved the emotional and physical symptoms of PMDD.

Although most trials of SRIs have examined the continuous administration of medication, the effectiveness of administering SRIs only during the luteal phase is being studied. Several controlled trials have documented the effectiveness of luteal phase dosing of SRIs, including fluoxetine, sertraline, and citalopram. In a comparison of continuous, partially intermittent (low-dose follicular and full-dose luteal) dosing and intermittent (full-dose luteal only) dosing of citalopram with placebo, all groups given active treatment experienced a significant reduction in premenstrual symptoms in comparison with those given placebo.

Other antidepressants are currently considered second-line therapies for PMS/PMDD because they are less well tolerated and cause more side effects. Clomipramine, a tricyclic antidepressant, is more effective than placebo. Other antidepressants, such as desipramine, maprotiline, and bupropion, are of limited efficacy, if any. In four of five controlled studies, alprazolam was more effective than placebo, particularly in the management of premenstrual anxiety symptoms. Clinicians should remain cautious when prescribing alprazolam because of the associated risk for tolerance and dependence.

If treatment with an SRI or second-line psychotropic agent is unsuccessful, hormonal therapies should be considered. Although oral contraceptives are used to treat mild to moderate premenstrual symptoms, only one controlled trial supports the efficacy of an oral contraceptive in combination with drosperinone in the treatment of moderate to severe symptoms. A meta-analysis of progesterone and progestogens in the management of PMS found no significant differences between active medications and placebo across studies. However, GnRH agonists, such as leuprolide, have been found to be effective in comparison with placebo. Because of the reduced tolerability of injectable medications, their cost, and their potential to cause menopause-like adverse effects, GnRH agonists are a third-line treatment strategy.

By using appropriate diagnostic tools to identify patients with PMS/PMDD, clinicians can improve their quality of life. A variety of available pharmacologic therapeutic interventions are available with good evidence of successful treatment in comparison with placebo. Enhanced physician, patient, and public education about PMS/PMDD should foster more systematic research in this area, which should ultimately lead to a better understanding of PMDD and the development of more specific therapeutics.

BIBLIOGRAPHY

American Psychiatric Association. *Diagnostic and statistical manual of mental disorders,* 4th ed—text revision. Washington, DC: American Psychiatric Press, 2000: 771–774.

Campbell EM, Peterkin D, O'Grady K, et al. Premenstrual symptoms in general practice patients: prevalence and treatment. *J Reprod Med* 1997;42:637–646.

Endicott J. Severe premenstrual dysphoria. *Journal of the American Medical Women's Association* 1998;53:170–175.

Eriksson E, Hedberg MA, Andersch B, et al. The serotonin reuptake inhibitor paroxetine is superior to the noradrenaline reuptake inhibitor maprotiline in the treatment of premenstrual syndrome. *Neuropsychopharmacology* 1995;12: 167–176.

Freeman EW, et al. Evaluation of a unique oral contraceptive in the treatment of premenstrual dysphoric disorder. *J Womens Health Gender-Based Med* 2001;10: 561–569.

Freeman EW, Rickels K, Sondheimer SJ, et al. Differential response to antidepressants in women with premenstrual syndrome/premenstrual dysphoric disorder. *Arch Gen Psychiatry* 1999;56:932–939.

Grady-Weliky TA. Premenstrual dysphoric disorder. *N Engl J Med* 2003;348: 433–438

Hylan TR, Sundell K, Judge R. The impact of premenstrual symptomatology on functioning and treatment-seeking behavior: experience from the United States, United Kingdom, and France. *J Womens Health Gender-Based Med* 1999; 8:1043–1052.

Jermain DM, Preece CK, Sykes FL, et al. Luteal phase sertraline treatment for premenstrual dysphoric disorder. *Arch Fam Med* 1998;8:328–332.

Kessel B. Premenstrual syndrome: advances in diagnosis and treatment. *Obstet Gynecol Clin North Am* 2000;27:625–639.

Mortola JF, Girton L, Beck L, et al. Diagnosis of premenstrual syndrome by a simple, prospective, and reliable instrument: the calendar of premenstrual experiences. *Obstet Gynecol* 1990;76:302–307.

Parry BL. Psychobiology of premenstrual dysphoric disorder. *Semin Reprod Endocrinol* 1997;15:55–68.

Pearlstein TB, Stone AB, Lund SA, et al. Comparison of fluoxetine, bupropion, and placebo in the treatment of premenstrual dysphoric disorder. *J Clin Psychopharmacol* 1997;17:261–266.

Prior JC. Perimenopause: the complex endocrinology of the menopausal transition. *Endocr Rev* 1998;19:397–428.

Rapkin AJ, Morgan M, Goldman L, et al. Progesterone metabolite allopregnenolone in women with premenstrual syndrome. *Obstet Gynecol* 1997;90: 709–714.

Schmidt PJ, Nieman LK, Danaceau MA, et al. Differential behavioral effects of gonadal steroids in women with and in those without premenstrual syndrome. *N Engl J Med* 1998;338:209–216.

Seippel S, Eriksson O, Grankvist K, et al. Physical symptoms in premenstrual syndrome are related to plasma progesterone and desoxycorticosterone. *Gynecol Endocrinol* 2000;14:173–181.

Steiner M, Korzekwa M, Lamont J, et al. Intermittent fluoxetine dosing in the treatment of women with premenstrual dysphoria. *Psychopharmacol Bull* 1997;33:771–774.

Steiner M, Steinberg S, Stewart D, et al. Fluoxetine in the treatment of premenstrual dysphoria. *N Engl J Med* 1995;332:1529–1534.

Su TP, Schmidt PJ, Danceau M, et al. Effect of menstrual cycle phase on neuroendocrine and behavioral responses to the serotonin agonist *m*-chlorophenylpiperazine in women with premenstrual syndrome and controls. *J Clin Endocrinol Metab* 1997;82:1220–1228.

Sundblad C, Hedberg MA, Eriksson E. Clomipramine administered during the luteal phase reduces the symptoms of premenstrual syndrome: a placebo-controlled trial. *Neuropsychopharmacology* 1993;9:133–145.

Thys-Jacobs S, Alvir JMJ, Fratarcangelo P. Comparative analysis of three premenstrual assessment instruments—the identification of premenstrual syndrome with core symptoms. *Psychopharmacol Bull* 1995;31:389–396.

Thys-Jacobs S, Starkey P, Bernstein D, et al. Calcium carbonate and the premenstrual syndrome: effects on premenstrual and menstrual symptoms. *Am J Obstet Gynecol* 1998;179:444–452.

Wang M, Hammarback S, Lindhe BA, et al. Treatment of premenstrual syndrome by spironolactone: a double-blind, placebo-controlled study. *Acta Obstet Gynecol Scand* 1995;74:803–808.

Wikander I, Sundblad C, Andersch B, et al. Citalopram in premenstrual dysphoria: is intermittent treatment during luteal phase more effective than continuous medication throughout the menstrual cycle? *J Clin Psychopharmacol* 1998;18:390–398.

Wyatt K, Dimmock P, Jones P, et al. Efficacy of progesterone and progestogens in the management of premenstrual syndrome: a systematic review. *BMJ* 2001;323:1–8.

Wyatt KM, Dimmock PW, Jones PW, et al. Efficacy of vitamin B_6 in the treatment of premenstrual syndrome: systematic review. *BMJ* 1999;318:1375–1381.

Yonkers KA, Halbreich U, Freeman E, et al. Symptomatic improvement of premenstrual dysphoric disorder with sertraline treatment. *JAMA* 1997;278:983–988.

CHAPTER 31
Uterine Leiomyomata

James Segars

Uterine *leiomyomata,* also called *fibroids* or *myomata,* are smooth muscle tumors of the uterus. Fibroids are the most common tumor of women. Except in extremely rare syndromes, fibroids do not occur in men, and no analogous condition exists in men. Fibroids are a considerable public health problem. In 1997, the Agency for Healthcare Research and Quality reported 213,718 discharges with a diagnosis of hysterectomy for fibroids at a mean cost of $9,041 per admission, for a total cost of $2.1 billion. In comparison, coronary bypass and graft procedures for women cost a total of $5.8 billion. Not including lost wages and other related expenses, billions of United States health care dollars are spent annually on the treatment of uterine fibroids.

Basic and clinical research on fibroids has been sparse or of poor quality. Research in the United States has been limited by a lack of public understanding of the condition, and few resources have been allocated to the study of the condition. As a result, the evidence-based medical management of fibroids lags behind that of other health problems of women. The management of fibroids advanced little in the 100 years prior to the past decade, and no preventive treatment or definitive cure of fibroids is available short of surgical excision.

EPIDEMIOLOGY AND PREVALENCE

In one study, 16% of predominantly white, asymptomatic women had fibroids on a screening ultrasonographic examination, and the percentage had increased to 27% after 2.5 years. Based on the results of a study of hysterectomy specimens, more than 70% of women have fibroid tumors of the uterus. Many of these are asymptomatic, but it is estimated that more than 25% of women experience symptoms related to fibroid tumors. The exact prevalence of fibroids is not known.

The prevalence of fibroids differs substantially between races; African-American and Caribbean-African women are two to three times more likely to undergo a hysterectomy for fibroids than Hispanic or white women. The lifetime likelihood that a black woman will have a hysterectomy approaches 22%, whereas it is 7% to 8% for a white woman. The rate of myomectomy is similarly increased in black women; it is 6%, in comparison with 1% in white women.

The prevalence of fibroids varies with age; fibroids are extremely rare before puberty, and fibroid disease is less prevalent in postmenopausal women. Fibroids are less common in women who have given birth, and it is possible that pregnancy is beneficial. Several epidemiologic studies have reported that the risk for fibroids increases with the body mass index. Cigarette smoking is associated with a reduced likelihood of fibroid disease. Hormonal contraception has been extensively studied, and it does not appear to have a consistent effect on fibroid growth or development. The results of at least one study suggest that the progestin contraceptive agent depot medroxyprogesterone acetate may reduce the incidence of fibroids. In contrast, hormonal replacement therapy with estrogen alone in postmenopausal women may increase the risk for hospitalization for fibroid-related disease. The incidence of fibroids is increased in the first-degree relatives of women with the disease.

ETIOLOGY

The exact cause of fibroids remains unknown. Histologically, fibroids are composed of nearly identical smooth muscle cells, but the nodules contain abundant fibrous tissue and collagen deposits and occasionally become calcified. The tumors are clonal, arising from single cells; in one uterus, different fibroids are derived from different clonal expansions. Chromosomal abnormalities are common in fibroids, but 40% of tumors do not exhibit chromosomal anomalies. Two high-mobility group proteins, HMGIC and HMGIY, are often overexpressed in fibroids. Fibroids are unlikely to undergo malignant transformation; malignant fibroids, leiomyosarcomas, are exceedingly rare (0.1%).

Considerable evidence suggests a role of gonadal steroids in the growth and development of uterine fibroids. Induction of a "medical menopausal state" with gonadotropin-releasing hormone (GnRH) agonists is associated with a reduction in fibroid size, which occurs in any state characterized by sustained low levels of circulating estrogen. The cells of normal uterine smooth muscle tissue undergo mitosis in the luteal phase of the menstrual cycle, so that the tissue from which fibroids arise is responsive to gonadal steroids. Gonadal steroids in combination with retinoids have been shown to initiate the development of myomata in a guinea pig model.

Although estrogens may promote the growth of fibroids, estrogen receptors are not overexpressed in fibroid tissues, nor have circulating estrogen levels been shown to be higher in women in whom fibroids develop. Two groups, one led by Tsibris and the other by Fukuhara, have suggested a role for the Wnt family of growth factor receptors and provided evidence implicating a number of proteins not previously associated with fibroids.

CLINICAL SYMPTOMS AND HISTORY

Fibroids most often present with pelvic pressure, menorrhagia, or menometrorrhagia. Fibroids often reach a size at which they cause symptoms of nocturnal frequency and urinary leakage; much more rarely, compression of the ureters leads to renal compromise. Women with large fibroids may note an increase in abdominal girth, or a hard mass in the lower abdomen may be accompanied by gastrointestinal symptoms, such as constipation. Fibroids may cause dyspareunia, infertility, or first-trimester miscarriage (see section " Leiomyomata and Pregnancy"). Obstetric complications of fibroids include second-trimester loss, intrauterine fetal growth retardation, preterm delivery, preterm labor, and placental abruption. The degree of symptomatology may bear no relation to the size of the fibroid; a small intracavitary uterine fibroid may cause substantial uterine bleeding, and a large pedunculated subserosal fibroid may remain asymptomatic.

Approximately one third of women with symptomatic fibroids experience abnormal uterine bleeding. Heavy menses (menorrhagia) or menometrorrhagia may be observed. The size of the myoma is not related to the amount of bleeding. Patients with persistently heavy menses not uncommonly present with iron deficiency anemia. In addition to ulceration of the surface of the fibroid, several other mechanisms have been suggested to explain the menorrhagia. Fibroids that enlarge and distort the uterine cavity cause a significant increase in the surface area of the uterine cavity, from 15 cm^2 to 200 cm^2, which results in a heavier flow. Studies of endometrial blood flow in women with fibroids have revealed venule ectasia and engorgement, which lead to greater endometrial blood loss. Buttram and Reiter reported that 81% of women reported a reduction in bleeding or relief of symptoms after myomectomy for bleeding.

Leiomyomata and Infertility

Fibroids have been identified as the sole cause of infertility in fewer than 10% of infertile patients. By obstructing the fallopian tube ostia, fibroids may prevent fertilization. Proving an association between fibroids and infertility is complicated because many factors are involved in establishing a pregnancy, and more than one of these may be causing a problem in an infertile couple. Furthermore, a randomized, controlled, life table analysis of fibroids and infertility has not been conducted. Most studies of the relationship between fibroids and infertility evaluate the effect of fibroids indirectly by assessing fertility after myomectomy. Based on current evidence, infertile women with fibroids may benefit from surgery when the myoma volume is more than 100 mL and at least one to five fibroids are present, but not more than five. Patients with submucous fibroids larger than 2 cm appear to benefit. A number of case series and a metaanalysis have suggested that slightly fewer than two thirds of women with otherwise unexplained infertility conceive after myomectomy.

Leiomyomata and Assisted Reproduction

The study of fibroids in women undergoing assisted reproduction allows a robust assessment of the effect of fibroids on fertility because pregnancy rates in assisted reproduction are high and pregnancies occur within a defined time interval. Studies of women undergoing assisted reproduction have clearly demonstrated that fibroids impair fertility. Farhi and colleagues reported a reduction in the number of embryos implanting in the uterus after assisted reproduction when the uterine cavity was distorted. In the study of Healy, pregnancy and implantation rates were lower in women with either intramural or submucous fibroids. In a metaanalysis by Pritts, an adverse effect of submucous fibroids was substantiated. In contrast, subserosal fibroids do not reduce pregnancy rates. Reports of clinical outcome after assisted reproduction in women with intramural fibroids are conflicting. Based on current information, if the uterine cavity is not distorted and the intramural fibroid is small (<1.9 cm), it may be reasonable to proceed with a cycle of assisted reproduction. If the woman does not become pregnant, then resection may be beneficial.

CLINICAL FINDINGS AND PHYSICAL EXAMINATION

The clinical assessment should include a physical examination with palpation of the lower abdomen. A careful bimanual examination is indicated, with particular attention given to the uterine contour. Even if the bimanual examination findings are normal, in cases of infertility, pregnancy loss, or vaginal bleeding, an ultrasonographic examination is in order because small fibroids may not be detected during the bimanual examination. For instance, a 1-cm intracavitary fibroid may cause repeated first-trimester loss. If the clinical examination suggests a mass or irregular uterine contour, an imaging study is indicated to confirm the presence of fibroids before treatment is initiated because other pelvic disease, such as ovarian tumors, may present with identical physical findings.

In clinical practice, fibroids may be located anywhere in the uterus, including the cervix and broad ligament. Large pedunculated subserosal fibroids may rarely become parasitic, detach from the uterus, and adhere to the bowel or other abdominal organs. The relationship between the symptoms and location is not precise, although fibroids in certain locations tend to present with characteristic symptoms.

IMAGING STUDIES

The preferred imaging study is a transvaginal ultrasonography with saline sonography. Fibroids typically appear as a sonolucent nodule on the ultrasonographic examination. The three most important facts about a fibroid are location, location, and location. In addition, an assessment of fibroid size, usually in centimeters, is helpful. If multiple fibroids are present, the location of each should be noted and documented.

The management of fibroid disease is impeded by the lack of a universal scoring system for fibroids that is related to clinical outcome. Similarly, it is difficult to compare studies of fibroids because scoring systems vary significantly. Tindall suggested a classification based on location: submucous, intramural, or subserous. More recently, the European Society of Hysteroscopy has agreed on a classification for submucous fibroids. Bajekal and Li have proposed a system for myoma classification that incorporates the previous classification schemes. A clinically useful classification based on saline sonography has also been proposed.

Myomata may be suspected if distortion of the uterine cavity is noted by hysterosalpingography. Fibroids suspected by hysterosalpingography should be confirmed by another imaging modality. Magnetic resonance imaging is an excellent modality for imaging fibroids, although it is more expensive than ultrasonography, and it offers the added capability of distinguishing between fibroids and adenomyosis. Computed tomography also clearly identifies fibroids and may be helpful in some cases.

Given the varied symptoms and almost infinite number of possible locations, the essential question to be answered is, Are the fibroid(s) identified causing the symptoms observed? In some cases, the answer is clear, as when an extremely large pelvic fibroid causes pelvic pressure and frequency; at other times, the association is more tenuous. The treatment should be based on the association between the fibroid and the symptom.

TREATMENT

Medical Therapy

The most common medical treatment for fibroids is the induction of menopause with GnRH agonists or, more recently, GnRH antagonists. A reduction in fibroid size correlates with a reduction in circulating estrogen levels, and a reduction of 30% has been reported. Medical treatment does not cause cell death within the tumors, and once therapy is halted, the fibroids return to their pretreatment size within 6 months. Therapy is limited by side effects such as hot flushes, vaginal dryness, and mood changes, and furthermore, continuation of therapy beyond 6 months results in significant bone loss. For these reasons, medical therapy is only a short-term solution. Treatment should be initiated for a specific length of time and with a clear purpose. It is possible that selective antiestrogens or progestins may offer alternative approaches, and antifibrotic medications such as pirfenidone are currently under evaluation.

Abdominal Myomectomy

For women who wish to preserve their fertility or their uterus, myomectomy is an option. Myomectomy by laparotomy is major surgery and carries risks for infection and bleeding. Although the goal of myomectomy is to avoid hysterectomy, hysterectomy is required in 1% to 2% of cases because of bleeding or complications. It should be noted that not all fibroids are circumscribed tumors, and it may be impossible to resect a diffuse adenofibroma involving a large portion of the uterus. Complications of myomectomy include adhesion formation and fibroid recurrence (see section "Recurrence after Myomectomy"). If the fibroid involves the uterine cavity, scarring may develop within the uterine cavity after myomectomy. Depending on the location of the excised fibroid and the incision of the uterine muscle, surgeons may recommend that a cesarean section be performed in subsequent pregnancies to avoid the catastrophe of uterine rupture during labor.

Hysteroscopic Myomectomy

In some cases, fibroids may be removed via hysteroscopy. The advantages of this approach are that it does not require an abdominal incision and can be performed on an outpatient basis. The fibroids amenable to hysteroscopic resection with current instruments are located predominantly within the uterine cavity and typically smaller than 1 to 2 cm in size. Larger myomata, or those with significant intramural components, are difficult to extirpate hysteroscopically. Complications of hysteroscopy include intravascular leakage of the distention medium, severe hyponatremia, and seizures. Newer hysteroscopic systems use a saline distention solution, thereby reducing the consequences of intravascular extravasation. Perforation of the uterus is a recognized complication and occasionally necessitates conversion of the procedure to a laparotomy or termination. As after all fibroid resections, fibroid recurrence requiring another operation is a risk. Because many submucous fibroids cause pregnancy loss, infertility, or bleeding problems and are located within the uterine cavity, they are often amenable to hysteroscopic surgery.

Laparoscopic Myomectomy

Since 1990, several groups have described the laparoscopic resection of fibroids. Several small, uncontrolled case series and a randomized clinical trial have been reported. With the current instruments, patients who are candidates for this procedure have fibroids no larger than 9 cm and one to three fibroids that are accessible via a laparoscope. For this reason, laparoscopy is better suited to excise subserosal and intramural fibroids. Spontaneous uterine rupture in pregnancy is rare, but a 1% incidence has been associated with laparoscopic fibroid resection. The contributing factors are not clear. In addition, although the data are very limited, a recurrence rate of 51% after laparoscopic resection has been reported, which is much higher than the recurrence rate after abdominal myomectomy. Therefore, laparoscopic resection has not gained wide acceptance.

Uterine Artery Embolization

Embolization of the uterine artery was introduced to treat myomata in 1995. Despite limited evidence of efficacy and a lack of randomized trials, the procedure has been applied in a large number of patients, reflecting the desire of many women to avoid hysterectomy. A catheter is passed into the uterine artery (not the vasculature of the myoma itself), and once it is distal to the gluteal structures, the embolic substance is injected. Overall, 40% to 69% shrinkage of myomata has been reported, but clinical success rates are 85%. Volume reduction of the entire uterus of 29% to 48% has been reported. Consensus appears to be evolving that pedunculated and subserosal fibroids do not respond well to embolization, reflecting a concern that the selection of patients and fibroids for the procedure are not well defined. For example, the Doppler sonographic appearance before embolization does not correlate with response.

Ovarian failure rates of up to 43% in women older than 45 years have been reported. Because of the possibility of permanent impairment of ovarian function, the technique is not recommended for women who desire future fertility. Amenorrhea is a late effect of impaired ovarian function, and ovarian reserve after embolization has not been tested sufficiently in current studies; therefore, it is possible that subtle ovarian impairment may be more common than has been reported. Because menopause is associated with a reduction in fibroid size, a relevant question is, Does impairment of ovarian function contribute to the reported response rate? Sepsis requiring emergency hysterectomy is an identified complication (2%), and at least one death from sepsis has occurred. Roughly 20% of women experience severe pain following embolization that often requires narcotics. Based on current information, the procedure is well suited to women in their 40s who are no longer interested in childbearing and in whom early induction of the menopause may not be problematic. More defined proof of efficacy and long-term follow up are needed.

Myolysis

Myolysis was first performed in the 1980s to avoid hysterectomy (see study of Donnez and colleagues). In this procedure, an instrument is inserted directly into the fibroid, and the myoma tissue is destroyed. In the first series, a neodymium:yttrium-aluminum-garnet (Nd:YAG) laser was used (n < 48), and a mean reduction of 41% at 6 months was reported. Later, a bipolar needle was used (n < 150) to achieve shrinkage of 30% to 50%. A later series reported an 88.5% reduction in myoma volume at 3 to 6 months. A mean reduction of 6% has been reported with cryomyolysis (n < 14), although a greater response was achieved in some cases. More recently, an endometrial laser intrauterine light procedure has been used for myolysis. To date, the follow-up, selection of patients and fibroids, and proof of efficacy are very limited because the current series are small. Based on existing information, use of this method must be restricted until the efficacy and long-term response are known. Shrinkage appears to be 30% to 50%, which is quantitatively similar to the results achieved with uterine artery embolization. The technique is not advised for women interested in childbearing.

Recurrence after Myomectomy

Six studies of abdominal myomectomy in which life table analysis was performed revealed cumulative recurrence rates of 27% to 44.2% at 3.6 to 8.5 years of follow-up. Fauconnier and colleagues emphasized that these recurrence rates represented a minimum because a loss of study patients to follow-up (censored patients) resulted in an underestimation of the recurrence rate. Fedele and colleagues reported that 29% of patients had persistent myoma 6 months after myomectomy. This begs the question, Does recurrence represent persistence of multiple myomata or the growth of new myomata after surgery? In a study of women with apparently normal findings by ultrasonography after myomectomy, Vavala and colleagues reported a 15% recurrence rate by ultrasonography at 3 years. This finding suggests that recurrence may represent both persistent myomata and de novo growth of small seedling myomata. In support of this conclusion, the likelihood of recurrence has been shown to increase with the number of myomata removed. Pregnancy after myomectomy has been reported to lower the risk for recurrence.

Hysterectomy

Hysterectomy is a definitive surgical solution. Hysterectomy may be indicated in cases in which the symptoms are significant and the woman no longer desires fertility. Hysterectomy may also be indicated if the uterus is extremely large or virtually replaced with fibroids, or if the uterus is rapidly enlarging and sarcoma is a concern. Mortality in the United States after hysterectomy is less than 0.1%. In some instances, laparoscopy may be used to secure vascular pedicles, thus permitting a vaginal hysterectomy, a method known as *laparoscopically assisted vaginal hysterectomy*.

LEIOMYOMATA AND PREGNANCY

It is generally accepted that 1% to 3.9% of pregnancies are complicated by fibroids, and a prevalence of 2.4% has been reported by Salvador and other investigators. In most cases, the size of fibroids remains the same or decreases during pregnancy, although they may grow or degenerate, causing pain. Their location determines whether fibroids may be associated with bleeding during pregnancy or miscarriage. Rates of first-trimester loss of 40% and rates of second-trimester loss of 7% to 17% have been observed. In pregnancies in which a live birth was achieved, significantly higher rates of preterm delivery were noted in patients with myomata than in controls (21.1% in a myoma group vs. 3.9% in a group undergoing amniocentesis). In addition, fibroids are associated with abruptio placentae, abnormal fetal presentation, and cesarean section. Because of the risks associated with intervention, treatment during pregnancy is usually directed to the management of obstetric complications, such as preterm labor, rather than surgery.

CONCLUSION

The precise cause and prevalence of fibroids remain unclear despite the immense burden this condition places on the U.S. health care system. Given the protean nature of the symptoms and an almost infinite number of locations, the principal objective of clinical evaluation is to map the location of the fibroids accurately. Treatment should be based on the association between the location of the fibroid, the symptoms, and the patient's age and plans for childbearing.

BIBLIOGRAPHY

Bajekal N, Li TC. Fibroids, infertility, and pregnancy wastage. *Hum Reprod Update* 2000;6:614–620.

Braude P, Reidy J, Nott V, et al. Embolization of uterine leiomyomata: current concepts in management. *Hum Reprod Update* 2000;6:603–608.

Buttram VC, Reiter RC. Uterine leiomyomata: etiology, symptomatology, and management. *Fertil Steril* 1981;36:433–445.

Cramer SF, Patel D. The frequency of uterine leiomyomas. *Am J Clin Pathol* 1990;94:435–438.

DeWaay DJ, Syrop CH, Nygaard IE, et al. Natural history of uterine polyps and leiomyomata. *Obstet Gynecol* 2002;100:3–7.

Donnez J, Squifflet J, Polet R, et al. Laparoscopic myolysis. *Hum Reprod Update* 2000;6:609–613.

Dubuisson J-B, Fauconnier A, Babaki-Fard K, et al. Laparoscopic myomectomy: a current view. *Hum Reprod Update* 2000;6:588–594.

Farhi J, Ashkenazi J, Feldberg D, et al. Effect of uterine leiomyomata on the results of in vitro fertilization treatment. *Hum Reprod* 1995;10:2576–2578.

Fauconnier A, Chapron C, Babaki-Fard K, et al. Recurrence of leiomyomata after myomectomy. *Hum Reprod Update* 2000;6:595–602.

Fedele L, Parazzini F, Luchini L, et al. Recurrence of fibroids after myomectomy: a transvaginal ultrasonographic study. *Hum Reprod* 1995;10:1795–1796.
Fukuhara K, Masatoshi K, Kita M, et al. Secreted frizzled related protein 1 is overexpressed in uterine leiomyomas, associated with high estrogenic environment, and unrelated to proliferative activity. *J Clin Endocrinol Metab* 2002;87: 1729–1736.
Healy DL. Impact of uterine fibroids on ART outcome. *Environ Health Perspect* 2000;108:845–847.
Lumbiganon P, Rugpao S, Phandhu-fung S, et al. Protective effect of depot-medroxyprogesterone acetate on surgically treated uterine leiomyomas: a multicentre case-control study. *Br J Obstet Gynaecol* 1995;103:909–914.
Morton C. Genetics of uterine leiomyomas. *Am J Pathol* 1998;153:1015–1020.
Myers ER, Barber MD, Gustilo-Ashby T, et al. Management of uterine leiomyomata: what do we really know? *Obstet Gynecol* 2002;100:8–17.
Pritts EA. Fibroids and infertility: a systematic review of the evidence. *Obstet Gynecol Surv* 2001;56:483–491.
Rosati P, Bellati U, Exacoustos C, et al. Uterine myoma in pregnancy: ultrasound study. *Int J Gynaecol Obstet* 1989;28:109–117.
Salvador E, Bienstock J, Blakemore KJ, et al. Leiomyomata uteri, genetic amniocentesis, and the risk of second trimester spontaneous abortion. *Am J Obstet Gynecol* 2002;186:913–915.
Schwartz SM, Marshall LM, Baird DD. Epidemiologic contributions to understanding the etiology of uterine leiomyomata. *Environ Health Perspect* 2000; 108:821–827.
Sudick R, Husch K, Steller J, et al. Fertility and pregnancy outcome after myomectomy in sterility patients. *Eur J Obstet Gynecol Reprod Biol* 1996;65:209–214.
Tindall VR. *Jeffcoate's principles of gynaecology,* 5th ed. Boston: Butterworth-Heinemann, 1987:415–445.
Tsibris JCM, Segars J, Coppola D, et al. Insights from gene arrays on the development and growth regulation of uterine leiomyomata. *Fertil Steril* 2002;78: 114–121.
Tulandi T, Sammour A, Valenti D, et al. Ovarian reserve after uterine artery embolization for leiomyomata. *Fertil Steril* 2002;78:197–198.
Vavala V, Lanzone A, Monaco A, et al. Postoperative GnRH analog treatment for the prevention of recurrences of uterine myomas after myomectomy: a pilot study. *Gynecol Obstet Invest* 1977;43:251–254.
Vercellini P, Maddalena S, De Giorgi D, et al. Abdominal myomectomy for infertility: a comprehensive review. *Hum Reprod* 1998;13:873–879.

CHAPTER 32
Genital Prolapse

Gunhilde M. Buchsbaum

Genital prolapse, or *pelvic organ prolapse,* is broadly defined as a loss of support to any of the pelvic organs. It can be thought of as a vaginal herniation. The terms in which genital prolapse are described depend on the part that has lost support (Fig. 32.1). A loss of support of the anterior vaginal wall with herniation of the bladder is termed a *cystocele.* A herniation of the rectum through a support defect of the posterior wall is a *rectocele.* A protrusion of the small bowel through the vagina is termed an *enterocele.* These defects may occur in isolation or in combination. Of 237 women who presented in a 2-year period to the gynecologic service at Johns Hopkins Medical Center with prolapse, 33% had predominantly an anterior compartment pelvic organ prolapse (cystocele), 19% a posterior compartment prolapse (rectocele), and 11% an apical prolapse. In 88 patients (37%), no single location was more severely affected than another. In most of the patients (51%), stage 2 genital organ prolapse was diagnosed. Complete loss of support of the vagina and uterus is called *procidentia.*

ETIOLOGY

Some degree of genital relaxation is noted in most women. In most cases, however, it is asymptomatic. Only 10% to 20% of women experience symptoms, which usually develop when prolapse reaches the hymen or beyond. Despite its high prevalence in women, however, little is known about the risk factors and causes of pelvic organ prolapse.

Trauma to the pelvic floor at the time of vaginal delivery is thought to be a major risk factor for the development of genital prolapse. Information to support this assumption is limited. Harris and colleagues reported a series of 748 women presenting to a specialty clinic with urinary incontinence or pelvic organ prolapse. Pelvic organ prolapse was diagnosed in 233 of them, 8.3% of whom were nulliparous, as are approximately 10% of women beyond their childbearing years. Swift evaluated 497 clinic patients ages 18 to 82 years and found that the complexity and severity of pelvic organ prolapse increase with age. Whereas 21% of subjects older than 70 years had pelvic organ prolapse beyond the hymen, none of the women younger than 30 years had that degree of pelvic organ prolapse.

Because the population of elderly women is increasing, it is expected that women with symptomatic genital prolapse will be seen more often. Although rare, two other conditions of genital prolapse should be mentioned. Neonatal uterine prolapse usually develops during the first days of life. It is successfully treated with temporary placement of a support device. Prolapse during pregnancy usually occurs in multiparous women who had some degree of prolapse before pregnancy. Prolapse beyond the hymen should be treated as soon as it is detected with a support device.

In a retrospective analysis of risk factors, Swift and colleagues compared women who had severe pelvic organ prolapse with women who did not have genital prolapse. They found that advancing age, the vaginal delivery of large babies, previous hysterectomy, and previous surgery for prolapse were the strongest etiologic predictors of severe pelvic organ prolapse. Obesity, chronic obstructive pulmonary disease, and diabetes mellitus were not independent risk factors for genital prolapse.

It is thought that any force that exerts stress on the pelvic support structures may lead to pelvic organ prolapse over time. (However, as mentioned in the preceding paragraph, Swift and colleagues did not find this to hold true for obesity and chronic obstructive pulmonary disease.) Other stressors are chronic constipation, heavy lifting, and walking upright. Genital prolapse is rare in quadrupeds.

ANATOMY

The pelvic floor is supported by a muscular plate, the levator ani, and by the fibromuscular connective tissue overlying the muscles of the pelvis and enveloping the vagina (Fig. 32.2). Condensations of this fibromuscular connective tissue, also referred to as the *endopelvic fascia,* support the vagina laterally to the arcus tendineus of the pelvic fascia and at the apex to the uterosacral ligaments.

The levator ani muscle acts as a hammock that supports the bladder, vagina, and rectum. When a woman is standing, this plate is nearly horizontal. Tonic contraction of the slow twitch muscles of the levator ani pulls the rectum and vagina forward, creating a nearly horizontal axis of both the vagina and rectum and effectively closing the levator hiatus. The levator hiatus is the opening through which the urethra, vagina, and rectum pass. Fibers of the levator ani insert around the urethra, vagina, and anus, providing additional support.

DIFFERENTIAL DIAGNOSIS

The differential diagnosis of genital prolapse is short. Most protrusions or bulges of the vagina are indeed a type of genital pro-

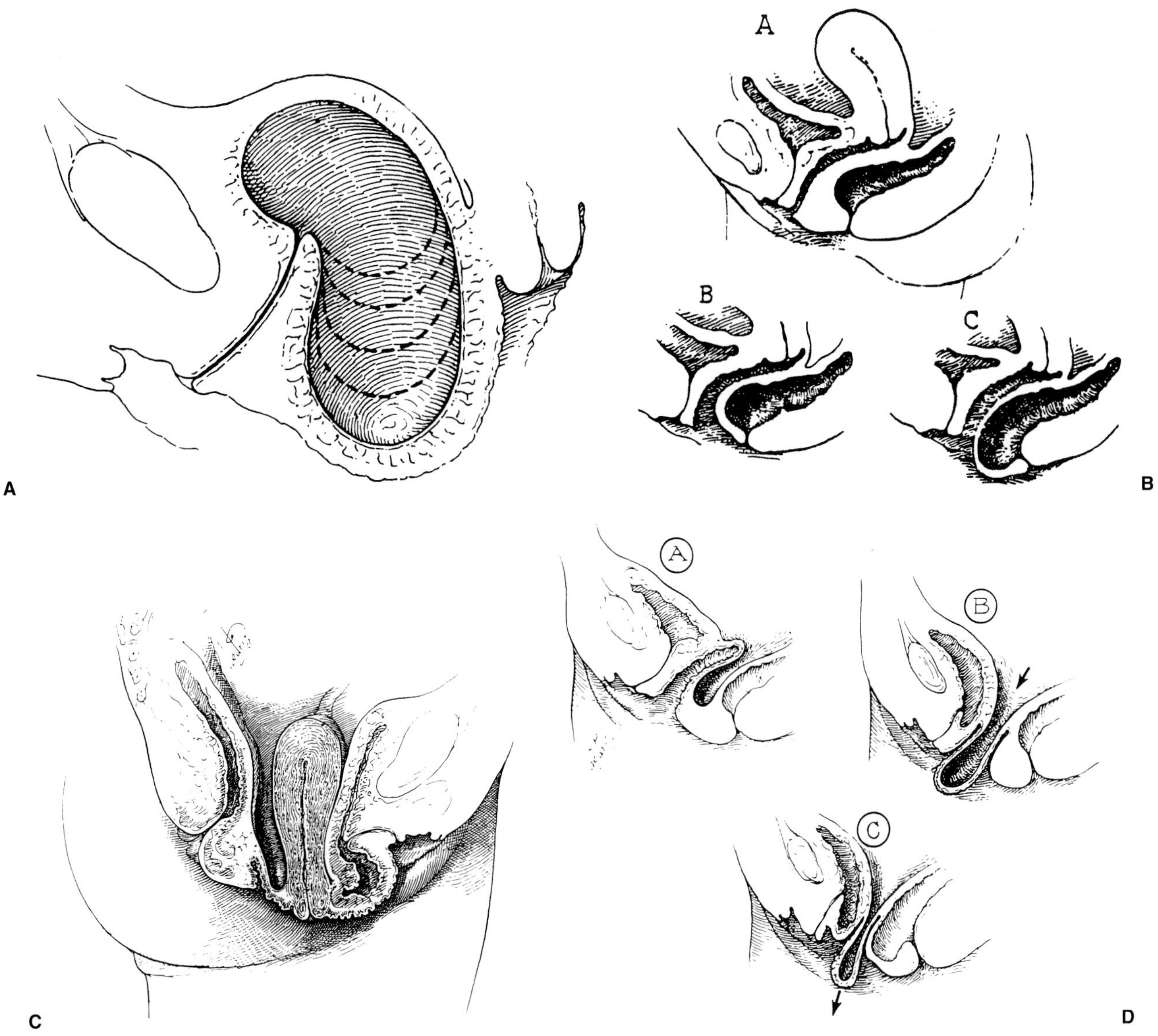

FIG. 32.1. **A:** Varying degrees of posterior distention-type cystocele are shown by the *broken lines.* **B:** A normal relationship between vagina, perineum, and rectum is depicted in *A.* A major perineal defect is seen in *B;* no rectocele is present, but restoration of the perineal body is indicated. A major perineal defect with rectocele is shown in *C;* in this circumstance, perineorrhaphy should be accompanied by an appropriate posterior colporrhaphy. **C:** Uterovaginal or sliding prolapse. An enterocele, but no rectocele, is present. The uterosacral ligaments are long and strong. Note the position of the uninvolved anterior rectal wall. (Adapted from Nichols DH, Randall CL, eds. *Vaginal surgery,* 3rd ed. Baltimore: Williams & Wilkins, 1989, with permission.) **D:** *A* shows posterior enterocele without eversion of the vagina. *B* shows pulsion enterocele, in which the upper vagina is everted and the enterocele sac follows the everted vault. Cystocele and rectocele are minimal. *C* shows traction enterocele, with eversion of the vagina, enterocele, cystocele, and rectocele. (From Nichols DH. *Obstetrics and gynecology.* New York: Elsevier Science, 1972:257, with permission.)

lapse. However, it is important to differentiate between types of prolapse.

A bulge of the anterior vaginal wall may also be a vaginal or suburethral cyst, a urethral diverticulum, or a fibroid. A cyst has a characteristic feel and does not collapse with pressure. A urethral diverticulum may be tender to palpation. With digital compression, one can sometimes express the contents through the urethra. A fibroid feels like a firm mass.

As previously mentioned, genital prolapse disorders include prolapse of any of the three compartments of the vagina—the anterior wall, posterior wall, and apex. They also include prolapse of the perineum and rectum. Mucosal prolapse, polyps, or other lesions may cause tissue to protrude through the anus. Rectal prolapse is concentric, whereas polyps are not. Also, polyps have no rugae.

It is helpful for the primary care physician to be able to identify the different types of vaginal prolapse. Again, a prolapse of the anterior vaginal wall is also referred to as a *cystocele,* and one of the posterior wall is called a *rectocele.* In an *enterocele,* small bowel is present within the genital prolapse. An enterocele is not always detected by physical examination alone. Enteroceles are further classified as pulsion or traction enteroceles, and cystoceles are similarly classified as pulsion or traction cystoceles. These differentiations are of clinical importance only when surgical correction of the specific defect is being considered.

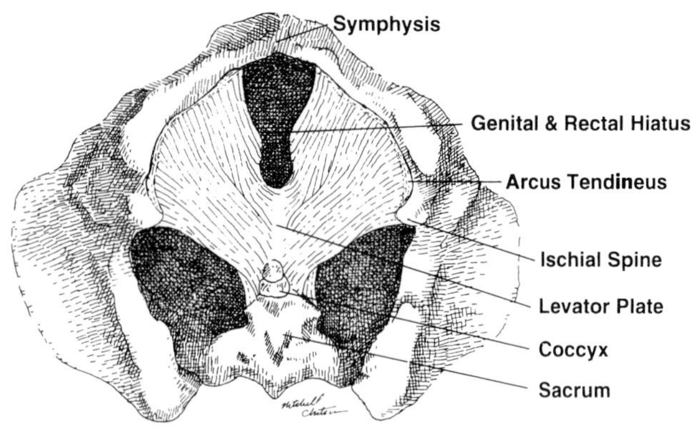

FIG. 32.2. Diagrammatic representation of the levator ani muscles in a nulliparous woman showing the levator plate, levator cruris, and prerectal fibers, which course between the rectum and the posterior vaginal wall. (Adapted from Nichols DH, Milley PS. Clinical anatomy of the vulva, vagina, lower pelvis, and perineum. In: Sciarra JJ, ed. *Gynecology and obstetrics,* vol 2. Philadelphia: JB Lippincott, 1993:1, with permission.)

CLINICAL SYMPTOMS AND HISTORY

It is crucial to ask a patient presenting for a routine examination if she is aware of any protrusion from her vagina because prolapse can be entirely missed during an examination performed with the patient in the dorsal lithotomy position. Many women do not voluntarily describe a prolapse because they are concerned about being thought of as abnormal.

In most women, genital prolapse remains asymptomatic until it extends beyond the hymen. At that time, the patient may feel a bulge, usually when wiping or washing. Some women experience low back pain and pelvic pressure, although in the study of Heit and associates, low back pain and pelvic pressure did not correlate with the severity of genital prolapse in their cohort of 152 women.

Women with progressive prolapse of the anterior wall, or cystocele, may experience difficulty urinating that worsens as the day goes on. Typically, they describe urinary urgency and frequency associated with small voids during the daytime. They usually void best at night and early in the morning, when the prolapse is reduced and the obstruction caused by the prolapse is relieved. In extreme cases, women with severe prolapse are unable to void at all unless the prolapse is reduced.

It is important to inquire about urinary symptoms and incontinence. In some women with prolapse, urge-related incontinence or overactive bladder develops when the prolapse irritates the bladder. In other women, voiding dysfunction develops, and they note urinary hesitancy, prolonged or intermittent flow, and a need to change position to void. In still others, prolapse actually relieves stress incontinence (loss of urine during activity, coughing, and lifting) if a cystocele or a large rectocele obstructs the urethra. Recurrent urinary tract infection may be the sequela of chronically large post void residuals and in some patients is the only presenting symptom.

A woman with rectocele often has difficulty defecating. She must frequently push down on the back wall of the vagina to evacuate the rectal vault because part of the stool becomes trapped within the prolapsed rectum. On the other hand, some women with rather large rectoceles are asymptomatic, and not all women with genital prolapse experience symptoms that correlate with compartment-specific defects. In the study of Ellerkman and associates correlating presenting symptoms with the location and severity of pelvic organ prolapse, more severe prolapse was weakly or moderately associated with specific symptoms.

Sexual dysfunction is common in women with pronounced genital prolapse. One of three patients with genital prolapse reports that the condition affects their sexual relations "moderately" or "greatly." Although sexual activity is decreased in women with genital prolapse, the stages of sexual excitement are not found to be different from those in women without prolapse.

In women with long-standing genital prolapse extending beyond the hymen, ulcers may develop on the dependent parts of the protrusion. Pelvic organ prolapse may progress slowly during years or decades or quickly within just months.

CLINICAL AND PHYSICAL EXAMINATION FINDINGS

During the examination of a patient with prolapse, it is important to see the prolapse at its worst. Examine the woman with prolapse initially in the upright position. Ask her to perform a Valsalva maneuver or whatever will produce the prolapse. A prolapse of any compartment of the vagina feels taut when fully distended. Ask the patient to confirm that what you see is indeed the worst protrusion she experiences. Note how far the anterior and the posterior vaginal walls protrude. In a woman with a uterus, check the location of the cervix. In a woman without a uterus, evaluate the distance of the apex from the introitus during a Valsalva maneuver. Reduce the prolapse and ask the patient to cough; note any urine loss.

Examine the patient again in the dorsal lithotomy position. Insert a speculum and observe how far the vaginal apex or cervix descends when the patient bears down. Note also the leading part of the prolapse—that is, does the anterior or posterior vaginal wall or the apex protrude the farthest? Perform a Papanicolaou smear and cultures if indicated. Then, take the speculum apart to evaluate the anterior and posterior vaginal walls separately. Use the posterior blade of the speculum to depress the posterior vaginal wall gently and fully visualize the anterior wall. While the patient is bearing down, withdraw the speculum and observe the descent of the anterior vaginal wall. Rotate the posterior blade of the speculum to elevate the anterior wall and expose the posterior wall of the vagina. Observe how far the vaginal wall descends. A rectal exam is helpful to evaluate the posterior wall for a rectocele.

Various methods have been devised to describe prolapse. The one most widely used by gynecologists in the past was that of Baden and Walker. In 1996, the International Continence Society proposed a new system to standardize the terminology for describing genital prolapse (Table 32.1). The three compartments of the vagina (the anterior and posterior walls and the

TABLE 32.1. Staging of Genital Prolapse According to the International Continence Society Terminology

Stage 0	No prolapse. Points Aa, Ap, Ba, and Bp are all at −3, and either point C or point D is no less than the total vaginal length (TVL) −2.
Stage 1	Criteria for stage 0 are not met, but the most distal portion of the prolapse is more than 1 cm above the level of the hymen.
Stage 2	The most distal portion of the prolapse is no more than 1 cm proximal or distal to the hymen.
Stage 3	The most distal portion of the prolapse is more than 1 cm below the plane of the hymen but protrudes no further than 2 cm less than the TVL in centimeters.
Stage 4	Essentially complete eversion of the lower genital tract.

apex) are evaluated. Two points are defined for each of these sites. These are points Aa and Ba on anterior vaginal wall, points Ap and Bp on the posterior vaginal wall, and points C and D for the apex (Fig. 32.3). Also measured for a reference is the total vaginal length. Point Aa is 3 cm proximal to the urethral meatus on the anterior vaginal wall, and point Ap is 3 cm proximal to the hymen on the posterior vaginal wall. The location of these points is noted with reference to the hymen and measured in centimeters. Protrusions beyond the hymen are noted as positive values. The values can range from –3 in a patient without prolapse to +3 in one with maximal prolapse. Points Ba and Bp are at the most distal portion of the anterior and posterior walls, respectively. Point C is the most distal part of the cervix or, in its absence, of the vaginal cuff. Point D is the location of the posterior cul-de-sac. This point is measured only when a cervix is present. It helps to distinguish between true uterovaginal prolapse and cervical elongation. The difference between points C and D is an estimate of the cervical length in centimeters. This system is valuable in assessing whether a prolapse is progressing over time and for research purposes.

Next, perform a bimanual and rectovaginal examination as usual to evaluate for pelvic masses and confirm the findings of the prior examination by palpation. This is also the time to instruct the patient how to perform pelvic floor muscle exercises or Kegel exercises. If they are done properly, you should note an elevation of the levator ani, which in turn pushes up the examiner's fingers. Many women perform a Valsalva maneuver when asked to contract their pelvic floor muscles. This should be discouraged because it may worsen the problem rather than relieve it.

Lastly, the post void residual urine should be determined. An 8F intermittent catheter is generally well tolerated. This helps to detect voiding dysfunction, which may be caused by the prolapse. One should not diagnose a voiding dysfunction solely on the basis of one large post void residual. A large post void residual should be confirmed at a second visit, when the patient is catheterized after she has voided ad libitum rather than on command. The urine obtained is used to rule out a urinary tract infection.

LABORATORY AND IMAGING STUDIES

Unless surgical intervention is planned to correct the genital prolapse, few studies are indicated. A urine dip stick test should be performed on all patients, especially those with a history of urinary tract infection. Women with a large post void residual volume on repeated examination should be evaluated for hydronephrosis and hydroureter. The baseline renal function should be checked in patients with evidence of reflux. Before surgery, however, a urodynamic evaluation is indicated for all patients with prolapse beyond the hymen to evaluate for occult stress urinary incontinence. Such urinary incontinence becomes apparent after the prolapse is reduced. This situation can be prevented if urinary incontinence is detected preoperatively and a concomitant incontinence repair is performed.

TREATMENT

Pessary

Only symptomatic prolapse requires treatment, except in a patient with asymptomatic urinary retention, reflux, or chronic ulceration. In general, the options for the treatment of genital prolapse include a variety of surgical approaches and nonsurgical management with a pessary.

The conservative management of genital prolapse is often considered as an option for women who are not surgical candidates, are very old, or are awaiting surgery. However, it is an option for any woman with symptomatic prolapse who desires treatment. For some of these women, surgical repair may also be an option, for others not. Conservative management is an alternative to surgery that should be presented to any woman who may benefit. Cundiff and colleagues conducted a survey of members of the American Urogynecologic Society. Of the respondents, 77% said they used pessaries as a first-line treatment for genital prolapse, whereas 12% reserved it for women who were not candidates for surgery. When these physicians were questioned further about which pessaries they used for different types of pro-

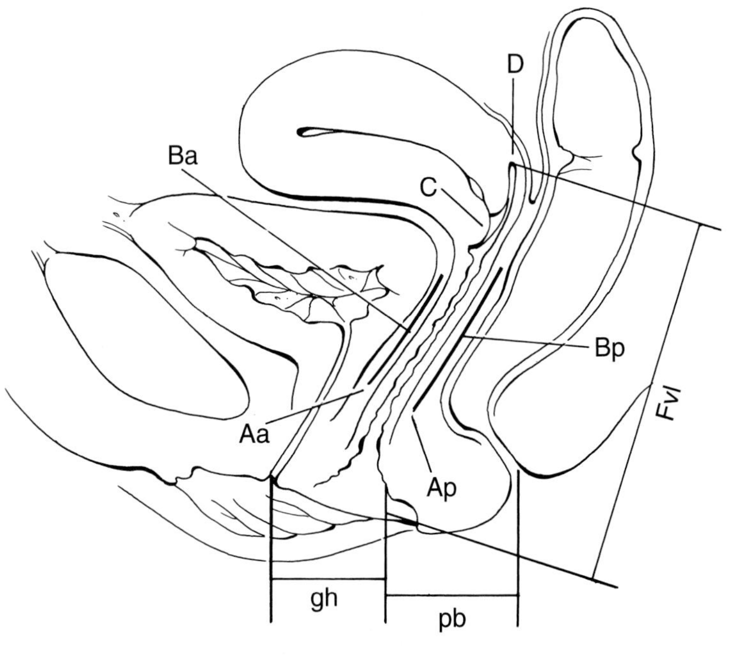

FIG. 32.3. The six points, genital hiatus *(gh)*, perineal body *(pb)*, and total vaginal length *(tvl)* are used to quantify prolapse. (Adapted from International Continence Society. *The standardization of terminology of female pelvic organ prolapse and pelvic floor dysfunction.* Bristol, UK: International Continence Society, 1994, with permission.)

lapse, 21% said they used the same pessary for all support defects, whereas 78% tailored management to the specific type of prolapse. A trend to the use of pessaries for specific defects was noted, but no clear consensus. In fact, no good clinical study has evaluated the optimal pessaries for different types of defects.

Very little information is available about how many patients with prolapse can be successfully managed conservatively, and about how many of those who can be successfully fitted find it a satisfactory long-term solution. Wu and colleagues reported about 110 women with symptomatic genital prolapse. Of these, 81 (74%) were fitted successfully. According to their life table analysis, two of three women who used a pessary for 1 month will still be using it after 12 months, and 53% will still be using it after 3 years. Sulak and colleagues obtained similar long-term results. Fifty percent of their patients who were fitted with a pessary for prolapse reduction continued to use the pessary. One of four proceeded to surgical correction, and 21 of 101 chose no treatment.

Although a large variety of pessaries are available, most clinicians find a small assortment sufficient (Fig. 32.4). Anterior wall support defects with or without a mild apical component are usually well corrected by a support pessary with diaphragm. Examples of such pessaries are the ring, Smith, and Hodge pessaries. A predominantly apical defect, with or without cystocele and rectocele, is well reduced with a Gellhorn pessary. Cube pessaries or doughnuts may be used if a Gellhorn pessary cannot be retained because the sides of a cube pessary work like suction cups, adhering to the walls of the vagina. Isolated posterior defects are often not satisfactorily reduced with a pessary, although one may want to try a space-occupying pessary, such as a doughnut.

A well-fitted pessary reduces the prolapse and its associated symptoms satisfactorily and is not otherwise noticed. In other words, the woman should not be aware of a foreign body within her vagina. Once a pessary is properly fitted, frequent follow-up is not necessary for a woman who can take care of the pessary herself. A woman who cannot remove and insert her pessary should be evaluated every 3 to 6 months. More frequent follow-up does not improve outcome. The most frequent adverse reaction to a pessary is odorous vaginal discharge. Alnaif and Drutz obtained vaginal cultures from 44 pessary users and matched controls. They observed bacterial vaginosis in 32% of the pessary users and 10% of the controls. The development of vaginal erosions can be decreased by the topical treatment of vulvovaginal atrophy. Severe complications, such as vesicovaginal or rectovaginal fistulae and urosepsis, are rare and usually associated with neglect of the pessary.

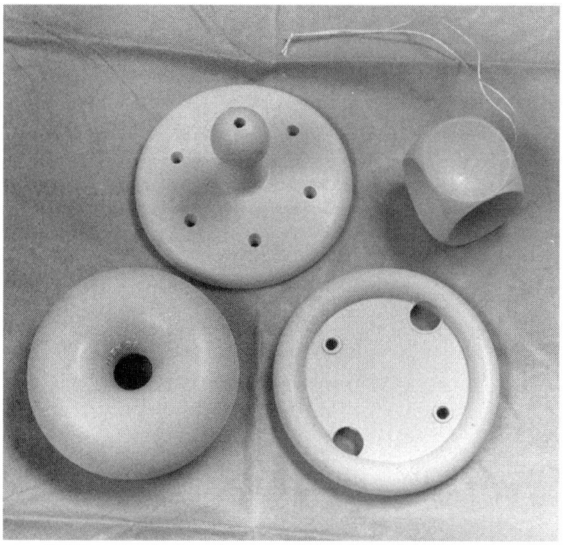

FIG. 32.4. Examples of commonly used pessaries.

When properly selected, pessaries are safe for the long-term management of genital prolapse in women who prefer conservative management or are not surgical candidates. Women with concomitant stress urinary incontinence, however, usually will continue with conservative long-term management because incontinence often worsens after prolapse reduction, when the urethral obstruction caused by the prolapse is relieved. Surgery is usually necessary to alleviate both problems—genital prolapse and stress urinary incontinence.

Surgical Management

The surgical management of prolapse should aim to repair all areas of support defects. Genital prolapse can be corrected laparoscopically via a vaginal or abdominal route, or via a combination of the vaginal and abdominal routes. Synthetic or autologous fascia and dermal allografts have been used to reinforce surgical repairs. The success rates of these approaches are usually reported in case series with varying numbers of patients and lengths of follow-up. No randomized prospective studies have compared the success rates of any of the repairs. Unfortunately, genital prolapse frequently recurs after surgery. Most studies quote success rates between 80% and 90%, although failure rates above 30% have been reported.

Most women undergoing surgery for prolapse reduction undergo reconstructive surgery—that is, surgery that aims to restore normal anatomy and function. Complete vaginal reconstruction is required for women with procidentia or total vaginal eversion after hysterectomy. For women with massive prolapse who are medically unstable and cannot undergo reconstructive surgery or are not interested in retaining the potential for vaginal intercourse, an obliterative procedure of the vagina may offer a good surgical alternative. This can be performed under local or regional anesthesia with few complications and a relatively quick recovery time. In Le Fort colpocleisis, the vagina is partially obliterated and the uterus left in place. In women without a uterus, colpectomy results in reported cure rates between 89% and 100%.

Cervical and uterine pathology must be excluded when a Le Fort colpocleisis is considered. Any woman with prolapse beyond the hymen should be evaluated for occult stress urinary incontinence because it has been observed in 20% to 30% of women with advanced genital prolapse.

PREVENTION

Many specialists advise their patients to avoid any activity that will increase intra-abdominal pressure, such as heavy lifting and coughing, and to attempt to prevent constipation. Others advise their patients to perform pelvic floor muscle exercises. Some even advocate elective cesarean section. Although a general health benefit is derived from preventing constipation and treating a persistent cough, no evidence indicates that these implementing these measures or avoiding vaginal delivery prevents the development or progression of pelvic organ prolapse.

BIBLIOGRAPHY

Alnaif B, Drutz HP. Bacterial vaginosis increases in pessary users. *Int Urogynecol J Pelvic Floor Dysfunct* 2000;11:219–222.

Barber MD, Visco AG, Wyman JF, et al. Sexual function in women with urinary incontinence and pelvic organ prolapse. *Obstet Gynecol* 2002;99:281–289.

Beecham CT. Classification of vaginal relaxation. *Am J Obstet Gynecol* 1980;136: 957–958.
Bump RC, Mattiasson A, Bo K, et al. The standardization of terminology of female pelvic organ prolapse and pelvic floor dysfunction. *Am J Obstet Gynecol* 1996;175:10–17.
Cundiff GW, Weidner AC, Visco AG, et al. A survey of pessary use by members of the American Urogynecologic Society. *Int Urogynecol J Pelvic Floor Dysfunct* 1999;10:407–408.
Ellerkmann RM, Cundiff GW, Melick CF, et al. Correlation of symptoms with location and severity of pelvic organ prolapse. *Am J Obstet Gynecol* 2001;185: 1332–1337.
Harris RL, Cundiff GW, Coates KW, et al. Urinary incontinence and pelvic organ prolapse in nulliparous women. *Obstet Gynecol* 1988;92:951–954.
Heit M, Culligan P, Rosenquist C, et al. Is pelvic organ prolapse a cause of pelvic or low back pain? *Obstet Gynecol* 2002;99:23–28.
Karram MM, Sze EHM, Walters MD. Surgical treatment of vaginal vault prolapse. In: Walters MD, Karram MM, eds. *Urogynecology and reconstructive pelvic surgery*, 2nd ed. St. Louis: Mosby, 1999:235–256.
Miller DS. Contemporary use of the pessary. In: Sciarra JJ, ed. *Gynecology and obstetrics*, vol 1. Philadelphia: Lippincott-Raven, 1997:1–12.
Poma PA. Nonsurgical management of genital prolapse: a review and recommendations for clinical practice. *J Reprod Med* 2000;45:789–797.
Roberge RJ, Mc Candish MM, Dorfsman ML. Urosepsis associated with vaginal pessary use. *Ann Emerg Med* 1999;33:581–583.
Rogers GR, Villarreal A, Kammerer-Doak D, et al. Sexual function in women with and without urinary incontinence and/or pelvic organ prolapse. *Int Urogynecol J Pelvic Floor Dysfunct* 2001;12:361–365.
Sulak PJ, Kuehl TJ, Shull BL. Vaginal pessaries and their use in pelvic relaxation. *J Reprod Med* 1993;38:919–923.
Swift SE. The distribution of pelvic organ support in a population of female subjects seen for routine gynecologic health care. *Am J Obstet Gynecol* 2000;183: 277–285.
Swift SE, Pound T, Dias JK. Case-control study of etiologic factors in the development of severe pelvic organ prolapse. *Int Urogynecol J Pelvic Floor Dysfunct* 2001;12:187–192.
Weber AM, Abrams P, Brubaker L, et al. The standardization of terminology for researchers in female pelvic floor disorders. *Int Urogynecol J* 2001;12:178–186.
Wu V, Farrell SA, Baskett TF, et al. A simple protocol for pessary management. *Obstet Gynecol* 1997;90:990–994.

CHAPTER 33

Environmental and Occupational Hazards Involving Reproduction

Richard K. Miller

Because of the complexity of assessing and understanding environmental and occupational exposures, providers of reproductive health care often overlook these issues in evaluating their patients. However, as we know, a number of such exposures have been associated with early menopause (tobacco), adverse pregnancy outcomes (anesthetic gases, cadmium, lead, methylmercury, radiation, solvents such as ethanol, toluene, and gasoline), and male infertility (dibromochloropropane, lead). Thus, it is important for each health care provider to identify environmental and occupational exposures as they relate to reproduction (Table 33.1).

In New York State, screening pregnant women for exposure to lead has sensitized all providers to identifying environmental and occupational exposures during pregnancy, not only to lead but also to many other substances. The health care provider and employer must appropriately identify risks and work with experts in the fields of occupational medicine and toxicology, so that the patient can be counseled about risk for these exposures to date and so appropriate action can be planned.

TABLE 33.1. Human Reproductive Toxicants/Teratogens/Fetal Toxicants

Angiotensin-converting enzyme inhibitors	Misoprostol
Androgens	Narcotics
Anesthetic gases[a]	Polychlorinated biphenyls[a]
Cadmium[a]	Phenobarbital
Cancer chemotherapy[a]	Phenytoin
Cocaine	Retinoids
Dibromochloropropane (DCBP)[a]	Solvents (gasoline, toluene)[a]
Diethylstilbestrol[a]	Tetracycline
Ethanol[a]	Thalidomide
Heat[a]	Tobacco[a]
Radioactive iodine	Trimethadione
Lead[a]	Valproate
Methylmercury[a]	Warfarin (Coumadin)
	X-irradiation[a]

[a]Potential environmental or occupational exposures.

The goal of this chapter is to facilitate communication and understanding among patients, employers, and health care providers, all of whom are critical to the process of managing exposures (Fig. 33.1).

CASE STUDY: MRS. MARGARET

To illustrate the importance of environmental and occupational assessments, a case study is provided.

An obstetrician identified that a patient, Mrs. Margaret, had symptoms related to exposures in the workplace. Mrs. Margaret was referred by both her obstetrician and her employer to a reproductive toxicologist at a regional teratogen information service working within a prenatal genetics division.

Mrs. Margaret (born July 19, 1979) is a primigravida whose last menstrual period was September 28. A pregnancy test was performed on December 1. Mrs. Margaret was seen on December 8 by the consultant after being referred by her obstetrician and her employer.

Medication and Nutrition

Mrs. Margaret is currently taking prenatal vitamins. She indicates a history of cigarette smoking. Before becoming pregnant, she smoked on average one and one-half packs per day. Since October 2, she has smoked no more than 10 cigarettes per day. Mrs. Margaret consumes a typical American diet. She does not eat swordfish or liver. She does eat tuna, but only one meal per week. Her home was built after 1980.

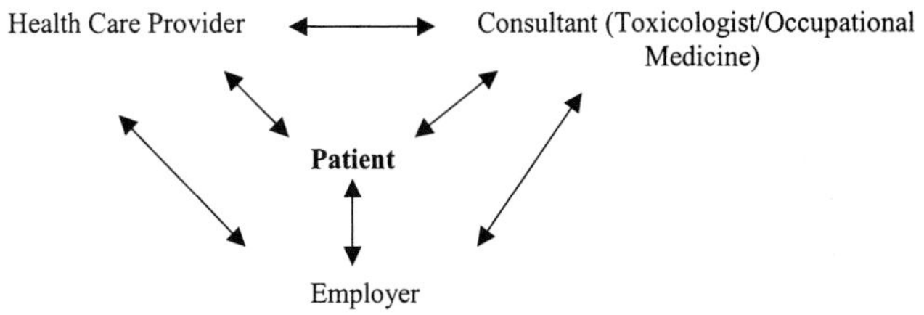

FIG. 33.1. Paradigm for understanding how occupational exposures affect reproductive health. Patient is at the center of the triangle formed by the health care provider, consultant, and employer.

Occupation

Mrs. Margaret has been a press worker since the age of 18 years. She has worked for The Packaging Company for the past 2 years. Her workday begins at 7 a.m. and is completed by 3 p.m. Approximately 20% of her time is devoted to mixing colored inks and delivering them to the presses. She prepares the inks for all three shifts. The remaining 80% of her workday is devoted to clerical and computer work, performed in the same mixing room within the plant. This room was built in October to increase her work efficiency. The mixing room does have exhaust and air supply fans; however, the supply air is drawn from the press area, not from external sources. She performs all these tasks by herself. She is also responsible for cleaning all metal parts and components involved in dye preparation in addition to the actual mixing process. According to Mrs. Margaret and The Packaging Company, the products with which she comes in direct contact are the following:

Diamond Type Wash (2815208), Ashland Chemical Inc.	
Acetone 67-64-1	25%
Aliphatic petroleum distillates (64742-89-8)	75%
Hammer Deglazer (2286498), Ashland Chemical Inc.	
Aliphatic hydrocarbons (Stoddard type) 8052-41-3	10%–30%
Aromatic petroleum distillates 84742-96-6	68%
Surfactant 68131-40-8	1%–10%

Typically, Mrs. Margaret does not wear protective gloves or a solvent mask when washing the instruments or during the mixing process. Mrs. Margaret is the only woman in the workplace. Since the middle of November, her symptoms of nausea, dizziness, sweating, and vomiting have become substantially worse. Within 5 minutes after entering her office/mixing room, she becomes sick and vomits, even though the fans have been on all night. She has lost her appetite during the past few weeks, especially at lunch.

What Are Her Risks? What Are the Recommendations? What Additional Information Is Required to Make a Recommendation?

CHECKLIST FOR EXPOSURE FACTORS

1. Are any of her symptoms associated with the workplace or exposure area only, or are her symptoms more severe in the workplace or exposure area than at home or in other locations? How often or persistent are the symptoms (related only to the workplace, only to pregnancy)?
2. To what substances or conditions is the patient being exposed? Is she using protective equipment? Has documentation from Manufacturer Safety Data Sheets been requested?
3. What is the amount of the time the patient is exposed to these substances or conditions in terms of duration per day or per week? Are monitoring data (personal and air sampling) available for the substances of concern? Is ventilation adequate?
4. Do other male or female workers report similar or other symptoms resulting from workplace/environmental exposures?
5. Do home environment, hobbies, spouse's work, and diet create exposures of concern for the patient?

Let us explore the description of the patient according to the preceding checklist.

1. Mrs. Margaret certainly demonstrates symptoms (nausea, vomiting shortly after arriving at work, symptoms she did not have before she became pregnant). She does not use protective equipment, nor has she been fitted for any protective equipment.
2. Mrs. Margaret's exposures have been to solvents (as listed previously according to the Material Safety Data Sheets). Nausea and vomiting are associated with exposure to solvents, as is headache (migraine type). The difficulty is that a number of these symptoms are similar to those associated with morning sickness of pregnancy.
3. The amount of her exposure to solvents is unknown. Monitoring of solvents is not available from the employer. Twenty percent of the time, Mrs. Margaret is mixing inks and dyes and cleaning up; 80% of the time, she is at her computer in the very same room. The airflow in the room appears to be good, but the air is not fresh. Mrs. Margaret asked another (male) employee to mix her dyes; however, she still could not remain in the room without experiencing multiple symptoms. We know that exposure to high levels of solvents such as ethanol, toluene, and gasoline (see section "Solvents") can lead to reproductive problems. At issue is her actual level of exposure.
4. She is the only woman working at the plant, and none of her male coworkers have had any of the same symptoms in the printing area or in the ink room where she works.
5. Other factors:

Her home was built after 1980 and on city water—no lead issue.
Her husband is a computer programmer—no exposure issues to be brought home.
She does not eat a great deal of predator fish—no methylmercury issue.
She does not eat liver—no vitamin A toxicity issue.
She does not eat ethnic foods or candies (imported)—no lead issue.
Her diet is compromised by vomiting, principally at work, but she also experiences nausea to other odors (diesel fumes), although not as severe.

EVALUATION AND RECOMMENDATIONS

1. Request of employer: Monitor Mrs. Margaret's work area for the specific solvents of concern.
2. What are the effects of solvents in general, and specifically of these agents? The health care provider can turn to two computerized services for information: REPROTOX (an on-line information system developed by the Reproductive Toxicology Center, Bethesda, Maryland) and TERIS (a teratogen information system provided by the University of Washington, Seattle, Washington). Both of these services can be accessed directly or through a teratogen information service such as OTIS (Organization of Teratology Information Services) or a regional poison control center. With solvents, the issue can usually be judged based on the response as an initial index. Often, smelling the solvent establishes exposure and perhaps toxicity. For example, toluene can be detected by its odor at 3 ppm; however, it is regulated at 25 ppm. As a guideline, Motherisk published in the *Journal of the American Medical Association* a small study indicating that pregnant women who have symptoms caused by solvent exposures are at greater risk for delivering children with birth defects than pregnant women who do not have such exposures. Even though the range of solvents and types of birth defects have not been determined, the principle of symptoms secondary to exposures must be kept in mind during a clinical evaluation. Such symptoms can constitute a reason to remove a patient from a workplace or environmental exposure.
3. Request of employer: Pending the results of solvent monitoring, relocate Mrs. Margaret to an alternate work area

without solvent exposures so that she can continue her computer work. Recommend that another employee work with the inks and solvents. If alternate work areas are not available, Mrs. Margaret may have to consider other options (e.g., medical disability).

4. Recommendations to employee concerning exposures after receipt of the monitoring data for solvents:
   a. Because the levels indicated by the monitoring data are well below the Occupational Safety and Health Administration permissible exposure limits, the employer wants Mrs. Margaret to return to work. However, as is widely known, some pregnant woman exhibit exaggerated responses to noxious odors. Some of these odors may not be a problem before the pregnancy, but can cause extreme nausea and vomiting during pregnancy.
   b. Such appears to be the case for Mrs. Margaret. Even though to anesthetic gases, especially nitrous oxide, during all tpes of surgery the solvent levels are not within a toxic range, the odors are causing a rapid response during her pregnancy that prevent her from conducting her normal duties.
   c. Mrs. Margaret has to leave the workplace within a few minutes after exposure, an advantage in regard to her pregnancy. It is important to establish with the patient that the background risk for loss of pregnancy is approximately 20%, and for birth defects, it is approximately 3%. The concern for Mrs. Margaret is how the risk to date will affect her baby. Because her exposures to low levels of solvents have been relatively brief, it is unlikely that her risk for having a child with birth defects has been increased significantly above the background risk. This has to be communicated to the patient, so that she understands that a risk for birth defects still exists but is unlikely to be associated with the workplace exposure.
   d. Because of the patient's continued symptoms during workplace solvent exposures and an inability of the employer to provide her with an alternate work area during this pregnancy, Mrs. Margaret is to be released on medical disability.

This case study shows that substantial effort may be required in both understanding and resolving environmental and occupational exposures that may affect reproductive success. Such evaluations can be applied to a woman who is not pregnant and her male partner concerning reproductive risks associated with exposures. Additional evaluations of male and female reproductive function can be undertaken as noted elsewhere in this textbook.

As previously mentioned, it is important to have access to both animal and human data regarding exposures of concern for an individual patient and the possible toxic effects on mother, father, and baby. Few exposures are to just one chemical. Mixtures are typical, and considerable judgment is required to estimate the degree of interaction.

Brief descriptions of selected solvents, metals, and other agents that pose occupational and environmental health risks are discussed here. The reader is referred to REPROTOX, TERIS, and MEDLINE for additional information about other agents. Often, a regional teratogen information service can provide current information and assistance in interrupting exposures associated with reproductive risk.

SOLVENTS

Solvents are among the most complex and numerous substances that cause reproductive risks in both male and female workers. Additionally, workers are often not sure of the specific agents to which they are exposed because they are unaware of the chemical composition of the products they use. Material Safety Data Sheets provide information about the solvents in a product. Thus, workers in industries that use glue (manufacturers of shoes) or metal cleaners (manufacturers of orthotics, cleaners of large metal surfaces such as subway cars) may be exposed to a solvent such as toluene. Workers in dry cleaning establishments, microelectronics clean rooms, and chemistry laboratories may be exposed to other substances.

It is known that solvents can be associated with loss of pregnancy, birth defects, and male infertility. The difficulty of assessing the risk to the patient lies in determining the exposure. For example, toluene causes birth defects and loss of pregnancy when the mother is exposed to excessive doses during pregnancy, as in sniffing glue. Occupational exposures may be substantially smaller. However, when after only 2 hours at work an employee starts to vomit, becomes dizzy, hallucinates while using a metal cleaner, and takes aspirin because of "painful" headaches, prompt action must be taken. The health care provider should remove the worker/patient immediately from the workspace until it can be determined that the exposure is minimal and that either physical barriers are in place or the exposure is to nonsymptomatic levels. It may be most appropriate to recommend the services of an industrial hygienist to the employer. Other consequences of exposure in adults are renal acidosis, peripheral neuropathy, decreased brain size, and muscle weakness. Male reproductive toxicity has been reported in humans and rodents at levels of 1,000 ppm.

Chronic exposure to ethanol, gasoline, glycol ethers, and combinations of solvents causing maternal toxic symptoms has been associated with birth defects and loss of pregnancy. However, additional studies including large numbers of patients with detailed exposure information are required to prove this association.

METALS

Lead, mercury, and cadmium are metals that may cause reproductive risk. Additional information can be found in the 1992 article by Paul and in REPROTOX.

Lead

Lead continues to be a health risk for everyone. It is a product of our industrialized society. The objective is to minimize exposures. Fortunately, lead has been removed from gasoline; however, it remains in our older buildings and homes, soil, and water. It becomes quite a problem when older homes are remodeled because fine particles are produced. Lead is often found in pottery and dishes that have been decorated with lead-based paints. Contaminated food and various products (especially ethnic foods and candies, home-distilled liquor, traditional folk remedies, cosmetics not sold in stores, crayons, lead candle wicks) are other sources. Many exposures today occur in occupations and environments in which lead continues to be used (soldering in the electronics, jewelry, and stained glass industries; scrapping and painting; manufacture and recycling of lead glass; foundries; manufacture and installation of plumbing; auto repair; manufacture of batteries and fire arms; firing ranges, ceramics; bridge and ship building and repair; lead abatement). Urine drinkers may have elevated levels of lead.

It has been known for centuries that exposure to lead can compromise spermatogenesis in men and cause pregnancy loss

TABLE 33.2. Relationship Between Blood Levels and Various Biologic Effects of Lead

Biologic effect	Blood level (µg/dL)
Gastrointestinal colic	>80
Acute encephalopathy	>80
Anemia	>80
Chronic renal disease	>60
Altered spermatogenesis	>35
Peripheral neuropathy	>30
Increased erythrocyte protoporphyrin	>20–25
Increased δ-aminolevulinic acid dehydratase	>20
Increased blood pressure	? Threshold
Developmental delays in offspring	? Threshold

in women. At one time, lead was considered an abortifacient. Reproductive toxicity occurs when blood levels of lead are in excess of 35 µg/mL (Table 33.2). However, developmental effects are noted with much lower levels of lead. Cord blood levels of lead in excess of 10 µg/mL have been associated with cognitive developmental changes in children.

New York State requires that all pregnant women be screened in an effort to reduce lead exposure in children, beginning with the embryo/fetus (Table 33.3). It should be noted that different actions are recommended based on the maternal blood levels. In a case heard before the U.S. Supreme Court (Johnson Controls), a workplace standard was established based on the fact that women were being excluded from specific areas of a workplace because they were being exposed to lead. The point was made that the manufacturer (employer) was protecting the unborn from lead exposures. The Court ruled that women cannot be excluded from a workplace where they are exposed to lead while men are allowed to work there because lead causes reproductive toxic effects in both women and men, although at different concentrations. The ruling was that the manufacturers had to reduce lead exposures to levels acceptable for both sexes, a worthy objective. Many companies using lead today believe they have reduced exposures below those leading to levels in excess of 10 µg/mL, but based on experience, when women are screened, their levels can be in excess of 20 µg/mL. Thus, monitoring employees is critical. If the company is not monitoring, then the health care provider should obtain a blood lead level and make recommendations based on the values listed in Table 33.3.

TABLE 33.3. New York State Action Levels for Lead Poisoning in Pregnant and Postpartum Women

Blood lead level	Action
0–9 µg/dL	Provide information on sources of lead and how to avoid.
10–19 µg/dL (mildly elevated)	Retest blood lead level to determine if lead is increasing. If increasing, seek consultation with TIS or regional resource centers. If no upward trend, repeat blood lead testing near term.
20–44 µg/dL (moderately elevated)	Retest blood lead level to determine if lead is increasing. If increasing, seek consultation with TIS or other regional resource centers. If decreasing, seek consultation for further risk reduction.
≥45 g/dL	Retest blood level; consult with a regional lead poisoning prevention center. Provide counseling on possible sources. Refer to local health agency. Consult TIS.

TIS, teratogen information service.

Infertility in men, loss of pregnancy in women, and birth defects in children are possible outcomes. It should be noted that growth restriction and neurobehavioral effects caused by prenatal exposures have been well documented in humans. However, no series of cases have confirmed an association of structural malformations in humans with prenatal lead exposure, as they have in animal studies.

The treatment for excess levels of lead consists of (a) identifying and eliminating the source of lead exposure and (b) administering chelation therapy depending on the patient's blood level (Table 33.3) and symptoms. However, chelation is often contraindicated during pregnancy because additional free lead is drawn from body depots (e.g., bone), so that levels in tissues and in the embryo/fetus are actually increased.

Mercury

It is important to determine the form of mercury (elemental, inorganic, and organic) to which a patient is being exposed because the different forms have different sites of action and effects in adults, pregnant women, and their offspring. Thus, when a health care provider is investigating possible environmental, therapeutic, and occupational exposures to mercury, the form of the metal is critical.

ELEMENTAL MERCURY

The major concern with elemental mercury is exposure via inhalation. Typical exposures occur in dental offices and in the home or workplace when sources of elemental mercury are spilled. In both situations, the cleanup can either eliminate the mercury or increase the exposure. In too many instances, the homeowner or employee uses a vacuum cleaner to clean up a broken thermometer or spilled beads of mercury. *Never use a vacuum cleaner!* Sources of heat should never be used to remove elemental mercury! They vaporize the mercury, which is then inhaled. In cases of potential exposure, measuring the levels of mercury is important in evaluating the risk.

Elemental mercury is not readily transmitted through the human placenta to the embryo/fetus. Dental amalgams have been associated with release of mercury, especially during the first 30 days. However, no adverse reproductive effects have been associated with amalgams to date. The levels of mercury in the blood of dental workers appears to be twice those in the blood of unexposed controls. Studies have not identified any increase risks for infertility or birth defects in dental workers in comparison with others. In one study of dental workers, an apparent 1.8-fold increase in risk for loss of pregnancy was noted for dental workers who performed more than 50 mercury amalgams per week. Exposures may be related to how the workers prepare the amalgams, whether they use physical protection (gloves), and how they clean the work area.

INORGANIC MERCURY

A number of medicinal products used as disinfectants, treatments for syphilis, or abortifacients contain mercury. In two case reports of women continually exposed to high levels of inorganic mercury during pregnancy, the offspring appeared to be normal. Thus, limited human information is available concerning exposure to inorganic mercury and its effects on reproductive outcome.

ORGANIC MERCURY

Organic mercury (especially methylmercury) is toxic to humans, especially the unborn. People are typically exposed to methylmercury through food (large predator fish such as swordfish, shark, and tuna). Contaminated fish from polluted streams and waters are also a source of exposure, as was noted in Minamata Bay, Japan, where the fetal methylmercury syndrome was first identified. Other products are rarely involved except in the case of unusual toxic exposures to animals (e.g., pigs fed contaminated food products). Levels tend to be lower in smaller predator fish and in smaller fish lower in the food chain (e.g., sardines). Alternatively, food can be contaminated when grain is treated with methylmercury as a fungicide. This occurred in the 1970s in Iraq, where toxicity developed in adults and neurologic impairments in their offspring.

The World Health Organization has recommended a level of organic mercury of 5 ppm in hair, which is 10-fold less than the observed toxic dose in adults. Interestingly, the toxic dose for the fetus in utero is closer to 10 ppm. It is recommended that predator fish be ingested in no more than one meal (0.50 lb) per week. During pregnancy, limiting intake further is prudent. Many people today try to limit their intake of red meat and consume more predator fish. In one case report, consuming predator fish in at least three meals per week resulted in hair levels of approximately 18 ppm in a mother and elevated levels well above 5 ppm in her newborn. This is understandable because consuming one meal of shark raises the hair level of mercury beyond the level of 5 ppm recommended by the World Health Organization for 30 days. The biologic half-life of methylmercury in persons who eat fish is approximately 50 days.

Studies demonstrate that methylmercury rapidly enters breast milk and is transmitted to the suckling infant, causing neurologic impairments. Interestingly, much like lead, methylmercury tends to produce neurologic defects rather than gross structural defects.

Interest has focused on thimerosal (mercury), which has been used as a preservative in vaccines and other products since the 1930s. This is metabolized to ethylmercury. It is feared that the vaccines and preservatives cause autism in children. Multiple forms of evidence indicate that mercury is a contributing factor to autism in children. Autism is an embryopathy occurring early in pregnancy that is related to exposures to teratogens (e.g., thalidomide) and gene expression (e.g., *HOXA1* and *HOXB1* mutants).

Cadmium

Cadmium, like lead, is widely distributed in industrial societies. Besides occupational exposures, some of the most common exposures are from tobacco smoke, old and poorly plated cookware (a silver-plated pitcher containing an acid-based drink such as lemonade), and ingested shellfish and kidney. Exposures can lead to acute distress (gastritis), such as when cadmium leeches into "grandma's lemonade," and 2 to 4 μg of cadmium can accumulate in a cigarette smoker consuming one pack per day. It is well established that cadmium levels are significantly increased in the placenta of women who smoke during pregnancy. In both animal and human in vitro studies, the human placenta appears to be more sensitive to the toxic effects of cadmium than the kidney. The kidney is commonly thought to be organ at risk for occupational exposure in welders, workers in foundries and cadmium battery factories, and smelters. Two case reports identified cadmium intoxication in women who taught welding. They lost multiple pregnancies and could not carry a child beyond the second trimester. Thus, occupational exposures to renally toxic doses of cadmium appear to alter reproductive function in women. A higher incidence of Itai-Itai disease has been reported in postmenopausal women. The half-life of cadmium in the body is 30 years.

Even though multiple animal studies have demonstrated that high doses of cadmium cause testicular toxicity, human data are limited. No clear association of occupational exposures to cadmium and testicular toxicity has been shown. One study did suggest an association between cadmium and varicocele-associated infertility. More work is required to confirm such as association.

OTHER EXPOSURES

Anesthetic gases, heat, and x-rays are discussed in the following sections. Both health care workers and their patients are exposed to gases, chemicals, and infectious agents. We consider occupational exposures to anesthetic gases and x-rays rather than patient exposures.

Anesthetic Gases

Continual exposure to anesthetic gases, especially nitrous oxide, during all types of surgery by operating room staff has been reported to be associated with pregnancy loss. However, other studies did not confirm this association. Such results may reflect important differences in study design that led to less bias in collection. Thus, it is suspected that some factor in the operating room environment increases the risk for spontaneous abortion. During dental procedures, ambient nitrous oxide concentrations of 700 ppm have been measured. The Occupational Safety and Health Administration limits are 25 ppm. Exposure of female dental personnel to nitrous oxide in unscavenged workplaces has been associated with an increased risk for spontaneous abortion (relative risk, 2.6; 95% confidence interval, 1.3–5.0). No increase in risk after exposure to nitrous oxide was noted when scavenging equipment was used. In a questionnaire study of Swedish midwives, the use of nitrous oxide in more than 50% of their deliveries was not associated with an increased risk for spontaneous abortion, although the same authors subsequently reported that nitrous oxide exposure was associated with a lower birth weight and an increased number of infants small for their gestational age.

The data are insufficient to draw conclusions about congenital defects in children of operating room staff. In addition, the current use of operating room anesthetic gas scavengers results in much lower levels of exposure than were noted in earlier studies, which demonstrated an association (REPROTOX).

The fertility of rats is adversely affected by exposure to nitrous oxide. In a telephone questionnaire study of dental assistants who had been pregnant within the past 4 years, calculation of time to pregnancy, which estimates fertility, demonstrated a reduction in per-cycle fecundity in association with nitrous oxide exposure. Finally, issues of male fertility related to workplace exposures to anesthetic gases have not been reported.

Radiation

For more than half a century, risks for impaired reproduction related to diagnostic, therapeutic, occupational, and environmental exposures to x-rays have been a concern. Diagnostic and therapeutic exposures of patients comprise the largest percentage of exposures, but people working in the health care professions and those working with radioactivity and in nuclear plants are also concerned about exposure to radiation.

Often, gamma radiation is the principal exposure of concern; however, exposure to lower-energy alpha and beta radiation also be a concern, especially if radioactive isotopes (^{14}C, ^{32}P, ^{3}H) are ingested by persons working with them. For this reason, it is forbidden to eat, drink, or smoke in a laboratory while radioactive materials are being used. Wearing protective clothing, such as gloves and laboratory coats, is critical. Lead aprons must be worn when gamma radiation is used (e.g., x-rays, ^{125}I, ^{131}I). Concerns for patients include actual exposure and the risk associated with the exposure. Determining this risk may be difficult without the input of an experienced health physicist.

Microcephaly and mental retardation were associated with exposure to doses of ionizing radiation of 50 rad or more in Hiroshima and Nagasaki. However, these exposures cannot be readily compared with the low linear energy transfer (LET) filtered radiation used in diagnostic radiology. In a clinical assessment of reproductive risk, the National Council on Radiation Protection (1979) stated that the risk for malformations at 5 rad or less was negligible in comparison with the other risks associated with pregnancy.

Besides reproductive and developmental problems, cancer has been associated with exposure to ionizing radiation. Human studies suggest that intrauterine exposure to x-rays increases the relative risk for leukemia and other childhood cancers by approximately 40%. Based on an extensive review, the overall risk for malformations and cancer in fetuses irradiated by 1 rad in utero during the first 4 months of gestation is between 0 and 1 per 1,000.

As reported in REPROTOX, occupational exposures of orthopedic surgeons to x-rays or of nuclear power plant employees to low-level ionizing radiation were not associated with an increased risk for congenital abnormalities or childhood malignancies in their children. However, in a more recent study of stillborn offspring of male radiation workers at a nuclear reprocessing plant, a small but statistically significant increase in the incidence of stillbirths was found in association with increased occupational exposure to external radiation. The available data do not demonstrate a causal relationship, but additional data from a future study may help to clarify this issue.

An adverse outcome occurred in 34 (30%) of 114 pregnancies in women who had received abdominal irradiation as children for embryonal renal tumor (Wilms tumor): 17 perinatal deaths and 17 low-birth-weight infants. In contrast, only 2 (3%) of 77 pregnancies in the wives of male irradiated patients had an adverse outcome. In another report, the risk for an adverse reproductive outcome was increased in women who had been exposed to ionizing radiation in the management of adolescent idiopathic scoliosis. Within this cohort, a reduction in birth weight appeared to be related to the dose of radiation received. These findings suggest that radiation therapy during childhood may cause somatic damage to abdominopelvic structures that later interferes with pregnancy. In 17,393 women treated with irradiation for skin hemangiomata at the age of 18 months or younger, the mean ovarian dose was 6 rad and the maximum dose was 855 rad. No clear dose-related adverse effects on reproduction were discovered in the exposed population.

From these reports, it can be concluded that ionizing radiation can be a reproductive and developmental toxicant. The National Council on Radiation Protection cutoff of 5 rad appears to be a useful threshold in the evaluation of reproductive and developmental risk.

SUMMARY

In assessing the effect of environmental/occupational exposures on reproduction, it is critical to define possible exposures and then attempt to assess the risk. Selected agents have been reviewed. For anyone seeking information about exposures and reproductive health, REPROTOX and TERIS, in addition to the other references listed in Table 33.4, are excellent resources. However, as noted in Fig. 33.1, establishing a good working relationship with experts in the field and with teratogen information services (OTIS), occupational medicine programs, prenatal genetics programs, and poison control centers is also essential. Often, the woman or women with repeated loss of pregnancy become the "canaries in the mine shaft," portending problems in the workplace or environment. However, pregnant women should not be the reason for identifying a problem in the workplace or environment, although much too often they are. Usually, signs and symptoms in other workers indicate a risk but are often overlooked. In closing, Dr. Anthony Scialli's statement is quoted to reinforce the concept that protecting reproductive health is good business for everyone:

> It appears prudent, in spite of the lack of consistency among studies, to limit chemical exposures at work through the use of standard safety procedures, including adequate ventilation, the use of protective clothing and gloves, and the avoidance of eating, drinking, and smoking in the work environment. These recommendations may be just as important for the protection of the general health of the worker as for his or her reproductive health.

TABLE 33.4. Resources for Occupational and Environmental Exposures

Amudar MO, Doull J, Klassen CD. *Casarett and Doull's toxicology.* New York: Pergamon Press, 1991.
ENTIS—European Network of Teratology Information Services, www.ENTISORG.org.
MEDLINE—National Library of Medicine, www.nlm.nih.gov/medlineplus.
New York State Department of Health. *Lead poisoning prevention guidelines for prenatal care providers* (publication no 2535, December 1995).
OTIS—Organization of Teratology Information Services, www.OTISPREGNANCY.org. Telephone: (866) 626-OTIS or (866) 626-6847 (free consulations with teratogen information specialists).
Paul M. *Occupational and environmental reproductive hazards: a guide for clinicians.* Baltimore: William & Wilkins, 1992.
Reproductive Toxicology, www.elsevier.com/locate/reprotox.
REPROTOX—www.reprotox.org. Telephone: (301) 657-5984; e-mail: reprotox@capu.net (access through membership or via Micromedics).
Scialli AR. Pregnancy and the workplace. *Semin Perinatol* 1993;19:18.
Scialli AR. *A clinical guide to reproductive and developmental toxicology.* Boca Raton, FL: CRC Press, 1992.
Teratology Society, www.teratology.org.
Teratology (birth defects journal). Hoboken, NJ: Wiley-Liss.
TERIS—Teratology Information Services and *Shepard's catalogue of teratogenic agents, http://depts.washington.edu/~terisweb/teris/* (access directly through membership or through Micromedics).
Working P. *Toxicology of the male and female reproductive systems.* New York: Hemisphere Publishing, 1992.

ACKNOWLEDGMENTS

This work was supported in part by National Institute of Environmental Health Sciences (NIEHS) Grant No. ES01247 to PEDECS (Perinatal Environmental and Drug Exposure Consultation Service–an NIEHS/New York Teratogen Information Service) as part of the University of Rochester Environmental Health Sciences Center (ES01247). We acknowledge the invaluable resources of REPROTOX, TERIS, and MEDLINE, in addition to the editorial support of Mrs. Jacqulyn White.

BIBLIOGRAPHY

Axelsson G, Ahlborg G Jr, Bodin L. Shift work, nitrous oxide exposure, and spontaneous abortion among Swedish midwives. *Occup Environ Med* 1996;53:374.

Bellinger D, Leviton A, Waternaux C, et al. Longitudinal analysis of prenatal and postnatal lead exposure and early cognitive development. *N Engl J Med* 1987; 316:1037.

Benoff S, Hurley IR, Barcia M, et al. A potential role for cadmium in the etiology of varicocele-associated infertility. *Fertil Steril* 1997;67:336.

Bodin L, Axelsson G, Ahlborg G Jr. The association of shift work and nitrous oxide exposure in pregnancy with birth weight and gestational age. *Epidemiology* 1999;10:429.

Brent RL, ed. National Council on Radiation Protection Proceedings. Pre- and post-conception reproductive effects of exposures to radiation. *Teratology* 1999;59:182.

Brent RL, Chambers CD, Chernoff CF, et al. Pregnancy outcome following gestational exposure to organic solvents: a response. *Teratology* 1999;60:328.

Cordier S, Bergeret A, Goujard J, et al. Congenital malformations and maternal occupational exposure to glycol ethers. *Epidemiology* 1997;8:355.

Correa A, Gray RH, Cohen R, et al. Ethylene glycol ethers and risks of spontaneous abortion and subfertility. *Am J Epidemiol* 1996;143:707.

Eisenmann CJ, Miller RK. Placental transport, metabolism and toxicity of metals. In: Chang LW, ed. *Toxicology of metals*. Boca Raton, FL: CRC Press, 1996:1003.

Hunter AGW, Thompson D, Evans JA. Is there a fetal gasoline syndrome? *Teratology* 1979;20:75.

Jensen TK, Hjollund NHI, Henriksen TB, et al. Does moderate alcohol consumption affect fertility? Follow-up study among couples planning first pregnancy. *BMJ* 1998;317:505.

Jones K, Smith DW, Streissguth AP, et al. Outcome in offspring of chronic alcoholic women. *Lancet* 1974;1:1076.

Khattak S, K-Moghtader G, McMartin K, et al. Pregnancy outcome following gestational exposure to organic solvents: a prospective controlled study. *JAMA* 1999;281:1106.

Mason HJ. Occupational cadmium exposure and testicular endocrine function. *Hum Exp Toxicol* 1990;9:91.

Miller RK. Lead screening of pregnant women in New York State: role of a teratogen information service. *Teratology* 1997;55:102.

Mole RH. The biology and radiobiology of in utero development in relation to radiological protection. *Br J Radiol* 1993;66:1095.

National Council on Radiation Protection and Measurements. *Medical radiation exposure of pregnant and potentially pregnant women*. NCRP report no 54.32, 1979.

Ono A, Kawashima K, Sekita K, et al. Toluene inhalation induces epididymal sperm dysfunction in rats. *Toxicology* 1999;139:193.

Otake M, Schull WJ. In utero exposure to A-bomb radiation and mental retardation: a reassessment. *Br J Radiol* 1984;57:409.

Paul M, eds. *Occupational and environmental reproductive hazards*. Baltimore: Williams & Wilkins, 1993.

REPROTOX. *Anesthesia* (no 1008); *Cadmium* (no 1373); *Heat* (no 1099); *Lead* (no 1116); *Mercury* (no 1123); *Solvents* (no 1198); *X-rays* (no 1221).

Rowland AS, Baird DD, Shore DL, et al. Nitrous oxide and spontaneous abortion in female dental assistants. *Am J Epidemiol* 1995;141:531.

Rowland AS, Baird DD, Weinberg CR, et al. Reduced fertility among women employed as dental assistants exposed to high levels of nitrous oxide. *N Engl J Med* 1992;327:993.

Schuyt HC, Brakel K, Oostendorp SGLM, et al. Abortions among dental personnel exposed to nitrous oxide [Letter]. *Anaesthesia* 1986;41:82.

Stodgell CJ, Ingram JL, Hyman SL. The role of candidate genes in unraveling the genetics of autism. *Int Rev Res Ment Retard* 2000;23:57.

Wilkins-Haug L. Teratogen update: toluene. *Teratology* 1997;55:145.

PART 4

Endocrine Problems

CHAPTER 34
Thyroid Disease

David F. Gardner

Functional and anatomic disorders of the thyroid are the most common nondiabetic endocrine conditions encountered in the ambulatory setting. Because virtually all thyroid disorders occur more commonly in women than in men, it is critical that every primary care physician who cares for significant numbers of female patients has a basic understanding of the presentation, diagnosis, and management of these conditions. This chapter focuses on the most common thyroid disorders encountered in the outpatient setting—hyperthyroidism, hypothyroidism, and goiter.

The normal adult thyroid consists of two lobes connected by the thyroid isthmus and weighs 15 to 20 g. It is located in the lower neck, anterior to the trachea, between the cricoid cartilage superiorly and the suprasternal notch inferiorly. The major secretory products of the thyroid are the iodinated amino acids thyroxine (T_4) and triiodothyronine (T_3), with most of the circulating T_3 (approximately 85%) derived from deiodination of T_4 in peripheral tissues. The metabolic effects of thyroid hormones are myriad, and a complete discussion is beyond the scope of this chapter. Most important, however, are their stimulation of the basal metabolic rate and mitochondrial oxidation, effects on plasma membranes, and stimulation of protein synthesis in a wide variety of organ systems. Thyroid hormones are critical during early childhood as evidenced by the devastating effects of thyroid hormone deficiency in the neonate (i.e., cretinism) and on normal growth in children.

The major factor regulating thyroid hormone secretion is thyroid-stimulating hormone (TSH, thyrotropin), which stimulates thyroid hormone synthesis and release and thyroid growth and vascularity. TSH secretion is regulated by the stimulatory effect of thyrotropin-releasing hormone from the hypothalamus and the negative feedback of circulating thyroid hormones that inhibit TSH secretion directly and indirectly via inhibition of thyrotropin-releasing hormone release. This classic negative feedback loop is responsible for the tight regulation of circulating T_4 and T_3 levels in normal individuals. After the release of thyroid hormones into the systemic circulation, they are tightly bound to circulating binding proteins, most importantly thyroxine-binding globulin (TBG). More than 99% of circulating T_4 and T_3 is protein bound and therefore biologically inert. It is only the free fractions of these hormones that are biologically active and available to tissues, and it is the free hormone concentration that is regulated by TSH secretion. A variety of nonthyroidal conditions may result in abnormalities in the serum TBG concentration, which in turn affect *total* T_4 but not *free* T_4 concentrations. The most common causes of increased TBG levels are estrogen therapy (e.g., oral contraceptives or postmenopausal estrogens), acute hepatitis, and a genetic TBG excess syndrome. The most common causes of TBG deficiency are the nephrotic syndrome, chronic androgen and/or glucocorticoid therapy, chronic nonthyroidal illness, and a genetic TBG deficiency syndrome.

HYPERTHYROIDISM

Hyperthyroidism (or thyrotoxicosis) is a clinical syndrome of diverse etiologies that have in common an increase in circulating thyroid hormone concentrations. The clinical signs and symptoms reflect the effects of these excess thyroid hormone levels on various organ systems.

Etiology

The diverse causes of hyperthyroidism are summarized in Table 34.1. The first five conditions on this list—Graves disease, toxic multinodular goiter, solitary hyperfunctioning nodule, subacute thyroiditis, and exogenous thyroid hormone excess—account for more than 95% of the patients with hyperthyroidism seen in the primary care setting. The rest of these conditions are quite rare, with the possible exception of iodine-induced thyrotoxicosis, which may occur after intravenous iodinated contrast administration or after ingestion of iodine-containing medications, such as amiodarone. The most common cause of hyperthyroidism in the United States is Graves disease, a systemic disorder occurring most frequently in women between the ages of 20 and 50. It is characterized by hyperthyroidism, diffuse thyroid enlargement, and often dra-

TABLE 34.1. Causes of Hyperthyroidism

Graves disease
Toxic multinodular goiter
Solitary hyperfunctioning nodule
Subacute thyroiditis
Exogenous thyroid hormone (iatrogenic or factitious)
TSH-secreting pituitary tumor
Trophoblastic tumors (e.g., choriocarcinoma)
Struma ovarii
Metastatic follicular thyroid carcinoma
Iodine induced

TSH, thyroid-stimulating hormone.

matic extrathyroidal manifestations involving the eyes (opthalmopathy), skin (dermopathy), and digits (acropachy). There is a considerable body of evidence supporting an autoimmune basis for Graves disease, and, in fact, the direct stimulus for thyroid hyperfunction is a circulating antibody against the TSH receptor. This antibody has been referred to as thyroid-stimulating immunoglobulin or thyrotropin receptor antibody.

Differential Diagnosis

The constellation of clinical findings, summarized below, along with a goiter, provides strong evidence for hyperthyroidism in most patients. Other disorders requiring consideration include psychiatric disorders such as anxiety, panic attacks, and bipolar states; substance abuse (cocaine and amphetamines); overdoses with β-adrenergic agonists or anticholinergic agents; and pheochromocytoma.

Clinical Symptoms

Although symptoms will vary from patient to patient, the following are most often reported: nervousness, increased sweating, heat intolerance, tremulousness, fatigue, palpitations, dyspnea, weight loss despite an increased appetite, hair loss, and ocular symptoms, particularly eye irritation associated with Graves ophthalmopathy. Menstrual cycle abnormalities may include anovulation, amenorrhea, oligomenorrhea, and menometrorrhagia. The term "masked" or "apathetic" hyperthyroidism describes the occasional hyperthyroid patient who does not manifest many of the classic symptoms of the disorder. These patients are usually elderly and present with unexplained weight loss, muscle weakness, atrial fibrillation, and heart failure. The diagnosis is often overlooked because these patients lack the more typical symptoms of adrenergic overactivity and may in fact appear hypothyroid.

Clinical Findings

The typical hyperthyroid patient is hyperactive and appears to have lost weight. Speech may be rapid and rambling, and facial features may reflect anxiety and apprehension. Other important physical findings include a resting tachycardia (occasionally associated with atrial fibrillation); warm, smooth, moist skin; thyroid enlargement; fine tremor of the hands; and hyperactive deep tendon reflexes. Pulses are often bounding, the cardiac apical impulse is typically hyperdynamic, and there may be a systolic flow murmur. Hair often becomes fine in texture and easily falls out, occasionally resulting in significant alopecia. The nails may become soft and the distal margins separated from the nailbed (onycholysis). The nature of the thyroid enlargement depends on the etiology of the hyperthyroidism. Enlargement will be diffuse in Graves disease, nodular in toxic multinodular goiter, and tender in subacute thyroiditis. The absence of a goiter in a hyperthyroid patient suggests factitious hyperthyroidism or the extremely rare disorder, struma ovarii. Increased blood flow through an enlarged thyroid in a patient with Graves disease may result in a bruit or palpable thrill. Lid lag and lid retraction, resulting in a characteristic stare, may be seen in all hyperthyroid patients. Infiltrative eye signs (exophthalmos, conjunctival inflammation and swelling, and extraocular muscle palsies) are specific for Graves disease. Patients with long-standing untreated hyperthyroidism may manifest signs of a proximal myopathy with frank proximal muscle wasting.

Laboratory and Imaging Studies

Definitive diagnosis of hyperthyroidism is based on the demonstration of elevated thyroid hormone levels and a suppressed serum TSH concentration. An algorithm for the diagnosis of hyperthyroidism is shown in Fig. 34.1. Virtually all patients with hyperthyroidism will have a suppressed serum TSH, and, therefore, a serum TSH determination is the best *screening* test for the detection of this disorder. The only exception to this rule is the extremely rare patient with a TSH-secreting pituitary tumor. The finding of a low serum TSH should be followed by a determination of the free T_4 concentration, because not all patients with suppressed TSH levels are hyperthyroid. A normal TSH level, however, is very strong evidence against the diagnosis of hyperthyroidism. Measurement of the total T_4 should not be substituted for a free T_4 determination, because alterations in serum thyroid hormone binding proteins, particularly TBG, may increase the total T_4 concentration without affecting the free T_4. In most clinical laboratories, the free T_4 concentration is estimated using the free T_4 index, which is calculated from the total T_4 concentration and the T_3 resin uptake.

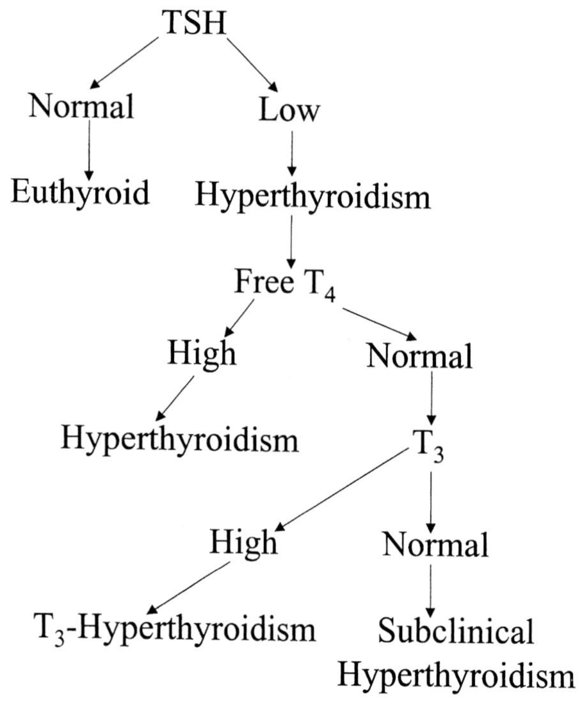

FIG. 34.1. Diagnosis of hyperthyroidism.

In addition, there are now generally available direct free T_4 immunoassays. An occasional hyperthyroid patient with a low TSH level will have a normal serum free T_4 concentration, and this patient should be further assessed with a serum T_3 determination. Hyperthyroidism with a normal free T_4 level and elevated T_3 has been called T_3-hyperthyroidism (or T_3-thyrotoxicosis) and accounts for 4% to 5% of all patients presenting with hyperthyroidism. Patients with normal serum free T_4 and T_3 concentrations and suppressed TSH levels are said to have "subclinical hyperthyroidism."

Radionuclide studies should not play a role in the *initial* diagnosis of hyperthyroidism, although they may be of value in defining the etiology of the hyperthyroid state. Most patients with Graves disease and toxic nodular goiters will have elevated 24-hour radioactive iodine uptakes. A suppressed radioactive iodine uptake suggests subacute thyroiditis, factitious hyperthyroidism, iodine contamination (e.g., after administration of an iodinated contrast agent), or struma ovarii.

Treatment

Therapy varies with the etiology of the hyperthyroidism. Exogenous hyperthyroidism responds to adjustment or cessation of thyroid hormone therapy. Patients with TSH-producing pituitary tumors, trophoblastic hyperthyroidism, struma ovarii, and metastatic follicular carcinoma require therapy directed at the primary neoplasm. Subacute thyroiditis is a self-limited disorder in most patients, usually requiring only symptomatic treatment with a beta-blocker. The most common forms of hyperthyroidism—Graves disease, toxic multinodular goiter, and the solitary hyperfunctioning nodule—may be treated with antithyroid drugs that inhibit thyroid hormone synthesis or thyroid ablation with radioactive iodine or surgery.

Pharmacologic therapy for hyperthyroidism includes the thiourea agents propylthiouracil (PTU) and methimazole (Tapazole) and β-adrenergic blocking agents (see below). The major action of the thioureas is inhibition of thyroid hormone synthesis. In addition, PTU, but not methimazole, inhibits the conversion of T_4 to T_3 in peripheral tissues. The usual starting dose of PTU is 300 mg/d, given in divided doses three times a day. The starting dose of methimazole is 30 mg/d, and it can be administered once daily. After 3 to 4 weeks of therapy, the doses of these drugs often require downward adjustment to prevent the development of hypothyroidism. Restoration of the euthyroid state generally takes 6 to 8 weeks. Antithyroid drugs effectively lower thyroid hormone concentrations in virtually all patients with hyperthyroidism if given in sufficient doses. Side effects of the thioureas include rash, hepatic dysfunction, arthralgias, a lupuslike syndrome, and, rarely, agranulocytosis. Agranulocytosis occurs in 0.2% to 0.4% of patients and is reversible with cessation of the drug.

β-Adrenergic blocking drugs, although having no direct effects on thyroid hormone secretion, effectively reverse many of the signs and symptoms of hyperthyroidism. Both cardioselective and nonselective beta-blockers decrease symptoms of nervousness, palpitations, sweating, and tremor and improve the patient's overall sense of well-being. A reasonable starting dose for a cardioselective agent is 50 mg atenolol every morning and for a nonselective agent, 20 mg propranolol three to four times per day. Because beta-blockers do not reverse many of the adverse tissue effects of hyperthyroidism, they should only be considered adjuncts to more specific therapies that lower circulating thyroid hormone concentrations.

Radioactive iodine is the treatment of choice for hyperthyroidism in adults in many centers because it is effective, safe, and convenient to administer. The effectiveness of therapy has been convincingly demonstrated, with 85% to 90% of patients cured by a single dose. Acute complications are rare, and the only proven long-term complication is hypothyroidism. There is some evidence, however, that radioactive iodine may worsen ophthalmopathy in some patients with Graves disease. A common concern of patients and physicians is the potential for carcinogenesis or induction of genetic damage in the recipients of radioactive iodine, particularly women of childbearing age. To date, there is no evidence that such damage occurs, nor is there any evidence to suggest an adverse effect on future fertility. In fact, it is now common to administer radioactive iodine to patients of all ages, including adolescents and young adults. Many clinicians, however, remain concerned about these issues and limit radioiodine treatment to patients beyond their childbearing years. The administration of radioactive iodine is absolutely contraindicated in pregnancy.

The role of surgery in the management of hyperthyroidism is limited. Possible surgical candidates include children, adolescents, and pregnant women not responding to or having an adverse reaction to antithyroid drugs and patients refusing radioactive iodine treatment. Complications of thyroid surgery include hypoparathyroidism, recurrent laryngeal nerve damage resulting in hoarseness, and hypothyroidism. All patients should have hyperthyroidism controlled with antithyroid drugs and iodine before surgical intervention.

The management of hyperthyroidism in patients with Graves disease must take into account a unique characteristic of this disorder—the occurrence of spontaneous remissions. The exact incidence of remissions is disputed, with estimates ranging from 20% to 50%. It is the occurrence of these remissions that has led to the considerable controversy regarding the *best* treatment for Graves disease. Probably the single most important factor in determining therapy is the age of the patient. Most experienced clinicians favor a trial of antithyroid drugs in children and adolescents, whereas radioactive iodine is the treatment of choice in patients beyond their reproductive years. Thus, it is the management of hyperthyroidism in young adults that is most problematic. The decision to use antithyroid drugs versus ablative therapy with radioactive iodine must be made on an individual basis, with the patient's understanding of the alternatives and the physician's personal experience being the determining factors. Definitive long-term therapy for patients with a toxic multinodular goiter or a solitary hyperfunctioning nodule should be radioactive iodine, although some of these patients may require short-term therapy with antithyroid drugs to manage acute hyperthyroid symptoms before radioactive iodine.

Pregnancy

Hyperthyroidism is a relatively uncommon complication of pregnancy, with estimates ranging from 0.1% to 0.4%. In most women the etiology is Graves disease. The most significant complication of hyperthyroidism in pregnancy is spontaneous abortion. Other concerns include gestational hypertension, preeclampsia, preterm delivery, cardiac arrhythmias, and rarely thyroid storm at the time of delivery. Fetal complications include intrauterine growth retardation, prematurity, stillbirth, and neonatal hyperthyroidism, a potentially life-threatening complication in the newborn. The treatment of choice for hyperthyroidism in pregnancy is the antithyroid drug PTU. Most pregnant hyperthyroid women can be controlled with doses of 300 mg/d or less, in divided doses, with no adverse effects on the fetus. Just as in nonpregnant patients, the dose of PTU should be progressively titrated down so that the euthyroid state is maintained with the lowest dose possible. Methimazole has been associated with a rare scalp defect, aplasia cutis, and should be avoided. Radioactive iodine is absolutely contraindicated in pregnancy, and in the rare patient with a serious adverse reaction to PTU, surgery during the second trimester is the management option of choice.

HYPOTHYROIDISM

Hypothyroidism is a clinical syndrome of diverse etiologies that have in common a decrease in circulating thyroid hormone concentrations. The clinical signs and symptoms reflect the effects of these decreased thyroid hormone levels on various organ systems. It is a common disorder, occurring most frequently in women between the ages of 40 and 60. The overall incidence is about 1% in women and 0.1% in men. The prevalence of the disorder increases with age and may be as high as 6% in women over the age of 60. If subclinical hypothyroidism is included, some studies have documented a prevalence approaching 15% in elderly women. The term myxedema is often used synonymously for hypothyroidism, but, in fact, it is a clinical presentation only seen in the most severely hypothyroid patients.

Etiology

Causes of hypothyroidism fall into four general categories: loss of functioning thyroid tissue, inhibition of thyroid hormone synthesis, TSH and thyrotropin-releasing hormone deficiency ("central" etiologies), and the rare thyroid hormone resistance syndromes. The various specific causes of hypothyroidism are summarized in Table 34.2. The most common cause of hypothyroidism in adults in the United States is autoimmune thyroiditis (Hashimoto disease, chronic lymphocytic thyroiditis). Hypothyroidism is also common after radioactive iodine therapy for hyperthyroidism and after thyroid surgery for goiter, hyperthyroidism, and thyroid cancer. From a global perspective, iodine deficiency remains the most common cause of hypothyroidism, but this is a rare occurrence in industrialized societies like the United States. In some patients, even after thorough investigation, the cause of hypothyroidism remains obscure. A number of disorders are associated with an increased risk of hypothyroidism, and these conditions are summarized in Table 34.3. Patients with any of these conditions should be screened periodically for the development of hypothyroidism.

TABLE 34.2. Causes of Hypothyroidism

Loss of functioning thyroid tissue
Autoimmune thyroiditis (Hashimoto disease)
Thyroidectomy
Irradiation
Radioactive iodine
External-beam irradiation for nonthyroid malignancy
Thyroid agenesis, dysgenesis
Replacement of thyroid tissue by systemic disease (sarcoidosis, amyloidosis)
Idiopathic
Inhibition of thyroid hormone synthesis
Iodine deficiency
Iodine excess (in susceptible individuals)
Antithyroid drugs (PTU and methimazole)
Inherited biosynthetic defects
Environmental goitrogens (e.g., turnips, casava)
Drugs (e.g., lithium, amiodarone)
Secondary causes
Pituitary disease (TSH deficiency)
Hypothalamic disease (TRH deficiency)
Thyroid hormone resistance syndromes (rare)

PTU, propylthiouracil; TRH, thyrotropin-releasing hormone; TSH, thyroid-stimulating hormone.

TABLE 34.3. Disorders Associated with Increased Risk of Hypothyroidism

Addison disease
Pernicious anemia
Type 1 diabetes mellitus
Autoimmune polyendocrine deficiency syndrome
Rheumatoid arthritis, scleroderma, systemic lupus erythematosus
Celiac disease, primary biliary cirrhosis
Chromosomal disorders (Turner, Klinefelter, Down syndromes)

Differential Diagnosis

The symptoms of hypothyroidism, summarized below, are often nonspecific and therefore may be confused with depression, anemia, fibromyalgia, chronic fatigue syndrome, and a host of other chronic illnesses. It is important to remember that hypothyroidism represents a wide spectrum of clinical severity, ranging from profound myxedema to its most subtle form, subclinical hypothyroidism. The former is readily recognized by its dramatic clinical presentation, whereas the latter is often diagnosed only when the patient undergoes laboratory screening at the time of a routine physical examination.

Clinical Symptoms

Typical symptoms include weakness, fatigue, sleepiness, cold intolerance, weight gain, constipation, dry skin, hair loss, hoarseness, and nonspecific muscle aches, stiffness, and cramps. Menstrual disturbances are common and are characterized by anovulation, oligomenorrhea, and menorrhagia. Psychiatric manifestations may be prominent. These may include depression, progressive cognitive impairment, memory loss, decreased libido, and impaired attention and abstract thinking. Frank psychosis with agitation and delusions, although uncommon, has also been reported.

Clinical Findings

Findings on physical examination suspicious for hypothyroidism include bradycardia, dry cool skin, coarse brittle nails, and hair loss, the latter sometimes associated with significant alopecia. Additional findings may include thinning of the eyebrows and facial puffiness, often with prominent periorbital edema. In more severe cases there may be thickening of the tongue, slow speech, and hoarseness of the voice. The hands and feet may swell, and the lower extremities may demonstrate nonpitting peripheral edema ("myxedema"). The thyroid may be enlarged, nodular, normal in size and configuration, or completely absent, depending on the etiology of the hypothyroidism. Neurologic findings include delayed relaxation of the deep tendon reflexes (pseudomyotonia), decreased muscle strength, carpal tunnel and other nerve entrapment syndromes, decreased hearing, and significant cognitive impairment with poor memory and concentration, especially in the elderly.

A spectrum of more uncommon presentations should raise the suspicion of underlying hypothyroidism, when no other etiologies for these findings are readily apparent. These include unexplained new onset diastolic hypertension; galactorrhea; sleep apnea; cardiomegaly ("myxedema heart"); serous effusions of the pleural, pericardial, and peritoneal spaces; and psychiatric manifestations, including dementia and psychosis. Unexplained laboratory abnormalities attributable to hypothyroidism may include anemia, elevated creatine kinase levels, hypercholesterolemia, and hyponatremia.

Laboratory and Imaging Studies

Because most patients with hypothyroidism have *primary* hypothyroidism (i.e., hypothyroidism due to intrinsic thyroid disease), the test with the highest sensitivity and specificity is the serum TSH concentration. Fig. 34.2 provides an algorithm for the diagnosis of hypothyroidism. An elevated TSH level should be followed by a determination of the free T_4, and the combination of an elevated TSH and low free T_4 is diagnostic of primary hypothyroidism. However, patients with milder degrees of hypothyroidism may have an elevated serum TSH with a free T_4 in the normal range. This combination of laboratory findings has been referred to as "subclinical hypothyroidism." This term is misleading, however, because many patients with even mild thyroid failure may have symptoms that resolve with appropriate thyroid hormone therapy. The one situation in which screening for hypothyroidism with a serum TSH level can be misleading is the uncommon patient with "secondary" hypothyroidism due to pituitary or hypothalamic disease. In these patients, the serum TSH level may be normal or low despite clinical hypothyroidism and a low free T_4 concentration. Thus, patients with convincing clinical evidence for hypothyroidism who do not have an elevated serum TSH should be further screened with a free T_4 measurement. The combination of a low free T_4 and normal or low TSH indicates underlying pituitary or hypothalamic disease, and these patients should be referred for more detailed endocrinologic and radiologic investigation.

Measurement of the serum T_3 concentration is of little value in the evaluation of hypothyroidism, because many patients with well-documented hypothyroidism will have T_3 levels in the normal range. In addition, many patients with low T_3 levels are not hypothyroid but may have a significant nonthyroidal illness impairing T_4 to T_3 conversion or may be taking a drug that impairs this peripheral conversion (e.g., glucocorticoids, beta-blockers, etc.). Radioactive iodine uptakes and scans are not useful in the diagnosis of hypothyroidism and should be avoided. Adjunctive studies may help in defining the etiology of hypothyroidism. In particular, the presence of thyroid peroxidase antibodies (previously called thyroid microsomal antibodies) is diagnostic of autoimmune thyroiditis. Patients with this disorder are at increased risk for other endocrine autoimmune disorders, including Addison disease, type 1 diabetes mellitus, and premature ovarian failure, and for nonendocrine autoimmune connective tissue disorders, such as systemic lupus erythematosus and rheumatoid arthritis.

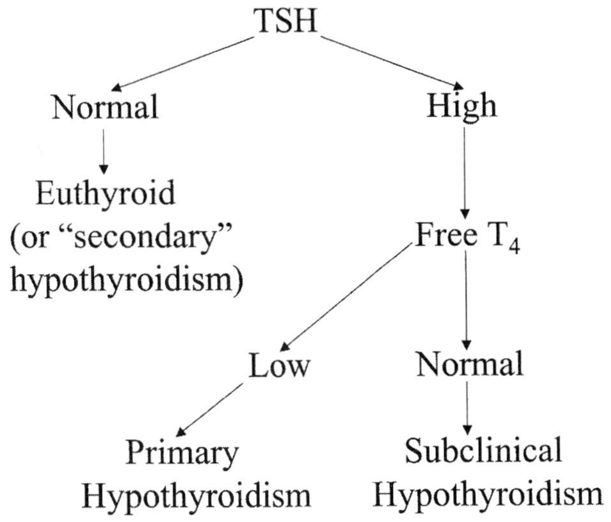

FIG. 34.2. Diagnosis of hypothyroidism.

Treatment

The goals of therapy in hypothyroidism are to reverse the signs and symptoms of the disorder, restore the serum TSH and free T_4 into the normal range, and avoid overtreatment. Replacement therapy should be in the form of T_4, not T_3. T_3 is rapidly absorbed from the gastrointestinal tract and has a much shorter half-life than T_4 (24–36 hours compared with 7 days), resulting in wide swings in serum T_3 concentrations after oral administration. T_4 administration is associated with stable serum T_4 and T_3 levels and is the treatment of choice for both primary and secondary hypothyroidism. The appropriate dose of T_4 will vary from patient to patient, but a reasonable estimate in most patients is 1.65 μg/kg body weight. The usual starting dose in young healthy patients is 50 to 100 μg/day, depending on the severity of the hypothyroidism—that is, patients with higher TSH levels should receive higher initial doses of T_4 replacement. Titration of the replacement dose is based on serial TSH measurements at 6- to 8-week intervals, with the goal being restoration of the TSH into the normal range. Elderly patients and those with underlying heart disease should be started on a low initial dose of T_4, 25 to 50 μg/d, because of the risk of precipitating an ischemic cardiac event with initial full replacement doses. The dose of T_4 replacement can then be gradually titrated upward until an appropriate clinical and biochemical response is achieved. Most hypothyroid patients will be adequately replaced with a total daily T_4 dose in the range of 75 to 125 μg, but there are many patients who will require doses outside this range. Although restoration of normal serum TSH and T_4 concentrations may be achieved fairly rapidly, resolution of clinical signs and symptoms frequently lags behind, often taking 2 to 4 months after restoration of normal thyroid function. Once normal thyroid function is restored, follow-up thyroid studies should be obtained at yearly intervals for 1 to 2 years and then every 2 to 3 years, unless the patient develops symptoms suspicious for thyroid dysfunction.

Replacement therapy in patients with secondary hypothyroidism, due to hypothalamic or pituitary disease, is more problematic, because the serum TSH concentration does not provide useful information regarding the appropriateness of the replacement dose. In these patients, the goal should be a serum free T_4 in the mid-normal range, but adjustments based on the patient's *clinical* response are often necessary.

A recent publication suggests that the combination of T_4 and T_3 is superior to T_4 alone in the treatment of hypothyroidism. This conclusion was based on improvements in some measures of cognitive performance and mood scores in a small group of patients treated for 5 weeks on each regimen. Although these findings are interesting and provocative, they need confirmation in larger groups of patients treated for longer periods of time before the routine use of T_3 can be recommended. In addition, if a T_3 preparation is used, it should be a "slow release" formulation to avoid the wide swings in T_3 concentrations observed with currently available preparations. Slow release T_3 preparations are not yet commercially available.

A potential risk associated with chronic thyroid hormone therapy is progressive bone demineralization and the development of osteoporosis. However, this is not a significant concern in patients who are appropriately replaced—that is, have serum TSH and free T_4 levels within the normal range. Overtreatment with thyroid hormone does increase the risk of bone loss and some cardiac complications, particularly atrial fibrillation, and should be strenuously avoided.

Pregnancy

Two important issues in the management of the hypothyroid pregnant patient require the clinician's close attention. The first relates to the observation that the T_4 dose needed to maintain the euthyroid state will increase in 50% to 70% of hypothyroid women during pregnancy. Although individual dose increases will vary considerably, the average dose increase needed to maintain a normal serum TSH concentration will range from 30% to 50%. Patients should be monitored in the mid–first trimester (6–7 weeks of gestation) and then in the middle of subsequent trimesters until the completion of pregnancy. Any change in the replacement dose requires a follow-up TSH determination in 6 to 8 weeks.

The second important issue concerning hypothyroidism in pregnancy is the potential adverse effects of maternal hypothyroidism on the neuropsychological development of the offspring. Several recent studies suggest that maternal hypothyroidism impairs the intellectual development of the newborn, but there is no consensus at this time as to whether all women should be screened for hypothyroidism before or shortly after conception. Certainly women at high risk should be screened (i.e., women with goiters, other autoimmune diseases, strong family history of thyroid disease, etc.), but more information is needed before universal screening can be recommended. The critical importance of monitoring pregnant women with known hypothyroidism for increased T_4 dose requirements during pregnancy has already been discussed.

GOITERS AND NODULES

Goiter is a nonspecific term indicating enlargement of the thyroid gland. Thyroid enlargement may be focal, involving a single lobe or portion of a lobe, or diffuse, involving the entire thyroid gland. Patients may be hypothyroid, hyperthyroid, or euthyroid. Classification of thyroid anatomy is based on physical examination and/or thyroid imaging studies such as ultrasound or radionuclide scanning. Diffuse goiter typically refers to a gland that is relatively smooth and symmetrically enlarged, although mild asymmetry is often present. This is the typical appearance of the thyroid gland in patients with Graves disease. Nodular goiters are characterized by focal areas of enlargement that may be solitary or multiple. The hyperthyroid patient with a solitary hyperfunctioning nodule will typically present with a single nodule, as will many patients with underlying thyroid neoplasms, both benign and malignant. Multinodular goiters typically involve both lobes, and they may progressively enlarge to cause significant obstructive symptoms, including dysphagia and respiratory compromise, although these symptoms are uncommon. When goiters are associated with hyperthyroidism, they are frequently referred to as "toxic" goiters, whereas "nontoxic" goiters refer to patients who are either euthyroid or hypothyroid.

The exact prevalence of goiter in the United States is uncertain, but it is clearly the most common of all thyroid disorders, increasing with age and affecting large numbers of patients above the age of 50. Women are affected five to six times more frequently than men. The prevalence of nodular thyroid disease in the adult population is 4% to 7%, and if ultrasound examination is used to detect nodules, the prevalence exceeds 50% in patients over the age of 60.

Etiology

From a global perspective, iodine deficiency remains the most common cause of goiter. Endemic goiter refers to a goiter occurring in a region where more than 10% of the population is affected. The common etiologic factor in most cases is iodine deficiency, and daily iodine intake of less than 50 μg/d may result in progressive thyroid enlargement. Average daily iodine intake in the United States is 100 to 200 μg/d. Sporadic goiter arises in nonendemic areas as a result of factors that do not affect the general population, and this is the most common form of goiter in the United States. Although the specific cause of goiter in any given patient may be elusive, the common denominator is believed to be some factor that prevents the production of adequate amounts of thyroid hormone, resulting in chronic TSH stimulation and thyroid enlargement. The resulting increase in thyroid mass may at least temporarily result in the production of normal quantities of thyroid hormones and maintenance of the euthyroid state.

Clinical Symptoms and Signs

Goiters are often asymptomatic and only detected as incidental findings on routine physical examination. The clinical presentation may be related to thyroid dysfunction, and it is the symptoms of hyperthyroidism or hypothyroidism rather than the goiter itself that brings the patient to medical attention. Many patients, however, do have significant local symptomatology. They may report a sensation of fullness or tightness in the neck; dysphagia; respiratory distress, including stridor associated with tracheal compression, hoarseness, pain, and tenderness (usually associated with thyroiditis or hemorrhage into a nodule); and rarely the superior vena cava syndrome. The latter is uncommon and is typically seen in association with a large goiter at the thoracic inlet. Often, goiters are detected incidentally at the time of radiographic studies performed for other purposes. Common examples include chest computed tomography (CT) that extends into the lower neck, Doppler ultrasound examinations aimed at detecting carotid artery disease, and cervical spine imaging studies such as CT and magnetic resonance imaging (MRI).

Careful physical examination will often provide a clue as to the etiology of the goiter. Diffuse thyroid enlargement associated with hyperthyroidism is almost always related to underlying Graves disease and much more rarely to a TSH-secreting pituitary tumor or trophoblastic tumor producing large amounts of human chorionic gonadotropin. Most nodular goiters are readily recognizable on neck examination, although the number of nodules detected is often significantly less than those ultimately seen on radiologic studies such as ultrasound. Thyroid tenderness and asymmetric enlargement is the hallmark of subacute thyroiditis. Firm rubbery enlargement of the thyroid is typical of Hashimoto disease, whereas stony hard thyroid enlargement should raise the suspicion of an anaplastic thyroid cancer or the extremely rare disorder, Riedel thyroiditis. Solitary thyroid nodules most often represent benign thyroid neoplasms, but the differential diagnosis is wide and includes thyroid malignancies, cysts, lymphocytic thyroiditis, and colloid nodules. More than 50% of patients with solitary nodules on physical examination will have multiple nodules detected on an ultrasound examination.

Laboratory and Imaging Studies

The first step in the laboratory evaluation of a goiter should be thyroid function tests, and a screening serum TSH determination should be sufficient for most patients. Because Hashimoto disease (chronic lymphocytic or autoimmune thyroiditis) is the most common cause of goiter in younger women, thyroid antibody studies may be helpful in patients suspected of having this disorder. The best current test is the anti-thyroid peroxidase antibody (formerly called anti-microsomal antibody). For patients with a solitary nodule, the most useful diagnostic test is a fine needle aspiration biopsy, and this is discussed in more detail below.

A variety of thyroid imaging modalities are available, including radionuclide scanning, ultrasonography, CT, and MRI. Most patients *do not* require thyroid imaging at the time of initial evaluation, although uncertain findings on physical examination may justify further anatomic assessment. In most patients the imaging study of choice should be a thyroid ultrasound because it is the least expensive, provides an excellent reproducible assessment of size, and does not require intravenous contrast. Ultrasound may also be useful in guiding fine needle aspiration biopsy of small or difficult to palpate thyroid nodules. Radioactive iodine imaging is useful in the diagnosis of a solitary hyperfunctioning ("hot") nodule and also helps define which nodules in a multinodular goiter are hyperfunctioning versus hypofunctioning. The major indication for CT or MRI of the thyroid is in patients with very large diffuse or multinodular goiters to determine the extent of the goiter, especially substernal extension, and to assess the degree of airway compromise associated with tracheal compression. Imaging findings in these patients will often facilitate the decision as to whether or not to proceed with thyroid surgery.

A common dilemma in the outpatient setting is the appropriate management of the patient presenting with a solitary thyroid nodule. Although the overwhelming majority of these nodules are benign (>90%–95%), the presence of a localized growth in the thyroid generates concern in both the patient and physician regarding an underlying thyroid malignancy. This concern often results in overly extensive and expensive diagnostic evaluations. If thyroid function tests are normal, the most appropriate next diagnostic study should be a fine needle aspiration biopsy rather than any imaging studies. Fine needle aspiration biopsy is a safe, accurate, relatively inexpensive diagnostic procedure, with excellent sensitivity and specificity in terms of distinguishing benign from malignant lesions. The one exception to proceeding initially to fine needle aspiration biopsy is the patient with a low serum TSH in whom the possibility of a hyperfunctioning nodule is significantly increased. In such a patient, the most appropriate diagnostic study after thyroid function testing is a radioactive iodine thyroid scan. If the nodule is hyperfunctioning ("hot") compared with surrounding normal thyroid tissue, the risk of malignancy is extremely low, and the focus of management is treating the hyperthyroidism, usually with radioactive iodine.

Treatment

The management of patients with goiters and nodules will vary with the underlying etiology and thyroid function. In patients with goiters associated with hypothyroidism, therapy with T_4 is usually sufficient and will often result in a diminution in the size of the goiter. Therapy for goiters associated with hyperthyroidism has been reviewed above. The most problematic situation is the patient with a euthyroid goiter, where options include simple observation, a trial of thyroid hormone suppression therapy, surgery, and radioactive iodine ablation. Considerable controversy remains regarding the efficacy of thyroid hormone suppression therapy in patients with a nodular goiter. Several studies suggest that T_4 is no more effective than placebo, whereas others have documented benefit in terms of shrinking the goiter. In one 5-year trial, T_4 suppression therapy did not significantly shrink thyroid nodules, but it did prevent further growth and the appearance of new nodules. In general, the more long-standing and larger the goiter, the less likely it is to respond to suppression therapy. The major risk of suppression therapy is the induction of hyperthyroidism. In many patients with nodular goiters, thyroid function is autonomous and therefore not TSH dependent, and the administration of T_4 will result in hyperthyroidism. Therefore, all patients started on suppression therapy should have thyroid function studies rechecked in 6 to 8 weeks. The goal should be suppression of the TSH into the low end of the normal range—that is, 0.3 to 0.6 μU/mL in an assay with a lower limit of normal of 0.3 μU/mL.

Surgery is usually reserved for patients with one of the following: (a) significant local neck symptoms such as dysphagia or respiratory difficulty, (b) patients in whom progressive growth of the goiter is documented on physical examination or serial ultrasound examinations, (c) patients who insist on removal of the goiter for cosmetic reasons, and (d) patients believed to be at significant risk for an underlying malignancy on the basis of a suspicious fine needle aspiration biopsy. Asymptomatic patients with a stable goiter at low risk for malignancy generally do not require surgical intervention. The role of radioactive iodine in the management of patients with large euthyroid goiters has expanded considerably in recent years. Large doses of radioiodine have been shown to cause a significant reduction in the size of some goiters and should be considered in elderly patients and patients with serious confounding medical illnesses who require a reduction in thyroid size but are poor surgical candidates.

SCREENING FOR THYROID DYSFUNCTION

Although patients with overt hyperthyroidism and hypothyroidism are usually readily detected by a careful history and physical examination, there remains a significant subset of the population with milder degrees of thyroid dysfunction in whom clinical manifestations are subtle and often overlooked. Estimates of the prevalence of subclinical hypothyroidism in the general population range from 5% to 17%, and for subclinical hyperthyroidism, 0.1% to 6%. Both hypothyroidism and hyperthyroidism can be accurately diagnosed with generally available laboratory studies, and both conditions are readily treatable. As previously discussed, the serum TSH concentration remains the most reliable test to diagnose the common forms of hypothyroidism and hyperthyroidism in the ambulatory care setting. Recently, the American Thyroid Association recommended that all adults be screened for thyroid dysfunction with a serum TSH determination, beginning at age 35 and every 5 years thereafter. Although this recommendation represents the consensus opinion of experts in the field and is not necessarily evidence based, it appears reasonable based on an earlier cost-effectiveness analysis that showed that the cost of screening for hypothyroidism was comparable with other commonly accepted screening studies, such as those for breast cancer and hypertension. The data supporting routine screening for hyperthyroidism is not nearly as compelling, related primarily to the lower prevalence of this disorder. A normal serum TSH concentration in an otherwise healthy ambulatory patient has a high negative predictive value in ruling out significant thyroid dysfunction.

Certain groups of patients are particularly susceptible to thyroid dysfunction, and it is reasonable to screen these patients at an earlier age and at more frequent intervals. On the basis of a recent report demonstrating impaired cognitive function in the offspring of women with even mild hypothyroidism during pregnancy, some experts are now advocating routine screening of women for hypothyroidism prepartum or early in the first trimester of pregnancy. A definitive recommendation in this regard has not been made, but it is certainly reasonable to screen women at significant risk for hypothyroidism either before or early during their pregnancy.

BIBLIOGRAPHY

Davies TF, ed. Symposium: autoimmune thyroid disease. *Endocrinol Metab Clin North Am* 2000;29:239–449.

Gharib H. Changing concepts in the diagnosis and management of thyroid nodules. *Endocrinol Metab Clin North Am* 1997;26:777–800.

Greenspan SL, Greenspan FS. The effect of thyroid hormone on skeletal integrity. *Ann Intern Med* 1999;130:750–758.

Ladenson PW, Singer PA, Ain KB, et al. American Thyroid Association guidelines for detection of thyroid dysfunction. *Arch Intern Med* 2000;160:1573–1575.

Mandel SJ, Cooper DS. The use of antithyroid drugs in pregnancy and lactation. *J Clin Endocrinol Metab* 2001;86:2354–2359.

Ross DS, ed. Symposium: assessment of thyroid function and disease. *Endocrinol Metab Clin North Am* 2001;30:245–528.

Singer PA, Cooper DS, Daniels GH, et al. Treatment guidelines for patients with thyroid nodules and well-differentiated thyroid cancer. *Arch Intern Med* 1996;156:2165–2172.

Singer PA, Cooper DS, Levy EG, et al. Treatment guidelines for patients with hyperthyroidism and hypothyroidism. *JAMA* 1995;273:808–812.

Smallridge RC, ed. Symposium: thyroid disease in pregnancy and the postpartum period. *Thyroid* 1999;9:629–748.

Smallridge RC, Ladenson PW. Hypothyroidism in pregnancy: consequences to neonatal health. *J Clin Endocrinol Metab* 2001;86:2349–2353.

CHAPTER 35
Adrenal Diseases

Lynnette K. Nieman

The cortex of the adrenal gland is comprised of three layers that produce distinct families of steroids. The outermost layer, the glomerulosa, secretes aldosterone and other mineralocorticoids, which regulate salt and water metabolism by promoting sodium reabsorption and potassium excretion in the kidney. The fasciculata, or middle layer, secretes cortisol and other glucocorticoids, which regulate energy balance and multiple intracellular processes. The innermost layer, the reticularis, secretes androgenic compounds such as testosterone, androstenedione, and dehydroepiandrosterone (DHEA). The adrenal medulla secretes the catecholamines epinephrine and norepinephrine, which affect vascular tone and cardiac output. Adrenal gland diseases may involve underproduction or overproduction of products from one or more cortical layers or the medulla and are considered in this way below.

DISORDERS OF THE ADRENAL CORTEX

Adrenal Insufficiency

Primary adrenal insufficiency reflects destruction of the entire adrenal cortex and results in loss of both glucocorticoid and mineralocorticoid activity. By contrast, secondary adrenal insufficiency reflects an inability of the hypothalamic-pituitary unit to deliver corticotropin-releasing hormone (CRH) and/or corticotropin (ACTH), thus reducing trophic support to otherwise normal glands. As a result, only cortisol production decreases, because mineralocorticoid production is not very ACTH dependent.

Autoimmune destruction is the most common etiology of primary adrenal insufficiency in the United States and may occur alone or in association with autoimmune polyglandular syndromes. Infections cause about 15% of primary adrenal insufficiency and typically include tuberculosis, systemic fungal diseases (histoplasmosis, coccidiomycosis, blastomycosis), and acquired immunodeficiency syndrome–associated opportunistic infections such as cytomegalovirus. These glands tend to be large on computed tomography (CT), whereas those affected by autoimmune destruction are small. Adrenal tissue may be replaced by bilateral metastases (most commonly primary carcinoma of the lung, breast, kidney, or gut, or primary lymphoma) or by hemorrhage, leading to insufficient steroidogenesis.

The congenital adrenal hyperplasias are a disparate group of diseases caused by a genetic deficiency of one of the enzymes needed for adrenal steroidogenesis. Patients with nearly complete deficiency of an enzyme required for cortisol synthesis present in childhood with adrenal insufficiency and salt-wasting crisis. This is most problematic in patients with mutation of the 21-hydroxylase (CYP21) or 11β-hydroxylase (CYP11) gene. The increase in ACTH levels caused by cortisol deficiency drives the intact steroidogenic pathways so that there is excessive production of the steroids just proximal to the enzymatic block, 17α-hydroxyprogesterone and 11-deoxycortisol, respectively, in 21-hydroxylase and 11β-hydroxylase deficiency. Because of the increased levels of precursor steroids, adrenal androgen levels increase. As a result, severely affected girls may be virilized in utero. Girls and women with nonclassic congenital adrenal hyperplasias have greater enzyme activity so that cortisol production is adequate, but increased ACTH values cause hyperandrogenism after puberty.

The characteristic clinical presentation of acute primary adrenal insufficiency includes orthostatic hypotension, circulatory collapse, fever, hyperkalemia, hyponatremia, and hypoglycemia. These features are most likely to be caused by hemorrhage, metastasis, or acute infection. The typical history and clinical findings of chronic primary adrenal insufficiency include a longer history of malaise, fatigue, anorexia, weight loss, salt craving, joint and back pain, and darkening of the skin, especially in the creases of the hands, extensor surfaces, recent scars, buccal and vaginal mucosa, and nipples. Associated biochemical features include hyponatremia, hypoglycemia, and hyperkalemia.

Suppression of the hypothalamic-pituitary-adrenal axis by exogenous or endogenous glucocorticoids is the most common cause of secondary adrenal insufficiency. Until full recovery occurs, up to 18 months after discontinuation of medication, the patient should receive supplemental steroids at times of physiologic stress (see below). Secondary adrenal insufficiency also may result from structural lesions of the hypothalamus or pituitary gland that interfere with CRH production or transport or with corticotrope function. This includes tumors, destruction by infiltrating disorders, x-ray irradiation, and lymphocytic hypophysitis.

Biochemical testing confirms the diagnosis of adrenal insufficiency. In acute adrenal insufficiency, a serum cortisol value generally is normal or subnormal, an inappropriate value for the state of hypotension, in which cortisol values are usually well above 18 μg/dL. In chronic adrenal insufficiency there is controversy about the best diagnostic test. Many use the cortisol response to exogenous ACTH as a gold standard test of adrenal steroidogenic ability. Others propose insulin-induced hypoglycemia and lower doses of the ACTH stimulation test, especially in patients with mild or recent secondary adrenal insufficiency who may respond to pharmacologic doses of ACTH. However, because there is no commercial formulation of ACTH for the lower dose tests, the product must be diluted and delivered on site, leading to concerns about accuracy of the administered dose and the validity of the results. Insulin testing has significant risks in patients without normal counter-regulatory processes and in those with coronary artery disease or epilepsy.

In the classic test, 250 μg of ACTH (cosyntropin) is given intravenously or intramuscularly, at any time of day. This supraphysiologic dose of ACTH is a maximal stimulus to the adrenal gland, so that the peak cortisol response measured 30 to 60 minutes later is greater than 18 μg/dL. Lower values indicate adrenal insufficiency.

Primary and secondary adrenal insufficiency may be distinguished by measurement of plasma ACTH. In primary adrenal insufficiency, ACTH levels generally are above the normal range and may exceed the normal range before the cortisol response to ACTH stimulation is subnormal. Additionally, hyperkalemia and elevated renin values are characteristic of primary but not secondary adrenal insufficiency.

Therapy of adrenal insufficiency should provide physiologic replacement of steroids. Glucocorticoid replacement is best achieved by administering 12 to 15 mg/M^2 of hydrocortisone daily in one or two oral doses. Ideally, the morning dose is given as soon after waking as possible; for individuals who feel extremely fatigued in the morning before the agent is absorbed, a strategy of taking the medication 30 minutes before arising may be helpful. Although many patients do well with a single dose, others complain of pronounced fatigue in the afternoon and evening. For them, a split-dose regimen, in which about one third of the daily dose is given around 4 p.m., may be useful.

Other glucocorticoids may be used for daily replacement therapy. Prednisone, 5 to 7.5 mg daily, has the advantage of a long half-life and may be particularly helpful in patients with afternoon or evening fatigue. Hydrocortisone offers the advantage of multiple dose tablets, which allows for fine adjustment and splitting of the daily dose.

Patients with primary adrenal insufficiency also should receive mineralocorticoid as Florinef 50 to 300 μg/d. This dose should be adjusted until plasma renin activity is in the normal range. If no mineralocorticoid is given, often the dose of hydrocortisone or other steroid with mineralocorticoid activity is increased to reduce hyperkalemia or salt craving. The problem with this approach is that the amount of glucocorticoid increases beyond physiologic replacement, so that the patient becomes cushingoid. These patients should be encouraged to salt their food and not limit salt intake.

Patients with primary adrenal insufficiency also have decreased serum DHEA levels. Replacement of DHEA at a 50-mg daily dose improves overall well-being and self-reported scores for fatigue, depression, and anxiety. In women but not men, there is improvement in sexual interest and the level of satisfaction with sex.

In suspected acute adrenal insufficiency, hydrocortisone is the treatment of choice because it has both glucocorticoid and mineralocorticoid activity. Treatment with intravenous saline for volume expansion, glucose for hypoglycemia, and intravenous hydrocortisone, 100 mg, is started immediately after placement of an intravenous line and withdrawal of blood for documentation of the cortisol value.

All patients receiving chronic glucocorticoid replacement therapy should be instructed that they must take glucocorticoids as prescribed and that failure to take or absorb the medication will lead to adrenal crisis and possibly death. They should obtain a medical information bracelet or necklace that identifies this requirement (Medic Alert Foundation, Turlock, CA). It is important to educate patients and their families about glucocorticoid adjustment during physiologic stress conditions, including emergency administration of intramuscular glucocorticoid using a kit containing prefilled syringes with injectable steroid.

The daily oral glucocorticoid dose is usually doubled for "stressful" physiologic conditions such as fever, nausea, and diarrhea, although few data support this strategy. Additionally, this practice may lead to chronic overmedication by the patient because of a liberal interpretation of what constitutes physical stress. Thus, education of when and how to change the dose of steroid should be reinforced periodically, preferably with written material, and the dangers of excessive steroid use should be emphasized. If the patient is vomiting, has severe diarrhea, or has collapsed, intramuscular glucocorticoids should be given before transport a medical facility.

Generally, the daily glucocorticoid dose is increased in conditions such as surgery in proportion to the amount of stress. Thus, during maximally stressful situations (adrenal crisis, major surgery, trauma, or labor and delivery) the daily hydrocortisone dose will be 100 to 300 mg. (Few data support the need for this 10-fold physiologic replacement dose, as opposed to mere replacement, but the safety of not following this practice has not been established.) For more moderate stress, such as that of cholecystectomy, the dose is reduced to 75 to 100 mg hydrocortisone on the day of surgery, and the dose is tapered more rapidly. Patients undergoing minimal stress such as tooth extraction or short operative orthopedic procedures may not require any additional supplementation.

Clinical assessment is the best way to judge whether the glucocorticoid dose is correct. Symptoms of adrenal insufficiency improve on adequate therapy. In primary adrenal insufficiency, plasma ACTH levels decrease but remain elevated in the range of 100 to 200 pg/mL. Renin values, however, normalize completely and may be used to judge the adequacy of mineralocorticoid replacement. Although hydrocortisone is metabolized to cortisol, plasma cortisol values should not be used to monitor therapy, because clearance from the bloodstream is rapid and circulating values are low for most of the day. Urine free cortisol (UFC) does not reflect adequate replacement, because the increase in plasma cortisol levels after a single daily dose may exceed corticosteroid-binding globulin capacity, resulting in excessive urine levels and overestimation of integrated cortisol levels.

Monitoring for clinical features such as development of a cushingoid habitus or weight gain is the best way to monitor for glucocorticoid excess. The development of osteopenia may be the only sign of subtler overreplacement. In women, DHEA replacement increases testosterone levels, so that hirsutism, acne, or other signs of androgen excess may suggest overreplacement.

Hypercortisolism

Cushing syndrome is a symptom complex that reflects excessive tissue exposure to cortisol. The diagnosis cannot be made without both clinical features and biochemical abnormalities. Thus, clinical features consistent with the syndrome prompt biochemical screening.

Clinical features of Cushing syndrome (Table 35.1) reflect the amount and duration of exposure to excess cortisol. Not all patients have all features, and patients with mild or intermittent cortisol excess usually have fewer features than those with very high glucocorticoid production. Because these signs and symptoms are common in the general population, the diagnosis may be confused with psychiatric disorders, the metabolic syndrome, anovulation, simple obesity, fibromyalgia, or acute illness. However, because worsening hypercortisolism may precipitate hypertension, glucose intolerance, infections, psychiatric disturbance, impaired cognition, and hypercoagulability, it is important to identify this treatable disorder so as to prevent its associated morbidity and mortality. Cushing syndrome is unusual in pregnancy, as hypercortisolism is more likely to cause anovulation and infertility.

Because clinical features do not reliably identify patients with Cushing syndrome, screening tests must be used to establish the diagnosis. However, the commonly used screening tests have less than optimal diagnostic accuracy. If clinical features are mild, the risk of a false-positive test is high and the risk of morbidity is low. In this setting, the certainty of the diagnosis may increase if screening is deferred until additional clinical signs or symptoms appear. Because Cushing syndrome tends to progress over time, the absence of progression mitigates against the diagnosis.

Screening is most likely to be positive in patients with signs that are most typical of glucocorticoid excess, including abnormal fat distribution in the supraclavicular and temporal fossae, proximal muscle weakness, wide (>1 cm) purple striae, or new irritability, decreased cognition, and decreased short-term memory. Testing is also indicated for a patient with multiple clinical features that have progressed over time. Such temporal change may provide an important clue. For example, oligomenorrhea is more suggestive of Cushing syndrome if it marks a change from previous normally timed menses than if it has been present since menarche. Old photographs help document physical changes.

UFC excretion over 24 hours is an excellent test for the diagnosis of Cushing syndrome. However, UFC excretion also may be increased in psychiatric disorders (depression, anxiety disorder, obsessive-compulsive disorder), chronic pain, severe exercise, alcoholism, uncontrolled diabetes, and morbid obesity. In these so-called pseudo-Cushing states, it is thought that central brain mechanisms stimulate CRH release, with subsequent activation of the entire hypothalamic-pituitary-adrenal axis. Cortisol negative feedback inhibition on CRH and pituitary ACTH release restrains the resulting hypercortisoluria to less than fourfold normal. Thus, if UFC excretion greater than normal is used to indicate Cushing syndrome, many patients with pseudo-Cushing states would be falsely diagnosed with the disorder. Conversely, patients with Cushing syndrome may have normal UFC by immunoassay because of intermittent hypercortisolism or altered renal metabolism of cortisol. If UFC is only mildly elevated and clinical features are minimal, it is best to treat any pseudo-Cushing state and to remeasure UFC with the expectation that it will normalize. Conversely, if UFC is normal but clinical suspicion is high, repeated UFC might disclose intermittent hypercortisolism.

Because of antibody cross-reactivity, immunoassays measure cortisol and its metabolites as well as structurally similar steroids. Techniques such as liquid chromatography-mass spectroscopy are becoming the new gold standard method for measurement of urine cortisol because they distinguish cortisol from these other compounds, so that the normal range is lower and more specific.

The 1-mg overnight dexamethasone suppression test (DST) is a simple screening test involving administration of dexamethasone, 1 mg, orally between 11:00 p.m. and midnight and measurement of plasma cortisol between 8:00 a.m. and 9:00 a.m. the following morning. The best criterion for interpretation is debated; recent proposals to decrease it to less than 1.8 μg/dL (50 nmol/L) will increase sensitivity but decrease specificity, giving more false-positive results. There is up to a 30% false-positive rate in chronic illness, obesity, psychiatric disorders, and normal individuals.

The 2-day 2-mg DST discriminates patients with a pseudo-Cushing state if plasma cortisol endpoints of 1.4 or 2.2 μg/dL are used. The test involves taking dexamethasone, 500 μg, orally every 6 hours for eight doses beginning at noon and measuring plasma cortisol at 8:00 a.m., 2 hours after the last dose. The test has excellent sensitivity (90%–100%) and specificity (97%–100%) for discriminating Cushing syndrome but has the disadvantage of high cost and the requirement for excellent patient compliance. The immediate subsequent administration of CRH (1 μg/kg body weight intravenously) and measurement of cortisol 15 minutes later increased the sensitivity and specificity to 100% in a small study of 58 patients. Values greater than 1.4 μg/dL indicate Cushing syndrome. Although this combined dexamethasone–CRH test has a very high diagnostic accuracy, it has the disadvantages of the 2-day DST and the added cost of CRH testing. Because of these drawbacks, in the United States these tests usually are reserved for patients with ambiguous or confusing results on UFC or the 1-mg DST. CRH is available commercially (ACTHREL, Ferring Corp.) with approved label-

TABLE 35.1. Frequency of Clinical Signs and Symptoms of Cushing Syndrome

Sign/symptom	Percent of 70
Decreased libido	100
Obesity or weight gain	97
Plethora	94
Round face	88
Menstrual changes	84
Hirsutism	81
Hypertension	74
Eccymoses	62
Lethargy, depression	62
Striae	56
Weakness	56
Electrocardiographic changes or atherosclerosis	55
Dorsal fat pad	54
Edema	50
Abnormal glucose tolerance	50
Osteopenia or fracture	50
Headache	47
Backache	43
Recurrent infections	25
Abdominal pain	21
Acne	21
Female balding	13

ing by the U.S. Food and Drug Administration (FDA) for the differential diagnosis of Cushing syndrome. Use of the agent in the dexamethasone–CRH test represents an off-label use.

Any dexamethasone test may give false results in patients with abnormal metabolic clearance of the drug. Agents that induce the cytochrome P450–related enzymes (alcohol, rifampin, phenytoin, and phenobarbital) increase dexamethasone clearance, whereas renal or hepatic failure retards dexamethasone clearance. If these medications cannot be discontinued, measurement of a dexamethasone level can determine if its clearance has been altered.

Measurement of plasma cortisol at midnight distinguishes pseudo-Cushing states from Cushing syndrome with 95% diagnostic accuracy using a cutpoint of more than 7.5 μg/dL for the diagnosis of Cushing syndrome. Measurement of salivary cortisol at bedtime or midnight works as well as the plasma cortisol. However, the cutpoints used in the various studies are different, suggesting that the assays are different, so that salivary cortisol assays must be validated before they are used for this purpose.

The causes of Cushing syndrome may be divided broadly into ACTH-dependent (85%) and -independent (15%) forms (Table 35.2). Primary adrenal disorders with autonomous activation suppress ACTH, whereas in primary ACTH excess disorders, the adrenal gland responds passively to ACTH. The two forms can be distinguished by measurement of ACTH, which is usually less than 10 pg/mL in primary adrenal disorders (adenoma, cancer, and rare bilateral hyperplasia). In this setting, patients undergo adrenal imaging to identify the site(s) of adrenal abnormality. Values greater than 10 pg/mL are found in corticotrope tumors (termed Cushing disease) and ectopic ACTH-secreting tumors. These patients must undergo a complex set of biochemical and radiographic tests to discriminate between these etiologies, ideally under the direction of an experienced endocrinology team. Although inferior petrosal sinus sampling is the best test, the 8-mg DST, the CRH stimulation test and magnetic resonance imaging of the pituitary also may be useful. The identification of an ectopic ACTH-secreting tumor relies on imaging studies. By contrast, pituitary magnetic resonance imaging often is normal in Cushing disease and is not required to establish that diagnosis.

The optimal treatment of Cushing syndrome is surgical resection of the lesion that is producing excessive ACTH or cortisol. In ACTH-dependent Cushing syndrome, if this is unsuccessful or cannot be done, bilateral adrenalectomy is an option. Medical therapy also may be used for patients with occult ectopic ACTH-secreting tumors, and pituitary irradiation may be used to treat Cushing disease.

Hyperaldosteronism

Primary adrenal hyperaldosteronism presents as spontaneous hypokalemia with hypertension. The diagnosis also should be considered in patients with hard-to-control hypertension. However, hyperaldosteronism can result from nonadrenal causes, as a result of elevated renin values, which stimulate aldosterone secretion. As a result, the diagnosis rests on demonstration of an increased ratio of aldosterone to plasma renin activity (>20) when the aldosterone value is more than 15 pg/mL. Having made the diagnosis, one must differentiate between the two adrenal etiologies: hyperplasia or an adenoma. Adrenal CT may show nonfunctioning nodules and falsely suggest an adenoma. Salt loading with oral or intravenous sodium and upright posture, respectively, suppresses and stimulates aldosterone in normal individuals. Patients with hyperplasia tend to retain these responses, but there is significant overlap between patient groups. The best diagnostic test involves measurement of cortisol and aldosterone in adrenal venous effluent and a peripheral vein before and after administration of ACTH. Cortisol is used to evaluate catheter placement in the adrenal veins, because levels from the two sides should be similar. When an adenoma is present, the aldosterone-to-cortisol ratio on one side is usually at least 10-fold greater than the other, which may be similar to the periphery, indicating suppression. Bilateral hyperplasia tends to produce similar values on each side. Surgical resection is the treatment for adenomas. Hyperplasia is treated with the mineralocorticoid antagonist spironolactone.

Hyperandrogenism

Women with excess circulating androgens or increased sensitivity to androgens present with complaints of hirsutism, acne, and/or anovulation/infertility. When testosterone is secreted in great excess, women may virilize and show deepened voice, clitoromegaly, a masculinized body habitus, and alopecia. As part of the hyperandrogenic anovulation syndrome, women may develop features of the metabolic syndrome, with hyperlipidemia, hypertension, and visceral obesity.

The adrenal causes of hyperandrogenism, congenital adrenal hyperplasia, Cushing disease, adrenal cancer, and androgen-producing adrenal adenoma are uncommon. Most women have no clear-cut etiology (idiopathic hirsutism) or polycystic ovary syndrome. Rarely, androgen-secreting ovarian tumors, hyperprolactinemia, glucocorticoid resistance, or exogenous drugs cause hyperandrogenism. Idiopathic hirsutism generally presents with a long history of hirsutism

TABLE 35.2. Etiology of Cushing Syndrome

Exogenous	Endogenous

Most common cause of Cushing syndrome
  Prescribed glucocorticoids (oral, intramuscular, or inhaled)
  Or ACTH-driven
May be factitious or iatrogenic
	ACTH independent—autonomous adrenal activation (20%)
	  Adrenal carcinoma (40%–50%)
	  Adrenal adenoma (40%–50%)
	  Rare causes: primary pigmented nodular adrenal disease, McCune-Albright syndrome, massive macronodular adrenal disease
	ACTH dependent—adrenal activation by excessive ACTH (80%)
	  Ectopic ACTH secretion (20%)
	  Corticotrope adenoma (80%)
	  Ectopic CRH secretion (rare)

ACTH, corticotropin; CRH, corticotropin-releasing hormone.

alone, whereas tumors, which are associated with more severe hyperandrogenism, tend to have a shorter history and signs of progressive virilization.

Laboratory findings may help to exclude idiopathic hirsutism, in which androgen levels are normal. This condition likely represents increased sensitivity of the hair follicle to normal circulating androgen levels. Patients with other forms of hyperandrogenism usually have increased serum levels of testosterone, dehydroepiandrosterone sulfate (DHEAS), or androstenedione. The type of androgen secreted in excess may provide an etiologic clue. In general, the ovary secretes excess testosterone, and the adrenal secretes excess DHEA and DHEAS, whereas androstenedione excess may be caused by pathology in either organ. DHEA and DHEAS are weak androgens but can be converted to androstenedione and then testosterone in the adrenal glands and hair follicles. As DHEA and DHEAS levels decline through adult life, these values must be interpreted with age-specific normal ranges. Although a tumor is more likely if DHEAS is greater than 500 μg/dL or testosterone is greater than 200 ng/mL, it is not excluded at lower levels. Imaging identifies nearly all adrenal tumors but may miss a small intraovarian one. UFC may be elevated in patients with virilizing adrenal carcinoma or Cushing disease (see above) and in those with glucocorticoid resistance. By contrast, androgen-secreting adrenal adenomas do not have glucocorticoid excess. Measurement of prolactin is helpful if menstrual abnormalities, galactorrhea, or other features of prolactinoma are present but is not likely to be abnormal in their absence. Women suspected of having nonclassic forms of congenital adrenal hyperplasia should undergo measurement of precursor and product hormones before and after ACTH to confirm the diagnosis.

Treatment of hyperandrogenism varies according to the cause. Adrenal and ovarian tumors are best resected. Although adrenal carcinoma may be metastatic at the time of initial resection, continued removal of other lesions provides the best duration of survival, because there is no effective chemotherapy. Late-onset congenital adrenal hyperplasia is treated by glucocorticoids to normalize ACTH and hence androgen levels (typically dexamethasone 0.125–0.375 mg at bedtime).

In addition, local therapy such as electrolysis or antiandrogen therapy may be needed to address androgen action at the hair follicle. Although it is not labeled by the FDA for this purpose, there is a long experience in the United States with the use of spironolactone at a daily dose of 75 to 200 mg. This antiandrogen also has antimineralocorticoid and diuretic properties, so that side effects include polymenorrhea, symptoms of hypovolemia, and, rarely, hypokalemia. Because of the polymenorrhea, oral contraceptives are a useful adjunctive therapy. Oral contraceptives also reduce androgen levels when given alone by suppressing gonadotropins, thus reducing ovarian androgen production, and by increasing hepatic synthesis of sex hormone-binding globulin, thus reducing the biologically active free testosterone level. Recently, investigators have shown that the insulin sensitizers such as metformin improve insulin resistance, allowing ovulation in some women with polycystic ovary syndrome. This approach does not have FDA approval, however.

DISORDERS OF THE ADRENAL MEDULLA

Pheochromocytoma

The excess catecholamine production by a pheochromocytoma classically presents as a triad of episodic headache, sweating, and tachycardia. Nearly all patients are hypertensive, but paroxysmal hypertension only occurs in about 50%. Patients may have other symptoms, including papilledema, pallor, dilated cardiomyopathy, orthostatic hypotension, and anxiety attacks. Depending on the spectrum of signs and symptoms, the differential diagnosis includes panic disorder, hyperthyroidism, and other causes of hypertension, headache, or heart disease. Sympathomimetic drugs (amphetamines, epinephrine, phenylpropanolamine, and monoamine oxidase inhibitors taken with tyramine-containing foods) may precipitate hypertension that mimics the symptoms of pheochromocytoma.

The diagnosis of pheochromocytoma is made by measurement of plasma or urine catecholamines or metabolites such as metanephrine in a patient not taking medications that elevate these values. Having made the diagnosis, CT and/or magnetic resonance imaging is obtained to locate the tumor(s), which are usually in the adrenal medulla or the abdomen (95%) but which may occur anywhere in the sympathetic ganglia. Occasionally, iodine-123 meta-iodobenzylguanidine, which is taken up by these cells, may be needed to localize the tumor. Bilateral pheochromocytomas are more likely in the associated familial disorders, von Hippel-Lindau syndrome, and multiple endocrine neoplasia type 2. However, a large fraction of patients with nonsyndromic pheochromocytoma have a germ-line mutation, so that screening the patient and family may be reasonable.

Treatment of pheochromocytoma is surgical. Because manipulation of the tumor may release large quantities of catecholamines, an experienced surgical and anesthesiology team is necessary to reduce morbidity.

PREGNANCY AND DISORDERS OF THE ADRENAL GLAND

Infertility is common in patients with cortisol and androgen excess because of the resultant anovulation. If a woman with Cushing syndrome becomes pregnant, miscarriage is more common, and hypertension may complicate the pregnancy. Generally, these women should receive medical or surgical treatment of hypercortisolism to improve pregnancy outcome. Similarly, women with extreme androgen excess may virilize a female fetus, so that treatment of the condition before pregnancy is important. Dexamethasone treatment to prevent virilization of a female fetus should be considered before pregnancy is attempted if salt-losing classic congenital adrenal hyperplasias is suspected. Women with adrenal insufficiency who take hydrocortisone may require an increased dose of the agent in late pregnancy to compensate for corticosteroid-binding globulin increases and sequestration of cortisol and should receive stress doses of hydrocortisone at the time of delivery. Women with pheochromocytoma should undergo surgical therapy before attempting pregnancy to avoid hypertensive crisis.

BIBLIOGRAPHY

Azziz R, Carmina E, Sawaya ME. Idiopathic hirsutism. *Endocr Rev* 2000;21:347–362.

Borst GC, Michenfelder HJ, O'Brian JT. Discordant cortisol responses to exogenous ACTH and insulin-induced hypoglycemia in patients with pituitary diseases. *N Engl J Med* 1982;302:1462–1464.

Coursin DB, Wood KE. Corticosteroid supplementation for adrenal insufficiency. *JAMA* 2002;287:236–240.

Derksen J, Nagesser SK, Meinders AE, et al. Identification of virilizing adrenal tumors in hirsute women. *N Engl J Med* 1994;331:968–973.

Graber AL, Ney RL, Nicholson WE, et al. Natural history of pituitary-adrenal recovery following long-term suppression with corticosteroid. *J Clin Endocrinol Metab* 1965;25:11–16.

Grinspoon SK, Biller BM. Clinical review 62: laboratory assessment of adrenal insufficiency. *J Clin Endocrinol Metab* 1994;79:923–931.

Hunt PJ, Gurnell EM, Huppert FA, et al. Improvement in mood and fatigue after dehydroepiandrosterone replacement in Addison's disease in a randomized, double blind trial. *J Clin Endocrinol Metab* 2000;85:4650–4656.

Legro RS. Polycystic ovary syndrome: long-term sequelae and management. *Minerva Ginecol* 2002;54:97–114.
Lenders JW, Pacak K, Walther MM, et al. Biochemical diagnosis of pheochromocytoma: which test is best? *JAMA* 2002;287:1427–1434.
Merke DP, Camacho CA. Novel basic and clinical aspects of congenital adrenal hyperplasia. *Rev Endocr Metab Disord* 2001;2:289–296.
Moghetti P. Advances in the treatment of polycystic ovary syndrome. *Expert Opin Invest Drugs* 2001;10:1631–1640.
Neumann HP, Bausch B, McWhinney SR, et al. Germ-line mutations in nonsyndromic pheochromocytoma. *N Engl J Med* 2002;346:1459–1466.
New MI. Minireview: 21-hydroxylase deficiency congenital adrenal hyperplasia. *J Steroid Biochem Mol Biol* 1994;48:15–22.
Newell-Price J, Trainer P, Besser M, et al. The diagnosis and differential diagnosis of Cushing's syndrome and pseudo-Cushing's states. *Endocr Rev* 1998;19:647.
Nieman LK. The evaluation of ACTH-dependent Cushing's syndrome. *The Endocrinologist* 1999;9:93–98.
Nieman LK. Cushing syndrome. In: *DeGroot's textbook of endocrinology.* Philadelphia: WB Saunders, 2000.
Nieman LK. Diagnostic tests for Cushing's syndrome. *Ann N Y Acad Sci* 2002;970: 112–118.
Nieman LK, Rother KI. Glucocorticoids for postnatal treatment of adrenal insufficiency and for the prenatal treatment of congenital adrenal hyperplasia. In: Meikle AW, ed. *Contemporary endocrinology: hormone replacement therapy:* Totowa, NJ: Humana Press, 1999:221–230.
Papanicolaou DA, Mullen N, Kyrou I, et al. Nighttime salivary cortisol: a useful test for the diagnosis of Cushing's syndrome. *J Clin Endocrinol Metab* 2002;87: 4515–4521.
Papanicolaou DA, Yanovski JA, Cutler GB Jr, et al. A single midnight serum cortisol measurement distinguishes Cushing's syndrome from pseudo-Cushing states. *J Clin Endocrinol Metab* 1998;83:1163–1167.
Plotz CM, Knowlton AI, Ragan C. The natural history of Cushing's syndrome. *Am J Med* 1952;13:597–614.
Taylor RL, Machacek D, Singh RJ. Validation of a high-throughput liquid chromatography-tandem mass spectrometry method for urinary cortisol and cortisone. *Clin Chem* 2002;48:1511–1159.
Tordjman K, Jaffe A, Trostanetsky Y, et al. Low-dose (1 mcg) adrenocorticotrophin (ACTH) stimulation as a screening test for impaired hypothalamo-pituitary-adrenal axis function: sensitivity, specificity and accuracy in comparison with the high-dose (250 mcg) test. *Clin Endocrinol (Oxf)* 2000;52:633–640.
Yanovski JA, Cutler GBJ, Chrousos GP, et al. Corticotropin-releasing hormone stimulation following low-dose dexamethasone administration: a new test to distinguish Cushing's syndrome from pseudo-Cushing's states. *JAMA* 1993; 269:2232–2238.
Young WF Jr. Pheochromocytoma and primary aldosteronism: diagnostic approaches. *Endocrinol Metab Clin North Am* 1997;26:801–827.

CHAPTER 36
Ovarian Endocrine Disorders

Richard S. Legro

ETIOLOGY

Ovarian endocrine disorders result from both hyperfunction and hypofunction of the ovary. Hyperfunction of the ovary results primarily in androgen excess disorders, whose clinical presentations range from ovulatory dysfunction to frank virilization. Of these, polycystic ovary syndrome (PCOS), or unexplained hyperandrogenic chronic anovulation, is probably the most common. Hypofunction of the ovary results most commonly from premature ovarian failure (POF). This chapter briefly overviews androgen excess disorders and then examines POF.

ANDROGEN EXCESS STATES

Differential Diagnosis

Other causes of androgen excess include an androgen secreting tumor, exogenous androgens, Cushing syndrome, and nonclassic congenital adrenal hyperplasia (CAH). Hyperthecosis may represent the most severe presentation (in terms of hyperandrogenism) of PCOS (see Chapter 37). Other rare conditions depending on the presentation are acromegaly and cases of extreme androgen excess and insulin resistance due to mutations in genes directly involved in insulin action, such as the insulin receptor mutations in the Rabson-Mendenhall syndrome and leprechaunism. Women with PCOS have mild elevations of circulating prolactin, and this appears to be an epiphenomena rather than a cause of the excess circulating androgens. Also, other differential diagnoses of androgen excess in an adult female are the use of exogenous androgens, for example, anabolic steroids in a body builder, or an overdose of androgens in a postmenopausal women.

Others have defined PCOS on the basis of the morphology of the ovary (Fig. 36.1). Polycystic ovaries are found in a wide variety of unrelated disorders, including in up to 30% of women with normal menses and normal circulating androgens. The differential diagnosis of polycystic ovaries is extensive, with some syndromes having little overlap with hyperandrogenic chronic anovulation. There have been reports to suggest that polycystic ovaries per se may identify a group of women with some further stigmata of reproductive and metabolic abnormalities found in the endocrine syndrome of PCOS, but the data have not been consistent. It is important to note that not all women with the endocrine syndrome of PCOS have polycystic-appearing ovaries and that polycystic ovaries alone should not be viewed as synonymous with PCOS.

Nonclassic CAH, often referred to as late-onset CAH (see Chapter 35), can present in adult females with anovulation and hirsutism and is due almost exclusively to genetic defects in the steroidogenic enzyme, 21-hydroxylase (CYP21) (as opposed to other steroidogenetic enzymes that are only rarely mutated). In asymptomatic women who harbor mutations, this has been referred to as cryptic CAH. This high rate of mutation in this autosomal gene is due to its location near the human leukocyte antigen complex on chromosome 6, an area of frequent recombination. Nonclassic CAH is estimated to be present in less than 1% of unselected hirsute women. Because of the lack of 21-hydroxylation and minimal lyase activity of CYP17, the metabolite 17α-hydroxyprogesterone (17-OHP) accumulates. Because of the lack of cortisol synthesis, corticotropin (ACTH) levels increase, resulting in overproduction and accumulation of cortisol precursors, which in turn are shunted to androgen biosynthetic pathways. Phenotype is largely due to the amount of functional enzymatic activity of the allelic variants. For instance, those with salt-wasting CAH tend to have no recognizable enzymatic activity, whereas those with simple virilizing CAH tend to have around 2% activity and those with nonclassic CAH have 10% to 20% activity.

Clinical Symptoms and a History

There is a wide variety of presenting complaints for androgen excess, including infertility, obesity, menstrual disorders, and hirsutism. In women with PCOS, long-term health problems must also be considered. Chronic anovulation, hirsutism, and obesity are associated with endometrial cancer. There are no systematic prospective studies of the prevalence of endometrial hyperplasia/neoplasia in a population with PCOS or conversion rates over time. No routine screening recommendations can be made at this time. PCOS is also associated with insulin resistance and many metabolic sequelae such as impaired glucose tolerance, diabetes, and dyslipidemia (see Chapter 37).

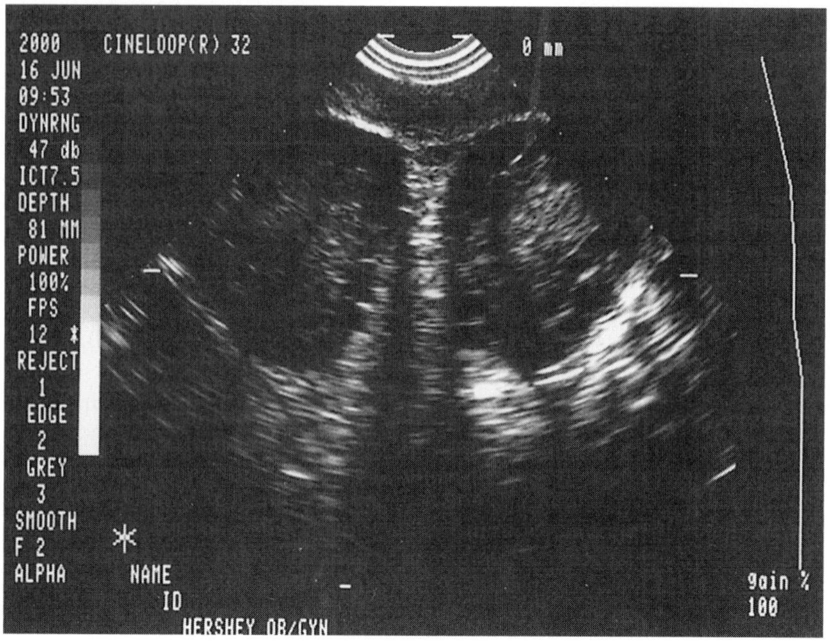

FIG. 36.1. Transvaginal ultrasound view of bilateral polycystic ovaries.

PCOS was once thought to be exclusively a disorder of reproductive-aged women, but that notion is fading. The earliest recognized PCOS phenotype to date is that of premature pubarche characterized by elevated dehydroepiandrosterone sulfate (DHEAS) levels and hyperinsulinemia. These girls are at high risk to develop the full PCOS phenotype. It is important to note that age can modify the phenotype and serum androgen levels decline, menstrual irregularity improves steadily in the fourth and fifth decades of life, and polycystic ovary morphology may resolve. A clear postmenopausal PCOS phenotype has not been established.

Clinical Findings and the Physical Examination

History and physical are essential to making a diagnosis of the underlying cause of oligo-ovulation. A family history of diabetes and cardiovascular disease (especially first-degree relatives with premature onset: males <55 years and females <65 years) is an important part of the history. Physical examination should carefully check the patient for signs of hyperandrogenism, including balding, acne, excess midline body hair, and clitoromegaly. Signs of insulin resistance on physical examination such as obesity, a centripetal fat distribution, and the presence of acanthosis nigricans (Fig. 36.2) should be recorded (see Chapter 37).

Coexisting signs of Cushing syndrome, including a moon facies, buffalo hump, abdominal striae, centripetal fat distribution, and hypertension, should be documented and cause further screening. Because Cushing syndrome has an extremely low prevalence in the population (1 in a million) and screening tests do not have 100% sensitivity/specificity, routine screening of all women with hyperandrogenic chronic anovulation for Cushing syndrome is not indicated. Cortisol excess can be screened with a 24-hour urine for free cortisol (which better quantifies excess cortisol production than random spot blood levels). Values for urinary free cortisol more than 300 μg/d are virtually diagnostic for Cushing syndrome. Intermediate elevations require further testing.

A pelvic examination should be performed because 90% of ovarian tumors present with unilateral enlargement. A transvaginal ultrasound examination, increasingly an office-based examination, should be able to identify ovarian masses more than 1 cm in diameter, although physiologic follicular and cystic developments throughout the normal menstrual cycle, especially a corpus luteal cyst, can masquerade as more serious pathology.

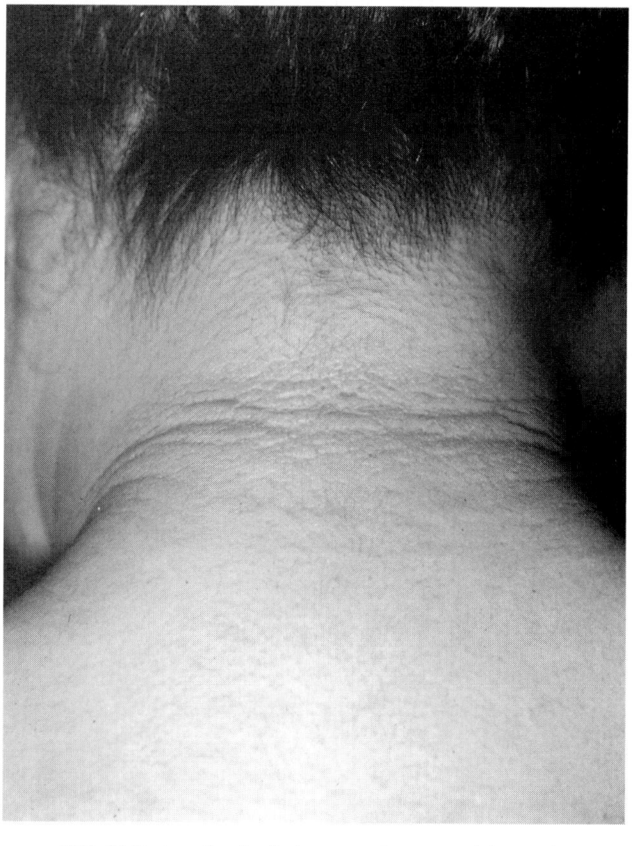

FIG. 36.2. Acanthosis nigricans on the nape of the neck.

Laboratory and Imaging Studies

The best circulating androgen to measure to document unexplained androgen excess is uncertain. A testosterone and/or bioavailable/free testosterone are useful for documenting ovarian hyperandrogenism (see Chapter 37). A DHEAS may be useful in cases of rapid virilization (as a marker of adrenal origin), but its utility in common hirsutism assessments is questionable.

Androgen secreting tumors, primarily of ovarian and secondarily of adrenal origin, are invariably accompanied by elevated circulating androgen levels. However, there is no absolute level that is pathognomonic for a tumor, just as there is no minimum androgen level that excludes a tumor. In the past, testosterone levels greater than 2 ng/mL and DHEAS levels greater than 700 μg/dL were regarded as suspicious for a tumor of, respectively, ovarian and adrenal etiology, but these cutoffs display poor sensitivity and specificity. In one study, less than 10% of women with a total testosterone level greater than 250 ng/dL had a tumor. Nonetheless, they are useful to quantify the amount of circulating androgen excess and potential source.

A prolactin level can identify prolactinomas that secrete massive amounts of prolactin that may stimulate ovarian androgen production, but this is an extremely rare cause of hyperandrogenic chronic anovulation. A serum thyroid-stimulating hormone level is also useful given the protean manifestations and frequency of thyroid disease in a female population with menstrual disorders.

Nonclassic CAH due to CYP21 mutations can be screened for with a fasting 17-OHP level in the morning. A value less than 2 ng/mL is normal, and recently cutoffs as high as 4 ng/mL have been proposed if obtained in the morning and during the follicular phase. Values above this cutoff or values above 2 ng/mL obtained at a random time during the day or during the menstrual cycle should be screened with an ACTH stimulation test. This is performed in the early morning by giving 250 μg of Cortrosyn, a synthetic form of ACTH, intravenously after baseline 17-OHP analysis and then obtaining a 1-hour value. Results may be interpreted according to the nomogram of New and associates (1983), but more commonly a cutoff 1-hour value of 17-OHP less than 10 mg/mL excludes nonclassic CAH. Although the yield is low, all patients with unexplained androgen excess should be screened for nonclassic CAH due to CYP21 mutations, because this diagnosis has a different prognosis, a different treatment regimen, and requires genetic counseling regarding the risks of congenital transmission.

Inappropriate gonadotropin secretion has been one of the characteristic signs of PCOS since assays were available to characterize it. These are rarely used because of the lack of sensitivity (>50% of women with no detectable gonadotropin abnormality), especially in obese women. The suppression of luteinizing hormone levels by increasing obesity reduces the usefulness of gonadotropin levels as diagnostic criteria in PCOS.

Treatment

Treatment of ovarian endocrine disorders involves surgery, if a tumor (androgen or cortisol producing) is diagnosed, dopaminergic agents if hyperprolactinemia is diagnosed, and low dose glucocorticoids if nonclassic CAH is diagnosed. PCOS poses treatment challenges, and there are different strategies depending on short-term goals, such as ovulation induction, or long-term goals, such as ovarian suppressive therapy (see Chapter 37). There is no evidence-based schema to guide the initial and subsequent choices of treatment methods. The goal of long-term suppressive therapy is to improve hyperandrogenic stigmata and prevent the development of endometrial hyperplasia. A variety of agents has been used to achieve ovarian and adrenal suppression in women with androgen excess. Additional benefits that may occur from such treatment include cycling/suppression of the endometrium, and thus a decreased chance for endometrial hyperplasia/carcinoma, and increased circulating levels of sex hormone-binding globulin (SHBG) and decreased bioavailable androgen. This increase in SHBG thus works synergistically with decreased androgen production to improve hyperandrogenism in PCOS.

Ovarian and adrenal suppression can be achieved through negative feedback of potent sex steroids, such as progestin or combined oral contraceptive therapy at the hypothalamic-pituitary axis or by direct pituitary inhibition of gonadotropin production and release by gonadotropin-releasing hormone (GnRH) agonists. Adrenal suppression can be achieved through inhibition of the hypothalamic-adrenal axis by potent glucocorticoids. Additionally, synthetic progestins may serve as androgen receptor antagonists (such as cyproterone acetate) or competitive inhibitors of 5α-reductase.

ORAL CONTRACEPTIVES

Oral contraceptives have been the mainstay of long-term management of PCOS. Individual combinations due to varying doses/combinations may offer varying risk-to-benefit ratios. For instance, varying progestins have been shown to have varying effects on circulating SHBG levels, but whether that translates into a clinical benefit is uncertain. The best oral contraceptive for women with PCOS is unknown, although arguably the pill containing a progestin with a favorable antiandrogenic profile, such as cyproterone acetate or drospirenone, is the best theoretical choice.

Oral contraceptives in the larger population have been associated with a significant reduction in endometrial cancer risk (50% decrease), a benefit that persists for at least 10 years after stopping. In the larger population, oral contraceptive use has not been associated with an increased risk of developing type 2 diabetes. Suppression of androgens with the oral contraceptive pill was associated with a significant elevation in circulating triglycerides and in high-density-lipoprotein cholesterol in the largest study of women with PCOS of the longest duration (3 years). No studies have suggested that women with PCOS experience an increased number of cardiovascular events through the use of oral contraceptives. The World Health Organization Scientific Group reported that myocardial infarction is rare in nonsmoking reproductive-aged women nor did it increase the risk of either ischemic or hemorrhagic stroke.

PROGESTINS

There are minimal data to guide the use of progestins in PCOS. A recent Cochrane Database Systematic review of the use of progestins and estrogen–progestin combinations to control anovulatory bleeding found no randomized trials. Both depot and intermittent oral medroxyprogesterone acetate (10 mg for 10 days) have been shown to suppress pituitary gonadotropins and circulating androgens in women with PCOS. The frequency of induced cycles and the type of cyclic oral progestin therapy that prevents endometrial cancer in women with PCOS is unknown. Extrapolating from the postmenopausal hormone replacement literature, monthly treatment for a minimum of 10 days and perhaps longer are optimal.

INSULIN SENSITIZING AGENTS

Drugs developed initially to treat type 2 diabetes have also been used to treat PCOS. Although drugs exhibiting a variety of mechanisms may improve diabetes, most published studies have focused on agents that improve peripheral insulin sensitivity with a lowering of circulating insulin levels. These drugs (metformin and thiazolidinediones) do not increase insulin secretion, as do sulfonylureas, and therefore rarely are associated with hypoglycemia, a risk in a fasting normoglycemic population. These drugs are often referred to under the rubric "insulin sensitizing agents," although there are both interclass differences (i.e., effect on weight between biguanides and thiazolidinediones) and intraclass differences (i.e., prevalence of hepatotoxicity between troglitazone and rosiglitazone) that discourage lumping.

Nonetheless, improving insulin sensitivity is associated with a decrease in circulating androgen levels, an improved ovulation rate, and an improvement in glucose tolerance. It is difficult to separate the effects of improving insulin sensitivity from that of lowering serum androgens, as any "pure" improvement in insulin sensitivity can raise SHBG and thus lower bioavailable androgen. These agents include metformin, thiazolidinediones, and an experimental insulin sensitizer drug d-*chiro*-inositol. None of these agents is currently approved by the U.S. Food and Drug Administration for the treatment of PCOS or for related symptoms such as anovulation, hirsutism, or acne.

OVARIAN DRILLING/DIATHERMY

The value of laparoscopic ovarian drilling/diathermy as a primary treatment for subfertile women with anovulation (failure to ovulate) and PCOS is undetermined according to a Cochrane review. There is insufficient evidence to determine a difference in ovulation or pregnancy rates when compared with gonadotrophin therapy as a secondary treatment for clomiphene-resistant women. Multiple pregnancy rates are reduced in those women who conceive after laparoscopic drilling/diathermy. None of the various drilling/diathermy techniques had any obvious advantages. The results of the ovarian drilling/diathermy may in some cases also be temporary, and ovarian drilling/diathermy does not appear to improve metabolic abnormalities in PCOS with insulin sensitivity and dyslipidemia unaffected post-procedure. Thus, the benefit and the role of surgical therapy in ovulation induction in women with PCOS is uncertain.

LIFESTYLE INTERVENTIONS

Multiple studies in women with PCOS have shown that weight loss can improve the fundamental aspects of the endocrine syndrome of PCOS: Lower circulating androgen levels and cause spontaneous resumption of menses. These changes have been reported with a weight loss as small as approximately 5% of the initial weight. Other reported benefits include decreased circulating insulin levels, a decrease in unbound testosterone levels largely mediated through increases in SHBG, and decreases in circulating luteinizing hormone levels.

OTHER TREATMENTS

A metaanalysis found no studies of adequate power to confirm the benefit of pulsatile GnRH to induce ovulation in PCOS. This method has been used sparingly because of difficulty in obtaining pumps and maintaining venous access. An aromatase inhibitor, letrozole, has in one small study been reported to improve ovulation and result in pregnancy. Ketoconazole, an oral synthetic antifungal imidazole derivative that inhibits gonadal and adrenal steroidogenesis, has been used as an adjunctive agent in inducing ovulation with gonadotropins. Octeotride, a somatostatin analogue, has also been used as an adjunctive agent in ovulation induction. Antiopioid blockade with naltrexone has shown varying results. No benefit has been found using dexamethasone alone nor was there any relationship of ovulation to circulating DHEAS levels.

Pregnancy

Ovulation induction in women with PCOS is potentially dangerous due to the recruitment of multiple follicles. It is also prone to failure given the underlying obesity and insulin resistance of the syndrome. Women with polycystic ovaries and PCOS are at marked increased risk for ovarian hyperstimulation syndrome. Ovarian hyperstimulation syndrome has been reported in women with PCOS who have had low-dose gonadotropin protocols, received GnRH alone, and even in a PCOS woman who conceived spontaneously. Hyperinsulinemic women with PCOS may be at even increased risk for excessive follicular recruitment with gonadotropin stimulation. Ovulation induction in PCOS has been shown to lead to a higher multiple pregnancy rate than treatment of other types of anovulatory infertility.

Many studies have reported increased pregnancy loss rates in women with PCOS with a range of 30% to 50%. Most of these reports involved nonobese women and were associated with hypersecretion of luteinizing hormone. Elevated androgens have been associated with recurrent miscarriage. Obesity may also be an independent adverse predictor of pregnancy wastage. Other stigmata of PCOS, such as polycystic ovaries, have not been associated with recurrent miscarriage. These data must be interpreted in the light of the high spontaneous loss rate of 30% in the general population and the early pregnancy detection bias that these studies entail. Women with PCOS appear to be at increased risk for complications of pregnancy, including gestational diabetes and hypertensive disorders, so this would be additional reason to avoid multiple pregnancy in this subgroup of women.

PREMATURE OVARIAN FAILURE

Etiology and Differential Diagnosis

POF is a rare disorder whose upper limits of age overlap with the population undergoing natural menopause. Definitions in the past have included age limits of less than 35 or less than 40. About 1% of the population will undergo menopause before the age of 40, and 95% of the population will experience menopause between the ages of 44 and 56. The likelihood of an idiopathic or unknown etiology tends to increase with age. An early presentation of ovarian failure tends to identify a more severe etiology (i.e., genetic or contributing metabolic abnormality). Genetic abnormalities include loss of the X chromosome (Turner syndrome; 45,XO represents the most severe example) or key portions (ovarian determining genes appear to be on the short arm Xp) or loss of key genes involved in ovarian function that may be located on the X chromosome or other autosomes. Genetic defects in other genes may allow toxic metabolites to accumulate; this may be the case with galactosemia, due to mutation in galactose-1-phosphate uridyltransferase. Rare mutations in key genes involved in ovarian follicular development, such as gonadotropin genes or receptors, may give the phenotype of ovarian failure. Acquired causes may include autoimmunity, leading to follicular depletion or the development of inactivating antibodies to key proteins in the reproductive axis. Iatrogenic causes, such as the use of chemotherapy or radiation for a variety of clinical diseases (cancers, lupus, etc.) or inadvertent destruction of the ovary or its blood supply at the time of surgery, may also be the culprit.

Finally, environmental agents (the best example is smoking) may lower the age of natural menopause through cytotoxic effects.

Clinical Findings and the History and Physical Examination

More severe forms of POF present at the time of adrenarche and pubarche with delayed puberty or primary amenorrhea. The stigmata of Turner syndrome—short stature, webbed neck, low-set ears, low posterior hairline, high-arched palate, cubitus valgus, and widely spaced nipples, may be present. Some patients with Turner syndrome have a later onset of POF and present with secondary sexual development and a history of previous menstrual bleeding. Less severe forms can present with secondary oligomenorrhea or amenorrhea, combined with other menopausal symptoms of estrogen deficiency (vasomotor symptoms, sexual dysfunction, etc.). A family history of premature ovarian failure is also a clear risk factor.

POF may in some of its manifestations be a temporary situation, with periodic recovery of ovarian function and even spontaneous conceptions. The fluctuating nature of these cases and factors that promote reawakening of ovarian function are poorly understood.

Laboratory and Imaging Studies

Persistent follicle-stimulating hormone levels in the menopausal range identify women with POF. Therefore, serial levels may be indicated. This also helps to eliminate the possibility of a false-positive elevated follicle-stimulating hormone level due to a mid-cycle ovulatory surge. Karyotype is most likely to identify chromosomal abnormalities in a younger population, but some mild Turner variants, due to small deletions, may present late in reproductive life, so the upper limit of age in which to pursue a karyotype is indeterminate. Patients with Turner syndrome or variants need additional diagnostic testing to evaluate for cardiac abnormalities such as coarctation of the aorta, renal abnormalities, thyroid disease, and diabetes mellitus. To a lesser extent, endocrine abnormalities due to loss of function have been reported in women with idiopathic POF, purportedly due to autoimmunity. However, the yield of routing screening appears to be low, with an incidence of thyroid disease less than 10% and of diabetes less than 3%. The chance of parathyroid failure or adrenal failure appears to be very low, so that screening serum calcium and phosphate levels or an ACTH stimulation test of adrenal reserve is not cost effective. Clinical testing for antibodies directed against the ovary or adrenal has not been validated, and their utility tends to rest in the eye of the assay holder. Routine ovarian biopsy is not indicated or useful.

Treatment

The main goal of treatment is correction of estrogen deficiency, either as replacement for those women who experienced some period of ovarian function or as initiation for sexual development for those with more severe forms of ovarian failure. Sexually infantile women need stimulation of breast growth with low-dose estrogen therapy. The effects of estrogen for this purpose may be hindered by the presence of the potent progestins contained in low-dose oral contraceptives. In general, hormonal replacement therapy is preferable to the use of oral contraceptives for POF. Hormone replacement therapy is not risk free; there is still an appreciable increase in clotting events in user compared with nonusers. Hormone replacement therapy also does not suppress ovulation, so the periodic return of ovarian function may result in pregnancy, although the overall chance of this is extremely rare. Other modes of contraception may be necessary in those who do not desire this option.

Pregnancy

In patients with POF, conception is rare and treatments apocryphal. Suppression of the reproductive axis with either oral contraceptives or GnRH agonist therapy has been associated with rebound ovulation but not pregnancy. This diagnosis often results in overtreatment to the benefit of the clinician and the detriment of the patient. Oocyte or embryo donation remain the mainstay of treatment for these women to deliver an infant (delivery rates for oocyte donation approach 40% nationally). Pregnancy in women with POF does not pose additional obstetric risks.

The prevention or preservation of ovarian function has become an increasing possibility for those women undergoing chemotherapy or radiation therapy. Transposition of the ovaries out of the radiated field has been used. Additionally, suppression of the ovaries during chemotherapy with oral contraceptives or a GnRH agonist may protect against cytotoxic damage. Finally, ovarian cryopreservation for either future in vitro use or autotransplantation offers promising preliminary results but still is a long way from routine clinical care.

ACKNOWLEDGMENTS

This work was supported by PHS grants U54 HD34449 The National Cooperative Program in Infertility Research (NCPIR), K24 HD01476, a General Clinical Research Center (GCRC) grant MO1 RR 10732 to Pennsylvania State University, and U10 HD 38992 The Reproductive Medicine Network.

BIBLIOGRAPHY

Franks S. Polycystic ovary syndrome. *N Engl J Med* 1995;333:853–861.

Chang PL, Lindheim SR, Lowre C, et al. Normal ovulatory women with polycystic ovaries have hyperandrogenic pituitary-ovarian responses to gonadotropin-releasing hormone-agonist testing. *J Clin Endocrinol Metabolism* 2000;85:995–1000.

Loucks TL, Talbott EO, McHugh KP, et al. Do polycystic-appearing ovaries affect the risk of cardiovascular disease among women with polycystic ovary syndrome? *Fertil Steril* 2000;74:547–552.

Dahlgren E, Friberg LG, Johansson S, et al. Endometrial carcinoma: ovarian dysfunction—a risk factor in young women. *Eur J Obstet Gynecol Reprod Biol* 1991;41:143–150.

Ibanez L, Potau N, Virdis R, et al. Postpubertal outcome in girls diagnosed of premature pubarche during childhood: increased frequency of functional ovarian hyperandrogenism. *J Clin Endocrinol Metab* 1993;76:1599–1603.

Elting MW, Korsen TJ, Rekers-Mombarg LT, et al. Women with polycystic ovary syndrome gain regular menstrual cycles when ageing. *Hum Reprod* 2000;15:24–28.

Koivunen R, Laatikainen T, Tomas C, et al. The prevalence of polycystic ovaries in healthy women. *Acta Obstet Gynaecol Scand* 1999;78:137–141.

Waggoner W, Boots LR, Azziz R. Total testosterone and DHEAS levels as predictors of androgen-secreting neoplasms: a populational study. *Gynecol Endocrinol* 1999;13:394–400.

New MI, Lorenzen F, Lerner AJ, et al. Genotyping steroid 21-hydroxylase deficiency: hormonal reference data. *J Clin Endocrinol Metabolism* 1983;57:320–326.

Robinson S, Rodin DA, Deacon A, et al. Which hormone tests for the diagnosis of polycystic ovary syndrome? *Br J Obstet Gynaecol* 1992;99:232–238.

Arroyo A, Laughlin GA, Morales AJ, et al. Inappropriate gonadotropin secretion in polycystic ovary syndrome: influence of adiposity. *J Clin Endocrinol Metab* 1997;82:3728–3733.

Chasen-Taber L, Willett WC, Stampfer MJ, et al. A prospective study of oral contraceptives and NIDDM among U.S. women. *Diabetes Care* 1997;20:330–335.

Hickey M, Higham J, Fraser IS. Progestogens versus oestrogens and progestogens for irregular uterine bleeding associated with anovulation. Cochrane Database of Systematic Reviews. Issue 2, 2001.

Nestler JE, Jakubowicz DJ, Reamer P, et al. Ovulatory and metabolic effects of d-

chiro-inositol in the polycystic ovary syndrome. *N Engl J Med* 1999;340:1314–1320.
Farquhar C, Vandekerckhove P, Arnot M, et al. Laparoscopic "drilling" by diathermy or laser for ovulation induction in anovulatory polycystic ovary syndrome [review]. Cochrane Database of Systematic Reviews 2000;(2): CD001122.
Lemieux S, Lewis GF, Ben-Chetrit A, et al. Correction of hyperandrogenemia by laparoscopic ovarian cautery in women with polycystic ovarian syndrome is not accompanied by improved insulin sensitivity or lipid-lipoprotein levels. *J Clin Endocrinol Metab* 1999;84:4278–4282.
Huber-Buchholz MM, Carey DG, Norman RJ. Restoration of reproductive potential by lifestyle modification in obese polycystic ovary syndrome: role of insulin sensitivity and luteinizing hormone. *J Clin Endocrinol Metab* 1999;84:1470–1474.
Mitwally MF, Casper RF. Use of an aromatase inhibitor for induction of ovulation in patients with an inadequate response to clomiphene citrate. *Fertil Steril* 2001;75:305–309.
Fulghesu AM, Villa P, Pavone V, et al. The impact of insulin secretion on the ovarian response to exogenous gonadotropins in polycystic ovary syndrome. *J Clin Endocrinol Metab* 1997;82:644–648.
Rai R, Backos M, Rushworth F, et al. Polycystic ovaries and recurrent miscarriage—a reappraisal. *Hum Reprod* 2000;15:612–615.
Guerrero NV, Singh RH, Manatunga A, et al. Risk factors for premature ovarian failure in females with galactosemia. *J Pediatr* 2000;137:833–841.
Hoek A, Schoemaker J, Drexhage HA. Premature ovarian failure and ovarian autoimmunity. *Endocr Rev* 1997;18:107–134.
van Kasteren YM, Hundscheid RD, Smits AP, et al. Familial idiopathic premature ovarian failure: an overrated and underestimated genetic disease? *Hum Reprod* 1999;14:2455–2459.
Kim TJ, Anasti JN, Flack MR, et al. Routine endocrine screening for patients with karyotypically normal spontaneous premature ovarian failure. *Obstet Gynecol* 1997;89(5 Pt 1):777–779.
Blumenfeld Z, Haim N. Prevention of gonadal damage during cytotoxic therapy. *Ann Med* 1997;29:199–206.

CHAPTER 37
Polycystic Ovary Syndrome

Maria J. Iuorno, Jean-Patrice Baillargeon, and John E. Nestler

The polycystic ovary syndrome (PCOS), also known as Stein-Leventhal syndrome, is the most common form of female factor infertility in the Western World, affecting approximately 5% to 10% of reproductive-aged women. In the last 15 years, current knowledge regarding the etiology and treatment of this disease has burgeoned, and it is now recognized as both a reproductive and metabolic disorder. In fact, there is growing evidence that women with PCOS suffer not only from infertility and reproductive disorders but are also at significantly increased risk for type 2 diabetes mellitus and cardiovascular disease. This chapter aims to assist the primary care physician in the diagnosis of PCOS and to delineate the goals of therapy.

DEFINITION AND ETIOLOGY

The most widely accepted criteria for the diagnosis of PCOS are derived from the conference sponsored in 1990 by the National Institute of Child Health and Human Development (NICHD) These criteria are in order of importance: (a) clinical and/or biochemical hyperandrogenism (i.e., hirsutism or increased free or total testosterone), (b) chronic anovulation or oligomenorrhea (often defined as fewer than or equal to six menstrual periods per year), and (c) exclusion of other etiologies (see Differential Diagnosis, below).

Although the clinical and laboratory characteristics of PCOS are established, the underlying etiology of this disorder is still unclear, and its molecular and physiologic mechanisms have yet to be fully characterized. In fact, currently there are no satisfactory animal models for this disease, underscoring the complex constellation of genetic and environmental factors that play a role in its development. Nonetheless, certain aspects of the genetics, prevalence of comorbidities, and underlying pathophysiology have been studied, and some of these relevant findings are discussed here.

Genetics

PCOS demonstrates familial clustering. Studies formally evaluating the heritability of PCOS among female first-degree relatives strongly suggest an autosomal-dominant inheritance pattern, albeit without complete penetrance of expression. Kahser-Miller et al. examined 78 mothers and 50 sisters of 93 women with PCOS and found that as many as 35% of mothers and 40% of sisters of women with PCOS also had the syndrome. It is equally important to note that family histories of women with PCOS may not only display a clustering of PCOS in female family members but also a history of type 2 diabetes mellitus in both female and male relatives of the prepositus. Furthermore, a positive family history of type 2 diabetes confers higher risk to the prepositus for developing diabetes herself. Although various genetic markers and variant alleles related to insulin signaling, gonadotropins, and ovarian androgen production have been identified or studied, no one single gene or gene pattern has yet to be attributed to this disease with great prevalence.

Insulin Resistance and Hyperinsulinemia

Insulin resistance is defined as decreased glucose utilization by the body's tissues in response to insulin. Insulin resistance is frequently accompanied by a compensatory hyperinsulinemia and can sometimes progress to relative pancreatic insulin insufficiency, resulting in glucose intolerance (impaired glucose tolerance [IGT] or overt type 2 diabetes). Insulin resistance is highly prevalent among women with PCOS. Studies of both lean and obese women with PCOS document the presence of insulin resistance, as determined by the hyperinsulinemic-euglycemic clamp analysis, the gold standard for measuring insulin sensitivity. This finding emphasizes the near universality of insulin resistance among women with PCOS.

PCOS is also associated with clinical markers of insulin resistance, such as the skin lesion acanthosis nigricans and obesity, in both adolescents and adults. Although certain molecular mechanisms for insulin resistance (i.e., abnormal serine phosphorylation of the insulin receptor, abnormal GLUT-4 transport mechanisms, etc.) have been identified in a limited number of women with PCOS, a clearly major and prevalent molecular defect in insulin signaling has yet to be identified.

Numerous studies suggest that hyperinsulinemia of insulin resistance plays a direct role in stimulating ovarian androgen production in PCOS. In the ovary, the theca cell produces testosterone via an enzyme called cytochrome P450c17. Studies indicate that insulin can directly stimulate this enzyme in the ovary and thereby increase testosterone production. Insulin can also enhance stimulation of ovarian testosterone production by luteinizing hormone (LH). These effects may be due to both increased circulating insulin levels and/or increased "gain" in ovarian theca cell response to insulin for the production of testosterone.

In addition to its direct effects on the ovary, hyperinsulinemia can increase the availability of circulating free testosterone in PCOS. In normal women, 99% of circulating testosterone is bound to a protein called sex hormone-binding globulin

(SHBG), which is produced primarily by the liver. Less than 1% of testosterone is free or unbound in normal women, and it is held that free testosterone is the biologically active form of the hormone. Hyperinsulinemia increases circulating free testosterone in PCOS by directly and independently suppressing hepatic production of SHBG. Therefore, most women with PCOS have relatively low measurable serum SHBG and increased free testosterone concentrations.

Finally, insulin may also contribute to anovulation in PCOS by affecting gonadotropin secretion. In animal models, insulin has been demonstrated to increase secretion of LH from the anterior pituitary. Insulin could also affect ovulation through interactions with the intraovarian insulin-like growth factor system.

Obesity and Other Associated Risks

OBESITY

In addition to the insulin resistance intrinsic to PCOS, many women with PCOS suffer an additional burden of insulin resistance secondary to obesity. At least 50% to 80% of women with PCOS are obese. This also implies that at least 20% of women with PCOS are lean, yet studies have shown that these lean women are also insulin resistant. Obesity is clearly associated with increased risk for chronic health problems later in life, such as cardiovascular disease and type 2 diabetes mellitus. Multiple studies now indicate that women with PCOS are at significantly increased risk for both, especially in those with family history of type 2 diabetes mellitus in a first-degree relative.

TYPE 2 DIABETES MELLITUS

Women with PCOS are at increased risk for both IGT (defined as a plasma glucose >139 and <200 mg/dL at 2 hours during a 75-g dextrose oral glucose tolerance test) and type 2 diabetes mellitus. Notably, 35% to 50% of women with PCOS will have either IGT or type 2 diabetes by the age of 35. The prevalence of type 2 diabetes in women with PCOS is approximately 10%, and the prevalence of IGT is even higher, at 40%.

IGT is recognized as a major risk factor for the development of type 2 diabetes, and the rate of conversion from IGT to frank type 2 diabetes mellitus is from 1% to 5% per year. Therefore, women with PCOS are at extremely high risk for the development of type 2 diabetes. In fact, among premenopausal women with previously diagnosed type 2 diabetes mellitus, the prevalence of PCOS has been found to be greater than 25%. The risk for developing type 2 diabetes in a woman with PCOS is further augmented and particularly high if she has a positive family history for type 2 diabetes mellitus.

CARDIOVASCULAR DISEASE

The syndrome of insulin resistance consists of increased risk of type 2 diabetes mellitus, coronary artery disease, dyslipidemia (low serum high-density-lipoprotein [HDL] cholesterol and high triglycerides), and hypertension. This clustering of disorders has been termed "syndrome X" or the "dysmetabolic syndrome."

Women with PCOS often display features of the dysmetabolic syndrome, such as hyperinsulinemia, hypertension, propensity for abdominal obesity, and low serum HDL cholesterol. The presence of the dysmetabolic syndrome is now recognized as a major cardiac risk factor by the third consensus conference of the National Cholesterol Education Program, and the dysmetabolic syndrome was recently assigned a separate ICD-9 code (277.7).

Although no long-term prospective studies are yet published that directly evaluate cardiovascular mortality in women with PCOS, multiple studies have evaluated surrogate endpoints such as carotid intimal thickness and nitrous oxide–mediated vasodilatation. The findings of these studies strongly support the idea that women with PCOS are at significantly increased risk for cardiovascular disease. In addition, because women with PCOS have increased prevalence of obesity, low serum HDL cholesterol, and hypertension, they often display multiple risk factors for the development of coronary artery disease.

DIFFERENTIAL DIAGNOSIS

The differential diagnosis for PCOS is listed in Table 37.1. The list includes the differential for women who present with a history of chronic oligomenorrhea or anovulation in the presence of hirsutism. The evaluation of these women includes testing for the presence of nonclassic congenital adrenal hyperplasia (due most commonly to adrenal 21-hydroxylase enzyme deficiency) and for the presence of androgen-secreting tumors of the adrenal or ovary. Both are relatively rare disorders compared with PCOS. In addition, all women with secondary amenorrhea should have a baseline laboratory evaluation to exclude thyroid disease and hyperprolactinemia. If hirsutism is the primary complaint or finding but chronic anovulation or oligomenorrhea is absent, the diagnosis of idiopathic familial hirsutism should be entertained. However, it should be noted that up to 10% of women with PCOS may have regular monthly menstrual cycles that on further evaluation were documented to be anovulatory. Anovulation can be documented by the presence of an inappropriately low midluteal serum progesterone level (<2.5 ng/mL).

TABLE 37.1. Differential Diagnosis and Laboratory Values for Hirsutism Associated with Oligomenorrhea[a]

Diagnosis	Diagnostic laboratory values[b]
Polycystic ovary syndrome	Total testosterone >50 ng/dL or free testosterone >0.90 ng/dL
Nonclassic congenital adrenal hyperplasia (21-hydroxylase deficiency)	17α-hydroxyprogesterone >200 ng/dL (value greater than 200 ng/dL merits referral to an endocrinologist for further tests)
Androgen-secreting adrenal tumors or ovarian tumors	Dehydroepiandrosterone sulfate (DHEAS) >700 ng/dL
Cushing syndrome	24-hour urinary free cortisol >50 μg/dL

[a]In addition, all patients with oligomenorrhea should be evaluated for thyroid disease and prolactinoma (see text).
[b]To convert total testosterone and free testosterone to nmol/L, multiply by 3.467; to convert 17α-hydroxyprogesterone to nmol/L, multiply by 0.03026; to convert DHEAS to μmol/L, multiply by 2.714; to convert free cortisol to nmol/L, multiply by 27.59.

CLINICAL SYMPTOMS OR HISTORY

Patients with PCOS often present with menstrual abnormalities, most commonly oligomenorrhea (frequently defined as six or fewer menstrual periods per year). The presence of oligomenorrhea may begin early after menarche or later in the reproductive years. Patients with PCOS may also present with a history of dysfunctional uterine bleeding or menometrorrhagia. The latter occurs due to a lack of increased concentrations of midcycle progesterone resulting in endometrial hyperplasia and persistent heavy bleeding patterns.

Hirsutism is also a common complaint among women with PCOS and is defined as increased terminal body hair growth in unwanted areas, such as the face, back, down the inner thigh, or on the torso above the umbilicus. Not all women with PCOS are hirsute, however, and evidence suggests that certain ethnicities (Asians, Northern Europeans) are less prone to hirsutism despite prominent elevations in serum testosterone levels. In addition to hirsutism, PCOS patients may also complain of persistent adult acne (or severe acne during adolescence) or alopecia, both driven by excess testosterone.

An obstetric history is often revealing as well. Women with PCOS may have prior history of infertility and may have required fertility treatments in the past. Many of these women also have a history of early pregnancy loss, as some studies report that women with PCOS are at increased risk for first-trimester miscarriage. Finally, women with PCOS may reveal a history of gestational diabetes during prior pregnancies. A family history may be strongly positive for type 2 diabetes mellitus in both male and female family members and may also be positive for symptoms of PCOS in female family members.

PHYSICAL FINDINGS

Most of the physical findings are associated with either hyperandrogenism or insulin resistance and are not specific to PCOS. Of note, increased serum testosterone levels can produce hirsutism, alopecia, or persistent adult acne. A pelvic examination may be abnormal, revealing palpable enlarged ovaries or even clitoromegaly. The presence of clitoromegaly, however, is usually accompanied by extremely high androgen levels (serum testosterone >200 ng/dL) and may be associated with a condition called hyperthecosis. The presence of clitoromegaly also necessitates the exclusion of an ovarian or adrenal androgen-secreting tumor.

Because most women with PCOS are also insulin resistant, obesity, particularly abdominal obesity (waist circumference >33 inches), is a highly prevalent finding among women with the disorder. In addition, due to insulin resistance, acanthosis nigricans, a raised velvety hyperpigmented plaque found in the supranuchal area or the axilla, is often seen. Finally, many of these women will display clinical hypertension at a relatively young age, likely due to their insulin resistance or hyperinsulinemia.

LABORATORY FINDINGS

Table 37.1 summarizes some of the common laboratory values evaluated to both confirm the presence of PCOS and to exclude other causes of hirsutism or chronic oligomenorrhea.

Before evaluation, women should withhold hormonal contraceptive therapy for at least 4 months because endogenous pituitary and gonadal hormones will be suppressed in the presence of exogenous estrogens or progestins. For the diagnosis of PCOS, a number of laboratory values and assessments have been used in a combined fashion, such as the ratio of LH to follicle-stimulating hormone, total testosterone, free testosterone, and SHBG. Current literature suggests that in an unselected population of women evaluated for oligomenorrhea and hirsutism, the presence of an elevated free testosterone (>1 ng/dL) and a low SHBG (<37 nmol/L) was 87% sensitive and 87% specific in identifying the presence of PCOS.

Notably, although an increased ratio of LH to follicle-stimulating hormone greater than 2.5 is relatively specific for the presence of PCOS, it is not very sensitive, particularly in obese women with PCOS. The LH value can also be acutely suppressed if measured within 2 weeks of a recent ovulation. It is also important to note that a pelvic ultrasound finding of anatomically polycystic ovaries is neither a sensitive nor specific test to diagnose PCOS, because as many as 20% of normal women will have this finding. It is for this reason that the presence of polycystic ovaries is not included in the NICHD conference's defining criteria for the diagnosis of PCOS (see Definition and Etiology, above).

Because women with PCOS are at increased risk for type 2 diabetes and cardiovascular disease and frequently suffer from dyslipidemia and hypertension, they should be evaluated by a 75-g dextrose 2-hour oral glucose tolerance test and a lipid profile. It is unknown how frequently these tests should be repeated, but given the high risk, every 2 to 3 years does not seem unreasonable and would be consistent with American Diabetes Association guidelines for populations at risk.

TREATMENT

The treatment of women with PCOS can be divided into three major categories: (a) chronic management of oligomenorrhea and other health-related issues, (b) treatment of hirsutism, and (c) treatment of infertility.

Chronic Management of Oligomenorrhea

ORAL CONTRACEPTIVES

Historically, treatment of oligomenorrhea in PCOS has been based on the use of oral contraceptives or other reproductive hormonal drugs. Hormonal contraceptives often provide regular menses and reduce the incidence of endometrial hyperplasia in affected women. However, they may also have the disadvantages of increasing serum triglycerides, worsening insulin resistance, and inducing glucose intolerance in these women. It is therefore advisable to monitor for the presence of these adverse effects as much as possible while a patient is being treated with hormonal contraceptives.

Because women with PCOS are insulin resistant and have increased propensity for dyslipidemia and hypertension, highly progestational or progestin-only type drugs (such as Depo-Provera) are less advocated. Rather, monophasic oral contraceptives with low androgenic potential such as Demulen 1/35 (35 μg ethinyl estradiol plus 1 mg ethynodiol) or Yasmin 28 (drospirenone/ethinyl estradiol) are preferable. Persistent dysfunctional bleeding despite the use of oral contraceptives or despite the use of intermittent medroxyprogesterone therapy for 7 days may merit further evaluation and treatment by a gynecologist for the presence of endometrial hyperplasia, fibroids, or endometrial cancer.

INSULIN-SENSITIZING DRUGS

Recently, insulin-sensitizing drugs such as metformin or thiazolidinediones (rosiglitazone or pioglitazone) have become a viable option for the treatment of PCOS. These drugs have the advantage of reducing insulin resistance in these women and therefore do not exacerbate and often improve dyslipidemia and hypertension.

With respect to hyperandrogenism, use of insulin-sensitizing drugs improves menstrual frequency and monthly ovulation by as much as 50% or more in PCOS, permitting a woman who is seeking pregnancy to spontaneously ovulate and conceive. These drugs may also enhance overall fertility in PCOS. Metformin has been shown to reduce serum free testosterone from 40% to 70% in both lean and obese women with PCOS, which is related in part to an increase in serum SHBG. Reduction in serum insulin with these drugs is accompanied by a generous increase in SHBG and therefore a reduction in free testosterone.

Neither metformin nor the thiazolidinediones cause hypoglycemia in nondiabetic individuals; both can ameliorate blood glucose control in women with IGT or type 2 diabetes mellitus. Patients with history of renal insufficiency (serum creatinine >1.6 mg/dL), significant congestive heart failure, or increased liver function tests greater than 2.5 times normal are not candidates for metformin. Similarly, patients with elevated liver function tests or congestive heart failure are not candidates for thiazolidinediones.

Overall, metformin should be considered the preferred insulin-sensitizing drug in the typical premenopausal woman with PCOS because it is a U.S. Food and Drug Administration category B drug safe for use in pregnancy, whereas the thiazolidinediones are category C drugs associated with teratogenicity in animal models.

Metformin can be administered in doses from 1,500 to 2,000 mg/d in two divided doses. This dose is usually achieved gradually over 3 to 4 weeks to avoid the side effects of diarrhea or gastrointestinal distress. Thiazolidinediones, such as pioglitazone or rosiglitazone, can be administered as recommended in diabetic individuals. Once these drugs have been initiated, it is advisable to monitor the patient's serum total and free testosterone at 3- to 4-month intervals to assess response to therapy. A menstrual diary is also helpful. Most patients will have considerable improvement in menstrual frequency after 3 to 4 months of therapy, though this may take longer in some.

DIET AND WEIGHT LOSS

Just as the insulin-sensitizing drugs help to improve menstrual frequency and hyperandrogenemia in women with PCOS, so does weight loss, with its attendant improvement in insulin sensitivity. Multiple studies have demonstrated that even mild weight loss (5%–10%) accomplished by hypocaloric diets (1,000–1,400 kcal/d) and exercise significantly increases insulin sensitivity, improves menstrual frequency, reduces serum free testosterone (and increases SHBG), and improves ovulation and conception rates.

For those women who are morbidly obese (body mass index >40 kg/m^2), some studies suggest that insulin-sensitizing drugs alone may not be adequate to reduce hyperandrogenism and that weight loss becomes a prerequisite to successful therapy. In addition, at least one study has demonstrated that the combined use of metformin with weight loss therapy can be additive in terms of reducing insulin resistance, adiposity, and serum testosterone levels. Given that these women are also at high risk for the development of type 2 diabetes mellitus and coronary artery disease, it seems reasonable to advocate weight loss as adjunctive therapy for prevention of these chronic diseases and for treatment of symptoms of PCOS.

A recent development has been the frequent use of low carbohydrate diets for weight loss. However, the use of such diets should be limited because many of these diets are also composed of high saturated fats, which can both exacerbate insulin resistance and increase the risk for the coronary artery disease.

Hirsutism

In addition to local cosmetic methods (such as electrolysis or depilatories), hirsutism may be treated using an antiandrogen. Antiandrogens block hair growth by competitively binding to the dihydrotestosterone and testosterone receptor at the hair follicle. These drugs can improve both the hirsutism and acne associated with PCOS. Among the most commonly used of the antiandrogens is the diuretic spironolactone, which is an aldosterone antagonist with high affinity for the dihydrotestosterone receptor. It also acts as a weak inhibitor of testosterone biosynthesis. Spironolactone is commonly administered in dosages of 50 to 100 mg twice daily and can lead to modest to moderate reductions in hirsutism and acne. Its primary side effect is dysfunctional menstrual bleeding. It also has a potential for teratogenicity, and an oral contraceptive is usually recommended as concurrent therapy.

In addition to spironolactone, the drugs finasteride and flutamide have been used in the United States to treat hirsutism. Both drugs should not be used in pregnancy because of risk of teratogenicity. Flutamide is used less frequently because of its increased cost and side effects. Rarely, flutamide has been associated with liver toxicity. Finasteride is a 5-reductase inhibitor, and its mechanism of action is to inhibit the conversion of testosterone to dihydrotestosterone. Finasteride, given at a dose of 5 mg daily, provides modest reduction of hirsutism over 6 months time.

Finally, eflornithine hydrochloride is a new prescription cream that can be applied twice daily to the face to slow facial hair growth. Because it can be applied only to the face, it offers no benefit for other sites of excess hair growth, and it can sometimes exacerbate acne.

Fertility

Treatment of infertility in PCOS is usually managed by a reproductive endocrinologist or gynecologist. Usually, treatment is initiated with clomiphene citrate in gradually increasing doses to induce ovulation. Current data suggest that concomitant use of metformin with clomiphene citrate increases the success rate of ovulation induction and increases pregnancy rates. Women who fail to conceive despite successful induction of ovulation with clomiphene citrate alone or with artificial insemination merit further evaluation for uterine or anatomic abnormalities. In women who fail other methods, in vitro fertilization is frequently used.

ACKNOWLEDGMENTS

Supported by NCRR M01RR00065-37S1 (to M. J. I.) and K24HD40237 (to J. E. N.).

BIBLIOGRAPHY

Azziz R, Ehrmann D, Legro RS, et al. Troglitazone improves ovulation and hirsutism in the polycystic ovary syndrome: a multicenter, double blind, placebo-controlled trial. *J Clin Endocrinol Metab* 2001;86:1626–1632.

Balen AH, Conway GS, Kaltsas G, et al. Polycystic ovary syndrome: the spectrum of the disorder in 1,741 patients. *Hum Reprod* 1995;10:2107–2111.

Carmina E, Lobo RA. Do hyperandrogenic women with normal menses have polycystic ovary syndrome? *Fertil Steril* 1999;71:319–322.

Chang RJ, Nakamura RM, Judd HL, et al. Insulin resistance in nonobese patients with polycystic ovarian disease. *J Clin Endocrinol Metab* 1983;57:356–359.

Coleman MP, Key TJ, Wang DY, et al. A prospective study of obesity, lipids, apolipoproteins, and ischaemic heart disease in women. *Atherosclerosis* 1992;92:177–185.
Dunaif A, Segal KR, Futterweit W, et al. Profound peripheral insulin resistance, independent of obesity, in polycystic ovary syndrome. *Diabetes* 1989;38:1165–1174.
Ehrmann DA, Sturis J, Byrne MM, et al. Insulin secretory defects in polycystic ovary syndrome: relationship to insulin sensitivity and family history of non-insulin-dependent diabetes mellitus. *J Clin Invest* 1995;96:520–527.
Escobar-Morreale HF, Asuncion M, Calvo RM, et al. Receiver operating characteristic analysis of the performance of basal serum hormone profiles for the diagnosis of polycystic ovary syndrome in epidemiological studies. *Eur J Endocrinol* 2001;145:619–624.
Fedorcsak P, Storeng R, Dale PO, et al. Obesity is a risk factor for early pregnancy loss after IVF or ICSI. *Acta Obstet Gynaecol Scand* 2000;79:43–48.
Gokmen O, Senoz S, Gulekli B, et al. Comparison of four different treatment regimes in hirsutism related to polycystic ovary syndrome. *Gynecol Endocrinol* 1996;10:249–255.
Korytkowski MT, Mokan M, Horwitz MJ, et al. Metabolic effects of oral contraceptives in women with polycystic ovary syndrome. *J Clin Endocrinol Metab* 1995;80:3327–3334.
Legro RS, Kunselman AR, Dodson WC, et al. Prevalence and predictors of risk for type 2 diabetes mellitus and impaired glucose tolerance in polycystic ovary syndrome: a prospective, controlled study in 254 affected women. *J Clin Endocrinol Metab* 1999;84:165–169.
Moghetti P, Castello R, Negri C, et al. Metformin effects on clinical features, endocrine and metabolic profiles, and insulin sensitivity in polycystic ovary syndrome: a randomized, double-blind, placebo-controlled 6-month trial, followed by open, long-term clinical evaluation. *J Clin Endocrinol Metab* 2000;85:139–146.
Muderris II, Bayram F, Guven M. A prospective, randomized trial comparing flutamide (250 mg/d) and finasteride (5 mg/d) in the treatment of hirsutism. *Fertil Steril* 2000;73:984–987.
Nestler JE, Barlascini CO, Matt DW, et al. Suppression of serum insulin by diazoxide reduces serum testosterone levels in obese women with polycystic ovary syndrome. *J Clin Endocrinol Metab* 1989;68:1027–1032.
Nestler JE, Jakubowicz DJ. Decreases in ovarian cytochrome P450c17α activity and serum free testosterone after reduction in insulin secretion in women with polycystic ovary syndrome. *N Engl J Med* 1996;335:617–623.
Nestler JE, Jakubowicz DJ. Lean women with polycystic ovary syndrome respond to insulin reduction with decreases in ovarian P450c17α activity and serum androgens. *J Clin Endocrinol Metab* 1997;82:4075–4079.
Nestler JE, Powers LP, Matt DW, et al. A direct effect of hyperinsulinemia on serum sex hormone-binding globulin levels in obese women with the polycystic ovary syndrome. *J Clin Endocrinol Metab* 1991;72:83–89.
Pasquali R, Gambineri A, Biscotti D, et al. Effect of long-term treatment with metformin added to hypocaloric diet on body composition, fat distribution, and androgen and insulin levels in abdominally obese women with and without the polycystic ovary syndrome. *J Clin Endocrinol Metab* 2000;85: 2767–2774.
Reaven GM. Banting lecture 1988: role of insulin resistance in human disease. *Diabetes* 1988;37:1595–1607.
Talbott EO, Guzick DS, Sutton-Tyrrell K, et al. Evidence for association between polycystic ovary syndrome and premature carotid atherosclerosis in middle-aged women. *Arterioscler Thromb Vasc Biol* 2000;20:2414–2421.
Zawadzki JK, Dunaif A. Diagnostic criteria for polycystic ovary syndrome: towards a rational approach. In: Dunaif A, Givens JR, Haseltine FP, et al., eds. *Polycystic ovary syndrome.* Boston: Blackwell Scientific, 1992:377–384.

CHAPTER 38
Parathyroid Disease

Diane M. Biskobing and Angela Novy

Primary hyperparathyroidism is the most common cause of hypercalcemia, with a 3:1 predominance in women. The average age at diagnosis is in the sixth decade, with an incidence of 1 in 500 to 1 in 1,000. Overall, the prevalence in women is estimated to be 0.45%, but in women over the age of 70 the prevalence may be as high as 2% to 3.6%. Because the only curative therapy for primary hyperparathyroidism is surgery, careful assessment of the asymptomatic patient should be done to determine whether surgery is indicated.

Serum calcium levels are tightly regulated by parathyroid hormone (PTH) and 1,25-dihydroxyvitamin D. PTH secretion from the parathyroid glands is controlled by extracellular calcium via a calcium receptor. As serum calcium falls, PTH secretion is increased and vice versa. PTH then acts on the bones to increase bone resorption and release of calcium into the extracellular fluid. In addition, PTH has two effects on the kidneys that increase serum calcium: Renal tubular reabsorption of calcium is increased and activity of the 1-hydroxylase enzyme is stimulated, increasing production of 1,25-dihydroxyvitamin D. The major action of 1,25-dihydroxyvitamin D is to increase gastrointestinal absorption of calcium and phosphorous.

ETIOLOGY

Primary hyperparathyroidism is due to inappropriate secretion of PTH despite elevated serum calcium. Most patients have a solitary benign parathyroid adenoma (80%–85%). Four-gland hyperplasia (10%–15%), multiple adenomas (2%), and carcinoma (<1%) are much less common.

The exact etiology for sporadic parathyroid adenomas is not known. Adenomas have been found to be of clonal origin, suggesting a genetic defect within the parathyroid cell. Several candidate genes have been proposed, but there are likely multiple genetic mutations that result in clonal growth. The adenomas exhibit an altered set point for feedback inhibition of PTH secretion. The remaining three glands display normal function.

Four-gland parathyroid hyperplasia is most frequently seen in association with hereditary forms of primary hyperparathyroidism. The most common etiology of hereditary primary hyperparathyroidism is multiple endocrine neoplasia type 1 (MEN-1)—consisting of anterior pituitary, parathyroid, and pancreatic tumors. Inheritance is autosomal dominant, with primary hyperparathyroidism being the most common feature. The genetic defect has recently been localized to the long arm of chromosome 11.

Multiple endocrine neoplasia type 2A (MEN-2A), also inherited as an autosomal-dominant trait, is characterized by medullary thyroid carcinoma, pheochromocytomas, and hyperparathyroidism due to parathyroid hyperplasia. Hyperparathyroidism, however, in distinction from MEN-1, is the least common manifestation, with only 10% to 30% developing overt hypercalcemia. Many more patients have been reported to have hyperplasia on pathologic specimens but do not have clinical hypercalcemia.

Other familial causes of hyperparathyroidism include the hyperparathyroidism-jaw tumor syndrome and familial isolated hyperparathyroidism. The hyperparathyroidism-jaw tumor syndrome has an autosomal-dominant inheritance and is characterized by early onset parathyroid tumors with severe hypercalcemia and fibroosseous jaw tumors. There is controversy whether familial isolated hyperparathyroidism is a distinct entity from the other familial syndromes. Several kindreds with familial hypercalcemia have been reported, but many of these were later classified as MEN-1 or hyperparathyroidism-jaw tumor syndrome.

DIFFERENTIAL DIAGNOSIS

The differential diagnosis of hypercalcemia is extensive (Table 38.1). Most cases of hypercalcemia seen in the primary care setting are due to either primary hyperparathyroidism or malignancy. All other causes account for less than 10% of cases. Initially, the differential diagnosis can be narrowed with measurement of intact PTH. Primary hyperparathyroidism is characterized by elevated intact PTH in the setting of high cal-

TABLE 38.1. Differential Diagnosis of Hypercalcemia

Elevated PTH
Primary hyperparathyroidism
Familial hypocalciuric hypercalcemia
Suppressed PTH
Hypercalcemia of malignancy
Humoral hypercalcemia of malignancy
Lytic bone lesions
Granulomatous disease
Sarcoidosis
Tuberculosis
Histoplasmosis
Coccidiomycosis
Leprosy
Endocrine disorders
Thyrotoxicosis
Adrenal insufficiency
Pheochromocytoma
VIPoma
Drugs
Vitamin D
Thiazide diuretics
Lithium
Vitamin A
Aminophylline
Miscellaneous
Immobilization
Renal failure
TPN
Milk-alkali syndrome

PTH, parathyroid hormone; TPN, total parenteral nutrition.

cium. Familial hypocalciuric hypercalcemia can also present with mildly elevated calcium and PTH. This autosomal-dominant syndrome is characterized by low urinary calcium excretion in the setting of mildly elevated calcium that does not respond to parathyroidectomy. The genetic defect has recently been identified as a mutation in the calcium receptor gene in the parathyroid and renal tubular cells. All other causes of hypercalcemia are associated with suppressed PTH levels.

Hypercalcemia of malignancy is the most likely etiology for hypercalcemia with a low PTH. Humoral hypercalcemia of malignancy due to PTH-related peptide secretion by the tumor is seen with tumors of the lung, esophagus, head and neck, renal cell, ovary, and bladder. Hypercalcemia resulting from lytic bone lesions is most commonly associated with multiple myeloma and breast cancer. Other causes of hypercalcemia characterized by a suppressed PTH are much less common. Granulomatous disease such as sarcoidosis is associated with ectopic production of 1,25-dihydroxyvitamin D. Hypercalcemia is occasionally seen in thyrotoxicosis but much less frequently associated with adrenal insufficiency, pheochromocytoma, and a vasoactive intestinal polypeptide tumor.

Occasionally, an elevated PTH level is found in the absence of hypercalcemia. Primary hyperparathyroidism can rarely be associated with high normal calcium. When calcium levels are in the low to low normal range, other etiologies leading to secondary hyperparathyroidism need to be considered. Chronic renal failure results in elevated phosphorus and decreased production of 1,25-dihydroxyvitamin D, leading to decreased gastrointestinal absorption of calcium and decreased serum calcium. PTH levels become elevated in response to the low serum calcium and elevated phosphorus. This is a fairly obvious cause for secondary hyperparathyroidism; however, other causes may be less evident. Hepatobiliary disease can lead to decreased production of 25-hydroxyvitamin D and secondary hyperparathyroidism. Occult nutritional vitamin D deficiency can result in secondary hyperparathyroidism. If vitamin D deficiency is diagnosed and ultraviolet radiation exposure and nutritional intake appear to be adequate, further workup for malabsorption is indicated.

CLINICAL SYMPTOMS AND HISTORY

Albright described classic symptoms of primary hyperparathyroidism nearly 70 years ago. He described a series of patients who presented with nephrolithiasis, bone lesions, and a proximal neuromyopathy. Today, in contrast, patients rarely present with these classic symptoms because the diagnosis of hypercalcemia is often an incidental laboratory finding. Approximately 25% of patients develop nephrolithiasis. However, most patients now present with much more subtle symptoms or are asymptomatic.

The bone disease most clearly associated with primary hyperparathyroidism is osteitis fibrosa cystica characterized by bone cysts and brown tumors. However, patients now rarely present with this advanced manifestation of hyperparathyroidism. More commonly seen is evidence of excessive bone remodeling demonstrated by development of osteoporosis. Classically, PTH excess results in cortical bone loss demonstrated by low bone density in the wrist. However, more recently, trabecular bone loss leading to osteoporosis in the spine has been described in a subset of patients with hyperparathyroidism. A long-term study of patients with primary hyperparathyroidism in Rochester, Minnesota showed increased risk for vertebral, forearm, rib, and pelvic fractures.

Neurologic dysfunction such as proximal myopathy, which resolved after parathyroid surgery, was clearly demonstrated in the early patients with advanced disease. Currently, patients presenting with mild hyperparathyroidism do not exhibit evidence of myopathy. Other nonspecific symptoms, such as cognitive impairment, depression, fatigue, and weakness, have been historically associated with hyperparathyroidism. Yet, controversy exists over the extent to which these other neuropsychiatric symptoms can be attributed to primary hyperparathyroidism. Several studies have failed to show that these symptoms are more common in hyperparathyroidism or change significantly after parathyroidectomy.

In addition, other signs and symptoms previously described as features of hyperparathyroidism have not been shown to be clearly associated with the disease. Hypertension is found more frequently in patients with primary hyperparathyroidism. However, it is unclear whether the hypercalcemia is causative or coincidental because most patients remain hypertensive after surgical cure of hyperparathyroidism. Left ventricular hypertrophy has also been associated with primary hyperparathyroidism in the past but is rarely seen today in mild hyperparathyroidism. Previously peptic ulcer disease was reported to be associated with hyperparathyroidism. However, there is no clear evidence of an increased prevalence of peptic ulcers associated with primary hyperparathyroidism, outside the setting of MEN-1 syndrome. Pancreatitis also has been reported in the past with increased frequency in those with primary hyperparathyroidism; currently it is rarely seen because calcium elevations tend to be very mild.

Signs and symptoms due to hypercalcemia, regardless of the etiology, are most often dependent on the degree of calcium elevation. Constipation is the most common gastrointestinal complaint of patients with hypercalcemia. Increasing levels of calcium may also result in nausea, vomiting, and abdominal pain. Pancreatitis occurs with extreme elevations of calcium. Hypercalcemia leads to polyuria as a result of interference with vasopressin stimulated free water reabsorption. This places the hypercalcemic patient at risk for volume depletion and worsening hypercalcemia. Cardiac effects of marked hypercalcemia include shortened QT intervals. Central nervous system effects are dependent on the degree of elevation. Mild increases in calcium are associated with fatigue but can progress to altered mental status and eventually coma.

CLINICAL FINDINGS AND PHYSICAL EXAMINATION

Findings on physical examination in patients with mild primary hyperparathyroidism are minimal. A normal physical examination is consistent with a diagnosis of primary hyperparathyroidism. Enlarged parathyroid adenomas are not usually palpable in the neck except in the case of parathyroid carcinoma.

LABORATORY AND IMAGING STUDIES

Once hypercalcemia is confirmed, initial testing should begin with an intact PTH level, which will determine the focus of further testing (Fig. 38.1). If PTH is elevated, 24-hour urine calcium and creatinine should be measured as well as concurrent serum creatinine. From these values, the fractional excretion of calcium can be determined. If fractional excretion of calcium is low (<0.01), then familial hypocalciuric hypercalcemia is likely and further evaluation is not warranted. Surgery is not recommended in patients with familial hypocalciuric hypercalcemia because hypercalcemia persists after parathyroidectomy. If urine calcium excretion is high, then primary hyperparathyroidism is confirmed. Bone mineral density testing should be done to aid in the decision whether to recommend surgery.

Low PTH should lead to an evaluation for other causes of hypercalcemia as listed in Table 38.1 and Fig. 38.1. The clinical presentation will likely suggest one or more of the potential causes of hypercalcemia. 25-Hydroxyvitamin D and 1,25-dihydroxyvitamin D levels may be helpful in confirming suspicion of vitamin D toxicity or increased 1,25-dihydroxyvitamin D production by granulomas. Further laboratory evaluation such as thyroid function tests, cortisol, serum protein electrophoresis, or PTH-related peptide levels should be obtained on a case-by-case basis.

Imaging studies are not necessary to confirm the diagnosis of primary hyperparathyroidism nor have they been done routinely to locate the adenoma before parathyroidectomy. The standard operative procedure for parathyroidectomy has been bilateral neck exploration with identification of all four parathyroid glands and frozen section before excision of the parathyroid adenoma. When an experienced parathyroid surgeon does bilateral neck exploration, imaging studies have not been shown to increase the long-term success rate of parathyroidectomy or decrease morbidity.

However, with the current advent of less invasive surgical procedures and shorter hospital stays, the issue of preoperative imaging has once again come to the forefront. Several centers now perform preoperative imaging with neck ultrasound or sestamibi scanning to localize the lesion before unilateral neck exploration. If a single lesion is identified by ultrasound or a single focus of uptake is seen on sestamibi scanning, the success rate of unilateral neck exploration has been reported to be sim-

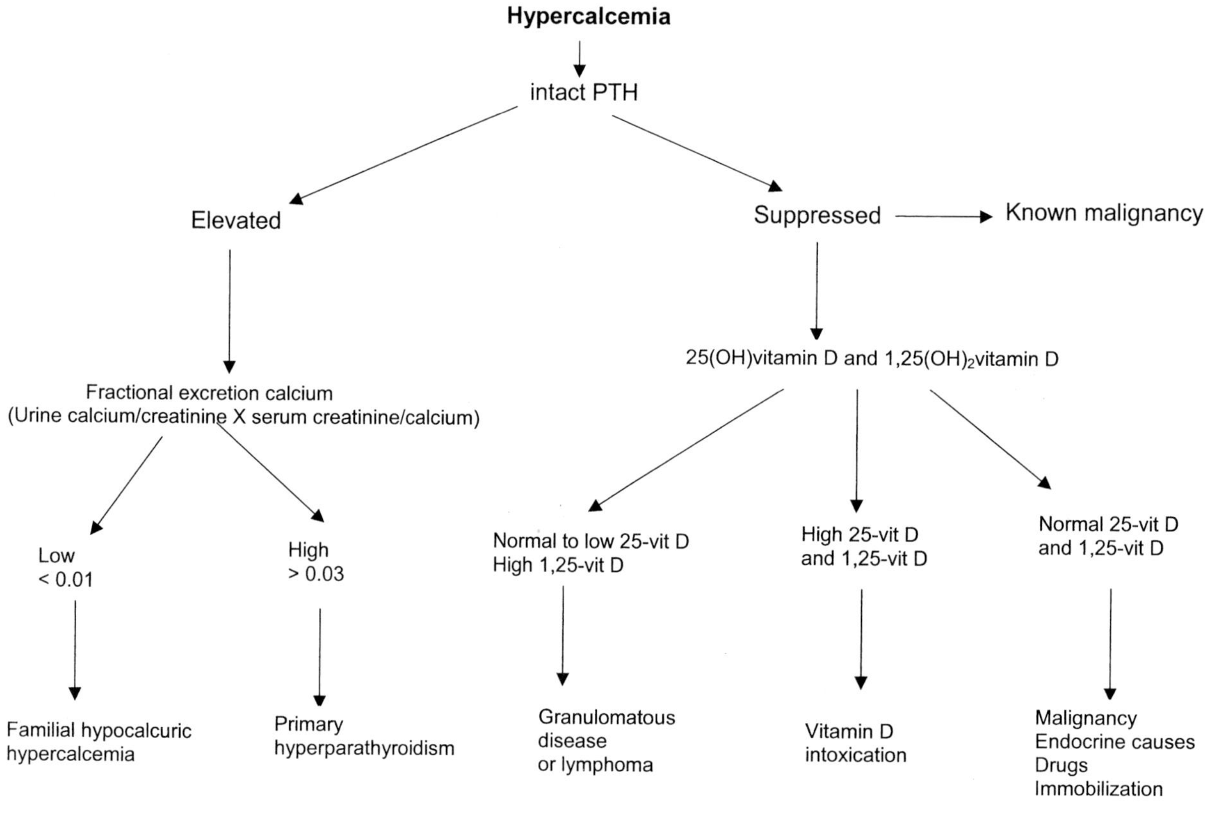

FIG. 38.1. Laboratory evaluation of hypercalcemia.

ilar to bilateral neck exploration. The most accepted indication for sestamibi scanning is to localize a lesion in a patient with recurrent or persistent hypercalcemia if the first neck exploration was not curative.

TREATMENT

Decisions concerning the management of primary hyperparathyroidism should be made in conjunction with an endocrinologist. Once a diagnosis of primary hyperparathyroidism is confirmed, the patient should be referred to an endocrinologist to consider whether surgery is indicated. The only effective treatment currently is parathyroidectomy by an experienced surgeon. Surgical cure is seen in greater than 95% of patients after the first neck exploration. The best guarantee that a patient will experience minimal complications with a surgical cure is to refer to an experienced parathyroid surgeon. Successful parathyroidectomy leads to resolution of classic symptoms of hyperparathyroidism. In addition, patients with lumbar spine osteoporosis show significant improvement in bone mineral density after surgery.

Debate continues in the surgical community over the best surgical technique for parathyroidectomy. Bilateral neck exploration has been the gold standard, with excellent success rates and minimal morbidity. However, the question now arises whether minimally invasive unilateral neck exploration with preoperative imaging is more cost effective and efficient while achieving similar success rates as the standard procedure. In the centers with the most experience, success rates for cure of hypercalcemia are greater than 90% and complications have been reported to be less than bilateral neck exploration. However, because some unilateral explorations have to be converted to bilateral procedures, these procedures should only be performed by surgeons experienced with bilateral exploration. In addition, surgeons specializing in minimally invasive parathyroid surgery are currently not available in many communities.

Because many patients are asymptomatic at presentation, surgery may not be indicated in all patients. In 2002 the National Institutes of Health held a consensus conference to update recommendations for the management of asymptomatic primary hyperparathyroidism. At that conference it was agreed that all patients with classic symptoms of hyperparathyroidism should have parathyroidectomy. Criteria for surgical management of asymptomatic patients were updated from the 1990 recommendations. Parathyroidectomy was recommended for the following indications: (a) age less than 50, (b) serum calcium greater than 1 mg/dL above the upper limit of normal, (c) 24-hour urine calcium excretion greater than 400 mg/d, (d) bone density of the distal radius, lumbar spine, or hip more than 2.5 standard deviations below peak bone mass (T score < -2.5); (e) creatinine clearance reduced by more than 30% compared to age-matched controls.

For those patients who have osteoporosis and refuse surgery or are not surgical candidates, medical therapy should be considered. Oral phosphate was used in the past to lower serum calcium levels. The mechanism may be twofold: increasing the calcium × phosphorus product and inhibition of 1,25-dihyrdroxyvitamin D production. Because of concern over metastatic calcification and deleterious effects on renal function, however, oral phosphorus is now rarely used in the treatment of hyperparathyroidism. Hormone replacement therapy has been shown to slightly but significantly decrease serum calcium levels and improve total body, spine, hip, and forearm bone marrow density. Raloxifene has recently been reported to have similar effects in a small number of patients. Alendronate has also been demonstrated to improve bone marrow density at all sites. However, those treated with alendronate did not show a long-term change in serum calcium levels. Calcium initially decreased after 6 months but rebounded back to baseline by 24 months. PTH, on the other hand, increased in response to the decreased calcium and reached a new equilibrium. A new class of drugs, the calcimimetics, may become available in the near future for medical management of hyperparathyroidism. These agents target the calcium-sensing receptor on the parathyroid cells, increasing their sensitivity to extracellular calcium and decreasing PTH secretion.

Since the development of these guidelines, more information has been collected on the natural history of hyperparathyroidism in asymptomatic patients, who do not have surgery. Silverberg and colleagues published results of a 10-year study of primary hyperparathyroidism with or without surgery. Overall, in a group of 52 untreated patients, serum calcium, urine calcium, and PTH remained stable. Approximately 20% developed biochemical evidence of progression with either marked hypercalcemia (calcium >12 mg/dL) or hypercalciuria (urine calcium >400 mg/d). No one developed a clinically symptomatic complication such as nephrolithiasis. Because there was no predictor of which patient would progress, routine monitoring of these patients is necessary.

PREGNANCY

Primary hyperparathyroidism in women of childbearing age is estimated to be 8 cases per 100,000 population per year. The exact incidence of hyperparathyroidism in pregnancy is unknown because it rarely occurs. As in all cases of primary hyperparathyroidism, the diagnosis is made when elevated calcium is found in association with an inappropriately normal or elevated PTH. After 21 weeks' gestation the volume of maternal plasma increases, thus lowering the serum albumin level. Although ionized calcium is accurate, the total serum calcium level is falsely low in the presence of hypoalbuminemia. Failure to make the appropriate calcium correction could result in delaying or missing the diagnosis.

The symptoms of primary hyperparathyroidism and hypercalcemia in a pregnant woman are the same as those in a nonpregnant person, yet the complications can be more severe due to the pregnancy. Even in an asymptomatic mother, hypercalcemia can lead to neonatal tetany, stillbirth, and spontaneous abortion. Early studies of pregnant women reveal the following complications associated with primary hyperparathyroidism: neonatal tetany (~30%–50%), stillbirth, spontaneous abortion or neonatal death (~25%), and occasional maternal death. In addition, low birth weight, prematurity, and intrauterine growth retardation are reported to occur more commonly in mothers with hyperparathyroidism. The hypercalcemia may also lead to secondary illnesses such as nephrolithiasis, pancreatitis, urinary tract infections, hypertension, and seizures, all of which can lead to complications of the pregnancy. Evaluation and treatment of these illnesses may need to be altered due to possible effects of radiologic procedures and medications on the fetus. A team of physicians, including obstetrics, endocrinology, neonatology, and surgery, is required for the best possible outcome.

Throughout the pregnancy, close monitoring is required because the mother may progress to acute hyperparathyroid or hypercalcemic crisis. This is defined as serum calcium greater than 14 mg/dL, with nausea, vomiting, weakness, and mental status changes potentially progressing to uremia, coma, and death of the mother and/or fetus. It is also important to monitor for worsening hypercalcemia in the mother after delivery. Elevated levels of 1,25-dihydroxyvitamin D combined with the cessation of calcium shunting across the placenta to the fetus and the loss of the extra plasma volume may lead to an acute elevation in calcium. On the contrary, the newborn is at risk for hypocalcemic tetany several hours after birth because of suppression of its own parathyroid glands. This condition usually persists for 3 to 5 months but can be permanent. Treatment consists of supplementary calcium, dietary phosphate restriction, and vitamin D supplementation.

Primary hyperparathyroidism in pregnancy can be managed medically or surgically. Before 1970, surgical treatment of hyperparathyroidism in the pregnant patient was usually performed after delivery. Most of those who have reviewed the small body of literature on cases of hyperparathyroidism in pregnancy have concluded that the risk of obstetric complications is greater in those who did not have curative surgery during the pregnancy. Kelly combined all reported cases from 1930 to 1990. Of a total of 109 reported cases, 70 cases were treated medically and 39 cases were treated surgically, primarily during the first or second trimester. Of the 70 cases treated medically, 53% of the infants developed complications, including 16% with neonatal death. In the 39 cases that underwent parathyroid surgery, the complication rate was only 12.5% and the neonatal death rate was 2.5%. Generally, reports of poor fetal outcome due to surgery primarily involve those that took place during the third trimester. The current National Institutes of Health guidelines for all patients with hyperparathyroidism recommend that all those under 50 years old, including women of childbearing age, have parathyroid surgery. If the diagnosis is made during pregnancy, the treatment of hyperparathyroidism should be individualized based on the symptoms, the severity of the disease, and the gestational age. Generally, surgery should be performed after stabilization of the patient and preferably in the second trimester after organogenesis in the fetus has been completed. In asymptomatic mothers diagnosed in the third trimester and in women with conditions that preclude surgery, medical treatment can be provided until after delivery. Medical treatments during pregnancy include oral phosphates, hydration and furosemide, calcitonin, corticosteroids, and intravenous magnesium sulfate. Mithramycin is contraindicated in pregnancy because of bone marrow, liver, and renal toxicity. Bisphosphonates are contraindicated in pregnancy because they may cause abnormalities in fetal bone development. Close monitoring of calcium levels is required to avoid an acute crisis. In summary, the consequences of hyperparathyroidism during pregnancy incurred by the mother and fetus are significant, making recognition and appropriate management vital.

BIBLIOGRAPHY

Bilezikian JP, Potts JT, Fuleihan GE, et al. Sumary statement from a workshop on asymptomatic primary hyperparathyroidism: a perspective for the 21st century. *J Bone Mineral Res* 2002;17(Suppl 2):N2–N11.

Howe JR. Minimally invasive parathyroid surgery. *Surg Clin North Am* 2000;80: 1399–1426.

Kelly TR. Primary hyperparathyroidism during pregnancy. *Surgery* 1991;110: 1028–1034.

Kort KC, Schiller HJ, Numann PJ. Hyperparathyroidism and pregnancy. *Am J Surg* 1991;177:66–68.

Murray JA, Newman WA, Dacus JV. Hyperparathyroidism in pregnancy: diagnostic dilemma? *Obstet Gynecol Surv* 1997;52:202–205.

Potts J, ed. Proceedings of the NIH consensus development conference on diagnosis and management of asymptomatic primary hyperparathyroidism. *J Bone Mineral Res* 1991;6[Suppl]:2.

Silverberg SJ. Natural history of primary hyperparathyroidism. *Endocrinol Metab Clin North Am* 2000;29:451–464.

Silverberg SJ, Bilezikian JP, Bone HG, et al. Therapeutic controversies in primary hyperparthyroidism. *J Clin Endocrinol Metab* 1999;84:2275–2285.

Strewler GJ. Medical approaches to primary hyperparathyroidism. *Endocrinol Metab Clin North Am* 2000;29:523–539.

CHAPTER 39
Diabetes Mellitus

John N. Clore

DEFINITION AND CLASSIFICATION

Based on evidence linking threshold levels of plasma glucose concentration and diabetic complications, diagnostic criteria for diabetes mellitus have recently undergone review. Diabetes mellitus is currently defined as a plasma glucose level greater than 126 mg/dL (7 mM) after an overnight (10- to 12-hour) fast or a random plasma glucose greater than 200 mg/dL (11.1 mM) (Table 39.1). In most cases, the diagnosis can be made without need for formal glucose tolerance testing. However, a plasma glucose value greater than 200 mg/dL at 2 hours after a 75-g oral glucose tolerance test is also diagnostic. In all cases, confirmation of the result is required before a diagnosis of diabetes can be made. Individuals with fasting plasma glucose values between 110 and 125 mg/dL are at high risk for the development of diabetes (prediabetes) and should be followed closely.

Diabetes mellitus is a heterogeneous group of conditions with hyperglycemia as the common clinical manifestation. Type 1 diabetes mellitus (previously referred to as insulin-dependent diabetes mellitus) is an autoimmune disease characterized by

TABLE 39.1. Diagnostic Criteria for Diabetes Mellitus, Impaired Glucose Tolerance (IGT), and Gestational Diabetes Mellitus (GDM)

	Diabetes mellitus[a]	IGT[a]	GDM[b]
Fasting plasma glucose	≥126 mg/dL	≥110, <126 mg/dL	≥95 mg/dL
1-h OGTT	—		>180 mg/dL
2-h OGTT	>200 mg/dL	≥140, <200 mg/dL	>155 mg/dL
Random	>200 mg/dL		

[a]Values for glucose tolerance testing are after a 75-g oral glucose load.
[b]Values for a 3-h glucose tolerance testing are after a 100-g oral glucose load. A positive diagnosis of GDM is made when two or more thresholds are met or exceeded.
OGTT, oral glucose tolerance test.

absolute insulin deficiency, whereas type 2 diabetes (previously referred to as non–insulin-dependent diabetes mellitus) is characterized by both insulin resistance and a relative impairment in insulin secretion. As discussed below, this change in classification places emphasis on mechanism rather than treatment. In addition to these most common forms of diabetes, hyperglycemia may be observed secondary to either genetic abnormalities in insulin secretion or action or drug-induced insulin resistance. The reader is referred to the report of the Expert Committee of the American Diabetes Association for a full listing of conditions and/or drugs found in this category. Gestational diabetes mellitus (GDM) is retained as a distinct category and is discussed in detail below.

Type 1 diabetes accounts for approximately 6% to 10% of all persons with diabetes. Autoimmunity plays a significant role in its etiology. In response to unknown environmental stimuli in genetically susceptible individuals, an immunologic response results in complete destruction of pancreatic beta cells and subsequent insulin deficiency. Susceptibility is strongly associated with certain human leukocyte antigen genes, with human leukocyte antigen alleles DR3/4 most commonly found. Antibodies to insulin and components of the beta cell (e.g., islet cell antibodies, (ICA), glutamic acid decarboxylase, (GAD_{65}) are also produced and may be detected in plasma of most individuals at the time of diagnosis. Type 1 diabetes is most often diagnosed in children, but the condition may occur in young adults and in the elderly.

Type 2 diabetes, which makes up 85% to 90% of diabetes in the United States, is not linked with human leukocyte antigen. In this form of diabetes, impaired insulin secretion and insulin action are present in varying degrees. Evidence for a genetic component to type 2 diabetes is overwhelming, including concordance rates of nearly 100% in monozygotic twins. Current research has focused on defects in insulin action, leading to impaired carbohydrate storage in skeletal muscle and liver. Impaired insulin action in adipose tissue, leading to increased circulating levels of free fatty acids and release of cytokines derived from adipose tissue which antagonize insulin action, also appear to be important. However, the genes responsible for type 2 diabetes remain unknown. Several genetic mutations have been found in individuals with the relatively rare condition termed maturity onset of diabetes in young. These mutations are not observed in individuals with type 2 diabetes. Although the genetic factors responsible for the development of type 2 diabetes mellitus remain unknown, environmental factors leading to increased obesity are clearly linked to the 50% increase in the prevalence of diabetes observed from 1990 to 2000. Perhaps the greatest evidence for this effect is the marked increase in the prevalence of type 2 diabetes in obese adolescents and young adults as well as in adults. Established risk factors for the development of type 2 diabetes include family history, obesity, ethnicity, and a prior history of GDM (Table 39.2).

Gestational diabetes is genetically heterogeneous. In most cases, gestational diabetes represents a preclinical form of type 2 diabetes, but it is important to realize that pregnancy may also unmask type 1 diabetes. Screening for GDM is routinely performed at 24 to 28 weeks' gestation using a 50-g oral glucose tolerance test. Plasma glucose values greater than 140 mg/dL at 1 hour identify high-risk individuals (80% sensitivity). Some authorities advocate a threshold of more than 130 mg/dL at 1 hour (90% sensitivity). Diagnostic values are provided in Table 39.1.

Because of the clear relationship between GDM and risk for type 2 diabetes, an alternative to universal screening was recently suggested. In this schema, low risk individuals, defined as those younger than 25 years, of normal body weight, without a family history of diabetes mellitus, and not in ethnic groups known to be at increased risk (Hispanic-Americans, African-Americans, Native-Americans, Asian-Americans), would not be screened. All other women would undergo screening as outlined above.

TABLE 39.2. Persons Who Should Be Screened for Diabetes

Persons with a strong family history of diabetes
Markedly obese persons (body mass index > 25 kg/m²)
Persons in high-risk populations (African-American, Latino, Native-American, Asian-American, Pacific Islander)
Persons with hypertension
Women with a history of stillbirth, neonatal death, large-for-gestational-age infant (over 9 lb), toxemia of pregnancy, and glycosuria (if known)
All pregnant women between 24 and 28 wk
Patients with recurrent genital, urinary tract, and skin infections

CLINICAL SYMPTOMS AND HISTORY

Regardless of the type of diabetes mellitus, the clinical presentation of diabetes mellitus is closely linked to plasma glucose concentration. In the patient with incipient type 1 diabetes, as the capacity for insulin secretion falls, progressive hyperglycemia is observed. This may manifest as fatigue, frequent vaginal yeast infections, polydipsia/polyuria, and visual changes. As the degree of insulin deficiency becomes more severe, involuntary weight loss is observed. This is initially due to increased protein breakdown. However, if the diagnosis of diabetes is delayed further and absolute insulin deficiency results, increased breakdown of adipose tissue will be observed. This may lead ultimately to the hepatic oxidation of free fatty acids and the production of ketones (diabetic ketoacidosis). In persons with type 2 diabetes mellitus, manifestations are generally confined to those of hyperglycemia because insulin secretion is inadequate to maintain normal glucose levels but is usually more than sufficient to prevent ketoacidosis. Significant weight loss is infrequently observed in persons with type 2 diabetes mellitus and may often be a valuable discriminator between types 1 and 2 diabetes.

The long-term consequences of hyperglycemia are manifest as both microvascular and macrovascular complications. Because mild hyperglycemia may be undetected for many years, it is estimated that individuals with type 2 diabetes have had their disease for 5 to 10 years at the time of diagnosis. Thus, complications are often found at the time of initial diagnosis. In contrast, the diagnosis of type 1 diabetes is usually more fulminant, and complications are found less often at initial presentation. Microvascular complications related to diabetes mellitus include retinopathy, nephropathy, and neuropathy. Each is related to both degree and duration of hyperglycemia and occurs with equal frequency in types 1 and 2 diabetes mellitus. Early eye and kidney disease are often asymptomatic and require focused evaluation (see below). On the other hand, clinical symptoms occur commonly in individuals with diabetic neuropathy. For individuals with symptoms of peripheral neuropathy, paresthesias, pain, and/or numbness may occur, often in the feet or hands. Involvement of parasympathetic fibers of the gastrointestinal system may result in postprandial bloating (gastroparesis) or, more commonly, constipation. Finally, sexual dysfunction may also be a manifestation of diabetic neuropathy in women.

Hypotheses proposed to explain the link between microvascular complications and hyperglycemia include intracellular accumulation of sorbitol, increased protein kinase C activity, and accumulation of advanced glycosylation end products. Clinical trials designed to test these hypotheses are ongoing. Importantly, large clinical trials in patients with types 1 and 2 diabetes have clearly demonstrated that both the development and progression of microvascular disease can be reduced by approximately 25% for every 1% reduction in glycosylated hemoglobin A_{1c} (HbA_{1c}). These studies strongly implicate hyperglycemia as the common pathogenetic basis for microvascular disease and support more aggressive treatment strategies.

Macrovascular complications, including coronary artery disease, peripheral vascular disease, and cerebral vascular disease, occur two to four times more frequently in women with diabetes compared with nondiabetic women. Moreover, the risk of a first myocardial event in persons with diabetes mellitus is equivalent to the risk of a second cardiac event in a person without diabetes but with documented cardiac disease. Evidence in support of tighter glucose control to prevent macrovascular complications is less compelling than that for microvascular disease. However, attention to other modifiable risk factors is essential (see below).

PHYSICAL EXAMINATION

In women without an established diagnosis of diabetes mellitus, the history and physical examination should be focused on identification of risk factors for diabetes, including family history, obesity, ethnicity, and a prior history of either GDM or large infants (>4,000 g) (Table 39.2). The presence of risk factors should prompt a more extensive evaluation similar to that of the patient with a known diagnosis of diabetes. In all patients, an assessment of lifestyle will provide invaluable information that can guide the clinician in the development of an individualized treatment strategy with a higher likelihood of success. The initial examination of a patient with diabetes mellitus should be focused on the detection of diabetic complications and as such will be comprehensive. Height and weight should be assessed and body mass index calculated (kg/m^2). Supine and upright blood pressures should also be performed with the initial visit to detect hypertension and orthostasis. Hypertension in the patient with diabetes is defined as a blood pressure greater than 130/80. The presence of orthostasis with an increase in pulse suggests dehydration, whereas orthostasis without a change in pulse suggests cardiac autonomic dysfunction and should alert the clinician to the likelihood of other autonomic abnormalities.

The head and neck examination should include a funduscopic examination and thyroid palpation (thyroid abnormalities occur commonly in patients with diabetes mellitus). Detection of absent respiratory variation during the cardiac examination may also suggest autonomic dysfunction. Abdominal examination is focused on evidence for hepatomegaly and skin changes suggestive of secondary causes of diabetes (e.g., glucocorticoid excess). In addition, the skin examination may reveal acanthosis nigricans (a marker of insulin resistance) or lipohypertrophy (a common cause of altered insulin absorption and erratic blood sugars in patients who have used insulin). Examination of the feet should be a routine component of the examination and focuses on skin changes (e.g., blisters, infection, calloses, cracking) as well as neurologic assessment. The latter should include an assessment of vibratory (128-Hz tuning fork) and light touch (5.07 monofilament) sensation to detect early diabetic neuropathy. It has been estimated that as many as 55% of persons presenting with type 2 diabetes already have evidence of neuropathy.

LABORATORY EVALUATION

The routine laboratory evaluation recommended for patients with diabetes is shown in Table 39.3. For the purposes of assessing glucose control, the percentage of hemoglobin that has undergone nonenzymatic glycosylation (HbA_{1c}) should be performed every 3 to 4 months. The rate of formation of HbA_{1c} is directly proportional to the average concentration of glucose within the erythrocyte. In a patient with a normal erythrocyte life span, the values accurately reflect average blood sugar for the previous 2 to 3 months and provide invaluable information to direct treatment. For example, an HbA_{1c} of 7% (normal, 4%–6%) indicates an average blood sugar of approximately 150 mg/dL; an HbA_{1c} of 9% indicates an average blood glucose of approximately 230 mg/dL. In patients with a hemolytic process (e.g., sickle cell disease, glucose-6-phosphate dehydrogenase [G6PDH] deficiency), the HbA_{1c} value will be significantly lowered and is not useful. HbA_{1c} should not be used as a diagnostic test.

Measurement of urinary albumin excretion should also be performed to assess the presence or absence of early kidney damage (microalbuminuria). The test had previously been performed on a 24-hour urine and definitions of normal (<20 μg/min), microalbuminuria (20–200 μg/min), and macroalbuminuria (>200 μg/min) were established. However, measurement of a simultaneous microalbumin and creatinine concentration on a spot urine sample with a microalbumin (μg)-to-creatinine (mg) ratio greater than 30 μg/mg has been shown to have similar predictive value. An assessment of

TABLE 39.3. Recommended Laboratory Determinations in Individuals with Diabetes Mellitus

Test	Normal values	Treatment change needed	Frequency
HbA1c	4%–6%	>7%	3 mo
Lipid profile			
LDL	<100 mg/dL	>100 mg/dL	Annual[a]
Triglycerides	<150 mg/dL	>150 mg/dL	
Microalbumin	<30 μg/mg creatinine	>30 μg/mg creatinine	Annual
TSH	0.3–4 μU/mL	>10 μU/mL	Initial

[a]Testing frequency assumes target values. If LDL is greater than target, more frequent assessment may be appropriate with medication dosage adjustment.
LDL, low density lipoprotein; TSH, thyroid stimulating hormone.

serum lipids should be performed at least annually, again to direct treatment in this high-risk group of women. Finally, all patients with diabetes mellitus should be referred for a dilated funduscopic examination.

TREATMENT

The treatment of diabetes is predicated first on the type of diabetes. In all patients, lifestyle modification is an essential component of a successful treatment strategy. However, a prescription for an 1,800-calorie diet and a recommendation to exercise three times a week is unlikely to succeed. Attention to lifestyle issues such as when and what the patient eats provides important clues to modifiable habits. Opportunities to exercise should be explored. In many cases, the involvement of a diabetes educator in the overall treatment regimen will lead to greater understanding and commitment by the patient and enhance the likelihood of success. Instruction in self-monitoring of blood glucose provides a powerful tool for empowerment and is also recommended.

The current dietary recommendations for persons with diabetes include 40% to 60% carbohydrate, 30% fat (<10% saturated fat), and 20% protein. Several recent changes in the recommendations for persons with diabetes should be noted. Caloric intake should be individualized based on current weight. Goals in obese women with diabetes may include weight loss of 5% to 7% to enhance insulin sensitivity. It is also now recognized that glycemic control is related more to the total amount of carbohydrate rather than the type of carbohydrate. Thus, simple sugars are no longer restricted. However, they should be substituted for other carbohydrates rather than added to overall carbohydrate intake to maintain glucose control. Previous diet plans for patients with diabetes also emphasized a high fiber diet. However, in most cases, the amounts of fiber necessary to alter metabolic control are poorly tolerated and are not encouraged. Finally, the use of snacks in the overall meal plan should *not* be considered routine. In most patients with diabetes, the addition of snacks is unnecessary and diverts attention from a more careful examination of the medical prescription.

The advantages of exercise in the patient with diabetes mellitus are several. First and foremost, regular aerobic exercise provides cardiovascular benefit in individuals with increased risk for macrovascular disease and should be encouraged. In addition, acute exercise promotes glucose uptake and storage, thereby contributing to improved day-to-day glycemic control. Exercise also appears to provide benefit in a weight reduction program through the enhancement of weight maintenance. In all cases, patients should be assessed for preexisting cardiovascular disease before beginning an exercise program. In most cases, history and a resting electrocardiogram are sufficient. In others, a more thorough evaluation may be necessary.

With regard to medical management, the past 10 years have seen the addition of a wide array of insulins and oral medications for diabetes that provide opportunity to tailor treatment to the individual. As shown in Table 39.4, oral medications include insulin secretagogues, insulin sensitizers, and enzyme blockers. Each has its place in the treatment of type 2 diabetes mellitus. However, it should be pointed out that none of these agents is approved for use during pregnancy (see below). Sulfonylureas, metformin, and thiazolidinediones result in a similar reduction in HbA_{1c} when used as monotherapy in patients with type 2 diabetes. Moreover, when HbA_{1c} values exceed 7% to 8%, the addition (but not the substitution) of a second agent has been shown to lower HbA_{1c}, often to within target ranges less than 7%. When the combination of two agents is unsuccessful, clinicians may either add a third oral agent or consider insulin therapy. It is increasingly appreciated that diabetes mellitus is a progressive disease characterized by loss of insulin secretory capacity. Unfortunately, our reluctance to initiate insulin therapy early has, in many cases, led to prolonged and unnecessary elevations in HbA_{1c} in patients with type 2 diabetes.

Insulin is a requirement for patients with type 1 diabetes. It is often required for patients with type 2 diabetes and women with GDM who have consistently elevated fasting plasma glucose levels or an elevated postprandial glucose level despite diet therapy. In most instances, insulin regimens should begin with long-acting insulin given at bedtime (~0.2 units/kg) to control blood glucose overnight. This may include either neutral protamine Hagedorn (NPH) insulin or the longer acting insulin analogue, glargine insulin (Table 39.5). The bedtime

TABLE 39.4. Oral antihyperglycemic Medications

Drug	Mechanism of action	HbA1c efficacy[a]	Adverse effects
Sulfonylureas Glyburide Glimepiride Glipizide	Insulin secretagogue	1%–2%	Hypoglycemia
Nonsulfonylureas Nataglinide Repaglinide	Insulin secretagogue	1%–2%	Hypoglycemia
Metformin	Insulin sensitizer (liver)	1%–2%	Diarrhea Lactic acidosis[b]
Thiazolidinediones Pioglitazone Rosiglitazone	Insulin sensitizer (Adipose tissue and skeletal muscle)	0.5%–2%	Edema Hepatotoxicity[c]
α-Glucosidase inhibitors Acarbose Miglitol	Decreased carbohydrate absorption	0.5%–1%	Flatulance

[a]When used as monotherapy.
[b]Metformin is contraindicated in patients with hepatic or renal disease (creatinine >1.5 mg/dL).
[c]Routine monitoring of liver enzymes is recommended.

TABLE 39.5. Insulin Preparations

Insulin	Peak action	Duration of action
Short acting		
Regular	2 h	6–8 h
Lispro[a]	1 h	3–4 h
Aspart[a]	1 h	3–4 h
Intermediate acting		
NPH	4–6 h	12–14 h
Lente	4–6 h	12–14 h
Long acting		
Ultralente	6–8 h	12–18 h
Glargine[a]	Minimal	18–24 h

[a]Insulin analogs. These insulins are not currently approved for use in pregnancy.

insulin is titrated to achieve the target fasting plasma glucose. In nonpregnant women on oral medication, the bedtime insulin is usually added to the oral treatment regimen. If the HbA_{1c} remains above target (>7%) with this combination strategy, the oral medications should be discontinued and a more comprehensive insulin regimen initiated. Ideally the insulin regimen should reflect the lifestyle of the patient rather than require rigidity in mealtimes and content. For example, a short-acting insulin may be added with each meal. Although this approach increases the number of injections required, enhanced flexibility is often seen as superior to more traditional regimens used. In many cases, the dosage of insulin used is adjusted based on the carbohydrate intake for the meals. For example, one unit of short-acting insulin is given for every 10 to 15 g of carbohydrate in the meal. In nonpregnant women with diabetes, target plasma glucose values are generally less than 120 mg/dL before meals and at bedtime and less than 180 mg/dL after the meal.

CONSIDERATIONS IN PREGNANCY

During normal gestation, the fasting glucose level decreases the first few weeks of pregnancy and reaches its lowest level by the 12th week of gestation. Thereafter, the levels remain unchanged until delivery. This decrease is about 15 mg/dL in the pregnant woman who has fasted overnight, compared with a nonpregnant woman. In contrast to nonpregnant women, pregnant women respond to a meal with an increased postprandial glucose level. This is thought to facilitate glucose transport to the fetus across the placenta. Insulin levels in a basal state are no different from those in nonpregnancy during the first and second trimesters, but they increase by 50% in the third trimester. This increase in insulin despite maintenance of plasma glucose reflects the insulin resistance of pregnancy. These changes are related, at least in part, to the effect of increased estrogen and progesterone in pregnancy.

In women with diabetes, pregnancy outcome is closely related to glucose control. Poor glucose control is associated with a marked increase in macrosomia (17% vs. 5%), congenital anomalies (3% vs. 1.8%), and hyperbilirubinemia (16.5 vs. 8.2%) (Table 39.6). Women with diabetes should ideally receive special preconceptual and prenatal care to maintain glucose control well within that seen in normal pregnant patients. Before pregnancy, the diabetic woman should be evaluated for general medical status and for signs of retinopathy, nephropathy, hypertension, and ischemic heart disease. An ophthalmologic examination, an electrocardiogram, and renal function tests should be performed. Patients with type 2 diabetes should be told to stop oral hypoglycemia medication and begin insulin. The goal is to have near-normal HbA_{1c} before conception.

Experts in the management of complicated high-risk pregnancies and diabetic control should follow women closely during pregnancy. By maintaining euglycemia with mean blood glucose levels below 100 mg/dL, perinatal mortality is reduced. The target maternal glucose to maintain in pregnancy is the blood glucose seen in normal pregnancy: This means that fasting plasma glucose levels should be 60 to 80 mg/dL. The mean diurnal glucose level should be 85 mg/dL, and postprandial levels should rarely exceed 120 mg/dL. If insulin is required, the strategy is often the same as that used for intensive insulin therapy in nonpregnant women using a combination of basal insulin to control preprandial glucose and boluses of short-acting insulin for meals. Daily insulin requirements should be expected to fall slightly in the first trimester and then increase progressively through the remainder of the pregnancy to levels, approaching two- to threefold higher than prepregnancy requirements. Self-monitoring of blood glucose is essential to achieve tight control. Composition of the diet will depend on body habitus at the time of conception and should be individualized. A birth weight in excess of 4,000 g or a birth weight above the 90th percentile of gestational age occurs in 30% of all diabetic pregnancies. These infants have a higher morbidity and mortality. Among these infants, the incidence of diabetes in later life is markedly increased. Macrosomia can be prevented by tight glucose control during pregnancy. The fetus of a diabetic mother requires careful surveillance, including ultrasound and antenatal fetal heart rate testing and biophysical scores. An insulin-requiring diabetic woman must give birth in a hospital with expert professional staff capable of caring for her and her newborn.

In women with GDM, most will revert to euglycemia after delivery. However, they should be reminded that their risk for development of type 2 diabetes is nearly 50%. Prevention strategies, including diet and exercise, have now been shown to significantly reduce this risk. In women with preexisting diabetes who had been treated successfully with oral agents, these agents may be resumed unless the mother plans to nurse. All oral hypoglycemics appear in breast milk and should not be given as long as the mother is breast-feeding.

TABLE 39.6. Complications in Newborn of Diabetic Mother

Significant macrosomia
Birth trauma
- Hypoglycemia
- Hypocalcemia and hypomagnesemia
- Polycythemia
- Hyperbilirubinemia
- Respiratory distress syndrome
- Intrauterine chronic hypoxia leading to neonatal asphyxia
- Cardiomyopathy

BIBLIOGRAPHY

American Diabetes Association. Report of the expert committee on the diagnosis and classification of diabetes mellitus. *Diabetes Care* 1997;20:1183–1197.

American Diabetes Association. Standards of medical care for patients with diabetes mellitus. *Diabetes Care* 2002;25:S33–S49.

The Diabetes Control and Complications Trial Research Group. The effect of intensive treatment of diabetes on the development and progression of long-term complications in insulin-dependent diabetes mellitus. *N Engl J Med* 1993;329:977–986.

Escalante P, Alpizar S. Changes in insulin sensitivity, secretion and glucose effectiveness during menstrual cycle. *Arch Med Res* 1999;30:19–22.
Franz MJ, Bantle JP, Beebe CA, et al. Evidence-based nutrition principles and recommendations for the treatment and prevention of diabetes and related complications. *Diabetes Care* 2002;25:148–198.
Haffner SM, Lehto S, Ronnemaa T, et al. Mortality from coronary heart disease in subjects with type 2 diabetes and in nondiabetic subjects with and without prior myocardial infarction. *N Engl J Med* 1998;339:229–234.
Harris MI, Klein R, Welborn TA, et al. Onset of NIDDM occurs at least 4–7 yr before clinical diagnosis. *Diabetes Care* 1992;15:815–819.
Inzucchi SE. Oral antihyperglycemic therapy for type 2 diabetes: scientific review. *JAMA* 2002;287:360–372.
Jovanovic L, Knopp RH, Brown Z, et al. Declining insulin requirement in the late first trimester of diabetic pregnancy. *Diabetes Care* 2001;24:1130–1136.
Jovanovic L, Pettitt DJ. Gestational diabetes mellitus. *JAMA* 1928;286:2516–2518.
Knowler WC, Barrett-Connor E, Fowler SE, et al. Reduction in the incidence of type 2 diabetes with lifestyle intervention or metformin. *N Engl J Med* 1907; 346:393–403.
Mokdad AH, Ford ES, Bowman BA, et al. Diabetes trends in the U.S.: 1990–1998. *Diabetes Care* 2000;23:1278–1283.
UK Prospective Diabetes Study Group. Effect of intensive blood glucose control with metformin on complications in overweight patients with Type 2 diabetes (UKPDS 34). *Lancet* 1998;352:854–865.
UK Prospective Diabetes Study Group. Intensive blood glucose control with sulphonylureas or insulin compared with conventional treatment and risk of complications in patients with type 2 diabetes (UKPDS 33). *Lancet* 1998;352: 837–853.

CHAPTER 40
Hirsutism

Richard S. Legro

ETIOLOGY OF HIRSUTISM

Hirsutism is defined as excess body hair in undesirable locations and as such is a subjective phenomenon that makes both diagnosis and treatment difficult. Hirsutism should be viewed much as polycystic ovaries, as a sign rather than a diagnosis. Most commonly hirsutism is associated with androgen excess, or what is referred to as androgen-dependent hirsutism. This tends to be a midline predominant hair growth.

The pilosebaceous unit is the common skin structure that gives rise to both hair follicles and sebaceous glands and are found everywhere on the body except the palms and soles. The density is greatest on the face and scalp (400–800 glands/cm^2) and lowest on the extremities (50 glands/cm^2). The number of pilosebaceous units does not increase after birth (about 5 million), but they can become more prominent through activation and differentiation. Before puberty the body hair is primarily fine, unpigmented, vellus hair. After puberty and stimulated by increased androgens, some of these hairs (mainly midline hair) are transformed into coarser, pigmented, terminal hairs. A similar mechanism may explain the increase in acne with puberty with increased sebum production by the sebaceous glands. Hair in some regions of the body undergoes conversion to terminal hair without androgen exposure, such as the eyebrows, lashes, and scalp.

After a period of active growth (anagen), the hair follicle enters a resting phase (telogen) of varying length. The period of transition from anagen to telogen is sometimes referred to as catagen. During this transition the hair shaft separates from the dermal papillae at the base. The period of anagen varies from 3 years on the scalp to 4 months on the face. For corresponding parts of the skin, men have longer anagens than women do, which may be partially due to higher circulating androgen levels.

Androgen excess is most visible in its effects on the pilosebaceous unit. Hirsutism occurs when androgens stimulate the transformation of fine, unpigmented, vellus hair to coarse, pigmented, thickened, terminal hair. This is thought to be mediated by the intracellular actions of enzymes 17-ketosteroid reductase, which converts androstenedione to testosterone, and 5α-reductase, which converts testosterone to dihydrotestosterone (DHT; 5–10 times as potent as testosterone). Paradoxically, androgens can exert opposite effects in hair follicles on the scalp, causing conversion of terminal follicles to vellus-like follicles and leading to male pattern baldness characterized by frontal and temporal balding. Androgens can also cause increased sebum production and abnormal keratinization in the pilosebaceous unit, contributing to the development of acne. There are ethnic and genetic differences that can ameliorate the effects of androgen excess in the periphery as demonstrated by Asian women with polycystic ovary syndrome (PCOS) who are not hirsute.

DIFFERENTIAL DIAGNOSIS

The differential diagnosis overlaps substantially with ovarian endocrine disorders (see Chapter 36). Idiopathic, familial, and iatrogenic (medications) causes may be more common in hirsutism. Androgen-independent hirsutism may be a familial tendency (familial hypertrichosis) or due to medications, such as cyclosporin, diazoxide, and minoxidil. These medications often result in hypertrichosis, a generalized increase in body hair rather than the midline development of marked terminal hair growth. Idiopathic hirsutism was coined to identify the presence of hirsutism in eumenorrheic women with normal circulating androgens, but this may reflect our limited ability to assess androgen action in the peripheral compartment. When thoroughly investigated for androgen excess, most idiopathic cases disappear.

Virilization in adult women is a rare disorder. It includes the common signs of acne and hirsutism but is also accompanied by other peripheral effects such as temporal balding, clitoromegaly, deepening of the voice, breast atrophy, and changes in body contour. Amenorrhea may occur in a premenopausal woman. Virilization is never "idiopathic," and all cases need to be investigated until a cause if discovered. PCOS or the adult forms of nonclassic congenital adrenal hyperplasia rarely cause virilization.

CLINICAL SYMPTOMS AND HISTORY

Hirsutism due to PCOS frequently develops early in the maturation process, at adrenarche or menarche. Associated signs of androgen excess are acne and female pattern balding. Virilization is often characterized by the rapidity of onset of symptoms, which often leads to a speedy evaluation and diagnosis, whereas the more lingering forms may be overlooked until there is marked masculinization.

CLINICAL FINDINGS AND PHYSICAL EXAMINATION

Androgen-dependent hair is midline hair: on the upper lip, chin, and cheeks, intermammary hair, and hair in the escutcheon, inner thighs, and lower back into the intergluteal area. Methodology of the assessment of hirsutism and response to treatment

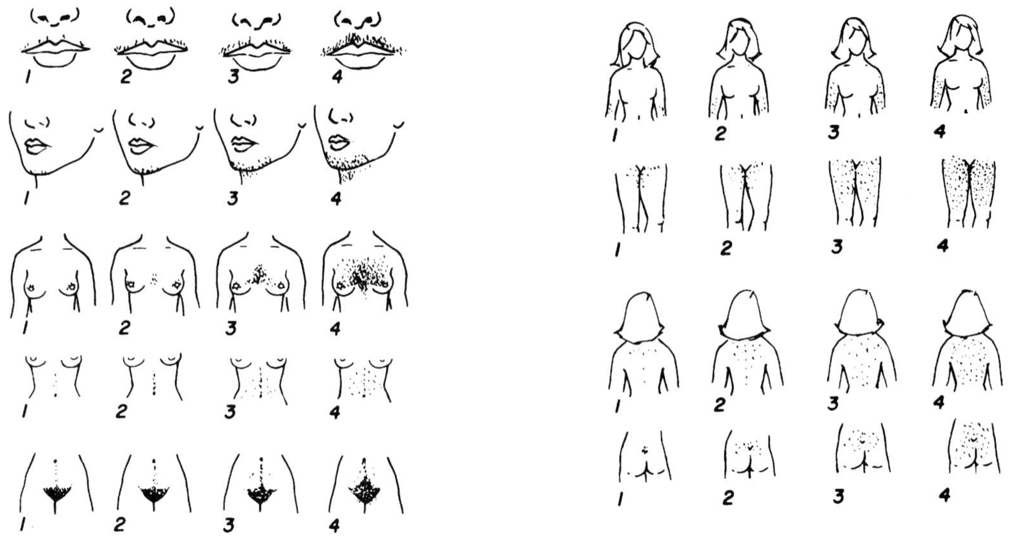

FIG. 40.1. Ferriman-Gallwey scoring system of hirsutism. (From Hatch R, Rosenfield RL, Kim MH, et al. Hirsutism: implications, etiology, and management. *Am J Obstet Gynecol* 1981;140:815–830, with permission.)

have been poorly validated. Hirsutism scores are notoriously subjective, and even the most frequently used standard of subjective hirsutism scores, the modified Ferriman-Gallwey score, relies excessively on non-midline nonandrogen-dependent body hair to make the diagnosis (Fig. 40.1). A subjective scale is important for discriminating unwanted excess hair with a diffuse distribution (hypertrichosis) from hirsutism. The best discrimination between a control population and a hirsute population has been found using the sum of the scores for four regions: upper lip, chin, lower abdomen, and thighs. Another confounder of the assessment of hirsutism are the often robust mechanical means women use to remove hair, thus "improving" the amount of hirsutism viewed by a subjective observer.

Virilization presents with a variety of peripheral effects. Balding, especially with centripetal balding and frontal recession, is more characteristic of androgenic alopecia in men as opposed to the more indolent presentation of androgenic alopecia in women with a generalized thinning of the crown region. A deepening of the voice has been reported in women with androgen-secreting tumors or undergoing exogenous androgen treatment (this does not necessarily improve after removal of the androgen excess). Increase in the size of the larynx is one factor in the voice change. Clitoromegaly is defined as a clitoral index greater than 35 mm^2 (the clitoral index is the product of the sagittal and transverse diameters of the glans of the clitoris). In a normal woman these diameters are in the range of 5 mm each. The degree of clitoral enlargement correlates with the degree of androgen excess. Androgens can lead to body composition changes, especially in the upper body, with increased muscle mass and decreased fat mass. This is accompanied by breast atrophy.

LABORATORY AND IMAGING STUDIES

Workup in many cases may mirror that of androgen excess in ovarian endocrine disorders (see Chapter 36). The degree of androgen excess that can result in hirsutism most commonly has its source in increased production (or intake) of androgens. However, other factors such as the potency of the androgen produced (DHT > testosterone > androstenedione > dehydroepiandrosterone), the amount of androgen that is free or weakly bound in serum and thus bioavailable (sex hormone-binding globulin [SHBG] preferentially binds more potent androgens than estrogens) and the peripheral metabolism of androgens (primarily the intracellular production of DHT from precursors) all factor in the phenotype of hirsutism. Both the adrenal glands and ovaries contribute to the circulating androgen pool in women. The adrenal preferentially secretes weak androgens such as dehydroepiandrosterone or its sulfated "depot" form dehydroepiandrosterone sulfate (up to 90% of adrenal origin).

These hormones, in addition to androstenedione (often elevated in PCOS women), may serve as prohormones for more potent androgens such as testosterone or DHT. The ovary is the preferential source of testosterone, and it is estimated that 75% of circulating testosterone originates from the ovary (mainly through peripheral conversion of prohormones by liver, fat, and skin but also through direct ovarian secretion). Androstenedione, largely of ovarian origin, is the only circulating androgen that may be higher in premenopausal women than men, yet its androgenic potency is only 10% of testosterone. DHT is the most potent androgen, though it circulates in negligible quantities and results primarily from the intracellular 5α-reduction of testosterone. In the past, measurement of 3α-androstanediol glucuronide, a peripheral metabolite of DHT, was used as a circulating marker of androgen excess in the skin (hirsutism and acne), but its clinical use is negligible. Some authors have piloted the use of prostate-specific antigen as a serum marker of response to therapy, but results with this have been mixed.

It is important to note that factors other than androgens may contribute to the development of hirsutism. Hyperinsulinemia that accompanies many benign forms of virilization can also stimulate the pilosebaceous unit either directly or indirectly by contributing to hyperandrogenemia. Screening for glucose tolerance may be indicated in many women with hirsutism.

TREATMENT

Most medical methods, although improving hirsutism, do not produce the rapid and clear results patients desire. In general, combination therapies appear to produce better results than single-agent approaches, response with medical therapies often take 3 to 6 months to notice improvement, and adjunctive mechanical removal methods are often necessary. Hirsutism scales are often used but remain problematic to institute into both research and clinical practice. Other assessments of hirsutism have included measurement of hair shaft diameter, hair follicle density, growth rate, and weight of shaved hair from a given area.

Trials have been hampered by the above methodology concerns and by small numbers of subjects. For instance, although spironolactone has had a long and extensive use as an antiandrogen and multiple clinical trials have been published showing a benefit, the overall quality of the trials and small numbers enrolled have limited the ability of a metaanalysis to document its benefit in the treatment of hirsutism. There have been fewer studies of acne and even fewer with androgenic alopecia, so in general treatment for hirsutism is extrapolated to the treatment of other stigmata of hyperandrogenism at the pilosebaceous unit.

Lifestyle Modifications

For obese patients with hirsutism, weight loss is frequently recommended as a potential benefit. Increases in SHBG through improved insulin sensitivity from weight loss may lower bioavailable androgen levels. In one study, about 50% of these women who lost weight experienced improvement in their hirsutism.

Ornithine Decarboxylase Inhibitors

Ornithine decarboxylase is necessary for the production of polyamines and is also a sensitive and specific marker of androgen action in the prostate. Inhibition of this enzyme limits cell division and function. Recently, a potent inhibitor of this enzyme, eflornithine, has been tested and found to be effective as a facial cream against hirsutism and has been approved by the U.S. Food and Drug Administration for this indication. It is given as a 13.9% cream of eflornithine hydrochloride and applied to affected areas twice a day for a minimum of 4 hours each. In clinical trials 32% of patients showed marked improvement after 24 weeks compared with 8% of placebo treated. Benefit was first noted at 8 weeks. It is pregnancy category C and appears to be well tolerated. A variety of adverse skin conditions occurred in 1% of subjects.

Androgen Suppressive Therapies

Women with documented hyperandrogenemia would theoretically benefit most from this form of therapy. Suppressing the ovary has been achieved with oral contraceptives, depot progestins, or gonadotropin-releasing hormone (GnRH) analogue treatment. Oral contraceptives both inhibit ovarian steroid production, through lowering of gonadotropins, and raise SHBG, through their estrogen effect, thus further lowering bioavailable testosterone. They also may inhibit DHT binding to the androgen receptor and 5α-reductase activity and increase hepatic steroid clearance (due to stimulation of the P-450 system). These myriad actions contribute to improving hirsutism. There are theoretical reasons for choosing an oral contraceptive using a progestin with antiandrogenic properties, but few studies showed a clinical difference between different types of progestins. One such compound, drospirenone, is now available in a combination oral contraceptive in the United States. Although a triphasic oral contraceptive containing norgestimate has been shown to improve acne and received a U.S. Food and Drug Administration indication for this, other pills also offer similar results.

A GnRH agonist may cause greater lowering of circulating androgens, but comparative trials against other agents and combined agent trials have been mixed and have not shown a greater benefit to one or the other or combined treatment. A GnRH agonist given alone results in unacceptable bone loss. Glucocorticoid suppression of the adrenal also offers theoretical benefits, but deterioration in glucose tolerance is problematic for PCOS women, and long-term effects such as osteoporosis are significant concern.

Insulin-Sensitizing Agents

It is difficult to separate the effects of improving insulin sensitivity from that of lowering serum androgens, because any "pure" improvement in insulin sensitivity can raise SHBG and thus lower bioavailable androgen. Given the long onset of action for improving hirsutism, longer periods of observation are needed. In the largest and longest randomized trial to date of these agents, troglitazone in a dose-response fashion was found to significantly improve hirsutism in PCOS women without lowering total testosterone (benefit presumably achieved through significantly lowering free testosterone).

Antiandrogens

ANDROGEN RECEPTOR ANTAGONISTS

These compounds antagonize the binding of testosterone and other androgens to the androgen receptor. Therefore, as a class they are teratogenic and pose risk of feminization of the external genitalia in a male fetus should the patient conceive. Spironolactone, a diuretic and aldosterone antagonist, also binds to the androgen receptor with 67% of the affinity of DHT. It has other mechanisms of action, including inhibition of ovarian and adrenal steroidogenesis, competition for androgen receptors in hair follicles, and direct inhibition of 5α-reductase activity. The usual dose is 25 to 100 mg twice a day, and the dose is titrated to balance efficacy with avoiding side effects. There is a dose-response effect and a long period of onset, 6 months or more. About 20% of women will experience increased menstrual frequency, and this is one reason for combining this therapy with the oral contraceptive. Other side effects include polyuria, orthostatic hypotension, nausea, and fatigue. Because it can cause and exacerbate hyperkalemia, it should be used cautiously in patients with renal impairment. The medication also has potential teratogenicity as an antiandrogen, although exposure has rarely resulted in ambiguous genitalia in male infants. Acne has also been successfully treated with spironolactone. Thus, much of the treatment basis is empiric.

Flutamide is another nonsteroidal antiandrogen that has been shown to be effective against hirsutism. The most common side effect is dry skin, but its use has rarely been associated with hepatitis. A dose of 250 mg/d is given. There is greater risk of teratogenicity with this compound, and contraception should be used as with all antiandrogens.

5α-REDUCTASE INHIBITORS

There are two forms of the enzyme 5α-reductase: type 1, predominantly found in the skin, and type 2, predominantly found in the prostate and reproductive tissues. Both forms are found in the pilosebaceous unit and may contribute to hirsutism, acne, and balding. Finasteride inhibits both forms and is available as a 5-mg tablet for the treatment of prostate cancer and a 1-mg tablet for the treatment of male alopecia. It has been found to be effective for the treatment of hirsutism in women. Finasteride is better tolerated than other antiandrogens but has the highest and clearest risk for teratogenicity in a male fetus, and adequate contraception must be used. Randomized trials have found that spironolactone, flutamide, and finasteride all have similar efficacy in improving hirsutism.

Other Agents

Minoxidil has mild efficacy in increasing hair growth in women with alopecia. Ketoconazole is an inhibitor of the P-450 enzyme system and thus inhibits androgen biosynthesis but has hepatotoxicity.

Depilatory Methods

Mechanical hair removal (shaving, plucking, waxing, depilatory creams, electrolysis, and laser vaporization) can control hirsutism and often are the front line treatment used by women. Laser vaporization is receiving increasing attention. Hair is damaged using the principle of selective photothermolysis with wavelengths of light well absorbed by follicular melanin and pulse durations that selectively thermally damage the target without damaging surrounding tissue. Patients with dark hair and light skin are ideal candidates, and it appears to be most effective during anagen.

Surgical Options

Surgery, consisting of total abdominal hysterectomy and bilateral salpingo-oophorectomy, is not a usual initial treatment option for androgen excess but may be indicated in some cases of refractory ovarian hyperandrogenism. The role of ovarian drilling, if any, in the treatment of hirsutism is uncertain.

PREGNANCY

Severe hirsutism and even virilization that occurs during pregnancy has its own unique differential, including benign ovarian sources such as hyperreactio luteinalis (i.e., gestational ovarian theca-lutein cysts) or luteomas and extremely rare fetoplacental sources such as aromatase deficiency, resulting in androgen excess due to the placental inability to convert precursor androgens into estrogens. Pregnancy, with its estrogen excess and estrogen-mediated increase in SHBG (and thus free androgens), may be a respite from the fertile soil of androgen excess that stimulates hirsutism.

ACKNOWLEDGMENTS

This work was supported by PHS grants U54 HD34449, The National Cooperative Program in Infertility Research (NCPIR), K24 HD01476, a GCRC grant MO1 RR 10732 to Pennsylvania State University, and U10 HD 38992, The Reproductive Medicine Network.

BIBLIOGRAPHY

Azziz R, Ehrmann D, Legro RS, et al. Troglitazone improves ovulation and hirsutism in the polycystic ovary syndrome: a multicenter, double-blind, placebo-controlled trial. *J Clin Endocrinol Metab* 2001;86:1626–1632.

Azziz R, Ochoa TM, Bradley EL Jr, et al. Leuprolide and estrogen versus oral contraceptive pills for the treatment of hirsutism: a prospective randomized study. *J Clin Endocrinol Metab* 1995;80:3406–3411.

Carmina E, Koyama T, Chang L, et al. Does ethnicity influence the prevalence of adrenal hyperandrogenism and insulin resistance in polycystic ovary syndrome? *Am J Obstet Gynecol* 1992;167:1807–1812.

Carr BR, Breslau NA, Givens C, et al. Oral contraceptive pills, gonadotropin-releasing hormone agonists, or use in combination for treatment of hirsutism: a clinical research center study. *J Clin Endo Metab* 1995;80:1169–1178.

Derksen J, Moolenaar AJ, Van Seters AP, et al. Semiquantitative assessment of hirsutism in dutch women. *Br J Dermatol* 1993;128:259–263.

Eil C, Edelson SK. The use of human skin fibroblasts to obtain potency estimates of drug binding to androgen receptors. *J Clin Endocrinol Metab* 1984;59:51–55.

Fruzzetti F, De Lorenzo D, Ricci C, et al. Clinical and endocrine effects of flutamide in hyperandrogenic women. *Fertil Steril* 1993;60:806–813.

Groves TD, Corenblum B. Spironolactone therapy during human pregnancy. *Am J Obstet Gynecol* 1995;172:1655–1656.

Hatch R, Rosenfield RL, Kim MH, et al. Hirsutism: implications, etiology, and management. *Am J Obstet Gynecol* 1981;140:815–830.

Helfer EL, Miller JL, Rose LI. Side-effects of spironolactone therapy in the hirsute woman. *J Clin Endocrinol Metab* 1988;66:208–211.

Lee O, Farquhar C, Toomath R, et al. Spironolactone versus placebo or in combination with steroids for hirsutism and/or acne. *Cochrane Database of Systematic Reviews* 2000;(2):CD000194.

McCann PP, Pegg AE. Ornithine decarboxylase as an enzyme target for therapy. *Pharmacol Therap* 1992;54:195–215.

Moghetti P, Castello R, Magnani CM, et al. Clinical and hormonal effects of the 5 alpha-reductase inhibitor finasteride in idiopathic hirsutism. *J Clin Endocrinol Metab* 1994;79:1115–1121.

Moghetti P, Tosi F, Tosti A, et al. Comparison of spironolactone, flutamide, and finasteride efficacy in the treatment of hirsutism: a randomized, double-blind, placebo-controlled trial. *J Clin Endocrinol Metab* 2000;85:89–94.

Negri C, Tosi F, Dorizzi R, et al. Antiandrogen drugs lower serum prostate-specific antigen (psa) levels in hirsute subjects: evidence that serum psa is a marker of androgen action in women. *J Clin Endocrinol Metab* 2000;85:81–84.

Pasquali R, Antenucci D, Casimirri F, et al. Clinical and hormonal characteristics of obese amenorrheic hyperandrogenic women before and after weight loss. *J Clin Endocrinol Metab* 1989;68:173–179.

PART 5

Cardiovascular Disease

CHAPTER 41
Hypertension

George F. Aziz and Wen-Chih Wu

Hypertension, defined as a systolic blood pressure of 140 mm Hg or greater or a diastolic blood pressure of 90 mm Hg or greater, is a common disease among women in the United States. The prevalence varies from less than 2% for white women under age 25 to more than 70% for elderly African-American women. The prevalence of high blood pressure increases with age and is greater for African-American women than for white women. In young adulthood and early middle age, the prevalence of high blood pressure is greater for men than for women; thereafter, the reverse is true. Nonfatal and fatal cardiovascular diseases, as well as renal disease and all causes of mortality, increase progressively with higher levels of both systolic and diastolic blood pressure. It is important to screen for and treat even mildly elevated blood pressure, because the risk for end-organ damage with stroke, myocardial infarction, and renal dysfunction rises with increased blood pressure. Furthermore, treatment of hypertension has been shown to reduce this risk.

FACTORS ASSOCIATED WITH HYPERTENSION

Excess weight is associated with hypertension in women, as is the distribution of body fat. Hypertension is more frequently associated with intra-abdominal upper body obesity, as compared with obesity of the hips and buttocks. Insulin resistance is also associated with hypertension, independent of weight and age. Type II diabetes occurs twice as frequently in hypertensive patients, compared with matched normotensive patients.

Race is associated with different patterns of hypertension in Americans. African-Americans have a higher prevalence of hypertension and a higher proportion of uncontrolled hypertension, as well as a higher incidence of stroke, renal failure, and heart involvement. The risk of end-stage renal disease is much greater for hypertensive African-Americans than for hypertensive whites. Response to medications may also vary by race.

Sodium and potassium intake may be significant factors in some salt-sensitive patients, including African-Americans, the elderly, and first-degree relatives of hypertensive patients. Several studies have indicated a relation between low calcium intake and elevated blood pressure. Calcium supplementation may lower blood pressure in some patients, particularly those who consume less than the recommended daily doses for calcium.

DIFFERENTIAL DIAGNOSIS

Many patients are falsely labeled hypertensive as a result of transient anxiety, recent intake of stimulants, or use of inappropriate blood-pressure measuring equipment. As many as 20% of patients classified as hypertensive have "white coat hypertension" and manifest increases in blood pressure only in the physician's office. Many of these patients display normal blood pressures when tested outside the physician's office or in less stressful situations. Thus, home monitoring and 24-hour ambulatory monitoring of blood pressure are important adjuncts to physician values in determining the true state of hypertension. In ambulatory monitoring, the patient wears a blood-pressure cuff and a recording monitor for 24 hours. Activities and emotions are also recorded during this time. Studies indicate that ambulatory blood-pressure readings may correlate better with certain complications of high blood pressure, specifically left ventricular hypertrophy, than do office or home values.

Many patients who present with apparent hypertension have only transiently elevated values due to recent ingestion of various drugs. Theophylline preparations, corticosteroids, over-the-counter asthma preparations (e.g., ephedrine), and over-the-counter common cold preparations containing phenylpropanolamine or pseudoephedrine can also raise blood pressure. Nonsteroidal antiinflammatory drugs reportedly raise blood pressure an average of 5 to 8 mm Hg and are commonly used by ambulatory patients who may have borderline blood-pressure elevations. Cyclosporine and estrogen-containing compounds, including birth control pills, may raise blood pressure, as may nasal decongestants, appetite suppressants, erythropoietin, tricyclic antidepressants, monoamine oxidase inhibitors, certain illicit drugs, and herbal remedies.

Blood pressure should be determined precisely and should be measured in such a way that the values obtained represent the patient's usual levels. Patients should be seated with their arm bared and supported at heart level. They should not have smoked or ingested caffeine within 30 minutes before the measurement. Patients should be allowed to rest quietly for 5 minutes before blood-pressure determinations are made.

A blood-pressure cuff of appropriate size must be used for women (the bladder within the cuff should encircle 80% of the arm). Oversized cuffs can underestimate blood pressure; undersized cuffs may overestimate it. Measurements should be taken with the mercury sphygmomanometer, a recently calibrated aneroid manometer, or an electronic device. Systolic and diastolic pressures should be recorded, with the diastolic value being the disappearance of the Korotkoff sound. At least two readings separated by 2 minutes should be averaged. If the first two readings differ by more than 5 mm Hg, additional readings should be obtained and averaged to yield a more representative value.

The diagnosis of hypertension should not be based on a single measurement. Ideally, the patient is seen on at least two subsequent visits 1 to 4 weeks after the initial readings are made, unless the initial readings are stage 3 (see below). The time of the patient's visits should vary to ensure a spectrum of times during the day. The patient's three initial visits should be divided between morning, midday, and afternoon.

LEVELS OF HYPERTENSION

Hypertension is graded to ensure appropriate therapy and follow-up. The following classifications have been established by the Joint National Committee on Detection, Evaluation, and Treatment of High Blood Pressure:

- Less than 130/85 mm Hg: normal
- 130 to 139/85 to 89 mm Hg: high normal
- 140 to 159/90 to 99 mm Hg: hypertension stage 1
- 160 to 179/100 to 109 mm Hg: hypertension stage 2
- Greater than 180/110 mm Hg: hypertension stage 3.

EVALUATION

Once the patient has been identified as hypertensive, it is important to consider whether she has primary or secondary hypertension. Most hypertensive patients have primary essential hypertension. Fewer than 10% have secondary causes, and most of these patients have kidney disease. The history should include questions regarding types of medications, including over-the-counter preparations, herbal remedies, and illegal drugs such as cocaine. The physical examination should attempt to identify patients who have abdominal or flank masses suggestive of polycystic kidneys. It should also identify abdominal bruits that may indicate renovascular disease. Delayed or absent femoral pulses and decreased blood pressure in the lower extremities may be compatible with aortic coarctation. Truncal obesity with purple striae may denote Cushing syndrome. Tachycardia, tremor, orthostatic hypotension, sweating, and pallor may indicate a pheochromocytoma.

The clinician must then identify the target organ disease or dysfunction. This requires assessment of the fundi, kidneys, and heart in all hypertensive patients. In addition, cardiovascular risk factors must be identified. Coronary artery disease and stroke are more likely to occur where hypertension exists with other risk factors, including hypercholesterolemia, family history, cigarette smoking, diabetes, obesity, and sedentary lifestyle. The presence of cardiovascular risk factors, in addition to the degree of blood-pressure elevation, determines the absolute risk level and therefore how aggressively blood pressure may need to be reduced.

Medical History

The evaluation begins with a complete medical history. Historical data should include information regarding family history of hypertension, premature coronary heart disease, stroke, diabetes mellitus, dyslipidemia, and cigarette smoking. Symptoms of cardiovascular disease, pending stroke or transient ischemic attack, renal disease, diabetes, dyslipidemia, or gout should be sought. It is also important to identify how long and to what degree the patient's blood pressure has been elevated. Information regarding physical activity, recreational drug use, sodium intake, consumption of alcohol, level of fat in the diet, and recent changes in weight is also important, as are questions regarding the patient's psychosocial status. The information gained may affect the subsequent level of control with treatment and may identify issues preventing adequate control. The history should also include questions about the patient's use of medications or herbal remedies that could raise the blood pressure, as listed earlier.

Physical Examination

The physical examination for hypertensive patients should include multiple blood pressure determinations separated by 2 minutes with the patient either supine or seated and after the patient has been standing for at least 2 minutes. Blood pressure should be taken in both arms, with the higher value used as a baseline. The examination should include estimates of height, weight, and variation from ideal body weight. A critical part of the examination is the funduscopic examination. This attempts to identify arteriolar narrowing, arteriovenous nicking, hemorrhages, exudates, or even papilledema. It includes examination of the neck for carotid bruits, distended veins, and enlarged thyroid indicative of metabolic disease.

The examination of the heart should include an estimate of the point of maximal impulse and should identify clicks, murmurs, arrhythmias, and additional heart sounds, including S_3 and S_4 gallops. Examination of the lungs should identify rales or evidence for bronchospasm. Examination of the abdomen should identify bruits, enlarged organs (particularly the kidneys), and the presence or absence of an abnormal aortic pulsation. The examination of the extremities is intended to identify diminished or absent peripheral pulses, bruits, or edema. A neurologic examination appropriate to the patient's condition should be performed. If evidence of hypertensive encephalopathy exists, then a full neurologic examination with mental status determination is appropriate.

Laboratory Evaluation

Routine laboratory studies in patients presenting with hypertension should include urinalysis, complete blood cell count, fasting blood glucose, creatinine clearance, potassium, fasting lipid profile with total cholesterol, high-density lipoprotein, and triglyceride levels. An electrocardiogram should be done on all patients to provide a baseline.

More extensive evaluations for secondary causes of hypertension include creatinine clearance, microalbuminuria, 24-hour urinary protein, serum calcium, uric acid, glycosylated hemoglobin, thyroid-stimulating hormone, echocardiography, arterial ultrasonography, measurement of ankle/arm index, plasma renin activity, and urinary sodium. These evaluations may be appropriate in the settings of severe hypertension or suspected secondary hypertension:

- Females less than age 25 with marked hypertension should be evaluated for renovascular etiology.
- Patients with evidence of advanced atherosclerosis with new-onset hypertension should be evaluated for renovascular hypertension.
- Patients with spontaneous or low-dose diuretic-induced persistent hypokalemia should be evaluated for aldosteronism.
- Patients with headache, flushing, diaphoresis, and marked blood-pressure lability should be evaluated for pheochromocytoma.
- Patients with previously well-controlled hypertension whose blood pressures begin to rise.
- Patients with stage 3 hypertension should be evaluated for renovascular hypertension.
- Patients with sudden onset hypertension.
- Patients who have resistant hypertension (hypertension not amenable to conventional therapy) should be evaluated for renovascular hypertension or other secondary causes.

Evaluation of Renovascular Hypertension

Renovascular disease is a rare cause of hypertension, occurring in fewer than 5% of hypertensive patients. Because it is potentially curable, the diagnosis should be considered in (a) young white women with hypertension who may have fibromuscular hyperplasia, (b) older hypertensive patients with hypertension of recent onset or those refractory to therapy, (c) patients who have evidence of advanced atherosclerotic disease or abdominal bruits, (d) patients with accelerated or resistant hypertension, (e) patients with recurrent "flash" pulmonary edema, (f) patients with renal failure of uncertain cause, and (g) patients with acute renal failure precipitated by antihypertensive medications, especially angiotensin-converting enzyme (ACE) inhibitors or angiotensin II receptor blockers (ARB).

Evaluation of renovascular causes of hypertension should be considered only in patients who are candidates for surgical or angioplastic correction of renal artery stenosis. The presence of renal artery stenosis can be initially determined noninvasively by duplex ultrasonography, magnetic resonance angiography, or computed tomographic angiography. Nuclear imaging with technetium-labeled pentetic acid to determine the total glomerular filtration rate and the glomerular filtration rate to each kidney is valuable as an adjunct to these noninvasive tests. The indications to proceed with renal revascularization (via surgical or percutaneous techniques) are controversial.

Not all stenotic lesions are functionally significant; therefore, split renal vein renin determinations after administration of ACE inhibitor are useful in predicting responses to surgery or angioplasty. Revascularization alone is rarely sufficient to control hypertension in these settings, and antihypertensive medical therapy is typically needed after revascularization. The likelihood of cure of hypertension is highest in patients with resistant hypertension and fibromuscular dysplasia. The ideal candidate for renal artery revascularization will be further clarified as more trials concerning this issue are completed.

TREATMENT

Complications, including stroke, heart failure, and myocardial infarction, are common in hypertensive patients. Several studies, including the Veterans Administration Cooperative Study, have shown a decrease in mortality and morbidity when patients whose diastolic blood pressures exceeded 104 mm Hg had their pressures lowered with drugs, lifestyle changes, or both. The most striking benefits from treatment of mild hypertension come from prevention of stroke rather than from reductions in myocardial infarction. However, metaanalyses of randomized trials indicate that the rates of fatal and nonfatal myocardial infarction are decreased by about 20% when mild to moderate hypertension is treated. Another metaanalysis of randomized trials indicated a 42% reduction in stroke from a diastolic reduction of just 5 to 6 mm Hg. A similar reduction in diastolic blood pressure effected a 14% decrease in coronary heart disease during 6 years of follow-up. Ideally, blood pressure should be maintained below 140/90 mm Hg if tolerated. Treatment to lower levels may be desired, in certain instances, to prevent stroke, maintain renal function, or attenuate heart failure progression. In the presence of diabetes mellitus the goal of therapy should be 130/80 mm Hg.

Because the goal of therapy is to reduce or modify cardiovascular risk factors, the intensity of treatment is predicated by the patient's perceived risk and presence of cardiovascular disease. To that end, patients can be stratified into three major categories of cardiovascular risk based on the presence of risk factors or cardiovascular disease (Table 41.1). Risk group A is defined as patients with hypertension who do not have clinical cardiovascular disease or risk factors; risk group B includes patients with hypertension who do not have clinical cardiovascular disease but have one or more risk factors, excluding diabetes mellitus; risk group C includes patients with hypertension who have clinical cardiovascular disease and/or diabetes mellitus. The intensity of therapy for hypertension, particularly the need for pharmacologic therapy, is governed by the patient's risk category and stage of hypertension (Table 41.2). Pharmacologic therapy is always instituted in conjunction with lifestyle modification.

Diet and Lifestyle Changes

Lifestyle modifications may be adequate to control hypertension. These initiatives are consistent with good general health and, in some instances, with reduction in cardiovascular risk. In many instances, they are adequate to control mild to moderate hypertension (stage 1 or 2). Even if lifestyle modifications are not adequate to control elevated blood pressure, they are still important adjuncts to therapy for all levels of hypertension.

TABLE 41.1. Components of Cardiovascular Risk Stratification in Patients with Hypertension

Major risk factors	Target organ damage/ clinical cardiovascular disease
Smoking	Heart diseases
Dyslipidemia	Left ventricular hypertrophy
Age >60 y	Angina/prior myocardial infarction
Sex (men and postmenopausal women)	Prior coronary revascularization
	Heart failure
Family history of cardiovascular disease	Stroke or transient ischemic attack
Women under age 65 or men under age 55	Nephropathy
	Peripheral arterial disease
	Retinopathy

Adapted from The sixth report of the Joint National Committee on prevention, detection, evaluation, and treatment of high blood pressure. *Arch Intern Med* 1997;157:2413–2446, with permission.

TABLE 41.2. Risk Stratification and Treatment

Blood pressure stages (mm Hg)	Risk group A	Risk group B	Risk group C
High–normal (130–139/85–89)	Lifestyle modification	Lifestyle modification	Drug therapy[a]
Stage 1 (140–159/90–99)	Lifestyle modification (up to 12 months)	Lifestyle modification[b] (up to 6 months)	Drug therapy
Stages 2 and 3 (≥160/≥100)	Drug therapy	Drug therapy	Drug therapy

[a]For those with heart failure, renal insufficiency, or diabetes.
[b]For patients with multiple risk factors, clinicians should consider drugs as a part of initial therapy.
Adapted from The sixth report of the Joint National Committee on prevention, detection, evaluation, and treatment of high blood pressure. *Arch Intern Med* 1997;157:2413–2446, with permission.

Body mass index (weight in kilograms divided by height in meters) over 27 and excess fat in the upper part of the body (waist circumference greater than 85 cm [34 inches] in women) have been associated with increased risk for hypertension, dyslipidemia, diabetes, and coronary disease. Weight reduction should be recommended for all patients who meet these criteria. A blood-pressure reduction usually occurs early, with a weight loss of as small as 10 pounds. Furthermore, weight reduction improves the effect of pharmacologic therapy for hypertension and reduces cardiovascular risk factors. An individualized weight reduction program, which includes caloric restriction and increased exercise, is helpful; however, recidivism is common. Pharmacologic therapy for obesity should be avoided in these patients because many of these agents increase blood pressure, are associated with valvular heart disease, or cause pulmonary hypertension.

Moderation of alcohol intake is recommended for all patients with hypertension. Alcohol can raise blood pressure and can also cause resistance to antihypertensive therapy. Patients should be counseled to drink no more than 1 oz of ethanol (8 oz of wine or 24 oz of beer) in a 24-hour period.

Regular aerobic exercise is important in achieving fitness, helping to lower blood pressure and reducing the risk of cardiovascular disease and all causes of mortality. Unfit normotensive patients have a 20% to 50% increased risk of developing hypertension when compared with their more active and fit counterparts. Moderately intense physical exercise at 40% to 60% of maximal oxygen consumption can lower a hypertensive patient's systolic blood pressure by 10 mm Hg. For most sedentary patients, brisk walking 30 to 45 minutes three to five times per week will achieve these goals. It may also help promote weight loss and minimize other cardiovascular risks. However, patients with known cardiac disease or other more serious health problems should undergo a thorough examination before proceeding with even moderate exercise.

Dietary changes, with limitation of saturated fat and total calories, should be recommended for patients who have elevated lipids and for those above ideal body weight. The Dietary Approaches to Stop Hypertension diet has been shown to be effective in preventing and treating hypertension (more information regarding this diet is available on line through *www.nhlbi.nih.gov*). In addition, sodium restriction seems prudent. Patients who reduce their daily sodium intake to less than 2.4 g of sodium, or about 6 g of sodium chloride, may be able to reduce their systolic blood pressure by up to 5 to 10 mm Hg. African-American women and elderly women seem to benefit most from reductions in dietary sodium chloride. Dietary counseling to achieve this level of sodium reduction is usually required. Sodium avoidance may be adequate in and of itself to control stage 1 hypertension but also benefits patients treated with antihypertensive medications. Although there is an association between dietary potassium and calcium intake in the prevention and control of blood pressure, formal supplementation is not recommended. Patients should ingest the usual daily allowance of these substances, preferably from food sources. Diuretics that enhance hypokalemia may complicate hypertensive therapy. In addition, patients with renal impairment or those who are taking ACE inhibitors or ARBs should avoid high-potassium regimens. Although much has been written about magnesium supplementation in hypertensive patients, there are no convincing data to justify recommending an increased magnesium intake in an effort to lower blood pressure. Similarly, claims of near-magical effects of garlic and onion supplements in lowering blood pressure have not been confirmed in controlled trials.

Smoking cessation is critical for patients with essential hypertension. Although smoking cessation may not significantly lower blood pressure, it reduces the cardiovascular risks in hypertensive patients. Smoking has a multiplicative effect when combined with hypertension in increasing coronary and vascular risks. Smoking cessation agents contain lower amounts of nicotine and usually will not raise blood pressure and may be used as adjuncts to counseling and behavioral interventions.

Many patients with hypertension suffer from variable levels of anxiety. In some cases, stress plays a role in inducing and maintaining hypertension. Stress reduction and management are appropriate goals to maximize the quality of life, but there is little evidence that behavior modification and stress management are effective in controlling hypertension. For certain patients, however, antianxiety therapy may be an appropriate adjunct to hypertension treatment.

Drug Therapy

If blood pressure remains at or above 140/90 mm Hg despite vigorous efforts at lifestyle modification, pharmacologic agents should be started. This is especially true in patients who have target organ dysfunction, cardiovascular disease, or other cardiovascular disease risk factors (Table 41.2). If patients do not have target organ dysfunction or other risk factors and pressures are 149/94 mm Hg or below, they may be observed for another 3 to 6 months with nonpharmacologic therapy. These patients should be observed closely and not lost to follow-up, because blood pressure in these patients often rises and may lead to target organ dysfunction before appropriate therapy is initiated.

Various agents in multiple drug classes effectively lower blood pressure. Table 41.3 describes medications, dosages, and

TABLE 41.3. Oral Antihypertensive Agents

Drug	Usual dose range total[a] (mg/d)	Side effects[b]
Diuretics (partial list)		Short term: increases in cholesterol and glucose levels; biochemical abnormalities: decreases potassium, sodium, and magnesium levels, increases uric acid and calcium levels; rare blood dyscrasias, photosensitivity, pancreatitis, hyponatremia
Chlorthalidone	12.5–50 (1)	
Hydrochlorothiazide	12.5–50 (1)	
Indapamide	1.25–5 (1)	(Less or no hypercholesterolemia)
Metolazone	2.5–10 (1)	
Loop diuretics		
Bumetanide	0.5–4 (2–3)	(Short duration of action, no hypercalcemia)
Ethacrynic acid	25–100 (2–3)	(Only nonsulfonamide diuretic, ototoxicity)
Furosemide	40–240 (2–3)	(Short duration of action, no hypercalcemia)
Torsemide	5–100 (2)	
Potassium-sparing agents		Hyperkalemia
Amiloride hydrochloride	5–10 (1)	
Spironolactone	25–100 (1)	(Gynecomastia)
Triamterene	25–100 (1)	
Adrenergic inhibitors		
Peripheral agents		
Guanadrel	10–75 (2)	(Postural hypotension, diarrhea)
Guanethidine monosulfate	10–150 (1)	(Postural hypotension, diarrhea)
Reserpine	0.05–0.25 (1)	(Nasal congestion, sedation, depression, activation of peptic ulcer)
Central alpha-agonists		Sedation, dry mouth, bradycardia, withdrawal hypertension
Clonidine hydrochloride	0.2–1.2 (2–3)	(More withdrawal)
Guanabenz acetate	8–32 (2)	
Guanfacine hydrochloride	1–3 (1)	(Less withdrawal)
Methyldopa	500–3,000 (2)	(Hepatic and "autoimmune" disorders)
Alpha-blockers		Postural hypotension
Doxazosin mesylate	1–16 (1)	
Prazosin hydrochloride	2–30 (2–3)	
Terazosin hydrochloride	1–20 (1)	
Beta-blockers		Bronchospasm, bradycardia, heart failure, may mask insulin hypoglycemia, impaired peripheral circulation, insomnia, fatigue, decreased exercise tolerance, hypertriglyceridemia
Acebutolol	200–800 (1)	
Atenolol	25–100 (1–2)	
Betaxolol	5–20 (1)	
Bisoprolol fumarate	2.5–10 (1)	
Carteolol hydrochloride	2.5–10 (1)	
Metoprolol tartrate	50–300 (2)	
Metoprolol succinate	50–300 (1)	
Nadolol	40–320 (1)	
Penbutolol sulfate	10–20 (1)	
Pindolol	10–60 (2)	
Propanolol hydrochloride	40–480 (2)	
Timolol maleate	20–60 (2)	
Combined alpha- and beta-blockers		Postural hypotension, bronchospasm
Carvedilol	12.5–50 (2)	
Labetalol	200–1200 (2)	
Direct vasodilators		Headaches, fluid retention, tachycardia
Hydralazine hydrochloride	50–300 (2)	(Lupus syndrome)
Minoxidil	5–100 (1)	(Hirsutism)
Calcium antagonists		
Nondihydropyridines		Conduction defects, worsening of systolic dysfunction, gingival hyperplasia
Diltiazem hydrochloride	120–360 (1–2)	(Nausea, headache)
Mibefradil dihydrochloride	50–100 (1)	(No worsening of systolic dysfunction; contraindicated with terfenadine, astemizole, and cisapride)
Verapamil hydrochloride	90–480 (1–2)	(Constipation)
Dihydropyridines		Edema of the ankle, flushing, headache, gingival hypertrophy
Amlodipine	2.5–10 (1)	
Felodipine	2.5–20 (1)	
Isradipine	5–20 (1–2)	
Nicardipine	60–90 (2)	
Nifedipine	30–120 (1)	
Nisoldipine	20–60 (1)	

(continued)

TABLE 41.3. (*continued*)

Drug	Usual dose range total[a] (mg/d)	Side effects[b]
Angiotensin-converting enzyme inhibitors		Common: cough; rare: angioedema, hyperkalemia, rash, loss of taste, leukopenia
Benazepril hydrochloride	5–40 (1–2)	
Captopril	25–150 (2–3)	
Enalapril maleate	5–40 (1–2)	
Fosinopril sodium	10–40 (1–2)	
Lisinopril	5–40 (1)	
Moexipril	7.5–15 (1–2)	
Quinapril hydrochloride	5–80 (1–2)	
Ramipril	1.25–20 (1–2)	
Trandolapril	1–4 (1)	
ARBs		Angioedema (very rare), hyperkalemia
Losartan potassium	25–100 (1–2)	
Valsartan	80–320 (1)	
Irbesartan	150–300 (1)	

[a]Values in parentheses are frequency per day. These dosages vary from those listed in the *Physician's Desk Reference* (51st edition), which may be consulted for additional information.
[b]The listing of side effects is not all inclusive, and side effects are for the class of drugs except where noted in parenthesis.
Adapted from The sixth report of the Joint National Committee on prevention, detection, evaluation, and treatment of high blood pressure. *Arch Intern Med* 1997;157:2413–2446, with permission.

dosing intervals. Several factors should be taken into consideration when selecting an initial antihypertensive drug, including efficacy, cost, compliance, adverse effects, organ involvement, and atherosclerotic risk factor modification. About half of all patients can be expected to respond to monotherapy. When a second drug from a different class is added, 70% to 90% of patients achieve blood-pressure control.

Confusion may exist as to when to add a second agent rather than substituting a different drug for the initial one. In patients who respond to the initial medication with a reduction in blood pressure of 15 mm Hg systolic or 10 mm Hg diastolic but who do not achieve their goal blood pressure, additive therapy is recommended. If, at maximum tolerated doses, the initial drug used in monotherapy did not result in significant reduction in blood pressure, then substituting a different class of drug is often effective. Newer agents that offer combinations of two different classes of drugs are attractive in these settings. Two drugs from a similar class are generally not recommended for routine control of blood pressure. The addition of a third medication, frequently a diuretic, is not uncommon to control stage 3 hypertension. Frequently, adding a second or third medication not only facilitates the desired further decrease in blood pressure but also deals with the side effects of the two others. For example, diuretics may be used as a second or third class of drug when hypertension is not yet under adequate control and significant edema has occurred as a result of certain classes of medications, such as calcium antagonists. Diuretics may also be used to control the mild potassium elevations that may occur with the use of ACE inhibitors or ARBs in certain patients.

In many patients, it is undesirable to reduce the diastolic blood pressure below 80 mm Hg because of the J-curve phenomenon. In this hypothesis, it is believed that lowering diastolic blood pressure too much may increase the risk of coronary heart disease, possibly by lowering diastolic perfusion pressure in the coronary circulation. However, an increase in mortality in this setting is probably not caused by reduced diastolic blood pressure specifically but by underlying coronary artery disease and subsequent hypoperfusion. The clinician must carefully weigh the risks of myocardial ischemia and cerebral hypoperfusion that can occur with overly aggressive intervention. In the absence of target organ dysfunction or system failure symptoms, a less aggressive approach may be appropriate. In the case of stage 3 hypertension, the goal of therapy should be to reduce blood-pressure levels *toward* normal but not necessarily *to* normal. In general, it is safe to reduce blood pressure under these circumstances to about 160/90 mm Hg.

When therapy in stage 1 and 2 hypertension has been deemed necessary, monotherapy is recommended. Diuretics and beta-blockers have been studied extensively and shown to reduce cardiovascular morbidity and mortality and thus are preferred for initial drug therapy. Thiazide diuretics effectively reduce stroke, myocardial infarction, and cardiovascular mortality in patients with mild to moderate hypertension. They tend to be inexpensive. However, they may worsen insulin resistance, cause hypokalemia, and affect lipid status. Beta-blockers are particularly useful in young white females who are hyperadrenergic. They may be less effective in older African-American women.

Many clinical settings exist that make the choice of an agent from another class more compelling because of the potential favorable or adverse effects on the comorbid conditions. For example, ACE inhibitors are desirable as initial therapy in patients with congestive heart failure and hypertension, whereas beta-blockers are not desired in patients with concomitant bronchospastic disease and hypertension. Table 41.4 summarizes considerations to individualize therapy. The optimal agent should provide 24-hour efficacy with daily dosing. A clinician must always be attentive to potential drug interactions when initiating therapy for hypertension (Table 41.5). Figure 41.1 provides an algorithm that helps the clinician address considerations in therapy initiation and modification.

Therapeutic regimens for stage 3 hypertension consist of starting with medications as for stage 1 and 2 hypertension and adding a second or third agent if necessary. The intervals

TABLE 41.4. Considerations for Individual Drug Therapy

Indication	Drug therapy
Compelling indications unless contraindicated	
Diabetes mellitus (type 1) with proteinuria	ACE inhibitor
Heart failure	ACE inhibitor, diuretics
Isolated systolic hypertension (elderly)	Diuretics (preferred), calcium antagonists (long acting dihydropyridine)
Myocardial infarction	Beta-blockers, ACE inhibitors
May have favorable effects on comorbid conditions	
Angina	Beta-blockers, calcium antagonists
Atrial tachycardia and fibrillation	Beta-blockers, calcium antagonists (nondihydropyridine)
Cyclosporine-induced hypertension	Calcium antagonists
Diabetes mellitus (type 1 or 2) with proteinuria	ACE inhibitor (preferred), calcium antagonist
Diabetes mellitus (type 2)	Low-dose diuretics
Dyslipidemia	Alpha-blockers
Essential tremor	Beta-blockers
Heart failure	Carvedilol, losartan potassium
Hyperthyroidism	Beta-blockers
Migraine	Beta-blockers, calcium antagonists
Myocardial infarction	Diltiazem hydrochloride, verapamil hydrochloride
Osteoporosis	Thiazides
Preoperative hypertension	Beta-blockers
Renal insufficiency (caution in renovascular hypertension and creatinine >3 mg/dL)	ACE inhibitors
May have unfavorable effects on comorbid conditions	
Bronchospastic disease	Beta-blockers
Depression	Beta-blockers, central α-agonists, reserpine
Dyslipidemia	Beta-blockers, diuretics (high dose)
Gout	Diuretics
Second- or third-degree heart block	Beta-blockers, calcium antagonists (nondihydropyridine)
Heart failure	Beta-blockers (except carvedilol), calcium antagonists (except amlodipine, felodipine)
Liver disease	Labetalol, methyldopa
Peripheral vascular disease	Beta-blockers
Pregnancy	ACE inhibitors, ARBs
Renal insufficiency	Potassium-sparing diuretics
Renovascular disease	ACE inhibitors, ARBs

ACE, angiotensin-converting enzyme.
Adapted from The sixth report of the Joint National Committee on prevention, detection, evaluation, and treatment of high blood pressure. *Arch Intern Med* 1997;157:2413–2446, with permission.

between redocumentation of blood pressure and changes in the regimen should be decreased. In some cases, it may be necessary to use more than one agent for initial therapy. In patients whose diastolic pressure exceeds 120 mm Hg, more aggressive therapy may be required. If significant target organ dysfunction is present, these patients may benefit from hospitalization and consultation.

Follow-Up of Hypertensive Patients

After patients have been diagnosed with hypertension, follow-up at appropriate intervals is required. Recommendations for follow-up based on the initial set of blood-pressure measurements are outlined in Table 41.6. Although patients should be started on the lowest dosages listed in Table 41.3 to minimize side effects, increases in dosage may be required to effect adequate control. The clinician should not be discouraged if the patient does not initially respond to pharmacologic therapy. One may increase the medication to the next dosage level and subsequently to maximal dosages over several weeks to months. This presumes that the patient has tolerated the medication well in terms of not having significant adverse effects. If the patient does not tolerate a low dose of an initial therapeutic agent, she certainly will not tolerate a higher dose. Under these circumstances, it may be appropriate to switch to an alternative drug. If the agent is well tolerated but blood-pressure control is inadequate, the dosage should be increased over several weeks to months to achieve a maximally recommended and tolerated dose. When therapy is inadequate to control blood pressure, the clinician should consider the possibility of secondary hypertension as well as causes for the lack of responsiveness to therapy as listed in Table 41.7.

When patients have been well controlled on antihypertensive medications, attempts should be made to decrease the dosage of these medications or their number, or both. When blood pressure has been effectively controlled during at least four visits over a 1-year period, a deliberate slow withdrawal of medication is prudent. The patient must continue lifestyle modifications. Many patients can be maintained under adequate control with a small dosage of a single medication; if multiple drugs had been used, many patients can be maintained with monotherapy.

HYPERTENSION IN SELECTED SITUATIONS

Isolated *systolic hypertension* is frequently seen in elderly women. When systolic hypertension without diastolic hypertension occurs in younger females, it indicates a hyperdynamic circulation and may predict future diastolic elevations. When

TABLE 41.5. Selected Drug Interactions with Antihypertensive Therapy

Class of agent	Increase efficacy	Decrease efficacy	Effect on other drugs
Diuretics	Diuretics that act on different sites in the nephron (e.g., furosemide + thiazides)	Resin binding agents NSAIDS Steroids	Diuretics raise serum lithium levels Potassium-sparing agents may exacerbate hyperkalemia due to ACE inhibitors
Beta-blockers	For hepatically metabolized agents 1. Cimetidine 2. Quinidine 3. Food	NSAIDS Withdrawal of clonidine agents that induce hepatic enzymes, including rifampin and phenobarbitol	Propanolol hydrochloride induces hepatic enzymes to increase clearance of drugs with similar metabolic pathways Beta-blockers may mask and prolong insulin-induced hypoglycemia Heart block may occur with nondihydropyridine calcium antagonists Sympathomimetics cause unopposed α-adrenoreceptor mediated vasoconstriction Beta-blockers increase angina inducing potential of cocaine
ACE inhibitors	Chlorpromazine or clozapine	NSAIDS Antacids Food decreases absorption (moexipril)	ACE inhibitors may raise serum lithium levels ACE inhibitors may exacerbate hyperkalemic effect of potassium sparing agents
Calcium antagonists	Grapefruit juice Cimetidine or ranitidine	Agents that induce hepatic enzymes, including rifampin and phenobarbitol	Cyclosporine levels increase with diltiazem hydrochloride, mibefradil dihydrochloride, or nicardipine hydrochloride but not felodipine, isradipine, or nifedipine Nondihydropyridines increase levels of other drugs metabolized by the same hepatic enzyme system, including digoxin, quinidine, sulfonylureas, and theophylline Verapamil hydrochloride may lower serum lithium levels
Alpha-blockers			Prazosin may decrease clearance of verapamil hydrochloride
Central α-agonists and peripheral neuronal blockers		Tricyclic antidepressants (and probably phenothiazines) Monoamine oxidase inhibitors Sympathomimetics or phenothiazines antagonize guanethidine monosulfate or guanadrel sulfate	Methyldopa may increase serum lithium levels Severity of clonidine hydrochloride withdrawal may be increased by beta-blockers Many agents used in anesthesia are potentiated by clonidine hydrochloride

Adapted from The sixth report of the Joint National Committee on prevention, detection, evaluation, and treatment of high blood pressure. *Arch Intern Med* 1997;157:2413–2446, with permission.

the systolic blood pressure consistently exceeds 160 mm Hg even though the diastolic blood pressure is less than 90 mm Hg, therapy should be considered. Younger patients without evidence of target organ dysfunction should be continued on lifestyle modification and close observation.

Pseudohypertension is occasionally encountered in elderly patients with rigid brachial arteries. Because the sphygmomanometer cuff cannot compress the brachial artery, artificially high readings are obtained. This condition should be suspected in elderly women who have not previously been hypertensive and who manifest no evidence of target organ dysfunction despite very high blood pressures. This condition can be confirmed by palpation of a radial artery pulse despite inflation of a blood pressure cuff to pressures well above expected systolic pressure.

Hypertension emergencies are an important category to consider but are beyond the scope of this chapter. The primary care physician should seek appropriate consultation and referral for these patients.

Hypertensive encephalopathy results from excessive perfusion of the brain when its autoregulatory mechanism is exceeded and is a hypertension emergency. Sodium nitroprusside administration may be used to reduce blood pressure over 3 to 4 hours to 160/100 mm Hg; however, blood pressure should not be reduced by more than 25% of initial levels.

Use of several *illicit drugs,* including cocaine, crack, amphetamines, phencyclidine hydrochloride, or diet pills, may acutely raise blood pressure. Frequently, the patient presents with stroke, seizures, myocardial infarction, or encephalopathy (all of which constitute a hypertension emergency). Sodium nitroprusside is the treatment of choice. Phentolamine is an alternative therapy. Beta-blockers should be avoided because of the potential for coronary spasm as a result of unopposed α-adrenergic receptor activation.

Most women experience a slight rise in blood pressure with use of *oral contraceptives.* However, their blood pressure usually does not rise out of the normal range. Hypertension may be as much as three times more common in women taking oral contraceptives for more than 5 years than in those never exposed to oral contraceptives. Risks of hypertension appear to increase with duration of use, age, and increased body mass. In general, oral contraceptives should be avoided in women over the age of 35 if they cannot stop smoking. Most of the cardiovascular deaths attributable to oral contraceptives have occurred in

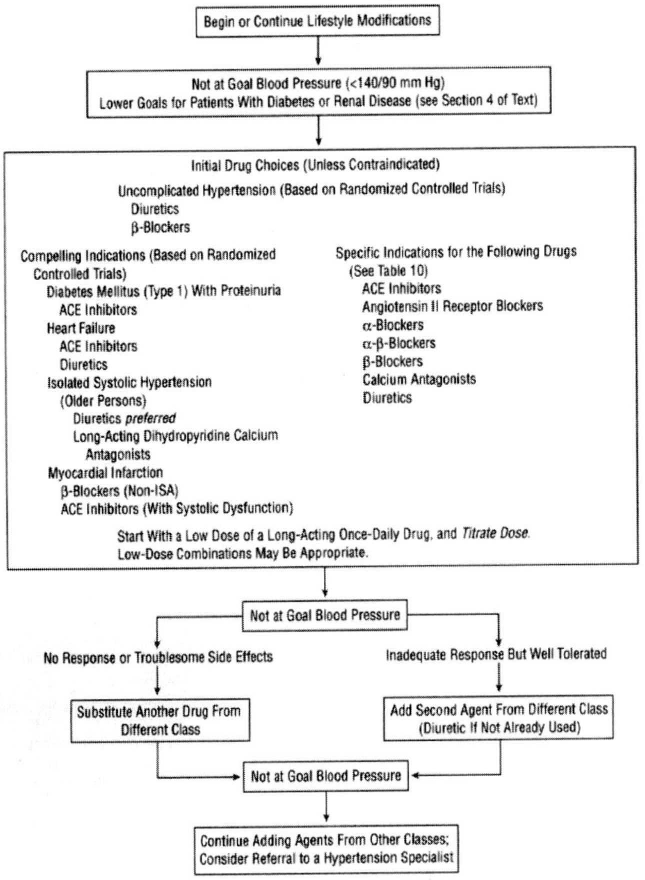

FIG. 41.1. An algorithm for treatment selection for hypertension. (Adapted from the sixth report of the Joint National Committee on prevention, detection, evaluation, and treatment of high blood pressure. *Arch Intern Med* 1997;157:2413–2446, with permission.)

women over age 35 who have continued to smoke. Hypertension among women taking oral contraceptives should result in discontinuation of these drugs and close monitoring of subsequent blood pressure. If no other suitable form of contraceptive therapy is available and the risk of pregnancy in a particular patient is greater than the risk of hypertension, then oral contraceptive therapy may be continued in conjunction with pharmacologic therapy for hypertension. Hormonal replacement therapy with estrogen compounds in postmenopausal women has generally not been associated with the development of hypertension. These patients, however, should have blood-pressure levels determined 1 month and 6 months after starting therapy.

Hypertension and diabetes mellitus increase the risk of cardiovascular events fourfold in women. These patients are also at increased risk of retinopathy and nephropathy. Several trials have demonstrated improved outcomes in these patients with lower target blood pressure levels; therefore, the American Diabetes Association recommends treatment target to be systolic less than 130 mm Hg and diastolic less than 80 mm Hg. With regards to lifestyle modification, the American Diabetes Association recommends exercise testing before beginning a vigorous exercise program for all diabetic patients over the age of 35. Stress testing is not recommended for patients planning to undergo low or moderate levels of exercise, such as walking.

CONSIDERATIONS IN PREGNANCY

It is important to diagnose and treat hypertension during pregnancy effectively, because it may result in life-threatening consequences for mother and fetus. The criteria for diagnosing hypertension in pregnancy are blood-pressure measurements of greater than 140/90 mm Hg. According to a classification recommended by the National High Blood Pressure Education Program's Working Group Report on High Blood Pressure in Pregnancy, hypertension in pregnancy may be placed in one of four categories: chronic hypertension, preeclampsia–eclampsia, preeclampsia superimposed on chronic hypertension, and gestational hypertension.

Chronic hypertension is hypertension observed before pregnancy or diagnosed before the 20th week of gestation. Hypertension that is diagnosed during pregnancy and continued postpartum is also classified as chronic hypertension. Women with hypertension of several years' duration and evidence of end-organ damage should be advised that pregnancy might accelerate their end-organ dysfunction. In patients with renal dysfunction, the risk of fetal loss is 10-fold when hypertension is present during pregnancy, compared with when it is not. The patient's prepregnancy medication may be continued, with the

TABLE 41.6. Recommendations for Follow-up Based on Initial Blood Pressure Measurements[a]

Initial blood pressure		Follow-up recommended
Systolic	Diastolic	
<130	<85	Recheck in 2 yr
130–139	85–89	Recheck in 1 yr
140–149	90–99	Confirm within 2 mo
160–179	100–109	Evaluate or refer to source of care within 1 mo
≥180	≥110	Evaluate or refer to source of care immediately or within 1 wk depending on the clinical situation

[a]If any systolic and diastolic categories are different, follow recommendations for shorter time to follow-up. Modify schedule of follow-up based on reliable information about prior blood pressure measurements, known risk factors, or target organ disease.

Adapted from The sixth report of the Joint National Committee on prevention, detection, evaluation, and treatment of high blood pressure. *Arch Intern Med* 1997;157:2413–2446, with permission.

TABLE 41.7. Causes of Inadequate Responses to Therapy

Class	Examples
Pseudoresistance	"White coat" hypertension Pseudohypertension in older patients Use of inappropriately sized cuff
Volume overload	Excess salt intake Progressive renal damage Fluid retention from reduction of blood pressure Inadequate diuretic therapy
Drug-related costs	Doses too low Wrong type of diuretic Inappropriate combinations Rapid inactivation Drug actions and interactions Sympathomimetics Nasal decongestants Appetite suppressants Cocaine and other illicit drugs Caffeine Oral contraceptives Adrenal steroids Licorice Cyclosporine, tacrolimus Erythropoietin Antidepressants Nonsteroidal antiinflammatory drugs
Associated conditions	Smoking Increasing obesity Sleep apnea Insulin resistance/hyperinsulinemia Ethanol intake >1 oz./d Anxiety-induced hyperventilation or panic attacks Chronic pain Intense vasoconstriction (arteritis) Organic brain syndrome (e.g., memory deficit)

Adapted from The sixth report of the Joint National Committee on prevention, detection, evaluation, and treatment of high blood pressure. *Arch Intern Med* 1997;157:2413–2446, with permission.

exception of ACE inhibitors and ARBs, which can cause serious neonatal problems, including renal failure and death. For patients who were not previously on a medication and who do not respond to rest and moderate sodium restriction, antihypertensive drug therapy should be instituted when the systolic blood pressure is 150 mm Hg or greater or the diastolic blood pressure is 100 mm Hg or greater. The presence of target organ damage requires pharmacologic therapy. Aggressive pressure-lowering regimens are discouraged to avoid compromising the uteroplacental blood flow. Methyldopa has been used extensively in pregnancy, is considered safe, and is the agent of choice. Beta-blockers are as effective as methyldopa in lowering blood pressure, but their safety in early pregnancy has been questioned. The use of diuretic agents during pregnancy is only recommended in the setting of continuing prepregnancy agents; they are not recommended in preeclampsia. Hydralazine is the first-line parenteral agent because of its long history of safety and efficacy.

Preeclampsia is a state of gestational blood pressure elevation associated with proteinuria and edema and frequently with abnormalities of coagulation and liver function. Preeclampsia must be recognized, because it may evolve to eclampsia. It should be noted that women who have a systolic blood pressure rise of more than 30 mm Hg or a diastolic blood pressure rise of more than 15 mm Hg but do not meet the criteria for hypertension in pregnancy warrant close observation for signs of eclampsia. The diagnosis of preeclampsia superimposed on chronic hypertension may be difficult to distinguish from worsening chronic hypertension, because there are no established criteria for the former syndrome. It is recommended to maintain a high clinical suspicion of this syndrome. Further details regarding preeclampsia and eclampsia can be found in appropriate obstetric texts.

Gestational or transient hypertension involves blood pressure elevations that usually occur after the 20th week of pregnancy and disappear after delivery. Often these patients are overweight and have a family history of hypertension, and they often become hypertensive in later years. They must be observed closely during pregnancy, with frequent determinations of blood pressure, as well as detection of urinary protein, serum uric acid, creatinine clearance, blood urea nitrogen, hemoglobin, hematocrit, and coagulation profiles to identify progression to preeclampsia. Methyldopa or beta-blockers are usually effective in lowering blood pressure if nonpharmacologic efforts are unsuccessful and the diastolic blood pressure remains above 100 mm Hg.

With regards to hypertensive women who are breast-feeding, the clinician may withhold medication and undergo close monitoring of women with stage 1 hypertension. Methyldopa, hydralazine, propanolol, and labetalol (but not other beta-blockers) are recommended agents in lactating hypertensive women. ACE inhibitors and ARBs should be avoided. Given the paucity of data, lactating women and their infants should be closely monitored for adverse effects.

REFERRAL OF HYPERTENSIVE PATIENTS

Primary care physicians should feel comfortable in managing most patients with hypertension, but referral of patients to a hypertension specialist, either a cardiologist or a nephrologist with an interest in hypertension, is appropriate in the following situations:

- Refractory blood-pressure elevations despite multiple trials with maximal-dose agents in a combination of two or more of these medications in different classes
- Strong suspicion of renovascular hypertension
- Evidence of ongoing target organ dysfunction or organ system deterioration (e.g., evidence of myocardial ischemia or infarction, progressive left ventricular dysfunction with or without acute pulmonary edema, hypertensive encephalopathy, transient ischemic attack, cerebrovascular accident, progressive proteinuria, deterioration of blood urea nitrogen and creatinine clearance, and other end-organ dysfunctional agents)
- Any patient whose blood pressure has been reasonably well controlled but who has intolerable side effects despite attempts at multiple alternative agents.

Patients suspected of having aldosteronism, pheochromocytoma, or other endocrine states resulting in hypertension should be referred to an endocrinologist for definitive diagnosis and treatment. Hypertension in pregnancy is a serious complication and mandates referral to or consultation with a perinatologist or obstetrician experienced in the management of hypertensive diseases of pregnancy.

BIBLIOGRAPHY

ALLHAT Officers and Coordinators for the ALLHAT Research Group. Major outcomes in high-risk hypertensive patients randomized to angiotensin-convert-

ing enzyme inhibitor or calcium channel blocker versus diuretic. The Antihypertensive and Lipid-Lowering Treatment to Prevent Heart Attack Trial (ALLHAT). *JAMA* 2002;228:2981–2997.
American Diabetes Association. Treatment of hypertension in adults with diabetes. *Diabetes Care* 2002;25:71–73.
Appel LJ, Moore TJ, Obarzanek E, et al. A clinical trial of the effects of dietary patterns on blood pressure. Dash Collaborative Research Group. *N Engl J Med* 1997;336:1117–1124.
Aviv A. The roles of cell Ca^{2+}, protein kinase C, and the $Na(^{+})$-H^{+} antiport in the development of hypertension and insulin resistance. *J Am Soc Nephrol* 1992;3: 1049.
Burker EJ, Fredrikson M, Rifai N, et al. Serum lipids, neuroendocrine, and cardiovascular responses to stress in men and women with mild hypertension. *Behav Med* 1994;19:155.
Choo MH. Problems and solutions in diagnosing systemic hypertension. *Ann Acad Med Singapore* 1990;19:113.
Collins R, Peto R, MacMahon S, et al. Blood pressure, stroke, and coronary heart disease. Part 2. Short-term reductions in blood pressure: overview of randomized drug trials in their epidemiological context. *Lancet* 1990;335:765.
Conde-Agudelo A, Lede R, Belizan J. Evaluation of methods used in the prediction of hypertensive disorders of pregnancy. *Obstet Gynecol Surv* 1994;49:210.
Constantino RS. Hypertension. *Primary care for women.* Philadelphia: Lippincott Williams & Wilkins, 1996.
Croog SH, Elias MF, Colton T, et al. Effects of antihypertensive medications on quality of life in elderly hypertensive women. *Am J Hypertens* 1994;7:329.
Drory Y, Pines A, Fisman EZ, et al. Exercise response in young women with borderline hypertension. *Chest* 1990;97:298.
Eison H, Phillips RA, Ardeljan M, et al. Differences in ambulatory blood pressure between men and women with mild hypertension. *J Hum Hypertens* 1990;4: 400.
Enstrom I, Lindholm LH. Blood pressure in middle-aged women: a comparison between office-, self-, and ambulatory recordings. *Blood Press* 1992;1:240.
Epstein FH. The hypertensive patient beyond blood pressure. *J Hum Hypertens* 1992;6:459.
Falkner B. Differences in African Americans and whites with essential hypertension: biochemistry and endocrine. *Hypertension* 1990;15:681.
Greene J. NSAIDS and blood pressure: five not-so-silly millimeters. *Intern Med Alert* 1994;16:169.
Hall PM. Hypertension in women. *Cardiology* 1990;77:25.
Hansson L, Zanchetti A, Carruthers SG, et al. Effect on intensive blood-pressure lowering and low dose aspirin in patients with hypertension: principal results of the Hypertension Optimal Treatment (HOT) randomized trial. *Lancet* 1998;351:1755–1762.
Jamerson K, Julius S. Predictors of blood pressure and hypertension: general principles. *Am J Hypertens* 1991;4:5985.
Karpanou EA, Vyssoulis GP, Georgoudi DG, et al. Ambulatory blood pressure changes in the menstrual cycle of hypertensive women: significance of plasma renin activity values. *Am J Hypertens* 1993;6:654.
Knott C. The treatment of hypertension in pregnancy: clinical pharmacokinetic considerations. *Clin Pharmacokinet* 1991;21:233.
Langford HG, Davis BR, Blaufox D, et al. Effect of drug and diet treatment of mild hypertension on diastolic blood pressure: the TAIM Research Group. *Hypertension* 1991;17:210.
Manhem K, Jern C, Pilhall M, et al. Cardiovascular responses to stress in young hypertensive women. *J Hypertens* 1992;10:861.
Mann SJ. Systolic hypertension in the elderly: pathophysiology and management. *Arch Intern Med* 1992;152:1977.
Mann SJ, Pickering TG. Detection of renovascular hypertension. *Ann Intern Med* 1992;117:845.
Mundal HH, Nordby G, Lande K, et al. Effect of cold pressor test and awareness of hypertension on platelet function in normotensive and hypertensive women. *Scand J Clin Lab Invest* 1993;53:585.
O'Brien E, O'Malley K, Mee F, et al. Ambulatory blood pressure measurement in the diagnosis and management of hypertension. *J Hum Hypertens* 1991;5:23.
Os I, Nordby G. Hypertension and the metabolic cardiovascular syndrome: special reference to premenopausal women. *J Cardiovasc Pharmacol* 1992;20:515.
Parodi O, Neglia D, Sambuceti G, et al. Regional myocardial blood flow and coronary reserve in hypertensive patients: the effect of therapy. *Drugs* 1992;44:48.
Phillips RA. Etiology, pathophysiology, and treatment of left ventricular hypertrophy: focus on severe hypertension. *J Cardiovasc Pharmacol* 1993;21:555.
Report of the National High Blood Pressure Education Program Working Group on High Blood Pressure in Pregnancy. *Am J Obstet Gynecol* 2000;183:S1–S22.
Safian RD, Textor SC. Renal artery stenosis. *N Engl J Med* 2001;344:431–442.
The sixth report of the Joint National Committee on prevention, detection, evaluation, and treatment of high blood pressure. *Arch Intern Med* 1997;157: 2413–2446.
Verdecchia P, Porcellati C. Defining normal ambulatory blood pressure in relation to target organ damage and prognosis. *Am J Hypertens* 1993;6:2075.
Yusuf S, Sleight P, Pogue J, et al. Effects of an angiotensin-converting-enzyme inhibitor, ramipril, on cardiovascular events in high-risk patients: the Heart Outcomes Prevention Evaluation Study Investigators. *N Engl J Med* 2000; 342:145–153.

CHAPTER 42
Chest Pain

Patricia G. Fitzpatrick

The evaluation of chest pain is a common and diagnostically challenging problem facing primary care physicians. The potential etiologies are numerous, and the diagnosis relies on a careful history and physical examination to direct further investigation. Serious disorders such as acute myocardial infarction and unstable angina must be recognized and treated expediently. In the remainder of patients, the process of determining the presence or absence of coronary artery disease and the associated prognosis requires assessment of a variety of factors, including the patient's presentation, risk factor evaluation, pretest probability of disease, physical examination, and response to a therapeutic trial of medication or preliminary diagnostic testing. The difficulty in arriving at a diagnosis is compounded by the marked variation in presentation that is seen among patients who are later documented to have coronary artery disease.

Cardiac disease is the leading cause of death in men and women, with about 550,000 deaths annually in the United States. More than half of these deaths occur in women, and most of these are related to coronary artery disease. In addition, although mortality associated with cardiac disease has declined in recent years, the rate of decline has been less rapid in women. Until recently, chest pain, the usual manifestation of coronary disease, has been perceived as a relatively benign process in women, because when studied angiographically up to 50% of women presenting with "angina" have been shown to have no or minimal coronary artery disease. However, in women of advanced years, classic angina pectoris carries the same prognosis as in their male counterparts, with similar or greater associated morbidity and mortality.

DIFFERENTIAL DIAGNOSIS

Angina pectoris is a term first used by Heberden in the 18th century to describe a strangulation or choking sensation, triggered by exertional effort and relieved with rest. The differential diagnosis of chest pain is extensive, and some of the more common etiologies are listed in Table 42.1. Obtaining a detailed accurate history is the most important way to assess the significance and likely causes of chest pain. Chest pain is the most common manifestation of coronary artery disease; however, more vague symptoms such as fatigue, dyspnea on exertion, or no discomfort, such as in silent ischemia, may predominate. The chest discomfort of angina pectoris is typically not "painful" but rather is a pressure, squeezing, or tightness in the chest, occurring with or without associated symptoms such as shortness of breath, diaphoresis, nausea, and lightheadedness. Characterization of factors, such as location and quality of the discomfort, its intensity and duration, associated symptoms, and factors that precipitate or relieve symptoms, aid in the categorization of chest pain as typical angina, atypical angina, or nonanginal pain (Table 42.2).

Esophageal Disorders

Gastroesophageal reflux is relatively common and can cause inflammation of the esophageal mucosa. Patients also may develop esophagitis in other ways (Barrett esophagitis, lower esophageal sphincter disorders). Symptomatically, patients may experience retrosternal burning; however, this discomfort

TABLE 42.1. Differential Diagnosis of Chest Pain

Cardiac causes
- Myocardial infarction/acute ischemic syndromes (including coronary artery spasm or Prinzmetal angina)
- Mitral valve prolapse
- Aortic valvular stenosis
- Pericarditis
- Hypertrophic cardiomyopathy
- Microvascular angina (or syndrome X)

Pulmonary causes
- Pulmonary embolism ± infarction
- Pneumothorax
- Bronchitis, pneumonia, carcinoma
- Pleuritis

Esophageal causes
- Esophagitis, reflux, or other causes
- Esophageal spasm
- Esophageal motility disorders
- Esophageal rupture
- Tumor, foreign body
- Zenker diverticulum

Other gastrointestinal causes
- Cholecystitis, cholelithiasis
- Pancreatitis
- Peptic ulcer disease

Musculoskeletal/chest wall causes
- Costochondritis (including Tietze syndrome)
- Fracture, neoplasm, osteomyelitis
- Manubriosternal or episternal arthralgia
- Cervicothoracic spinal disorders
- Thoracic outlet obstruction
- Cystic mastitis

Miscellaneous causes
- Aortic dissection/aneurysm
- Hyperventilation syndrome
- Anxiety states

is nonradiating and continuous, is often precipitated by eating or swallowing certain foods and aggravated by lying down, is not related to exertion, and is relieved with food or antacids. *Esophageal spasm* may be relieved by sublingual nitroglycerin, but other features more typical for esophageal pain usually help differentiate this from a cardiac source. A diagnosis of hiatal hernia or gastroesophageal reflux does not exclude the diagnosis of coronary artery disease because the two disorders occur concomitantly in approximately 10% of patients.

Other Gastrointestinal Causes of Chest Pain

Biliary colic, caused by a rapid increase in biliary pressure due to obstruction of the bile or cystic duct, causes symptoms that may be confused with angina pectoris. The discomfort is usually constant, with a longer duration than typical angina (hours), and is more prominent in the right upper quadrant, although it may radiate to the substernal area as well as the epigastrium, left abdomen, and scapula. It typically occurs spontaneously, although there may be a history of dyspepsia or fatty food intolerance, and usually resolves spontaneously as well. *Peptic ulcer* discomfort usually is an epigastric or substernal burning that persists for hours; it is typically aggravated by lack of food or by foods with high acidity and is relieved with antacids or food.

Musculoskeletal Disorders and Chest Wall Syndromes

Costochondritis is a common musculoskeletal disorder that can mimic angina pectoris. It is characterized by localized superficial discomfort, which is aggravated by movement and palpation of the costochondral junctions, and typically is relieved by antiinflammatory medication and rest. *Tietze syndrome*, where there is actual swelling of the costochondral junction, is uncommon. Other uncommon musculoskeletal disorders also may produce symptoms similar to angina but are usually easily differentiated by a careful history and physical examination. *Cystic mastitis* is a common cause of chest wall pain, reproduced by pressure over tender areas of breast tissue.

Pulmonary Disorders

Pulmonary embolism typically causes a substernal chest discomfort that may be confused with angina, but usually the predominant symptom is dyspnea. It often occurs spontaneously, without association with exertion. With *pulmonary infarction* there may be a pleuritic component to the pain, so that deep inspiration aggravates symptoms, and a pleural rub may be heard on auscultation. Duration of symptoms is often prolonged and usually relieved with rest over time. Patients with severe *pulmonary hypertension* may describe chest pain similar to angina but typically have findings on physical examination (parasternal lift, palpable or loud pulmonary component of the second heart sound) and electrocardiography (right ventricular hypertrophy) that distinguish this from true angina.

Functional or Psychogenic Chest Pain

Often referred to as Da Costa syndrome or neurocirculatory asthenia, the functional or psychogenic chest pain accompanying this anxiety state is typically localized to the left chest and is characterized as a prolonged, dull, persistent ache with intermittent sharp stabbing pain of brief duration accompanied by

TABLE 42.2. Features of Typical Angina and Noncardiac Chest Pain[a]

Feature	Angina	Noncardiac pain
Location of pain	Substernal, diffuse, often radiates	Localized
Quality of pain	Dull, constricting, deep weight on chest; burning band across chest	Sharp, shooting, knife-like, jabbing
Intensity and duration	Steady, with gradual changes in intensity, typically lasts 5–15 min	Fluctuates in intensity, with rapid changes, lasts seconds to hours
Provoking factors	Physical or emotional stress	Single movement or action, related to meal
Relief	After several minutes of rest and/or nitroglycerin	Often spontaneously, within seconds or after prolonged rest, usually not by nitroglycerin

[a]Atypical angina may have features of both noncardiac chest pain and typical angina, with the noncardiac features usually more prominently weighed in consideration of the differential diagnosis.

fatigue, emotional strain, lightheadedness, and breathlessness and has little relationship to exertion. Its response to intervention is variable but sometimes is helped by rest, exercise, analgesics, or anxiolytic medications.

Cardiovascular Disorders Unrelated to Coronary Artery Disease

Mitral valve prolapse is one of the most common cardiac valvular abnormalities, affecting 5% to 10% of the population, resulting from a variety of abnormalities of the mitral valve apparatus. It is more common in women. Chest discomfort is a common symptom in mitral valve prolapse and is typically prolonged, not associated with exertion, may be associated with intermittent sharp stabbing pain, and typically resolves spontaneously. Chest pain also may accompany other valvular disorders, with or without associated coronary artery disease, such as *severe aortic stenosis*, where coronary blood flow is reduced or unable to provide adequate supply to the hypertrophied muscle. Typically, dyspnea is a more prominent feature in aortic stenosis compared with coronary artery disease. The pain of *acute pericarditis* also may resemble angina; however, it is usually sudden in onset, prolonged and severe, with pleuritic components, such that it is aggravated by inspiration, cough, reclining, and is relieved by sitting forward. A pericardial friction rub, when auscultated, aids in the diagnosis. *Aortic dissection* is typically characterized by severe persistent retrosternal discomfort radiating to the back. A history of hypertension is usually present. *Microvascular angina* (also called *syndrome* X) has been identified in a subset of patients with typical—and sometimes atypical—angina who have normal epicardial vessels at angiography and an abnormally increased coronary vascular resistance when atrially paced after the administration of intravenous ergonovine. This affects women disproportionately more than men. Symptoms often are characteristic of angina, although there may be more rest pain, prolonged pain, and a variable response to nitrates. Electrocardiographic changes may be present at rest and are frequent after exercise or pharmacologic stress testing. Effective treatment usually involves a standard antianginal regimen, and the long-term prognosis is excellent for most patients. *Cocaine abuse* also must be considered in the differential diagnosis of chest pain. Cocaine can trigger intense coronary artery spasm, with or without superimposed thrombus formation, resulting in unstable angina pectoris or myocardial infarction.

HISTORY

In determining the probability of coronary artery disease, it is important to risk stratify the patient using a variety of clinical factors, including description of symptoms as discussed earlier, age, gender, risk factors associated with heart disease, and physical findings. Evaluation of chest pain, however, can be particularly challenging in women (Fig. 42.1). Even when women present with symptoms of typical angina, defined as chest pressure or tightness, substernal in nature with or without radiation to the jaw, neck, or left arm, with a duration of 2 to 15 minutes, studies of the natural history of disease, such as the Framingham Heart Study, have demonstrated a low frequency of evolution to myocardial infarction when compared with men (14% in women with angina versus 25% of men with angina). Part of this discrepancy may be related to the policy of equating symptoms of angina with the presence of coronary artery disease in women. In the Coronary Artery Surgery Study Registry, only 50% of women believed to have angina had evidence of coronary disease compared with 83% of men. Women have a higher prevalence of conditions that can mimic atherosclerotic heart disease, such as coronary artery spasm, mitral valve prolapse, and microvascular angina, which adds to the complexity of diagnostic evaluation. However, when symptomatic women are stratified by age, the probability of disease increases. For example, the subset of women in the Framingham Heart Study aged 60 to 69 years with typical angina symptoms had a prognosis similar to that of men. Thus, the occurrence of coronary disease is much more age dependent in women compared with men, with a low prevalence of coronary disease in those aged 35 to 44 year, whereas by 75 years of age, morbidity related to coronary disease is similar in men and women (Table 42.3).

Major risk factors for the development of cardiac disease have undergone extensive study. However, most of these studies have focused on men. Whereas women tend to have a lower

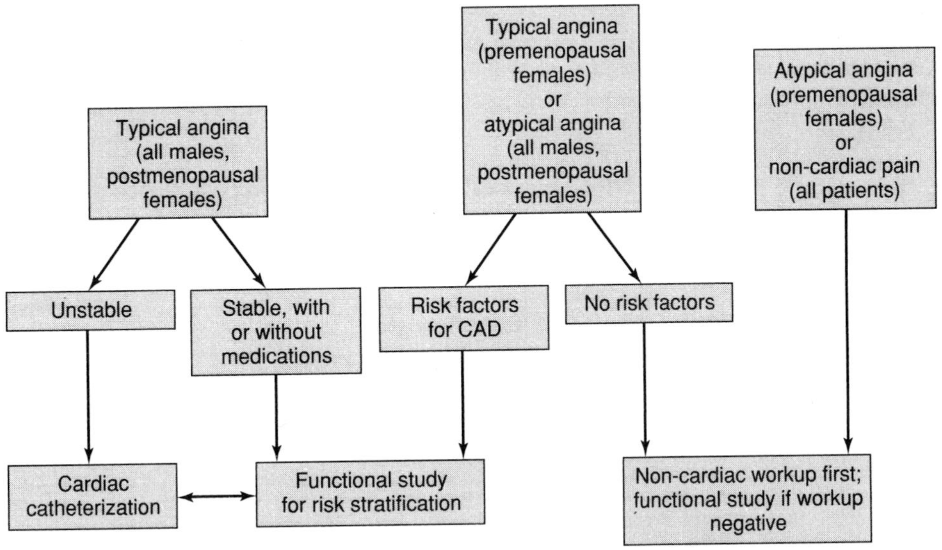

FIG. 42.1. Strategy for evaluation of chest pain. CAD, coronary artery disease.

TABLE 42.3. Use of Probability Analysis in the Diagnosis of Coronary Artery Disease[a]

Age	Nonanginal chest pain		Atypical angina		Typical angina	
	Male	Female	Male	Female	Male	Female
Pretest likelihood of disease (%)						
30–39 yr	5	1	22	4	70	26
60–69 yr	28	19	67	54	94	91
Posttest likelihood of disease (%)						
With ST depression 0–0.5 mm						
30–39 yr	1	0	6	1	24	7
60–69 yr	8	5	32	21	79	69
With ST depression 1.0–1.5 mm						
30–39 yr	10	2	38	8	83	42
60–69 yr	45	33	81	72	97	95
With ST depression 2.0–2.5 mm						
30–39 yr	38	8	76	33	96	79
60–69 yr	81	72	96	93	99	99

[a]*Typical angina:* (a) pressure or squeezing discomfort, substernal with or without radiation to jaw, neck or left arm, lasting 2–15 min and (b) precipitated by exertion or stress and relieved by rest. *Atypical angina:* (a) or (b) but not both. *Nonanginal chest pain:* neither (a) nor (b).

Modified from Diamond GA, Forrester JS. Analysis of probability as an aid in the clinical diagnosis of coronary artery disease. *N Engl J Med* 1979;300:1350, with permission.

prevalence of classic cardiac risk factors for coronary artery disease, differences in risk profile, changes with age, and the influences of potential risk factors unique to women have only recently been examined (Table 42.4). Major risk factors affect men and women in similar ways, with some interesting differences. Diabetes mellitus, for example, is more prevalent in women, and the risk of developing coronary artery disease is higher in female diabetics compared with male diabetics. As a consequence, the prevalence of coronary artery disease is similar in male and female diabetics, even when younger premenopausal women are compared with men of similar age. The recently described metabolic syndrome (hypertriglyceridemia, obesity, hyperinsulinemia, hypertension, and low high-density lipoprotein) confers a heightened risk of coronary artery disease

TABLE 42.4. Risk Factors for Coronary Artery Disease

	Men		Women
Major risk factors			
Age	45 yr or older		55 yr or older or premature menopause
Family history		MI or sudden death in first-degree relative before age 55 yr (men) or 65 yr (women)	
Current cigarette smoking			Combination of smoking and oral contraceptive use increases risk of MI
Hypertension		BP 140/90 mm Hg or greater or taking antihypertensive medications	
Diabetes mellitus	Age <45, more common in men		Age >45, more common in women More prevalent in women; confers risk of CAD equal to men across all age groups
Lipid disorders	Total cholesterol >200, HDL <35, LDL >130 Total cholesterol and LDL tend to stabilize at age 45		Total cholesterol >200, HDL <50, LDL >130 Total cholesterol and LDL tend to rise at age 45 yr and exceed levels of men beyond age 55 yr; HDL levels run higher than men but drop slightly after menopause
Other factors			
Metabolic syndrome[a]	Relative risk (≥3 factors) of CAD = 2.39		Relative risk (≥3 factors) of CAD = 5.9
Obesity			
Stress			
Sedentary lifestyle			More prevalent in women
hs-CRP	Low risk value <1.0, high risk >3.0		

[a]*Metabolic syndrome:* obesity, hypertriglyceridemia, hyperinsulinemia, hypertension, and low HDL.

BP, blood pressure; CAD, coronary artery disease; HDL, high-density lipoprotein; LDL, low-density lipoprotein; MI, myocardial infarction.

and death, especially in women. Novel risk factors for heart disease, especially inflammatory markers and genetic markers, are being avidly investigated. High sensitivity C-reactive protein has emerged as one inflammatory marker that enhances risk assessment in men and women. Contributions of certain potential risk factors unique to women, such as oral contraceptive use, pregnancy, hysterectomy with or without oophorectomy, menopause, and the mechanisms by which they may confer risk or benefit, are currently under investigation.

PHYSICAL EXAMINATION

In patients with coronary artery disease and angina pectoris, the physical examination may be entirely normal. The focus of the examination is directed toward differentiating the probable causes of chest pain and searching for evidence that may help to corroborate a suspicion of coronary artery disease. The presence of a corneal arcus on inspection of the eyes is known to correlate with increased levels of cholesterol and low-density lipoprotein. Xanthelasmas, which are deposits of lipid intracellularly in the skin, correlate with increased triglyceride levels and a deficiency of high-density lipoprotein. The blood pressure may be elevated, chronically or acutely, in patients with angina. Peripheral arterial disease often is a clue to more extensive atherosclerosis and is frequently present in coronary artery disease. The cardiac examination can provide useful information in the differential diagnosis of chest pain. A sustained cardiac impulse on palpation often is seen in patients with left ventricular dysfunction. The presence of a heart murmur can help distinguish the pain associated with aortic stenosis or hypertrophic cardiomyopathy. Transient apical systolic murmurs may indicate papillary muscle dysfunction in the presence of ischemia. A third or fourth heart sound may be heard in patients with angina pectoris. A midsystolic click with or without a late systolic murmur is characteristic of mitral valve prolapse. A continuous murmur over the precordium is uncommon but may be attributed to turbulent flow across a stenotic proximal coronary artery.

LABORATORY STUDIES

Appropriate laboratory testing is directed by the results of the history and physical examination. Several studies are available to determine the presence or absence of coronary artery disease.

Electrocardiogram

A resting electrocardiogram (ECG) is normal in at least one third of patients with angina pectoris. Evidence of prior myocardial infarction or nonspecific ST-T wave changes, particularly if these changes were not present on a previous ECG, aid in the diagnosis. Ambulatory ECG recordings may be useful in detecting ST segment depression associated with ischemia, which frequently occurs in the absence of symptoms.

Exercise Electrocardiography

The exercise tolerance test is most useful when there is at least an intermediate pretest probability of coronary artery disease. However, in general, up to 30% to 40% of results in women may be falsely positive (compared with a 10% rate in men), depending on the population being tested. Several factors reduce the diagnostic accuracy of exercise testing in women. Factors that reduce the specificity of the test are the lower incidence of coronary artery disease in premenopausal women and the higher prevalence of mitral valve prolapse with its nonspecific electrocardiographic changes, electrocardiographic changes with hyperventilation, and vasospasm. Factors that reduce the sensitivity of the test are a higher incidence of single-vessel disease in women and the tendency for women to attain a lower cardiac workload with exercise testing compared with men. A normal finding on exercise study in women is useful; a normal finding has a high negative predictive value for the absence of coronary artery disease. In addition, the exercise tolerance test is valuable in assessing the severity and prognosis of the disease, as judged by duration of exercise, symptom provocation, blood pressure response to exercise, and extent and duration of electrocardiographic changes with exercise.

Radionuclide Angiography

Radionuclide imaging performed during exercise and/or with pharmacologic intervention improves the sensitivity and specificity of routine stress testing for the detection of coronary artery disease and provides additional prognostic value. In women with perfusion abnormalities and atypical chest pain, the sensitivity is increased to 85%, whereas with typical angina the sensitivity is 93%. Recognition of breast attenuation artifact and use of newer agents, such as technetium-99 sestamibi, has improved the specificity rate to 91%. Women have been shown to have a greater incidence of side effects during pharmacologic testing with agents such as dipyridamole or adenosine. This is believed to be related to the greater proportion of adipose tissue and smaller intravascular volume of distribution in women compared with men, even though doses are weight adjusted. Further study is necessary.

Stress Echocardiography

Echocardiography can be used to detect regional changes in contractility during stress (exercise or pharmacologic) compared with rest. This has become an established diagnostic tool for assessing the presence of coronary artery disease. Studies have demonstrated sensitivity rates of 79% to 88% and specificity rates of 84% to 93% in groups of women with moderate pretest probability of disease. The predictive accuracy of the technique also appears to be preserved for single-vessel versus multivessel disease.

Coronary Angiography

Coronary angiography generally is restricted to patients who have symptoms refractory to medical therapy, patients who are believed to be at high risk for a coronary event based on noninvasive testing, or patients who are unable to undergo risk stratification in any other way. Several studies show that women tend to be referred for diagnostic angiography less often than men, even when they have classic symptoms of angina and equivalent electrocardiographic changes on stress testing, perfusion defects on nuclear imaging, or both, with higher subsequent morbid event rates. This referral pattern is largely age dependent, with an estimated 17.5% decline in angiography after myocardial infarction for every 10-year age increase in women.

TREATMENT

Once the cause of chest pain has been elucidated through a careful history, physical examination, and supplemental laboratory studies, the treatment can be more specifically directed. Treatment of nonanginal chest pain is not covered here. Treatment of coronary artery disease generally is divided into medical therapy versus revascularization with either coronary artery bypass surgery or angioplasty.

Medical Therapy

Standard treatment of angina pectoris involves the use of nitrates, beta-blockers, calcium channel blockers, and aspirin. Aspirin, in doses of 81 to 160 mg/d or 325 mg every other day, has been shown to decrease the incidence of death and nonfatal myocardial infarction in both men and women. Nitrates have a dual action of increasing oxygen supply and reducing oxygen demand, resulting in relief of anginal symptoms. These are useful in patients with fixed-threshold angina, where symptoms are predictably reproduced with certain types of activity, as well as with variable-threshold angina, where vasospasm may play a more important role in producing angina. Sublingual nitroglycerin or inhaled spray is used to treat individual episodes. When angina occurs more than two to three times per week or when silent ischemia is documented, longer acting nitrates often are used, either in a transdermal preparation or orally. A 10- to 12-hour nitrate-free interval (usually overnight) is useful in limiting nitrate tolerance and improving effectiveness. Intravenous preparations are available for use in unstable angina.

Beta-blockers are particularly useful in effort-related angina. These work by inhibiting the effects of circulating catecholamines on β-adrenergic receptors, thereby reducing heart rate and contractility, resulting in reduced myocardial oxygen demand, particularly during periods of activity or excitement. Use of beta-blockers in the setting of bradyarrhythmias, significant depressive illness, asthma, severe diabetes mellitus, severe peripheral vascular disease, or when a strong vasospastic component to the angina is suspected may be limited by side effects. Calcium channel blockers work by causing relaxation of vascular smooth muscle in both the systemic and coronary arteries. Entry of calcium into myocardial cells is opposed, resulting in a negative inotropic effect. Generally, if vasospasm is suggested and the heart rate is normal, calcium channel blockers are preferred over beta-blockers, whereas if arrhythmias or tachycardia at rest or with exertion are present, beta-blockers may be more effective. Simultaneous use of beta-blockers and calcium channel blockers, in addition to nitrates, often is needed to control anginal symptoms but should be done cautiously due to the risk of severe bradycardia, atrioventricular block, hypotension, and congestive heart failure.

Observational studies have suggested a 30% to 50% decrease in the incidence of coronary artery disease in postmenopausal women when they are treated with hormone replacement therapy. Recently, randomized controlled trials of combination estrogen and progesterone have been completed. The secondary prevention trial Heart and Estrogen/progestin Replacement Study showed no benefit of hormone replacement therapy in postmenopausal women with heart disease followed over a period of 6.8 years. The primary prevention study, Women's Health Initiative, demonstrated an increased risk of coronary events in treated patients versus placebo (excess of seven more cardiac events/10,000 person years) and an excess of risk overall, leading to premature termination of this arm of the Women's Health Initiative after a mean follow-up of 5.2 years. The estrogen alone arm of the study, which includes women who have had hysterectomies, continues.

Aggressive cholesterol lowering, particularly with statins, has been shown to alter vascular tone favorably and may have a direct effect on control of symptoms. Other agents, such as the histamine antagonist cyproheptadine, may be useful in Prinzmetal angina, and angiotensin-converting enzyme inhibitors have been successfully used in unstable angina. There are relatively little data on the usefulness of medical therapy in women versus men with angina pectoris, nor has relative effectiveness of combination therapy been examined by gender.

Revascularization

Revascularization generally should be considered for any patient who has acceptable coronary anatomy for revascularization and either fails a trial of medical management or has markers for high risk of a major cardiac event on noninvasive testing (Table 42.5). The choice of angioplasty versus coronary artery bypass surgery (CABG) depends on the extent, distribution, and severity of disease; left ventricular function; other comorbid disease; and physician and patient preference.

Percutaneous transluminal coronary angioplasty (PTCA) has been available since the early 1980s as an alternative treatment to CABG in selected patients with refractory angina who have suitable coronary anatomy. Advances in technology, including atherectomy, stents, and brachytherapy, have broadened the indications for the procedure, although typically PTCA is recommended in patients with normal or mildly depressed left ventricular function, with focal stenoses involving one or more vessels. Women presenting for PTCA tend to be older, with a higher prevalence of congestive heart failure, more severe symptoms of angina, and more cardiac risk factors compared with their male counterparts. In the early registry of patients undergoing PTCA, women tended to have lower procedural success rates, with higher rates of complications, including mortality. It was believed that much of this difference could be explained by the higher risk profile of women presenting for PTCA. Over subsequent years this gender gap has narrowed. Vessel size appears to be a major determinant of outcome, with smaller vessel size implicated in adverse outcomes. Long-term follow-up of PTCA patients reports no differences in survival, rates of myocardial infarction, or occurrence of severe angina, although women seem

TABLE 42.5. Stress Test Markers of High Risk for Cardiac Event

Electrocardiographic criteria
Failure to complete 6.5 METS or attain HR >120 beats/min
ST depression >2 mm
Flat or decreasing blood pressure response to exercise
ST depressions that persist >6 min postexercise
ST depressions that occur in multiple leads
Exercise-induced ventricular tachycardia
ST elevation in leads without Q waves
Radionuclide criteria
New redistribution defects at low workload (≤6.5 METS or HR ≤20 beats/min)
Multiple redistribution defects
Increased lung uptake of isotope
Redistribution defects remote from an infarct zone
Redistribution defect in a zone of non-Q wave MI
Increase in cardiac pool of isotope
Echocardiographic criteria
Ejection fraction ≤35%
Multiple new wall motion defects
New wall motion defects at low workload (≤6.5 METS or HR ≤20 beats/min)
Exercise increase in ejection fraction <5%

HR, heart rate; METS, metabolic equivalents; MI, myocardial infarction.

more likely to have ongoing anginal symptoms and to be treated with antianginal medications.

CABG has been shown to improve survival in patients with left main three-vessel coronary artery disease or with significant left ventricular dysfunction. As with PTCA, women who present for CABG tend to be older, with more severe and more unstable anginal symptoms, although left ventricular function is more often preserved with fewer diseased vessels compared with men. Women have more comorbid disease preoperatively and a higher operative mortality compared with men, with a relative risk of 1.5 to 2.5 in most studies. These differences may be related to differences in age, comorbid disease, body surface area, more urgent procedures and coronary artery size. Recent evidence suggests that adverse outcomes are related to the higher incidence of left ventricular hypertrophy and hypertensive heart disease and subsequent higher rates of postoperative congestive heart failure in women compared with men. Symptomatically, women seem to have similar long-term results after CABG, with no apparent differences in 5- or 10-year survival based on gender. Clearly, ongoing study of treatment options in women, with an emphasis on earlier recognition of disease, management of comorbid conditions, and use of techniques to improve acute revascularization outcomes is needed.

CONSIDERATIONS IN PREGNANCY

Whereas shortness of breath and fatigue are common manifestations of the major hemodynamic alterations that occur during pregnancy, chest pain and ischemic heart disease are unusual in women of childbearing potential and when seen typically occur in women older than 35 years of age. Aortic dissection is a rare cause of chest pain that can occur in pregnancy. When necessary, diagnostic evaluation using exercise tolerance testing at a submaximal level usually can be performed safely. The effects of radionuclide isotopes, such as thallium or sestamibi, on the unborn fetus have not been well studied and should be avoided when the diagnosis can be made another way. When the baseline ECG finding is not normal, stress echocardiography may provide additional information safely. Cardiac catheterization and angiography should be avoided if the patient is medically stable, because of the radiation exposure to the fetus.

For treatment of angina pectoris during pregnancy, calcium channel blockers are generally recommended. Beta-blockers can depress uterine contraction and cause bradycardia, hypotension, and hypoglycemia in the newborn and should be avoided. When required for stabilization of symptoms, β_1-selective blockers are preferred. Labetalol, which is both an α-adrenergic receptor antagonist and a nonselective β-adrenergic receptor antagonist, has been shown to be safe when used in pregnancy for chronic hypertension. Labetalol is another potential option when uncontrolled hypertension is present and is a factor precipitating episodes of angina pectoris. Nitrates are relatively ineffective in the presence of the marked vasodilation and decreased peripheral vascular resistance already present during pregnancy.

BIBLIOGRAPHY

Ayanian JZ, Epstein AM. Differences in the use of procedures between women and men hospitalized for coronary artery disease. *N Engl J Med* 1991;325:221.

Bell MR. Coronary artery disease in women: the safety and efficacy of coronary angioplasty. *Cardiovasc Rev Rep* 1995;7:15.

Cannon RO III, Camici PG, Epstein SE. Pathophysiological dilemma of syndrome X. *Circulation* 1992;85:883.

DeSanctis RW. Clinical manifestations of coronary artery disease: chest pain in women. *Cardiovasc Rev Rep* 1994;5:10.

Diamond GA, Forrester JS. Analysis of probability as an aid in the clinical diagnosis of coronary artery disease. *N Engl J Med* 1979;300:1350.

Eysmann SB, Douglas PS. Coronary heart disease: therapeutic principles. In: Douglas PS, ed. *Cardiovascular health and disease in women.* Philadelphia: WB Saunders, 1993:43.

Eysmann SB, Douglas PS. Reperfusion and revascularization strategies for coronary artery disease in women. *JAMA* 1992;268:1903.

Jacobs AK, Johnston JM, Haviland A, et al. Improved outcomes for women undergoing contemporary percutaneous coronary intervention: a report from the National Heart, Lung, and Blood Institute Dynamic Registry. *J Am Coll Cardiol* 2002;39:1606–1614.

Kannel WB, Wilson PWF. Risk factors that attenuate the female coronary disease advantage. *Arch Intern Med* 1995;155:57.

Lerner DJ, Kannel WB. Patterns of coronary heart disease morbidity and mortality in the sexes: a 26-year follow-up of the Framingham population. *Am Heart J* 1986;117:383.

Matthews KA, Wing RR, Kuller LH, et al. Influence of the perimenopause on cardiovascular risk factors and symptoms of middle-aged healthy women. *Arch Intern Med* 1994;154:2349.

Nambi V, Hoogwerf BJ, Sprecher DL. A truly deadly quartet: obesity, hypertension, hypertriglyceridemia, and hyperinsulinemia. *Cleve Clin J Med* 2002;69: 985–989.

O'Connor GT, Morton JR, Diehl MJ, et al. Differences between men and women in hospital mortality associated with coronary artery bypass graft surgery. *Circulation* 1993;88:2104–2110.

Pearson TA, Mensah GA, Alexander RW, et al. Markers of inflammation and cardiovascular disease: application to clinical and public health practice—a statement for healthcare professionals from the Centers for Disease Control and Prevention and the Americal Heart Association. *Circulation* 2003;107:499–511.

Pepine CJ. Angina pectoris. In: Freed M, Grines C, eds. *Essentials of cardiovascular medicine.* Birmingham, MI: Physicians' Press, 1994:54.

Rutherford JD, Braunwald E. Chronic ischemic heart disease. In: Braunwald E, ed. *Heart disease: a textbook of cardiovascular medicine,* 4th ed. Philadelphia: WB Saunders, 1992:1292.

Vittinghoff E, Shlipak MG, Varosy PD, et al. Risk factors and secondary prevention in women with heart disease: the Heart and Estrogen/Progestin Replacement study. *Ann Intern Med* 2003;138:81–89.

Wenger NK. Coronary heart disease: diagnostic decision-making. In: Douglas PS, ed. *Cardiovascular health and disease in women.* Philadelphia: WB Saunders, 1993:25.

Williams MJ, Marwick TH, O'Gorman D, et al. Comparison of exercise echocardiography with an exercise score to diagnose coronary artery disease in women. *Am J Cardiol* 1994;74:435.

Writing Group for the Women's Health Initiative Investigators. Risks and benefits of estrogen plus progestin in healthy postmenopausal women: principal results from the Women's Health Initiative randomized controlled trial. *JAMA* 2002;288:321–333.

CHAPTER 43
Angina and Myocardial Infarction

Gary M. Katzman

CAD in women is a serious entity, accounting for significant morbidity and mortality, yet its impact traditionally has been underappreciated by both the general population and the health care profession. Whereas in the United States breast cancer will affect one in nine women over the course of a lifetime, some 500,000 women each year will suffer a myocardial infarction (MI), and coronary artery disease (CAD) is responsible for one third of all female deaths. CAD, which clinically may manifest as angina, MI, congestive heart failure (CHF), or lethal arrhythmia, generally is a result of flow-limiting atherosclerosis, an insidious process that develops over decades, probably starting in childhood. Pathophysiologically, the disease is the same among genders, but providers of women's primary care must be alert to the very different epidemiology, clinical presentation, treatment strategies, and outcome in women compared with men. The diagnosis of CAD is more challenging in women, who especially at a younger age are more apt to have an "atypical" presentation.

In addition, noninvasive testing has inherent limitations in women, making correct test selection of paramount importance. Coronary disease tends to be more debilitating in women, thus warranting a good understanding of the risk factors, presentation, and diagnostic and treatment modalities.

ATHEROSCLEROSIS

Atherosclerotic coronary disease is the most important cause of both anginal chest pain and the acute coronary syndromes, including unstable angina and MI. Over the course of years, endothelial injury from hypertension, smoking, diabetes, and hypercholesterolemia lead, via the interaction of platelet and leukocyte derived agents, to the development of fibrous plaques. The stable fibrous plaque is a complex dynamic intimal collection of lipid-laden macrophages, surrounded by an extracellular matrix of proteoglycans, collagen, and elastin. As macrophages engulf low-density lipoprotein (LDL) cholesterol (thus becoming foam cells) and die, an inflammatory cascade is initiated within the plaque, which eventually leads to an increase in the density of fibrous material. Smooth muscle cell proliferation also may play a major role in the initiation of plaque formation. The fibrocalcific coronary plaque may then remain stable for years.

Risk Factors

The traditional and noncontroversial coronary risk factors include family history, hypertension, diabetes, hypercholesterolemia, and smoking. Men and women share these risk factors; however, the relative importance of each one may be different between genders. In addition, the presence or absence of one or more risk factors does not guarantee the existence or absence of clinically significant disease. A history of premature coronary disease in first-degree relatives, that is, clinically apparent disease in a male before age 50 years or in a female before age 60 years, is a strong independent risk factor.

Hypercholesterolemia is a well-established coronary risk factor in women. Most primary prevention studies in the past had excluded women. LDL levels generally are lower in women than in men, and high-density lipoprotein (HDL) tends to be higher until menopause, when levels of both "bad" cholesterol (LDL) and "good" cholesterol (HDL) approach those of men. This change in cholesterol levels at menopause coincides with the increase in risk for coronary disease. Low HDL may be a stronger predictor of coronary disease in women than in men. Recent secondary prevention studies have included women and definitely demonstrate a protective benefit in cholesterol lowering in postmenopausal women. In the Cholesterol and Recurrent Events trial, which evaluated the utility of cholesterol lowering in people with only mildly elevated cholesterol levels after MI, those treated with pravastatin had a significant reduction in all endpoints (death, reinfarction, and revascularization). In the 576 women randomized in this trial, the benefit of statin therapy was more dramatic than in men, with a 46% reduction in coronary events compared with a 20% reduction in men.

In women estrogen levels decline at menopause. This decrease in estrogen is associated with a rise in LDL and decline in HDL. In addition, exogenously administered estrogen has a favorable effect on lipid levels. Thus, it would seem intuitive that in postmenopausal women estrogen replacement should be first-line therapy for primary and secondary prevention. And actually, this has been the standard of care for several years, supported by observational nonrandomized studies. Recently there has been a great change in the understanding of postmenopausal hormone replacement therapy. In the Heart and Estrogen/Progestin Replacement Study Follow-up, over a 6.8-year period there was no statistically significant decrease, compared with placebo, in the rate of the combined primary endpoint (nonfatal MI and cardiovascular death) in postmenopausal women with clinically manifest coronary disease randomly assigned to take 0.625 mg of conjugated estrogen plus 2.5 mg of medroxyprogesterone acetate. In 2002 the Women's Health Initiative Controlled Trial, which was intended to evaluate over an 8.5-year period the utility of estrogen/progestin in primary prevention of coronary heart disease, was stopped early after 5.2 years when it was found that women randomized to the treatment arm had a 29% increase in the incidence of coronary events, predominantly nonfatal MIs. The results of these studies underscore the importance of randomized prospective evaluation.

Hypertension is a significant risk factor for coronary disease in women and should be aggressively treated. Although essential hypertension is the most common etiology in women under age 40, consideration should be given to the possibility of renal artery stenosis from fibromuscular dysplasia, which has a strong female preponderance. Oral contraceptives can also elevate blood pressure. Diabetes not only is a serious risk factor, but the combination of diabetes and smoking is a particularly dangerous combination, especially in women. A diabetic woman with chest pain warrants prompt evaluation.

Smoking, unlike all other coronary risk factors, is completely avoidable. Women who smoke are at greater risk for the development of coronary disease than male smokers. The coronary risk is proportional to the amount smoked, with absolutely no evidence that smoking "light" brands is less atherogenic. There is benefit to smoking cessation at any age, with the incidence of first coronary event declining to that of a nonsmoker after 4 years.

ANGINA

Angina is caused by myocardial oxygen supply and demand mismatch. Understanding this simple concept is critical, because evaluation of the etiology and subsequent treatment of angina depends on identifying inciting factors. The epicardial coronary arteries are rich in smooth muscle cells, which in conjunction with an intact endothelial layer and via local regulatory agents are able to autoregulate their diameter to meet demand. Epicardial coronary arteries have a certain degree of flow reserve. Depending on the needs of the body, the coronary circulation can vasodilate, increasing myocardial flow by fourfold. In the presence of an atherosclerotic plaque, the section of coronary artery downstream has the ability to dilate to maintain adequate flow. As a plaque approaches 70% of the coronary diameter (or 50% in the left main coronary), during times of increased demand, the coronary segment and thus the myocardial region distal to the stenosis may become supply deficient. This leads to myocardial dysfunction and most commonly is manifest symptomatically as angina. Evaluation of patients with angina should always include a search for factors that increase myocardial demand and decrease supply. Common conditions that increase demand include untreated hypertension, hyperthyroidism, fever, cardiac tachyarrhythmias, and aortic stenosis. On the supply side, anemia, hypoxemia, and hyperviscosity syndromes can bring about angina.

Angina classically is described as a midsternal pressure or heavy sensation, brought on predictably by exertion or emotional upset and relieved within a few minutes of rest and/or use of nitroglycerin. Often there is associated neck, jaw, or arm pain. There are many variations in this pattern. Not uncommonly, the anginal equivalent is effort-induced epigastric discomfort or heartburn, shortness of breath, or even jaw or arm pain in the absence of chest discomfort. Exertional shortness of

TABLE 43.1. New York State Heart Association Functional Classification of Angina

Functional class	Clinical status	Approximate exercise tolerance (METs)[a]
Class I	Symptoms with unusual activity, little impairment	7 or more
Class II	Symptoms with moderate activity, capable of light work	5–6
Class III	Symptoms with daily activities, capable of sedentary work	3–4
Class IV	Symptoms at rest, severely disabled	1–2

[a]Physical work is often expressed in METs. 1 MET = 3.5 mL of oxygen uptake/kg body weight/min and is the metabolic cost of standing quietly at rest.

breath may be the only clue in a diabetic. Generally, pain lasting for seconds or hours is not angina. Patients must not simply be questioned about "pain," because anginal discomfort is often quite subtle and thus could be missed. Although most women present with classic angina, disproportionately more women than men may report "atypical" symptoms. This may partially account for the lower percentage of women referred for cardiac testing. A possible explanation for an atypical presentation is the older age at presentation and accompanying greater number of comorbidities in women. The New York State Heart Association classification is useful shorthand for describing the clinical status of a patient with chronic angina (Table 43.1).

Evaluation of Angina in the Ambulatory Setting

Once a thorough history is taken, a focused cardiovascular physical examination should be performed. Although there may be clues to the presence of coronary disease, the physical examination usually is rather unremarkable, sometimes entirely normal. Hypertension may be present. Diminished peripheral pulses and carotid or abdominal bruits are an indication of peripheral vascular disease, which often coexists with coronary disease. Resting tachycardia, an enlarged or displaced cardiac point of maximal impulse, or an S_4 gallop all suggest chronic left ventricular dysfunction. Xanthelasma generally is a result of significant hypercholesterolemia. Examination of a patient during an anginal episode may reveal transient tachycardia, hypertension, cardiac gallop, and an apical systolic murmur consistent with mitral regurgitation as a result of ischemic papillary muscle dysfunction.

The resting electrocardiogram (ECG) may also be normal (Fig. 43.1) but should be obtained in all patients with chest discomfort. Left ventricular hypertrophy and evidence for distant or even recent MI can be discerned from the ECG. During

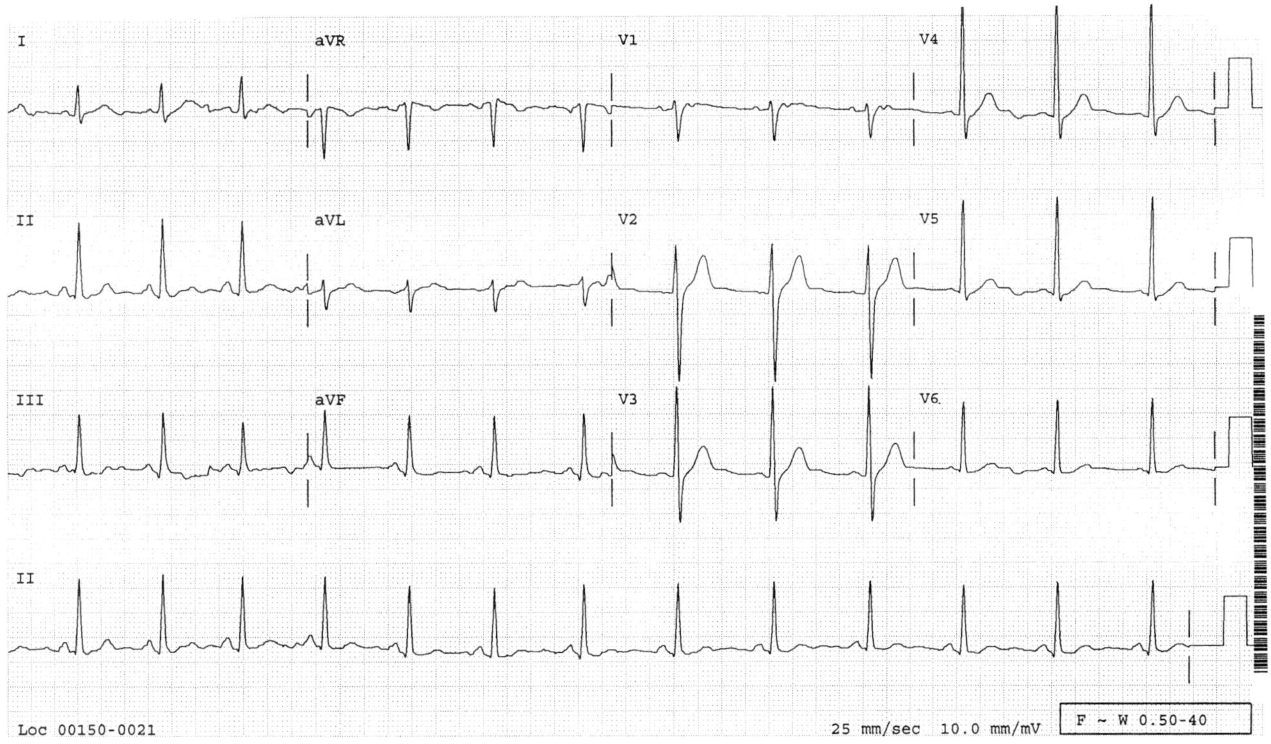

FIG. 43.1. Electrocardiogram in a 51-year-old perimenopausal woman with a history of hypertension and hypercholesterolemia. The patient presented with exertional chest pain for 6 weeks. The tracing meets the criteria for high voltage. Heart catheterization showed an 80% focal narrowing of the proximal segment of the left anterior descending coronary artery.

angina, most patients have identifiable ischemic ST or T wave abnormalities, usually ST depressions that normalize once the ischemia has resolved. These so-called dynamic electrocardiographic changes correlate well with the presence of underlying flow limiting coronary disease.

Diagnostic testing is required in patients believed to have coronary disease to confirm or exclude the diagnosis and to better define the severity of the disease. In some contexts, the immediate referral to a cardiologist for heart catheterization is appropriate. This is the case when the patient's symptoms clearly represent unstable angina. When it is unclear whether the patient's chest discomfort is secondary to flow-limiting coronary disease or if the symptoms are chronic, unchanging, and mild, noninvasive diagnostic testing should be considered.

The exercise treadmill test is the most commonly used form of stress testing in the ambulatory setting. A standardized treadmill protocol is used, usually the Bruce protocol, which incrementally increases cardiac workload by adjusting the treadmill speed and incline (Table 43.2). Ideally, the heart rate should increase to 85% predicted age adjusted maximum. Ischemic ST depression occurring with exercise, particularly when associated with typical symptoms, strongly correlates with the presence of CAD. Patients with severe disease tend to have marked ST depression at fairly low levels of exercise. A drop in blood pressure or serious ventricular arrhythmias with exercise may indicate severe, often multivessel disease. The location of ST depressions does not correlate with the myocardial region at risk. Occasionally, ST elevations are present during exercise, the location of which does tend to correlate with the ischemic myocardial region. ST segment elevations may be present with severe coronary ischemia or with vasospasm (Prinzmetal angina).

Exercise treadmill testing is not 100% accurate. The overall sensitivity rate for exercise testing in detecting CAD is about 60% to 70%, with a test specificity rate of 75% to 90%. Factors that lower test accuracy include inability to exercise to target heart rate; the presence of baseline electrocardiographic abnormalities, such as left ventricular hypertrophy and bundle branch blocks; and a variety of medications, most commonly digoxin. False-positive results may occur in patients with mitral valve prolapse, and some healthy individuals have confounding ST abnormalities with hyperventilation.

The diagnostic accuracy of stress testing is largely dependent on the pretest probability of disease, which in turn is dependent on the prevalence of disease in the population. It is useful to think of three probability groups within a population to determine the utility of stress testing: low probability (less than 15% chance), intermediate probability (15%–85%), and high probability (greater than 85% chance). Stress testing is most helpful in patients who fall into the intermediate group. In a 25-year-old female marathon runner with episodic, sharp, nonexertional chest discomfort, 1 mm of ST depression during an exercise stress test is likely to represent a false positive. Alternatively, a 70-year-old diabetic female with a strong family history of CAD who complains of predictable effort-induced midsternal pressure with radiation down the left arm has a high probability of having coronary disease, and a negative stress result is likely to represent a false negative. Stress testing is only a tool and should always be considered in the context of each particular patient.

Stress testing is significantly less accurate in women than in men. The false-positive rate in treadmill testing is higher in women, resulting in lower specificity. This likely is due to the lower pretest probability in premenopausal women. The overall sensitivity of treadmill testing is also lower in women. This can be explained by the older age at onset of coronary disease in women and thus the greater likelihood of being unable to reach target heart rate on the treadmill.

Limitations in the sensitivity and specificity of treadmill testing led to the introduction of radionuclide imaging. The combination of exercise and nuclear imaging has dramatically improved the diagnostic accuracy of stress testing. The simple concept is that uptake of radiotracer depends on the presence of intact coronary blood flow and myocyte viability. At peak exercise, a cardioselective radioisotope (most commonly either thallium or sestamibi) is administered intravenously. A gamma camera scans the heart in multiple planes, absorbing radiation. This radiation is converted into electrical signals, which then are converted by a computer into visual images. Exercise images are compared with those at rest. Ischemic regions of myocardium appear as "cold" spots on stress images. In recent years, single photon emission computed tomography has largely replaced planar imaging in most noninvasive laboratories. The sensitivity and specificity of radionuclide stress testing approach 90% and are similar in men and women. As with treadmill testing alone, the pretest probability in any patient undergoing radionuclide stress imaging must be considered carefully.

Recently, exercise stress echocardiography has gained popularity as an alternative to radionuclide imaging. This test uses the detection of ischemic-induced left ventricular wall motion abnormalities by echocardiography to detect coronary disease. In experienced centers, stress echocardiography has similar sensitivity with perhaps slightly higher specificity than nuclear imaging. A stress echocardiography has the added advantage of being able to evaluate for other causes of chest pain, such as aortic stenosis, hypertrophic cardiomyopathy, and mitral valve prolapse. The presence of a pericardial effusion may be a clue to concomitant pericarditis.

Patient may be either unable to exercise on a treadmill or have significant baseline electrocardiographic abnormalities (most commonly left bundle branch block) that preclude exercise stress testing. In these patients, other forms of noninvasive

TABLE 43.2. Bruce Treadmill Protocol: 3-Min Stages

Stage	Speed (mph)	Grade (%)	Workload (METs)
½[a]	1.0	5	3
I	1.7	10	5
II	2.5	12	7
III	3.4	14	9
IV	4.2	16	13
V	5.0	18	16

[a]The standard Bruce protocol begins at stage 1. However, the protocol is sometimes modified to start at a lower level of exercise for elderly patients or in patients with limited physical ability to walk at an incline.
METs, 1 MET = 3.5 mL oxygen uptake/kg body weight/min.

testing can be used, including dipyridamole (Persantine) or adenosine radionuclide scanning and dobutamine echocardiography. Both dipyridamole and adenosine cause normal coronary segments, but not stenotic ones, to dilate, increasing blood flow severalfold in the normal regions. This disparity between flow in normal and stenotic segments becomes apparent after radioisotope injection. Dipyridamole and adenosine are contraindicated in patients with a significant history of asthma. Chronic obstructive pulmonary disease without bronchospasm is not a contraindication. Dobutamine radionuclide imaging can be a useful, albeit somewhat less accurate, modality in asthmatic patients who are unable to exercise and have poor echocardiographic "windows" due to body habitus. All nonexercise forms of stress testing lack the advantage of supplying information about exercise tolerance, which in the setting of coronary disease has significant prognostic implications. Patients should always be encouraged to exercise unless contraindicated.

When coronary disease is likely, based on clinical presentation or stress testing, it usually is appropriate to refer the patient to a cardiologist for further evaluation. The cardiologist can help decide the appropriateness of diagnostic heart catheterization with coronary angiography. Angiography is done to confirm the diagnosis, define prognosis, and assess the need for coronary bypass surgery. The decision to perform angiography is influenced by many factors, including (a) the individual patient's lifestyle and activity level, (b) the patient's age and comorbidity, (c) the severity and stability of the angina, and (d) the likelihood of severe disease, especially triple-vessel disease or left main coronary disease, where bypass surgery is likely to positively affect mortality. Although heart catheterization generally is a very safe routine procedure, it does carry some risks, including dye allergy, nephrotoxicity, stroke, MI, and death. Patients must understand the benefits and risks well in advance of an elective heart catheterization.

There is a well-established gender gap in the treatment of women with coronary disease. After an abnormal stress test, women are less likely to be referred for coronary angiography, even though the prognosis of an abnormal stress result is worse in women than in men. Women have a higher incidence of coronary events after an abnormal stress test and have as much to gain from revascularization when appropriate. Although the reasons for this gender bias are uncertain, it may in part be because of the older age and greater potential comorbidity in women at presentation. In addition, physicians may perceive CAD to be less serious in women, as evidenced by the lower percentage of women prescribed beta-blockers and aspirin. Women are more likely than men to undergo cardiac surgery for an unstable or emergency condition, rather than more electively. This may contribute to the higher mortality rate in women than men for bypass surgery

Treatment

The treatment of angina involves a three-pronged approach. First, risk factors should be identified and corrected. Smoking cessation and hyperlipidemia management is a good starting point. Second, conditions that increase demand, such as hypertension, tachyarrhythmias (most commonly atrial fibrillation), and valvular disease, must be treated appropriately. Often, temporary limitation of exertional activities is necessary. Patients should learn to recognize anginal precipitants and avoid them. Isometric exercise should be substituted for aerobic physical conditioning, which, via the development of peripheral collateral circulation and increased energy utilization efficiency, may allow for a greater amount of physical activity within the anginal threshold. Third, anemia and hypoxemia decrease myocardial oxygen supply and require correction.

Medical therapy plays a central role in the treatment of angina (Table 43.3). Beta-blockers are very effective and are considered first-line therapy, unless contraindicated because of bronchospasm, symptomatic bradycardia, or severe decompensated CHF. Beta-blockers work by slowing the heart rate, lowering blood pressure, and decreasing the myocardial sympathetic drive. A history of asthma is not an absolute contraindication to beta-blocker use. Low to medium doses of highly β_1-selective beta-blockers generally are well tolerated in asthmatics.

In patients who cannot tolerate beta-blockers, calcium channel blockers are a reasonable alternative. Negatively inotropic

TABLE 43.3. Antianginal Medications for Chronic Angina

Medication class	Mode of action	Other benefits	Side effects
Aspirin	Antiplatelet agent to reduce risk of intracoronary clot and MI	Decrease in neurologic events with carotid disease. Reduces risk of recurrent MI	GI side effects and bleeding
Beta-blockers, e.g., metoprolol, atenolol, propranolol, nadolol	Decrease cardiac workload by decreasing HR, BP, and contractility during exercise	Post-MI decreases risk of recurrent MI and death; antiarrhythmic and antihypertensive	Negative inotropic effect may worsen CHF if LV dysfunction is severe May cause bronchospasm, fatigue depression, bradycardia, and can worsen claudication or mask hypoglycemia
Calcium blockers, e.g., diltiazem, verapamil, amlodipine, nifedipine	Decrease myocardial oxygen demand; increase coronary flow by vasodilatation	Antihypertensives; some (verapamil and diltiazem) are used for supraventricular arrhythmias	Hypotension; worsening CHF (should not be used if serious LV dysfunction); bradycardia with verapamil and diltiazem; constipation, flushing, and peripheral edema
Long-acting nitrates, e.g., isosorbide dinitrate or isosorbide mononitrate PO, or transdermal nitroglycerin patches	Vasodilators; prevent coronary spasm; increase collateral and subendocardial flow; decrease venous return to lower intracardiac pressures	May help CHF symptoms by lowering intracardiac pressures	Headache, postural hypotension; tachyphylaxis can occur, therefore must have a nitrate-free interval

BP, blood pressure; CHF, congestive heart failure; GI, gastrointestinal; HR, heart rate; LV, left ventricular; MI, myocardial infarction.

cardioselective calcium channel blockers should be avoided if either severe left ventricular dysfunction or significant bradycardia is present. Recently, newer peripherally acting calcium channel blockers, such as amlodipine, have gained popularity as an adjunct in treating angina.

Nitroglycerin preparations are a mainstay of therapy for stable angina. Predominantly through venodilation, nitroglycerin decreases preload and thus the myocardial work requirement. Nitrates generally are very effective at promptly relieving angina. Chest discomfort that is not relieved by a few sublingual nitroglycerines spaced 5 minutes apart should prompt the seeking of emergency help. Likely, chest discomfort that does not respond to nitrates and lasts more than 20 minutes either represents noncardiac pain or a potential MI. Long-acting oral nitroglycerin preparations are helpful in preventing angina. As long as the particular regimen allows for a nitrate-free period, tolerance does not develop. Some patients find prophylactic use of sublingual nitroglycerin or nitroglycerin spray before exertion quite helpful in preventing angina. The use of long-acting nitrates does not obviate the need for sublingual nitroglycerin in the setting of an anginal attack.

Patients should be encouraged not to hesitate in using nitroglycerin if their symptoms are mild or if they are uncertain whether their discomfort is anginal in nature. Nitrates are not addictive. The immediate side effects of nitrates include headache and lightheadedness. Long-acting nitrates are less likely to cause these symptoms. Nitroglycerin has a relatively short shelf life, and patients should routinely be reminded to renew their supply every few months to ensure potency.

Aspirin, an antiplatelet agent, has a well-established role in preventing coronary events, such as unstable angina and MI in patients with coronary disease and in those who have risk factors. In addition, in the event of MI, aspirin has proven benefit in significantly reducing mortality. Aspirin should be dosed between 75 and 325 mg daily. Enteric-coated preparations help to prevent gastric irritation and are favored in the chronic setting.

A common practice among patients with coronary disease is to attempt "working through" episodes of angina. This should always be discouraged. At the onset of chest discomfort, all physical activity should cease, because the presence of angina indicates underlying coronary ischemia and accompanying left ventricular dysfunction. Depending on the degree of coronary disease, prolonged untreated ischemia can precipitate frank CHF or ventricular arrhythmia. Angina probably represents the "tip of the ischemic iceberg." As can be eloquently demonstrated during exercise stress echocardiography, in the setting of ischemia, the onset of angina generally follows the development of stress-induced wall motion abnormalities and electrocardiographic changes.

Women and their partners may hesitate to inquire about the safety of maintaining an active sexual life. Sexual intercourse is generally not a problem if the patient can tolerate a flight of stairs or exercise to a heart rate of 120 betas/min. Nitroglycerin may be used prophylactically before sexual activity.

Unstable Angina and the Acute Coronary Syndromes

Chronic stable angina and unstable angina are two very different conditions. Chronic stable angina refers to predictable effort-related chest discomfort, the pattern of which may remain unchanged for years. Generally, this pattern of chest discomfort implies an underlying stable fibrocalcific coronary plaque. Unstable angina, on the other hand, is by definition angina of recent onset, increasing frequency, or occurring at rest. Any of these three symptom patterns may be a warning sign of impending MI and thus requires prompt aggressive evaluation and therapy, often in the inpatient setting. Often, unstable angina eventually proves to be secondary to a coronary plaque that simply has attained critical mass. "Acute coronary syndrome" is, perhaps, a more useful term that has evolved in recent years and encompasses unstable angina and acute MI. An acute coronary syndrome essentially describes a dynamic process, central to which is plaque disruption with resultant platelet activation and aggregation. This may lead to vessel occlusion, which if not treated emergently causes myocardial necrosis. A patient with a stuttering course of resting angina and accompanying dynamic electrocardiographic changes likely is in the midst of an acute coronary syndrome. Within the diseased coronary segment, thrombosis is competing with thrombolysis. This may go on for hours or days. Overall, patients presenting with unstable angina go on to infarct 10% of the time, with a 5% mortality.

The initial approach to a patient with an acute coronary syndrome is the same as that for chronic stable angina. A search for inciting stressors, such as uncontrolled hypertension, fever, or profound anemia, must quickly be done. Medications to decrease myocardial demand are administered. Beta-blockers, aspirin, and heparin compounds positively influence mortality. Recently, it has become clear that low-molecular-weight heparin is superior to unfractionated heparin in preventing adverse cardiac outcome, with no significant increase in major bleeding complications. Platelet inhibitors, such as the IIb/IIIa agents and adenosine-mediated platelet aggregation inhibitors (i.e., clopidogrel), are useful adjuncts that in the appropriate setting can lower mortality and should be considered. There is no role for thrombolytic agents in acute coronary syndromes, unless ST elevation is present.

Patients should never be admitted to the hospital to "rule out" MI. The appropriate course is to admit for intensive monitoring and treatment of the coronary syndrome. Once the patient is stable, which generally should not be entirely evident for the first 24 hours, then risk stratification can begin.

A non-Q wave MI generally is the result of transient coronary thrombus formation, which has lysed before causing extensive or transmural damage. The occurrence of a non-Q wave MI portends a lower in-hospital mortality but a higher 1-year mortality than Q wave transmural MI, thus necessitating aggressive treatment and risk stratification.

MYOCARDIAL INFARCTION

An MI usually occurs due to thrombus formation at the site of intracoronary atherosclerotic plaque; vasospasm and coronary emboli are rare causes. Plaque rupture is the initial event. A complex cascade of events follows, the result being occlusive intracoronary thrombus with complete cessation of blood flow. The amount of permanent myocardial damage depends on many factors, such as the location of the thrombus, the presence of collateral coronary circulation, the intensity of therapy to decrease myocardial demand, and the time it takes to reestablish flow in the vessel.

Women presenting with an MI should be managed as aggressively as men. Decisions regarding initial therapy, management of complications, and post-MI risk stratification should involve the input of a cardiologist.

Diagnosis

Patients presenting with an acute MI must be evaluated immediately, because survival depends on prompt appropriate triage and therapy. The classic MI usually is described as chest pressure or pain, sometimes radiating to the arms or neck, and often accompanied by diaphoresis, nausea, and dyspnea. Some patients present with less typical symptoms. Epigastric discomfort or "heartburn" may indicate an acute MI. Syncope can herald the beginning of an MI, usually affecting the inferior wall of the heart. The history and physical should be brief and focused, and when the diagnosis is obvious, therapy should never be delayed. Consideration should always be given to other potentially life-threatening cardiovascular emergencies, including pulmonary embolus and aortic dissection.

The physical examination during an acute MI generally will reveal evidence for heightened sympathetic drive and cardiac dysfunction, but occasionally the examination can seemingly be normal. Hypertension and tachycardia usually are present, except in the setting of an inferior wall MI, where bradycardia and hypotension may be seen. An S_3 gallop indicates significant left ventricular dysfunction. Mitral regurgitant murmurs commonly are present and likely are caused by papillary muscle dysfunction. Jugular venous distension and rales indicate CHF. If the infarct is extensive, frank cardiogenic shock, with hypotension, poor distal pulses, and altered mental function may ensue. Other causes of cardiogenic shock include the development of a ventricular septal defect or papillary muscle rupture with subsequent severe mitral regurgitation. Patients presenting late may have accompanying pericarditis, as evidenced by a rub. A differential in peripheral arm pulses suggests an aortic dissection, which can affect the coronary arteries (most commonly the right coronary artery), causing ST elevations.

An ECG should be obtained simultaneously with the history and physical. The presence of significant ST segment elevation in two or more contiguous leads is diagnostic of acute MI (Fig. 43.2). ST segment elevation in leads II, III, and aVF, often with reciprocal ST segment depression in the anterior precordial leads, is seen with inferior MI, usually from occlusion of the right coronary artery. ST segment elevation in the anterior precordial leads generally is seen with occlusion of the left anterior descending artery and results in an anterior wall infarct (Fig. 43.3). Sometimes, left bundle branch block is the only electrocardiographic clue to anterior wall MI. Occlusion of the circumflex artery may be more subtle; ST segment elevation may occur in leads I and aVL or in the inferior leads. ST segment depressions anteriorly may represent a posterior wall infarct.

In patients who present with suspected acute MI and a nondiagnostic ECG, a repeat tracing should be obtained several minutes later. Thrombosis is a dynamic process, and thus classic ST elevations may not be apparent immediately.

An acute MI is confirmed on blood sampling by demonstration of a dynamic increase in the blood concentration of cardiac markers of necrosis. If MI is suspected but the ECG is nondiagnostic, initial therapy should never wait until laboratory confirmation. Traditionally, the most commonly used marker has been creatinine kinase (CK), specifically its cardiac isoform (MB), which is present in high concentration within the cardiac myocyte. CK-MB blood levels begin to rise 6 hours after the onset of MI and peak at about 24 hours. By 72 hours CK-MB levels return to baseline. CK levels should be checked every 8 hours. Obviously, the CK level may be normal at the time of patient presentation, limiting its utility somewhat.

Recently, cardiac troponins, which are contractile proteins only found within the myocardium, have become the gold standard blood marker of MI. Troponin levels begin to rise in the blood between 4 and 6 hours after the onset of necrosis and peak between 24 and 48 hours. Troponins have the distinct advantage of remaining detectable in the blood for up to 10 days, thus making it possible to diagnose MI several days after a coronary event. The high sensitivity of troponin as a cardiac marker does come at some cost. Occasionally, the troponin level

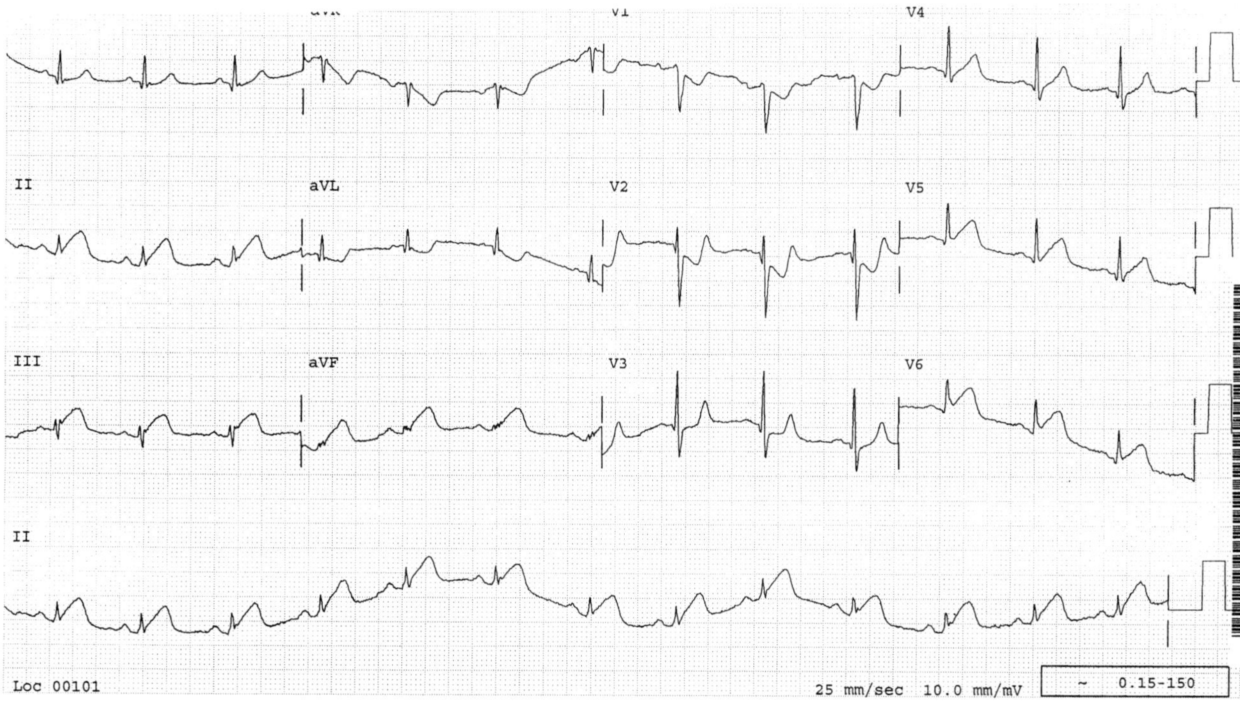

FIG. 43.2. Electrocardiogram in a 47-year-old diabetic woman with 4 hours of epigastric burning and nausea. The tracing shows ST segment elevation in leads II, III, and aVF and reciprocal ST segment depression in leads V_2 and V_3. An emergent heart catheterization revealed a totally occluded proximal right coronary artery.

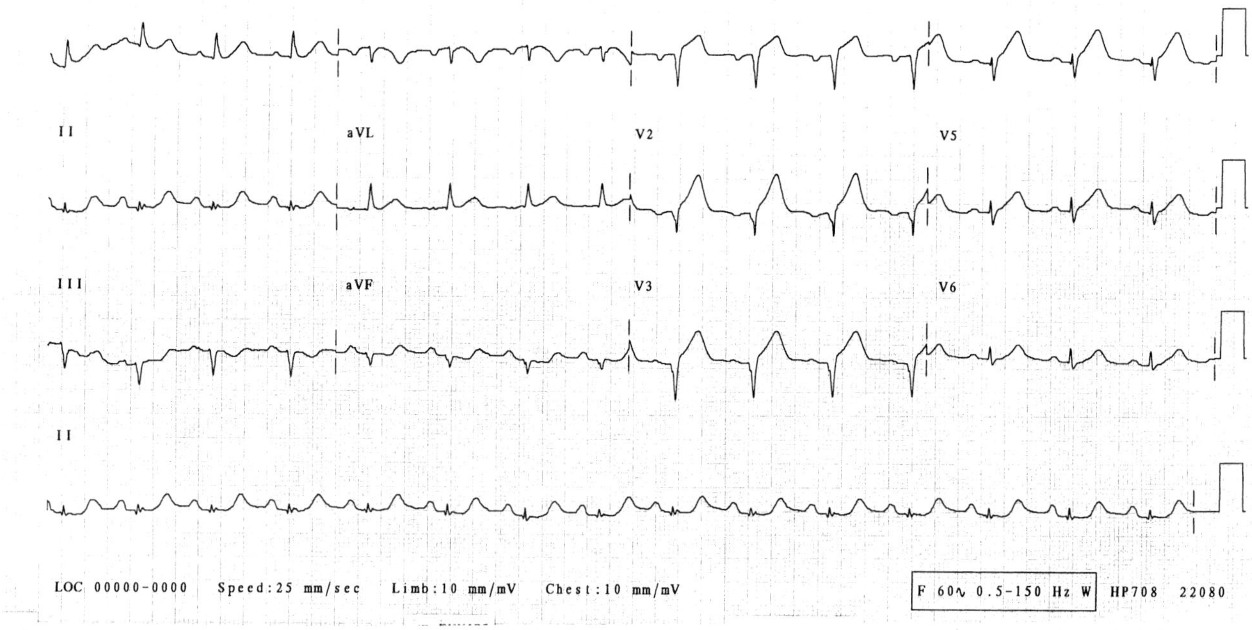

FIG. 43.3. Electrocardiogram in a 60-year-woman with hypertension and diabetes. The tracing shows ST segment elevation in leads V_2–V_4. The patient suffered ventricular fibrillation shortly after this tracing was recorded. Emergent heart catheterization showed a 99% stenosis in the midregion of the left anterior descending coronary artery.

may be slightly elevated in the setting of unstable angina, but this generally does not pose a significant diagnostic dilemma. Actually, the presence of an elevated troponin level in unstable angina predicts a high likelihood of underlying significant flow-limiting coronary disease.

Treatment

The primary goal in the treatment of MI is the timely reestablishment of coronary flow. Quicker reperfusion correlates positively with smaller infarct size and lower mortality. Before settling on the mode of reperfusion strategy, a clearly defined protocol of medical therapy must be initiated. Table 43.4 lists the most common adjunctive medications administered for acute MI.

Ideally, patients should chew and swallow a 325-mg aspirin before arrival in the emergency department. If given in the emergency department, baby aspirins are used because they taste better. A patient who swallows an enteric-coated aspirin before calling rescue should be given another nonenteric-coated dose, chewed and swallowed. Aspirin alone has been shown in numerous landmark trials to significantly reduce mortality from MI.

Heparin compounds are routinely administered for acute MI. Their use has always been somewhat controversial, as far as mortality benefit. In the years before thrombolytic therapy and primary angioplasty, heparin had been shown to reduce reinfarction rates and mortality. As aspirin and thrombolytic use came into vogue, the precise benefit of heparin became less clear. In the modern era of treatment, the proven benefit of heparin primarily is as an adjunct to tissue plasminogen activator. Heparin prevents reocclusion of the infarct artery.

Weight-adjusted low-molecular-weight heparin has become the standard of care in the treatment of unstable angina. The role of low-molecular-weight heparin in acute MI has yet to be firmly established but is in the process of intensive investigation.

Beta-blockers are important in the treatment of acute MI. Unless contraindicated by significant bradycardia, active bronchospasm, or CHF, intravenous metoprolol should be given in an effort to slow the heart rate and lower the blood pressure. Generally, three 5-mg doses of metoprolol spaced 5 to 10 minutes apart is adequate. Beta-blockers reduce infarct size, lower the rate of reinfarction, and decrease short-term mortality.

In addition to the above medications, all patients having an MI should be administered supplemental oxygen, nitroglycerin, and analgesia, most commonly morphine. As the above measures are being instituted, serious consideration of the modality of reperfusion therapy must begin, because the benefits of reperfusion are greatest within the first hour of an infarct and drop off significantly with each passing hour. The two treatment strategies include thrombolysis and primary angioplasty.

Thrombolysis was the first widely used method of reestablishing coronary flow. The use of thrombolytics reduces mortality by upward of 30%. Thrombolytics should be initiated in a timely fashion. Although the greatest benefit is in treatment within the first hour, some survival benefit is still present if thrombolytics are given even up to 12 hours after the onset of symptoms. The overall rate of achieving normal coronary flow in the infarct vessel is about 60%. There is an inherent risk of serious bleeding with thrombolytics, and several contraindications preclude their use. Patients who present with uncontrolled hypertension should not receive thrombolytics. Often it is difficult to know if an elevated blood pressure on presentation is merely secondary to MI-induced heightened sympathetic drive or chronic. Active or recent significant bleeding is a contraindication. A history of stroke, transient ischemic attack, recent head trauma, and cancer preclude the use of thrombolytics. Patients who have unwitnessed syncope may have unknowingly hit their head and should not receive thrombolytics. The use of thrombolytics in the setting of unsuspected aortic dissection carries a high risk of mortality from cardiac tamponade. Pregnancy is a contraindication, but menstrual bleeding does not appear to be a contraindication to thrombolytics.

TABLE 43.4. Adjunctive Therapies in Acute Myocardial Infarction

Therapy	Commonly used doses	Benefits	Cautions and comments
Aspirin	325 mg PO given with lytic therapy, then qd	Improved mortality (alone or with lytic therapy); prevention of rethrombosis and recurrent MI	Contraindicated if true aspirin allergy; can cause bleeding and GI side effects
Oxygen	2–4 L/min; need to monitor oxygen sats and increase if needed in CHF	Improved oxygenation, esp. in CHF	Caution in patients with COPD who can develop carbon dioxide retention
Nitroglycerin	Initially given in sublingual form, then in IV form starting at 20–30 μg/min	Increases venous capacitance to lower intracardiac pressures; coronary vasodilatation; may be esp. useful for CHF or hypertension	IV dosage rate is adjusted according to BP and pain relief
Morphine	2–5 mg IV q 5–30 min	Anxiolytic and analgesic; decreases preload and afterload and thereby decreases myocardial oxygen consumption; good in CHF	Caution to avoid respiratory depression and hypotension
Beta-blockers (metoprolol)	5 mg IV q 5 min for three doses, then 50 mg PO q 8–12 h for 48 h, then 100 mg PO bid	Reduce long-term mortality after MI and may reduce acute mortality when used with lytic drugs; reduce reinfarction incidence; reduce HR and cardiac oxygen consumption; may have antiarrhythmic effect	Contraindicated if hypotension, bradycardia, heart block, or severe LV dysfunction
IV heparin	In conjunction with lytic drug, bolus with 5,000–10,000 U, then start IV drip at 800–1,000 U/h; titrate to APTT of 60–80 s; continue for about 48 h	Helps prevent coronary reocclusion; in cases of large, usually anterior MIs, helps prevent LV thrombus	Usual bleeding precautions; must monitor for thrombocytopenia; in case of large anterior MI, coumadin is indicated for 4–6 mo after heparin is stopped to prevent LV thrombus
ACE inhibitors (e.g., captopril, enalapril, lisinopril)	Depends on patients BP and EF; if BP is low in patient with poor EF, start at low doses.	Started within 24 h after MI, appears to reduce mortality. After MI, prevents LV remodeling, dilatation, especially with anterior infarcts and severe LV dysfunction. Reduces afterload to treat CHF	Must avoid hypotension, monitor renal function and potassium. Cough is a common but nonserious side effect

APTT, activated partial thromboplastin time; ACE, angiotensin-converting enzyme; BP, blood pressure; CHF, congestive heart failure; COPD, chronic obstructive pulmonary disease; EF, ejection fraction; GI, gastrointestinal; HR, heart rate; LV, left ventricular; MI, myocardial infarction; sats, saturation levels.

It is not always possible to tell clinically if thrombolytic therapy has opened up the culprit vessel. The presence of continued chest pain, persistent ST elevation, or hemodynamic instability at 90 minutes after thrombolytic administration should prompt consideration for "rescue" angioplasty. Conversely, the presence of sudden resolution of chest discomfort and ST elevation, usually with reperfusion arrhythmia, is a good sign that flow has been reestablished. Accelerated idioventricular rhythm is the classic reperfusion arrhythmia and does not generally require treatment.

By far the most dreaded complication of thrombolytic therapy is intracranial bleeding. The overall incidence of intracranial bleeding with the use of thrombolytics is between 0.5% and 1% and is somewhat more likely to occur in women. This may be due to lower body weight. Unfortunately, intracranial bleeding portends a poor prognosis. In women, as in men, the risk of major bleeding is offset by the benefit of reestablishing coronary flow.

Primary percutaneous angioplasty, performed by an interventional cardiologist, involves the inflation of a small balloon across the culprit coronary stenosis. Generally, a metallic stent is left in place. The success rate in restoring normal blood flow is in the vicinity of 90%, without a significant risk of intracranial bleeding.

Historically, one of the great controversies in cardiology has been that of which modality of reperfusion, thrombolysis or primary angioplasty, is superior. An in-depth discussion of the debate is beyond the scope of this chapter, but some generalizations can be made. Both reperfusion modalities are effective in limiting infarct size and lowering mortality. Recent evidence supports probable superiority of primary angioplasty if it can be done within the first 90 minutes, preferably even earlier. Patients who present with symptoms that have been ongoing for more that a couple hours lose this angioplasty benefit. In small medical centers where angioplasty is not readily available and quick transfer to an angioplasty center is not feasible, thrombolytic therapy is superior. It is likely that this situation will become less of a factor, because recent studies have demonstrated the safety of primary angioplasty in centers without emergency cardiovascular surgery backup. Cardiogenic shock is one circumstance where primary angioplasty is superior to thrombolytic therapy.

Complications

Potential complications in patients with acute MI include persistence of coronary occlusion after thrombolytic therapy, CHF, cardiogenic shock, left ventricular aneurysm formation, arrhythmias, and pericarditis.

CHF is a common complication of acute MI and is the result of poor systolic pumping function of the heart or can be due to myocardial "stiffness" as a result of ischemia. Diuretics, oxygen, nitrates, and morphine are the mainstays of therapy in the acute setting. Angiotensin-converting enzyme inhibitors, by decreasing mortality, play a central role in the long-term treatment of patients with significant left ventricular function, with or without CHF. Digoxin helps alleviate the symptoms of CHF by increasing cardiac output, but there is no proven mortality benefit. Recently, it has become clear that beta-blockers, which have a proven benefit in reducing mortality in patients with MI, actually lead to improvement in left ventricular function when used in the long term. They should be avoided in the setting of acute CHF.

Cardiogenic shock, defined as persistent poor cardiac output, with accompanying hypotension and inadequate end-organ tissue perfusion, confers a poor prognosis. Most patients presenting in cardiogenic shock generally have had damage to at least 40% of their left ventricular mass and have mortality upward of 70%. A minority of shock cases is secondary to mechanical complications, such as papillary muscle rupture, and necrosis-mediated ventricular septal defect. Ventricular free wall rupture is a particularly ominous entity. These mechanical complications carry with them a mortality rate of about 90% if not recognized and surgically treated early but fortunately are less common in the age of reperfusion therapy. Patients with MI should be examined frequently for the development of new murmurs, because they can herald a mechanical complication. Echocardiography is very helpful in distinguishing the etiology of cardiogenic shock.

Sometimes cardiogenic shock is the result of infarction of the right ventricle or the inferior left ventricular wall with right ventricular involvement. A clue to right ventricular infarction is the presence of the constellation of hypotension, elevated right-sided pressure (neck vein distension), and relatively clear lung fields. Generally, nitroglycerin administration results in profound hypotension. The goal in patients with right ventricular infarction is reperfusion. In these patients, the hypotension responds to vigorous fluid resuscitation, in combination with inotropic agents (i.e., dobutamine).

Left ventricular aneurysm formation is another potential complication of MI. Aneurysms most commonly occur after an anterior wall MI, when a large area of scarred myocardium becomes permanently dyskinetic. Thrombus may form within the aneurysm, and therefore anticoagulants are indicated. Ventricular arrhythmia and CHF are common complications of aneurysm formation, but rupture generally does not occur. This is in contrast to the so-called false aneurysm in which spontaneous rupture is a high likelihood. False aneurisms, in fact, represent a tear in the myocardium with temporary walling off of the hemorrhage by the pericardium. False aneurysms represent a surgical emergency.

Pericarditis can occur 12 hours to 10 days after an MI. Clinically it manifests as a sharp pleuritic chest discomfort and often is accompanied by an evanescent pericardial friction rub. Occasionally, a pericardial effusion can be seen on echocardiography. Post-MI pericarditis generally responds well to nonsteroidal antiinflammatory drugs, such as ibuprofen. Once pericarditis is diagnosed, heparin should be discontinued. Thrombolytics should never be given if there is a suspicion of pericarditis.

A variety of rhythm disturbances, including bradycardias and tachycardias, may complicate acute MI. The decline in MI mortality over the last several decades is partially due to recognition and appropriate treatment of potentially fatal arrhythmias. Patients should have continuous central telemetry monitoring for at least 48 hours. Ventricular fibrillation is most likely to occur within the first few hours of presentation and is fatal without immediate electrical defibrillation. Fortunately, ventricular fibrillation early after an MI does not influence long-term prognosis. Most commonly, intravenous lidocaine is used in the short term to prevent further ventricular fibrillation. In a significant departure from the past, lidocaine is no longer used prophylactically in MI patients.

Nonsustained ventricular tachycardia is common after acute MI, and much investigation has taken place to learn which patients with nonsustained ventricular tachycardia are at risk for sudden death. It is well established that the presence of nonsustained ventricular tachycardia within the first 48 hours of an MI does not impact on long-term prognosis, with respect to sudden death. In patients with an ejection fraction less than 40% who have nonsustained ventricular tachycardia after 48 hours, mortality is significantly lower with the surgical implantation of an electrical defibrillator. Recent evidence suggests that implantation of a defibrillator may improve mortality in any patient who has had an MI and has an ejection fraction less than 30%, regardless of the presence or absence of nonsustained ventricular tachycardia.

Sinus bradycardia is particularly common with inferior MI because of heightened vagal tone. This requires treatment only if accompanied by hypotension. Atropine generally is effective.

Some form of atrioventricular (AV) block occurs in about 20% of patients with acute MI. Prolongation of the PR interval or first-degree heart block requires no therapy. There are two types of second-degree heart block, type I (Wenckebach) and type II. Wenckebach is manifest on ECG as progressive PR prolongation followed by a nonconducted P wave and is common with inferior wall MI. This is usually transient and resolves spontaneously. Type II second-degree heart block represents the sudden AV nonconductance of a P wave and is more ominous, signaling possible complete or third-degree heart block. Complete heart block is manifest on ECG as dissociation between P waves and the QRS complex and may be accompanied by profound hemodynamic instability, depending on the origin of the QRS complex within the ventricle. When complete heart block occurs with inferior wall MI, it is the result of the combination of heightened vagal tone and edema in the AV node. Although it often is well tolerated, temporary pacing usually is required. The complete heart block virtually always resolves spontaneously; however, it may take up to 2 weeks. Third-degree AV block in the setting of anterior wall MI is the result of extensive necrosis in the vicinity of the bundle of His and generally does not resolve, necessitating a permanent pacemaker. Patients who develop bundle branch blocks after acute MI must also be monitored closely for the development of complete heart block.

Supraventricular arrhythmias are not uncommon after acute MI and include atrial fibrillation, atrial flutter, and atrial tachycardia. The presence of these arrhythmias alone does not have any mortality ramifications but may be indicative of significant left ventricular dysfunction or electrolyte imbalance. Atrial fibrillation and flutter are often seen with post-MI pericarditis. Heart rate control and consideration of cardioversion are important, because prolonged tachycardia can lead to infarct extension. Adenosine is highly effective in terminating supraventricular tachycardia.

Hospital Convalescence and Post-Myocardial Infarction Evaluation

The greatest mortality and morbidity risk in the hospital is immediately after the MI; thus, monitoring in a coronary care unit for the first 48 to 72 hours should be routine. Even patients who have had a small infarct and look "well" should be monitored closely. In the absence of CHF or recurrent ischemia, patients can begin gradual ambulation within 48 hours.

Once therapy has been initiated and patients demonstrate stability, serious thought must then be given to prevention of future coronary events. Risk factor modification, including smoking cessation, weight reduction, aggressive cholesterol-lowering therapy, and treatment for hypertension, all are important factors in reducing the risk of another MI. The hospital setting is an especially good place to start discussing smoking cessation.

The most important immediate task for the physician managing a post-MI patient is determining the risk of future MI or death. Statistically, patients who appear to be at highest risk for recurrent MI or death in the year after an MI are those who either have severe left ventricular dysfunction or those who have evidence of ongoing ischemia, that is, viable myocardium that is in jeopardy. Two strategies for post-MI evaluation of risk include a conservative and an early invasive approach. The conservative strategy involves observation for recurrent angina at rest or with hallway ambulation, followed by low-level stress testing before hospital discharge and a full stress test 6 weeks later. In this approach, heart catheterization and revascularization are reserved for either recurrent angina or ischemia on stress testing. The early invasive strategy involves routine heart catheterization after MI. Perhaps the most popular misconception is that younger "healthier" patients should have routine heart catheterization, reserving stress testing for older infirm patients. Physicians often are most concerned about missing another MI in younger patients. Actually, the reverse is true. Older patients are at higher risk for future MI or death after MI. Another misconception is that coronary angiography will predict the patient's risk for future events. Patients very often request heart catheterization out of concern for having another MI. The chance of having another MI probably is more closely related to ongoing risk factors, including smoking, hypercholesterolemia, and hypertension, rather than the presence of coronary lesions. The existence of coronary lesions does not necessarily predict future events. Retrospective observational studies have shown that MI more commonly occurs on the substrate of moderate severity coronary lesions, ones that may not even cause angina or show up on stress testing. The explanation for this is that MI is caused by plaque instability, not plaque severity.

The United States and Canada historically have had significantly different practice patterns with regard to invasive versus conservative strategy; the rate of angiography with subsequent angioplasty or bypass surgery are threefold and fourfold higher, respectively, in the United States. Despite these differences, the 1-year mortality is not statistically different between countries.

A general set of guidelines has evolved based on factors that are considered high risk. In MI patients who have not been treated with primary angioplasty, recurrent angina, CHF, ejection fraction less than 40%, ventricular arrhythmia, and age greater than 70 should prompt consideration for early angiography to assess the appropriateness of revascularization by angioplasty or bypass surgery. Diabetics should strongly be considered for early invasive strategy.

The same principles of risk stratification can be applied to patients who have had unstable angina or non-Q wave MI. A conservative strategy is a reasonable starting point. Angiography should strongly be considered in patients with significant left ventricular dysfunction, ventricular arrhythmia, and diabetes. Patients presenting with elevations in troponin should also be considered for angiography.

Recent studies looking at the benefit of early invasive versus conservative strategy have included significant numbers of women. The results indicate that women are just as likely as men to benefit from early invasive strategy when deemed prudent, based on the above-mentioned risk factors.

Patients should be encouraged to enroll in cardiac rehabilitation programs after MI, generally beginning 6 weeks after discharge from the hospital. These programs are designed to individualize exercise regimens to facilitate attainment of maximal functional capacity. These rehabilitation programs also provide patient education on risk factor modification, and psychosocial support.

The emotional stress of an MI on the patient and family can be great. Disbelief, denial, fear, depression, anxiety, and anger are common responses to MI. Women often have nurturing roles within their family, and the changes within the family dynamics during a women's convalescence may cause significant stress. Family members may be fearful and therefore overprotective or may use denial to deal with the situation. Cardiac rehabilitation should involve education of the family. Often, because women have MIs at an older age, they are more likely than men to be living alone and may have less family support. Reassurance, education, and encouragement of physical reconditioning can restore the patient's sense of well-being, confidence, and self-worth after a potentially life-threatening event such as an MI.

CORONARY DISEASE AND MYOCARDIAL INFARCTION IN PREGNANCY

Clinically apparent coronary disease is rare during pregnancy. Although the presence of underlying atherosclerotic disease should be considered, a well-known phenomenon of coronary dissection, especially in the peripartum period, exists. The left anterior descending coronary artery is most often involved. Coronary vasospasm is another cause of acute MI in pregnancy and sometimes occurs in the setting of pregnancy-induced hypertension.

The evaluation and management of coronary disease in pregnancy must take into consideration the minimization of risk to both the mother and fetus. Both cardiac catheterization and nuclear imaging expose the fetus to radiation. There are no randomized prospective studies looking at the best method of evaluation of chest pain in pregnant women. Exercise stress echocardiography probably is the safest noninvasive means for evaluating anginal chest pain in pregnancy.

The treatment of acute MI in pregnancy is controversial. Thrombolytics have been given without detrimental consequences to the fetus. Coronary angiography and angioplasty have been done safely, though efforts should be made to delay exposing the fetus to radiation until beyond the first trimester. Adjunctive medications, such as beta-blockers and low dose aspirin, are believed to be safe during pregnancy. Hypotension should be avoided.

BIBLIOGRAPHY

Braunwald E. *Heart disease: a textbook of cardiovascular medicine.* Philadelphia: WB Saunders, 1997:1704.

Braunwald E, et al. ACC/AHA 2002 guideline update for the management of patients with unstable angina and non-ST-segment elevation myocardial infarction: a report of the American College of Cardiology/American Heart Association Task Force on Practice Guidelines (Committee on the management of Patients with Unstable Angina). *Circulation* 2002;106:1893–1900.

The Clopidogrel in Unstable Angina to Prevent Recurrent Events Trial Investigators. Effects of clopidogrel in addition to aspirin in patients with acute coronary syndromes without ST-segment elevation. *N Engl J Med* 2001;345:494–502.

Fragmin and Fast Revascularization during instability in CAD (FRISC II) Investigators. Invasive compared with non-invasive treatment in unstable CAD: FRISC II prospective randomised multicentre study. *Lancet* 1999;354: 708–715.

Gibbons R, et al. ACC/AHA 2002 guidelines update for the management of patients with chronic stable angina—summary article: a report of the American College of Cardiology/American Heart Association Task Force on Practice Guidelines (Committee to Update the 1999 Guidelines for the Management of Patients with Chronic Stable Angina). *Circulation* 2003;107:149–158.

Grady D, Herrington D, et al. Cardiovascular disease outcomes during 6.8 years of hormone therapy: heart and estrogen/progestin replacement study follow-up (HERS II). *JAMA* 2002;288:49–57.

Leppert PC, Howard FM. *Primary care for women.* Philadelphia: Lippincott-Raven, 1996.

Rossouw J, et al. Risks and benefits of estrogen plus progestin in healthy postmenopausal women: principal results from the women's health initiative randomized controlled trial. *JAMA* 2002;288:321–333.

Sacks F, Pfeffer M, et al. The effect of pravastatin on coronary events after myocardial infarction in patients with average cholesterol levels. Cholesterol and Recurrent Events Trial investigators. *N Engl J Med* 1996;335:1001.

Wenger N, Speroff L, Packard B. Cardiovascular health and disease in women (proceedings of a NHLBI conference). Greenwich, CT: LeJacq Communications, 1993:61.

CHAPTER 44

Peripheral Vascular Disease

Cynthia K. Shortell

Peripheral vascular disease encompasses disorders of the arterial, venous, and lymphatic systems. The incidence and manifestations of these disorders frequently differ according to gender. Some vascular diseases, such as atherosclerosis obliterans, have affected predominantly males in the past, but with the increase of smoking and stressful lifestyles, these diseases have become more prevalent in women. Other diseases, such as aneurysm formation, are more common in men than in women for unknown reasons. Finally, some disorders, such as thromboangiitis obliterans and Takayasu disease, are seen virtually exclusively in one gender or the other. This chapter provides an overview of peripheral vascular diseases and elucidates those aspects of disorders that are unique to women.

BASIC CONSIDERATIONS

Clinical Evaluation of the Patient with Vascular Disease

The object of the vascular history is to determine whether the patient has a disorder of the arterial, venous, or lymphatic system. A history of intermittent claudication of the upper or lower extremity is suggested by the presence of crampy pain with a fixed degree of exertion, such as walking two blocks. The discomfort is located just distal to the level of the arterial occlusion; thus, calf cramps suggest disease in the superficial femoral artery. Cramps in the absence of exertion are not likely to be vascular in etiology. More severe degrees of ischemia result in rest pain, characteristically affecting the toes or instep and relieved by dependency. The sudden onset of pain is suggestive of acute arterial occlusion. True ischemic rest pain must be distinguished from other pain syndromes, such as diabetic neuropathy, in which the patient typically experiences burning on the plantar surface of the foot. Finally, the patient should be questioned regarding the presence of nonhealing sores or ulcers and the location of these lesions determined; lesions of the toes and feet suggest arterial disease, whereas perimalleolar lesions suggest a venous etiology. If aneurysmal disease is suspected, the patient should be questioned for a history of abdominal, back, and flank pain, as well as the presence of "blue toes," suggestive of embolic events.

Symptoms of atherosclerotic cerebrovascular disease include the classic hemispheric complaints of transient monocular blindness (amaurosis fugax), hemiparesis or hemiparesthesia, dysphasia, and dysarthria, as well as nonhemispheric symptoms such as blurred vision, ataxia, and syncope.

Patients with venous disorders may present with acute or chronic complaints. The sudden onset of pain, swelling, and cyanosis of an extremity is highly suggestive of deep venous thrombosis. Patients with varicose veins should be questioned regarding the presence of pain, rupture, and superficial phlebitis. Chronic venous insufficiency is characterized by skin pigmentation, edema, and chronic ulceration.

Physical examination of the patient with vascular disease begins with observation of the skin, noting the presence of pallor, dependent rubor, and digital ulceration suggestive of arterial disease, as well as cyanosis, pigmentation, swelling, and malleolar ulceration suggestive of venous disorders. Isolated painful blue toes indicate an embolic process. Auscultation for bruits over the aorta and its major branches may suggest areas of disease but are not diagnostic of the presence of stenosis. The patient should next be examined for the presence of all pulses, which should be graded from 1+ to 4+, indicating a diminished-to-aneurysmal quality. Aneurysms of the aorta and popliteal arteries are detected by palpation of the epigastrium and popliteal fossa, respectively.

Noninvasive and Invasive Evaluation of the Vascular System

If vascular disease is suspected on the basis of the clinical history and physical examination, noninvasive vascular screening is indicated. Segmental measurement of the blood pressure in the lower extremity provides information regarding the location and severity of arterial disease; a drop in pressure is indicative of occlusive disease proximal to the level of measurement. Duplex evaluation of the carotid arteries and venous systems can determine the presence of a stenosis or valvular incompetency, respectively, with a very high degree of accuracy. Ultrasound is used to identify and quantify aneurysmal changes, usually involving the infrarenal abdominal aorta. Arteriography is usually reserved for patients in whom operative intervention is planned, because it confers the added risk of arterial puncture and contrast administration.

ARTERIAL DISEASES

Associated Conditions

Patients with significant peripheral vascular disease are rarely without associated medical conditions. Some of these disorders, such as hypertension, tobacco abuse, and diabetes, are etiologic factors associated with atherosclerosis obliterans, whereas other disorders have a shared etiology with atherosclerosis (e.g., coronary artery disease and chronic obstructive pulmonary disease). These concomitant disease processes are significant because they influence the management of patients with peripheral vascular disease. Individuals with severe underlying medical conditions such as coronary artery disease may pose an unacceptable operative risk, precluding consideration for elective procedures such as revascularization for claudication. Alternatively, underlying disease may require additional medical or surgical therapy (e.g., coronary artery bypass grafting) before proceeding with nonelective surgery such as repair of a large abdominal aortic aneurysm. Finally, in elderly or terminally ill patients, it may be determined that the patient is likely to die of other underlying medical conditions before succumbing to her vascular problem, rendering intervention by the vascular surgeon futile.

All patients in whom major operative intervention is being considered should be screened for coronary artery disease, even those who are asymptomatic. The most appropriate screening test has not yet been established, but dipyridamole thallium and dobutamine stress echocardiogram have both been successfully used. Pulmonary function tests should be obtained in all smokers.

It important to keep in mind that peripheral vascular disease is a symptom of the more global disorder of atherosclerotic disease. As such, many patients have other manifestations of systemic atherosclerosis, such as coronary artery disease and cerebrovascular disease. It is sobering to consider that as a result of these associations, the presence of peripheral vascular disease confers a substantial reduction in long-term survival. This effect is proportional to the degree of peripheral vascular disease: Patients with moderate disease at the time of presentation have a 5-year survival rate of 65%, whereas those with severe disease at the time of presentation have a 5-year survival rate of only 35%.

Aortoiliac and Lower Extremity Occlusive Disease

The incidence of lower extremity peripheral vascular disease is estimated at 1.5% of all women under age 59 years and 5% of all women over age 60 years. Of these individuals, 25% will require revascularization and 5% will eventually undergo amputation. Small artery syndrome is a variant of atherosclerotic occlusive disease seen exclusively in slightly built women with a heavy smoking history. These patients experience premature disease onset and an accelerated course and should be treated aggressively with operative intervention and smoking cessation.

The most common presenting symptom of lower extremity occlusive disease is intermittent claudication. Patients experience cramping pain involving the muscle groups immediately distal to the obstructed arterial segment; thus, thigh and calf claudication are typically experienced by patients with iliac and superficial femoral artery occlusions, respectively. Symptoms are highly reproducible and consistent with respect to walking distance in a given individual. Night cramping is typically seen in elderly and pregnant women and may be due to a variety of factors but is not vascular in origin. Other conditions involving the lower extremity that are frequently confused with arterial occlusive disease include lumbar disc disease and spinal stenosis. The differential diagnosis is primarily based on a careful history, because older patients may have objective evidence of both disease processes. The major differences between true claudication and pseudoclaudication are outlined in Table 44.1.

Rest pain is the next clinical step in the progression of lower extremity occlusive disease. The pain is characteristically located in the toes, forefoot, and instep and may awaken the patient at night. Relief is obtained by dangling the feet or walking briefly. Symptoms of this severity usually indicate occlusive lesions involving two or more arterial segments, such as iliac and superficial femoral arteries. The differential diagnosis includes diabetic neuropathy, in which patients experience burning pain in the soles of the feet that is unrelieved by dependency and is often in the presence of normal pedal pulses. Ischemic ulceration and gangrene represent the ultimate progression of peripheral vascular disease. Lesions are typically found at the tips of toes or over pressure points (such as the metatarsal heads) in contrast to venous ulcerations, which are pretibial or perimalleolar.

If lower extremity occlusive disease is suspected on the basis of the history and physical examination, the patient is referred for arterial noninvasive evaluation, with segmental blood pressure recordings at the high thigh, low thigh, calf, and ankle levels. The ratio between the highest brachial pressure and the ankle pressure is referred to as the ankle–brachial index and is 1.0 or slightly higher in normal individuals. Claudicants and patients with single-level disease usually have an ankle–brachial index between 0.5 and 0.75, whereas patients with rest pain and ulceration will usually have an ankle–brachial index between 0 and 0.3.

The treatment of intermittent claudication due to superficial femoral occlusion involves smoking cessation, exercise, and cilostazol in patients who have no history of congestive heart failure. In patients with aortoiliac lesions (Fig. 44.1), surgical intervention may be recommended, because these individuals are theoretically at risk for retrograde aortic and renal artery thrombosis if progression to complete occlusion occurs. Patients with rest pain and gangrene should undergo revascularization; this may be performed in conjunction with toe amputation. Amputation of the affected digit without appropriate bypass surgery is unlikely to heal and may lead to progressively higher levels of amputation. Arteriography is reserved for patients undergoing surgery and is performed before the operation to provide the surgeon with information regarding the origin and termination of the bypass graft. Aortoiliac occlusive disease requires replacement of the diseased arterial segments using a prosthetic graft originating from the infrarenal aorta and terminating at the common femoral arteries bilaterally (aortobifemoral bypass). Patency of these grafts is 80% to 90% at 5 years. An alternative for short, isolated, partial iliac artery occlusions is percutaneous balloon dilatation (angioplasty) and arterial stenting; in properly selected patients, the results of iliac stenting approach that of surgical repair. Infrainguinal disease is treated with a bypass graft beginning at the common femoral artery and extending beyond the occlusive process to the popliteal, tibial, or pedal arteries. Saphenous vein is the preferred conduit, but prosthetic material is acceptable when the distal anastomosis is above the knee joint. Patency of infrainguinal grafts depends on location and conduit but is between 45% and 75% at 5 years. Angioplasty has not been as successful for arteries below the femoral level. Primary amputation is reserved for patients with irreversible extensive gangrene, for nonambulatory patients, and for patients in whom major surgery poses an unacceptable risk.

Cerebrovascular Disease

Symptoms of cerebrovascular insufficiency are classified as either hemispheric or nonhemispheric, based on whether they correspond to carotid territory or vertebrobasilar territory disease, respectively. Hemispheric, or carotid distribution, symptoms include contralateral weakness and numbness of the upper and lower extremities and face, dysphasia, and ipsilateral monocular blindness (amaurosis fugax). Nonhemispheric, or vertebrobasilar, symptoms typically involve disorders of gait and vision, including blurred vision, double vision, ataxia, dysarthria, and symptoms of brainstem ischemia such as drop attacks, vertigo, and dizziness. The severity of the event is further classified based on the clinical duration: Transient ischemic attacks are defined as symptoms lasting less than 24 hours,

TABLE 44.1. Claudication versus Pseudoclaudication

	Intermittent claudication	Pseudoclaudication
Symptoms	Cramping pain	Paresthesias, weakness, radicular pain
Location	Buttock, thigh, calf	Buttock, thigh, calf
Symptomatic occurrence	With walking only (exercise)	Walking, sitting, standing
Symptomatic relief	Stop walking	Change position

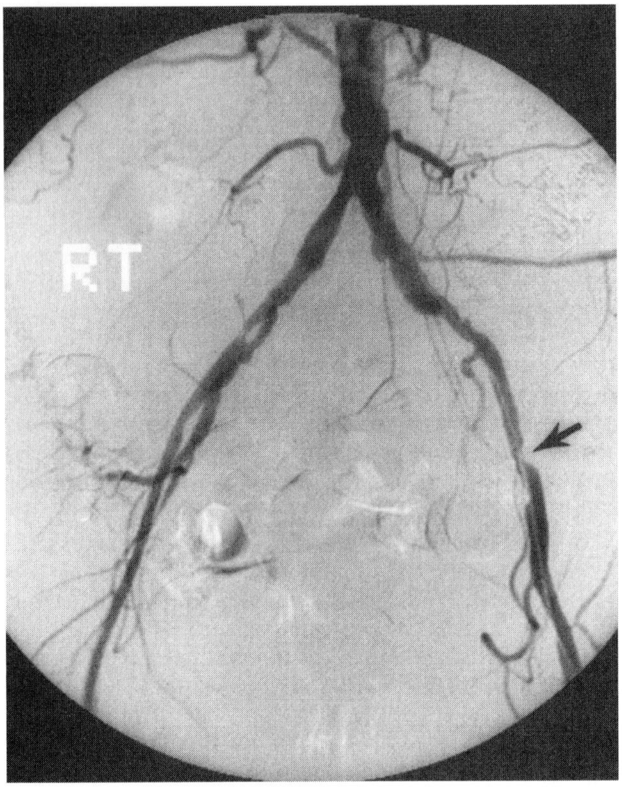

FIG. 44.1. Intra-arterial aortogram of a patient with left leg ischemia demonstrates diffuse disease of both iliac systems, with a severe stenosis of the left iliac artery *(arrow)*.

reversible ischemic neurologic deficits as symptoms lasting between 24 hours and 2 weeks, and a completed stroke as any deficit persisting for longer than 2 weeks.

There are two possible etiologies for symptoms due to cerebrovascular disease: embolization and flow reduction. Embolic phenomena occur in a hemispheric distribution and are a result of detachment of debris from atherosclerotic plaque located in the proximal internal carotid artery (Fig. 44.2). Flow-related symptoms are nonhemispheric in nature, are much less common, and are due to a global reduction in blood flow to the

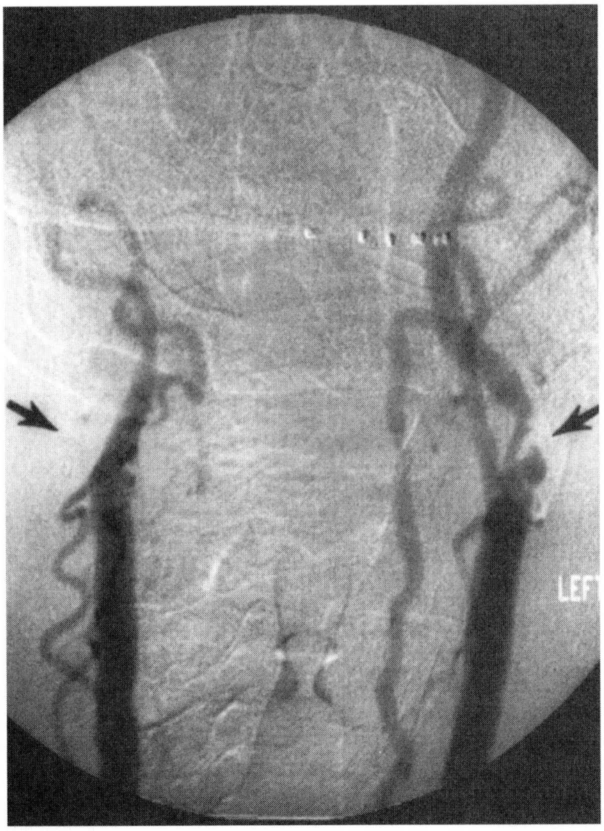

FIG. 44.2. Arteriogram of a patient with left eye amaurosis fugax demonstrates stenosis and complex plaque in the left internal carotid artery and complete occlusion of the right internal carotid artery *(arrows)*.

brain. Flow-related symptoms are usually due to disorders other than cerebrovascular disease that result in intracerebral hypoxia, such as cardiac arrhythmias and obstructive lung disease, because the collateral flow to the brain is usually adequate to compensate hemodynamically for even severe vascular lesions.

A special case of flow-related symptoms occurs with the subclavian steal syndrome. In this situation, lesions of the subclavian artery proximal to the origin of the vertebral artery result in a pressure gradient that causes reversal of flow in the vertebral artery and diversion of blood away from the brain, especially under circumstances where blood flow to the arm is increased, such as with exercise. Treatment is only indicated in symptomatic patients.

In patients with hemispheric or nonhemispheric symptoms, as well as in those with asymptomatic bruits, the first screening test for determining the presence or absence of cerebrovascular disease is the duplex study, combining B-mode ultrasound and Doppler analysis. This is an extremely sensitive means of identifying stenosis of the carotid arteries and determining the direction of flow in the vertebral arteries. After duplex evaluation, the decision regarding further workup and treatment is determined by the presence or absence of symptoms. If no lesion is detected, other etiologies should be considered, including cardiac emboli, lesions of the aortic arch and great vessels (rare), hypertensive strokes, and migraine equivalents. If the patient is asymptomatic, operative intervention is appropriate only if the stenosis is severe (80%–99%). If the patient is symptomatic, surgery should be considered if the stenosis is greater than 50%, although this remains controversial. Patients with crescendo transient ischemic attacks or thrombus in the internal carotid artery constitute a surgical emergency. Surgery is not indicated for patients with complete occlusions of the carotid artery and should be delayed for 6 weeks after a completed stroke with a positive head computed tomography (CT). Operative intervention consists of internal carotid artery endarterectomy, a procedure that carries a 2% risk of perioperative stroke in asymptomatic patients and up to a 5% risk of stroke in patients presenting with symptoms preoperatively.

Visceral Ischemic Syndromes

The intestinal tract receives its blood supply from three major arterial systems: the celiac axis, the superior mesenteric artery, and the inferior mesenteric artery. A rich plexus of collaterals connects these vascular beds; therefore, occlusion of only one of these vessels rarely results in visceral ischemia, with the exception of acute occlusion of the superior mesenteric artery.

Chronic mesenteric ischemia is typically seen in patients with advanced atherosclerosis of the coronary and peripheral vascular systems. Clinical features include weight loss, severe postprandial abdominal pain, and diarrhea. The diagnosis is confirmed by arteriographic evaluation and treatment consists of bypass grafting from the aorta to the involved arteries, usually superior mesenteric, celiac, or both.

Acute mesenteric ischemia may be due to one of four causes. Treatment is based on diagnosis of the underlying pathology using clinical and arteriographic findings. Regardless of the etiology, the clinical picture is similar—sudden onset of severe abdominal pain, with pain out of proportion to physical findings. With progression of bowel ischemia, leukocytosis, fever, and eventually peritonitis are found. Superior mesenteric artery thrombosis occurs in patients with underlying chronic superior mesenteric artery stenoses. Treatment consists of revascularization by either surgical or interventional means, after arteriographic evaluation. Embolic occlusion of the superior mesenteric artery, usually from a cardiac source, is treated with embolectomy. In patients with both thrombotic and embolic occlusions, the decision regarding bowel resection is made after blood flow is reestablished. Mesenteric venous thrombosis is seen in patients with hypercoagulable states and can be treated with either anticoagulation or venous bypass, with bowel resection as needed. Nonocclusive mesenteric ischemia is due to vasospasm and occurs in patients with severely compromised cardiac output and splanchnic vasoconstriction. It may be associated with the use of digitalis preparations or vasopressor agents. Treatment involves discontinuation of responsible medications and improvement in the underlying condition and may also include intra-arterial papaverine administration in selected cases.

The existence of celiac artery and superior mesenteric artery compression syndromes is controversial, but they almost exclusively involve women and so deserve mention. The celiac axis compression syndrome is characterized by abdominal pain and is due to compression of the celiac artery by the median arcuate ligament, as determined arteriographically. The superior mesenteric artery syndrome, or cast syndrome, is characterized by duodenal obstruction and is caused by compression of the duodenum by the superior mesenteric artery. This syndrome is seen in patients with rapid severe weight loss or in patients immobilized in body casts and is diagnosed by upper gastrointestinal series. Operative intervention may be appropriate in very selected cases.

Renovascular Hypertension

Although hypertension is a commonly encountered medical disorder, renovascular disease is rarely the cause, especially in women (<0.5%). Conversely, the presence of benign (i.e., not causing hypertension or renal insufficiency) renal artery stenosis is relatively high, particularly in patients with underlying vascular disease. Renovascular hypertension should be suspected in patients in whom the onset of hypertension is sudden, occurs at an unusually early (younger than 30 years) or late (over 55 years) age, or is difficult to control using standard medications. Causes include atherosclerosis obliterans and, in women between the ages of 25 and 50, fibromuscular dysplasia. The diagnosis is confirmed with renal artery duplex evaluation. If a lesion is detected, its severity and significance with regard to hypertension and renal function must be evaluated with arteriography, followed by renal vein renin determination and split renal function tests, respectively. If the lesion is found to be responsible for either hypertension or diminished renal function, treatment is appropriate. The treatment of choice for atherosclerotic nonorificeal lesions and for most fibromuscular dysplastic lesions is angioplasty. Lesions not amenable to angioplasty are treated with renal artery bypass grafting in acceptable risk patients. Surgical options include renal endarterectomy, aortorenal bypass, splenorenal bypass, and hepatorenal bypass, and treatment is individualized to reflect the patient's health and anatomy.

Arterial Aneurysms and Dissections

An aneurysm is defined as a localized dilatation of an artery to at least twice its normal size in a given patient. Aneurysms are more common in men than women and rare in individuals under age 50 years. The natural history of arterial aneurysms is expansion over time, and they are rarely benign. Complications include rupture, embolization, and compression of adjacent structures; the relative frequency depends on the type and location of the aneurysm. Aneurysms are classified as true or false. True aneurysms are dilatations that involve all three layers of the arterial wall, develop spontaneously, and are usually fusiform in shape. False aneurysms occur when the full thickness of the arterial wall is disrupted and extravasation of blood is contained by the adventitia and surrounding soft tissue structures. They are usually saccular in shape. The treatment of true aneurysms depends on their size, location, and the patient's health, whereas repair is almost always indicated for false aneurysms because of their unstable structure. The etiology of most aneurysms is atherosclerotic degeneration, although the exact mechanism by which atherosclerosis leads to aneurysm formation is uncertain. A genetic susceptibility to aneurysm formation is believed to play an important role in most patients. This is particularly true in women. When aneurysmal disease occurs in women, all first-degree relatives should be screened for the disorder after age 50 years. Congenital defects in the arterial wall, such as Ehlers-Danlos and Marfan syndromes, may be a cause of aneurysm formation, as may acquired defects such as vasculitis due to Takayasu disease and polyarteritis nodosa. Infection, once a common factor in aortic aneurysm formation in the form of syphilitic aortitis, is now a rare cause of aneurysmal degeneration, with the most common agent being salmonella in primary infections. Trauma remains an important cause of aneurysm formation and may result in the development of either true aneurysms, in the case of repetitive blunt trauma, or false aneurysms, in the case of penetrating trauma due to violent or iatrogenic causes (e.g., catheterization). A special case of traumatic aneurysm formation is postoperative separation of a vascular graft from the native artery, resulting in false aneurysm formation.

Thoracic aortic aneurysms have decreased in incidence with the advent of treatment for syphilis. The most common type of thoracic aneurysm involves the descending thoracic aorta. Most patients with this disorder are asymptomatic, and the diagnosis is made unexpectedly as an incidental finding on a chest x-ray. When they occur, the most frequently noted symptoms are upper back pain, chest pain, and hoarseness. The prognosis of untreated thoracic aortic aneurysms is surprisingly poor (25% survival at 3 years); therefore, operative intervention is indicated for patients with aneurysms larger than 6 cm whose life expectancy exceeds 2 years. Urgent intervention is indicated for rapid expansion, larger size, symptomatic aneurysms, and severely hypertensive patients.

Abdominal aortic aneurysms are the most commonly encountered form of aneurysmal disease. They are usually asymptomatic, especially if small in size, and may be discovered by the patient or by the primary care practitioner on physical examination. When present, symptoms usually consist of pain in the abdomen, back, flanks, or groin or may be related to embolization of debris from the inside of the aneurysm to distal structures (blue toe syndrome). Physical examination may fail to reveal the aneurysm if it is small or if the patient is obese. Conversely, intraabdominal masses overlying a normal aorta, such as a pancreatic carcinoma, may transmit an exaggerated aortic pulse and be confused with an aneurysm. If the diagnosis of abdominal aortic aneurysm is suspected based on clinical or physical findings, the screening test of choice is abdominal ultrasound. This test provides accurate information regarding the presence and size of the aneurysm and is also an excellent modality with which to follow aneurysm size in patients in whom observation is elected. If rupture is suspected, however, ultrasound is inadequate and abdominal CT should be obtained. Similarly, abdominal CT is required in preparation for operative intervention because it provides important additional anatomic details to the surgical team (Fig. 44.3). The goal of operative intervention is the prevention of complications and preservation of life; the mortality for elective abdominal aortic aneurysm repair is 3%, as compared with 50% to 75% for ruptured aneurysms. The indications for operative repair include symptoms of pain or embolization, rapid expansion (greater than 1 cm in a year), and size greater than 5 cm in an otherwise healthy patient. In poor-risk patients, the risk of rupture (Table 44.2) must be weighed against the individual patient's estimated operative risk. Elective repair should always be preceded by a thorough evaluation for cardiac, pulmonary, and carotid artery disease, because these disorders are often encountered in patients with abdominal aortic aneurysms and may be asymptomatic. Operative repair consists of graft replacement of the aneurysmal portion of the aorta, usually from the infrarenal abdominal aorta to its bifurcation. Placement of either the aortic cross-clamp or the graft itself above the level of the renal arteries significantly increases the operative morbidity and mortality of the procedure. In recent years the use of endovascular grafts to repair infrarenal aortic aneurysms has become increasingly frequent. Difficulty with short- and long-term complications, such as leakage around the graft, graft

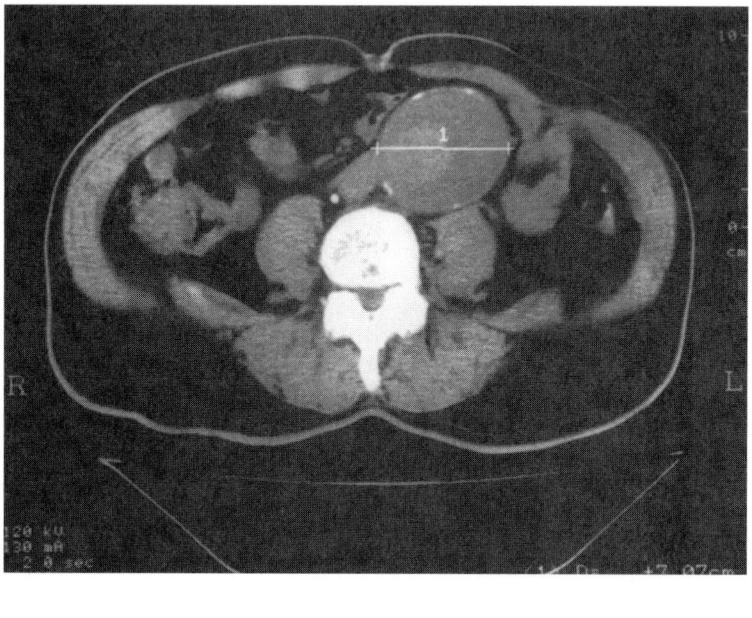

FIG. 44.3. Abdominal computed tomography demonstrates a large infrarenal abdominal aortic aneurysm with intraluminal thrombus.

TABLE 44.2. Risk of Rupture of Abdominal Aortic Aneurysm with Increasing Size

Aneurysm size	5-Year risk of rupture[a]
4 cm	10%
5 cm	20%
6 cm	30%
7 cm	50%
8 cm	80%

[a]Percentages based on estimates from a variety of sources.

migration, and rupture of aneurysms despite endografting, has limited their use to date. As technologic advances in this area occur, it is likely that endovascular grafting will be applicable to a greater number of patients. At present, it is especially valuable in very high-risk patients with large aneurysms.

Thoracoabdominal aneurysms consist of a number of anatomic patterns of aneurysms involving all or part of the thoracic and abdominal aorta. They confer a much higher mortality, both with and without surgery, than either thoracic or abdominal aneurysms alone because of the involvement of great vessels and visceral vessels in many cases and their high rate of rupture. Repair should be undertaken only in those centers that specialize in care of these patients; even in the most experienced hands the incidence of perioperative complications such as stroke, paraplegia, renal failure, myocardial infarction, and gut ischemia is high.

Aneurysms of the iliac arteries are rarely seen in isolation but are frequently associated with abdominal aortic aneurysms. They rarely cause symptoms until rupture occurs or is imminent. When larger than 3 cm in diameter, they should always be repaired, either alone or in conjunction with aortic aneurysm repair.

Aneurysmal degeneration may also occur in virtually any of the visceral arteries, including hepatic, celiac, gastroduodenal, and superior mesenteric. The most common visceral artery to become aneurysmal is the splenic artery, of interest because this is the only site in which aneurysmal degeneration is much more common in women than in men. Splenic artery aneurysms rarely cause symptoms before rupture, with the highest rate of rupture seen during the third trimester of pregnancy. Under these circumstances, maternal and fetal mortality is very high; hence any splenic artery aneurysm larger than 2 cm detected in a woman of childbearing age should be repaired electively. The popliteal and femoral arteries are also relatively common sites for aneurysm formation, particularly in individuals with abdominal aortic aneurysms, and repair is almost always indicated to avoid complications. Both of these lesions are extremely rare in women, however.

Arterial dissection may occur in any location but is most common in the thoracic aorta and is rare in other segments of the aorta and its branches. The lesion is initiated by an intimal tear in the vessel, followed by separation of the layers of the media and creation of a false arterial channel. This process should not be confused with aneurysm rupture, because the vessel is not initially aneurysmal but only becomes aneurysmal over time due to the weakness of the arterial wall caused by dissection. The clinical signs and symptoms of aortic dissection reflect two simultaneous events: The expansion of the artery and surrounding structures results in severe chest and upper back pain, whereas occlusion of arterial branches to the heart, brain, intestines, kidneys, and extremities by the false channel results in ischemia to these organs. Most patients are severely hypertensive as well. The diagnosis is made on the basis of chest x-ray, electrocardiogram, chest CT, and arteriogram. Dissections are classified based on the relationship to the great vessels: Type I begins at the level of the aortic root and extends throughout the descending thoracic aorta, type II begins at the aortic root and extends to the origin of the innominate artery, and type III begins distal to the left subclavian artery and involves the descending thoracic aorta. Patients with types I and II dissections should undergo immediate operative repair because of the danger to the coronary and cerebral circulation. Type III dissections may be managed medically, at least in the acute phase, with aggressive antihypertensive therapy and monitoring in the intensive care unit, provided that perfusion to vital organs and extremities is not impaired by the dissection channel.

Acute Peripheral Arterial Occlusion

The classic signs and symptoms of acute arterial occlusion are described by the "six Ps": pain, pulselessness, paresthesias, pallor, paralysis, and poikilothermy (cold temperature). In reality, however, symptoms may vary greatly from patient to patient depending on the arterial anatomy and collateral blood supply to the extremity. The patient with acute thrombosis of a previously stenotic artery often has extensive collateral circulation to the extremity and may experience minimal or no symptoms. By contrast, the patient with sudden occlusion of a previously normal artery is unlikely to have developed significant collaterals and will probably experience severe limb-threatening ischemia as described by the six Ps. As noted, acute arterial occlusion is either thrombotic or embolic in nature, with 90% of emboli to the lower extremity and virtually all emboli to the arm originating from a cardiac source. Thrombotic occlusion usually occurs in the setting of preexisting atherosclerosis but may also be a result of traumatic or iatrogenic injury. The diagnosis is made initially based on the history and physical examination, and an attempt is made to assess the etiology. Normal pulses in the contralateral extremity, absence of a history of claudication, and the presence of atrial fibrillation or valvular heart disease suggest an embolic etiology, whereas abnormal contralateral pulse examination, a history of preexisting vascular disease, and the absence of cardiac pathology suggest a thrombotic cause. Regardless of the etiology, the patient is immediately heparinized to prevent antegrade and retrograde propagation of the thromboembolic process. Embolic occlusions are treated with simple embolectomy, whereas thrombotic occlusions require bypass grafting, as thrombectomy alone is doomed to reocclusion. If the degree of ischemia is severe or if the etiology is clearly embolic, the patient is taken directly to the operating room. If doubt exists as to the nature and location of the occlusion, however, and the patient's condition permits, arteriography is performed to aid in planning the operation. In patients with embolic occlusions, heparin should be continued postoperatively and a thorough search made for the source of the embolus.

An alternative treatment option in patients without severe ischemia is the use of intra-arterial thrombolytic agents, often in conjunction with mechanical thrombectomy devices, to dissolve the offending thrombus. Proponents argue that reduction in the clot volume may reduce the frequency and magnitude of operative interventions required in these patients, but this has yet to be proved.

Vasculitides

The systemic vasculitides encompass a wide variety of inflammatory disorders involving large, medium, and small arteries throughout the body. The inflammatory process may be mediated by immune complex deposition, complement activation, or cellular mechanisms, and the classification of these disorders (Table 44.3) is based in part on these distinctions.

Polyarteritis nodosa is a necrotizing vasculitis involving medium-sized arteries and affecting women slightly less often than men. The disease may be devastating, with multisystem involvement, although survival is now 80% at 5 years with the use of steroids and cyclophosphamide. In the hypersensitivity vasculitides, the inciting agent may be a pharmacologic agent, an immunization, or a chemical agent. The most important entity in this group is the vasculitis associated with underlying medical (usually connective tissue) disorders, such as systemic lupus erythematosus, rheumatoid arthritis, and scleroderma, which affect primarily women. In these patients, the most frequently involved sites are the distal digital arteries, and digital ulceration and even gangrene may result. The vasculitis of the patient with Wegener granulomatosis consists of an inflammation of the small- and medium-sized arteries, with major involvement of the respiratory and renal circulations. Women are affected less often than men (2:3). Treatment with steroids and cyclophosphamide has improved the prognosis considerably.

Giant cell arteritis consists of two distinct clinical syndromes characterized by identical vascular histopathology (giant cell infiltration of the vessel wall). Both are much more common in women than men. Temporal arteritis is seen in patients over 50 years of age and is characterized by symptoms of temporal headache and tenderness (unilateral or bilateral), visual disturbances, and jaw claudication. Diagnosis is made by the laboratory finding of an elevated erythrocyte sedimentation rate and by temporal artery biopsy; treatment consists of steroid administration. Takayasu disease affects young women (adolescent to 35 years) and usually begins as a systemic illness with fever, sweats, and malaise. The disorder affects large arteries, including the pulmonary circulation and the ascending and descending aorta and branches, especially the great vessels. The inflammatory process may lead to either stenosis or aneurysm formation. The diagnosis is made based on an elevated erythrocyte sedimentation rate, as well as the clinical and arteriographic findings of vascular disease. Biopsy is rarely possible because of the inaccessible nature of the involved vessels. Treatment is medical, with steroids and cyclophosphamide, unless the arterial pathology mandates surgical intervention.

Raynaud Disease

This vasospastic disorder affecting the digits of the upper and lower extremities is seen almost exclusively in women. It may be classified as either primary, when it occurs in the absence of an underlying systemic disease, or secondary, when it occurs in the setting of an underlying systemic disease, usually a connective tissue disorder.

In patients with Raynaud disease, the digits are extremely sensitive to cold exposure and undergo an excessive vasoconstrictor response under conditions of cold. The classic three phases consist of pallor with cold exposure, followed by cyanosis with initial rewarming, and concluding with a hyperemic rubor. Not all patients exhibit all of these phases, however. The diagnosis is suspected based on clinical findings and is confirmed in the vascular laboratory with measurement of digital pressures and waveforms before, during, and after cold immersion. In patients with Raynaud disease, digital pressures and waveforms are markedly dampened with cold exposure. Reduced digital artery pressures before cold immersion are suggestive of fixed occlusion and an underlying connective tissue disorder with associated vasculitis. This finding or a history of systemic symptoms should prompt a search for underlying pathology. In addition to the overall implications of an underlying disorder, the prognosis with regard to the digital lesions differs between the primary and secondary forms of the disease.

Patients with primary Raynaud disease virtually never develop ischemic ulceration or tissue loss, whereas patients with secondary Raynaud disease may develop painful digital lesions, including permanent cyanosis, ulceration, and even gangrene resulting in tissue loss. Treatment of the primary form of Raynaud disease consists of cold avoidance and, in severe cases, the use of calcium channel blockers or sympatholytic agents. In patients with secondary Raynaud disease, treatment of the underlying cause is paramount. Other medical and surgical modalities, including cervical sympathectomy, are of limited benefit.

TABLE 44.3. Classification of Vasculitides

Necrotizing vasculitis
Classic polyarteritis nodosa
Allergic granulomatosis
Hypersensitivity vasculitis group
True hypersensitivity vasculitis
Henoch-Schönlein purpura
Vasculitis with mixed cryoglobulinemia
Vasculitis with connective tissue disorder
Wegener granulomatosis group
Classic and limited Wegener granulomatosis
Lymphomatoid granulomatosis
Benign lymphocytic angiitis
Giant cell arteritis
Temporal arteritis
Takayasu arteritis

Thoracic Outlet Syndrome

Thoracic outlet syndrome refers to a group of disorders producing symptoms in the neck, shoulder, and upper extremity due to compression of neurologic, venous, and arterial structures as they exit the thoracic cavity. The disorder is more common in women than men because of the less well-developed shoulder girdle muscles.

The neurologic syndrome is the most common (95%) and results from compression of the brachial plexus by a variety of muscular, fibrous, and skeletal anomalies. The clinical features of neurologic thoracic outlet syndrome include pain and paresthesias of the neck, occiput, and upper extremities, which is exacerbated by activity, particularly elevation of the arm above shoulder level. Symptoms may be precipitated by a seemingly minor injury or may develop spontaneously and occur in the distribution of either the radial or ulnar nerves, depending on whether the upper or lower portion of the brachial plexus is impinged upon by the responsible structures. Physical examination reveals tenderness over the supraclavicular area, the back of the neck, and the shoulder. Of the many "maneuvers" reported, only the elevated arm stress test is actually helpful in diagnosing the syndrome; pulse obliteration with elevation and abduction occurs in 50% of normal patients and is not diagnostic. To perform the elevated arm stress test, the patient stands with the arms held at 90 degrees of abduction and external rotation and is asked to open and close both hands for 3 minutes. Normal individuals do not experience discomfort with this maneuver; reproduction of symptoms on the affected side is considered diagnostic of thoracic outlet syndrome. The mainstay of diagnosis is a careful history and physical examination, although a chest x-ray is indicated to rule out a cervical rib. Other diagnostic modalities, such as nerve conduction studies, are not helpful. The differential diagnosis includes carpal tunnel syndrome, which is characterized by median nerve involvement, and cervical disc disease, in which pain is radicular in nature, is not exacerbated by activity, and is not associated with tenderness on physical examination. Treatment of neurologic thoracic outlet syndrome is initially conservative, with exercises to strengthen the shoulder girdle muscles and thus relieve pressure on structures exiting the chest. If this is unsuccessful, surgical intervention is used, removing a cervical rib when present or, more commonly, removing the first rib to decompress the thoracic outlet.

When structures within the thoracic outlet compromise venous outflow, thrombosis of the subclavian vein may occur (Paget-von Schröetter syndrome, effort thrombosis). This often occurs in the setting of repetitive physical activities, such as weight-lifting or pitching, and is most common in muscular young men. The clinical findings include swelling, cyanosis, and pain of the affected arm, with prominent cutaneous venous collaterals visible around the shoulder. Treatment consists of heparinization and elevation; if more aggressive therapy is desired based on the severity of symptoms or the patient's occupation, surgical or medical (thrombolytic) clot removal in conjunction with first rib resection should be used.

Arterial thoracic outlet syndrome is the least common (1%) and most serious of the various forms of thoracic outlet syndrome. The etiology is chronic compression of the subclavian artery by one of the bony structures of the thoracic outlet, either a cervical rib or clavicular fracture. If diagnosed early, simple removal of the offending structure is adequate therapy. If, however, the process becomes chronic, the artery is injured and aneurysm formation and embolization occur. Under these circumstances, repair of the aneurysm and removal of the offending bony structure are required.

VENOUS DISORDERS

Venous Thromboembolism

This is covered completely in Chapter 91 and so is not mentioned further here.

Chronic Venous Insufficiency and Varicose Veins

The venous circulation is comprised of a deep system, including the femoral, popliteal, and tibial veins; a superficial system comprised of the greater and lesser saphenous veins draining into the deep system; and a set of perforating veins directing blood from the superficial to the deep system within the calf. All these veins contain valves at regular intervals designed to facilitate forward flow and prevent retrograde flow and venous hypertension. Malfunction of the valves at any level may result in venous insufficiency and varicose veins; patients with varicose veins often have intrinsic degeneration of the venous wall in addition to the above-mentioned factors.

Varicose veins may range in severity from mild cosmetic defects to large, tortuous, bulging lesions. Symptoms vary from none to throbbing, aching, and itching, particularly after long periods of standing, during menses, and during pregnancy, when venous pressure is increased by compression of the iliac veins. As noted earlier, the etiology of varicose veins includes hereditary factors within the vessel wall, greater saphenous valvular insufficiency, and pregnancy. The diagnosis of greater saphenous incompetence can be made using venous duplex scanning. Initial treatment consists of elastic compression stockings. If these fail to control the patient's symptoms, high ligation and stripping of the greater saphenous system and excision of individual varicosities is highly effective. Sclerotherapy (injection) using hypertonic saline is effective only for spider veins and very small varicosities. Endovenous thermal ablation of the saphenous vein and branches may soon be available on a more widespread basis and represents a less invasive means of obliterating the greater saphenous vein than standard surgical techniques.

With long-standing valvular incompetence in the deep and superficial systems and perforators, changes of chronic venous stasis occur. These begin as thickening of the skin with pigmentation secondary to hemosiderin deposits and progress to ulceration, edema, and cellulitis that may be difficult to eradicate. If ulcers occur and greater saphenous incompetence is prominent, high ligation and stripping may be helpful. If perforator incompetence is predominant, subfascial endoscopic ligation of perforators may be beneficial. Otherwise, as in most patients, the mainstay of therapy is the heavyweight elastic compression stocking, used in conjunction with meticulous wound care and strict bed rest with leg elevation in the acute period.

LYMPHEDEMA

Lymphedema is defined as a swelling of the extremities due to inadequate lymphatic drainage and can be classified as either primary or secondary. The primary lymphedemas are further classified based on the patient's age at onset, with earlier age at onset correlating with a more severe clinical picture. Milroy disease (familial lymphedema) usually presents in the first decade of life, lymphedema praecox presents in early adolescence, and lymphedema tarda presents after puberty. In all primary lymphedemas, intrinsic anatomic abnormalities of the lymphatics are causative, including lymphatic aplasia, hypoplasia, or hyperplasia with valvular reflux. Secondary lymphedemas are due to obstruction of previously normal lymphatics by tumor, infection, radiation, or surgical interruption.

Clinically, lymphedema can be differentiated from venous stasis disease by physical examination. In patients with venous disorders, pigmentation and ulceration are prominent; by contrast patients with lymphedema have no pigmentation or ulceration. Swelling of the dorsum of the foot and scaling and redundant skin involving the entire extremity are characteristic of lymphedema and absent in patients with venous disease. Recurrent cellulitis is more common in patients with lymphedema and may become quite troublesome. If the diagnosis still remains in doubt, lymphangiography or lymphoscintigraphy may be used, but they add little to the management of these patients.

Treatment of lymphedema involves elevation and elastic compression stockings. In more severe cases, the Lymphapress, a graded compression device, may be helpful. Medical therapies have not been proven to be effective and diuretics may actually be harmful. In the most incapacitating cases, operative therapy, consisting of resection of large quantities of subcutaneous tissue and skin grafting, has been of benefit.

BIBLIOGRAPHY

DeWeese JA. Vascular surgery. In: Dudley H, Carter DC, eds. *Rob and Smith's operative surgery*, 4th ed. London: Butterworths, 1985.

Fields WS, Lemak NA. Joint study of extracranial arterial occlusion. *JAMA* 1976;235:2734.

Goldman L, Calder DL, Nussbaum SR, et al. Cardiac risk assessment in non-cardiac procedures. *N Engl J Med* 1977;297:846.

Moore W, ed. *Vascular surgery: a comprehensive review.* Philadelphia: WB Saunders, 1993.

North American Symptomatic Carotid Endarterectomy Trial Collaborators. Beneficial effect of carotid endarterectomy in symptomatic patients with high-grade carotid stenosis. *N Engl J Med* 1991;325:445.
Rutherford RB, ed. *Vascular surgery*. Philadelphia: WB Saunders, 1989.
Sanders RJ, Haug C. Subclavian vein obstruction and thoracic outlet syndrome: a review of etiology and management. *Ann Vasc Surg* 1990;4:397.
Szilagyi DE, Smith RF, DeRusso FJ, et al. Contribution of abdominal aortic aneurysmectomy to prolongation of life. *Ann Surg* 1966;164:678.
Symposium on Vascular and Endovascular Surgery: 2001. Massachusetts General Hospital, Boston, May 10–12, 2001.
Wolf PA, Kannel WB, Dawber TR. Prospective investigation: the Framingham Study and the epidemiology of stroke. *Adv Neurol* 1978;19:107.
Young JR, Graor RA, Olin JW, et al., eds. *Peripheral vascular diseases*. St. Louis: Mosby-Year Book, 1991.

CHAPTER 45
Cardiac Arrhythmias

Roy S. Wiener

At rest, the healthy cardiac cell membrane maintains an electrically negative cell interior relative to the extracellular space. During the action potential, the transmembrane voltage becomes depolarized (i.e., the cell interior becomes electrically positive). A phase of gradual repolarization occurs next and is followed by return of the cell to its resting state. Heart cells exhibit refractoriness—in other words, time must elapse for recovery before the next activation can occur. The action potential has two primary functions: it triggers contraction and it mediates intracardiac conduction.

Normally, the sinus node paces the heart. Next, the atria contract, inscribing the P wave on the electrocardiogram (ECG). During the PR interval, conduction to the ventricles occurs slowly through the atrioventricular (AV) node and then rapidly through the His-Purkinje system (HPS). The ventricles contract synchronously, inscribing a narrow QRS complex. The T wave represents the return of the ventricle to its resting electrical state.

One mechanism that produces premature beats and tachycardias is increased automaticity in cells that normally exhibit pacemaker activity. A second cause is triggering; during or after repolarization, repetitive reactivation occurs. The most common etiology is reentry; a cardiac substrate supports circular conduction of activation with transmission out of the circuit to the atria or ventricles or both. If the myocytes are no longer refractory when excitation returns to its starting point, the tachyarrhythmia may become sustained. Bradycardias occur when there is a decrease in the automaticity of pacemaker cells or block in the conduction system.

ETIOLOGY

Arrhythmia may arise in the setting of underlying disease or with no known cause. It may be the most clinically important part of a patient's illness or of secondary importance. Many conditions contribute to the onset or exacerbation of arrhythmias. When evaluating and managing patients, these factors should be systematically explored.

First, one should establish whether there is structural heart disease, such as coronary artery disease, myocardial infarction, cardiomyopathy, valvular dysfunction, or pericarditis. Underlying disease may trigger arrhythmia or amplify its consequences. For example, supraventricular tachycardia is generally well tolerated in a normal heart but frequently causes serious hemodynamic decompensation in the presence of left ventricular dysfunction or coronary artery disease.

Noncardiac precipitants include hypertension, thyroid disease, anemia, infection, fever, hypoxia, pulmonary disease or embolism, sleep apnea, the postoperative state, and changes in autonomic tone. In some women, arrhythmias can begin or worsen with pregnancy, phases of the menstrual cycle, or menopause. Vagal discharge may lead to sinus bradycardia, sinus pauses, and AV block; increased sympathetic tone, anxiety, or emotional stress can precipitate tachycardias. Acid-base derangement and abnormal levels of potassium, magnesium, and calcium should be excluded.

β-Adrenergic agonists, theophylline, and anticholinergic agents cause premature beats and tachycardia, whereas calcium antagonists and β-adrenergic blockers are associated with bradycardias and conduction block. Paradoxically, antiarrhythmic agents may worsen existing arrhythmias or trigger new ones. Diuretics act indirectly by inducing electrolyte abnormalities. Digoxin, at both therapeutic and toxic levels, may cause premature beats, tachycardias, and AV block. One should specifically inquire about nonprescription and illicit drugs, especially cocaine. Drug discontinuation can also be arrhythmogenic, either by removal of a therapeutic effect or by inducing a withdrawal syndrome. This is frequently noted when β-adrenergic blockers are abruptly discontinued. Alcohol, tobacco, and caffeine commonly precipitate ectopy and tachycardias.

HISTORY

Asymptomatic arrhythmias may be found when taking the pulse, examining the heart, or recording an ECG on a patient who is being routinely evaluated. Palpitations, syncope, and lightheadedness suggest arrhythmia; however, these symptoms also have other causes. Chest pain, dyspnea, and fatigue may also occur during rhythm disturbance, but these symptoms are even less specific. Symptom severity may correlate loosely with some arrhythmias; one patient may be distressed by rare premature beats whereas another may be oblivious to frequent ectopy.

Palpitations are not precisely defined, although the term is often used to refer to a sensation that the heartbeat is abnormally strong, fast, slow, or irregular. The patient should be urged to describe her sensations in detail. Premature ventricular contractions (PVCs) may be felt as a flip-flop sensation, as a skipped beat, or as a hyperdynamic postectopic beat. Regular tachycardias are often felt as a steady pounding in the chest, whereas atrial fibrillation is sensed as an irregular heartbeat. Hyperdynamic states characterized as palpitations include normal pregnancy, anxiety, panic disorder, thyrotoxicosis, anemia, and increased sympathetic tone.

Syncope or lightheadedness may occur when either tachycardia or bradycardia induces hypotension that compromises cerebral perfusion. Common etiologies not directly related to arrhythmia include vasodepression, orthostatic hypotension (especially drug related), and aortic stenosis (see Chapter 48). Vertigo may be characterized as a sensation of lightheadedness (see Chapter 104). Seizure is usually of primary neurologic origin, but cortical ischemia secondary to arrhythmia and hypotension may also trigger convulsive activity (see Chapter 105).

Ischemic chest pain may result if the hemodynamic consequences of arrhythmia are severe enough to compromise the balance between myocardial oxygen supply and demand. This is most commonly seen when there is coexisting coronary artery disease, aortic stenosis, or left ventricular hypertrophy. At rapid heart rates, even patients with otherwise normal hearts may experience anginal-type discomfort; other patients note chest pain of uncertain mechanism. Dyspnea may result when arrhythmia induces heart failure and pulmonary congestion. A patient with cardiomyopathy who is well compensated in sinus rhythm may develop fatigue and exercise intolerance when atrial fibrillation supervenes.

Symptoms may be ongoing if the patient presents with a chronic arrhythmia or during a paroxysm. Prompt definitive treatment is needed if abnormal mentation, severe dyspnea, or angina is due to arrhythmia. If the symptoms have remitted, one should document the frequency, duration, and precipitants of the episode, as well as the presence of the triggering factors noted above.

PHYSICAL EXAMINATION

If arrhythmia is present during evaluation, the first priority is to confirm that the vital signs are stable. Once it is established that the patient is not in imminent danger, the examination may provide evidence for associated disease or may suggest the ECG diagnosis. The general appearance may suggest pulmonary disease, a thyroid disorder, or cardiac failure. Hypotension is seen with hypovolemia, pump failure, or medication effects. Resting sinus tachycardia commonly occurs with hyperthyroidism; bradycardia suggests sinus node dysfunction, conduction block, or medication effects. Ectopic beats usually cause skips or weak beats against a background of regularity; a randomly irregular pulse suggests atrial fibrillation. Elevated jugular venous pressure, rales, and peripheral edema raise the issue of heart failure. Irregular cannon *a* waves in the jugular venous waveform suggest AV block or ventricular tachycardia (VT). Cardiac examination may reveal abnormal heart sounds, murmurs, gallops, or rubs indicative of valvular disease, left ventricular failure, or pericarditis. Neurologic examination may reveal abnormal reflexes or muscle weakness suggestive of thyroid disease.

LABORATORY AND IMAGING STUDIES

A 12-lead ECG with a long rhythm strip should be obtained, ideally during arrhythmia. Single-lead monitor strips are often inadequate for determining true QRS duration and defining P waves. During ECG analysis, one needs to identify and focus on the relation between atrial and ventricular activity, irregularity, prematurity, and pauses. Esophageal or intracardiac recording is occasionally necessary for diagnosis. Carotid sinus massage or other vagal stimuli may uncover atrial activity by transiently slowing tachycardias or decreasing AV conduction. Carotid sinus massage is performed with ECG monitoring; it is contraindicated in the presence of a carotid bruit, and caution is advised in the elderly. Drugs may be used for diagnostic purposes; for example, adenosine can transiently decrease AV conduction and uncover flutter waves that are obscured by QRS complexes and T waves. Electrolytes, thyroid function, and drug levels should be checked.

Syncope or hemodynamic instability generally requires inpatient monitoring. Frequent benign symptoms may be evaluated with ambulatory ECG recording; a carefully recorded diary is essential. Occasional episodes may be captured with ECG event recorders. One type is placed on the chest when symptoms start; a continuously acquiring loop monitor is useful for episodes that are very brief or lead rapidly to syncope. Rarely, it is useful to surgically implant a small monitor that can be externally activated to store the ECG.

Echocardiography and exercise testing may be performed to investigate whether structural heart disease is present. Cardiac catheterization may be needed for diagnosis or when percutaneous or surgical intervention is contemplated. An electrophysiologic study (EPS) uses electrode catheters to measure and stimulate intracardiac activity. It is used when arrhythmia has not been documented despite significant symptoms, to evaluate drug efficacy, and to map arrhythmogenic foci in preparation for ablation. EPS is also indicated to determine the need for an implantable cardioverter-defibrillator (ICD) in patients at high risk of sudden death.

TREATMENT

It is optimal to obtain a diagnostic ECG of the arrhythmia before initiating therapy. When possible, the best approach is to remove precipitating factors. Occasional, benign, and mild symptoms are often managed with reassurance and observation. For more frequent and serious arrhythmias, the goals include prevention of recurrence and control of symptoms while improving, or at least not worsening, survival. Caution is necessary, because some drugs have been documented to increase mortality when given to patients with structurally abnormal hearts.

Antiarrhythmic drugs have been grouped by the Vaughan-Williams classification, which categorizes agents on the basis of their predominant electrophysiologic effects. Because the mechanisms of many drugs are complex, this system is imperfect but widely used. Class I agents (sodium channel blockade) are subgrouped by their effect on action potential duration. Class IA drugs (quinidine, procainamide, and disopyramide) treat both supraventricular and ventricular arrhythmias. These drugs are now used infrequently. Class IB drugs (lidocaine, mexiletine, tocainide, and phenytoin) are effective for ventricular arrhythmias; use of these agents is also relatively uncommon. Class IC drugs (flecainide, propafenone, and moricizine) are active against supraventricular and ventricular arrhythmias.

Class II drugs (β-adrenergic receptor blockade) are effective in decreasing the ventricular response in atrial fibrillation and for arrhythmias triggered by increased sympathetic tone or exercise. They can also be used to suppress supraventricular tachycardias and ectopic beats. Long-acting cardioselective agents such as atenolol and metoprolol are often preferred.

Class III drugs (potassium channel blockade and prolongation of refractoriness) may have significant adverse effects. Amiodarone and sotalol are active against both ventricular and atrial arrhythmias. Ibutilide and dofetilide are relatively new agents that are used to treat atrial fibrillation.

Class IV drugs (calcium channel blockade) are used for atrial arrhythmias. Verapamil converts and prevents reentrant supraventricular tachycardia. Diltiazem, both orally and as a continuous infusion, is used to slow the ventricular response in atrial fibrillation and flutter.

Digoxin is used to control the ventricular response in atrial fibrillation. Atropine is a vagolytic used to treat bradycardia and AV block. Adenosine blocks AV node conduction, leading to conversion of reentrant supraventricular tachycardias.

Electrical cardioversion terminates arrhythmias by depolarizing the heart and allowing sinus rhythm to reemerge. It is used emergently for VT and ventricular fibrillation and hemodynamically unstable supraventricular arrhythmias. It is also frequently used for elective conversion of atrial fibrillation and flutter.

Pacemakers are commonly used for bradyarrhythmias and occasionally for treatment of tachycardias. Transcutaneous and temporary transvenous pacemakers are used emergently; permanent leads are attached to subcutaneously implanted generators for long-term therapy. Most patients receive dual-chamber pacemakers that mimic normal cardiac physiology, preventing symptoms caused by loss of normal AV synchrony.

ICDs are frequently used to prevent sudden death from malignant ventricular arrhythmias. They are usually implanted with transvenous lead systems connected to small units that contain both the power source and programmable circuitry. Episodes of VT may be terminated with rapid pacing sequences; if unsuccessful or in the presence of ventricular fibrillation, a shock is delivered. ICDs also provide pacing for bradycardia that occurs spontaneously or after cardioversion.

Radiofrequency current delivered via electrode catheters is used for ablation of accessory pathways, supraventricular tachycardia, and some forms of VT. Surgical methods for control of atrial fibrillation and resection of ventricular arrhythmogenic foci are used occasionally in specialized centers.

SPECIFIC ARRHYTHMIAS

Atrial Arrhythmias

Normal sinus rhythm is defined as rates between 60 and 100 beats/min, with a P wave morphology consistent with sinus origin. Sinus bradycardia (<60 beats/min) is usually benign in otherwise healthy people unless the rate is low enough to cause hypotension or lightheadedness. Sinus tachycardia (>100 beats/min) is generally a response to a physiologic drive such as fever, anemia, exercise, hypovolemia, hypoxia, anxiety, pain, hyperthyroidism, impaired left ventricular function, shock, pheochromocytoma, or drug effect. Identification and treatment of the underlying cause is indicated.

Sinus arrhythmia denotes periodic variations in sinus rate, often related to the respiratory cycle. Atrial rhythm occurs when an ectopic atrial focus, characterized by an abnormal P wave, paces the heart. Wandering atrial pacemaker is similar, with several P wave morphologies appearing. These arrhythmias are generally benign and do not require further investigation or treatment.

Premature atrial contractions (PACs) occur when an atrial focus discharges, usually leading to an early beat with an abnormal P wave morphology and a normal QRS. However, if the HPS is partially refractory at the time that the premature depolarization reaches it, a wide QRS complex resembling a PVC will be inscribed (Fig. 45.1). If the conduction system is completely refractory, conduction to the ventricles will not occur and no QRS will be inscribed. This is a common and benign cause of pauses; thus, an early P wave should be carefully sought when a pause is evaluated. The patient with frequent PACs is at increased risk for supraventricular tachycardias. PACs arise in both normal and diseased hearts; occasionally, they are the presenting manifestation of significant cardiac dysfunction. In the absence of structural heart disease, reassurance is appropriate and treatment is usually not necessary.

Supraventricular Tachycardias

AV nodal reentrant tachycardia (AVNRT) is commonly seen in both structurally normal and diseased hearts. It is regular with rates usually between 120 and 220 beats/min. Atrial activation is retrograde; inverted P waves with a short RP interval may be noted but are often not seen due to superimposition on the QRS complex (Fig. 45.2). Acute episodes may convert spontaneously or with vagal maneuvers; if not, adenosine is the drug of choice. Prevention of recurrent episodes can be attempted with β-adrenergic blockers, verapamil, diltiazem, digoxin, or class IA/IC/III agents. However, radiofrequency catheter ablation is frequently used as a curative procedure that eliminates the need for medication.

AV reentrant tachycardia (AVRT) is common and occurs in the presence of a congenital accessory pathway connecting atrium to ventricle. It usually occurs when a circuit combines antegrade AV node and retrograde bypass tract transmission; preexcitation on the baseline ECG is variably seen. AVRT is regular at 140 to 250 beats/min, and the abnormal P wave is usually seen after the QRS with a relatively long RP interval. Management is as for AVNRT, except that use of digoxin is avoided in the presence of an accessory pathway.

Atrial tachycardia is caused by abnormal automaticity or triggering in an atrial focus with subsequent AV conduction; because the AV node is not part of the arrhythmia mechanism, AV block may occur. The P wave morphology in atrial tachycardia differs from the P wave of sinus rhythm. This arrhythmia is relatively uncommon and is usually seen in the presence of structural heart disease or digoxin toxicity. It is managed with AV blocking agents or primary antiarrhythmic drugs if the underlying causes cannot be controlled. Multifocal atrial tachycardia is a chaotic rhythm with multiple P wave morphologies that often vary from beat to beat; it is usually associated with poorly controlled pulmonary disease and generally resolves as the underlying illness improves.

In atrial fibrillation, atrial electrical activity becomes disorganized and fine or coarse irregularity of the ECG baseline is seen instead of P waves. The AV node is bombarded by an incoming 400 to 600 impulses per minute and conducts to the ventricle at a rate of 140 to 180 beats/min (Fig. 45.3). Slower ventricular responses suggest drug effect or intrinsic conduction system disease. The loss of atrial systole may lead to hemodynamic deterioration of marginally compensated patients. Stasis of blood in the atrium predisposes to thrombus formation and embolic events, especially strokes. Atrial fibrillation frequently occurs in association with underlying disease, but lone (idiopathic) atrial fibrillation is also common. Common noncardiac causes that are amenable to treatment include hyperthyroidism and alcohol use. The prevalence of atrial fibrillation is age dependent; it is relatively uncommon in the young but is present in more than 6% of women older than 80 years.

In both chronic and paroxysmal atrial fibrillation, ventricular rate may be controlled with β-adrenergic or calcium channel blockers and digoxin. If atrial fibrillation has been present for less than 48 hours, cardioversion may be performed. If atrial fibrillation has been present for more than 48 hours, anticoagu-

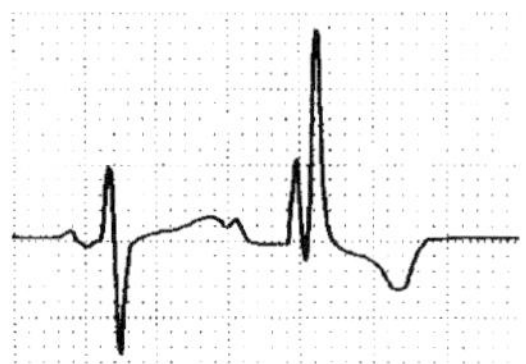

FIG. 45.1. Premature atrial contraction (with aberrant conduction).

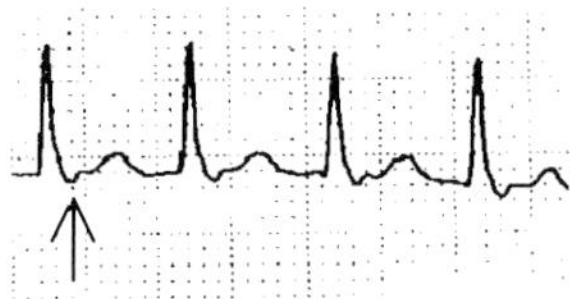

FIG. 45.2. Atrioventricular nodal reentrant tachycardia with retrograde P wave *(arrow)*.

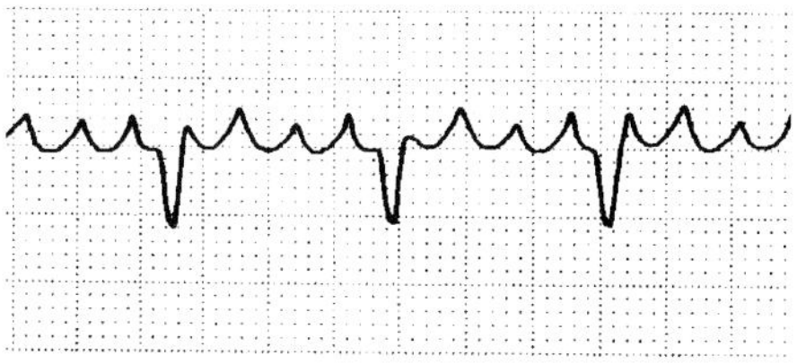

FIG. 45.3. Atrial flutter with 4:1 conduction.

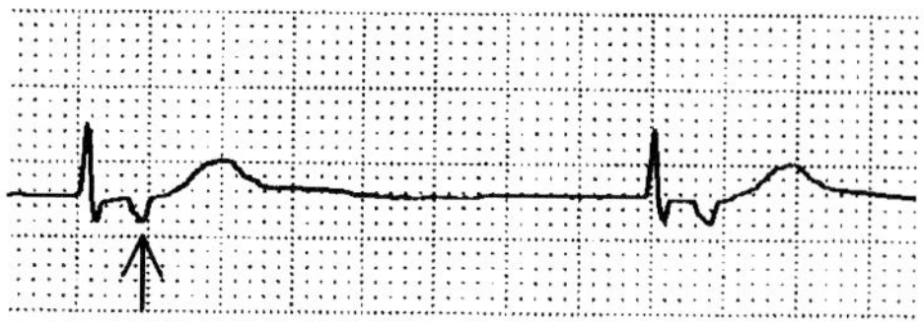

FIG. 45.5. Junctional rhythm with retrograde P wave *(arrow)*.

lation with warfarin to international normalized ratio of 2.0 to 3.0 for 3 weeks before and 4 weeks after the conversion is indicated to decrease the risk of embolic events. Alternatively, if transesophageal echocardiography does not detect intracardiac thrombus, immediate cardioversion followed by 4 weeks of anticoagulation may be performed.

Factors that favor maintenance of sinus rhythm include short duration of atrial fibrillation, absence of marked left atrial dilation, and control of an identified underlying cause. Class IA/IC/III antiarrhythmics have been used to prevent recurrence, but 1-year success rates are at best about 50% and drug toxicity is a significant concern. Recent clinical trials that compared therapy designed toward rate control in atrial fibrillation with strategies to maintain sinus rhythm found similar outcomes for both approaches as measured by incidence of mortality and stroke. Patients with a rapid ventricular response in atrial fibrillation who cannot be successfully managed with medications may undergo permanent pacemaker implantation followed by AV node ablation.

Clinical research has established that when atrial fibrillation occurs in association with risk factors, the incidence of stroke is significantly increased. The Sixth American College of Chest Physicians Consensus Conference on Antithrombotic Therapy developed guidelines that can reduce this risk. History of prior stroke, transient ischemic attack, systemic embolism, hypertension, poor left ventricular function, age more than 75 years, rheumatic mitral valve disease, or prosthetic valve confer a high risk for stroke. Ages 65 to 75 years, diabetes mellitus, and coronary artery disease confer a moderate risk for stroke. Patients who have any high-risk factor or more than one moderate-risk factor should be treated with warfarin. Patients who have one moderate-risk factor may be treated with either warfarin or aspirin. Patients without any risk factors are treated with aspirin.

Atrial flutter occurs when reentry within the atrium cycles at about 250 to 350 beats/min, usually accompanied by 2:1 AV conduction in the absence of medications or conduction abnormalities (Fig. 45.4). It is usually seen in association with structural heart disease and should be suspected when evaluating a regular narrow QRS rhythm at 150 beats/min. Atrial activity classically has a sawtooth pattern in the inferior leads but may resemble a normal P wave in lead V_1. Flutter waves blending into the QRS complex, and ST-T wave are easily missed by the unwary, leading to misdiagnosis as sinus tachycardia, AVNRT, or AVRT. Ventricular rate control, maintenance of sinus rhythm, and anticoagulation issues in atrial flutter are generally handled as in atrial fibrillation.

Junctional Rhythms

Premature junctional contractions arise from the AV node and present as early beats with normal QRS morphology but without a preceding P wave. Treatment and evaluation is as for PACs. AV node cells normally pace at about 45 beats/min, with junctional rhythm emerging as an escape during sinus arrest or AV block (Fig. 45.5). Accelerated junctional rhythms (60–120 beats/min) appear when this focus becomes faster than the sinus rate, usually secondary to structural heart disease or digoxin toxicity; they are usually well tolerated and treatment is directed at underlying cause.

Ventricular Arrhythmias

PVCs arise from a ventricular focus and are characterized by wide QRS beats without a preceding P wave and usually with a subsequent pause (Fig. 45.6). They are commonly seen with and without underlying heart disease. In otherwise normal patients, they do not have prognostic significance and do not require treatment. If PVCs are associated with severely symptomatic palpitations despite reassurance, a trial of β-adrenergic blockers is reasonable. In patients with structural heart disease, an association between frequency and complexity of ventricular ectopy with mortality has been noted. However, pharmacologic attempts at PVC suppression in this setting have demonstrated worsened rather than improved survival.

VT is defined as three or more ventricular beats in a row at a rate from 100 to 250 beats/min; 30 seconds duration is commonly considered the division between nonsustained and sustained VT (Fig. 45.7). VT is usually reentrant and associated with structural heart disease, especially coronary artery disease and cardiomyopathy. Symptoms are sometimes absent but may range from palpitation and brief lightheadedness to syncope and death. When evaluating a wide QRS tachycardia, hemodynamic stability does not exclude the diagnosis of sustained VT. In ventricular fibrillation, ventricular activity is severely disorganized, with the ECG demonstrating fine or coarse irregularity without QRS complexes. Death is immediate without prompt electrical defibrillation.

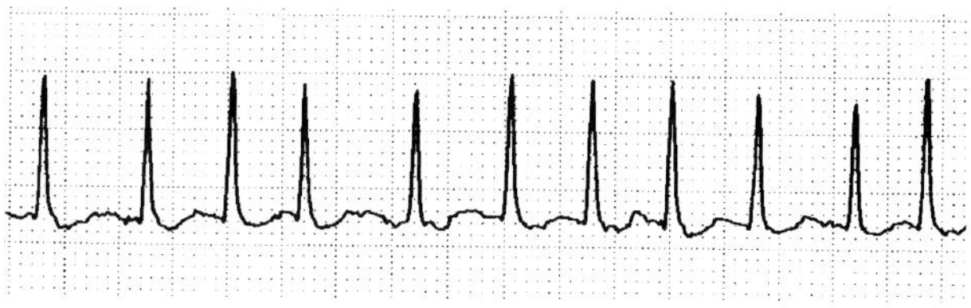

FIG. 45.4. Atrial fibrillation with rapid ventricular response.

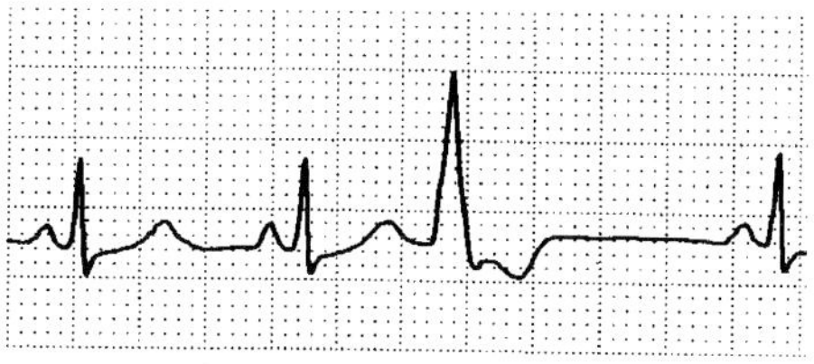

FIG. 45.6. Ventricular premature contraction followed by compensatory pause.

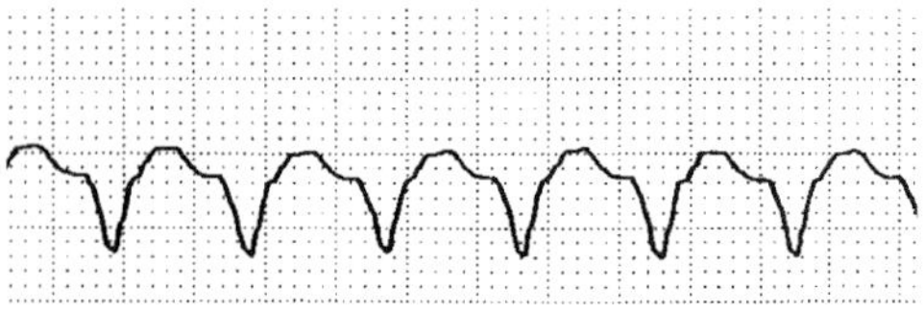

FIG. 45.7. Ventricular tachycardia.

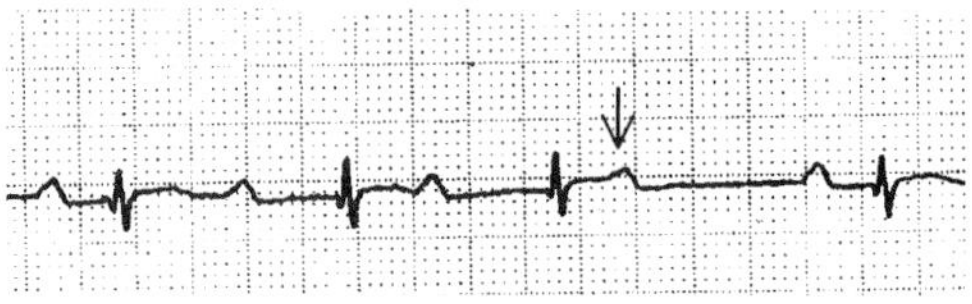

FIG. 45.9. Mobitz I, second-degree, atrioventricular block; blocked P wave superimposed on T wave *(arrow)*.

In the acute setting, sustained VT and ventricular fibrillation are treated with immediate defibrillation. When these arrhythmias occur in the initial phase of acute myocardial infarction, long-term antiarrhythmic drug treatment is not usually required. Otherwise, ICD implantation is appropriate for most patients who survive cardiac arrest or who have sustained VT inducible at EPS. ICDs also improve survival in the setting of coronary artery disease, spontaneous nonsustained VT, impaired systolic function, and sustained VT inducible at EPS. The MADIT II trial suggested that ICDs improve survival in similar patients even in the absence of documented VT. Sotalol and amiodarone are the most commonly used drugs for suppression of serious ventricular arrhythmias.

Idioventricular rhythm (20–40 beats/min) arises from spontaneous pacemaker activity in ventricular cells. A wide QRS bradycardia emerges as an escape rhythm in association with failure of sinus and junctional escape rhythms or HPS block. The patient is usually unstable; a pacemaker is indicated. Accelerated idioventricular rhythm (40–100 beats/min) is a similar rhythm at a faster rate; it is commonly seen during acute myocardial infarction and generally does not require treatment (Fig. 45.8).

Bradycardias

Sinus pauses are noted when the expected P wave fails to appear on time; they may be terminated by return of sinus function or junctional/ventricular escape beats. Severity ranges from short pauses without clinical significance to long periods of asystole associated with syncope. Pacemaker placement is indicated for symptoms or long pauses not due to reversible causes.

AV block is initially characterized by severity. In first-degree AV block, all P waves conduct to the ventricle, but the PR interval is more than 0.2 seconds. In second-degree AV block, some P waves conduct and some are blocked. In third-degree AV block, no P waves conduct and junctional or ventricular escape rhythms emerge. When diagnosing AV block it is important to confirm that the P waves are not premature and fail to conduct because of physiologic refractoriness.

Second-degree AV block has several subtypes. Mobitz I (Wenckebach) is characterized by PR interval lengthening before and shortening after the blocked P wave (Fig. 45.9). Usually, block is at the AV nodal level and responds to atropine, QRS width is normal, and a stable junctional escape focus emerges if third-degree AV block develops. Mobitz II usually demonstrates PR interval constancy before and after the blocked P wave. Block is typically in the HPS, QRS width is usually prolonged, and unreliable, slow, idioventricular rhythms emerge if progression to third-degree AV block occurs (Fig. 45.10).

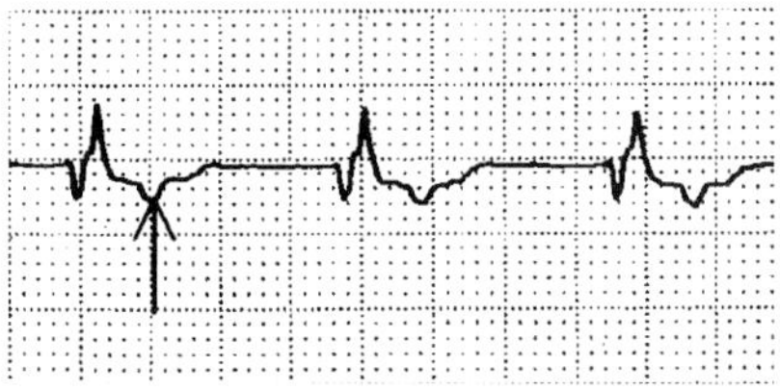

FIG. 45.8. Accelerated idioventricular rhythm with retrograde P waves *(arrow)*.

AV conduction ratios of 2:1 or higher and third-degree AV block may occur with either AV nodal or HPS pathology; the clinical situation and QRS width suggest the site of the lesion. AV nodal block is generally better tolerated due to presence of junctional escape rhythms.

Etiologies of AV block include myocardial infarction (inferior, Mobitz I; anterior, Mobitz II), cardiomyopathy, calcification or fibrosis of the conduction system, and medications. A pacemaker is indicated if symptoms occur or if HPS pathology is likely.

ARRHYTHMIA SYNDROMES

Sick sinus or bradycardia-tachycardia syndrome, usually seen in the elderly, is characterized by bradycardia and pauses, often in association with episodes of atrial tachyarrhythmia (Fig. 45.11). AV nodal and ventricular escape mechanisms may also be abnormal. Pacing and antiarrhythmic drugs therapy are often necessary. In carotid sinus hypersensitivity, stimulation of the carotid baroreceptor is followed by an exaggerated vagal response characterized by bradycardia or vasodepression. A dual-chamber pacemaker is usually effective in preventing recurrent symptoms.

Wolff-Parkinson-White syndrome is associated with arrhythmias due to the presence of a congenital accessory bypass tract that connects atrium and ventricle. Antegrade conduction through the bypass tract inscribes a delta wave on the ECG, indicating preexcitation of the ventricle and creating a short PR interval/lengthened QRS duration. Orthodromic reciprocating tachycardia (AVRT; see above) occurs when a circuit is formed antegrade through the AV node and retrograde through the bypass tract. Occasionally, the reentry goes antegrade through the bypass tract and retrograde up the AV node (antidromic reciprocating tachycardia), inscribing a wide preexcited QRS complex. Atrial fibrillation in association with an accessory pathway that conducts antegrade with a short refractory period can lead to rapid ventricular rates that degenerate into ventricular fibrillation and death. Patients who experience tachycardias associated with Wolff-Parkinson-White syndrome

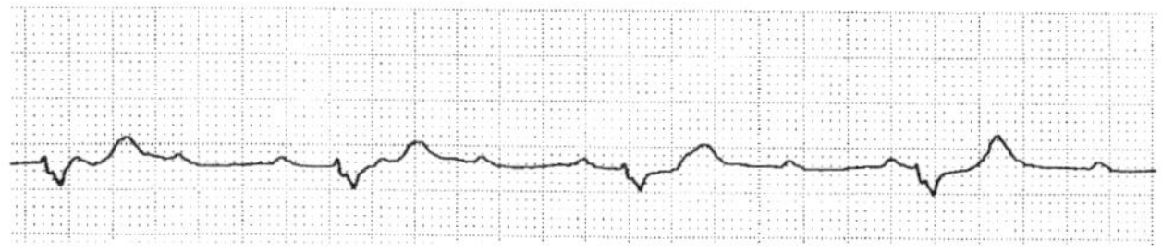

FIG. 45.10. Sinus tachycardia with third-degree atrioventricular block.

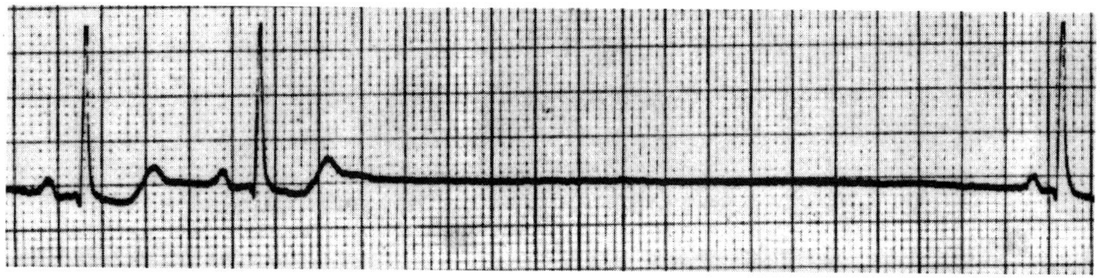

FIG. 45.11. Sinus pause characteristic of sick sinus syndrome.

are best managed with radiofrequency ablation, thus avoiding the inconvenience and side effects of antiarrhythmic drugs.

Wide QRS tachycardia may be due to either VT or supraventricular tachycardia with bundle branch block/aberrant conduction. Evidence of AV dissociation or a previous history of myocardial infarction favors the diagnosis of VT. If the QRS morphologies during the tachycardia and in sinus rhythm are completely or nearly identical, a supraventricular origin is more likely. Guidelines based on 12-lead ECG patterns are also helpful in differentiating between the two possibilities.

Long QT interval syndrome may be congenital or secondary to drugs, electrolyte abnormalities, severe bradycardia, and abnormal nutritional states. When the QT interval is prolonged, the patient is at significant risk of developing torsades de pointes, a polymorphous VT with QRS complexes that fluctuate in size and direction in an oscillating pattern (Fig. 45.12). This arrhythmia often causes syncope or death. Causal antiarrhythmic drugs include class IA/C agents, sotalol, ibutilide, dofetilide, and amiodarone. Other drugs that have been implicated include chlorpromazine, thioridazine, tricyclic antidepressants, erythromycin, pentamidine, and trimethoprim/sulfamethoxazole. Hypomagnesemia, hypocalcemia, and hypokalemia can trigger torsades de pointes; these electrolyte disturbances may be the etiology in cases associated with liquid protein diets and anorexia nervosa. Bradyarrhythmias trigger torsades de pointes by inducing rate related QT prolongation. Treatments include discontinuation of the inciting drug, correction of electrolyte abnormalities, magnesium sulfate, and pacing.

Mitral valve prolapse is often associated with palpitations; these are usually benign. However, occasionally significant arrhythmias requiring evaluation and treatment occur.

Bundle branch block occurs when conduction through these segments of the HPS fails. A characteristic pattern of QRS complex prolongation occurs. Left bundle branch block is usually associated with and may be the presenting manifestation of significant underlying structural heart disease. Right bundle branch block may occur with or without associated cardiac disease; extensive investigation is not required if the clinical evaluation is benign. Progression to AV block requiring pacing occurs in a small percentage of patients with bundle branch block.

CONSIDERATIONS IN PREGNANCY

In pregnancy, cardiac output, blood volume, and heart rate increase, blood pressure falls; and the hormonal milieu changes. Positional compression of the inferior vena cava and abdominal aorta can induce sudden changes in central blood volume. These factors may trigger exacerbation of previously experienced arrhythmias or onset of new ones.

Pharmacologic treatment is avoided whenever possible, especially in the first trimester, because controlled trials measuring adverse fetal effects are not generally available. Drug levels and effects may vary due to changes in intravascular volume, plasma protein binding, metabolism, and absorption. When predicted efficacy is similar, it is best to use older drugs that have been found to be safe over longer periods of experience. Most antiarrhythmic drugs, except amiodarone, appear to be safe for breast-feeding of infants.

Cardioversion and pacing have been used during pregnancy without untoward effects to mother or fetus. In late pregnancy, efficacy of cardiopulmonary resuscitation may be improved by tilting the patient toward her left side, thus decreasing vascular compression from the uterus. If it appears that resuscitation will be unsuccessful and the fetus is of viable age, cesarean section should be initiated within 15 minutes of arrest.

Mild sinus tachycardia is normally seen during pregnancy. Premature atrial and ventricular contractions are frequently detected and generally do not require further evaluation or treatment. Some women have first onset of supraventricular tachycardia in pregnancy; those with a prior history, especially in the setting of Wolff-Parkinson-White syndrome, commonly experience increased frequency and severity of episodes. Rare patients develop continuous automatic atrial tachycardia that resolves after delivery. Episodes of AVNRT/AVRT are approached with vagal maneuvers. First-line drug therapy is adenosine, which is safe, effective, and rapidly metabolized. If recurrent episodes are sufficiently frequent or severe, digoxin (AVNRT only), β-adrenergic blockers, verapamil, quinidine, and procainamide have been used safely and effectively. Digoxin is the first choice for ventricular rate control in atrial fibrillation. Other options are cardioselective β-adrenergic blockers, verapamil, or diltiazem. Heparin is the preferred

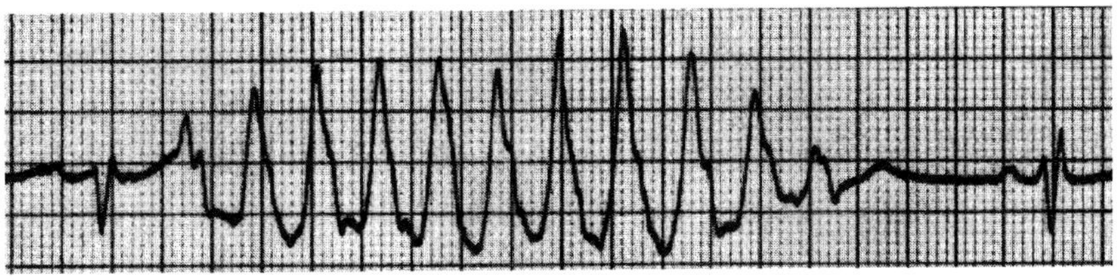

FIG. 45.12. Torsades de pointes.

method of anticoagulation due to the teratogenicity of warfarin.

VT during pregnancy is rare; initially, the presence or absence of associated cardiac disease should be established. Sustained episodes may be treated with intravenous lidocaine or procainamide. Patients with structurally normal hearts and episodic VT usually respond to β-adrenergic blockers. When identifiable cardiac pathology is present, treatment proceeds as in the nongravid state. Type IA agents are usually tried first; second-line agents are sotalol and propafenone. Amiodarone is avoided in pregnancy unless necessary.

Bradycardias are uncommon during pregnancy. Occasionally, congenital third-degree AV block is encountered; these patients may require temporary or permanent pacing.

BIBLIOGRAPHY

Albers GW, Dalen JE, Laupacis A, et al. Antithrombotic therapy in atrial fibrillation. *Chest* 2001;119:194S–206S.

Elkayam U, Gleicher N, eds. *Cardiac problems in pregnancy: diagnosis and management of maternal and fetal disease,* 3rd ed. New York: Wiley-Liss, 1998.

Fuster V, Rydén LE, Asinger RW, et al. ACC/AHA/ESC guidelines for the management of patients with atrial fibrillation: executive summary. *J Am Coll Cardiol* 2001;38:1231–1265.

Kusumoto FM, Goldschlager N. Device therapy for cardiac arrhythmias. *JAMA* 2002;287:1848–1852.

Prystowsky EN, Klein GJ. *Cardiac arrhythmias: an integrated approach for the clinician.* New York: McGraw-Hill, 1994.

CHAPTER 46
Cardiac Murmurs

Laura J. von Doenhoff

The finding of a heart murmur on physical examination in a patient not known to have cardiac disease may generate anxiety in the patient and prompt consternation in the physician. Today's informed patient may press for detailed information about the implications of the heart murmur. Her dentist, knowing that a murmur exists, may insist on guidance regarding periprocedural antibiotic prophylaxis. Furthermore, the recent availability of high-quality echocardiography has resulted in additional pressure on the physician to characterize and diagnose the murmur definitively. Most contemporary physicians practice in a litigious climate. There is no single approach to this clinical problem. The strategy for workup is governed by the characteristics of the murmur and other individual factors, including the patient's age, overall health, symptoms, and level of anxiety.

This chapter gives a practical approach to the evaluation and management of heart murmurs. This is intended to be a guide for primary care clinicians in the outpatient setting and not a detailed discussion of valvular or congenital heart disease. The technique of auscultation is briefly described; various murmurs are then discussed in approximate order of prevalence.

PHYSICAL EXAMINATION: A BRIEF GUIDE TO THE TECHNIQUE OF AUSCULTATION

The patient should be placed comfortably in the supine position with the head of the bed elevated to about 30 or 45 degrees. The precordium should be palpated with the entire palm to locate the left ventricular impulse and to feel for any thrills (vibrations accompanying a murmur). The patient should then assume the left decubitus position; the left ventricular impulse again should be located and palpated. In this position, the bell of the stethoscope should be lightly placed over the left ventricular impulse and the deep-pitched apical sounds appreciated. These include the first heart sound (S_1), any third heart sound (S_3), the fourth heart sound (S_4), and any mitral diastolic rumble. Auscultation should proceed with the diaphragm of the stethoscope held to the left ventricular impulse, listening for higher pitched sounds at the apex, such as systolic murmurs. With the patient supine again, auscultation with the diaphragm should proceed from the apex, inching upward toward the base of the heart. One should listen not only in the traditional tricuspid, pulmonic, and aortic areas but also over the sternum and clavicles, because bony structures transmit high-pitched sounds well. At the base of the heart, attention should be paid to the second heart sound and to higher pitched murmurs (e.g., aortic stenosis [AS] or aortic sclerosis, mitral regurgitation [MR], pericardial rubs). Ultimately, the patient should sit up, leaning forward, as the examiner listens with the diaphragm for the high-pitched sounds of rubs and aortic regurgitant murmurs. It may be necessary for the patient to hold expiration. Finally, the patient should stand to allow for characterization of the murmurs of mitral valve prolapse (MVP) and hypertrophic obstructive cardiomyopathy and (in some patients) to obtain full closure of the second heart sound.

Murmurs have been historically classified as grade 1 (barely audible), grade 2 (faint), grade 3 (moderately loud), grade 4 (accompanied by a thrill), grade 5 (audible with the stethoscope held partly off the chest), and grade 6 (audible with the stethoscope held entirely off the chest). The patient's body habitus greatly affects the transmission of heart sounds to the chest wall surface. Obesity, increased anteroposterior chest dimension, hyperinflated lungs, and pulmonary adventitious sounds impede cardiac auscultation.

CLINICAL FINDINGS

Systolic Murmurs

FLOW MURMURS (EJECTION MURMURS, INNOCENT MURMURS)

This broad category comprises systolic murmurs heard in the absence of any identifiable disease and connotes a benign process. There is no meaningful distinction between flow, ejection, and innocent murmurs. It is not always possible to pinpoint the valvular etiology of these murmurs, even by echocardiography; rarely, if ever, is it necessary to do so. These murmurs often are described as either aortic flow murmurs or pulmonic flow murmurs, depending on the location. They relate to the volume of blood flow, or turbulence, or both.

No symptoms are referable to flow murmurs. Benign systolic murmurs can occur in the setting of hyperdynamic or high-output physiology such as anemia, fever, anxiety, hypertension, and exertion. They also are associated with the increased stroke volume that occurs with pregnancy, obesity, athletic conditioning, and bradycardia.

On auscultation they are systolic, characteristically "crescendo-decrescendo" or "diamond shaped" in their volume profile, relatively low pitched, sometimes musical, often faint (grade 1, 2, or 3, depending on the hemodynamic conditions), and sometimes evanescent. It is typical for the murmur to come and go with serial examinations, depending on the patient's hemodynamic state, and this evanescence may be a tip-off that the murmur is a flow murmur. (On the other hand, the mitral regurgitant murmur associated with MVP also may vary, but usually more clearly with position rather than with hemodynamic state.) The murmur may be most prominent at the upper or lower left sternal border or at the apex. Flow murmurs are common in the young (35 years of age or younger) patient.

Cardiorespiratory (cardiopulmonary) murmurs are soft systolic murmurs that are evident only during inspiration and disappear in expiration or when the breath is held. These murmurs may be of somewhat higher pitch and thus may resemble regurgitant murmurs, except for their phasic nature. They are benign.

If the examiner is confident that the murmur fits these descriptions, then no further workup and no treatment is necessary. Serial auscultation is helpful in confirming the murmur's characteristics and sometimes in establishing its evanescent nature. If an echocardiogram were ordered, results would be benign; it might show an increased stroke volume and (in obese, pregnant, or athletic patients) increased chamber sizes. No valvular disease would be manifest. This point of view concurs with recent work done on outpatients, predominantly women, which suggests that healthy young women (up to 35 years of age) with soft systolic murmurs (up to grade 2) rarely have significant valvular abnormalities on echocardiogram.

AORTIC SCLEROSIS

Aortic sclerosis refers to the deposition of calcium, visible on echocardiogram, on an otherwise normal, mobile, tricuspid aortic valve. Calcification typically begins in the seventh or eighth decade; it occurs earlier in patients with hypertension, abnormal calcium metabolism, and other conditions. No symptoms are referable to it. It reflects a hemodynamically insignificant degree of AS.

The murmur is systolic and crescendo-decrescendo but often somewhat harsher and louder (grade 2 or 3) than the previously described flow murmur. It may have a musical quality, but unlike hemodynamically significant AS, high-frequency components are not predominant. The murmur peaks in early to midsystole. The second heart sound is not obscured. It may be best heard at the base of the heart (over the sternum or at the left sternal border). Typically, it is a constant rather than an evanescent finding. The auscultatory findings in some patients may be hard to differentiate from greater degrees of AS and from MR. In such patients, echocardiography can be helpful. Management depends on the results of the echocardiogram.

In the past, aortic sclerosis was thought to be a benign indolent condition. More recent reviews suggest that it may be a marker of generalized atherosclerotic cardiovascular disease. It is now evident that the risk factors for development of aortic valvular sclerosis resemble the risk factors for atherosclerotic vascular disease: age, hypertension, dyslipidemia, smoking, renal disease, and inflammation. Moreover, it is now known that the process in the aortic valve, like the vascular process, is a dynamic one. Aortic valvular calcium accumulates at variable, but sometimes rapid, rates. Whether the process can be slowed, arrested, or reversed is a topic of great current interest.

AORTIC STENOSIS

By the eighth and ninth decades of life, calcification of a previously relatively normal aortic valve in a woman may have progressed to a hemodynamically significant lesion. The rate of progression is variable, probably depending on the above risk factors and individual characteristics.

Hemodynamically significant AS may also occur in noncalcified valves. In approximately 2% of the population the aortic valve is bicuspid or otherwise dysplastic. These patients are more often male than female. The pathognomonic clinical sign of a bicuspid aortic valve is an early systolic ejection click, which corresponds to the "doming" of a pliable valve.

The noncalcified, bicuspid, or dysplastic valve may or may not be significantly stenotic early in life. These valves calcify more quickly than do structurally normal tricuspid aortic valves; by midlife, the valves that were not already stenotic may become so. As the bicuspid aortic valve calcifies and stiffens, the click may disappear.

AS that is moderate may cause few, if any, symptoms. AS that is severe may cause dyspnea or lightheadedness on exertion. The classic triad of angina, syncope, and congestive heart failure occurs late in the disease process. Patients with severe AS may have no cardiac symptoms, especially if their activities are limited for other reasons. The electrocardiogram and the chest roentgenogram may show cardiac enlargement.

On auscultation, the systolic murmur of AS is best heard at the base, that is, over the sternum, over the right clavicle, at the upper right sternal border (the aortic area), or along the left sternal border. It is typically harsh and wheezy or grinding but can be musical. Both high- and low-frequency audio components are present. The timing of the peak of the murmur may help to differentiate mild to moderate AS (early to midsystolic peak) from severe AS (late systolic peak, occasionally obscuring the second heart sound). The milder the stenosis, the more the situation resembles the previously discussed aortic sclerosis.

The murmur of AS commonly radiates to the carotid arteries, especially the right carotid, and can be confused with an arterial (carotid or subclavian) bruit. A bruit should be loudest over the affected artery and almost inaudible at the base of the heart. When a diastolic murmur (that of aortic regurgitation [AR]) is also heard, this finding may help localize the systolic murmur to the aortic valve.

The finding of a murmur suggestive of AS warrants echocardiography. In most cases, the aortic valve area, gradient, and other indicators of severity, as well as an estimate of left ventricular function, are available from the echocardiogram. Patient management depends on the results of the echocardiogram and may involve cardiology referral. Periprocedural antibiotic prophylaxis is in order if the aortic valve is thought to be bicuspid. Recommendations are less firm for calcified tricuspid valves and less firm when there is uncertainty about whether the valve is bicuspid or tricuspid.

Rarely, the stenosis is subaortic rather than valvular and is due to a congenital fibrous subaortic "collar" or membrane. This is known as discrete subaortic stenosis. In childhood, this can be a serious progressive lesion requiring surgical resection; when it presents in adulthood, it is typically milder and more slowly, if at all, progressive. The systolic murmur may be indistinguishable from that of valvular AS. The subaortic jet can deform the aortic cusps, causing AR. Echocardiography can fully characterize this lesion, which warrants periprocedural antibiotic prophylaxis for the indicated procedures and perhaps cardiology referral.

MITRAL VALVE PROLAPSE

MVP, also known as Barlow syndrome and the click-murmur syndrome, most often is suspected in young female patients. Traditional estimates of its incidence in the general population range from 5% to 15%; a more current estimate, using a strict echocardiographic definition, is 1.3%. It is an autosomal-dominant congenital trait. It is equally common in men and women, but women may be more symptomatic from it. A history of palpitations, atypical chest pain, cold hands and feet, migraine headaches, other neurologic phenomena, or panic attacks may prompt a search for MVP. On the other hand, many patients are asymptomatic and are found to have a click or characteristic murmur on physical examination.

The pathologic mechanism in classic cases involves elongation, redundancy, and thickening of the mitral leaflets related to myxomatous degeneration. In systole the leaflets billow, resulting in the characteristic click. Overclosure or faulty coaptation of the leaflets in systole results in regurgitation into the left atrium.

Much has been made of the tall, thin, asthenic habitus associated with this lesion, but in everyday practice MVP can be found in a variety of body types. It is notably prevalent in patients with a marked pectus excavatum. Typically, the electrocardiogram and chest roentgenogram are normal when the lesion is not hemodynamically significant.

The classic auscultatory findings are a systolic click (literally a high-pitched clicking, "clucking," or snapping sound) followed by an apical regurgitant murmur crescendoing toward the second heart sound. Classically, the click moves earlier in systole and the murmur becomes longer when the patient stands up, because with that maneuver the left ventricular chamber becomes smaller and the disproportion between the small left ventricular chamber and redundant mitral valve increases. In everyday practice, things are less classic. Patients shown by echocardiography to have MVP with significant MR may have no murmur, even when the body habitus is slender. The murmur may be present but, for some reason, is more outflow (diamond shaped and deep pitched) than regurgitant (higher pitched, narrow in frequency range, "whooshy," crescendo or holosystolic, occasionally musical) in character. A coexisting aortic systolic murmur may mask the regurgitant murmur. When the MR is marked, the murmur may be harsh enough to mimic aortic sclerosis or stenosis. The click may be absent.

The presence of a click or multiple clicks, with or without a murmur, indicates a high likelihood of MVP. Other possibilities include that the click is tricuspid in origin (indicating tricuspid valve prolapse) or aortic in origin (the click may be an aortic ejection sound accompanying a bicuspid aortic valve). The latter sound classically occurs earlier in systole than a mitral click and may be associated with the diastolic blow of AR. It is also important not to mistake the sequence of S_4–S_1 for the sequence of S_1–click. This commonly happens in hypertensive patients whose S_4 can be loud. The fourth and first heart sounds are deep pitched; the click is high pitched. A split S_1 also can mimic the S_1–click sequence. Again, both the mitral and tricuspid components of the split S_1 are deep pitched.

As the regurgitation associated with MVP progresses, the murmur becomes more prominent and assumes an increasingly classic regurgitant character (either crescendo or holosystolic in nature). The click may become relatively less prominent.

Three questions typically arise when MVP is suspected:

1. *Is MVP present?* The finding of a distinctly mitral click, sometimes followed by a regurgitant murmur, is the most powerful clinical indicator of MVP. More often, however, the findings are less clear-cut, and echocardiography is needed to answer this question. Establishing a diagnosis of MVP may provide an etiology for the patient's chest pain, palpitations, and other symptoms. Refuting the diagnosis of MVP may allow discontinuation of periprocedural antibiotics currently taken by the patient.

2. *Does it require periprocedural antibiotic prophylaxis against infective endocarditis?* Recent work suggests that the greatest risk of endocarditis occurs in those MVP patients whose mitral leaflets are thickened to 5 mm or more, as measured on the echocardiogram. These patients should as a rule receive antibiotic prophylaxis. Other patients, some with a distinct click, may have normal or minimally increased leaflet thickness. The latter group should be labeled as having "nonclassic" or "normal-variant" prolapse and in the absence of other compelling findings should not receive antibiotic prophylaxis.

Other factors conferring risk of infective endocarditis after a procedure such as dental cleaning include male gender, age 45 or greater, and the presence of mild or greater MR. These factors can color the decision regarding prophylaxis. It should be noted that the overall risk of endocarditis in MVP, as compared with the risk in other congenital heart conditions, is low.

3. *Is the MR hemodynamically significant?* The clinical examination can underestimate the severity of the regurgitation accompanying MVP. Patients with only a click and no murmur can sometimes be found on the echocardiogram to have mild, moderate, or, rarely, even severe MR. Patients with an unimpressive regurgitant murmur can sometimes be found on the echocardiogram to have severe MR, cardiac chamber enlargement, and depressed ventricular function. Many patients with significant MR are surprisingly asymptomatic, which is to say that they are unaware of any exertional dyspnea or palpitations.

Thus, whenever MVP is suspected clinically, careful echocardiography is warranted. Patient management depends on the results of the echocardiogram and may involve cardiology referral.

MVP receives attention as a syndrome affecting the young, but as a congenital condition, it is lifelong and equally prevalent in the elderly. As noted, the click may become less prominent with age, possibly because of progressive calcification of the mitral apparatus restricting leaflet motion. The regurgitant murmur may coexist with or may be masked by the murmur of aortic sclerosis, but the need to offer antibiotic prophylaxis only increases with age. As the patient ages, the auscultatory findings may be harder to sort out and the echocardiogram may have increasing usefulness.

HYPERTROPHIC CARDIOMYOPATHY

Hypertrophic cardiomyopathy with or without obstruction (the former previously known as idiopathic hypertrophic subaortic stenosis) originally was described in young patients with rare severe familial disease. Currently we have come to understand its greater prevalence as a mild familial disease and as an acquired disease. The latter is characteristically associated with hypertensive patients, often elderly women with small hyperdynamic left ventricles. Exertional dyspnea may be present, especially if there is tachycardia. The electrocardiogram and chest roentgenogram may show left ventricular hypertrophy.

When a murmur is present it suggests dynamic subaortic obstruction. This obstruction, which can be shown on echocardiogram as a subvalvular pressure gradient, is variable with hemodynamic factors such as heart rate, hydration, and blood pressure. If there is a high degree of obstruction at rest (common when there is tachycardia or dehydration), then the systolic murmur may be harsh and on occasion indistinguishable from the murmur of valvular AS. If the patient is elderly, then calcification of the aortic valve and cardiac skeleton is likely and the murmur of aortic sclerosis (or even significant AS) will be superimposed, confounding the picture.

When lesser degrees of this dynamic subaortic obstruction are present and when significant aortic valvular calcification is absent, diagnosis is facilitated by taking advantage of the change in hemodynamics that occurs with position. That is, the left ventricle becomes smaller when the patient stands. The murmur, which may be soft and "whooshy" with the patient seated (and either holosystolic or late systolic or, perhaps, diamond shaped), becomes more prominent when the patient stands. If late systolic at rest, it may become holosystolic. This is in contrast to the behavior of valvular AS but similar to the behavior of the classic murmur of MVP. The latter condition may be indistinguishable from hypertrophic cardiomyopathy on physical examination.

Echocardiography is warranted when hypertrophic cardiomyopathy is suspected. Patient management depends on the results of the echocardiogram and may involve cardiology referral. Hypertrophic cardiomyopathy with obstruction requires antibiotic prophylaxis.

PAPILLARY MUSCLE DYSFUNCTION

Women who sustain a myocardial infarction, particularly one involving the inferior wall and inferoseptal papillary muscle, may develop MR as a result of dysfunction of the papillary muscle apparatus necessary for the active closure of the mitral valve. Failure of the myocardial wall to contract in and around the papillary muscle can result in incomplete leaflet coaptation and leakage. Acute ischemia without infarction can give the same result, causing transient MR that resolves after resolution of the ischemia. The clinical history, electrocardiogram, and echocardiogram as a whole would paint the picture of ischemia or infarction. The murmur is systolic and regurgitant in character. Most believe that it does not warrant periprocedural antibiotic prophylaxis.

PULMONIC STENOSIS

Hemodynamically significant valvular pulmonic stenosis is a congenital lesion that is usually corrected or ameliorated in childhood. Mild degrees of it often persist after surgical or balloon procedures into adulthood. In other cases, the congenital lesion is mild from birth, and unsuspected.

In mild pulmonic stenosis, the patient is typically asymptomatic. The electrocardiogram and chest roentgenogram may be normal. More severe degrees of pulmonic stenosis may give rise to exertional dyspnea, and the electrocardiogram and chest roentgenogram may show right ventricular hypertrophy or enlargement.

The systolic murmur is likely to be most prominent at the upper left sternal border (the pulmonic area). It is outflow in character, sometimes coarse, and often grade 3 or 4. As with most right-sided cardiac sounds, it increases on inspiration. It may be associated with a pulmonic ejection sound, which is an early systolic click caused by the doming of a pliable valve. (Paradoxically, the pulmonic ejection sound decreases on inspiration.) There may be an associated diastolic murmur, that of pulmonic regurgitation, particularly in patients who have undergone procedures to lessen the pulmonic stenosis; this is also most prominent at the upper left sternal border. There may be a left parasternal lift when significant right heart enlargement is present.

Pulmonic stenosis and regurgitation do not require periprocedural antibiotic prophylaxis. Lesions confined to the right side of the heart, which functions at pressures much lower than the left side of the heart, typically do not require prophylaxis.

VENTRICULAR SEPTAL DEFECT

Most congenital hemodynamically significant defects in the interventricular septum are corrected in childhood. Many smaller defects close spontaneously in infancy. Those that persist into adulthood are typically perimembranous and hemodynamically insignificant, but they require vigilant periprocedural antibiotic prophylaxis. A ventricular septal defect is among the lesions at highest risk of infection during bacteremic procedures.

Ventricular septal defect is rarely a cause of a systolic murmur in an adult. Typically, the patient is asymptomatic. The electrocardiogram and chest roentgenogram may be completely normal. The murmur is prominent (often grade 3 or 4) and will have drawn attention throughout the patient's life. It is holosystolic, regurgitant, and loud. The smaller the actual defect, the higher the velocities (seen by Doppler echocardiography) across it, and the harsher the murmur.

Echocardiography is warranted if ventricular septal defect is suspected. When ordering the test, it is crucial to specify what is being sought, because the routine echocardiographic examination may not include a thorough search for a ventricular septal defect.

Diastolic Murmurs

AORTIC REGURGITATION

The most common cause of a diastolic murmur is AR. This may be the result of an anatomic abnormality of the aortic valve itself, as when the valve is bicuspid or otherwise dysplastic, redundant, calcified, or affected by rheumatic disease. It can also result from enlargement of the aortic root; this occurs in hypertension, myxomatous degeneration, and rarely in syphilis.

Mild degrees of AR typically cause no symptoms. Patients with more marked regurgitation, or with uncontrolled hypertension, may report exertional dyspnea. The electrocardiogram and chest roentgenogram results are normal in mild degrees and may show left ventricular enlargement when the AR is substantial. Marked aortic root enlargement can be seen on the chest roentgenogram.

The diastolic murmur of AR is easy to overlook on physical examination. As mentioned earlier, it is best heard over or alongside the sternum as the patient sits up, leaning forward, during expiration. Its intensity and length generally vary with the severity of the regurgitation. What shows on echocardiogram as trace or mild AR usually is inaudible, even on careful listening. More severe degrees of AR are likely to be audible, depending on the body habitus. Severity generally correlates with pulse pressure (the difference between systolic and diastolic blood pressure).

The murmur is a blow that begins immediately after the second heart sound and that usually has a tambour quality. On occasion, a tambour quality of the second heart sound itself may be the only tip-off to the presence of AR. The blow is decrescendo and high pitched and may occupy any length of diastole. When the aortic root is substantially enlarged, the blow may be loudest to the right of the sternum.

Significant degrees of AR usually are accompanied by a forward systolic aortic flow murmur, even in the absence of significant AS. On the other hand, hemodynamically significant AS commonly coexists with AR. The murmur of AR can be confused with an unusually loud murmur of pulmonic regurgitation, with the murmur of patent ductus arteriosus (PDA), and occasionally with a multicomponent pericardial rub.

Echocardiography is warranted when AR is suspected or when any clearly diastolic murmur is heard. It can delineate the severity of the AR and provide measurements of the aortic root and left ventricle. Patient management depends on the results of the echocardiogram and may involve cardiology referral.

Periprocedural antibiotic prophylaxis may not be necessary when the AR is due to aortic root enlargement or valve sclerosis, when the valve itself is minimally abnormal. Bicuspid aortic valves, on the other hand, are at high risk of infection during bacteremic procedures and warrant prophylaxis.

MITRAL STENOSIS

Now much less common than in the preantibiotic era but still prevalent in some geographic areas, rheumatic mitral stenosis (MS) is suspected clinically much more often than it is found on echocardiogram. In many patients labeled as having it on the basis of a history of a febrile childhood illness, the diagnosis can be refuted by echocardiography. The typical patient with true MS is an older woman with few symptoms or, in more severe disease, exertional dyspnea and general fatigue.

The auscultatory findings are easy to misinterpret, in part because they are infrequently encountered by the clinician. Making the diagnosis requires careful listening at the cardiac apex and at the left sternal border, with the patient lying on her left side. The most striking finding is usually the accentuated first heart sound. This can be considered the focal point for the entire cadence of MS, which consists of presystolic accentuation, loud S_1, S_2, prominent opening snap, and deep-pitched diastolic rumble. Familiarity with the entire cadence and listening for it as a whole help to establish the diagnosis. The systolic murmur of MR, occurring between S_1 and S_2, often accompanies the findings. As the mitral valve calcifies with age and the stenosis progresses, the auscultatory findings may become more difficult to appreciate.

Echocardiography is warranted whenever MS is suspected and whenever a past diagnosis of it was made on clinical grounds alone. Patient management depends on the results of the echocardiogram and may involve cardiology referral.

Rarely, MS is congenital rather than rheumatic. In the postantibiotic era, the incidence of congenital MS relative to rheumatic MS has increased, especially in young patients. The implication, however, is the same. Echocardiography, which can differentiate the congenital from the rheumatic etiology, is warranted. MS requires periprocedural antibiotic prophylaxis. Rheumatic MS in young patients also requires nonprocedural, daily, antibiotic prophylaxis to prevent disease recurrence.

Abnormal Second Heart Sound

ATRIAL SEPTAL DEFECT

Failure of the interatrial septum to close during embryonic development can result in a variety of anatomic malformations. Ostium primum defects are often associated with other intracardiac problems and are typically identified and corrected in childhood. Ostium secundum defects may be large and identified early or relatively small and undetected until adulthood.

Symptoms of ostium secundum defects may be minimal. The patient may notice exertional dyspnea or palpitations. The chest roentgenogram typically shows right heart enlargement and increased pulmonary vascularity. The electrocardiogram usually shows right bundle branch block and right axis deviation. Atrial arrhythmias may be present. In fact, any patient with right bundle branch block and atrial arrhythmias should be suspected of having atrial septal defect (ASD).

On physical examination, there may be a right ventricular lift at the lower left sternal border. A systolic murmur is usually present; echocardiography has shown that tricuspid regurgitation, increased pulmonic flow, and MVP all are common in ASD. But the striking auscultatory finding is persistent splitting of the second heart sound rather than any murmur.

In the normal patient, the pulmonic component of the second heart sound (P_2) is delayed on inspiration but superimposed on its aortic component (A_2) in expiration, allowing full closure of S_2. It may be necessary for the patient to hold expiration and stand for S_2 to close completely. In ASD, wide fixed splitting of S_2, equal in inspiration and expiration, has classically been described. In everyday practice, what holds true more often in ASD is that P_2 is louder and more delayed than normal. The delay of P_2 may be greater on inspiration than expiration, yielding persistent rather than fixed splitting of S_2. In either case, S_2 cannot be made to close fully.

Confounding factors include the fact that right bundle branch block itself—as well as idiopathic benign right heart enlargement—delays P_2. The suspicion of ASD warrants echocardiography, which clarifies the anatomy. Patient management depends on the results of the echocardiogram. Cardiology referral and transesophageal echocardiography may be necessary.

Murmurs that Are Both Systolic and Diastolic

PERICARDIAL RUB

The visceral and parietal layers of the pericardial sac can become inflamed after viral infection, after transmural myocardial infarction, as a result of a systemic connective tissue disease, or for other reasons. When the two inflamed pericardial surfaces move against each other, a rubbing sound is created. Pericardial effusion often accompanies the inflammation. Large effusions may eliminate the rub by preventing contact between the two pericardial layers. The patient may present with pleuritic chest pain.

The classic rub is a three-component high-pitched scratching sound, with one component in systole and two in diastole. The rub often changes or disappears over a matter of hours. One or both diastolic components may disappear, allowing the rub to mimic a systolic murmur.

Pericardial rubs may be best heard over the sternum with the patient leaning forward in expiration. It may also be useful to have her lie on her left side while the examiner listens at the cardiac apex. Pleural rubs may accompany or mimic pericardial rubs; the former relate clearly to respiratory motion and the latter to cardiac motion.

The chest roentgenogram most often is normal but may show cardiomegaly if a moderate or large effusion is present. The electrocardiogram may show characteristic repolarization changes. Echocardiography is not warranted unless there is hemodynamic compromise, persistent pleuritic pain, or uncertainty in diagnosis. When performed, the echocardiogram may or may not show pericardial fluid. Management, in the absence of hemodynamic compromise (tamponade), is directed at the inflammation causing the patient's symptoms and any underlying condition; management is not generally affected by echocardiographic findings.

PATENT DUCTUS ARTERIOSUS

PDA is a congenital lesion that is not common, but the consequences of overlooking it are substantial. When the normal fetal connection between the pulmonary artery and the descending thoracic aorta fails to close after birth, a left-to-right shunt develops. Systolic and diastolic shunting and turbulence are detectable by Doppler study of the pulmonary artery.

These patients can be asymptomatic or can report low-grade exertional dyspnea and palpitations. The chest roentgenogram and electrocardiogram results most often are normal, as the amount of the shunt is typically small.

The murmur is continuous, that is, both systolic and diastolic. Classically, this harsh "machinery" murmur is heard at the upper left sternal border or inferior to the left clavicle. It is loudest in late systole and early diastole, with a late diastolic silent interval. The murmur can be subtle. The diastolic component of it can be mistakenly attributed to aortic or pulmonic regurgitation. The diastolic component can be absent, leaving only a systolic murmur. If the body habitus is large, the murmur can be inaudible.

The finding of any diastolic murmur warrants echocardiography, as does any suspicion of PDA. When ordering the test, it is critical to specify what is being sought, because the routine echocardiographic examination may not include a thorough search of the pulmonary artery for disturbed flow signaling the presence of PDA.

A continuous murmur also can be the result of a fistula between a coronary artery and coronary vein as well as aberrant origin of a coronary artery from the pulmonary artery. These rarer conditions usually are distinguished from PDA by means of transesophageal echocardiography or arteriography.

Cardiology referral is warranted in all three of these conditions. PDA, in particular, is highly correctable in the young. Uncorrected PDA leaves the patient at high risk of bacterial endarteritis after bacteremic procedures. Antibiotic prophylaxis is crucial.

VENOUS HUM

Venous hum, a benign murmur, is included here for differentiation from PDA. It is heard most often in children and young adults, especially those with hyperdynamic circulation. Typically, the venous hum, although both systolic and diastolic, is deeper pitched, softer, and more nearly continuous than the machinery murmur of PDA. It may be louder in diastole. The venous hum is best heard in the medial aspect of the supraclavicular fossa, especially on the right; it can radiate inferiorly. It is typically obliterated with pressure on the ipsilateral internal jugular vein.

CONSIDERATIONS IN PREGNANCY

The primary hemodynamic alteration in pregnancy is the increase in circulating blood volume, usually to about 50% above the prepregnant state. Accordingly, echocardiography can demonstrate a slight increase in the size of all four cardiac chambers. Cardiac stroke volume increases. Thus, systolic flow murmurs are exceedingly common. It is not clear how soon after delivery the changes return to normal. Cardiac chamber enlargement may persist for 6 months or more and may partly reflect the unreversed maternal weight gain.

Cardiac valvular lesions that restrict cardiac output can become a management problem in the pregnant patient; thus, AS and MS require vigilance by the primary care provider and the cardiologist. Most other cardiac valvular lesions do not present a problem, apart from excessive volume overload produced by the combination of pregnancy and significant valvular regurgitation.

A mammary souffle can be heard late in pregnancy and early in the postpartum period of lactating women. It is high pitched, late systolic, or continuous and heard anywhere on either breast. It reflects arterial blood flow to the breast.

SUMMARY

The stethoscope is not obsolete. The careful clinician develops good judgment in selecting patients for echocardiography referral and cardiology consultation. At times, however, even the seasoned practitioner is confounded by a particular heart murmur. Echocardiography is a powerful, increasingly sophisticated, increasingly useful diagnostic tool that should be sought whenever the murmur cannot be adequately characterized. The appropriate and cost-effective use of echocardiography and of cardiology consultation is a goal for all clinicians involved in the primary care of women.

BIBLIOGRAPHY

Agmon Y, Khandheria BK, Meissner I, et al. Aortic valve sclerosis and aortic atherosclerosis: different manifestations of the same disease? *J Am Coll Cardiol* 2001;38:827–834.

Bates B. *A guide to physical examination and history taking,* 6th ed. Philadelphia: JB Lippincott, 1994.

Beppu S, Suzuki S, Matsuda H, et al. Rapidity of progression of aortic stenosis in patients with congenital bicuspid aortic valves. *Am J Cardiol* 1993;71:322–327.

Feigenbaum H. *Echocardiography,* 5th ed. Philadelphia: Lea & Febiger, 1994.

Fink BW. *Congenital heart disease: a deductive approach to its diagnosis.* Chicago: Year Book Medical Publishers, 1975.

Fink JC, Schmid CH, Selker HP. A decision aid for referring patients with systolic murmurs for echocardiography. *J Gen Intern Med* 1994;9:479.

Freed LA, Levy D, Levine RA, et al. Prevalence and clinical outcome of mitral-valve prolapse. *N Engl J Med* 1999;341:1–7.

Hickey AJ, MacMahon SW, Wilcken DEL. Mitral valve prolapse and bacterial endocarditis: when is antibiotic prophylaxis necessary? *Am Heart J* 1985;109: 431–435.

Otto CM, Lind BK, Kitzman DW, et al. Association of aortic-valve sclerosis with cardiovascular mortality and morbidity in the elderly. *N Engl J Med* 1999;341: 142–147.

Palta S, Pai AM, Gill KS, et al. New insights into the progression of aortic stenosis. Implications for secondary prevention. *Circulation* 2000;101:2497–2502.

Perloff JK. *The clinical recognition of congenital heart disease,* 4th ed. Philadelphia: WB Saunders, 1994.

Stewart BF, Siscovick D, Lind BK, et al. Clinical factors associated with calcific aortic valve disease. *J Am Coll Cardiol* 1997;29:630–634.

Topol EJ, Traill TA, Fortuin NJ. Hypertensive hypertrophic cardiomyopathy of the elderly. *N Engl J Med* 1985:312:277–283.

CHAPTER 47
Bacterial Endocarditis Prophylaxis

Winnie W. K. Sia

Infective endocarditis causes significant morbidity and mortality. It is estimated that 4,000 to 8,000 new cases of endocarditis occur per year in the United States. Most cases of endocarditis are from bacterial infections, although fungal infections can also occur. Many efforts have therefore focused on antibiotic prophylaxis against bacteremia in preventing infective endocarditis. Currently, it is standard practice to administer antimicrobial prophylaxis before dental or other bacteremia-associated procedures to individuals believed to be at risk for developing endocarditis. The rationale for giving antibiotic prophylaxis to prevent bacterial endocarditis is based on several observations. First, about one fourth of patients with endocarditis have preexisting cardiac abnormalities. Valvulitis or turbulent flow leads to sterile platelet-fibrin thrombi that may be a nidus for infection during bacteremia. Second, 25% to 50% of endocarditis cases occur in temporal association with invasive medical procedures. Third, bacteremias resulting from medical procedures generally are caused by organisms with predictable sensitivity patterns. Thus, it is reasonable to attempt to prevent some cases of endocarditis by using antibiotics before procedures that are associated with bacteremia in individuals at risk. However, one must weigh the risk of allergic reactions, antibiotic resistance, and cost against the potential benefit to the individual patient. Failure to consider the above principles will lead to overuse of antimicrobial therapy, development of antimicrobial resistance, risk of adverse drug effects, and excessive cost.

The American Heart Association (AHA) published guidelines on the prevention of bacterial endocarditis. These recommendations are based on case-control studies on small numbers of patients, case reports assuming a causal relation mainly due to the temporal relation between a health care procedure and the infection, animal studies/models, *in vitro* studies of bacteriology of endocarditis, and expert opinion. There are no prospective human studies. However, considering the impressive risk reduction demonstrated in case-control studies, positive results from animal studies, and the significant mortality and morbidity associated with infective endocarditis, routine antibiotic prophylaxis in those at risk seems justifiable.

Although it is important to prescribe antibiotics for individuals at risk for endocarditis, primary care providers should avoid routine antibiotic prescription for those at low or negligible risk for infective endocarditis, especially if the anticipated procedure carries minimal risk of bacteremia. Drug anaphylaxis, inducing antibiotic resistance in bacterial organisms, and cost of drug therapy are disadvantages that outweigh the potential benefit, if any, in low-risk individuals. It is estimated that 6% of all cases of endocarditis could have been prevented by administration of prophylaxis. This means that extensive use of antibiotic prophylaxis can prevent 240 to 480 cases per year in the United States. Therefore, use of antibiotics should be targeted at high- and moderate-risk individuals with cardiac conditions undergoing procedures that produce endocarditis prone bacteremia.

PRINCIPLES OF PROPHYLAXIS RECOMMENDATIONS

The three principles that guide the prevention of infective endocarditis are as follows:

1. To identify at-risk patients in the high- and moderate-cardiac risk categories
2. To identify procedures or events that induce bacteremia caused by organisms that have a predilection for endocardium
3. To choose antibiotics that target the most likely culprit organisms caused by the procedure.

For individuals with cardiac lesions in the high- and moderate-risk groups, endocarditis prophylaxis is recommended for procedures at risk for bacteremia. In certain respiratory, gastrointestinal, or genitourinary tract procedures in which prophylaxis is normally not recommended, prophylaxis is considered optional for high-risk cardiac individuals. For low- or negligible-risk individuals undergoing low-risk procedures, prophylaxis should not routinely be administered.

The 1997 AHA recommendations are provided in the following sections as guidelines, yet they should be tailored to the individual patient.

SPECIFIC CARDIAC DEFECTS AND THE RISK FOR ENDOCARDITIS

Antibiotic use for bacterial endocarditis prophylaxis is recommended for high- and moderate-risk cardiac categories but not for the negligible-risk group. Estimates of risk of endocarditis for specific cardiac defects are based on the frequency with which these conditions are found in patients with documented endocarditis. The conditions for each risk category are listed in Table 47.1. High-risk cardiac conditions include prosthetic cardiac valves, previous bacterial endocarditis, complex cyanotic congenital heart disease, and surgically constructed systemic pulmonary shunts or conduits. For the moderate-risk category, the congenital cardiac conditions include the following uncorrected conditions: patent ductus arteriosus, ventricular septal defect, primum atrial septal defect, coarctation of the aorta, and bicuspid aortic valve.

Mitral valve prolapse (MVP) is common, and the need for prophylaxis is controversial. Only a small percentage of MVP patients develops complications at any age. Because the mitral valve leaflet closure depends on the valve apparatus and the size of the end-systolic ventricle, which is variable and dynamic, dehydration and tachycardia are common causes of intermittent MVP. The risk of endocarditis is not increased in patients with a normal mitral valve without regurgitation on Doppler studies nor with minimal mitral regurgitation on a normal mitral valve and motion. However, structurally normal but prolapsing mitral valves from larger regurgitant orifices should receive prophylactic antibiotics, based on cost-to-benefit analysis. Patients with MVP and an audible regurgitant murmur or echocardiographic findings of thickened redundant valvular tissue seem to be at highest risk. Antibiotic prophylaxis is also recommended for patients with myxomatous mitral valve degeneration with regurgitation.

TABLE 47.1. Cardiac Conditions Associated with Endocarditis

Endocarditis prophylaxis recommended
High-risk category
Prosthetic cardiac valves, including bioprosthetic and homograft valves
Previous bacterial endocarditis, even in the absence of heart disease
Complex cyanotic congenital heart disease (e.g., single ventricle states, transposition of the great arteries, tetralogy of Fallot)
Surgically constructed systemic pulmonary shunts or conduits
Moderate-risk category
Most other congenital cardiac malformations (other than above and below)
Acquired valvular dysfunction (e.g., rheumatic heart disease)
Hypertrophic cardiomyopathy
Mitral valve prolapse with valvular regurgitation and/or thickened leaflet[a]
Endocarditis prophylaxis not recommended
Negligible-risk category (no greater risk than the general population)
Isolated secundum atrial septal defect
Surgical repair of atrial septal defect, ventricular septal defect, or patent ductus arteriosus (without residua beyond 6 mo)
Previous coronary artery bypass graft surgery
Mitral valve prolapse without valvular regurgitation[a]
Physiologic, functional, or innocent heart murmurs
Previous Kawasaki disease without valvular dysfunction
Previous rheumatic fever without valvular dysfunction
Cardiac pacemakers (intravascular and epicardial) and implanted defibrillators

[a]See text for further details.

Reproduced with permission. *Prevention of Bacterial Endocarditis.* © 1997, American Heart Association.

BACTEREMIA-PRODUCING PROCEDURES

Procedure-related bacteremias occur soon after the procedure and usually are short-lived. The incidence of positive blood cultures is highest 30 seconds after a tooth extraction. Dental procedures cause bacteremias usually for less than 10 minutes. This is the basis for the preprocedure antibiotic dose, which should be administered close in timing to the procedure at a dose that provides adequate serum levels to last for hours after the procedure. Not all procedures cause the same frequency or intensity of bacteremia nor are they associated with bacteria prone to adhere to endothelium. Therefore, surgical and dental procedures are stratified into categories for which prophylaxis recommendations are made.

When considering the need for prophylaxis based on the planned procedure, three questions should be asked: Is the procedure associated with significant rates of bacteremia? Are the organisms likely to cause endocarditis? Is there reasonable clinical evidence that the procedure has been associated with endocarditis? Rates of bacteremia associated with specific procedures are given in Table 47.2.

TABLE 47.2. Representative Rates of Bacteremia after Various Dental, Diagnostic, and Therapeutic Procedures[a]

Procedure and site	Incidence rate (range)
None (spontaneous bacteremia)	<1 (0–3)
Oral cavity	
Tooth extraction	60 (18–85)
Periodontal surgery	88 (60–90)
Brushing teeth or irrigation	40 (7–50)
Tonsillectomy	35 (33–38)
Respiratory tract	
Tracheal intubation	<10 (0–16)
Nasotracheal suctioning	16
Bronchoscopy	
Rigid bronchoscope	15
Flexible bronchoscope	0
Genitourinary tract	
Catheter insertion or removal	13 (0–26)
Dilation of strictures	28 (19–86)
Normal delivery	3 (1–5)
Gastrointestinal tract	
Upper gastrointestinal endoscopy	4 (0–8)
Transesophageal echocardiography	1 (0–17)
Endoscopic retrograde cholangiopancreatography	5 (0–6)
Barium enema	10 (5–11)
Colonoscopy	5 (0–5)
Sigmoidoscopy	
Rigid sigmoidoscopy	5
Flexible sigmoidoscopy	0
Proctoscopy	2
Hemorrhoidectomy	8
Esophageal dilation	45
Vascular system	
Cardiac catheterization	2 (0–5)

[a]Ranges are given, if available. Insufficient data were available to calculate the incidence rate of bacteremia after the removal of tympanostomy tubes or cesarean section.
From Durack DT. Prevention of infective endocarditis. *N Engl J Med* 1995; 332:38, with permission.

TABLE 47.3. Dental Procedures and Endocarditis Prophylaxis

Endocarditis prophylaxis recommended[a]
- Dental extractions
- Periodontal procedures including surgery, scaling and root planning, probing, and recall maintenance
- Dental implant placement and reimplantation of avulsed teeth
- Endodontic (root canal) instrumentation or surgery only beyond the apex
- Subgingival placement of antibiotic fibers or strips
- Initial placement of orthodontic bands but not brackets
- Intraligamentary local anesthetic injections
- Prophylactic cleaning of teeth or implants where bleeding is anticipated

Endocarditis prophylaxis not recommended
- Restorative dentistry[b] (operative and prosthodontic) with or without retraction cord[c]
- Local anesthetic injections (nonintraligamentary)
- Intracanal endodontic treatment; post placement and buildup
- Placement of rubber dams
- Postoperative suture removal
- Placement of removable prosthodontic or orthodontic appliances
- Taking of oral impressions
- Fluoride treatments
- Taking of oral radiographs
- Orthodontic appliance adjustment
- Shedding of primary teeth

[a]Prophylaxis is recommended for patients with high- and moderate-risk cardiac conditions.
[b]This includes restoration of decayed teeth (filling cavities) and replacement of missing teeth.
[c]Clinical judgment may indicate antibiotic use in selected circumstances that may create significant bleeding.
Reproduced with permission. *Prevention of Bacterial Endocarditis.* © 1997, American Heart Association.

Dental and Oral Procedures

Current recommendations by the AHA for prophylaxis related to dental and surgical procedures are listed in Table 47.3. Because poor dental hygiene can lead to bacteremia even in the absence of a procedure, all high-risk patients should maintain good oral health. Antibiotic prophylaxis is recommended for all dental procedures likely to cause gingival bleeding from hard or soft tissues, such as periodontal surgery, scaling, and professional teeth cleaning. If a series of procedures is required, a 9- to 14-day interval between procedures should be observed to avoid the emergence of resistant organisms. Ill-fitting dentures may result in oral ulcers, which can also lead to bacteremia. Antiseptic mouth rinses, such as chlorhexidine hydrochloride and povidone-iodine, applied immediately for about 30 seconds before dental procedures, may reduce the incidence or magnitude of bacteremia.

Respiratory, Gastrointestinal, and Genitourinary Tract Procedures

Current AHA recommendations for respiratory, gastrointestinal, and genitourinary procedures are listed in Table 47.4. Surgical procedures involving respiratory mucosa may lead to bacteremia for which prophylaxis is recommended in high- and moderate-risk cardiac categories. Rigid bronchoscopy may lead to mucosal injury and may warrant antibiotic prophylaxis, whereas flexible bronchoscopy is unlikely to cause such damage. Endotracheal intubation is not an indication for prophylaxis.

The instrumented gastrointestinal tract seems to be a less common portal of entry for endocarditis-causing organisms than the oral cavity or urinary tract. Endoscopy with or without gastrointestinal biopsy is not sufficient to warrant antibiotic prophylaxis. In addition, barium studies of the gastrointestinal tract and liver biopsy also are believed to be procedures at low risk for bacteremia. However, prophylaxis is indicated for esophageal stricture dilatation, sclerotherapy of esophageal varices, instrumentation of obstructed biliary tree, cholecystectomy, and surgical operations that involve intestinal mucosa in high-risk cardiac patients and is optional for moderate-risk cardiac patients.

Surgery or instrumentation of the genitourinary tract may cause bacteremia but primarily when infection is present. Therefore, prophylaxis is recommended for procedures such as urinary catheterization only if an infection is present. Similarly, most obstetric and gynecologic procedures, such as dilation and curettage, therapeutic abortion, cervical brushings or biopsy, sterilization procedures, cesarean delivery, and insertion or removal of intrauterine devices, do not require prophylaxis unless infection is present (Table 47.4). Prophylaxis is optional in high-risk patients for vaginal delivery and vaginal hysterectomy but is not routinely warranted in uncomplicated vaginal delivery. The American College of Obstetricians and Gynecologists in the June 1992 *Technical Bulletin* recommended endocarditis prophylaxis for a broader range of indications, but the bulletin was withdrawn in 1999 and there has been no updated American College of Obstetricians and Gynecologists guidelines on this topic.

TABLE 47.4. Other Procedures and Endocarditis Prophylaxis

Endocarditis prophylaxis recommended
- Respiratory tract
  - Tonsillectomy and/or adenoidectomy
  - Surgical operations that involve respiratory mucosa
  - Bronchoscopy with a rigid bronchoscope
- Gastrointestinal tract[a]
  - Sclerotherapy for esophageal varices
  - Esophageal stricture dilation
  - Endoscopic retrograde cholangiography with biliary obstruction
  - Biliary tract surgery
  - Surgical operations that involve intestinal mucosa
- Genitourinary tract
  - Prostatic surgery
  - Cystoscopy
  - Urethral dilation

Endocarditis prophylaxis not recommended[b]
- Respiratory tract
  - Endotracheal incubation
  - Bronchoscopy with a flexible bronchoscope, with or without biopsy[b]
  - Tympanostomy tube insertion
- Gastrointestinal tract
  - Transesophageal echocardiography[b]
  - Endoscopy with or without gastrointestinal biopsy[b]
- Genitourinary tract
  - Vaginal hysterectomy[b]
  - Vaginal delivery[b]
  - Cesarean section
  - In uninfected tissue
    - Urethral catheterization
    - Uterine dilation and curettage
    - Therapeutic abortion
    - Sterilization procedures
    - Insertion or removal of intrauterine devices
- Other
  - Cardiac catheterization
  - Implanted cardiac pacemakers, implanted defibrillators, and coronary stents
  - Incision or biopsy of surgically scrubbed skin
  - Circumcision

[a]Prophylaxis is recommended for high-risk patients; it is optional for moderate-risk patients.
[b]Prophylaxis is optional for high-risk patients.
Reproduced with permission. *Prevention of Bacterial Endocarditis.* © 1997, American Heart Association.

TABLE 47.5. Prophylactic Regimens for Dental, Oral, or Respiratory Tract or Esophageal Procedures for Adult Patients

Situation	Drug and dosing regimen
Standard general prophylaxis	**Amoxicillin** 2.0 g orally 1 h before procedure
Unable to take oral medications	**Ampicillin** 2.0 g IM or IV within 30 min before procedure
Allergic to penicillin	**Clindamycin** 600 mg orally 1 h before procedure **or cephalexin**[a] or **cefadroxil**[a] 2.0 g 1 h before procedure **or azithromycin** or **clarithromycin** 500 mg orally 1 h before procedure
Allergic to penicillin and unable to take oral medications	**Clindamycin** 600 mg IV within 30 min before procedure **or Cefazolin**[a] 1.0 g IV within 30 min before procedure

IM, intramuscularly; IV, intravenously.
[a]Cephalosporins should not be used in individuals with urticaria, angioedema, or anaphylaxis to penicillins.
Reproduced with permission. *Prevention of Bacterial Endocarditis.* © 1997, American Heart Association.

PROPHYLACTIC REGIMENS

Antibiotic prophylaxis should be initiated shortly before a procedure in sufficient doses to ensure adequate serum levels, and it should not be continued beyond 6 to 8 hours after the procedure. This is because most procedure-related bacteremia is transient. If a patient is already on an antibiotic that is used for endocarditis prophylaxis, it is important to choose an antibiotic from a different class instead of increasing the dose of the current antibiotic. If possible, consider delaying the procedure until at least 14 days after the completion of the current antibiotic to avoid bacterial resistance.

Regimens for Dental, Oral, Respiratory Tract, or Esophageal Procedures

Streptococcus viridans (α-hemolytic streptococci) is the most common cause of bacterial endocarditis after dental, respiratory tract, and esophageal procedures, and therapy should be specifically directed at these organisms. Standard oral regimens are outlined in Table 47.5. A single dose of amoxicillin is the recommended standard prophylactic regimen. The newly recommended dose of 2.0 g of amoxicillin should be administered 1 hour before the anticipated procedure. A second dose is no longer necessary because the serum levels have been shown to last for 6 to 14 hours against most oral streptococci. Ampicillin is recommended as a parenteral agent for individuals who are unable to take or absorb oral medications. For individuals allergic to penicillins, clindamycin is one recommended alternative. Other alternatives are listed in Table 47.5. Erythromycin is no longer recommended because of gastrointestinal upset. An alternative drug to ampicillin or amoxicillin should be given to individuals on chronic penicillin for rheumatic fever prevention, because the oral cavity may be colonized with penicillin-resistant streptococci.

Regimens for Genitourinary and Nonesophageal Gastrointestinal Procedures

Bacterial endocarditis after genitourinary or gastrointestinal procedures most often is caused by *Streptococcus faecalis* (enterococcus). Although Gram-negative bacilli or anaerobic bacteremia may occur after such procedures, these organisms rarely cause endocarditis. Therefore, antibiotic regimens for genitourinary or gastrointestinal procedures should be directed against enterococci (Table 47.6). The AHA continues to recommend parenteral antibiotics in patients at highest risk, with an alternative oral regimen for moderate-risk patients. For procedures in which prophylaxis is not routinely recommended, it is optional to administer in high-risk patients.

Prevention of all cases of bacterial endocarditis is not possible. Infections do occur, even with optimal prophylaxis. The current AHA recommendations are meant be reasonable guidelines for practicing physicians. However, the individual physician should exercise clinical judgment when tailoring prophylaxis to a specific patient. Physicians and dentists should be aware of endocarditis signs and symptoms, such as unexplained fever, myalgia, arthralgia, lethargy, malaise, night chills, and weakness, in those at risk for developing endocarditis. Most cases of procedure-related endocarditis occur within 2 weeks of the procedure.

TABLE 47.6. Prophylactic Regimens for Genitourinary/Gastrointestinal (Excluding Esophageal) Procedures for Adult Patients

Situation	Drug and dosage regimen[a]
High-risk patients	**Ampicillin** 2.0 g IM or IV **plus gentamicin** 1.5 mg/kg (not to exceed 120 mg) within 30 min of starting procedure; 6 h later, **ampicillin** 1 g IM/IV **or amoxicillin** 1 g orally
High-risk patients allergic to ampicillin/amoxicillin	**Vancomycin** 1.0 g IV over 1–2 h **plus gentamicin** 1.5 mg/kg (not to exceed 120 mg) within 30 min of starting procedure; complete injection/infusion within 30 min of starting procedure
Moderate-risk patients	**Amoxicillin** 2.0 g orally 1 h before procedure, **or ampicillin** 2.0 g IM/IV within 30 min of starting procedure
Moderate-risk patients allergic to ampicillin/amoxicillin	**Vancomycin** 1.0 g IV over 1–2 h; complete infusion within 30 min of starting procedure

IM, intramuscularly; IV, intravenously.
[a]No second dose of vancomycin or gentamicin is recommended.
Reproduced with permission. Prevention of Bacterial Endocarditis. © 1997, American Heart Association.

BIBLIOGRAPHY

American College of Obstetricians and Gynecologists. Cardiac disease in pregnancy: ACOG technical bulletin 168. Washington, DC: American College of Obstetricians and Gynecologists, 1992.

Baker TH, Hubbell R. Reappraisal of asymptomatic puerperal bacteremia. *Am J Obstet Gynecol* 1967;97:575.

Dajani AS, Taubert KA, Wilson W, et al. Prevention of bacterial endocarditis: recommendations of the American Heart Association. *JAMA* 1997;277:1794–1801.

Durack DT. Prevention of infective endocarditis. *N Engl J Med* 1995;332:38.

Greenman RL, Bisno AL. Prevention of bacterial endocarditis. In: Kaye D, ed. *Infective endocarditis*. New York: Raven Press, 1992:465.

Seaworth BJ, Durack DT. Infective endocarditis in obstetric and gynecologic practice. *Am J Obstet Gynecol* 1986;154:180.

Sugrue D, Blake S, Troy P, et al. Antibiotic prophylaxis against infective endocarditis after normal delivery: is it necessary? *Br Heart J* 1980;44:499.

CHAPTER 48
Syncope

Paul C. Gordon

Syncope is a temporary loss of consciousness due to impaired cerebral perfusion. Because the brain is critically dependent on blood glucose for metabolic fuel, interruption of cerebral blood flow leads to syncope in as little as 8 to 10 seconds. Syncope is a common clinical problem, accounting for 3% of emergency department visits and 1% of hospital admissions. The annual cost of evaluating and treating syncope is estimated to be $800 million dollars. Syncope is more common in elderly patients, because cerebral blood flow declines with aging. Two thirds of patients presenting with syncope are over age 60. In this population, syncope occurs at an annual rate of approximately 6%, with a recurrence rate of 30%.

Typically, a fall in systolic blood pressure below 70 mm Hg or a mean pressure of 30 to 40 mm Hg results in syncope. Other accompanying factors may include pallor, sweating, loss of consciousness, and shallow breathing. The patient is usually motionless but is not incontinent. The syncopal episode may or may not vary with posture, depending on the etiology. Consciousness is regained once cerebral perfusion is restored. Considerable morbidity can occur, particularly in elderly patients, when trauma is sustained due to this abrupt loss of consciousness.

ETIOLOGY

Although autoregulation occurs in the cerebral vasculature, cerebral perfusion is critically dependent on systemic arterial blood pressure, which in turn is related to the product of the cardiac output and systemic vascular resistance. The cardiac output is governed by the product of the heart rate and stroke volume, which in turn is regulated by preload, afterload, and cardiac contractility. Thus, a reduction in systemic blood pressure may be produced by an abnormality anywhere in the chain of neural mechanisms for peripheral vascular control, that is, the carotid, aortic, ventricular, and atrial baroreceptors that carry afferent impulses to the medulla; the central vasomotor centers in the medulla that receive afferent impulses and transmit efferent impulses; cortical and spinal efferent tracts; and peripheral sympathetic or parasympathetic nerves. Additionally, a fall in blood pressure may depend on mechanical factors that normally limit pooling of blood in the peripheral veins, intravascular blood volume, and the heart's ability to maintain cardiac output. These etiologic factors divide the important causes of syncope into five broad categories (Table 48.1).

TABLE 48.1. Causes of Syncope

Cause	Prevalence (approximate)
Cardiac	
Arrhythmias	15%
Bradyarrhythmias	
Complete heart block	
Sick sinus syndrome	
Pacemaker malfunction	
Tachyarrhythmias	
Supraventricular tachycardia	
Ventricular tachycardia	
Torades de pointes (long QT syndrome)	
Anatomic (obstruction or impairment of blood flow)	5%
Vascular	
Orthostatic hypotension	10%
Hypovolemia/blood loss	
Primary autonomic failure	
Secondary neurogenic	
Drug induced	
Reflex mediated	25%
Neurally mediated (vasovagal)	
Carotid sinus hypersensitivity	
Situational	
Metabolic/endocrine	2–3%
Neurologic disease	10%
Migraine	
Seizure	
Transient ischemic attack	
Psychogenic	2%
Anxiety/panic disorder	
Hysterical	
Unknown	30%

Cardiac Syncope

Cardiac syncope results from disturbances of heart rate and rhythm, obstruction to blood flow, and/or impaired ventricular function. Disturbances of rate and rhythm may result from either asystole due to conduction abnormalities, severe bradycardia, or tachyarrhythmias of atrial and ventricular origin. Arrhythmic disorders are common causes of syncope, accounting for approximately 15% of cases.

More than 50,000 new cases of complete heart block occur annually in the United States, and it is estimated that 50% of these patients experience syncope. Complete heart block in the elderly is most often degenerative in etiology (sick sinus syndrome), including Lev and Lenegre diseases. Rarely, degenerative diseases (Friedreich ataxia, progressive muscular dystrophy, myotonic dystrophy, and Duchenne dystrophy), infectious diseases (Lyme disease, diphtheria, syphilis, toxoplasmosis, mumps, rheumatic fever, Chagas disease), valvular heart disease (endocarditis or postvalve replacement), tumor infiltration, endocrine and metabolic disorders (gout with mate deposition in the conduction system, hypo- and hyperthyroidism, hemochromatosis, Addison disease), trauma, electrolyte disturbances (hyperkalemia, acidosis, and hypomagnesemia), or infiltrative diseases (sarcoidosis and amyloidosis) may cause complete heart block. Coronary artery disease, especially with an acute myocardial infarction, can result in transient heart block. In addition, toxicity from sinoatrial and atrioventricular (AV) nodal blocking drugs such as digitalis, beta-blockers, and dihydropyridine calcium channel blockers—usually in the setting of an underlying sick sinus syndrome—can cause complete heart block.

When syncope occurs in pacemaker-dependent patients, pacemaker malfunction should be considered. Generator failure or lead fracture can lead to failure of the pacemaker to capture. In patients with single-chamber pacemakers, the lack of AV synchrony may produce the *pacemaker syndrome* due to compromised ventricular filling and reduced cardiac output, or a vasodepressor response may occur due to reflex vasodilation produced by atrial contraction and distention occurring against closed AV valves.

Syncope rarely results from supraventricular tachyarrhythmias such as atrial fibrillation, atrial flutter, atrial tachycardia, AV nodal reentry tachycardia, or Wolff-Parkinson-White syndrome (rapid conduction of atrial impulses to the ventricles or AV reentry tachycardia due to an accessory Kent bundle bypass tract). The rapid heart rate shortens the ventricular diastolic filling time, reducing cardiac output and leading to a fall in blood pressure and syncope. Most patients with supraventricular tachyarrhythmia present with lightheadedness or palpitations, and syncope rarely occurs unless there is accompanying cardiac outflow obstruction (aortic stenosis or hypertrophic cardiomyopathy with left ventricular outflow obstruction) or the ventricular rate is extremely fast (Wolff-Parkinson-White syndrome with atrial fibrillation or flutter and one-to-one conduction from the atrium to the ventricle through the bypass tract).

In patients with impaired left ventricular function from any cause (especially coronary artery disease and prior myocardial infarction) or during an acute myocardial infarction, self-terminating ventricular tachycardia is a life-threatening cause of cardiac syncope. Syncope (from either AV nodal block or ventricular tachycardia) has been reported to be the presenting symptom of myocardial infarction in 7% of patients over age 65. Rarely, ventricular tachycardia occurs in patients with apparently normal hearts. In some patients, ventricular tachycardia is provoked by stress or exercise due to a release of catecholamines. Ventricular tachyarrhythmias may also be caused by metabolic abnormalities such as hypokalemia or hypomagnesemia; drugs such as phenothiazines, antidepressants, or antiarrhythmic agents; and illicit drugs such as cocaine. In young patients, right ventricular dysplasia may produce an isolated right ventricular cardiomyopathy and cause syncope due to ventricular tachycardia. The Brugada syndrome is an inheritable disorder characterized by ST-segment elevation in the right precordial leads and a right bundle branch block seen on the electrocardiogram (ECG) that is associated with reentrant ventricular tachycardia.

Polymorphic ventricular tachycardia or torsades de pointes may occur in patients with the long QT syndrome and may cause syncope or sudden death. Congenital causes of the long QT syndrome include the Romano-Ward syndrome and Jervell and Lange-Nielsen syndromes associated with congenital deafness. Acquired long QT syndrome may be induced by type IA (quinidine, procainamide, disopyramide) or type III (sotalol, dofetilide) antiarrhythmic agents, tricyclic antidepressants (amitriptyline), pentamidine, phenothiazines, trimethoprim/sulfamethoxazole, or intravenous erythromycin. Repolarization abnormalities by hypokalemia, ischemia, myocarditis, severe bradycardia, and central nervous system disease (subarachnoid hemorrhage) can lengthen the QT interval and predispose to torsades de pointes.

Anatomic obstruction to blood flow accounts for 5% of the cases of syncope. Depending on the severity of obstruction to flow, symptoms may occur at rest or only with exercise. Peripheral arteriolar vasodilation of the muscle beds occurs during exercise and results in a drop in systemic vascular resistance. This normally produces a compensatory increase in cardiac output and arterial blood pressure. However, if there is significant obstruction to outflow, the cardiac output cannot increase sufficiently to compensate for the decline in systemic vascular resistance. Consequently, arterial blood pressure may fall and result in cerebral hypoperfusion and syncope. Common causes of obstruction to flow are aortic stenosis and hypertrophic cardiomyopathy. Patients with aortic stenosis have a fixed valvular orifice area and therefore cannot increase the cardiac output based on demands posed by exercise. Patients with hypertrophic cardiomyopathy may have fixed or dynamic outflow tract obstruction precipitated by conditions that increase contractility, decrease left ventricular diastolic chamber dimensions (hypovolemia or tachyarrhythmias such as atrial fibrillation), or decrease afterload.

Other conditions that lead to obstruction to outflow include pulmonic stenosis (valvular, subvalvular, and supravalvular) and supravalvular aortic stenosis. Obstruction to ventricular inflow may occur in a patient with an atrial myxoma or thrombus. The latter is an ominous complication of a mechanical prosthetic valve. Primary pulmonary hypertension, pulmonary peripheral branch stenosis, pulmonary emboli, cardiac tamponade, mitral or tricuspid stenosis, a malfunctioning prosthetic aortic or mitral valve, cor triatriatum, tetralogy of Fallot, and Eisenmenger syndrome (with pulmonary hypertension) are other conditions associated with syncope due to obstruction to blood flow.

Vascular Causes of Syncope

Syncope may result from reduced effective circulating blood volume produced by conditions such as hemorrhage, dehydration, or after hemodialysis. Postural hypotension is a common cause of syncope (8%–10% of cases). When a person stands, the decrease in cardiac output and blood pressure produced by peripheral venous pooling is usually compensated by reflex tachycardia and vasoconstriction mediated by sympathetic stimulation. Usually, these intact compensatory mechanisms produce only a transient systolic blood pressure drop of 5 to 15 mm Hg, and the diastolic pressure tends to rise. In patients with orthostatic hypotension, however, there is a more profound and persistent decline of systolic pressure (>20–30 mm Hg), with or without a concomitant drop (>10 mm Hg) in diastolic pressure. Orthostatic hypotension is more prevalent (30%–50% incidence) in elderly (>75 years) patients, particularly in those receiving cardiovascular or psychotropic drugs.

Orthostatic hypotension may be an idiopathic disorder. The Bradbury-Eggleston syndrome is characterized by postural hypotension without a compensatory tachycardia, hypohidrosis, impotence, and disturbed sphincter control. It is due to primary degeneration of the autonomic nervous system (primary autonomic insufficiency). Patients often develop postprandial hypotension and presyncope as well as visual impairment while standing or walking. These symptoms become progressive, occurring more frequently in the morning while suddenly assuming an upright posture. Another idiopathic disorder that causes postural hypotension is the Shy-Drager syndrome (multiple system atrophy), characterized by autonomic failure with involvement of the extrapyramidal tracts and basal ganglia (parkinsonism) and ataxia. Familial dysautonomia (young people with severe autonomic failure with loss of sweating, fixed dilated pupils, fixed heart rate, and bladder and bowel dysfunction) is associated with postural hypotension.

Secondary postural hypotension may occur in association with diseases that affect the peripheral, autonomic, or central nervous system. Such disorders include diabetes mellitus, uremia, pyridoxine deficiency, multiple sclerosis, tabes dorsalis, pernicious anemia, Parkinson disease, syringomyelia, and alcoholism and Wernicke encephalopathy.

Most antihypertensive agents may cause postural hypotension, particularly in the setting of dehydration and hypovolemia exacerbated by diuretic administration. The agents that provoke the greatest postural hypotension are ganglionic blockers, depletors of catecholamines (such as reserpine), and drugs that block the release of catecholamines (such as guanethidine). These agents have largely been replaced by others in clinical practice. Alpha-blockers, such as prazosin, terazosin, and doxazosin, are used for both hypertension and prostatic and have a profound first-dose effect that can result in syncope. Tranquilizers, sedatives, hypnotics, or antidepressants may cause hypotension by depressing the vasomotor center. Calcium channel blockers and nitrates, often used in the treatment of angina, may produce hypotension. Postural hypotension may also occur in association with the administration of agents such as tricyclic antidepressants (especially nortriptyline) and bromocriptine. Cardiovascular deconditioning after prolonged recumbency, space flight, or illness—particularly in the elderly—may produce orthostatic hypotension.

Reflex-mediated syncope is composed of a trigger (the afferent limb) and a response (the efferent limb) consisting of increased vagal tone and a withdrawal of peripheral sympathetic tone leading to bradycardia, vasodilation, and ultimately hypotension and syncope. It accounts for approximately 25% of all cases of syncope. The specific triggers distinguish these causes of syncope.

Neurally-mediated syncope (vasovagal hypotension or vasodepressor syncope, including the common "faint") is the most common (~55%) cause of syncope in otherwise healthy young people. It is characterized by the abrupt onset of hypotension with or without bradycardia. Triggers associated with the development of neurally-mediated syncope are those that either reduce ventricular filling or increase catecholamine secretion. It is often precipitated by the sight of blood or loss of blood through trauma, surgery, or phlebotomy or by pain or stress. It is more likely to occur in the upright position, associated with hunger and fatigue, particularly in a crowded hot room. Warning signs suggestive of autonomic nervous system overactivity usually occur before syncope: yawning, pallor, sighing, hyperventilation, epigastric discomfort, nausea, diaphoresis, blurred vision, impaired hearing, and unawareness. These clinical phenomena result from a paradoxical reflex that is initiated when ventricular preload is reduced. This causes a decreased cardiac output and blood pressure that is sensed by arterial baroreceptors, which in turn increases catecholamine levels, leading to a vigorously contracting volume-depleted ventricle. Mechanoreceptors or C-fibers within the heart are activated by the vigorous contraction, which results in a "paradoxical" withdrawal of peripheral sympathetic tone and an increase in vagal tone, causing vasodilation and bradycardia with a fall in total peripheral vascular resistance that is not adequately compensated for by a rise in cardiac output. Assuming a sitting or recumbent position (with legs elevated) usually alleviates the symptoms, and syncope can often be aborted.

Carotid sinus hypersensitivity may produce syncope through inappropriate or excessive activation of vasomotor reflexes. Afferent impulses from the carotid sinuses travel via the glossopharyngeal nerve to the vasomotor and cardioinhibitory centers in the medulla. The efferent limb of the carotid sinus reflex is formed by vagal and cervical sympathetic fibers. Increased pressure on the walls of the carotid arteries leads to an increased frequency of afferent stimulation of the vasomotor center, thereby increasing parasympathetic outflow, reducing sympathetic outflow, and causing systemic vasodilation and bradycardia. The vagal or cardioinhibitory type is the most common form of carotid sinus hypersensitivity, occurring in about 70% of patients. Here, bradycardia, sinus arrest, AV block, or even asystole may occur to produce dizziness, presyncope, and syncope. The second or vasodepressor type (5%–10% of patients) is characterized by marked hypotension without significant bradycardia or AV block. The mixed type includes both cardioinhibitory and vasodepressor responses (20%–25%). Carotid sinus hypersensitivity usually occurs in the elderly and is more common in men than in women. However, the mere presence of carotid sinus hypersensitivity does not prove that it is the cause of syncope. Atherosclerosis, hypertension, diabetes mellitus, and local pathologic changes such as scars, lymph nodes, and tumors involving the carotid body predispose to carotid sinus hypersensitivity. Turning of the head or pressure on the carotid sinus area (tight collar or necktie) may precipitate an episode of syncope.

Situational syncope is mediated via the autonomic nervous system reflex mechanisms that lead to a vasodepressor response and syncope. Examples include syncope during micturition, cough, deglutition, defecation, and acute pain states. Micturition syncope is usually caused by rapid emptying of the bladder, which causes reflex vasodilation and decreased cerebral blood flow; this may be further accentuated by the effects of a Valsalva maneuver during voiding. Deglutition syncope can occur in patients with or without esophageal disease. Defecation syncope has been attributed to a reflex mechanism such as a prolonged Valsalva maneuver, leading to decreased cardiac output or reduced cerebral perfusion from a rapid increase in cerebrospinal fluid pressure. Trigeminal neuralgia with paroxysmal pain in the posterior pharynx or external auditory canal is occasionally accompanied by syncope secondary to vasodilation and bradycardia. Postprandial hypotension may occur in elderly patients with impaired baroreflex function due to the inability to compensate for pooling of blood in the splanchnic circulation after meals. In patients with chronic obstructive pulmonary disease, cough or tussive syncope is triggered by vagally mediated hypotension and bradycardia produced by prolonged, excessive, violent coughing. In these patients, the propensity for syncope is exacerbated by the decreased venous return produced by the marked increase in intrathoracic pressure from coughing. Oculovagal syncope after ocular compression; sneeze syncope; instrumentation syncope occurring during endoscopy, bronchoscopy, or insertion of intrauterine devices; diver's or submersion syncope; Jacuzzi syncope; weightlifter's syncope; and trumpet-player's syncope have all been described as causes of situational syncope.

Metabolic and Endocrine Disturbances

A reduction of plasma volume, altered adrenergic function, or vasodilation may occur with certain metabolic and endocrine disturbances and may produce hypotension and syncope. Disorders of this type include diabetes mellitus, primary systemic amyloidosis, and acute porphyria. Hypotension due to hypovolemia is seen in adrenal insufficiency, hypoaldosteronism, and salt-wasting nephritis. Altered vascular responses to catecholamines may occur in Addison disease, and angiotensin levels may be diminished in conditions in which plasma renin activity is low. Postural hypotension is common in pheochromocytoma due to depletion of plasma volume. In addition, epinephrine release may mediate vasodilation. Serotonin-secreting tumors (the carcinoid syndrome) and electrolyte disturbances such as hypokalemia are other disorders that may produce syncope. Hypoglycemia is often accompanied by signs of sympathetic nervous system overstimulation such as restlessness, tachycardia, and confusion. It may ultimately lead to loss of consciousness that begins gradually but may be prolonged and even progress to coma. The onset of the episode may be 3 to 5 hours after a meal, when there is a reactive surge of insulin, or after a prolonged fast if caused by an islets of Langerhans tumor.

Neurologic/Cerebrovascular

Neurologic problems such as migraines, seizures, or transient ischemic attacks are uncommon causes of syncope and account for less than 10% of syncopal episodes. Transient ischemic attacks are usually due to atherosclerosis of the cerebral vessels that produces ischemia, resulting in transient neurologic deficits. Neurologic deficits usually affect motor, sensory, visual, or speech faculties. They impair consciousness only when the transient ischemic attack or stroke (territory at risk) is large or when it involves the brainstem. Epileptic seizures often last longer, begin suddenly in any position with or without aura, and are associated with biting injury to the lips, injury to the body from falling, urinary incontinence, and postictal confusion and somnolence.

Psychogenic Syncope

Anxiety disorders, hysterical fainting, and panic disorders are other conditions that can be associated with syncope (~2% of cases). Anxiety disorders may produce attacks in which a patient may have dizziness due to reduced cerebral perfusion produced by prolonged hyperventilation. These episodes are not posture dependent and consequently cannot be remedied by assuming a supine position. Fainting on a hysterical basis is not accompanied by hemodynamic abnormalities attributable to changes in heart rate or blood pressure.

HISTORY

The history and the physical examination are the critical part of the initial evaluation of a patient with syncope, establishing the diagnosis in up to 50% of patients presenting with syncope. The examiner must determine the onset, frequency, and duration of premonitory symptoms; the circumstances surrounding the attacks (e.g., relation to meals, alcohol ingestion, cough, micturition, defecation, or movements of the head and neck); associated symptoms such as nausea, vomiting, chest pain, or dyspnea; medications used; and the presence of potentially predisposing disorders such as diabetes mellitus, chronic illness with weight loss, prolonged bed rest, blood loss, or plasma volume depletion.

A cardiac arrhythmia is suggested by an abrupt onset, without premonitory symptoms or signs, leading to a precipitous fall and major injury. Exertional syncope is associated with cardiac outflow obstruction, global myocardial ischemia, or tachyarrhythmias. Relation to meals, alcohol or drug ingestion, cough, swallowing, micturition, defecation, posture, abdominal pain, or a surgical procedure suggests situational syncope. Syncope with head rotation or tight collars suggests carotid sinus hypersensitivity. Premonitory symptoms (e.g., yawning, nausea, epigastric discomfort, pallor, diaphoresis) usually precede neurally-mediated syncope. Transient ischemic attacks are associated with vertigo, dysarthria, diplopia, and other motor or sensory symptoms. Syncope with arm exercise might suggest subclavian steal (from increased retrograde vertebral artery blood flow distal to a proximal subclavian artery stenosis to "steal" blood from the vertebrobasilar cerebral circulation).

Recovery from syncope is usually prompt; a seizure is followed by prolonged postictal somnolence and confusion. Atypical tonic or clonic motor activity may accompany syncope during ventricular tachycardia or fibrillation and complicates the clinical distinction of syncope from seizures.

A detailed medication history is important. First-dose syncope is associated with alpha-blockers (prazosin or terazosin), angiotensin-converting enzyme inhibitors (captopril), or nitroglycerin. Postural hypotension is associated with many antihypertensive agents and diuretics may cause hypovolemia, orthostasis, and subsequent syncope. Some drugs may be proarrhythmic (i.e., torsades de pointes), such as type IA and III antiarrhythmic agents, phenothiazines, and tricyclic antidepressants. Drugs that affect the sinus node or AV node such as methyldopa, beta-blockers, and digoxin may aggravate either carotid sinus hypersensitivity or chronic conduction system disease, resulting in complete heart block.

PHYSICAL EXAMINATION AND CLINICAL FINDINGS

A complete physical examination is necessary. Orthostatic vital signs should be obtained in every patient with syncope. Blood pressure and heart rate should be obtained in the supine, sitting, and standing positions. Recordings should be obtained immediately on standing and after several minutes. Evaluation of blood pressure in both arms and the legs, as well as recognition of bruits in the carotid, subclavian, supraorbital, and temporal vessels, may identify patients with vascular disorders such as Takayasu disease, aortic dissection, or the subclavian steal syndrome. A careful cardiac examination may detect signs of aortic stenosis, idiopathic hypertrophic subaortic stenosis, mitral valve prolapse, or pulmonary hypertension. Cyanosis, clubbing, and other signs of congenital heart disease should be sought.

Carotid sinus massage should be done as part of the workup of any patient with syncope. The presence of carotid bruits or cerebrovascular disease is considered a relative contraindication to carotid sinus massage, because it can cause contralateral hemiparesis. This test may be done in an office setting, provided intravenous access is established and atropine is available before doing the test. Carotid sinus pressure is applied separately on each side for 5 seconds, with ECG and blood-pressure monitoring in the sitting position. A pause of 3 seconds or longer or a systolic blood-pressure drop of more than 50 mm Hg without symptoms (or 30 mm Hg with symptoms) is abnormal. A positive test confirms carotid sinus hypersensitivity only if other causes of syncope can be excluded.

Stool testing for occult blood is needed to evaluate gastrointestinal bleeding. This test is particularly important in patients who are orthostatic. A thorough neurologic examination should be performed to exclude focal deficits suggesting a transient ischemic attack or stroke.

LABORATORY AND IMAGING STUDIES

In up to 50% of patients with syncope, no specific cause is found despite an extensive initial evaluation. Hospitalization is advisable when the syncopal episode has resulted in serious injury or when the initial evaluation suggests a serious underlying disorder (e.g., a cardiac arrhythmia or myocardial ischemia). Routine blood tests have a low diagnostic yield (except in appropriate clinical circumstances) but include a complete blood count to evaluate for anemia and infection; electrolyte, blood urea nitrogen, and creatinine levels to evaluate volume and metabolic status; drug and alcohol levels; and cardiac enzyme levels to rule out a myocardial infarction. Electroencephalography and computed tomography have a low diagnostic yield in patients with syncope who have a nonfocal neurologic examination, a negative neurologic history, and no carotid bruits. When a diagnosis of partial complex seizures is suspected in patients with recurrent syncope, a sleep-deprived electroencephalography with nasopharyngeal leads may be helpful. A chest x-ray is not very helpful unless congestive heart failure, pericardial effusion, or mitral stenosis is suspected. Ventilation/perfusion lung scanning or computed tomographic angiography are not routine but would be diagnostic if a pulmonary embolism is suggested by the history and physical examination.

In the evaluation of syncope, the presence of structural heart disease (coronary artery disease, congestive heart failure, valvular heart disease, or congenital heart disease) has emerged as the most important factor predicting the risk of death and the likelihood of arrhythmias. An ECG should be obtained routinely to evaluate for the presence of ischemia or infarction, arrhythmia, ventricular hypertrophy, conduction abnormalities, preexcitation from Wolf-Parkinson-White syndrome, or the long QT syndrome. Echocardiography should also be performed to help confirm or exclude the diagnosis of structural heart disease and left ventricular dysfunction, thus directing further testing and risk stratifying the patient. With a normal ECG and echocardiogram, it is unlikely that a recurrent syncopal episode will be associated with an increased mortality.

Monitoring in a telemetry unit is helpful if a serious arrhythmia is suspected. If the suspicion of a serious arrhythmia is lower, 24-hour ambulatory Holter monitoring is cost effective and advisable. Two 24-hour Holter monitoring tests performed during the course of the evaluation or a single 48-hour Holter monitoring test increases the sensitivity of detection of significant arrhythmias. If recurrent syncopal episodes are rare, capturing the cardiac rhythm during a syncopal spell may be possible by prolonged ambulatory transtelephonic monitoring with patient-activated event recorders that may be worn for months at a time. This may help differentiate arrhythmic from nonarrhythmic syncope and has been shown to be very useful in patients with unexplained syncope. The advantage of loop recorders is that their digital or solid-state memory loops can be activated after the syncopal event and can retrieve information about the cardiac rhythm during the preceding 4 minutes. Implantable event recorders can be placed subcutaneously in the chest for up to 2 years to monitor for arrhythmias as the cause of infrequent episodes of syncope.

Exercise testing may be performed to provoke arrhythmias or hypotension in patients with exertional syncope or suspected coronary artery ischemia. However, this test is rarely diagnostic. Exertional syncope in young patients should be evaluated by echocardiography to exclude aortic stenosis, hypertrophic cardiomyopathy, or mitral stenosis. Cardiac catheterization may be warranted if the echocardiogram or stress test is abnormal or if an anomalous origin of the left coronary artery from the right sinus of Valsalva coursing between the aorta and pulmonary artery is suspected (young athlete with recurrent syncope without other cardiac cause). If a patient presents with syncope and a cardiac abnormality is detected as the cause during the initial workup, referral to a cardiology subspecialist is appropriate due to the relatively high 1-year mortality (20%–30%) from the underlying cardiac cause.

Invasive electrophysiologic studies are warranted when the suspicion for cardiac syncope remains high in the face of a nondiagnostic noninvasive evaluation. Electrophysiologic tests are useful in diagnosing conduction abnormalities of the sinus node, AV node, and the His-Purkinje system. In addition, an attempt is made to provoke supraventricular and ventricular arrhythmias through electrical stimulation. Patients with underlying structural heart disease and unexplained syncope by noninvasive testing are the best candidates for electrophysiologic studies, because they have a relatively high 1-year mortality (18%–30%).

Of all patients referred for electrophysiologic testing to evaluate syncope of undetermined origin, only one third of patients will have a presumptive diagnosis established. Clinical factors identified as predictors of a positive response on electrophysiologic studies include impaired ventricular function, male sex, prior myocardial infarction, bundle branch block, and nonsustained ventricular tachycardia. The two thirds of patients with a negative response to an electrophysiologic study are considered to be at low risk of sudden cardiac death. However, in patients with severely impaired ventricular function, especially those with an idiopathic dilated cardiomyopathy, electrophysiologic studies are less predictive, and unexplained syncope in these patients even with a negative electrophysiologic study for inducible arrhythmias should be treated with an automatic implantable cardioverter-defibrillator.

Most patients without structural heart disease have neurally mediated syncope. Tilt-table testing is recommended in patients with recurrent syncope, for severe episodes (those associated with major injury or accidents), or for those with high-risk occupations such as airline pilots. An upright tilt of 60 to 80 degrees is done for 10 to 60 minutes using a tilt table with a foot board for weightbearing. An intravenous infusion of isoproterenol or nitroglycerin may be given to enhance the test's sensitivity. A positive result (bradycardia, hypotension, or both) involves the reproduction of symptoms on the tilt table, and in the absence of pharmacologic provocation the specificity of the test for vagally or neurally mediated syncope is 90%. Fig. 48.1 summarizes the general approach in the diagnostic evaluation of syncope.

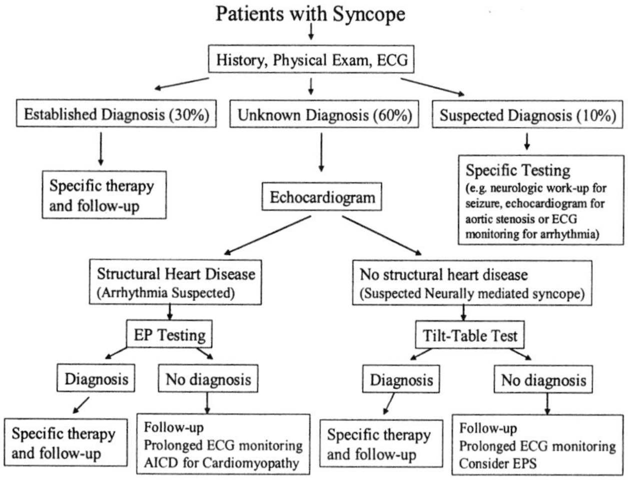

FIG. 48.1. General approach to the patient with syncope. EP(S), electrophysiology (study); AICD, automatic implantable cardioverter-defibrillator.

TREATMENT

The prognosis and treatment of syncope largely depend on the etiology. The 1-year mortality is 20% to 30% for cardiac syncope, 5% for noncardiac causes, and up to 10% for unexplained syncope. Simple measures involving the removal of offending agents may be effective for situational or reflex syncope. Postprandial syncope may be treated by eliminating hypotensive drugs before meals and resting in a supine position after meals.

Simple measures that may be taken to treat postural syncope include wearing support stockings or pantyhose, eliminating offending vasodilators, minimizing volume depletion, and using high-salt diets or mineralocorticoids (fludrocortisone). Beta-blockers (propranolol or pindolol) reduce sympathetic nervous system discharge and have been advocated for some patients with idiopathic orthostatic hypotension. Clonidine is reportedly beneficial in postganglionic idiopathic orthostatic hypotension. Vasopressor agents such as ephedrine, phenylephrine, ergotamine, or hydroxyamphetamine seldom help.

Bradyarrhythmic causes of syncope such as AV block, His-Purkinje disease, sick sinus syndrome, or the cardioinhibitory carotid sinus syndrome are generally treated with a pacemaker. However, this should be done only after removing agents that may cause sinus node or AV nodal block. Treatment of malignant tachyarrhythmias is usually guided by invasive electrophysiologic testing with radiofrequency ablation of bypass tracts in the Wolf-Parkinson-White syndrome and placement of an automatic implantable cardioverter-defibrillator for inducible ventricular tachycardia. Supraventricular tachyarrhythmias may be treated with beta-blockers, calcium channel blockers, or antiarrhythmic agents, but ventricular tachycardia is generally treated with automatic implantable defibrillators, with antiarrhythmic drug therapy reserved as an adjunct to an automatic implantable cardioverter-defibrillator to suppress frequent symptomatic episodes of ventricular tachycardia.

In the acquired long QT syndrome, withdrawal of the offending drug or correction of the metabolic or electrolyte abnormalities is usually successful. Alternatively, patients may be treated with beta-blockers for idiopathic or congenital long QT syndrome. Those who fail drug therapy may be considered for left cervicothoracic sympathectomy (stellectomy), permanent pacing, or implantation of an automatic implantable defibrillator.

The treatment of cardioinhibitory carotid sinus syncope generally includes permanent pacemaker implantation, preferably a dual-chamber model. Treatment for vasodepressor carotid sinus syncope, on the other hand, has been unsatisfactory, with limited success being reported with dihydroergotamine, ephedrine, irradiation, or surgical denervation of the carotid sinus. Syncope due to aortic stenosis is an ominous prognostic indicator and is considered an indication for surgical valve replacement.

Patients with idiopathic hypertrophic subaortic stenosis may be treated with beta-blockers, calcium channel blockers, or both. Because syncope and sudden death frequently occur with strenuous exertion in these patients, strenuous exercise should be avoided. Rapid atrial fibrillation in these patients is usually highly symptomatic and can cause syncope due to the loss of the atrial contribution to ventricular filling and the decreased left ventricular diastolic filling period. Hence, aggressive rate control should be instituted promptly, followed by pharmacologic or electrical cardioversion. If medical treatment is ineffective in preventing chest pain or syncope in these patients, a dual-chamber pacemaker with appropriate selection of an AV interval and timing of ventricular contraction may be considered. Alternatively, alcohol septal ablation or surgical myomectomy of the hypertrophied septum with or without mitral valve replacement may be considered. Although these therapies may improve symptoms of angina or syncope in these patients, they have not been shown to improve mortality. Patients with familial hypertrophic cardiomyopathy with a family history of sudden cardiac death or with a high-risk gene mutation may benefit from electrophysiologic studies with placement of an automatic implantable cardioverter-defibrillator.

Treatment of patients with neurally-mediated syncope begins with a careful history to determine precipitating factors. Initial therapy for infrequent episodes includes avoidance of precipitating factors, moderate increased salt intake, and avoiding volume depletion. First-line medications for treating more frequent episodes include beta-blockers and increased salt intake (>3 g/d). Serotonin reuptake inhibitors, midodrine, and fludrocortisone may be tried if beta-blockers are not effective. Permanent pacemaker implantation may be indicated in refractory cases who have a predominant cardioinhibitory (bradycardia or asystole) response on tilt-table testing.

SYNCOPE IN PREGNANCY

To manage heart disease during pregnancy, the clinician must understand the circulatory and respiratory adaptations to the normal gravid state. The increase in maternal blood volume starts early in pregnancy, peaks at 32 weeks, and plateaus until term, resulting in an increase of about 40% to 50% over pregestational level. The increase in intravascular volume in pregnancy sets the stage for a rise in cardiac output, which increases 30% to 50% over pregravid values. Most of this increase occurs in the first trimester due to an increase in stroke volume, with the peak at 20 to 24 weeks. As pregnancy advances, heart rate continues to rise and stroke volume declines. Cardiac lesions that cause right or left ventricular obstruction to blood flow (e.g., aortic stenosis, mitral stenosis, pulmonic stenosis, and pulmonary hypertension) are poorly tolerated during pregnancy because of the inability to raise cardiac output adequately to meet the increased hemodynamic demands. Thus, syncope may arise for the first time during pregnancy as a result of either unsuspected or previously only moderately obstructive lesions, due to the vascular changes outlined above.

Infrequently, bradycardic hypotensive syncope occurs in the supine position (supine hypotensive or uterocaval syndrome)

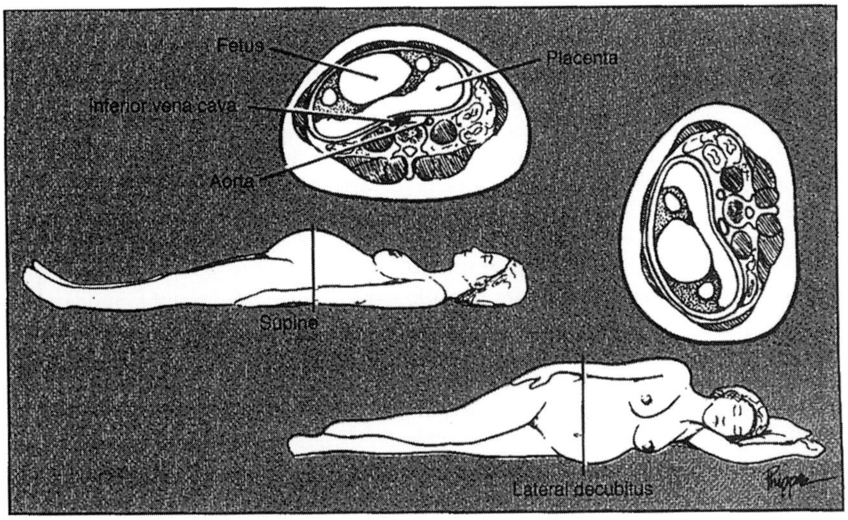

FIG. 48.2. Supine hypotensive syndrome of pregnancy. Venocaval compression of the inferior vena cava and abdominal aorta by the gravid uterus can lead to decreased venous return, leading to a reduced cardiac output and syncope in the supine position. Turning the patient on her side alleviates symptoms. (From Elkayam U, Gleicher N. *Cardiac problems in pregnancy,* 2nd ed. New York: Alan R. Liss, 1990:61, with permission.)

during the latter part of pregnancy when the gravid uterus compresses the inferior vena cava and the abdominal aorta. This dramatic event is promptly reversed by turning the patient on her left side. The bradycardia may be attributed to a selective vasovagal baroreceptor response to inferior caval compression (Fig. 48.2).

Supraventricular and ventricular arrhythmias and orthostatic hypotension also are important causes of syncope during pregnancy. Arrhythmias during pregnancy fall into two categories: benign rhythm disturbances that occur during an otherwise normal uncomplicated gestation and disturbances in rhythm associated with certain cardiac diseases that prevail in women of childbearing age. Sinus arrhythmia, occasionally sinus bradycardia or tachycardia, and atrial or ventricular premature beats are relatively common benign occurrences. The sensation of "skipped beats" during pregnancy is more likely to be caused by atrial than by ventricular premature beats. Regardless of their site of origin, sporadic premature beats are of no clinical importance if they are not subjectively disturbing and if the patient is appropriately reassured. Even bigeminy or trigeminy is generally unimportant in the pregnant woman without organic heart disease. However, multiform ventricular beats or episodes of ventricular tachycardia, especially near term, should arouse suspicion of peripartum cardiomyopathy.

Arrhythmias during pregnancy may or may not produce syncope, depending on the patient's ventricular rate and volume status. The most common arrhythmia during pregnancy is paroxysmal AV nodal reentry tachycardia. This is a relatively common rhythm disturbance, with a peak incidence in women of childbearing age. Those with a prior history are likely to have recurrences during the third trimester of pregnancy.

BIBLIOGRAPHY

Abboud FM. Neurocardiogenic syncope. *N Engl J Med* 1993;328:1117–1119.
Ailings M, Wilde A."Brugada" syndrome: clinical data and suggested pathophysiological mechanism. *Circulation* 1999;99:666–673.
Bachinsky WB, Linzer M, Weld L, et al. Usefulness of clinical characteristics in predicting the outcome of electrophysiologic studies in unexplained syncope. *Am J Cardiol* 1992;69:1044–1049.
Benditt DG, Ferguson DW, Grubb BP, et al. Tilt table testing for assessing syncope. *J Am Coll Cardiol* 1996;28:263–275.
Calkins H, Shyr Y, Frumin H, et al. The value of the clinical history in the differentiation of syncope due to ventricular tachycardia, atrioventricular block, and neurocardiogenic syncope. *Am J Med* 1995;98:365–373.
Calkins H, Zipes DP. Hypotension and syncope. In: Braunwald E, Zipes D, Libby P, eds. *Heart disease,* 6th ed. Philadelphia: WB Saunders, 2001:932.
Connolly SJ, Sheldon R, Roberts RS, et al. The North American Vasovagal Pacemaker Study (VPS): a randomized trial of permanent cardiac pacing for the prevention of vasovagal syncope. *J Am Coll Cardiol* 1999;33:16–20.
Elkayam U. Pregnancy and cardiovascular disease. In: Braunwald E, Zipes DP, Libby P, eds. *Heart disease,* 6th ed. Philadelphia: WB Saunders, 2001:2172.
Kapoor WN. Syncope. *N Engl J Med* 2000;343:1856–1862.
Kapoor WN, Fortunato M, Hanusa BH, et al. Psychiatric illnesses in patients with syncope. *Am J Med* 1995;99:505–512.
Knight BP, Goyal R, Pelosi F, et al. Outcome of patients with nonischemic dilated cardiomyopathy and unexplained syncope treated with an implantable defibrillator. *J Am Coll Cardiol* 1999;33:1964–1970.
Krahn AD, Klein GJ, Yee R, et al. Use of an extended monitoring strategy in patients with problematic syncope. *Circulation* 1999;99:406–410.
Morillo CA, Camacho ME, Wood MA, et al. Diagnostic utility of mechanical, pharmacological, and orthostatic stimulation of the carotid sinus in patients with unexplained syncope. *J Am Coll Cardiol* 1999;34:1587–1594.
Morillo CA, Eckberg DL, Ellenbogen KA, et al. Vagal and sympathetic mechanisms in patients with orthostatic vasovagal syncope. *Circulation* 1997;96:2509–2513.
Nyman JA, Krahn AD, Bland PC, et al. The costs of recurrent syncope of unknown origin in elderly patients. *Pacing Clin Electrophys* 1999;22:1386–1394.
Soteriades ES, Evans JC, Larson MG, et al. Incidence and prognosis of syncope. *N Engl J Med* 2002;347:878–885.
Sra JS, Jazayeri MR, Avitall B, et al. Comparison of cardiac pacing with drug therapy in the treatment of neurocardiogenic (vasovagal) syncope with bradycardia or asystole. *N Engl J Med* 1993;328:1085–1090.
Sutton R, Peterson MEV. The clinical spectrum of neurocardiogenic syncope. *J Cardiovasc Electrophysiol* 1995;6:569.

CHAPTER 49
Hyperlipidemia

Ara Sadaniantz

Cardiovascular disease has become the most common cause of death and chronic illness worldwide. Coronary artery disease (CAD) is the number one cause of death in the United States and the leading cause of death in women over age 65. The etiology of atherosclerotic vascular disease is multifaceted, ranging from hereditary vessel wall microenvironmental factors to cultural contributions such as nutrition, lack of physical activity, and influence of television and mass media. Among these contributing factors, hyperlipidemia is recognized as a major risk for arterial disease that now can be effectively treated. Nearly half of the 600,000 deaths occurring annually due to coronary heart disease are associated with hyperlipidemia.

Hyperlipidemia is caused by multiple factors, including poor nutrition, hereditary enzyme deficiencies, diabetes mellitus, obesity, and sedentary lifestyle. Except for hereditary issues, these factors may be effectively altered through personal choice and determination. There are also vast differences in population-based total cholesterol levels among different countries and cultures that in turn are closely related to cardiovascular event rates (Fig. 49.1). Lipid abnormalities, which include an elevation of either total serum cholesterol, low-density lipoprotein (LDL) cholesterol, and triglycerides or any combination thereof, are relatively common among American women. Childhood obesity has also reached epidemic proportions in United States.

Serum lipids are composed of various fractions consisting of cholesterol and triglycerides bound in lipoprotein transport molecules. These subfractions include LDL cholesterol, also known as atherogenic or "bad" cholesterol; high-density lipoprotein (HDL) or "good" cholesterol; and very-low-density lipoprotein cholesterol, predominantly triglycerides. Chylomicrons and intermediate-density lipoprotein are subfractions beyond the scope of this discussion.

Hypercholesterolemia, particularly an elevated LDL cholesterol level and a diminished HDL cholesterol level, is strongly correlated with the genesis of CAD. Some risk factors for CAD cannot be modified, such as age, male gender, hereditary predisposition of vessel wall, and infectious predisposition to vessel wall injury. However, other risk factors, such as hyperlipidemia, hypertension, smoking, and diabetes, can easily be diagnosed and modified.

The incidence of CAD is much lower in premenopausal women than in postmenopausal women and men of the same age. The incidence in women is approximately equivalent to that of men 10 to 15 years younger. The risk of CAD rises in postmenopausal women and approaches the incidence in men by age 70.

Risk factors for CAD in women are similar across all cultures and races. However, age-adjusted mortality from CAD has not declined as dramatically in African-American women as it has in white women over the past several decades. It is speculated that limited access to medical care, higher smoking rates, and less nutritious diets are the cause of this disparity. The most effective way to reduce the incidence of CAD in the entire population in terms of cost and outcome is to reduce the prevalence of modifiable risk factors (Table 49.1).

Modifying hypercholesterolemia is of great importance in reducing the risk of coronary heart disease. The incidence of CAD is directly related to levels of LDL and inversely related to levels of HDL. Studies of middle-aged men with mildly to moderately elevated total cholesterol levels have documented that for each 1% reduction in LDL levels and 1% increase in HDL levels, there is an associated 2% to 3% reduction in CAD. It is thought that a similar relation exists in women, although data are less certain.

In addition to the risk of CAD, the overall risk of vascular disease in general rises with hypercholesterolemia or low HDL levels. Peripheral vascular disease, retinopathy, renal disease, and central nervous system disease, such as stroke, are also influenced by serum cholesterol levels. In addition, hypertriglyceridemia with values above 200 mg/dL, predominantly in the very-low-density lipoprotein fraction, is commonly associated with reduced levels of HDL cholesterol and vascular risk. There is still debate about whether an elevated serum triglyceride level by itself is an independent risk factor for CAD. However, current recommendations are to treat specifically if triglycerides are 500 mg/dL or higher. Triglyceride values higher than this level are frequently associated with xanthelasma and pancreatitis.

DIAGNOSIS

Hyperlipidemia is diagnosed only by serum lipid levels. Physical signs of hyperlipidemia, such as xanthelasma on the eyelids and extensor tendons, cannot be used in a clinical setting for accurate diagnosis or treatment endpoints.

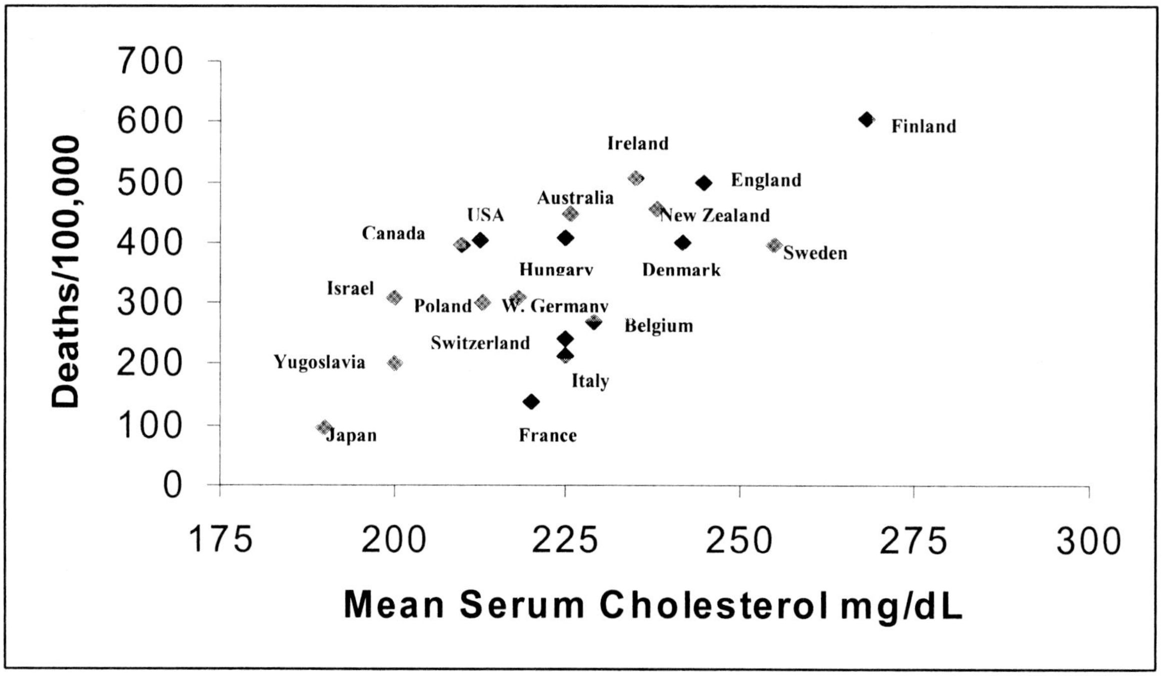

FIG. 49.1. Coronary artery disease mortality rate versus serum cholesterol. (From Simons LA. Interrelations of lipids and lipoproteins with coronary artery disease mortality in 19 countries. *Am J Cardiol* 1986;57:5G, with permission.)

TABLE 49.1. Risk Factors for Cardiac Heart Disease

Modifiable	
Cigarette smoking	
Hypertension (≥140/90 mm Hg or on antihypertensive medication)	
Obesity	
Physical inactivity	
Diabetes mellitus	
Premature menopause without estrogen replacement therapy	
Nonmodifiable	
Age and gender	
Men ≥45 yr	
Women ≥55 yr	
Family history of premature coronary heart disease	
Father <55 yr	
Mother <65 yr	

A negative risk factor is the presence of high high-density lipoprotein cholesterol (≥60 mg/dL). In the presence of high high-density lipoprotein cholesterol, one risk factor is subtracted.

From Mattson C, Koentopp C, Jackson K. Treatment of high blood cholesterol. *Clin Pharm Rev* 1995, volume 1, with permission.

Tables 49.2 and 49.3 show Adult Treatment Panel III suggested lipid levels, which in turn allows the diagnosis of hyperlipidemia. HDL is considered protective at values of 60 mg/dL or greater. LDL values are considered acceptable if a patient with fewer than two coronary heart risk factors has a value of 160 mg/dL or less. If the patient has no coronary heart disease but has two or more risk factors for CAD, then optimal LDL levels are less than 130 mg/dL. If the patient has known CAD, desirable LDL levels are less than 100 mg/dL.

However, it is difficult to categorically apply these numbers to all patients on either the high or low end. Certainly an 86-year-old woman free from CAD with an LDL of 180 mg/dL is a very different patient from a 19-year-old sedentary obese woman with an LDL of 159 mg/dL. Therefore, the numbers presented in Tables 49.2 and 49.3 need to be interpreted on an individual patient basis. Adult Treatment Panel III guidelines recommend a fasting lipid profile for all patients aged 20 and older every 5 years, even if the subject has no risk factors. Many authorities recommend that lipoprotein levels should be performed after a 9- to 12-hour fast. Yet it is generally acceptable to measure a nonfasting lipid panel. If either total cholesterol is greater than 200 or HDL less than 40 mg/dL, a full fasting lipid profile is suggested, particularly if triglycerides are elevated. Furthermore, because lipid levels relate to CAD risk assessment on a continuum, in an individual patient a fasting or random lipid level may be of small importance.

Current practice emphasizes coronary heart disease risk status as a guide to the type and intensity of cholesterol-lowering therapy. Patients with coronary heart disease or other atherosclerotic disease are at highest risk, and lower target levels for LDL should be established. In addition, age 55 or older is a major coronary heart disease risk factor in women. Drug therapy should be individualized in premenopausal women with high LDL levels who are otherwise at low risk for coronary heart disease. The decision to treat "high LDL" in premenopausal woman with high HDL is even more controversial, and treatment needs to be individualized based on all risk factors. Postmenopausal women with hyperlipidemia have a high risk for coronary heart disease, so in general pharmacologic treatment is recommended. More attention must be paid to HDL levels as a coronary heart disease risk factor. HDL and LDL levels should be included in all cholesterol determinations. A high HDL level should be viewed as a negative risk factor for CAD and should be considered when selecting drug therapy.

THERAPY

As well-randomized clinical studies accumulate, the question has shifted from whether we should reduce serum cholesterol concentration to how low the cholesterol should be. The answer depends in part on whether the patient has established CAD (Fig. 49.2). CAD mortality is significantly reduced in the patient with established CAD when cholesterol is reduced. Yet the rate of CAD mortality remains quite flat in patients without established CAD over a wide range of serum cholesterol concentration. Currently, well-randomized studies are in progress to improve our understanding of how low LDL should be, especially in patients with established CAD.

Diet and Exercise

Diet and risk factor modification are in order if HDL levels are less than 35 mg/dL and the patient has no other associated lipid

TABLE 49.2. LDL Cholesterol Goals and Cutpoints for Therapeutic Lifestyle Changes and Drug Therapy in Different Risk Categories

Risk category	LDL goal (mg/dL)	LDL level at which to initiate therapeutic lifestyle changes (mg/dL)	LDL level at which to consider drug therapy (mg/dL)
CHD or CHD risk equivalents (10-yr risk >20%)	<100	≥100	≥130 (100–129: drug optional)[a]
Two + risk factors (10-yr risk ≤20%)	<130	>130	10 year risk 10–20%: ≥130 10 year risk <10%: ≥160
Zero to 1 risk factor[b]	<160	≥160	≥190 (160–189: LDL lowering drug optional)

[a]Some authorities recommend use of LDL lowering drugs in this category if an LDL cholesterol level of <100 mg/dL cannot be achieved by therapeutic lifestyle changes. Others prefer use of drugs that primarily modify triglycerides and high-density lipoprotein, e.g., nicotinic acid or fibrate. Clinical judgment also may call for deferring drug therapy in this subcategory.

[b]Almost all people with 0–1 risk factors have a 10-yr risk <10%; thus, 10-yr risk assessment in people with 0–1 risk factors is not necessary.

CHD, coronary heart disease; LDL, low-density lipoprotein.

From Expert Panel on Detection, Evaluation, and Treatment of High Blood Cholesterol in Adults. Executive Summary of The Third Report of The National Cholesterol Education Program (NCEP) Expert Panel on Detection, Evaluation, And Treatment of High Blood Cholesterol In Adults (Adult Treatment Panel III). *JAMA* 2001;285(19):2486–2497, with permission.

TABLE 49.3. ATP III Classification of LDL, Total, and HDL Cholesterol (mg/dL)

LDL cholesterol	
<100	Optimal
100–129	Near or above optimal
130–159	Borderline high
160–189	High
≥190	Very high
Total cholesterol	
<200	Desirable
200–239	Borderline high
≥240	High
HDL cholesterol	
<40	Low
≥60	High

ATP, adult treatment panel; LDL, low-density lipoprotein; HDL, high-density lipoprotein.
From Expert Panel on Detection, Evaluation, and Treatment of High Blood Cholesterol in Adults. Executive Summary of The Third Report of The National Cholesterol Education Program (NCEP) Expert Panel on Detection, Evaluation, And Treatment of High Blood Cholesterol In Adults (Adult Treatment Panel III). *JAMA* 2001;285(19):2486–2497, with permission.

abnormalities, if HDL levels are low and LDL levels are high, or if there are triglyceride abnormalities. For patients failing nonpharmacologic therapy, drug therapy should follow. Treatment recommendations are summarized in Table 49.2 and discussed in the next section.

When a patient is determined to be hyperlipidemic, the first intervention should be a careful nutritional history. The challenge for the practicing physician is to select an appropriate diet, among many "authoritative protocols" such as American Heart Association Step I and II, Atkins diet, Mediterranean diet, Weight Watchers diet, and others. The decision needs to be individualized to the patient and available resources. An obese and hyperlipidemic patient must attempt to lose weight. This combination can be most challenging to effectively treat. Weight loss and exercise promote a reduction of cholesterol levels and have other beneficial effects as well, including reduced triglycerides, increased HDL levels, lowered blood pressure, and a decreased risk of diabetes.

Nutrition

The emphasis on reduction of serum cholesterol level to reduce CAD and related clinical events is very important. Dietary therapy to reduce serum cholesterol levels has focused on fat intake. Unfortunately, many guidelines, public information sources, and commercial food sources have promoted the concept of low fat intake without any significant emphasis on total caloric intake. When fat is removed from the diet, it is generally replaced with carbohydrates, resulting in higher calories per portion, an imbalance of nutritional value, a false sense of security, and a hungry individual. This in turn causes higher triglycerides, higher total and LDL cholesterol, obesity, and a higher risk of diabetes mellitus.

In the now classic Lyon Diet Heart Study, 600 men and women were randomized to a specific Mediterranean diet versus no dietary advice. After 104 weeks there was no change in total cholesterol, triglyceride, lipoproteins, apoproteins, weight, or blood pressure between the groups. But 20 deaths occurred in the control group compared with 8 in the experimental (Mediterranean diet) group. Therefore, we can safely assume that the type of food one eats affects the risk of cardiovascular death independent of lipid levels. On the other hand, in epidemiologic studies, the French and Albanian paradox are real, and despite high fat intake in France and the lower social economic status of Albania, both populations enjoys a low CAD risk. It seems that a Mediterranean or Indo-Mediterranean diet may be more heart healthy than the Step I and II National Cholesterol Education Program prudent diet.

A balanced diet is the best approach. One should limit fat intake, but it makes little sense to replace a small scoop of genuine ice cream with a huge serving of fat-free, sugar-loaded, artificial, frozen concoction. Olive oil should be used when possible as a replacement for other fats. All attempts should be made to include complex carbohydrates such as beans, rice, root vegetables, fruits, and green vegetables and to avoid processed carbohydrates touted as low-fat healthy food for breakfast and snacks. Modest amounts of proteins are essential for healthy living and balance. Most importantly, total calorie intake needs to be watched carefully and to equal daily calorie expenditure for a person of ideal body weight. With the over-

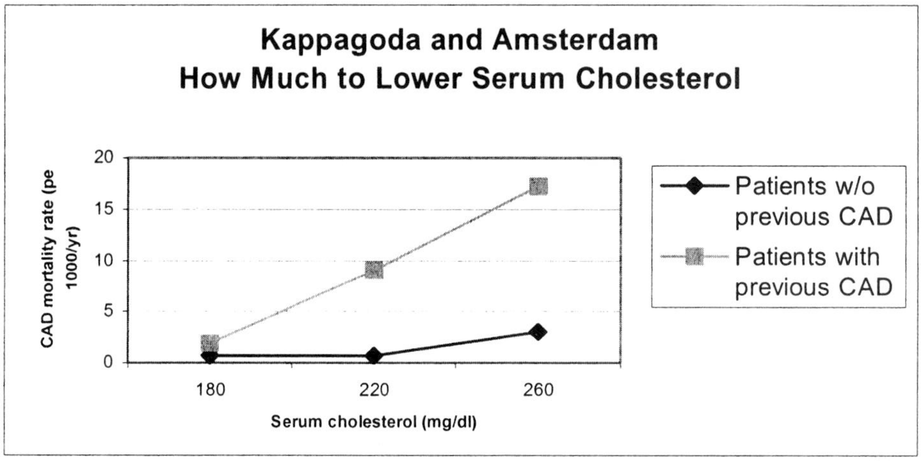

FIG. 49.2. Relationship between coronary artery disease (CAD) mortality rate and serum cholesterol. The patients with previous evidence of CAD have a steeper relationship compared with those without. These data were obtained from the Lipid Research Clinics Program Prevalence Study, in which patients received no lipid lowering treatment (6). (From Kappagoda CT, Amsterdam EA. How much to lower serum cholesterol: is it the wrong question? *J Am Coll Cardiol* 1999;34:289–292, with permission.)

weight patient, the daily caloric intake must be less than expenditure to achieve weight loss.

The importance of "empty calories" associated with sugar and highly refined grains needs to be emphasized. In the milling process of flour, 60% to 90% of vitamin B_6, vitamin E, folate, and other nutrients are lost. Some food products are fortified with thiamin, riboflavin, and niacin. But it is suspected that many other micronutrients are lost and not replaced. Therefore, it is best to avoid empty calories even when fortified.

There are good and bad carbohydrates. The glycemic index of carbohydrates (low for beans and high for glucose, instant rice, and bread) is a significant determinant for plasma HDL. Patients who consume food low in glycemic index have higher HDL levels. Total cholesterol intake should be restricted to less than 200 mg/d. The services of a registered dietitian or other qualified nutritional expert are usually necessary to achieve compliance with this intensive diet.

Exercise is an effective adjunctive therapy for lowering cholesterol and minimizing cardiac risk factors. Aerobic exercise, achieving a maximal heart rate of 60% to 80% of the age-adjusted pulse rate, for 30 to 45 minutes every other day is adequate. Exercise also promotes weight loss, in addition to its other beneficial effects. Patients at risk for CAD should be screened before starting a regular exercise regimen. Vigorous exercise also increases beneficial HDL levels.

Pharmacologic Treatment

It is important to think in terms of primary and secondary prevention once the diagnosis of hyperlipidemia is made. If healthy eating, weight loss, and exercise do not result in adequate control of cholesterol or triglyceride levels, drug therapy may be appropriate. Primary prevention of coronary heart disease regardless of risk factors should be considered for patients with an LDL level of 190 mg/dL or greater. If a patient with more than two other cardiac risk factors has an LDL value above 160 mg/dL, drug therapy should be instituted. Diabetes should be considered a very serious risk factor, and in these patients LDL should be aggressively reduced.

As an example of primary prevention, the Air Force/Texas Coronary Atherosclerosis Prevention Study evaluated the effect of lovastatin on patients free from coronary heart disease and with "average" lipid levels. Total cholesterol was 221 ± 21 mg/dL and LDL 150 ± 17 mg/dL. There were 997 women in the study. At the end of the study there was a 37% relative reduction in acute major cardiovascular events (fatal or nonfatal myocardial infarction, unstable angina, or sudden cardiac death) with lovastatin compared with placebo.

Secondary prevention is of paramount importance because 18% of men and 35% of women with coronary heart disease have another coronary event within 6 years after the first heart attack. Multiple randomized studies have shown a significant benefit of lipid reduction in patients with known vascular disease.

Secondary prevention is the attempt to lower cholesterol in patients who have already developed coronary heart disease. In general, the goal for LDL should be 100 mg/dL or less in these patients. If the patient has an LDL level greater than 100 mg/dL, then earnest diet and exercise therapy should be initiated. If LDL level is greater than 130 mg/dL, then aggressive drug therapy is appropriate.

There are four major categories of drugs used to lower cholesterol, triglycerides, or both and to raise HDL cholesterol: bile acid sequestrants, niacin, β-hydroxy-β-methylglutaryl-coenzyme A (HMG-CoA) reductase inhibitors (statins), and other drugs (fibric acid derivatives, probucol, ezetimibe [Zieta]). Table 49.4 lists certain drug effects on lipoproteins.

The selection of pharmacologic agent for a given patient must be individualized based on comorbid conditions, the type of lipid abnormality, patient preference, tolerance, and cost. The process is probably similar to selecting an antihypertensive medication. A brief description of the currently available pharmaceutical agents follows.

BILE ACID SEQUESTRANTS

Bile acid sequestrants, such as colestipol and cholestyramine, are effective and safe in lowering total cholesterol and LDL levels by up to 15% to 30% while raising HDL levels by 3% to 5%. These medications are particularly effective in primary prevention when therapy is required in premenopausal women with moderately elevated LDL levels. They may also be used in more severe forms of hypercholesterolemia in combination with other drugs. These medications are generally safe. They are not absorbed from the gastrointestinal tract and therefore lack systemic effects. Constipation and bloating are common but can be minimized by the use of fiber-based stool softeners. Psyllium may reduce gastrointestinal symptoms; even when used alone, psyllium may reduce cholesterol by up to 5% to 10%. Sequestrants may decrease the absorption of certain oral medications, such as HMG-CoA reductase inhibitors, thiazide diuretics, digoxin, fat-soluble vitamins, and anticoagulants. All other medications taken coincidentally should be taken 1 hour before or 4 hours after the sequestrant dose. Sequestrants are generally most effective and best tolerated when taken before or with meals.

β-HYDROXY-β-METHYLGLUTARYL-COENZYME A REDUCTASE INHIBITORS

All HMG-CoA reductase inhibitors are relatively similar in efficacy at lower doses. These agents cause a decrease in the total cholesterol level of 20% to 40% and an increase in HDL of 5% to

TABLE 49.4. Drug Effects on Lipoproteins

Drug	Total cholesterol and LDL	HDL	Triglycerides
Niacin	↓ 15–25%	↑ 15–35%	↓ 20–50%
Sequestrants	↓ 15–30%	↑ 3–5%	0% or slight ↑
HMG-CoAs	↓ 20–40%	↑ 5–15%	↓ 10–20%
Gemfibrozil	↓ 10–15%	↑ 10–15%	↓ 20–50%
Probucol	↓ 5–15%	↓ 20–30%	0%
Zetia	↓ 15–20%	↓ 2–4%	↓ 5–10%

HDL, high-density lipoprotein; LDL, low-density lipoprotein; HMG-CoAs, β-Hydroxy-β-methylglutaryl-coenzyme A. Modified from Mattson C, Koentopp C, Jackson K. Treatment of high blood cholesterol. *Clin Pharmac Rev* 1995, volume I, with permission.

15%. They may also decrease triglycerides by 10% to 20%. When used as monotherapy, this class of drug is most effective when taken in the evening. These medications are well tolerated by most patients. Gastrointestinal intolerance, with gas, bloating, and constipation, is usually mild and subsides over time. Myopathy is rare, occurring in less than 0.1% of patients. Myopathy becomes much more common when this class of drug is used in combination with cyclosporine, niacin, and gemfibrozil. Abnormal liver function studies occur infrequently and generally resolve completely when the dose is reduced or discontinued.

Prolonged prothrombin times have been reported when HMG-CoA therapy is initiated. Long-term safety data on the use of these drugs are limited, so they should probably be avoided in primary prevention in young females. In severe hypercholesterolemia or if secondary prevention is required, the use of an HMG-CoA reductase inhibitor with a sequestrant drug or niacin has been shown angiographically to reduce progression and increase regression of coronary artery lesions. But this change is relatively small. The true effect of cholesterol reduction results in a very significant reduction in clinical events, strongly suggesting stabilization of coronary plaques. Because abnormal liver function studies may develop, HMG-CoA reductase inhibitors are contraindicated during pregnancy and nursing and in patients with liver disease.

NICOTINIC ACID

Nicotinic acid is effective in lowering total cholesterol and triglyceride levels and raising levels of HDL. Niacin may lower cholesterol 15% to 25% and lower triglycerides 20% to 50%. HDL levels may rise as much as 15% to 35% in patients treated with niacin. Nicotinic acid has several side effects, including flushing, pruritus, gastrointestinal disturbances, liver toxicity, hyperuricemia, and hyperglycemia. Patients should be started on low-dose short-acting or immediate-release preparations. Dosage of niacin should start at 250 mg/d and should gradually be increased over several-week intervals to a daily maximal dosage of 1,500 to 3,000 mg. Low-dose aspirin or a nonsteroidal drug given 60 minutes before the morning dose may mitigate flushing and pruritus when therapy is begun or when the dosage is increased. Niacin given with meals reduces gastrointestinal disturbances.

Niacin should be avoided or used with great caution in patients with a history of gout, peptic ulcer disease, liver disease, and non–insulin-dependent diabetes and in elderly patients. Postural hypotension may occur in patients, particularly elderly women, who are taking antihypertensive drugs because of an additive vasodilatory effect. Sustained-release preparations of niacin should be avoided, because they have been associated with an increased incidence of hepatic dysfunction. Because of its significant effect on LDL, HDL, and triglycerides, nicotinic acid is particularly valuable in treating high blood cholesterol levels in patients with low HDL levels or in the treatment of combined hyperlipidemia. It is quite effective in the treatment of hypertriglyceridemia.

OTHER MEDICATIONS

Fibric acid drugs, such as gemfibrozil, lower cholesterol 10% to 15% and raise HDL 10% to 15% as well. They also lower triglyceride levels by 20% to 50%. This class of medication is most effective in lowering triglyceride levels, particularly in patients with familial dysbetalipoproteinemia (type III hyperlipoproteinemia). These drugs also may be effective when used in combined therapy and particularly when used in diabetic patients with elevated triglycerides.

Gemfibrozil is generally well tolerated but occasionally causes gas or mild indigestion. Gemfibrozil use increases the risk of developing cholesterol gallstones. It can also potentiate the effect of warfarin. Because gemfibrozil has a relatively low impact on total cholesterol and LDL levels, it is generally reserved for use in diabetics and combination drug therapy. Unfortunately, when it is used in conjunction with other medications, particularly HMG-CoA reductase inhibitors, the risk of myositis increases. However, a careful periodic history and liver function tests and creatine phosphokinase at appropriate intervals (every 2–6 months depending on the patient) will minimize the risk of myositis and hepatitis.

The enthusiastic estrogen replacement therapy of 1980 through 1990 was recently shown to be of no significant value in large, well-randomized, prospective studies. Hence, at this time there is no evidence to start a woman on estrogen replacement therapy prophylactically to prevent CAD. It is possible that in the future, different combinations or selective estrogen types may be helpful in postmenopausal women to reduce the risk of CAD.

Ezetimibe (Zetia) is a newer pharmacologic agent available to reduce serum cholesterol levels. Its mechanism of action differs from those of other classes. It inhibits the absorption of cholesterol by acting at the brush border of the small intestine. It does not seem to interact with anticholesterol agents in other classes in a negative fashion, and when given concurrently it further reduces serum cholesterol levels.

COMBINATION THERAPY

When pharmacologic monotherapy, in conjunction with diet and exercise, has failed to yield the desired result, combination drug therapy may be used. It may also be considered if the desired results are achieved but the patient is poorly tolerant of the medication used or the lifestyle imposed by therapy. Combining medications from several lipid-lowering drug classes at lower doses is generally better tolerated, more efficacious, and may increase compliance with the regimen compared with higher dose single-agent therapy. In addition, it may be more cost effective to use lower doses of two medications than to use a high dose of a single medication, although this depends on the medications involved. When combination therapy is required, hepatic and renal functions must be monitored. Common combinations include a bile acid sequestrant with either niacin or an HMG-CoA reductase inhibitor. HMG-CoA reductase inhibitors have also been successfully combined with gemfibrozil, but this combination increases the risk of severe myopathy.

Alcohol

Alcohol in moderation may favorably influence lipid levels. "Moderation" is defined as a daily amount not exceeding 2 oz of hard liquor, two 6-oz glasses of wine, or two 12-oz glasses of beer. Several studies have documented a lowering of total cholesterol and an increase in HDL. Some studies have indicated that this benefit occurs only if the calories from alcohol are substituted for other calories, particularly those that contain fat. If alcohol is ingested in addition to a regular caloric load, benefits may also accrue in terms of diminished CAD despite persistently elevated cholesterol levels. This phenomenon has been found in certain populations that ingest large quantities of red wine. Some researchers believe the phenol dye created in the production of red wine may be a scavenger for free radicals that ultimately diminishes arterial endothelial damage. In any event, some populations ingesting red wine, despite a high fat intake, are relatively protected from CAD. It is not known if this principle is applicable in all populations.

Alcohol increases triglyceride levels and may increase the risk of CAD in patients prone to hypertriglyceridemia, particularly when triglyceride levels alone are viewed as a cardiac risk factor. It seems prudent to recommend the ingestion of low-dose alcohol if patients desire alcohol as part of their daily consumption and if the alcohol is substituted for other calories in a still nutritionally sound diet.

HYPERTRIGLYCERIDEMIA

Elevated serum triglyceride levels are positively correlated with coronary heart disease in univariate analysis but are not as strongly predictive when other cardiac risk factors are added. There is an association between hypertriglyceridemia, low HDL levels, and very atherogenic forms of LDL. This seems to be the case in women with diabetes and in certain familial combined hyperlipidemias. Patients with triglyceride levels above 500 to 1,000 mg/dL have an increased risk of acute pancreatitis.

Nonpharmacologic therapy, with weight reduction in overweight patients and alcohol avoidance and enhanced physical activity for all patients, is generally required. A strict trial of carbohydrate reduction is recommended in all patients with high triglycerides. Drug therapy should be considered when triglyceride levels are elevated in association with familial combined hyperlipidemia or in diabetic patients with high triglyceride levels. Fibric and nicotinic acid medications are generally used in this situation and are also used to prevent acute pancreatitis in patients with triglyceride levels above 1,000 mg/dL. Increased triglyceride levels may be a signal for alcohol abuse, diabetes mellitus, obesity, and hypothyroidism. A careful history and clinical evaluation are warranted.

SECONDARY DYSLIPIDEMIA

Diabetes mellitus, chronic renal failure, nephrotic syndrome, and hypothyroidism commonly cause secondary dyslipidemia. Diabetes mellitus is frequently accompanied by an elevated triglyceride level and a low HDL level. It is important to treat diabetic women in this category aggressively, because diabetes seems to negate any benefit of the premenopausal state. Tight control of diabetes and correction of the hypothyroid state generally improve the lipid abnormality. Nephrotic syndrome is usually associated with hypertriglyceridemia and generally can be controlled with nonpharmacologic therapy.

SEVERE FORMS OF HYPERCHOLESTEROLEMIA

Severe elevations of cholesterol occur in a number of conditions. Familial hypercholesterolemia occurs in 1 in 500 people and is characterized by marked elevations of LDL. Severe polygenic hypercholesterolemia manifests as LDL levels exceeding 220 mg/dL. It occurs in about 1% of the adult population and is commonly associated with premature coronary heart disease. Familial combined hyperlipidemia is characterized by elevations of total cholesterol, triglycerides, or both in different members of the same family. It occurs in about 1% of the population and causes premature coronary heart disease. In any female presenting with these severe forms of hypercholesterolemia, family screening is mandatory to detect other members at risk who may benefit from therapy.

CHOLESTEROL IN THE ELDERLY

The risk of CAD and cardiovascular death is much lower among premenopausal women compared with men. However, after menopause there is a sharp rise in the incidence of both CAD and cardiovascular death. The role of lipid abnormality among postmenopausal women is well established, but the effect of cholesterol level on prevalence of CAD among women after age 65 is more nebulous.

Data for octogenarian women is even more sparse. In an observational study among patients with documented CAD (26% women), if statin therapy was initiated in the hospital, follow-up mortality was reduced in all age groups (<65, 65–70, >80). In the Prosper Study, in patients aged 70 to 82 where 52% were women, those patients with known vascular disease or high risks for CAD pravastatin treatment for 3 years had a reduced risk of CAD death, but there was an increase in the incidence of cancer death. All-cause mortality, however, was unchanged. In a community-based study of 724 patients aged 85 and older where 72% were women, higher cholesterol concentration was associated with longevity due to lower mortality from cancer and infection.

CONSIDERATIONS IN PREGNANCY

Fatty streak formation begins during fetal life. The progression during childhood of fatty streaks to adult CAD is clear. Pathologic findings unquestionably demonstrate that antepartum risk factors strongly influence the severity of vascular lesions in children and young adults. The FELIC Study demonstrated that maternal serum cholesterol level during pregnancy causes changes in fetal aortic fatty streaks. Lesions progressed strikingly faster in children with hyperlipidemic mothers. Hence, there is good reason for dietary lipid-lowering intervention for the expectant hyperlipidemic mother. At this time, drug intervention during pregnancy is not suggested because the risk and benefit of such intervention has not been studied. Currently, cholesterol-reducing drugs are not recommended during pregnancy.

REFERRAL

Most patients with a lipid disorder can be safely managed by the primary care provider. However, referral to a lipid specialist, commonly a cardiologist or an endocrinologist with an interest in lipids, should be considered if the goals of therapy are not achieved. Referral should also be considered if control is adequate but the patient does not tolerate the medication and lifestyle changes well. For certain noncompliant patients, referral to a specialist is a strong signal that the condition is serious and requires attention.

SUMMARY

The goal of treatment of hyperlipidemia is to reduce the incidence of coronary heart disease and vascular disease. The primary care provider must identify patients at risk for hyperlipidemia-induced coronary heart disease and must reduce the prevalence of other modifiable risk factors that can lead to enhanced coronary disease. Patients must be advised of the need for lipid control, but the clinician must weigh the potential adverse effects of medications against the potential gains.

Hypercholesterolemia is a chronic disease that frequently requires lifelong dietary and drug therapy. Because patients often do not feel any symptoms from hyperlipidemia, it is sometimes difficult to ensure compliance with medications that may cause adverse effects. The clinician must educate the patient in this regard and provide motivation and credibility relative to the importance and benefits of ongoing therapy.

BIBLIOGRAPHY

Assmann G, Carmena R, Cullen P, et al., for the International Task Force for the Prevention of Coronary Heart Disease. Coronary heart disease: reducing the risk—a worldwide view. *Circulation* 1999;100:1930–1938.

De Lorgeril M, Salen P, Martin J-L, et al. Mediterranean dietary pattern in a randomized trial: prolonged survival and possible reduced cancer rate. *Arch Intern Med* 1998;158:1181–1187.

De Lorgeril M, Salen P, Martin J-L, et al. Mediterranean diet, traditional risk factors, and the rate of cardiovascular complications after myocardial infarction (final report of the Lyon Diet Heart Study). *Circulation* 1999;99:779–785.

Denke MA. Individual responsiveness to a cholesterol-lowering diet in postmenopausal women with moderate hypercholesterolemia. *Arch Intern Med* 1994;154:1977.

The Esprit Team: Cherry N, Gilmour K, Hannaford P, et al. Oestrogen therapy for prevention of reinfarction in postmenopausal women: a randomised placebo controlled trial. *Lancet* 2002;360:2001–2008.

Hulley S, Grady D, Bush T, et al., for the Heart and Estrogen/progestin Replacement Study (HERS) Research Group. Randomized trial of estrogen plus progestin for secondary prevention of coronary heart disease in postmenopausal women. *JAMA* 1998;280:605–613.

Irons BK, Snella KA, McCall K, et al. Update on the management of dyslipidemia. *Am J Health-System Pharmac* 2002;59:1615–1625.

Johnson CL, Rifkind BM, Sempos CT, et al. Declining serum total cholesterol levels among U.S. adults. The National Health and Nutrition Examination Surveys. *JAMA* 1993;269:3002.

Kant AK, Schatzkin A, Graubard BI, et al. A prospective study of diet quality and mortality in women. *JAMA* 2000;283:16:2109–2115.

Kappagoda CT, Amsterdam EA. How much to lower serum cholesterol: is it the wrong question? *J Am Coll Cardiol* 1999;34:1:289–292.

Larsen ML, Illingworth DR. Drug treatment of dyslipoproteinemia. *Med Clin North Am* 1994;78:225.

Napoli C, Glass CK, Witztum JL, et al. Influence of maternal hypercholesterolaemia during pregnancy on progression of early atherosclerotic lesions in childhood: Fate of Early Lesions in Children (FELIC) study. *Lancet* 1999;354: 1234–1241.

National Cholesterol Education Program. Summary of the second report of the National Cholesterol Education Program (NCEP) Expert Panel on Detection, Evaluation, and Treatment of High Blood Cholesterol in Adults (Adult Treatment Panel II). *JAMA* 1993;269:3015.

Pitt B, Waters D, Brown WV, et al., for the Atorvastatin Versus Revascularization Treatment Investigators. Aggressive lipid-lowering therapy compared with angioplasty in stable coronary artery disease. *N Engl J Med* 1999;341: 70–76.

Sacks FM, Pfeffer MA, Moye LA, et al., for The Cholesterol and Recurrent Events Trial Investigators. The effect of pravastatin on coronary events after myocardial infarction in patients with average cholesterol levels. *N Engl J Med* 1996; 335:14:1001–1009.

Scandinavian Simvastatin Survival Study Group. Randomised trial of cholesterol lowering in 4444 patients with coronary heart disease: the Scandinavian Simvastatin Survival Study (4S). *Lancet* 1994;344:1383–1389.

Sempos CT, Cleeman JI, Carroll MD, et al. Prevalence of high blood cholesterol among U.S. adults: an update based on guidelines from the second report of the National Cholesterol Education Program Adult Treatment Panel. *JAMA* 1993;269:3009.

Singh RB, Dubnov G, Niaz MA, et al. Effect of an Indo-Mediterranean diet on progression of coronary artery disease in high risk patients (Indo-Mediterranean Diet Heart Study): a randomised single-blind trial. *Lancet* 2002;360:1455–1461.

Stampfer MJ, Sacks FM, Salvini S, et al. A prospective study of cholesterol, apolipoproteins, and the risk of myocardial infarction. *N Engl J Med* 1991; 325:373.

Waters DD, Alderman EL, Hsia J, et al. Effects of hormone replacement therapy and antioxidant vitamin supplements on coronary atherosclerosis in postmenopausal woman: a randomized controlled trial. *JAMA* 2002;288: 2432–2440.

Willett WC. Diet and health: what should we eat? *Science* 1994;264:532–537.

CHAPTER 50
Heart Failure in Women

Nadine Sauvé and Margaret A. Miller

Heart failure (HF) is a relatively common health problem, causing a tremendous amount of morbidity, mortality, hospitalizations, and cost worldwide. It was just recently recognized as a major health issue for women, with epidemiologic data showing higher prevalence of HF in elderly women compared with men. Research has recently exploded with treatment opportunities for patients suffering from HF. There are clear gender differences in types of HF, etiologies, prognosis, and even response to treatment. Unfortunately, women were underrepresented in trials, and data about women are often lacking or incomplete. People are now recognizing the particularities of HF in women, and there is a trend toward including more women in trials and studying them specifically.

DEFINITIONS

HF is the final common pathway of numerous cardiac diseases and systemic disorders affecting the heart. HF is the *clinical syndrome* resulting from the inability of the heart to provide enough perfusion to tissues and/or the compensatory mechanisms developed to fulfill those requirements. HF is divided into different types.

Systolic versus Diastolic

Systolic HF is secondary to myocardial loss of contractile capacity. Causes include myocardial infarction, viral myocarditis, or end-stage valvulopathy. In most trials, systolic dysfunction was defined as echocardiographic measurement of ejection fraction (EF) below 40%. In *diastolic* dysfunction (DD), the myocardium is unable to relax appropriately (restrictive cardiomyopathy or acute ischemia) *or* something is preventing it from filling normally (constrictive pericarditis, hypertensive cardiomyopathy). The diagnosis of DD is controversial. Some experts believe that the classic findings of HF syndrome with a normal EF of the left ventricle on imaging done within 72 hours from the episode should be enough. A study showed that when those two criteria are present, echocardiogram or left heart catheterization confirmed the diagnosis of DD in 94% and 92% of cases, respectively. The diagnosis is supported by the underlying clinical conditions likely associated with DD: elderly patient, hypertension, recent onset tachyarrhythmia contributing to HF episode, and evidence of coronary artery disease. Systolic dysfunction and DD can exist concomitantly.

Low Output versus High Output

In *low-output* HF, the heart is responsible for tissue hypoxic state. In *high-output* HF, the needs of peripheral tissues are so high that even a normal heart cannot fulfill them. This is found with hyperthyroidism, anemia, and pregnancy but also with rare disorders like Beri-Beri, severe Paget disease, or arteriovenous fistulae. From a clinical standpoint, it is often not possible to distinguish one from the other.

PATHOPHYSIOLOGY

The numerous mechanisms used by the body to compensate for failing cardiac output are responsible for the clinical manifestations of HF. They are initially helpful in restoring and maintaining arterial pressure and cardiac output but with time become exaggerated and harmful.

In response to any type of myocardial injury causing either systolic dysfunction or DD, the activation of various neurohumoral systems are seen, including the sympathetic nervous system, the renin-angiotensin-aldosterone system, and increased production of the antidiuretic hormone, atrial natriuretic peptide, and brain natriuretic peptide (BNP). Other substances like endothelium factors (endothelin, nitric oxide) and cytokines, including tumor necrosis factor, are also implicated.

These neurohumoral factors result in peripheral vasoconstriction that will try to maintain arterial pressure by redistribution of blood flow to vital organs. Increased myocardial contractility and heart rate will maintain cardiac output. Volume expansion also contributes by increasing venous return and elevating end-diastolic volume. This will, based on the Frank-Starling mechanism, result in a rise of stroke volume.

Unfortunately, the balance of beneficial and deleterious effects of these adaptations is clearly negative with chronicity. The increased left ventricular afterload induced by high peripheral resistance contributes to deterioration of myocardial function. Ischemia is worsened by catecholamine-stimulated contractility and tachycardia. Elevated end-diastolic pressure is transmitted retrogradely to the pulmonary and systemic vasculature, contributing to pulmonary and peripheral edema. Maladaptive hypertrophic remodeling, fibrosis, and apoptosis promoted by catecholamines and angiotensin II contribute to further deterioration of the myocardial function.

EPIDEMIOLOGY

Six percent to 10% of people older than 65 years suffer from HF in North America. Globally, prevalence seems to be equal in women and men, although among patients older than 70 years the prevalence of HF in women is higher than in men. According to a recent report from the Framingham Heart Study, in the last 50 years the incidence of HF has decreased among women but not in men, probably due to a more aggressive treatment of hypertension, the principal cause of HF in women. Survival after the onset of HF has improved in both sexes. In the United States and Canada, HF is the number one diagnosis for hospitalization and cost.

ETIOLOGY

Underlying Causes

For *systolic* HF, the two major etiologies are hypertension and coronary artery disease. Less frequent ones are outlined in Table 50.1. For *diastolic* dysfunction, the vast majority of patients do not have a defined myocardial disease. The most common identified causes are hypertension (hypertrophic nonobstructive cardiomyopathy), ischemic heart disease, hypertrophic obstructive cardiomyopathy, and restrictive cardiomyopathy, mainly infiltrative diseases (Table 50.1). Aging is believed to be a contributing factor in many.

There is a clear gender difference with etiology of HF. A hypertensive woman is more at risk to develop HF than a man with the same degree of hypertension. Coronary artery disease is less frequently a cause of HF in white women and is more frequently in cause in African-American women compared with men. However, when a woman does sustain a myocardial infarction, her risk of HF is higher. Women with HF are more likely to have diabetes, obesity, or valvular heart disease than men. Peripartum cardiomyopathy is particular to women and is discussed later. Anthracycline chemotherapy for breast cancer should always be considered in exposed patients. Finally, more women than men have an unknown cause of left ventricular dysfunction. It is of paramount importance to try to establish precisely the cause of HF because treatment and prognosis is directly dependent of etiology.

TABLE 50.1. Etiologies of Systolic Myocardial Dysfunction

Hypertension
Coronary artery disease
Valvulopathy
Cardiomyopathy
Idiopathic dilated
Alcohol
Viral myocarditis
Toxic (chemotherapy)
Parasitic myocarditis (Chagas disease)
Infiltrative
Hemochromatosis
Amyloidosis
Connective tissue disease
Sarcoidosis
Metabolic (hypothyroidism)
Diabetes
Persistent tachyarrhythmia
Chronic high-output heart failure (hyperthyroidism, anemia)

Precipitating Causes

Acute disturbances that place an additional load on the fragile heart are often responsible for the first or recurrent HF decompensations. The most frequent precipitating factors are listed in Table 50.2. Specifically applicable to women in childbearing ages, pregnancy can precipitate failure in a previously compen-

TABLE 50.2. Precipitating Causes of Heart Failure Exacerbations

High output
Infection or fever
Anemia
Hyperthyroidism
Pregnancy
Emotional stress
Exercise
Substance abuse
Arteriovenous shunt, Paget disease
Volume overload
Excessive sodium or water intake (IV or PO)
Salt-retaining drugs (corticosteroids, nonsteroidal antiinflammatory drugs)
Renal failure
Decreased myocardial function
Tachyarrhythmia or bradyarrhythmia
Hypertension
Hypoxemia
Ischemia
Pulmonary embolism
Ethanol
Metabolic disturbances (hypocalcemia, hyper/hypoglycemia)
Medications (beta-blockers, nondihydropyridine calcium channels blockers, chemotherapeutic agents)
Noncompliance to heart failure therapy

sated heart. It is very important to meticulously look for those factors because their treatment can drastically modify the course of the acute episode and the prognosis.

EVALUATION AND DIAGNOSIS

The two parts in the evaluation of a patient suspected of HF are confirming the presence of the syndrome and looking for its etiology. Unexpectantly, when a diagnosis of HF is posed clinically in a woman, there is less chance than in a man that the echocardiogram will confirm a myocardial dysfunction. DD is then suspected to be the underlying pathologic finding. Some data suggest that women presenting with HF are less likely to be evaluated by echocardiogram, referred to the hospital, or seen by specialists.

History

Symptoms can be divided in antegrade or retrograde, depending if they result from low cardiac output or increased ventricular end-diastolic pressure, respectively. *Retrograde symptoms* from the *left side* of the heart are well recognized. Dyspnea is the most frequent symptom. Initially only with activity (interstitial edema increases the workload of the respiratory muscles already depleted in oxygen by the low cardiac output), dyspnea can progress and occur with minimal activity or even at rest. Then, orthopnea, nocturnal cough, and paroxysmal nocturnal dyspnea may appear because of redistribution of fluid from the abdomen and lower extremities to the chest during recumbency. Others factors, such as ventilatory center depression and diminished myocardial function by reduced adrenergic stimulation during sleep, may also contribute. The patient usually will need to sit or stand for 30 to 45 minutes before symptoms attenuate. Lower extremity edema or anasarca is a retrograde symptom from the *right side* of the heart. Hepatic congestion causing abdominal pain and fullness from ascites is also frequently described. This may result in anorexia.

Antegrade symptoms are less well recognized, because they are less specific, but are certainly a major cause of morbidity. Asthenia and weakness are reputed to be secondary to the limited capacity of the failing heart to deliver oxygen to the exercising muscles. Particularly in the elderly patient, hypoxemia and reduced cerebral perfusion can cause cognitive difficulties.

Physical Examination

These symptoms will translate into various signs, depending on severity. Respiratory distress, with tachypnea and cyanosis, is seen is severe cases. Cheyne-Stokes respiration (cyclic pauses alternating with tachypnea) can be seen with severe prolongation of the circulation time from the lung to the brain. Tachycardia is frequent, if not blocked by medication. Arrhythmia (e.g., atrial fibrillation) can be perceived on physical examination. Blood pressure is characterized by diminished pulse pressure and increased diastolic pressure because of systemic vasoconstriction. Hypotension is an ominous sign. Hepatojugular reflux followed by frank jugular vein distension are right heart's retrograde classic signs. Further down, hepatomegaly with tender and pulsatile liver can be seen, sometimes so severe that ascites and icterus (from hepatic dysfunction and hepatocellular hypoxia) can appear. At the heart level, an S_3 or S_4 can be heard with eccentric or concentric hypertrophy, respectively. Murmurs from the etiologic valve anomaly or from the secondary mitral or tricuspidal regurgitation that comes with the heart dilation can be heard. The apex is usually displaced laterally and enlarged in systolic dysfunction and only sustained in diastolic failure from hypertrophic myocardium. Coarse crepitants, sometimes with wheezing (cardiac asthma), are typical of pulmonary edema. Dullness to percussion at the lung bases can reveal pleural effusions (right side more than left side). Cardiac cachexia is a late finding.

The New York Heart Association (NYHA) classification is useful to the clinician for prognostic purposes and to guide therapy, because benefits of medication in studies are reported according to these classes:

Class I: Symptoms of HF only at levels that would limit normal individuals.
Class II: Symptoms of HF with ordinary exertion.
Class III: Symptoms of HF on less than ordinary exertion.
Class IV: Symptoms of HF at rest.

Women are found to have more symptoms and signs of HF, especially edema, exercise intolerance, an S_3, and jugular vein distension. This could be partially explained because DD causes more symptoms and women have a higher prevalence of DD; this is also true for systolic dysfunction and so is not well elucidated. For women, their absolute number of hospitalizations, annual admission rate, and duration of stay is higher. Contributing factors proposed include older age, more comorbidities, and the fact that they live alone more often than men.

Chest X-Ray

A chest x-ray can confirm the presence of pulmonary edema and eliminate some other causes of dyspnea. In acute settings, cephalization of pulmonary vessels and peribronchovascular edema are usually present first and then progress to septal lines. Frank alveolar edema comes next. Pleural effusion is more a subacute finding. Cardiomegaly is seen with ventricular enlargement. Cardiac silhouette and valvular calcifications can help identify the underlying anomaly.

Electrocardiogram

Most patients with systolic dysfunction have an abnormal electrocardiogram (left ventricular hypertrophy, ischemic signs, left bundle branch block, etc.). The negative predictive value of a normal electrocardiogram is 98% for systolic dysfunction. Arrhythmia can also be detected.

Blood and Urine Testing

Complete blood count, electrolytes (including calcium and magnesium), blood urea nitrogen, serum creatinine, glucose, blood lipids, liver function tests, thyroid-stimulating hormone, and a urinalysis are considered the baseline initial workup. If any other specific etiology is suspected from personal or familial history and physical examination, they should then be sought: hemochromatosis screening (iron saturation and ferritin), antinuclear antibody, rheumatoid factor, serum and urinary protein electrophoresis (amyloidosis), and urinary metanephrines or vanillylmandelic acid (pheochromocytoma). Human immunodeficiency virus serology is recommended by some without strong data. Recently, BNP has been advocated to help differentiate cardiogenic from noncardiogenic dyspnea. In both systolic dysfunction and DD, ventricular cells will secrete BNP stimulated by high ventricular filling pressure and the serum level will increase. This can be an early finding in asymptomatic patients with left ventricular dysfunction. BNP could even become the first paraclinic test to rule out HF as the cause of nonspecific dyspnea or effort intolerance in the future.

Transthoracic Echocardiogram

Two-dimensional transthoracic echocardiogram with Doppler flow studies is probably the most useful diagnostic tests. It can assess ventricular function and ventricular hypertrophy, chamber size, valvular function, and any septal defects. One false belief is that regional wall motion abnormalities are compatible with coronary artery disease. In fact, it can be seen in 50% to 60% of idiopathic dilated cardiomyopathy. Transthoracic echocardiogram can also identify pericardial thickening, abnormal myocardial texture (amyloidosis), right ventricle size and function, and pulmonary artery pressure.

Radionuclide Ventriculography

This test can also assess global and segmental ventricular contractility and dilation of both left and right heart but does not provide any information about valves, hypertrophic walls, pericardium, or pulmonary artery pressure. It can be useful in patients not optimally evaluated by transthoracic echocardiogram (e.g., pulmonary disorders, morbid obesity).

Cardiac Catheterization

According to the American College of Cardiology and the American Heart Association (ACC/AHA), cardiac catheterization is required for every patient considered a candidate for revascularization who has *known or suspected* coronary artery disease. The author's opinion is that *every* patient with an *unexplained* cardiomyopathy should be catheterized because it is by far the more frequent etiology in North America and treatment of coronary artery disease can impact directly on prognosis.

Noninvasive Myocardial Imaging

Non-invasive myocardial imaging, with or without stress, can be considered in patients with known coronary artery disease but no clinical clues of active ischemia to detect ischemia and assess viability of the myocardium if candidates for revascularization. Noninvasive myocardial imaging is also recommended by the ACC/AHA to diagnose coronary artery disease, although no strong data support this. One option could be to reserve these noninvasive tests when no revascularization is considered in a patient, but finding coronary heart disease would change medical management.

Endomyocardial Biopsy

Also very controversial, endomyocardial biopsy can be done if inflammatory or infiltrative disease is strongly suspected. The diagnostic yield remains low because these diseases are often patchy and pathology nonspecific. This test should not be considered routine.

PREVENTION

The current HF guidelines recommend aggressive treatment of hypertension, diabetes, and lipid disorders according to their respective guidelines. They also suggest avoidance of smoking and alcohol and drug abuse. Angiotensin-converting enzyme inhibitors (ACEIs) should be started according to the HOPE study in every patient over age 55 years with coronary or peripheral vascular disease or stroke or diabetics (with one other cardiovascular risk factor) for significant primary or secondary prevention of cardiovascular mortality. Supraventricular tachyarrhythmias should be treated, as well as thyroid disease. All susceptible patients should be periodically assessed for signs and symptoms of HF and evaluated by transthoracic echocardiogram if present. For asymptomatic patients, noninvasive evaluation of left ventricular function is more controversial but still recommended with strong family history of cardiomyopathy or for patients receiving cardiotoxic intervention. It should not be use routinely in other patients.

TREATMENT

There are three essential components in the management of HF. First, the underlying etiology should be treated. Every patient with ischemic heart disease must be evaluated for possible revascularization by angioplasty or bypass surgery *if* the underlying myocardium is demonstrated viable. There is a clear benefit to survival in patients with angina with bypass surgery. Valvuloplasty or valvular replacement surgery are also options in HF from valvular disease before irreversible cardiac injury or pulmonary hypertension occur. Hypertension must be controlled with agents that are appropriate for the type of HF (systolic or diastolic). Alcoholic cardiomyopathy can regress with decreased consumption. Treatment of dysthyroidism and arrhythmias is also necessary. Hereditary hemochromatosis occurs in 0.5% to 1.0% of whites. Phlebotomy early in the course of the disease can reverse the pathologic changes in the myocardium.

Second, precipitating factors should be corrected. Anemia is worth mentioning here because it is frequent in chronically ill patients. Some preliminary data on a small group revealed that correction of anemia with erythropoietin and iron supplements to hemoglobin over 12 g in severe HF patients (NYHA class III–IV) could improve mortality, left ventricular EF, need for diuretics, and hospitalization duration. The rest of the potential precipitating factors are listed in Table 50.2 and should be sought and corrected when possible. Finally, HF should be treated and further deterioration of cardiac function prevented.

Lifestyle Modifications

Salt restriction, by avoiding salt-rich food and salt added at the table, is more important than water restriction. A very severe diet with less than 2 g of sodium per day is rarely necessary. Water restriction is mainly reserved for the hyponatremic patient or those who are clearly exacerbated with increased intake. Limited ethanol intake is suggested to all HF patients, and abstinence is essential for ethanol-induced HF. Vaccination for influenza annually and against pneumococcus in every HF patient is part of routine care. The old recommendation to HF patients to avoid exercise has been challenged in the past decade. Some studies have shown the reversal of skeletal muscle abnormalities with decreased sympathetic nervous system activation and improvement in exercise tolerance and clinical status with cardiac rehabilitation exercise programs. A decrease in clinical events has also been suggested, but there are still no good data on mortality. No change in EF has been reported after training, which confirms the finding that exercise performance does not perfectly correlate with EF. An individualized program of exercise training should be offered to all stable NYHA class I to III patients starting with an exercise test. Aerobic and resistance training are recommended. It is known that women are less often referred for cardiac rehabilitation, although they benefit from it.

Drug Therapy

Women were clearly underrepresented in major trials on HF, with an estimated zero to 32% proportion only. The data available on women for each class of medication are presented in each section. Small numbers, retrospective subgroup analysis, and more frequent discontinuation of drugs in women must be taken into account to interpret those results. Awaiting new data specifically about women, the results of most studies are generalized to them.

To understand the rationale of HF treatment, we must understand the *two mechanisms* by which drug therapy is beneficial in these patients:

1. By counteracting the compensatory mechanisms that are deleterious on the long term. This includes the *sympathetic nervous system* with the use of beta-blockers and the *renin-angiotensin-aldosterone system* with ACEIs (block conversion of angiotensin I to angiotensin II, a potent vasoconstrictor), angiotensin II receptor blockers (ARBs; block the action of angiotensin II on receptor AT I, which is responsible for vasoconstriction, sodium retention, proliferation, as opposed to receptor AT II, which is responsible for vasodilatation, antiproliferative effect and against apoptosis), and spironolactone (a direct antagonist of aldosterone effect). *Volume retention* should also be reduced with the use of diuretics.
2. By increasing myocardial contractility with inotropic agents (digoxin).

VASODILATORS

ACEIs improve survival in all degrees of myocardial dysfunction (EF <40%), including asymptomatic patients. They also improve symptoms. There is concern that ACEIs and ARBs are less effective in women than men, but it is uncertain at this point if this is purely an effect of underenrollment with insufficient statistical power to demonstrate benefit. ACEIs are clearly the first line of treatment and should be part of the arsenal against HF in *all* patients with an EF less than 40% (class I–IV) unless side effects or contraindication preclude their use. This is probably a class effect, but using the agents and doses that have been well studied is recommended. The "start low, go slow" rule applies (Table 50.3). This can be hastened in the inpatient setting under direct surveillance but is recommended no more rapidly than every 7 to 14 days as an outpatient. The highest dose has been clearly proven better than a lower dose.

Hypotension, acute renal failure, and hyperkalemia should be followed closely (before and 7–14 days after each increment of dose). A certain increase in creatinine is possible and tolerated (up to 2.4 mg/dL or 220 μmol/L according to some experts) because the benefit on mortality clearly outweighs the risk. The major side effect is cough, caused by inhibition of bradykinin breakdown by the same enzyme, mandating discontinuation in 5% of patients. Contraindications to ACEIs are progressive or severe renal failure (creatinine ≥2.4 mg/dL or 220 μmol/L), hyperkalemia (≥5.0–5.5 mEq/L), bilateral stenosis of the renal arteries, hypotension (systolic blood pressure <80–85 mm Hg), and angioedema.

Studies have failed to demonstrate superiority of *ARBs* over ACEIs. In fact, we still do not have the proof that they are equivalent to ACEIs, although most experts believe so. Even if no data exist comparing them with hydralazine–nitrates combination, they are currently considered *second* line for patients who are intolerant (mostly intractable cough) to ACEIs. The combination of an ACEI and an ARB was evaluated recently in a multicenter trial. There was no benefit to mortality from the combination, but it decreased hospitalizations and symptoms and improved EF, NYHA class, and quality of life. There was one concern that addition of an ARB to an ACEI *with* a beta-blocker could increase mortality. This needs to be evaluated further, so for now caution is required.

Adding an ARB to an ACEI can be considered in very symptomatic patients not currently taking a beta-blocker. Extreme caution is warranted in combining an ACEI, an ARB, and spironolactone because this was not previously evaluated and confers a very high risk of hyperkalemia. Contraindications for ACEIs and ARBs are the same. Side effects, except for cough, and follow-up during adjustments of therapy are identical to ACEIs. Starting and objective doses are found in Table 50.3.

The combination of *hydralazine and isosorbide dinitrate* has been shown to decrease mortality and improve symptoms to some extent, although it is not as powerful as an ACEI. It can be

TABLE 50.3. Recommended Starting and Objective Dosing of Major Heart Failure Drugs

Drug	Starting dose	Maintenance dose
ACEI		
Captopril	6.25 mg tid	25–50 mg tid
Enalapril	2.5 mg q day	10 mg bid
Lisinopril	2.5 mg q day	5–20 mg q day
Perindopril	2 mg q day	4 mg q day
Ramipril	1.25–2.5 mg q day	2.5–5 mg bid
Trandolapril	1 mg q day	4 mg q day
Beta-blockers		
Bisoprolol	1.25 mg q day	10 mg q day
Carvedilol	3.125 mg bid	25–50 mg bid
Metoprolol[a]	6.25–12.5 mg bid	100 mg bid
Metoprolol XL	12.5–25 mg q day	200 mg q day
ARB		
Losartan	25 mg q day	50 mg q day
Valsartan	40 mg bid	160 mg bid
Others		
Hydralazine	25 mg tid	100 mg tid
Isosorbide dinitrate	10 mg bid or tid	40 mg bid or tid
Isosorbide mononitrate[a]	30 mg q day	120 mg q day

[a]Drugs not studied directly in heart failure trials. Doses suggested by experts.
ACEI, angiotensin-converting enzyme inhibitors; ARB, angiotensin II receptor blockers.

used in the cases where ACEIs and ARBs are contraindicated. We have no evidence in women to confirm this. Hypotension and reflex tachycardia are the major side effects. Starting and objective doses are found in Table 50.3. Combination of an ACEI or ARB with hydralazine and/or nitrates in persistently symptomatic patients can also be attempted.

BETA-BLOCKERS

Beta-blockers are now clearly part of the treatment of all NYHA class II and III patients. It should be carefully considered in stabilized class IV patients, but data are conflicting. According to the ACC/AHA and Canadian guidelines, NYHA class I should also be considered, especially post-myocardial infarction. Pooled data on beta-blocker trials confirmed the mortality benefit in women, which seems to be equivalent to men. They decrease mortality anywhere from 20% to 65%.

Carvedilol, bisoprolol, and metoprolol should be used preferentially because they are the drugs studied so far. Carvedilol, a β_1-, β_2-, and α_1-blocker, is the most likely to cause hypotension. Beta-blockers with intrinsic sympathomimetic activity should be avoided. Contraindications are severe bronchospasm and advanced heart block, and caution is required with bradycardia below 60 beats/min. Prior stabilization of the patient's condition for at least 4 weeks is mandatory. Patients should be euvolemic at the initiation of therapy. The "start low, go slow" rule also applies. Doses should be doubled if tolerated every 2 to 3 weeks up to the dose shown in Table 50.3.

An initial pharmacologic effect (negative inotropy) can cause deterioration of symptoms with hypotension, pulmonary congestion, and peripheral edema that can be helped by adjusting diuretic and/or vasodilators. If too severe, beta-blockers should be decreased to the previous step but not completely stopped if possible, and the patient should be restabilized (sometimes 2–12 weeks are necessary) before a new attempt to increase dosage is made. It may take a few attempts to finally succeed. With time (up to 1 year), the biologic effect of beta-blockers in HF will occur (depression of adrenergic system) and the patient will then feel better. The highest dose similar to the study doses should be aimed for if tolerated. If hypotension is preventing introduction or increase in beta-blockers dose, a moderate dose of both ACEIs and beta-blockers is probably better than the maximal dose of each alone, although this has not been studied and is based on expert opinions only.

DIURETICS

The only reason to start a diuretic other than spironolactone in HF is clear clinical demonstration of fluid overload. Loop diuretics are usually necessary. Addition of a thiazide or potassium-sparing diuretic is sometimes useful in refractory cases to potentiate the effect of the loop diuretic by blocking sodium reabsorption at a different level (distal or collecting tubule, respectively). Diuretics should be titrated down as ACEIs are increased. One should remember that ACEIs also have a significant effect on water and sodium balance either directly or through increased cardiac inotropy and renal perfusion. A common mistake is to maintain a high dose of diuretic, lowering blood pressure and preventing escalating doses of "mortality-affecting drugs" (ACEIs and beta-blockers).

Spironolactone is considered apart in this category. It was recently proven that a small dose of 25 mg/d was capable of dramatically decreasing mortality (30%) in NYHA class III to IV patients on ACEI therapy. The outcomes were not specified for the 27% of female participants. It is believed to do so by preventing the toxic effect of aldosterone on remodeling and fibrosis of the heart and blood vessels and by decreasing arrhythmia by increasing potassium level. The major side effect is hyperkalemia when combined with an ACEI, and this needs to be followed regularly (at least 5 days after introduction). Contraindications are creatinine over 2.5 mg/dL (225 μmol/L) or potassium over 5.0 mEq/L.

DIGOXIN

There is clearly no benefit to mortality from digoxin, but a clear benefit to symptoms and number of hospitalizations has been demonstrated in populations of men and women. Digoxin may be added to any patient with NYHA class II to IV who is still symptomatic on ACEIs. Another indication of digoxin is to control ventricular rate in patients with chronic or paroxysmal atrial fibrillation. Initial dose depends on patient renal function (0.0625–0.25 mg/d) with initial follow-up of serum level, the toxic level being close to the therapeutic interval. This may be especially true in women where mortality was increased by 4.2% in a post-hoc analysis, potentially due to higher serum levels for the same dose compared with men. These findings are not strong enough for experts to believe we should abandon digoxin in all women, but this raises the issue that digoxin levels should be monitored more closely in women and that they can have higher levels than men on equivalent doses. According to the DIG trial, around 0.7 μg/L is ideal; 1.0 μg/L or more could be detrimental, predisposing patients to arrhythmias. Once adjusted, there is no need to repeat serial blood levels unless risk factors are present (renal failure, noncompliance) or symptoms of toxicity are present (nausea, arrhythmia, cognitive dysfunction). The dose should be halved if amiodarone is started due to their interaction. We should be aware that stopping digoxin abruptly can cause exacerbation of HF symptoms.

OTHER INOTROPIC AGENTS

Dobutamine, amrinone, and milrinone have been used in acute settings for decompensated HF. There is no role to date in the long-term management of HF because of the potential adverse effect on survival.

The two major objectives of pharmacologic treatment of HF are to *decrease mortality* (ACEI/ARB or combination hydralazine-dinitrate, beta-blockers, spironolactone) and to *improve symptoms* (ACEI, ARB, or hydralazine-dinitrate, beta-blockers, digoxin, diuretics). Table 50.4 is a good summary of indications for drug therapy in all stages of systolic HF.

Other Therapies

PACEMAKERS

Cardiac resynchronization with atrial-synchronized biventricular pacing may improve symptoms, quality of life, exercise capacity and EF and decrease hospitalization in HF patients with dilated left ventricle, EF less than 35%, and NYHA class III to IV *with* an intraventricular conduction delay (QRS ≥130 ms). In an ongoing study, major complications during installation have been reported in 1.2% of patients and technical failure in 8%.

DEVICES

Extracorporeal and implantable left ventricular assist devices are approved for support of the patient in acute decompensation, patients with expected short-term recovery (viral myocarditis), or as a bridge to heart transplant only.

CARDIAC SURGERY

Mitral valve repair is considered beneficial in certain cases of idiopathic dilated cardiomyopathy with secondary mitral

TABLE 50.4. Therapeutic Agents Summary According to the NYHA Classification

	NYHA class			
	I	II	III	IV
ACE inhibitor*	All	All	All	All
BB	Consider	All	All	Consider if stable
Spironolactone			All	All
Digoxin		If symptoms	If symptoms	If symptoms
Diuretics		If fluid retention	If fluid retention	If fluid retention

ACE, angiotensin-converting enzyme; BB, beta-blockers; NYHA, New York Heart Association.
*Or ARB, if ACEI not tolerated.

regurgitation in NYHA class III or IV patients before transplant is considered.

CARDIAC TRANSPLANT

Cardiac transplant can improve survival and quality of life in severe HF. Only 20% of transplant recipients are women. Coronary artery disease and idiopathic dilated cardiomyopathy are less frequent in women and HF is more frequent in elderly women, which can partially explain this low percentage of transplants. The criteria are strict and include NYHA class IV, failed maximal medical therapy, no surgical options (bypass), poor 1-year survival, reproducible maximal oxygen uptake during exercise of less than 15 mL/kg/min, and good rehabilitation capacity. No other serious disease should be present. The small number of donors limits the use of this very effective approach.

COMPLICATIONS

Arrhythmias

Atrial fibrillation occurs frequently (10%–50%) with HF. Losing the atrial systole, responsible for 20% to 25% of the cardiac output, can be dramatic in these patients. Mortality is increased in HF patients with atrial fibrillation. The major goal is to control the ventricular response with beta-blockers, amiodarone, digoxin, or atrioventricular nodal ablation with permanent pacemaker insertion. Restoration of sinus rhythm is desirable in some patients who do not tolerate atrial fibrillation well. Antiarrhythmic drugs of class 1 are contraindicated in HF patients because of increased mortality in this setting. However, all these patients, either in chronic or paroxysmal atrial fibrillation, should be anticoagulated to prevent thromboembolic events if no contraindication is present.

Ventricular Arrhythmia

Ventricular tachycardia or ventricular fibrillation are responsible for approximately one half of HF deaths. Beta-blockers have been shown to reduce sudden death in HF patients, so this is another good reason to include beta-blockers in HF treatment. For symptomatic ventricular tachycardia or survivors of ventricular fibrillation, the treatment of choice is an implantable cardiac defibrillator. If the patient is not a candidate, beta-blockers and amiodarone are alternatives. Asymptomatic nonsustained ventricular tachycardia should be evaluated by electrophysiological studies in every patient with an EF of 35%. If ventricular tachycardia/ventricular fibrillation is inducible during electrophysiological studies and the patient is a good candidate for an implantable cardiac defibrillator, this is the procedure of choice. Amiodarone is, again, an alternative in patients who are not candidates for an implantable cardiac defibrillator, but this is much more controversial and should be discussed with an electrophysiologist. A provocative recent trial on implantable cardiac defibrillator in all post-myocardial infarction patients with an EF below 30% showed benefit to survival. The cost effectiveness of this alternative is clearly an issue. The ACC/AHA does not recommend routine use of ambulatory electrocardiographic monitoring for the detection of asymptomatic ventricular arrhythmia in HF patients.

Thromboembolic Complications

Women with HF are believed to be more at risk than men to suffer from pulmonary embolism, and clinical suspicion should always be present. Coumadin is clearly indicated in every cardiomyopathy patient with atrial fibrillation, patients who had previous cardioembolic manifestations, or those with has a well-documented intracavitary thrombus. It is more controversial in patients in sinus rhythm. Although some recommend that EF below 30% warrants coumadin therapy, this is based on weak data. A recent Cochrane systematic review did not recommend routine anticoagulation in HF patients in sinus rhythm. Whether the risk-to-benefit ratio is different in women is unknown. Aspirin has not been shown so far to reduce thromboembolic risk in these patients. An ongoing prospective trial should answer this question.

DIASTOLIC DYSFUNCTION

This topic is particularly pertinent for women because about 50% of HF in women is due to DD. Although representing 20% to 40% of overall patients with HF, DD has never been studied in multicenter, randomized, controlled trials. There are no data on asymptomatic DD. For symptomatic DD, recommendations are based on small studies and expert opinions from clinical experience and pathophysiologic concepts.

There are three major objectives in treating diastolic HF. First, symptoms should be reduced. We can reduce pulmonary congestion in diastolic HF by reducing end-diastolic pressure. Slowing down the heart rate to 60 to 70 beats/min at rest with beta-blockers or nondihydropyridine–calcium channel blockers (diltiazem or verapamil) can help accomplish this. It is a particularly important factor in patients with atrial fibrillation. Some experts encourage restoration of sinus rhythm in this situation. Beta-blockers and calcium channel blockers are also believed to cause regression of left ventricular hypertrophy. Decreasing total blood volume with diuretics and decreasing central blood volume (preload) with nitrates are also helpful. Although most of these are the same drugs used in systolic HF, they are not used for the same purpose. Beta-blockers will be better tolerated in DD and do not need to be started at very small doses and titrated as slowly. Diuretics must be used more cautiously because the problem is mostly misdistribution more than global overload of fluid. They can be very useful acutely, but long-term use should be evaluated carefully. There is probably no indication for positive inotropic agents in diastolic HF, and they may in fact aggravate the problem by increasing ischemia and heart rate and inducing arrhythmias. There is a lot of controversy over the benefit of digoxin in decreasing symptoms in the Digitalis Investigation Group trial, but data were incomplete and a recent review underlines a possible risk for increase DD with its use.

The second objective is to limit neurohumoral activation. ACEIs, ARBs, and aldosterone antagonists can help by improving fluid retention and central and systemic volume and minimizing remodeling of the left ventricle (hypertrophy, fibroblast activity, interstitial fibrosis) and functional myocardial stiffness (intracellular calcium handling). They therefore can help to decrease symptoms and to improve exercise capacity in patients with DD. Two trials (PEP-CHF and CHARM) are ongoing to define the role ACEIs and ARBs in DD. Other vasodilators are not indicated and can even be detrimental by inducing reflex tachycardia and drastically reducing blood pressure, stroke volume, and cardiac output.

The third major objective in treating diastolic HF is to correct the underlying pathologic disease causing the DD. Attention should be directed to hypertension, ischemia, valvulopathy, and any other underlying disease.

REFERRAL TO A SPECIALIST

Any patient that has a systolic dysfunction and is a candidate for revascularization should be referred to a cardiologist to be evaluated for cardiac catheterization. All patients without an obvious etiology for systolic dysfunction or DD, especially hypertrophic or infiltrative disease, should also be referred. Arrhythmias, especially ventricular, should be referred to an electrophysiologist. Severe HF that does not respond to standard therapy should be evaluated for optimization of treatment, possible participation in ongoing trials on new treatments and evaluation for heart transplant.

ACUTE TREATMENT OF HEART FAILURE

Nonspecific treatment of HF and specific treatment of its potential precipitating factor should be started, if possible, simultaneously. The first step is to ensure oxygenation. Sitting the patient up with dependent legs and a 100% nonrebreathing mask should be done first, followed by, if not sufficient, noninvasive positive pressure ventilation or endotracheal intubation with mechanical ventilation. Then diuretics should be given intravenously. Furosemide is the drug of choice, being powerful and rapid. A bladder catheter is needed to measure diuresis accurately and immediately. The initial dose depends on renal function and previous exposure to diuretics. Furosemide 20 to 40 mg intravenously is a good start, and the dose should be doubled every 20 to 30 minutes until a good diuresis is obtained (>250–300 mL). If a dose of furosemide does not produce a satisfactory response, it should not be repeated but instead doubled until the threshold dose required is found.

Vasovenodilators such as intravenous or sublingual nitroglycerine and intravenous morphine are useful in decreasing preload and afterload and lowering end-diastolic volume. If these measures do not improve the patient's symptoms, intravenous inotropic agents can be started. The edematous patient with slow progression of symptoms is likely to have systolic dysfunction and volume overload. In this case, diuretics will be the most useful and should be repeated every 8 to 12 hours for several days. In the rapidly occurring "flash" pulmonary edema (minutes to hours) with mild or no peripheral edema, the patient is probably euvolemic but has misdistribution of its volume. Preload modifiers agents like nitroglycerine will be most useful and diuretics will help acutely but should be repeated only as needed after the initial recuperation.

FOLLOWING HEART FAILURE PATIENTS

The key to good treatment is close contact and communication between health care providers and patients. This permits early detection of deterioration and quick response and adjustment of treatment. Patients should be educated about their disease, the symptoms and signs of deterioration, and have a clear emergency plan if this occurs (whom to call, how to increase diuretics, when to present to hospital). They should weigh themselves daily and keep a diary. Measuring weight, renal function, and electrolytes regularly and with each change of medication is mandatory. Recently, adding BNP to the blood workup for routine follow-up has been shown to facilitate tighter control of HF.

CONSIDERATIONS IN PREGNANCY

There are many changes in cardiovascular physiology during pregnancy. Blood volume increases by 30% to 50%, starting as early as the sixth week, reaching its maximum around the 26th to 28th weeks, and plateaus in the third trimester. Cardiac output increases by as much as 40%. This dramatic change is produced by an increase in preload and stroke volume early on and maintained by increased heart rate late in pregnancy. Systemic vascular resistance drops by 25% to 30%. Blood pressure decreases during pregnancy, reaching its nadir in the second trimester. Central venous pressure, pulmonary capillary wedge pressure, and pulmonary artery pressure remain the same. Colloid oncotic pressure is decreased with hypoalbuminemia. Pregnancy is clearly a hyperdynamic state. Labor and delivery also drastically alter hemodynamic steady state. Contractions result in tachycardia and hypertension and increase preload by approximately 500 mL, increasing cardiac oxygen consumption. Sudden hypotension can occur with epidural analgesia or blood loss. Caesarean section can also be stressful for the heart because of increased blood loss and possibility of rapid introduction of analgesia/anesthesia. A normal heart adapts easily to these changes, but a patient with an underlying cardiac anomaly may decompensate into HF.

The diagnosis of HF is similar to that of a nonpregnant patient. Clinically, some physiologic changes of pregnancy can be mistaken as manifestations of HF. Some degree of tachycardia, low arterial pressure, high jugular vein pressure, third heart sound, displaced and enlarged apex, systolic functional flow murmur, and lower extremity edema can all be seen normally in late pregnancy. Mild electrocardiographic changes and increase pulmonary markings on chest x-ray due to mammary tissue are possible. Transthoracic echocardiogram is the diagnostic tool of choice, as is the stress echocardiogram, if required.

Because women are having babies later in life, all the etiologies and precipitating factors quoted in Tables 50.1 and 50.2 are to be considered. However, there are some specific considerations related to pregnancy. The initial prenatal visit is often the first real contact with health care providers, so undiagnosed anomalies like congenital heart disease or ignored rheumatic valvulopathy may be discovered then. Second, pregnancy and delivery are a major hemodynamic stress. In general, regurgitant valvular lesions are better tolerated than stenotic lesions. A surgically repaired septal defect or cyanotic congenital heart problems are usually well tolerated if there is no severe systolic dysfunction, pulmonary hypertension, or hypoxemia and cyanosis. For endocarditis prophylaxis, some experts recommend antibiotic prophylaxis at delivery (vaginal or cesarean section) for high and moderate risk valvulopathies because of the high-output state that may increase the risk. Third, some diseases or conditions are specifically associated with pregnancy. Peripartum cardiomyopathy is a severe disorder causing systolic left ventricular dysfunction, occurring usually toward the end of the pregnancy or during the postpartum period. It is a dilated cardiomyopathy caused by a myocarditis of unknown etiology, possibly immunologic, and is associated with high risk of thromboembolism and arrhythmia. Treatment is the same as previously described except that hydralazine and nitrates should be used in pregnant women because ACEIs are contraindicated during pregnancy (renal failure in the fetus). ACEIs should be substituted after delivery and are compatible with breast-feeding. Antepartum thromboprophylaxis with heparin is recommended and can be changed to coumadin postpartum. If EF is lower than 35% or a thrombus is seen, therapeutic heparin is recommended by experts. Fifty percent of patients are markedly improved after 6 months of evolution. Although the EF may return to normal on a standard echocardiogram, some patients still have a suboptimal response to hemodynamic stress demonstrated by a dobutamine stress echocardiogram. Fifty percent remain with a variable degree of ventricular dysfunction and symptoms. Some will need transplant. Counseling for future pregnancies is controversial. If complete recovery occurred, as demonstrated by a normal dobutamine echocardiogram, there is a good chance of an uneventful future pregnancy. If dobutamine echocardiogram is abnormal, the patient should be aware of potential deterioration with future pregnancy. Patients with persistent left ventricular dysfunction have the highest risk of death in subsequent pregnancies, and they should be counseled against future pregnancy.

A few final factors should be considered when facing a pregnant or immediate postpartum woman with pulmonary edema. Abundant fluids are often given to these laboring and hypoalbuminemic women. Tocolytic agents like terbutaline and magnesium sulfate may contribute to some cases of pulmonary edema either through a direct endothelial effect or because of the fluid associated with their use. Preeclampsia with capillary leak syndrome, decreased myocardial function, and decreased albumin with urinary protein loss is a frequent intervening factor. Infection, especially pyelonephritis, through a suspected pulmonary endothelial dysfunction, is often the cause.

Treatment of acute pulmonary edema in a pregnant woman is essentially the same. Sitting position, oxygen (oxygen saturation desired over 95% if pregnant to protect the fetus), stopping the offending agent (e.g., intravenous fluids), and morphine are all appropriate. Small dose of diuretics (10–20 mg) in these furosemide-naive patients is required. Nitroglycerine can be used but is rarely needed in noncardiogenic causes of pulmonary edema.

PROGNOSIS

The prognosis of HF varies according to the etiology of the underlying heart disease and to the presence or absence of a precipitating factor. Overall, women with HF have a better prognosis, mainly because a greater amount of them have normal left ventricular function. The general annual mortality is 10% to 15% in systolic HF, 5% to 8% in diastolic HF, and 1% for age-matched control subjects. An increasing amount of data suggest that the mortality is in fact equal in patients older than 70 years for systolic and diastolic HF patients. However, in the SOLVD registry where all patients had low EF, mortality in white women was higher than mortality in white men and mortality in African-American women was equivalent to African-American men. For both genders, in systolic dysfunction specifically, annual mortality is less than 5% in asymptomatic patients but up to 30% to 80% in NYHA class IV patients.

CONCLUSION

HF needs to be taken seriously in women. It is at least as frequent as in men and carries a dark prognosis. Women have been disadvantaged in trials and in clinical practice, although they seem to benefit from pharmacologic and nonpharmacologic interventions. Treatment should be focused on the two major objectives in all HF patients: to decrease mortality and improve symptoms. Starting early in evolution can make a difference.

BIBLIOGRAPHY

Abraham WT, Westby FG, Smith AL, et al. Cardiac resynchronization in chronic heart failure. *N Engl J Med* 2002;346:1845–1853.

Albero GW, et al. Antithrombotic therapy in atrial fibrillation. Sixth ACCP Consensus Conference on Antithrombotic Therapy. *Chest* 2001;119[Supp 1]: 194S–206S.

The Antiarrhythmics versus Implantable Defibrillators (AVID) Investigators. A comparison of antiarrhythmic-drug therapy with implantable cardioverter defibrillators in patients resuscitated from near-fatal ventricular arrhythmia. *N Engl J Med* 1997;337:1576–1583.

Belardinelli R, Georgiou D, Cianci G, et al. Randomized controlled trial of long-term moderate exercise training in chronic heart failure: effects on functional capacity, quality of life, and clinical outcome. *Circulation* 1999;99:1173–1182.

Beta-Blocker Evaluation of Survival Trial Investigators. A trial of beta-blocker bucindolol in patients with advanced chronic heart failure. *N Engl J Med* 2001; 344:1659–1667.

Bolling SF, Pagani FD, Deeb GM, et al. Intermediate-term outcome of mitral reconstruction in cardiomyopathy. *J Thorac Cadiovasc Surg* 1998;115:381–388.

Bourassa MG, Gurne O, Bangdiwala SI, et al. Natural history and current practices in heart failure. *J Am Coll Cardiol* 1993;22[Suppl]:14A–19A.

Buxton AE, Lee KL, Fisher JD, et al. A randomized study of the prevention of sudden death in patients with coronary artery disease. Multicenter Unsustained Tachycardia Trial Investigators. *N Engl J Med* 1999;341:1882–1890.

2001 Canadian Cardiovascular Society Consensus Guideline Update for the Management and Prevention of Heart Failure. *Can J Cardiol* 2001;17[Suppl E]: 5E–25E.

Cohn JN, Jonhson G, Ziesche S, et al. A comparison of enalapril with hydralazine-isosorbide dinitrate in the treatment of chronic congestive heart failure. *N Engl J Med* 1991;325:303–310.

Cohn JN, Tognoni G, Valsartan Heart Failure Trial Investigators. A randomized trial of the angiotensin-receptor blocker valsartan in chronic heart failure. *N Engl J Med* 2001;345:1667–1675.

Connolly SJ, Gent M, Roberts RS, et al. Canadian implantable defibrillator against amiodarone. *Circulation* 2000;101:1297–1302.

Dao Q, Krishnaswamy P, Kazanegra E, et al. Utility of B-type natriuretic peptide in the diagnosis of congestive heart failure in an urgent care setting. *J Am Coll Cardiol* 2001;37:379–385.

Davie AP, Francis CM, Love MP, et al. Value of the ECG in identifying heart failure due to left ventricular systolic dysfunction. *BMJ* 1996;312:222.

The Digitalis Investigation Group. The effect of digoxin on mortality and morbidity in patients with heart failure. *N Engl J Med* 1997;336:525–533.

Dries DL, Rosenberg YD, Waclawiw MA, et al. Ejection fraction and risk of thromboembolic events in patients with systolic dysfunction and sinus rhythm: evidence for gender differences in the studies of left ventricular dysfunction trials. *J Am Coll Cardiol* 1997;29:1074–1080.

Gandhi SK, Powers JC, Nomeir AM, et al. The pathogenesis of acute pulmonary edema associated with hypertension. *N Engl J Med* 2001;344:17–22.

The Heart Outcomes Prevention Evaluation Study Investigators. Effects of an angiotensin-converting-enzyme inhibitor, ramipril, on cardiovascular events in high-risk patients. *N Engl J Med* 2000;342:145–153.

Hunt SA, Baker DW, Chin MH, et al. ACC/AHA guidelines for the evaluation and management of chronic heart failure in the adult: executive summary: a report of the American College of Cardiology/American Heart Association Task Force on Practice Guidelines (Committee to Revise the 1995 Guidelines for the Evaluation and Management of Heart Failure). *Circulation* 2001;104:2996–3007.

Krum H, Sackner-Bernstein JD, Goldsmith RL, et al. Double-blind, placebo-controlled study of the long term efficacy of carvedilol in patients with severe chronic heart failure. *Circulation* 1995;92:1499–1506.

Lee RV, Rosene-Montella K, Barbour LA, et al., eds. *Medical care of the pregnant patient*. Women's Health Series. Philadelphia: American College of Physicians, 2001.

Levy D, Kenchaiah S, Larson SD, et al. Long-term trends in the incidence of and survival with heart failure. *N Engl J Med* 2002;347:1397–1402.

Lip GYH, Gibbs CR. Anticoagulation for heart failure in sinus rhythm: a Cochrane systematic review. *Q J Med* 2002;95:451–459.

Lip GYH, Gibbs CR. Antiplatelet agents versus control or anticoagulation for heart failure in sinus rhythm: a Cochrane systematic review. *Q J Med* 2002;95:461–468.

Luann RG. Women and heart failure. *Heart Lung* 2001;30:87–97.

McKelvie RS, Teo KK, McCartney N, et al. Effects of exercise training in patients with congestive heart failure: a critical review. *J Am Coll Cardiol* 1995;25: 789–796.

Moss AJ, Hall WJ, Cannom DS, et al. Improved survival with an implanted defibrillator in patients with coronary disease at high risk for ventricular arrhythmia. Multicentre Automatic Defibrillator Implantation Trial Investigators. *N Engl J Med* 1996;335:1933–1940.

Moss AJ, Zareba W, Hall WJ, et al. Prophylactic implantation of a defibrillator in patients with myocardial infarction and reduced ejection fraction. *N Engl J Med* 2002;346:877–883.

Packer M, Poole-Wilson P, Amstrong PW, et al. Comparative effects of low and high doses of the angiotensin-converting inhibitor, lisinopril, on morbidity and mortality in chronic heart failure. ATLAS Study Group. *Circulation* 1999; 100:2312–2318.

Petrie MC, Dawson NF, Murdoch DR, et al. Failure of women's hearts. *Circulation* 1999;99:2334–2341.

Pitt B, Poole-Wilson P, Segal R, et al. Effect of losartan compared with captopril on mortality in patients with symptomatic heart failure: randomised trial—the Losartan Heart Failure Survival Study ELITE II. *Lancet* 2000;355: 1582–1587.

Pitt B, Zannad F, Remme WJ, et al. The effect of spironolactone on morbidity and mortality in patients with severe heart failure. Randomized Aldactone Evaluation Study Investigators. RALES. *N Engl J Med* 1999;341:709–717.

Rathore SS, Wang Y, Krumholz HM. Sex-based differences in the effects of digoxin for the treatment of heart failure. *N Engl J Med* 2002;347:1403–1411.

Silverberg DS, Wexler D, Sheps D, et al. The effect of correction of mild anemia in severe, resistant congestive heart failure using sub-cutaneous erythropoietin and intravenous iron: a randomized controlled study. *J Am Coll Cardiol* 2001; 37:1775–1780.

Troughton RW, Frampton CM, Yandle TG, et al. Treatment of heart failure guided by plasma amino-terminal brain natriuretic peptide (N-BNP) concentrations. *Lancet* 2000;355:1126–1130.

Wenger NK. Women, heart failure, and heart failure therapies. *Circulation* 2002; 105:1526–1528.

Yamaguchi S, Tsuiki K, Hayasaka M, et al. Segmental wall motion abnormalities in dilated cardiomyopathy: hemodynamic characteristics and comparison with thallium-201 myocardial scintigraphy. *Am Heart J* 1987;113:1123–1128.

Zile M, Brutsaert D. New concepts in diastolic dysfunction and diastolic heart failure. Part II. Causal mechanisms and treatment. *Circulation* 2002;105: 1503–1508.

Zile MR, Brutsaert DL. New concepts in diastolic dysfunction and diastolic heart failure. Part I. Diagnosis, prognosis, and measurements of diastolic function. *Circulation* 2002;105:1387–1393.

Zile MR, Gaasch WH, Carroll JD, et al. Heart failure with a normal ejection fraction: is measurement of diastolic function necessary to make the diagnosis of diastolic heart failure? *Circulation* 2001;104:779–782.

CHAPTER 51

Secondary Prevention for Coronary Artery Disease

Douglas M. Burtt

Coronary atherosclerotic heart disease (ASHD) is the leading cause of disability and death in the United States in both men and women. In individuals under age 40, men are more often affected by ASHD than women; beyond age 70 the incidence of ASHD in males and females is identical. In men, the peak incidence of clinical manifestations occurs at ages 50 to 60; in women, it occurs at ages 60 to 70.

TABLE 51.1. Risk Factors for the Development of ASHD

Risk factor	Applicable to women?
Cigarette smoking	+++
Diabetes mellitus	+++
Blood lipid abnormalities (↑ LDL, ↓ HDL, ↑ Lp(a))	++
Family history of early ASHD (<50 in men, <60 in women)	++
Hypertension (>140/90)	+
Male gender	–
Advanced age	++ (especially postmenopausal without HRT)

HDL, high-density lipoprotein; HRT, hormone replacement therapy; LDL, low-density lipoprotein.

The classic risk factors for the development of ischemic heart disease (Table 51.1) include a positive family history (particularly coronary disease occurring before age 50), diabetes mellitus, blood lipid abnormalities (including elevated low-density lipoprotein [LDL] cholesterol levels, decreased high-density lipoprotein [HDL] cholesterol levels, and increased lipoprotein(a) levels), hypertension, cigarette smoking, age, and male gender. Other factors of less certain importance include obesity, physical inactivity, and personality type. Patients with clinical manifestations of coronary disease before age 50 tend to have several predisposing risk factors, but this is often not the case in older individuals. In patients with no previous ASHD, active modification of risk factors is termed *primary prevention*. In patients with *known ASHD*, management and control of risk factors or treatment with medication proven in clinical trials to reduce cardiovascular morbidity or mortality is termed *secondary prevention*.

PATHOPHYSIOLOGY

Knowledge concerning the pathophysiology of atherosclerosis and of acute coronary syndromes has advanced dramatically over the past two decades. Abnormal lipid metabolism or excessive intake of cholesterol and saturated fats, especially when superimposed on a genetic predisposition, initiates the atherosclerotic process. The initial pathologic finding is the fatty streak, a subendothelial accumulation of lipids and lipid-laden macrophages or "foam cells." LDLs are the major atherogenic lipids. HDLs, in contrast, are protective and probably assist in the mobilization of LDLs from arterial walls, returning them to the liver. The pathogenetic role of other lipids, including triglycerides, is less clear, although elevated levels of lipoprotein(a) are also associated with increased risk of ASHD. LDLs undergo *in situ* oxidation, which makes them more difficult to mobilize as well as locally cytotoxic.

Subsequent steps in atherogenesis include altered endothelial function (associated with inhibition of endothelium-derived relaxing factor production), disruption of the endothelium, adherence of platelets and release of platelet-derived growth factor and other growth factors, cell proliferation, and formation of the mature fibrous plaque (Fig. 51.1). These processes are usually slowly progressive over decades. However, the behavior of atherosclerotic plaques may also progress abruptly, particularly in immature plaques, resulting in unstable coronary atherosclerotic syndromes.

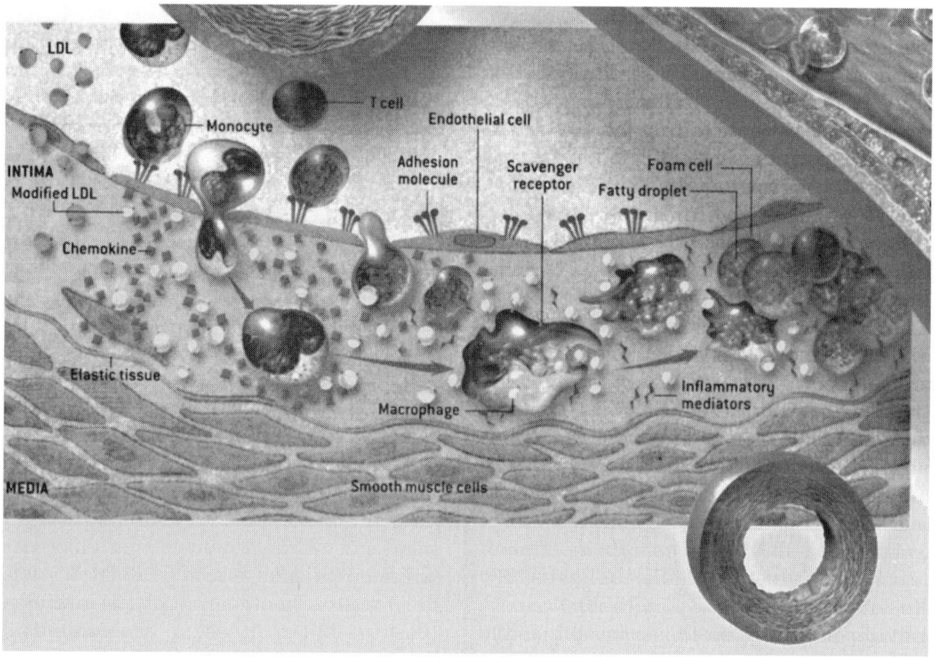

FIG. 51.1. Birth of a plaque. (1) Excess low-density lipoprotein (LDL) particles accumulate in the artery wall and undergo chemical alterations. The modified LDLs then stimulate endothelial cells to display adhesion molecules, which latch onto monocytes (central players in inflammation) and T cells (other immune system cells) in the blood. The endothelial cells also secrete "chemokines," which lure the snared cells into the intima. (2) In the intima, the monocytes mature into active macrophages. The macrophages and T cells produce many inflammatory mediators, including cytokines (best known for carrying signals between immune system cells) and factors that promote cell division. The macrophages also display so-called scavenger receptors, which help them ingest modified LDLs. (3) The macrophages feast on LDLs, becoming filled with fatty droplets. These frothy-looking fat-laden macrophages (called foam cells) and the T cells constitute the fatty streak, the earliest form of atherosclerotic plaque.

Plaque ulceration, fracture, or hemorrhage can initiate a cascade of further injury, platelet adherence, and thrombus formation that can either heal (often with more severe luminal obstruction) or cause unstable ischemic syndromes, as described below (Fig. 51.2). "Soft," lipid-laden, but nonocclusive plaques are particularly susceptible to rupture, initiating a series of events leading to thrombotic occlusion. These are often the "culprit lesions" in young persons with acute myocardial infarction (AMI) or sudden death as their first manifestation of coronary disease, and this abrupt progression explains why most infarctions do not occur at the site of a preexisting critical stenosis. Similarly, the relatively greater reduction in clinical events than lesion severity in lipid-lowering treatment trials is probably explained by the regression, stabilization, or prevention of these early nonfibrotic lesions.

OVERVIEW: PREVENTION OF ISCHEMIC HEART DISEASE

Reducing certain modifiable risk factors, such as smoking and hyperlipidemia, can both prevent coronary disease (primary prevention) and delay its progression and complications after it has become manifest (secondary prevention). Treatment of lipid abnormalities has been shown to delay the progression of atherosclerosis and in some cases to provide regression. More importantly, many studies have shown lipid reduction therapy to significantly reduce the incidence of acute coronary events in patients with previously documented ASHD.

Another preventive measure that has proven efficacy in both primary and secondary prevention is aspirin prophylaxis. Aspirin (80 mg/d) in males over age 50 significantly reduces the incidence of myocardial infarction. Whether this approach should be used for women in the general population or only in those at higher risk is unclear, and the optimal dosage of aspirin is unknown. A reasonable approach would be to administer 80 mg/d or 325 mg every other day in women with known ASHD (secondary prevention). Other platelet inhibiting agents, such as ticlopidine and clopidogrel, have recently been shown to have similar efficacy to aspirin, and in at least one trial comparing clopidogrel and aspirin, clopidogrel had slightly superior efficacy in patients with documented atherosclerosis. The value of other platelet-inhibiting agents and dietary supplements, such as fish oil or omega-3 fatty acids, is uncertain. Because LDL oxidation may be a necessary step in trapping LDL particles in the vessel wall, antioxidant therapy has been advocated as a preventive measure. Suggestive data are available for vitamin E, but more information is required before this approach can be recommended to the general public.

Reduction of elevated blood pressure has been shown to reduce the risk of myocardial infarction. Guidelines for the treatment of hypertension in patients with and without other coronary risk factors are outlined in Table 51.2, which includes all guidelines from the American Heart Association/American College of Cardiology 2001 update for the secondary prevention for patients with coronary and other vascular diseases. The beneficial role of exercise is accepted, at least insofar as regular aerobic exercise can favorably affect the total cholesterol-to-HDL ratio. Recent data confirm that the combination of dietary modification of fat intake coupled with regular aerobic exercise can consistently reduce serum LDL levels. The decrease in the number of coronary deaths over the last two decades is due in large part to better control of ASHD risk factors, but probably also reflects improvements in medical therapy: quicker presentation to the hospital; the role of coronary care units; better treatment of angina, arrhythmias, and

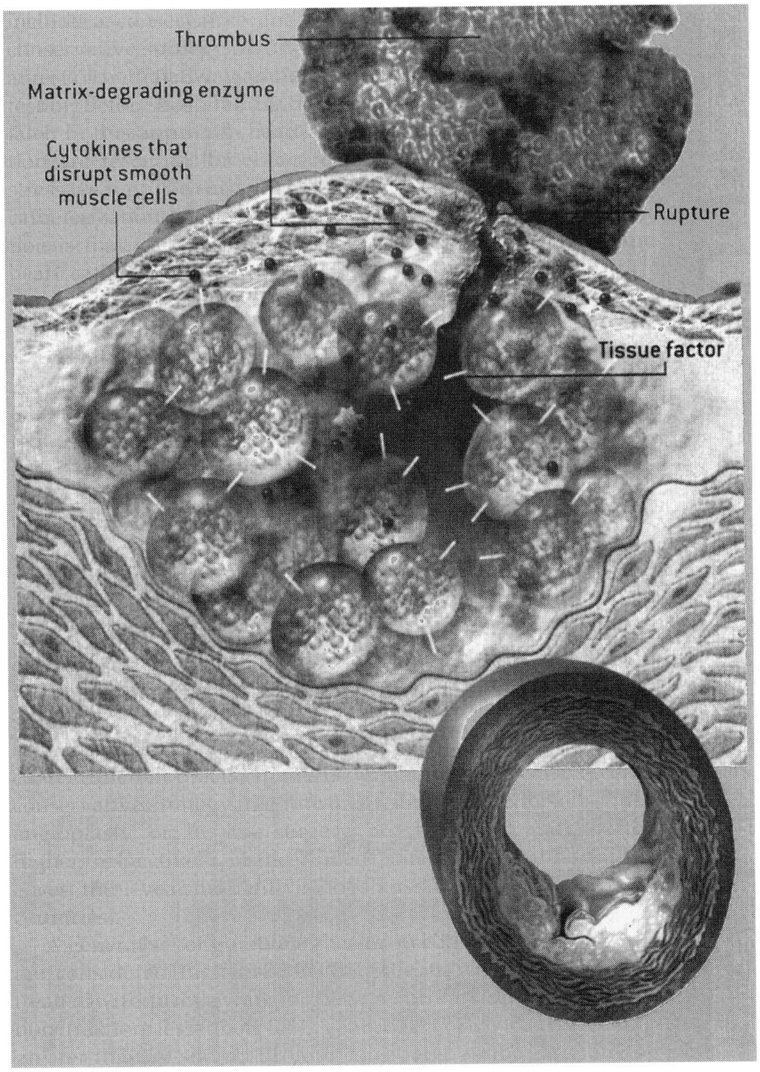

FIG. 51.2. Inflammatory substances secreted by foam cells can dangerously weaken the cap by digesting matrix molecules and damaging smooth muscle cells, which then fail to repair the cap. Meanwhile, the foam cells may display tissue factor, a potent clot promoter. If the weakened plaque ruptures, tissue factor will interact with clot-promoting elements in the blood, causing a thrombus, or clot, to form. If the clot is big enough, it will halt the flow of blood to the heart, producing a heart attack—the death of cardiac tissue.

heart failure; and improved survival after early coronary revascularization in many patients.

PATHOPHYSIOLOGY OF CORONARY SYNDROMES

Advanced coronary atherosclerosis and even complete coronary occlusion may remain clinically silent. There is only a modest correlation between the degree of clinical symptoms and the anatomic extent of disease. The best means of determining the exact location, morphology, and extent of narrowing is coronary arteriography, although ischemia can be recognized and assessed by other less invasive tests. Myocardial ischemia may be provoked by either increased myocardial oxygen requirements (exercise, mental stress, or spontaneous fluctuations in heart rate and blood pressure) or decreased oxygen supply (caused by plaque rupture or progression, thrombus formation, coronary vasospasm, anemia, or hypoxia). Abnormal endothelial function appears to play a role in the fluctuating threshold for ischemia; impaired release of endothelium-derived relaxing factor may permit unopposed vasoconstriction and facilitate platelet adhesion.

Most studies indicate that in stable angina pectoris, increased oxygen demand is the most frequent mechanism. For this reason, much of the medical therapy directed at stable angina works via reduction of myocardial oxygen demand, by reduction of heart rate and blood pressure (e.g., beta-blockers, calcium channel blockers). In contrast, the acute coronary syndromes of unstable angina and myocardial infarction are most often caused by plaque disruption, platelet plugging, and coronary thrombosis. Of interest is the predilection for these episodes to occur in the early morning or shortly after rising. The increased incidence of myocardial infarction shortly after rising may reflect the daily circadian rhythm of epinephrine and norepinephrine levels that are highest at that time. Concomitantly, increased levels of platelet aggregateness occur in the setting of increased levels of these sympathetic amines.

The ultimate outcome—whether or not the vessel becomes occluded (or whether thrombolysis occurs and the plaque is stabilized)—may be determined primarily by levels of platelet activation and levels of local vasoreactivity, although other factors undoubtedly are involved. Thus, current therapy of acute coronary syndromes is primarily directed toward inhibition of platelet activity (aspirin, ADP-binding inhibitors and GPIIb/IIIa inhibitors) and early treatment with thrombolysis

TABLE 51.2. AHA/ACC Secondary Prevention for Patients with Coronary and Other Vascular Disease: 2001 Update

Goals	Intervention recommendations
Smoking Complete cessation	Assess tobacco use. Strongly encourage patient and family to stop smoking and to avoid second-hand smoke. Providence counseling; pharmacologic therapy, including nicotine replacement and buproprion; and formal smoking cessation programs as appropriate.
BP control <140/90 mm Hg or <130/85 mm Hg if heart failure or renal insufficiency <130/80 mm Hg if diabetes	Initiate lifestyle modification (weight control, physical activity, alcohol moderation, moderate sodium restriction, and emphasis on fruits, vegetables, and low-fat dairy products) in all patients with blood pressure ≥130 mm Hg systolic or 80 mm Hg diastolic. Add blood pressure medication, individualized to other patient requirements and characteristics (i.e., age, race, need for drugs with specific benefits) ***if*** blood pressure is not <140 mm Hg systolic or 90 mm Hg diastolic ***or*** if blood pressure is not <130 mm Hg systolic or 85 mm Hg diastolic for individuals with heart failure or renal insufficiency (<80 mm Hg diastolic for individuals with diabetes).
Lipid management Primary goal: LDL <100 mg/dL	Start dietary therapy in all patients (<7% saturated fat and <200 mg/d cholesterol) and promote physical activity and weight management. Encourage increased consumption of omega-3 fatty acids. Assess fasting lipid profile in all patients and within 24 h of hospitalization for those with an acute event. If patients are hospitalized, consider adding drug therapy on discharge. Add drug therapy according to the following guide: LDL < 100 mg/dL (baseline or on-treatment): Further LDL-lowering therapy not required; Consider fibrate or niacin (if low HDL or high TG) LDL 100–129 mg/dL (baseline or on-treatment): Therapeutic options: Intensify LDL-lowering therapy (statin or resin[a]); Fibrate or niacin (if low HDL or high TG); Consider combined drug therapy (statin + fibrate or niacin) (if low HDL or high TG) LDL ≥130 mg/dL (baseline or on-treatment): Intensity LDL-lowering therapy (statin or resin[a]); Add or increase drug therapy with lifestyle therapies
Secondary goal: If TG ≥200 mg/dL, then non-HDL[b] should be <130 mg/dL	If TG ≥150 mg/dL or HDL <40 mg/dL: Emphasize weight management and physical activity. Advise smoking cessation. If TG 200–499 mg/dL: Consider fibrate or niacin *after* LDL-lowering therapy[a] If TG ≥500 mg/dL: Consider fibrate on niacin *before* LDL-lowering therapy[a] Consider omega-3 fatty acids as adjunct for high TG
Physical activity 30 min 3–4 days per week Optimal: daily	Assess risk, preferably with exercise test, to guide prescription. Encourage minimum of 30–60 min of activity, preferably daily, or at least three or four times weekly (walking, jogging, cycling, or other aerobic activity) supplemented by an increase in daily lifestyle activities (e.g., walking breaks at work, gardening, household work). Advise medically supervised programs for moderate- to high-risk patients.
Weight management BMI 18.5–24.9 kg/m^2	Calculate BMI and measure waist circumference as part of evaluation. Monitor response of BMI and waist circumference to therapy. Start weight management and physical activity as appropriate. Desirable BMI range is 18.5–24.9 kg/m^2. When BMI ≥ 25 kg/m^2, goal for waist circumference is ≤40 inches in men and ≤35 inches in women.
Diabetes management HgA_{Ic} <7%	Appropriate hypoglycemic therapy to achieve near-normal fasting plasma glucose, as indicated by HgA_{Ic}. Treatment of other risks (e.g., physical activity, weight management, blood pressure, and cholesterol management).
Antiplatelet agents/ anticoagulants	Start and continue indefinitely aspirin 75–325 mg/d if not contraindicated. Consider clopidogrel 75 mg/d or warfarin if aspirin contraindicated. Manage warfarin to international normalized ratio = 2.0–3.0 in post-MI patients when clinically indicated or for those not able to take aspirin or clopidogrel.
ACE inhibitors	Treat all patients indefinitely post-MI; start early in stable high-risk patients (anterior MI, previous MI, Killip class II [S_3 gallop, rales, radiographic CHF). Consider chronic therapy for all other patients with coronary or other vascular disease unless contraindicated.
Beta-blockers	Start in all post-MI and acute ischemic syndrome patients. Continue indefinitely. Observe usual contraindications. Use as needed to manage angina, rhythm, or blood pressure in all other patients.

[a]The use of resin is relatively contraindicated when TG > 200 mg/dL.
[b]Non-HDL cholesterol = total cholesterol minus HDL cholesterol.
ACE, angiotensin-converting enzyme; BMI, body mass index; BP, blood pressure; CHF, congestive heart failure; HDL, high-density lipoprotein; HgA_{Ic}, major fraction of adult hemoglobin; LDL, low-density lipoprotein; MI, myocardial infarction; TG, triglycerides.

and/or acute coronary intervention when total vessel occlusion occurs.

Some episodes of myocardial ischemia are painful, causing angina pectoris; others are completely silent. Many silent episodes are brought on by emotional and mental stress. In patients with diagnosed coronary disease, as evidenced by prior myocardial infarction or angina, silent ischemic episodes have the same prognostic import as symptomatic ones. The prognosis for patients with only silent ischemia is not well established, nor is the potential benefit of preventing silent ischemia.

ANGINA PECTORIS

Angina pectoris is usually due to ASHD (see Chapter 43).

Circumstances that Precipitate and Relieve Angina

Angina occurs most commonly during activity and is relieved by resting. Exertion that increases both heart rate and blood pressure, such as walking rapidly, walking uphill, or heavy lifting, precipitates attacks most consistently. The amount of activity required to produce angina may be relatively consistent under comparable physical and emotional circumstances or may vary from day to day. It usually is more prominent after meals, during excitement, or on exposure to cold. The threshold for angina is often lower in the morning or after strong emotion; the latter can provoke attacks in the absence of exertion. In addition, discomfort may occur during sexual activity, at rest, or during sleep as a result of coronary spasm.

Effect of Nitroglycerin

The diagnosis of angina pectoris is strongly supported if sublingual nitroglycerin invariably shortens an attack and if prophylactic nitrates permit greater exertion or prevent angina entirely. Most patients do not have a risk profile markedly different from that of the general population.

Coronary Vasospasm and Angina with Normal Coronary Arteriograms

Although most symptoms of myocardial ischemia result from fixed stenosis of the coronary arteries or thrombosis or hemorrhage at the site of lesions, some ischemic events may be precipitated by coronary vasoconstriction. Spasm of the large coronary arteries with resulting decreased coronary blood flow may occur spontaneously or may be induced by exposure to cold, emotional stress, or vasoconstricting medications (e.g., ergot derivative drugs). Spasm may occur both in normal and stenotic coronary arteries and may be silent or result in angina pectoris. Even myocardial infarction may occur as a result of spasm in the absence of visible obstructive coronary heart disease, although most instances of coronary spasm occur in the presence of some degree of coronary stenosis.

Electrocardiogram Interpretation

The resting electrocardiogram (ECG) is entirely normal in about one fourth of patients with angina. Exercise testing is the most useful noninvasive procedure for evaluating the patient with angina.

The usual ECG criterion for a positive test is 1 mm (0.1 mV) horizontal or downsloping ST segment depression (beyond baseline) measured 80 ms after the J point. By this criterion, 60% to 80% of patients with anatomically significant coronary disease have a positive test, but 10% to 20% of those without significant disease are also positive. False-positive results are uncommon when 2 mm or more of ST depression is present. Additional prognostic information is obtained from the time of onset and duration of the ECG changes, their magnitude and configuration, blood-pressure and heart-rate changes, the total duration of exercise, and the presence of associated symptoms. In general, patients exhibiting more severe ST segment depression (2 mm) at low workloads (less than 6 minutes on the Bruce protocol) or heart rates (70% of age-predicted maximum), especially when the duration of exercise is limited or when hypotension occurs during the test, have more severe disease and a poorer prognosis. Depending on symptom status, age, and other factors, such patients may require referral for coronary arteriography and possible revascularization. On the other hand, less positive tests in asymptomatic patients are often false-positive results. Therefore, exercise testing results that do not conform to the clinical picture should be confirmed by stress scintigraphy or stress echocardiography.

Scintigraphic Assessment of Ischemia

Nuclear medicine studies may provide additional information about the presence, location, and extent of coronary disease. Myocardial perfusion scintigraphy provides images in which radionuclide uptake is proportional to blood flow at the time of injection. These data provide information regarding the extent and location of ischemia and of prior infarction. The extent of ischemia, the presence of abnormal cavity dilation, and/or increased lung uptake correlate directly with prognosis. In addition, gated nuclear studies can quantitate left ventricular systolic function, which is also directly linked to prognosis.

Echocardiography

Echocardiography can image the left ventricle and reveal segmental wall motion abnormalities, which may indicate ischemia or prior infarction. It is a convenient and safe technique for assessing left ventricular function. Echocardiograms performed before and immediately after upright exercise can reveal exercise-induced segmental wall motion abnormalities as an indicator of location and extent of ischemia. In experienced laboratories, the increment in test accuracy compared with routine stress testing is comparable with that obtained with scintigraphy, although a higher proportion of tests are technically suboptimal. Pharmacologic stress with incremental doses of intravenous dobutamine (2–4 mg/kg/min; start at 10 μg/kg/min) can be used as an alternative to exercise.

Coronary Angiography

Selective coronary arteriography remains the most definitive diagnostic procedure for coronary artery disease. Although invasive, it can be performed with low mortality (about 0.1%) and morbidity (1%–5%), but the cost is high, and with currently available noninvasive techniques it is usually not indicated solely for diagnosis. Currently accepted indications for coronary arteriography are summarized in Table 51.3.

Coronary arteriography allows direct visualization of the location, severity, and morphology of stenoses. Narrowing greater than 50% of the luminal diameter is considered clinically significant, although most lesions producing ischemia are associated with narrowing in excess of 70%. This information has important prognostic value, because mortality rates are progressively higher in patients with one-, two-, and three-vessel disease and in those with left main coronary artery obstruction (ranging

TABLE 51.3. Reasons to Perform Coronary Arteriography

- Patients being considered for coronary artery revascularization because of limiting stable angina who have failed to improve on an adequate medical regimen or who have intolerable side effects on medical therapy.
- Patients in whom coronary revascularization is being considered because the clinical presentation (e.g., unstable angina, postinfarction angina) or noninvasive testing suggests high-risk disease.
- Patients with aortic valve disease who also have angina pectoris to determine whether the angina is due to accompanying coronary disease. Coronary angiography is also performed in asymptomatic older patients undergoing valve surgery so that concomitant bypass may be done if the anatomy is propitious.
- Patients who have had coronary revascularization with subsequent recurrence of symptoms to determine whether bypass grafts or native vessels are occluded or whether intervention sites have restenosed.
- Patients with cardiac failure in whom a surgically correctable lesion, such as left ventricular aneurysm, mitral regurgitation, or reversible ischemic dysfunction, is suspected.
- Patients surviving sudden death or with symptomatic or life-threatening arrhythmias in whom coronary artery disease may be a correctable cause.
- Patients with chest pain of uncertain cause or cardiomyopathy of unknown cause.

from 1% per year to 25% per year). Among stable patients, 20%, 30%, and 50% have one-, two-, and three-vessel involvement, respectively; left main disease is present in 10%. In those with strongly positive exercise ECGs or scintigraphic studies, three-vessel or left main disease may be present in 75% to 95%, depending on the criteria used. Coronary arteriography also shows whether the obstructions are amenable to bypass surgery or percutaneous coronary intervention (PCI; angioplasty, stent placement, debulking procedures, or combined strategies).

Left Ventricular Angiography

Left ventricular angiography is usually performed at the same time as coronary arteriography. Global and regional left ventricular function is visualized and quantified, including degree of mitral regurgitation if present. Left ventricular function is the single most important determinant of prognosis in stable coronary disease and of the risk of bypass surgery.

Medical Therapy of Angina Pectoris

GENERAL GUIDELINES

Other than modification of coronary risk factors, optimization of medical therapy for patients with established ASHD remains a key factor in secondary prevention. Because angina may be aggravated by uncontrolled hypertension, left ventricular failure, tachyarrhythmias, anemia, and hypoxia, medical therapy directed at correction of these precipitating factors should always be optimized. Other precipitants, such as strenuous activity, cold temperatures, and emotional states, should be similarly avoided, when possible.

SPECIFIC MEDICAL THERAPY

Sublingual Nitroglycerin. Nitroglycerin, 0.15 to 0.6 mg sublingually, or nitroglycerin aerosol, 0.4 to 0.8 mg, in addition to being used to treat episodes of angina, can be used effectively when taken 1 to 5 minutes before activities that are likely to precipitate angina. Sublingual isosorbide dinitrate (2.5–5 mg) acts slightly longer than sublingual nitroglycerin.

Long-Acting Nitrates. Long-acting nitrate preparations include isosorbide dinitrate (10–40 mg every 6 hours or controlled-release 40–80 mg every 8–12 hours), isosorbide mononitrate (10–20 mg orally twice daily or 60–120 mg once daily in a sustained-release preparation), nitroglycerin ointment (7.5–30 mg applied two times daily), and transdermal nitroglycerin patches that deliver nitroglycerin at a predetermined rate (usually 0.2–0.8 mg/24 h). The main limitation to chronic nitrate therapy is tolerance, which occurs to some degree in most patients. The degree of tolerance can be limited by using a regimen that includes at least an 8- to 10-hour period without nitrates. Isosorbide dinitrate given three times daily, with the last dose after dinner, is one commonly used approach. Isosorbide mononitrate, because it is the active metabolite of the dinitrate, has more consistent bioavailability and allows for a once or twice daily regimen that may improve patient compliance. Transdermal preparations should be applied in the morning and removed overnight in most patients. Nitrate therapy is often limited by headache, although other side effects include nausea, dizziness, and hypotension.

Beta-Blockers. Beta-blockers reduce anginal frequency and severity by reducing myocardial oxygen requirements during exertion and stress. This is accomplished by reducing the heart rate, myocardial contractility, and, to a lesser extent, blood pressure. Beta-blockers are the only *antianginal* agents that have been demonstrated to prolong life in patients with coronary disease after myocardial infarction. They are at least as effective as alternative agents in studies using exercise testing, ambulatory monitoring, and symptom assessment. As a result, they should be considered as first-line therapy in most patients with chronic angina.

In the United States, only propranolol, metoprolol, nadolol, atenolol, and carvedilol are approved for angina. Nonetheless, all available beta-blockers appear to be effective for angina, although those with intrinsic sympathomimetic activity, such as pindolol, are less desirable because they may exacerbate angina in some patients and have not been effective in secondary prevention trials. The major contraindications are bronchospastic disease, bradyarrhythmias, and overt heart failure. Patients with chronic controlled heart failure, however, have also been shown to have an improved long-term prognosis when treated with some beta-blockers, especially carvedilol. Beta-blockers can be categorized based on several factors, including lipid solubility, duration of action, and β_1 selectivity. The less lipid-soluble beta-blockers, including atenolol, nadolol, and bisoprolol, cross the blood–brain barrier less readily and have been shown to cause less cognitive dysfunction as a result. The more β_1-selective beta-blockers include metoprolol, atenolol, and bisoprolol, with bisoprolol acting as the most β_1-specific beta-blocker to date, allowing its cautious use in patients with varying degrees of concomitant pulmonary disease.

Calcium Entry-Blocking Agents (Calcium Channel Blockers). Verapamil, diltiazem, nifedipine, nicardipine, and amlodipine are chemically and pharmacologically heterogeneous agents that prevent angina by reducing myocardial oxygen requirements and by inducing coronary artery vasodilation. Isradipine and felodipine are not approved in the United States for angina but probably are about as effective as nifedipine and other dihydropyridine agents. These agents lessen myocardial oxygen demand by reducing blood pressure, left ventricular wall stress, and, in the case of verapamil and diltiazem, resting or exercise heart rate. Although these agents are all potent coronary vasodilators, it is unclear whether they improve myocardial blood flow in most patients with stable exertional angina. In those with coronary vasospasm, however, the calcium entry blockers may be the agent of choice.

Most calcium channel blockers have negative inotropic, chronotropic, and dromotropic properties *in vitro*, but the reflex sympathetic response may obscure these effects *in vivo* (except in the presence of beta-blockade or severely depressed left ventricular function). Several newer calcium channel blockers of the dihydropyridine class, including felodipine and amlodipine, have less negative inotropic action, and recent data confirm relative safety in utilizing amlodipine in patients with stable congestive heart failure. Unlike the beta-blockers, calcium channel blockers have not reduced mortality postinfarction and in some cases have been shown to increase ischemia and mortality rates. This appears to be the case with some dihydropyridines and with diltiazem and verapamil in patients with AMI and clinical heart failure or moderate to severe left ventricular dysfunction. Thus, calcium blockers should not be used as the initial antianginal medication in most patients. Although all have been shown to be efficacious for angina, not all preparations and agents are approved for this indication.

COMBINATION THERAPY

Patients remaining symptomatic when given one class of antianginal agent should be treated with combination therapy. A combination of a beta-blocker and a long-acting nitrate or a beta-blocker and a calcium channel blocker (other than verapamil, where the risk of atrioventricular block or heart failure is higher) is the most appropriate combination. A few patients have a further response to a regimen including all three agents.

PLATELET-INHIBITING AGENTS

Coronary thrombosis is responsible for most episodes of myocardial infarction and many unstable ischemic syndromes. Several studies have demonstrated the benefit of antiplatelet drugs after unstable angina and infarction with significant reductions in future events including acute coronary syndromes and stroke. Therefore, unless contraindicated, small doses of aspirin (162–325 mg/d or 325 mg every other day) should be prescribed for all patients with angina and status post-AMI. For patients with acetylsalicylic acid or aspirin (ASA) sensitivity, the use of clopidogrel 75 mg/d by mouth is as effective in the prevention of recurrent acute ischemic coronary syndromes.

Prognosis

The prognosis of angina pectoris has improved with advances in the understanding of its pathophysiology and in pharmacologic therapy. Mortality rates range from 1% to 25% per year depending on the number of vessels diseased, the severity of obstruction, the status of left ventricular function, and the presence of complex arrhythmias. In patients with stable symptoms and normal left ventricular ejection fractions (≥55%, depending on the laboratory), the mortality rate is less than 4% per year. However, the outlook in individual patients is unpredictable, and nearly half of cardiovascular deaths occur suddenly. Therefore, risk stratification is often attempted. Patients with accelerating symptoms have a worse prognosis than those with stable symptoms. Among stable patients, those whose exercise tolerance is severely limited by ischemia (<6 minutes on the Bruce treadmill protocol) and those with extensive ischemia by exercise ECG or scintigraphy have more severe anatomic disease and a poorer prognosis.

Over 90% of patients can be rendered pain free with revascularization measures. Patients who do not become ischemia free on medical therapy should have early coronary arteriography and revascularization. Controlled trials have not shown any reduction in infarction rates with coronary artery bypass grafting (CABG) compared with medical therapy, but an improved survival has been shown with CABG in patients with left main stenosis of at least 70% or moderately reduced left ventricular function and multivessel disease. Many patients treated medically ultimately need revascularization for recurrent or uncontrolled symptoms. Depending on the stringency of the definition of unstable angina, 10% to 30% of patients have an early infarction, and the 1-year mortality rate is 10% to 20%. Even in the absence of chest pain, many patients with "silent" episodes of ST segment depression or, less commonly, elevation on ambulatory monitoring have a worsened prognosis.

Because recurrent episodes, infarction, and sudden death may occur after relief of unstable angina, additional evaluations should be performed in patients who have been stabilized, consisting of early exercise or pharmacologic stress testing to identify high-risk subsets for further invasive evaluation or coronary arteriography. The choice should be individualized based on the patient's age and general health, as well as the severity of symptoms and signs of ischemia. The artery responsible for the ischemia can usually be determined from echocardiographic or scintigraphic changes during exercise or electrocardiographic changes during episodes of chest pain, and the "culprit" lesion is often amenable to PTCA. If revascularization is not performed, long-term management is the same as for stable angina pectoris.

Indications for Revascularization

The indications for coronary artery revascularization in patients with stable angina pectoris are often debated. There is general agreement that otherwise healthy patients who meet specific criteria as shown in Table 51.4 are reasonable candidates for revascularization.

In addition, many cardiologists argue that patients with stable anginal symptoms should be revascularized if they have anatomically critical lesions (90% proximal stenoses, especially of the proximal left anterior descending artery) or physiologic evidence of severe ischemia (early positive exercise tests, large exercise-induced thallium scintigraphic defects, or frequent episodes of ischemia on ambulatory monitoring). This trend toward aggressive intervention has accelerated in parallel with the growing availability of coronary interventions. Although this subgroup of patients is at increased risk, it has not been proven that their prognosis is better after coronary revascularization by either surgery or coronary intervention. In many, a trial of medical therapy is warranted to determine whether symptoms and other evidence of ischemia improve.

TABLE 51.4. Indications for Coronary Artery Revascularization in Patients with Stable Angina Pectoris

- Persistent unacceptable symptoms despite medical therapy to its tolerable limits.
- Left main coronary artery stenosis greater than 70% (with or without symptoms).
- Multivessel disease involving the LAD coupled with left ventricular dysfunction (ejection fraction ≤45% or previous transmural infarction).
- Previously unstable angina where, after symptom control by medical therapy, continued ischemia is manifest on exercise testing or monitoring.
- Postmyocardial infarction patients with persistent angina or ischemia during noninvasive testing, particularly if they have received thrombolytic treatment.

LAD, left anterior descending.

NONMEDICAL THERAPY OF ANGINAL SYNDROMES

Coronary Artery Bypass Grafting

CABG can be accomplished with a very low mortality rate (1%–3%) in otherwise healthy patients with preserved cardiac function. However, the mortality rate of this procedure has increased slightly in recent years because the proportion of high-risk and older patients is growing. Increasingly, younger patients with focal lesions of one or several vessels are undergoing coronary angioplasty as the initial revascularization procedure.

Grafts using one or both internal mammary arteries (usually to the left anterior descending artery or its branches) provide the best long-term results in terms of patency and flow. Segments of the saphenous veins from the leg or the radial artery from the arm are also anastomosed between the aorta and the coronary arteries distal to the obstructions. One to five distal anastomoses are commonly performed. After successful surgery, symptoms generally improve significantly. The need for antianginal medications diminishes, and left ventricular function may improve.

The operative mortality rate is increased in patients with poor left ventricular function (left ventricular ejection fraction < 35%) or those requiring additional procedures (valve replacement or repair or ventricular aneurysmectomy). Patients over age 70, patients undergoing repeat procedures, or those with important noncardiac disease (especially renal insufficiency, diabetes, or poor general health) also have higher operative mortality and morbidity rates, and full recovery is slower. Thus, CABG should be reserved for more severely symptomatic patients in this group. Early (1–6 months) graft patency rates average 85% to 90% (higher for internal mammary grafts), and subsequent graft closure rates are about 4% per year. Early graft failure is common in vessels with poor distal flow; late closure is more common in patients who continue smoking and those with treated hyperlipidemia. Antiplatelet therapy with aspirin, and possibly clopidogrel, improves graft patency rates. Vigorous treatment of blood lipid abnormalities is necessary, with a goal for LDL cholesterol of less than 100 mg/dL and for HDL cholesterol more than 45 mg/dL.

Repeat CABG or angioplasty is sometimes necessitated by progressive native vessel disease and graft occlusions. Reoperation is technically demanding and less often fully successful than the initial operation.

Percutaneous Coronary Interventions (PCI)

Coronary artery stenoses can be effectively dilated by inflation of a balloon under high pressure most often accompanied by the implantation of an intracoronary stent. This procedure is performed in the cardiac catheterization laboratory under local anesthesia either at the same time as diagnostic coronary arteriography or at a later time. The mechanism of dilation is rupture of the atheromatous plaque, with subsequent resorption of intraluminal debris and remodeling of the arterial wall.

This procedure was at one time reserved for proximal single-vessel disease, but now it is widely used in multivessel disease with multiple lesions, although only rarely in left main disease. Intervention, especially stent placement, is also effective in CABG stenoses. Optimal lesions for intervention are relatively proximal, noneccentric, free of plaque dissection, and removed from the origin of large branches. With continued improvement in interventional devices, however, experienced operators can manipulate the balloon catheter across about 98% of approachable lesions and successfully dilate more than 97% of those. The major early complication after stent placement is subacute thrombosis; however, this risk has been reduced to less than 0.5% with the use of combination antiplatelet therapy post-stent (aspirin plus clopidogrel or ticlopidine), coupled with optimized stent deployment using techniques including intracoronary ultrasound. Current guidelines require that these procedures be done in a laboratory where surgery is available on short notice, although studies are ongoing to test the feasibility of primary stenting for AMI without immediate surgical backup available.

In the United States, the number of interventional procedures now exceeds that of CABG operations, but the justification for some of these is inconclusive. One small controlled study showed PTCA to be superior to medical therapy for symptom relief but not for preventing infarction or death. Controlled studies of interventional therapy versus either medical treatment or CABG in multivessel disease are not yet available.

The major limitation of coronary intervention has been restenosis, which occurs in the first 6 months in 15% to 50% of vessels dilated depending primarily on vessel size, lesion length, and the presence or absence of diabetes mellitus. Most in-stent restenoses can be successfully treated with redilation of the stenotic site, followed by adjuvant local radiation therapy or "brachytherapy," resulting in a low incidence of recurrent restenosis. Recently, the U.S. Food and Drug Administration approved the use of drug-eluting stents shown to have a dramatically reduced incidence of restenosis by virtue of inhibiting post-stent intimal smooth muscle hyperplasia.

Results

The mortality and infarction rates with PCI and CABG are generally comparable in stable angina. Recovery after PCI is obviously faster, but the intermediate-term success rate of CABG is higher, because of restenosis associated with PCI. The increasing popularity of PCI primarily reflects its lower cost, shorter hospitalization, the perception that CABG is best done only once and can be reserved for later, and the preference of patients for less invasive treatment. These arguments make PCI the procedure of choice for revascularization of single-vessel disease, although this is usually indicated only when symptoms are refractory to medical treatment or when medication side effects are intolerable. The situation is less clear with multivessel disease. Several randomized studies comparing PCI and CABG in patients with two- or three-vessel disease have been reported. In general, mortality and nonfatal infarction rates have not differed between treatments. However, PCI patients have required substantially more subsequent revascularizations. The early cost savings with PCI usually disappear over 1 to 3 years because of this higher reintervention rate. The recent introduction of brachytherapy for treatment of in-stent restenosis and, more importantly, of drug-eluting stents promises to further reduce the requirement for repeat intervention, however. In general, the excellent outcome of many patients treated medically has made it difficult to show an advantage with either revascularization approach, except in patients who remain symptom limited, are intolerant of medications, or have left main lesions or multivessel disease and left ventricular dysfunction.

UNSTABLE ANGINA

Most clinicians use the term *unstable angina* to denote an accelerating or crescendo pattern of chest discomfort or where previously stable angina occurs with less exertion or at rest, lasts longer, or is less responsive to medication (see Chapter 43).

Treatment

Treatment of unstable angina should be multifaceted and vigorous. Patients should be hospitalized, maintained at bed rest or limited activity, and monitored on telemetry. Sedation and supplemental oxygen is usually administered. The systolic blood pressure is usually maintained at 100 to 120 mm Hg, except in previously severe hypertensive patients. Most patients should be given beta-blockers, titrating to a heart rate of 50 to 60 beats/min, unless severe heart failure or other medical contraindications are present.

Medical therapy for unstable angina is virtually identical to therapy for stable angina, except that shorter acting parenteral agents may sometimes be required. Antiplatelet therapy with aspirin is always indicated, with the use of clopidogrel or ticlopidine in patients with contraindication to aspirin. Parenteral GP2B-3A inhibitors have been shown to be effective in patients with acute coronary syndromes, including non-Q wave myocardial infarction. Intravenous heparin, titrated to a partial thromboplastin time of 50 to 70, or weight-adjusted, subcutaneous, low-molecular-weight heparin are both effective in reducing the risk of AMI in acute coronary syndromes. Other effective parenteral agents in acute coronary syndromes include intravenous nitroglycerin, which can be rapidly titrated to symptoms or blood pressure in a closely monitored setting. Although the data on efficacy of calcium channel blockers are less extensive and less favorable than with beta-blockers, these agents are sometimes used especially when alterations in coronary vasomotor tone are thought to play a role in an unstable ischemic syndrome.

Perhaps the most important tool used in the management of acute coronary syndromes, particularly when symptoms are prolonged, associated with ST segment deviation, and are refractory to medical therapy, is early coronary angiography with an eye toward early PCI or CABG. High-grade, ulcerated, and even thrombotic stenosis responds extremely well to pretreatment with GP2B-3A inhibitors, aspirin, and clopidogrel, followed by urgent stent placement. This approach usually results in immediate abolition of symptoms with high acute success rates and low morbidity and mortality.

ACUTE MYOCARDIAL INFARCTION

The initial manifestation of ASHD in many patients is AMI. Most patients with AMI will be candidates for early intervention with either thrombolysis or with primary PCI. In addition, patients who initially fail thrombolytic therapy may be candidates for "salvage" PCI. The diagnosis and treatment of AMI are covered separately in Chapter 43.

Perhaps the most important issue to be settled after AMI is that of residual ischemia and jeopardized myocardium, that is, the risk of recurrent AMI over the 12 months after the initial presentation. Those patients at higher risk of recurrence are those most likely to benefit from revascularization before hospital discharge.

Because of the increasing use of thrombolytic therapy and accumulating experience with acute PCI, the indications for revascularization are rapidly evolving. Postinfarction patients who appear likely to benefit from early revascularization if the anatomy is appropriate are outlined in Table 51.5. Patients who survive infarctions without complications, have preserved left ventricular function (ejection fraction 50%), and have no exercise-induced ischemia have an excellent prognosis and do not require invasive evaluation.

TABLE 51.5. Post-MI Patients Most Likely to Benefit from Early Revascularization

- Those who have undergone thrombolytic therapy and have residual symptoms or electrocardiographic or enzymatic evidence of recurrent ischemia.
- Those with left ventricular dysfunction (ejection fraction 30%–40%) and evidence of residual ischemia.
- Those with non–Q-wave infarction and evidence of residual (more than mild) ischemia.
- Those with strongly positive exercise tests and multivessel disease.

The value of revascularization in the following groups is less clear:

- Those treated with thrombolytic agents, with little evidence of reperfusion or residual ischemia.
- Those with left ventricular dysfunction but no detectable ischemia.
- Those with preserved left ventricular function who have mild ischemia and are not symptom limited.

Therapy After Myocardial Infarction: Secondary Prevention

After AMI the modification of coronary risk factors, adjustments in lifestyle, and specific medical therapies may all be considered integral parts of secondary prevention. Postinfarction management should begin with identification and modification of risk factors. Treatment of hyperlipidemia and smoking cessation both clearly reduce risk of recurrent infarction. Guidelines for dietary modification and medical therapy of hyperlipidemia are covered in detail below. In addition, blood-pressure control, weight loss, and regular aerobic exercise are recommended after AMI (Table 51.2).

Many drugs have been studied after AMI, and some have been shown to be beneficial in preventing death or reinfarction. However, their usefulness in the era of thrombolysis and revascularization is not entirely clear. Beta-blockers have been shown to improve survival rates, primarily by reducing the incidence of sudden death in high-risk patients. Beta-blockers should be given to such patients, except those with overt heart failure, but are of limited value in uncomplicated patients with small infarctions and normal exercise tests. No advantage of one preparation over another has been demonstrated, except that those with intrinsic sympathomimetic activity have not proved beneficial in postinfarction patients.

Calcium channel blockers have not been shown to improve prognosis overall, but both diltiazem and verapamil may reduce mortality rates in selected patients with preserved left ventricular function. Diltiazem may help to prevent reinfarction after non-Q wave infarction.

Antiplatelet agents are clearly beneficial; low-dose aspirin or clopidogrel 75 mg/d is recommended in all patients after AMI. Warfarin anticoagulation for 3 months reduces the incidence of arterial emboli after large anterior infarctions and, according to the results of at least one study, may improve long-term prognosis, but an additive benefit to aspirin after 6 months has not been confirmed.

Specific antiarrhythmic therapy with agents other than beta-blockers has not been shown to be effective, except in patients with symptomatic arrhythmias; in fact, class IC agents increase the mortality rate in postinfarction patients. However, several small studies and a metaanalyses have indicated that low-dose amiodarone may be beneficial. Post-AMI patients with low ejection fractions (≤30%) and either wide QRD complexes (≥0.14 seconds) or nonsustained ventricular tachycardia appear to benefit from placement of an implantable defibrillation device. Although cardiac rehabilitation programs and exercise training can be of considerable psychological and emotional benefit, it is unknown whether they alter prognosis after AMI.

Specific Medical Therapy After Acute Myocardial Infarction

ANGIOTENSIN-CONVERTING ENZYME INHIBITORS

Patients who sustain substantial myocardial damage during AMI often experience subsequent progressive left ventricular dilation and dysfunction, leading to clinical heart failure and reduced long-term survival. A recent trial demonstrated that in patients with ejection fractions less than 40%, captopril (25–50 mg three times daily commencing 3–16 days postinfarction) prevents left ventricular dilation and the onset of heart failure and also reduces the mortality rate. Similar data have been collected with ramipril. Although two large trials found a benefit from treating unselected patients beginning on admission, it is unclear whether or not this occurs in patients without left ventricular dysfunction and whether there is any advantage to starting treatment very early, while the patient may be hemodynamically unstable.

MEDICAL TREATMENT AND DIETARY MODIFICATION FOR LIPID DISORDERS

Serum lipoproteins are important mainly because of their relation to atherosclerotic vascular disease, especially coronary heart disease. Several clinical trials showing that lowering high blood cholesterol reduces the incidence of coronary heart disease have given impetus to nationwide campaigns to reduce serum cholesterol levels. It is important to target LDL concentrations to less than 100 mg/dL for secondary prevention. There is convincing evidence that this is effective in women. Current therapies have been associated with reduction in total mortality as well (see Chapter 49).

LIPOPROTEINS AND ATHEROGENESIS

The plaques found in the arterial walls of patients with atherosclerosis contain large amounts of cholesterol, providing a clue that serum cholesterol might be an important factor in their development. Epidemiologic studies have established that the higher the level of LDL cholesterol, the greater the risk of ASHD; conversely, the higher the level of HDL cholesterol, the lower the risk of coronary heart disease. This is true in men and women, in different racial and ethnic groups, and at all adult ages. It is also true in patients without previously manifest ASHD (primary prevention) and in those with documented ASHD (secondary prevention).

Because most cholesterol in serum is LDL cholesterol, high total cholesterol levels are also associated with an increased risk of coronary heart disease. As a general approximation in men, each 10-mg/dL increase in cholesterol (or LDL cholesterol) increases the risk of coronary heart disease by about 10%; each 5-mg/dL increase in HDL reduces the risk by about 10%. The effect of HDL cholesterol is greater in women, but the effects of total and LDL cholesterol are smaller. All these relations diminish with age.

THERAPEUTIC EFFECTS OF LOWERING CHOLESTEROL

Beneficial effects on the risk of coronary heart disease have been seen with the bile acid-binding resins, with gemfibrozil, with niacin, with statins, and from dietary reduction of cholesterol. In patients who already have coronary heart disease, the net benefits of cholesterol lowering are clearer, with reductions in the progression of coronary atherosclerosis, fewer subsequent coronary events, less mortality from coronary heart disease, and perhaps a reduction in mortality from all causes. The important exceptions among current therapies are the fibric acid derivatives (clofibrate and gemfibrozil), which have not shown benefits in the secondary prevention of coronary heart disease, and probucol, which has not been studied with clinical endpoints. Several studies have also shown that cholesterol lowering actually causes regression of atherosclerotic plaques in some women. This effect appears to occur throughout the range of LDL cholesterol levels; the lower the LDL, the greater the regression.

The net benefits from cholesterol lowering depend on the underlying risk of coronary heart disease and of other disease. In patients with manifest atherosclerosis, morbidity and mortality rates associated with coronary heart disease are high.

LOW CHOLESTEROL AND OTHER DISEASES

Although high cholesterol levels are associated with an increased risk of coronary heart disease, low cholesterol levels (especially <160 mg/dL) are associated with an increased risk of mortality from other causes, including cancer, respiratory disease, injuries and accidents, and liver disease. The biologic explanation for this excess mortality is unknown. Some studies have suggested that low cholesterol represents a preclinical manifestation of the underlying disease (e.g., an undiagnosed malignancy). Other analyses have found that the increase in risk persists for at least several years. Thus, the net effect is that the overall relation between cholesterol and mortality is somewhat bow-shaped, with mortality rates highest in those with either low or high cholesterol levels.

SECONDARY CONDITIONS THAT AFFECT LIPID METABOLISM

Several factors, including drugs, can influence serum lipid levels (Table 51.6). These are important for two reasons: Abnormal lipid levels (or changes in lipid levels) may be the presenting sign of some of these conditions, and correction of the underlying condition may obviate the need to treat an apparent lipid disorder. Diabetes and alcohol use, in particular, are commonly associated with high triglyceride levels that decline with improvements in glycemic control or reduction in alcohol use, respectively. It is unnecessary to rule out each of these secondary causes, but the clinician should consider each possibility.

TREATMENT OF HIGH LOW-DENSITY LIPOPROTEIN CHOLESTEROL

Reduction of LDL cholesterol is just one part of a program to reduce the risk of cardiovascular disease. Other measures, including smoking cessation and hypertension control, are also of central importance. Less well studied but potentially of great value is raising the HDL cholesterol level. Several healthy habits have more than one benefit. Quitting smoking, for example, reduces the effect of other cardiovascular risk factors (e.g., a high cholesterol level); it may also increase the HDL cholesterol level. Exercise (and weight loss) may reduce the LDL cholesterol level and increase the HDL cholesterol level. Modest alcohol use (1–2 oz/d) also raises the HDL level and appears to have a salutary effect on coronary heart disease rates. The clinician may not wish to recommend alcohol use to patients, but its safe use in moderation does not need to be discouraged.

DIET

Dietary modifications play a central role in most algorithms for treatment of elevated lipid levels. The primary recommendation is to reduce the consumption of total dietary fat to less than 30% of total calories, which should be set at the level required

TABLE 51.6. Secondary Causes of Lipid Abnormalities

Cause	Associated lipid abnormality
Obesity	Increased triglycerides, decreased HDL cholesterol
Sedentary lifestyle	Decreased HDL cholesterol
Diabetes	Increased triglycerides, increased total cholesterol
Alcohol use	Increased triglycerides, increased HDL cholesterol
Hypothyroidism	Increased total cholesterol
Hyperthyroidism	Decreased total cholesterol
Nephrotic syndrome	Increased total cholesterol
Chronic renal insufficiency	Increased total cholesterol, increased triglycerides
Hepatic disease (cirrhosis)	Decreased total cholesterol
Obstructive liver disease	Increased total cholesterol
Malignancy	Decreased total cholesterol
Cushing disease (for steroid use)	Increased total cholesterol
Oral contraceptives	Decreased LDL cholesterol, increased HDL cholesterol, increased triglycerides
Diuretics	Increased total cholesterol, increased triglycerides
Beta-blockers[a]	Increased total cholesterol, decreased HDL

[a]Beta-blockers with intrinsic sympathomimetic activity, such as pindolol and acebutolol, as well as the combination α_1, beta-blocker carvedilol do not adversely affect lipid levels.
HDL, high-density lipoprotein; LDL, low-density lipoprotein.

to achieve and then maintain ideal body weight. Most Americans currently eat 35% to 40% of calories as fat. In someone eating 2,000 kcal/d, 30% of calories as fat would correspond to about 67 g of fat (one pat of butter or margarine contains 15 g). Many clinicians without special expertise and interest in dietary therapy find it advantageous to refer patients to a dietitian. This may be especially helpful if stringent diets (20% calories as fat, with 7% as saturated fat) are prescribed.

In particular, saturated fats (mainly found in animal products, including meats and dairy products) should be reduced to at most 10% of calories. Most dietary fat intake should be divided between polyunsaturated fats (such as those found in many vegetable oils) and foods rich in *cis*-monounsaturated fats, such as olive oil. *Trans*-monounsaturated fats (as found in margarine) should be limited. The effect of cholesterol-lowering diets varies considerably from individual to individual, suggesting that genetic or other factors influence diet responsiveness. Overall, most studies of free-living patients have shown that low-fat diets result in only modest changes in serum cholesterol levels, with reductions in both the LDL and HDL fractions of a few mg/dL. In contrast, several studies have shown that optimization of dietary fat intake coupled with regular exercise affects both LDL and HDL levels favorably.

Soluble fiber, as found in oat bran or psyllium, may reduce LDL cholesterol levels by about 5%. Insoluble fiber (e.g., that found in wheat bran) does not affect lipid levels. Diets should also be rich in antioxidant vitamins, which are found primarily in fruits and vegetables.

PHARMACOLOGIC AGENTS

If the decision to treat a patient with an LDL-lowering drug is made, the clinician must select an appropriate agent based on the safety, efficacy, cost, and effect on other lipid levels (Tables 51.2 and 51.7) and set a goal for treatment (see Chapter 49). Current recommendations do not include drug use to treat low HDL levels in patients who do not also have high LDL levels. As with all therapies for chronic conditions, the therapeutic goal is best approached slowly and steadily, watching carefully for side effects and encouraging continued compliance with nonpharmacologic measures. Combinations of drugs may be necessary. Once the goal is reached, the lipid profile should be monitored every 6 to 12 months, with consideration given to periodic reductions in drug dose or even drug holidays. With the exception of niacin (available generically for a few dollars per month), all these drugs are expensive and may cost more than $100 per month. Moreover, they may need to be given for decades.

Niacin (Nicotinic Acid). Niacin has been associated with a reduction in total mortality. Long-term follow-up of a secondary prevention trial of middle-aged men with previous myocardial infarction disclosed that about 52% of those previously treated with niacin had died, compared with 58% in the placebo group. This favorable effect on mortality was not seen during the trial itself, although there was a reduction in the incidence of coronary heart disease in patients with previous myocardial infarction or stable angina.

Niacin reduces the production of very-low-density lipoprotein particles, with secondary reduction in LDL and increase in HDL cholesterol levels. The average effect of niacin is to reduce LDL levels by about 10% to 15% and triglyceride levels by up to 50%, while increasing HDL levels by 10%. It is best to begin at a low dose (at 500 mg/d, using the vitamin preparations of niacin), slowly increasing to the therapeutic range (1,000 mg two to three times a day with meals). Niacin causes a prostaglandin-mediated flushing; some patients complain of hot flashes or pruritus. This problem can usually be ameliorated by pretreatment with aspirin (325 mg 30 minutes before each dose) or other nonsteroidal antiinflammatory agents. Niacin may exacerbate gout and peptic ulcer disease and may provoke hyperglycemia in patients with diabetes. Hepatitis is an important side effect, perhaps especially among patients treated with a sustained-release preparation, which is also more expensive.

TABLE 51.7. Effects of Selected Cholesterol-lowering Drugs

Drug	ASHD events	Long-term safety	Effects on LDL	Effects on HDL	Effects on triglycerides	Regression of ASHD
Niacin	Reduced	+	↓	↑	↓	Yes, with resins
Cholestyramine	Reduced	+	↓	+/−	↑	Yes, with niacin
Statins	Reduced	?	↓↓	Slight ↑	↓	Yes
Gemfibrozil	Reduced	?	Slight ↓	↑	↓↓	Not proven

HDL, high-density lipoprotein; LDL, low-density lipoprotein.

Whether routine monitoring of liver function tests helps to avoid this side effect is unknown.

Bile Acid-Binding Resins (Cholestyramine, Colestipol). Treatment with these agents reduces the incidence of coronary events (such as myocardial infarction) in middle-aged men by about 20%, with no conclusive effect on total mortality. The resins work by binding bile acids in the intestine. The resultant reduction in the enterohepatic circulation causes the liver to increase its production of bile acids, using hepatic cholesterol to do so. Thus, hepatic LDL receptor activity increases with a decline in plasma LDL levels. The triglyceride level tends to increase slightly in some patients treated with bile acid-binding resins; they should be used with caution in those with elevated triglycerides and probably not at all in patients who have triglyceride levels above about 500 mg/dL. The clinician can anticipate a reduction of 20% to 30% in LDL cholesterol, with minor changes in the HDL level.

The usual dose of cholestyramine is 8 to 16 g of resin per day in divided doses with meals, mixed in water, or, more palatably, juice. The prepackaged 4-g doses are more expensive than the bulk form. Doses of colestipol are 20% higher (the packets each contain 5 g of resin).

These agents often cause gastrointestinal symptoms such as constipation and gas. They may interfere with the absorption of fat-soluble vitamins (thereby complicating the management of patients receiving warfarin) and may bind other drugs in the intestine. Concurrent use of psyllium may ameliorate the gastrointestinal side effects.

β-Hydroxy-β-Methylglutaryl-Coenzyme A Reductase Inhibitors (Lovastatin, Pravastatin, Simvastatin, Atorvastatin). The effects of these agents in preventing coronary heart disease have been reassuring: Simvastatin has reduced death by 30%. They work by inhibiting the rate-limiting enzyme in the formation of cholesterol. Cholesterol synthesis in the liver is reduced, with a compensatory increase in hepatic LDL receptors (presumably so that the liver can take more of the cholesterol that it needs from the blood) and a reduction in the circulating LDL cholesterol level of up to 35%. There are also modest increases in HDL levels and decreases in triglyceride levels.

Doses of all statins range from 10 to 80 mg/d. These agents are usually given once a day in the evening (most cholesterol synthesis occurs overnight); at the high end of the dose ranges, twice-a-day dosing may be used. Side effects include myositis; the incidence may be higher in patients concurrently taking fibrates or niacin. Manufacturers recommend monitoring liver and muscle enzymes. Several agents (notably erythromycin and cyclosporine) reduce the metabolism of these agents.

Fibric Acid Derivatives (Gemfibrozil, Clofibrate). In the largest clinical trial that used clofibrate, there were significantly more deaths, especially due to cancer, in the treatment group than in the control. Although still available, clofibrate is rarely used given the availability of its equally effective relative, gemfibrozil. Gemfibrozil reduced coronary heart disease rates in hypercholesterolemic middle-aged men free of coronary disease in the Helsinki Heart Study, perhaps only among those who also had high triglyceride levels. Among men with previous myocardial infarction, however, gemfibrozil increased overall mortality as well as that due to coronary heart disease. Clinicians should also be aware of the trend toward increased numbers of cancer deaths among subjects treated with gemfibrozil in the Helsinki Heart Study.

The fibrates reduce the synthesis and increase the breakdown of very-low-density lipoprotein particles, with secondary effects on LDL and HDL levels. They reduce LDL levels by about 10% and triglyceride levels by about 40% and raise HDL levels by about 20%. The usual dose of gemfibrozil is 600 mg twice a day. Side effects include cholelithiasis, hepatitis, and myositis. The incidence of the latter two conditions may be higher among patients also taking other lipid-lowering agents. Given that clofibrate caused a statistically significant increase in cancer mortality, it should not be used.

Probucol. The effects of probucol on coronary heart disease, as well as its long-term safety, are unknown. It reduces the deposition of LDL into xanthomas in humans (and into atherosclerotic plaques in rabbits). The mechanism of action is unclear. It apparently reduces the amount of oxidized LDL (it was originally used as an industrial antioxidant). Probucol reduces LDL levels by 10% to 15% but has the potentially important adverse effect of lowering HDL levels by up to 10%. It also may be cardiotoxic. Probucol, if used at all, should be reserved for patients with a clear genetic disorder who have failed other therapies.

HIGH BLOOD TRIGLYCERIDES

Patients with very high levels of serum triglycerides are at risk for pancreatitis. The pathophysiology is uncertain, because some patients with very high triglyceride levels never develop pancreatitis. Most patients with congenital abnormalities in triglyceride metabolism present in childhood; hypertriglyceridemia-induced pancreatitis that first presents in adults is more commonly due to an acquired problem in lipid metabolism.

Although there are no clear triglyceride levels that always result in pancreatitis, most clinicians are uncomfortable with levels above 1,000 mg/dL. The risk of pancreatitis may be more related to the triglyceride level after consumption of a fatty meal. Because postprandial increases in triglycerides are inevitable if fat-containing foods are eaten, fasting triglyceride levels in persons prone to pancreatitis should be kept well below that level.

The primary therapy for high triglyceride levels is dietary, avoiding alcohol and fatty foods. Control of secondary causes of high triglyceride levels may also be helpful. In patients with persistent elevations in the pancreatitis range despite adequate dietary compliance—and certainly in those with a previous episode of pancreatitis—therapy with a triglyceride-lowering drug (e.g., niacin, in doses as described above) is indicated.

Whether patients with elevated triglycerides (>250 mg/dL) and no other lipoprotein abnormalities are at increased risk of atherosclerotic disease is unknown. Some of these patients may belong to families with a genetic disorder known as familial combined hyperlipidemia. This disorder is characterized by various lipid abnormalities in different family members: Some have high cholesterol levels, some high triglyceride levels, and some both. It appears that the common link is an abnormality in one of the LDL-associated apoproteins (B-100) and that this may be a coronary risk factor. However, the effect on coronary heart disease risk of treating an isolated high triglyceride level in these patients is unknown. Some authorities recommend treating an isolated high triglyceride level in patients with known coronary heart disease, reasoning that such patients are likely to have some abnormality in lipid metabolism. Treatment is primarily nonpharmacologic, with an emphasis on weight loss, a low-fat diet, avoidance of excess alcohol, and exercise.

OTHER PHARMACOLOGIC AGENTS

All patients whose risk from coronary heart disease is considered high enough to warrant pharmacologic therapy of an elevated LDL cholesterol should be given aspirin prophylaxis at a dose of about 325 g every other day, unless there are contraindications such as aspirin sensitivity, bleeding diatheses, or active peptic ulcer disease. Current data suggest that the effect of aspirin in reducing the risk of coronary heart disease is equal to or even greater than that of cholesterol lowering.

SPECIAL CONSIDERATIONS IN WOMEN

Hormonal Therapy in Women

The direct effects of estrogen on the vasculature promote increased levels of endothelial-derived nitrous oxide, resulting in vasodilation and may also be inhibit the development and progression of ASHD. However, some of the nonvascular effects of estrogen may offset its beneficial vascular effects. There are currently no estrogens with relative vascular selectivity.

Treatment of postmenopausal women with oral estrogen replacement therapy is associated with a 15% reduction in LDL levels and a 15% increase in HDL levels. These lipid effects appear to be responsible for about one third to one fourth of the possible benefit of postmenopausal estrogens on reducing coronary heart disease. The addition of a progestin to the hormone regimen, however, may diminish the beneficial effect on lipids.

In May 2002, the Women's Health Initiative trial of daily *combined* therapy with estrogen and progestin in postmenopausal women was terminated early due to an increased risk of breast cancer as well as a slightly increased risk of AMI in the hormone therapy group. Several other studies had previously raised concerns that combined therapy with estrogens and progestins increased the risk of venous thromboembolism, gallbladder disease, stroke, and breast cancer, although the risk of AMI was not clearly worsened. Conversely, studies looking at the use of *estrogen alone* (usually reserved as treatment for women with previous hysterectomy due to the increased risk of endometrial cancer with estrogen alone) have documented slower progression of subclinical atherosclerosis when compared with placebo.

Current recommendations for the use of both oral contraceptives in younger women and hormone replacement therapy in postmenopausal women should include advice to avoid cigarette smoking. Many experts advise against long-term use of hormone replacement therapy because the increased risks of venous thromboembolism, stroke, and breast cancer outweigh the potential benefits. In women status post-hysterectomy, estrogen use alone should be considered for hormone replacement therapy.

Occurrence of Acute Myocardial Infarction in Premenopausal Women

Mortality from coronary artery disease in women in the United States below age 30 is negligible: it is 10 per 100,000 and doubles by age 45. The total incidence of symptomatic coronary disease exceeds 50 per 100,000 at age 40 and increases rapidly thereafter. Predisposing factors are diabetes, hypertension, hypercholesterolemia, or a positive family history.

Cigarette smoking contributes significantly to the incidence of coronary disease in young women. Counseling young women against cigarette smoking is a major responsibility of all health professionals. Sudden death from coronary heart disease is strongly related to cigarette smoking in women.

Oral contraceptives act synergistically with other atherogenic risk factors, particularly cigarette smoking, that predispose to coronary thrombosis. Low-dose ("third-generation") oral combination contraceptive pills apparently do not significantly increase the risk of atherosclerosis in young females.

On occasion, the occurrence of angina pectoris and myocardial infarction in persons with angiographically normal coronary arteries has been recognized. Coronary artery spasm and coronary embolism are two possible mechanisms. The syndrome is more likely to occur in young women than in men.

SPECIAL CONSIDERATIONS: PREGNANCY

Coronary artery disease is uncommon during pregnancy, but chest pain is not. Usually it is mild and transient and disappears with reassurance. Often its cause is unclear, but thoracic distortion resulting from elevation of the diaphragm and flaring of the ribs is a common explanation. In addition, esophageal reflux occurs more commonly during pregnancy. Similar chest pain, although not otherwise typical, may be associated with prolapse of the mitral valve.

Effects of Pregnancy

Some of the changes in the circulation that occur during pregnancy may affect the adequacy of oxygen supply to the myocardium. For example, an increased myocardial oxygen consumption would be expected as a result of the changes in heart rate, left ventricular size, and cardiac output. In patients who begin pregnancy with anemia, the hemodilution that usually accompanies pregnancy may require further increases in cardiac work and myocardial oxygen consumption. Additionally, the fall in systemic vascular resistance that accompanies normal pregnancy may divert blood flow from a coronary artery that has been narrowed by atherosclerotic changes. Finally, exercise during pregnancy leads to a greater increase in oxygen consumption than does similar exercise in a nonpregnant patient, and the oxygen requirements of the myocardium for the same workload are probably increased.

On the other hand, vasodilation occurs in some parts of the body during pregnancy, and the total peripheral resistance is lower than in the nonpregnant state. The decline in peripheral resistance reduces the magnitude of the increase in work required of the heart, and the vasodilation of pregnancy may involve the coronary vasculature. The hypothesis is that the balance between myocardial oxygen need and coronary blood flow is unfavorably altered by pregnancy in patients with coronary artery disease. Some evidence suggests that coronary artery spasm is particularly common in pregnancy, and this cause of myocardial hypoxia deserves attention when the anginal syndrome occurs in a young pregnant woman in the absence of factors that predispose to premature coronary atherosclerosis.

The incidence of symptomatic coronary atherosclerosis in pregnant women appears to be increasing, perhaps because of increased cigarette smoking by women. Additionally, the use of β-adrenergic drugs for the treatment of premature labor is associated with a significant incidence in angina pectoris. The actions of these compounds (terbutaline and ritodrine are the most commonly used) include increases in heart rate and myocardial contractility. Despite an increase in cardiac output, diastolic blood pressure often falls, jeopardizing coronary perfusion. As a result, myocardial hypoxia may occur, especially in women with coronary artery disease.

Chest pain that resembles angina pectoris in location and radiation, when induced by a β-adrenergic agonist, usually disappears promptly when the drug is stopped. These drugs should not be used unless a carefully directed history and physical examination raise no suspicion of heart disease. A pretreatment ECG should be normal, and the occurrence of chest pain during administration of the drug dictates prompt cessation.

The prognosis of a myocardial infarction that occurs during pregnancy depends in part on the time in gestation when it occurs. When myocardial infarction occurs in the first 7 months of pregnancy, death in association with pregnancy is unusual. Eleven of the reported 13 deaths associated with pregnancy occurred among women who suffered a myocardial infarction in the last trimester of pregnancy or during labor. Pregnancy imposes an increased risk to patients with well-documented myocardial ischemia. If a firm diagnosis of myocardial ischemia is made, pregnancy is contraindicated, because evidence indicates that the risk of maternal death is approximately doubled during pregnancy and the postpartum period.

In planning and implementing medical management, angina pectoris should be seen as a syndrome that is usually precipitated by the superimposition of several burdens. Removal or mitigation of one or more of these burdens may restore the balance between myocardial oxygen supply and demand. In general, obesity, anxiety, and physical activity can be controlled or altered. Smoking and exposure to hot humid environments are prohibited. In addition, such complicating conditions as hypertension, anemia, hyperthyroidism, and infection must be corrected. Medical management may include sublingual nitroglycerin, calcium channel blockers, or β-adrenergic blocking drugs. If episodes of angina pectoris continue, and especially if they increase in frequency or severity despite medical management, mechanical intervention should be considered. If possible, from the fetal standpoint, surgery is best delayed until at least the 12th to 16th week of pregnancy, when organogenesis is nearly complete. Other precautions that are helpful from the fetal standpoint include

- Performing surgery under normothermic or modestly hypothermic states when possible
- Maintaining extracorporeal circulation at a high flow level
- Instituting fetal monitoring with an obstetric team on standby (if fetal maturity is appropriate)
- Ensuring that the efflux from the coronary sinus does not circulate so as to affect the fetus
- Having a highly experienced cardiac surgeon perform the operation.

Modest rotation of the mother into the left lateral decubitus position should also be done to prevent impedance of flow through caval and aortic compression.

Thrombolytic therapy, the mainstay for treatment of early myocardial infarction in the nonpregnant patient, may potentiate significant bleeding in the mother and fetus. Angioplasty may be more hazardous because of the possible predisposition of the pregnant patient to coronary artery dissection. Even cardiac resuscitation may become more complex, necessitating emptying the uterus, if no response occurs to initial attempts within minutes. Finally, multiple medications used in treatment may affect uterine tone and adversely affect the fetus.

Many recommend that interruption of pregnancy be considered with the hope of prompt symptomatic improvement. Both angioplasty and bypass surgery require coronary angiography and thus pose an added risk for the fetus. When pregnancy has been completed (or interrupted), careful evaluation for long-term management is essential.

When a myocardial infarction occurs during pregnancy, its management should be the same as in nonpregnant patients. If bed rest is necessary, anticoagulation with heparin is probably desirable to minimize the risk of thromboembolism, but anticoagulation should be discontinued as soon as mobilization is possible.

If congestive failure, shock, arrhythmias, or ischemic pain persists after a myocardial infarction despite treatment with beta-blockers, long-acting nitrates, and calcium channel blockers, termination of pregnancy before the fourth month is recommended. After the fourth month, the hazards of interruption are probably similar to those of continuing pregnancy. If none of these complications persists, interruption of pregnancy is not justified.

Myocardial infarction in pregnancy is rare. It is frequently overlooked as a diagnostic possibility in the young pregnant patient with chest pain (often ascribed to gastrointestinal causes). The chest pain history should be closely taken. If the pain is not classic for reflux esophagitis or if it is atypical or crescendo in nature, the potential of a cardiac origin should be entertained. At the very least, an ECG should be obtained and a cardiology consultation considered. In the patient who has had an ischemic event, consultation among the cardiologist, anesthesiologist, and obstetrician should be obtained as early as possible. Labor presents multiple physiologic changes that must be addressed in the patient with left ventricular dysfunction. Pharmacologic manipulations are central to the management of these patients, and the use of the pulmonary artery catheter to adjust several parameters may yield the best outcome. It is hoped that the mortality associated with myocardial infarction can be lowered using these new technologies.

SUMMARY

The pathophysiology, diagnostic methods, clinical syndromes, and treatment of ASHD were reviewed. Specific measures for primary and secondary prevention, with emphasis on the latter, were detailed. These secondary prevention measures include the modification of coronary risk factors (Table 51.2), medical and interventional treatment during and after acute coronary syndromes, and the use of pharmacologic agents documented to reduce recurrent events in patients with known ASHD. Finally, a review of some of the recent still controversial data regarding hormonal therapy in women and some special considerations in pregnancy were addressed.

BIBLIOGRAPHY

Amsterdam EA, Hyson D, Kappagoda CT. Nonpharmacologic therapy for coronary artery atherosclerosis: results of primary and secondary prevention trials. *Am Heart J* 1994;128:1344.

Bedinghaus J, Leshan L, Diehr S. Coronary artery disease prevention: what's different for women? *Am Fam Pract* 2001;63:1393–1400.

Blankenhorn DH, Azen SP, Kramsch DM, et al. Coronary angiographic changes with lovastatin therapy—the Monitored Atherosclerosis Regression Study (MARS). *Ann Intern Med* 1993;119:969–976.

Blankenhorn DN, Nessim SA, Johnson RL, et al. Beneficial effects of combined colestipol-niacin therapy on coronary atherosclerosis and coronary venous bypass graft. *JAMA* 1987;257:3233–3240.

Canner PL, Barge GK, Wenger NK, et al., for the Coronary Drug Projects Research Group. Fifteen-year mortality in coronary drug patients: long-term benefit with niacin. *J Am Coll Cardiol* 1986;8:1245–1255.

Denton TA, Fonarow GC, Labresh KA, et al. Secondary prevention after coronary bypass: the American Heart Association "Get With the Guidelines" Program. *Ann Thorac Surg* 2003;75:758–760.

Despres JP, Lamarche B. Low-intensity endurance exercise training, plasma lipoproteins and the risk of coronary heart disease. *J Intern Med* 1994;236:7.

Gaziano JM. Antioxidant vitamins and coronary artery disease risk. *Am J Med* 1994;97[Suppl 3A]:18S.

Grodstein F, Clarkson TB, Manson JE. Understanding the divergent data on postmenopausal hormone therapy. *N Engl J Med* 2003;348:645–650.

Haskell WL, Alderman EL, Fair JM, et al. Effects of intensive multiple risk factor reduction on coronary atherosclerosis and clinical cardiac events in men and women with coronary artery disease. The Standford Coronary Risk Intervention Projects. *Circulation* 1994;89:975–990.

Herrington DM, Reboussin DM, Brosnihan B, et al. Effects of estrogen replacement on the progression of coronary artery atherosclerosis. *N Engl J Med* 2000;343:522–529.

Hess DB, Hess LW. Management of cardiovascular disease in pregnancy. *Obstet Gynecol Clin North Am* 1992;19:679.

Heyden S. Polyunsaturated and monounsaturated fatty acids in the diet to prevent coronary heart disease via cholesterol reduction. *Ann Nutr Metab* 1994;38:117.

Hoffman RM, Garewal HS. Antioxidants and the prevention of coronary heart disease. *Arch Intern Med* 1995;155:241.

Hulley S, Grady D, Bush T, et al. Randomized trial of estrogen plus progestin for secondary prevention of coronary heart disease in postmenopausal women. Heart and Estrogen/Progestin Replacement Study (HERS) Research Group. *JAMA* 1998;280:605–613.

Just H, Frey M. Role of calcium antagonists in progression of arteriosclerosis: evidence from animal experiments and clinical experience. *Basic Res Cardiol* 1994;1[Suppl 89]:177.

LaRosa JC. Dyslipoproteinemia in women and the elderly. *Med Clin North Am* 1994;78:163.

Lavie CJ, Milani RV, Littman AB. Benefits of cardiac rehabilitation and exercise training in secondary coronary prevention in the elderly. *J Am Coll Cardiol* 1993;22:678.

Mendelsohn ME, Karas RH. The protective effects of estrogen on the cardiovascular system. *N Engl J Med* 1999;340:1801–1811.

Metcalfe J, McAnulty JH, Ueland K. *Burwell and Metcalfe's heart disease and pregnancy: physiology and management*. Boston: Little, Brown, 1986:295.

Nolan TE, Hankins GD. Myocardial infarction in pregnancy. *Clin Obstet Gynecol* 1989;32:71.

Pitt B, Mancini GBJ, Ellis SG, et al., for the PLACI Investigators. Pravastatin limitation of atherosclerosis in the coronary arteries (PLAC-I): reduction in atherosclerosis progression and clinical events. *Am J Cardiol* 1995;26: 1133–1139.

Ridker PM, Hennekens CH, Buring JE, et al. C-reactive protein and other markers of inflammation in the prediction of cardiovascular disease in women. *N Engl J Med* 2000;342:836–843.

Robinson JG, Leon AS. The prevention of cardiovascular disease: emphasis on secondary prevention. *Med Clin North Am* 1994;78:69.

Rosenson RS, Frauenheim WA, Tangney CC. Dyslipidemia and the secondary prevention of coronary heart disease. *Disease-a-Month* 1994;40:369.

Sacks FM, Pasternak RC, Gibson CM, et al., for the Harvard Atherosclerosis Reversibility Project (HARP). Effect on coronary atherosclerosis of decrease in plasma-cholesterol concentrations in normocholesterolaemic patients. *Lancet* 1994;344:1182–1186.

Sacks FM, Pfeffer MA, Moye LA, et al. The effect of pravastatin on coronary events after myocardial infarction in patients with average cholesterol levels. *N Engl J Med* 1996;335:1001–1009.

Sacks FM, Rouleau JL, Moye LA, et al. Baseline characteristics in the cholesterol and recurrent events (CARE) trial of secondary prevention in patients with average serum cholesterol levels. *Am J Cardiol* 1995;75:621.

The Scandinavian Simvastatin Survival Study Group. Randomised trial of cholesterol lowering in 4,444 patients with coronary heart disease: the Scandinavian Simvastatin Survival Study (4S). *Lancet* 1994;344:1383–1389.

Scottish Intercollegiate Guidelines Network. Secondary Prevention of Coronary Heart Disease following Myocardial Infarction: A National Clinical Guideline. Available at the SIGN Web site: *www.sign.ac.uk*.

Seed M. Postmenopausal hormone replacement therapy, coronary heart disease and plasma in lipoproteins. *Drugs* 1994;47[Suppl 2]:25.

Solomon CG, Dluhy RG. Rethinking postmenopausal hormone therapy. *N Engl J Med* 2003;348:579–580.

Tanis BC, VanDenBosch MAAJ, Kemmeren JM, et al. Oral contraceptives and the risk of myocardial infarction. *N Engl J Med* 2001;345:1787–1793.

Truswell SA. Review of dietary intervention studies: effect on coronary events and on total morality. *Aust N Z J Med* 1994;24:98.

Williams MA, Fleg JL, Ades PA, et al. Secondary prevention of coronary heart disease in the elderly (with emphasis on patients ≥ 75 years of age): an American Heart Association Scientific statement from the Council on Clinical Cardiology Subcommittee on Exercise, Cardiac Rehabilitation and Prevention. *Circulation* 2002;105:1735–1743.

Wood DA. Cholesterol lowering does have a role in secondary prevention. *Br Heart J* 1995;73:4.

PART

6

Respiratory Problems

CHAPTER 52
Pneumonia

Sarah Nicklin and William L. Miller

Pneumonia, infection of the normally sterile lung parenchyma of the lower respiratory tract, remains a commonly encountered, difficult to diagnose, and serious illness in primary care. Unfortunately, there are very little available data specific to women regarding this common condition. Pneumonia is the sixth leading cause of death and the most common infectious disease cause of death in the United States. There are an estimated 2 to 5.6 million cases of community-acquired pneumonia (CAP) diagnosed each year, with 500,000 to 1.1 million being hospitalized. Incidence increases in winter and at the extremes of age. In the northern hemisphere, CAP affects about 12 of 1,000 people a year overall, with incidence by age as follows: less than age 1 year, 30 to 50 per 1,000 per year; aged 15 to 45 years, 1 to 5 per 1,000 per year; aged 60 to 70 years, 10 to 20 per 1,000 per year; and aged 71 to 85 years, 50 per 1,000 per year. The mortality rate from pneumonia varies from less than 1% to 5% in the outpatient setting to 12% to 14% overall among those hospitalized. The rate increases in certain subgroups, including bacteremic patients and those from nursing homes, rising to near 40% among those severely ill and requiring intensive care.

ETIOLOGY AND DIFFERENTIAL DIAGNOSIS

Over 100 microorganisms have been implicated as causative in CAP and include bacteria, viruses, atypical bacteria, mycobacteria, and fungi. Prospective studies attempting to identify causes of CAP have failed to do so in 40% to 60% of cases and have identified at least two organisms in 2% to 20%.

The most common etiology identified in almost all studies is *Streptococcus pneumoniae*. Other bacterial and atypical pathogens identified include *Haemophilus influenzae, Mycoplasma pneumoniae, Chlamydia pneumoniae, Staphylococcus aureus, Streptococcus pyogenes, Neisseria meningitidis, Moraxella catarrhalis, Klebsiella pneumoniae, Legionella* species, and other Gram-negative organisms. Anaerobic oropharyngeal flora may be seen in aspiration pneumonia, though more recent studies have isolated *S. pneumoniae, S. aureus, H. influenzae,* and Enterobacteriaceae in community-acquired aspiration and Gram-negative bacteria, including *Pseudomonas aeruginosa,* in hospital-acquired aspiration. Other etiologies vary in frequency depending on specific epidemiologic factors and include *Chlamydia psittaci* (psittacosis), *Coxiella burnetii* (Q fever), and *Francisella tularensis* (tularemia). *Bacillus anthracis,* the bacterial cause of anthrax, does not usually cause pneumonia, but rather its pulmonary manifestation is inhalation anthrax, characterized by hemorrhagic necrosis of the thoracic lymph nodes, hemorrhagic mediastinitis, and, occasionally, a necrotizing pneumonia at the site of entry. Tuberculosis can present as a pulmonary infiltrate. In one prospective study, pulmonary infiltrates developed in 27% of 517 new tuberculin converters followed for more than 5 years.

Viral causes of pneumonia include influenza virus (varies by season), respiratory syncytial virus, adenovirus, parainfluenza virus, and varicella. Hantavirus does not cause pneumonia but rather a pulmonary syndrome characterized by a noncardiogenic pulmonary edema, hemodynamic compromise, and high mortality.

Fungal pneumonias are caused by fungi endemic to certain geographic areas and should be considered in people who live or travel in those areas. They include histoplasmosis and blastomycosis in the Mississippi and Ohio River basins and coccidioidomycosis in the southwestern United States and parts of Latin America. Cryptococcal infection usually presents as meningitis, and isolated pneumonia is rare. *Pneumocystis carinii,* now considered a fungus, should be considered in immunocompromised patients, especially those with acquired immunodeficiency syndrome or on corticosteroids. Aspergilli, Zygomycetes, and other fungi rarely cause pneumonia unless neutropenia, diabetic ketoacidosis, or profound immunodeficiency is present.

The differential diagnosis of respiratory and systemic symptoms and signs suggestive of pneumonia is quite broad and includes infectious and noninfectious etiologies. Among these are chemical pneumonitis from aspiration, bronchitis, sinusitis, asthma, chronic obstructive pulmonary disease, congestive heart failure (CHF), pulmonary embolus, pneumothorax, malignancy (primary or metastatic), bronchial obstruction from neoplasm or foreign body, vasculitis, inflammatory disorders, toxin exposure, hypersensitivity to environmental agents, and alveolar hemorrhage, as in Goodpasture syndrome. In patients, such as the elderly, presenting with systemic rather than respiratory symptoms of pneumonia, the differential diagnosis is greatly expanded and includes sepsis; infections of other organ systems; myocardial infarction; cerebrovascular accident; toxins, including medications; and neurologic and endocrine disorders.

CLINICAL SYMPTOMS AND HISTORY

Women with CAP present with a large number of possible symptoms. Respiratory symptoms may include cough (productive or not), dyspnea, chest pain (pleuritic or not), and hemoptysis. Other symptoms may include fatigue; malaise; fever; chills or rigors; headache; myalgias; diaphoresis, especially night sweats; generalized weakness; anorexia; and abdominal pain. In the elderly, common presenting symptoms may only consist of confusion, worsening of an underlying chronic illness, and/or falls. Unfortunately, no specific symptom or combination of symptoms on history can confirm the diagnosis of pneumonia. One review of the literature found that no single item in the clinical history, even when combined with physical examination, raised the odds of pneumonia high enough to confirm the diagnosis without a chest radiograph.

A focused history can give many clues to potential etiologies and prognosis of CAP in primary care. Medical history of respiratory diseases such as asthma, chronic obstructive pulmonary disease or restrictive pulmonary disease, CHF, and dementia should be gathered. Medication history may provide clues to potential etiologies, for example, recent antibiotics, immunosuppressants, and sedatives, the last of which increase the risk of aspiration, especially in the elderly. Exploration of personal history should include use or abuse, including amount and duration, of tobacco, alcohol, and other recreational drugs. Exposure to children in day care or to hospitalized patients may increase chances of exposure to resistant organisms. Family history should include information about contagious diseases, like tuberculosis, and hereditary pulmonary conditions like asthma, cystic fibrosis, and α_1-antitrypsin deficiency.

Occupational history should investigate potential exposure to infectious agents and hazardous substances. *C. psittaci* (psittacosis) is seen in patients with a history of regular contact with birds. *C. burnetii* (Q fever) should be considered in patients with pneumonia who report contact with farm or newborn animals. *F. tularensis* (tularemia) can be transmitted by vectors like the dog tick or the Lone Star tick or by handling infected rabbits, hares, squirrels, or rodents. Toxin exposures to be considered include asbestos, silicon, coal, beryllium, iron oxide, and others. Details should include severity and duration of exposure and protective measures used during the exposure.

CLINICAL FINDINGS AND PHYSICAL EXAMINATION

Examination of the chest can be performed through the usual steps of inspection, palpation, percussion, and auscultation. Inspection includes the pattern of respiration, the rate, depth, regularity, and any distress; symmetry of chest wall expansion; and retractions. Palpation includes palpating the chest wall for tenderness and crepitus (soft tissue and bony) and testing for vocal fremitus. Percussion may reveal dullness, which can be caused by atelectasis, consolidation, pleural effusion, pleural thickening, or neoplasm. Finally, auscultation assesses the intensity of normal breath sounds, the transmission of spoken words, and the presence of adventitious sounds in all areas of the chest. Tubular or bronchial breath sounds, normally heard only over the trachea, may be heard in the peripheral lung fields in areas of lung consolidation. The principal abnormal sounds in CAP are crackles (formerly rales). Computer analyses of lung sounds identified distinct findings in each of four diseases: idiopathic pulmonary fibrosis, chronic obstructive pulmonary disease, CHF, and pneumonia. Patients with pneumonia tended to have more coarse crackles, most of which were pan-inspiratory, which differed from the findings in other conditions. It has been suggested that auscultation should be performed with the patient breathing at normal tidal volumes, because inspiration from lower lung volumes (i.e., residual volume) can yield abnormal auscultatory findings in as many as 50% of normal subjects. Data on the accuracy of physical examination findings are limited but suggest that a single physical examination finding or combination of findings reliably predicts the presence or absence of pneumonia. One review of the literature on diagnosing pneumonia by history and physical examination found that clinicians frequently disagree about the presence or absence of individual findings on chest examination of patients with CAP, as well as other respiratory illnesses, and that individual signs have inadequate test characteristics to rule in or rule out the diagnosis.

One prospective study of 52 male patients in the emergency department of a Veterans Affairs medical center looked at the accuracy of various physical examination techniques in diagnosing pneumonia and compared interobserver reliability of the techniques among three examiners. The study found that physical examination of the chest is not sufficiently accurate to confirm or exclude the diagnosis of pneumonia (confirmed or excluded with chest radiographs) and that interobserver agreement was highly variable for different physical examination findings. The most valuable examination findings in detecting pneumonia were unilateral crackles in the upright position and crackles in the lateral decubitus position. Another study also found that auscultation of each lung in the lateral decubitus position may be a more sensitive technique for detecting crackles in patients with pneumonia.

More helpful, perhaps, are that absence of vital sign abnormalities and presence of asthma make pneumonia significantly less likely, though they are not sufficient to rule it out. An evidence- and quality-based review of four prospective studies and a validation study concluded that absence of vital sign abnormalities (heart rate, 100 beats/min; respiratory rate, 24 beats/min; or oral temperature, 100.4°F [38°C]) and chest examination abnormalities suggestive of focal consolidation (e.g., crackles, egophony, fremitus) sufficiently reduced the likelihood of pneumonia to the point where further diagnostic testing is ordinarily not necessary. Of note, presence or absence of sputum is not determinate.

Clinical prediction rules can guide the selection of patients in whom to pursue further diagnostic testing such as chest radiograph. One study identified temperature higher than 37.8°C (100°F), pulse more than 100 beats/min, crackles, decreased breath sounds, and the absence of asthma as multivariate predictors of radiographically confirmed pneumonia. Another found that temperature higher than 37.8°C (100°F), pulse more than 100 beats/min, or respiration more than 20/min were 97% sensitive in predicting chest radiographic infiltrates. These prediction rules were found to be more sensitive than physician judgment alone. The Institute for Clinical Systems Improvement, in their guideline on CAP, recommends obtaining a chest radiograph, especially if two or more of the following five signs are present: temperature more than 37.8°C (100°F), pulse more than 100 beats/min, decreased breath sounds, crackles, and respiratory rate more than 20/min (Fig. 52.1). They note, however,

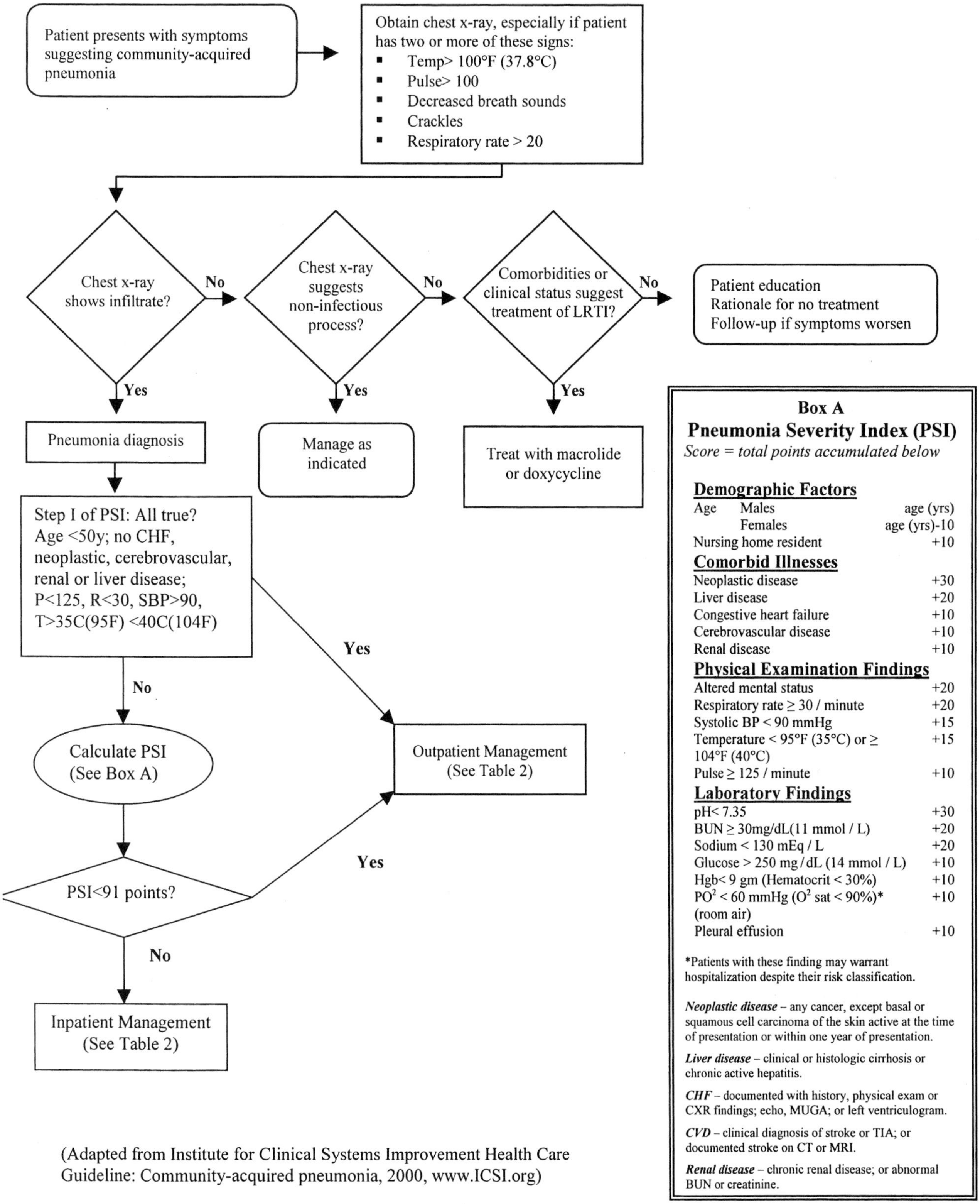

FIG. 52.1. Decision making in patients with possible pneumonia.

that even among patients with four or five of these signs, up to 45% may not have pneumonia confirmed radiographically. Thus, clinical judgment, and possibly a chest radiograph, is essential in deciding whether or not antibiotic treatment is appropriate. Because no combination of history and physical examination findings have been identified that reliably predict or confirm the diagnosis of pneumonia itself, clinical findings cannot be relied on to diagnose a particular etiology for CAP.

LABORATORY AND IMAGING STUDIES

Chest radiography

Chest radiograph or roentgenogram has long been, and still is, considered the gold standard for diagnosing pneumonia. Unfortunately, the evidence to support this faith is not conclusive. Most studies require radiographic confirmation of infiltrate on chest radiograph to make the diagnosis of pneumonia; therefore, we do not have good data on the false-negative rate of a chest radiograph as it relates to the diagnosis of pneumonia. Nonetheless, false-negative results are known by all clinicians and have been attributed to dehydration, *P. carinii* pneumonia (PCP), neutropenia, and evaluation during the first 24 hours.

The role of dehydration was investigated in a retrospective study of 125 patients. It documented progression of radiographic findings of pneumonia in patients who were dehydrated on admission (elevated blood urea nitrogen) and were hydrated (higher fluid volume administered), suggesting that dehydration may mask radiographic findings of pneumonia. A retrospective review of 93 patients with PCP found that 39% had a falsely negative chest radiograph at presentation, which corresponded to a less severe clinical course. Evidence does not support the supposition that neutropenia increases the likelihood of a falsely negative chest radiograph.

In one study that provided some data on the false-negative chest radiograph rate, investigators did both chest radiograph and high-resolution computed tomography of the chest in patients with clinical symptoms and signs suggestive of CAP. Of 47 patients enrolled, 18 had pulmonary infiltrates by both chest radiograph and computed tomography. An additional eight with a negative chest radiograph had infiltrates on computed tomography, resulting in a false-negative rate for chest radiograph of 28%, or 1 of 4. Information on hydration status, duration of symptoms, and absolute neutrophil counts were not provided.

Another perspective on the question of false-negative chest radiograph rates in pneumonia is offered by data from three studies on interobserver variation on chest radiograph interpretation in patients with clinical presentations consistent with pneumonia. One prospective multicenter study assessed interobserver reliability between two staff radiologists at a university hospital. The radiologists read chest radiographs of 282 adults with symptoms or signs of pneumonia and a pulmonary radiographic infiltrate documented by a local study site radiologist. They were not in agreement about the presence or absence of infiltrate in 15% (1 of 7) of chest radiographs of adults who had already been diagnosed with CAP. Another prospective multicenter study conducted as part of the Pneumonia Patient Outcomes Research Team investigation had a radiology panel of three radiologists look specifically at the radiographic findings of 2,287 patients who had already met study inclusion criteria that included one or more clinical symptoms suggestive of pneumonia and radiographic evidence of pneumonia determined by a local study site radiologist. The discordance rate was 12% (1 of 8). A third study, this one retrospective, found that of 93 patients with PCP, initial chest radiograph interpretations by two radiologists were discordant for the presence or absence of infiltrates in 12, a discordance rate of 13% (1 of 8). All these data suggest that given a clinical picture consistent with pneumonia, chest radiograph may be falsely negative in 12% to 28% of patients (1 of 4 to 1 of 8).

Chest radiography does have value in addition to aiding in diagnosis of pneumonia; it may be helpful as a predictor of mortality and in diagnosing other conditions. Previous studies have suggested that multilobar infiltrates are significantly associated with mortality. Better recent evidence from a multicenter, prospective, cohort study of radiographs of 1,906 patients with CAP, analyzed by multivariate analysis, found the presence of bilateral pleural effusions to be the only independent predictor of short-term (30-day) mortality. Chest radiography can help to differentiate pneumonia from other conditions that may mimic it and may identify other or coexisting conditions, including lung abscess, tuberculosis, bronchial obstruction, and pneumothorax. Like history and physical findings, radiographic features cannot be used reliably to determine the etiology of pneumonia with adequate sensitivity and specificity.

Other Diagnostic Testing

Once the clinical diagnosis of pneumonia is made, further diagnostic evaluation should only be considered with an understanding of three key points: in more than 50% of cases, a specific etiology is never identified; in a significant number of cases, coinfection may exist with both bacterial and atypical pathogens and focused therapy may not cover both; and if diagnostic testing results in delay of appropriate therapy, outcome may be adversely effected.

Most studies have concluded, and most guidelines have concurred, that sputum Gram stain and culture are not of sufficient value to guide therapy, so there is little to be gained from obtaining them routinely. The American Thoracic Society guideline of 2001 offered a practical and evidence-based approach. Given the limitations of routine sputum analysis, the need for therapy to begin expeditiously, and to cover a wide range of likely organisms to improve outcomes, it is recommended that sputum be obtained only when a drug-resistant pathogen or an organism not covered by usual empiric therapy is suspected. Gram stain should not be used to focus initial therapy but could be used to broaden therapy to include organisms seen that are not covered by initial empiric therapy. Also, it should be used to guide interpretation of sputum culture results because sensitivity and specificity of culture results alone are poor.

A sputum sample from the lower respiratory tract that is not significantly contaminated by oral secretions should have fewer than 10 squamous epithelial cells and greater than 25 neutrophils per low-power field. A metaanalysis of sputum Gram stain in community-acquired pneumococcal pneumonia found that sensitivity and specificity varied so dramatically in different settings that results could be misleading and thus its use might even be hazardous. One prospective study of adults hospitalized with CAP without comorbidity found that sputum Gram stain and culture had no value in management.

Sputum studies offer greater potential benefit when used selectively in certain patients. Direct staining (non-Gram stain methods) and/or specialized cultures may be diagnostic for infections such as *Mycobacterium* species, *Legionella* species, fungi and *P. carinii*. Bacterial culture of sputum may be helpful in patients deemed to be at higher risk of organisms, like drug-resistant pneumococci, other resistant pathogens, or *S. aureus*. If legionella is suspected because of the presence of abdominal pain, headache, confusion, bradycardia, and/or elevated liver enzymes, in addition to cough, fever, and pulmonary infiltrates, legionella culture should be specifically requested on respiratory secretions, which may be clear and watery, so usual sputum adequacy criteria do not apply. For evaluation of mycobacterial infection, three sputum samples collected on three separate days are required for staining and culture for acid-fast bacilli. Newer methods have decreased average time to recovery and identification of acid-fast organisms in culture to 10 to 12 days and susceptibility testing to just 5 days. If fungal infection is suspected, sputum should be sent for fungal stain and culture. If PCP is suspected, sputum should be sent for direct fluorescent antibody testing.

Routine laboratory tests (complete blood counts and differential, chemistries including serum electrolytes, hepatic enzymes, and renal function tests) are of limited value for determining the etiology of pneumonia but can have prognostic significance. Thus, these routine tests can help in the decision about whether or not to hospitalize a patient with pneumonia.

Blood cultures are positive in only 4% to 18% of patients hospitalized with CAP, with pneumococcus isolated most commonly. In patients treated with antibiotics before blood cultures are drawn, fewer than 5% are positive. False-positive results further confound interpretation and diminish the usefulness of this diagnostic test. A retrospective study of blood cultures from 517 nonimmunosuppressed patients with CAP admitted to the hospital found 25 (4.8%) had growth of contaminants and 34 (6.6%) were positive for pathogens. Antibiotic therapy was changed for seven patients (1.4% of study patients) at a cost of $34,122 or $66 per patient, casting doubt on both the cost effectiveness and the clinical utility of the test. A prospective study of adults hospitalized with CAP without comorbidity found that blood cultures had no value in management. However, in more severely ill patients and patients with comorbidity, obtaining blood cultures should be considered, because two sets drawn before antibiotic treatment is begun may help identify bacteremia and diagnose a resistant pathogen (overall yield 11%).

All hospitalized patients should have oxygen saturation assessed by pulse oximetry. Arterial blood gas should be obtained in any patient with severe illness or chronic lung disease to determine both the level of oxygenation and the degree of carbon dioxide retention.

Antigen tests are available for testing urine and sputum for pneumococcus and legionella and for testing serum for pneumococcus. Clinical usefulness is limited for urinary antigen tests. Sensitivity of the pneumococcal urinary antigen test varies from 75% to 95% and specificity, from 71% to 94%. Urine enzyme immunoassay can be done to detect *Legionella pneumophila* serogroup 1 antigen, but sensitivity varies from 70% to 90% and it does not detect the other 62 serovariants. A new kit for detecting more serotypes was recently developed, but its performance has yet to be evaluated. Sensitivity of the sputum and serum tests is so low that they have little value in the clinical setting.

Serologic tests are also of limited usefulness, and their routine use is not recommended. Acute and convalescent antibody titers that detect fourfold changes in levels are helpful, making diagnoses retrospectively and for epidemiologic purposes, but do not help guide therapy. Serologic testing is not recommended for legionella because antibodies develop slowly and many people who live in endemic areas may have elevated titers. When testing for mycoplasma, IgM may be lacking in adults, and cold agglutinins lack sufficient sensitivity and specificity to be used as diagnostic tools.

Various nucleic acid detection and amplification methods, such as DNA probes and polymerase chain reaction, are being investigated for diagnostic use in respiratory tract infections and are beginning to become commercially available. However, most aspects of this methodology have not been fully standardized, so clinical use is limited. Nucleic acid amplification methods are already in use for laboratory evaluation of certain mycobacterial specimens.

Viral cultures are not useful in the initial evaluation of patients. During appropriate seasons, however, testing respiratory secretions for influenza by rapid detection methods, which have sensitivities of 70% to 90%, followed by culture of specimens negative by rapid testing may help to guide decisions about the use of antiviral agents for treatment and provide useful data for the community.

Invasive diagnostic tests are sometimes performed in complicated or severely ill patients, though the benefits of such efforts have not been proven. Thoracentesis can be performed when pleural effusion is present and the fluid evaluated, though sensitivities of many tests on pleural fluid (Gram stain, culture, cytology) are low. Bronchoscopy is sometimes necessary to obtain specimens via brushings or bronchoalveolar lavage or for identification and/or biopsy of an obstructing lesion. Transtracheal aspirate is low yield and risks generally outweigh benefits. Transthoracic needle aspiration is a potential alternative to bronchoscopy in severely ill or immunocompromised patients with nonresolving focal infiltrate in whom noninvasive methods have been nondiagnostic.

The logical conclusion, after reviewing the relative usefulness of various diagnostic and testing strategies, is that, contrary to conventional medical teaching, there are no reliable objective findings: Clinical judgment is essential.

TREATMENT

Treatment of pneumonia is largely empiric, and each geographic area has its own unique microbiologic (and antibiotic resistance) patterns that cannot be sufficiently elucidated in studies of one area or another. It is incumbent upon clinicians to know these patterns for their own areas (data available from hospital and other microbiologic laboratories) and to adjust their prescribing accordingly.

Evidence from retrospective studies demonstrates that prompt administration of antibiotics improves survival, and empiric therapy should cover both bacterial and atypical pathogens. A multicenter cohort review of 14,069 patients hospitalized with pneumonia demonstrated that administering antibiotics within 8 hours and collecting blood cultures within 24 hours of arrival to the hospital were associated with lower 30-day mortality. A review of 39 cases of *Legionella* pneumonia found that delay in initiation of erythromycin therapy is associated with increased mortality. For the 10 people who died, median delay between diagnosis of pneumonia and start of erythromycin was 5 days (range, 1–10 days) and for those who survived it was 1 day (range, 1–5 days). A review of 12,945 inpatients with pneumonia demonstrated that three initial antibiotic regimens were associated with lower 30-day mortality: a second-generation cephalosporin plus macrolide, a nonpseudomonal third-generation cephalosporin plus macrolide, or a fluoroquinolone alone. Use of a β-lactam/β-lactamase inhibitor plus macrolide and an aminoglycoside plus another agent were associated with increased 30-day mortality.

Once the diagnosis of CAP has been made, the next critical step is the treatment decision: where (outpatient or inpatient; if inpatient, intensive care unit or not) and with what antibiotic(s)? Clinicians tend to overestimate the risk of death in patients with CAP, and there is marked regional variation in rates of hospital admission for these patients. Clinical prediction rules are one way to standardize risk assessment.

The key to treatment of CAP is deciding which risk group a patient is in, which will determine whether she can be treated as an outpatient or needs to be hospitalized and, if so, whether she will need intensive care. Various groups, notably the American Thoracic Society, the Infectious Diseases Society of America, the British Thoracic Society, the Canadian Infectious Disease Society together with the Canadian Thoracic Society, and the Institute for Clinical Systems Improvement, have all recently published guidelines on the management of CAP. Each has a strategy for risk stratifying patients that include assessment of clinical severity, comorbid conditions, risk factors, and demographic characteristics. Patients are then put into risk groups and antimicrobial therapy recommended based on what pathogens are believed to be likely in that group. These guidelines are based on expert opinion and published data and have not been validated with outcome studies.

The Pneumonia Patient Outcomes Research Team developed and validated a prediction tool for stratifying adults with CAP into five risk classes according to their risk of death within 30 days and other clinically relevant major outcomes (subsequent admission to the hospital or intensive care unit, length of stay, and time to usual activities) as a tool to aid in decision making about outpatient treatment or hospital admission. Studies that have used it refer to it as the Pneumonia Severity Index (PSI). Patients were not included if they had been discharged from an acute care hospital in the previous 10 days or if they were known to be positive for human immunodeficiency virus.

The PSI is designed in two steps to parallel clinical decision-making processes. Step 1 allows identification of a subgroup of patients at low risk of adverse outcome based solely on history and physical examination findings, thus obviating the need for further testing. The 11 variables in step 1 found to increase risk are as follows: age older than 50 years, any of five coexisting illnesses (neoplastic disease, CHF, cerebrovascular disease, renal disease, and liver disease), and any of five physical examination findings (pulse rate >125/min, respiratory rate >30/min, systolic blood pressure <90 mm Hg, temperature <35°C [95°F] or >40°C [104°F], and altered mental status). If none is present, the patient is assigned to the lowest risk class, class I. Step 2 adds selected demographic, laboratory, and radiographic data (male sex, nursing home residence, blood urea nitrogen >30 mg/dL, glucose >250 mg/dL, hematocrit <30%, sodium <130 mmol/L, partial pressure of arterial oxygen <60 mm Hg, arterial pH <7.35, and pleural effusion). Variables are assigned point values to calculate which risk class (II thru V) patients fall into. Those in risk class I or II are candidates for outpatient treatment, those in risk class III are potential candidates for outpatient treatment or brief inpatient observation, and those in classes IV and V should be hospitalized. The authors offer the caveat that other psychosocial and medical factors will contribute to the decision about whether outpatient therapy is appropriate for any given patient. These factors include patient preferences, ability to maintain oral intake, substance abuse, psychiatric or cognitive impairment, ability to carry out activities of daily living and other factors that might impact ability to adhere to prescribed therapy. Other factors include immunosuppression and severe neuromuscular disease, which may increase likelihood of poor prognosis. Nonetheless, it is estimated that use of this rule could reduce hospital admissions by 25% to 31% and reduce length of stay for another 13% to 19% with hospitalization briefly for observation, without jeopardizing health and quality of care. The safety and efficacy of this prediction tool has been validated in other studies.

Evaluation and management decision making regarding patients presenting with possible pneumonia, including use of the PSI, is depicted in Fig. 52.1. Modifying factors that increase the risk of infection with certain pathogens are depicted in Table 52.1. Organisms and initial empiric therapy for patients with CAP in various risk categories are depicted in Table 52.2.

Few nonpharmacologic interventions commonly prescribed to hasten recovery from pneumonia (e.g., early mobilization, chest percussion and postural drainage, deep breathe and cough) have been shown to improve outcomes. One exception is bottle blowing that, together with early mobilization, was shown in a prospective randomized trial of 145 adults hospitalized with CAP to reduce hospital stay by 1.4 days from 5.3 to 3.9 days compared with early mobilization alone. The technique involves sitting up and blowing bubbles in a bottle containing 10 cm water through a plastic tube 20 times on 10 occasions daily. No adverse effects were reported.

Viral etiologies of pneumonia include influenza and varicella. Treatment of influenza with neuroaminidase inhibitors shortens the duration of symptoms by 1 day if administered within 48 hours of symptom onset, but they do not have much role in the treatment of pneumonia associated with influenza because it generally develops beyond 48 hours from symptom onset. Pneumonia in patients with influenza is treated as bacterial secondary infection with the same antimicrobial guidelines as CAP. Varicella can be complicated by pneumonia, a serious and potentially life-threatening complication that occurs more commonly in adults and in immunocompromised persons. Among adults, it is estimated to occur in 1 in 400 cases of infection. It generally appears 3 to 5 days into the course of illness and is associated with tachypnea, cough, dyspnea, and fever. Chest radiographs usually reveal nodular or interstitial pneumonitis. Treatment should be initiated with intravenous acyclovir as soon as the diagnosis is made.

Fungal pneumonia must be treated promptly with antifungals like amphotericin B, fluconazole, or itraconazole, depending on the clinical context. Surgical interventions are required as part of treatment more often than in pneumonia of other etiologies.

Aspiration pneumonia must be distinguished from aspiration pneumonitis, the latter being a self-limited chemical inflammatory condition that tends to resolve in 48 hours. Thus, contrary to the need for prompt antibiotic administration in CAP, patients with aspiration should be observed for 48 hours, and empiric therapy with broad-spectrum antibiotics should be

TABLE 52.1. Modifying Factors that Increase the Risk of Infection with Specific Pathogens

Penicillin-resistant and drug-resistant pneumococci
Age >65 y
β-Lactam therapy within the last 3 mo
Alcoholism
Immune-suppressive illness (including therapy with corticosteroids)
Multiple medical comorbidities
Exposure to a child in a daycare center
Enteric gram negatives
Residence in a nursing home
Underlying cardiopulmonary disease
Multiple medical comorbidities
Recent antibiotic therapy
Pseudomonas aeruginosa
Structural lung disease (bronchiectasis)
Corticosteroid therapy (>10 mg prednisone per day)
Broad-spectrum antibiotic therapy for >7 days in the past month
Malnutrition

Source: American Thoracic Society Guidelines. Community-acquired pneumonia in adults. *Am J Respir Crit Care Med* 2001;163:1732, with permission.

TABLE 52.2. Usual Organisms and Initial Therapy in Patients with Pneumonia[a]

Usual organisms	Initial therapy
Outpatients, no cardiopulmonary disease, no modifying factors	
S. pneumoniae	Advanced generation macrolide: azithromycin or clarithromycin[b]
M. pneumoniae	
C. pneumoniae (alone or as mixed infection)	***or***
H. influenzae	Doxycycline[c]
Respiratory viruses	
Miscellaneous (*Legionella* spp., *M. tuberculosis,* endemic fungi)	
Outpatient, with cardiopulmonary disease and/or other modifying factors	
S. pneumoniae (including DRSP)	β-Lactam (oral cefpodoxime, cefuroxime, high-dose amoxicillin, amoxicillin/clavulanate; or parenteral ceftriaxone followed by oral cefpodoxime)
M. pneumoniae	
C. pneumoniae	
Mixed infection (bacteria plus atypical pathogen or virus)	***plus***
	Macrolide or doxycycline[c]
H. influenzae	***or***
Enteric gram-negatives	Antipneumococcal fluoroquinolone (used alone)
Respiratory viruses	
Miscellaneous (*M. catarrhalis, Legionella* spp., aspiration (anaerobes), *M. tuberculosis,* endemic fungi)	
Inpatients, no cardiopulmonary disease, no modifying factors	
S. pneumoniae	Intravenous azithromycin alone
H. influenzae	If macrolide allergic or intolerant: Doxycycline and a β-lactam
M. pneumoniae	
C. pneumoniae	***or***
Mixed infection (bacteria plus atypical pathogen)	Monotherapy with an antipneumococcal fluoroquinolone
Viruses	
Legionella spp.	
Miscellaneous *(M. tuberculosis,* endemic fungi, *P. carinii)*	
Inpatients, cardiopulmonary disease and/or modifying factors	
S. pneumoniae (including DRSP)	Intravenous β-lactam (cefotaxime, ceftriaxone, amoxicillin/sulbactam, high-dose ampicillin)
H. influenzae	
M. pneumoniae	***plus***
C. pneumoniae	Intravenous or oral macrolide or doxycycline
Mixed infection (bacteria plus atypical pathogen)	***or***
Enteric gram-negatives	Intravenous antipneumococcal fluoroquinolone alone
Aspiration (anaerobes)	
Viruses	
Legionella spp.	
Miscellaneous *(M. tuberculosis,* endemic fungi, *P. carinii)*	
***ICU-admitted patients, no risks for* Pseudomonas aeruginosa**	
S. pneumoniae (including DRSP)	Intravenous β-lactam (cefotaxime, ceftriaxone)
Legionella spp.	***plus either***
H. influenzae	Intravenous macrolide (azithromycin)
Enteric gram-negative bacilli	***or***
S. aureus	Intravenous fluoroquinolone
M. pneumoniae	
Respiratory viruses	
Miscellaneous (*C. pneumoniae, M. tuberculosis,* endemic fungi)	
***If risks for* P. aeruginosa**	**Combination antipseudomonal antibiotic therapy required**

[a]Excludes patients at risk for human immunodeficiency virus.
[b]Erythromycin is not active against *H. influenzae* and advanced generation macrolides are often better tolerated.
[c]Many isolates of *S. pneumoniae* are resistant to tetracycline; use only if patient cannot take macrolides.
ICU, intensive care unit.
Source: American Thoracic Society/Guidelines. Community-acquired pneumoniae in adults. *Am J Respir Crit Care Med* 2001;163:1735, with permission.

initiated if the condition persists. Antibiotics with specific anaerobic activity are not routinely needed unless a patient has severe periodontal disease, putrid sputum, or evidence of lung abscess or necrotizing pneumonia on chest radiograph. Evidence does not support the use of corticosteroids; thus they are not recommended.

PREVENTION

Data on the efficacy of pneumococcal vaccine for prevention of pneumococcal pneumonia or pneumonia in general is mixed, with some studies showing limited or no effect, and others showing improvement in patient-oriented outcomes. The U.S. Preventive Services Task Force recommends pneumococcal vaccine for all immunocompetent individuals 65 years and older or otherwise at increased risk for pneumococcal disease. It states there is insufficient evidence to recommend for or against pneumococcal vaccine for high-risk immunocompromised individuals but states recommendations for vaccinating these persons may be made for other reasons, including high incidence and case-fatality rates of pneumococcal disease and minimal adverse effects from the vaccine. One fifth of healthy elderly adults (mean age, 71 years) do not have an antibody response to vaccination. Routine revaccination is not recommended but can be considered in immunocompetent individuals at highest risk for morbidity and mortality from pneumococcal disease who were vaccinated more than 5 years previously.

Influenza vaccination of the elderly has been shown to reduce significantly the risk of influenza and associated complications, including hospitalization, pneumonia, and death. Similarly, immunization of health care workers in geriatric medical long-term care sites has been shown to reduce significantly influenza-like illness and total mortality. The U.S. Preventive Services Task Force recommends it be administered annually to anyone age 65 and older; anyone 6 months of age and older who resides in a chronic care facility or suffers from a chronic cardiopulmonary, metabolic, immunosuppressive, or renal disorder or hemoglobinopathy; and health care workers of high-risk patients. Neuraminidase inhibitors are also effective for the prevention of influenza and may be started at the time of vaccination and continued for 2 weeks or used daily throughout flu season for patients in whom the vaccine is contraindicated (i.e., those with allergy to egg protein).

Lifestyle modification is another strategy for prevention of pneumonia, and data exist on the degree to which alcohol, smoking, and excessive weight gain increase risk of CAP in middle-aged and older adults. Among women, physical activity has been found to decrease the risk of CAP. In the elderly, modifiable risk factors for pneumonia include witnessed large volume aspiration, which could be decreased by formal swallowing evaluation and prescribed feeding to minimize aspiration risk, and sedative medication, use of which could be decreased by alternative management strategies for anxiety and disruptive behavior. Tube feeding increases rates of aspiration pneumonia and should be avoided whenever possible.

SUMMARY RECOMMENDATIONS

In summary, the diagnosis and care of pneumonia in women remains a difficult challenge for the primary care clinician. Four principles, based on the literature reviewed above, can help guide decision-making: (a) *diagnose with judgment* (clinically ill, crackles, comorbidity, judicious use of chest radiograph), (b) *treat early* with antibiotics, (c) *treat locally* based on antibiotic susceptibility patterns, and (d) *use the PSI* to help decide where to provide care.

CONSIDERATIONS IN PREGNANCY

Pneumonia, though rare in pregnancy, is the most common cause of fatal nonobstetric infection in pregnancy and the peripartum period. In considering pneumonia in pregnancy, one must consider the impact of pregnancy on pneumonia as well as the impact of pneumonia on pregnancy for both mother and fetus.

Changes in maternal physiology and immune function in pregnancy theoretically increase the risk of pneumonia to the mother. Physiologic changes include decreased functional residual capacity, increased oxygen consumption, and increased lung water. Changes in immune function include decreased lymphocyte proliferative response, decreased natural killer cell activity, and decreased helper T-cell numbers. Hormones increased in pregnancy may additionally inhibit cell-mediated immunity. These changes are seen most in the second and third trimesters. Despite these theoretical concerns, current limited evidence suggests there is, in general, no significant difference in susceptibility to or severity of pneumonia in pregnant and nonpregnant women. Recent studies suggest a pneumonia incidence of 0.44 to 2.7 per 1,000 deliveries with 0% to 4% mortality, similar to incidence and mortality rates in nonpregnant adults aged 15 to 45 years.

The same, however, cannot be said of the effects of maternal pneumonia on the fetus. These effects include preterm delivery, poor fetal growth, and perinatal loss. Preterm delivery occurs in 4% to 43% of cases, even with antibiotic and supportive therapy. Also, infants of mothers with pneumonia have significantly lower birth weights and higher frequency of low birth weight (2,500 g or less). Increased fetal loss is likely due to prematurity and fetal stress from hypoxemia, maternal sepsis, and impaired uteroplacental circulation.

Risk factors for development of pneumonia in pregnancy have been identified and include anemia (hematocrit <30%), asthma, antepartum corticosteroids to enhance fetal lung maturity, and tocolytics, which can precipitate pulmonary edema and thus are contraindicated in patients with known pneumonia. Smoking, human immunodeficiency virus, cystic fibrosis, and other pulmonary, systemic, or immunocompromising conditions also increase risk, as they do in nonpregnant women.

Misdiagnosis and delay in diagnosis of pneumonia are common in pregnancy. Misdiagnoses range from 10.5% to 20% and include initial diagnoses of pyelonephritis, appendicitis, and preterm labor with no precipitating cause. Indications for chest radiograph are the same in pregnant as in nonpregnant women, and it should not be withheld to avoid radiation exposure to the fetus. Differential diagnosis of alveolar infiltrate in pregnancy includes pulmonary edema secondary to preeclampsia or tocolytics, aspiration, and, very rarely, choriocarcinoma with pulmonary metastases.

Pathogenesis of pneumonia in pregnancy has not been rigorously investigated, but existing data suggest the same pathogens occur with similar frequency as in nonpregnant adults with CAP. Pneumonia caused by bacterial or atypical pathogens appears to present with similar features and severity as in nonpregnant adults and, similarly, clinical features cannot reliably predict pathogenesis so empiric treatment is indicated.

No antimicrobial agents are approved for use in pregnancy by the U.S. Food and Drug Administration, though some data do exist. The potential risks and benefits of their use must be discussed and informed consent obtained. Available data on antimicrobial agents in pregnancy are summarized in Table 52.3. Teratogenicity rates must be compared with the background rate of major malformations in the general population of 2% to 3%. Empiric antibiotic coverage for pneumonia caused by bacterial and atypical organisms should be initiated as soon as possible with the safest antibiotics that will cover likely organisms (e.g., for CAP, a third-generation cephalosporin such as ceftriaxone or cefotaxime and a macrolide such as azithromycin; a macrolide is a reasonable alternative to a tetracycline to cover Q fever). Oxygen should be administered to maintain an arterial partial pressure of oxygen at or above 70 mm Hg to maintain adequate fetal oxygenation. The supine position should be avoided during treatment, with preference for a left lateral recumbent position to optimize uteroplacental perfusion. Careful attention should be paid to this if pneumonia is complicated by respiratory failure requiring mechanical ventilation. Elective delivery has not been shown to improve maternal respiratory function or condition and thus is not indicated. Pneumococcal vaccine is not recommended in pregnant or breast-feeding women.

Viral pneumonia in pregnancy is usually caused by influenza or varicella. Three types of influenza virus cause human disease, A, B, and C, but influenza epidemics are usually due to influenza A. Since 1958, influenza epidemics have not

TABLE 52.3. Safety in Pregnancy and Lactation of Selected Antimicrobial Agents Used to Treat Pneumonia

Class of antibiotic	Evidence regarding adverse effects	Safety in human pregnancy (FDA pregnancy risk category)	Safety in breast-feeding (lactation risk category[a])
Antibacterial agents			
Penicillins and amoxicillin/ clavulanic acid	Widely used without evidence of problems.	Good (B)	Good (L1, most; L2, Ticarcillin, Piperacillin; L3, Methicillin)
Cephalosporins	Widely used without evidence of problems.	Good (B)	Good (L1 and L2)
Macrolides	Widely used without evidence of problems. Most data on erythromycin (estolate may cause maternal hepatitis), less data on clarithromycin or azithromycin.	Good (B) (clarithromycin, C)	Good (L1, Erythromycin; L2, azithromycin, clarithromycin)
Aminoglycosides	No published reports on fetal nephropathy, case reports of irreversible bilateral congenital deafness after maternal gentamicin. Ability of premature infants to eliminate gentamicin dependent on gestational age.	Potential risk of nephropathy and ototoxicity. Maternal plasma levels should be carefully monitored if clear indication exists for use (D).	Moderately safe (L2 and L3)
Sulphonamides	May cause kernicterus if given in late pregnancy. Of 2,296 newborns exposed to cotrimoxazole during the first trimester, 126 (5.5%) major birth defects were observed, 98 expected.	Avoid. Insufficient information on high doses. Theoretical risk of neural tube defects with cotrimoxazole due to folate antagonist activity.	Moderately safe (L2 and L3)
Quinolones	Arthralgia and tendonitis reported in adults but none after in utero exposure in human pregnancy.	Insufficient evidence of safety (C)	Most moderately safe (L3, most; L4, ciprofloxacin)
Tetracyclines	Administration in the second or third trimesters can cause yellow-brown staining and banding of the teeth of the child and reversible growth retardation of the long bones.	Avoid, especially at or after 12 weeks (D)	Moderately safe for short-term use (L2, tetracycline; L3, doxycycline—short term; L4, doxycycline—chronic use)
Metronidazole	Conflicting data. Some epidemiologic studies suggest increased risk of malformations, stillbirths and low-birth-weight infants. Other studies totalling exposure to over 3,000 newborns have found no increase in congenital anomalies.	Unclear (B—contraindicated in first trimester)	Good (L2)
Antiviral agents			
Amantadine	Limited preclinical data in animals showed a possible association with cleft palate. In a study of 64 pregnancies, five births with defects were reported.	Insufficient evidence of safety (C)	Moderately safe (L3)
Zanamivir	No information in humans. In animals high doses were not associated with malformation.	Insufficient evidence of safety. Theoretically safer than amantadine (C).	Hazardous (L4)
Ribavirin	Teratogenic or embryolethal in nearly all animal species.	Avoid (X)	Hazardous (L4)
Acyclovir	Prospective register (1984–1999) with data on 1,246 pregnancies showed no increase in birth defects compared with the general population.	Recommended when risk . from untreated infection is greater than risk of possible adverse effects (e.g., life-threatening varicella infections (B).	Good (L2)
Antifungal agents			
Amphotericin B	Case reports of fetal toxicity involving anemia, transient acidosis with uremia, and respiratory failure.	Use if benefit outweighs risk of fetal toxicity (usually maternal toxicity also present) (B, intravenous; C, oral)	Safety not established
Itraconzole	Embryotoxic and teratogenic in laboratory animals. Of 198 women exposed during the first trimester, 3.2% major malformations were seen.	Best avoided. Manufacturer recommends contraception for one menstrual cycle after stopping treatment (C).	Good (L2)
Fluconzale	Embryotoxic and teratogenic in high doses in rats. Multiple congenital abnormalities reported with high dose use in humans. Possible dose dependent teratogenicity.	Avoid (C)	Good (L2)

[a]See Appendix A.
Source: Lim WS, Macfarlane JT, Colthorpe CL. Pneumonia and pregnancy. *Thorax* 2001;56:398, with permission.

been associated with increase morbidity or mortality in pregnant women. Influenza A virus can traverse the placenta, but whether it can cause congenital anomalies is unclear. Efficacy and safety of amantadine and newer neuraminidase inhibitors have not yet been determined so their routine use cannot be recommended. Influenza vaccine is recommended after completion of the first trimester for women who will be in the second or third trimester of pregnancy during flu season. This is not so in the United Kingdom where it is recommended only for pregnant women who meet other Department of Health criteria for influenza immunization.

Varicella infection occurs in 0.7 of 1,000 pregnancies. Clinical manifestations of varicella pneumonia are no different in pregnancy. It should be treated with intravenous acyclovir, for which benefits appear to outweigh risks. Fetal effects from varicella are variable and related to the timing of infection. Pneumonia caused by other viruses, such as rubeola, mononucleosis, and hantavirus, has been reported in pregnancy but the incidence is unknown. Safety in pregnancy and lactation of selected antimicrobial agents used to treat pneumonia are summarized in Table 52.3.

APPENDIX: LACTATION RISK CATEGORIES

L1 Safest: Drug that has been taken by a large number of breast-feeding mothers without any observed increase in adverse effects in the infant. Controlled studies in breast-feeding women fail to demonstrate a risk to the infant, and the possibility of harm to the breast-feeding infant is remote. Or the product is not orally bioavailable in an infant.

L2 Safer: Drug that has been studied in a limited number of breast-feeding women without an increase in adverse effects in the infant, and/or, the evidence of a demonstrated risk that is likely to follow use of this medication in a breast-feeding woman is remote.

L3 Moderately Safe: There are no controlled studies in breast-feeding women; however, the risk of untoward effects to a breast-fed infant is possible, or, controlled studies show only minimal nonthreatening adverse effects. Drugs should be given only if the potential benefit justifies the potential risk to the infant.

L4 Hazardous: There is positive evidence of risk to a breast-fed infant or to breast milk production, but the benefits from use in breast-feeding mothers may be acceptable despite the risk to the infant (e.g., if the drug is needed in a life-threatening situation or for a serious disease for which safer drugs cannot be used or are ineffective).

L5 Contraindicated: Studies in breast-feeding mothers have demonstrated a significant and documented risk to the infant based on human experience, or, it is a medication that has a high risk of causing significant damage to an infant. The risk of using the drug in breast-feeding women clearly outweighs any possible benefit from breast-feeding. The drug is contraindicated in women who are breast-feeding an infant.

Source: Hale T. *Medications and mothers' milk,* 9th ed. Amarillo: Pharmasoft Publishing, 2000:15–16, with permission.

BIBLIOGRAPHY

Albaum MN, Hill LC, Murphy M, et al. Interobserver reliability of the chest radiograph in community-acquired pneumonia. *Chest* 1996;110:343–350.

American Thoracic Society Guidelines. Community-acquired pneumonia in adults. *Am J Respir Crit Care Med* 2001;163:1730–1754.

Atlas SJ, Benzer TI, Borowsky LH, et al. Safely increasing the proportion of patients with community-acquired pneumonia treated as outpatients: an interventional trial. *Arch Intern Med* 1998;158;1350–1356.

Baik I, Curhan GC, Rimm EB, et al. A prospective study of age and lifestyle factors in relation to community-acquired pneumonia in U.S. men and women. *Arch Intern Med* 2000;160:3082–3088.

Bartlett JG, Dowell SF, Mandell LA, et al. Guidelines from the Infectious Diseases Society of America: practice guidelines for the management of community-acquired pneumonia in adults. *Clin Infect Dis* 2000;31:347–382.

Barton S, Jones G, Amore LGC, et al. *Clin Evid* 2001;6:1171–1180.

Bjorkqvist M, Wiberg B, Bodin L, et al. Bottle-blowing in hospital-treated patients with community-acquired pneumonia. *Scand J Infect Dis* 1997;29:77–82.

Fine MJ, Auble TE, Yealy DM, et al. A prediction rule to identify low-risk patients with community-acquired pneumonia. *N Engl J Med* 1997;336:243–250.

Fine MJ, Smith MA, Carson CA, et al. Efficacy of pneumococcal vaccination in adults: a meta-analysis of randomized controlled trials. *Arch Intern Med* 1994;154:2666–2677.

Finucane TE, Bynum JP. Use of tube feeding to prevent aspiration pneumonia. *Lancet* 1996;348:1421–1424.

Gennis P, Gallagher J, Falvo C, et al. Clinical criteria for the detection of pneumonia in adults: guidelines for ordering chest roentgenograms in the emergency department. *J Emerg Med* 1989;7:263–268.

Gleason PP, Meehan TP, Fine JM, et al. Associations between initial antimicrobial therapy and medical outcomes for hospitalized elderly patients with pneumonia. *Arch Intern Med* 1999;159:2562–2572.

Gonzales R, Bartlett JG, Besser RE, et al. Principles of appropriate antibiotic use for treatment of uncomplicated acute bronchitis: background. *Ann Intern Med* 2001;134:521–529.

Hale T. *Medications and mothers' milk,* 9th ed. Amarillo: Pharmasoft Publishing, 2000:15–16.

Hasley PB, Albaum MN, Li Y, et al. Do pulmonary radiographic findings at presentation predict mortality in patients with community-acquired pneumonia? *Arch Intern Med* 1996;156:2206–2212.

Heckerling PS, Tape TG, Wigton RS, et al. Clinical prediction rules for pulmonary infiltrates. *Ann Intern Med* 1990;113:664–670.

Institute for Clinical Systems Improvement. Health Care Guideline: community-acquired pneumonia. July 2000. Available at *www.icsi.org/guide/Pneum.pdf.*

Lim WS, Macfarlane JT, Colthorpe CL. Pneumonia and pregnancy. *Thorax* 2001; 56:398–405.

Marik PE. Aspiration pneumonitis and aspiration pneumonia. *N Engl J Med* 2001;344:665–671.

Marrie TJ, Lau CY, Wheeler SL, et al. A controlled trial of a critical pathway for treatment of community-acquired pneumonia. *JAMA* 2000;283:749–755.

Meehan TP, Fine MJ, Krumholz HM, et al. Quality of care, process, and outcomes in elderly patients with pneumonia. *JAMA* 1997;278:2080–2084.

Metlay JP, Kapoor WN, Fine MJ. Does this patient have community-acquired pneumonia? Diagnosing pneumonia by history and physical examination. *JAMA* 1997;278:1440–1445.

Opravil M, Marincek B, Pope T, et al. Shortcomings of chest radiography in detecting *Pneumocystis carinii* pneumonia. *J Acquir Immune Defic Syndr* 1994;7:39–45.

Reed WW, Byrd GS, Gates RH, et al. Sputum gram's stain in community-acquired pneumococcal pneumonia: a meta-analysis. *West J Med* 1996;165:197–204.

Saubolle MA, McKellar PP. Laboratory diagnosis of community-acquired lower respiratory tract infection. *Infect Dis Clin North Am* 2001;15:1025–1045.

Skerrett SJ. Diagnostic testing for community-acquired pneumonia. *Clin Chest Med* 1999;20:531–548.

Syrjala H, Broas M, Suramo I, et al. High resolution CT for the diagnosis of community-acquired pneumonia. *Clin Infect Dis* 1998;27:358.

Theerthakarai R, El-Halees W, Ismail M, et al. Nonvalue of the initial microbiological studies in the management of nonsevere community-acquired pneumonia. *Chest* 2001;119:181–184.

U.S. Preventive Services Task Force. *Guide to clinical preventive services,* 2nd ed. Baltimore: Williams & Wilkins, 1996.

Vergis EN, Brennen C, Wagener M, et al. Pneumonia in long-term care: a prospective case-control study of risk factors and impact on survival. *Arch Intern Med* 2001;161:2378–2381.

CHAPTER 53
Acute Bronchitis

Raymond O. Powrie

ETIOLOGY

Five percent of adults self-report an episode of acute bronchitis each year, and up to 90% of persons with bronchitis seek medical attention for their symptoms. Acute bronchitis therefore accounts for nearly 10 million visits to the doctor each year in the United States alone, making it one of the most common reason that patients in the United States seek medical care.

Ninety percent of cases of acute bronchitis are viral in origin. The typical pathogens responsible for acute bronchitis are respiratory viruses. Influenza A and B, parainfluenza, corona virus, adenovirus, rhinovirus, and respiratory syncytial virus (particularly in households with children) are all known to cause acute bronchitis, but identification of the particular pathogen responsible for an individual case is rarely clinically necessary.

Bacterial causes of acute bronchitis are uncommon and usually not important to identify early in routine clinical practice. Only *Mycoplasma pneumoniae*, *Chlamydia pneumoniae* (TWAR), and *Bordetella pertussis* and parapertussis have been identified as bacterial causes of acute bronchitis, and these organisms account for no more than 5% to 10% of all cases. There is no evidence that *Streptococcus pneumoniae*, *Haemophilus influenzae*, or *Moraxella catarrhalis* cause acute bronchitis in patients without underlying lung disease.

DIFFERENTIAL DIAGNOSIS

The most important differential diagnosis of acute bronchitis is pneumonia, a far more serious diagnosis that, unlike acute bronchitis, will generally require close monitoring and antibacterial therapy. Pneumonia should be suspected and chest radiographs obtained in the setting of cough occurring in association with fever, tachycardia (heart rate >100 beats/min), tachypnea (resting rate >24 beats/min), and/or the finding of crackles on pulmonary auscultation. Purulent sputum is a typical feature of acute bronchitis and does not in itself suggest the presence of pneumonia.

Cough lasting beyond 3 weeks is not usually acute bronchitis and should be labeled chronic or persistent cough. Chronic or persistent cough has a broader differential diagnosis that includes gastroesophageal reflux disease, postnasal drip, occupational diseases, and asthma. Chronic bronchitis is a separate and distinct entity defined as daily cough and sputum production lasting for at least 3 months in 2 consecutive years. Cough due to asthma will often be associated with wheezing on examination and/or the suggestion of obstructed flow on spirometry. Worsening at night and/or on exposure to cold air should make one consider this diagnosis, but, again, only after cough has persisted for longer than 3 weeks. Postnasal drip syndrome related to both acute bacterial sinusitis and allergic rhinitis is also an important cause of persistent cough that warrants consideration. The sensation of postnasal drainage, the need to frequently clear the throat or the presence of persistent mucopurulent nasal secretions, may suggest this diagnosis. Finally, gastroesophageal reflux should also be considered as a cause of persistent cough without fever, sputum, or constitutional symptoms. The associated presence of heartburn or a sour taste in the mouth may suggest this diagnosis.

CLINICAL SYMPTOMS AND HISTORY

Acute bronchitis is defined clinically as an acute respiratory illness of 2 to 3 weeks duration in which persistent productive cough is the predominating symptom and pneumonia has been ruled out. The cough of acute bronchitis is generally associated with other upper respiratory tract symptoms (pharyngitis, rhinorrhea, or laryngitis) and constitutional complaints (malaise, myalgias, or fatigue). Acute bronchitis is a diagnosis of exclusion that should only be made if there is not adequate evidence to support alternative diagnoses such as asthma, pneumonia, sinusitis, and allergic rhinitis.

The illness generally begins with 1 to 5 days of fever, myalgia, and malaise that corresponds to the initial proliferation of the infectious agent in the tracheobronchial epithelium and the associated host inflammatory response. This stage is followed by a protracted period of bronchial hyper-responsiveness characterized by cough, phlegm production, and wheezing. Fever is not common during this phase of the illness.

CLINICAL FINDINGS AND PHYSICAL EXAMINATION

The examination of patients with acute viral bronchitis should reveal a normal pulse, respiratory rate, and blood pressure. Temperature may be elevated in the early days of the illness. Chest auscultation should be either normal or reveal some wheezing. Crackles should not be heard on lung auscultation in patients with acute bronchitis.

Mycoplasma and *Chlamydia* are most commonly seen as causes of acute bronchitis in young adults and typically cause a 2- to 6-week illness of low-grade fever, cough, laryngitis, and pharyngitis.

Pertussis, although still an uncommon cause of acute bronchitis, may also present as a persistent cough in adults and may be a more important cause of acute bronchitis than has been previously recognized. A diagnosis of pertussis in adults is less likely to present as the classic "whooping cough" familiar to pediatricians and is therefore difficult to distinguish from other causes of acute bronchitis in adults. One study from San Francisco found that 12% of adults presenting with chronic cough persisting for at least 2 weeks had evidence of pertussis and that this diagnosis was not specifically suspected by the evaluating physician in any of the patients. Primary immunization for pertussis is not 100% protective and what protection it does provide begins to wane by 3 years after immunization and is often absent by 10 years.

LABORATORY AND IMAGING STUDIES

Complete blood counts and blood cultures are rarely necessary in acute bronchitis, but, if obtained, these tests should always be normal. The chest x-ray, if obtained, is normal in acute bronchitis. Some portion of patients with acute bronchitis will have a demonstrable decrease in their forced expiratory volume that may persist as long as 6 weeks after presentation but will not otherwise have a history suggestive of asthma.

Pneumonia should be suspected and chest radiographs obtained in the setting of cough with fever, in association with tachycardia (heart rate >100 beats/min), tachypnea (resting rate > 24 beats/min), and/or the finding of crackles on pulmonary auscultation. The absence of all these features has good predictive value that pneumonia is not present, and therefore a chest x-ray is not generally necessary in previously healthy patients presenting with cough, but none of the other features, that has been present for less than 3 weeks. A chest x-ray may still be advisable in the absence of tachycardia, tachypnea, or crackles on lung auscultation in patients who have had a significant exposure to influenza; patients who are over the age of 65; or those patients who have known chronic obstructive pulmonary disease, congestive heart failure, or immunosuppression.

Identifying which specific respiratory virus is responsible for a case of acute bronchitis may be done by obtaining acute and convalescent serology. However, such testing is not clinically useful and should rarely if ever be carried out.

Cases of acute viral bronchitis due to influenza may be identified by rapid (10–20 minutes) and sensitive tests using nasal swabs. However, the use of nasal swabs for the diagnosis of influenza and/or the use of antiviral agents in an otherwise healthy young population presenting with bronchitis and no evidence of pneumonia is not presently routinely recommended. Symptomatic and supportive treatment in these cases is generally all that is needed. However, influenza nasal swab testing may be of benefit if done within the first 48 hours of an acute bronchitis among the elderly, immunosuppressed, or institutionalized—a population for whom the use of antiviral medications to ameliorate the course of this disease is justifiable.

In practice, although laboratory confirmation of bacterial causes of acute bronchitis such as *Mycoplasma* or *Chlamydia* might be done with serology, it is rarely necessary because acute bronchitis caused by these organisms is usually self-limited and antibiotics likely only mildly shorten the course of the illness. If confirmatory testing is deemed appropriate, alternatives to serology to diagnose *Mycoplasma* include cultures of pharyngeal washings for cell wall–deficient organisms and antigen detection with polymerase chain reaction (PCR). A cold agglutinin titer exceeding 1:64 is suggestive of *Mycoplasma* but is very nonspecific. Alternatives to serology to diagnose *Chlamydia pneumoniae* include culture on McCoy cells or PCR.

Testing to identify pertussis as a cause of acute bronchitis is difficult and should therefore generally only be done in the setting of a known outbreak. The diagnosis of pertussis is established by culture using the "cough plate" method, nasopharyngeal aspirate, or PCR. However, cultures are relatively insensitive, and PCR is not readily available.

TREATMENT

Ninety percent of patients with acute bronchitis have a viral illness and require no more than reassurance and symptomatic treatment. Patients with acute bronchitis do not benefit from antibiotics because bacteria are rarely responsible. Nine randomized controlled trials of three different antibiotics for acute bronchitis have been published. Only four of these studies suggested any clinical benefit of antibiotic use in this setting. Three major metaanalyses of these trials have each shown that antibiotic use for acute bronchitis does not impact duration of illness, activity, or loss of work. Criticisms based on some minor methodologic weaknesses in some of these trials were addressed in a recent study comparing the use of azithromycin to vitamin C capsules in acute bronchitis. This study carefully examined the clinical outcomes most relevant to patients: health-related quality of life and return to usual daily activities. No difference in outcomes were seen between the azithromycin and the vitamin C groups. Unfortunately, despite overwhelming evidence now that antibacterials are not helpful in the setting of acute bronchitis, this illness remains the number one cause of antibiotic misuse in the world today.

Providers often complain that they prescribe antibiotics for acute bronchitis because they believe their patient will not be satisfied if they do not receive antibiotics for this condition. The evidence suggests otherwise. Although it does appear that patients do *expect* antibiotics when they present to a provider with acute bronchitis, they do so mostly because they have received antibiotics for this indication in the past. Research suggests the patient satisfaction can be readily achieved without antibiotics by a careful explanation of the nature of the illness, by referring to it as a "chest cold" rather than as "bronchitis," and by emphasizing that it will last 10 to 14 days regardless of treatment. Studies also suggest that patients are more likely to feel satisfied without an antibiotic if the risks of antibiotic resistance are presented as a personal rather than a public health issue. The patient should be specifically told that unnecessary antibiotic use and subsequent antibiotic resistance may place the patient at personal future risk.

Symptomatic Treatment

Several randomized control trials have found that patients with acute bronchitis receive some symptomatic benefit from treatment of cough with inhaled bronchodilators (albuterol, one to two puffs every 4 hours), although it remains unclear which patients are most likely to benefit from this intervention. More recently, a metaanalysis found that β_2-agonists were not effective for the treatment of acute bronchitis or cough of less than 4 weeks duration in children or in adults unless airflow obstruction was present. This treatment might therefore be best reserved for those patients with a history suggestive of reactive airway disease in the past.

Although cough medicines are commonly used for acute bronchitis, the literature is not convincing on their efficacy for acute bronchitis. Nonetheless, use of agents such as dextromethorphan, guaifenesin, or codeine to try to suppress the cough of acute bronchitis is greatly preferable to the inappropriate use of antibiotics from a public health perspective. Reassurance and time remain our best options for these patients, coupled with the use of nonsteroidal antiinflammatory drugs and/or acetaminophen for patients with systemic complaints.

Treatment of influenza-related cases of bronchitis warrants some particular discussion. Rapid (10–20 minutes) and sensitive tests are now available for the diagnosis of influenza, which may present as a bronchitis-like illness. The ability to rapidly diagnose influenza using nasal swabs is useful in determining whether to institute antiviral therapy. Amantadine, rimantadine, and the newer neuraminidase inhibitors zanamivir and oseltamivir all have proven efficacy to treat influenza. However, for these agents to be effective they need to be initiated within 48 hours of the onset of the illness (see Chapter 52). The rapid diagnosis and treatment of influenza-related bronchitis is particularly important in patients over age 65 or patients who have underlying immunosuppression, congestive heart failure, or chronic obstructive pulmonary disease for whom a particularly high risk of influenza pneumonia presenting atypically always will warrant careful consideration.

Acute bronchitis caused by *Mycoplasma* or *Chlamydia* is treated with a 14-day course of erythromycin 500 mg four times a day or oral azithromycin 500 mg once daily for 1 day and then 250 mg once daily for 4 days. Pertussis is treated with erythromycin (250–500 mg four times a day for 7–14 days). Unless initiated in the first 7 days of illness, antibiotic treatment does not appear to shorten the course of this infection. However, antibiotics may have a role in decreasing spread of the organisms to others.

PREGNANCY

The etiology, incidence, course, and treatment of acute bronchitis is not significantly changed by pregnancy. Available safety data suggest the use of albuterol, dextromethorphan, guaifenesin, and codeine for acute bronchitis is justifiable in pregnancy. In the rare cases of acute bronchitis caused by pertussis, *Chlamydia*, or *Mycoplasma*, use of erythromycin or azithromycin is justifiable but the use of clarithromycin or the fluoroquinolones should not be considered first line during the reproductive years because of possible harmful fetal effects. Pregnant women may be at increased risk of influenza and should therefore be encouraged to get the influenza vaccine in the second or third trimester if pregnant during the influenza season. However, use of nasal swabs for identification of influenza in cases of acute bronchitis presenting during pregnancy is unlikely to be helpful because the older antiinfluenza agents (amantadine or rimantadine) are known not to be safe in pregnancy and the newer neuraminidase inhibitors zanamivir (inhaled) and oseltamivir (oral) remain unstudied in human gestation. Prevention of influenza with the use of the vaccine in pregnant women remains our best option. Symptomatic and supportive treatment is all that can be recommended for those cases of acute influenza bronchitis that do occur during pregnancy.

BIBLIOGRAPHY

Advisory Committee on Immunization Practices. Prevention and control of influenza: recommendations of the Advisory Committee on Immunization Practices (ACIP). *MMWR Morb Mortal Wkly Rep* 1995;44(RR-3):l.

Bent S, Saint S, Vittinghoff E, et al. Antibiotics in acute bronchitis: a meta-analysis. *Am J Med* 1999;107:62–67.

Berquist SO, Bernander S, Dahnsjo H, et al. Erythromycin in the treatment of pertussis: a study of bacteriologic and clinical effects. *Pediatr Infect Dis J* 1987; 6:458.

Boldy DA, Skidmore SJ, Ayres JG. Acute bronchitis in the community: clinical features, infective factors, changes in pulmonary function and bronchial reactivity to histamine. *Respir Med* 1990;84:377.

Brickfield FX, Carter WH, Johnson RE. Erythromycin in the treatment of acute bronchitis in a community practice. *J Fam Pract* 1986;23:119–122.

Campbell LA, Perez-Melgosa M, Hamilton DJ, et al. Detection of *Chlamydia pneumoniae* by polymerase chain reaction. *J Clin Microbiol* 1992;30:434.

Christie CDC, Marx ML, Marchant CD, et al. The 1993 epidemic of pertussis in Cincinnati. *N Engl J Med* 1994;33:16.

Denny FW, Clyde WA, Glenzen WP. *Mycoplasma pneumoniae* disease: clinical spectrum, pathophysiology, epidemiology, and control. *J Infect Dis* 1971;123:74.

Dular R, Kajioka R, Kasatlya S. Comparison of Gen-Probe commercial kit and culture technique for the diagnosis of *Mycoplasma pneumoniae* infection. *J Clin Microbiol* 1988;26:1068.

Dunlay J, Reinhardt R, Roi LD. A placebo-controlled, double-blind trial of erythromycin in adults with acute bronchitis. *J Fam Pract* 1987;25:137–1141.

Evans AT, Husain S, Durairaj L, et al. Azithromycin for acute bronchitis: a randomized double-blind controlled trial. *Lancet* 2002;359(9318):1648–1654.

Faehy T, Stocks N, Thomas T. Quantitative systematic review of randomized control trials comparing antibiotic with placebo for acute cough in adults. *BMJ* 1998;316:906–910.

Franks P, Gleiner JA. The treatment of acute bronchitis with trimethoprim and sulfamethoxazole. *J Fam Pract* 1984;19:185–190.

Freestone C, Eccles R. Assessment of the antitussive efficacy of codeine in cough associated with common cold. *J Pharm Pharmacol* 1997;49:1045.

Gaydos CA, Quinn TC, Eiden JJ. Identification of *Chlamydia pneumoniae* by DNA amplification of the 16S rRNA gene. *J Clin Microbiol* 1992;30:796.

Gonzales R, Bartlett JG, Besser RE, et al. Principles of appropriate antibiotic use for treatment for uncomplicated acute bronchitis: background. *Ann Intern Med* 2001;134:521–529.

Gonzales R, Sande M. What will it take to stop physicians from prescribing antibiotics in acute bronchitis. *Lancet* 1995;345:665.

Gonzales R, Steiner JF, Lum A, et al. Decreasing antibiotic use in ambulatory practice: impact of a multidimensional intervention on the treatment of uncomplicated acute bronchitis in adults. *JAMA* 1999;281:1512.

Gonzales R, Steiner JF, Sande MA. Antibiotic prescribing for adults with colds, upper respiratory tract infections, and bronchitis by ambulatory care physicians [see comments]. *JAMA* 1997;278:901.

Gonzales R, Wilson A, Crane LA, et al. What's in a name? Public knowledge, attitudes, and experiences with antibiotic use for bronchitis. *Am J Med* 2000;108:83–85.

Hayden FG, Treanor JJ, Fritz RS, et al. Use of the oral neuraminidase inhibitor Oseltamivir in experimental human influenza: randomized controlled trials for prevention and treatment. *JAMA* 1999;282:1240.

He Q, Viljanen MK, Arvilommi H, et al. Whooping cough caused by *Bordetella pertussis* and *Bordetella parapertussis* in an immunized population. *JAMA* 1998; 280:635.

Henkinson D. Duration of effectiveness of pertussis vaccine: evidence from a 10-year community study. *BMJ* 1998;296:612.

Henry D, Ruoff GE, Rhudy J. Effectiveness of short-course therapy with cefuroxime axetil in treatment of secondary bacterial infections of acute bronchitis. *Antimicrob Agents Chemother* 1995;39:2528.

Hoppe JE. Methods for isolation of *Bordetella pertussis* from patients with whooping cough. *Eur J Clin Microbiol Infect Dis* 1988;7:616.

Hueston WJ. A comparison of albuterol and erythromycin for the treatment of acute bronchitis. *J Fam Pract* 1991;33:476–480.

Hueston WJ. Albuterol delivered by metered dose inhaler in acute bronchitis. *J Fam Pract* 1994;39:437–440.

Irwin RS, Curley FJ, French CL. Chronic cough: the spectrum and frequency of causes, key components of the diagnostic evaluation, and outcome of specific therapy. *Am Rev Respir Dis* 1990;141:640.

Irwin RS, Zawacki JK, Curley FJ, et al. Chronic cough as the sole presenting manifestation of gastroesophageal reflux. *Am Rev Respir Dis* 1989;140:1294.

King DE, Williams CW, Bishop L, et al. Effectiveness of erythromycin in the treatment of acute bronchitis. *J Fam Pract* 1996;42:601–605.

Kuhn JJ, Hendley JO, Adams KF, et al. Antitussive effect of guaifenesin in young adults with natural colds: objective and subjective assessment. *Chest* 1982;82:713.

MacKay DN. Treatment of acute bronchitis in adults without underlying lung disease. *J Gen Intern Med* 1996;11:557.

Martinex-Frias M-L, Rodriques-Pinilla E. Epidemiologic analysis of prenatal exposure to cough medicines containing dextromethorphan: no evidence of human teratogenicity. *Teratology* 2001;63:38–41.

Meade BD, Bollen A. Recommendations for use of the polymerase chain reaction in the diagnosis of *Bordetella pertussis* infections. *J Med Microbiol* 1994;41:51.

Mello CJ, Irwin RS, Curley FJ. Predictive values of character, timing and complications of chronic cough in diagnosing its cause. *Arch Intern Med* 1996;156:997.

Monto AS, Robinson DP, Herlocher ML, et al. Zanamivir in the prevention of influenza among healthy adults. *JAMA* 1999;282:31.

Nennig ME, Shinefield HR, Edwards KM, et al. Prevalence and incidence of adult pertussis in an urban population. *JAMA* 1996;275:1672.

Orr PH, Scherer K, MacDonald A, et al. Randomized placebo-controlled trials of antibiotic for acute bronchitis: a critical review of the literature. *J Fam Pract* 1993;36:507.

Pasternack MS. Pertussis in the 1990s: diagnosis, treatment, and prevention. *Curr Clin Top Infect Dis* 1997;17:24–36.

Scherl ER, Riegler SL, Cooper JK. Doxycycline in acute bronchitis: a randomized double-blind trial. *J Ky Med Assoc* 1987;85:539–541.

Smucny JJ, Becker LA, Glazier RH, et al. Are antibiotics effective for the treatment of acute bronchitis? A meta-analysis. *J Fam Pract* 1998;47:453–460.

Smucny JJ, Flynn CA, Becker LA, et al. Are beta2-agonists effective treatment for acute bronchitis or acute cough in patients without underlying pulmonary disease? A systematic review. *J Fam Pract* 2001;50:945.

Snow V, Mottour-Pilson C, Gonzales R. Principles of appropriate antibiotic use for treatment for uncomplicated acute bronchitis: background. *Ann Intern Med* 2001;1–14:518–520.

Stott NC, West RR. Randomized controlled trial of antibiotics in patients with cough and purulent sputum. *BMJ* 1976;2:556–559.

Tukiainen H, Kurttunen P, Silvasti M, et al. The treatment of acute transient cough: a placebo-controlled comparison of dextromethorphan and dextromethorphan-beta 2 sympathomimetic combination. *Eur J Respir Dis* 1986;69:95.

Uldurn SA, Jensen JS, Sondergard-Anderson J, et al. Enzyme immunoassay for detection of immunoglobin M (IgM) and IgG antibodies to *Mycoplasma pneumoniae*. *J Clin Microbiol* 1992;30:1198.

Verheij T, Hermans J, Mulder J. Effects of doxycycline in patients with acute cough and purulent sputum: a double-blind placebo-controlled trial. *Br Gen Pract* 1994;44:400–404.

Williamson HA. A randomized, controlled trial of doxycycline in the treatment of acute bronchitis. *J Fam Pract* 1984;19:481–486.

Wirsing von Konig CH, Postels-Multani S, Bogaert H, et al. Factors influencing the spread of pertussis in households. *Eur J Pediatr* 1998;157:391.

CHAPTER 54
The Common Cold

Elizabeth Hyde and William L. Miller

Caring for the patient suffering with the common cold is a quintessential example of the craft of primary care. It requires that clinicians negotiate a plan of care with patients, avoid antibiotic use, provide meaningful symptom relief, and discern serious illness and complications. This must be done efficiently and effectively. This can be primary care at its finest. The common cold is the most common acute infectious syndrome in humans and is experienced by most persons on several occasions during a lifetime. Although very rarely the cause of permanent disability or death, the common cold disrupts the everyday function of millions of people each year.

Common colds have a significant economic impact on society. In the United States more than $2 billion dollars is spent annually on cough and cold preparations. Antibiotic costs account for one third of the treatment expense for the common cold. The cold is the most common reason for time lost from work or school. More than 250 million days are lost from work or school per year, at an estimated cost of about $5 billion per year. About half of all acute care illness visits to the primary care physician are for the common cold. Yet, less than 2 of every 10 people with a cold go to the doctor.

EPIDEMIOLOGY AND ETIOLOGY

The *common cold* is a colloquial term for a category of acute infectious illnesses involving the upper respiratory tract (anything above the alveoli), with nasal congestion as a predominant symptom. A more accurate and inclusive term is acute upper respiratory infection (AURI). AURI usually presents with generalized symptoms involving most of the upper respiratory tract, but often symptoms localize to specific anatomic areas. The infectious syndrome is labeled accordingly as laryngitis, sinusitis, bronchitis, pharyngitis, or otitis. Traditionally, the common cold has been considered to have a viral etiology; whereas the presence of focal inflammation has often been seen as an indication of bacterial infection, necessitating an antibiotic. It is now clear that AURIs are characterized by a mix of common viruses and bacteria, initially triggered by a viral infection. Thus, attempts to clinically differentiate viral from bacterial infection are no longer helpful. The misbelief that focal inflammation has a bacterial source has been one factor in the epidemic overprescription of antibiotics for AURI. Primary care practitioners serve a vital role in the management of this epidemic through the appropriate use of antibiotics. More important in this regard is the recognition of the occasional serious bacterial complication of an AURI that does require antibiotic therapy. The common cold itself is caused by a mix of common virus and bacteria.

Investigators have identified over 200 viruses that initiate AURI. The overall incidence of AURI remains fairly constant throughout the year, with some increase in the fall, winter, and spring. However, there is much seasonal variation in regards to which virus is most prevalent. Knowledge of this seasonal variation is an important part of epidemic surveillance and management. Single-stranded RNA viruses trigger most colds. About 30% of these are caused by over 100 strains of rhinovirus, and the more than 60 strains of coronavirus account for another 15% to 20%. Rhinovirus is prevalent year long with a small peak in June, whereas coronavirus is more prevalent February through May. Fall, winter, and spring are the seasons for parainfluenza and the related respiratory syncytial virus. Parainfluenza 3 is responsible for some childhood croup, and parainfluenza 1 commonly causes laryngitis, especially in late fall and early winter. Acute bronchiolitis and additional cases of childhood croup are caused by respiratory syncytial virus. About 10% of colds are related to the 41 strains of double-stranded DNA adenoviruses. This group of viruses is capable of epidemic outbreaks and, along with enterovirus, can cause "summer camp" flu. Adenovirus is also associated with the syndrome of pharyngoconjunctival fever. Cultures failed to identify a causative agent in 35% of patients diagnosed with AURI. Table 54.1 shows the seasonal prevalence of AURI-related viruses.

Some cases of AURI are associated with bacterial growth. Most of these behave similarly to viral AURI and resolve without antibiotic treatment. Less than 2% of sinus infections are caused by significant bacterial overgrowth, and 69% of these resolve without antibiotic treatment in about 14 days. Between 5% and 10% of cases of acute bronchitis also have a bacterial etiology and yet still resolve without antibiotic treatment. *Streptococcus pneumoniae, Haemophilus influenzae,* and *Moraxella catarrhalis* are the most common bacteria isolated from infected maxillary sinuses, middle ear aspirates, and bronchial washings. *Bordetella pertussis, Mycoplasma pneumoniae,* and *Chlamydia pneumoniae* are occasional infectious agents found in cases of acute bronchitis.

Adults average 2 to 4 common colds per year, and children average 6 to 10. Families with large numbers of children or in crowded living conditions have an average of 7 to 10 colds in a year. The transmission of AURI occurs as a result of exposure to respiratory droplets containing virus or through hand-to-mouth contact. Simple procedures such as frequent hand washing and covering the mouth when coughing or sneezing can significantly reduce transmission. Although peak viral shedding typically occurs when symptoms are most prominent, viral shedding can occur for extended periods of time before and after symptoms. For practical infection control, children should not return to school or adults to work until they are fever free for 24 hours. It is important for clinicians to be alert for cluster outbreaks of more virulent illnesses, which should be reported to local Health Departments. Community outbreaks that occur in group settings can require aggressive preventive measures because health care workers and day care workers can be important vectors for viral transmission.

CLINICAL PRESENTATION

The typical common cold has a predictable course. This is most helpful for patients to know. A popular false belief is that a cold lasting more than 3 days is more serious and may require antibiotics. Clarifying expectations can not only alleviate

TABLE 54.1. Seasonal Prevalence of ARI Viruses

Virus	Winter	Spring	Summer	Fall
Rhinovirus	Prevalent	Prevalent	Prevalent	Prevalent
Coronavirus	Peak incidence	Peak incidence	Prevalent	Prevalent
Adenovirus	Prevalent	Prevalent	Prevalent	Prevalent
Respiratory syncytial virus	Peak incidence	Prevalent	Prevalent	
Parainfluenza 1	Prevalent		Peak incidence	
Parainfluenza 3	Peak incidence	Peak incidence	Prevalent	Peak incidence
Influenza	Peak incidence			Prevalent
Enterovirus			Peak incidence	

ARI, acute respiratory infection.

patients' worry but also provide parameters for patients to help them identify more serious infection. Presence or absence of purulent sputum did not change outcomes in AURI. AURIs resolve spontaneously within 2 weeks. In a study of the natural history of rhinovirus infections, although most patients had symptom resolution in 10 days, 25% were still symptomatic after 14 days and the range of symptoms was 1 to 33 days. After successful transmission, the virus incubates in the body for 2 to 5 days. Subsequently, the patient experiences 2 to 5 days of peak symptoms involving some combination of congestion, facial pressure, fever, sore throat, cough, and malaise. Typically, these symptoms do not fully resolve for an additional 5 to 14 days. In addition, some respiratory viruses leave the patient with a dry irritating cough lasting up to 4 weeks. Research from patients voluntarily inoculated with rhinovirus shows that nasal secretions progress from clear and thin to thick and purulent, finally thinning and resolving as the body overcomes the infection. Thus, purulence of nasal secretions is not a marker for bacterial infection.

Not everyone with symptoms of an AURI seeks care from a primary care practitioner. Only 10% to 20% of adults with colds visit the doctor, and they come with characteristics and expectations that differ from those adults practicing self-care. Those who come to the doctor for a cold tend to lack access to over-the-counter medications, to have completed less schooling, to live in more overcrowded conditions, to have missed more than 3 days of work because of illness, and to feel more unhappy. Several studies have explored the reasons that patients visit a health care provider. Patients with the common cold go to the doctor for reassurance (80%), for pain and symptom relief (80%), and for an antibiotic (60%). Two decades ago, only 30% of patients visiting the doctor expected to get an antibiotic. Studies that crossed broad ethnic, socioeconomic, and cultural groups found that presently 60% of patients with symptoms of the common cold expect an antibiotic. Physicians share some responsibility for this because the strongest predictor of expectations for antibiotics is previous experience receiving antibiotics for the common cold.

EVALUATION

In evaluating the patient who presents with nasal discharge, stuffy nose, sneezing, scratchy throat, cough, malaise, chills, facial pressure, and/or headache, the role of the physical examination is to listen to the patient's symptoms, confirm the diagnosis of AURI, and rule out the unusual cause or rare complication. It is not as critical to discern a viral versus bacterial etiology as it is to correctly identify and support those patients whose host defenses are or could be overwhelmed. Common findings on physical examination include mild erythema and edema of nasal, middle ear, and pharyngeal mucosa along with mild sinus tenderness, lymphadenopathy, and low-grade fever. Purulent nasal discharge or phlegm is not indicative of bacterial infection.

The discerning clinician will evaluate the complaint of common cold to rule out evidence of significant host compromise or serious illness. A very small number of patients with AURI develop complications associated with serious bacterial infection. Compelling symptoms and signs of bacterial infection include abrupt onset of severe symptoms, periorbital findings, fever over 103°F, and "camel-back" fever or second sickness pattern. The camel-back fever metaphor refers to the double-humped camel and describes a pattern of fever, fever resolution, and fever return, usually accompanied by more significant malaise or focal complaint. In the absence of other more compelling findings, persistent complaint beyond 14 days is not a clear indication of bacterial infection. Cough, otitis media with effusion, and runny nose can persist well past 2 weeks. Occasionally, patients will present with the common cold because they are concerned about upcoming elective surgery. They should be counseled to avoid elective surgery because, at least in children, the rate of postoperative complications is four to seven times higher in patients with AURI.

DIFFERENTIAL DIAGNOSIS

Focal inflammation of the upper respiratory tract can have serious causes other than infection. Inflammation alone can cause serious illness as in unrecognized asthma, allergic rhinitis, or bronchial hyperreactivity. Pharyngitis can be the presenting symptom of agranulocytosis, indicating severe systemic illness. Inhalation of a foreign body can cause unilateral breath sounds, stridor, or simple inflammatory cough in the absence of fever and malaise. Chronic exposure to irritants from hobbies or the workplace can cause inflammation of the upper respiratory tract. Tuberculosis and latent human immunodeficiency virus presenting with *Pneumocystis carinii* pneumonia remain present in every community in the United States. All patients should be asked about recent weight loss and dyspnea on exertion. Exacerbation of congestive heart failure may present with cough, malaise, and a distinct nocturnal pattern of dyspnea and orthopnea. Table 54.2 highlights some of the "red flags" that signal a reason to look beyond the diagnosis of AURI.

TREATMENT

Successful treatment of the common cold includes providing specific symptom relief and directly addressing the patient's actual reason for coming to the provider. It also includes spe-

TABLE 54.2. Symptoms Suggestive of Significant Illness Requiring Further Evaluation

Periorbital edema with extraocular movement pain	Tachypnea
Dental abscess or focal, enlarged, tender lymph node	Tachycardia
Second sickness pattern or camel-back fever pattern	Fever over 103°F
Unilateral breath sounds	Dehydration
Sudden onset severe malaise	Paroxysmal nocturnal dyspnea
Unexplained weight loss, anorexia, night sweats	Dyspnea on exertion, particularly in a young person with an unremarkable lung examination
	Orthopnea

cific instructions for symptom relief and the promotion of good self-care skills. Work and school issues should be addressed. The use of antibiotics should be discussed openly with patients.

Antibiotic resistance due to the misuse of antibiotics in medicine and in agriculture is a serious public health epidemic. Primary care practitioners are a vital part of epidemic management. Avoiding the inappropriate use of antibiotics is a national health priority that has proven refractory to attempts at educating both patients and clinicians. Public health initiatives to provide clear guidelines for antibiotic use in AURI infections are an important part of the fight against antibiotic resistance. Excellent consensus guidelines clarify the appropriate use of antibiotics in the treatment of specific and nonspecific upper respiratory tract infections in adults. These guidelines were developed through the sponsorship of the Centers for Disease Control and Prevention (CDC) by a panel of physicians representing internal medicine, family medicine, emergency medicine, and infectious disease. Their development occurred as a result of the epidemic of antibiotic-resistant *S. pneumoniae*. In analyzing antibiotic sources at the community level, antibiotics prescribed for AURI are the primary source. Studies show that the occurrence of antibiotic resistant *S. pneumoniae* drops when the use of antibiotics for upper respiratory infection falls. Each one of the CDC consensus guidelines repeats the same message: Antibiotics are not indicated for the treatment of uncomplicated specific or nonspecific AURI.

Uncomplicated AURI includes uncomplicated otitis, sinusitis, non-strep pharyngitis, and bronchitis. In all these, the likelihood of harm from antibiotic treatment approaches the likelihood of benefit. Acute bronchitis provides a good example of this. There is no role for antibiotics in the treatment of acute bronchitis. In the absence of unilateral abnormal breath sounds, known chronic obstructive lung disease, or systemic indications of compromise such as tachycardia, tachypnea, and high fever, the CDC guidelines do not recommend treatment with antibiotics. Once again, purulent sputum is not an indication for treatment. The very young and the very old are most likely to get antibiotics for an AURI. Patients who use tobacco or have tonsillar exudates or purulent secretions are also more likely to receive antibiotics unnecessarily.

To achieve reductions in antibiotic use, clinicians must find common ground with patients and adequately address their most worrisome issues. One effective technique to reduce antibiotic use is to provide a diagnostic name that closely matches the most worrisome complaint but avoids the use of words like sinusitis, otitis, or bronchitis. More acceptable words include face cold, cold in the ears, and chest cold. Another effective technique for reducing antibiotic use is to negotiate with patients to "give their bodies a chance" to heal the infection. In this scenario, patients are actually given an antibiotic prescription at the initial visit and asked to delay filling the prescription for 5 to 7 days. Research indicates that patients given this treatment plan do not fill a substantial number of prescriptions.

In the inevitable case that a patient with the common cold leaves the office with a prescription, the most narrow-spectrum antibiotics specific to the three most likely causes of significant bacterial infection should be used. Amoxicillin, trimethoprim/sulfamethoxazole, and doxycycline are all acceptable choices and provide adequate coverage of *S. pneumoniae, H. influenzae,* and *M. catarrhalis*. For treatment of AURI, none of these antibiotics should be used for more than 5 days. Tetracycline can cause skin sensitivity to sun, and patients should be counseled to use sunscreen. Antibiotics particularly rapid to the development of community levels of resistance, such as quinolones, should be avoided.

Despite clear guidelines for not using antibiotics in the context of AURI, most patients who present to the doctor's office for the common cold still leave with a prescription. The CDC estimates that following the consensus guidelines would avoid approximately 50 million unnecessary antibiotics per year. In a large study using direct observation of clinical encounters to explore why patients get antibiotics, 68% of patients with AURI complaints received antibiotics. Eighty percent of those encounters did not meet CDC criteria for antibiotic prescriptions. Patients receiving antibiotics made direct requests for them, reported previous relief with antibiotics, appealed to life circumstances, implied a diagnosis, and/or conveyed worrisome symptom severity. Clinicians in these situations rationalized their prescribing by reporting reasons and diagnoses that were medically acceptable. One initiative to reduce inappropriate antibiotic use is to develop strategies for addressing each of these five patient scenarios.

Primary care physicians must also address some of their own misconceptions and uncertainties about the use of antibiotics for the common cold. Two of these fears have been labeled the "chagrin factor" and the "fudge factor." The chagrin factor refers to physicians' fear that patients will choose a different practice if not given antibiotics. This is a classic demonstration of the power of anecdotes over evidence. Nearly every clinician can remember an example of this, although the data indicate it is a rare occurrence in practice. This is not unlike the fudge factor. In one study, the physicians did not know the patient's actual reason for the visit in 26% of AURI-related encounters. In these situations, the physicians "fudged" toward chagrin; they worried that the patients might want antibiotics and would be upset if they did not get them. Physicians will often point to the presence of sinus tenderness, discolored nasal discharge, or postnasal drainage as explanations for prescribing antibiotics, even though evidence demonstrates that these are not clinically useful discriminators.

If the cycle of inappropriate antibiotic use for AURI is to be broken, physicians must change the way they handle the clinical encounter. This means identifying and addressing the patient's actual reason for the visit, identifying those symptoms that are most bothersome to the patient, and providing clear instructions for relief. The issue of work or school should be addressed and appropriate written notes and excuses provided as needed. Most important, the patient and the practitioner must consciously and collaboratively negotiate the use of antibiotics. Patients who leave the office satisfied actually had more rapid symptom resolution than patients who were not satisfied. The strongest factor in patient satisfaction appears to be whether or not the physician addressed the patients concerns, not the use of antibiotics.

SPECIFIC SYMPTOM RELIEF

A major reason for patient visits for the common cold is to get information and advice about symptom relief. Providing this comfort is closely associated with patient satisfaction. A dizzying array of over-the-counter medications can make symptom relief seem complex and overwhelming to patients. Drug-to-drug interactions are also a valid source of concern. Patients should be taught about the safe and appropriate use of antipyretics and analgesics because these medications form the cornerstone of symptom relief. Many patients are reluctant and confused about using acetaminophen and nonsteroidal antiinflammatory drugs (NSAIDs). It is important to find out which of the over-the-counter NSAIDs the patient is using and then give instructions for their safe and appropriate use, including adequate doses at correct dose intervals and when to stop regular use. Risks associated with their use include potential for gastrointestinal upset and ulcer formation, as well as renal toxicity from overdosing. Acetaminophen avoids most of these side effects but has no antiinflammatory activity.

Many symptoms of the common cold are relieved with moist warm air. There are multiple sources; a warm-air humidifier, hot compresses, steam treatments, chicken soup, and hot drinks help to relieve congestion and soothe inflammation. Normal saline nose drops provide some relief for facial congestion and avoid the irritating side effects of decongestants or the sedation of antihistamines.

Asking the patient to identify the symptom that is most bothersome allows the clinician to give more specific instructions for relief. Suggestions for specific symptom relief are presented in Table 54.3. Table 54.4 provides an overview of over-the-counter medications available for symptom relief. Sneezing and a runny nasal discharge are successfully relieved with a first-generation antihistamine, taking advantage of their strong anticholinergic effects. These medications are well tolerated and have low potential for drug-to-drug interactions. Their major disadvantage is sedation, which can be useful for night relief but disrupt function and even safety during the day. The complaint of facial pressure, plugged ears, or sinus pain is best relieved with an antiinflammatory. Facial pressure is not well relieved with decongestants. Topical decongestants may provide some daytime comfort, but patients must be counseled to limit their use to 3 days to avoid rebound congestion. Systemic decongestants have the potential for sympathetic stimulation and can cause sleep disruption. Symptom relief for facial pressure may include instructions in steam treatments and the benefits of warm compresses.

Sore throat as the most prominent symptom requires a review of the clinical criteria for group A β-hemolytic *Streptococcus*. Patients who do not meet these criteria do not need an antibiotic. These patients should be instructed to drink very hot or very cold fluids and to use anesthetic lozenges.

Cough is an irritating and complex complaint that frequently prompts a visit. For chest colds it is important to teach patients the importance of good coughing. Many patients are relieved to hear that cough can perform an important function in clearing the lungs. Patients should be instructed to take a warm shower on rising and then go into a cooler room to cough. Coughing is most effective after three or four slow deep breaths. Pulmonary hygiene is a sensible part of chest cold care. Cough suppression medications should be reserved for the cough that disrupts sleep or is dry and convulsive. Over-the-counter dextromethorphan is as effective as, and safer than, codeine, although it can cause an upset stomach. Codeine syrups will cause sedation and constipation. If codeine or other opiate is prescribed, then patients should be given a specific plan for preventing and managing the side effect of constipation. Neither medication will suppress some coughs. Benzonatate offers an alternative for dry coughs that is effective for some people. Recent research indicates that some patients will experience a wheezy reactive airway in response to the common cold. These patients will experience relief with a short course of bronchodilator therapy. Water is more effective as an expectorant

TABLE 54.3. Suggestions for Specific Symptom Relief

Generalized malaise
Antiinflammatory agents taken regularly for 72 h
Give specific written instructions including dose, timing, and instructions to stop after 72 h
Rest
Echinacea purpurea
Zinc lozenges
Fever
Antipyretics
Give specific written instructions including dose, timing, and instructions to stop after 72 h
Warn patients about over-the-counter medications that already contain antipyretic medications and the potential for unintentional overdose
Plenty of fluids
Runny nose
Humidified air, hot liquids
First-generation antihistamines (warn about sedation side effect)
Stuffy nose
Normal saline nose drops
Humidified air, hot liquids, warm compresses
+/– First-generation antihistamines
+/– Topical nasal decongestants
Warn about potential for rebound congestion if used for more than 3 days
Cough
Humidified air, lozenges with menthol, hot drinks
Guafenesin as effective as water for expectorant
Dextromethorpan and codeine not effective
Nausea and constipation side effects must be addressed
Benzonatate may be effective for some irritative coughs
With reactive airway, consider short course (3 days) of β-agonist
Ear pain
Antiinflammatory
Give specific written instructions including dose, timing, and instructions to stop after 72 h
Humidified air
Sore throat
Anesthetic lozenges
Hot or cold liquids

TABLE 54.4. Guidelines for Over-the-Counter Cold Medicines

Category and name	Doses	Strengths	Maximum daily dose	Precautions	Pregnancy and lactation	Contained in combination formula brand names
Decongestants						
Pseudoephedrine				**Medications** MAOIs TCA	Avoid first trimester Poor fetal reserve	Actifed, Benadryl Cold, Chlor-Trimeton, Novafed, Seldane D, Sudafed
Short Acting	60 mg q4–6h	30 mg, 60 mg	240 mg	Beta-blockers		Comhist, Dimetane, Dristan, Histaforte, Naldecon, Ru-Tuss
Long Acting	120 mg q12h	15 mg/mL, 30 mg/5 mL		**Medical conditions** CAD, BPH, HTN,		
Phenylephrine	10 mg q4–6h 20 mg q8–12h		60 mg	Hypothyroidism		
Topical				Use of these agents for longer than 3–4 days can cause rebound nasal congestion	Avoid first trimester	
Short Acting	2 drops q3h	0.05% sol/20 mL				Privine
Naphazoline HCl	2 sprays q4–6h	0.05% spray/12 mL 0.25%, 0.5%, 1% sol in 15–30 mL				Neo-Synephrine, Nostril, Vicks, Sinex
Phenylephrine HCl	2–3 drops or sprays q4h					Afrin, Dristan, Neo-Synephrine,
Long-Acting						Vicks Neo-Synehrine, Otrivin
Oxymetazolin HCl	2 drops q12h	0.025%, 0.05 drops 0.05%/15–30 mL spray				
Xylometazoline HCl	2–3 drops q8–10h	0.05%–0.1%/15 mL spray 0.05–0.1%/15 mL sol				
Antihistamines						
Chlorpheniramine maleate	2–4 mg q6–8h 8 mg q12h	2, 4, 8 mg		**Medications** TCA, MAOIs **Medical conditions**	Avoid first trimester and during lactation	
Bromphenairamine maleate	2–4 mg q6–8h 12 mg q12h 25–50 mg q6–8h	2, 4, 12 mg 12.5, 25, 50 mg		BPH Angle closure Glaucome		
Diphenhydramine HCl						
Clemastine fumarate	12.5–50 mg q6h	12.5, 25, 50 mg				
Pyrilamine maleate	1.25–2.5 mg q4–6h	1.25, 2.5 mg				
Tripolodine HCl						
Antitussives						
Dextromethorpan	10–20 mg q4–8h 30 mg q8h	 10, 15.30 mg	120 mg 120 mg	**Medications** MAOIs **Medical Conditions** Avoid with continued high dose use in asthmatics with COPD	Avoid first trimester and during lactation	Benylin, Cerose-DM, Conar, Delsym, Naldecon-DM, Pertussin, Robitussin DM, Tussar, Vicks Actifed-WC, Calcidrine
Codeine Sulfate	30 mg q6–8h		600 mg			Dimetane-DC, Naldecon-CY Nucofed, Pediacof, Robitussin-Noahistane-DH, AC/DAC, Triaminic, Tussar-2
Hydrocodone bitartate	30 mg q6–8h					Hydrocodone, Hycomine Hycuss, P-V-Tussin, Ru-Tuss Tussionex
Benzonatate (Tessalon)	100 mg q6–8h					Breosin, Deconsal, Entex, Glycotuss, Glytuss, Humibid, Hytuss, Naldecon, Robitussin
Expectorants						
Guaifenesin	100–600 mg		2,400 mg		Avoid during pregnancy	

BPH, benign hypertrophy; CAD, coronary artery disease; COPD, chronic obstructive pulmonary disease; MAOIs, monoamine oxidase inhibitors; TCA, trycyclic antidepressants.

than guaifenesin. Symptom relief advice should be specific to the patient's worst symptom and sensitive to potential drug interactions, insurance coverage, and cost.

COMPLEMENTARY AND ALTERNATIVE MEDICINE

Many patients will also have questions about the use of complementary and alternative therapies for the care and prevention of AURI. Effective, safe, and gentle complementary treatments for the symptoms of the common cold exist. Some of these medications have symptom relief responses that match or even outdo common over-the-counter medications for the common cold. Zinc gluconate and zinc acetate lozenges reduce the intensity and duration of symptoms 1 to 3 days sooner than patients taking placebo. Lozenges should be started at first sign of the cold, taken every 2 hours, and dissolved completely by sucking. Zinc will interfere with the absorption of fluoroquinolones and tetracycline. Patients should take no more than 40 mg of zinc a day and stop as soon as the cold is over.

Data supporting the use of Echinacea for the common cold is uneven. Several botanical forms of Echinacea are used medicinally. Metaanalysis of data on Echinacea has been confounded by the various botanical preparations used. In addition, different commercial companies have preparations with different concentrations of phenolic compounds. Most data are based on Echinacea purpurea. More than half the studies on Echinacea suggest that use resulted in a reduction in days of symptoms or, at least, a reduction in symptom intensity. Research shows that Echinacea does not prevent colds. It also appears to weaken host immune responses if taken for more than 8 weeks. Echinacea is contraindicated in pregnant women, in women trying to conceive, or in breast-feeding women. For the otherwise healthy individual with symptoms of the common cold, Echinacea purpurea taken as soon as symptoms begin and stopped when symptoms subside is likely to be as effective as any over-the-counter medications.

Vitamin C clearly improves immune function. Yet, data to show its beneficial effect specifically on the common cold are weak. Pooled analysis of available data on vitamin C showed that people who took vitamin C were just as likely to catch a cold as those who took the placebo. In a study involving nearly 3,000 patients, vitamin C did not shorten the length of the cold, but it did ease discomfort for about 25% of patients. Vitamin C is generally safe and well tolerated. There is no contraindication to it use for the common cold.

Finally, a visit for the common cold offers the clinician a window of opportunity for promoting patient self-care skills. The common cold is often the window of opportunity to help people stop smoking. Even the recommendation to exercise regularly can reduce the symptoms of a cold. Women who exercised regularly cut the number of days they were sick with a cold in half. The visit is a chance to teach patients about hand washing, the natural history of AURI, and the appropriate safe use of over-the-counter medications. Table 54.4 shows an overview of over-the-counter cold medications and dosage guidelines.

The care of the common cold offers the clinician a chance to have an impact on the health of the individual, the family, and the community. Excellent care requires that primary care practitioners work collaboratively with patients to address their concerns, relieve their symptoms, prevent the development of antibiotic resistance, and develop strategies for self-care. This requires compassion, empathy, and skill.

CONSIDERATIONS IN PREGNANCY

Often, women will experience more colds than usual when they are pregnant. Homes with small children are reservoirs for the common cold, and nursing mothers need specific instructions about return to work when ill, plus appropriate paperwork. Mastitis and pyelonephritis can both present as generalized malaise that can be mistaken for the common cold. Depression and violence can also present as nonspecific malaise and are more common in pregnant and nursing women. The risk of complications from influenza are elevated in pregnancy, and clinicians should take the opportunity to immunize women in the second and third trimesters of pregnancy.

During the first trimester, it is advisable to avoid all cough and cold medications because their teratogenic effects are not well understood. Codeine, first-generation antihistamines, and pseudoephedrine have been associated with birth anomalies. Rest, extra fluids, nasal saline, and warm moist air will all help to comfort symptoms safely. Acetaminophen at the recommended doses appears to be safe during the first trimester. Caution is still advised in the use of over-the-counter cold medicines during the second and third trimesters, but all standard cold medications can be used at low doses except for NSAIDs. NSAIDS can potentially aggravate bleeding and are associated with premature closure of the ductus arteriosus during the third trimester. All cold medicines appear in low amounts in breast milk and can affect the infant's behavior but appear to be relatively safe. The first-generation antihistamines, because of their anticholinergic activity, may inhibit milk production in lactating women. Echinacea and zinc are not recommended. There are several excellent references that detail medication use during pregnancy and lactation that should be reviewed (see Bibliography).

BIBLIOGRAPHY

Barrett B, Vohmann M, Calabrese C. Echinacea for upper respiratory infection. *J Fam Pract* 1999;48:628–635.

Bensenor IM, Cook NR, Lee IM, et al. Active and passive smoking and risk of colds in women. *Ann Epidemiol* 2001;11:225–231.

Braun BL, Fowles JB, Solberg L, et al. Patient beliefs about the characteristics, causes, and care of the common cold: an update. *J Fam Pract* 2000;49:153–156.

Bridges CB, Fukuda K, Cox NJ, et al. Advisory Committee on Immunization Practices. Prevention and control of influenza. Recommendations of the Advisory Committee on Immunization Practices (ACIP). *MMWR Morb Mortal Wkly Rep* 2001;50:1–44.

Cohen MM, Cameron CB. Should you cancel the operation when a child has an upper respiratory tract infection? *Anesth Analg* 1991;72:282–288.

Colgan R, Powers JH. Appropriate antimicrobial prescribing: approaches that limit antibiotic resistance. *Am Fam Phys* 2001;64:999–1004.

Couchman GR, Rascoe TG, Forjuoh SN. Back-up antibiotic prescriptions for common respiratory symptoms: patient satisfaction and fill rates. *J Fam Pract* 2000;49:907–913.

Douglas RM, Chalker EB, Treacy B. Vitamin C for preventing and treating the common cold. *The Cochrane Library*. Oxford: Update Software, 2000:2.

Dowell J, Pitkethly M, Bain J, et al. A randomized controlled trial of delayed antibiotic prescribing as a strategy for managing uncomplicated respiratory tract infection in primary care. *Br J Gen Pract* 2001;51:200–205.

Dowell SF, Schwartz B, Phillips WR. Appropriate use of antibiotics for URIs in children. Part II. Cough, pharyngitis, and the common cold. The Pediatric URI Consensus Team. *Am Fam Phys* 1998;58:1335–1342.

Gwaltney JM Jr. Epidemiology of the common cold. *Ann N Y Acad Sci* 1980;353: 54–60.

Hale T. *Medications and mothers' milk*. Amarillo: Pharmasoft, 2000.

Marshall S. Zinc gluconate and the common cold: review of randomized controlled trials. *Can Fam Phys* 1998;44:1037–1042.

Melchart D, Linde K, Fischer P, et al. Echinacea for preventing and treating the common cold. *The Cochrane Library*. Oxford: Update Software, 2000:2.

Mossad SB, Macknin ML, Medendorp SV, et al. Zinc gluconate lozenges for treating the common cold: a randomized, double-blind, placebo-controlled study. *Ann Intern Med* 1996;125:81–88.

Ressel G, Centers for Disease Control and Prevention, American College of Physicians, American Society of Internal Medicine, et al. Principles of appropriate

antibiotic use. Part II. Nonspecific upper respiratory tract infections. *Am Fam Phys* 2001;64:510.
Ressel G, Centers for Disease Control and Prevention, American College of Physicians, American Society of Internal Medicine, et al. Principles of appropriate antibiotic use. Part V. Acute bronchitis. *Am Fam Phys* 2001;64:1098–1100.
Schroeder K, Fahey T. Systematic review of randomized controlled trials of over the counter cough medicines for acute cough in adults. *BMJ* 2002;324:329–339.
Scott JG, Cohen D, DiCicco-Bloom B, et al. Antibiotic use in acute respiratory infections and the ways patients pressure physicians for a prescription. *J Fam Pract* 2001;50:853–858.
Singh M. Heated, humidified air for the common cold. *The Cochrane Library*. Oxford: Update Software, 2002:1.
Smucny JJ, Flynn CA, Becker LA, et al. Are beta2-agonists effective treatment for acute bronchitis or acute cough in patients without underlying pulmonary disease? A systematic review. *J Fam Pract* 2001;50:945–951.
Snow V, Mottur-Pilson C, Cooper RJ, et al. Principles of appropriate antibiotic use for acute pharyngitis in adults. *Ann Intern Med* 2001;134:506–508.
Snow V, Mottur-Pilson C, Hickner JM, et al. Principles of appropriate antibiotic use for acute sinusitis in adults. *Ann Intern Med* 2001;134:495–497.
Solberg LI, Braun BL, Fowles JB, et al. Care-seeking behavior for upper respiratory infections. *J Fam Pract* 2000;49:915–920.
Taverner D, Bickford L, Draper M. Nasal decongestants for the common cold. *The Cochrane Library*. Oxford: Update Software, 2002:2.

CHAPTER 55
Asthma

Anthony J. Fedullo

Asthma is a common chronic respiratory disease, affecting about 5% of adults. It is characterized by reversible airway obstruction, traditionally thought to be due to bronchial muscle hyperreactivity. More recently, inflammation within the airway has been recognized as an important component of obstruction. Asthma can be severe: In 15% to 20% of patients with asthma, the disease limits their activity, and more than 50% of patients with asthma seek help from a health care provider each year. The prevalence and severity of the disease have reportedly increased in the United States recently, particularly in urban areas. This may reflect changes in the urban environment or inadequacies in health care delivery, prevention, and treatment in these areas. An increase in asthma deaths has also been observed, attributed in part to the overuse or abuse of β-agonist medication, but very likely also having a basis in poor care and control of asthma.

The prevalence of asthma does not differ greatly among adult men and women. In childhood and early adolescence, boys are more often affected; women predominate among the elderly. The prevalence of asthma is highest in childhood, but it can appear at any age. Adult-onset asthma or recurrence of asthma in adults after teenage remission is not unusual. The prevalence varies among racial and ethnic groups: African-Americans have a higher prevalence of asthma than do whites.

ETIOLOGY

The precise etiology of asthma is unknown, but it may have a basis in atopy or allergy. Asthmatics have higher rates of reaction to the antigens used in skin testing than do nonasthmatics. Asthmatics also more commonly have a history of other atopic disorders (e.g., hay fever, allergic rhinitis, eczema). Fifty percent or more of asthmatics have nasal allergic symptoms as well, and about one third of patients with allergic rhinitis have had episodes of asthma. Asthmatics often have a family history of atopy. The history need not include asthma itself, but many asthmatics have relatives with other allergic disorders, such as hay fever.

Although asthma has a link to allergic conditions, it is not a purely allergic disorder. Allergy is not the major precipitating factor in many asthmatics. Asthma is often exacerbated by cold air, emotional states, and airborne irritants such as cigarette smoke that do not act by allergic mechanisms.

The exact nature of the relation between asthma and allergy remains uncertain, but more is known about the basic mechanisms causing symptoms once asthma is present. Asthma has long been considered a disease of airway hyperreactivity, whereby bronchial smooth muscle contraction would constrict airways, causing the airflow limitation and wheezing associated with the disease. Evidence of bronchial smooth muscle hyperreactivity in asthmatics is found in the increased bronchial constriction occurring with cholinergic agents such as methacholine and with β-sympathomimetic antagonists or blockers such as propranolol. These agents are contraindicated in asthma. Similarly, anticholinergic agents such as atropine and ipratropium and sympathomimetic agents such as epinephrine and albuterol are used therapeutically.

Emphasis has been placed recently on a mechanism of airway obstruction in asthma that is not primarily related to smooth muscle hyperreactivity. Inflammation is increasingly being seen as a predominant factor in asthma, causing excessive mucous hypersecretion, mucous cell and mucous gland hyperplasia, and edema and inflammatory infiltration of the airway wall. This mechanism explains the mucous secretion and productive cough that often accompany asthma in the absence of infection. Evidence of inflammation is seen in the mucous-packed airways of patients who die with severe asthma, as well as the finding of active inflammatory cells in bronchoalveolar lavage specimens from asthmatics. The degree of inflammation does not seem to be related to whether asthma is triggered by allergic or nonallergic factors.

Many mediators can cause the inflammatory changes in the airways and bronchoconstriction, although the prime role of any particular one has not been identified. Mast cells and histamine release, prostaglandins and leukotrienes, macrophages, eosinophils, and lymphocyte products all play a role. Specific agents against these or other mediators may someday be available for therapy. At present, nonspecific antiinflammatory agents such as corticosteroids, cromolyn, and nedocromil play an important role in asthma therapy.

The basic mechanisms of inflammation and bronchoconstriction remain uncertain, but asthma attacks or exacerbations are triggered by fairly well-defined clinical variables. Allergens remain a prominent factor in inducing an asthma attack. Seasonal allergens such as trees, grass, or weeds are a factor in many asthma attacks, as are the more subtle influences of allergens such as the ubiquitous dust mite or molds containing *Aspergillus* species. Removal or avoidance of these environmental factors or desensitization to specific allergens is a prominent part of asthma therapy. Air pollution has been associated with asthma exacerbation. Ozone and sulfur dioxide cause an increase in airway resistance and obstruction; this may play a role in the increased prevalence of asthma in cities. The relation between *occupational triggers* and asthma is often made by obtaining a history of exacerbation with exposure to the offending agent (e.g., certain wood dusts in hobbyists or carpenters; chemicals such as toluene diisocyanate used in the plastics industry; flour or animal excreta in flour ["baker's asthma"]). *Viral respiratory infections*, but not bacterial ones, are common precipitants of asthma attacks. *Cold air* and *exercise* are common asthma triggers. The mechanism is thought to be due to cooling and dehydration of the airway mucosa, causing the release of inflammatory mediators. Outdoor jogging in cold, dry, winter air is more likely to cause an asthma exacerbation than is swimming in a heated indoor pool. *Emotional factors* can trigger episodes of acute asthma. The mechanism is uncertain, but anger, anxiety, and unresolved conflicts have been recognized as triggers for asthma exacerbation.

Nocturnal exacerbation of asthma is common. Nocturnal awakening with asthma usually occurs between 2 a.m. and 5 a.m. and is thought to be due to circadian differences in ventilation and mediator release. In many asthmatics, nocturnal awakening is a prominent part of their symptomatology. Nocturnal awakening may also represent inadequate daytime asthma control. Many asthmatics can tolerate considerable declines in pulmonary function and not complain of daytime symptoms. The physiologic increase in airway resistance at night may then more easily trigger symptoms as the airways become further narrowed.

There is an interesting relation between asthma and the *menstrual cycle.* Premenstrual worsening of asthma occurs in about a third of women. Studies of airway function do not show large declines in pulmonary function, and the mechanism of the symptomatic exacerbation is uncertain. Fluid retention and changes in circulating progesterone have been suggested, but no convincing physiologic correlates to this clinical observation have been found. *Pregnancy* can affect the severity or frequency of asthma. The complex hormonal and psychological effects of pregnancy must be related to this phenomenon, but the specifics are uncertain. About one third of pregnant asthmatics have worse asthma during pregnancy, one third have improved disease, and one third are unaffected. Good control of asthma is important in pregnancy to ensure adequate fetal oxygenation.

Some asthmatic patients are sensitive to *ingested* material. In adults, this is an uncommon trigger of asthma but should be recognized. Shellfish can produce severe bronchoconstriction. Sulfites, contained in some alcoholic beverages or used in the preservation of foods such as salads, may exacerbate asthma. The mechanism is uncertain, but it is less likely to be allergenic than due to the release of endogenous sulfur dioxide through the airway mucosa. Tartrazine yellow, a food coloring, has been associated with asthma induction. This is thought to be due to effects on prostaglandin metabolism and production.

Drugs can exacerbate or trigger asthma. Any agent that produces anaphylaxis can cause airway edema and wheezing. β-Sympathomimetic blockers, often used in the therapy of hypertension and angina, can affect bronchomotor tone, resulting in enhanced bronchoconstriction. Asthmatics should not take these drugs systemically. Some asthmatics are sensitive even to eye drops that contain them. A few asthmatics are sensitive to aspirin and other antiinflammatory agents. In these asthmatics, the disease is usually of adult onset, with nasal polyposis and rhinitis. The mechanism is thought to be the changes in prostaglandin metabolism and production induced by these drugs. Acetaminophen does not share these effects and can be used safely by asthmatics.

Animal proteins from *pets and dust mites* can be prominent asthma triggers. They can permeate a home and cause asthma in the absence of a pet, indeed even long after a pet has been removed.

These and other possible asthma triggers must be considered when interviewing the asthmatic. Important parts of asthma therapy are recognizing asthma triggers and avoiding them (or instituting prophylactic treatment if avoidance is impossible). This is as important as providing medical therapy for the symptoms.

DIFFERENTIAL DIAGNOSIS

The differential diagnosis of asthma involves the symptoms of cough, shortness of breath, and wheezing. Upper airway obstruction can cause these symptoms; this should be considered in patients who do not have a prior history of asthma. Epiglottitis, for example, should be considered in a patient who has dysphagia and painful swallowing; it is not a disease confined to children. Involvement of the cricoarytenoid joint in rheumatoid arthritis can also present with upper airway narrowing and wheezing, as can laryngeal carcinoma. Stridorous wheezing from an upper airway abnormality should be considered an emergency. The residual airway may be very small (millimeters) by the time wheezing and shortness of breath from an upper airway cause become apparent. These upper airway causes are much less common than asthma but should be considered in adults who have wheezing and shortness of breath without a prior history of asthma. Clues to an upper airway cause for wheezing include a wheeze heard prominently over the central airways in the neck, a predominantly inspiratory component to the wheezing (stridor) rather than the predominantly expiratory wheezing in asthma, and arterial blood gas measurements that show a normal or near-normal oxygen level (taking into account the inspired oxygen concentration) relative to the degree of respiratory distress exhibited.

Congestive heart failure can present with wheezing due to compression of the small airways by interstitial edema. This diagnosis is usually apparent from other physical findings and from the chest x-ray. Pulmonary embolism can sometimes have associated wheezing due to the release of bronchoconstricting mediators.

HISTORY

Patients with asthma complain of intermittent cough, shortness of breath, and wheezing. All these symptoms need not be present in each patient; some patients with asthma have cough as their only complaint. The symptoms are episodic and intermittent, vary in intensity, and are often related to particular events such as exercise, cold air, or exposure to allergens. Patients may describe their asthma as a tightness or heaviness in the chest. This complaint in older asthmatics suggests angina as a differential diagnosis. Nocturnal awakening with shortness of breath and wheezing is common and may suggest congestive heart failure. Symptoms may be chronic in patients who are not adequately treated or who have underlying chronic bronchitis or emphysema, but even in these patients, the symptoms vary in intensity when an asthmatic component is present, depending on exposure to exacerbating factors.

The relation of symptoms to asthma severity as measured by pulmonary function tests is imprecise: Some patients have symptoms with only slight airway obstruction, and others have few symptoms with severe obstruction. Many patients have no symptoms until airway function, as measured by the forced expiratory volume in 1 second (FEV_1), falls by 30% to 40%. The absence of symptoms, therefore, does not necessarily indicate adequate treatment. Pulmonary function may still be quite abnormal, leaving the patient susceptible to recurrent symptoms.

PHYSICAL EXAMINATION AND CLINICAL FINDINGS

Patients with asthma may have a normal examination, in keeping with the intermittent and episodic nature of the disease.

During an asthma attack, findings of airway obstruction such as a prolonged expiratory time or expiratory wheezing are found. These findings can be made more obvious by asking the patient to take a deep breath and perform a forced expiration. The intensity of wheezing is not a good marker for the severity of asthma: Slight obstruction may cause easily audible wheezing because of the large volume and velocity of air moving through obstructed airways. A cough may be present and may sound congested or "moist." As asthma increases in severity, evidence of tachypnea and respiratory distress becomes evident. Wheezing may not be as prominent because severe obstruction may allow little airflow. An increased pulsus paradoxus (>20 mm Hg) also reflects more severe asthma. Predominantly inspiratory wheezing suggests upper airway obstruction, and rales and a gallop rhythm suggest congestive heart failure.

LABORATORY AND IMAGING STUDIES

During asthma attacks, pulmonary function tests show a decreased peak expiratory flow (PEF) and a decreased FEV_1, particularly when compared with the forced vital capacity (FVC). Inexpensive PEF measuring devices are available. Measuring the PEF helps patients with asthma monitor their own disease and allows recognition of the early phases of an exacerbation. Reduced PEF and a reduced FEV_1/FVC ratio are nonspecific for asthma and are also found in bronchitis and emphysema. The clinical findings should allow the physician to distinguish emphysema and chronic bronchitis from asthma. Bronchitis and emphysema have chronic symptomatology and evidence of chronic airway obstruction, in contrast to the intermittent and episodic nature of asthma. However, it is sometimes difficult to separate these entities, and they often coexist, particularly in the older patient who has smoked heavily.

One useful characteristic of asthma on pulmonary function tests is improvement after the use of bronchodilator medication. A 15% to 20% improvement in the FEV_1 suggests the presence of reversible airway obstruction, characteristic of asthma. Sometimes the improvement is seen predominantly in the FVC; this is also considered evidence of bronchodilator responsiveness. Absence of bronchodilator response on pulmonary function testing does not exclude asthma, because when patients are severely obstructed, a single treatment with bronchodilator medication may not produce benefit.

If the patient has intermittent symptoms but at the time of the examination or pulmonary function testing has no wheezing or normal airway function, asthma challenge tests can be used. The challenge test most frequently done in pulmonary function laboratories is the inhalation of serial concentrations of methacholine. A positive test is a 20% fall in FEV_1 from baseline. Some laboratories use cold air inhalation or exercise as a challenge. Occasionally, specific challenges are done with agents involved in occupational exposures. However, there is often little need for this in the presence of a history, suggesting occupational asthma, and the tests are poorly standardized as to the dose of the agent.

The chest x-ray in asthma is usually normal or shows hyperinflation if the obstruction is severe. Allergic bronchopulmonary aspergillosis, which may affect a few asthmatics, may show infiltrates on chest x-rays, representing mucous impaction.

An increased number of eosinophils on the complete blood count may be seen, but the absence of this finding does not exclude asthma. Immunoglobulin E levels are elevated in many asthmatics. Very high levels (>1,500 ng/mL) suggest allergic bronchopulmonary aspergillosis. Asthmatic patients may have skin test hyperreactivity to antigens, but the antigens causing skin reactions do not correlate well with those that cause symptomatic asthma exacerbation.

TREATMENT

There are two goals of asthma therapy: control symptoms so that the patient is asymptomatic at rest and can perform normal daily activities and keep the PEF normal. This is particularly important in the difficult-to-control patient. Treating to symptom relief only can leave a considerable deficit in pulmonary function and can predispose to symptomatic asthma episodes when the patient is exposed to triggering factors.

Treatment of asthma must be tailored to the patient. Avoidance of inciting factors, when possible, is the first step in treatment. Smoking, for example, should be avoided. Some asthmatics are bothered by pets, and removing the animals may be helpful. It often takes a considerable amount of time for the house to be cleaned of all animal products, because animal proteins may be in the carpets and upholstered furniture. Removing mold in the environment and careful cleaning with regard to dust mites are useful. Some asthmatics are sensitive to sulfites in alcoholic beverages, others to aspirin and nonsteroidal antiinflammatory agents, and still others to exposures at work. To avoid or minimize these and other agents triggering asthma, they must first be identified by obtaining a careful history regarding exacerbating factors.

Mild asthmatics with infrequent exacerbations may be treated with medium duration inhaled β_2-agonists, two puffs by a metered-dose inhaler. Of the many agents in this class, a commonly used one is albuterol. These agents may be used at the onset of a mild asthma attack or preferably are used prophylactically against factors that consistently result in symptoms and may be given every 2 hours for a few doses.

In patients with more than mild asthma (exacerbations more than a few times a week or exacerbations that last more than an hour or two each), the next step in therapy is to add an inhaled antiinflammatory agent administered by a metered-dose inhaler two to four times daily, not used just when symptoms occur. In children, cromolyn is often chosen; in adults, inhaled corticosteroids are usually the first choice. Latest generation corticosteroids such as fluticasone and budesonide are of high potency. In normal doses they have no systemic side effects, but if used above recommended doses they can be absorbed enough to cause corticosteroid related side effects and adrenal suppression.

If on this regimen the patient still has a few attacks of asthma a week, each episode lasting more than a few hours, or has nocturnal asthma, inhaled β-agonists can be taken on a regular basis to achieve better control. Albuterol can be given four times daily, or longer acting β-agonists (such as formoterol or salmeterol) can be given twice a day, Additional use of albuterol beyond this (two or three times daily as needed) may be allowed, but beyond that, additional agents are probably necessary, or the patient should seek more definitive care for a refractory attack. It should be noted that the long-acting β-agonists are not intended for treatment of acute attacks; they are used to maintain better overall control and to avoid exacerbations. The frequent use of inhaled β-agonist medication has been associated with increased mortality in asthma, although this phenomenon may reflect mortality due to uncontrolled asthma in which the patient overused the β-agonist rather than seeking more definitive care.

Inhaled β-agonists and inhaled corticosteroids are available in dry powder preparations, separately or combined for convenience, as well as the traditional liquid aerosol. This is predominantly a matter of patient preference; some believe the dry inhalation systems are less prone to patient delivery error and the irritative effects of the aerosol.

If further therapy is needed to control symptoms, ipratropium, an anticholinergic bronchodilator available in a metered-dose inhaler, may be prescribed. Its use is often advocated in the patient with chronic obstructive pulmonary disease who has a bronchospastic component, but it is efficacious in asthma and has no side effects.

The role and positioning of oral leukotriene antagonists (montelukast and zafirlukast) in asthma is uncertain. Some suggest adding it after intermittent β-agonists have been tried before inhaled steroids; it may be used after all inhaled regimens have been tried, avoiding systemic side effects and believing inhaled corticosteroids are equally efficacious. Theophylline preparations are not often used in asthma currently, given their side effects and limited efficacy.

Antibiotics are not routinely administered to younger patients with asthmatic exacerbations. In older patients with underlying chronic obstructive pulmonary disease, acute bacterial bronchitis is more common and may be associated with exacerbations of dyspnea and wheezing. Antibiotics are frequently given in this case.

It is important to aggressively treat asthma that does not respond well to a maintenance therapeutic regimen. Episodes of acute asthma will require treatment by more frequent doses of shorter acting β-agents, but if that becomes necessary every few hours without response, or with a transient and increasingly poor response, this should be recognized within a day or 2 so that a course of oral corticosteroids can be offered. Patients must be instructed to alert their physician to this change and not to use increasingly frequent doses of β-agonist inhalers. The course of steroids can be relatively short if exacerbations that become refractory to routine medication are treated early (within a few days of determining their refractoriness). For example, 40 to 50 mg prednisone given once daily for 3 or 4 days and stopped without tapering can result in amelioration of asthma sufficient to allow control to be again achieved with inhaled medication. If, in a refractory exacerbation, the use of oral corticosteroids is avoided for weeks, the inflammatory component, with mucous hypersecretion and mucosal cell hypertrophy, becomes so prominent that a much longer course of corticosteroids, and even hospitalization, may become necessary. The increasing mortality in asthma may reflect avoidance in definitive therapy of refractory exacerbations, hesitancy to use corticosteroids promptly, and overuse of inhaled β-agonists.

Many patients with asthma visit the emergency department or require hospitalization. These patients have acute severe attacks or attacks that have not responded well to outpatient therapy, including a trial of corticosteroids. Unless the patient responds very well in the emergency department, consultation with physicians trained in general internal medicine, pulmonary medicine, or allergy and immunology (depending on the practice patterns in the area) is useful. These specialists can help determine the need for hospitalization, can help manage these often very ill patients, and can give advice on the postdischarge outpatient regimen.

For the very ill patient in the emergency department or one who requires admission, a patient under age 40 may receive subcutaneous epinephrine or terbutaline; this can be repeated every 20 minutes for three doses. Intravenous corticosteroids are started at a dosage of 40 to 60 mg methylprednisolone every 6 to 8 hours. Inhaled β-agonists are given via nebulization four to six times daily. As the patient improves, intravenous corticosteroids are stopped and the patient is switched to oral prednisone 40 to 60 mg/day, to be tapered over a few days, and the nebulized β-agonist is changed to a metered-dose inhaler.

The use of chronic corticosteroids is sometimes necessary in severe asthma. Because of the side effects associated with long-term use of corticosteroids, it is useful to embark on this therapy in conjunction with help from consulting physicians. Patients who need long-term corticosteroid therapy for control of asthma should be on a maximal regimen of less toxic drugs and should take the lowest dose of corticosteroid to provide asthma control, preferably on an every-other-day basis.

Skin testing and desensitization are controversial in the management of patients with asthma. This therapy should not be offered routinely. Many asthmatics do not have trigger factors that are allergic in nature, and even among asthmatics who have allergic asthma, the results of desensitization are often marginal. Most asthmatics can be treated successfully with inhaled agents, and desensitization adds little to their need for medications or asthma control. Desensitization should be considered only in asthmatics who are difficult to control and have strong seasonal or allergic components to their asthma, as evaluated by history and observation. Before initiating this, the patient should be on a maximal inhaled bronchodilator regimen, perhaps with the use of theophylline as well, and should have the environment investigated thoroughly to avoid exacerbating agents whenever possible.

CONSIDERATIONS IN PREGNANCY

Asthma is the most common chronic disease affecting pregnant women. About 5% to 7% of women of childbearing age have asthma. About equal proportions of women have their asthma improve, worsen, or remain unchanged during pregnancy. Asthma in subsequent pregnancies behaves similarly.

The major risk to the fetus results from maternal hypoxemia. Hypoxemia, which can be significant even in mild asthma, can threaten fetal oxygenation. Respiratory alkalosis from asthma-induced hyperventilation can produce fetal vasoconstriction, further compromising oxygen delivery to the fetus. Poorly controlled asthma in pregnancy has measurable adverse effects on fetal outcome. Epidemiologic studies have shown an increase in preterm births and increased neonatal mortality. Some studies suggest an increased incidence of preeclampsia in women with asthma.

Asthma, although it may not limit the woman's activity, carries a serious risk to the fetus because of the low blood oxygen values. Treatment of asthma in pregnancy is not significantly different than that previously outlined. Epinephrine is avoided because of its constrictive effects on the vasculature, but inhaled β_2-agonists, inhaled corticosteroids and other inflammatory agents, theophylline, and even courses of oral corticosteroids should be used as the clinical circumstances warrant. The goal is asthma control and normalization of pulmonary function tests, just as it is in the nonpregnant woman.

To reiterate, very mild asthmatics may be treated as needed with inhaled β-agonists. Asthmatics with more than a few episodes of asthma weekly or episodes lasting more than an hour should begin regular therapy with inhaled corticosteroids. If control is not achieved, regular β_2-agonist use or therapy with a sustained-release theophylline preparation should be instituted. A short course of oral corticosteroids can be used for refractory exacerbations. More severe asthma requiring emergency department visits or hospitalization can be treated with intravenous corticosteroids and bronchodilators given by nebulization.

Consultative help in the care of the pregnant asthmatic is often useful. In addition to assistance in medical management, it offers the opportunity to reinforce patient education regarding the need for good control of asthma and medication compliance, and it can help ease the concern patients feel about taking medication during pregnancy.

BIBLIOGRAPHY

Bailey WC. Symposium on asthma. *Clin Chest Med* 1984;5:557.

Chan-Yeung M, Lam S. Occupational asthma. *Am Rev Respir Dis* 1986;133:686.

Corticosteroids: their biologic mechanisms and application to the treatment of asthma. *Am Rev Respir Dis* 1990;141[Suppl]:S1.

Frazier CA, ed. *Occupational asthma.* New York: Van Nostrand Reinhold, 1980.

Holgate S. Mediator and cytokine mechanisms in asthma. *Thorax* 1993;48:103.

Lang DM, Polansky M. Patterns of asthma mortality in Philadelphia from 1969 to 1991. *N Engl J Med* 1994;331:1542.

Management of asthma during pregnancy. U.S. Department of Health and Human Services, Public Health Service, National Institutes of Health. NIH Publication No. 93-3279, September 1993.

Martin RJ. Asthma. *Semin Respir Critical Care Med* 1994;15:97.

Pauli BD, Reid RL, Munt PW, et al. Influence of the menstrual cycle on airway function in asthmatic and normal subjects. *Am Rev Respir Dis* 1989;140:358.

Practical guide for the diagnosis and treatment of asthma. NIH Publication No. 97-4053, October 1997.

Rakel RE, Cockcroft DW, Lieberman P, et al. Improved management of asthma: putting today's knowledge to use. *J Respir Dis* 1994;15:S1.

Scanlon PD, Beck KC. Methacholine inhalation challenge. *Mayo Clin Proc* 1994; 69:1118.

CHAPTER 56
Tuberculosis

Anthony J. Fedullo

Disease caused by *Mycobacterium tuberculosis* has been known to humankind for thousands of years. Archaeologic evidence of bony disease and descriptions of the clinical syndrome from literate societies indicate its long-standing problem as a human pathogen. Tuberculosis (TB) as a disease is impacted by the social and economic environment. Urbanization of civilization has resulted in increasing acquisition and death rates from the disease. In the late 1800s, the rates of TB in urban areas approached 300 to 400 per 100,000, far above levels in the country. Decline in TB acquisition and mortality began before the antibiotic era, due to improvements in urban crowding, public hygiene, and increased public health awareness with identification of cases and isolation. In the 1940s, streptomycin was shown to be an effective agent in the treatment of TB. Shortly after its introduction, however, organisms resistant to its use as a single agent appeared, a lesson that remains pertinent to TB therapy today. In the early 1950s, isoniazid was introduced, and by 1985 the number of annually reported patients had fallen from 84,000 in 1953 to 22,000, most of whom had reactivation of previously acquired disease. This decline hid some disturbing statistics, however. TB still was distressingly common in some urban communities and among minorities and immigrant groups. Adverse socioeconomic conditions, drug dependency and abuse, and rising rates of human immunodeficiency virus (HIV) infection led to an increase in TB in certain segments of the urban population. There were 4,000 to 5,000 more cases of TB in 1991 than the cases reported in 1984, many due to recent acquisition of disease rather than reactivation of remotely acquired disease, and the increase is predicted to continue. In addition to the increase in the prevalence of disease, strains of mycobacteria resistant to multiple antibiotics have emerged, due to poor compliance with medications and importation of resistant strains from areas where single-drug therapy has fostered resistance.

ETIOLOGY

There are more than 50 species in the genus *Mycobacterium*. The pathogenic *M. tuberculosis* complex includes four of these, *M. tuberculosis, Mycobacterium bovis, Mycobacterium africanum,* and *Mycobacterium microti.* Most clinical disease in this group is caused by *M. tuberculosis,* and the term tuberculosis bacillus henceforth refers to this organism unless noted otherwise.

Mycobacterium species other than *M. tuberculosis* can cause disease. *Mycobacterium avium* complex (which includes *M. avium* and *M. intracellulare), M. kansasii, M. scrofulaceium, M. fortuitum,* and *M. chelonae* can cause human disease. These organisms are not usually transmitted from individual to individual but are likely acquired from soil or water. These and other mycobacteria can colonize individuals without causing infection or disease, so their presence alone does not necessarily indicate the need for treatment.

M. tuberculosis is acquired by inhalation of infected aerosol particles containing the organism. Although deposition of a few organisms in the alveolus can produce infection, TB infection is not acquired by all persons who come into contact with patients who are excreting bacilli in their sputum. It is estimated that even with close contact, only one of three persons become infected, and with casual contact the likelihood of acquiring TB is much lower. Proximity, circulation of air, and crowding are important factors in increasing the likelihood of acquiring TB. The amount of bacilli shed in the sputum is a risk factor for acquiring TB. Individuals who have negative sputum stains for acid-fast bacilli but are positive on culture are much less infectious than those with positive stains. Patients become noninfectious, even if their sputum is still stain positive, within 2 weeks of initiation of therapy. Transmission of organisms can be decreased by avoiding open coughing. The major risk of acquiring TB is in instances in which the disease is not suspected and the patient is coughing into a poorly ventilated environment or is in close contact with other individuals. This may occur in the community before the patient is recognized as requiring medical attention or in the hospital if TB is not considered in the differential diagnosis.

After inhalation of tuberculous bacilli, local defense mechanisms in the lung such as macrophages and lymphocytes attack the organism in a fairly nonspecific fashion. If the organism survives, it multiplies locally. Under ideal circumstances, the organism can replicate every 24 hours, but the usual rate of growth is much slower than this due to continuing local defense mechanism. During the first month of infection, local reaction in the lung may cause tuberculous pneumonia with adjacent lymph node involvement. This can often be asymptomatic or only minimally symptomatic. During this same interval of time, TB is spread hematogenously throughout the body to areas such as the lung apices, kidney, and meninges, becoming foci for later reactivation. After 1 to 2 months of this process, specific cell-mediated immunity develops and attacks the mycobacteria within the lung and wherever hematogenously dispersed. This usually results in containment of the infection and is manifest on the x-ray occasionally by a small calcified focus. During this interval, the tuberculin skin test becomes positive as a marker of infection. If the disease cannot be contained by the specific immune response, disseminated disease occurs with multiple areas of TB throughout the lung (miliary TB) and involves other organs such as the meninges, kidneys, and bone. Dissemination occurs more frequently in infants and very young children, those who have specific immunocompromise, such as patients with immunologic malignancies or HIV infection, and in individuals who are nonspecifically immunocompromised, such as by old age or malnutrition.

Ordinarily, tuberculous infection is contained rather than disseminated. This sets the stage for reactivation TB, which is the most common presentation of clinical disease. Risk of reactivation disease is at its highest in the first few years after acquisition of infection and may be 3% to 5% in that interval. After that time, the risk is lower, perhaps 0.1% to 0.2% yearly. The specific mechanisms favoring reactivation are unknown, but change in the local and systemic immune status relative to the organisms present in the lung tilt in favor of the organism, and tuberculous bacilli begin to multiply in these areas. In the lung, these areas are usually in the posterior part of the upper lobes of the lung, although it can occur in other areas as well. When the organism begins to grow, the body's immune response often leads to an inflammatory lesion with local necrosis, leading to the cavitary disease that on chest x-ray is characteristic in about half of patients with reactivation pulmonary disease. Reactivation may take place in other areas where the tuberculous bacilli has been disseminated. Approximately 10% to 20% of reactivation TB may occur in areas outside of the lung parenchyma, although many of these are accompanied by parenchymal reactivation as well. The genitourinary tract, bones and joints, meninges, and gastrointestinal tract are among the areas where reactivation disease may be seen.

DIFFERENTIAL DIAGNOSIS

The differential diagnosis of TB can be broad, depending on the phase of the disease. For example, it is in the differential diagnosis of pneumonia, particularly if symptoms are chronic and nonresolving with routine antibiotic therapy. If pulmonary TB is associated with cavitary disease on chest x-ray, anaerobic lung abscess, fungal infections of the lung, and noninfectious causes such as malignancy, Wegener granulomatosis need to be considered. If TB presents with a pleural effusion, the effusion is often large and unilateral. This differential diagnosis would include malignancy and a parapneumonia effusion or empyema associated with another bacterial infection. When TB occurs in nonpulmonary sites, fever without apparent cause can be a predominant manifestation, and other causes of persistent fever such as malignancy, bacterial endocarditis, and other occult infections need to be considered.

HISTORY

The history relevant to the acquisition of TB can be divided into that which occurs during primary infection and that which can occur with reactivation. Primary infection was usually seen in children when the disease was more endemic in the population. Now, it is often a disease of adults. The primary infection is often asymptomatic. About 25% of patients will have symptoms such as fever, cough, and fatigue. If an x-ray is taken during this time, a midlung zone infiltrate may be seen that is noncavitary and is not specific for TB. This presentation is similar to that of any bacterial pneumonia, and because a natural history is most often toward containment of the infection and resolution of symptoms, the possibility of TB may not be considered further.

Pleural involvement is usually a manifestation of primary TB, although it can occur in reactivation disease. Disease may occur from rupture of a subpleural focus of TB into the pleural space and usually occurs within weeks to months of acquisition of the infection. Symptoms are nonspecific and include fever, pleuritic chest pain, and shortness of breath if the pleural effusion is large. Lymph node enlargement, usually not painful, may be a symptom of primary disease, and fever and systemic symptoms may be slight.

Occasionally, the primary infection is not locally contained, and progressive primary TB ensues. The immunocompromised population, particularly patients with HIV infection with low CD4 counts, are susceptible to progressive disease. Persistent fever, cough, and fatigue and a nonresolving or worsening clinical course and x-ray despite routine antibiotic therapy should raise the question of TB.

Primary infection, although usually locally contained by the immune system, may present as widely disseminated or miliary disease. Immunosuppression predisposes to this form of TB, and young children, the elderly, and those weakened by malnutrition are also at increased risk, Fever may be the predominant symptom, and disseminated TB is still a prominent cause of "fever of unknown origin." Evidence of dissemination may not be visible on the chest x-ray in the early part of the illness. Because the infection is widely spread, symptoms such as headache or lethargy may indicate meningeal involvement, abdominal pain may indicate intestinal or peritoneal involvement, and pyuria or hematuria may indicate genitourinary tract involvement.

Reactivation pulmonary disease may present with symptoms of cough, hemoptysis, and fever or more subtle symptoms such as fatigue, anorexia, weight loss, and night sweats. Symptoms may be very slight in reactivation pulmonary disease; an occasional cough may be all that is present. Pleural involvement, again usually a manifestation of primary acquisition of infection, may be seen in reactivation disease, so that shortness of breath or pleuritic chest pain may be presenting manifestations.

Reactivation of TB in bone is seen in about 10% of individuals with reactivation disease. Pain is the most common complaint and will be localized at the area of involvement. Any bone can be affected, but the vertebrae are involved in about half the cases. If not diagnosed, vertebral destruction can occur, and symptoms of weakness and paralysis may then occur. Genitourinary reactivation TB may be associated with dysuria, hematuria, or flank pain. Some patients will have fever or weight loss.

Reactivation in the nervous system often takes the form of meningeal involvement from rupture of a caseous focus into the subarachnoid space. Symptoms may include headache, lethargy, or other changes in mental status. Fever is often, but not invariably, present.

Reactivation TB in the gastrointestinal tract occurs in about 5% of cases of extrapulmonary TB. The peritoneum is most often affected; symptoms are abdominal pain or swelling. The ileocecal bowel may be involved, with symptoms of crampy abdominal pain related to intestinal obstruction.

Cardiovascular reactivation TB is relatively uncommon. It may manifest itself as symptoms of pericarditis, related to rupture of a tuberculous focus from the lung into the adjacent pericardium. Shortness of breath and orthopnea may relate to a pericardial effusion related to TB.

Rare manifestations of extrapulmonary involvement from reactivation may include hoarseness related to laryngeal involvement, skin ulcerations, and involvement of the adrenal glands, with symptoms of Addison disease.

Disseminated TB, although usually a manifestation of primary infection that is not controlled by the immune system, can occasionally occur as part of the reactivation process, particularly in patients who are immunocompromised. These patients, in addition to the systemic complaints of fatigue and weight loss, may have symptoms pointing to extrapulmonary sites of dissemination, such as headache and cranial neuropathies suggestive of meningitis, or symptoms related to anemia or to bone marrow involvement.

PHYSICAL EXAMINATION AND CLINICAL FINDINGS

Physical findings are often nonspecific for the diagnosis of TB. Evidence of consolidation on chest x-ray, lymphadenopathy, or tenderness to percussion over the area of bone pain, pericardial rub, and abdominal tenderness are not diagnostic of tuberculous involvement of these organs. These findings may be useful to help pinpoint the site of involvement in a patient in whom TB is suspected, but rarely will the findings on physical examination be diagnostic.

LABORATORY AND IMAGING STUDIES

The tuberculin purified protein derivative (PPD) test is used to diagnose infection with *M. tuberculosis*. It is not useful in determining whether a patient who is clinically ill has active disease, because patients who are tuberculin positive may have other causes of their acute symptomatology. Similarly, a negative PPD does not exclude active TB, because of possible malnutrition, immunosuppression, or other factors leading to cutaneous anergy.

The tuberculin test is used to define tuberculous infection so that prophylaxis may be given to avoid later reactivation. The Mantoux intradermal injection of 5 tuberculin units (TU) of PPD (0.1 mL) is used and is given to patients who are increased risk of acquiring tuberculous infection or who will be at increased risk of reactivation. Such individuals include close contacts of infectious cases; patients with HIV infection; patients with fibrotic disease on chest x-ray consistent with untreated TB; persons with medical conditions that may increase the risk of TB, such as prolonged therapy with greater than 20 mg of prednisone daily or other chronic immunosuppressive therapy; residents of long-term care nursing homes; health care workers; individuals born in areas with a high prevalence of TB (e.g., Latin American, Asia, Africa); patients with diseases known to increase the risk of reactivation TB, such as silicosis, malnutrition, and chronic renal failure; and medically underserved low income populations. It is not recommended that patients who do not have a high likelihood of having been infected or acquiring infection be routinely skin tested. Therefore, not all patients coming to a practice for the first time should have tuberculin skin tests as a routine part of initial laboratory assessment, because tuberculin skin tests may be falsely positive from exposure to nontuberculous mycobacteria. In a population at low risk for acquiring TB, the chance of false positivity of a skin test becomes close to that of true positivity, with the risk that unnecessary isoniazid prophylaxis will be given.

Skin test positivity is measured by the degree of induration at the injection site measured at 48 to 72 hours. Reactions greater than or equal to 5 mm are positive in individuals with HIV infection, individuals who are close contacts of infectious cases, and individuals with stable fibrotic lesions on chest x-ray, consistent with contained, although advanced, primary infection. A PPD whose induration is greater or equal to 10 mm is positive for adults in the other risk situations listed earlier, such as prolonged therapy with steroids, immigrants from areas endemic for TB, the medically underserved, and residents of long-term care facilities. For other individuals, a PPD greater than or equal to 15 mm is considered positive. Pregnancy is not thought to affect the reactivity of the PPD, so the values noted above remain valid. For individuals who are tested at regular intervals with PPD because of risk of exposure (e.g., health care workers), a 10 mm or greater increase in induration within a 2-year period in those under age 35 years and a greater than 15 mm increase for those over 35 years of age is considered positive.

In cases of suspected active TB, laboratory examination may reveal an elevated blood cell count, low serum albumin reflecting malnutrition, an elevated sedimentation rate, and, occasionally, hyponatremia from inappropriate secretion of antidiuretic hormone. The latter is nonspecific, however, and is found in many pulmonary inflammatory disorders.

The chest x-ray shows infiltrates in the apical or posterior segment of an upper lobe in most instances, although the superior segment of the lower lobe may be involved as well. Lower lobe disease, although rare, can occur, and its presence on an x-ray should not exclude consideration of TB in the differential diagnosis. Cavitation occurs in about half of the patients with reactivation disease. Cavitation is less likely to be seen in patients with HIV infection, because cavitation is due in part to the inflammatory reaction against the organism. Occasionally, TB can appear as a solitary pulmonary nodule (a tuberculoma), mimicking the chest x-ray appearance of a primary lung cancer.

In bone disease, the x-ray may show bony destruction or erosion. Gastrointestinal TB of the ileocecal area can occur, and contrast studies showing narrowing and irregularity of the lumen can be mistaken for regional enteritis.

The major laboratory test in TB is identification of the organism on culture or smear. Routine examination of material for bacterial pathogens does not reveal tuberculous organisms unless the appropriate stain is requested for "acid-fast organism." If these stains are performed, the mycobacteria are stained red against a blue background. In most instances of TB, except in immunocompromised individuals, the acid-fast organisms are not plentiful, and the slide must be examined carefully. In as much as 20% to 30% of pulmonary TB, the acid-fast bacilli smear is negative. Many of these smears will ultimately grow out acid-fast organisms on culture, but this may take weeks. Bronchoscopy with brushings, washings, and lavage can be useful in patients if routine sputum is smear negative, because specimens from bronchoscopy have a higher yield for the organism.

The ultimate diagnostic test for TB is growth of the organism in culture. If TB is suspect, special culturing must be requested, because TB will not grow in routine media. It will take TB 3 to 6 weeks to grow. Biochemical tests are performed to confirm that the organism is *M. tuberculosis* and not other mycobacteria. After growth of the organism, tests for drug susceptibility should be performed in all isolates.

The Bactec System is a relatively new method for identifying *M. tuberculosis* that has shortened the time required to identify the organism. The organism is detected by measuring metabolic radioactive carbon dioxide production when colonies are still too small to be visible; by this technique organisms can be identified in 4 to 8 days. Once a *Mycobacterium* is identified, the Bactec System may selectively provide nutrients to identify which *Mycobacterium* is present. Drug susceptibility testing can also be done.

TREATMENT

There are two aspects to treatment of TB: prophylactic treatment of tuberculous-infected individuals and treatment of active disease. Prophylactic treatment with isoniazid is offered to patients who have been infected with TB but do not have active disease. The goal of therapy is to reduce risk of reactivation disease. Drug resistance is not considered a significant problem with single-drug therapy for prophylaxis because the infective load of organisms is small. Standard therapy is 12 months of isoniazid 300 mg/d, although 6 months of therapy may be adequate. Patients are offered therapy based on their risk factor and size of the tuberculin test induration, as discussed in the previous section. For example, persons with HIV infection, close contacts of persons with newly diagnosed infectious TB, and patients with stable fibrotic upper lobe disease consistent with previous TB who have a PPD greater than or equal to 5 mm should be treated. A PPD greater than 10 mm is considered an indication for treatment in residents of long-term care facilities, health care workers, immigrants from endemic areas, the medically underserved, children under 4 years of age, and patients with diseases increasing the risk of TB. In a patient without risk factors, a PPD of 15 mm or more is positive.

If a PPD is positive as defined above, consideration needs to be given to instituting prophylactic treatment. It is useful to seek expert advice here, but in general, patients with positive PPDs who have HIV infection, those who are close contacts of patients with active disease, recent convertors of PPD from negative to positive within 2 years (defined as ≥10 mm change in size for those under 35 years of age and 15 mm change for those over 35), those with certain medical conditions such as treatment with immunosuppressive therapy or prolonged corticosteroid therapy, endstage renal disease, and poorly controlled diabetes should be considered.

Treatment with isoniazid is expected to reduce the risk of developing reactivation TB by between 65% (for a 6-month course of therapy) and 75% (for a 12-month course). It is administered as a single daily dose, and has some mild gastrointestinal upset associated with it. However, the major risk is isoniazid hepatitis, which can be severe and has caused death. The rate of isoniazid hepatitis seems to increase with age. It is rare under the age of 35 and occurs at a rate of 1% to 2% for patients in their 60s. Because of the isoniazid, patients receiving this medication should be questioned at monthly intervals for symptoms and signs of hepatitis; if signs are present, the patient should have liver function tests obtained at that time. About 20% of patients receiving isoniazid develop asymptomatic abnormalities of liver function, with aspartate aminotransferase rising two- to threefold. Thus, monitoring liver function at intervals is prudent. Although asymptomatic rises in liver function are not strictly a cause for discontinuing therapy, many physicians will discontinue isoniazid if aspartate aminotransferase rises four- to fivefold.

Another form of prevention, which is not used in the United States, is vaccination with bacillus Calmette-Guérin, an attenuated strain of *M. bovis*. Protection from vaccination has been variably reported from 10% to 50% and does not seem to provide immunity beyond 15 to 20 years. Because the goal of bacillus Calmette-Guérin is to prevent infection, it has not been offered in the United States, because most active cases of TB have risen as reactivation disease in individuals who were infected in the past. However, with TB spreading more rapidly in some populations, more interest may appear in the future in preventing primary infection. At present, however, bacillus Calmette-Guérin vaccine is recommended only for infants and children who are at high risk of being exposed for long periods to others with untreated TB or are being exposed to individuals who have resistant organisms. Such situations could arise, for example, among socially economically deprived children living in areas where TB is epidemic.

Treatment of active TB is an area in which expert help should always be sought. The appearance of multiple drug–resistant TB has made it imperative that treatment must involve at least two effective drugs so that further resistance will not develop. In practice this means four drugs may be started while the culture and sensitivity results are pending. Drugs that are considered for first-line use in TB include isoniazid, rifampin, pyridoxine, ethambutol, and streptomycin. The major side effect of isoniazid is hepatitis, the incidence of which increases with age, being 1.2% for patients aged 35 to 50 years and about 2.3% for patients aged 50 to 64 years. Incidence does not increase much above age 65 years. Peripheral neuropathy is another complication of isoniazid, and the drug should be given with pyridoxine 50 mg/d.

Rifampin, like isoniazid, is bactericidal for *M. tuberculosis*. The drug has few side effects, the most common being gastrointestinal upset. Usual dosing for adults is 600 mg/d. In doses greater than 10 mg/kg/d some patients may experience a flulike illness and thrombocytopenia. Rifampin is excreted in bodily fluids and colors them orange. This is not harmful but is alarming to patients if they are not forewarned.

Pyrazinamide is another bactericidal antibiotic. Liver toxicity is associated with its use as well, but it does not seem to cause increased liver injury when used in combination with other potentially hepatotoxic drugs such as isoniazid and rifampin. Heparinemia may occur, although acute gout is uncommon.

Ethambutol is a bactericidal agent. The most serious side effect is retrobulbar neuritis with changes in vision, including changes in color vision acuity. This complication is unusual, however, occurring in less than 1% of individuals given a dose of 15 mg/kg/d. The 25-mg/kg/d dose of ethambutol is associated with a higher frequency of neuritis, but there is rarely a reason to use ethambutol at this dose.

Streptomycin is another bactericidal agent. It requires parenteral therapy and can be used in twice-weekly dosing regimens when given at a dose of 25 to 30 mg/kg. Dosage must be adjusted if there is any renal impairment. Ototoxicity and vestibular toxicity are side effects of the drug. Second-line antibiotics effective against TB include paraaminosalicylic acid, ethionamide, capreomycin, cycloserine, and ciprofloxacin.

To treat TB successfully, the drug should be taken for the appropriate period of time, which is usually many months, and on a regular basis so that irregular use does not promote drug resistance. The American Thoracic Society has advocated initial therapy with isoniazid, rifampin, ethambutol, and pyrazinamide until sensitivities return. If the mycobacterium is susceptible to these agents, ethambutol is discontinued and the other drugs maintained for 8 weeks, followed by 16 weeks of isoniazid and rifampin. Twice-weekly dosing is an option in the second phase of treatment with isoniazid and rifampin, a regimen useful in populations in whom compliance with medication is a problem, because it makes administration under direct observation easier.

When TB is susceptible to the agents used, patients usually become noninfectious within 2 weeks. The sputum cultures are usually negative by 2 months. Acid-fast organisms may occasionally be found in a sputum specimen for some time after that. Patients do not necessarily need to be hospitalized for 2 weeks of therapy and if compliant with medication and cough hygiene may be discharged to their home. They have often spent sufficient time at home before diagnosis, in which case infection of family members may already have occurred. If it has not, avoiding close contact and using cough precautions may not result in much further infection risk for the week or two of treatment it takes to become noninfectious. However, in individuals who will have close contact with others or who will be in situations in which they will be exposed to many people and may be unable to avoid this, such as homeless shelters or chronic care facilities, at least the initial 2 weeks of therapy until they are not infectious should be administered in an environment that allows isolation from others.

Extrapulmonary TB is treated similar to the pulmonary disease, except that the therapeutic course tends to be a bit longer, perhaps 9 to 12 months, because there is not much experience with the shorter courses of chemotherapy that have evolved for the treatment of pulmonary disease.

SPECIAL CONSIDERATIONS IN PREGNANCY

Prophylactic treatment with isoniazid in a pregnant patient with a positive skin test usually is delayed until after the first trimester if the PPD conversion was recent (within 2 years) or after delivery if the date of conversion is longer than that or is unknown.

In active TB, therapy must be initiated during pregnancy. It is not thought that the risk to the fetus from either the disease or therapy warrants therapeutic abortion. Drugs that are used include isoniazid, ethambutol, and rifampin, all of which have been used safely in pregnancy, although rifampin has been associated with isolated reports of fetal malformation. Streptomycin and other aminoglycosides are avoided because of associated fetal hearing and vestibular impairment. There are limited data regarding teratogenicity of pyrazinamide, and it is not used in pregnancy in the United States, although it has been recommended in other countries. Breast milk will contain only small quantities of antituberculous drugs, and breast-feeding can be done while the mother is on therapy.

If the mother is on therapy and thought not to be contagious at delivery, the family members should be carefully checked to make sure there is no reservoir of TB to affect the newborn. The infant is begun on isoniazid prophylaxis, and tuberculin testing is done at 4 to 6 weeks of age. If negative, the test is repeated at 3 to 4 months and again at 6 months, and if negative at 6 months, isoniazid can be discontinued.

If the mother at the time of delivery has active pulmonary disease that has not yet been treated, then the infant should not have contact with the mother until sufficient therapy has been given to reduce the chance of infection, usually about 2 weeks. The child is also begun on isoniazid prophylaxis and skin tested at the intervals described above.

If the mother has widely disseminated disease with hematogenous spread and multiple organ involvement (miliary TB), the infant may not only be at risk for infection after birth as when the mother has only pulmonary TB but may have acquired congenital active TB. Clinical evidence of disease in the infant warrants treatment for active TB with a multiple drug regimen.

In all situations involving treatment of TB, including during pregnancy, it is wise to seek expert consultative help.

NONTUBERCULOUS MYCOBACTERIA

Organisms other than *M. tuberculosis* can cause human disease. As mentioned earlier, these mycobacteria include the *M. avium* complex, (*M. avium* and *M. intracellulare*), *M. kansasii, M. chelonae,* and *M. scrofulaceum*. Other mycobacteria can cause human disease as well. These mycobacteria have been isolated from soil, water, and animals but are not thought to be transmitted human to human. They may be colonizers of the human respiratory tract, and their presence identified on culture does not always mean clinical disease. Most individuals who have disease from these organisms have preexisting pulmonary disease such as preexisting cavitary lesions, chronic obstructive pulmonary disease, and interstitial fibrosis. When these organisms cause disease, it is similar in clinical presentation to that caused by *M. tuberculosis*. In the immunocompromised patient, however, particularly those with HIV infection and low CD4 counts, *M. avium* and *M. intracellulare* can cause rapidly progressive pulmonary disease and disease that is widely disseminated hematogenously.

These organisms appear similar to *M. tuberculosis* on acid-fast smears, and they are distinguished from TB only by culture. These organisms, particularly the *M. avium* complex, may be resistant to multiple drugs, and multiple-drug regimens are often necessary for effective treatment.

It is useful to have advice from a specialist when nontuberculous mycobacteria are isolated from the sputum or when they are suspected of causing disease in immunocompromised individuals. In immunocompetent individuals, consultants can be helpful in deciding whether the organisms represent colonization or true infection. In cases of disseminated or extensive pulmonary disease in the patient with acquired immunodeficiency syndrome or HIV infection, the consultant may provide diagnostic help (e.g., bronchoscopy) and help in choice of antimicrobial agents.

BIBLIOGRAPHY

American Thoracic Society. Diagnosis and treatment of disease caused by nontuberculous mycobacteria. *Am Rev Respir Dis* 1990;142:940.

American Thoracic Society. Treatment of tuberculosis and tuberculosis infection in adults and children. *Am Rev Respir Dis* 1994;149:1359.

American Thoracic Society/Centers for Disease Control. Diagnostic standards and classification of tuberculosis. *Am Rev Respir Dis* 1990;142:725.

American Thoracic Society/Centers for Disease Control and Prevention. Targeted tuberculin testing and treatment of latent tuberculosis infection. *Am J Resp Crit Care Med* 2000;161:S221.

Barnes PF, Barrows SA. Tuberculosis in the 1990s. *Ann Intern Med* 1993;119:400.

Bass JB, ed. Mycobacterial disease. *Semin Respir Med* 1988;9:1.

Bass JB, Farer LS, Hopewell PC, et al. Treatment of tuberculosis and tuberculosis infection in adults and children. *Am J Respir Crit Care Med* 1994;149:1359.

Snider DE, guest ed. Mycobacterial diseases. *Clin Chest Med* 1989;10:297.

Snider DE Jr, Caras GJ. Isoniazid-associated hepatitis deaths: a review of available information. *Am Rev Respir Dis* 1992;145:494.

Snider DE, Layde PM, Johnson MW, et al. Treatment of tuberculosis during pregnancy. *Am Rev Respir Dis* 1980;122:65.

Vallejo JG, Starke JR. Tuberculosis and pregnancy. *Clin Chest Med* 1992;13:693.

CHAPTER 57
Chronic Obstructive Pulmonary Disease

Anthony J. Fedullo

Chronic obstructive pulmonary disease (COPD) is a category of disorders characterized by airflow obstruction. Asthma, bronchitis, and emphysema are the major diseases in this category. Asthma has been included in this category, but there is a tendency to separate it from the more chronic and irreversible causes of obstructive pulmonary disease. Bronchospasm, however, can coexist with bronchitis and emphysema; recognizing a coexisting bronchospastic component in these disorders is important, because it provides an avenue for therapy. The emphasis in this chapter is on emphysema and bronchitis; asthma was discussed in Chapter 55.

COPD is the fourth leading cause of death in the United States among those over age 45 and the highest cause of mortality with an avoidable cause, cigarette smoking. In addition to mortality, COPD also causes significant morbidity. Patients are often limited and disabled by dyspnea. The roughly 6 million Americans with COPD make up 5% of office visits and about 10% to 15% of hospitalizations.

Because emphysema occurs after many years of cigarette smoking, most patients present with this disease between ages 55 and 70. COPD has traditionally been considered a disease of older men, but women are equally susceptible and by the late 1980s had a prevalence similar to that of men. More disturbing is the fact that the prevalence of COPD has been stable or declining in men but continues to rise in women, probably reflecting their later development of cigarette smoking.

ETIOLOGY

The main cause of chronic bronchitis and emphysema is cigarette smoking. This evidence is based on epidemiologic studies that attribute 80% to 90% of cases of emphysema and chronic bronchitis to cigarette smoking. There is a strong epidemiologic relation between cigarette smoking and COPD, but only about 15% of smokers develop clinically significant COPD, although a larger number have airway obstruction on pulmonary function tests.

The precise mechanism by which cigarette smoking causes COPD is uncertain. Destruction of lung tissue by products of inflammation plays a role in emphysema by reducing the connective tissue framework that helps to maintain airway integrity and patency. When the supporting framework is not present, airway collapse and limitation of airflow occur. Inhaled irritants are thought to play a role in producing the mucosal hypertrophy and mucous hypersecretion characteristic of chronic bronchitis. These changes result in airway narrowing and airflow limitation.

There are other risk factors in addition to cigarette smoking. The best-defined one is α_1-antitrypsin deficiency, a genetic disorder. Antitrypsin and other serum antiproteases prevent digestion of lung connective tissue by the proteolytic enzymes that are released by inflammatory cells. Patients heterozygous for the gene responsible for α_1-antitrypsin production have levels of α_1-antitrypsin sufficient to protect the lung and do not have an increased rate of emphysema. Homozygous-deficient persons, however, are at risk for developing early emphysema. Nonsmokers with homozygous α_1-antitrypsin deficiency may not develop significant or symptomatic COPD until well into later life, but smokers with the deficiency may develop severe emphysema by age 30 or 40. α_1-Antitrypsin deficiency is responsible for only 1% to 3% of cases of emphysema in the United States, but because of the genetic implications and the availability of replacement enzyme, this must be considered, particularly in younger patients with advanced emphysema.

Other risk factors include a poorly understood familial clustering of the disease, not related to a known genetic defect. Air pollution in urban areas or dust exposure in the workplace increases the incidence of chronic bronchitis but is usually not a factor in clinically significant COPD.

Childhood respiratory infections may increase the risk of developing COPD. Maternal smoking can adversely affect the respiratory status of children living in the home, can increase childhood respiratory infections and bronchial hyperresponsiveness, and perhaps can predispose to COPD.

The effects of airway obstruction include increased work of breathing, which is partly responsible for the dyspnea patients feel. The airway obstruction also decreases the high peak flow rates that allow coughing to clear secretions, predisposing to atelectasis and recurrent chest infection. Destruction of the alveolar–capillary interface in emphysema results in a greater proportion of each breath occurring without gas exchange (increased dead space) and leads to the need for increased ventilatory effort to excrete carbon dioxide. When increased ventilation and the work of breathing it requires can no longer be easily accomplished, carbon dioxide retention develops. Alveolar ventilation to lung capillary perfusion mismatching leads to hypoxemia. Hypoxemia, particularly with a partial pressure of oxygen (P_{O_2}) below 55 to 60 mm Hg, leads to pulmonary hypertension and the development of cor pulmonale (right-sided heart failure due to pulmonary disease), with peripheral edema.

Patients with advanced COPD often cannot fulfill their ventilatory needs in acute infections such as bronchitis or pneumonia. Partial pressure of carbon dioxide (P_{CO_2}) elevation and respiratory acidosis ensue, and the patient may require mechanical ventilation.

DIFFERENTIAL DIAGNOSIS

Because COPD may cause dyspnea and right-sided heart failure, the differential diagnosis includes disorders that cause these findings in smokers or former smokers of middle age or older. Left ventricular heart failure with secondary right-sided heart failure in this age group is often a consideration. Moreover, COPD and left ventricular dysfunction often coexist, both contributing to dyspnea. Pulmonary vascular disease (e.g., primary pulmonary hypertension or chronic thromboembolic disease) can cause dyspnea with evidence of right-sided heart failure. Anemia may cause dyspnea but usually does not do so with mild to moderate exertion until the hematocrit level is quite low (often in the upper teens or low 20s) and, unless severe enough to cause heart failure, usually is not accompanied by edema. Large pleural effusions (e.g., those associated with malignancy) can cause dyspnea. Obesity is a common cause of complaints of shortness of breath with exertion and may be associated with peripheral edema due to stasis. Other parenchymal lung diseases, such as interstitial lung disease, can cause dyspnea and cor pulmonale. Rarer causes of dyspnea include neuromuscular diseases that inhibit adequate ventilation, such as amyotrophic lateral sclerosis.

Dyspnea in a smoker does not necessarily implicate COPD as a cause, because only about 15% of smokers develop significant COPD. An evaluation still must be done to prove the presence of COPD and to evaluate other potential causes of dyspnea.

HISTORY

Patients with COPD have dyspnea or reduced exercise ability as their prominent complaint. COPD progresses slowly in smokers who are susceptible, but lung function must be reduced considerably before symptoms become noticeable. Early in the disease, many patients decrease their activity level so that they do not perceive any disability or discomfort with exercise. Dyspnea is a subjective complaint, and patients may begin to perceive it only when activities at work or around the home become associated with an uncomfortable shortness of breath. Sometimes the onset of shortness of breath is related to an acute respiratory infection or occurs after a surgical procedure, at which time the decreased respiratory function, muscle weakness, and deconditioning make the symptoms more noticeable.

Nocturnal awakening with dyspnea or orthopnea can occur in COPD but more often reflects asthma or congestive heart failure. In exacerbations of COPD, when the patient is more breathless, many patients want to sit fairly upright: In that position, the chest wall configuration, the positioning of the diaphragm, and respiratory muscle use minimize airflow limitation.

Sputum production is characteristic of chronic bronchitis and defines the disease (3 months of cough for 2 consecutive years). COPD is often associated with wheezing because of the decreased expiratory flow rates. Wheezing does not necessarily mean that a reversible bronchospastic component is present, but asthma can coexist with bronchitis and emphysema. Symptoms that suggest an asthmatic component are intermittent or episodic increases in shortness of breath with wheezing, unrelated to other causes such as acute chest infection or congestive heart failure. Symptomatic relief with bronchodilators also points to a bronchospastic component. It is useful to recognize a reversible bronchospastic component because even mild degrees of bronchospasm may significantly affect a person with an already severe fixed obstructive disease, such as emphysema.

PHYSICAL EXAMINATION AND CLINICAL FINDINGS

Early in the disease, when dyspnea is experienced only during moderate exertion, the physical examination reveals little. Auscultation over the trachea during a forced expiration after a full breath often reveals airflow to last more than 4 or 5 seconds, suggesting airway obstruction. Wheezing, either at rest or with forced expiration, may also be heard, although this may be due to asthma, not emphysema or bronchitis. With more advanced disease, dyspnea may be observed with ambulation, and an increased resting respiratory rate may be noticed. As the disease progresses and airflow continues to decline, the cough sounds weak and cannot easily raise mucus adequately. Dyspnea at rest and the use of accessory muscles of respiration may be obvious. Pursed-lip breathing may be seen; it may be a mechanism to enhance airway patency and minimize obstruction to airflow.

Elevated jugular venous pressure and peripheral edema suggest cor pulmonale secondary to hypoxemia. The degree of hypoxemia does not correlate well with the severity of airflow obstruction, so cor pulmonale is not necessarily a marker of severe disease. Cyanosis may be seen, but many observers find it difficult to detect. A certain amount of desaturated hemoglobin is required for cyanosis to be visible; hence, it is not as obvious in anemic patients and may be due to circulatory causes rather than hypoxemia. The absence of cyanosis does not rule out significant COPD or even significant hypoxemia.

In advanced COPD, weight loss occurs because the work of breathing accounts for a higher proportion of basal metabolism and because the patient experiences shortness of breath with minimal activities such as eating or with gastric distention after a meal. Depression and anxiety due to disabling disease further contribute to poor appetite and weight loss.

Many patients with advanced COPD become depressed, anxious, and dependent. This is understandable in a slowly progressive disease with the symptom of shortness of breath that eventually progresses to the sense of near suffocation. These patients are often elderly and often lack strong coping mechanisms or outlets.

The terms "pink puffer" and "blue bloater" have been used to describe the stereotypical characteristics of patients with emphysema and bronchitis, respectively. These terms describe extremes of presentation and have a demeaning depersonalized connotation. It is true, however, that some patients with COPD, particularly those with emphysema, resist carbon dioxide retention. To keep their P_{CO_2} low or normal, these emphysematous patients must ventilate, so they appear to "puff." Oxygenation tends to be better, partly because of their lower P_{CO_2} and partly because they are usually not obese and have no airway secretions to cause atelectasis; hence, they are "pink." On the other hand, the obese patient with chronic bronchitis and atelectasis has more hypoxemia and is "bluer." Because of the obesity and peripheral edema from cor pulmonale due to the hypoxemia, the patient appears "bloated." These characteristics cannot be used to quantify the severity of COPD. It is better to characterize each patient through clinical examination, pulmonary function studies, and arterial blood gas analysis.

LABORATORY AND IMAGING STUDIES

The major characteristic of COPD is airflow obstruction as determined by pulmonary function tests, which should be a routine part of the evaluation of a patient with dyspnea. The fundamental abnormality seen on these tests in COPD is a decrease in the forced expiratory volume in 1 second (FEV_1), particularly as a percentage of the forced vital capacity (FVC). Normal values on pulmonary function tests are derived from population surveys and depend on age, sex, and height. In general, however, most patients in the middle years of life or older exhale 75% of their vital capacity in the first second; hence, the FEV_1/FVC ratio is 75%. In COPD, the FEV_1 declines at a faster rate than the roughly 40 mL/y that occurs due to aging alone. Therefore, an abnormal FEV_1/FVC ratio in a smoker in early middle age suggests that significant problems will occur in the ensuing years, as airway function continues to decline. An abnormal FEV_1/FVC ratio defines the presence of obstructive lung disease. An abnormal FEV_1/FVC ratio is also seen in asthma, but in pure asthma this is reversible with therapy.

Correlation of pulmonary function test results with symptoms is not strict, but generally the FEV_1/FVC ratio may fall to 50% without causing much dyspnea, particularly in older persons who do not exert themselves. As the ratio falls below 50%, most patients note dyspnea with exertion such as climbing stairs, rapid walking, or walking up hills. As the ratio falls to 35%, patients become symptomatic with slight exertion, the cough becomes less effective, and it is difficult to clear mucus well. When the ratio falls under 35%, patients are often symptomatic at rest or with minimal exertion and begin to have frequent emergency department visits or hospitalizations. Respiratory failure may complicate pneumonia or acute bronchitis as the ratio falls below 25%. Symptoms, however, are often a poor guide to the extent of pulmonary dysfunction, and pulmonary function tests are far more accurate in quantifying disease.

Pulmonary function tests do not need to be done frequently. Smokers and patients with dyspnea should have tests performed as part of the initial evaluation. Tests should be done when the patient is at a stable baseline, and they may be rechecked in 1 or 2 years to give some estimate as to the rate of progression. Some smokers can be motivated to stop smoking when they are shown their declining pulmonary function and are told that disability from emphysema may ensue.

The chest x-ray in emphysema may show hyperinflation, bullae, and a flattened diaphragm, but often it is normal. The chest x-ray cannot be relied on to detect COPD or to quantify its severity.

Oxygen levels on arterial blood gas analysis also do not correlate well with the severity of disease; they may be normal even in severe lung disease. On the other hand, P_{CO_2} elevation occurs late in the disease and often signifies an FEV_1 under 35%

of predicted. Polycythemia may be present when the P_{O_2} falls below 50 to 55 mm Hg, but the hematocrit level rarely exceeds 55% to 60%.

α_1-Antitrypsin levels can be obtained when significant airway obstruction occurs in a nonsmoker or a smoker under age 45 or when a chest x-ray shows bullae in a young person, particularly when the bullae are in the lung bases and when there is a familial history of early emphysema.

TREATMENT

The most important therapeutic intervention in COPD is to stop smoking. This is often difficult but very worthwhile. With smoking cessation, bronchitis usually disappears within 2 months and the accelerated decline in pulmonary function stops. Nicotine replacement therapy can be useful in smoking cessation but is not the sole answer. The successful smoking cessation program involves a committed patient and a physician who continuously counsels and encourages her. Some believe that a useful tactic before stopping smoking entirely is to withdraw to five cigarettes daily. The patient often reduces her nicotine addiction by this step, feels some pride in decreasing to this level from her usual 20 or more cigarettes a day, and perhaps can more easily discontinue from that point completely. Much of the damage induced by cigarette smoke has a dose relationship, so although smoking cessation is the essential ultimate goal, reducing cigarette consumption is a valid intermediate step. Self-help groups, hypnosis, and acupuncture have had some success.

The next most important therapy is a trial of bronchodilator medication. A 15% to 20% improvement in the FEV_1 10 to 15 minutes after administration of an inhaled bronchodilator suggests that these medications will be useful. However, a lack of improvement in the FEV_1 does not rule out the use of bronchodilators, because in some patients, improvement will occur after days of therapy, rather than at once. Most patients with COPD should be given an inhaled β_2-agonist such as albuterol (two puffs four times a day) or an anticholinergic medication such as ipratropium (two puffs four times a day). Some believe that ipratropium is more beneficial in COPD than β_2-agonists, but most patients who have reversible airway obstruction respond to either in a fairly similar manner. Depending on the severity of the associated bronchospastic component, some patients benefit from routine use of inhaled corticosteroids.

Theophylline is falling out of favor in the treatment of COPD. Older patients commonly have adverse side effects when theophylline levels rise above 15 µg/mL, and many medications and superimposed acute medical processes (e.g., a viral infection) can alter theophylline's kinetics.

Short courses of systemic corticosteroids can be given for bronchospastic exacerbations refractory to other medication. Systemic corticosteroids should be used with great caution in patients with COPD and only if there is proof, based on pulmonary function testing, that benefit occurs. Patients on higher doses of steroids often feel euphoric and improved, even though there is no change in pulmonary function. Unfortunately, this effect is not long lasting, but the initial subjective benefit often commits the patient to long-term use.

Long-term use of oral corticosteroids is not recommended in COPD. There are some who believe a small number of patients derive benefit, perhaps by exerting a maximal bronchodilator effect beyond that obtained by the usual bronchodilator drugs. Before entertaining this therapy, the patient should receive maximal therapy for COPD without corticosteroids and then undergo pulmonary function testing. A dose of 30 to 40 mg/d of prednisone is then given for 1 to 2 weeks, and the pulmonary function tests are repeated. An improvement of 25% or more suggests that the patient will benefit from chronic corticosteroid use. In that case, the steroid dose is reduced gradually as long as the benefit is maintained; ideally, an alternate-day regimen can be achieved. Because of the long-term side effects of corticosteroids, including respiratory and peripheral muscle weakness (which increase dyspnea and decrease exercise tolerance), the advice of a pulmonary medicine consultant is often helpful before committing to their use.

Antibiotics are used when acute bronchitis occurs. They are usually prescribed at the onset of symptoms. Although half of these infections are nonbacterial, treating all symptomatic patients empirically without waiting for culture results has benefit in decreasing the duration of symptoms and the frequency of hospitalization. The antibiotics could include trimethoprim/sulfamethoxazole, doxycycline, amoxicillin, or amoxicillin with clavulanate if there is a high community incidence of β-lactamase-producing *Haemophilus influenzae.*

Broader spectrum and more expensive antibiotics are usually unnecessary. Even if some of these have broader coverage of "atypical" organisms such as mycoplasma or chlamydia, they seem to provide no better clinical response. If there is no response within a week, a sputum culture is taken to check for resistant organisms. Patients who have recently been in the hospital, perhaps within 1 to 2 months, may become colonized with resistant organisms; these patients in particular should be cultured if they fail to respond to an initial course of antibiotics. Patients with COPD should receive a yearly influenza vaccination; pneumococcal vaccination is also recommended.

Mucolytic agents are generally not useful in COPD patients. The cough is ineffective in patients with severe COPD not because the mucus is thick but because the reduction in airflow reduces the adequacy of cough.

Emphysema due to α_1-antitrypsin deficiency can be treated with a weekly intravenous infusion of human α-proteinase inhibitor. Therapy with this enzyme is expensive and is only given to patients who are homozygous for the deficiency gene. Patients who are heterozygous for α_1-antitrypsin deficiency have adequate levels of the enzyme to prevent emphysema.

Oxygen therapy should be given to patients who have a room air resting P_{O_2} of below 55 mm Hg (saturation 85%) or a P_{O_2} between 55 and 59 mm Hg (saturation 85%–89%) when accompanied by polycythemia and cor pulmonale. Oxygen should be given for about 18 hours/d. Patients generally use oxygen all night while sleeping and whatever part of the day they can while at home sitting or resting. Patients do not need portable oxygen 24 hours a day unless their P_{O_2} is very low (perhaps 40–45 mm Hg). Patients with COPD have decreased exercise ability, and a portable oxygen system that they wheel or carry may limit their ability to get out of the home and do routine activities. The goal of oxygen therapy is to reduce the effects of hypoxemia (e.g., cor pulmonale, polycythemia); this goal is achieved when using oxygen 16 to 18 hours daily. Dyspnea is not an indication for oxygen unless it is accompanied by a low P_{O_2} because the dyspnea of COPD is more related to the increased work of breathing due to the disease itself than it is due to the oxygen deficiency.

Oxygen may also need to be considered when a patient with marginal oxygenation changes altitude from a site near sea level to one above 5,000 to 8,000 feet. At these levels, the oxygen level in the air is reduced by 10% to 20%, which may result in hypoxemia severe enough to cause cor pulmonale. Oxygenation during airline flights—cabins are pressurized to the equivalent of 5,000 to 8,000 feet above sea level—can be arranged if prior notice is given to the airline. Surgical therapy, such as bullectomy or lung volume reduction surgery, are not clearly known to be efficacious, and consultation with a specialist is recommended if this is entertained.

Multidisciplinary pulmonary rehabilitation programs that involve education, emotional support, and exercise conditioning seem to be efficacious in exercise tolerance and improving symptoms of dyspnea and fatigue. Even if these programs are not available, patients with COPD need attention to nutrition, depression, and in particular the maintenance of activity, which helps avert muscle deconditioning and thus helps avoid further exercise intolerance.

Patients with chronic and severe dyspnea who have had no relief with other medication and whose lifespan is limited can obtain symptomatic relief with opiates, particularly when care is directed to a comfort-oriented focus as the condition becomes terminal. Because of their potential to depress respiration, opiates and sedatives should be used with great caution in acute exacerbations of COPD or in COPD patients with agitation and confusion (which may occur because of changes in oxygen or carbon dioxide levels). In acute instances of mental status change, opiates and steroids should not be given without checking arterial blood gas measurements and determining that the deterioration in COPD is not the primary cause.

Patients with severe COPD are prone to respiratory failure with acute exacerbations. They often need intensive care unit admission and perhaps mechanical ventilation. Patients with COPD with their first episode of respiratory failure have a fairly high chance of leaving the ventilator in a relatively short time and being discharged home. As COPD becomes severe, exacerbations become more frequent, and the quality of life deteriorates, the likelihood of successful weaning from a ventilator drops. In severe disabling COPD, the difficult issues of whether to continue aggressive care or perform recurrent resuscitation should be openly discussed with the patient.

CONSIDERATIONS IN PREGNANCY

Because COPD is a disease of older persons, smoking women of childbearing age rarely have significant disease unless they are deficient in α_1-antitrypsin. Smoking in pregnancy has adverse effects. Smoking a pack a day or more may double the risk of delivering an infant weighing less than 2,500 g. The growth-retarding effects of smoking are seen at all gestational ages and are probably due to fetal hypoxemia, related to the carbon monoxide in cigarette smoke and to placental vasoconstriction from nicotine exposure. Smoking increases the risk of preterm delivery, spontaneous abortion, placental abruption, and placenta previa. Smoking has not been associated with an increased risk of congenital defects.

Exposure of the child to cigarette smoke after delivery has been associated with an increased frequency of respiratory illnesses, bronchoreactivity, and bronchitis. There is conflicting evidence on whether childhood exposure to smoking in the home predisposes to respiratory disease in adult life.

BIBLIOGRAPHY

Guyatt GH, Townsend M, Pugsley SO, et al. Bronchodilators in chronic airflow limitation: effects on airway function, exercise capacity, and quality of life. *Am Rev Respir Dis* 1987;135:1069.

Hodgkin JE, ed. Chronic obstructive pulmonary disease. *Clin Chest Med* 1990;11:363.

Kellner R, Samet J, Pathak D. Dyspnea, anxiety, and depression in chronic respiratory impairment. *Gen Hosp Psychiatry* 1992;14:20.

Mahler DA. Evaluation of chronic dyspnea. *Clin Pulmon Med* 1994;1:208.

National Institutes of Health, National Heart, Lung, and Blood Institute. Global initiative for chronic obstructive lung disease. NIH Publication no. 2701A, 2001.

Rovner MS, Stoller JK. Therapy for alpha 1-antitrypsin deficiency: rationale and strategic approach. *Clin Pulmon Med* 1994;1:135.

Standards for the diagnosis and care of patients with chronic obstructive pulmonary disease (COPD) and asthma. Official statement of the American Thoracic Society. *Am Rev Respir Dis* 1987;136:225.

CHAPTER 58

Lung Cancer

Anthony J. Fedullo

Each year, 160,000 cases of lung cancer are diagnosed and 140,000 lung cancer patients die. Lung cancer is the most common cause of cancer death in men and has replaced breast cancer as the leading cause of cancer death among women. Whereas the incidence of lung cancer among men has reached a plateau, the rate in women has continued to rise, probably due to their increased cigarette smoking. Survival in lung cancer is poor. Five-year survival rates are 10% to 15%. At time of presentation, approximately 70% of patients with non–small cell lung cancer (NSCLC) are not candidates for curative surgical resection, and small cell lung cancer (SCLC), although responding initially to chemotherapy, is rarely cured. Lung cancer, however, is a preventable disease: 85% to 90% of cases result from cigarette smoking.

ETIOLOGY

Cigarette smoking is a predominant cause of lung cancer. In the 1950s, a study of British doctors showed an increased risk of lung cancer associated with tobacco use, particularly cigarettes. In 1964, the report of the U.S. Surgeon General on smoking and health demonstrated a correlation of smoking and lung cancer sufficiently strong to argue convincingly for a causal relationship. Historically, a rise in lung cancer was seen after the increase in smoking in the male population during World War I. Women began to increase their smoking later, during World War II and after, and their increase in lung cancer soon followed.

A relationship exists between the number of cigarettes smoked and the risk of developing lung cancer. For the 25% to 35% of the adult population who smoke cigarettes, one-pack-a-day smokers have a death rate of 120 per 100,000 individuals, whereas in those who smoke over one pack a day the rate rises to about 250 deaths per 100,000. Using filtered cigarettes decreases the risk relative to unfiltered cigarettes, but the risk reduction is not as great as expected, because smokers of filtered cigarettes tend to inhale more deeply and frequently or smoke more cigarettes. This behavior may be related to a need to achieve certain nicotine levels.

Many carcinogenic substances have been found in cigarette smoke. Although it is uncertain which of these is the predominant cause of cancer, this question has little relevance in view that cessation of cigarette smoking would avoid all of them. Nicotine is not the carcinogenic substance but is the substance that has addictive or habituating potential for cigarette smokers, leading them to continue the habit and leading to some of the withdrawal symptoms associated with smoking cessation.

Concern has arisen recently about risk associated with passive or "second-hand" cigarette smoking. There is evidence that spouses of smokers have a slightly higher risk of lung cancer than persons who live in a totally smoke-free environment. The risk is small compared with active cigarette smoking but probably is real. Casual or infrequent contact with cigarette smoke should not cause great concern among nonsmokers, but it is appropriate to segregate smokers from nonsmokers because any added risk, however small, should not be inflicted on nonsmoking individuals.

Whereas cigarette smoking is a predominant cause of lung cancer, it is not the sole cause. It has been well recognized that exposure to certain carcinogens in the occupational setting is associated with lung cancer. Asbestos is a substance with a fairly strong association, although it is particularly dangerous when combined with cigarette smoking. To be a carcinogen, the asbestos fibers must be in inhalable form. Encapsulated or contained asbestos, such as found in intact insulation products, provides no great risk. Great concern by the general public regarding asbestos in the environment is probably unwarranted. Exposure to chromium, certain nickel compounds, and organic compounds such as coal tars, soots, and diesel exhaust also has been associated with an increase in cancer. Women had generally been spared from many of these due to the prominent role of men in occupations where these substances are found. However, as women enter the workplace more broadly, they may be exposed as well. For example, concern has been raised about diesel engine school buses as a new health hazard for women in that many women are drivers.

Radon decay products are one possible cause of lung cancer that has received much attention and that is ubiquitous in the environment. The U.S. Environmental Protection Agency (EPA) has released standards for indoor exposure to radon, and most sales of homes require radon measurement as a contingency clause for the sale. Given the widespread possible exposure to radon and patients' concern about it publicity over the issue, some discussion is warranted.

Radon is a gas that is a decay product from naturally occurring uranium and radium found in rock, and its radioactive decay sequence generates carcinogenic alpha particles, such as isotopes of polonium and lead. These attach to dust particles, are respirable, and can be mutagenic to airway mucosal cells. It is these intermediate decay products, not radon itself, that are carcinogenic. The increased risk of lung cancer related to radon exposure was first identified in uranium miners, but radon may also be found in home environments. Radon gas enters homes through the ground. Certain areas of the United States have rock structures more predisposed to emit radon, but radon entry can occur in any location. Radon levels are negligible where there is adequate ventilation, so levels on the first floor are much lower than in basements.

Radon can be measured by charcoal-containing canisters, placed in a closed basement for a few days, that trap radon gas. Because radon levels can vary widely in any individual home based on soil moisture, wind speed and direction, atmospheric pressure, and basement ventilation, a more precise measurement can be taken using a tracking device that records the radon decay products. This allows measurements to be made for 1 to 12 months, providing an average reading that is a better estimate of risk.

The EPA has made recommendations for action based on levels. If the short-term screening shows a level of 4 to 8 pCi/L, no action needs to be taken. Between 8 and 20 pCi/L, it is recommended that the tracking device take long-term measurements for a span of about 6 to 12 months. If short-term levels are above 20 but below 200, measurements should be taken for 3 months. If levels on long-term measurement are above 8 pCi/L or if initial screening levels are above 200, prompt remediation should be considered. Remediation involves venting the area below the foundation to the outside atmosphere and may cost $2,000 to $6,000.

The risk of lung cancer in the general public from radon exposure is uncertain. Estimates of the risk are extrapolated from information on uranium miners and do not control other variables well. No literature convincingly demonstrates that the average individual has significant risk from exposure to radon. The EPA has estimated that radon causes 13,000 cases of lung cancer a year, but most of these are in cigarette smokers with the radon acting as a cocarcinogen. Although persistently high radon levels are reason for concern, the levels set by the EPA are considered by many to be too stringent. The nonsmoking general population should not worry excessively about lung cancer due to exposure to radon.

CLASSIFICATION

Lung cancer can be divided into two types: small cell ("oat cell") carcinoma and NSCLC. NSCLC includes squamous cell carcinoma, adenocarcinoma, large cell undifferentiated carcinoma, bronchoalveolar cell carcinoma (a variant of adenocarcinoma), and mixed types. These can be recognized microscopically, but the major clinical importance is that in NSCLC, surgery is the primary curative therapy. SCLC, on the other hand, is considered at time of diagnosis not to be surgically curable except in the rare instances where it presents as a peripheral nodule. At the time of diagnosis, 50% of SCLCs have metastasized to the bone marrow, and almost all have metastasized to lymph nodes within the mediastinum. Therapy for SCLC is chemotherapy in which there is often a good remission rate, although not many long-term survivors.

DIFFERENTIAL DIAGNOSIS

The symptoms associated with lung cancer are often nonspecific. Differential diagnostic possibilities are usually raised by findings on chest x-ray.

A solitary pulmonary nodule may be due to infectious processes such as tuberculoma, histoplasmoma and nocardiosis, vascular malformations, benign tumors such as hamartomas, and bronchial carcinoids. Rheumatoid nodules, Wegener granulomatosis, and metastatic malignancy may present with solitary nodules, although the usual pattern is multiple.

Mediastinal enlargement may be due to lymphoma, and lymphoma also presents as a parenchymal mass. Irregular infiltrative or masslike lesions also can be seen in tuberculosis, actinomycosis, and histoplasmosis. Lipoid pneumonia, pulmonary sequestration, "rounded atelectasis," and aneurysmal dilatation of central vessels also can have patterns on x-ray that resemble bronchogenic cancer.

HISTORY

Lung cancer may be asymptomatic until it is far advanced and uncurable. Hemoptysis in a cigarette smoker, even when associated with an acute bronchitis, warrants a chest x-ray. If the chest x-ray finding is negative, studies suggest that 3% to 8% of these individuals have an occult intrabronchial lesion that will be found at bronchoscopy. Cough can be a symptom of lung cancer, but most studies investigating causes of chronic cough have found carcinoma to be low on the list. Recurrent pneumonia in the same anatomic area of the lung may suggest a partially obstructing endobronchial lesion predisposing to infection. Whereas there are other causes of recurrent chest infection, recurrent infections in the same part of the lung in a cigarette smoker warrants referral to a specialist for evaluation. Shortness of breath may be a complaint caused by an obstructed airway or a malignant pleural effusion. Systemic symptoms of weight loss, anorexia, and malaise can be presenting manifestations and often indicate advanced disease. Pain is not a manifestation of lung cancer in its early stage. The lung parenchyma does not contain pain receptors, and only when the tumor involves the pleura or adjacent structures does pain become a symptom.

Unfortunately, many of the presenting complaints in lung cancer represent disseminated or advanced intrathoracic disease that prohibits resection. For example, hoarseness from compression of the recurrent laryngeal nerve implies mediastinal involvement that precludes surgery. Similarly, bone pain and focal neurologic complaints referable to metastases make the disease inoperable. Central nervous system involvement is common in lung cancer. It has been suggested that 10% of patients with squamous cell carcinoma have asymptomatic central nervous system metastases, and symptomatic metastases to the central nervous system may be the presenting manifestation in 15% of patients.

Given the late presentation of lung cancer in an often uncurable state, it is natural to ask whether *screening* for lung cancer is useful. Studies show that chest x-rays performed yearly or every other year, as well as regular sputum cytologic study, do not affect the overall mortality from lung cancer. Therefore, screening for lung cancer by these methods is not recommended as a public health measure. Nonetheless, many physicians obtain chest x-rays yearly or every other year in their patients who are heavy cigarette smokers, hoping to find early evidence of carcinoma, which does not become symptomatic until it is far advanced. Screening by computed tomography (CT) in smokers has been a recent topic of discussion, with the goal being to identify nodules that are invisible on chest x-ray. Because many of these are benign, the initial CT is followed by another some months later, and any nodule changing in size is removed as a cancer suspect. As with other screening strategies for lung cancer, there is not sufficient evidence that this affects mortality or any other outcome at this time, and it cannot be recommended as a routine strategy.

PHYSICAL EXAMINATION

Evidence of a focal wheeze on auscultation of the chest may point to a focal endobronchial lesion. The presence of digital clubbing, although not specific for lung cancer, is consistent with it. Evidence of disseminated disease should be sought so that diagnosis and staging can be made with the least invasive procedure. Enlarged lymph nodes in the supraclavicular area may be found. They can be aspirated for diagnosis and cell type, and if no small cell malignancy is found, this will also stage the disease, excluding curative surgery. Neurologic examination may show signs of focal deficits, consistent with metastatic disease to the brain. Patient complaints of bone tenderness should be evaluated by palpation and percussion to detect focal tenderness and guide imaging studies to detect metastases. Tumors growing in the apex of the lung may involve the cervical sympathetic ganglia and lead to Horner syndrome. Compression of the mediastinal vessels may produce the superior vena cava syndrome, which is characterized by elevated venous pressure with facial plethora, edema of the arm and upper body, and collaterals on the chest wall. The superior vena cava syndrome is a serious complication of lung cancer, usually requiring emergent treatment because brain edema can occur, causing mental status change and coma. Elevated jugular venous pressure also may be caused by a malignant pericardial effusion, which requires urgent intervention if cardiac output is affected.

Blood work may show hypercalcemia. This may not be due to a bony metastases but can be hormonally produced and does not necessarily indicate inoperability.

IMAGING STUDIES

Chest x-ray findings for lung carcinoma may be normal. In cigarette smokers with hemoptysis, a small percentage of patients with a normal finding on chest x-ray have an endobronchial lesion observed on bronchoscopy. Usually, the chest x-ray shows a mass lesion. In some cases, a peripheral nodule is found. These are usually adenocarcinomas, are almost always asymptomatic, and often are found incidentally. If the lesion has not changed in size for a 2-year interval of time, it is unlikely to be lung cancer and can be followed by x-rays over the next 1 to 2 years. If the nodule is new, or at least not known to be old, the risk of carcinoma in a cigarette smoker is sufficiently high to warrant aggressive investigation, usually by exploratory thoracotomy. Patterns of calcification in a pulmonary nodule are rarely diagnostic of benignity. Needle aspiration of these lesions rarely convincingly yield a benign origin and, if results are negative, do not exclude malignancy.

The more common x-ray presentation of lung cancer is evidence of a central mass lesion or irregular infiltrate, hilar enlargement, lobar atelectasis, or mediastinal adenopathy, because cancer arises at the site of carcinogen deposition in these central airways and spreads to adjacent lymph nodes. Approximately 20% to 25% of these central lesions are small cell carcinoma, another quarter is adenocarcinoma, and a third is squamous cell. The remainder is large cell undifferentiated or mixed type.

Pleural effusions can be seen in lung cancer as well. This may be due to pleural involvement with a tumor but also can be due to local lymphatic obstruction without pleural involvement. In NSCLC, pleural effusions with malignant cells exclude operability, whereas pleural effusions that are cytologically negative for malignancy still allow the possibility of curative resection.

A third pattern of lung cancer on x-ray is seen in the relatively rare form of lung cancer, called bronchoalveolar cell carcinoma. This is a variant of adenocarcinoma in which the malignant cells palisade along alveolar structures, assuming an infiltrative appearance on chest x-ray and resembling a pneumonia or other primary alveolar process.

A CT of the chest is obtained as part of an evaluation of a patient with suspected lung cancer. The CT is useful in defining the presence and extent of mediastinal adenopathy. Lymph nodes under 2 cm, especially if they occur in a few discreet areas, have about a 50% chance of being benign. Lymph nodes greater than 2 to 3 cm, particularly diffusely involving the mediastinum, have a much higher chance of being malignant. Whereas the CT cannot be definitive regarding malignancy in these nodes, the CT definition of the mediastinal anatomy allows this area to be approached by fine needle aspiration or mediastinoscopy to both diagnose and stage the disease, perhaps sparing the need for a thoracotomy.

A recent imaging modality used in the evaluation of lung cancer is positron emission tomography (PET). This technique measures metabolic activity using a positron emitting marker of glucose metabolism. In pulmonary nodules over about 1 cm in size, it has a sensitivity and specificity of 95% and 85%, respectively, for carcinoma. Whether or not this is sufficient to alter the approach to nodules that are new (or not known to be old) in a smoker of cancer age is uncertain, because many believe these nodules should be resected regardless of radiologic or PET appearance. Medicare has approved reimbursement for PET for evaluation of solitary nodules, finding it cost effective relative to routine surgery on all nodules.

PET also has better sensitivity and specificity in mediastinal staging than CT, but again the importance of this is uncertain in that definitive staging requires tissue confirmation. PET may detect unsuspected distant metastases, saving the patient unnecessary attempts at curative surgery. One study reported this to take place in 11% of patients. There are false positives (any metabolically active tissue, e.g., inflammation) and false negatives (small or microscopic metastatic lesions), and the true clinical overall value of PET for distant metastases is therefore uncertain. PET in lung cancer is a technique in evolution. It is recommended that clinical consultation around its use be sought, especially from clinicians dealing with the management of patients with lung cancer and not just those interested in the imaging aspects.

It is not recommended that patients routinely have bone scans and CTs of the brain. Bone pain, bone discomfort, and neurologic symptoms or findings on examination, however, should lead to investigation of these areas. The older and more infirm the patient, the more likely one is to search for evidence of inoperability by bone scan or brain CT before thoracotomy.

An important laboratory examination in a patient with suspected lung cancer is pulmonary function testing. Chronic obstructive pulmonary disease increases the risk of postoperative complications and, if severe, may prohibit thoracic surgery and resection of lung. Pulmonary medicine and thoracic surgery consultants usually are involved in deciding fitness for operability. However, as a rule of thumb, if after resection the residual forced expiratory volume in 1 second is less than 700 mL, surgery usually is not considered to be an option.

TREATMENT

At presentation, perhaps only one fourth or one third of lung cancer patients have potential for curative treatment because of metastatic disease, mediastinal involvement, or poor pulmonary function. The specific diagnostic and therapeutic approach to the patient with lung cancer usually is multidisciplinary. A physician must be able to help guide the patient through the evaluative process and then through the options for treatment, thoracic surgery, medical oncology, or radiation oncology, depending on the typing and staging of the disease. A pulmonologist often plays this role, although the primary care physician can do so if there is an understanding of the concepts that determine the available options.

The peripheral nodule smaller than 4 cm in diameter occurs in some patients with lung cancer but is a favorable finding. At presentation, depending on size, the cure rate can be as high as 60% to 80% for these lesions. Therefore, in a cigarette smoking patient older than 40 years of age for whom the diagnostic workup is usually fairly slight, old chest x-rays should be sought; a lesion unchanged for 2 years is unlikely to be cancer and can be followed by serial chest x-rays. Bronchoscopy has a low yield in diagnosing these peripheral nodules. Moreover, they rarely are small cell cancers, and a positive diagnosis of NSCLC does not change the need for eventual surgery if the patient is otherwise a candidate for curative resection. It has been suggested that bronchoscopy may detect an occult synchronous primary lesion in a more central airway, but that likelihood is so small that routine bronchoscopy is not warranted. Fine needle transthoracic aspiration of the nodule often can make the diagnosis of lung cancer. However, in a patient who is otherwise a candidate for curative resection, this does not affect the need to undergo surgery. Because a negative result on fine needle aspiration does not give sufficient confidence to rule out malignancy, the fine needle aspirate is rarely useful in specifically diagnosing other conditions.

The preoperative diagnosis of malignancy in a solitary nodule by needle or bronchoscopy is useful in patients who refuse surgery, cannot tolerate surgery, or have convincing clinical evidence of metastatic disease. A CT of the chest is useful to detect mediastinal adenopathy not visible on chest x-ray. Obtaining a biopsy on these nodes by needle aspiration or mediastinoscopy is useful before surgery because mediastinal involvement with tumor would make resection of the nodule unnecessary. The evaluation should include pulmonary function testing to determine operative risk or ability to undergo resection, and good clinical history and physical examination should be performed to determine bone or central nervous system metastases. In the absence of such symptoms, bone scans and brain CTs usually are not routinely obtained. If there is no evidence for metastatic or mediastinal disease from these relatively simple studies and the patient can tolerate surgery based on pulmonary function tests and other medical conditions, then referral to thoracic surgery for thoracotomy follows. Some of these lesions, if sufficiently peripheral, can be removed by thoracoscopy; this is an option left to the individual thoracic surgeon.

In individuals who are extremely elderly, refuse surgery, or have pulmonary function abnormalities prohibiting surgery, a nonsurgical diagnosis should be made. Needle aspiration is usually preferred, although, depending on the location of the nodule in the chest, fluoroscopic-guided bronchoscopy may be useful as well. If there is no evidence of mediastinal or metastatic spread, then the patient can be referred to radiation oncology for curative radiation therapy. The cure rate with full-dose radiation therapy for a solitary pulmonary nodule under 3.0 to 4.0 cm in diameter may be as high as 25%.

The more common presentation of lung cancer is a central mass, for which the prognosis, 15% survival at 5 years, is much poorer than is the case with a peripheral nodule. The focus of the evaluation is to define reasons that will avoid unnecessary thoracotomy. Flexible fiberoptic bronchoscopy is performed because it has a high yield in diagnosing the lesions that arise in the central airways; of equal importance, it can diagnose the 20% to 25% of lesions that are SCLC, and hence, require chemotherapy rather than surgery. Bronchoscopy also is be useful in showing the extent of the tumor in the airway, defining what degree of resection is necessary, and excluding operability when it involves the carina or subcarinal lymph nodes, which can be aspirated transbronchially. Patients should be interviewed and examined carefully. A supraclavicular node often can be aspirated by needle, and this provides a diagnosis as well as staging, saving an unnecessary thoracotomy. Complaints of bone pain may lead to a bone scan that would reveal foci of metastatic disease. Similarly, eliciting neurologic symptoms leading to a brain CT showing lesions consistent with metastatic disease would stage the disease clinically, even if the brain rarely undergoes biopsy for confirmation. The CT of the chest may show mediastinal adenopathy not visible on chest x-ray, which could be approached by possible needle aspiration or mediastinoscopy. If the evaluation reveals no demonstrable metastatic disease and no evident spread to the mediastinum, the patient is referred for thoracotomy. Unfortunately, in large central lesions, many patients who undergo exploration with curative intent are found to be inoperable because of mediastinal extension or invasion diagnosed only at the time of good visualization at thoracotomy.

For patients with NSCLC who are inoperable for cure, alternative therapy does not provide great benefit. Chemotherapy offers some survival advantage to patients with advanced NSCLC, but in studies comparing the best routine supportive care with multidrug chemotherapeutic drug regimens, median survival is increased from 4 to 8 months at best, and the toxicity is significant.

Radiation therapy for otherwise unresectable NSCLC does not have a curative role. It is used in palliation to shrink lesions that encroach on the airway and to palliate bony metastases or intracranial lesions. Endoscopically delivered laser resection also is used for palliation when the tumor mass encroaches on a central airway such as the trachea and causes severe dyspnea with imminent suffocation.

In SCLC chemotherapy is the preferred treatment. It results in remission of disease in most patients, lasting as long as 12 to 24 months. The cure rate remains low despite remission, and 5-year cures are rare.

OTHER LUNG CANCERS

In addition to bronchogenic carcinoma, other cancers can arise primarily in the thorax. Carcinoid tumors rise in the airway, can occur at any age, and are unrelated to cigarette smoking. Because of their location in the airway, the presenting manifestations may be recurrent pneumonia in distal lung, cysts, or evidence of persistent atelectasis on chest x-ray. These lesions have some malignant potential and are not truly "benign" adenomas, as they are often labeled. The malignant potential is low, but they can metastasize to regional lymph nodes and even distantly.

Mesothelioma is a primary malignancy of the pleura. It has been strongly related to asbestos exposure and has been predominantly a disease of men working in asbestos-related industries. Mesothelioma presents with recurrent pleural effusion that is often hemorrhagic, thickened pleura on x-ray, and persistent chest wall pain from intercostal nerve involvement. Although they often grow slowly, these lesions are uncurable by either chemotherapy or surgery.

CONSIDERATIONS IN PREGNANCY

Primary bronchogenic carcinoma is unusual in patients younger than 35 years of age. Occasionally, a chest x-ray in a pregnant woman shows a small peripheral nodule that is not known to be old or unchanged because there are no previous x-rays for comparison. In people younger than 35 years of age, even cigarette smokers, these have a low likelihood of being malignant, approximately 5%. Even if the lesion was malignant, there is little evidence that waiting some months will result in a marked deterioration in the probability of cure. It has been estimated, although the data are poor, that every month of waiting may reduce the likelihood of survival by 1%. Patient preference and attitudes relative to the pregnancy play a significant role in how these situations are handled.

Because of the less aggressive malignant behavior of carcinoid tumors, definitive treatment can be deferred until after delivery, unless there are mitigating circumstances such as persistent hemoptysis or uncontrollable pneumonia due to airway obstruction.

BIBLIOGRAPHY

Bains MS. Surgical treatment of lung cancer. *Chest* 1991;100:826.

Eddy DM. Screening for lung cancer. *Ann Intern Med* 1989;111:232.

Erasmus JJ, Paltz EF. Positron emission tomography imaging of the thorax. *Clin Chest Med* 1999;20:715.

Figlin RA, Holmes EC, Petrovich A, et al. Lung cancer. In: Haskell CM, ed. *Cancer treatment,* 3rd ed. Philadelphia: WB Saunders, 1990.

Harley NH, Harley JH. Potential lung cancer risk from indoor radon exposure. *CA Cancer J Clin* 1990;40:265.

Marino P, Pampallona S, Preatoni A, et al. Chemotherapy vs. supportive care in advanced non-small-cell lung cancer: results of a meta-analysis of the literature. *Chest* 1994;106:861.

Matthay RA, guest ed. Lung cancer. *Clin Chest Med* 1993;14:1.

Ost D, Fein A. Evaluation and management of the solitary pulmonary nodule. *Am J Respir Crit Care Med* 2000;162:782.

Samet JM, Nero AV Sounding board: indoor radon and lung cancer. *N Engl J Med* 1989;320:591.

CHAPTER 59
Cough

Anthony J. Fedullo

Studies examining the etiology of chronic cough have variously defined it as a cough that has been present for longer than 3 to 8 weeks. This time period generally excludes coughs that are due to acute processes such as pneumonia or bronchitis. Chronic cough is a common problem, estimated to be responsible for 30,000,000 physician visits yearly. Whereas a wide variety of disorders can cause cough, the etiology often is determined by history, physical examination, or therapeutic trials directed to its common causes. Radiographic procedures, endoscopic examination, or blood tests play only a minor role in the diagnostic evaluation.

ETIOLOGY AND DIFFERENTIAL DIAGNOSIS

Cough is a protective mechanism, clearing mucus and irritative substances from the lung and guarding against inhalation and retention of foreign material. Submucosal cough receptors richly innervate the pharynx, posterior pharynx, and the airways. Irritation of these, as well as cough receptors on the pleural, pericardial, and diaphragmatic surfaces, can trigger cough.

Cough can be triggered by mechanical stimulation or by irritating fumes. The stimulus is transferred to a cough center in the medulla, and efferent pathways then initiate cough. Coughing involves taking a breath to fill the lungs completely. The glottis is closed while the chest, abdominal muscles, and diaphragm begin to contract, generating intrathoracic pressure. The glottis then opens, letting out an explosive rush of air, clearing the offending material. An effective cough depends on an alert central nervous system, ability to draw a deep breath, ability to close the glottis, and sufficient muscle strength to exert forceful contraction. When irritating stimuli continually trigger the cough receptors or when the receptors become overly sensitive, chronic cough results.

Chronic cough may be productive of purulent sputum ("moist"), indicative of active inflammation and mucous production. Coughs may be nonproductive ("dry") or productive only of small amounts of thin mucus, suggesting persistent noninflammatory irritation of cough receptors. Whereas causes of cough may overlap in these areas, they provide a useful clinical distinction in investigating cough.

Chronic bronchitis from cigarette smoking is a common cause of productive cough. Most studies evaluating chronic cough have excluded cigarette smokers from analysis, but these patients do not exclude themselves from physicians' offices. It is surprising how frequently cigarette smokers present to the physician complaining of long-standing cough without considering smoking as an etiology. Some of these patients may have their coughs exacerbated by viral or bacterial infections and may need intermittent antibiotic treatment for the latter. However, the irritating effect of cigarette smoke produces chronic inflammatory change and mucous production, and the cough will not resolve unless cigarette smoking is stopped.

Among nonsmokers, the duration of productive cough after an *acute respiratory infection* such as bronchitis or pneumonia may exceed the 3 to 8 weeks that many studies use to define chronic cough. Patients with cough after an acute respiratory infection usually have the cough slowly improve over 2 to 8 weeks, and as long as the cough is improving, no further diagnostic evaluation or treatment is needed. However, on occasion, postinfectious cough can continue for many months, becoming nonproductive of mucus. It is not clear why some patients develop a *persistent postinfectious cough.* Triggering of latent asthma is a possibility, as well as upper respiratory infection causing postnasal drip, both of which may cause the chronic cough. Severe or persistent coughing during the acute phase of the infection may traumatize the trachea and larynx, making the cough receptors hypersensitive and irritable to any stimulation. Some evidence of hyperirritability is found if the patient communicates that voice use causes the cough and that the cough is triggered by mildly irritating odors or smells that had not caused cough previously.

Bronchiectasis may cause chronic productive cough, often accompanied by large quantities of purulent sputum. Bronchiectasis is a dilatation of bronchioles, usually resulting from previous chest infection that has destroyed surrounding and supporting lung parenchyma. Tuberculosis was a prominent cause in the past, but childhood respiratory illnesses and adult bacterial pneumonias are more frequent causes. The cough in bronchiectasis is characterized by chronic or recurrent sputum production; is often related to body position because the bronchiectatic segment drains into more normal airways, triggering cough; and is often most productive in the morning, when the secretions that accumulate overnight are cleared. Bronchiectasis can be marked by intermittent febrile illnesses with infiltrates on chest x-ray, because the chronic presence of purulent secretions predispose to pneumonia.

Chronic respiratory infections, in addition to bronchiectasis, also cause a chronic productive cough. Tuberculosis can cause chronic cough with sputum production. Often, systemic symptoms such as weight loss, fatigue, fever, and night sweats are present, but in the earlier stages these may be absent. *Cystic fibrosis* can first appear in early adulthood and can present with productive cough.

Chronic coughs that are nonproductive or only produce small amounts of mucus are more common than coughs that are productive of purulent mucus. *Postnasal drip* is probably the most common cause of chronic cough. Mucous production may be present but is relatively slight compared with the amount produced in the coughs previously discussed, and the patient and physician can recognize that the mucus is being cleared from the posterior pharynx rather than arising from a source deep within the chest. The etiology of a cough associated with postnasal drip is probably irritation of cough receptors in upper airway structures from postnasal drainage. Because postnasal drip is a common problem, it is not clear why it causes cough in some patients, but it may be that a preceding respiratory infection has sensitized the upper airway to be more sensitive to an irritant phenomenon.

In studies examining chronic cough, *asthma* is the second most common etiology. Cough can be the sole manifestation of asthma; wheezing may not be heard on examination, and the patient may not complain of shortness of breath. The cough of asthma may be triggered by factors such as exercise or cold air, may occur nocturnally, and although it usually does not produce mucus, may do so if a significant inflammatory component is present.

Gastroesophageal reflux may cause a chronic cough. This may occur due to reflex bronchoconstriction from acid reflux into the esophagus or from reflux to the level of the pharynx with laryngeal irritation and aspiration. Esophageal pH monitoring demonstrates the temporal relationship of cough to reflux, although not all studies show this association. Only one half of patients with cough from gastroesophageal reflux, identified by pH monitoring or response to specific therapy, do not have reflux symptoms. Reflux may occur in the upright position, so that although gastroesophageal reflux may cause or exacerbate cough during sleep, it can also be a cause of cough during waking hours.

Postnasal drip, asthma, and gastroesophageal reflux can coexist to play a role in chronic cough. In studies evaluating the etiology of chronic cough, many patients have two or more of these disorders, which need to be treated before cough is improved.

Cough sometimes persists for many months after otherwise uncomplicated respiratory infections. This has been referred to as *postinfectious persistent cough.* Whereas viral respiratory infection may trigger asthma or cause postnasal sinus drainage, these are not the cause of postinfectious cough, as demonstrated by negative results on bronchoprovocation testing and lack of response to treatment trials. The etiology of postinfectious cough may be persistent trauma or irritation of the upper airway from the mechanical effects of coughing itself. Patients often notice that the cough is triggered by using the voice and that slight hoarseness or loss of voice strength occurs. The vocal cords may appear edematous and inflamed on examination.

Drugs can cause cough. Cough may occur in 5% of patients taking *angiotensin-converting enzyme inhibitor* medication. The cough may begin long after the medication is initiated or arise after a change in dose. The mechanism that causes these coughs is unknown, but it does not seem related to bronchial hyperreactivity caused by the agent.

In addition to these common causes of nonproductive cough, *bronchogenic carcinoma* can present with a nonproductive cough. A normal finding on chest x-ray does not exclude cancer; in smokers with hemoptysis, a small percentage of patients have an endobronchial lesion on bronchoscopy with a normal chest x-ray result. Irritation of the *diaphragm,* such as by subphrenic masses or infections, can cause cough; processes involving the *pericardium* also can cause cough, such as pericarditis, although other manifestations of pericarditis are rarely absent. *Pleural effusions,* which are apparent on examination or on the chest x-ray, may have cough as a symptom. *Interstitial lung disease* can have cough as a prominent symptom, but x-ray abnormalities are usually present. *Recurrent aspiration* can be a cause of cough, particularly in patients who have had cerebrovascular accidents and disruption of the normal swallowing mechanism. This cough is likely triggered by recurrent aspiration of saliva and may be more prominent during meals when food also is aspirated. *Congestive heart failure* can cause cough, particularly with exercise or nocturnally. This can be confused with cough associated with asthma, which can occur under similar circumstances. A rare cause of chronic cough is due to a reflex from irritation of the *external ear canal,* such as from ingrown hairs, foreign material, or external otitis.

A relatively rare cause of chronic cough, to be considered after the above are excluded, is lymphocytic or eosinophilic bronchitis (not related to asthma). In these conditions the bronchial mucosa is infiltrated with these inflammatory cells. The condition responds very well to corticosteroids. Because the etiology in unknown, it may be that this condition reflects a prolonged inflammatory response to irritants or to infectious agents and is a variant of postinfectious chronic cough.

Finally, a cough may have a *psychogenic* or *habitual* cause. Some patients persistently have a throat-clearing slight cough that does not respond to therapy for postnasal drip. Other patients have dry cough triggered under circumstances of stress or anxiety. Before ascribing cough to this cause, organic etiologies should first be excluded.

HISTORY

The history relating to a patient complaining of cough often is far more helpful in elucidating the cause than are laboratory tests or other interventions beyond a simple chest x-ray. It should first be determined whether the cough is predominantly productive of mucopurulent material or is nonproductive. In a cigarette smoker, a chronic productive cough often is due to irritative bronchitis; in a nonsmoker, bronchiectasis should be considered. Sputum production in bronchiectasis often is greatest on awakening in the morning, when retained secretions are cleared, and the cough of bronchiectasis may be exacerbated by the change in secretions as they empty from the bronchiectatic areas into areas of normal lung having intact cough reflexes. Relationship to a recent respiratory infection should be noted. A productive cough may last for several weeks after an acute respiratory infection. Persistent systemic symptoms of malaise, fever, night sweats, or fatigue raise the question of an indolent infection such as tuberculosis. Productive cough may be a manifestation of occupational-related respiratory irritants, and the relationship of cough to these exposures should be identified.

The presence of hemoptysis in a cigarette smoker suggests the possibility of a bronchogenic carcinoma. Cigarette smokers with hemoptysis and normal chest x-ray findings have an approximately 5% chance of having an endobronchial lesion accounting for an abnormality that is not visible on x-ray. Hemoptysis also may suggest the possibility of indolent infection, particularly tuberculosis. These patients often have systemic symptoms, such as fever and malaise, to suggest infection, but may not, and evidence of parenchymal infiltrates or cavities of tuberculosis are found only when a chest x-ray is obtained.

In patients with a nonproductive cough and who are well except for their complaint of cough, the most common diagnoses are postnasal drip, asthma, gastroesophageal reflux, persistent postinfection cough, or, frequently, a combination of two or more of these. Approximately one half of patients with postnasal drip are asymptomatic. They have no nasal discharge or pharyngeal sense of drainage and, therefore, the exclusion of these findings on history does not exclude the diagnosis. Similarly, asthmatics with a primary complaint of cough may not notice wheezing or shortness of breath. Gastroesophageal reflux causing cough is silent in at least half of the patients who are believed to have cough on that basis, and conversely, the presence of reflux symptoms are common and do not necessarily implicate reflux as the cause of the cough. Persistent postinfectious cough is identified by its relationship to a previous respiratory infection. Once mucous production associated with the acute infection has stopped, usually within a few weeks, these coughs become dry and are associated with a tickling or "raw" sensation in the upper airway, exacerbation of cough by using the voice, and often a change in voice quality.

Historical information also helps in determining the etiology of less common causes of dry nonproductive cough. Cough with exertion or occurring nocturnally with orthopnea or paroxysmal nocturnal dyspnea may point to congestive heart failure as the etiology, although nocturnal asthma can have similar characteristics.

Hypersensitivity pneumonitis is a symptom complex of fever, cough, and shortness of breath that occurs on exposure to organic antigens such as thermophilic *Actinomyces, Aspergillus* species, or other antigens. This disease has several names that are associated with the specific exposures, such as farmer lung, bird fancier disease, and humidifier lung. Patients usually have symptoms of shortness of breath, fever, and cough, but occasionally cough may be the predominant complaint. If a history of exposure is not obtained, these patients can go on to develop chronic interstitial fibrosis with permanent loss of lung function.

A complete drug history should be obtained. Drugs such as nitrofurantoin, thiazide diuretics, amiodarone, bleomycin, and methotrexate cause pulmonary infiltrates. These are generally associated with dyspnea, but cough may be the initial symptom. Angiotensin-converting enzyme inhibitors, which are commonly used in adults for treating hypertension or congestive heart failure, are frequently associated with causing a cough. These drugs do not cause pulmonary infiltrates or other manifestations such as cough, wheezing, or shortness of breath. The cough may begin some months or even longer after initiation of the drug, and patients may notice the onset after switching from one drug in the family to another. Cough is usually described as an irritating dry cough accompanied by a tickling or raw sensation in the upper airway. The exact mechanism for the cough is uncertain, but the cough is not due to asthma induction by the medication. The cough resolves on cessation of the drug; it takes days to see some effect but may take weeks for the cough to resolve fully.

PHYSICAL EXAMINATION AND CLINICAL FINDINGS

Auscultation of the chest may be helpful. In patients with asthma, a prolonged expiratory time or wheezing may be heard. In patients with interstitial fibrosis, dry rales may be heard, and moister rales may be heard in patients with congestive heart failure. A focal wheeze with expiration suggests the possibility of an obstructing endobronchial lesion. Localized evidence of consolidation suggests a pulmonary infiltrative process such as pneumonia, and dullness and decreased breath sounds suggest a pleural effusion. Focal rales or rhonchi suggest the presence of bronchiectasis.

Examination of the pharynx and upper airway may show evidence of postnasal drainage. However, this is a common and nonspecific finding, so its presence does not implicate postnasal drip as the cause of cough.

An S_3 gallop on examination of the heart and pedal edema may suggest congestive heart failure as a cause of the cough. With some patients, examination of the ear canal elicits brisk cough, and in these sensitive individuals, pathologic elements in the ear canal such as external otitis or irritating hairs may be an etiology of the cough.

LABORATORY AND IMAGING STUDIES

A chest x-ray is a useful part of the evaluation of a patient with chronic cough. A chest x-ray shows most carcinomas that are associated with a chronic cough. Abnormalities suggesting chronic infection, such as tuberculosis, interstitial lung disease, hypersensitivity pneumonitis, or congestive heart failure, may be found. Bronchiectasis sometimes produces findings on chest x-ray such as thickened bronchial walls or cystic spaces, which can suggest that diagnosis. Mediastinal masses, pericardial disease, and pleural effusions also can be seen when either the history or physical examination does not reveal them.

Most of the time, however, the chest x-ray does not give positive results in patients who have a chronic cough, particularly if the cough is not productive and the patient is otherwise feeling well. If the history suggests that asthma may be present, then pulmonary function tests should be performed to demonstrate airway obstruction. If airway obstruction is absent and asthma is still suspected, then a methacholine challenge to induce asthma can be performed. If cough is productive and purulent, then a sputum culture is useful to demonstrate bacterial infection in bronchiectasis, which may require specific antibiotic treatment as therapy.

Bronchoscopy has only a limited role in evaluating patients with cough, with the exception of smokers with hemoptysis. It is usually considered only after interventions directed toward the common etiologies of chronic cough have not benefited the patient.

TREATMENT

Even after careful and complete history, physical examination, chest x-ray, and sputum culture, the etiology of cough often is not precisely determined. In these patients, a program of staged treatment directed toward the most common causes of cough serves both a treatment and diagnostic purpose. Because postnasal drip is the most common cause of chronic cough, the initial step is treatment with an antihistamine/decongestant preparation. With this therapy, cough may improve within weeks, but occasionally months may be needed for the cough to completely resolve. As long as the patient shows some improvement, this therapy can be continued. If there is no improvement after weeks of therapy or if some improvement has occurred but the cough persists, further evaluation is warranted. Because asthma in most studies has been shown to be the next most common cause of chronic cough, a trial of inhaled albuterol, two puffs four times daily for 1 to 2 weeks, is given. If the cough responds promptly, this confirms asthma as an etiology, and asthma treatment can be continued. If the cough is not better or is only partially better, pulmonary function tests with bronchoprovocation challenge should be performed. If results are positive, a short trial of prednisone, 20 to 30 mg/d for 1 week, can be used to treat asthma that has been refractory to bronchodilators. If the pulmonary function tests and bronchoprovocation tests give negative results and there is a history of onset of cough after respiratory infection, then the same dose of steroids can be given to treat "postinfectious persistent cough." The antiinflammatory action of steroids works fairly effectively in coughs of this nature, often stopping the cough completely or ameliorating it significantly.

If cough is not improved, then patients are treated for gastroesophageal reflux with a histamine blocker, along with routine antireflux measures, such as avoidance of caffeine, alcohol, and chocolate; avoidance of eating before sleep; and raising the head of the bed by 15 to 20 cm (6–8 inches). If the cough is not improved after a few weeks of this therapy, some authorities suggest 24-hour esophageal pH monitoring, and if reflux is present, treatment with histamine Z blockers should be continued, with the addition of omeprazole.

After this staged approach, most patients who meet the entry criteria, that is, having a nonproductive cough lasting for more than 1 to 2 months and no other symptoms, have the cough relieved. Cough recurs in a few of these but responds again to therapeutic trials.

In patients who continue to have a nonproductive cough after this sequence of treatment, bronchoscopy is indicated to evaluate the possibility of an endobronchial lesion and to obtain secretions. If no abnormality is found and the cough still persists, another trial of corticosteroids and an inhaled bronchodilator could be performed, with reconsideration of the more uncommon causes of cough. It is best to consider causes such as bronchiectasis, tuberculosis, congestive heart failure, interstitial lung disease, and drug-related cough before empirically embarking on what may be a many-week course of a graded treatment trial, so that if no benefit is achieved, the former have already been carefully considered.

While specific therapy is being attempted, nonspecific treatment for cough can be helpful when the cough is severe, annoying, and disturbs sleep. Soothing treatment for upper airway irritation from coughing itself can be useful. Over-the-counter preparations, cough drops and lozenges, and home remedies can provide relief. More potent cough suppression in the form of medications containing opiates or opiate analogues can be useful. They often allow sleep when the cough is nonproductive and irritating. During the daytime, however, cough suppression by these medications may cause drowsiness. Cough-suppressant medications usually do not affect cough to such a degree that the ability to assess the response to progressive trials of various medications is lost.

CONSIDERATIONS IN PREGNANCY

The etiology of the cough may produce effects that pertain to pregnancy. Cough due to asthma, for example, can result in hypoxemia even when there is minimal shortness of breath, and in pregnant patients with cough, it is useful to ensure that arterial blood oxygen tension or oxygen saturation by oximetry is normal. The greatest consideration in pregnancy and cough is to make sure that a systemic disease is not causing the cough and to ensure that the cough is not associated with hypoxemia. Coughing itself is associated with increased intraabdominal pressure because of the contraction of the abdominal and the thoracic musculature. The pressure increase is usually not so large as to cause any mechanical problems to the fetus or placenta. Urinary incontinence with coughing can occur and may be exacerbated in pregnancy. In late pregnancy, whether the sudden loud sound of cough disturbs the fetus in any psychologic or developmental way is unknown but seems unlikely.

Medications used in the sequential approach to cough, as described earlier, may need to be modified in pregnancy. It may be prudent to avoid vasoconstrictive decongestants, such as pseudoephedrine, that are used to treat postnasal drip. Among antihistamines, diphenhydramine, brompheniramine, loratadine, and cyproheptadine are category B agents. Bronchoprovocation challenge with methacholine is not advised in the pregnant asthma suspect. Antacids and H_2 blockers for gastroesophageal reflux are not contraindicated in pregnancy and are rated as category B drugs, except for nizatidine, which is category C. There is insufficient experience with omeprazole in pregnancy, and it is a category C drug. Treating asthma in pregnancy is advisable to avoid hypoxemia, and most agents, including systemic corticosteroids, can be used safely. Fiberoptic bronchoscopy, if necessary, can be performed safely. Short-term use of opiates for cough suppression is safe in pregnancy.

BIBLIOGRAPHY

Corrao WM. Chronic cough: when to take the less traveled path. *J Respir Dis* 1993;14:273.

Corrao WM, Braman SS, Irwin RS. Chronic cough as the sole presenting manifestation of bronchial asthma. *N Engl J Med* 1975;292:555.

Doan T, Patterson R, Greenberger PA. Cough variant asthma: usefulness of a diagnostic-therapeutic trial with prednisone. *Ann Allergy* 1992;69:505.

Ing AJ, Ngu MC, Breslin AB. Chronic persistent cough and gastrooesophageal reflux. *Thorax* 1991;46:479.

Irwin RS, Curley FJ. The treatment of cough: a comprehensive review. *Chest* 1991;99:1477.

Irwin RS, Curley FJ, French CL. Chronic cough: the spectrum and frequency of causes, key components of the diagnostic evaluation, and outcome of specific therapy. *Am Rev Respir Dis* 1990;141:640.

Lee SY, Cho JY, Shim JJ, et al. Airway inflammation as an assessment of chronic nonproductive cough. *Chest* 2001;120:1114.

Poe RH, Harder RV, Israel RH, et al. Chronic persistent cough: experience in diagnosis and outcome using an anatomic diagnostic protocol. *Chest* 1989;95:723.

Poe RH, Israel RH, Utell MJ, et al. Chronic cough: bronchoscopy or pulmonary function testing? *Am Rev Respir Dis* 1982;126:160.

Pratter MR, Banter T, Akers S, et al. An algorithmic approach to chronic cough. *Ann Intern Med* 1993;119:977.

PART

7

Gastrointestinal Problems

CHAPTER 60

Gastrointestinal Bleeding

Edward Feller

Gastrointestinal (GI) bleeding encompasses a spectrum from sudden, trivial, or massive hemorrhage to slow occult (inapparent) oozing due to a wide variety of upper GI (UGI) sites (esophagus, stomach, duodenum) and colonic sources (lower GI [LGI]). Rarely, bleeding originates from the small bowel. UGI lesions are much more common than colonic, accounting for 75% of acute bleeding episodes. More than 350,000 hospitalizations occur yearly in the United States for UGI bleeding. Hematemesis is defined as vomiting of blood, indicating a source proximal to the ligament of Treitz. Melena reflects rectal passage of black or tarry stool. Hematochezia connotes passage of red blood rectally. Occult bleeding refers to that which is not apparent to the patient. Physicians refer to obscure bleeding as being either occult or acute but which persists or recurs after a negative initial colonoscopy and UGI endoscopy.

ETIOLOGY

Upper Gastrointestinal Bleeding

Peptic ulcer disease of the duodenum or stomach is the most common etiology of acute UGI bleeding, accounting for about half of all cases. Approximately 300,000 admissions for UGI hemorrhage occur yearly in the United States. Major risk factors for ulcers and bleeding complications are *Helicobacter pylori* infestation, use of nonsteroidal antiinflammatory drugs (NSAIDs), excess gastric acid, and anticoagulation (Table 60.1). Complications of ulcers, including bleeding, are more common in the elderly. Gastric or duodenal erosions, gastritis, or duodenitis may also occur in the spectrum of ulcer disease. *H. pylori* eradication is mandatory in all patients with peptic ulcer disease to reduce risk of both recurrence and its major complication (bleeding).

In most urban environments, esophagogastric variceal bleeding due to portal hypertension is the second most common cause of acute bleeding, found in 10% to 15% of cases. Hepatitis C virus infection and alcoholic liver disease are the most frequent etiologies of portal hypertension and variceal hemorrhage. Physicians must be aware that varices can also occur in the small bowel, colon, and rectum. As many as 50% of patients with known portal hypertension who bleed do so from etiologies other than varices, most commonly peptic ulcer disease. Portal hypertension is also associated with a possible "congestive" gastropathy or colopathy associated with minor and major bleeding. Women have a lower incidence of both alcoholism and hepatitis C infection than men. Ethanol itself is not generally a direct irritant to the UGI mucosa. Mallory-Weiss mucosal tears at the gastroesophageal junction are lacerations that are common after repeated vomiting or retching. Nausea and vomiting associated with pregnancy increases the risk.

Arteriovenous malformations (angiodysplasia), more common in the colon, do occur in the UGI tract and may be responsible for about 5% of acute UGI bleeding episodes. Rarely, bleeding is due to a Dieulafoy lesion (an aberrant mucosal arteriole eroding into the lumen of the digestive tract, especially the stomach), hemosuccus pancreaticus or hemobilia (bleeding

TABLE 60.1. Causes of Acute UGI Bleeding

Common
Gastric/duodenal ulcer
Gastric/duodenal erosions
Mallory-Weiss (mucosal) tear
Esophageal varices
Uncommon
Esophagitis
Carcinoma (esophagus, stomach, duodenum)
Submucosal tumor (e.g., leiomyoma)
Dieulafoy lesion
Rare
Aortoenteric fistula
Hemobilia
Esophageal rupture
Nasal/pharyngeal bleeding

from the pancreatic or bile ducts), gastric antral vascular ectasias ("watermelon stomach"), or aortoduodenal fistula.

NSAIDs are a common cause of bleeding from ulcers or erosions that may uncommonly occur in the small bowel or colon. NSAID use may not be reported by patients. Bisphosphonates, commonly used for postmenopausal osteoporosis prophylaxis, are associated with UGI bleeding from both gastric ulcer and pill-associated erosive esophagitis. Stress-induced ulcers, gastritis, or gastric erosions are common sources of UGI bleeding in intensive care units. The two primary risk factors for hemorrhage in this setting are respiratory failure and coagulopathy.

Lower Gastrointestinal Bleeding

Colonic sources are one third as common as upper sites. Assigning an exact etiology to a specific source is impossible in some cases of LGI bleeding, in which "proven," "potential," or "possible" bleeding sites (diverticula, hemorrhoids, etc.) are encountered. Visible rectal bleeding can be perianal due to hemorrhoids or anal fissure, both of which may cause pain, itching, or rectal pressure. These local anal disorders are the most common etiologies of minor rectal bleeding, especially in younger patients. Age is a prime determinant of the likelihood of different bleeding sources. Colonic bleeding increases with age, reflecting the increased frequency of common sources of large bowel bleeding in the elderly. Diverticular bleeding is responsible for 25% to 50% of cases of major acute rectal hemorrhage in older individuals. Diverticula, acquired lesions of aging, are pouch-like protrusions of the colonic muscle wall. At age 40, less than 5% of the population has diverticula; the prevalence increases to 30% to 40% at age 60 and 60% to 70% at age 85. Less than 10% of individuals with diverticula develop GI bleeding. Because diverticular bleeding is arteriolar in origin, diverticular hemorrhage is classically abrupt, painless, and major. Alternative diagnoses must be considered when bleeding is occult or minor. Associated acute inflammation (diverticulitis) is typically absent.

Angiodysplasia, resulting from dilated submucosal vessels, is also more common in the elderly. These vascular ectasias, especially in the right colon, account for 20% to 30% of cases of LGI bleeding in the geriatric population. Because bleeding is venous, angiodysplasia may manifest as major hematochezia or more minor hemorrhage, including occult blood loss with or without iron deficiency anemia. Meckel diverticulum must be considered in patients younger than age 25. Colon cancer is rare in younger women, but malignancy is the underlying lesion in as many as 10% of bleeding patients older than age 50. Other diagnostic possibilities include inflammatory bowel disease or ischemic colitis. At any age, a history of chronic liver disease indicates possible portal hypertensive-associated bleeding: Varices may occur in the small bowel, colon, or rectum as well as being esophageal or gastric and may manifest as melena or hematochezia.

Infectious etiologies, including *Campylobacter jejuni, Escherichia coli* 0157:H7, and *Entamoeba histolytica* are considerations in selected patients. *Clostridia difficile* toxin-induced pseudomembranous colitis occasionally presents as rectal bleeding rather than as bloody or nonbloody diarrhea and is possible in any patient having received antibiotics in the preceding 2 months. Less common causes, considered in selected patients, are radiation colitis or vasculitis.

CLINICAL SYMPTOMS

Acute GI bleeding may present as hematemesis, melena, or hematochezia. Vomiting of red blood or of blackish material resembling coffee grounds signifies an UGI site. The passage of blood from the rectum may originate from any part of the GI tract. Hematochezia may be the only complaint in approximately 10% of patients ultimately determined to have a rapidly bleeding UGI source. Melena typically signifies blood loss greater than 100 mL. Melena generally originates from the UGI tract but can result from a bleeding lesion as distal as the right colon. Black stools must be differentiated from the greenish-black color of orally ingested iron or the black stool produced by use of bismuth compounds. In rare circumstances, a patient may confuse vaginal bleeding with a GI source.

A rapid evaluation of possible etiology, site, and severity of hemorrhage is required. Patients with GI bleeding must be assessed for signs of hemodynamic compromise, including fatigue, dizziness, postural complaints, palpitations or chest pain, dyspnea from inadequate blood flow, and poor oxygenation. The presence of complicating factors increases the patient's risk (e.g., age, comorbid illness, anticoagulant use, congenital or acquired clotting disorders) and must be documented. A careful medication history is vital. Some patients may not reveal NSAID use. Even low-dose aspirin use increases bleeding risk, especially when administered concomitantly with NSAIDs. The initial evaluation assesses the magnitude of bleeding and need for resuscitative efforts. Clinical history and examination may not reliably distinguish between UGI and LGI sites in patients presenting with rectal bleeding. Evidence indicates that patient or physician description of the color and quantity of blood loss may be subjective and erroneous. In elderly patients, preexisting dyspepsia may be less common, pain may be less frequent and poorly localized, and clinical details may be impaired by cognitive defects. Syncope in the geriatric age group should raise the possibility of GI bleeding.

PHYSICAL EXAMINATION

The initial assessment of patients with acute GI bleeding requires evaluation of hemodynamic stability. Resuscitative efforts are the primary goal. Because the extent and rapidity of bleeding may not be evident, any evidence of shock or hypotension must be rapidly sought. A careful measurement of postural vital signs revealing tachycardia or decreased blood pressure may be the first indication of major hemodynamically significant hemorrhage. Postural changes in pulse and blood pressure are influenced by underlying cardiovascular status, age, and the rapidity and magnitude of bleeding. Postural hypotension of greater than 10 mm Hg correlates with at least a 15% to 20% reduction in circulating blood volume. Conjunctival pallor, dryness of mucous membranes, tachypnea, or labored respiration supports the impression of hypovolemia. Cutaneous stigmata of portal hypertension or advanced liver disease (jaundice, spider angiomata, ascites, hepatosplenomegaly) are clues for possible variceal bleeding with major management and prognostic implications. The presence of skin ecchymoses suggests anticoagulation or an acquired clotting disorder potentiating bleeding. Useful information is supplied by the presence of an abdominal mass or clinical evidence suggesting chronic liver disease (hepatosplenomegaly, ascites, increased collateral circulation on the anterior abdominal wall). When present, tenderness may be a clue to peptic ulcer disease, inflammatory bowel disease, or mesenteric ischemia. Rectal examination should be performed and may provide information to diagnose perianal pathology such as hemorrhoid or anal fissure. Rectal carcinoma may be palpated on digital examination. Documentation of stool color and magnitude of bleeding may also guide management and determine whether bleeding is from the upper or lower tracts.

LABORATORY EVALUATION

Hemoglobin determination is vital. In an acute bleeding episode, the initial hemoglobin or hematocrit may not reflect the magnitude of bleeding because equilibration with extravascular fluid may take 6 to 24 hours. Red blood cell indices are generally normochromic, normocytic in acute hemorrhage. A decrease in the mean cell volume or mean corpuscular hemoglobin may correlate with acute bleeding superimposed on a chronic source of blood loss and iron deficiency. GI bleeding may also occur in the context of other disorders producing a concomitant vitamin B_{12} or folate deficiency. Hemorrhage from additional sites, including intraperitoneal or from major muscle groups, may coexist. Leukocytosis may accompany acute bleeding, but when present, consideration of active inflammation or infection is prudent. Coagulation status should be assessed, measuring the platelet count, prothrombin time, and partial thromboplastin time.

Stratification of risk in GI bleeding helps predict rebleeding, the need for surgery, and the level of care required. Adverse prognostic features include advancing age, tachycardia, hypotension or shock, orthostatic change in vital signs, anticoagulation, coexisting illnesses, active bleeding at initial evaluation, history of chronic liver disease or malignancy, onset of bleeding in a hospitalized patient, hemoglobin less than 8 g/dL, and rebleeding. Endoscopic predictors of increased risk are presence of esophageal varices, malignant etiology, and stigmata of recent hemorrhage (arterial bleeding, visible vessel in a lesion, or adherent clot).

TREATMENT

Initial management of acute bleeding is focused on resuscitation and the need for replacement of decreased circulating blood volume. Large-caliber intravenous catheters should be inserted for vascular access. Finding fresh blood or coffee ground material on placement of a nasogastric tube localizes the site to the UGI tract. A negative nasogastric aspirate for blood has been reported in up to 25% of cases of documented acute UGI bleeding. Clinically important UGI bleeding may have occurred despite finding no blood on aspiration, because bleeding may have stopped, tube placement may be suboptimal, or no reflux of blood into the stomach from a duodenal bleed is present.

The need for blood transfusion depends on hemodynamic status, magnitude of bleeding, the presence of cardiorespiratory or systemic symptoms, the pattern of hemoglobin change on repeat measurement, and comorbidity. In the patient with a normal initial hemoglobin and stable vital signs without evidence of active bleeding, transfusion may be withheld. Sustained and rapid hemorrhage or hemoglobin less than 10 g/dL with orthostatic change in vital signs or hypotension requires urgent transfusion. Guidelines for transfusion must include providing a reserve if hemorrhage continues or recurs and relief or prevention of symptoms of myocardial ischemia in patients at risk. A target hemoglobin of 10 g/dL may be appropriate in patients with cardiovascular disease.

UGI endoscopy is the diagnostic procedure of choice in known or suspected acute UGI bleeding. Urgent endoscopy is indicated in the presence of hemodynamic instability as resuscitative efforts proceed. Endoscopy is highly accurate in identifying the site and nature of bleeding lesions from the esophagus to the descending duodenum. The ability to achieve hemostasis via a variety of thermal or injection techniques may reduce the rebleeding rate, transfusion requirement, and need for surgery and increase survival. Endoscopic criteria also help stratify risk, informing management decisions concerning need for hospitalization and determination of the intensity of surveillance needed (intensive care unit care). Mortality from variceal hemorrhage is as high as 30% in the initial hospitalization. Endoscopic ligation of varices is the preferred treatment compared with sclerotherapy of varices; the former is associated with a lower rebleeding rate, reduced mortality, and less local complications and achieves obliteration of varices in fewer therapy sessions compared with variceal sclerosis. Contrast (barium) radiographs of the UGI tract are contraindicated in acute bleeding, because contrast will obscure visualization for subsequent endoscopy, arteriography, or surgery. Tagged red blood cell scans using technetium-labeled red blood cells are controversial because of insensitivity in some studies for the detection of bleeding and poor correlation with findings at surgery.

Pharmacologic therapy with antisecretory agents reduces the risk of ulcer rebleeding and hastens healing. The preferred regimen is use of a proton pump inhibitor (PPI), which dramatically reduces acid output. Omeprazole (20 mg orally every 12 hours or its equivalent) decreases rebleeding rates. The availability of parenteral formulations of PPIs has facilitated management. Histamine H_2 receptor antagonists are also used but have less effect on acid reduction and less clinical benefit than PPIs in reducing rebleeding. Ulcer recurrence is markedly decreased by eradication of *H. pylori*, if present, and discontinuation of NSAIDs. Among patients with *H. pylori* infection and a history of UGI bleeding who are taking low-dose aspirin, eradication of the organism is equivalent to treatment with a PPI in preventing recurrent hemorrhage.

Patients with acute LGI bleeding should undergo colonoscopy after oral purgatives unless massive hemorrhage is present or clinical suspicion is most indicative of a perianal source (minor bleeding in a hemodynamically stable patient, especially less than age 40). In the latter case, flexible sigmoidoscopy may be preferred. In massive hematochezia, a rapidly bleeding UGI site must be considered; in this circumstance, patients should have UGI endoscopy before colonic evaluation. Actively bleeding colonic diverticula can occasionally be treated by thermal coagulation techniques or epinephrine injection. The former modality will obliterate angiodysplastic lesions. Barium contrast roentgenograms have no role in initial assessment of acute LGI bleeding. Angiography must be considered as the initial test in patients with massive hemorrhage. Persistent, massive, or recurrent bleeding requires surgical evaluation with an attempt at preoperative localization, except in the rare case of potentially exsanguinating hemorrhage.

ACUTE BLEEDING IN PREGNANCY

The maternal hematocrit may not reliably indicate the magnitude of bleeding because of differing effects of intravascular fluid accumulation and an increase in total erythrocyte mass during pregnancy. Because of the use of ionizing radiation, UGI radiography is contraindicated during pregnancy. Data suggest that yearly in the United States, conditions normally associated with an indication for UGI endoscopy occur in 12,000 pregnant women. Case series of small numbers of patients undergoing UGI endoscopy suggest that endoscopy is relatively safe during pregnancy when the clinical information to be gained is vital. One series of 20 patients found no serious complications in the 19 patients with known outcomes. Colonoscopy during pregnancy should typically be reserved for uncontrolled hemorrhage. Unconfirmed evidence suggests teratogenicity of diazepam sedation for endoscopy.

OCCULT GASTROINTESTINAL BLEEDING

The American Gastroenterological Association characterizes occult GI bleeding as the presence of a positive fecal occult blood test or iron deficiency anemia without visible evidence of blood loss apparent to patient or physician. Obscure bleeding is defined as bleeding of unknown cause that presents or recurs after an initially negative evaluation, including colonoscopy and UGI endoscopy. Patients with GI blood loss of less than 100 mL/d may not have melena or hematochezia. The fecal occult blood test depends on the property of guaiac to turn blue upon oxidation by hemoglobin in the presence of the reagent hydrogen peroxide. The probability of a positive fecal test for occult blood depends on the quantity of blood in stool. Physicians must be aware that orally administered iron does not cause positive guaiac-based fecal occult blood tests, although the black or dark-green color of iron-containing stool may be mistaken for the blue of a true-positive test.

Etiology

A prime concern in adults is to detect or exclude colon carcinoma or advanced benign large bowel polyps. Underlying lesions in occult bleeding, however, may be located anywhere from the mouth to the rectum. Tumors of the esophagus, stomach, or small bowel may also produce bleeding. Rarely, bleeding may be due to metastatic malignancy or erosion of a contiguous tumor into the GI tract. Inflammatory lesions are a common cause of bleeding. Peptic ulcer, esophagitis, and inflammatory bowel disease must be considered. A careful medication history is vital, with NSAIDs as the most common drug implicated. Other medications have been associated with UGI inflammation, including oral potassium chloride tablets, calcium channel blockers, and bisphosphonates (used commonly in prevention of postmenopausal osteoporosis). Neither warfarin anticoagulation nor aspirin prophylaxis of cardiovascular disease should be considered sufficient to produce occult bleeding.

The small bowel is responsible for bleeding in less than 10% of cases. The most common small intestinal lesions are vascular ectasias, followed by small bowel tumors and NSAID-related small bowel ulceration. Celiac sprue, a common cause of iron malabsorption, may also cause occult bleeding. In young adults, tumors are a more common small bowel cause for bleeding. In the elderly, bleeding vascular ectasia and tumors (carcinoma, adenomas) are frequent sources. Rare causes include long distance running (which is associated with decreased splanchnic blood flow and possible ischemic colitis or gastritis). Esophageal varices and colonic diverticula, common sources of acute blood loss, do not cause occult bleeding. Patients with portal hypertension, however, may have occult bleeding from a congestive gastropathy. Rarely, epistaxis, bleeding from the gums, oral lesions, or misdiagnosed hemoptysis will be responsible.

Occult blood loss in premenopausal women represents a distinct and controversial group. Iron deficiency may be as high as 10% in this group, with iron deficiency anemia present in 5%. In addition to GI blood loss, decreased iron stores in younger women may reflect menstrual losses, dietary factors, possible iron loss with pregnancy and lactation, or iron malabsorption. Endoscopic evaluation in the setting of iron deficiency anemia in premenopausal women has been associated with a 12% yield for relevant GI pathology, including peptic ulcer and gastric and colonic malignancy. Results suggest the need for endoscopic evaluation in premenopausal women with anemia not clinically consistent with menstrual losses, the presence of a positive fecal occult blood test, hemoglobin less than 10 g/dL, or suggestive abdominal complaints. The threshold for GI assessment of younger women is higher than that for older patients. Iron deficiency anemia in premenopausal women should be attributed to menorrhagia with caution and evaluation individualized.

Symptoms

Patients may be identified by a positive fecal occult blood test during routine physical examination, as part of screening for colon cancer, or during evaluation of abdominal complaints. Occult blood loss in the absence of anemia causes no symptoms other than any associated with specific underlying pathology. In this setting, the clinical history is directed toward medications injurious to the GI tract, any complaints referable to the digestive system, or symptoms of malignancy or other potential disorders capable of producing bleeding. The patient with anemia secondary to chronic GI blood loss may have multiple complaints, including weakness, fatigue, headache, irritability, dyspnea, or chest pain. Symptoms may appear or be exacerbated by exercise or the standing position.

Physical Examination

No abnormalities are found, in general, in the patient with incidentally discovered occult bleeding. Occasional patients will have evidence of the causative disorder. Stigmata of chronic liver disease or an abdominal mass or tenderness are possible findings. The patient with iron deficiency anemia may have signs reflecting the effect of chronic blood loss depending on cardiovascular status, age, and magnitude and duration of bleeding. Tachycardia, tachypnea, postural change in pulse or blood pressure, and conjunctival pallor may be present.

Laboratory Evaluation

Documentation of fecal occult blood loss requires evaluation. Hemoglobin must be measured to determine if anemia exists. If present, anemia due to iron deficiency is generally confirmed by a decreased serum ferritin level. Occasional patients will require a bone marrow biopsy to differentiate between various types of anemia (Table 60.2).

Colonoscopy is the most accurate and widely used modality to evaluate the large bowel in patients with occult bleeding. Colonoscopy has the advantages of directly visualizing large bowel mucosa and the ability to biopsy suspect lesions, remove colonic adenomas, and ablate angiodysplasia. Air–contrast barium enema has a higher false-negative rate for both colon carcinoma and benign large bowel polyps but is indicated when technical performance of colonoscopy is suboptimal or incomplete. In younger women, a less invasive preferred evaluation may be air–contrast barium enema complemented by flexible sigmoidoscopy rather than colonoscopy. Similarly, choice of barium enema may be appropriate based on individualized risk of conscious sedation, general patient condition, or comorbid conditions. Younger individuals may also be considered initially for a brief empiric trial of treatment directed against hemorrhoids and anal fissure. Preliminary data suggest that computed tomographic-assisted colonoscopy (virtual colonoscopy) may eventually become a practical modality for diagnosis in this setting. Colonoscopy is generally the first diagnostic test because the imperative in unexplained, asymptomatic, occult bleeding, especially in older patients, is to exclude colon cancer or advanced adenoma. Collected series indicate that a negative colonoscopy

TABLE 60.2. Occult GI Bleeding: Differential Diagnosis

Inflammatory lesions
Esophagitis
Peptic ulcer
Celiac disease
Inflammatory bowel disease
Tumors
Carcinoma
Large bowel adenoma
Small bowel tumor (benign, malignant)
Vascular
Ischemic colitis
Angiodysplasia
Congestive gastropathy/colopathy (due to portal hypertension)
Dieulafoy lesion
Gastric antral vascular ectasia
Infectious
Non-GI origin
Epistaxis
Hemoptysis
Oral source
Hemobilia/hemosuccus pancreaticus

should be followed by UGI endoscopy with a yield for clinically relevant pathology of 25% to 40%.

When the source of iron deficiency anemia remains unclear after both colonoscopy and UGI endoscopy, small bowel pathology must be considered. Contrast radiographs of the small intestine are insensitive for mucosal abnormalities but may document a mass lesion. Endoscopic evaluation of the small bowel by enteroscopy should be considered after negative colonoscopy and UGI endoscopy in patients with persistent symptoms, failure of iron-replacement therapy, and in those in whom occult bleeding has recurred after a symptom-free interval. Small bowel angiodysplasia is the most common finding in this setting. Wireless capsule endoscopy, producing photos of the small intestine, may assume greater diagnostic prominence in the future.

Treatment

Iron replacement with oral ferrous sulfate is indicated in cases of iron deficiency anemia. Specific treatment is that of the underlying disorder.

Occult Bleeding in Pregnancy

Local perianal lesions (hemorrhoids and rectal fissures) may be more common in the gravid state. The increased incidence of reflux esophagitis in pregnancy may be associated with occult bleeding. Peptic ulcer disease and its complications are not more common during pregnancy. Diagnostic evaluation by endoscopy is generally reserved for biopsy of suspected malignancy and selected cases of occult GI blood loss producing severe iron deficiency anemia.

BIBLIOGRAPHY

American Society of Gastrointestinal Endoscopy. An annotated algorithmic approach to upper gastrointestinal bleeding. *Gastrointest Endosc* 2001;53:853–858.

American Society of Gastrointestinal Endoscopy. An annotated algorithmic approach to acute lower gastrointestinal bleeding. *Gastrointest Endosc* 2001;53:859–863.

Bini EJ, Micale PL, Weinshel EH. Evaluation of the gastrointestinal tract in premenopausal women with iron-deficiency anemia. *Am J Med* 1998;105:281–286.

Bond JH. Rectal bleeding: is it always an indication for colonoscopy? *Am J Gastroenterol* 2002;97:223–224.

Cappell MS. The safety and efficacy of gastrointestinal endoscopy during pregnancy. *Gastroenterol Clin North Am* 1998;27:37–71.

Chan FKL, Chung SC, Suen BY, et al. Preventing recurrent upper gastrointestinal bleeding in patients with *Helicobacter pylori* infection who are taking low-dose aspirin or naproxen. *N Engl J Med* 2001;341:967–973.

Chan FKL, Sung JJ. The medical care of patients with gastrointestinal bleeding after endoscopy. *Gastroenterol Clin North Am* 1997;7:671–682.

Freeman ML. Stigmata of hemorrhage in bleeding ulcers. *Gastrointest Endosc Clin North Am* 1997;7:559–583.

Hay JA, Maldonado L, Weingarten SR, et al. Prospective evaluation of a clinical guideline recommending hospital length of stay in upper gastrointestinal tract hemorrhage. *JAMA* 1997;278:2151–2156.

Hernandez-Diaz S, Rodriguez LA. Association between nonsteroidal anti-inflammatory drugs and upper gastrointestinal tract bleeding/perforation: an overview of epidemiologic studies published in the 1990s. *Arch Intern Med* 2000;160:2093–2099.

Imperiale TF, Birgisson S. Somatostatin or octreotide compared with H2 antagonists and placebo in the management of acute nonvariceal hemorrhage: a meta-analysis. *Ann Intern Med* 1997;127:1062–1071.

Jensen DM, Machicado GA, Jutabha RJ, et al. Urgent colonoscopy for the diagnosis of severe diverticular hemorrhage. *N Engl J Med* 2000;342:28–82.

Laine L, Peterson WL. Bleeding peptic ulcer. *N Engl J Med* 1994;331:717–727.

Lau JY, Sung JJ, Lee KK, et al. Effect of intravenous omeprazole on recurrent bleeding after endoscopic treatment of bleeding peptic ulcers. *N Engl J Med* 2000;343:310–316.

Longstreth GF. Epidemiology of hospitalization for acute upper gastrointestinal hemorrhage: a population-based study. *Am J Gastroenterol* 1995;90:206–210.

McGuire HH Jr. Bleeding colonic diverticula: a reappraisal of natural history and management. *Ann Surg* 1994;220:653–656.

Rockey DC. Occult gastrointestinal bleeding. *N Engl J Med* 1999;341:38–45.

Schoenfeld PS, Butler JA. An evidence-based approach to the treatment of esophageal variceal bleeding. *Crit Care Clin* 1998;14:441–455.

Zuccarro G. Management of the adult patient with acute lower gastrointestinal bleeding. *Am J Gastroenterol* 1998;93:1202–1208.

Zuckerman GR, Prakash C. Acute lower intestinal bleeding: clinical presentation and diagnosis. *Gastrointest Endosc* 1998;48:606–616.

Zuckerman GO, Prakask C, Askin MP, et al. AGA technical review on the evaluation and management of occult and obscure gastrointestinal bleeding. *Gastroenterology* 2000;118:201–221.

CHAPTER 61

Gastroesophageal Reflux Disease

Sripathi R. Kethu and Edward Feller

Gastroesophageal reflux disease (GERD) is one of the most common gastrointestinal disorders seen by the primary care physician. Nearly everyone experiences heartburn or acid regurgitation at some point. GERD encompasses a spectrum of disorders; the presenting symptoms and signs may vary widely. It is best defined as chronic symptoms or mucosal damage produced by the abnormal reflux of gastric contents into the esophagus. Reflux esophagitis denotes a subset of patients with GERD symptoms and endoscopic evidence of inflammation. Not all patients with symptoms of heartburn have esophagitis on upper endoscopy. Patients with nonerosive reflux disease have heartburn complaints with a normal endoscopic examination of the esophagus.

EPIDEMIOLOGY

At least 20% of people in the United States suffer from heartburn or acid regurgitation once a week, and 7% experience symptoms daily. It is estimated that over 25% of American adults ingest antacids more than twice a month. Most of these heavy users of antacids suffer from reflux, and many experience relief with this therapy. GERD is often considered to be a disorder of advancing age. Indeed, persons over age 50 are much more likely to require medical attention for symptoms or complications of reflux than younger individuals. However, GERD may occur in any age group, including young children. Although there is no reported difference in the rate of GERD complaints between men and women, up to 75% of pregnant women experience heartburn. Males are more likely than females to be affected with some of the complications of GERD, such as esophagitis or Barrett esophagus. GERD occurs in all demographic groups.

Some patients with GERD develop local complications such as esophagitis, esophageal ulcer, stricture, or cancer. Fewer develop extraesophageal complications, including asthma, laryngitis, and pneumonitis. Worldwide, it is estimated that the evaluation and treatment of GERD is responsible for $2 to $3 billion per year in medical costs.

An iceberg model is often used to describe populations with GERD. Most persons with GERD make up the hidden base of the iceberg, experiencing only mild symptoms and rarely seeking medical care. Just below the surface is a smaller group whose symptoms are frequent and severe enough to require medical attention, although complications are uncommon. The tip of the iceberg represents the small proportion of patients with GERD who have severe chronic symptoms commonly associated with complications such as esophagitis, stricture, bleeding, or cancer. They invariably require medical care.

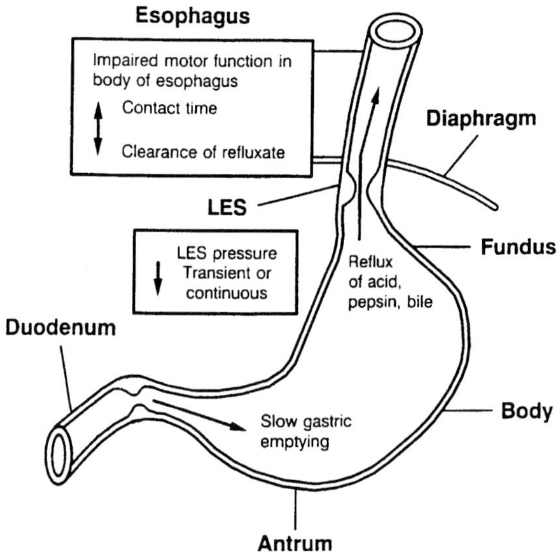

FIG. 61.1. Mechanisms involved in the development of gastroesophageal reflux disease. (Adapted from Wolfe MM. Pathophysiology and clinical implications of gastroesophageal reflux disease. Pract Gastroenterol 1994;18:S10, with permission.)

ETIOLOGY

GERD is a spectrum of disorders in which there is reflux of acid and other noxious substances from the stomach into the esophagus. This causes symptoms such as heartburn or acid regurgitation with or without associated damage to the esophageal mucosa. Nearly everyone has episodes of gastroesophageal reflux, usually after eating; they are considered a normal physiologic occurrence and are usually not perceived by the individual. When the contact between gastric secretions and the esophageal mucosa is unusually long or protective mechanisms are overwhelmed, GERD may develop.

Many factors determine whether someone develops GERD, including (a) antireflux barrier, (b) esophageal clearance, (c) the potency of refluxate, and (d) esophageal mucosal defenses. Abnormalities in any one of these can lead to epithelial damage (Fig. 61.1).

Reflux of gastric contents into the esophagus is usually prevented by barrier mechanisms, the most important of which is the lower esophageal sphincter (LES). This ring of smooth muscle is 2.5 to 3.5 cm long and is located at the gastroesophageal junction, just below the diaphragm. (When a hiatal hernia is present, the gastroesophageal junction and the LES extend above the diaphragm.) The sphincter relaxes in response to swallowing a bolus of food, allowing the food to pass into the stomach. Once the food passes, the LES reverts back to a pressure high enough to prevent gastric contents from refluxing back into the esophagus. Several factors—drugs, hormones, and foods—may affect LES tone and lead to inappropriate relaxation (Table 61.1). This allows gastric contents to enter the esophagus more frequently or in greater amounts, exacerbating reflux in susceptible persons.

Hormones may affect the tone of the LES. Oral contraceptives and other estrogen–progesterone supplements decrease LES pressure. This effect is probably related to the progesterone content of the drugs, although estrogen may also play a priming role. Heartburn is more common in the latter parts of the menstrual cycle and pregnancy. This effect is due at least partially to a hormonally mediated decrease in the sphincter pressure.

Many foods decrease LES pressure. Chocolate is a notorious promoter of reflux and probably adversely affects the sphincter because of its methylxanthine content. Carminatives such as spearmint and peppermint also relax the LES; onions may have a similar effect. Fatty foods are particularly effective in increasing esophageal acid exposure. This effect is related to two mechanisms induced by fat ingestion: reduction in the LES pressure and delayed gastric emptying. Although coffee has a bad repu-

TABLE 61.1. Factors Causing Diminished LES Pressure

Drugs
Anticholinergics
Calcium channel blockers
Nitrates
α-Adrenergic antagonists
β_2-Adrenergics
Methylxanthines
Prostaglandins
Meperidine
Diazepam
Morphine
Barbiturates
Angiotensin-converting enzyme inhibitors
Cardioselective β_1-antagonists
Oral contraceptives and hormonal supplements
Foods
Chocolate
Carminatives (spearmint and peppermint)
Onions
Fat
Alcohol
Nicotine
Systemic disorders
Scleroderma
Mixed connective tissue disease
Pregnancy

tation when it comes to GERD, its effect on the LES is unknown. Recent studies seem to indicate that coffee promotes GERD by direct irritation of the esophageal mucosa and by increasing acid production, not by reducing LES pressure. Alcohol and nicotine both relax the LES and promote esophageal reflux. Certain diseases are associated with a chronically diminished LES tone, including scleroderma and mixed connective tissue disease. GERD frequently complicates these systemic disorders and may be particularly severe.

Esophageal clearance—the ability of the esophagus to empty or neutralize gastric contents—is important in the prevention of GERD. Primary peristalsis is stimulated by swallowing and secondary peristalsis by esophageal distention. Together these actions clear much of the refluxed material; the rest is neutralized by swallowed saliva. Persons with GERD have prolonged esophageal clearance times, increasing the duration of contact of refluxed gastric contents with esophageal mucosa. Reflux frequency correlates less well with tissue damage than does duration of reflux. This distinction is best illustrated in esophageal motor disorders such as scleroderma, where there is diminished peristaltic function, resulting in impaired esophageal clearance and GERD. An impaired flow of saliva affects the rate of neutralization of the refluxate. Salivary flow diminishes at night, making this a vulnerable time for GERD. Chronic xerostomia, seen in Sjögren syndrome, or diminished salivary flow due to cigarette smoking or the use of anticholinergic drugs promotes esophageal acid exposure.

The potency of the material that refluxes into the esophagus also affects the development of GERD. Hydrogen is probably the final mediator of tissue injury, but additional substances such as pepsin, bile, and food hyperosmolality may also play a role. Most people with GERD have normal or slightly elevated basal levels of gastric acid secretion; some have gastric hypersecretion.

The esophageal mucosal defense mechanisms, although not well understood, undoubtedly play an important role in the prevention of GERD. The esophagus has several defenses against cellular acidification, a process that leads to tissue injury. The superficial layer of squamous epithelium of the esophageal mucosa, the stratum corneum, is a "tight" epithelium that deters back diffusion of hydrogen ions and other toxic substances into the mucosa. This defense can be overcome when a high concentration of hydrochloric acid is perfused into the esophageal lumen. Acidification of the surface cells occurs, they become ballooned and necrotic, and esophagitis results.

Foods promote reflux in several ways. Many affect LES pressure, as noted above. Other foods, such as coffee, beer, and milk, are potent stimuli of gastric acid secretion. Still others may directly irritate the esophageal mucosa, such as orange juice, tomato drinks, and perhaps coffee.

Increase in gastric and intra-abdominal pressure may exceed the ability of even a normal LES to keep gastric contents within the stomach. For example, an association exists between morbid obesity and GERD. In obese people, the gastroesophageal pressure gradient, not the absolute LES pressure, determines reflux. Tight clothing, ascites, pregnancy, or obesity encourage reflux during sphincter relaxation.

At different times during the past 50 years, hiatal hernia has been thought to be either synonymous with GERD or an insignificant bystander. Current understanding suggests that hiatal hernia may be a factor in the development of GERD. Along with the smooth muscle LES, the striated muscle crural diaphragm is a component of the antireflux barrier. In the setting of a hernia, the anatomic relation between the diaphragm and the LES is altered, potentially weakening the antireflux barrier. A hernia may potentiate reflux by increasing the frequency of transient LES relaxations. In addition, acid clearance by the esophagus may be impaired when a hiatal hernia is present.

Other factors may play a role in the development of GERD. Delayed gastric emptying as a result of mechanical, hormonal, or neurologic factors predisposes to more frequent episodes of reflux. Exercise, such as jogging, may induce reflux by decreasing LES pressure. Although *Helicobacter pylori* is a common etiology of gastritis and peptic ulcer, no difference in frequency of this infection exists in individuals with and without GERD. Eradication of *H. pylori* does not ameliorate heartburn or affect esophageal mucosal healing.

In summary, the consistent event in the development of GERD is the movement of gastric contents from the stomach into the esophagus. If the refluxed material is particularly injurious, or if there is perturbation of either the antireflux barrier or mucosal defenses, or diminished esophageal clearance is present, GERD may occur.

CLINICAL FEATURES

Symptoms

GERD encompasses a spectrum of symptoms (Table 61.2). The most common symptom, reported by over half of affected patients, is heartburn. Also called pyrosis, this is classically described as a retrosternal burning sensation. It may radiate, wave-like, from the epigastrium up to the neck or, less commonly, into the back or the arms. Sometimes the discomfort is limited to the epigastric area or the throat.

Heartburn is an intermittent symptom, usually occurring within an hour after meals (particularly if they are large or high in fat), during exercise, or with bending or lying down. It is usually relieved quickly with antacids, although the beneficial effect may not persist. Heartburn is thought to be caused by the stimulation of nerve endings in the esophageal epithelium by refluxed acid.

Heartburn may be associated with regurgitation, the return of gastric or esophageal contents into the pharynx. The fluid may be described as bitter or sour. It most commonly occurs when the person is lying down or bending over. Some individuals are awakened at night. Vomiting is less common, generally effortless, and is not associated with nausea or abdominal contractions when related to GERD.

Water brash or hypersalivation is the spontaneous appearance of fluid in the mouth. It is secondary to the esophagosali-

TABLE 61.2. Clinical Features of GERD

Heartburn: Most common symptom of GERD, experienced by over 75%
Regurgitation: Nearly as common as heartburn
Vomiting: "Effortless" when associated with GERD
Water brash: Increase in salivary flow; salty or bland tasting
Dysphagia: Difficulty swallowing due to acid-induced dysmotility
Odynophagia: Painful swallowing; uncommon in uncomplicated GERD
Chest pain: May mimic cardiac pain
Globus sensation: Persistent lump or tickle in the throat
Hoarseness: Related to laryngeal inflammation from acid reflux
Cough: Manifestation of laryngeal or pulmonary disease from GERD
Asthma: 50% of adults with asthma have associated GERD
Pneumonia: Possible complication of GERD

GERD, gastroesophageal reflux disease.

vary reflex, the stimulation of salivary secretion that occurs with reflux. The fluid is described as salty or bland tasting.

Dysphagia occurs in about one third of patients with GERD. This is a sensation that the passage of food is delayed or becomes stuck as it moves from the pharynx to the stomach. Dysphagia may be due to a peptic stricture from acid reflux with tissue damage. Mucosal inflammation without persisting luminal narrowing may induce spasm with subsequent dysphagia. An abnormal sensory perception within the esophagus or an associated motility disorder may play a role in this symptom. Progressive dysphagia over weeks or months that is worse for solids than liquids, in the setting of GERD, suggests the development of a peptic or malignant stricture.

Odynophagia refers to pain with swallowing. The pain is usually localized to the retrosternal area and is a rare complaint with uncomplicated GERD. Odynophagia invariably indicates a severe inflammatory process. It is more common in the setting of infectious esophagitis and pill-induced esophagitis than in GERD.

Chest pain distinct from heartburn or odynophagia may occur as a result of GERD. It is the only symptom in 10% of patients with this disorder. The pain may be gripping or knife-like and usually occurs in the retrosternal area. The pain is not always related to swallowing but may be triggered by the ingestion of very hot or cold liquids. It may radiate to the abdomen, back, neck, or arm and can be severe. Pain of esophageal origin may be difficult to distinguish from angina. As many as half of the patients with chest pain who have normal coronary angiograms may have GERD as a cause of their symptoms. The cause of chest pain in individuals with GERD is unclear. It may be an extension of heartburn or secondary to acid-induced esophageal spasm.

Globus sensation is almost constant perception of a lump, fullness, or tickle in the throat. It is unrelated to swallowing and is occasionally seen as a manifestation of GERD. The mechanism for this symptom is not well understood, although psychological factors may be important.

Complications

The complications of GERD reflect the mucosal injury or esophagitis that occurs in some patients. Approximately 50% of patients with heartburn may have no esophagitis on upper endoscopy, leading to the term nonerosive reflux disease. In these patients, low-grade inflammation may be detected only histologically. Red streaks or erosions extending proximally up the esophagus are the earliest changes of esophagitis. As the damage progresses, the injury becomes more confluent, eventually involving the entire circumference of the esophageal lumen. Edema, hyperemia, and friability of the mucosa may develop, with progression to deep ulceration. Histologic findings range from increased height of the papillae and basal cell hyperplasia as the earliest changes to infiltration of the mucosa by acute and chronic inflammatory cells.

Bleeding may occur from reflux-induced erosions or ulcerations of the esophageal mucosa. The bleeding is often insidious and can eventually lead to an iron deficiency anemia. Frank hemorrhage is rare and is usually due to an esophageal ulcer. A stricture of the esophagus, narrowing of the lumen, is a complication that results from chronic inflammation or ulceration of the esophageal mucosa. Continued mucosal damage with partial healing leads to fibrosis and narrowing of the lumen of the esophagus. Strictures are more common in the elderly, in those with Barrett esophagus, and in patients with scleroderma. Most patients who develop strictures have a history of heartburn, although as many as 25% of patients present without a history suggestive of GERD. Certain drugs may increase the tendency to develop strictures in the setting of GERD, including potassium tablets, doxycycline, quinidine, and nonsteroidal antiinflammatory drugs. The most common presenting symptom of a stricture is slowly progressive dysphagia. In the case of a reflux-induced stricture, the dysphagia is initially for solid food, particularly meat. If left untreated, patients may eventually have difficulty with soft foods and liquids as well. Reflux-induced strictures are usually short and located in the distal esophagus (Fig. 61.2). Sudden esophageal obstruction, usually due to meat impaction, may also occur.

The most severe histologic consequence of chronic GERD is Barrett esophagus, in which squamous epithelium is replaced with metaplastic columnar epithelium. Intestinal metaplasia represents a premalignant lesion of esophageal adenocarcinoma. This metaplastic change may involve a small portion of the distal end of the esophagus or may involve the entire organ. Patients with Barrett esophagus may have more severe reflux, although the symptoms may be indistinguishable from those without Barrett esophagus. In fact, up to one third of patients with Barrett esophagus have no symptoms of reflux. The

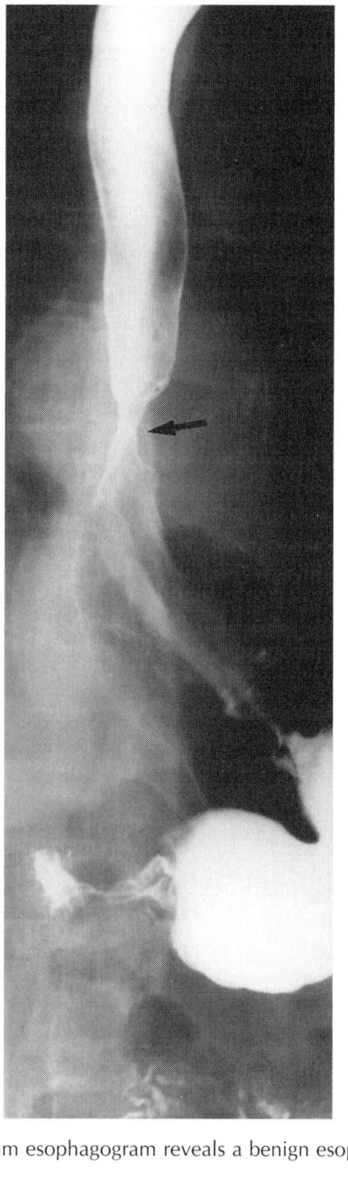

FIG. 61.2. Barium esophagogram reveals a benign esophageal stricture *(arrow)*.

esophageal mucosa may be relatively insensitive to pain in these patients. The frequency of Barrett esophagus in the general population is unknown. In patients with long-standing GERD undergoing endoscopy, the prevalence is 5% to 12%. In patients with more severe GERD, such as those with strictures or scleroderma, Barrett esophagus reportedly occurs in as many as 40%. Barrett esophagus is more common in men than in women. The significance of Barrett mucosa lies in its malignant potential, because the columnar epithelium is more likely to develop adenocarcinoma. The risk of developing esophageal adenocarcinoma in patients with Barrett esophagus is 0.5% per year. Increased risk of cancer is associated with the length of the Barrett esophagus and the presence of dysplasia.

Extraesophageal Manifestations

Extraesophageal disorders that may develop as a result of GERD include signs and symptoms related to the oropharynx, larynx, and respiratory tract. Laryngeal symptoms due to GERD include hoarseness, a persistent nonproductive cough, a sensation of pressure deep in the throat, and the need to clear the throat continually. These otolaryngologic symptoms may be due to direct tissue injury by refluxed gastric contents. Classic symptoms of reflux or esophagitis are often minimal in these patients. Nocturnal reflux may be the key to the development of laryngeal disorders, perhaps related to a diminution of the upper esophageal sphincter tone at night. Refluxed acid might then reach the proximal esophagus and regurgitate into the hypopharynx. A diagnostic clue may be the appearance or exacerbation of symptoms in the morning after a night in the recumbent position.

GERD appears to exacerbate or potentiate asthma in some patients. As many as 50% of adult patients with asthma may have GERD. The exact mechanisms responsible for the pulmonary manifestations of reflux are not well understood. Two possible mechanisms have been proposed. First, recurrent microaspiration of gastric contents into the lungs, resulting in acid-induced injury and bronchoconstriction. A second potential cause is vagally mediated reflex bronchoconstriction occurring when acid refluxes into the esophagus. In some cases, the association may be due to a shared risk factor, such as smoking. As is seen with laryngeal disease, many persons with asthma and GERD have minimal reflux symptoms or esophagitis. Although endoscopic or pH monitoring may identify asthmatics with GERD, neither method proves that cause and effect exists. Symptoms that may suggest reflux-related asthma include onset of asthma at a late age; nocturnal cough or wheezing; asthma that is exacerbated after meals, exercise, or the supine position; and asthma that is exacerbated by bronchodilators (which may reduce LES tone). Collected data suggest that treatment of GERD may improve respiratory symptoms in selected patients with asthma.

GERD may be the cause of 10% to 40% of cases of chronic cough. Acid stimulation of esophageal nerve endings may activate cough centers. These patients may not complain of heartburn; thus, diagnosis may be missed or delayed unless clinical suspicion is present. Recurrent pneumonia, bronchitis, and possibly pulmonary fibrosis have also been proposed to be complications of GERD.

NATURAL HISTORY

GERD is generally a chronic condition, most often requiring long-term therapy. Symptoms are heterogeneous without clear relation between symptoms and either the amount of reflux or the degree of mucosal injury within the esophagus. For example, a 3-year follow-up study of patients with endoscopically mild esophagitis indicated that only 5% progressed to a more severe type of esophagitis, 50% had no changes, and 45% spontaneously healed.

DIFFERENTIAL DIAGNOSIS

Several gastrointestinal and nongastrointestinal disorders may mimic GERD. Although typical symptoms of GERD are generally quite characteristic, it is sometimes necessary to distinguish them from those related to cholelithiasis, peptic ulcer, gastritis, infectious or pill esophagitis, dyspepsia, coronary artery disease, and esophageal motor disorders.

Some patients may have chest pain that is difficult to distinguish from angina. Pain may even radiate into the jaw or arms and be exacerbated by exertion. Because both GERD and coronary artery disease are common disorders of middle age, some women have symptoms of both, resulting in difficulty distinguishing between the two. If coronary ischemia is a potential diagnosis, a cardiac evaluation should be performed before gastrointestinal studies are considered.

Dyspepsia refers to a heterogeneous group of symptoms defined as pain or discomfort in the upper abdomen, which may be accompanied by an array of complaints, including fullness, bloating, distention, eructation, indigestion, early satiety, and nausea. Although dyspepsia is commonly due to a structural lesion such as peptic ulcer or gastric cancer, more than half of all patients do not have any detectable organic cause.

Pill and infectious esophagitis are usually associated with significant odynophagia, which is rare in uncomplicated GERD. Infectious esophagitis can be seen in immunocompromised persons and is commonly caused by *Candida albicans*, the herpes simplex virus, and cytomegalovirus. *Candida* is associated with a cheesy exudate on the surface of the mucosa of the esophagus; herpes and cytomegalovirus typically cause multiple punctate ulcerations. Medications such as bisphosphonates (alendronate and risedronate), potassium chloride, quinidine, and tetracycline may cause single deep ulcers, usually at a level where the pill may transiently hang up, such as the aortic arch. Most other disorders that could be clinically confused with GERD can be excluded or documented with upper endoscopy, an upper gastrointestinal series, and biliary ultrasonography.

DIAGNOSIS

The diagnosis of GERD may be established in several ways. In most cases, a careful history elicits symptoms that are sufficient to confirm a diagnosis of GERD. Heartburn or regurgitation that occurs after meals or is exacerbated by the recumbent position and relieved by antacids is the typical symptom of GERD. In most persons, no further diagnostic testing is required.

Further investigation is warranted in patients with heartburn associated with "alarm" symptoms such as recent weight loss, dysphagia, odynophagia, guaiac-positive stools, or anemia. Atypical symptoms or persistent problems despite therapy are also indications to pursue the diagnosis. Choice of the initial diagnostic test depends entirely on what question needs to be answered—whether the presence of reflux is in question or if investigation is required to detect and treat complications.

Barium Esophagogram

When a double-contrast technique is used, cases of moderate and severe esophagitis may be demonstrated, especially if ulcerations are present. When compared with upper endoscopy, however, contrast radiographs have only 50% sensitivity in detecting mucosal injury. The demonstration of reflux by this study has questionable significance. In one representative study, for example, the sensitivity of barium radiography in demonstrating reflux was only 26% when compared with ambulatory pH monitoring. The barium esophagogram remains a useful initial examination in a patient with dysphagia because of its ability to detect subtle strictures, assess esophageal peristaltic function, and provide necessary information to plan possible endoscopic evaluation and therapy.

Upper Endoscopy

Upper endoscopy is considered if studies to document the complications of GERD are required. Endoscopy provides direct visualization of the esophageal mucosa and has a high sensitivity and specificity in detecting mucosal injury. Endoscopic findings in patients with GERD include erythema, edema, friability, exudate, erosions, ulcerations, strictures, and Barrett epithelium. Endoscopic biopsy is the most sensitive test to document tissue injury. However, endoscopy is an insensitive test to demonstrate the presence of reflux.

Twenty-Four–Hour Ambulatory pH Monitoring

Twenty-four–hour ambulatory esophageal pH monitoring remains the gold standard for detecting reflux but is unnecessary in most patients. For this study, a small pH electrode is passed transnasally and positioned in the lower esophagus. Intraesophageal pH is recorded continuously over 24 hours by a portable recorder that is attached to the patient's belt or a shoulder strap. The percentage of time that the pH in the distal esophagus is less than 4.0 is a good criterion for GERD, although some overlap occurs between normal persons and those with GERD. Patients with typical symptoms and documented esophagitis do not need to undergo this study. This test is useful in patients who do not respond to therapy or who have atypical chest pain, pulmonary symptoms, unexplained hoarseness, or when confirmation of GERD is required before antireflux surgery.

Esophageal Manometry

Esophageal manometric studies can measure LES pressure and esophageal peristalsis but are of limited value in diagnosing GERD. The measurement of esophageal motility may be necessary, however, if disorders such as achalasia or scleroderma must be excluded. If a patient with GERD is being considered for surgical therapy, motility studies help verify the presence of effective peristalsis within the esophagus, which should be confirmed to avoid postoperative dysphagia.

TREATMENT OPTIONS

The goals of treatment of GERD are to control symptoms, to heal esophagitis, and to prevent relapse and complications.

Lifestyle Modifications

Lifestyle modifications should be part of the initial management in almost everyone with GERD, whether it is mild or severe. They include elevating the head of the bed by using 6-inch blocks under the legs at that head-end or a foam wedge under the pillow or mattress, avoiding recumbency for 3 hours after meals, smoking cessation, decreasing fat intake, avoiding tight-fitting garments, restricting alcohol and chocolate intake, losing weight if necessary, and avoiding drugs that potentially decrease LES pressure (Table 61.3). These modifications promote the esophageal clearance of acid and minimize episodes of reflux.

Pharmacologic Therapy

ANTACIDS AND ALGINIC ACID

Antacids increase gastric pH, deactivate pepsin, and may increase LES pressure through gastric alkalinization. Alginic acid forms a foamy layer on the surface of gastric secretions and creates a barrier between acid and the esophageal mucosa. Antacids and alginic acid have been shown to be more effective than placebo in relieving symptoms of GERD. In two open-label studies, combined antacid–alginic acid use led to an improvement in symptoms in 80% of subjects with GERD. Data indicate that healing of erosive esophagitis is correlated directly with the proportion of a 24-hour period in which the pH of the stomach remains above 4. However, patients should be cautioned against excessive use of such medication because they mask the development of worsening disease or complications. Moreover, many patients may have already used over-the- counter preparations before seeking medical care, necessitating prescription medications for acid-suppressive therapy.

HISTAMINE H_2 RECEPTOR ANTAGONISTS

Many patients with mild occasional symptoms respond well to lifestyle changes and intermittent antacid or alginic acid therapy. Those with persistent symptoms or a complication of GERD, however, generally require acid-suppressive therapy. The histamine H_2 receptor antagonists (H2-RAs) inhibit gastric acid secretion by blocking the H_2 receptors on the parietal cell. The H2-RAs marketed in the United States are cimetidine, ranitidine, famotidine, and nizatidine (Table 61.4). When these agents inhibit gastric acid production, the material refluxed from the stomach is less harmful to the esophageal mucosa.

Several clinical trials have investigated the efficacy of H2-RAs in GERD. The design and results of these studies vary, but pooled data indicate that approximately 60% of persons with GERD have a significant reduction in symptoms after treatment with standard doses of H2-RA for 6 to 12 weeks. However, symptom resolution does not correlate well with the healing of esophagitis. Healing rates are inversely proportional to the severity of esophagitis. Higher and more frequent doses of H2-RAs than standard doses may be necessary in severe cases. H2-RAs are safe: The reported incidence of adverse reactions is about 4%. Cimetidine may bind reversibly to the cytochrome P-450 microsomal enzymes of the liver, resulting in drug interac-

TABLE 61.3. Lifestyle Modifications for Gastroesophageal Reflux Disease

Elevate the head of the bed 6–8 inches.
Avoid eating for 3 h before retiring.
Stop smoking.
Reduce alcohol consumption.
Eat small meals.
Lose weight if necessary.
Avoid tight clothes.
Avoid dietary fat, chocolate, coffee (caffeinated and decaffeinated), tea, carminatives, and cola.
Avoid drugs that decrease LES pressure.

TABLE 61.4. Acid-Suppressive Therapy for Gastroesophageal Reflux Disease

Medication	Dosage
Histamine H_2 receptor antagonists	
Cimetidine (Tagamet, generic)	400–800 mg 2–4 times/d
Ranitidine (Zantac, generic)	150–300 mg 2–4 times/d
Famotidine (Pepcid, generic)	20–40 mg 1–2 times/d
Nizatidine (Axid)	150–300 mg 1–2 times/d
Proton pump inhibitors	
Omeprazole (Prilosec)	20 mg once/d
Lansoprazole (Prevacid)	15–30 mg once/d
Rabeprazole (Aciphex)	20 mg once/d
Pantoprazole (Protonix)	40 mg once/d
Esomeprazole (Nexium)	20–40 mg once/d

tions with theophylline, warfarin, phenytoin, and benzodiazepines. Caution should be used when cimetidine is combined with one of these drugs. Other H2-RAs may also bind to the cytochrome P-450 system, although with less affinity. Other potential side effects include central nervous system disturbances (<0.2%) and hepatotoxicity. Isolated cases of hematologic side effects have been noted. Cimetidine has weak antiandrogenic activity, and rare instances of gynecomastia, impotence, and hyperprolactinemia have been reported.

PROTON PUMP INHIBITORS

Proton pump inhibitors (PPIs) inhibit the activity of H^+/K^+-ATPase ("proton pump"), the final common step of acid secretion by the parietal cell. Five PPIs are currently available in the United States—omeprazole, lansoprazole, rabeprazole, pantoprazole, and esomeprazole (Table 61.4). PPIs lead to a prolonged and profound inhibition of gastric acid production. They have significantly stronger inhibitory effect on acid secretion than that of H2-RAs. For example, composite data from more than 50 studies demonstrated that healing rates of esophagitis with H2-RAs is approximately 50%; with PPIs the healing rates are over 85%. Therefore, PPIs are considered to be the most effective medical therapy for controlling symptoms of GERD and for healing esophagitis. PPIs are generally considered safe. Previous concerns raised about the reports of the development of carcinoid tumors in rats has not been reported in humans after more than 10 years of use. Asymptomatic decrease in vitamin B_{12} levels has been reported with the use of PPI. Omeprazole decreases the metabolism of warfarin, phenytoin, and diazepam.

PROKINETIC AGENTS

Prokinetic drugs reduce reflux by increasing LES pressure and enhancing esophageal peristalsis, gastric emptying, and esophageal acid clearance. Bethanechol, a cholinergic agonist, enhances LES pressure and increases the flow of saliva. When used in a dose of 25 mg four times a day, bethanechol improves symptoms of GERD compared with placebo. It is seldom used in the management of GERD because of the high frequency of side effects such as flushing, blurry vision, abdominal cramps, and urinary frequency. Metoclopramide, a dopamine antagonist and a cholinergic agonist, has effects similar to those of bethanechol in increasing LES pressure. Although metoclopramide is effective in reducing esophageal reflux, it is recommended for short-term use only because of frequent neuropsychiatric side effects, particularly in elderly patients. Another dopamine antagonist, domperidone, causes fewer side effects than metoclopramide and may control symptoms as effectively as H2-RAs. Domperidone is not available in the United States.

Cisapride releases acetylcholine at the myenteric plexus, increases the amplitude of esophageal peristalsis and LES pressure, and promotes gastric emptying. It provides similar rates of symptomatic relief of GERD and healing of esophagitis as H2-RAs. Several reports of serious cardiac arrhythmias caused by cisapride have resulted in a decision by the U.S. Food and Drug Administration to remove it from the U.S. market in July 2000. Cisapride is still available from the manufacturer based on a limited-access protocol.

SITE-PROTECTIVE AGENTS

Sucralfate, a salt of aluminum hydroxide and sucrose octasulfate, is sometimes useful in the treatment of esophagitis. It works locally, binding to damaged epithelium, and possibly acts as a barrier to the noxious effects of acid and pepsin. Studies have not shown sucralfate to be uniformly effective in GERD. Although its systemic absorption is minimal, sucralfate must be used cautiously if at all in patients with renal disease, in whom aluminum toxicity may occur.

Surgical Therapy

Antireflux surgery to reestablish a competent LES has undergone a revolution with the introduction of laparoscopic techniques. Laparoscopic Nissen fundoplication is the most common procedure performed for GERD. This operation involves wrapping the upper part of the stomach (fundus) around the lower esophagus, thus forming an antireflux barrier. Considerable controversy exists regarding which patients should be referred for surgery. Several factors need to be considered before surgical referral. First and foremost is proper patient selection. Patients should have clear understanding of the risks and benefits of the surgery. Although surgery has proven to be at least as effective, if not superior to, medical therapy in the short-term, long-term follow-up studies have demonstrated conflicting results. A substantial number of patients experience recurrence of symptoms requiring additional medical therapy after antireflux surgery. Complications from the surgery include dysphagia, gastric ulceration, postoperative plication breakdown and inability to belch (gas bloat syndrome), and a mortality rate of 0.3% to 0.5%. Results also depend on the surgeon's experience, particularly for a laparoscopic procedure.

The decision to have antireflux surgery should be individualized. Provided the patient is a good surgical candidate, fundoplication may be considered in three situations: (a) in the patient with symptomatic esophagitis who has failed optimal medical therapy, (b) in the patient who desires a permanent solution to avoid taking life-long medication, or (c) in the patient who is intolerant to PPI therapy. Patients with poor or absent esophageal peristalsis (and thus at risk of severe dysphagia post-fundoplication), patients with highly functional symptoms, and elderly patients are considered poor candidates for surgery.

Endoscopic Therapy

Endoscopic therapy for GERD is in a developmental phase. Four basic types of endoscopic therapy exist: endoscopic suturing, radiofrequency ablation, injection therapy, and bulking procedures. Three devices have received U.S. Food and Drug Administration approval. However, there is concern about their usage in the absence of long-term data on efficacy or safety. In addition, other currently available medical or surgical therapies have already proven to be effective with long-term safety data.

DIAGNOSTIC AND THERAPEUTIC APPROACH

Initial Management

The patient with symptoms of GERD is traditionally approached in a stepwise fashion (Fig. 61.3). Most patients who present with recurrent uncomplicated heartburn should first be instructed in lifestyle modifications and the use of antacids or alginic acid. An empiric course of an H2-RA in a standard dose for 3 to 4 weeks is also appropriate.

If the patient does not respond to these measures, then a once-daily morning dose of PPI therapy can be administered. Alternatively, some experts recommend directly prescribing PPI as the initial therapy. The rationale behind this approach is that half of the patients with GERD have erosive disease that may eventually require PPI therapy. In addition, this approach not only relieves patient symptoms most effectively and rapidly, but also confirms the diagnosis of GERD if the patient responds to PPI therapy. Any patient with treatment-resistant symptoms or alarm features should be referred to a gastroenterologist for further evaluation.

If endoscopy is performed and reveals evidence of esophagitis characterized by erosions or ulcerations, PPI therapy should be given for at least 6 to 8 weeks in an attempt to heal mucosal disease. Among the PPIs, esomeprazole has been shown to be marginally superior to other PPIs in healing erosive esophagitis. Because the relapse rate in patients with erosive esophagitis is as high as 90% at 12 months, maintenance therapy of some type is recommended to minimize the rate of relapse and to prevent complications. This may include H2-RAs in at least standard doses or a PPI. Once the drug is stopped, the patient is monitored for recurrence of symptoms. If they recur quickly, continued chronic acid suppression with either an H2-RA or a PPI at the minimally effective dose is often needed.

One challenging issue is managing patients with nocturnal symptoms who do not respond to twice a day PPI therapy. Limited data suggest that adding a bedtime H2-RA might be effective in reducing nocturnal acid breakthrough. However, tachyphylaxis to H2-RAs with ineffective acid suppression develops in some patients when these agents are used long term. One way to avoid this tolerance is to use H2-RAs at bedtime on an as-needed basis. Younger women with recurrent symptoms, facing a lifetime of taking drugs for GERD, may consider surgical therapy.

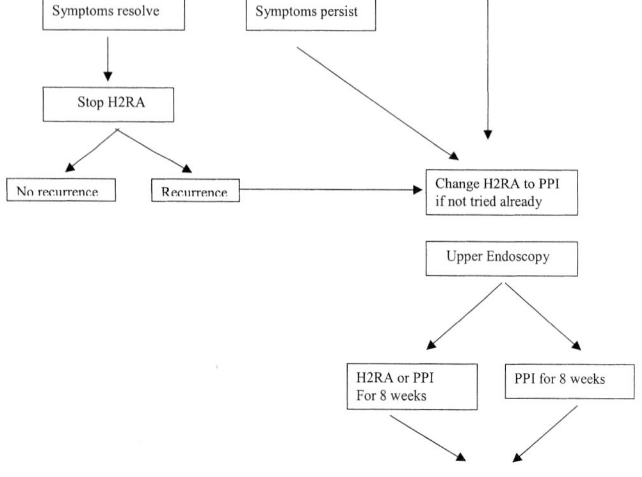

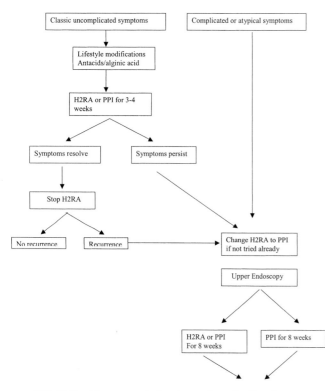

FIG. 61.3. Management of gastroesophageal reflux disease.

Maintenance Therapy

Many patients with GERD ultimately require long-term, perhaps lifetime, therapy. Once the mucosal disease has healed, long-term PPI therapy is needed to prevent recurrence because underlying mechanisms promoting reflux persist. However, in patients with no esophagitis on endoscopy, symptom control can be achieved either with the lowest dose of H2-RA or a PPI. To identify the few patients who remain asymptomatic after initial therapy, an attempt should be made to stop therapy in all patients who respond completely to initial treatment.

Recent studies support the use of "on-demand" therapy (on an as-needed basis, after the onset of symptoms) in patients who require long-term maintenance. Patients are instructed to resume therapy once symptoms recur and to stop treatment when they have been free of symptoms for at least 24 hours. This approach substantially reduces the costs of long-term therapy and is a particularly attractive option in patients with no evidence of esophagitis on endoscopy.

TREATMENT OF COMPLICATIONS

Stricture

Dilatation by tapered rubber dilators (bougienage) or a balloon is the most common approach to the treatment of esophageal strictures. About 40% of patients with a stricture respond to one dilatation. Strictures of the esophagus may recur, requiring periodic dilatations. This procedure is not risk free, and the complication rate is about 0.5%. Therefore, patients should be placed on chronic PPI therapy to prevent recurrence of stricture formation.

Barrett Esophagus

Barrett esophagus must be managed as both severe GERD and as a premalignant lesion. Aggressive medical therapy usually reduces symptoms and may prevent or reduce the development of strictures, but it is unknown if treatment reverses Barrett epithelium. Generally, patients who are over the age 40 with long-standing (arbitrarily, 5 years) GERD are recommended to have an upper endoscopy to screen for the presence of Barrett esophagus. Depending on the presence or absence and degree of dysplasia, the frequency of surveillance endoscopy is decided thereafter. Patients who have Barrett esophagus with high-grade dysplasia are generally recommended to have esophageal resection surgery, provided the patient is fit for surgery.

Extraesophageal Complications

The management of the extraesophageal complications of GERD, particularly laryngeal, pharyngeal, and pulmonary diseases, includes aggressive treatment of reflux, often with PPIs. The subsequent response of asthma, hoarseness, or cough to this therapy is usually the best evidence that the problem is a complication of GERD.

CONSIDERATIONS IN PREGNANCY

Pregnancy has a major effect on gastrointestinal motility and thus predisposes some women to develop GERD. Heartburn is reported by as many as 75% of pregnant women. Although it may occur during any trimester, heartburn most commonly develops at 5 months of gestation, becoming more pronounced as the pregnancy progresses. It is at its worst during the final months. Symptoms are usually mild. Complications occur rarely, possibly because GERD in pregnancy is usually an acute pregnancy-related symptom without chronic underlying pregravid esophagitis. In most cases, heartburn ceases soon after delivery. Subsequent pregnancies are often associated with recurrent GERD symptoms.

The etiology of GERD in pregnancy has been extensively studied. The LES pressure progressively diminishes during pregnancy, and by 36 weeks' gestation nearly all women have a low LES pressure (Fig. 61.4). This pressure returns to normal in the postpartum period. The decrease in pressure appears to be an effect of progesterone on the smooth muscle, although estrogen may be required for a priming effect. As the uterus enlarges, the increased intraabdominal pressure may further compromise an already weakened LES.

The clinical features of GERD in pregnancy do not differ from those in the general population: Heartburn and regurgitation are the predominant symptoms. Some patients complain of isolated nausea as heartburn equivalent. Referral to a gastroenterologist and endoscopy are rarely needed and should be reserved for patients in whom the diagnosis is unclear or treatment is ineffective or when complications such as bleeding occur. When needed, endoscopy is safe for both mother and the fetus with careful monitoring of maternal blood pressure, pulse oximetry, and conscious sedation. Medications commonly used in endoscopy, including meperidine, midazolam, and diazepam, are probably safe, especially after the first trimester. The U.S. Food and Drug Administration has not approved use of these medications for this indication in pregnancy. Histologic esophagitis may be seen, but severe erosive esophagitis is rare. On occasion, 24-hour pH studies are needed to confirm the diagnosis. Contrast barium radiographs should be avoided because of the teratogenic potential.

Mild symptoms in pregnant women may respond well to lifestyle modification. Small meals, not eating for several hours before retiring, avoiding stooping and bending, or lying down within several hours of a meal and elevating the head of the bed should be the initial recommendations. If pharmacologic intervention is required, aluminum, calcium, or magnesium-containing antacids are deemed safe based on teratogenic studies in animals; however, a small percentage are absorbed and may also interfere with iron absorption. Women receiving iron preparations should have antacids administered at an interval of several hours from supplemental iron. Sodium bicarbonate should be avoided, because it may cause a metabolic alkalosis and fluid overload in both mother and fetus. Alginic acid contains magnesium trisilicate and is not safe in pregnancy because of reports of fetal respiratory distress, nephrolithiasis, and cardiovascular impairment. Sucralfate, a surface-acting mucosal protectant, appears to be safe because of its limited systemic absorption; this drug has been reported to be effective in relieving heartburn symptoms in one small controlled trial in pregnancy.

If symptoms are refractory to nonsystemic therapy, an H2-RA may be required. This class of drugs crosses the placenta

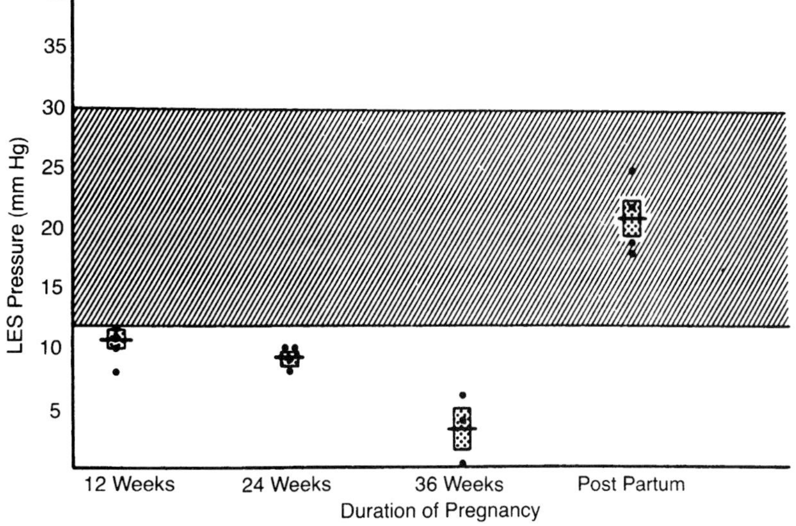

FIG. 61.4. Lower esophageal sphincter pressure recorded in four volunteer women during pregnancy and the postpartum period. Lower esophageal sphincter pressure declined progressively during pregnancy but returned to normal in the postpartum period. (From Van Thiel DH, et al. Heartburn of pregnancy. *Gastroenterology* 1997;72: 666–678, with permission.)

and is secreted in breast milk. Animal studies do not reveal evidence of teratogenicity, and although the H2-RAs have not been studied prospectively in humans, anecdotal experience with cimetidine and ranitidine suggests that they are safe. A combined study assessing two cohorts, one of 1,179 pregnancies in the United Kingdom and the other of 1,057 pregnancies in Italy, found no major risk of fetal malformations when mothers had used cimetidine, ranitidine, or omeprazole during pregnancy. Although all the available H2-RAs belong to pregnancy category B (animal studies show no risks, but human studies are inadequate or animal studies show some risk not supported by humans), few studies of famotidine use in pregnancy exist, and conflicting reports of nizatidine toxicity in experimental animal studies indicate that other H2-RAs should be used in pregnancy. Information concerning safety of PPIs is also limited. High doses of omeprazole (pregnancy category C) have been associated with fetal toxicity and pregnancy disruption in animals. Other available PPIs (lansoprazole, rabeprazole, pantoprazole, and esomeprazole) belong to pregnancy category B. However, given the absence of conclusive long-term safety data in pregnancy, the use of PPIs should be restricted to endoscopically documented complicated GERD that is not responsive to H2-RAs.

BIBLIOGRAPHY

Arora AS, Castell DO. Medical therapy of gastroesophageal reflux disease. *Mayo Clin Proc* 2001;76:102–106.

DeVault KR, Castell DO. Practice and parameters committee of the American College of Gastroenterology. Updated guidelines for the diagnosis and treatment of gastroesophageal disease. *Am J Gastroenterol* 1999;94:1434–1442.

Field SK, Sutherland LR. Does medical antireflux therapy improve asthma in asthmatics with gastroesophageal reflux? A critical review of the literature. *Chest* 1998;114:275–283.

Ing AJ. Cough and gastroesophageal reflux. *Am J Med* 1997;103:91S–96S.

Kahrilas PJ. Diagnosis of symptomatic gastroesophageal reflux disease. *Am J Gastroenterol* 2003;98:S15–S23.

Orlando RC. Pathogenesis of gastroesophageal reflux disease. *Gastroenterol Clin North Am* 2002;31:S35–S44.

Pope CE. Acid-reflux disorders. *N Engl J Med* 1994;331:656.

Richter JE. Gastroesophageal reflux disease during pregnancy. *Gastroenterol Clin North Am* 2003;32:235–261.

Sampliner RE and The Practice Parameters Committee of the American College of Gastroenterology. Updated guidelines for the diagnosis, surveillance, and therapy of Barrett's esophagus. *Am J Gastroenterol* 2002;97:1888–1895.

Spechler SJ. Barrett's esophagus. *N Engl J Med* 2002;346:836–842.

Szaka LA, DeVault KR, Murray JA. Diagnosing gastroesophageal reflux disease. *Mayo Clin Proc* 2001:76:97–101.

Waring JP. Surgical and endoscopic treatment of gastroesophageal reflux disease. *Gastroenterol Clin North Am* 2002;31:S89–S109.

CHAPTER 62
Peptic Ulcer Disease

Sripathi R. Kethu and Edward Feller

Gastritis and peptic ulcer disease (PUD) comprise a clinical and pathologic spectrum of injury to the upper gastrointestinal (GI) tract. Ulcers represent circumscribed mucosal damage extending into the submucosa, whereas gastritis and erosions are superficial and are confined to the mucosa. These conditions overlap clinically, without specific symptom patterns to allow easy distinction. More commonly, patients present to the primary care provider with symptoms of dyspepsia regardless of the presence or absence of PUD. Hence, it is important to discuss dyspepsia before the discussion of PUD.

DYSPEPSIA

Dyspepsia represents a heterogeneous group of symptoms defined as pain or discomfort that may be accompanied by an array of complaints, including fullness, bloating, distention, eructation, indigestion, early satiety, and nausea. Pain is characteristically upper abdominal and may be meal related. Although the true prevalence of dyspepsia is unknown, it is estimated that up to 5% of family practice consultations are for dyspepsia.

Etiology and Differential Diagnosis

The relationship of dyspepsia with PUD may be confusing because laypersons and health professionals may term symptoms of dyspepsia as PUD. Dyspepsia can also be due to gastroesophageal reflux disease (GERD), malignancy, disorders of motility, lactose intolerance, irritable bowel syndrome, pancreaticobiliary disorders, emotional conditions, or secondary to the use of specific medications. Functional dyspepsia refers to symptoms for which clinical evaluation has not yielded a specific organic cause. Thus, it is a diagnosis of exclusion requiring evaluation before being termed "functional" or "nonulcer" dyspepsia. Because dyspepsia is so common, it may coexist with underlying illness such as PUD, GERD, or irritable bowel syndrome.

Clinical history is essential in assessing dyspepsia. A useful distinction exists in delineating three general patterns of dyspeptic complaints: (a) acid-like dyspepsia, in which symptoms are described as burning, hunger-like, or gnawing pain; (b) dysmotility-like dyspepsia, in which distention, eructation, early satiety, fullness, and nausea predominate; and (c) reflux-type dyspepsia, where discomfort may rise in the chest, be exacerbated by recumbency, or be associated with sour taste in the mouth. These three categories, however, exhibit considerable overlap and predict poorly the underlying diagnosis when assessed by endoscopic findings. PUD is found on investigation of up to 25% of patients complaining of dyspepsia. Although it is impossible to distinguish gastric and duodenal ulcers by symptoms alone, the pain of both gastric and duodenal ulcers is typically epigastric, episodic, and often worse at night. Some patients report that food ingestion precipitates pain. Symptoms are often temporarily relieved with food or antacids in the case of duodenal ulcer; in contrast, food may precipitate gastric ulcer pain. Associated symptoms such as anorexia, nausea, or vomiting may suggest a diagnosis of a gastric ulcer or pyloric stenosis. Gastric malignancy, which accounts for less than 2% of the cases of dyspepsia, may also present with similar symptoms.

A careful medication history is essential. Nonsteroidal anti-inflammatory drugs (NSAIDs) are the most common offending agents causing dyspepsia. Other medications linked to dyspepsia include bisphosphonates (commonly used for prophylaxis and treatment of postmenopausal osteoporosis), corticosteroids, iron preparations, digitalis, potassium supplements, narcotics, colchicine, theophylline preparations, β-hydroxy-β-methylglutaryl coenzyme A reductase inhibitors ("statins") used to treat hypercholesterolemia, niacin, and antibiotics, particularly macrolides, metronidazole, and ampicillin. Hormonal influences associated with dyspepsia are hormone replacement therapy, oral contraceptives, and pregnancy.

Functional or nonulcer dyspepsia represents up to 60% of all dyspeptic complaints. Functional dyspepsia and PUD share overlapping complaints; clinical differentiation by history is commonly not possible. Functional dyspepsia applies to symptoms for which a specific organic illness has not been documented by medical evaluation. By definition, this diagnosis is one of exclusion. In 1999, one expert panel defined nonulcer dyspepsia as excluding symptoms relieved by defecation or being associated with a change in stool character, frequency, or form (thus excluding irritable bowel syndrome). A variable number of these patients may have nonerosive reflux disease, excess intradigestive gas, motility disorders, irritable bowel syndrome, visceral hypersensitivity, or emotional disorders.

Evaluation

All patients with persistent dyspepsia require a thorough history and physical examination to determine the cause. For many patients, dietary, lifestyle, or medication changes may alleviate symptoms. Because the underlying cause of dyspeptic complaints ranges from excess gas to peptic ulcer or malignancy, alarm symptoms must be sought and investigated, when present. Anemia, weight loss, any evidence of GI bleeding, early satiety, or dysphagia must be evaluated. New onset of complaints, especially in patients older than age 45, or clear worsening of chronic complaints must be assessed. The most accurate first test for dyspepsia is upper endoscopy, which visualizes the mucosa for ulcer, other inflammation, erosive esophagitis, or malignancy and at the same time allows biopsy for histologic diagnosis and/or documentation of *Helicobacter pylori* infection. Contrast dye (barium) radiographs are less sensitive and specific compared with upper endoscopy and can be used as an alternative to endoscopy. Right upper quadrant ultrasonography can be done if there is suspicion for pancreaticobiliary disease as evidenced by the history or abnormal liver enzymes. Selected patients with risk factors for gastroparesis will also require gastric emptying study. For younger patients and those without alarm symptoms, an empiric 4- to 6-week trial of acid-lowering therapy should be considered before diagnostic evaluation.

H. pylori infection is the major risk factor for the development of PUD. The association of *H. pylori* with nonulcer dyspepsia is uncertain. Collective evidence suggests no clear role of the organism in causation of functional dyspepsia. In a younger woman or one in whom no worrisome features are present, some authorities recommend a "test and treat" strategy for *H. pylori* before any diagnostic evaluation. The rationale for this approach is the high prevalence of *H. pylori* in the population, the efficacy of eradication in the subgroup of dyspeptic patients who do have underlying PUD, and the symptomatic improvement in a variable proportion of patients with nonulcer dyspepsia. The benefits of this approach, whether measured by symptom relief or cost-benefit analysis, remain unproven. Failure of symptomatic relief or presence of alarm symptoms warrants consideration of upper endoscopy.

Management of Functional (Nonulcer) Dyspepsia

Once the cause of dyspepsia is established, management involves treating the underlying disorder. The most challenging task is managing patients with functional dyspepsia. *H. pylori* eradication therapy for patients who do not have an ulcer may result in symptomatic improvement in some (approximately in 15% of patients) over placebo. However, most patients will remain symptomatic after eradication therapy, thus requiring other therapies.

Patient education and reassurance are vital for optimal management. Excluding serious disease may have important benefits for physical and emotional well-being. Avoidance of potential precipitating factors, including coffee, smoking, NSAIDs, alcohol, carbonated beverages, and foods that exacerbate symptoms, must be discussed. An exploration of psychosocial influences including depression and anxiety will be useful in selected patients, with individualization of any needed psychopharmacologic therapy. Long-term management of nonulcer dyspepsia may require periodic reassessment and more aggressive evaluation if the clinical situation changes.

American Gastroenterology Association guidelines recommend an empiric trial of 4 to 6 weeks of antisecretory treatment with histamine H_2 receptor antagonists (H2-RA) or proton pump inhibitors (PPI) in the young patient with dyspepsia and ulcer-type symptoms without alarm symptoms and who are *H. pylori* negative. Endoscopy should be considered if symptoms persist. Dyspeptic patients with distention or bloating, especially after meals, may have impaired gastric emptying. A prokinetic agent such as metoclopramide at a dosage of 5 to 10 mg 30 minutes to 1 hour before meals and at bedtime for 4 to 6 weeks to enhance antral contractility may be useful. Antidepressants such as amitriptyline 50 mg at bedtime or antispasmodics such as dicyclomine 10 to 20 mg every 8 hours are adjunctive agents for symptom relief in some patients. A subgroup will have complaints that overlap with irritable bowel syndrome or noncardiac chest pain. The former may experience symptom relief with antispasmodic agents. The benefit of individual drugs should be weighed against the side-effect profile and cost. Alternative therapies such as acupuncture, cognitive behavioral therapy, and hypnotherapy have been reported anecdotally to be beneficial.

PEPTIC ULCER DISEASE

A peptic ulcer is a circumscribed mucosal injury generally found in the stomach or duodenum. In contrast to gastritis, which is superficial, an ulcer extends through the muscularis mucosae. Any portion of the GI tract exposed to aggressive factors such as acid or pepsin, including the esophagus and small bowel, may be involved. Injury occurs when the normal mucosal defense mechanisms are overwhelmed. The stomach is protected by a bicarbonate-rich layer bathing the mucosa and an anatomic structure with tight mucosal junctional complexes between mucosal cells (functioning) to maintain mucosal blood flow and to protect against hydrogen ion. The lifetime risk of PUD in the United States is approximately 10%, with a male-to-female ratio of 1.3:1 for a duodenal ulcer and 1:1 for a gastric ulcer. Duodenal ulcer occurs more commonly between ages 25 and 55, whereas gastric ulcer affects a slightly older population (ages 40–70). In the United States, 500,000 new cases of PUD occur yearly.

Etiology and Risk Factors

H. pylori colonization is the cause of most peptic ulcers, followed by NSAIDs. Cigarette smoking injures the gastric mucosa and interferes with mucosal protective factors by decreasing prostaglandin production and inhibiting acid-stimulated bicarbonate production. Smoking not only doubles the ulcer risk but also retards ulcer healing and increases the risk of bleeding. A threefold increase in risk occurs in first-degree relatives of individuals with documented PUD. This increase may represent similar environmental exposure to such factors as *H. pylori* or genetic influences. Coffee in its caffeinated and uncaffeinated forms commonly causes dyspepsia but is not directly linked to PUD. Specific foods may cause dyspepsia in some patients, but no data support diet, even highly spicy foods, as a risk factor for ulcer. Emotional stress has been linked classically to PUD. However, current data indicate that stressful circumstances are not sufficient to induce PUD. Such symptoms are properly termed "nonulcer dyspepsia" in most patients.

HELICOBACTER PYLORI-ASSOCIATED ULCERS

H. pylori is a Gram-negative, spiral, flagellate bacterium acquired in childhood that colonizes the antral gastric mucosa, causing chronic gastritis. The prevalence of *H. pylori* is between 20% and 50% in the western world, including the United States. However, *H. pylori* is much more prevalent in developing nations, colonizing as many as 90% of the population. In the United States, the prevalence is higher in the elderly, possibly reflecting the poor sanitary conditions that existed in the early part of the century, and is more common in African-Americans, Hispanics, and immigrants from Asia and Africa. Populations of low socioeconomic status also have higher infection rates, probably related to crowded living conditions.

Early studies in the United States indicated that *H. pylori* was detected in approximately 90% of duodenal ulcer patients and 60% with gastric ulcers. More recent estimates show a slightly lower prevalence of *H. pylori* in both duodenal and gastric ulcers, probably reflecting the relative increase in NSAID-associated ulcers.

Approximately 10% of all individuals with chronic gastritis due to *H. pylori* will eventually develop peptic ulcer disease. *H. pylori* infection is associated with a three- to sixfold increased risk of gastric cancer, leading to its designation by the World Health Organization as a carcinogen. *H. pylori* is also a major risk factor for the relatively rare mucosa-associated lymphoid tissue gastric B-cell lymphoma.

The exact pathophysiologic mechanism(s) by which *H. pylori* causes either duodenal or gastric ulcer and why only some infected individuals will develop clinically overt disease is not known. Duodenal ulcer is thought to result from increased gastric acid secretion secondary to increased gastrin release caused by *H. pylori*. Another proposed mechanism involves the ability of *H. pylori* to impair bicarbonate secretion in the duodenum, resulting in decreased buffering of gastric acid in the duodenum and eventual duodenal ulcer. In contrast to duodenal ulcer, gastric ulcer is associated with decreased acid production. Inflammation associated with chronic *H. pylori* colonization, in some cases, may lead to gastric atrophy (atrophic gastritis) and intestinal metaplasia of the gastric epithelium. Intestinal metaplasia may lead to hypochlorhydria, resulting in impaired mucosal defense that leads to gastric ulceration and possibly gastric cancer.

NONSTEROIDAL ANTIINFLAMMATORY DRUG-INDUCED ULCERS

Estimates indicate that 20% of Americans are treated with NSAIDs yearly, with a much higher percentage in the elderly. NSAIDs are responsible for most peptic ulcers in *H. pylori*-negative individuals. Peptic ulcer has been documented endoscopically in approximately 15% to 20% of chronic NSAID users. Comorbid factors increasing ulcer risk include age older than 60 years, prior ulcer history, high-dose NSAIDs, and concurrent administration of corticosteroids or anticoagulation. NSAIDs cause gastric ulcers much more commonly than duodenal ulcers. Up to 40% of NSAID-associated ulcers are asymptomatic. Data suggest that ulcers associated with NSAIDs are more likely to be refractory or complicated (bleeding, perforation, and obstruction). Surreptitious NSAID use is common.

The most important mechanism by which NSAIDs cause ulcers is by limiting prostaglandin production via the inhibition of the cyclooxygenase-1 (COX-1) enzyme. Prostaglandins are vital for the integrity of the mucosal barrier by producing mucus, increasing the generation of bicarbonate, decreasing acid production, and maintaining mucosal blood flow. The analgesic and antiinflammatory effects of NSAIDs result from the inhibition of the COX-2 isoenzyme. Nonselective NSAIDs cause inhibition of both COX-2 and COX-1, resulting in considerable GI toxicity. The more recently developed selective COX-2 inhibitors (such as celecoxib [Celebrex], rofecoxib [Vioxx], and valdecoxib [Bextra]) inhibit COX-2 to a much greater extent than COX-1, resulting in a better GI safety profile. COX-2 inhibitors reduce the risk of gastroduodenal ulcers by 60% to 75% compared with nonselective NSAIDs.

IDIOPATHIC (NON-*HELICOBACTER PYLORI*, NON-NONSTEROIDAL ANTIINFLAMMATORY DRUG) ULCERS

PUD is less common in the symptomatic patient who is both *H. pylori* negative and has not used NSAIDs. The subgroup of patients with truly idiopathic ulcers should not be confused with "unexplained" ulcers where 60% of patients may have a history of surreptitious NSAID use. False-negative testing for *H. pylori* also complicates establishing the true incidence of idiopathic ulcers. The exact pathogenic mechanism that causes idiopathic ulcers remains unknown. Genetic predisposition, defective mucosal defense mechanisms, and increased acid production have all been postulated.

Clinical Features

The natural history of PUD is variable, ranging from asymptomatic to fulminant, complicated or recurrent. Clinical signs and symptoms of PUD are nonspecific (Table 62.1). More than 80% of patients complain of upper abdominal pain; however, only 25% of patients with dyspepsia have PUD. Ulcer pain is characteristically described as burning, gnawing, or as a vague hunger-like discomfort felt in the epigastrium. Classically, patients describe discomfort before meals when the stomach is empty and relieved by food or antacid intake but also occurring in the postprandial period. Gastric ulcer pain is commonly described as occurring soon after food intake, whereas duodenal ulcer symptoms occur several hours after a meal. Considerable overlap exists, limiting the utility of this temporal distinction. Documented ulcers are discovered in occasional patients who describe pain in one of the upper abdominal quadrants with a dull, sharp, or crampy quality rather than burning in nature. Pain radiating to the back is also reported by some but is a nonspecific indicator. Population-based surveys indicate that only 15% to 30% of patients reporting typical ulcer-like dyspepsia will have PUD on investigation. GERD, also associated with food intake and acid release, may coexist in some patients with PUD. Food or antacids may relieve ulcer pain or nausea. Nocturnal symptoms may awaken some patients and symptoms usually wax and wane over a period of months.

The physical examination is usually normal in uncomplicated PUD. Epigastric tenderness on palpation may be present but is an unreliable sign. Stool test for occult blood is positive in up to one third of patients. Endoscopic surveillance studies suggest that approximately 2% of healthy adults may harbor asymptomatic ulcers. As many as one fifth of all ulcers will present with GI bleeding in the absence of prior abdominal complaints. Evidence suggests that both asymptomatic ulcers and ulcers presenting with bleeding may be more common in the elderly or in individuals taking NSAIDs. Some ulcers heal spontaneously or as a result of treatment and never recur. Other patients experience periodic exacerbations lasting weeks or months interspersed with symptom-free intervals of months to years. Ulcer healing and disappearance of symptoms are not synonymous with ulcer "cure." The natural history of variable exacerbations and remissions can be interrupted by specific therapeutic interventions, including eradication of *H. pylori* when present, avoidance of NSAIDs,

TABLE 62.1. Symptoms of Gastric and Duodenal Ulcers and Nonulcer Dyspepsia

Symptom	Gastric ulcer (%)	Duodenal ulcer (%)	Nonulcer dyspepsia (%)
Pain/discomfort	100	100	100
Features of pain			
Primary pain			
Epigastric	67	61–86	52–73
Right hypochondrium	6	7–17	4
Left hypochondrium	6	3–5	5
Frequently severe	68	53	37
Within 30 min of food	20	5	32
Gnawing pain	13	16	6
Increased by food	24	10–40	45
Clusters (episodic)	16	56	35
Relieved by alkali	36–87	39–86	26–75
Food relief	2–48	20–63	4–32
Occurs at night	32–43	50–88	24–32
Not related to food or variable	22–53	21–49	22–65
Radiation to back	34	20–31	24–28
Increased appetite		19	
Anorexia	46–57	25–36	26–36
Weight loss	24–61	19–45	18–32
Nausea	54–70	49–59	43–60
Vomiting	38–73	25–57	26–34
Heartburn	19	27–59	28
Nondyspeptic symptoms	2	8	18
Fatty food intolerance		41–72	53
Bloating	55	49	52
Belching	48	59	60

abstinence from smoking, or prophylactic use of acid-suppressing medication in selected cases.

Diagnostic Evaluation

Routine serum studies may not be helpful in establishing the diagnosis of PUD. Anemia, if present, is an important clue to the possibility of occult ulcer bleeding. Uncomplicated PUD is not associated with leukocytosis or abnormalities of hepatic enzymes. Any elevation should suggest an alternative diagnosis. Upper endoscopy is the gold standard in making a diagnosis of peptic ulcer. However, endoscopy is relatively expensive and invasive. Factors favoring early endoscopy in the dyspeptic patient being evaluated for possible ulcer include:

- Age older than 45 years
- Weight loss
- Evidence of occult/overt GI bleeding
- Nighttime pain
- Dysphagia
- Exacerbation of chronic complaints
- Poor response to acid suppression.

If none of the aforementioned alarm symptoms is present, double-contrast barium radiography may be considered. A radiographically documented ulcer (gastric or duodenal) mandates treatment with acid suppressive therapy, minimization of precipitating risk factors, and testing for the presence of *H. pylori*. Upper endoscopy is generally routine in radiographically identified gastric but not duodenal ulcers. In the former, biopsy excludes malignancy, while allowing for direct endoscopic testing for *H. pylori*, and may be useful in assessing ulcer healing.

Multiple invasive or noninvasive testing options exist for the diagnosis of *H. pylori* (Table 62.2). Testing for *H. pylori* is separated into modalities requiring gastric biopsies and those not requiring mucosal samples. The clinical context and the patient's need for endoscopy determine selection of the appropriate means of *H. pylori* diagnosis. For example, testing for serologic antibodies against *H. pylori* may be appropriate for the initial testing for *H. pylori*. However, serology is not useful to document effectiveness of eradication therapy directed against the organism because the antibody levels may decline unpredictably and may remain positive for months or years after *H. pylori* eradication. Patients with alarm symptoms and all patients above 45 years of age with dyspeptic symptoms should undergo endoscopy at which time *H. pylori* testing can be done by gastric mucosal biopsy. Confirmation of the eradication of *H. pylori* should be done 4 weeks after therapy by either the stool antigen test or the urea breath test.

Differential Diagnosis

PUD must be considered in any woman with episodic or persistent mid-abdominal pain. The vast majority of patients will complain of dyspepsia, but clinical evaluation may not distinguish PUD from nonulcer dyspepsia. A low sensitivity and specificity exists for various characteristics of abdominal pain in distinguishing PUD from a wide range of common organic or functional GI disorders. Esophageal, cardiac, biliary, or pancreatic pain may be localized to the epigastrium. Functional dyspepsia is major differential diagnostic consideration in all patients with upper abdominal pain (see Dyspepsia, above). Pain in GERD commonly rises up the chest and is associated with nausea, a sour taste in the mouth, or regurgitation symptoms. Dysphagia (the sensation of food sticking after swallowing) may occur and requires evaluation.

Biliary disease, more frequent in women, may be confused with PUD. Biliary pain tends to be discrete, episodic, sharp, and infrequent rather than daily as in PUD. Biliary colic or acute cholecystitis characteristically are severe, more prolonged than PUD pain, and not relieved by food ingestion or antacids. Irrita-

TABLE 62.2. Diagnosis of *H. Pylori*

Diagnostic test	Sensitivity (%)	Specificity (%)	Approximate cost in U.S. dollars[a]
Tests not requiring endoscopy			
Finger-stick blood test	70–85	75–90	10–20
Serum IgG antibody (ELISA) test	90–95	80–95	40–75
	90–95	88–98	50–100
Urea breath test (14C or 13C)[b]	89–98	87–95	60
Stool antigen test[c]			
Tests requiring endoscopy			
Rapid urease test	80–90	95–100	10–20
Histology (multiple biopsies)	92–95	98–99	150–250
Culture	60–98	100	100–200

[a]Cost of endoscopy not included.
[b]H2-RA and PPI should be stopped at least 2 weeks before initial testing.
[c]H2-RA and PPI should be stopped 1 week before initial testing.
ELISA, enzyme-linked immunosorbent assay; H2-RA, histamine H_2 receptor antagonist; PPI, proton pump inhibitor.

ble bowel syndrome overlaps symptomatically and may coexist with both PUD and nonulcer dyspepsia. Clues to the irritable bowel syndrome include association of symptoms with defecation and an altered pattern of defecation. Malignancy of the GI tract may present with symptoms identical to those of PUD. Gastric or pancreatic carcinoma must be considered in the patient older than age 45 years with persisting upper abdominal pain, especially when accompanied by weight loss, anorexia, increasing symptoms, or absence of relief from acid-suppressing medications. In older patients, the postprandial occurrence of pain from mesenteric ischemia may be confused with the symptoms of PUD. Ulcer-like symptoms and endoscopic abnormalities may occasionally be seen in gastric involvement of Crohn disease or sarcoidosis. Zollinger-Ellison syndrome should be suspected if the ulcers are multiple or in unusual locations, refractory to treatment, or if associated with diarrhea.

Treatment

Therapeutic trials using placebo controls indicate that 25% to 40% of endoscopically documented ulcers heal spontaneously. Specific treatment improves these results substantially. Once a firm diagnosis of PUD is made, eradication of *H. pylori*, if present, is mandatory and associated with a dramatic reduction in the risk of ulcer recurrence. Antiulcer medications are varied (Table 62.3). Antacids may confer symptomatic relief and are inexpensive but less effective than antisecretory drugs in inducing ulcer healing. Both histamine H_2 receptor antagonists (H2-RA) and proton pump inhibitors (PPI) inhibit acid secretion. H2-RAs act by blocking H_2 receptors on the gastric parietal cell. This class of drugs are well tolerated with a very low risk of side effects. PPIs bind to the acid secreting H^+/K^+-ATPase enzyme or "proton pump" on the surface of the parietal cell, inhibiting the final common pathway of the gastric acid production. PPIs have the advantage of inhibiting more than 90% of the 24-hour acid secretion compared with a 50% to 60% decrease with H2-RA use. Efficacy in both healing and relief of ulcer symptoms is greater with PPIs. Some patients may require more frequent or higher doses of PPI because of lack of 24-hour suppression of acid release by once daily dosing or inadequate acid suppression after each dose of a twice daily regimen. Sucralfate has similar ulcer healing rates as H2-RAs. The mechanism of action

TABLE 62.3. Treatment Options for Peptic Ulcer

Pharmacologic agents	Active ulcer (gastric or duodenal)	Prevention of NSAID-induced ulcer recurrence
Antisecretory agents		
Histamine H_2 receptor antagonists		
Cimetidine (Tagamet)	400 mg bid or 800 mg qhs	Double the dose that is indicated for active ulcer
Ranitidine (Zantac)	150 mg bid or 300 mg qhs	
Famotidine (Pepcid)	20 mg bid or 40 mg qhs	
Nizatidine (Axid)	150 mg bid or 300 mg qhs	
Proton pump inhibitors		
Omeprazole (Prilosec)	20 mg qd	20 mg qd
Lansoprazole (Prevacid)	30 mg qd	30 mg qd
Rabeprazole (Aciphex)	20 mg qd	20 mg qd
Pantaprazole (Protonix)	40 mg qd	40 mg qd
Esomeprazole (Nexium)	40 mg qd	40 mg qd
Cytoprotective agents (less commonly used)		
Sucralfate (Carafate)	1 g qid	Not effective
Misoprostol (Cytotec)	100–200 μg qid	200 μg qid or 400 μg bid

NSAID, nonsteroidal antiinflammatory drug.

of sucralfate is unknown; it probably coats the ulcer base, thereby promoting ulcer healing. The frequent dosing schedule and large tablet size of sucralfate may reduce patient compliance. Effectiveness of currently used antisecretory drugs limits utility of this agent. Misoprostol is a prostaglandin analog approved for preventing NSAID-induced ulcers. Because of its frequent side effects of abdominal cramping and diarrhea, compliance with misoprostol is a problem, particularly at high doses.

H. pylori eradication is indicated in all ulcer patients who are *H. pylori* positive. The recurrence rate of PUD after acid suppressing medication without maintenance antisecretory therapy may be as high as 50% to 60%. Continued prophylaxis with acid reduction therapy further reduces recurrence to 20% to 30%. Eradication of *H. pylori*, when present, dramatically decreases recurrence to as low as 3% to 5% over several years. Current recommended regimens are successful in eradicating the bacterium in 80% to 90% of cases. Selected *H. pylori* eradication regimens are summarized in Table 62.4. Confirmation of eradication is mandatory for complicated ulcers associated with bleeding, perforation, or obstruction or when symptoms persist. Treatment of idiopathic ulcers (those negative for *H. pylori* and without history of NSAID use) is difficult and often requires chronic maintenance antisecretory therapy, particularly for complicated ulcers.

Prevention

Ulcer recurrence is frequent with chronic use of NSAIDs or with persistent *H. pylori* infection. The incidence of antibiotic resistance to *H. pylori* is rising. If the patient has persistent symptoms after multidrug antibiotic therapy, eradication failure should be strongly suspected and noninvasive testing for *H. pylori* should be performed. If the initial diagnosis of the ulcer was made by radiography, endoscopic confirmation is indicated. Drugs that have clearly been shown to be superior to placebo in preventing NSAID-induced ulcers are PPIs and misoprostol. Double the standard pharmacologic doses of H2-RAs that are used for the treatment of active ulcers are also significantly better than placebo in preventing NSAID-induced gastroduodenal ulcers (Table 62.3). PPIs are generally preferred over H2-RAs because of efficacy, safety, and simplicity of the dosing schedule. Alternatively, COX-2 inhibitors can be used instead of nonselective NSAIDs in patients with risk factors for developing an ulcer. The benefit of COX-2 inhibitors can be undermined by the concurrent use of aspirin. In this situation, prophylactic antiulcer agents should be considered, as should prophylactic *H. pylori* eradication in patients who will require long-term NSAIDs.

Complications

HEMORRHAGE

Peptic ulcers may be the underlying etiology in up to one half of all acute episodes of upper GI bleeding, and approximately 10% to 20% of ulcer patients develop significant GI bleeding with overall mortality up to 10%. Routine surveillance of PUD patients includes tests to assess the presence of fecal occult blood and hematocrit monitoring. Patients generally present with either melena or hematemesis. Rarely, hematochezia may be the clinical expression of upper GI hemorrhage from a gastric or duodenal ulcer. GI bleeding may be the first clinical sign of previously asymptomatic ulcer disease. PUD may also manifest as occult GI bleeding or iron deficiency anemia. Endoscopy is indicated in all patients with clinically significant bleeding, both for diagnosis and therapy. High-dose oral or intravenous PPIs should be instituted before endoscopy if upper GI bleeding is suspected. All *H. pylori*-positive patients must have confirmation of eradication after therapy. There is evidence suggesting that patients with a history of complicated ulcer, such as bleeding, have a higher risk of a subsequent complication than the patients with uncomplicated PUD. In *H. pylori*-positive patients with a history of UGI hemorrhage who are taking low-dose aspirin, eradication of the organism is equivalent to PPI treatment for prophylaxis of recurrent bleeding.

PERFORATION

Ulcer perforation into the peritoneal cavity is a rare life-threatening complication. The incidence has not changed despite the decreasing prevalence of *H. pylori*, probably because the use of NSAIDs continues to increase. An increased risk of perforated ulcer has been reported in association with cocaine use, NSAIDs, and in the elderly. Sudden severe abdominal pain may occur, frequently associated with circulatory collapse and signs of peritoneal irritation, either in the context of prior ulcer history, abrupt exacerbation of stable symptoms, or as an initial event without previous ulcer problems.

OBSTRUCTION

Peripyloric ulcers arising from the distal stomach, pylorus, or proximal duodenal cap may obstruct the gastric outlet. Obstruction may occur in approximately 2% of patients with PUD. A typical presentation includes nausea and vomiting, early satiety, or weight loss, as manifestations of acute or

TABLE 62.4. Selected FDA-Approved *H. pylori* Eradication Regimens

Medication	Dosage
PPI[a] (omeprazole 20 mg bid; esomeprazole 40 mg qd; lansoprazole 30 mg bid) + amoxicillin 1 g + clarithromycin 500 mg	Each antibiotic bid for 10 days
PPI[a] (omeprazole 20 mg or lansoprazole 30 mg) + amoxicillin 1 g + metronidazole 500 mg	Each bid for 10–14 days
Rabeprazole[a] 20 mg + amoxicillin 1 g + clarithromycin 500 mg	Each bid for 10 days
Bismuth subsalicylate 525 mg + metronidazole 250 mg + tetracycline 500 mg[b]	Each qid for 2 weeks with an H2-RA or PPI for 4 weeks

[a]Although not yet FDA approved for this indication, pantoprazole can be substituted for other PPIs.
[b]In penicillin-allergic patients, use either this regimen or use PPI + clarithromycin + metronidazole.
H2-RA, histamine H_2 receptor antagonist; PPI, proton pump inhibitor.

chronic gastric retention. A subset of patients, typically older, may describe isolated weight loss, persistent abdominal pain, or episodic nausea and vomiting without a recognizable pattern. The availability of potent acid-suppressing medication has decreased the frequency of this complication, previously the most common cause of gastric outlet obstruction. Obstruction due to malignancy is becoming more common, statistically, as an etiology of this complication.

PREGNANCY AND PEPTIC ULCER DISEASE

There is no increased incidence of PUD noted in pregnancy. The decreased incidence of PUD during pregnancy reported in some studies is likely due to the patients being misdiagnosed as having GERD or related to the lack of large-scale studies investigating dyspeptic symptoms by endoscopy during pregnancy. The risk factors for the development of PUD are similar to the general population. Symptoms of PUD are reported to be less severe, possibly related to the maternal avoidance of precipitating agents such as NSAIDs, smoking, alcohol, and caffeine.

Differential diagnosis of dyspepsia during pregnancy should include PUD, GERD, nausea and vomiting of pregnancy, pancreatitis, acute cholecystitis, hepatitis, appendicitis, and acute fatty liver of pregnancy. GERD is extremely common during pregnancy, particularly in the last trimester. Pregnant women with GERD tend to have discomfort radiating to the chest, exacerbated by recumbency and associated with regurgitation. Nausea and vomiting of pregnancy are more common in the morning as opposed to PUD symptoms, which are most intense at night or after meals during the day. Gallstone formation is very common during pregnancy, leading to the risk of acute cholecystitis and pancreatitis. Pain from acute pancreatitis is typically sharp, radiating to the back associated with fever or leukocytosis. Amylase and lipase elevations confirm the diagnosis of pancreatitis and are not affected by pregnancy. Diagnosis of acute cholecystitis is made by the history of right upper quadrant pain associated with fatty food intolerance, fever, Murphy's sign on physical examination, and leukocytosis. Hepatitis of any etiology is suggested by the presence of right upper quadrant pain associated with hepatomegaly, jaundice, and marked elevation of serum transaminases. Appendicitis may have an atypical presentation with right upper quadrant or epigastric pain because the appendix may be displaced upward by the gravid uterus. Fatty liver of pregnancy is rare and occurs after 36 weeks of pregnancy. Diagnosis is suggested by the elevation of transaminases, serum bilirubin, hyperuricemia, lactic acidosis, and leukocytosis.

Before any invasive testing, pregnant women with dyspeptic symptoms should be advised regarding diet and lifestyle changes. Avoiding fatty foods, caffeine, NSAIDs, cigarette smoking, and alcohol help to relieve symptoms. When symptoms continue despite these measures, antacids, preferably containing aluminum or magnesium, can be prescribed safely. Sucralfate is a safer alternative compared with antisecretory therapy. A very conservative approach is needed in prescribing H2-RAs and PPIs in pregnancy, particularly during the first trimester, because there are no controlled trials evaluating the safety of these drugs in pregnant women. Misoprostol is absolutely contraindicated during pregnancy, because it is abortifacient in humans. If worrisome or persistent symptoms indicate the need for investigation, endoscopy is safer than radiography, which requires exposure of the fetus to ionizing radiation. Endoscopy in pregnancy should be reserved for cases in which the information to be obtained is deemed vital.

BIBLIOGRAPHY

American Society of Gastrointestinal Endoscopy. An annotated algorithmic approach to upper gastrointestinal bleeding. *Gastrointest Endosc* 2001;53:853–858.

Cappell MS, Garcia A. Gastric and duodenal ulcers during pregnancy. *Gastroenterol Clin North Am* 1998;27:169–195.

Chan FKL, Chung SCS, Suen BY, et al. Preventing recurrent upper gastrointestinal bleeding in patients with *Helicobacter pylori* infection who are taking low-dose aspirin or Naproxen. *N Engl J Med* 2001;344:967–973.

Chan FKL, Leung WK. Peptic-ulcer disease. *Lancet* 2002;360:933–941.

Gabriel SE, Jaakkimainen L, Bombardier C. Risks for serious gastrointestinal complications related to the use of non-steroidal anti-inflammatory drugs: a meta-analysis. *Ann Intern Med* 1991;115:787–796.

Graham DY. *Helicobacter pylori* infection in the pathogenesis of duodenal ulcer and gastric cancer: a model. *Gastroenterology* 1997;113:1983–1991.

Graham DY. Therapy of *Helicobacter pylori:* current status and issues. *Gastroenterology* 2000;118:1–8.

Quan C, Talley NJ. Management of peptic ulcer disease not related to *Helicobacter pylori* or NSAIDs. *Am J Gastroenterol* 2002;97:2950–2961.

Rockey DC. Occult gastrointestinal bleeding. *N Engl J Med* 1999;341:38–45.

Rostom A, Wells G, Tugwell P, et al. Prevention of NSAID-induced gastroduodenal ulcers (Cochrane review). In: The Cochrane Library, Issue 4. Oxford: Update Software, 2002.

Suerbaum S, Michetti P. *Helicobacter pylori* infection. *N Engl J Med* 2002;347:1175–1186.

Talley NJ, Stanghellini V, Heading RC, et al. Functional gastroduodenal disorders. *Gut* 1999;45[Suppl 2]:37–42.

Wolfe MM, Lichtenstein DR, Singh G. Gastrointestinal toxicity of nonsteroidal anti-inflammatory drugs. *N Engl J Med* 1999;340:1888–1899.

CHAPTER 63

Acute Liver Disease

György Baffy

The liver serves a complex physiologic role, and its acute disturbances manifest with various clinical symptoms and signs (Table 63.1). Acute liver disease may predominantly involve either the parenchymal function (hepatocellular injury) or the biliary excretory function (cholestatic injury), and this is reflected in pertinent laboratory and imaging changes.

The term *hepatocellular injury* refers to hepatocyte necrosis and the subsequent development of elevated serum transaminase levels. Transaminases include aspartate aminotransferase and alanine aminotransferase. The pattern and magnitude of increasing transaminase levels may give an initial guide to the differential diagnosis. Serum transaminases are highest and may reach values well over 1,000 U/L in patients with acute viral hepatitis, hepatotoxic injury (e.g., acetaminophen or mushroom poisoning), and ischemic/hypoxic liver damage. In contrast, acute alcoholic hepatitis typically presents with transaminase values less than 500 U/L. In the context of jaundice, serum transaminase values in this lower range are nonspecific for hepatocellular injury and may also occur due to biliary obstruction. Importantly, viral hepatitis may present with a cholestatic pattern of liver injury.

Cholestasis refers to impaired bile formation or bile flow and is characterized by elevated alkaline phosphatase, γ-glutamyltranspeptidase, and predominantly conjugated ("direct") bilirubin levels. This may be secondary to extrahepatic obstruction (most commonly from stones or a tumor) or due to intrahepatic causes. The latter can be subdivided into hepatocellular and canalicular dysfunction (e.g., viral, drug induced, sepsis) and diseases causing mechanical obliteration or obstruction of the intrahepatic ducts (e.g., primary biliary cirrhosis, primary sclerosing cholangitis).

TABLE 63.1. Manifestations of Acute Liver Disease

General symptoms
Anorexia, fatigue, malaise
Fever
Nausea/vomiting
Pruritus
Malabsorption, steatorrhea
Physical signs
Jaundice
Hepatomegaly
Abdominal tenderness
Hepatic encephalopathy
Laboratory findings ***("liver function tests")***
Hepatocellular integrity
Elevated serum ALT and AST
Hepatocellular metabolic capacity
Coagulopathy (low PLT, high PT, low fibrinogen)
Hypalbuminemia
Hyperbilirubinemia (mixed)
Hyperammonemia
Hepatocellular excretory function
Hyperbilirubinemia (mostly conjugated)
Elevated serum AP and γ-GT
Elevated serum bile acids

ALT, AST, alanine and aspartate aminotransferase, respectively; AP, alkaline phosphatase; γ-GT, gamma-glutamyl-transpeptidase; PLT, platelets; PT, prothrombin time.

ACUTE VIRAL HEPATITIS

The term *hepatitis* refers to any inflammatory process in the liver. The most common cause of acute hepatitis is viral infection. Acute viral hepatitis includes infection with the hepatotropic viruses A through E and other viruses such as adenoviruses, Coxsackie virus, cytomegalovirus, Epstein-Barr virus, and herpes simplex virus (HSV). Hepatitis in the latter cases is part of a systemic infection. The course of acute viral hepatitis is variable, from asymptomatic disease to fulminant liver failure that may necessitate liver transplantation. Although acute hepatitis A through D infections usually show the same clinical course in pregnant women, hepatitis E infection has been reported to have a mortality rate up to 20% during pregnancy. HSV hepatitis has also been associated with a worse outcome in pregnant patients, but the use of acyclovir has greatly improved the prognosis if the patient is diagnosed and treated promptly. In general, there is no specific treatment for acute viral hepatitis; the disease is fortunately self-limited in most cases.

Hepatitis A

Hepatitis A virus (HAV), a small RNA virus that belongs to the group of Picornaviridae, was recognized in 1973. HAV infection is highly contagious and is routinely transmitted by the enteric (fecal–oral) route. Acute hepatitis A tends to occur in developing countries with less advanced hygiene and sanitation practices. In such areas, most patients have anti-HAV antibodies by age 10. In other parts of the world, the prevalence of anti-HAV antibody increases with age, reaching 74% among individuals over 50 in the United States. Travelers to endemic areas and homosexuals with oral–anal sexual practices are at increased risk for acquiring HAV infection. Nearly 60% of all acute viral hepatitis cases in the United States are due to HAV infection.

The incubation period of HAV lasts 15 to 45 days. Viral shedding may occur before symptoms of acute illness develop. The brief viremic episode preceding the onset of jaundice accounts for the rare blood-borne transmission of HAV. The virus persists in the stool for a week or longer after disease onset. Symptoms generally include nausea, vomiting, and fever, but patients sometimes present with mild or subclinical infection when the infection may be recognized incidentally. Enzyme levels are elevated for about 8 weeks. Mortality, usually due to fulminant HAV hepatitis, is about 0.1%, although it may be higher in the elderly.

Acute hepatitis A is diagnosed by serologic testing for IgM anti-HAV antibodies (these usually persist for 6 months). The presence of IgG anti-HAV indicates past infection and immunity. Once antibodies occur, they persist for lifetime. Patients with HAV infection do not develop chronic hepatitis or a carrier state.

Treatment of acute hepatitis A is supportive. Patients are monitored for the development of fulminant hepatitis. Close contacts of the patient (household, sexual, day care, nursing home, etc.) should receive passive prophylaxis with HAV immune globulin as soon as possible (unless they have documented immunity to HAV), no later than 2 weeks after exposure. Preexposure prophylaxis with HAV vaccine is recommended for travelers going to areas where it is endemic. The introduction of routine active immunization against HAV remains controversial.

Hepatitis B

Hepatitis B virus (HBV), identified in 1989, is a DNA virus with a unique mode of replication by using its messenger RNA for reverse transcription. The 42-nm-large HBV has a coat and a nucleocapsid. The coat is made up of the surface antigen (HBsAg), whereas the nucleocapsid contains the partially circular DNA, the core antigen, the precore-derived or envelope antigen (HBeAg), and a DNA polymerase. The primary mode of horizontal HBV transmission is through blood and various body fluids. HBsAg can be detected in semen, saliva, sweat, tears, and breast milk. Intravenous drug abuse, heterosexual and homosexual promiscuity, and health care employment put one at high risk for HBV infection. This transmission mode dominates in developed industrial countries. Vertical transmission of HBV is most important in countries where chronic HBsAg carrier state reaches endemic levels. There is an estimated 350 million HBV carriers in the world. Passing HBV from a carrier mother to her newborn results in most new chronic HBV carriers.

The incubation period of HBV infection is between 1 and 4 months. Symptoms commonly include nausea and vomiting and extrahepatic manifestations such as arthralgias. Up to 70% of patients have subclinical infection or remain anicteric. The physical examination may find tender hepatomegaly. Transaminase levels usually return to normal within 1 to 2 months. The prothrombin time is the best prognostic predictor, and its prolongation by 2 seconds or more may suggest the development of subacute hepatic necrosis or fulminant hepatitis and demands close monitoring. Fulminant liver failure is an unusual outcome in about 0.1% to 0.5% of the cases. Acute HBV infection becomes chronic in about 5% in adults, but the rate is about 90% in newborn with perinatal HBV exposure (see below).

The diagnosis of acute HBV infection relies on the serologic detection of various HBV antigens and antibodies. HBsAg usually appears before the onset of clinical symptoms and remains detectable for up to 6 months. Its continued presence beyond this period implies chronic infection. Parallel persistence of transaminase elevations indicates chronic hepatitis B, whereas other HBsAg-positive patients become asymptomatic carriers. Recovery from acute HBV infection is indicated by the appearance of anti-HBs. This may occur before or after HBsAg becomes undetectable. The window period, with no HBV surface marker in the serum, requires detection of IgM anti-HBc to establish the diagnosis of acute hepatitis B. Anti-HBs may coexist in a significant number of HBsAg-positive individuals, only to indicate insufficient immune response and confirm the carrier status. It has become clear that anti-HBs, even in the absence of HBsAg, does not signify complete HBV clearance, because HBV DNA can be detected with the new and sensitive polymerase chain reaction assays and HBV may reactivate years later upon immunosuppression in many anti-HBs–positive cases. Moreover, acute hepatitis B in patients transplanted with anti-HBc–positive liver grafts revealed that low-level HBV infection is a significant problem. HBeAg has been regarded as a marker of HBV replication and infectivity. Seroconversion of HBeAg into anti-HBe occurs relatively early in acute HBV infection. However, HBeAg may persist for years in patients with chronic HBV infection. HBe seroconversion is a marker of successful antiviral therapy. HBeAg may also disappear spontaneously due to a precore mutation solely to reveal the emergence of HBe-negative chronic hepatitis B.

The treatment of acute hepatitis B is supportive. Sexual contacts and persons who have had percutaneous or mucosal exposure to the patient should receive HBV immune globulin (passive immunoprophylaxis) and HBV vaccine, unless they have immunity to HBV. Preexposure vaccination is recommended for persons with occupational risk, clients and staff in institutions, hemodialysis patients, populations in which HBV is endemic, and travelers to endemic areas. As a move toward the global eradication of HBV, universal HBV vaccination of all newborns in the United States has been recommended. Currently available recombinant HBV vaccines are very safe and effective.

Hepatitis C

Hepatitis C, previously termed non-A, non-B hepatitis, accounts for about 20% of acute hepatitis in the United States. It is caused by the hepatitis C virus (HCV), a small RNA virus closely related to the flaviviruses and pestiviruses. HCV, identified in 1989, has been the most common cause of transfusion hepatitis. Screening of blood products was initiated in 1990, and current methods dwarfed the HCV transmission risk to 1 in roughly 1 million. About 40% of patients with HCV are intravenous drug abusers, whereas another 40% who acquire HCV infection have no clear route of transmission. Sexual, occupational, household exposure, blood transfusions, and hemodialysis account for the rest. Importantly, about 80% of patients infected with HCV will develop chronic hepatitis. Cirrhosis and end-stage liver disease due to HCV is the leading cause of liver transplantation in the United States.

The incubation of HCV infection lasts about 2 months. The clinical presentation is usually insidious. Nausea and vomiting are common; jaundice, fever, and arthralgias occur less often. The symptoms may last up to 3 months. The most common manifestation is subclinical, with asymptomatic elevation of transaminases noted incidentally on routine screening. High-risk patients therefore may need periodic screening for HCV.

The diagnosis is based on detection of anti-HCV antibodies that usually appear within 6 to 8 weeks, preceding the onset of clinical symptoms. New generation anti-HCV assays are much more reliable, although false-positive and false-negative tests still occur. Detection of HCV RNA by various assays is more accurate and is routinely used for confirmation and to guide the antiviral therapy. Because HCV infection shows a very high chronicity, antiviral treatment of patients with acute HCV infection has been recommended. Pegylated interferon-α may be given for 6 months, combined with ribavirin if no response is seen after 12 weeks. Because of the large number of asymptomatic acute infections, however, this approach is rather uncommon. Postexposure treatment with antiviral agents after needlestick injury from known HCV-positive source may be initiated based on serial monitoring.

Hepatitis D

Hepatitis D occurs only as a coinfection with HBV or as a superinfection in HBsAg-positive patients. Hepatitis D virus (HDV) is a defective RNA virus requiring the presence of HBV for complete virion assembly and secretion. Acute HDV coinfection is indistinguishable from acute hepatitis B. Superinfection with HDV is usually severe, with a high mortality rate and chronicity. HDV is highly infectious; transmission is percutaneous and sexual. The diagnosis is made by detection of IgM anti-HDV that indicates acute infection. Interestingly, HBV replication is usually suppressed in patients with concomitant HDV infection (virus interference).

Hepatitis E

Hepatitis E resembles acute hepatitis A in many regards. It is caused by the hepatitis E virus (HEV), a small unenveloped RNA virus, structurally similar to the group of calciviruses. The transmission of HEV is predominantly fecal–oral. Contaminated water is generally thought to be the source of infection. The disease is prevalent in Mexico and certain Asian and African countries with outbreaks occurring in the monsoon season. HEV in the United States has been occasionally described in persons returning from endemic areas. Pregnant women with travel plans to affected countries should be advised.

The mean incubation period is 6 weeks with an abrupt onset of nausea, vomiting, fever, and jaundice. There are no associated extrahepatic features, and the infection never becomes chronic. Acute hepatitis E is generally mild, but high mortality has been reported in pregnancy (mother, up to 20%; fetus, up to 50%). The diagnosis is aided by the detection of IgM type anti-HEV antibodies. Serology is helpful in differentiating hepatitis E from acute fatty liver of pregnancy (AFLP). HEV vaccine is not yet available.

Herpes Simplex Hepatitis

Herpes simplex hepatitis due to HSV types 1 and 2 may be associated with a fulminant course during pregnancy, possibly because of the associated immunocompromised state. Patients usually present in the second or third trimester with symptoms of upper respiratory tract infection and fever. Characteristic vesicular oral–genital lesions are found in 30% of cases. Significant transaminase elevation typically occurs without jaundice. The diagnosis can be confirmed by serology, HSV polymerase chain reaction assay, or immunofluorescence from lesion scrapings. The fulminant hepatitis is often fatal. Acyclovir has improved the mortality rates and should be given promptly once the diagnosis is recognized.

DRUG-INDUCED ACUTE LIVER INJURY

Liver is the primary site of drug metabolism. Drug modification and detoxification mainly occurs by the cytochrome P-450 system located in the endoplasmic reticulum. Drug-induced liver disease can resemble virtually every known pathologic condition of the liver. Some drugs are known to be toxic to the liver, and the degree of injury is dose dependent (intrinsic or predictable hepatotoxins). The toxic effect usually results from the effect of a toxic drug metabolite (indirect). Other drugs may cause liver injury in an unpredictable fashion (idiosyncratic hepatotoxins). Genetic polymorphism of the P-450 system may account for idiosyncratic drug reactions and unpredictable serum drug levels. The two major patterns of injury caused by intrinsic and idiosyncratic drugs are hepatitis-like (cytotoxic) and cholestatic.

Although the list of direct hepatotoxic agents is limited (some notable examples being carbon tetrachloride, mushroom poisons, trichloroethylene, yellow phosphorus, galactosamine, aflatoxins, and methotrexate), the number of drugs potentially causing idiosyncratic liver injury is virtually endless. When searching for a culprit in drug-induced liver injury, every medication should be suspected. Several drugs may cause liver disease by a mixed mechanism (e.g., methyldopa, isoniazid, valproic acid, and amiodarone).

The pattern of liver injury caused by a given drug many times is typical. Most idiosyncratic reactions result primarily in hepatocellular injury. Acute drug-induced hepatitis is most often caused by acetaminophen, tetracyclines, valproic acid, antidepressants, and antiretroviral medications. Cholestasis is the characteristic lesion caused by oral contraceptives, estrogen replacement, anabolic steroids, chlorpromazine, erythromycin, and tolbutamide.

Drug-induced liver injury depends on a variety of host factors. Biotransformation capacity of the liver changes significantly with age, and certain drugs cause liver injury with an age preference. Tetracyclines have been associated with acute fatty liver in pregnancy.

The clinical manifestation of drug-induced acute liver injury depends on the primary underlying pattern of liver damage. In hepatocellular injury, the clinical picture is that of acute hepatitis, with nonspecific gastrointestinal symptoms and malaise. Jaundice may be present. Serum transaminase levels are typically high, many times surpassing the values seen in viral hepatitis. In difficult cases, liver biopsy should be performed. Typical histologic lesion of acute drug-induced liver injury is steatosis, necrosis, or both. In cholestatic injury, pruritus may precede the onset of jaundice, but anicteric reactions are also common. Serum alkaline phosphatase and γ-glutamyltranspeptidase levels are increased, and transaminases are moderately elevated (usually no more than 100–200 U/L). Liver biopsy reveals cholestasis with bile plugs and mixed cell portal inflammation.

The most important therapeutic measure is to discontinue the offending agent. This usually results in resolution of the symptoms and laboratory abnormalities within a few weeks. If significant coagulopathy and encephalopathy develop, these herald the onset of acute liver failure and the need of intensive and specialized care.

Veno-occlusive disease is a special condition characterized by subendothelial swelling and collagenization of the small hepatic veins, leading to hepatomegaly, ascites, and significant weight gain. The disease was originally described in patients who ingested the toxic pyrrolizidine alkaloids of bush teas in Jamaica. Azathioprine, cyclophosphamide, and other chemotherapeutics may also cause veno-occlusive disease. Mortality in veno-occlusive disease is high (up to 25% in moderate disease).

Oral contraceptives appear to increase the risk of hepatic adenomas, a trend being changed by the use of reduced amounts of estrogens. The risk increases in women older than age 30 years. Elevated estrogen levels may account for the rapid growth of hepatic adenomas occasionally seen in pregnancy. Complications that may arise from hepatic adenomas include rupture and hemorrhage, especially in adenomas more than 3 cm in diameter. Malignant transformation has been associated. Patients may present with abdominal pain, a palpable mass, or with shock secondary to rupture and hemoperitoneum. Large (>5 cm) and symptomatic adenomas may need resection, especially before a planned pregnancy, to avoid the risk of acute complications.

LIVER DISEASE AND PREGNANCY

Liver disease is rare in pregnancy. When it occurs, however, liver disease may have a significant impact on the mother, the fetus, or both. Based on their causal relationship with pregnancy, liver diseases can be classified into four major categories: (a) liver diseases that occur in pregnancy, but their course is mostly unaffected (coincidental); (b) liver diseases predisposed or worsened by pregnancy; (c) liver diseases that are specific to pregnancy; and (d) pregnancy occurring in women with underlying chronic liver disease or after liver transplantation. Most features of liver disease are not unique to pregnancy. They include jaundice, pruritus, abdominal pain, nausea, vomiting, and an array of biochemical abnormalities. The gestational age is an important guide to the differential diagnosis.

Liver Diseases Coincidental with Pregnancy

Viral hepatitis is the most common cause of jaundice during pregnancy in the United States. With the exception of hepatitis E (see above), the course of these infections in pregnant women and in other patients is essentially similar. There is no evidence that HAV is more common or more severe during pregnancy. Vertical transmission is rare, presumably because of the brief viremic episode. Similarly, the course of pregnancy is not different in acute hepatitis B or in the HBsAg carrier state. Vertical transmission of HBV, however, is a great risk to the newborn, resulting in chronic hepatitis B infection in about 90% of cases. Transmission occurs during delivery and the incidence is much higher if the mother is HBeAg positive. Infants born to mothers who are HBsAg positive should therefore receive hepatitis B immune globulin administered within 12 hours after birth along with the first dose of HBV vaccine. With prophylaxis, breast-feeding is allowed because no additional risk of HBV transmission was found. Routine HBsAg screening of all pregnant women is mandatory in the United States. Vertical transmission of HCV is rare but appears to be enhanced by the coexistence of HIV infection. Currently there are no data to assess if antiviral therapy reduces perinatal transmission of HCV. Breast-feeding does not seem to transmit HCV.

Liver Diseases Predisposed or Worsened by Pregnancy

Certain liver diseases show an aggravated course in the pregnant woman. Acute HEV and HSV hepatitis during pregnancy are such notable conditions, associated with high maternal mortality when occurring in the last trimester. Cholelithiasis may become symptomatic or deteriorate during pregnancy, most likely as a result of decreased biliary motility ("sluggish gallbladder") caused by elevated serum levels of progesterone. Because pregnancy is associated with a hypercoagulable state (probably due to increased levels of fibrinogen and factors VIII, IX, and XII), hepatic vein obstruction, known as Budd-Chiari syndrome, occurs more often in the pregnant woman. Typically, it presents close to term with rapid onset of abdominal pain, large and tender liver, and ascites. Budd-Chiari syndrome may be diagnosed with Doppler ultrasonography, computed tomography, or angiography. If left untreated, mortality in Budd-Chiari syndrome is high. Treatment options include anticoagulation, revascularization surgery (angioplasty, transjugular intrahepatic portosystemic shunt, or portal-systemic shunt), and, eventually, liver transplantation.

Liver Diseases Specific to Pregnancy

Several liver diseases occur only in pregnancy. The relationship of these to the gestational stage is rather specific, and with the exception of hyperemesis gravidarum (HG), they usually develop late in the third trimester. Three unique conditions of late pregnancy associated with hepatocellular disease, namely AFLP, preeclampsia, and HELLP syndrome (*h*emolysis, *e*levated *l*iver enzymes, and *l*ow *p*latelet count), present with similar symptoms and show significant clinical overlap. The definitive therapeutic intervention in these conditions is delivery itself, although all three may manifest postpartum (in about 30%) and may also recur in subsequent pregnancies.

HYPEREMESIS GRAVIDARUM

HG is an aggravated form of morning sickness with intractable nausea and vomiting that presents in early pregnancy. It occurs in 0.3% to 1% of all pregnancies.

Etiology. The causative factors of HG are unknown. A psychological etiology has been implicated but never proven. Hormonal changes associated with pregnancy have also been proposed as a cause of this disorder. Jaundice is likely due to impaired bilirubin excretion in the setting of malnutrition. Factors that appear to be associated with an increased risk for HG include high body weight preceding the pregnancy, nulliparity, and twin gestation. Factors associated with a decreased risk include advanced maternal age and cigarette smoking.

Clinical Presentation. HG is generally accompanied by loss of more than 5% of the prepregnancy body weight. Physical findings generally include orthostatic hypotension and decreased skin turgor, consistent with dehydration. Abdominal pain is usually absent; if present, it should prompt investigation of other causes such as peptic ulcer disease. Excessive salivation (ptyalism) is frequently noted. Hepatomegaly may be evident on the physical examination.

Laboratory Findings. Laboratory findings are consistent with dehydration: elevated specific gravity of the urine, increased blood urea nitrogen, increased hematocrit associated with hemoconcentration, and significant ketonuria or ketonemia may be seen. About 50% of patients have hepatic complications, including hyperbilirubinemia and elevated serum aminotransferase levels. Liver biopsy, if performed, may show central cholestasis and centrizonal vacuolization, likely related to malnutrition.

Differential Diagnosis. Conditions that may coincide with the pregnancy and lead to nausea and vomiting and dehydration and malnutrition should be considered. These include gastrointestinal disorders, such as gastroenteritis, peptic ulcer disease, pancreatitis, or appendicitis, and endocrine disorders, such as diabetic ketoacidosis, hyperthyroidism, or hyperparathyroidism.

Treatment. The disease generally responds well to supportive treatment. Intravenous fluid replacement is the mainstay of therapy. In severe cases, total parenteral nutrition may be required. Rarely, termination of pregnancy is necessary. Thiamine needs to be replaced to avoid Wernicke encephalopathy. Conditions that may provoke nausea and vomiting, such as spicy foods, strong odors, and quick positional changes, should be avoided. Antiemetic drugs are routinely applied. Mild nausea may be controlled with vitamin B_6 (pyridoxine) and antihistamines. Choices for severe nausea and vomiting include metoclopramide, promethazine, chlorpromazine, droperidol, and 5-HT3 serotonin receptor antagonists such as ondansetron. Caution is advised with phenothiazines because they may worsen the cholestasis. Corticosteroids have been used with success in cases of severe and refractory HG.

The mean birth weight of infants born to mothers is usually not affected, although it has been reported to be lower with severe HG cases. There is no evidence of increased risk of fetal deformity. The disease may recur in subsequent pregnancies.

INTRAHEPATIC CHOLESTASIS OF PREGNANCY

Intrahepatic cholestasis of pregnancy (ICP) is the second most common cause of jaundice in pregnancy, after viral hepatitis. It is responsible for about 20% of all jaundice cases that occur during pregnancy. ICP is associated with a benign maternal outcome but with a paradoxically high incidence of prematurity and stillbirth. The incidence of this disease varies geographically. It reportedly occurs in about 1% to 3% of pregnancies in Scandinavia (where it was first recognized by Ahlfeld in 1883) and 2% to 5% of those in Chile. In other sites, the overall incidence is reported to be 0.5% to 1% of pregnancies. It is rarely seen in Asians and blacks. There appears to be a familial predilection.

Etiology. The etiology is not completely understood, but genetic factors are obviously important based on the higher incidence in certain ethnic groups, the familial clustering, and the recurrence with subsequent pregnancies. There appears to be an abnormality of estrogen metabolism that may include defective transport through the hepatocyte canalicular membrane. A problem that is otherwise clinically insignificant may become evident only during periods of stress such as pregnancy, when estrogen levels become elevated. The role of estrogens was further supported by the higher occurrence of ICP in twin pregnancies. Administration of an oral contraceptive to susceptible patients may cause a similar cholestatic picture. Progesterone may be associated with ICP and should also be avoided in women with a history of ICP.

Clinical Presentation. ICP usually begins in the third trimester, although up to a third of patients present earlier. The primary symptom is pruritus, and it may be the only manifestation. Pruritus generally predominates on the palms and soles and may become intolerable. Itching may be followed by the development of anorexia, right upper quadrant abdominal pain, nausea, and vomiting. Weight loss may be significant. About 20% of patients develop jaundice, generally 2 to 4 weeks after the development of pruritus. The physical examination is notable for the absence of stigmata of chronic liver disease.

Laboratory Findings. Laboratory findings are consistent with a cholestatic picture. If checked, serum total bile acid concentrations are found to increase 10- to 100-fold above normal levels in ICP. The total bilirubin level is usually less than 5 mg/dL. Whereas the alkaline phosphatase level is elevated, γ-glutamyltranspeptidase levels are mostly normal—an unusual finding in other forms of cholestasis. Aminotransferase levels are normal or modestly elevated, with occasionally high values found. Patients may have overt steatorrhea because of bile salt malabsorption. This results in malabsorption of fat-soluble vitamins and can lead to a prolonged prothrombin time.

Differential Diagnosis. If the jaundice is severe, the differential diagnosis must be extended to viral hepatitis and biliary tract disease. The presence of jaundice without pruritus is atypical in ICP and should prompt investigations to rule out other causes. If the onset is near term or the patient has severe symptoms and any evidence of renal or hematologic insufficiency, other causes of jaundice must be evaluated, such as AFLP or HELLP syndrome. Failure of the pruritus to resolve postpartum and the continuing high alkaline phosphatase levels also suggest an alternative etiology of cholestasis.

Treatment. Treatment should focus on alleviating the pruritus and prevent maternal and fetal complications. Cholestyramine has been tried because it binds bile acids and estrogen, but it may cause malabsorption of fat-soluble vitamins and worsen the steatorrhea and hypoprothrombinemia. Currently, the best results have been found with administration of ursodeoxycholic acid (UDCA). UDCA increases bile flow and proved to be useful in the treatment of primary biliary cirrhosis. In recent randomized controlled trials, UDCA treatment in ICP resulted in significant improvement of pruritus and declining bilirubin and transaminase levels. No fetal toxicity was observed, even when higher UDCA doses were used. UDCA treatment is therefore appropriate in severe cases of ICP, with an average dose of 15 mg/kg/d.

ICP usually resolves within 1 to 2 weeks postpartum. It is, however, not a routine indication for premature delivery because the maternal prognosis is excellent and complications are rare. Increased formation of cholesterol gallstones has been described in the mother, and patients may be at increased risk for biliary tract disease. The sequelae are more ominous for the fetus, because increased incidence of fetal wastage, stillbirth, and prematurity may occur in up to 60% of cases. Transplacental toxicity of maternal bile acids has been postulated to account for these events. Interestingly, UDCA treatment appeared to correct placental bile acid transport rather than contributed to toxicity. Maternal vitamin K deficiency can lead to neonatal intracranial hemorrhage. For these reasons, patients with ICP may be placed on prophylactic subcutaneous or oral vitamin K. Patients should be warned that ICP usually returns in subsequent pregnancies as well as with medications containing estrogens or progesterone.

ACUTE FATTY LIVER OF PREGNANCY

AFLP is a rare condition characterized by fatty infiltration of the liver in the third trimester. Its estimated incidence is about one in 6,000 to 16,000 pregnancies. It is more common in the first pregnancy, with twin gestation, and with male infants, although AFLP can occur with any gestation.

Etiology. The cause of AFLP is unclear. Based on its similarity to liver diseases associated with Reye syndrome, Jamaican vomiting sickness, and hepatotoxicity induced by drugs like tetracycline, amiodarone, or valproate, a deficiency of mitochondrial fatty acid oxidation has been suspected in AFLP. Indeed, most infants from pregnancies complicated by AFLP show a mutation (Glu474Gln) in the gene of long-chain 3-hydroxyacyl coenzyme A dehydrogenase, a key enzyme of fatty acid oxidation. Because this defect is autosomal recessive, usually the mother is heterozygous for the disorder, with a homozygously affected fetus. Accumulation and toxicity of long-chain fatty acid metabolites produced by the fetus may be the cause of maternal liver disease. As part of the systemic mitochondrial dysfunction, the disease may also affect the nervous system, pancreas, muscle, and kidneys.

Clinical Presentation. Affected, usually nulliparous, women present in the third trimester (the earliest onset of AFLP has been documented in the 28th gestational week). Leading symptoms are nausea and vomiting, abdominal pain, anorexia, fever, lethargy, and jaundice. Abdominal pain may be generalized or localized to the right upper quadrant or epigastrium. These symptoms may mimic biliary tract disease, acute pancreatitis, or gastroesophageal reflux. Almost half the patients who develop AFLP have signs and symptoms of preeclampsia (see later). Some patients, however, may be asymptomatic, and AFLP is diagnosed incidentally by laboratory or imaging studies.

On physical examination, the patient appears ill. The liver size is normal or shrunken. Severely affected patients may show neurologic findings such as asterixis and confusion, symptoms consistent with elevated ammonia levels and hypoglycemia.

Laboratory Findings. Women with AFLP show abnormal liver function tests, with aminotransferase levels up to 1,000 U/L (in contrast to acute viral hepatitis, in which transaminases usually exceed this value). Jaundice is relatively late and moderate, with total bilirubin levels generally less than 10 mg/dL. Leukocytosis is common, with white cell counts higher than usually seen in pregnancy, but this is nonspecific. The peripheral blood smear may demonstrate microangiopathic abnormalities such as schistocytes. If significant thrombocytopenia is seen, the disease may have progressed into disseminated intravascular coagulation (DIC), characterized by thrombocytopenia, microangiopathic hemolysis, and coagulopathy. Reduction in fibrinogen levels may be relative because fibrinogen is normally elevated at the end of pregnancy. In severe disease with hepatic failure, hypoglycemia and hyperammonemia may ensue. Renal insufficiency complicates AFLP in up to 60% of cases.

Differential Diagnosis. The diagnosis is largely made on clinical grounds. If a liver biopsy is performed, microvesicular steatosis is a pathognomonic finding, but the severe coagulopathy often precludes this procedure. It is important to exclude other etiologies such as a drug reaction or drug overdose, viral hepatitis, and HELLP syndrome. HELLP syndrome is not a cause of fulminant liver failure, unlike AFLP. Pruritus in AFLP is unusual and should suggest ICP.

Treatment. Close fetal monitoring is necessary. Treatment is delivery usually followed by improvement within 2 to 3 days. Because of the significant coagulopathy, cesarean section is preferred. Treatment of the liver disease is supportive, including replacement of coagulation factors and close monitoring of encephalopathy and serum glucose levels. The management often requires placement in an intensive care unit and may include hemodialysis, mechanical ventilation, and parenteral nutrition. If there is no improvement within 24 to 48 hours of delivery, transfer to a tertiary center that has liver transplantation capability should be considered.

Although AFLP used to be almost universally fatal, the current mortality rate varies from 8% to 33%. This is probably due to increased recognition of AFLP in less severe cases, improved supportive measures, and better intensive care management. Fetal mortality varies from 14% to 66%. Occasionally, orthotopic liver transplantation becomes necessary for a patient who does not improve after delivery. There are reports in the literature with recurring cases of AFLP during subsequent pregnancies. Women with history of AFLP and their newborn infants should be tested for the Glu474Gln mutation of long-chain 3-hydroxy-acyl coenzyme A dehydrogenase.

PREECLAMPSIA AND HELLP SYNDROME

Preeclampsia is a triad of hypertension, proteinuria, and edema, becoming gradually apparent in the late second or the third trimester. When seizures occur in addition to these symptoms, the condition is called eclampsia. Preeclampsia–eclampsia is usually diagnosed in nulliparas and complicates about 5% of pregnancies. The disease is a source of significant maternal and fetal morbidity and mortality. Hepatic disease is only seen in severe cases of preeclampsia. HELLP syndrome is a variant of preeclampsia that develops in about 20% of affected women and was named after several additional findings (*h*emolysis, *e*levated *l*iver enzymes, and *l*ow *p*latelet count). The overlap between preeclampsia and HELLP is not complete, and only up to 70% of patients with HELLP syndrome are hypertensive.

Etiology. The pathomechanism of preeclampsia and eclampsia is not entirely understood, but it has been suggested that fibrin deposition is the primary event. An alternative hypothesis is that segmental vasospasm occurs, followed by initiation of platelet aggregation and fibrin deposition, leading to severe end-organ injury that includes the liver, kidneys, brain, or heart.

Clinical Presentation. Nausea and vomiting are common in preeclampsia, as is a history of malaise. Patients usually have significant weight gain and generalized edema. Severe hypertension may not be present. Hepatic complications in severe preeclampsia and HELLP syndrome include intraparenchymal infarction, subcapsular hemorrhage, and liver rupture. In these cases, the patient presents with sudden onset of epigastric or right upper quadrant pain, vomiting, and circulatory collapse.

Patients with HELLP syndrome tend to be older and multiparous. About one third of all HELLP cases will occur postpartum. Maternal mortality in severe preeclampsia is less than 1% in institutions that are familiar with the condition. Most cases of death are due to central nervous system catastrophes, with hepatic complications accounting for the rest. Fetal mortality may arise from placental abruption, prematurity, and intrauterine growth retardation. In HELLP syndrome, mortality rates up to 25% have been reported. Additional complications may include DIC, acute renal failure, and respiratory distress. Perinatal mortality in HELLP syndrome varies between 10% and 60%.

Laboratory Findings. Abnormal liver function tests may be seen in 20% to 30% of women suffering from preeclampsia, with transaminase levels usually two to four times normal. Transaminase levels tend to be higher in HELLP syndrome, and marked elevations can be seen with liver infarction, hemorrhage, or rupture. Jaundice is uncommon except for major hepatic complications. By definition, hemolysis must be present in HELLP syndrome (microangiopathic hemolytic anemia) with platelet counts generally less than 100,000. Overt DIC is more prevalent in HELLP syndrome.

Differential Diagnosis. As noted above, there is a significant overlap between AFLP, preeclampsia–eclampsia, and HELLP syndrome. All three conditions tend to occur in the third trimester, accompanied by nonspecific gastrointestinal symptoms and frequently abnormal liver function tests. Several clinical and laboratory features, however, may help differentiate these disorders from each other. Sudden onset, profound jaundice, hepatic encephalopathy, and a small liver are all characteristic of AFLP. The liver is usually normal in size or moderately enlarged in preeclampsia and HELLP syndrome. Hypoglycemia is a distinctive feature of severe AFLP. Very high transaminase levels in the typical setting are suggestive of hepatic infarction or hemorrhage rather than acute viral hepatitis. DIC may complicate any of these disorders, but it is least frequent in preeclampsia. Liver steatosis is most prominent in AFLP and may be picked up on ultrasound examination, but fatty liver can also be seen in preeclampsia. Liver biopsy is best avoided because of the general underlying coagulopathy. The differential diagnosis of HELLP syndrome includes other microangiopathic hemolytic disorders, including thrombotic thrombocytopenic purpura and the hemolytic uremic syndrome.

Treatment. Patients with HELLP syndrome who are close to term should be considered preeclamptic and delivered promptly. This includes patients who are at or beyond 34 weeks of gestation or if there is evidence of fetal lung maturity. Patients who are remote to term should be transferred to a tertiary care center for intensive fetal monitoring and for further assessment and stabilization of the maternal condition. General treatment guidelines include bed rest, lateral decubitus position (to improve cardiac hemodynamics), blood pressure control, and magnesium sulfate for seizure prophylaxis. Fetal lung maturity may be hastened with administration of steroids (dexamethasone). HELLP syndrome is not an absolute indication for cesarean section; patients who are presenting in labor can be allowed to deliver vaginally in the absence of any other obstetric contraindications. Intravenous dexamethasone at 12-hour intervals has been successfully used either antepartum or postpartum to precipitate maternal recovery. Preeclampsia and HELLP syndrome may recur in subsequent pregnancies, indicating specific predispositions to these disorders.

Hepatic rupture is the most feared complication of preeclampsia and HELLP syndrome. Patients who are in circulatory shock and present with shoulder pain, ascites, or pleural effusion need quick evaluation by computed tomography or magnetic resonance imaging to exclude subcapsular hematoma of the liver. Ultrasound examination is less reliable to detect these lesions. Generally, rupture of the liver involves the right lobe. It is often preceded by the development of a hematoma. There may be several hours of severe epigastric pain before progression to circulatory collapse. The finding of a ruptured subcapsular hematoma of the liver is an indication for laparotomy and aggressive blood product replacement. Treatment is optimally managed by an experienced liver trauma team and may occasionally include liver transplantation. Even with appropriate treatment, mortality is over 50% for the mother and the fetus. If the hematoma has not ruptured and the patient is not hypotensive, hepatic infarction and subcapsular hematoma can be managed conservatively with close monitoring and visualization with serial computed tomography or magnetic resonance imaging.

ACUTE LIVER FAILURE

Definition

Acute liver failure results from massive hepatocyte necrosis and is defined as the onset of severely impaired liver function with no preceding liver disease within 6 months after the initial symptoms. Acute liver failure may become manifest within a few days or weeks after the insult. Based on the rapidity of evolving clinical picture, further classification is possible. Fulminant hepatic failure is described if major signs of the failing liver (encephalopathy, coagulopathy, and jaundice) occur within 2 weeks. Subacute and late-onset acute liver failure will denote less speedy scenarios.

Etiology

The causes of acute liver failure are numerous (Table 63.2). HBV is responsible for about 75% of cases of acute liver failure. Acetaminophen overdose from suicide attempts, a leading cause of fulminant hepatic failure in the United Kingdom, is less prevalent in the United States. Acetaminophen is metabolized by the liver cytochrome P-450 enzyme system to a toxic metabolite, *N*-acetyl-*p*-benzoquinoneimine, which is responsible for the liver injury. *N*-acetyl-*p*-benzoquinoneimine is normally detoxified by glutathione. Because alcohol stimulates the cytochrome P-450 system and depletes the glutathione stores, it may decrease the threshold for acetaminophen toxicity. An area of controversy is whether lower doses of acetaminophen cause hepatocellular injury in certain patients. Although there have been reports with fatalities in cases with therapeutic acetaminophen doses and acute alcohol ingestion, it is unusual to have acute liver failure with acetaminophen doses less than 4 g/d. The drugs most commonly causing idiosyncratic reactions include halothane, antituberculotics, anticonvulsants, nonsteroidal antiinflammatory drugs, and certain antidepressants. If transaminase elevation is noted in patients taking these medications, the agent should be stopped promptly. Ingestion of *Amanita* mushrooms usually results in prolonged vomiting and diarrhea, with the development of fulminant hepatic failure and acute renal failure within 3 to 8 days.

There are less frequent causes of acute liver failure. Wilson disease usually manifests with a picture of chronic liver disease but occasionally presents as fulminant hepatic failure and necessitates liver transplantation. Reye syndrome and AFLP may cause fulminant hepatic failure that is characterized by microvesicular steatosis. Reye syndrome occurs in children, usually after an acute febrile illness, and is associated with salicylate use. Hypoglycemia may become a significant problem. Budd-Chiari syndrome may also cause acute liver failure. Ischemic hepatitis may occur due to hypoperfusion from heart failure, shock, and protracted surgery. Massive metastasis formation in the liver leading to acute liver failure most likely originates from small cell carcinoma, breast tumor, malignant melanoma, or lymphoproliferative malignancies.

TABLE 63.2. Major Causes of Acute Liver Failure

Acute viral hepatitis
Hepatitis viruses A to E
Other viral agents
Chemicals and toxins
Idiosyncratic drug reactions
Acetaminophen overdose
Mushroom poisoning
Industrial poisons
Metabolic
Reye syndrome
Wilson disease
Acute fatty liver of pregnancy
Vascular
Budd-Chiari syndrome
Ischemic liver injury
Miscellaneous
Massive metastatic disease
Sepsis
Heat stroke

Clinical and Laboratory Findings

The onset of acute liver failure is often nonspecific, with nausea, vomiting, and malaise. These symptoms may be followed by rapid deterioration, deep jaundice, coagulopathy, and encephalopathy leading to coma. Immediate hepatology consultation is advised and the patients should be transferred to a specialized unit, preferably with an expertise for liver transplantation, as soon as possible. Survival in acute liver failure varies between 20% and 70%, but it may be improved to over 80% if transplantation is available. Patients with the best chances for spontaneous recovery include those with fulminant viral hepatitis and acetaminophen toxicity. Survival without orthotopic liver transplantation is less likely in patients younger than 10 and older than 40. There are multiple criteria for orthotopic liver transplantation in acute liver failure, and these are based on various clinical and laboratory parameters (age, etiology, grade of encephalopathy, blood pH, prothrombin time, serum creatinine). Management of acute liver failure is an exceedingly complex task and is beyond the scope of this treatise.

BIBLIOGRAPHY

Abell TL, Riely CA. Hyperemesis gravidarum. *Gastroenterol Clin North Am* 1992;21:835–849.

Caraceni P, Van Thiel DH. Acute liver failure. *Lancet* 1995;345:163–169.

Cuthbert JA. Hepatitis A: old and new. *Clin Microbiol Rev* 2001;14:38–58.

Hoofnagle JH, Carithers RL Jr, Shapiro C, et al. Fulminant hepatic failure: summary of a workshop. *Hepatology* 1995;21:240–252.

Jacobson IM, Dienstag JL, Werner BG, et al. Epidemiology and clinical impact of hepatitis D virus (delta) infection. *Hepatology* 1985;5:188–191.

Klein NA, Mabie WC, Shaver DC, et al. Herpes simplex virus hepatitis in pregnancy. *Gastroenterology* 1991;100:239–244.

Knox TA, Olans LB. Liver disease in pregnancy. *N Engl J Med* 1996;335:569–576.

Krawczynski K, Aggarwal R, Kamili S. Hepatitis E. *Infect Dis Clin North Am* 2000;14:669–687.

Lee WM. Drug-induced hepatotoxicity. *N Engl J Med* 1995;333:1118–1127.

Lok AS, Gunaratnam NT. Diagnosis of hepatitis C. *Hepatology* 1997;26:48S–56S.

Moseley RH. Evaluation of abnormal liver function tests. *Med Clin North Am* 1996;80:887–906.

Orland JR, Wright TL, Cooper S. Acute hepatitis C. *Hepatology* 2001;33:321–327.

Reyes H, Simon FR. Intrahepatic cholestasis of pregnancy: an estrogen-related disease. *Semin Liver Dis* 1993;13:289–301.

Riely CA. Liver disease in the pregnant patient. *Am J Gastroenterol* 1999;94: 1728–1732.

Sherlock S. Hepatic adenomas and oral contraceptives. *Gut* 1975;16:753–756.

Stone JH. HELLP syndrome: hemolysis, elevated liver enzymes, and low platelets. *JAMA* 1998;280:559–562.

Zimmerman HJ, Lewis JH. Chemical- and toxin-induced hepatotoxicity. *Gastroenterol Clin North Am* 1995;24:1027–1045.

Zimmerman RK, Ruben FL, Ahwesh ER. Hepatitis B virus infection, hepatitis B vaccine, and hepatitis B immune globulin. *J Fam Pract* 1997;45:295–315.

CHAPTER 64
Chronic Liver Disease

Pierre M. Gholam

Chronic liver disease is usually diagnosed by the primary care physician. Early diagnosis is essential. Therefore, clinicians must recognize the clinical and biochemical features of the various entities that lead to progressive liver damage. Recent advances in the treatment of viral hepatitis and liver transplantation have led to new treatment options and improved outcomes. This chapter briefly describes the most common chronic liver diseases with emphasis on clinical presentation, diagnostic modalities, and treatment. Particular focus is placed on diseases that are more prevalent in women, as well as issues related to liver disease in pregnancy.

PRIMARY BILIARY CIRRHOSIS

Etiology and Pathophysiology

Primary biliary cirrhosis (PBC) is a chronic cholestatic liver disease characterized by progressive inflammatory destruction of bile ducts, fibrosis, and eventually cirrhosis. Although a clear etiology has not been identified, an autoimmune component is believed to play a key role in the causation of disease. This is supported by the fact that antimitochondrial antibodies are presents in over 90% of patients. In addition, PBC is associated with a variety of autoimmune diseases, such as Sjögren disease, Hashimoto thyroiditis, celiac disease, and scleroderma. PBC is primarily a disease of females (female-to-male ratio of 9:1). Presentation is usually in middle age.

Presentation, Diagnosis, and Workup

PBC usually presents with unexplained itching, fatigue, jaundice, or unexplained weight loss. Right upper quadrant discomfort is sometimes present. Cutaneous manifestations include xanthelasmas. Other associated symptoms could include xerostomia, xerophthalmia, arthritis, and Raynaud phenomenon.

Biochemical abnormalities include an elevated alkaline phosphatase and serum IgM levels. Antimitochondrial antibodies are positive in 90% of patients. Modest elevations in transaminases and an increased serum cholesterol further suggest the diagnosis. Jaundice, hypoalbuminemia, and signs and symptoms of portal hypertension are found in advanced disease.

When suspected, the diagnosis is confirmed by a liver biopsy, which will also provide information about the disease stage and the prognosis. Florid duct lesions are histologic hallmarks of the disease. Imaging studies and endoscopic retrograde cholangiopancreatography are rarely useful.

Treatment

Liver disease in PBC is currently treated with ursodeoxycholic acid (13–15 mg/kg/d), which results in the lowering of serum bilirubin, alkaline phosphatase, transaminases, and IgM. Some improvement in pruritus may be observed. Data suggest that ursodeoxycholic acid may extend the time to death or transplantation, as compared with placebo. There is no definitive evidence that ursodeoxycholic acid improves liver histology in PBC. The drug is safe and well tolerated, except diarrhea may occur but rarely results in cessation of treatment. Other regimens have included colchicine, methotrexate, and cyclosporine, which are significantly more toxic. Transplantation remains the only treatment option for patients with advanced disease.

Another important aspect of treatment centers around the prevention of osteoporosis that appears to be associated with the disease. Dual-energy x-ray absorptiometry bone scans need to be periodically checked and calcium/vitamin D plus bisphosphonate therapy instituted where appropriate. Fat-soluble vitamin deficiency may occur and requires supplementation. Finally, despite elevations in serum cholesterol, there does not appear to be an increased risk of coronary artery disease in patients with PBC.

AUTOIMMUNE HEPATITIS

Etiology and Pathophysiology

Autoimmune hepatitis is an unresolving inflammation of the liver of unclear etiology. Pathologic hallmarks are interface hepatitis and portal plasma cell infiltration. Although the exact cause of disease is unknown, it is believed to have a strong autoimmune component.

Presentation, Diagnosis, and Workup

Patients often complain of fatigue, arthralgias, and jaundice. Women are affected more than men (female-to-male ratio of 3.6:1), and all age and ethnic groups are reported. Hypergammaglobulinemia and autoantibodies are found. Differentiating autoimmune hepatitis from hepatitis C can be difficult; guidelines are listed in Table 64.1.

The workup includes clinical suspicion and determination of antinuclear antibodies, SMA, and anti-LKM1 antibodies. Autoimmune hepatitis has been classified into several subgroups (Table 64.2). Histologic features on liver biopsy that suggest the diagnosis of autoimmune hepatitis are key to the diagnosis.

Treatment

Treatment should be instituted in patients with transaminase levels greater than 10-fold normal or patients with serum transaminase levels that are 5-fold the upper limit of normal in conjunction with a serum γ-globulin level at least twice the upper limit of normal. Extensive necrosis also requires therapy. Decision to treat may be individualized in patients who do not fit any of the above situations. Treatment may not be indicated

TABLE 64.1. Differentiation Between Autoimmune Hepatitis and Hepatitis C

Features	Autoimmune hepatitis	Hepatitis C
Age	Young, middle aged	All
Sex	Female	Male and female
Symptoms	Jaundice, fatigue	None
Association with autoimmune diseases	+	–
Transaminase levels	>10 × normal	<10 × normal
Contact with blood	–	+
Histologic findings	Plasma cell infiltrate, rosetting	Portal lymphoid aggregates, bile duct damage and loss, steatosis
Response to steroids	+	–

TABLE 64.2. Classification of Autoimmune Hepatitis

Type	Hyperglobulinemia	Sex	ANA	ASMA	Anti-LKM1	Anti-SLA	HCV ab	Steroid response	Interferon response
1 (classic)	+	F	+	+	–	–	–[a]	+	–
2a	–	F	–	–	+	–	–	+	–
2b	–	M	Low titer	Low titer	Low titer	–	+	–	+[b]
3	+	F	–	–	–	+	–	+	–
Cryptogenic	+	F	–	–	–	–	–	+	–

[a]False-positive results may occur.
[b]Approach with caution, perhaps only after failure of steroids.
ANA, antinuclear antibodies; ASMA, anti-smooth muscle antibody; anti-LKM1, anti-liver-kidney microsomal antibody; anti-SLA, antisoluble liver antigen; M, male; F, female; HCV ab, hepatitis C antibody.

in patients with inactive cirrhosis, multiple comorbid conditions, or intolerance to treatment regimens.

Prednisone given with azathioprine induces clinical, biochemical, and histologic remission and is the standard of care. The optimal duration of treatment is unclear. However, although 90% of adults have improvements in the serum transaminase, bilirubin, and γ-globulin levels within 2 weeks, remission usually does not occur before 12 months. Histologic improvement often lags behind clinical and laboratory improvement by up to 6 months, and treatment should be continued for at least this period. Liver biopsy assessment before cessation of treatment can be helpful in patients who satisfy clinical and laboratory criteria for remission. If interface hepatitis is found in patients with normal serum transaminase and γ-globulin levels during therapy, these individuals have a high likelihood of relapse after cessation of treatment. Thus, extension of treatment in these patients can prevent relapse.

HEREDITARY HEMOCHROMATOSIS

Etiology and Pathophysiology

Hereditary hemochromatosis (HH) is a genetic condition resulting in increased intestinal absorption of iron resulting in primary iron overload. The excess iron that is absorbed is deposited in the parenchymal cells of the liver, heart, joints, pancreas, and other endocrine organs, causing inflammation and subsequent fibrosis and destruction, which results in chronic disease.

HH is an autosomal-recessive disorder. Recent estimates place the prevalence of the homozygous genotype at 1 in 250 whites in the United States, and about one in nine is a carrier, making it the most common known genetic disorder in the United States. Whites of northern European descent have a higher prevalence of the disease, although it has been reported in other ethnic groups. A total of 85% to 90% of patients of northern European descent with HH are homozygous for the C282Y mutation in the *HFE* gene. A second mutation, H63D, has also been frequently noted. A C282Y/H63D compound heterozygote status has been associated with an increased risk of iron overload.

Presentation, Diagnosis, and Workup

The clinical manifestations of HH usually do not appear until a person reaches ages 40 to 60 years, when sufficient iron has accumulated to cause organ damage. Women may manifest iron overload after menopause due to the relative protection of monthly menstrual blood loss. Use of alcohol and other hepatotoxic drugs lowers the ability of the liver to safely store iron and may accelerate the development of the hepatic sequelae of iron overload.

A common early sign of progressive iron overload is elevation of transaminases. Later, right upper quadrant pain, hepatomegaly, and arthropathy may occur. Other early signs and symptoms include impotence, amenorrhea, irritability, depression, and fatigue. Although liver disease is the most common complication of HH, the clinician should seek a history of arthritis, cirrhosis, diabetes, heart disease, and psychological and sexual dysfunction. Once cirrhosis is present, the risk of hepatocellular carcinoma is increased 200-fold in patients with HH compared with persons without the disorder.

When HH is suspected, transferrin saturation is a valuable initial test. If repeated analyses are persistently elevated (>50%) and cannot be explained by the presence of other medical conditions, a presumptive diagnosis of HH may be made. If the transferrin saturation is not elevated on follow-up testing but the serum ferritin concentration is, evaluation for causes of inflammation is warranted. Elevated serum ferritin levels not related to an acute-phase response correlate with excess iron stores.

Liver biopsy is the gold standard for diagnosis of HH with Perl stain showing evidence of hepatic iron overload. It also gives valuable prognostic information about the presence and extent of inflammation and fibrosis. Young patients less than 40 years of age who have a serum ferritin concentration of less than 750 ng/mL and normal liver enzyme levels may not need a liver biopsy for initiation of treatment.

Treatment

HH is treated with phlebotomy regardless of the presence or absence of clinical manifestations. The aim is to induce excess iron loss then maintenance of iron at normal body store levels. Induction involves removal of excess iron by taking 1 U (500 mL) of blood once or twice weekly until iron deficiency anemia develops (hemoglobin, 11 g/dL in women and 12 g/dL in men). This ensures elimination of excess iron stores. This is followed by maintenance of normal iron status by periodic phlebotomy. The frequency of phlebotomy should be individualized, but general guidelines include maintaining a serum ferritin concentration less than 50 ng/mL and a normal hemoglobin level. Iron chelating agents can be used in patients who are refractory or cannot tolerate repeated phlebotomies.

Genetic counseling is required in patients with HH. This can identify relatives who should be screened for the mutations causing HH. First-degree relatives should be genetically screened. Strict dietary restrictions are not indicated. Patients with cirrhosis should be screened for hepatocellular carcinoma with serum α-fetoprotein measurement and imaging at least every 6 months, because the risk for development of cancer is markedly increased.

WILSON DISEASE

Etiology and Pathophysiology

Wilson disease is an autosomal-recessive disorder of copper metabolism. A genetic defect in a metal transporter results in failure to excrete copper into bile. Copper accumulates in hepatocytes generating damage via reactive oxygen species. Release of copper from necrotic hepatocytes leads to damage of other tissues.

Presentation, Diagnosis, and Workup

The disease affects mostly young patients, with diagnosis being usually made in childhood and adolescence. Any patient with recurrent hepatic disease and unexplained neurologic symptoms should be suspected. Liver disease occurs in half of the patients. It may manifest as acute fulminant hepatitis, chronic active hepatitis, or cirrhosis. Acute episodes result in the release of copper in the bloodstream and hemolytic anemia with negative Coombs test. This is a life-threatening condition if not promptly corrected.

Neurologic manifestations may occur without liver disease and present in a large variety of ways, including resting and intention tremors, spasticity, rigidity, and chorea and dystonic reactions. Psychiatric disturbances are present in most patients and include psychoses and neuroses. The finding of Kayser-Fleischer ring denotes neurologic disease.

Classic diagnostic findings include a low serum ceruloplasmin level (<20 mg/dL), Kayser-Fleischer rings, and increased amounts of urinary copper. The latter two signs are also found in other cholestatic diseases, like PBC. About 5% of patients with Wilson disease present with a normal serum ceruloplasmin level. Diagnostic tests include determination of total serum copper, free serum copper and serum ceruloplasmin concentrations, and urinary copper excretion. Confirmation of diagnosis may be achieved by liver biopsy and histologic determination of copper content.

Treatment

Once diagnosis is firmly confirmed, lifelong treatment should start as soon as possible, regardless of the presence or absence of symptoms. Untreated disease uniformly progresses and is often fatal. The mainstay of treatment are copper chelating agents: D-penicillamine, trientine, or zinc. The most extensive experience is with penicillamine. Response is quite slow and may take up to 1 year for a maximum effect. Neurologic symptoms may worsen in the first months of treatment. After 2 weeks of penicillamine intake, patients often experience fever, rash, lymphadenopathy, neutropenia, and thrombocytopenia that respond to prednisone. Later side effects include proteinuria, nephrotic syndrome, and systemic lupus erythematosus. In these cases, penicillamine should be discontinued for a few months during which alternative copper chelators such as trientine or zinc should be started. The relative freedom from severe side effects has made zinc the increasing drug of choice for the treatment of Wilson disease. Free copper serum concentrations and urinary copper excretion should reach values below 10 μg/dL and 80 μg/d, respectively. A significant improvement of clinical symptoms and normalization of parameters of copper metabolism can be expected beyond 6 months after onset of therapy. Treatment may be accompanied by a copper-reduced diet and referral to a dietitian is appropriate. End-stage liver disease and fulminant hepatic failure are indications for liver transplantation. Neurologic symptoms may improve to varying extents but are not reversed.

CHRONIC VIRAL HEPATITIS

Many viruses can infect the liver; however, in this chapter we only discuss the two pandemics of chronic hepatitis B and C.

Chronic Hepatitis C Virus Infection

ETIOLOGY AND PATHOPHYSIOLOGY

Since its discovery in 1989, chronic hepatitis C virus (HCV) infection has come to be recognized as a worldwide epidemic. HCV is one of the most common causes of chronic liver disease and the leading indication for liver transplantation in the United States. HCV is a member of the Flaviviridae family and has been classified into six major genotypes that differ by 30% to 50% in their nucleotide sequences.

PRESENTATION, DIAGNOSIS, AND WORKUP

HCV is primarily transmitted parenterally. Known risk factors for HCV are intravenous drug use, blood and/or blood product transfusion before 1992, and needlestick injuries in health care workers. Sexual transmission remains controversial and probably accounts for less than 5% of cases. The risk is increased in subjects with a history of multiple sex partners and sexually transmitted diseases. Perinatal transmission of HCV occurs in approximately 3% to 5% of infants born to women infected with HCV. It is associated with high maternal viral load at time of delivery and HIV positivity. Acute infection is rarely clinically evident, and 60% to 85% of HCV-infected persons develop chronic infection.

Patients with chronic HCV infection are usually asymptomatic. The most common complaints are fatigue and abdominal pain. The diagnosis is generally made by the primary care physician after the identification of risk factors or abnormal transaminases. Routine screening is also performed by blood banks and life insurance companies. Baseline HCV antibody determination along with other viral hepatitis serologies and liver function tests will usually make the diagnosis. Normal liver enzymes are present in 25% to 30% of infected subjects and should not deter from pursuing the diagnosis. Because an estimated 25% to 35% of subjects clear virus spontaneously but remain HCV antibody positive, the widely available quantitative HCV RNA determination by polymerase chain reaction will confirm the presence of chronic infection. HCV genotyping will help in outlining treatment options because genotypes 1 (75%–80% of all infected U.S. patients) and 4 respond less well to treatment compared with genotypes 2 and 3. A liver biopsy offers valuable information about disease activity and the extent of inflammation and fibrosis and should be sought in patients considering treatment. It also offers prognostic information in patients who are not currently interested in or have contraindications to available treatment options.

TREATMENT

Patients with chronic HCV infection should be vaccinated against hepatitis A and B viruses, because acute infection with these viruses may result in worsening of disease. Combination treatment with pegylated interferon alfa and ribavirin is currently considered the therapy of choice for treatment-naive chronic HCV patients. This regimen leads to sustained viral responses of 42% to 51% in patients infected with HCV genotype 1 and 76% to 80% in those infected with genotypes 2 and 3. A course of 48 weeks of treatment is needed for genotype 1, whereas 24 weeks may be sufficient for genotypes 2 and 3. Interferon-based treatment may slow fibrosis progression even in the absence of viral clearance. Side effects of interferon and ribavirin are common and require close medical and psychiatric follow-up, including frequent patient visits and blood monitoring for known side effects. This results in significant patient dropout during treatment.

Patients who have cirrhosis may be considered for treatment if they can tolerate the side effects. Screening for hepatocellular carcinoma with serum α-fetoprotein and imaging every 6 months is essential in these patients. Decompensated liver disease remains a contraindication for antiviral treatment outside of clinical trials, and referral for transplantation evaluation should be obtained.

Chronic Hepatitis B Virus Infection

ETIOLOGY AND PATHOPHYSIOLOGY

Chronic hepatitis B virus (HBV) infection is another worldwide epidemic, affecting 1.25 million of the U.S. population and 350 million persons worldwide. HBV is transmitted by perinatal, percutaneous, and sexual exposure, as well as by close person-to-person contact, most likely from skin breaks. The risk of developing chronic HBV infection after acute exposure ranges from 90% in newborns of hepatitis B envelope antigen (HBeAg)–positive mothers to less than 10% in adults. Immunosuppressed persons are more likely to develop chronic HBV infection after acute exposure. A broad spectrum of disease states ranges from the inactive carrier with a positive hepatitis B surface antigen (HBsAg), HBeAg negative, anti-HBe positive, serum HBV DNA less than 10^5 copies/mL, and normal transaminases to the patient with active hepatitis and viral replication manifested by elevated transaminases, HBeAg positive, anti-HBe negative, serum HBV DNA less than 10^5 copies/mL, and ongoing necroinflammatory activity on liver biopsy. Spontaneous loss of HBeAg and detection of anti-HBe in a person who was previously HBeAg positive and anti-HBe negative is associated with decrease in serum HBV DNA to less than 10^5 copies/mL and remission of active hepatitis. Reactivation of active hepatitis in carriers also occurs.

PRESENTATION, DIAGNOSIS, AND WORKUP

Patients with chronic HBV infection are often asymptomatic. History should focus on identifying risk factors, including family and, most importantly, maternal history of HBV and hepatocellular carcinoma. Based on known risk factors the following groups should be screened for HBV infection: persons born in hyperendemic areas; men who have sex with men; injecting drug users; dialysis patients; human immunodeficiency virus (HIV)-infected individuals; pregnant women; family members, household members, and sexual contacts of HBV-infected persons; and persons diagnosed with sexually transmitted diseases and their sexual partners. Laboratory tests should include assessment of transaminases, markers of HBV replication (HBeAg/anti-HBe, HBV DNA by polymerase chain reaction), and tests for coinfection with HCV, hepatitis D virus, and HIV in those at risk.

TREATMENT

Transmission can be prevented by screening and vaccination of high-risk groups listed above. Health care workers and persons requiring frequent transfusions of blood products should also be vaccinated if not immune. Universal testing for HBsAg of all pregnant women near delivery and universal HBV vaccination of infants and children have significantly decreased the risk of vertical transmission of chronic hepatitis B. Vaccination for hepatitis A should be administered in HBV-infected patients who do not have immune titers.

Treatment strategies are aimed at viral suppression and, hopefully, the prevention of significant liver disease and its complications. The aim is to clear HBeAg, suppress HBV DNA, and normalize alanine aminotransferase. Treatment is generally offered to patients with elevated alanine aminotransferase and active viral replication manifested by elevated HBV DNA by polymerase chain reaction. In general, a liver biopsy is performed by most hepatologists as part of the treatment evaluation to know the extent of inflammation and fibrosis.

The current armamentarium for the treatment of HBV is expanding and includes interferon-α subcutaneously at 5 million units daily or 10 million units three times a week for 16 weeks and lamivudine given at 100 mg/d orally. Both result in a loss of HBeAg in about a third of patients and suppression of viral load, which appears to be reflected in a histologic improvement on liver biopsy. A small percentage of patients (1%–2%) may lose HBsAg at 1 year. Lamivudine has the advantage of being administered orally and does not have the numerous side effects associated with interferon. However, a substantial number of patients develop lamivudine-resistant mutant viruses over time, which may be accompanied by acute exacerbations of liver disease and rarely hepatic decompensation. It appears that these patients continue to benefit from treatment despite the mutations, possibly because of suppression of the wild-type virus. A recently introduced medication, adefovir, appears to be effective in suppressing the replication of lamivudine-resistant HBV mutants. The major concern with this new drug is nephrotoxicity.

A key aspect in the management of HBV-infected individuals is screening for hepatocellular carcinoma, which occurs even in the absence of cirrhosis due to the carcinogenic effect of the virus. Most authorities advocate measurement of serum α-fetoprotein along with an imaging modality at least every 6 months.

ALCOHOLIC LIVER DISEASE

Etiology and Pathophysiology

Alcoholic liver disease is probably the best studied entity among all chronic liver diseases. Alcoholism is a worldwide epidemic. As a result, alcoholic liver disease may be the most common cause of liver disease worldwide. Approximately 10% to 35% of heavy drinkers develop alcoholic hepatitis, and 10% to 20% develop cirrhosis. Critical factors in the development of cirrhosis are the daily amount of alcohol consumed and the duration of consumption, rather than the type of beverage consumed. Daily ingestion of at least six cans of beer, 6 ounces of whisky, or a quart of wine for at least 5 to 10 years may lead to cirrhosis. In addition, there is emerging evidence of genetic susceptibility to the toxic effects of alcohol. Alcohol is believed to injure the liver via depletion of glutathione, which protects against oxidative injury, generation of reactive oxygen species that results in cell membrane damage, and cytokine-mediated liver injury. Most patients with alcoholic liver disease develop simple fatty infiltration that is reversible with abstinence. A subset of these patients develop alcoholic steatohepatitis characterized by neutrophilic infiltration with characteristic Mallory bodies and ballooning degeneration mostly in the pericentral area. This can be reversible but often occurs in patients with significant baseline scarring. The end spectrum of alcoholic liver disease is micronodular cirrhosis and its sequelae of chronic liver disease, including portal hypertension.

Women are more susceptible than men to alcohol-induced liver disease with more modest levels of intake. Therefore, the clinician must have a higher index of suspicion for making this diagnosis in women.

Presentation, Diagnosis, and Workup

Frequent findings associated with chronic liver disease range from the asymptotic state to jaundice, palmar erythema, spider angiomas, parotid and lacrimal gland enlargement, clubbing of the fingers, splenomegaly and muscle wasting, Dupuytren contracture, ascites with or without peripheral edema, female escutcheon, gynecomastia, and testicular atrophy in men. A history of long-term alcohol use in the appropriate clinical setting clinches the diagnosis. Imaging modalities may show fatty hepatic infiltration or a nodular liver consistent with cirrhosis.

Patients with alcoholic liver disease often have asymptomatic hepatomegaly and mild elevation of liver function tests. Aspartate aminotransferase often is more than twice the alanine aminotransferase. An elevated alkaline phosphatase, γ-glutamyl transferase, and an elevated mean corpuscular volume also may be seen. These features are particularly helpful in identifying the occasional patient who denies alcohol intake on an initial interview. The findings may help direct further questioning in that area.

Treatment

The cornerstone of treatment is abstinence. Outpatient (Alcoholics Anonymous) and/or inpatient detoxification should be pursued. When achieved, abstinence often results in stabilization of disease. Patients with cirrhosis should be screened for hepatocellular carcinoma with α-fetoprotein and imaging. Vaccination against hepatitis A and B, if not already immune, is often done. Referral to a transplant center should be obtained.

NONALCOHOLIC FATTY LIVER DISEASE

Etiology and Pathophysiology

Nonalcoholic fatty liver disease is an increasingly recognized entity characterized by histologic features of alcoholic liver disease in subjects who consume no or little alcohol. This entity includes a spectrum of diseases ranging from simple fatty liver to pericentral inflammation and ballooning of hepatocytes, pericellular fibrosis associated with fatty infiltration, and sometimes Mallory bodies (nonalcoholic steatohepatitis) to severe fibrosis and cirrhosis. Subjects with cirrhosis may not have significant fatty infiltration pointing to the etiology and are often labeled as having "cryptogenic cirrhosis". Increased intrahepatic levels of fatty acids provide a source of oxidative stress, which may in large part be responsible for the progression from steatosis to steatohepatitis to cirrhosis. The underlying etiology appears to be insulin resistance, suggesting that nonalcoholic fatty liver disease may be the hepatic manifestation of the metabolic syndrome X.

Obesity, type 2 diabetes mellitus, and hyperlipidemia (usually hypertriglyceridemia) are frequently associated with nonalcoholic fatty liver disease. No clear gender or ethnic predisposition has been identified.

Presentation, Diagnosis, and Workup

Most patients with nonalcoholic fatty liver disease are asymptomatic. Fatigue and/or right upper quadrant discomfort are sometimes reported. Hepatomegaly is the most common positive finding on physical examination. Signs and symptoms of portal hypertension are seen in advanced liver disease.

Asymptomatic elevation of transaminase levels and radiologic findings of fatty liver and/or hepatomegaly suggest the diagnosis. Imaging studies provide information about the presence and extent of fatty liver disease, but the degree of inflammation and fibrosis, if at all present, can only be determined with a liver biopsy.

Treatment

The natural history and determinants of progression of nonalcoholic fatty liver disease remain poorly understood. There is evidence to suggest that patients found to have simple fatty liver on biopsy have the best prognosis, whereas features of steatohepatitis or more advanced fibrosis are associated with a worse prognosis. Therefore, a liver biopsy may provide some prognostic information or clarify the diagnosis when other entities are being considered. Adequate glycemic control and gradual weight loss may be helpful. No medication has been proven to be effective for treatment, although trials are ongoing.

OTHER CHRONIC LIVER DISEASES

In addition to the above, chronic liver disease can be caused by a variety of entities. Very briefly, some of the more common ones are discussed.

Primary sclerosing cholangitis is a progressive cholestatic liver disease associated with inflammatory bowel disease and affects mostly men. The risk for cholangiocarcinoma is markedly increased. No effective treatments are available, although ursodeoxycholic acid is often prescribed.

Granulomas in the liver can be caused by mycobacteria (MTB, MAI), most notably in immunosuppressed individuals. Sarcoidosis is another cause of granulomatous liver disease.

α_1-Antitrypsin deficiency is a rare genetic disease mostly diagnosed in children. In adults with the homozygous defect (PI ZZ), symptoms of chronic obstructive pulmonary disease predominate. This condition is frequently aggravated by cigarette smoking. The prevalence of associated chronic liver disease is 10% to 40% in these patients. The risk of cirrhosis becomes higher with advancing years, particularly in men. Liver disease appears to progress rapidly when diagnosed in adulthood.

LIVER TRANSPLANTATION

Liver transplantation has evolved from an experimental procedure to a highly successful treatment option in patients with chronic liver disease. This success, coupled with a lack of available organs, has meant an exponential increase in the numbers of candidates on the United Network for Organ Sharing liver transplant list. In most cases, the indication for transplantation is easily recognized by the referring physician. Occasionally, however, lesser known indications for transplantation may arise and should prompt referral for transplant evaluation. Such examples include severe osteopenia with pathologic fractures or refractory pruritus in patients with chronic cholestatic liver diseases such as PBC and primary sclerosing cholangitis. Severe protein calorie malnutrition and marked muscle wasting should also prompt referral. Finally, hepatocellular carcinoma (tumors of 5 cm or less in diameter in patients with multiple lesions, a single lesion, and no more than 3 lesions) without evidence of extrahepatic disease is an indication for liver transplantation at most centers.

Although long-term survival can vary depending on the etiology of chronic liver disease with viral illnesses invariably recurring, a 1-year survival rate of 80% to 90% can be expected at most experienced centers.

General contraindications to liver transplantation include compensated cirrhosis without complications, extrahepatic malignancy, active untreated sepsis, advanced cardiopulmonary disease, active alcoholism or substance abuse, and anatomic abnormalities precluding liver transplantation. HIV-positive patients are currently only being transplanted in clinical trial settings. Many centers do not have an age cutoff, and individual decisions are made based primarily on functional status. Severe obesity is associated with worse outcomes peri- and post-transplantation, and patients are encouraged to make efforts to lose weight as part of their evaluation. Potential candidates undergo rigorous clinical and psychiatric testing before consideration. Waiting times may vary based primarily on severity of disease.

In view of the chronic shortage of organs, new transplantation alternatives have emerged. Increasing numbers of patients are undergoing living related donor liver transplantation. This involves receiving a portion (usually the right hepatic lobe) of a relative or emotionally related healthy donor. Although the outcomes have been promising, this option is currently not offered to critically ill patients with end-stage liver disease who usually need whole cadaveric organs for a successful outcome. Donors undergo extensive psychiatric and clinical evaluation to assess suitability and ensure their actions are not motivated by financial or emotional pressures. Finally, the risk for healthy donors is not trivial, and donor deaths have occurred, raising ethical concerns.

Post-transplantation, recurrence invariably occurs in viral hepatitis. This is an increasingly problematic issue in HCV where disease progression is accelerated post-transplant, possibly due to the immunosuppressed state. The administration of HBV immunoglobulins and, more recently, nucleoside analogs in HBV-infected transplant recipients has significantly improved their long-term outcomes. Cholestatic, autoimmune, and metabolic disorders have also been reported to recur.

SPECIAL CONSIDERATIONS IN PREGNANCY

Physiologic changes during pregnancy can cause biochemical abnormalities seen in liver disease. Serum albumin concentrations decrease near the end of gestation because of an increase in plasma volume. Serum alkaline phosphatase increases during the second trimester of pregnancy and continues to rise to values two to four times normal by the end of gestation. This is caused by the leakage into the maternal circulation of placental alkaline phosphatase. Values for γ-glutamyl transferase, aspartate and alanine aminotransferases, and bilirubin are normally unchanged. Abnormalities in these parameters should arouse suspicion of hepatobiliary disease. In addition, spider nevi on the chest, back, and face and palmar erythema occur in up to 60% of pregnant women but disappear after delivery.

Pregnant women with known chronic liver disease need to be followed in a high-risk setting, and close monitoring of both mother and fetus is necessary. Close collaboration between the obstetrician and the hepatologist is necessary to ensure favorable maternal and fetal outcomes.

Chronic Autoimmune Hepatitis

Flare-up of chronic autoimmune hepatitis has been frequently reported during pregnancy. Women with chronic autoimmune hepatitis have a higher incidence of stillbirths and prematurity. Commonly used drugs to treat chronic autoimmune hepatitis such as prednisone and azathioprine have been shown in fairly large retrospective series to be safe to mother and fetus during pregnancy.

Chronic Viral Hepatitis

There is little evidence that pregnancy influences the clinical course of chronic hepatitis in general, unless cirrhosis is present (see below).

CHRONIC HEPATITIS C INFECTION

An Italian study reported a decreased risk of perinatal transmission of chronic HCV with cesarean section when compared with vaginal delivery. This area remains controversial, and the current state of knowledge does not support routine cesarean section in HCV-infected mothers. Infants born to HCV-infected mothers may initially be HCV antibody positive due to passive transfer of the antibody across the placenta. This antibody may be present during the entire first year of a newborn's life before disappearing, if no infection is present. Therefore, the determination of HCV infection in the newborn requires the demonstration of a positive HCV RNA in the serum. Breast-feeding by mothers with HCV infection is not associated with transmission of viral infection.

CHRONIC HEPATITIS B INFECTION

HBsAg-positive women who are pregnant should receive hepatitis B immune globulin. HBV vaccine is given to the newborn immediately after delivery. Infants need to complete the recommended vaccination schedule, and follow-up HBV serologic markers are checked at 1 year of age. HBIG and concurrent hepatitis B vaccine prevent perinatal transmission of HBV in 95% of cases.

Primary Biliary Cirrhosis

PBC usually occurs in older women; therefore, PBC and pregnancy rarely coexist. When this occurs, however, the course of PBC does not seem to be significantly altered. Pregnancy tends to increase cholestatic biochemical parameters in women with PBC. After delivery, these abnormalities return to their baseline values.

Cirrhosis

Cirrhosis is a cause of unexplained infertility, and women with this disease are often amenorrheic. However, when pregnancy occurs, women often sustain a normal pregnancy without any significant worsening of their baseline liver disease. There is evidence to suggest that cirrhotic women have higher rates of stillbirths and premature infants. The incidence of variceal hemorrhage is thought to be increased during pregnancy in cirrhotic women, although solid evidence supporting this is lacking. Some experts have even advocated termination of pregnancy if varices are diagnosed early in the course of pregnancy, although this is highly controversial. When variceal hemorrhage occurs, the first line of therapy should be endoscopic treatment, which has been demonstrated to be safe and efficacious.

Vasopressin is relatively contraindicated due to its effects on the uterus. The safety and efficacy of somatostatin and its analogs as well as beta-blockers have not been evaluated. Anecdotal reports have described the performance of a transjugular intrahepatic portosystemic shunt in pregnant women with acute variceal hemorrhage. Hepatic encephalopathy can be safely treated with lactulose or neomycin.

Wilson Disease

Wilson disease is often diagnosed at a young age. Therefore, coexistence with pregnancy is not uncommon. Women with this disorder should be maintained on their prepregnancy regimen during gestation. The largest experience is with penicillamine, and no significant increase in adverse effects in the newborn has been reported. Dose reductions may be necessary in the latter stages of gestation. Zinc therapy appears to be theoretically safer, although solid evidence to support this is lacking. Discontinuation of medication during pregnancy has been associated with worsening of liver disease.

BIBLIOGRAPHY

Angulo P. Nonalcoholic fatty liver disease. *N Engl J Med* 2002;18:1221–1231.

Czaja AJ, Freese DK. Diagnosis and treatment of autoimmune hepatitis. *Hepatology* 2002;36:479–497.

Kaplan MM. Primary biliary cirrhosis. *N Engl J Med* 1996;21:1570–1580.

Lee WM. Pregnancy in patients with chronic liver disease. *Gastroenterol Clin North Am* 1992;21:889–903.

Lok AS, McMahon BJ. Practice Guidelines Committee, American Association for the Study of Liver Diseases Chronic Hepatitis B. *Hepatology* 2001;34:1225–1241.

Seeff LB, Hoofnagle JH. National Institutes of Health Consensus Development Conference: management of hepatitis C: 2002. *Hepatology* 2002;36[5 Suppl 1]:S1–S2.

Sheinberg IH. Wilson's disease. *Harrison's principles of internal medicine,* 13th ed. New York: McGraw-Hill, 1994.

Wiesner RH, Rakela J, et al. Recent advances in liver transplantation. *Mayo Clin Proc* 2003;78:197–210.

Witte DL, Crosby WH, Edwards CQ, et al. Practice guideline development task force of the College of American Pathologists: hereditary hemochromatosis. *Clin Chim Acta* 1996;245:139–200.

CHAPTER 65

Gallstones and Cholecystitis

Sripathi R. Kethu and Edward Feller

Gallstones are twice as common in women than in men. Approximately 20% of women and 10% of men in the United States have gallstones by age 65. Most gallstones never cause symptoms and are discovered incidentally by imaging studies performed for indications other than biliary-type pain; as many as 60% to 75% of stones remain asymptomatic and less than 10% of patients with gallstones ever experience a complication. Mexican-American women and Native Americans, particularly Pima Indians in North America, have the highest prevalence rates, probably attributable to genetic predisposition. Increased risk is also seen in Chilean Indians, North Americans (among whites), and Northern Europeans. The lowest prevalence rates are reported from Asia and Africa.

RISK FACTORS AND PATHOPHYSIOLOGY

Gallstones are divided into two categories based on chemical composition. Cholesterol stones, either pure or mixed type, constitute approximately 70% of the gallstones in the western world, and the remainder are pigment stones. Female gender and increasing age are the most prominent risk factors for gallstones, with prevalence increased by twofold in women. The discrepancy is most marked in the under 40 age group but persists at all ages (Table 65.1). Stones are rare in children, except those with congenital hemolytic anemias. Women must be aware that hormone therapy, including oral contraceptives and hormone replacement therapy, increases the likelihood of biliary disease. Additive risk is present with obesity, sedentary lifestyle, and a family history of stones. Biliary sludge and gallstones form more rapidly and frequently with rapid weight loss associated with very low calorie diets or weight loss surgery.

In some patients, stone formation is preceded by the presence of biliary sludge or microlithiasis. This biliary sludge has now been implicated in many cases of biliary colic, acute cholecystitis, and "idiopathic" pancreatitis. Because it becomes supersaturated in bile, ceftriaxone use can result in sludge formation, precipitating with calcium. This problem is particularly common in critically ill hospitalized patients, in diabetes mellitus, and those on total parenteral nutrition where gallbladder hypomotility contributes to stasis. Coffee consumption and vitamin C are thought to be protective factors against formation of gallstones.

Excess unconjugated bilirubin is commonly produced by chronic hemolysis (e.g., sickle cell anemia), hypersplenism (e.g., cirrhosis), advanced age, and long-term total parenteral nutri-

TABLE 65.1. Risk Factors and Pathophysiology of Cholesterol Stones

Risk factor	Pathophysiologic mechanism
Excess cholesterol excretion into the bile	
Female gender	Estrogens increase dietary uptake of cholesterol by stimulating lipoprotein receptors
Age	Increased biliary secretion of cholesterol
Obesity	Increased biliary secretion of cholesterol
Oral contraceptives	Decreased conversion of cholesterol to cholesteryl esters
Rapid weight loss	Mobilization of tissue cholesterol
Decreased bile acid secretion	
Ileal disease or resection (e.g., Crohn disease)	Decreased absorption or excess loss of bile acids
Primary biliary cirrhosis	Decreased bile acid secretion due to cholestasis
Propensity for nucleation of cholesterol crystals	Excess secretion of pronucleating factors such as mucin and α_1-acid glycoprotein
Gallbladder hypomotility	
Total parenteral nutrition	
Fasting	Impaired motility leading to decreased gallbladder emptying and bile stasis
Pregnancy	
Obesity	
Octreotide	

tion. Brown pigment stones, which are common in Asia, are associated with chronic biliary infections and bile stasis. Bacterial hydrolysis of conjugated bile to unconjugated bile results in brown pigment stones. Risk factors for the formation of brown pigment stones include biliary strictures, parasitic infestation (e.g., *Clonorchis sinensis*), and duodenal diverticulum near the ampulla of Vater.

DIFFERENTIAL DIAGNOSIS

Biliary colic or cholecystitis must be considered in any woman with acute right upper quadrant or epigastric pain, with or without accompanying fever and leukocytosis. Most patients with acute cholecystitis or biliary colic will report prior attacks. A variety of recurrent episodic disorders may produce similar symptoms. Acute pancreatitis may present with overlapping history, risk factors, and physical examination. Dissemination of pain to involve the left side of the abdomen, duration of pain greater than 24 hours, and marked elevations of serum amylase and lipase are important discriminating findings suggesting pancreatitis. Clinicians must be aware that pancreatic inflammation may be secondary to a migrating gallstone obstructing or irritating the sphincter of Oddi at the ampulla of Vater. Hepatic disorders that may uncommonly masquerade as biliary disease include hepatitis (alcoholic, viral, drug induced, autoimmune), focal nodular hyperplasia, hepatic adenoma, and peliosis hepatis (a condition in which the liver lobule contains extrasinusoidal blood-filled spaces, associated with the use of oral contraceptives and anabolic steroids). The pain of hepatitis is typically an aching heaviness in the right upper quadrant, which is dull and constant, unlikely to be confused with the acuity of biliary colic or acute cholecystitis. Pain, however, may be prominent in hepatic inflammation, seen more frequently in alcoholic hepatitis than in viral disease.

Acute appendicitis may be confused with acute biliary disease because the location of either may be in the upper or lower quadrant as well as epigastric with an identical pain pattern. The former tends to be more rapidly progressive. Abdominal ultrasonography will demonstrate gallstones in 90% to 95% of cases of cholecystitis. Uncomplicated peptic ulcer disease typically presents with aching or burning upper abdominal pain of mild to moderate degree. Reflux esophagitis may be episodic, potentiated by hormones that increase heartburn by decreasing lower esophageal sphincter pressure. Association with food and use of acid-suppressing medication will be suggestive of the latter two disorders. An ulcer complication, including perforation or penetration, can mimic acute biliary disease with worrisome features of muscle guarding and signs of peritoneal irritation. Severe intermittent pain may characterize irritable bowel syndrome, a disorder more common in women. Clues to irritable bowel syndrome may be association of pain with bowel movements, change in bowel frequency or form, absence of symptoms during the night, and potential association with stress.

At times, renal disease due to nephrolithiasis or pyelonephritis produces anterior abdominal pain potentially confused with that of biliary disease. Urinalysis should be a routine test in the evaluation of abdominal pain. Right lower lobe pneumonia with pleuritic involvement may present without cough, dyspnea, or sputum production and may be confused with right upper quadrant pathology. The pain of myocardial infarction may be atypical in location and character. Careful assessment is required to exclude myocardial ischemia, especially in older women and those with cardiac risk factors.

Gynecologic disorders commonly mimic biliary colic. Gonococcal perihepatitis (Fitz-Hugh-Curtis syndrome) may manifest as right upper quadrant pain without clear pelvic complaints. Similarly, complications of an ovarian cyst, at times, are localized to the upper abdomen. Adnexal tenderness should be assessed to rule out gynecologic cause. Acute abdominal symptoms in women in childbearing years require a careful gynecologic and menstrual history as well as a pregnancy test.

CLINICAL MANIFESTATIONS

Fig. 65.1 shows the clinical manifestations of gallstones.

Asymptomatic Gallstones

Silent gallstones are commonly discovered on imaging procedures done for indications unrelated to possible biliary disease. An asymptomatic patient has a probability of 15% to 20% over 10 years for developing symptoms. Most patients with gallbladder stones are asymptomatic.

Biliary Colic

Biliary colic occurs in approximately two thirds of patients with symptomatic biliary diseases. Pain may be due to contraction of the gallbladder, which cannot empty because the cystic duct is transiently obstructed by a stone. This disorder is described classically as discrete attacks of rapid onset and right upper quadrant or epigastric pain lasting from several minutes to several hours. Some patients describe constant rather than colicky pain. The location may be atypical, with documented cases manifesting as pain in the right lower, left lower, or left upper quadrants. Location in the chest may simulate myocardial ischemia. Some patients describe radiation of pain to the shoulder or through to the back. Abdominal tenderness may be present, but signs of peritoneal irritation are absent.

Acute Cholecystitis

Acute cholecystitis indicates inflammation of the gallbladder wall typically caused by mechanical cystic duct obstruction by an impacted stone. Chemical irritation and secondary infection may contribute to clinical symptoms. Biliary colic may evolve into an attack of acute cholecystitis. Features suggesting acute cholecystitis rather than biliary colic are increased duration of

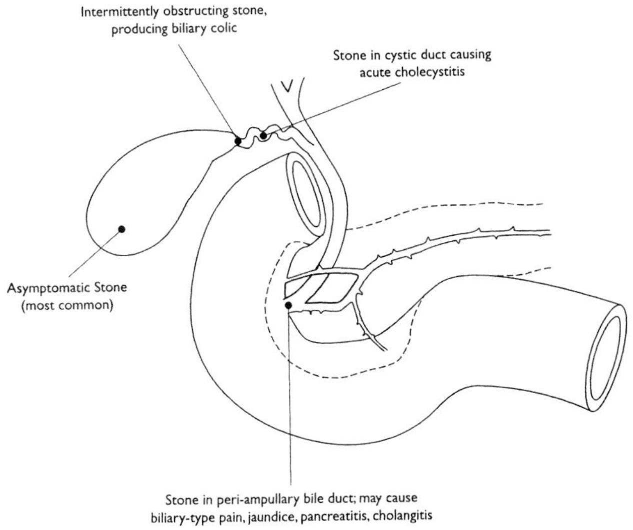

FIG. 65.1. Clinical manifestations of gallstones.

an attack of greater than 4 to 5 hours and the presence of fever and pronounced abdominal tenderness. Most patients report prior episodes consistent with biliary colic. Pain is typically felt in the right upper quadrant or epigastrium, but less classic descriptions of symptoms isolated to other parts of the abdomen or chest have been documented. Localized tenderness to palpation is generally found. Some patients have increased pain and cessation of respiratory effort when the right upper quadrant is palpated subcostally (Murphy's sign).

Chronic Cholecystitis

Repeated attacks of acute cholecystitis or biliary colic may produce chronic inflammatory changes to the gallbladder wall and cystic duct. The result is a poorly contracting, thickened, and fibrotic organ. Chronic cholecystitis may be asymptomatic or may progress to acute cholecystitis or may present with complications.

COMPLICATIONS

Choledocholithiasis

Gallstones may migrate from the gallbladder via the cystic duct and become trapped at the level of the sphincter of Oddi. These common bile duct stones occur in 10% to 15% of patients with gallstones. The incidence of bile duct stones increases with increasing age and with the presence of small gallstones, which are much more likely than large stones to traverse the cystic duct and be trapped above the sphincter of Oddi. Most common bile duct stones are mixed in composition or cholesterol stones and are initially formed in the gallbladder. Stones that form de novo in the common bile duct after cholecystectomy are generally pigment stones. Pigment stones are also more common in patients with hemolytic anemia or congenital or acquired ductal abnormalities. Common bile duct stones are more likely to be symptomatic than gallstones. Clinical features are due to biliary obstruction and subsequent increased biliary pressure. Varying combinations of pain, jaundice, and fever occur. Biochemically, elevation of serum alkaline phosphatase and bilirubin suggests this complication in the patient with biliary symptoms. Ultrasonography may reveal ductal dilatation, but obstruction, when partial, occurs without duct dilatation. Ultrasonography, though very accurate for detection of gallstones, is relatively insensitive for common bile duct stones.

Cholangitis

Ductal obstruction may trap bacteria above a stone, producing cholangitis with potential for bloodstream dissemination and septicemia. Charcot's triad of fever, pain, and jaundice may be inconsistent and can occur in up to 70% of patients. Rarely, cholangitis occurs in the setting of isolated fever without clinical clues to a biliary source. Cholangitis is more common in the setting of sudden obstruction by a stone than in gradual bile duct obstruction by a tumor. Physical examination reveals right upper quadrant tenderness. Leukocytosis with a left shift is seen, along with marked alkaline phosphatase, transaminases, and bilirubin elevations. Biliary obstruction is suspected when there is intrahepatic and extrahepatic biliary dilation on ultrasonography or computed tomography (CT). Bile and blood cultures are frequently positive for *Escherichia coli, Pseudomonas, Klebsiella,* and *enterococci.*

Gallstone-Induced Pancreatitis

Acute pancreatitis can result from a stone obstructing bile flow at the level of the sphincter of Oddi. Patients typically present with sudden severe upper abdominal pain, associated with nausea and vomiting. Amylase and lipase rise rapidly and normalize quickly within 1 to 2 days, because most often the stone is spontaneously passed through the bile duct into the duodenum, relieving the obstruction. The spectrum of clinical pancreatitis ranges from mild to severe with potential for organ failure and necrotizing pancreatitis.

Gangrene and Perforation

Prolonged impaction of a gallstone in the cystic duct may evolve into progressive gallbladder necrosis and gangrene with risk of perforation and peritonitis or may wall-off into an abscess. Rarely, secondary infection of cholecystitis occurs with gas-forming bacteria, including anaerobic *Streptococcus* and *Clostridia* species or *E. coli*. Gas in the gallbladder lumen or wall on imaging studies indicates this entity (emphysematous cholecystitis).

Gallstone Ileus

Rarely, a large gallstone may erode through the gallbladder wall, forming a fistula between gallbladder and duodenum (cholecystoduodenal fistula). Then the stone can travel through the fistula and become impacted in the small bowel, usually at the ileocecal valve, resulting in obstruction. The diagnosis can be made by either plain radiography or CT when there is air in the biliary tree in the presence of small bowel obstruction. Prompt laparotomy and stone extraction will relieve the obstruction.

Mirizzi Syndrome

Mirizzi syndrome is a rare cause of biliary obstruction caused when a gallstone that is impacted in the cystic duct or the neck of the gallbladder compresses the adjacent common bile duct. Diagnosis is usually made by ultrasonography that shows the impacted stone at the cystic duct with dilation of the proximal portion of the common hepatic duct and with normal caliber of the distal common bile duct.

LABORATORY FINDINGS

Patients who present with biliary colic with transient obstruction of the cystic duct may have normal laboratory studies. Patients with sustained cystic duct obstruction leading to acute cholecystitis often have mild to moderate leukocytosis. Mild elevation of transaminases, alkaline phosphatase, and bilirubin may also occur with acute cholecystitis. Substantial elevations, however, should raise the suspicion for bile duct obstruction by a stone and possibly cholangitis. Marked serum amylase and lipase elevation correlate with associated gallstone-induced pancreatitis. Mild pancreatic enzyme increases are seen occasionally in isolated biliary disease without pancreatitis.

RADIOGRAPHIC AND IMAGING STUDIES

Plain Radiography

Plain abdominal radiographs may detect gallstones when sufficient calcium is present. Approximately 50% of pigment stones and 10% to 15% of cholesterol or mixed stones can be detected by plain radiography.

Ultrasonography

Ultrasonography is the test of first choice in diagnosing cholelithiasis, with sensitivity and specificity more than 95%.

Ultrasonography is not only inexpensive and noninvasive, but also can be used safely in pregnant women because there is no risk of radiation exposure. Stones appear as movable high-amplitude shadows with post-acoustic shadowing. In acute cholecystitis, gallbladder wall thickening and pericholecystic fluid may be seen. Another sensitive and specific ultrasound finding is sonographic Murphy's sign: sudden cessation of breathing due to pain when the gallbladder is touched with the ultrasound transducer. The combination of gallbladder wall thickening, pericholecystic fluid, and sonographic Murphy's sign has a positive predictive value of more than 90% for acute cholecystitis in the absence of visualized cholelithiasis. Ultrasound also has the advantage of simultaneously imaging surrounding structures: gallbladder, bile ducts, pancreas, and liver. However, the sensitivity of ultrasonography in detecting common bile duct stones is only between 40% and 50%.

Hepatobiliary Scintigraphy

This study is useful to diagnose or to exclude acute cholecystitis when ultrasonography is inconclusive. This test involves, most commonly, intravenous administration of technetium 99m-labeled iminodiacetic acid analogs (HIDA). The compound has a high affinity for hepatic uptake and quickly concentrates in the gallbladder via bile. Normally the contrast reaches the gallbladder within 30 to 45 minutes, documented by the opacification of the gallbladder. If cystic duct obstruction or spasm is present, the radionuclide contrast fails to reach the gallbladder within a normal cutoff period of 90 minutes, indicating a diagnosis of acute cholecystitis. Certain conditions associated with bile stasis, including prolonged fasting, critical illness, and chronic cholecystitis, may result in a false-positive test. Therefore, films should be repeated after 4 hours to assess delayed gallbladder emptying, increases the sensitivity and specificity to more than 90% in diagnosing acute cholecystitis.

Computed Tomography

CT is not sensitive in diagnosing gallstones, and it is more expensive than ultrasonography. However, it is more accurate in detecting common bile duct stones and biliary obstruction. CT is particularly useful in detecting the exact site and the nature of obstructive jaundice when the clinical differentiation of obstruction due to biliary stones or tumor cannot be made.

Endoscopic Retrograde Cholangiopancreatography

Endoscopic retrograde cholangiopancreatography (ERCP) involves per-oral passage of a video endoscope through the esophagus, stomach, and into the region of the ampulla of Vater in the descending duodenum. A cannula is then introduced into the ampullary orifice to inject contrast dye to opacify the biliary and pancreatic ductal system. ERCP is not indicated to detect gallbladder stones or acute cholecystitis. This is the test of choice when a therapeutic intervention is desired, for example, when attempting to relieve an obstructed bile duct either by removing a stone or placing a stent through a biliary stricture. ERCP is invasive with risk of complications such as pancreatitis. ERCP can also be used when ultrasonography or CT is nondiagnostic in a case of cholestasis to rule out extrahepatic biliary obstruction.

Magnetic Resonance Cholangiopancreatography

This is a noninvasive and less expensive alternative to ERCP to image the biliary and pancreatic ducts. It is not recommended to diagnose gallbladder stones or cholecystitis. Magnetic resonance cholangiopancreatography has a high sensitivity and specificity of up to 90% in detecting bile duct stones and/or obstruction. This is particularly useful when there is low clinical suspicion for bile duct obstruction. However, if a high index of suspicion for biliary obstruction exists or if there is evidence of cholangitis, ERCP is preferred over magnetic resonance cholangiopancreatography, because the latter has no therapeutic potential in relieving obstruction.

TREATMENT

Asymptomatic Gallstones

Prophylactic cholecystectomy is not recommended in asymptomatic patients because of the low risk of developing symptoms or complications in this group. Exceptions to this recommendation include patients with high risk for gallbladder cancer (e.g., stones larger than 3 cm, calcified or "porcelain" gallbladder, Native Americans) or in certain groups of patients (e.g., sickle cell anemia, morbid obesity) when the procedure can be performed while undergoing abdominal surgery for another indication. In diabetics, the role of prophylactic cholecystectomy is controversial.

Symptomatic Gallstones

Patients with recurrent episodes of documented biliary colic, acute or chronic cholecystitis, choledocholithiasis, and gallstone-induced pancreatitis should all undergo laparoscopic cholecystectomy provided they are appropriate surgical candidates.

ACUTE CHOLECYSTITIS

Initial treatment of acute cholecystitis involves withholding oral feeding, intravenous hydration, and analgesics. Despite the lack of strong evidence of benefit, prophylactic antibiotics such as second-generation cephalosporins or a combination of ampicillin and gentamicin are generally recommended. Laparoscopic cholecystectomy is recommended in all patients who are at low surgical risk.

CHOLEDOCHOLITHIASIS AND CHOLANGITIS

Antibiotic therapy to cover Gram-negative enteric organisms, such as ciprofloxacin intravenously, a combination of ampicillin and gentamicin, or a third-generation cephalosporin, should be given immediately. Prompt biliary drainage, preferably by ERCP-assisted sphincterotomy and/or stent placement, is required in patients with evidence of cholangitis, biliary-type pain with a dilated common bile duct, or stones seen on ultrasonography or CT. In cases where ERCP has failed, radiologically assisted percutaneous drainage is recommended.

Surgical Treatment Options

Laparoscopic cholecystectomy is the procedure of choice for symptomatic gallstones. Generally, the complication rate is 2% to 4%. The most common adverse event is wound infection. Bile duct injuries occur in 0.2% to 0.5% of cases. Approximately 5% of laparoscopic cholecystectomies require conversion intraoperatively to open cholecystectomy. Open cholecystectomy is performed when laparoscopic cholecystectomy is technically difficult secondary to adhesions or when common bile duct stones cannot be removed by the laparoscopic method.

Medical Therapy

Ursodeoxycholic acid is a bile acid used to dissolve small (<1.5 cm) noncalcified (radiolucent) cholesterol stones. Ursodeoxycholic acid acts by not only decreasing cholesterol synthesis but also solubilizes the cholesterol, thereby dissolving the stones. This therapy is not effective for pigment stones. The usual dose of ursodeoxycholic acid is 8 to 10 mg/kg/d, divided two or three times a day. Although safe in the long term, this is an expensive and time-consuming therapy, often required for 1 to 2 years. Up to 50% of stones recur when therapy is stopped. Therefore, this therapy is reserved for patients with high surgical risk or who decline surgery.

Endoscopic Retrograde Cholangiopancreatography

ERCP is indicated for patients who have common bile duct stones with or without cholangitis and for gallstone-induced pancreatitis. Stones are removed endoscopically before cholecystectomy, so that common bile duct exploration can be avoided during surgery, resulting in less operative time and lower complications.

PREVENTION OF GALLSTONES

Women who undergo rapid weight loss either by very low calorie diets or after gastric bypass surgery have an increased risk of symptomatic gallstone disease (10%–20% in 16 weeks). In these situations, ursodeoxycholic acid 600 mg/d is effective in reducing the incidence of gallstones.

POSTCHOLECYSTECTOMY SYNDROME

Postcholecystectomy syndrome refers to the occurrence of abdominal symptoms after cholecystectomy. This term is a misnomer because the symptoms may or may not necessarily be related to the surgery itself. Clinicians should be aware that typical biliary symptoms are relieved in only 75% to 90% of patients after cholecystectomy. Persistent or recurrent symptoms are most commonly secondary to a retained or, less frequently, newly formed common bile duct stone. A motility disorder of the sphincter of Oddi may occur in 1% to 2% of patients postoperatively and mimic biliary colic. Sphincter of Oddi manometry performed at a tertiary care center will establish the diagnosis. Lack of resolution of abdominal symptoms may also be due to an incorrect diagnosis before cholecystectomy or occur as a complication of surgery. Postcholecystectomy diarrhea due to increased delivery of bile salts to the colon may be controlled by treatment with a bile salt-sequestering agent, such as cholestyramine 4 g two to three times a day.

GALLBLADDER DISEASE IN PREGNANCY

Pregnancy is strongly associated with gallstone formation. Approximately 2% to 4% of pregnant women are found to have gallstones, and approximately 30% have biliary sludge on routine ultrasonography. The risk of gallstone formation increases with number of pregnancies. However, only 5 to 10 per 10,000 (0.05%–0.1%) pregnant women present with symptomatic gallstone disease. During pregnancy, bile is supersaturated with cholesterol due to increased cholesterol secretion induced by estrogen. Gallbladder contraction in response to a standard meal is sluggish. Gallbladder hypomotility, related to progesterone's smooth muscle inhibitory action, potentiates lithogenesis. After pregnancy these changes reverse, leading to the disappearance of sludge and most small stones. The risk of gallstones increases with increasing parity, stones being found in 6.5% to 8.4% of nulliparous compared with 18.4% to 19.3% in multiparous women.

Clinical Manifestations and Differential Diagnosis

Clinical manifestations of gallstones are similar to those of nonpregnant women. Increasing uterine size as pregnancy progresses may shift the location of the appendix to the right upper quadrant, resulting in diagnostic confusion. Normal pregnancy may be associated with nausea, vomiting, leukocytosis, or elevations in serum transaminases or alkaline phosphatase. In addition to the conditions discussed above, the differential diagnoses of right upper quadrant pain specific to pregnancy include acute fatty liver of pregnancy, HELLP syndrome (*h*emolysis, *e*levated *l*iver enzymes, and *l*ow *p*latelet count), and preeclampsia. An increased, although rare, risk of hepatic rupture associated with pregnancy exists, typically in women with severe preeclampsia.

Imaging

Ultrasonography is the best and safest test in pregnancy because no risk of radiation exposure is present. The radiation exposure from hepatobiliary scintigraphy (HIDA) is equivalent to a plain film of the abdomen and is relatively contraindicated in pregnancy. CT is not recommended in pregnancy because of higher radiation exposure. Magnetic resonance cholangiopancreatography is generally safe but should be avoided in the first trimester, because data are lacking at this time.

Treatment Considerations

Pregnant women who present with biliary colic should be managed conservatively during pregnancy. However, patients with persistent symptoms or with complicated gallstone disease (acute pancreatitis, choledocholithiasis/cholangitis) should undergo laparoscopic cholecystectomy. Conservative management in acute pancreatitis, for example, can lead to a recurrent episode in about 70% of patients before term, leading to significant fetal loss. Coordination of care between the obstetric and surgical services is vital in managing these patients. Consideration of ERCP is reserved for the rare patient with persistent biliary obstruction, high likelihood of common bile duct stone, or fulminant cholangitis. Endoscopic ultrasonography is a safe and accurate means of imaging the bile duct to help select pregnant patients for ERCP. If possible, ERCP should be deferred until the second trimester due to the risk of ionizing radiation. Increased teratogenicity and fetal loss during the first trimester are present with laparoscopic cholecystectomy. Management must be individualized.

BIBLIOGRAPHY

Bateson MC. Gallbladder disease. *BMJ* 1999;318:1745–1748.

Chatzliannou SN, Moore WH, Ford PV, et al. Hepatobiliary scintography is superior to abdominal ultrasonography in suspected acute cholecystitis. *Surgery* 2000;127:609–613.

Cosenza CA, Saffari B, Jabbour N, et al. Surgical management of biliary gallstone disease during pregnancy. *Am J Surg* 1999;178:545–548.

Everhart JE, Khare M, Hill M, et al. Prevalence and ethnic differences in gallbladder disease in the United States. *Gastroenterology* 1999;117:632–639.

Fenster FF, Lonborg R, Thirlby RC, et al. What symptoms does cholecystectomy cure? Insights from an outcomes measurement project and review of the literature. *Am J Surg* 1995;169:533–538.

Johnston DE, Kaplan MM. Pathogenesis and treatment of gallstones. *N Engl J Med* 1993;328:412–421.
Nakeeb A, Comuzzie AG, Martin L, et al. Gallstones: genetics versus environment. *Ann Surg* 2002;235:842–849.
Ramin KD, Ramsey PS. Disease of the gallbladder and pancreas in pregnancy. *Obstet Gynecol Clin North Am* 2001;28:571–580.
Ransohoff DF, Gracie WA. Treatment of gallstones. *Ann Intern Med* 1993;119: 606–619.
Saini S. Imaging of the hepatobiliary tract. *N Engl J Med* 1997;336:1889–1894.
Schiffman ML, Kaplan GD, Brinkman-Kaplan V, et al. Prophylaxis against gallstone formation with ursodeoxycholic acid in patients participating in a very-low-calorie diet program. *Ann Intern Med* 1995;122:899–905.
Verson GT. Pregnancy and gallstones. *Hepatology* 1993;17:159–161.

CHAPTER 66
Pancreatitis

David S. Fefferman and Edward Feller

ACUTE PANCREATITIS

Etiology

Acute pancreatitis is an inflammatory disorder characterized by abdominal pain, usually associated with elevation of pancreatic enzymes in the serum. Approximately 250,000 patients with acute pancreatitis are hospitalized yearly in the United States, with 4,000 deaths. The two most common causes in the United States are gallstones and alcohol, which account for 70% to 80% of cases. Gallstone pancreatitis is more common in women, whereas alcohol-related disease has a male predominance.

GALLSTONES

Gallstones are the most common etiology of acute pancreatic inflammation in the United States, responsible for 30% to 50% of attacks (Table 66.1). Women are especially prone to biliary pancreatitis because estrogen increases biliary cholesterol secretion and stone formation by a rate of two- to threefold compared with men. Increased stone formation occurs irrespective of whether the estrogen is endogenous or exogenous in the form of oral contraceptives or replacement therapy. The elderly also have increased lithogenicity of bile due to age-related changes in bilirubin metabolism and gallbladder motility. Prolonged fasting and parenteral nutrition may also create an environment where sludge (microlithiasis) and small stones are more likely to form. Smaller gallbladder stones (less than 5 mm), rather than larger stones, are more likely to pass from the cystic duct into the common bile duct, subsequently becoming obstructed above the sphincter of Oddi. Sludge in the absence of stones may also traverse the biliary system to irritate or obstruct, potentially resulting in pancreatic inflammation. Although the prevalence of gallbladder stones is as high as 10% to 20% in younger women and increases to 25% to 30% after age 50, biliary pancreatitis occurs in less than 5% of persons with known stones. Stones remaining in the gallbladder, although prone to precipitate attacks of biliary colic or acute cholecystitis, do not cause pancreatitis. The mechanism of biliary-induced pancreatitis is unclear and may be due to reflux of bile into the pancreatic duct or due to obstruction at the ampulla of Vater by a stone migrating from the gallbladder to the periampullary common bile duct. Obstruction and subsequent ductal hypertension caused by continued flow of pancreatic secretions unable to bypass the blockage may lead to pancreatic enzyme autoactivation and inflammation.

TABLE 66.1. Causes of Acute Pancreatitis

Diagnosed by history and routine studies
Biliary stones
Alcohol
Hypercalcemia
Hypertriglyceridemia
Postoperative
Post-ERCP
Trauma
Specific infections
Medications
Pancreatic carcinoma
Diagnosis requires special investigations
Anatomic abnormalities
Ampullary stenosis
Pancreatic duct stone
Microlithiasis
Vasculitis
Genetic disorders
Autoimmune disease
Sphincter of Oddi dysfunction

ALCOHOL

Although alcohol is the second most common cause of acute pancreatitis, less than 10% of chronic alcoholics develop pancreatitis. Pancreatitis usually occurs after prolonged use (>10 years). The amount of ingestion required to induce an acute attack is thought by some authorities to be as much as three fourths of a bottle of wine or its equivalent per day. Newer concepts of pathogenesis suggest that individuals consuming smaller amounts of alcohol can develop acute and eventually chronic pancreatitis because of an inherited genetic susceptibility. In some, assessment of the contribution of alcohol may be difficult, because patients may be reluctant to divulge accurate ethanol intake. The mechanism by which alcohol causes pancreatitis is unknown. The most widely held theories include a direct toxic effect on pancreatic acinar cells and alcohol-induced precipitation of proteins that form the nidus for stones, resulting in pancreatic duct obstruction.

HYPERTRIGLYCERIDEMIA

Hypertriglyceridemia is a rare etiology of pancreatitis, implicated in 1% to 3% of cases. Pancreatic inflammation does not usually occur until the serum triglyceride level is greater than 1,000 mg/dL. This uncommon cause should be suspected when lactescent (milky) appearing serum is identified in patients with pancreatitis. The mechanism responsible is thought to be free fatty acid release from serum triglycerides by the action of pancreatic lipase. In addition to patients with hereditary hypertriglyceridemia, marked levels may be seen in association with alcoholism, diabetes mellitus, hypothyroidism, estrogen therapy, and pregnancy. Because of the risk of pancreatitis, estrogen use is not recommended in women with marked uncontrolled hypertriglyceridemia. Hypertriglyceride-related pancreatitis may be associated with a normal serum amylase due to the interference of the lipids with the laboratory assay of amylase.

HYPERCALCEMIA

Elevated serum calcium rarely causes pancreatitis. The mechanism is speculative; theories include obstruction from calcium precipitation in pancreatic ducts and calcium-induced activation of trypsinogen to the active form trypsin, resulting in autodigestion within the pancreatic parenchyma. The most common cause of calcium-related pancreatitis is hyperparathyroidism. Sarcoidosis, metastatic disease to bone, and vitamin D toxicity have all been implicated but are far less common.

INFECTIONS

Uncommonly, infections, including mumps, coxsackie, varicella-zoster, herpes simplex, aspergillus, mycoplasma, mycobacteria, and certain parasites, can be causative. The acquired immunodeficiency syndrome has been associated with an increased incidence of acute pancreatitis. Human immunodeficiency virus has also been associated with hyperamylasemia that is clinically asymptomatic and without evidence of pancreatic inflammation. Opportunistic infections in human immunodeficiency virus, including cytomegalovirus, herpes simplex, *Cryptosporidium*, and Microsporidia, may produce pancreatic inflammation.

MEDICATIONS

Over 100 drugs have been implicated in the causation of pancreatitis, either by a hypersensitivity reaction or by a metabolite producing a dose-related direct toxic injury. A careful medication history is necessary in every case. Clear associations have been reported for medications used in the treatment of human immunodeficiency virus, including didanosine and pentamidine. Hypersensitivity pancreatitis is reported in patients receiving azathioprine or 6-mercaptopurine. As noted above, women with endogenous hypertriglyceridemia have an increased risk of pancreatitis when receiving estrogen and tamoxifen, because these compounds increase lipogenesis. Treatment with metronidazole is also associated with an increased risk of acute pancreatitis.

GENETIC FACTORS

Gene mutations have been discovered in some patients previously considered to have unexplained or idiopathic acute or chronic pancreatitis. Abnormalities have been described for the cystic fibrosis transmembrane regulator (*CFTR*) gene and genes for cationic trypsinogen. The former abnormality may present as late as the sixth or seventh decade of life. Women with hereditary pancreatitis due to trypsinogen gene mutations typically have symptoms arising in childhood but may be delayed until the mid-30s. Recent data report such gene abnormalities in 13% to 40% of patients previously considered to have idiopathic pancreatitis. No gender predisposition exists. In patients whose alcohol intake is only moderate, genetic mutations may potentiate pancreatic inflammation, though the magnitude of this association remains speculative.

POSTOPERATIVE AND ISCHEMIC

The incidence and severity of acute pancreatitis are increased in shock or low-blood flow states. Decreased pancreatic perfusion may accompany acute or chronic mesenteric ischemia due to atherosclerosis, embolus, thrombosis, and postoperative states. Acute pancreatitis has been reported in up to one half of patients with shock after abdominal aortic aneurysm repair. Postoperative abdominal pain may be ascribed to typical postsurgical discomfort, may not be assessed correctly as pancreatitis, or may be masked by analgesics, sedatives, or confusion, especially in the elderly.

IDIOPATHIC

Despite thorough investigation, no obvious identifiable etiology is found in 10% to 30% of patients. In an unknown proportion of these cases, undiagnosed biliary lithiasis, unreported alcoholism, pancreatic duct abnormalities, or hereditary causes may be present. Rarely, pancreatic cancer produces pancreatitis via ductal obstruction. Patients with one attack of presumed idiopathic pancreatitis have a low risk (<5%) of a second episode in follow-up studies of several years duration. No consensus exists on the extent of testing which is appropriate if history, physical examination, and standard noninvasive imaging studies have failed to yield an etiology.

Detailed invasive investigation with endoscopic retrograde cholangiopancreatography (ERCP) and biliary manometry may not be needed after a single attack when common etiologies have been excluded, because the inherent risks of these invasive procedures are often higher than the 5% risk of recurrence. Investigation with magnetic resonance cholangiopancreatography may be an acceptable less invasive alternative to image the pancreatic and bile ducts. Similarly, in the absence of gallstones or suggestion of sludge, cholecystectomy may be deferred after a self-limited case of idiopathic pancreatitis. Some centers recommend empiric laparoscopic cholecystectomy after recurrence or after a single severe attack of unexplained pancreatitis. ERCP with possible biliary drainage for crystal determination and/or endoscopic ultrasound may reveal less common etiologies, including pancreatic duct stone, ampullary stenosis, a choledochal cyst, or pancreatic divisum (a controversial cause of pancreatitis resulting from failure of the embryonic dorsal and ventral pancreatic ducts to fuse). Motility disorders of the biliary system associated with sphincter of Oddi dysfunction are occasionally documented by sophisticated manometric studies in specialized centers.

Differential Diagnosis

The pain of pancreatitis is nonspecific and may be confused with a wide variety of intra-abdominal conditions that may also produce elevations of serum amylase and lipase. Acute biliary colic or cholecystitis is common in women and may present as episodic attacks of right upper quadrant or epigastric pain simulating pancreatic inflammation. Biliary colic or acute cholecystitis may progress to acute pancreatitis if a stone passes the cystic duct and becomes obstructed at the ampulla of Vater. Biliary colic tends to be of shorter duration and often waxing and waning in severity, although continuous pain lasting greater than 24 hours is more likely to be pancreatic in origin. Progression of an attack of presumed biliary pain to the left side of the abdomen suggests pancreatic inflammation. Because biliary pancreatitis is so common, evaluation of the gallbladder is mandatory in any woman presenting with clinical pancreatitis. Peptic ulcer disease or reflux esophagitis may present as mid-abdominal pain and may be difficult by history alone to differentiate from acute pancreatitis. In peptic ulcer disease, the pain tends to be more localized, related to food intake, and relieved by acid-suppressing medications. Perforated peptic ulcers are often associated with muscle guarding and signs of peritoneal irritation (rebound tenderness) on abdominal examination. Acute abdominal pain from a kidney stone will rarely be anterior and is classically nonlocalizing. Urinalysis should be routine in patients with acute abdominal pain. In older patients or those with risk factors for atherosclerosis or hypercoagulability, mesenteric ischemia may masquerade as pancreatitis with a clinically indistinguishable pain pattern and elevations of serum amylase and lipase. A ruptured ectopic pregnancy, acute salpingitis, or a ruptured ovarian cyst rarely may simulate the diffuse pain of pancreatitis and be associated with serum hyperamylasemia.

Clinical Symptoms and History

Abdominal pain is the cardinal complaint in 95% of patients with acute pancreatic inflammation. The pain of pancreatitis ranges from mild epigastric discomfort to excruciating diffuse pain associated with an acute abdomen and hemodynamic instability. The character of the pain is steady, often described as "boring," and may last as long as several days. An intermittent or colicky quality suggests an alternative diagnosis. The location is typically in the epigastrium or across the upper abdomen in a band-like fashion. The pain often radiates through to the back. The degree of pain does not appear to correlate with the severity of inflammation. Nearly all patients experience nausea and vomiting, with little or no amelioration after emesis. Patients may find relief leaning forward or with assumption of the fetal position with the knees flexed; in some, a recumbent posture exacerbates the pain.

Clinical Findings and Physical Examination

Findings on physical examination vary with the severity of the episode. Low-grade fever and tachycardia are common. Severe disease may be associated with signs of hypovolemia, hypotension, shock, or acute changes in mental status. Tachypnea or hypoxemia may be noted on presentation, associated with irritation of the diaphragm, pleural effusion, or the development of the acute respiratory distress syndrome in severe cases. The presence of scleral icterus suggests choledocholithiasis, underlying liver disease, or encasement of the distal intrapancreatic portion of the common bile duct in pancreatic edema. Upper abdominal tenderness ranges from mild or absent to severe with guarding and signs of peritoneal irritation (rebound or percussion tenderness). Hypoactive bowel sounds may indicate an adynamic ileus. Ecchymosis of the periumbilical area (Cullen's sign) or of the flank (Grey-Turner's sign) reflect abdominal hemorrhage, but both are rare and nonspecific. Cutaneous stigmata of chronic liver disease (jaundice, spider angiomata, ascites, increased collateral circulation on the anterior abdominal wall, hepatosplenomegaly) may be clues to an alcoholic etiology.

Laboratory Diagnosis

Although acute pancreatitis may be the most common explanation for serum elevations of amylase and lipase, a diverse range of other diseases, some with clinical features similar to those of pancreatic inflammation, are also associated with enzyme increases. The clinician must be aware that no biochemical gold standard exists for diagnosis and assessment of severity in pancreatitis.

The major limitation of amylase determination is poor specificity. Hyperamylasemia may occur in conjunction with inflammation or injury to the pancreas and biliary tract, intestines, salivary glands, genitourinary tract, and liver (Table 66.2). Elevated levels may occur from overproduction or from underexcretion during metabolic stresses, hypotension, hypoperfusion, trauma, acute or chronic renal failure, or metabolic acidosis or may be secondary to a variety of medications. Persistent asymptomatic elevations of both amylase and lipase occur in macroamylasemia or macrolipasemia, conditions in which the enzymes are bound to abnormal proteins that are too large for normal renal clearance. Determination of urinary amylase has no practical value except to exclude macroamylasemia. Salivary sources of amylase are common and may reflect inflammation or injury to the gland from mechanical forces, alcohol, or other toxins. In women, salivary hyperamylasemia is common in bulimics or anorexics who purge. Protracted vomiting from any cause may increase salivary amylase in serum.

Most difficult to distinguish is the serum amylase elevation accompanying intra-abdominal conditions clinically similar to pancreatitis. Intestinal perforation or mesenteric ischemia or infarction can produce leakage of luminal amylase from the gut into the bloodstream. Pancreatic enzymes may also be elevated in isolated biliary disease. Both amylase and lipase are increased in renal insufficiency due to failure of the kidney to clear enzymes normally from the serum. Severe metabolic acidosis may also be associated with a salivary hyperamylasemia.

TABLE 66.2. Conditions Associated with Hyperamylasemia

Acute pancreatitis
Pancreatic pseudocyst, abscess
Pancreatic carcinoma
Acute cholecystitis
Mesenteric infarction
Intestinal obstruction or perforation
Post-ERCP
Salivary disease
Renal failure
Metabolic acidosis
Anorexia-bulimia
Ruptured ectopic pregnancy
Salpingitis, tubo-ovarian abscess
Tumor hyperamylasemia

Serum lipase elevation, once considered specific for pancreatic inflammation, is also present in a wide variety of nonpancreatic conditions. Lipase may be increased in isolated biliary tract disease, renal insufficiency, metabolic acidosis, intestinal ischemia or infarction, and macrolipasemia. Advantages of lipase measurement are that it has a longer half-life than amylase, remaining elevated in serum longer than amylase, and has increased sensitivity for alcohol-induced pancreatitis. Normal amylase or lipase levels in the serum do not exclude pancreatic inflammation. Serum elevations in acute inflammation are transient, frequently returning to normal within 2 to 3 days after onset of an episode. Testing after enzyme levels have returned to normal may lead to misdiagnosis. Likewise, patients who have extensive destruction of the pancreatic parenchyma may be unable to produce amylase during acute inflammation. As many as one third of patients with chronic alcoholic pancreatitis with acute exacerbations of pain have a burned-out pancreas no longer able to manufacture enzymes despite acute inflammation.

Enzyme elevations that persist or become elevated after initial normalization should raise concern about a complication such as a pancreatic pseudocyst, abscess, necrosis, or blockage of the pancreatic duct. Serum levels of amylase and lipase do not correlate with the severity. A marked initial serum amylase level (>1,000 IU/L) is more commonly associated with biliary pancreatitis than an alcoholic etiology. Other markers have been shown to correlate with an increased risk of complicated disease. Hemoconcentration is a predictor of necrotizing pancreatitis and increased potential for organ failure. Data indicate that a hematocrit greater than 47% on admission plus a failure to decrease after 1 day suggest severe disease. Serum C-reactive protein is increased in acute inflammation such as severe pancreatitis; however, its peak elevation occurs at 2 to 3 days after onset of symptoms, limiting its clinical utility in early assessment. Other serum and urinary markers to assess the diagnosis and severity of acute pancreatitis have been evaluated, including immunoreactive trypsinogen, amylase isoenzymes, pancreatitis-associated protein, and various mediators of inflammation (tumor necrosis factors, interleukins). Though some are promising, none is helpful enough for routine laboratory assessment of pancreatitis.

Imaging Studies

Plain abdominal radiographs do not provide specific diagnostic information about pancreatic inflammation but may be helpful to exclude intestinal obstruction or perforation. The study may also document a "sentinal loop" or an adynamic ileus, which although common in severe disease are nonspecific findings. Chest radiography is abnormal in up to one third of patients, with abnormalities including atelectasis, elevated hemidiaphragm, pleural effusion, pneumonia, or evidence of acute respiratory distress syndrome in severe cases. Abdominal ultrasonography is routine in women presenting with a first attack of pancreatitis to detect gallbladder stones and assess the diameter of the common bile duct. Ultrasonography, although very accurate for gallstones and duct size, is insensitive for the diagnosis of common bile duct stones. During acute abdominal inflammatory processes, ileus or excessive bowel gas commonly obscures the pancreas and right upper quadrant, limiting the quality and utility of ultrasonography at admission in 25% to 35% of patients. In such circumstances, a repeat ultrasound is indicated after clinical resolution. Helical computed tomography (CT) is indicated to exclude other diagnoses, to evaluate for complications in severe cases when no improvement occurs after 48 hours, or to investigate acute deterioration. The use of intravenous contrast-enhanced CT (in the absence of renal dysfunction) will document pancreatic necrosis as unenhanced areas of parenchyma. In the patient with typical abdominal pain and enzyme elevation, CT may, at times, suggest an alternative diagnosis (such as mesenteric ischemia in the patient with imaging evidence of bowel wall thickening and a normal pancreas). After plain abdominal radiographs, most patients will have CT as the initial imaging study. Because of its greater sensitivity for gallbladder stones, eventual ultrasonography should be performed in women who have not had prior cholecystectomy.

Complications

Most cases of pancreatitis are mild, representing edematous disease. Ten percent to 15% are severe, with a high incidence of organ failure and necrotizing pancreatitis associated with an increased incidence of pancreatic and systemic complications and a mortality as high as 15% to 20%. Objective assessment of early prognostic signs may identify patients most likely to develop severe pancreatitis, require more intensive monitoring and intensive care unit transfer, or justify the use of additional modalities (e.g., prophylactic antibiotics). Scoring systems using clinical prediction rules (APACHE II, Ranson criteria, Bank, Agarwhal, and Glascow scores) and CT criteria have been used to predict severity. Clinical features assessing renal dysfunction, respiratory distress, circulatory collapse, and peritoneal irritation are as accurate as the many clinical prediction guidelines that have been promulgated. Contrast-enhanced CT will differentiate edematous from necrotizing pancreatitis. CT score using Balthazar's criteria will help stratify patients for prognostic purposes and serve as a baseline if deterioration or lack of resolution of an attack occur. Current recommendations are to obtain contrast-enhanced CT in patients predicted to have a severe attack, in patients not improving after 48 hours, or in patients whose clinical condition deteriorates. Of the clinical prediction guidelines studied, APACHE II may be the most accurate but is limited by its complexity to calculate. No current technique, including clinical assessment, accurately identifies most patients destined to have a severe clinical course.

EARLY COMPLICATIONS

The course of pancreatitis in the first few days is marked by the systemic effects of the inflammatory process and the potential for organ failure. Clinical and laboratory assessment is needed to monitor for respiratory distress syndrome, acute renal insufficiency, circulatory collapse, large fluid requirements, hypocalcemia, hypoglycemia, or hyperglycemia. As the inflammatory process spreads, peripancreatic inflammation may cause injury to nearby structures. Bowel necrosis, gastrointestinal bleeding, extension of the inflammatory process to involve the spleen and splenic vasculature, and mesenteric fat necrosis may occur in severe cases. Approximately half the deaths in pancreatitis occur in the first 2 weeks, mainly a consequence of multiorgan failure.

LATE COMPLICATIONS

After the first 7 to 10 days of an acute attack, the prognosis of pancreatitis is dominated by the potential for and consequences of infection. Mild edematous disease is very uncommonly complicated by infection, which may occur in 30% to 50% of patients with necrotizing pancreatitis. Balthazar and colleagues studied 88 patients with acute pancreatitis. Necrosis on CT is associated with as high as a 23% mortality and 82% morbidity compared with zero mortality and 6% morbidity without necrosis. Antibiotic prophylaxis with drugs achieving high concentration in pancreatic juice and inflamed or necrotic parenchyma (principally imipenem) have been associated with reduced infection rates from initially sterile pancreatic necrosis. Fulminant inflammation or ductal disruption may cause leakage of pancreatic juice with activated enzymes to form in the substance of the gland or in peripancreatic spaces. These initially amorphous fluid collections may wall-off, lined by reactive granulation tissue and encased by adjacent viscera, to form pseudocysts. These cysts may remain asymptomatic or produce a diverse range of complications, including extension into adjacent viscera and pain from continued cyst expansion, or become secondarily infected. Frank pancreatic abscesses may also form.

Treatment

Therapy for mild pancreatitis is supportive with hospitalization for intravenous fluids, pain control, and nothing by mouth status. Prognosis is excellent for rapid resolution without further therapy. Aggressive fluid resuscitation must be stressed, because third-space losses during pancreatic inflammation can be substantial and are often underestimated. There is no clear benefit from routine administration of acid-suppressing agents. Antibiotic prophylaxis is not indicated for mild to moderate pancreatitis by clinical or imaging criteria. Correction of the underlying etiology causing acute pancreatitis (biliary disease, hypercalcemia, hypertriglyceridemia, medication, etc.) is essential for long-term management and prevention of recurrence. When alcoholism is a factor, abstention must be stressed and appropriate multimodality treatment instituted. Infection is a secondary phenomenon, occurring principally from translocation of enteric bacteria; thus, it is theoretically preventable. Indications for prophylactic antibiotics include evidence of organ failure, Ranson's score more than 3, Apache II score more than 8, or patients with extensive necrosis (>30% of the gland) because they are at higher risk for developing infections.

Recent data support the preference for early enteral nutrition via a nasojejunal feeding tube in severe pancreatitis and in patients predicted to be unable to tolerate oral feedings for an extended period of time. Prolonged fasting may compromise gut function, blood flow, immune function, and protein synthesis. Using an enteral rather than a parenteral feeding route has been shown to enhance mucosal integrity as a barrier to bacterial translocation and to avoid the infectious and catheter-related complications of total parenteral nutrition. Patients with mild pancreatitis can be managed with initial intravenous hydration in the anticipation of rapid resumption of oral feeding.

Considerations in Pregnancy

Acute pancreatitis complicates pregnancy uncommonly, with a reported incidence ranging from 1 in 1,000 pregnancies to 1 in 10,000. In one population-based study, all cases occurred in the postpartum period. The minimally increased risk of pancreatitis in the gravid state is due primarily to biliary disease caused by increased lithogenesis induced by the elevated estrogen levels. Pregnancy also increases triglyceride levels, especially in the third trimester. Because gestational hyperlipidemia is mild, the risk of hypertriglyceridemic pancreatitis is typically present only in women with prepregnancy lipid disorders. Transabdominal ultrasonography is both safe and accurate in detection of stones within the gallbladder; however, it is less sensitive in detecting common duct stones. Routine use of CT is avoided because of the risks associated with fetal radiation exposure. Endoscopic ultrasonography is a safe and accurate method of assessing the common bile duct in the pregnant patient at high risk for choledocholithiasis. This technique is useful in selected patients, because ERCP requires exposure to ionizing radiation. The treatment of pancreatitis in pregnancy is similar to that for other etiologies. Maternal and fetal morbidity is low in mild pancreatitis, but an increased risk of spontaneous abortions and prematurity exists when necrotizing or severe pancreatitis is present. In women with biliary pancreatitis, cholecystectomy can be performed safely, especially during the second trimester. However, temporizing measures, including endoscopic sphincterotomy, have also been reported to be safe and effective, when required.

CHRONIC PANCREATITIS

In acute biliary pancreatitis, the pancreatic parenchyma and ducts are classically normal before an episode and generally return to normal with resolution of inflammation. Permanent chronic injury to the pancreas may occur with severe gallstone-induced acute disease, especially with necrotizing pancreatitis or duct disruption. However, biliary pancreatitis is generally considered to be an acute disease. Alcoholic pancreatitis, in contrast, occurs most frequently in a gland that is morphologically abnormal before and after an acute attack. In this sense, chronic alcoholic pancreatitis is an irreversible disorder of the pancreas defined by glandular destruction with inflammation and fibrosis. The disease is characterized by abdominal pain and pancreatic insufficiency marked by exocrine (acinar cell) and/or endocrine (islet cell) dysfunction. Most cases of biliary pancreatitis represent acute (possible recurrent) pancreatitis, whereas most cases of acute alcoholic pancreatitis represent chronic (relapsing) pancreatitis. Distinguishing between acute and chronic pancreatitis may be difficult in some patients when the clinical expression of the latter is recurrent attacks of acute pancreatic inflammation.

Etiology

Chronic heavy alcohol ingestion accounts for 70% to 80% of the cases worldwide. The risk increases with increasing ethanol intake; however, only 5% to 10% of chronic alcoholics develop chronic pancreatitis. Genetic influence and dietary factors are likely contributing factors responsible for some of the individual differences in susceptibility. Abstinence from alcohol retards progression in some patients. In addition to alcohol, less common etiologies of chronic pancreatitis include pancreatic duct obstruction, idiopathic chronic pancreatitis, hereditary pancreatitis, neoplasia, trauma, and cystic fibrosis (Table 66.3). Families with hereditary pancreatitis have an autosomal-dominant disorder related to mutations in a cationic trypsinogen gene. Rarely, chronic pancreatitis has been found in association with hyperparathyroidism, hyperlipidemia, abdominal radiation, and autoimmune diseases, including systemic lupus erythematosus and Sjögren disease. Tropical pancreatitis is rare in the Unites States and is believed to be related to dietary deficiencies or toxic ingestions. Idiopathic chronic pancreatitis, accounting for 10% to 30% of cases, exists in two distinct patterns, early-onset and late-onset disease. Both forms occur equally in men and women. The initial presentation of early-onset disease peaks at approximately age 20. This disorder is characterized predominantly by pain with pancreatic insufficiency that is slowly progressive over several decades. Late-onset idiopathic chronic pancreatitis peaks in the fifth to seventh decades. Pain is absent at presentation in 50% of patients. The clinical expression may be exocrine insufficiency (diarrhea, weight loss, or steatorrhea) and/or endocrine insufficiency (adult-onset diabetes mellitus). An unknown proportion of "idiopathic" cases may represent unrevealed ethanol excess or uninvestigated or as yet undiscovered genetic mutations.

Exocrine or endocrine deficiency (pancreatic insufficiency) can exist in the absence of pancreatic inflammation, principally resulting from the failure of release, activation, or poor mixing of pancreatic enzymes with the small bowel activating enzyme, enterokinase. Examples include Billroth II gastroenterostomy (with poor mixing of enzymes with ingested food possible), tumor blocking the pancreatic duct, cystic fibrosis, protein-calorie malnutrition, and Zollinger-Ellison syndrome (with intraluminal destruction of enzymes by excess acid).

Pathogenesis

A common feature of chronic pancreatitis is ductal obstruction. Chronic excess alcohol ingestion may induce hypersecretion of proteins from acinar cells without a concomitant increase in fluid and bicarbonate secretion from ductal cells. The result is formation of viscous debris of inspissated proteinaceous material. Precipitation of calcium carbonate in these protein plugs produces intraductal stones seen radiographically as radiolucent calcifications. Ductal plugs form in all types of chronic pancreatitis, but stones most commonly occur in patients with alco-

TABLE 66.3. Etiologies of Chronic Pancreatitis

Alcoholism (70%–80% of cases)
Genetic (mutations of CFTR gene, trypsinogen gene mutations)
Autoimmune disease
Duct obstruction (tumor, stone, congenital anomaly, stricture)
Hypercalcemia
Hyperlipidemia
Idiopathic (early and late-onset)
Tropical (rare in United States)
Pancreatic insufficiency without pancreatitis
Pancreatic resection
Gastric resection
Zollinger-Ellison syndrome
Severe protein-calorie malnutrition

hol-related disease. Alcohol also has a direct toxic effect on the pancreatic parenchyma. Some evidence suggests that repeated episodes of acute alcoholic pancreatitis may eventually culminate in irreversible changes to an initially normal gland. Conflicting data suggest that changes of chronic pancreatitis are present already at the first clinical episode of alcoholic pancreatitis. Gene mutations may be cofactors potentiating the development of alcoholic pancreatitis in an uncertain percent of cases, especially in patients with an unimpressive history of alcohol ingestion. Recent data indicate that 13% to 40% of patients with idiopathic chronic pancreatitis have mutations of the *CFTR* gene. Other gene mutations are likely to be implicated in the future.

Clinical Symptoms

The cardinal feature of chronic alcoholic pancreatitis is abdominal pain. The spectrum of disease in individual patients can be quite varied. Typically, in 70% to 80% of cases, patients experience intermittent episodes of pain with relative pain-free intervals. Others have pain that is chronic and unremitting, whereas some having acute on chronic exacerbations requiring hospitalization. For many patients, after a variable duration of time the pain subsides. One theory is that the pain is ameliorated as the pancreas becomes "burned out" due to progressive glandular destruction and fibrosis. Ten percent to 20% may have silent pancreatitis and present with weight loss associated with foul-smelling greasy stools (steatorrhea) resulting from protein maldigestion and fat malabsorption. Endocrine dysfunction and diabetes mellitus usually occur later in the disease. Patients with idiopathic pancreatitis, especially late-onset disease, commonly have no pain, presenting with isolated diabetes mellitus or evidence of fat malabsorption.

Differential Diagnosis

Acute attacks superimposed on underlying chronic pancreatitis need to be differentiated from the same diverse disorders potentially confused with acute pancreatitis. Pancreatic carcinoma may be particularly difficult to exclude in the patient with overlapping symptoms of pancreatic-type pain, weight loss, and jaundice. Because chronic pancreatitis may manifest as unexplained diarrhea, steatorrhea, adult-onset diabetes mellitus, or weight loss, identification of underlying complaints as being pancreatic in origin may require a high index of clinical suspicion.

Complications

Because chronic pancreatitis, especially that associated with alcohol, may manifest as recurrent acute attacks, the course of an episode is similar to that described for acute pancreatitis. Chronic disease may be complicated by pseudocyst formation, stenosis of the common bile duct, and vascular thrombosis of the portal, mesenteric, or splenic veins. Pancreatic ascites or pancreatic pleural effusion may occur. An increased risk of pancreatic carcinoma also exists in patients with chronic pancreatitis.

Laboratory and Imaging Studies

No gold standard exists for diagnosis. Serum amylase and lipase studies, vital in assessment of acute pancreatitis, are insensitive and generally unhelpful in chronic pancreatitis except during an acute exacerbation. Diagnosis may be simple in the alcoholic patient evaluated for acute abdominal pain with diabetes mellitus, malnutrition, and gross steatorrhea. However, clinically relevant deficiencies of pancreatic lipolytic and proteolytic enzymes do not occur until more than 90% of function is lost. Diabetes mellitus does not occur until 80% of islet cell function is destroyed. A spot stool specimen for fat and undigested muscle fibers will document steatorrhea and pancreatic maldigestion of proteins, respectively. Symptomatic deficiency of fat-soluble vitamins (A, D, E, K) and vitamin B_{12} are rare. Glucose intolerance is a late manifestation of alcoholic pancreatitis but present initially in 22% of patients with late-onset idiopathic chronic pancreatitis in a large Mayo clinic report.

Plain abdominal radiographs may demonstrate pancreatic calcifications in 30% to 50% of patients, especially with advanced disease. Imaging via CT or ultrasonography may demonstrate fluid collections, duct dilatation, pancreatic calcifications, atrophy, or enlargement. Imaging is not sensitive for the diagnosis of chronic pancreatitis but is more useful for detection of complications. Visualization of duct systems by ERCP commonly reveals early changes of disease, including duct dilatation, stricture, or secondary ductal proliferation. Some patients have a normal ERCP early in the disease process. Endoscopic ultrasonography permits visualization of the entire pancreas through the wall of the upper gastrointestinal tract, elucidating fine structural detail. Magnetic resonance imaging and magnetic resonance cholangiopancreatography are evolving noninvasive diagnostic technologies. Secretin hormonal stimulation of the pancreas, a test done at specialized centers, may detect exocrine insufficiency in up to 15% of patients with normal routine laboratory and imaging studies.

Treatment

Chronic pain is typically the dominant symptom requiring management. Pain in chronic pancreatitis may be intermittent or constant and unrelenting, ranging in severity from a mild discomfort to a debilitating complaint. Abstinence from alcohol must be stressed to forestall progressive destruction of the pancreas. A low-fat diet and nonnarcotic analgesia may be sufficient in some patients, especially early in the course of the disease. Pain is so highly variable that individualization of management is vital. An unclear proportion of patients become pain free after years of disease, possibly related to the onset of gross pancreatic insufficiency. Unfortunately, many have persisting pain requiring intermittent or continual use of narcotic analgesia. Options for pain control include an empiric trial of high-dose pancreatic enzymes. Oral administration of enzymes may induce feedback inhibition of pancreatic secretion, decreasing cholecystokinin-mediated pancreatic stimulation. Multiple enteric and nonenteric coated preparations with varying lipase content are available. Dosages require that several tablets be taken with each meal and snack. Attempts at short-term intermittent use combined with nonsteroidal antiinflammatory drugs will relieve pain in some patients. When nonsteroidal antiinflammatory drugs do not provide symptomatic relief in those with chronic unremitting symptoms, long-acting oral or patch form narcotic analgesics may be more effective and less habit forming than formulations that control pain for only several hours.

Surgery for pain relief in chronic pancreatitis, after failure of medical management, requires knowledge of pancreatic duct anatomy. When a dilated main pancreatic duct is present, decompression with a lateral pancreaticojejunostomy (Puestow procedure) is reported to relieve pain in up to 75% of cases with preservation of functioning pancreatic tissue. Inflammation involving the head of the pancreas may require pancreatic resection. Surgical and endoscopic techniques to remove pancreatic duct stones, dilate ductal strictures, and improve outflow via the ampulla of Vater benefit a variable percentage of patients, although no large long-term controlled trials of efficacy exist. Celiac plexus nerve block (via percutaneous or endoscopic ultrasound-directed injection) and splanchnic nerve interruption by thoracoscopic techniques have been used with some success. Investigational reports of total pancreatectomy with autograft islet transplantation have been beneficial to some patients with refractory pain and may become more widely used in the future.

STEATORRHEA

Reduction of fat intake may improve symptoms in patients with exocrine insufficiency of lipase. In those who fail dietary modifications, pancreatic lipase replacement is indicated through the use of a nonenteric coated preparations (Viokase) plus an acid-suppressing agent (histamine H_2 receptor antagonist or proton pump inhibitor) or through the use of an enteric coated formulation (Ultrase MT, Pancrease MT). Patient compliance with enzyme supplements may be a problem because multiple capsules need to be taken with every meal and with many snacks.

ENDOCRINE AND NUTRITIONAL TREATMENT

Diabetes mellitus in chronic pancreatitis is characterized by destruction of both insulin-secreting beta cells and glucagon-secreting alpha cells; thus, diabetes may be brittle and difficult to control. Many patients with this disease have multiple nutritional deficits due to the variable contribution of malnutrition from poor oral intake due to pain, effects of alcoholism, and the vitamin and nutrient deficits of pancreatic maldigestion. Efforts to relieve oxidative stress in chronic pancreatitis have used vitamins C and E, selenium, and methionine, but insufficient data exist to recommend this approach clinically.

Considerations in Pregnancy

The management of chronic pancreatitis in the pregnant woman is similar to that of the nonpregnant woman. Because of the possibility of major associated nutritional and caloric deficits associated with chronic pancreatitis, careful attention to diet, oral intake, and avoidance of alcohol must be stressed. Acute exacerbations are treated according to the same principles used in acute pancreatitis.

BIBLIOGRAPHY

Balthazar EJ. Acute pancreatitis: assessment of severity with clinical and CT evaluation. *Radiology* 2002;223:603–613.

Balthazar EJ, Robinson DL, Megibow AJ, et al. Acute pancreatitis: value of CT in establishing prognosis. *Radiology* 1990;174:331–336.

Bank S, Indaram A. Causes of acute and recurrent pancreatitis. *Gastroenterol Clin North Am* 1999;28:571–588.

Banks PA. Epidemiology, natural history, and predictors of disease outcome in acute and chronic pancreatitis. *Gastrointest Endosc* 2002;56[6 Suppl 2]:S226–S230.

Baron TH, Morgan DE. Acute necrotizing pancreatitis. *N Engl J Med* 1999;340: 1412–1417.

Clain JE, Pearson RK. Diagnosis of chronic pancreatitis: is a gold standard necessary? *Surg Clin North Am* 1999;79:829–845.

DiMagno EP. Gene mutations and idiopathic chronic pancreatitis: clinical implications and testing. *Gastroenterology* 2001;121:1508–1512.

Layer P, Yamamoto H, Kalthoff L, et al. The different courses of early- and late-onset idiopathic and alcoholic chronic pancreatitis. *Gastroenterology* 1994;107: 1481–1487.

Legro RS, Laifer SA. First-trimester pancreatitis: maternal and neonatal outcome. *J Reprod Med* 1995;40:689–695.

Levy MJ, Geenen JE. Idiopathic acute recurrent pancreatitis. *Am J Gastroenterol* 2001;96:2540–2555.

Maringhini A, Lankisch MR, Zinsmeister AR, et al. Acute pancreatitis in the post-partum period: a population-based case-control study. *Mayo Clin Proc* 2000; 75:361–364.

Mayer IE, Hussein H. Abdominal pain during pregnancy. *Gastroenterol Clin North Am* 1998;28:1–36.

Scolapio JS, Malhi-Chowla N, Ukleja A. Nutrition supplementation in patients with acute and chronic pancreatitis. *Gastroenterol Clin North Am* 1999;28:695–707.

Sharer N, Schwarz M, Malone G, et al. Mutations of the cystic fibrosis gene in patients with chronic pancreatitis. *N Engl J Med* 1998;339:645–652.

Steer ML, Waxman I, Freedman S. Chronic pancreatitis. *N Engl J Med* 1995;332: 1482–1490.

Steinberg W, Tenner S. Acute pancreatitis. *N Engl J Med* 1994;330:1198–1210.

Tham TC, Vandervoort J, Wong RC, et al. Safety of ERCP during pregnancy. *Am J Gastroenterol* 2003;98:308–311.

Warshaw AL, Banks PA, Fernandez-Del Castillo C. AGA technical review: treatment of pain in chronic pancreatitis. *Gastroenterology* 1998;115:765–776.

Windsor AC, Kanwar S, Li AG, et al. Compared with parenteral nutrition, enteral feeding attenuates the acute phase response and improves disease severity in acute pancreatitis. *Gut* 1998;42:431–435.

Yadav D, Agarwal N, Pitchumoni CS. A critical evaluation of laboratory tests in acute pancreatitis. *Am J Gastroenterol* 2002;97:1309–1318.

CHAPTER 67
Acute Gastroenteritis

Lucinda Anne Harris and Michelle Kang Kim

ETIOLOGY

Epidemiology

Gastroenteritis is a common disease usually of acute onset characterized by diarrhea and associated with the ingestion of infectious or chemical agents. Other gastrointestinal symptoms (nausea, vomiting, abdominal pain) or systemic symptoms (e.g., fever, anorexia, or myalgias) may be present. The disease can range in severity from a benign, self-limited, 24-hour syndrome to a more fulminant illness requiring hospitalization and even death.

This illness is of particular importance because of its significant morbidity and mortality around the world. Worldwide there are an estimated 3 to 5 billion illness episodes and 5 to 10 million deaths per year. Three million deaths are estimated to occur in children age 5 or younger. In the United States, the incidence of gastroenteritis is clearly underreported and difficult to estimate, because many patients do not seek medical attention. In 1997, 76 million patients became ill, 325,000 were hospitalized, and 5,000 people died in the United States alone.

Worldwide, children have the most acute infections, but the elderly in the Unites States are at greater risk of dying. Homosexual men are at risk for organisms associated with *gay bowel syndrome*, but being an adult female is a risk factor for gastroenteritis. Certain infections carry increased risk of morbidity and mortality during pregnancy.

The most common etiology of gastroenteritis is food-borne infections. Based on an annual surveillance report from the U.S. Centers for Disease Control and Prevention, the most common culture-confirmed infections were *Salmonella*, followed by *Campylobacter* and *Shigella*. Males had higher incidences of multiple surveyed pathogens, including *Cryptosporidium*, *Cyclospora*, *Listeria*, and *Escherichia coli* 0157:H7. Of note, men had a 27% increased rate of *Campylobacter* infection compared with women. When stratified according to age and sex, rates of *Salmonella* and *E. coli* 0157 infection were higher in women 20 years old and greater. Despite the above studies, viruses, especially the Norwalk virus, are the most common etiology behind food-borne infection in the United States. Norwalk virus alone is estimated to account for more than half of cases of gastroenteritis. Other entities, preformed toxins, medications, mushroom ingestion, and heavy metal ingestion, are rare causes of gastroenteritis. This chapter emphasizes infectious etiologies and important issues in the care of female patients, particularly when they are pregnant. Other etiologies are briefly discussed.

Risk Factors

Individuals at greatest risk of gastroenteritis are children, the elderly, pregnant women, and the immunocompromised. Individuals in nursing homes and hospitals—both residents and workers—are at increased risk. Travel to developing countries increases the risk of diarrheal illness in people of all ages. Enterotoxigenic *E. coli* is still the most common cause of traveler's diarrhea, although *Salmonella* and *Shigella* are also relatively common. Travel abroad was also implicated as a risk factor for *Campylobacter jejuni* in a 1999 study by the Centers for Disease Control and Prevention.

Pregnant women are known to be at increased risk of gastroenteritis, particularly with *Listeria* and hepatitis E. These infections also have more morbidity and mortality in pregnant women than in the general population. Female adults are at greater risk for gastroenteritis. This is not surprising when one considers that women are still the primary caretakers for children and for patients in institutional settings and as such their risk of exposure is greater. In addition, food-borne causes are the chief vector of disease. Women may be placed at increased risk because of their family role in food preparation. Inversely, women may be at lower risk of gay bowel syndrome, a term formerly used to describe diarrhea in patients infected with human immunodeficiency virus (HIV). However, sexual practices may also be implicated in the transmission of some gastrointestinal infections in this area as well. *Neisseria gonorrhoeae, treponema pallidum,* and *Chlamydia trachomatis* are but a few of the organisms that can be transferred to the gastrointestinal tract.

Other important factors to consider in gastroenteritis are immunocompromising conditions such as HIV and diabetes. Patients with HIV are at increased risk for opportunistic gastrointestinal infections like cytomegalovirus, herpes simplex virus, and *Mycobacterium avium intracellulare*. Also, acquired immunodeficiency syndrome patients frequently receive courses of antibiotics that change the flora of the gut, predisposing to bacterial overgrowth and bouts of gastrointestinal infection. In patients with diabetes, hypomotility may also cause a change in the flora of the intestine and may also result in decreased clearance of pathogens.

Medications should also be considered a risk factor. Steroids and other immunosuppressants affect susceptibility to a variety of organisms. These medications are used in a wide variety of diseases, such as inflammatory bowel disease, rheumatoid arthritis, and chronic pulmonary disease, and in patients on chemotherapy. Drugs that effect gut motility such as antidiarrheals or antibiotics that change intestinal flora may also play a role in the susceptibility of patients to various infections.

The defense system for gastroenteritis can also be weakened by conditions that affect the body's ability to protect itself, such as achlorhydria in the gastrointestinal tract or a history of gastric surgery. Anomalous enteric conditions such as fistulae, diverticulosis, and aperistaltic intestinal loops have all been implicated in increasing risk of enteric infections.

Modes of Transmission

Transmission of infectious agents—viral, parasitic, and bacterial—can occur via multiple modalities. Food-borne gastroenteritis is often the most common form of transmission and can involve contamination at any point along the chain in food growing, distribution, handling, or consumption. The medical literature is filled with many examples. For instance the epidemic of *Cyclospora*-associated diarrhea from raspberries in 1996 was traced to a water supply contaminated by human feces that was used to water plants. Improper processing of meat or inadequate disinfection of equipment can easily contaminate large quantities of meat before distribution. An outbreak of *Listeria monocytogenes* was attributed to chocolate milk from one dairy because of a contaminated milk storage tank. In restaurants or other establishments serving food, poor handwashing technique by food handlers can make food unsafe. In the home, failure to refrigerate food or to cook food thoroughly can easily allow pathogens to proliferate. The improper sharing and cleaning of cutting boards and utensils can also contaminate food. Any and all of these modes may have been the cause in the recent epidemic of Norwalk virus (2002) in the luxury cruise ship industry.

Less common forms of gastroenteritis exist. Ingestion of certain mushroom strains can cause gastroenteritis via toxins inherent in that food group. In addition, heavy metal intake (e.g., antimony, copper, and cadmium) can cause diarrhea. Some foods contain preformed toxins that cannot be rendered safe even with cooking, such as scromboid toxin and ciguatoxin in various seafoods. Finally, various medications, such as chemotherapeutic agents and antibiotics, can cause diarrhea either by directly damaging the intestine or allowing the proliferation of other bacteria (e.g., *Clostridia difficile*).

Transmission is often recurrent. Immunity is only short term if at all. Mothers may pass on some immunity to viruses to infants via breast-feeding that last about 3 months. Multiple strains of viruses exist, allowing patients to become infected again and again. Unfortunately, individuals are at risk of multiple infections with parasitic, bacterial, and viral causes throughout their lifetime.

Pathogenesis

Infectious agents can cause diarrhea by a number of mechanisms. These include *adherence, mucosal invasion, enterotoxin,* and/or *cytotoxin* production. The effect of these mechanisms results in decreased absorption or increased fluid secretion. Normally most of the fluid is absorbed in the small intestine. The colon generally completes this process. In diarrhea the increased fluid in the lumen overwhelms the body's ability to reabsorb the fluid. Hence, dehydration occurs with the concomitant loss of nutrients and electrolytes.

One can infer from this that organisms affecting the small intestine may produce far more dramatic diarrhea. Some bacteria produce *enterotoxins.* The prototype of this is *Vibrio cholera. Enterotoxigenic E. coli* is another example. These organisms work by generating enterotoxins that work directly on the secretory mechanisms of the cell usually via the adenylate cyclase-cyclic adenosine monophosphate. Sodium and water absorption is blocked, producing massive amounts of diarrhea. Enterotoxins may also stimulate emesis.

Some organisms produce *cytotoxins* (i.e., *Shigella,* enterohemorrhagic *E. coli, Vibrio parahaemolyticus, C. difficile*). The cytotoxin causes mucosal cell destruction and then an inflammatory infiltrate that results in bloody diarrhea. This is accompanied by a decreased absorptive capacity.

Shigella, Campylobacter, and enteroinvasive *E. coli* cause diarrhea by *enterocyte invasion* of the large bowel and terminal ileum. They then cause cell death and inflammatory diarrhea. *Yersinia* and *Salmonella* invade cells but do not cause cell death. They are, however, able to invade the lamina propria and go in to the bloodstream, causing enteric fever as in typhoid.

Diarrheal illnesses also occur because the host's ability to ward off the infection is overwhelmed. For *E. coli* over 100,000 organisms are needed. In the case of *Entamoeba histolytica* or *Giardia* as few as 10 cysts may cause infection. Some organisms (e.g., enterotoxigenic *E. coli, V. cholera*) also produce proteins that aid in their adherence to the intestinal wall, allowing them to displace normal flora. Other factors such as antibiotics may also change intestinal flora, allowing for the overgrowth of organisms such as *C. difficile.*

As mentioned above, other host factors such as gastric pH, hypomotility, anatomic changes and medications may also play a role in pathogenesis of gastroenteritis. More is understood about the pathogenesis of diarrhea than about other symptoms. For instance, vomiting is thought to be related to serotonin-stimulating chemoreceptor trigger zones in the lower brainstem. Some organisms, such as *Staphylococcus aureus* and *Bacillus cereus*, produce neurotoxins that when ingested cause severe vomiting.

DIFFERENTIAL DIAGNOSIS

The differential diagnosis for a patient with gastroenteritis depends largely on the symptoms upon presentation. Table 67.1 presents many of the organisms and toxins that can cause infectious diarrhea. However, the symptom constellation of nausea, vomiting, diarrhea, and abdominal pain may also raise a host of other possibilities. With predominantly proximal gastrointestinal symptoms such as nausea, vomiting, and upper abdominal pain, mechanical problems such as bowel obstruction and dysmotility such as gastroparesis in patients with diabetes or scleroderma should be considered. Hepatobiliary processes such as hepatitis, cholecystitis, biliary colic, and pancreatitis also have similar symptoms. In the appropriate clinical situation, nongastrointestinal etiologies should be ruled out (e.g., cardiac ischemia, cystic fibrosis, and urinary tract infections). Surgical history is also important, because gastric bypass surgery and short bowel syndrome from multiple surgical resections can cause diarrhea. A careful dietary history may raise the possibility of too much sorbitol, lactose, or high fructose corn syrup. With predominantly lower gastrointestinal symptoms and diarrhea, inflammatory bowel disease, radiation enteritis, and ischemic colitis can present very similarly to gastroenteritis. In a patient with severe abdominal pain, surgical processes such as appendicitis and cholecystitis should be ruled out.

In women, obstetric and gynecologic processes such as pregnancy, pelvic inflammatory disease, and tubo-ovarian processes should always be included in the differential. Irritable bowel syndrome is similarly an important consideration, given its increased prevalence in women. However, irritable bowel syndrome is generally a chronic disorder and never presents with bloody diarrhea. Nocturnal symptoms are also very rare. Other malabsorptive disorders such as celiac disease, eosinophilic gastroenteritis, tropical sprue, and Whipple disease are possible but generally have a more prolonged presentation than that of a patient with acute gastroenteritis. Carcinoid and other endocrine related tumors (vasoactive intestinal peptide [VIPoma]) may also be considered but are very rare and also have a more prolonged course.

CLINICAL SYMPTOMS AND HISTORY

History taking should not only determine the onset and duration of diarrhea but also the presence of accompanying symptoms, such as nausea, vomiting, fever, abdominal pain, nature of stools, blood, or mucus. Noninfectious causes should be suspected when diarrhea is present for longer than 2 to 3 weeks. Special attention should be paid to epidemiologic factors to identify patients at risk of further complications. These factors include not only the foods that were ingested, but time of ingestion, travel history, and illness in close contacts.

Certain symptoms may suggest particular etiologies. High persistent fever may suggest enteroinvasive organisms, although fever with diarrhea is fairly common in children. Vomiting implies proximal small bowel involvement and is particularly common in patients with *B. cereus* or *S. aureus* infection where there is preformed neurotoxin. Vomiting without diarrhea should particularly raise concern of intestinal obstruction and prompt evaluation for noninfectious causes. Abdominal pain with enteroinvasive organisms of the colon generally causes tenesmus or lower abdominal pain. Pain in patients over age 50, especially out of proportion to examination, should cause one to suspect ischemia. Right lower quadrant pain may suggest *Yersinia* because it can mimic appendicitis. Jejunoileal invasions seen in small bowel diarrheas often cause periumbilical pain and cramping. Cramping may also be a sign of electrolyte imbalance.

Patients should also be questioned about the form (solid, liquid), frequency, and nature (large or small volume, odor, color, and amount) of their stools. Rice water stools are suggestive of cholera. Blood and mucus suggest enteroinvasive organisms. Large-volume stools are associated with enteric infection, whereas small-volume stools suggest colonic organisms. Floaty, bulky, white stools are associated with malabsorption and small bowel pathology.

Assessing dehydration by asking about dizziness, lightheadedness, altered mentation, and diminished urine formation is important. The presence of these symptoms suggests more advanced dehydration and electrolyte loss. This can be particularly important in the elderly. When considering extraintestinal causes, medication use should be evaluated, particularly recent antibiotics or drugs associated with diarrhea, for example, colchicine, chemotherapy, magnesium-containing antacids, and quinidine. Recent radiation treatment, surgery, food and drug allergies, other endocrine or gastrointestinal disorders, or prior episodes of diarrhea should also be assessed.

Epidemiologic considerations include not only finding out where someone has traveled but inquiring about recent camping trips, hospital stays, or visits to similar institutions. Also, inquiries should be made about ingestion of raw or spoiled foods (e.g., seafood, eggs, meats, poultry, and dairy) as well as the health of close friends and family members and recent social events where everyone ate the same food. Homosexual men or couples practicing oral–anal intercourse may be more prone to get traditional organisms such as *Shigella, Campylobacter*, and entamoeba via the fecal–oral route. Anal receptive intercourse can lead to *N. gonorrhoeae, T. pallidum, C. trachomatis* and *herpes simplex* infection, causing diarrhea or tenesmus. In the severely immunocompromised patient with HIV (CD4 counts < 200), *cytomegalovirus, M. avium intracellulare, Isopora belli*, and *microsporidia* should all be considered.

CLINICAL FINDINGS AND PHYSICAL EXAMINATION

As with evaluation of any patient, the general appearance can give rapid insight into the severity of the illness. Vital signs remain an important initial part of this assessment: The presence or absence of fevers, tachycardia, weight loss, and orthostatics are key to determination of hydration status. Next, a thorough physical examination should be performed. Signs of

TABLE 67.1. Characteristics of Acute Illness Due to Infectious and Chemical Agents

Agent	Pathophysiology	Clinical symptoms	Incubation	Risk factors	Treatment
Bacteria					
Aeromonas	Enterotoxin, ? virulence factors	Diarrhea, cramps, vomiting, blood in stool. Hemolytic uremic syndrome, septicemia in the immunocompromised		Swimming in fresh water, meats, fish, produce, eggs	Quinolone, chloramphenicol, TMP/SMX, tetracycline only in severe cases
Bacillus cereus	Enterotoxin	Vomiting	2–16 h	Reheated rice	Supportive care
Campylobacter[a]	Invasion of small and large bowel, possible enterotoxin	Abdominal pain and diarrhea	1–7 days	Undercooked meat, foreign travel	Erythromycin
Clostridium botulinum	Neurotoxin	Vomiting, diarrhea, paralysis, respiratory distress	12–36 h	Canned goods, honey in infants	Antitoxin
Clostridium difficile	Suppression of normal flora by antibiotics, leading to cytotoxin and enterotoxin production in large bowel	Fevers and bloody diarrhea	1–10 days after start of antibiotics	Most commonly clindamycin or ampicillin	Metronidazole or vancomycin, cessation of causative antibiotic
Clostridium perfringens	Enterotoxin in large intestine	Watery diarrhea	8–16 h	Reheated meat	Supportive care
Enteroinvasive *Escherichia coli*	Invasion of large bowel	Fever, abdominal pain, diarrhea	1–7 days	Cheeses	TMP/SMX
Enterotoxigenic *Escherichia coli*	Enterotoxin	Watery diarrhea	1–2 days	Travel	Oral rehydration
Enteropathogenic *Escherichia coli*	Adherence to small bowel	Vomiting, watery diarrhea, may be persistent	1–2 days	Children	Oral rehydration
Enterohemorrhagic *Escherichia coli*[a]	Verotoxin in large bowel, most common species is 0157;H7	Bloody diarrhea	1–2 days	Undercooked ground beef	Supportive care, antibiotics may predispose to hemolytic uremic syndrome
Listeria[a]	Systemic infection	Diarrhea, can cause systemic symptoms, meningitis, vertical transmission to infant can occur	Days–6 wk	Unpasteurized dairy	Ampicillin, TMP/SMX, tetracycline, chloramphenicol, erythromycin, high-dose PCN-G
***Salmonella* species**	Small and large bowel invasion	Fever and diarrhea	12–48 h	Undercooked eggs and chicken	Antibiotics may prolong carrier state and excretion of organisms
Salmonella typhi[a]	Small bowel invasion, bacteremia	Slow onset of fever and constipation, followed by high fever, mental status changes, and abdominal pain	6–48 h	Previous gallbladder disease	Ceftriaxone, ciprofloxacin; ampicillin or ciprofloxacin to eliminate carrier state, vaccines available
***Shigella* species**[a]	Large bowel invasion	Fever, abdominal pain, diarrhea	12–48 h	Low bacterial burden causes disease	TMP/SMX
Staphylococcus aureus	Enterotoxin	Vomiting	1–8 h	Food-borne	None
Vibrio cholera	Enterotoxin in small intestine	Large-volume watery diarrhea	12 h–5 days	Contaminated food and water supplies	Aggressive rehydration, tetracycline
Vibrio parahemolyticus	Enterotoxin	Diarrhea and abdominal cramping	15–24 h	Contaminated seafood, seen in Japan	Supportive care
Yersinia[a]	Small and large bowel invasion	Fever and abdominal pain	3–7 days	Contaminated food	Doxycycline
Viruses					
Norwalk virus[a]	Small bowel invasion	Vomiting and diarrhea	1–3 days	Contaminated food and water, contained populations	Supportive care
Rotavirus	Small bowel invasion	Diarrhea	1–3 days	Young children	Supportive care
Adenovirus	Small bowel invasion	Diarrhea vomiting, fever	5–7 days	Children less than age 1 yr	Supportive care
Calcivirus	Small bowel invasion	Similar to rotavirus	3 days	Children and adults	Supportive care

Parasites					
Cryptosporidia	Colonization	Diarrhea self-limited in adults children, chronic in HIV	?2–7 days	Children and adults	?Paromomycin
Entamoeba histolytica	Invasion of large intestine	Diarrhea, can be chronic and bloody	Few days to months	Food- and water-borne, travel, person-to-person	Metronidazole or quinacrine
Giardia lamblia	Colonization, rare invasion of small intestine	Diarrhea, bloating, foul-smelling stool	1–4 wk	Water-borne, person-to-person	Metronidazole
Trichinella spiralis	Encysted organism in small intestine, large bowel invasion of cyst, migrate to muscle	Diarrhea, puffy eyes, achy muscles	2–28 days	Food-borne	Thiabendazole
Seafood					
Ciguatoxin	Cholinesterase-like toxin	Vomiting, diarrhea, warmth, blurred vision, muscle pains	1–6 h	Bottom-feeding fish, e.g., red snapper, barracuda	None
Scromboid, fish poisoning	Histamine intoxication	Flushing, headache, dizziness, burning mouth, diarrhea, urticaria, respiratory symptoms	Minutes to hours	Improperly stored fish like tuna, mackerel, mahi-mahi, bonito	None (can try Benadryl)
Mushrooms					
Muscarine	Muscarinic response	Colicky belly pain, nausea, vomiting, diarrhea, hypotension, miosis	Minutes to few hours	*Amanita muscaria*	Atropine SC or IV
Phalloidine (other toxins)	Diverse cytotoxins	Three stages Stage 1—nausea, abdominal pain, bloody diarrhea, weakness Stage 2—improvement (day 2–3) Stage 3—hepatic failure, delirium, death	6–15 h	*Amanita phalloides* and other *Amanita* species	None
Other heavy metals (antimony, copper, zinc, tin, iron, cadmium)	Upper gastrointestinal irritation	Metallic taste to food, nausea, vomiting or diarrhea	5 min to 8 h	Containers made of alloy that contains the heavy metal	None

[a]Indicates infection with special considerations during pregnancy.
PCN-G, penicillin-G; TMP/SMX, trimethoprim-sulfamethoxazole.

volume depletion such as dry mucous membranes or poor skin turgor may be present. In children one should look for depressed fontanelles, dry diapers, sunken eyes, and decreased tears. In patients with chronic diarrhea, signs of neural dysfunction or muscle wasting may be present. Abdominal examination should be performed with the objective of ruling out an acute abdomen. The examiner should be attuned to listening to bowel sounds and to ruling out masses, signs of perforation, or organomegaly. Children with appendicitis may present with diarrhea. Rectal examination should be done to rule out blood or mucus in the stool, tenesmus, fistulae, or fissures. Tenesmus can be associated with pelvic abscesses or irritable bowel disease and enteroinvasive infectious colitis. Fistulae and fissures may be associated with Crohn disease.

LABORATORY AND IMAGING STUDIES

Laboratory evaluation needs to be based on clinical condition. History, physical, and patient-specific risk factors should govern further diagnostic workup. Mild self-limited cases may require no diagnostic workup and only supportive care. Patients with severe dehydration, fever, and blood in the stool may warrant more thorough evaluation. Specific populations such as the elderly, immunocompromised, and pregnant women need to be evaluated more thoroughly because of their increased morbidity and mortality.

For those patients for whom further workup is deemed necessary, complete blood count and electrolytes should be performed to assess degree of dehydration. Examination of the stool for blood by Hemoccult and fecal leukocytes by Wright stain can be indicative of an invasive diarrhea. Fecal leukocytes are present in 80% to 90% of patients with *Shigella* or *Salmonella*. They are seen less reliably in *Campylobacter* or *Yersinia*. They can be seen in inflammatory bowel disease. Fecal leukocytes are absent with viruses, *Giardia*, enterotoxigenic *E. coli*, and toxigenic diarrheas. Stool culture (routine culture usually includes *Salmonella, Shigella, Campylobacter, Yersinia,* and *Aeromonas*) should be done if a bacterial source is suspected, particularly if there is bloody diarrhea or if the patient is a food handler or is immunocompromised. Patients who reside in a nursing home, who were recently hospitalized, or who have been on recent antibiotics should have stool sent for *C. difficile* toxin. One might consider sending stool for *E. coli* 0157:H7 in patients with bloody diarrhea or with recent ingestion of undercooked meat. The test and culture for *Vibrio* species must be specifically requested, because they are not part of a routine panel. In HIV-infected individuals or patients with a recent travel history, ova and parasites should also be included in the workup.

Food-borne viral gastroenteritis is not usually diagnosed, because no simple assay is available for detection of viruses. Electron microscopy is an expensive and insensitive technique. Polymerase chain reaction is sensitive and specific in its ability to test stool samples for viral genomic material. Both tools are prohibitively expensive; they are used in laboratories and public health departments and are not routinely available to clinicians. Enzyme-linked immunosorbent assays have not been reliable in routine clinical settings.

Luminal evaluation via flexible sigmoidoscopy or colonoscopy is generally not necessary in patients with gastroenteritis. However, in patients with *C. difficile* colitis, flexible sigmoidoscopy can quickly demonstrate pseudomembranes pathognomonic of the disease. Endoscopy can also aid in the differentiation between infectious and ischemic colitis; the latter will generally demonstrate discrete areas of involvement with sparing of segments in between. Additional situations in which colonoscopy is helpful are in acquired immunodeficiency syndrome patients where biopsies of the right colon can help to demonstrate cytomegalovirus. Also, if inflammatory bowel disease is a consideration, colonoscopy with intubation of the terminal ileum can frequently contribute useful information and look for generalized inflammation and classic mucosal changes for inflammatory bowel disease. Imaging studies of the colon are not believed to be helpful in the acute situation, unless there are signs of perforation or bowel obstruction or toxic megacolon.

TREATMENT

Most cases of gastroenteritis are self-limited. Treatment in the primary care setting is primarily symptomatic and should encompass two objectives. First, volume status should be optimized. Second, symptoms should be treated. Treatment of more severe infectious gastroenteritis involves not only rehydration and dietary changes but also use of antimotility agents and antibiotic therapy in selected situations. The noninvasive organisms, which tend to cause a large-volume diarrhea, lead to dehydration as the reabsorptive capacity of the large intestine is overcome by the fluid loss. The primary method of treatment is oral rehydration.

Oral rehydration is superior to intravenous replacement because this method incurs far fewer complications and can be used in the outpatient setting. Glucose-containing solutions are best because they take advantage of the coupling of glucose with sodium and water absorption in the enterocytes. Rehydration solutions should approximate plasma electrolyte concentrations as closely as possible. Food-based rehydration solutions, containing various cereals and grains, may also help to decrease the amount of diarrheal stools. Dietary changes that are recommended in cases of acute infectious gastroenteritis include avoidance of foods that may increase stool output. The most likely offenders include fatty, spicy, and high-fiber foods. Dairy products, alcohol, and caffeinated beverages may stimulate secretory mechanisms and increase stool output. The patient should be encouraged to consume juices, noncarbonated drinks, and soft foods. The BRATT (bananas, rice, apple juice, tea, and toast) diet has often been advocated as a home remedy for diet because these foods replete fluid losses and may be somewhat constipating.

Antimotility agents are believed to be effective in the treatment of noninvasive diarrhea but are not recommended in invasive disease or dysentery because of concern over prolonging or exacerbating the illness, as well as causing toxic megacolon. These medications have several effects, including decreasing fluid losses, decreasing small intestinal motor activity, and slowing transit time. Antimotility agents include opiates, loperamide, diphenoxylate, and bismuth subsalicylate. Opiates are believed to both decrease fluid output and increase mucosal fluid reabsorption. Loperamide has been found to bring about significant symptomatic improvement without the side effects of opiates. It works by decreasing intestinal motility and intestinal fluid secretion. It may also increase fluid and electrolyte absorption. Diphenoxylate may also be useful in reducing gut hyperperistalsis. Bismuth subsalicylate improves diarrhea for two reasons: the salicylate moiety has antisecretory effects and the bismuth moiety has antibacterial and antiinflammatory effects. Finally, this medication may reduce enterotoxin activity.

Antibiotics may be indicated in suspected invasive or parasitic diarrheal disease, especially with febrile dysentery. Other indications for antimicrobial therapy may include *C. difficile*, traveler's diarrhea, and particularly severe cases of salmonellosis. In cases of noninvasive watery diarrhea, antibiotic therapy is generally not warranted because these cases tend to be self-limited and show no symptomatic benefit from antibiotics.

CONSIDERATIONS IN PREGNANCY

The literature suggests that pregnant women are at risk for significant morbidity from gastroenteritis. Some studies have shown that gastrointestinal disease during pregnancy may be a risk factor for low-birth-weight infants. In one cohort study performed in Sweden, younger women were found to have an increased risk of gastroenteritis during pregnancy compared with older women. The presence of other children in the same household seemed to correlate with an increased incidence of gastroenteritis. In the same study, pregnant women working at day care centers with increased exposure to many children had increased susceptibility to infection. Despite this, only having three or more episodes of gastroenteritis during pregnancy seemed to correlate with an increased risk of preterm birth. This study did not demonstrate that gastroenteritis resulted in low-birth-weight infants. However, the study did not isolate the women with more severe diarrhea requiring hospitalization to see if their infants had lower birth weights. A prospective study, as they suggest, may be helpful in answering this question.

In terms of treatment of pregnant women, oral rehydration is usually the only treatment needed for the management of infectious diarrhea if it is self-limited. More persistent and severe cases may warrant intravenous fluids, antimotility agents, and antibiotic therapy. The bacterial, viral, and protozoal organisms that cause infectious diarrhea are not known to be teratogenic. Unfortunately, the toxicities of many antimicrobial agents to the mother, fetus, and newborn limit the number of options available in treating the pregnant patient.

Special clinical and treatment considerations for various infections in pregnancy are as follows:

1. *Shigella*—Bacteremia and toxemia are rare. In severe cases, ampicillin may be used because it is the only recommended antibiotic not associated with damage to the fetus or breast-feeding neonate. However, there is a high degree of ampicillin resistance. Resistant cases may require quinolone antibiotics, which can be teratogenic.
2. *Salmonellosis*—Antibiotics may also be indicated in the pregnant patient with positive blood cultures, fever, or a septic appearance. If antibiotics are to be considered, ampicillin or ceftriaxone are the drugs of choice. When given just before delivery, sulfa drugs, including trimethoprim/sulfamethoxazole, can lead to jaundice in the fetus and the breast-fed newborn. Quinolones should also be avoided because of teratogenic effects. *Salmonella typhi* poses some risk of maternal–fetal transmission despite antibiotic therapy.
3. *Campylobacter*—Mild campylobacteriosis does not appear to benefit from antibiotics. Erythromycin has been effective in culture-proven cases when used within the first 3 days of the clinical presentation. Pregnant women with IgA deficiency are at an increased risk of spontaneous abortion with this infection. Treatment of the pregnant patient with erythromycin (other than erythromycin estolate) and clindamycin may be provided in serious cases.
4. *Yersinia enterocolitica*—Antibiotics have not been shown to decrease the duration of the gastrointestinal symptoms but may be indicated in particularly severe infections. In these cases, the drug of choice is a third-generation parenteral cephalosporin, combined with an antipseudomonal aminoglycoside.
5. Enteroinvasive *E. coli* and enterohemorrhagic *E. coli* represent two pathogenic forms of *E. coli* that cause bloody diarrhea. Enteroinvasive *E. coli* is relatively rare and difficult to isolate in the United States. Enterohemorrhagic *E. coli* has typically been seen with food-borne outbreaks. This organism causes dysenteric stools with crampy abdominal pain but no fever. Patients with this infection may present less commonly with hemolytic uremic syndrome or thrombotic thrombocytopenic purpura. There is no clear evidence showing antibiotic therapy to be of benefit with these infections.
6. *Norwalk virus*—The infection typically lasts 1 week, although intestinal epithelial changes have been found to last for 8 weeks. Antibodies are produced after infection with this virus and appear to be transferred across the placenta. Newborns appear to be protected by passively acquired maternal antibodies for 3 months after birth.
7. *Listeria* is a rare cause of food poisoning syndromes and is notable for an extended incubation period of up to 6 weeks. This organism has a high rate of mortality compared with the more common pathogens. It tends to cause a more systemic syndrome with bacteremia, fever, and myalgias and has an increased incidence in pregnant or immunosuppressed patients. Findings of neurologic dysfunction on examination should be investigated for possible neurotoxin poisoning. The differential diagnosis includes seafood toxins, parasite toxins, *Clostridium botulinum* toxin, mushrooms, pesticides, and reactions to monosodium glutamate.

Besides primary prevention of infections by regulations governing sewage treatment, water purification, and food processing, emphasis must be given to secondary prevention. The inadequacy of primary prevention is seen in the fact that 50% of poultry sold in supermarkets is contaminated with *Salmonella* and/or *Helicobacter*. The following rules for food preparation and consumption are suggested to assist the primary practitioner to help patients prevent infection:

1. Perishable foods should be refrigerated as soon as possible after purchasing (within 1 hour) and not kept for long periods of time, even when refrigerated.
2. Avoid using raw foods in dishes that require no further cooking. Pregnant women should be instructed never to eat raw seafood or meats.
3. Thoroughly cleanse hands and all surfaces while preparing perishable foods. Use gloves or band-aids to handle food if there are open cuts.
4. Do not prepare perishable foods more than a day in advance and do not allow these foods to stand for several hours while warm.
5. Make sure all foods are cooked at high enough temperatures and for long enough periods of time when cooking and reheating. For meats, internal temperatures should be higher than 165°F and boiled foods should be boiled at least 15 minutes. Many reference cookbooks contain instructions for heating and cleaning foods. Keep hot foods hot (>140°F) and cold foods cold (<45°F).
6. Check to be sure that all serving dishes and cookware are safe for cooking and do not contain heavy metals.
7. Obtain foods from approved sources like Grade A pasteurized milk and USDA inspected meat and poultry.

It is the physician's responsibility to report suspected cases of contamination outside the home to the local health department. More care and instruction of patients in these vital areas will help to cut down on this worldwide and pervasive problem.

BIBLIOGRAPHY

Avery ME, Snyder JD. Oral therapy for acute diarrhea: the underused simple solution. *N Engl J Med* 1990;323:891–894.
Bennett WG. Acute gastroenteritis and associated conditions. In: Barker LR, ed. *Principles of ambulatory medicine,* 5th ed. Philadelphia: Lippincott Williams & Wilkins, 1999:307–318.
Bresee JS, Widdowson MA, Monroe SS, et al. Foodborne viral gastroenteritis: challenges and opportunities. *CID* 2002;35:748–753.
Centers for Disease Control and Prevention. 1999 Foodnet Annual Report. www.cdc.gov/foodnet/annual/1999.
Dalton CB, Austin CC, Sobel J, et al. An outbreak of gastroenteritis and fever due to *Listeria monocytogenes* in milk. *N Engl J Med* 1997;336:100–106.
Gerba CP, Rose JB, Haas CN. Sensitive populations: who is at greatest risk? *Int J Food Microbiol* 1996;30:113–123.
Goldsweig CD, Pacheco PA. Infectious colitis excluding *E. coli* 0157:H7 and *C. difficile. Gastroenterol Clin* 2001;30:709–733.
Herwaldt BL, Ackers M-L, et al. An outbreak of cyclosporiasis associated with imported raspberries. *N Engl J Med* 1997;336:1548–1556.
Kahn S, Orenstein SR. Eosinophilic gastroenteritis: epidemiology, diagnosis and management. *Paediatr Drugs* 2002;4:564–570.
Koopmans M, von Bonsdorff C-H, Vinje J, et al. Foodborne viruses. *FEMS Microbiol Rev* 2002;26:187–205.
Ludvigsson JF. Effect of gastroenteritis during pregnancy on neonatal outcome. *Eur J Clin Microbiol Infect Dis* 2001;20:843–849.
Mead PS, Slutsker L, Dietz V, et al. Food-related illness and death in the United States. *Emerg Infect Dis* 1999;5:607–625.
Peterson CA, Calderon RL. Trends in enteric disease as a cause of death in the United States, 1989–96. *Am J Epidemiol* 2003;157:58–65.

CHAPTER 68
Inflammatory Bowel Disease

William T. Chen and Samir A. Shah

Inflammatory bowel disease (IBD) includes two distinct disease entities: ulcerative colitis (UC) and Crohn disease (CD) (Table 68.1). Both are characterized by chronic intestinal inflammation with periodic exacerbations and a variety of local and systemic complications. These two idiopathic diseases affect approximately 1 million Americans and account for 700,000 physician visits per year and 100,000 hospitalizations per year. Despite limitations of our knowledge on the pathogenesis of IBD, a variety of therapeutic options is available for treatment. CD and UC pose specific problems for women in their reproductive years. In this chapter, we review the current knowledge about IBD with an emphasis on issues pertaining to women's health.

EPIDEMIOLOGY AND ETIOLOGY

Worldwide figures regarding the age distribution of UC and CD point to a peak incidence between the ages of 15 and 30 years, coinciding with the primary reproductive years of a woman. A second, but smaller peak, occurs between the ages of 60 and 80 years.

Epidemiologic data from North America and Europe reveal an essentially 1:1 female-to-male incidence ratio for UC across all age groups. Within the same population, the female-to-male incidence ratio for CD is tilted toward a greater female preponderance, ranging from 1:1 to 1.2:1.

The highest incidence of IBD has been reported in developed areas, including North America and northern Europe. Within these areas, there is an increased incidence in urban settings compared with rural areas. Increased incidence rates also have been noted in higher socioeconomic groups compared with lower socioeconomic groups. Although IBD can affect persons of any ethnic background, a higher frequency of IBD is seen in people of middle European Jewish ancestry.

There is a clear familial pattern of IBD. Studies have shown that the risk of IBD in first-degree relatives of an individual with IBD is 4 to 20 times greater than that the general population; the absolute risk of IBD among first-degree relatives has been estimated at 5% to 8%. If both parents have IBD, the risk of their child developing IBD is over 30%. Data collected on the concordance rates among monozygotic twins (44%–50% CD, 6%–14% UC) compared with dizygotic twins (7% CD, 3% UC) suggest a stronger genetic influence in the development of CD compared with UC.

The search for susceptibility genes had identified an area of linkage among familial clusters of CD (but not UC) on chromosome 16. A major advance in 2001 was the identification of the first gene linked to CD, initially called *NOD2* (nucleotide-binding oligomerization domain) located within the previously mapped IBD1 locus on chromosome 16. *NOD2* has been renamed *CARD15* (caspase-recruitment domain) and codes for a 1,040-amino acid protein expressed in monocytes and macrophages. It is involved in apoptotic signaling through activation of the neurofactor κB (NF-κB). This protein may serve to regulate NF-κB through the interaction with bacterial lipopolysaccharide and may be involved in macrophage apoptosis. Homozygotes for a variant of *CARD15* have a 20- to 40-fold increased risk for developing ileal CD compared with the general population. However, the penetrance of the homozygote and heterozygote carrier developing CD is only 1.7% and 0.003%, respectively. Identification of the *CARD15* gene is an important first step in the long journey to understanding IBD.

Environmental factors also play a role in the development of IBD. Smoking has a protective effect on the development of UC but is a risk factor for the development of CD. Another interesting observation is that appendectomy appears to have a protective effect on the development of UC. Nonsteroidal antiinflammatory drugs and acute infection have been reported to trigger IBD.

Murine models of IBD have added considerably to our understanding of the mucosal immune system and human IBD. In most murine models of colitis, the presence of the normal intestinal bacterial flora is required for disease development. Hence, the current pathogenesis of IBD is thought to be multifactorial, with a genetic predisposition, antigenic stimulation (perhaps by normal intestinal bacteria), leading to a dysregulated mucosal immune response and chronic intestinal inflammation.

CLINICAL PRESENTATION, DIFFERENTIAL DIAGNOSIS, AND EVALUATION

Ulcerative Colitis

UC affects the superficial (mucosal) layer of the rectum and colon and is characterized by continuous areas of inflammation starting at the rectum without intervening normal areas and a sharp transition to normal mucosa. Biopsies typically show a diffuse mucosal inflammatory infiltrate with crypt abscess and crypt branching (not seen in acute self-limited colitis or ischemic colitis) and decreased numbers of mucosal glands. When the rectum alone is involved, the term ulcerative proctitis is used; when the inflammation extends to the sigmoid/descending colon, the terms left-sided UC, distal colitis, or proctosigmoiditis are used; and when the inflammation

TABLE 68.1. Comparison of Crohn Disease and Ulcerative Colitis

	Crohn disease	Ulcerative colitis
Epidemiology		
Incidence	2–8/100,000	3–15/100,000
Prevalence	20–40/100,000	80–120/100,000
Female:male ratio	1:1 to 1.2:1	1:1
First peak incidence (age)	15–30	15–30
Second peak incidence	60–80	60–80
Higher in urban areas	Yes	No
Higher in higher socioeconomic levels	Yes	Possibly
Smoking	Increases risk	Decreases risk
Appendectomy	May increase risk	Decreases risk
Anatomic distribution		
Esophagus/stomach	Rare	0
Small bowel	30%–40%	0
Small and large bowel	40%–55%	0
Large bowel	15%–25%	100%
Rectum/rectosigmoid		40%–50%
Left colon (up to the splenic flexure)		30%
Entire colon (beyond the splenic flexure)		20%
Pathology		
Skip lesions	Yes	No
Cobblestoning	Yes	Rare
Discrete ulcerations	Yes	Yes
Pseudopolyps	Yes	Yes
Degree of involvement	Transmural	Mucosal
Cryptitis/crypt abscess	Yes	Yes
Noncaseating granulomas	Yes	No
Clinical presentation	Abdominal pain/cramping Rectal bleeding (uncommon) Diarrhea, nausea, vomiting Weight loss, anorexia, fevers Growth retardation in children	Rectal bleeding (>90%) Cramping Diarrhea, tenesmus Anorexia, fevers
Complications:	perianal disease/fistulae/abscesses Toxic megacolon Perforation not rare Obstruction Stricture Colon cancer Osteoporosis Bleeding Gallstones Kidney stones	 Toxic megacolon Perforation rare Obstruction rare Stricture rare Colon cancer Osteoporosis Bleeding
Extraintestinal manifestations	Perianal/perineal disease Arthritis Oral aphthous ulcers Erythema nodosum Pyoderma gangrenosum Ocular (uveitis, iritis, episcleritis) Primary sclerosing cholangitis (PSC)	 Arthritis Oral aphthous ulcers Pyoderma gangrenosum Erythema nodosum Ocular PSC

extends beyond the splenic flexure, the term pancolitis or extensive colitis is used. Rectal bleeding, diarrhea, tenesmus, weight loss, and abdominal cramping are the symptoms usually reported; weight loss and fever are less commonly reported and usually indicate more severe disease. Both the physical examination and laboratory findings are nonspecific, can be normal, and vary with the extent and severity of disease. Examination findings can include blood on rectal examination, abdominal tenderness, fever, pallor, tachycardia, postural hypotension, and signs of weight loss. Laboratory findings can include anemia, iron deficiency, elevated white blood cell count with a left shift, and elevated sedimentation rate/C-reactive protein. The extent of disease is important in selecting therapy and in determining long-term cancer risk. The diagnosis of UC requires integration of the clinical history, physical examination, laboratory parameters, and direct examination of the colonic mucosa by sigmoidoscopy or colonoscopy with biopsies for histology. Infectious colitis can present with bloody diarrhea, and therefore examination of the stool for *Shigella, Salmonella, Campylobacter, Aeromonas, Escherichia coli* 0157:H7, *Clostridia difficile* toxin, and *Entamoeba histolytica* to exclude infection is important. In older patients, smokers, and patients on oral contraceptive pills, ischemic bowel is critical to exclude and is easily done based on histology. Irritable bowel syndrome and microscopic colitis should also be considered in the differential diagnosis; however, these two disorders are not typically associated with rectal bleeding.

Crohn Disease

In contrast to UC, CD can affect any part of the gastrointestinal tract and is characterized by transmural inflammation and granuloma formation (but seen in <30% of biopsies with CD) with areas of intervening normal mucosa (hence the term "skip lesions"). This transmural inflammation can lead to fibrosis, obstruction, microperforation, fistulae, and abscess. A third of CD patients will have perianal disease, including perianal fistula. Approximately 80% of individuals with CD have small bowel involvement (usually the distal ileum). About 50% will have both ileal and colonic involvement (ileocolitis), 30% will have ileal involvement alone (ileitis), and only 20% will have disease limited to the colon (Crohn colitis). In addition, aphthous ulcers in the mouth and perianal fissures and/or fistulae are seen. Symptoms include crampy abdominal pain, diarrhea, fever, and weight loss. CD involving the distal colon can present similarly to UC. Staging the extent and location of the disease allows for selecting the optimal therapy and risk stratification for complications. The diagnosis of CD requires integration of history, examination, laboratory data, endoscopy, and histology but also uses radiologic examination, particularly small bowel follow-through or enteroclysis, computed tomography, and, recently, capsule endoscopy for small bowel disease. Barium enema is rarely used except when colonoscopy is not possible or when searching for colonic fistulae or strictures. Differential diagnosis include infection, malignancy (especially lymphoma), irritable bowel syndrome, collagen vascular diseases, microscopic colitis, and ischemic bowel disease.

Distinguishing UC from CD is usually straightforward (Table 68.1). However, in approximately 5% of patients, it is difficult to distinguish UC from CD; in these cases, the term indeterminate colitis is used. Although standard medical therapy may overlap for CD and UC, the surgical treatment options are distinct. Two laboratory tests may help distinguish UC from CD: perinuclear-staining antineutrophil cytoplasmic antibody is associated with UC, whereas anti-*Saccharomyces cerevisiae* antibody is associated with CD. Unfortunately, neither of these tests has adequate specificity nor sensitivity to definitively establish or exclude UC or CD.

Extraintestinal Manifestations

Both UC and CD have extraintestinal manifestations (Table 68.1). Among these manifestations are skin lesions (such as pyoderma gangrenosum and erythema nodosum), arthropathies (peripheral arthritis, ankylosing spondylitis, sacroiliitis), ocular involvement (episcleritis, scleritis, uveitis), and primary sclerosing cholangitis. The presence of these manifestations in the setting of nonspecific abdominal complaints may help guide the physician toward the diagnosis of IBD and distinguishing CD from UC. Primary sclerosing cholangitis and pyoderma gangrenosum are more commonly seen with UC, whereas erythema nodosum is more common with CD. Arthritis is the most common extraintestinal manifestation reported. Some of the extraintestinal manifestations are associated with active intestinal disease (i.e., peripheral arthritis, episcleritis, erythema nodosum), whereas others are independent of intestinal disease (ankylosing spondylitis, sacroiliitis, pyoderma gangrenosum, primary sclerosing cholangitis, and uveitis). Uveitis, ankylosing spondylitis, and sacroiliitis are associated with HLA-B27.

Advances in the understanding of the immune system have led to the concept of immune-mediated inflammatory disorders. This concept helps link the extraintestinal manifestations of IBD to the intestinal disease and supports the notion that IBD is a systemic disorder that affects primarily the intestines. Other immune-mediated inflammatory disorders include rheumatoid arthritis, multiple sclerosis, psoriasis, systemic lupus erythematosus, and type I diabetes mellitus. Hence, newer immune-based therapies may overlap in these immune-mediated inflammatory disorders; for example infliximab, a therapy directed against the cytokine tumor necrosis factor-α (TNF-α) is U.S. Food and Drug Administration (FDA) approved for CD and rheumatoid arthritis and is currently in clinical trials for psoriasis and UC.

TREATMENT

The goals of therapy for both UC and CD are to induce remission, maintain remission, and prevent complications, thereby improving quality of life. To achieve these goals, one must be familiar with the efficacy and safety profile of available treatments and be aware of convenience and cost of therapy to the patient. Engaging the patient in a collaborative model for a treatment plan and education with resources such as those available from the Crohn's and Colitis Foundation of America (www.ccfa.org) is vital.

Sulfasalazine and 5-Aminosalicylate

Sulfasalazine (Azulfidine) is a prodrug composed of sulfapyridine linked to 5-aminosalicylate (5-ASA) by an azo bond developed in the late 1930s for the treatment of rheumatoid arthritis; however, it was found to be effective for colonic IBD in doses ranging from 2 to 6 g/d. The 5-ASA moiety is the efficacious portion of sulfasalazine in treating UC and CD involving the colon. Sulfasalazine is minimally absorbed and travels unchanged to the proximal colon where luminal bacteria cleave the azo bond and release the 5-ASA from the sulfapyridine. Sulfapyridine is absorbed, metabolized by the liver, and subsequently excreted into the urine. The 5-ASA remains in the lumen of the colon until it is excreted in the stool. If 5-ASA is given orally, it is absorbed in the proximal small bowel and never reaches the distal intestine. This knowledge about the pharmacology of sulfasalazine has led to the development of new formulations of 5-ASA that target delivery to the affected areas of intestine.

The use of sulfasalazine, however, has been limited by a high rate of adverse side effects. These include headache, nausea, dyspepsia, anorexia, fever, rash, arthralgias, hemolysis, neutropenia, exacerbation of colitis, male infertility, and hypersensitivity reactions involving the lungs, liver, nerves, or pancreas. Most of the intolerance associated with sulfasalazine is attributed to high sulfapyridine serum levels (in a dose-dependent manner and therefore most patients will not tolerate more than 4g/d) and to allergic reactions to the sulfa moiety similar to that described with other sulfonamides. In addition, sulfasalazine interferes with folate absorption and therefore must be prescribed with folate supplementation.

TOPICAL 5-AMINOSALICYLATE

Researchers have demonstrated that 5-ASA is the active moiety in sulfasalazine by comparing the efficacy of 5-ASA enemas with sulfapyridine and sulfasalazine enemas in patients with

UC. The 5-ASA and sulfasalazine enemas had a 75% response rate by clinical and endoscopic criteria compared with 35% in the sulfapyridine group. Subsequent studies have demonstrated 5-ASA enemas in doses between 1 and 4 g/d to be effective in achieving clinical remission or improvement in 90% of patients with mild to moderate left-sided colitis. In addition, 5-ASA enemas (Rowasa) are effective in preventing relapse if used on a regular basis. For patients with ulcerative proctitis (inflammation up to 20 cm from the anus), 5-ASA suppositories (Canasa) are well tolerated and effective for induction of remission and maintenance of remission.

ORAL 5-AMINOSALICYLATE

Topical formulations of 5-ASA are useful in distal colitis but ineffective for ileal disease and inadequate alone to treat extensive colonic disease. The new oral 5-ASA agents use three different strategies to deliver 5-ASA to the distal small intestine and colon. The first coats 5-ASA with an acrylic resin that dissolves at pH greater than 6 (Asacol, Rowasa, Claversal, Salofalk). Of these, only Asacol is available in the United States and is used in 2.4- to 4.8-g/d doses. The second encapsulates the 5-ASA in ethylcellulose microspheres that gradually dissolve in the small and large intestine (Pentasa 3–4 g/d). The third links 5-ASA to another molecule via an azo bond, to another 5-ASA (Dipentum 1–3 g/d), or to 4-aminobenzoyl-β-alanine, an inert unabsorbed molecule (Colazal 6.75 g/d). The oral forms of delayed release 5-ASA and topical 5-ASA formulations are known generically as mesalamine (mesalazine in Europe). Olsalazine (Dipentum) is associated with diarrhea and therefore used less frequently than the other 5-ASA agents.

All three forms of oral 5-ASA have been shown to be efficacious in a dose-dependent manner in treating mild to moderately active UC and in maintaining remission. Combination therapy involving oral and rectal mesalamine formulations has been shown to produce earlier and more complete relief from rectal bleeding than either monotherapy in patients with left-sided UC. Furthermore, combination therapy is superior to oral mesalamine in preventing relapse in UC. Mesalamine has been shown to be of some benefit in individuals with mild to moderate active luminal CD and marginally effective in maintaining remission in patients with CD.

Most patients intolerant or allergic to sulfasalazine are able to tolerate mesalamine. Mesalamine does not have dose-dependent side effects. However, between 10% and 20% of these patients will experience reactions to mesalamine similar to those seen on sulfasalazine. In addition, patients allergic to aspirin should avoid the 5-ASA agents. Side effects reported with 5-ASA include rash, fever, diarrhea, exacerbation of colitis, pancreatitis, myocarditis, and nephritis.

How 5-ASA works in IBD remains unknown, although several mechanisms have been postulated. These include blocking the lipoxygenase pathway, acting as a free radical scavenger, inhibiting TNF-α, and suppressing the activation of NF-κB.

Corticosteroids

Corticosteroids are potent inhibitors of the inflammatory response via multiple nonspecific mechanisms, including inhibition of arachidonic acid release from cell membranes, cytokine release by immune cells, chemotaxis, and phagocytosis. Corticosteroids inhibit interleukin-2 transcription and messenger RNA production by preventing association of the AP-1 transcription factor with its corresponding binding site on a lymphocyte's interleukin-2 promoter. Glucocorticoids also recently have been shown to stimulate the production of the regulatory protein IκBα that binds to NF-κB, trapping it in the cytosol. NF-κB can activate many immunoregulatory genes in response to proinflammatory stimuli by translocating into the nucleus and acting as a transcription factor for these cytokine genes. Thus, inhibition of NF-κB activity by steroids may account for their multiple antiinflammatory effects.

TOPICAL STEROIDS

Topical hydrocortisone (Cortenema, Cortifoam), like topical 5-ASA, has been successfully used in treating active distal colitis. Appreciable systemic absorption has been demonstrated with topical hydrocortisone, leading to concern about chronic use. Therefore, topical steroids should not be used long term.

ORAL/PARENTERAL STEROIDS

For moderate to severe UC and CD unresponsive to 5-ASA drugs, systemic corticosteroids are the mainstay of therapy. Prednisone, prednisolone, or methylprednisolone are among the options available. For patients with severe disease, intravenous steroids are favored because oral absorption may be impaired. Hydrocortisone, prednisolone, and methylprednisolone have all been demonstrated to be effective. Methylprednisolone (48 mg/d) and prednisolone (60 mg/d) are equivalent to 300 mg of hydrocortisone; they can be given either as a continuous intravenous drip or in divided pulse doses. Higher doses have not been shown to be of benefit. Although effective in treating acute flares of both CD and UC, *corticosteroids are not effective in maintaining remission*. Furthermore, systemic side effects encountered with long-term steroid use have limited their use. Thus, once patients are recovering from a flare, intravenous steroids should be changed to an oral form (usually prednisone 40–60 mg/d) and slowly tapered while an alternate agent is used to maintain remission. If steroids are required to induce remission in CD, mesalamine is inadequate to maintain remission and therefore immunomodulators (see below) must be considered. The use of steroids should also prompt the clinician to consider osteopenia/osteoporosis (see below).

Budesonide (Entocort EC; 9 mg/d) is an enteric-coated steroid with a high first-pass metabolism in the liver. Studies suggest that it is as effective as traditional oral steroids but with fewer systemic side effects. As with other steroids, it has no role in maintenance therapy. Its long-term effects on bone metabolism and osteoporosis have not yet been adequately evaluated. The FDA approved budesonide in October 2001 for mild to moderate CD involving the ileum and/or right colon.

Immunomodulators

6-MERCAPTOPURINE AND AZATHIOPRINE

For patients with active IBD refractory to conventional treatment with sulfasalazine, corticosteroids, 5-ASA agents, and antibiotics, treatment with immunomodulators should be considered. Azathioprine (AZA) and 6-mercaptopurine (6-MP) are purine derivatives that are incorporated into DNA and inhibit DNA synthesis. AZA (Imuran) is metabolized in vivo to 6-MP (Purinethol), and its biologic effects are identical to those of 6-MP. Thus, both the mechanisms of action and the toxicities of these drugs are identical. Both drugs are used to prevent organ transplant rejection and to treat IBD and autoimmune hepatitis. AZA for IBD is used in doses of 2 to 2.5 mg/kg/d, whereas 6-MP is used in doses of 1 to 1.5 mg/kg/d.

6-MP is metabolized by three competing enzyme systems: Xanthine oxidase and thiopurine methyltransferase render inactive metabolites, whereas hypoxanthine-guanine phosphoribosyl-transferase produces ribonucleotides, including 6-thioguanine, that are incorporated into the DNA of rapidly dividing cells, causing cell death. Their exact mechanism of action is unknown but is thought to involve inhibiting T-helper lymphocyte activity. Metabolites of AZA/6-MP can now be measured (6-thioguanine, 6-methylmercaptopurine), making optimal dosing of these agents possible. Retrospective studies suggest that therapeutic 6-thioguanine levels are associated with response/remission, whereas high 6-methylmercaptopurine levels are associated with hepatotoxicity.

In 1980, a landmark study by Present and colleagues established the efficacy of 6-MP with a 70% response rate in individuals with steroid refractory CD. The mean treatment time required to achieve a response was 3.1 months. In addition to decreasing disease activity, 6-MP was found to have multiple beneficial effects in IBD, including steroid sparing, healing and closure of fistulae, and maintenance of remission in both CD and UC. Trials of AZA/6-MP in children and adolescents with IBD reported response rates similar to those seen in adults. Several studies have demonstrated the efficacy of 6-MP in chronic active UC.

An important side effect of AZA/6-MP is bone marrow depression in a dose-dependent fashion. Therefore, peripheral blood counts should always be monitored during therapy. A retrospective review of 396 patients treated with 6-MP found pancreatitis in 3.3%, fever and/or rash in 2%, bone marrow suppression in 2%, and drug-induced hepatitis in 0.3%. All reported toxicities were reversible with drug discontinuation. Additional side effects reported include nausea and drug-induced diarrhea. Theoretical concern for the increased risk of lymphoma while on immunomodulators was addressed in a recent retrospective study of 454 individuals with IBD: No increased risk was attributed to immunomodulator therapy. The cumulative experience of 60% to 80% efficacy and relative safety with AZA/6-MP makes these agents first-line therapies for refractory chronic active UC and CD in addition to steroid-dependent IBD and CD complicated by fistula(e).

METHOTREXATE

Methotrexate is an inhibitor of dihydrofolate reductase and has antiinflammatory and immunosuppressive effects. Side effects encountered with methotrexate treatment (given intramuscularly/subcutaneously at 15–25 mg weekly doses) in CD patients have included pneumonitis and abnormal liver transaminases. Methotrexate is reserved as a second-line immunomodulator for patients with CD who have failed treatment with AZA/6-MP. Methotrexate is used in refractory CD to induce remission, in CD patients dependent on steroids for steroid sparring, and for maintenance of remission in CD. Methotrexate is contraindicated in pregnancy.

CYCLOSPORINE

Cyclosporine A (CSA) is widely used as an immunosuppressant in organ transplantation for its selective effect on T-lymphocyte mediated immune responses. The CSA molecule enters the cytosol of T cells and binds to the cytosolic protein cyclophilin A. The CSA–cyclophilin complex in turn binds to calcineurin, inhibiting its phosphatase activity. Intravenous cyclosporine (4 mg/kg/d continuous infusion) led to dramatic improvement in 9 of 11 patients with severe steroid-refractory UC compared with no response in 9 patients treated with placebo. Avoidance of colectomy by using CSA in steroid refractory UC is clinically beneficial at least in the short term. However, the relapse rate is greater than 50% once CSA is tapered. Therefore, CSA should be used to induce remission with an attempt to transition a patient to more definitive maintenance therapy with AZA or 6-MP. With this approach, long-term efficacy (avoidance of colectomy) of up to 80% has been reported by one center. Given the potential side effects of CSA, its use should be reserved for centers with experience using the drug, done in the context of appropriate surgical consultation for colectomy. Side effects and drug interactions with CSA, some of which are life-threatening, include hypertension, paresthesias, nausea/vomiting, hirsutism, infection, seizures, and renal dysfunction. Prophylaxis against *Pneumocystis carinii* pneumonia during therapy with CSA is recommended.

INFLIXIMAB (ANTI-TUMOR NECROSIS FACTOR ANTIBODY)

TNF-α is a proinflammatory molecule with similar biologic action to interleukin-1. Studies have shown increased TNF-α and other proinflammatory cytokines in individuals with IBD and in animal models. Infliximab (Remicade) is a chimeric monoclonal antibody targeted against TNF-α. Randomized studies demonstrating the efficacy of infliximab given intravenously at a dose of 5 mg/kg in refractory luminal and fistulizing CD led to FDA approval of this drug in 1998. Trials of infliximab for maintenance of remission in luminal CD (ACCENT I) and fistulizing CD (ACCENT II) are now complete. Results from the ACCENT I trial reported in October 2001 suggest that infliximab given every 8 weeks for a year is safe and effective in maintaining remission and allows tapering of steroids. Results from ACCENT II suggest that as needed dosing is as effective as maintenance therapy for fistulizing disease initially responsive to infliximab. Infliximab is currently in trials for UC; trials of other cytokine-based therapies are underway. Long-term side effects (if any) of infliximab are not yet known. Anti-TNF therapy may reactivate quiescent tuberculosis, and therefore all patients should be assessed by history for tuberculosis exposure and with purified protein derivative testing and chest x-ray before receiving any anti-TNF therapy. Lymphomas and other cancers have been reported, but it is not yet clear whether these cancers can be attributed to the infliximab, other immunomodulatory drugs, or the underlying disease. Based on current data, infliximab does not appear to increase the risk for malignancy.

Antibiotics

Metronidazole is effective in treating active Crohn ileocolitis, colitis, and perianal disease but not in treating active UC. Ursing and colleagues demonstrated that metronidazole 400 mg twice daily was as effective as sulfasalazine in patients with Crohn ileocolitis and colitis. It was, however, not effective in individuals with isolated ileitis. Uncontrolled studies have shown metronidazole at doses between 10 and 20 mg/kg body weight per day for 2 months is effective in treating patients with perianal complications of CD. Gastrointestinal upset and peripheral neuropathy are the main adverse effects reported.

Ciprofloxacin has been shown to be effective in open trials for the treatment of perianal CD and active Crohn ileitis and ileocolitis. The mechanism of action for both metronidazole and ciprofloxacin is presumed to be related to an alteration of bowel flora. In addition, both have been found to have immune-modulating properties. Other antibiotics have been reported to have efficacy for treating CD in small uncontrolled reports.

Surgery

Ultimately, surgery may be required for a variety of reasons, including disease refractory to medical therapy and IBD complications such as cancer/dysplasia, stricture, obstruction, toxic megacolon, abscess, and perforation. For UC, total proctocolectomy is curative, and approximately 20% of UC patients go on to colectomy. The standard procedure, until recently, was proctocolectomy with ileostomy. Now, ileal pouch-anal anastomosis (IPAA) is the favored procedure, because of the advantages of no ostomy and bowel continence. Individuals with an IPAA can develop a nonspecific inflammation of the ileal pouch, known as pouchitis. Pouchitis can be recurring and chronic in nature but usually responds to antibiotics; the most commonly used antibiotics are ciprofloxacin and metronidazole. If pouchitis proves to be refractory to medical therapy, it may be due to CD. Endoscopic evaluation of the pouch should be performed, and if there is evidence of CD, treatment with infliximab may be of benefit. Unfortunately, surgical takedown of the CD-involved pouch and ileostomy is often required. Therefore, known CD is a contraindication to the pouch procedure.

With CD, the most common surgery involves resection of grossly diseased segments and primary anastomosis. Clinical recurrence rate of disease at the anastomotic site can be as high as 10% per year. Medical prophylaxis involving the use of 5-ASA, metronidazole, and/or immunomodulators can be considered in individuals with CD who are thought to be at greater risk for recurrence because of aggressive disease and/or previous surgeries. However, data on the efficacy of medical prevention of postoperative recurrence are lacking. It should be emphasized that smoking is a risk factor for early recurrence after surgery, and therefore all CD patients should be counseled on smoking cessation. Stricturoplasty for small bowel strictures has the advantage of preserving small bowel for absorption and is increasingly being performed. It is estimated that 70% to 80% of individuals with CD will need at least one surgery during their lifetime.

COLON CANCER RISK

Long-standing IBD is a known risk factor for colon cancer. Other risk factors for colon cancer in IBD include length of colon involved and the presence primary sclerosing cholangitis. Patients with ulcerative proctitis and Crohn ileitis are not at increased risk for colorectal cancer compared with the general population. The current recommendations are for screening colonoscopies every 1 to 3 years to begin after 8 to 10 years of pancolitis and after 12 to 15 years of left-sided disease. Annual colonoscopies are recommended after 20 years of the disease. Surveillance colonoscopies in these individuals should be performed while their disease is in remission with multiple biopsies taken (at least 33 for 90% confidence of detecting dysplasia). The identification of a dysplastic lesion or mass or confirmed high-grade dysplasia mandates colectomy. Many experts also advocate colectomy for confirmed low-grade dysplasia, although others would suggest close follow-up for low-grade dysplasia. Folic acid may reduce colon cancer risk in IBD and is reasonable to prescribe at 1 mg/day.

OSTEOPOROSIS

A major concern in individuals with IBD is the development of osteoporosis: 31% to 59% of individuals with IBD have low bone mass. The risk of osteoporosis is greater in individuals with CD because of malabsorption, secondary to ileal involvement or small bowel resections, leading to vitamin D deficiency. The risk of long-term corticosteroid use cannot be overemphasized; therefore, corticosteroid use should be avoided if possible. The increased levels of inflammatory mediators (such as interleukin-6) in IBD may also lead to increased bone turnover with higher risk for osteopenia and osteoporosis. The increased risk for osteoporosis makes screening a necessity in individuals with IBD. Assessment of the baseline bone mineral density of an individual at initial evaluation is recommended; currently, dual-energy x-ray absorptiometry is the test of choice. From the dual-energy x-ray absorptiometry, a T-score is calculated that represents the standard deviation of the individual's bone density compared with that of the peak bone mass of a gender-matched control. A T-score less than or equal to –2.5 is defined as osteoporosis. A T-score between –1 and –2.5 is defined as osteopenia. Because dual-energy x-ray absorptiometry will not differentiate between osteopenia and osteomalacia, a vitamin D level must also be obtained, especially in the setting of known ileal involvement or a history of small bowel resections. Depending on the initial evaluation, a combination of medical therapies, including calcium citrate, vitamin D, and bisphosphonates, can be used, often in conjunction with an endocrinologist. General measures that help prevent osteoporosis include regular weight-bearing exercises, avoiding excess alcohol, and smoking cessation.

INFLAMMATORY BOWEL DISEASE AND WOMEN'S HEALTH

Questions and concerns regarding sexuality, fertility, pregnancy, transmission of disease to offspring, and nursing are often raised by patients and their families. Fortunately, most women with IBD are able to conceive with healthy outcomes and no adverse impact on their disease.

FERTILITY

Data collected over the last 15 years indicate that the natural fertility rate of patients with inactive IBD is the same as that of the general population. In a study by the National Institutes of Health, 197 women with CD and 107 women with UC were compared with age- and race-matched neighbors. A reduction in fertility was found to be a function of patient choice rather than biologic impairment. Voluntary childlessness in IBD has been documented in several studies in England, and the lack of recognition of this situation may explain reports and studies in the 1980s that showed decreased fertility in women with IBD. In particular, this may be the explanation for the results of an oft-quoted study involving 275 women with CD from five European nations that showed a decreased in fertility associated with CD.

The reasons behind voluntary childlessness are multifold. Fears about disease reactivation, effect of medication on the fetus, and IBD inheritance by children clearly play a role. Finally, one cannot discount the role of antiquated (and incorrect) medical advice against conception.

Active disease does lead to decreased fertility in women with IBD. This reduced fertility has been demonstrated in women with active CD, as defined by both disease activity and the need for prior surgeries, but not in active UC. The exception is that the fertility in women with UC who have undergone IPAA appears to be reduced.

There is no evidence that IBD directly impacts on male fertility. However, sulfasalazine can cause a transient oligospermia and impaired sperm motility. This is fully reversible within 3 to 4 months of stopping the medication. It is vital to ask couples undergoing infertility evaluation if the male partner is on sulfasalazine before embarking on assisted reproduction. The newer 5-ASA drugs do not have this side effect and can be used instead.

EFFECT OF INFLAMMATORY BOWEL DISEASE ON PREGNANCY

Inactive IBD does not increase the incidence of spontaneous abortions, stillborns, or congenital malformations. In one population with UC over a 20-year span, over 80% of pregnancies in women whose UC was quiescent were normal. The incidence of congenital malformations was found to be comparable with that of the general population. Subsequently, a controlled study of 82 pregnancies of women with UC and CD culled from a similar population as the previous study showed no major effect on duration of pregnancy, mode of delivery, hypertension, or proteinuria.

An increased risk for preterm birth and low birth weights has been reported in IBD. In the same study of 82 pregnancies mentioned above, there was a small, but statistically significant, increase in the number of low-birth-weight deliveries in women with CD compared with control subjects, regardless of disease activity. However, the mean birth weights of cases were comparable with control subjects.

Three more recent studies also report significant increases in preterm delivery and low birth weights. Baird et al. reported an increased risk of preterm birth (defined as before 37 weeks' gestation) in women with CD (odds ratio 3.1) and in women with UC (odds ratio 2.7). Age of the woman and duration of disease were not significant predictors of preterm birth. Another study, analyzing 756 Swedish women with IBD (no distinction made between CD and UC), showed an increased risk of preterm birth (<33 weeks, odds ratio 1.81; <37 weeks, odds ratio 1.48) and birth weight (<1,500 g, odds ratio 2.15; <2,500 g, odds ratio 1.57). In the most recent controlled study to date, with a disease cohort of 155 women with CD and 107 with UC, only women with CD were noted to have an increased risk in preterm birth (odds ratio 2.3), low birth weight (odds ratio 3.6), and smallness for gestational age (odds ratio 2.3). Given the nature of the study design, none of the three studies addressed the impact of disease activity. But other investigations on disease activity and pregnancy reveal that the incidence of spontaneous abortion and stillbirth goes up significantly in women who have active disease during their pregnancies; up to 60% of women with active CD can develop complications during pregnancy. Therefore, health care providers must strongly advise patients to delay pregnancy until their disease is in remission.

Nutritional and immunologic deficiencies inherent to IBD may explain the above findings. Certainly folate, essential for neural tube development in the first trimester, must be supplemented at higher doses in pregnant women with IBD. Folate deficiency may be the result of the disease itself as well as medications. Ideally, supplementation with folic acid 1 mg daily should begin before conception. Adequate caloric intake to ensure proper weight gain can be a management challenge and may require further intervention.

Finally, the recommended method of delivery in most IBD patients remains controversial. Historically, there has been a higher rate of cesarean sections in women with IBD compared with the general population. One hypothesis that has been raised is that elevated prostaglandin levels in women with IBD or a disturbance in the neurologic mechanism of the smooth muscle could lead to altered labor, resulting in increased cesarean sections. Furthermore, one concern that has been raised is that vaginal delivery may lead to an increased risk of active perianal or perineal disease. One study based on questionnaires sent to members of the Crohn's and Colitis Foundation of America reported 18% of women with no preexisting perineal disease developing active perineal disease after vaginal delivery, often within 2 months postpartum. These results have not been replicated; in particular, another study showed that cesarean sections did not prevent women with CD from having a relapse in previously dormant perineal disease. Therefore, the mode of delivery needs to be individualized to each patient and her pregnancy. The presence of active perineal disease generally precludes vaginal delivery.

EFFECT OF PREGNANCY ON INFLAMMATORY BOWEL DISEASE

Pregnancy does not seem to affect the overall course of IBD. Pregnant women with inactive UC at the time of conception have relapse rates comparable with nonpregnant women. Nor does there appear to be an increase in relapse in the postpartum period. Similar results have been noted in data collected on women with CD. Studies from Europe and the United States revealed that over the course of pregnancy, approximately one third of women with inactive IBD at the time of conception relapse during the pregnancy, similar to the relapse rates of nonpregnant women over the course of a year. These studies were both control-matched studies and studies comparing the same cohort of women in both prepregnant and pregnant states. Observations have been made that IBD relapses are more common in the first trimester. However, this trend has been disputed in more recent literature; the discrepancy may be due to previously undocumented discontinuation of medication secondary to undue fears of the effects on the fetus.

Although there are several case reports of worsening complications during pregnancy in women with active IBD at the time of conception, larger studies reveal a more equivocal picture. In women with active UC at the time of conception, 45% worsened during the pregnancy, 25% improved, and 25% remained unchanged. The course of UC during a pregnancy does not accurately predict how the disease will behave in future pregnancies. In women with active CD at the time of conception, one third worsened during pregnancy, one third remained unchanged, and one third improved. Because it is more difficult to conceive during active disease, these trends may represent selection bias, and the true extent of the effect of pregnancy on active IBD may not be fully understood. Thus, the importance of achieving remission before conceiving a child must again be emphasized. To this end, appropriate medical management to achieve and maintain remission is vital (Table 68.2).

DIAGNOSTIC TESTING DURING PREGNANCY

A diagnostic dilemma may arise during the pregnancy of a woman with IBD—what testing can be done if a flare is suspected. The quandary becomes more acute in the symptomatic pregnant woman in whom the diagnosis of IBD has not been previously established. In the former scenario, if the clinical picture is consistent with an IBD flare, it is reasonable to empirically treat as such without endoscopic evaluation. Biochemical parameters that are often used to clarify the clinical presentation may be altered in pregnancy and must be interpreted cautiously. For example, due to hemodilution, both albumin and hemoglobin may be lower than expected, especially in the third trimester. The erythrocyte sedimentation rate may be slightly elevated during the course of a normal pregnancy.

Radiographic imaging may be problematic as well. Ultrasonography is a safe technique in pregnancy and may be able to assess the formation of abscesses as well as bowel wall thickening, which can be an indication of inflammation. Exposure of the fetus to x-rays obviously must be limited; however, the need for x-ray imaging may be unavoidable in situations such as suspected toxic megacolon or intestinal obstruction. In these situations, exposure to low-dose ionizing radiation (1–5 rad) is an acceptable risk. Studies indicate that such limited exposure

TABLE 68.2. IBD Medications in Pregnancy and Nursing[a]

Drug	Disease	Category	Use during pregnancy	Complications to fetus	Nursing
5-ASA	CD/UC	B	Yes	Interstitial nephritis	Yes[b]
Sulfasalazine	CD/UC	B	Yes[c]	Neural tube defects[d]	Yes[e]
Corticosteroids	CD/UC	B	Yes	Adrenal suppression[f]	Yes
Metronidazole	CD	B	Yes[g]	Unknown	Unknown
Ciprofloxacin	CD	C	Unknown	Arthropathy	Unknown
Azathioprine/6-mercaptopurine	CD/UC	D	Yes	Unknown	Unknown[h]
Cyclosporine[i]	UC	C	Unknown	Unknown	Unknown[h]
Methotrexate	CD	X	No	Fetal death/teratologic	No
Infliximab	CD	B	Unknown	Unknown	Unknown[h]

[a]Authors' recommendations regarding use based on currently available studies.
[b]Low levels of drug detected in human breast milk; unclear clinical significance.
[c]Causes transient oligospermia and decreased sperm motility.
[d]As a result of folate deficiency.
[e]Detected in human breast milk; theoretical concerns for kernicterus.
[f]In both mother and fetus.
[g]No data on long-term use.
[h]AZA and CyA present in human breast milk in low levels; very limited data on infliximab in breast milk.
[i]Use only by experienced centers/physicians.
5-ASA, aminosalicylic acid; BD, inflammatory bowel disease; CD, Crohn disease; CSA, cyclosporin; IUC, ulcerative colitis.

does not increase the risk of congenital malformation, mental retardation, or childhood leukemia.

Endoscopy should be considered during pregnancy *only if* it will substantially impact management. Based on multicentered studies, upper endoscopy and flexible sigmoidoscopy with biopsies may be performed safely; the second trimester may be the safest time to perform these procedures. Colonoscopy may be safe as well, but sufficient data are lacking and therefore cannot be recommended. Fetal heart monitoring should be performed during the procedures in the later stages of pregnancy. Medications used for sedation are generally considered safe. To decrease complications, an obstetrics consultation should be obtained before consideration of an endoscopy.

SURGERY DURING PREGNANCY

Despite small case reports regarding surgery during pregnancy, there is a lack of definitive data on safety to both the mother and the fetus. Surgery should be reserved for life-threatening situations, such as intestinal perforations. When emergent colectomies were performed on pregnant women with fulminant UC, fetal loss was as high as 50%. The data on less involved surgeries on pregnant women without IBD is less grim: 2% fetal loss in uncomplicated appendectomies and 5% in open cholecystectomies. However, it is difficult to extrapolate these data to women with IBD because of potential changes in anatomy from previous surgeries and inflammation. Elective surgery should be postponed until after delivery. The decision to proceed with surgery is fraught with potential catastrophe and, even in emergency situations, should be undertaken in a multidisciplinary fashion, with input from the gastroenterologist, surgeon, obstetrician, and neonatologist.

EFFECT OF SURGERY ON FERTILITY AND PREGNANCY

Women who have had ileostomies are capable of having normal pregnancies and deliveries. Some of the possible complications include transient stomal prolapse and intestinal obstruction. There can be significant nutritional issues and possible fetal effects raised in women with CD who have had intestinal resections: Data reveal an increased risk of prematurity beyond the risk of the IBD itself. Strict attention to potential nutritional deficits and even to the presence of short bowel syndrome is needed. There may even be a need for total parental nutrition in this population.

In recent years, extensive data have been collected on the effects of IPAA on fertility and sexual function. In the most recent study, data collected from four Scandinavian hospitals from 1982 to 1998 revealed a significant decrease in fecundity (defined as the biologic ability to conceive and often expressed as the probability of becoming pregnant per month with unprotected intercourse) after IPAA compared with women with UC before surgery and with a control population. These results mirror those from a prior study from the same group. Interestingly, the 1999 study also revealed a high rate of in vitro fertilization in women with IPAA, which suggests that voluntary childlessness was not an issue. This reduction in fertility may be attributable to the surgery, but the exact etiology is not so clear. In one case series of women with IPAA, one third had abnormal findings on hysterosalpingography. Thus, blockage of the fallopian tubes secondary to adhesions may be an important factor.

Another factor may be impairment of sexual function after IPAA. Dyspareunia has been reported in 7% to 26% of women after IPAA. However, there is conflicting evidence of improvement in sexual health after IPAA.

The effect of pregnancy on IPAA function has also been reported in the literature. Transient increases in stool frequency and fecal incontinence have been reported during pregnancy, with rapid returns to prepregnancy function soon after delivery. The route of delivery is debatable. Observations have been that although vaginal delivery is safe for women with IPAA, cesarean sections outnumber vaginal deliveries, probably because of concern about damage to the sphincter, pouch, and pudendal nerve.

ENTEROVAGINAL FISTULAE IN CROHN DISEASE

A problem that affects approximately 3% to 5% of women with CD, enterovaginal fistulae (EVF) can be difficult to diagnose and manage. A history of hysterectomy may increase the risk of EVF formation. Although diagnosis is easily made in situations where there is vaginal passage of gas and stool, EVF can mimic a chronic vaginal infectious process, with purulent vaginal discharge and suprapubic pain. Physical examination may reveal findings suggestive of EVF. Available imaging modalities to assess for the presence and extent of EVF include computed tomography, contrast radiography, and fistulograms, though each modality has its own limitations. Novel techniques to identify the presence of EVF include instilling dilute methylene blue into the rectum and determining dye staining of a previously placed vaginal tampon or an oral charcoal study producing staining of a vaginal tampon. Although surgery is the definitive treatment for EVF, it is not the best initial option in a pregnant woman. Data regarding the efficacy of infliximab is sparse; although approved by the FDA for enterocutaneous and perianal fistulae, there are no controlled trials investigating infliximab's potential role in EVF. O'Brien reported a case series of six patients, with four patients having complete resolution of EVF and all six improving symptomatically with infliximab.

MEDICAL THERAPY DURING PREGNANCY

It is vital to achieve and maintain remission in women with IBD before conception. Despite concerns about the effects of drugs on the fetus and nursing infant, by and large most medications used to treat IBD are safe for the mother and fetus/nursing infant.

As mentioned previously, sulfasalazine has a negative effect on male fertility. In addition, sulfasalazine inhibits absorption of folate and can exacerbate folate deficiency. Though sulfasalazine is known to cross the placental barrier and is found in significant amount in breast milk, there is no evidence that sulfasalazine itself increases abnormalities. In particular, theoretical concerns of jaundice and kernicterus have not been proven.

Extensive literature exists about the safety of mesalamine. Two prospective controlled studies of 123 and 165 pregnancies, respectively, show no increased risk in fetal malformation or spontaneous abortions compared with control subjects. There was no difference in outcomes whether a woman took mesalamine preconception or throughout pregnancy nor was there a significant difference in outcome in different doses of mesalamine. One case of interstitial nephritis in a newborn whose mother took 4 g/d mesalamine was documented, but a trend toward an increase risk of fetal nephrotoxicity has not been clearly demonstrated. Mesalamine, unlike sulfasalazine, is not associated with transient male infertility. On a practical note, the administration of enema preparations of mesalamine may be difficult and uncomfortable for a woman in the latter stages of pregnancy, and 5-ASA suppositories or oral formulations may be substituted.

Corticosteroids are very well tolerated in pregnancy and are the medical therapy of choice for women with moderate to severe IBD who fail mesalamine therapy. Much of the evidence for the safety of corticosteroids comes from experience with other diseases, such as asthma and rheumatoid arthritis. The largest series investigating corticosteroid use in pregnant women with IBD studied 168 women, with no significant increased risk for fetal malformations. Early reports of low birth weights may in fact be attributed to the disease and not the medication. Several theoretical concerns do require close monitoring during pregnancy if corticosteroids are used. Adrenal suppression due to chronic steroid use may require the use of increased supplemental dosing in the peripartum period. Prednisone or prednisolone at doses less than 30 mg daily minimally cross the placental barrier and have not been shown to result in neonatal adrenal insufficiency. Corticosteroids can be excreted in breast milk. Therefore, a 4-hour delay between administration of an oral dose and nursing should be recommended. Abnormal glucose metabolism and increased calcium excretion require close monitoring and possible calcium supplementation during pregnancy.

If antibiotics have been used routinely in the treatment of a woman's IBD, these should be substituted for alternate medical therapy before conceiving. Metronidazole crosses the placental barrier, and there have been conflicting animal studies on this antibiotic's teratogenetic effects. One large case-control study conducted by the World Health Organization showed no clinically significant increase in congenital malformations. A meta-analysis also suggested the safety of metronidazole in pregnancy. However, in these studies, metronidazole was used for the treatment of bacterial vaginosis for periods much less than that required for maintenance therapy for IBD. Ciprofloxacin has not been shown to increase the risk of congenital malformations in either animal studies or several small case series, including the use of long-term ciprofloxacin. There have been reports of arthropathy in young animals arising as a result of ciprofloxacin use during pregnancy. The lack of controlled human trials involving ciprofloxacin and the ready availability of drugs with more proven safety profiles makes it difficult to justify the use of antibiotics for maintenance therapy in pregnant women with IBD.

Immunomodulating drugs are being used more frequently to treat IBD and are a vital therapeutic option, particularly for patients with more aggressive disease. Although animal studies have suggested potential teratologic effects on the fetus, most human treatment literature supports the safety of using immunomodulators. AZA was studied in women who were kidney transplant recipients and was found to be safe in conjunction with pregnancy; rare case reports of spontaneous abortions, prematurity, jaundice, and congenital malformations should be noted. AZA use in pregnant women with IBD has been assessed in only one retrospective study, looking at 16 pregnancies in 14 women: no congenital malformations, altered development, childhood malignancies, or increased frequency of childhood infections were reported. 6-MP safety around pregnancy has been recently evaluated both in women and men with IBD. A large retrospective study reviewed the effects of 6-MP on the fetal outcomes in 79 women and 76 men and found no significant increases in spontaneous abortions, prematurity, congenital malformations, or neonatal infections. Given the current evidence, it seems reasonable to continue AZA and 6-MP after discussion with the individual patient. Because of the problems outlined in pregnancies in the setting of active disease, the safest course for woman and fetus may be to continue the medication with close obstetric follow-up. For women and men considering pregnancy and whose IBD has been maintained in remission by AZA or 6-MP for several years, a trial withdrawal of the medication before conception may be attempted. If possible, the drug should be held through the nursing period.

Cyclosporine use is usually reserved for severe or fulminant IBD. Despite the significant side-effect profile of cyclosporine on individuals, there is no clear evidence of an increase in fetal complications. Data collected from transplant patients note an increase in prematurity and low birth weights but not congenital malformations. These findings coincide with several case reports on the effect of intravenous cyclosporine on pregnant women with IBD. Perhaps the most important consideration before the use of cyclosporine is that the medication may allow a woman with fulminant IBD to delay surgery long enough to make cesarean section and surgery a viable option for both mother and child. There are no data on the safety of cyclosporine in actively nursing mothers.

Methotrexate is contraindicated in pregnancy and nursing and is the only Category X drug currently used to treat IBD. Infliximab's efficacy in CD has now been well established. What has yet to be clearly established is infliximab's safety in the setting of pregnancy. Data obtained from the manufacturer (as of 10/1/2001) revealed that of 54 documented pregnancy outcomes from women with exposure to infliximab, there were 36 live births, 10 miscarriages, and 8 therapeutic terminations. Of the 36 live births, there was 1 case of a preterm neonate who subsequently died at 3 weeks and 1 infant with teratology of Fallot who underwent surgical repair and has done well. The outcomes (live births, miscarriages, and therapeutic terminations) in the women treated with infliximab were consistent with those observed in a national cohort of healthy women. Although a promising trend, these data are insufficient to comment on the overall safety of infliximab in the pregnant woman. If a women prefers to delay pregnancy until infliximab is no longer present in the blood, pharmacokinetics of the antibody suggest that a washout period of 6 months is required. A single study of a 26-year-old nursing CD patient on infliximab failed to reveal any of the drug in the breast milk.

In most situations, a woman can receive medical treatment for IBD without adverse side effects on the well-being of her fetus/newborn. Aside from vitamin supplementation, there are no medications for IBD that fit into Category A drugs. However, most medications do fit into Category B, such as sulfasalazine, mesalamine, and corticosteroids. Recent studies support the safety of 6-MP and AZA. The only medication that has an absolute contraindication is methotrexate. The key is to tailor the drug regimen to the individual situation. The safety profiles of the newer cytokine-based therapies are not so clearly outlined. In these situations, it must be remembered that achieving and keeping a woman in remission may be the single most important goal in pursuing a normal course of pregnancy.

PSYCHOSOCIAL EFFECTS OF INFLAMMATORY BOWEL DISEASE ON WOMEN

One of the costs of IBD on an individual is quality of life. There is an increasing awareness and appreciation that proper recognition and management of the psychological and social aspects of IBD can contribute to the overall health of the individual.

The impact of IBD on sexual health is perhaps one of the many hidden costs of having the disease. One retrospective study reported significantly higher rates of sexual problems, including infrequent or no intercourse, even among women in stable relationships. Dyspareunia, abdominal pain, diarrhea, and fear of fecal incontinence are often cited as reasons for reduced sexual activity. Patients may be reluctant to volunteer information about sexual dysfunction to a physician; therefore, the burden falls on the health provider to facilitate discussions in an open and comfortable manner that may be beneficial. There is evidence that couples counseling can also be of significant help, and the primary care provider should be cognizant of the physical and emotional impact of IBD.

Beyond sexual and reproductive health, IBD can have a significant impact on the overall quality of life. One study reported that women with IBD are more likely to have significant premenstrual and menstrual complaints and changes in bowel habits during menses. This transient and cyclical cause of bowel changes must be taken into consideration before altering IBD management. There is also evidence of different gender perceptions of IBD. In a survey of men and women, women reported worse symptoms of IBD and more concern about the impact of IBD on self-image, attractiveness, having children, and feeling alone than men. An awareness of these issues should help guide the physician's approach and care for a woman with IBD.

BIBLIOGRAPHY

Alstead EM. Inflammatory bowel disease in pregnancy. *Postgrad Med J* 2002;78:23.

Andres PG, Friedman LS. Epidemiology and the natural course of inflammatory bowel disease. *Gastrointest Clin* 1999;28:255.

Baird DD, Narendranathan M, Sandler RS. Increased risk of preterm birth for women with inflammatory bowel disease. *Gastroenterology* 1990;99:987.

Bertschinger P, Himmelmann A, Risti B, et al. Cyclosporine treatment of severe ulcerative colitis during pregnancy. *Am J Gastroenterol* 1995;90:330.

Bomford JAL, Ledger JC, O'Keeffe BJ, et al. Ciprofloxacin use during pregnancy. *Drugs* 1993;45:461.

Brandt LJ, Estabrook SG, Reinus JF. Results of a survey to evaluate whether vaginal delivery and episiotomy lead to perineal involvement in women with Crohn's disease. *Am J Gastroenterol* 1995;90:1918.

Burtin P, Taddio A, Ariburnu O, et al. Safety of metronidazole in pregnancy: a meta-analysis. *Am J Obstet Gynecol* 1995;172:525.

Calkins BM, Linienfeld AM, Garland CF, et al. Trends in the incidence rates of ulcerative colitis and Crohn's disease. *Dig Dis Sci* 1984;29:913.

Cappell MS, Colon VJ, Sidhom OA. A study at 10 medical centers of the safety and efficacy of 48 flexible sigmoidoscopies and 8 colonoscopies during pregnancy with follow-up of fetal outcome and with comparison to control groups. *Dig Dis Sci* 1996;41:2353.

Counihan TC, Roberts PL, Schoetz DJ, et al. Fertility and sexual and gynecological function after ileal pouch-anal anastomosis. *Dis Colon Rectum* 1994;37:1126.

Czeizal AE, Rockenbauer M. A population-based case-control teratologic study of oral metronidazole treatment during pregnancy. *Br J Obstet Gynaecol* 1998;105:322.

D'Haens G, Rutgeerts P. Postoperative recurrence of Crohn's disease: pathophysiology and prevention. *Inflamm Bowel Dis* 1999;5:295.

Damgaard B, Wettergren A, Kirkegaard P. Social and sexual function following ileal pouch-anal anastomosis. *Dis Colon Rectum* 1995;38:286.

Diav-Citrin O, Park YH, Veerasuntharam G, et al. The safety of mesalamine in human pregnancy: a prospective controlled cohort study. *Gastroenterology* 1998;114:23.

Dominitz JA, Young JCC, Boyko EJ. Outcomes of infants born to mothers with inflammatory bowel disease: a population-based cohort study. *Am J Gastroenterol* 2002;97:641.

Farouk R, Pemberton JH, Wolff BG, et al. Functional outcomes after ileal pouch-anal anastomosis for chronic ulcerative colitis. *Ann Surg* 2000;231:919.

Firstenberg MS, Malangoni MA. Gastrointestinal surgery during pregnancy. *Gastroenterol Clin* 1998;27:73.

Francella A, Dyan A, Bodian C, et al. The safety of 6-mercaptopurine for childbearing patients with inflammatory bowel disease: a retrospective cohort study. *Gastroenterology* 2003;124:9.

Friedman S, Regueiro MD. Pregnancy and nursing in inflammatory bowel disease. *Gastroenterol Clin* 2002;31:265.

Hanauer SB, Feagan BG, Lichtenstein GR. et al. Maintenance infliximab for Crohn's disease: the ACCENT I randomized trial. *Lancet* 2002;359:1541.

Hensleigh PA, Kaufmann RE. Maternal absorption and placental transfer of sulfasalazine. *Am J Obstet Gynecol* 1977;127:443.

Hugot JP, Chamaillard M, Zouali H, et al. Association of NOD2 leucine-rich repeat variants with susceptibility to Crohn's disease. *Nature* 2001;411:599–603.

Juhasz ES, Fozard B, Dozois RR, et al. Ileal pouch-anal anastomosis function following childbirth. *Dis Colon Rectum* 1995;38:159.

Kane SV, Sable K, Hanauer SB. The menstrual cycle and its effect on inflammatory bowel disease and irritable bowel syndrome: a prevalence study. *Am J Gastroenterol* 1998;93:1867.

Katz JA, Lichtenstein GR, Keenan GF, et al. Outcome of pregnancy in women receiving Remicade (infliximab) for the treatment of Crohn's disease or rheumatoid arthritis. *Gastroenterology* 2001;120:A69.

Kornfeld D, Cnattingius S, Ekbom A. Pregnancy outcomes in women with inflammatory bowel disease—a population-based cohort study. *Am J Obstet Gynecol* 1997;177:942.

Lashner BA. Colorectal cancer surveillance for patients with inflammatory bowel disease. *GI Endosc Clin North Am* 2002;12:175.

Loftus EV, Tremaine WJ, Habermann TM, et al. Risk of lymphoma in inflammatory bowel disease. *Am J Gastroenterol* 2000;95:2308.

Lombardi DA, Feller ER, Shah SA. Medical management of inflammatory bowel disease in the new millennium. *Compr Ther* 2002;28:39.

Marteau P, Tennebaum R, Elefant E, et al. Foetal outcome in women with inflammatory bowel disease treated during pregnancy with oral mesalamine microgranules. *Aliment Pharmacol Ther* 1998;12:1101.

Maunder R, Toner B, de Rooy E, et al. Influence of sex and disease on illness-related concerns in inflammatory bowel disease. *Can J Gastroenterol* 1999;13:728.

Mayberry JF, Weterman IT. European survey of fertility and pregnancy in women with Crohn's disease: a case control study by European collaborative group. *Gut* 1986;27:821.

Miller JP. Inflammatory bowel disease in pregnancy: a review. *J R Soc Med* 1986;79:221.

Mogadam M, Dobbins WO, Korelitz BI, et al. Pregnancy in inflammatory bowel disease: effect of sulfasalazine and corticosteroids on fetal outcomes. *Gastroenterology* 1981;80:72.

Moody G, Probert CSJ, Srivastava EM, et al. Sexual dysfunction amongst women with Crohn's disease: a hidden problem. *Digestion* 1992;52:179.

Moody GA, Probert C, Jayanthi V, et al. The effects of chronic ill health and treatment with sulphasalazine on fertility amongst men and women with inflammatory bowel disease in Leicestershire. *Int J Colorect Dis* 1997;12:220.

Nielsen OH, Andreasson B, Bondesen S, et al. Pregnancy in Crohn's disease. *Scand J Gastroenterol* 1984;19:724.

O'Brien J. Medical management of rectovaginal fistula in patients with Crohn's disease (monograph). Princeton, NJ: Princeton Health Care Communications. *Ther Options for Crohn's Colitis* 2001.

Olsen KO, Joelsson M, Laurberg S, et al. Fertility after ileal pouch-anal anastomosis in women with ulcerative colitis. *Br J Surg* 1999;86:493.

Olsen KO, Juul S, Berndtsson I, et al. Ulcerative colitis: female fecundity before diagnosis, during disease, and after surgery compared with a population sample. *Gastroenterology* 2002;122:15.

Oresland T, Palmbad S, Ellstrom M, et al. Gynecological and sexual function related to anatomical changes in the female pelvis after restorative proctocolectomy. *Int J Colorect Dis* 1994;9:77.

Plevy SE. Corticosteroid-sparing treatments in patients with Crohn's disease. *Am J Gastroenterol* 2002;97:1607.

Podolsky DK. Inflammatory bowel disease. *N Engl J Med* 2002;347:417.

Porter RJ, Stirrat GM. The effects of inflammatory bowel disease on pregnancy: a case-controlled retrospective analysis. *Br J Obstet Gynaecol* 1986;93:1124.

Present DH, Korelitz BI, Wisch N, et al. Treatment of Crohn's disease with 6-mercaptopurine: a long-term, randomized, double-blind study. *N Engl J Med* 1980; 302:981–987.

Rogers RG, Katz VL. Course of Crohn's disease during pregnancy and its effect on pregnancy outcome: a review. *Am J Perinatol* 1995;12:262.

Sandborn WJ. A review of immune modifier therapy for inflammatory bowel disease: azathioprine, 6-mercaptopurine, cyclosporine, and methotrexate. *Am J Gastroenterol* 1996;91:423.

Subhani JM, Hamilton MI. The management of inflammatory bowel disease during pregnancy. *Aliment Pharmacol Ther* 1998;12:1039.

Trachter AB, Rogers AI, Leiblum SR. Inflammatory bowel disease in women: impact on relationship and sexual health. *Inflamm Bowel Dis* 2002;8:413.

Valentine JF, Sninsky CA. Prevention and treatment of osteoporosis in patients with inflammatory bowel disease. *Am J Gastroenterol* 1999;94:878.

CHAPTER 69
Irritable Bowel Syndrome

Jean Wang and Mark Donowitz

Irritable bowel syndrome (IBS) is a condition characterized by abdominal discomfort and abnormal bowel movement frequency or form. It was first given a name in 1944, and since then it has become one of the most common conditions seen by gastroenterologists and primary care physicians. IBS is a functional gastrointestinal (GI) disorder, which means by definition that no known identifiable structural or biochemical abnormalities are present to explain the symptoms. Categorization as a functional disorder does not imply that IBS is a psychiatric disorder, although symptoms can be influenced by psychological factors and stressful situations, and many patients with IBS have psychiatric diagnoses.

Most people with IBS do not seek medical care. In fact, it is estimated that only 30% of people with IBS ever come to the attention of a physician. The patients who do seek medical care often use health care more frequently and are more likely to also have multiple non-GI complaints. These most commonly include fibromyalgia, chronic fatigue syndrome, temporomandibular joint disorder, and chronic pelvic pain. They also are more likely to have had a history of hysterectomy.

The scope and prevalence of IBS is difficult to accurately determine because most patients with IBS never present to medical attention and there is no definitive biologic test to confirm the diagnosis. Epidemiologic studies estimate the overall prevalence of IBS in North America to be 10% to 15%. Women are more commonly affected than men (by a 2:1 ratio), and patients usually present between 30 and 50 years of age. IBS affects patients worldwide with similar prevalence.

The impact of IBS on health care in the United States is substantial, with a prevalence of approximately 15.4 million cases accounting annually for 3.7 million physician visits and $1.6 billion in total costs. The burden of disease to society associated with IBS is also significant due to absenteeism from work and decreased quality of life. Of note, IBS is associated with relatively low pharmaceutical costs ($80 million) compared with other chronic GI diseases such as gastroesophageal reflux disease ($6 billion), reflecting the lack of effective medications currently available for this indication.

ETIOLOGY

The mechanisms underlying IBS have not been explained, are likely multifactorial in nature, and probably involve abnormalities in the enteric nervous system. Understanding this condition is commonly called the last frontier of GI diseases.

The enteric nervous system refers to a complex network of neurons that controls the GI tract. It is closely related to the central nervous system and relies on many of the same neurotransmitters for transmitting signals. The enteric nervous system is comprised of two large ganglions of nerves. The myenteric (Auerbach) plexus resides between the muscle layers of the gut and contains the neurons that control motility. Meanwhile, the submucosal (Meissner) plexus contains motor fibers, which stimulate secretion and sensory cells that communicate with the myenteric plexus. Enterochromaffin cells lie in the GI epithelium and store 95% of the serotonin neurotransmitters in the body. It is thought that these enterochromaffin cells act as pressure transducers and secrete serotonin to initiate peristalsis in the setting of increased pressure (such as from a bolus of food). Over time, desensitization can occur, leading to decreased effect of the serotonin. Abnormalities in the enteric nervous system can likely explain most symptoms resulting from IBS.

Two main components of IBS are visceral hypersensitivity and abnormal GI motility, both of which are regulated in part by the enteric nervous system. Visceral hypersensitivity refers to the fact that IBS patients feel discomfort with lesser amounts of bowel distention compared with normal subjects. Studies have also shown that approximately 50% to 70% of IBS patients have lower than average thresholds for pain. IBS patients commonly complain of excess bloating and gas. Studies have shown, however, that these patients do not have elevated amounts of intestinal gas. Rather, they have abnormal pain at a given volume of gas. Ritchie and colleagues in the early 1970s inflated balloons in the rectums of patients. These patients exhibited pain at much lower balloon volumes and pressures than control subjects.

Numerous studies have studied the relationship of abnormal GI motility to IBS. Loss of the migrating motor complex in the small intestine and the presence of discrete clustered contractions and prolonged propagated contractions have been described. There have also been reports of exaggerated responses to stimuli, such as high-fat meals. However, no consistent motility profile seen in IBS patients can be used to confirm the diagnosis.

The close relationship between the enteric and central nervous systems is believed to play a large role in many functional GI disorders such as IBS. Brain–gut interactions are now being studied in functional brain imaging studies using positron emission tomography and functional magnetic resonance imaging. Autonomic dysfunction has also been found in some IBS patients and is being further investigated.

Psychological factors play a large role in patients who choose to seek medical care for IBS, which further supports the relationship of the enteric and central nervous systems to IBS. These patients are more likely to report significant life stresses and are more likely to have a history of physical, sexual, or emotional abuse. In addition, the prevalence of a coexisting psychological or psychiatric disorder is quite high, in the range of 40% to 90%. It is possible that the underlying cause of the psychiatric condition or its consequences may be linked to or also contribute to causing the IBS. However, not all patients with IBS have psychiatric diagnoses. For example, IBS patients who do not seek medical care for their symptoms have similar mental health profiles compared with the general population. Therefore, these studies suggest that psychological factors may influence which patients choose to seek health care for their symptoms and the severity of impact on the patient.

Some patients with acute bacterial enteritis (4%–31%) develop chronic IBS. The mechanism of how this occurs is still not clear. However, one possibility is that infiltration of inflammatory cells into the myenteric plexus during acute enteritis could then cause abnormalities in the enteric nervous system, thus leading to IBS symptoms. However, even here there is a link to psychological factors. Postinfectious enteritis IBS is more frequent in women, patients with a prolonged episode of acute diarrhea, and in patients with a psychiatric profile that includes anxiety, depression, somatization, or hypochondriasis. Clearly, much research is still needed to elucidate the pathophysiology underlying this complex syndrome.

DIAGNOSIS

The diagnostic evaluation for IBS is difficult because all standard laboratory tests are normal. However, the desire to "leave no stone unturned" can lead to unnecessary and costly testing (which is often repeated) while subjecting the patient to unneeded suffering, cost, and worry.

Before giving a patient the diagnosis of IBS, it is important to rule out organic GI disorders. The first step in the evaluation should involve excluding "alarm symptoms" (Table 69.1), such as onset of symptoms after age 50, fever, progressively worsening symptoms, nighttime symptoms, persistent diarrhea causing dehydration (requiring hospitalization), severe constipation causing fecal impaction, unexplained weight loss greater than 10 pounds, vomiting, occult blood in stools, rectal bleeding, anemia, abnormal physical examination other than mild abdominal tenderness, arthritis or dermatitis, recent antibiotic use, travel history to areas with endemic parasite diseases, and family history of inflammatory bowel disease, colon cancer, or celiac sprue.

Once these alarm symptoms have been excluded, the physician should then determine whether the patient meets the diagnostic criteria for IBS. There is currently no definitive biologic test available to diagnose IBS. Therefore, the diagnosis of IBS must be made based on clinical history and symptoms. Through the years, a number of diagnostic criteria have been developed for IBS. The Manning criteria were developed in 1978 but were criticized because of gender differences in the application of these criteria. Therefore, in 1990 the Rome I diagnostic criteria were published by a collaborative expert panel. These criteria were revised in 1999 and published as the Rome II criteria, which are the current diagnostic criteria for IBS (Table 69.2).

Patients presenting for the first time with symptoms suggestive of IBS deserve a careful and thorough initial evaluation to rule out other causes of diarrhea, constipation, or abdominal pain. Systemic causes of diarrhea should also be considered, such as diabetes mellitus and hyperthyroidism. However, once a complete evaluation has been performed that has not revealed an organic etiology, there is no need to repeat the studies and one may be reassured that the symptoms are likely due to IBS.

In patients with no alarm symptoms, applying the Rome II criteria has a very high positive predictive value of 98% for IBS based on clinical diagnosis after 2 years of follow-up. Therefore, the physician should be reassured that serious conditions have not been missed. In patients meeting the Rome II criteria, initial therapy should be given as outlined below. If the patient does not improve within 4 weeks, then additional evaluation should be performed as below.

TABLE 69.1. Alarm Symptoms that Need to be Excluded

Onset of symptoms after age 50
Fever
Progressively worsening symptoms
Night-time symptoms
Persistent daily diarrhea causing dehydration
Severe constipation causing fecal impaction
Unexplained weight loss greater than 10 pounds
Persistent vomiting
Occult blood in stools or rectal bleeding
Anemia
Abnormal physical examination other than mild abdominal tenderness
Arthritis or dermatitis
Recent antibiotic use
Travel history to areas with endemic parasite diseases
Family history of inflammatory bowel disease, colon cancer, or celiac sprue

TABLE 69.2. Rome II Diagnostic Criteria for Irritable Bowel Syndrome

At least 12 weeks, which need not be consecutive, in the preceding 12 months of abdominal discomfort or pain that has at least two of the following features:
Relieved with defecation
Onset associated with a change in frequency of stool
Onset associated with a change in form (appearance) of stool
Symptoms that cumulatively support the diagnosis of irritable bowel syndrome:
Abnormal stool frequency (defined as greater than three bowel movements per day or less than three bowel movements per week)
Abnormal stool form (lumpy/hard or loose/watery stool)
Abnormal stool passage (straining, urgency, or feeling of incomplete evacuation)
Passage of mucus
Bloating or feeling of abdominal distention

CLINICAL SYMPTOMS AND HISTORY

There is no single diagnostic physical finding, blood test, or x-ray that unquestionably confirms the diagnosis. Certain features, however, support the diagnosis. Therefore, a careful history is indispensable.

The age at onset is important to clarify with the patient. Symptoms generally, but not always, start between the ages of 30 and 50 years. Onset of symptoms after this period is concerning and deserves further evaluation. IBS symptoms are chronic but variable in severity. Symptoms can fluctuate over time. During initial presentation, symptoms can occur as frequently as 50% of the time, with pain one third of the time. Progressively worsening symptoms should be of concern and warrant further investigation. The patient who knows exactly the date of onset of symptoms usually does not have IBS. Rather, the onset of symptoms in IBS is gradual and vague.

The patient's abdominal pain should be characterized. In IBS, abdominal pain often is poorly localized but most frequently occurs in the middle or lower abdominal region. Very local abdominal pain can be a symptom of IBS, although abdominal wall entrapment syndromes must be considered. Many patients will have more than one site of pain. Descriptions of the pain may include crampy, burning, dull, sharp, steady, bloating, and knife-like. The pain typically does not radiate. It is commonly precipitated by meals and relieved by defecation. Bloating, belching, and flatus all are commonly present in IBS patients.

Stools can be described either as diarrhea or constipation or both alternating. It is important to have patients describe exactly what they mean by diarrhea or constipation. Many people believe if they do not have a daily bowel movement, they have constipation. In reality, normal stool frequency can range from three times a day to three times a week. Patients with constipation often have small "pellet-like" or "pencil-thin" stools resulting from spasm. In IBS, if the patient complains of diarrhea, the volume is small. Often, the patient states that the initial stool is formed, but subsequent stools are increasingly loose and eventually are liquid. A stool weight greater than approximately 300 g/d suggests a different diagnosis. Both the pain and diarrhea resolve during sleeping in IBS. If patients are being awakened at night by their symptoms, it is important to rule out organic GI disorders such as a secretory diarrhea or inflammatory bowel diseases. It is important to make the distinction between being awakened by pain and diarrhea versus being awakened for other reasons and then noticing pain and the need to evacuate. If the diarrhea continues during a 24-hour fasting state, this would be evidence against IBS and in favor of a secretory cause. However, maintaining a true 24-hour fast on an outpatient basis is difficult. Rectal bleeding suggests another diagnosis unless related to hemorrhoids or a fissure from straining and should be further evaluated with endoscopy.

A detailed surgical history, especially any abdominal surgery, needs to be obtained. Adhesions may cause symptoms that mimic IBS. Weight loss is important to ascertain. This is unusual in a patient with IBS unless there is concomitant depression. Unintentional weight loss of greater than 10 pounds should raise a red flag and be further evaluated.

An accurate record of family history with regard to inflammatory bowel diseases, colon cancer, or malabsorptive states such as sprue is important. Positive family history would warrant evaluation to exclude these disorders.

A good social history involving questions related to sexual and physical abuse is mandatory. One study found that patients with functional GI disorders were significantly more likely to have a history of rape or life-threatening physical abuse than patients with organic GI disorders. Patients are unlikely to volunteer this information unless specifically asked. In addition, a detailed travel history is necessary. Patients who have traveled to developing countries or areas with endemic parasitic diseases should be evaluated with more extensive stool studies to rule out infectious etiologies.

A list of all current and past medications, both prescribed and over the counter, is necessary. Multiple medications alter bowel motility and exacerbate symptoms. For example, antacids containing magnesium or aluminum can cause diarrhea or constipation, respectively. The patient also may be taking a laxative without realizing that it is contributing to the symptoms. For example, many health food products contain laxatives, fructose, or sorbitol.

A detailed dietary history is important. Patients should be instructed to keep a diary of their symptoms for 2 to 3 weeks and record types and quantities of food and liquids taken, time and severity of symptoms, and any associated environmental stressors. This will help identify potential associations of symptoms with food or stress, while allowing patients to participate in their care. Caffeinated products (including coffee, tea, and cola), carbonated products, and gas-producing foods may contribute to symptoms of bloating. Common gas-producing foods include broccoli, cabbage, Brussels sprouts, asparagus, cauliflower, and beans. Smoking, chewing gum, and eating quickly also cause more swallowed air, resulting in increased gas and bloating.

Lactose intolerance symptoms can mimic IBS and exacerbate its symptoms. About 40% of patients with IBS also have lactose intolerance. Lactose is present in a wide variety of foods; therefore, it is critical that labels be read to eliminate this sugar from the diet. Patients can be formally tested with a hydrogen breath test if there are any questions of intolerance to milk products or if they have already tried a nutritionist-guided lactose-free diet for about a week without response. Lactose intolerance affects over 90% of Asians and 60% to 80% of blacks, Ashkenazi Jews, and Native Americans. Sorbitol, which is a common sweetening agent used in "sugar-free" and other dietetic foods, also may contribute to symptoms. Normally, at least 90% of ingested sorbitol is absorbed in the small intestine by passive diffusion in which no enzyme is required. Ingestion of more than 30 g of sorbitol can cause osmotic diarrhea. Some individuals tolerate much less (approximately 10 g). Ten grams of sorbitol is present in four to five sugar-free mints (some varieties). Fructose also can cause significant abdominal distress. This sugar occurs naturally in fruits but also is added to a variety of processed foods. Symptoms seem to be related to the fermentation effect of colonic bacteria and malabsorbed carbohydrates. The combination of sorbitol and fructose can contribute to diarrhea and therefore should be eliminated from the diet on a trial basis.

CLINICAL FINDINGS AND PHYSICAL EXAMINATION

Patients with IBS have an unremarkable physical examination, with the exception of mild abdominal tenderness on palpation. However, a thorough abdominal examination should be performed at each visit to rule out abdominal masses or evidence of other organic GI disorders. If tympanitic bowel sounds, rebound tenderness, or boardlike rigidity are present, an obstruction or an acute abdomen should be suspected and a surgeon consulted immediately. Rectal examination should be performed to assess for masses or anal disease (hemorrhoids, fissures, fecal impaction, etc.) that could explain symptoms. Pelvic examination should be done if the patient's symptoms are primarily lower abdominal or pelvic in location. A fever is not part of IBS. The patient should also be carefully examined for any evidence of arthritis or dermatitis, and any signs of these should induce workup for associated GI inflammatory or immune-mediated conditions such as inflammatory bowel diseases or sprue.

LABORATORY AND IMAGING STUDIES

Screening studies are recommended to rule out anatomic, inflammatory, or infectious etiologies in patients who have a history of acute onset or worsening severity of symptoms, onset of symptoms at an older age, a family history of GI disorders such as inflammatory bowel diseases or colon cancer, or have no comorbid psychological or psychiatric disorders. The screening tests include a complete blood cell count, renal and liver function tests, thyroid-stimulating hormone, fasting blood glucose, and erythrocyte sedimentation rate. Serologies for celiac sprue (anti-gliadin IgA, anti-transglutaminase IgA, and anti-endomysial IgA) should be considered in patients with diarrhea-predominant symptoms and minimal pain. Stool Hemoccult should be performed to exclude evidence of GI bleeding, and positive evidence of occult blood in the stool should be further investigated with endoscopy. Patients with diarrhea should have their stool tested for ova and parasites at least three times. Stools should also be tested for *Clostridium difficile* toxin if there has been recent antibiotic exposure in the past 6 weeks. Colonoscopy should be performed in all patients over the age of 50 to screen for colon cancer and should be considered in younger patients based on clinical presentation (such as in cases of significant diarrhea).

TREATMENT

Treatment of IBS should be individualized and based on the patient's predominant symptoms and severity of illness. Patients with very mild symptoms may only want reassurance that their symptoms are not serious. Patients should be treated if they believe their IBS symptoms significantly impact their quality of life. Although there are prescription medications for treating IBS, their use is not necessary in all individuals and, at times, may be counterproductive. All drugs have side effects. Also, a high initial placebo effect causes patients to continue medications indefinitely when, in fact, these medications are not effective. Adequate medications for IBS have not yet been developed and are eagerly awaited by patients, physicians, and drug companies but will likely only come with increased understanding of the cause of the disorder. The foundation of treatment involves confidence in the diagnosis and a strong physician–patient relationship, which has been shown to reduce repetitive office visits. IBS is a chronic disorder, and therefore good communication is the key component. It is helpful to explain to the patient that IBS is a real disorder in which the intestine is especially sensitive to stimuli. It is necessary to determine the patient's understanding of the illness and concerns because some patients believe they may have cancer. It is definitely worthwhile to reassure the patient that IBS does not lead to cancer, require surgery, or shorten life expectancy.

It may be helpful to classify patients into one of the following three symptom-based subgroups for purposes of guiding treatment: constipation predominant; diarrhea predominant; and abdominal pain, gas, and bloating. However, it is important to note that many patients have alternating constipation and diarrhea.

For patients with constipation-predominant symptoms, increased fiber through diet (such as wheat bran, corn fiber) or supplements (such as psyllium) is the initial therapy. Fiber increases colonic transit time and relieves constipation. However, some patients have increased gas once fiber is consumed due to metabolism of fiber by intestinal bacteria, and about 15% cannot tolerate fiber at all. Therefore, it is recommended that fiber be started at a low dose and increased incrementally with the goal of 25 to 30 g/d. The fiber should be taken with a meal, usually breakfast. An insufficient dose of fiber is a frequent cause of failure; therefore, fiber intake should be quantitated and increased as tolerated. If necessary, a stool softener or osmotic laxative (such as magnesium citrate, milk of magnesia, sorbitol, lactulose, or polyethylene glycol) also can be used. Other laxatives can cause nerve or muscle damage to the gut with chronic use (e.g., senna, bisacodyl, etc.) and should not be used chronically.

If the constipation persists after 4 weeks of therapy, further investigation is warranted. Evaluation with thyroid function tests, glucose, calcium, magnesium, and colonoscopy should be considered. A colonic transit test using radiopaque markers with x-rays taken on days 4 and 7 after ingestion of 20 markers may be performed (known as the Sitzmark technique). Anorectal manometry, tests of rectal sensation and expulsion, and assessment of pelvic floor dysfunction are sometimes necessary. In contrast to IBS patients, patients with pelvic floor dysfunction predominantly have symptoms of straining and the sensation of rectal blockage, often requiring manual disimpaction to remove stool.

For patients with diarrhea-predominant symptoms, loperamide or diphenoxylate/atropine should be tried. Loperamide (Imodium) is the most commonly used agent and is available over the counter. It slows intestinal transit, enhances intestinal water absorption, and strengthens rectal sphincter tone. It is the safest agent for symptomatic relief and does not cross the blood–brain barrier. The prescribed dose is 2 to 6 mg up to three times a day for a maximum of 18 mg/d. Unlike patients with constipation-predominant symptoms, fiber has not been found to be consistently beneficial in patients with diarrhea-predominant symptoms. Patients with IBS often are sensitive to antidiarrheal agents, and sometimes a single dose causes constipation.

If the diarrhea persists after 4 weeks of therapy, the patient should be referred to a gastroenterologist for further evaluation. This will likely include 24-hour stool weight (while off medication) to confirm diarrhea, which is defined as greater than 200 g of stool per day. If this is the case, then stool electrolytes (sodium and potassium) should be checked to differentiate between a secretory or osmotic diarrhea. A stool or urine laxative screen should be done to exclude surreptitious laxative abuse. A 72-hour fecal fat collection is useful to rule out fat malabsorption. Upper endoscopy with small bowel biopsies may be performed to evaluate for celiac sprue, whereas colonoscopy with biopsies throughout the colon will be useful to rule out microscopic colitis. If lactose intolerance or bacterial overgrowth is suspected, an H_2 breath test should be done. A therapeutic trial with a lactose-free diet is also an adequate way to diagnose lactose intolerance.

Patients with abdominal pain, gas, and bloating as their primary symptoms should first be counseled on changing their diet to avoid gas-producing foods. These include fatty foods, alcohol, caffeine (coffee, tea, sodas), carbonated drinks, broccoli, cabbage, Brussels sprouts, asparagus, cauliflower, and beans. Smoking, chewing gum, and eating quickly also seem to cause more swallowed air, resulting in increased gas and bloating. If dietary modifications are not helpful, patients with predominantly gas and bloating symptoms can also try an α-galactosidase (Beano) or a simethicone preparation (e.g., Gas X, Phazyme). Patients who continue to have symptoms and do not have constipation may undergo a trial of antispasmodic medications, which act through anticholinergic effects and by enhancing intestinal smooth muscle relaxation. However, no currently available antispasmodic has consistently proven efficacy. Commonly used antispasmodics include dicyclomine (Bentyl) and hyoscyamine (Levsin). It is important to start treatment at a low dose and then increase it gradually. For example, dicyclomine can be started at 10 to 20 mg and may increased up to 40 mg orally four times a day. Hyoscyamine can be started at 0.125 mg and may be increased up to 0.25 mg orally four times a day. Unfortunately, sometimes efficacy is obtained only at a level at which side effects are more common. Potential side effects include urinary retention, constipation, dry mouth, and visual disturbances, due to the anticholinergic properties of these medications. These side effects should be discussed with the patient beforehand. The timing of the dosing is also crucial. Patients with postprandial symptoms should take the medication 30 minutes before meals. Meanwhile, patients who have unpredictable attacks of pain should use the medication on an as-needed basis up to four times per day. In some patients, these anticholinergic medications may appear to become less effective over time when used chronically.

If the symptoms persist despite the above measures, a flat plate x-ray of the abdomen during an acute episode of symptoms is recommended to exclude bowel obstruction. If the etiology is related to bowel obstruction, the x-rays should reveal bowel distention and air fluid levels. If the abdominal x-ray is negative and the patient remains symptomatic, further imaging studies such as small bowel follow-through, abdominal computed tomography, or pelvic ultrasound should be considered.

Antidepressant medication may be helpful for IBS because they appear to reduce the enhanced sensation of pain in IBS patients via the enteric nervous system, and effects are seen at doses that are subtherapeutic for the treatment of depression. Therefore, antidepressants at low doses (for instance, nortriptyline at 10–50 mg/d) should be considered and are underused in this condition. Common antidepressants used for therapy of IBS include tricyclic antidepressants such as nortriptyline. Although the use of tricyclic antidepressants for IBS are more established than selective serotonin reuptake inhibitors, tricyclic antidepressants have the potential for greater side effects. For example, tricyclic antidepressants may aggravate constipation because of their anticholinergic side effects. More recently, selective serotonin reuptake inhibitors such as paroxetine have also been shown to be effective for treatment of IBS in conjunction with psychotherapy.

The mechanism of action of antidepressants in improving IBS symptoms is likely due to several factors, but because we do not understand the pathobiology of IBS, how they work is not clear. However, we can postulate that the benefits of antidepressants in IBS are likely related to their effects on neurotransmitters, such as norepinephrine and serotonin, in the enteric nervous system. Other proposed theories by which antidepressants exert their effects involve treatment of any additional underlying psychiatric disorders, effects on GI motility, and reduction in pain perception. Patients should be warned that treatment effects can take 3 to 4 weeks before they are apparent. If patients do not respond to one antidepressant, other ones can be tried. Benzodiazepines are sometimes prescribed for patients who have anxiety contributing to their symptoms. However, studies have demonstrated rather weak benefits. Therefore, the physician should avoid prescribing benzodiazepines unless there is a strong anxiety component, and prescriptions should be given only on a limited basis. Careful discussion of the need for psychological or antidepressant treatment with the patient is critical for patients to follow through with the recommendation and prevent misunderstanding between the patient and physician.

New Therapies

New drug therapies are badly needed for IBS. However, until we better understand the pathobiology of the disease, we are unlikely to make major advances in treatment. In fact, it appears that drug companies are awaiting increased understanding of pathobiology before investing in major drug development in this area. New drug treatments of IBS have centered on 5-hydroxytryptamine (5-HT, serotonin), which plays a key role in peristalsis by acting on enteric neurons. For treatment of IBS with diarrhea-predominant symptoms, new medications targeted against 5-HT3 receptors are now being introduced. Alosetron hydrochloride (Lotronex) is a selective 5-HT3 antagonist that has been found to occasionally be effective in women with severe diarrhea-predominant symptoms. This agent works by slowing colonic transit and decreasing visceral hypersensitivity during colonic distention. However, this drug was temporarily withdrawn by the U.S. Food and Drug Administration (FDA) in 2000 because of postmarketing adverse effects, including severe constipation and acute ischemic colitis. Alosetron was reapproved by the FDA in 2002 and reintroduced into the market under restricted access guidelines for *women* with severe diarrhea-predominant symptoms in which conventional therapies have failed. Physicians who wish to prescribe alosetron must enroll in GlaxoSmithKline's prescribing program after attesting to their qualifications and acceptance of responsibilities. Meanwhile, patients who wish to take the medication must read a special four-page medication guide. Furthermore, both the prescribing physician and patient must sign a formal patient–physician agreement demonstrating an understanding of potential risks, assessment of the risk-to-benefit ratio, and dosing (details provided at www.lotronex.com). Alosetron should be started at 1 mg orally once a day. After 4 weeks, if the patient has tolerated the medication but is still having symptoms, the dosing can be increased to 1 mg orally twice a day. If after 4 weeks of treatment at 1 mg orally twice a day, the patient has not had adequate control of IBS symptoms, then the alosetron should be discontinued. Higher doses are not approved. Constipation is the most common adverse effect reported, and the medication should be stopped immediately if this occurs. Ischemic colitis is also an important potential complication associated with the use of alosetron. Ondansetron (Zofran), another 5-HT3 antagonist approved for severe vomiting, may be helpful in diarrhea-predominant patients, although it has not been FDA approved for this indication.

For patients with constipation-predominant symptoms, 5-HT4 receptor agonists have been mildly effective in randomized controlled trials, with 5% to 19% of patients taking tegaserod (Zelnorm) reporting significant improvement in global IBS symptoms compared with patients taking placebo. Tegaserod is a partial 5-HT4 agonist that was approved in 2002 for short-term treatment of female IBS patients with constipation-predominant symptoms. It acts by stimulating peristalsis, increasing intestinal transit, and reducing visceral sensitivity. Usual dosing is 6 mg orally twice a day, and it has no apparent serious side effects. Diarrhea is the most common adverse event. It is unclear whether its effects can be generalized to men, due to the small number of male patients included in the clinical trials.

Complementary and alternative therapies for IBS include relaxation therapy, hypnosis, biofeedback, cognitive therapy, and psychotherapy. These alternative therapies hold promise due to the close interplay between the brain and the gut (the so-called brain–gut connection) and its regulation of the enteric nervous system. Herbal remedies and probiotics could also have a role in patients with IBS and are also being evaluated, although it will be important to standardize what is being tested–for instance, some herbal preparations contain laxatives that would be expected to be less useful for diarrhea and IBS. Although hypnotherapy seems to have a positive effect in IBS, careful studies of these other alternative approaches are needed.

CONSIDERATIONS IN PREGNANCY

IBS in pregnancy has not been specifically studied. Treatment for pregnant patients with IBS is limited with regard to medications because of possible teratogenic effects. Conservative management is the rule, involving a high-fiber diet and eliminating lactose, sorbitol, fructose, caffeine, and gas-producing foods.

BIBLIOGRAPHY

Camilleri M. Testing the sensitivity hypothesis in practice: tools and methods, assumptions and pitfalls. *Gut* 2002;51[Suppl 1]:i34–i40.

Cash BD, Schoenfeld P, Chey WD. The utility of diagnostic tests in irritable bowel syndrome patients: a systematic review. *Am J Gastroenterol* 2002;97:2812–2819.

Chang L, Heitkemper MM. Gender differences in irritable bowel syndrome. *Gastroenterology* 2002;123:1686–1701.

Creed F, Fernandes L, Guthrie E, et al. The cost-effectiveness of psychotherapy and paroxetine for severe irritable bowel syndrome. *Gastroenterology* 2003;124: 303–317.

Donowitz M, Kokke FT, Saidi R. Evaluation of patients with chronic diarrhea. *N Engl J Med* 1995;332:725–729.

Drossman DA. Irritable bowel syndrome: how far do you go in the workup? *Gastroenterology* 2001;121:1512–1515.

Drossman DA, Camilleri M, Mayer EA, et al. AGA technical review on irritable bowel syndrome. *Gastroenterology* 2002;123:2108–2131.

Drossman DA, Corazziari E, Talley NJ, et al. *Rome II: the functional gastrointestinal disorders: diagnosis, pathophysiology, and treatment: a multinational consensus.* Mclean, VA: Degnon Associates, 2000.

Drossman DA, Li Z, Leserman J, et al. Health status by gastrointestinal diagnosis and abuse history. *Gastroenterology* 1996;110:999–1007.

Drossman DA, McKee DC, Sandler RS, et al. Psychosocial factors in the irritable bowel syndrome: a multivariate study of patients and nonpatients with irritable bowel syndrome. *Gastroenterology* 1988;95:701–708.

Drossman DA, Sandler RS, McKee DC, et al. Bowel patterns among subjects not seeking health care: use of a questionnaire to identify a population with bowel dysfunction. *Gastroenterology* 1982;83:529–534.

Fass R, Longstreth GF, Pimentel M, et al. Evidence- and consensus-based practice guidelines for the diagnosis of irritable bowel syndrome. *Arch Intern Med* 2001; 161:2081–2088.

Hahn B, Watson M, Yan S, et al. Irritable bowel syndrome symptom patterns: frequency, duration, and severity. *Dig Dis Sci* 1998;43:2715–2718.

Horwitz BJ, Fisher RS. The irritable bowel syndrome. *N Engl J Med* 2001;344: 1846–1850.

Jailwala J, Imperiale TF, Kroenke K. Pharmacologic treatment of the irritable bowel syndrome: a systematic review of randomized, controlled trials. *Ann Intern Med* 2000;133:136–147.

Kellow JE, Phillips SF. Altered small bowel motility in irritable bowel syndrome is correlated with symptoms. *Gastroenterology* 1987;92:1885–1893.

Manning AP, Thompson WG, Heaton KW, et al. Towards positive diagnosis of the irritable bowel. *Br Med J* 1978;2:653–654.

Neal KR, Hebden J, Spiller R. Prevalence of gastrointestinal symptoms six months after bacterial gastroenteritis and risk factors for development of the irritable bowel syndrome: postal survey of patients. *BMJ* 1997;314:779–782.

Olden KW. Diagnosis of irritable bowel syndrome. *Gastroenterology* 2002;122: 1701–1714.

Owens DM, Nelson DK, Talley NJ. The irritable bowel syndrome: long-term prognosis and the physician-patient interaction. *Ann Intern Med* 1995;122:107–112.

Peters GA, Bargen JA. The irritable bowel syndrome. *Gastroenterology* 1944;3: 399–402.

Ritchie J. Pain from distension of the pelvic colon by inflating a balloon in the irritable colon syndrome. *Gut* 1973;14:125–132.

Rodriguez LA, Ruigomez A. Increased risk of irritable bowel syndrome after bacterial gastroenteritis: cohort study. *BMJ* 1999;318:565–566.

Saito YA, Schoenfeld P, Locke GR III. The epidemiology of irritable bowel syndrome in North America: a systematic review. *Am J Gastroenterol* 2002;97: 1910–1915.

Sandler RS, Everhart JE, Donowitz M, et al. The burden of selected digestive diseases in the United States. *Gastroenterology* 2002;122:1500–1511.

Talley NJ, Spiller R. Irritable bowel syndrome: a little understood organic bowel disease? *Lancet* 2002;360:555–564.

Vanner SJ, Depew WT, Paterson WG, et al. Predictive value of the Rome criteria for diagnosing the irritable bowel syndrome. *Am J Gastroenterol* 1999;94: 2912–2917.

Viera AJ, Hoag S, Shaughnessy J. Management of irritable bowel syndrome. *Am Fam Physician* 2002;66:1867–1874.

Whitehead WE, Palsson O, Jones KR. Systematic review of the comorbidity of irritable bowel syndrome with other disorders: what are the causes and implications? *Gastroenterology* 2002;122:1140–1156.

CHAPTER 70
Diverticular Disease

Ramy Eid

Diverticulosis coli is the presence of diverticula in the colon. The term diverticular disease refers to the entire spectrum of asymptomatic to symptomatic disease associated with colonic diverticula. Clinical reports of diverticular disease were uncommon until the 20th century in economically developed Western societies. It is now clear that the incidence of diverticula rises within a population as it reduces its intake of dietary fiber. With the introduction of the roller process for milling wheat flour during the 1880s, dietary patterns changed, resulting in a widespread increase in the consumption of refined white flour. Conversely, the overall intake of fiber as bran decreased.

The true prevalence of diverticulosis coli is not known. In the United States and other developed countries, the prevalence approaches 10%. In addition to geographic location, age is an important factor. Autopsy reports suggest that it is found in up to one half of adults over the age of 60 and two thirds of individuals older than age 85 years. A slight preponderance in women has been reported in some studies. In Western nations, diverticular disease is predominantly left sided, whereas in Africa and Asia diverticulosis is usually right sided with prevalence less than 0.2%.

Whereas diverticula usually remain entirely asymptomatic, they may produce a wide variety of clinical presentations, ranging from mild abdominal discomfort and bowel irregularity to potentially life-threatening complications of acute inflammation, abscess formation, free perforation, obstruction, and bleeding.

ETIOLOGY

The decrease in consumption of dietary fiber produces a corresponding decrease in stool bulk. Consequently, higher intraluminal colonic pressures must be generated to ensure fecal transit. Two conditions must be present physiologically for diverticula to develop: a pressure gradient between the bowel lumen and the serosal surface and relative areas of weakness in the colonic wall caused by disordered colonic motility.

Most patients with sigmoid diverticula exhibit myochosis, which consists of thickening of the circular muscle layer, shortening of the taeniae, and luminal narrowing. There is no hypertrophy or hyperplasia of the bowel wall, but increased elastin deposition is found in the taeniae. Also, structural changes in collagen are similar to, but greater in magnitude than, those that occur as a result of aging. These changes may decrease resistance of the wall to intraluminal pressures. Colonic manometry has confirmed band-like or segmental high-pressure areas exceeding 90 mm Hg with slow waves cycling 12 to 18 times per minute in patients with diverticulosis coli. Within these high pressure segments, a pulsion-type diverticulum may develop through naturally occurring anatomic weak points where nutrient vessels penetrate the two antimesenteric taeniae. This is actually a pseudodiverticulum because the wall is composed of only the mucosal layer, lacking a true muscularis and serosa. This dietary hypothesis is well supported by additional observations that diverticular disease is distinctly rare among both lower socioeconomic populations, in whom dietary fiber intake remains high, and vegetarians.

Other lifestyle factors that might contribute to the pathogenesis of diverticular disease have been examined. There is no substantially increased risk associated with smoking, caffeine, or alcohol. On the other hand, an association has been noted between acute diverticulitis and obesity in men under age 40 years. Lack of vigorous exercise also may be a risk factor for diverticular disease. Structural changes in the colonic wall may also be responsible for the appearance of true diverticula at an early age in connective tissue disorders such as Ehlers-Danlos and Marfan syndromes and in autosomal-dominant polycystic kidney disease.

DIFFERENTIAL DIAGNOSIS

Many conditions, especially those associated with altered intestinal motility, may be confused with diverticular disease. The most common of these is irritable bowel syndrome, although the most important entity to consider is carcinoma. Both diverticular disease and carcinoma are common and are most frequently seen in elderly. Symptomatic diverticular disease can also mimic a variety of other diseases, such as acute appendicitis, ischemic colitis, pseudomembranous colitis, renal disease, cystitis, ovarian cyst, abscess or tumor, gallbladder disease, pancreatic disease, mucosal prolapse, small bowel obstruction, and peritonitis.

HISTORY

Most patients with diverticulosis coli have no or minor symptoms. Some patients have intermittent abdominal pain, bloating, excessive flatulence, and irregular defecation. Nausea, anorexia, the passage of pellet-like stools, or attacks of diarrhea may also be present.

Diverticulitis results from inflammation of a colonic diverticulum, and it is the most common complication of diverticulosis, occurring in 10% to 25% of patients. Diverticulitis is thought to be a result of fecal matter that has become inspissated within a diverticulum that will produce localized inflammation. This inflammatory process then proceeds to either a microperforation or a macroperforation. In case of a microperforation or uncomplicated diverticulitis, the most common symptoms include left lower quadrant pain and fever. The pain in this case is acute in onset, severe, and persistent. Associated symptoms may include nausea, vomiting, constipation, diarrhea, dysuria, and urinary frequency. A more complicated form of diverticulitis results from macroperforation. Either free perforation with generalized peritonitis or a walled off pericolonic abscess may occur. The septic process may erode into adjacent structures and produce a fistula. The most common fistula is colovesical presenting with recurrent urinary tract infections and pneumaturia; other common fistulae are colocutaneous, colovaginal, and coloenteric. Uncommon fistulae include those between the colon and ureter, uterus, fallopian tube, and perineum.

Diverticular bleeding is not due to an acute or chronic inflammatory process. As previously noted, the pseudodiverticula of diverticulosis coli occur at the site of anatomic penetration of nutrient vessels through the bowel wall. Should one of these nutrient vessels erode or simply rupture, painless lower intestinal bleeding ensues. The location of the leaking vessel and the rate of bleeding determine the patient's clinical course. The bleeding episode may be insignificant and self-limited or may be exsanguinating and life-threatening. Passed blood may be bright red but more commonly is maroon. Diverticular bleeding is one of the most common causes of lower gastrointestinal bleeding.

PHYSICAL EXAMINATION AND CLINICAL FINDINGS

For the patient experiencing only abdominal cramps and constipation, the physical examination is unremarkable, and only the patient's age may suggest the possibility of diverticulosis coli. Once inflammation arises within a diverticulum, the physical findings usually reflect both the extent and location of the process. Usually abdominal tenderness is present, characteristically in the left lower quadrant. When the inflammatory process is locally extensive or a contained abscess has developed, a tender abdominal mass is palpable and abdominal distension is common. A pelvic and rectal examination should be performed to define the mass. Further diagnostic studies are required to differentiate a diverticular abscess from a locally perforated neoplasm. A spiking fever usually occurs once an abscess has developed. Right lower quadrant tenderness usually results from diverticulitis in a redundant sigmoid colon or right-sided diverticulitis. Generalized tenderness and abdominal wall rigidity suggest free perforation and peritonitis.

If a fistula has developed, the patient may present with feculent vaginal discharge or chronic perineal soilage from colovaginal involvement, pneumaturia, or fecaluria from a colovesical fistula. If the patient presents with bleeding from diverticulosis coli, it is likely that no other unusual physical findings will be present.

DIAGNOSTIC STUDIES

Most patients with diverticulosis coli are asymptomatic and are identified only at the time of either screening colonoscopy or barium enema. In acute diverticulitis, the white blood cell count is usually elevated with a predominance of polymorphonuclear leukocytes. Urinalysis may reveal pyuria if the inflammatory process is adjacent to either the ureter or the bladder, and bacteriuria may suggest a colovesical fistula.

Computed tomography (CT) has become the optimal method of investigation in patients suspected of having acute diverticulitis. It is useful for diagnosis, assessment of severity, therapeutic intervention, and quantification of resolution of the disease. The sensitivity, specificity, positive, and negative predictive values of helical CT (with colonic contrast only) were 97%, 100%, 100%, and 98%, respectively, in a study that included 150 patients presenting to the emergency department with clinically suspected diverticulitis. Criteria suggestive of diverticulitis on CT include the presence of diverticula with increased soft tissue density within pericolic fat secondary to inflammation, thickening of the colonic wall, and soft tissue masses or fluid collections representing phlegmons or abscesses. CT can also identify the major complications of diverticulitis, including peritonitis, fistula formation (usually inferred from extraluminal air collections in the bladder, vagina, or abdominal wall), and obstruction. CT can be used as a therapeutic modality. Percutaneous drainage of localized abscesses can be done by CT guidance, thereby downstaging complicated diverticulitis, avoiding emergent surgery, and permitting single-stage elective surgical resection.

Contrast enema may play a complementary role to CT; it is safe in the acute phase if performed by the single contrast technique. Barium is absolutely contraindicated if peritonitis is present or perforation is suspected. Water-soluble contrast enemas are preferred and used even in the absence of these findings because an unexpected leak may be found.

Based on its relatively low cost, convenience, and noninvasive nature, high-resolution, graded, compression ultrasonography is a new method being used to evaluate diverticulitis. Characteristic findings include hypoechoic bowel wall thickening, presence of diverticula or abscesses, and hyperechogenicity surrounding the bowel wall, implying active inflammation. Reported sensitivities range from 85% to 98% and specificities from 80% to 98%. Although routine ultrasound may be useful in excluding pelvic and gynecologic pathology in elderly women, it remains a second-line diagnostic tool because it is operator dependent, and its utility is poorly defined.

In cases of diverticular bleeding, the early use of colonoscopy is warranted for the acutely bleeding but hemodynamically stable patient. In such patients, total colonoscopy is the procedure of choice. In expert hands bleeding sites have been identified in up to 85% of patients and these can be treated acutely. In patients with brisk bleeding, emergency angiography of the superior and inferior mesenteric arteries has become the initial procedure of choice; it is both specific and highly sensitive if the rate of bleeding is sufficient (0.5–1.0 mL/min). Nuclear scanning techniques may be useful to pinpoint the bleeding site in patients who experience a slower rate of bleeding.

MANAGEMENT

Good dietary habits at a young age may prevent the later development of diverticula and their complications. This includes the consumption of natural grain breads, fruits with high fiber content, beans, and leafy vegetables. Many patients find it difficult to ingest the needed 20 to 30 g of fiber per day from dietary foods. The addition of bulk-forming agents in the form of bran or psyllium provides effective supplements to dietary fiber.

Acute Diverticulitis

UNCOMPLICATED DIVERTICULITIS

Patients can be treated on an outpatient basis if they have minimal symptoms or signs of inflammation, no peritoneal signs, and have the ability to take oral fluids. A clear liquid diet is recommended, and broad-spectrum oral antibiotics such as metronidazole and ciprofloxacin are continued for 7 to 10 days. Two exceptions to this approach are immunosuppressed patients and diabetics, who should not be treated as outpatients.

If signs of significant inflammation are present, then the patient needs to be hospitalized for bowel rest, intravenous fluids, and broad-spectrum intravenous antibiotics Antibiotic choice should include agents that are effective against common enteric organisms (both aerobes and anaerobes). If pain medication is required, parenteral meperidine hydrochloride is an appropriate analgesic because it has been shown to decrease intraluminal pressure. Improvement in most patients occurs in the first 48 to 72 hours, diet is resumed, and the patient may be discharged to complete a 7- to 10-day course of oral antibiotics as an outpatient. A high-fiber diet supplemented with psyllium is often recommended. Barium enema or preferably colonoscopy is usually performed 4 to 6 weeks after resolution of symptoms to exclude other diagnostic considerations such as colonic neoplasia.

Only 20% to 30% of patients have a recurrent episode of diverticulitis. If the patient suffers a second attack of diverticulitis requiring antibiotic treatment, surgical treatment should be considered. Diverticulitis is relatively uncommon in patients under 40 years of age, and there seems to be a male predominance in this age group. A more aggressive course of the disease has been reported in young patients. Elective surgery should be considered after only one episode of diverticulitis in a young patient.

Several surgical options are available; the choice is dictated by the acuteness of the disease or its complications and the experience of the surgeon. These options include resection and primary anastomosis, resection with sigmoid colostomy and closure of the rectal stump (Hartman procedure), transverse colostomy and drainage, and laparoscopic colectomy.

COMPLICATED DIVERTICULITIS

Formation of abscesses, fistulae, or free perforation into the abdominal cavity with subsequent peritonitis may complicate acute diverticulitis. The management of diverticular abscesses should be individualized to their size and complexity. Small pericolic abscesses can be often be treated with antibiotics and bowel rest. For distant abscesses or unresolving abscesses, drainage is indicated. CT-guided percutaneous drainage of abdominal abscesses will often eliminate the need for a two-stage procedure with colostomy, instead allowing for temporary palliative drainage and a subsequent single-stage resection in 3 to 4 weeks.

When a diverticular phlegmon or abscess extends or ruptures into an adjacent organ, fistulae may occur. This is a relatively frequent complication of diverticulitis and has been reported in 5% to 33% of diverticular disease patients requiring an operation. A colovesical fistula is the most common type, occurring more often in men than women with sex ratios ranging from 2:1 to 6:1. This gender difference is attributed to the protection the bladder is given by the uterus. Treatment of fistulae require control of sepsis followed by preoperative bowel preparation and a single-stage operative resection with fistula closure and primary anastomosis.

Acute free perforation requires aggressive preoperative resuscitation and emergency laparotomy. Guidelines for emergency operations for patients who have generalized peritonitis secondary to perforated diverticulitis include limiting the extent of resection to the perforated segment, irrigating the abdominal cavity and drainage of any residual infected cavities, and creating a temporary proximal diverting colostomy.

Antibiotics should be continued until evidence of infection has resolved. Enteral nutrition may be started with return of colostomy function. If the patient's course is complicated and prolonged, then total parenteral nutrition should be instituted. Once the patient has totally recuperated from such an operation (usually several months), colostomy closure may be considered.

Bleeding Diverticulosis Coli

In most patients with diverticular hemorrhage, the bleeding stops spontaneously. For patients who continue to bleed and have their bleeding confirmed angiographically, a trial of selective intra-arterial vasopressin is indicated. This can be temporarily effective in controlling the hemorrhage, but rebleeding occurs in up to half of these patients after withdrawal of vasopressin. Emergency surgery is indicated in the treatment of persistent or recurrent bleeding. Appropriate segmental colectomy yields a very low rebleeding rate. Subtotal colectomy may be needed and remains the preferred option in cases where the bleeding site is not isolated.

CONSIDERATIONS IN PREGNANCY

Because diverticular disease primarily afflicts postmenopausal women, it rarely, if ever, complicates pregnancy. However, if patients of childbearing age do develop symptomatic diverticulitis, they should be managed just like anyone else. Both the patient and her physician should not be surprised if her course is of a virulent nature that might require surgical intervention at some future time. If diverticulitis (or one of its complications) does develop during pregnancy, the patient should be treated aggressively with antibiotics. Obviously, if surgery is required, the risk to the pregnancy is significant and the patient's obstetrician should be closely involved in the patient's care.

BIBLIOGRAPHY

Aldoori WH, Giovannucci EL, Rimm EB, et al. A prospective study of alcohol, smoking, caffeine, and the risk of symptomatic diverticular disease in men. *Ann Epidemiol* 1995;5:221.

Aldoori WH, Giovannucci EL, Rimm EB, et al. Prospective study of physical activity and the risk of symptomatic diverticular disease. *Gut* 1995;36:276.

Farrel RJ, Farrell JJ, Morrin MM. Diverticular disease in the elderly. *Gastroenterol Clin* 2001;2.

Hachigian MP, Honickman S, Eisenstat TE, et al. Computed tomography in the initial management of acute left-sided diverticulitis. *Dis Col Rectum* 1992;35: 1123.

Konvolinka CW. Acute diverticulitis under age forty. *Am J Surg* 1994;167:562.

Liberman MA, Phillips EH, Carroll BJ, et al. Laparoscopic colectomy vs. traditional colectomy for diverticulitis: outcome and costs. *Surg Endosc* 1996;10:15.

Neff CC, van Sonneberg E, Casola G, et al. Diverticular abscesses: percutaneous drainage. *Radiology* 1987;163:15.

Painter NS, Burkitt DP. Diverticular disease of the colon: a deficiency of Western civilization. *Br Med J* 1971;2:450.

Rao PM, Rhea JT, Novelline RA, et al. Helical CT with only colonic contrast material for diagnosing diverticulitis: prospective evaluation of 150 patients. *AJR Am J Roentgenol* 1998;170:1445.

Rege RV, Nahrwold DL. Diverticular disease. *Curr Probl Surg* 1989;26:133.

Scheff RT, Zuckerman G, Harter H, et al. Diverticular disease in patients with chronic renal failure due to polycystic kidney disease. *Ann Intern Med* 1980;92:202.

Sleisenger & Fordtran's gastrointestinal and liver disease, 7th ed. 2002:2100–2112.

Smajda C, Sbai I, Tahrat M, et al. Elective sigmoid colectomy for diverticulitis: results of a prospective study. *Surg Endosc* 1999;13:645.

Stabile BE, Puccio E, van Sonneberg E, et al. Preoperative percutaneous drainage of diverticular abscesses. *Am J Surg* 1990;159:99.

Stevenson AR, Stitz RW, Lumley JW, et al. Laparoscopically assisted anterior resection for diverticular disease. *Ann Surg* 1998;227:335.

Stollman N, Raskin J. Diagnosis and management of diverticular disease of the colon in adults. *Am J Gastroenterol* 1999;94:3110.

Wess L, Eastwood MA, Wess TJ, et al. Cross linking of collagen is decreased in colonic diverticulosis. 1995;37:91.

Yacoe ME, Jeffrey RB Jr. Sonography of appendicitis and diverticulitis. *Radiol Clin North Am* 1994;32:899.

Zielke A, Hasse C, Nies C, et al. Prospective evaluation of ultrasonography in acute diverticulitis. *Br J Surg* 1997;84:385.

CHAPTER 71
Constipation

Harlan G. Rich

Constipation is one of the most common digestive complaints in the general population, accounting for an estimated 2.5 million physician visits per year. The cost of evaluating and treating these patients is substantial. A methodical approach in the primary care setting should help to provide symptomatic relief, exclude serious or life-threatening disease, and minimize unnecessary testing.

The primary physiologic functions of the colon are to absorb fluid and electrolytes flowing into it from the small intestine and to store the residual fecal material until an acceptable time arises to allow for defecation. The frequency of bowel movements varies among healthy individuals, from three stools per day to three stools per week. A bowel habit that is "normal" for one patient (size, shape, consistency, frequency), however, may not be "normal" for another. One patient's description of "constipation" may be consistent with another patient's concept of normal bowel function.

Patient's definitions of constipation may include straining to pass fecal material, passing hard stools, infrequent passage of stools, or an inability to defecate at will. A generally accepted definition is passing fewer than three stools per week. The consensus diagnostic criteria for functional constipation, developed by an international panel of experts, is met by having two or more of the following symptoms for at least 12 (not necessarily consecutive) weeks:

- Straining in greater than 25% of defecations
- Lumpy or hard stools in greater than 25% of defecations
- Sensation of incomplete evacuation in greater than 25% of defecations
- Sensation of anorectal obstruction or blockade in greater than 25% of defecations
- Manual maneuvers to facilitate greater than 25% of defecations
- Less than three defecations per week.

These definitions assume no structural or biochemical explanation for the symptoms. Note also that using this classification, patients may be diagnosed as constipated even with daily bowel movements.

The epidemiology of constipation varies based on the definition used and on whether constipation is self-reported or measured in a clinical research center. The prevalence of constipation in the United States is estimated at 2% to 3% of the general adult population and is reported to be as high as 20% to 30% in persons age 70 and older. Females are twice as likely to report constipation as males. The difference in prevalence persists from middle to old age.

In the primary care setting, a complaint of constipation needs to be investigated to determine the nature and severity of the problem. If the patient's bowel habits are not out of the realm of normal, education may be all that is necessary, because reassurance removes significant anxiety. If the initial assessment suggests gastrointestinal tract dysfunction, further evaluation is required to determine the nature of the problem and to provide appropriate therapy.

ETIOLOGY

The etiology of constipation can be broken down into extracolonic and colonic causes. The extracolonic causes include metabolic, endocrine, neurologic, and motor disorders and drug therapies that decrease colonic motility. The colonic causes are divided into structural and functional causes. The structural group includes obstructive processes and intestinal aganglionosis (i.e., Hirschsprung disease). The functional causes are subdivided into two broad categories, slow colonic transit and anorectal dysfunction, and have no anatomic correlates.

Metabolic abnormalities associated with constipation include uremia, hypokalemia, hypomagnesemia, porphyria, amyloidosis (causing a neuropathy), diabetes, and hypercalcemia. Endocrine disorders associated with constipation include hypothyroidism, pseudohypoparathyroidism, pheochromocytoma, glucagon-producing tumors, and disorders that lead to hypercalcemia (e.g., primary hyperparathyroidism, milk alkali syndrome, disseminated bony metastasis). Neurologic causes of constipation include lesions of the central and peripheral nervous systems. Central lesions include cerebral tumors, injury secondary to cerebrovascular accident, Parkinson disease, and multiple sclerosis. The peripheral nervous system disorders associated with constipation include autonomic neuropathy, lumbosacral spine injury, meningomyelocele, or sacral nerve (parasympathetic) injury. Motor disorders include amyloidosis, scleroderma, myotonic dystrophy, and dermatomyositis.

Many medications can lead to constipation. The most commonly implicated include narcotic analgesics, muscle relaxants, calcium or aluminum-containing antacids, diuretics, medications used to treat Parkinson disease, antidepressants, monoamine oxidase inhibitors, antipsychotics, calcium or iron supplements, anticholinergics, and calcium channel blockers. Chronic laxative abuse, particularly with hydroxymethylanthraquinone-containing agents such as senna and cascara, has been thought to cause damage to the myenteric plexus of the colon and subsequent dysmotility and constipation.

Obstructive processes may be extrinsic or intrinsic to the lumen of the colon. Extraluminal obstruction may be caused by extrinsic tumors, chronic volvulus, or hernias. Intraluminal obstruction of the colon and rectum may be caused by benign or malignant tumors or benign strictures related to inflammation (diverticular or ischemic) or after surgical reconstruction. Descending perineum syndrome (descent or "ballooning" of the perineum below the level of the ischial tuberosities with straining, often associated with impaired straightening of the rectoanal angle) and rectocele may both be seen after childbirth and can lead to obstructed defecation. Lesions of the anal canal, including stenosis, tumors, anal fissures, intussusception, and mucosal prolapse, can all play a role in constipation. Hemorrhoids are not a cause of constipation, although some argue that hemorrhoids can be worsened by chronic constipation.

Slow transit constipation may be associated with dietary or cultural phenomena or abnormal colonic motility. Motility studies may show decreased propagation of contractions and retention of feces in the right colon or increased uncoordinated contractions in the distal colon that functionally reduce normal transit. The etiology is unknown, but muscular, neurologic, or even psychological problems may play a role.

Anorectal (also known as defecatory or pelvic floor) dysfunction may be associated with normal or delayed colonic transit and is notable for storage of fecal residue in the rectum. For defecation to proceed smoothly, there must be coordination between the rectum and the anus. As the rectum contracts to expel the stool, the anus must relax to open the rectal outlet and allow passage of the fecal mass. Failure of this coordination leads to anorectal dysfunction and constipation. Failure of the rectum to contract is known as rectal inertia; failure of the anus to relax is called outlet obstruction. Anismus describes the failure of the anal sphincters to relax; anorectal dyssynergia is used to indicate a failure to relax or inappropriate contraction of the puborectalis and external anal sphincter muscles during defecation. Rarely, patients will have features of both slow transit constipation and anorectal dysfunction. Evacuatory dysfunction needs to be ruled out before any consideration is made about surgical therapy for intractable constipation (see below).

Numerous factors may account for the increased prevalence of functional constipation seen in women. Studies have suggested that female patients with slow transit constipation may have diminished sex hormone levels during each of the phases of the menstrual cycle and altered patterns of secretion of gut regulatory peptides. Constipation has been reported as a consequence of hysterectomy, although the mechanism (altered hormonal levels, iatrogenic pelvic nerve injury, psychological) is unclear. Women with idiopathic constipation have been shown to have significantly increased levels of anxiety, depression, and somatization, as well as impaired intimate relations. Several studies have correlated specific "biopsychosocial" factors with constipation in both males and females, including low income, low educational level, low caloric intake, low activity level, and an increased number of medications taken. A history of childhood, physical, or sexual abuse is present in many of these patients and has been independently associated with poorer health status and increased visceral and/or psychological perception of "normal" gut stimuli. Other studies suggest that psychological factors may influence gut function via an effect on extrinsic autonomic neural pathways.

HISTORY

A good history provides the foundation for all further evaluation and therapy. Because constipation is a symptom, an accurate description of the problem from the patient's point of view is crucial. For instance, is the chief complaint straining at stools, but with a normal number of bowel movements? Is infrequent defecation the greatest concern? Does the patient have the urge to defecate? Does she ignore or postpone defecation? Does she self-digitate or put pressure on her perineum to evacuate? Does the patient have episodic diarrhea, and if so what is the relation to diet or laxative use? Has she lost weight, or does she have abdominal pain? The nature of the stool (e.g., hard or soft, small or large, brown or bloody or melenic) should be determined. Accurate documentation of the patient's typical bowel habits (e.g., timing, frequency, amount of time spent straining, usual result) is required. This is best accomplished via the maintenance of a symptom diary.

One of the most important points in the history is the onset of constipation. If it has been since birth, a congenital abnormality, idiopathic megarectum, or Hirschsprung disease should be considered. If the patient is middle aged and the symptoms are chronic (>2 years), it is less likely that significant pathology is to blame. However, if the onset was less than 2 years before presentation, the risk of a partially obstructing colonic malignancy should be considered. The patient should also be interviewed to determine whether any association exists between episodes of childbirth (leading to pelvic floor injury) and the onset of constipation.

The patient's diet (particularly the amount and sources of fiber in the diet) and use of medications (especially laxatives, enemas, or suppositories) are also important. Prescribed and over-the-counter medications (including agents obtained in health food stores or from nontraditional medical providers) should be reviewed, with potential constipating agents noted.

A thorough review of systems may help to rule out systemic or neurologic disorders with constipation as a secondary effect. A history of abuse should be carefully elicited by sensitive questioning, particularly in patients in whom a diagnosis of functional constipation is suspected or confirmed.

PHYSICAL EXAMINATION AND CLINICAL FINDINGS

The physical examination is as important as the history. A complete examination is useful to rule out other medical problems contributing to or causing constipation. In particular, stigmata of systemic diseases (e.g., hypothyroidism) or metabolic abnormalities should be noted.

Examination of the abdomen should note the presence and activity level of bowel sounds. Palpable masses may indicate a near-obstructing lesion. Lower quadrant tenderness may indicate an active inflammatory process such as diverticulitis. Hard formed stool may sometimes be palpated in the colon. Hernias may cause partial obstruction, can present with the complaint of constipation, and should be sought on physical examination. Femoral hernias are more common in women than in men and may be overlooked on a cursory examination.

Examination of the anus, rectum, and perineum may be the most revealing part of the examination. Perineal innervation may be investigated by assessing perianal sensation and anal reflex contraction to light stroking or scratching of the perianal skin. Gross examination of the anus may show it to be patulous, asymmetric, or lax, suggesting a neurologic disorder. It may also show evidence of local trauma such as abrasions or multiple fissures. Both of these signs have been linked to sexual abuse and may lead to direct questioning. Digital examination of the anus and rectum assesses the content of the rectal vault and helps to rule out mass lesions, fissures, or hemorrhoids. Anal fissures cause enough pain and swelling that patients refrain from defecating, causing a functional outlet obstruction and hardening of the stools, which worsens the problem. Fecal impaction can quickly convince the physician of the diagnosis of constipation.

The digital examination can give a reasonable assessment of sphincter function and basic anorectal coordination. The patient is asked to bear down as if to strain against stool, and the physician notes the behavior of the internal and external anal sphincters. If the normal anorectal reflex is present, straining should lead to contraction of the external sphincter and relaxation of the internal anal sphincter. If the patient contracts the puborectalis and external anal sphincters instead, a diagnosis of anismus can be considered. Descent of the perineum below the ischial tuberosities with straining may help confirm a diagnosis of descending perineum syndrome. A pelvic examination should be performed to rule out a rectocele.

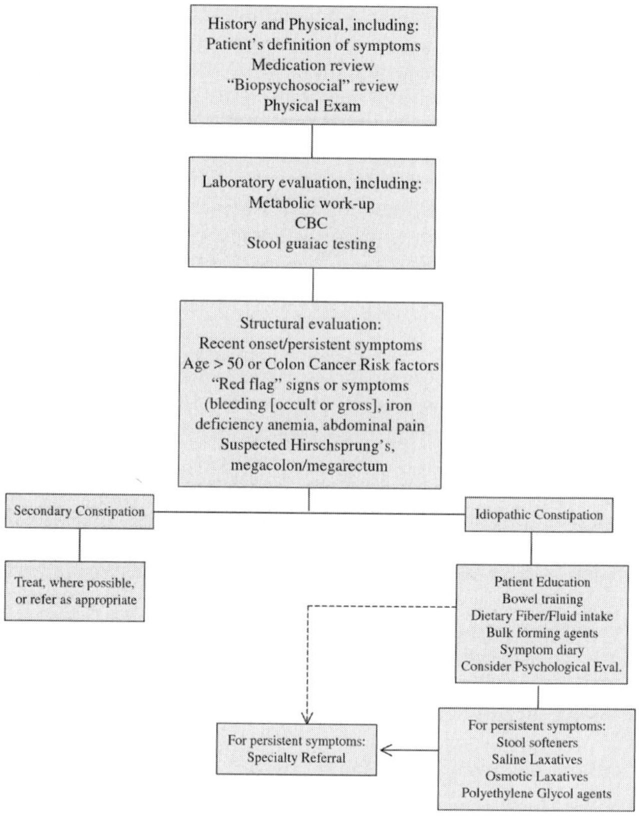

FIG. 71.1. Suggested evaluation and management of patients with constipation in the primary care setting.

LABORATORY AND IMAGING STUDIES

Laboratory and imaging studies used in the evaluation of constipation in the primary care setting are relatively few and simple (Fig. 71.1). However, for patients who fail routine management and have no identifiable anatomic pathology, the number of studies used for evaluation increases greatly, as does their complexity.

Laboratory studies useful in the evaluation of patients with constipation include serum chemistries (important to rule out diabetes, hypokalemia, hypomagnesemia, hypercalcemia, and uremia) and thyroid function tests. A blood count with red blood cell volume is done to rule out a microcytic anemia.

Studies of the gastrointestinal tract can be divided into anatomic/structural and functional studies. Anatomic studies address mechanical obstructions, pseudoobstruction, and histologic disease (aganglionosis [Hirschsprung disease]). They are indicated in the initial evaluation of all patients older than age 30 who are presenting with new onset of symptoms (<2 years) if unexplained by other causes. Anatomic studies are also indicated if gross or occult rectal blood is found during a routine examination or by history. These studies can be either endoscopic or radiographic. Sigmoidoscopy (which may be performed in the primary care office setting) or colonoscopy allows direct visualization and tissue biopsy. Colonoscopy is preferred in patients with evidence of gastrointestinal blood loss, iron deficiency anemia, or who are otherwise appropriate for colon cancer screening (whether average or high risk). Barium enema may also be a suitable study, offering a similar sensitivity but less specificity due to the inability to gather histologic data. When megacolon or megarectum is suspected by history, barium enema is the better examination. Some centers prefer Gastrografin or other water-soluble agents to minimize problems with evacuation of the contrast after the study.

Once this initial evaluation is completed, a tentative diagnosis can be assigned and treatment initiated. The response to medical management, such as behavioral and dietary changes, should be carefully assessed in patients who have no anatomic or secondary causes of constipation. If there is no response, the addition of supplemental bran fiber or bulking agents should be tried. A small percentage of patients may fail this trial and are classified as refractory to treatment. Further workup by a specialist is then in order. This evaluation involves the assessment of colonic motility and pelvic floor function and must be done in an organized fashion for best results. Fig. 71.2 is a simplified outline of evaluation and treatment options.

A colonic marker transit study can objectively confirm the patient's subjective complaints and documents slow colonic transit. Twenty to 30 radiopaque markers are ingested, and their passage through the colon is monitored by serial abdominal flat plates over a 5-day period. An abnormal transit time is greater than 72 hours. Serial abdominal films may show segmental transit variations (generalized slow transit, left colonic dysfunction, or pelvic floor/rectal dysfunction). The marker transit test is a safe, reliable, and reproducible measure of colonic transit time and is sufficient to rule out colonic dysmotility. A normal study may provide some overall reassurance about colonic function. If the transit time is normal and the patient has no symptoms of defecatory dysfunction (e.g., excessive straining, digital disimpaction), a trial with bulking agents or a colonic cleansing agent is made. If the colonic transit is increased and the patient fails to respond to a therapeutic trial or if the patient has concurrent symptoms of obstructed defeca-

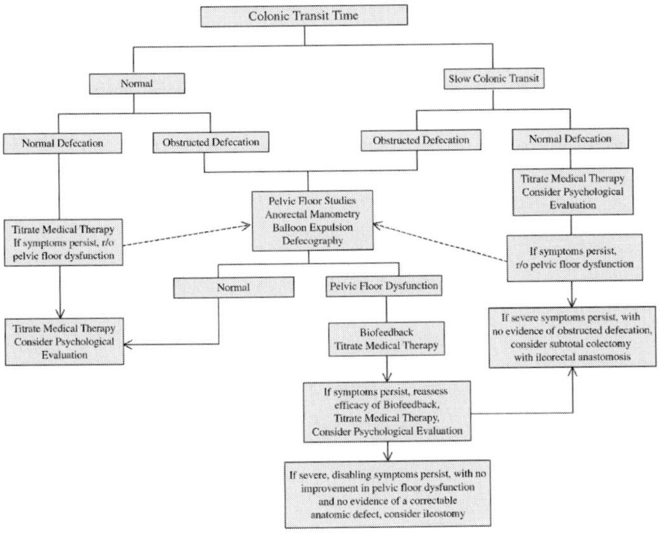

FIG. 71.2. Suggested evaluation and management of patients without secondary or anatomic causes of constipation who are refractory to conservative treatment.

tion, the patient should be evaluated for evidence of pelvic floor dysfunction. Psychological evaluation may be helpful in further assessment of patients with no clearly defined functional abnormalities.

The complex nature of the anatomy and function of the pelvic floor and anus is reflected in the number and diversity of studies designed to describe and quantify their integrated function. A diagnosis of pelvic floor dysfunction is confirmed when two or more of the following studies are abnormal.

Anorectal manometry is done using a catheter placed through the anus and into the rectum. Resting, straining, and squeeze pressures from the rectal and anal canals are measured. Sensation and the rectoanal inhibitory response can be assessed via balloon distension. This test may be helpful to exclude Hirschsprung disease and to provide support for a diagnosis of pelvic floor dyssynergia.

The *balloon expulsion test* helps to screen for pelvic floor dysfunction or anismus. A balloon is inserted into the rectum and filled with 50 mL of warm water. The patient's ability to expel the balloon is tested with and without the addition of weight to the balloon. Normal patients spontaneously pass the balloon. Some patients with defecatory disorders cannot expel the balloon spontaneously or require a significant amount of weight to be added to expel the balloon.

Defecography allows an anatomic and functional evaluation of the process of defecation and is reserved primarily for patients with suspected obstructed defecation or pelvic floor dysfunction. The evacuation of barium paste is monitored fluoroscopically. The anorectal angle, which normally straightens upon defecation, may fail to open or actually narrow in patients with pelvic floor dyssynergia. Pelvic floor descent may be decreased in patients with anismus (impaired pelvic floor relaxation) or increased in patients with descending perineum syndrome. Rectal prolapse, rectal intussusception, and rectocele may be visualized by this technique. When done in conjunction with a barium enema, other structural anomalies can be excluded.

Electromyography can evaluate pudendal nerve activity in the puborectalis muscle and the anal sphincter during straining. Surface electrodes measure global activity and are generally used in conjunction with manometry. Concentric needle electromyography is a more highly specialized form of testing and can selectively evaluate the external sphincter and pelvic floor muscles. These studies can demonstrate abnormal continued electrical activity in the external anal sphincter during straining, confirming the diagnosis of anismus.

TREATMENT

The treatment offered to a patient complaining of constipation is guided by the initial evaluation. If the patient is found to have normal bowel habits, teaching and reassurance may reduce distress. The initial evaluation will help rule out structural or metabolic abnormalities requiring specific treatment. Patients with secondary causes of constipation should be treated medically, where possible, or surgically, as appropriate. For the remaining patients, including those with secondary causes that lack specific therapy (e.g., amyloidosis), a care plan for functional constipation can be formulated. If the patient uses laxatives, a trial without them is important to assess baseline bowel function.

Education is of utmost importance. This starts with a discussion of toilet training and bowel habit. Patients should be encouraged not to suppress the urge to defecate, because doing so promotes constipation. Patients should try to defecate after a specific meal, establishing a routine. Increased activity may also be important, because physically active people tend to experience less constipation than people who are sedentary.

An increase in dietary fiber to 20 to 35 g/d, together with adequate fluid intake, is a very effective way to eliminate constipation. This can usually be accomplished by eating raw fruits and vegetables, along with whole grain breads and breakfast cereals. Increased dietary fiber results in increased water retention and subsequently increased stool weight. This usually provides larger and softer stools, which are more easily passed. Many people find it difficult to attain this goal for dietary fiber. Adding 20 g of wheat bran to the daily diet guarantees sufficient dietary fiber.

If the patient finds dietary adjustments too difficult or distasteful, bulking agents can be added instead of natural fiber. These include psyllium, methylcellulose, malt soup extract, and polycarbophil. A total of 4 to 12 g/d significantly increases stool bulk. For most patients seen in routine practice, the addition of a bulking agent leads to the resolution of constipation, but for some organic causes of constipation (obstruction or megacolon/megarectum), bulking agents actually worsen the symptoms. Patients with pelvic floor dysfunction may also not see any benefit.

Patients should not expect immediate results from either of these maneuvers. Fiber intake may need to be gradually increased to minimize bloating or flatulence; these symptoms usually abate after several days. Patients may also need to titrate their fiber intake up or down to an acceptable bowel habit.

Numerous other laxative preparations exist, but ideally their use should be confined to short-term trials in an effort to clean out the bowel. Osmotic agents include both saline laxatives and nonabsorbed sugars. Saline laxatives include magnesium citrate, magnesium hydroxide (milk of magnesia), magnesium sulfate, and the sodium phosphates. Most of these should be avoided in patients with CHF, renal failure, or other sodium avid states. The nonabsorbed sugars include lactulose, lactitol, sorbitol, and mannitol. These agents provide an osmotic load that leads to increased water retention in the colon and subsequently in the stool. The overall effect is increased water retention, with subsequent increased bulk and softness of the stools. The nonabsorbed sugars are also metabolized in the gut lumen to form short-chain fatty acids. Bacterial metabolism may lead to the production of intestinal gas, an undesirable side effect. The salts and the nonabsorbed sugars are harmless when used in moderation, but long-term frequent use is unwarranted without further workup of the etiology of the constipation.

Polyethylene glycol is manufactured both with and without added salts. The "pure" form (e.g., Miralax) functions as an osmotic agent; the preparations with added salts (e.g., Colyte, Nulytely, GoLYTELY) are isoosmotic and function as oral washout solutions. Either form can be used with success; 250 to 500 mL can be given orally at night.

Emollient laxatives work by increasing the mixture of fatty and aqueous substances in the stool. These are detergents such as docusate sodium and are sometimes referred to as stool softeners. Although they are probably not harmful, their benefit is dubious and has not been proven in clinical studies. Lubricant laxatives generally rely on mineral oil in some form and can be taken orally or as a retention enema. Routine oral use can result in decreased absorption of the fat-soluble vitamins and subsequent problems. Stimulant laxatives work by stimulating the smooth muscle of the colon to contract and by causing increased secretory activity in the colon. These include bisacodyl, cascara sagrada, castor oil, and senna. Concerns have been raised that the anthraquinone derivatives (senna, cascara) may injure the enteric nervous system. Stimulant laxatives are highly effective in the short term, but the side-effect profile and these other concerns suggest they have no role in the long-term management of constipation.

In the past, prokinetic agents such as metoclopramide or cisapride were used to treat constipation, often with disappointing results. Tegaserod maleate, a type 4 5-hydroxytryptamine receptor agonist, was approved by the U.S. Food and Drug Administration in July 2002 for use in patients with constipation-predominant irritable bowel syndrome. This agent appears to increase gastrointestinal transit and reduce symptoms of visceral hypersensitivity, including pain and bloating, and has a favorable safety profile.

Patients with pelvic floor dysfunction and normal colonic transit times may benefit from conservative treatment with electromyographic biofeedback. Success in correcting inappropriate pelvic floor contraction and restoring normal coordination is reported in over 70% to 80% of patients in intensive programs. Success rates are lower for patients with descending perineum syndrome. Some studies support the use of concurrent psychotherapy or training in relaxation techniques. There is little to no morbidity associated with this approach.

Conservative therapy in slow colonic transit constipation will fail in a small percentage of patients. Patients who have undergone an aggressive protracted trial of dietary and medical therapy and who have severe disabling symptoms may be considered for subtotal colectomy with ileorectal anastomosis. Anorectal dysfunction and pseudoobstruction should be excluded. Some authorities also recommend evaluating patients for and excluding those with evidence of total gastrointestinal tract dysmotility. Patients must be aware that surgery may improve their bowel habit but may not necessarily relieve other symptoms (e.g., pain, bloating). In skilled hands, this operation has a low morbidity and mortality; results have shown most patients having three or four stools per day for the first 2 years and two to three stools per day after this. Recurrence rates of constipation are very low. With appropriate patient selection, excellent results can be expected. In large tertiary referral centers, only 5% of patients are ultimately referred for operative management.

Some patients with significant pelvic floor dysfunction and normal colonic transit times may fail biofeedback and suffer severely from their constipation. Those who fail should continue with conservative management and undergo psychological evaluation. Very rarely, patients with a markedly impaired quality of life may be treated via creation of an ileostomy.

Patients with prolonged colonic transit time and pelvic floor dysfunction may be the most difficult to treat. Most authorities suggest that the pelvic floor dysfunction should be addressed first. Patients with mucosal or rectal prolapse, rectocele, or intussusception can be considered for surgical repair. Some reports suggest that these do not affect the outcome of conservative management, nor that surgical repair consistently improves patient outcomes. Patients with persistent symptoms should have a psychological evaluation followed by a therapeutic trial of biofeedback. If constipation persists and is thought to be secondary to slow colonic transit, conservative therapy should be attempted. If this fails, the patient can be referred for subtotal colectomy with ileorectal anastomosis. Success rates in these patients are lower than in patients with colonic inertia alone, related primarily to continuing problems with obstructed defecation.

The evaluation and treatment of patients with intractable constipation must be done carefully, with strict adherence to the plan and careful interpretation of test results. If patients with slow colonic transit or pelvic floor dysfunction are carefully selected, surgical intervention or biofeedback has a high likelihood of success. An integrated approach is important in these patients. Patients with psychological problems underlying constipation frequently have persistent symptoms postoperatively; consideration may be given to excluding them from this treatment option.

CONSIDERATIONS IN PREGNANCY

Abnormalities of motility have been reported in most segments of the gastrointestinal tract of pregnant women. These contribute to common complaints such as nausea, vomiting, heartburn, and the high incidence of gallstones and biliary tract disease. The prevalence of constipation in pregnancy has been reported to be between 11% and 38%. Constipation may develop during pregnancy related to behavioral, physiologic, or mechanical processes.

Behavioral changes may include decreased fluid intake (particularly in association with hyperemesis), decreased fiber intake, and decreased physical activity. Physiologic changes may contribute to constipation, particularly in the second and third trimesters. Estrogen and progesterone levels rise progressively through pregnancy. Progesterone alone has been demonstrated to reduce the force of contraction in colonic circular and longitudinal smooth muscle. Several studies suggest that elevations of both estrogen and progesterone lead to a prolongation of colonic transit time. The mechanism by which this occurs may relate to alterations in calcium flux across cell membranes or to an increase in the release of nitric oxide from inhibitory nonadrenergic noncholinergic neurons within the myenteric plexus. Motilin levels decrease through the second and third trimester and normalize in the postpartum period. Motilin is known to stimulate the interdigestive migrating motor complex and stimulates smooth muscle contraction of most segments of the gut. Levels have also been reported as diminished in patients with idiopathic constipation. Delayed transit may lead to increased fluid and electrolyte absorption and desiccated stools.

Mechanical factors may include pressure on the rectosigmoid by the gravid uterus or pressure on the anal canal by engorged hemorrhoids. Pressure of the fetal head against the rectum may also play a role either during pregnancy or later as a contributor to pelvic floor dysfunction. Intestinal obstruction has been reported secondary to adhesions, intestinal volvulus, and malignancy. Colon cancer has been reported in pregnant women with an incidence of between 1 in 13,000 to 1 in 50,000 live births, with a preponderance of rectal tumors. Symptoms may be indistinguishable from those attributable to the pregnancy, and the diagnosis is often made at a later stage of disease.

The evaluation of pregnant patients complaining of constipation should be done in the same manner as in nonpregnant patients. A careful history is taken and a physical examination performed. Prior history of constipation, diet, and medications should be assessed. Thyroid function tests, electrolytes, and serum calcium level may be useful. Digital rectal examination should be performed, and stool tested for occult blood. If an obstructing lesion is suspected, evaluation of the rectum and colon by endoscopy is performed rather than using a radiologic procedure. Sigmoidoscopy appears to be safe in stable patients with appropriate indications. Colonoscopy has been performed safely in pregnancy but requires a higher level of monitoring and significant alterations from the "standard" technique. It is usually reserved for urgent indications or as an alternative to colonic surgery.

Treatment begins with patient education and behavioral changes that may lead to more regular bowel habits. Dietary fiber and liquid intake is maximized. Bran or wheat fiber supplements or other bulking agents can be added to maintain regularity, are often effective, and are safe in pregnancy. Emollient agents such as docusate sodium (Colace) are used extensively in pregnancy, with no reported significant adverse effects. Lactulose is poorly absorbed from the gut lumen, rated safe in pregnancy, and was found to be very effective in a multicenter study. Saline hyperosmotic laxatives (containing citrate, magnesium, phosphate, or sulfate ions) may be effective but can result in maternal sodium retention. Hypernatremia, hypokalemia, hypermagnesemia, hyperphosphatemia, hypocalcemia, dehydration, metabolic acidosis, tetany, renal failure, and death have all been reported related to improper or excessive use. Polyethylene glycol based laxatives (e.g., Miralax) are minimally absorbed and may be effective but are rated pregnancy Category C because of a lack of data on safety. Lubricant laxatives such as mineral oil should not be used routinely, because they lead to decreased maternal absorption of the fat-soluble vitamins. This has reportedly resulted in neonatal coagulopathy, resulting in hemorrhage. Stimulant laxatives may cause abdominal cramping and have been associated with premature labor.

Because the pelvic floor musculature plays an important role in constipation, strengthening and protection of the pelvic floor may be helpful. Biofeedback-assisted Kegel exercises have been shown to increase the number of bowel movements each week. These are performed routinely and on a long-term basis for the best chance of success.

BIBLIOGRAPHY

Camilleri M, Thompson WG, Fleshman JW, et al. Clinical management of intractable constipation. *Ann Intern Med* 1994;121:520.

Cappell MS, Colon VJ, Sidhom OA. A study at ten medical centers of the safety and efficacy of 48 flexible sigmoidoscopies and eight colonoscopies during pregnancy with follow-up of fetal outcome and with comparison to control groups. *Dig Dis Sci* 1996;41:2353.

Devroede G. Constipation. In: Sleisenger MH, Fordtran JS, Scharschmidt BF, et al., eds. *Gastrointestinal disease: pathophysiology, diagnosis, and management,* 5th ed. Philadelphia: WB Saunders, 1993:837.

Diamant NE, Kamm MA, Wald A, et al. AGA technical review on anorectal testing techniques. *Gastroenterology* 1999;116:735.

Drossman DA, Leserman J, Nachman G, et al. Sexual and physical abuse in women with functional or organic gastrointestinal disorders. *Ann Intern Med* 1990;113:828.

Drossman DA, Zhiming L, Andruzzi E, et al. U.S. householder survey of functional gastrointestinal disorders: prevalence, sociodemography, health impact. *Digest Dis Sci* 1993;38:1569.

Emmanuel AV, Mason HJ, Kamm MA. Relationship between psychological state and level of activity of extrinsic gut innervation in patients with a functional gut disorder. *Gut* 2001;49:209.

Jewell DJ, Young G. Interventions for treating constipation in pregnancy (Cochrane Review). In: *The Cochrane Library,* Issue 4. Oxford: Update Software, 2002.

Jost WH, Schrank B, Herold A, et al. Functional outlet obstruction: anismus, spastic pelvic floor syndrome, and dyscoordination of the voluntary sphincter muscles: definition, diagnosis, and treatment from the neurologic point of view. *Scand J Gastroenterol* 1999;34:449.

Knowles CH, Martin JE. Slow transit constipation: a model of human gut dysmotility: review of possible aetiologies. *Neurogastroenterol Motil* 2000;12:181.

Lau CW, Heymen S, Alabaz O, et al. Prognostic significance of rectocele, intussusception, and abnormal perineal descent in biofeedback treatment for constipated patients with paradoxical puborectalis contraction. *Dis Colon Rectum* 2000;43:478.

Lennard-Jones JE. Clinical management of constipation. *Pharmacology* 1993;47 [Suppl 1]:216.

Leroi AM, Berkelmans I, Denis P, et al. Anismus as a marker of sexual abuse: consequences of abuse on anorectal motility. *Dig Dis Sci* 1995;40:1411.

Locke GR, Pemberton JH, Phillips SF. AGA technical review on constipation. *Gastroenterology* 2000;119:1766.

Mason HJ, Serrano-Ikkos E, Kamm MA. Psychological morbidity in women with idiopathic constipation. *Am J Gastroenterol* 2000;95:2852.

Pemberton JH, Rath DM, Ilstrup DM. Evaluation and surgical treatment of severe chronic constipation. *Ann Surg* 1991;214:403.

Pfeifer J, Agachan F, Wexner SD. Surgery for constipation. *Dis Colon Rectum* 1996;39:444.

Pikarsky AJ, Singh JJ, Weiss EG, et al. Long-term follow-up of patients undergoing colectomy for colonic inertia. *Dis Colon Rectum* 2002;44:179.

Shafik A. Constipation: pathogenesis and management. *Drugs* 1993;45:528.

Shah S, Nathan L, Singh R, et al. E2 and not P4 increases NO release from NANC nerves of the gastrointestinal tract: implications in pregnancy. *Am J Physiol Regul Integr Comp Physiol* 2001;280:R1546.

Talley NJ, Weaver AL, Zinsmeister AR, et al. Functional constipation and outlet delay: a population-based study. *Gastroenterology* 1993;105:781.

Thompson WG, Longstreth GF, Drossman DA, et al. Functional bowel disorders and functional abdominal pain. *Gut* 1999;45[Suppl II]:1143.

Walter S, Hallböök O, Gotthard R, et al. A population-based study on bowel habits in a Swedish community: prevalence of faecal incontinence and constipation. *Scand J Gastroenterol* 2002;37:911.

West L, Warren J, Cutts T. Diagnosis and management of irritable bowel syndrome, constipation, and diarrhea in pregnancy. *Gastroenterol Clin North Am* 1992;21:793.

CHAPTER 72

Colorectal Cancer in Women

Edward A. Pensa, Neil R. Greenspan, and Samir A. Shah

Colorectal cancer is a common and often fatal disease, posing a significant threat to the health of women. According to estimates from the National Cancer Institute, there were 75,700 women diagnosed with colorectal cancer in the United States in 2002 and 28,800 deaths. Colorectal cancer accounts for 11% of all cancer fatalities in American women and is the third most common cause of female cancer mortality, after lung and breast cancer.

The incidence of colorectal cancer rises markedly with advancing age. Although the lifetime risk of developing colon cancer is almost 6% for women in the United States, 90% of cases are diagnosed after the age of 50. There is significant variability in the frequency of colorectal cancer among different ethnic groups, with African-American women having an annual incidence of disease almost twice that of Hispanic women (44.7 cases per 100,000 individuals vs. 23.2 cases per 100,000) and significantly greater than white female (36.3 cases per 100,000).

The prognosis for colorectal cancer is primarily dependent on the anatomic stage at diagnosis. The 5-year survival for patients with localized disease is 94%, as compared with 70% for regional disease and 9% for metastatic disease. Although the annual incidence of colorectal cancer has remained fairly stable, death rates have been decreasing by about 2% per year for American women since 1984.

ETIOLOGY

Most colorectal cancers arise from benign adenomatous polyps. The progression from normal mucosa to adenomatous tissue to cancer generally occurs over many years and results from an accumulation of acquired genetic alterations. These genetic changes primarily involve the activation of oncogenes, which impart a growth advantage to specific cell lines, and the loss of tumor-suppressor genes, which regulate cellular differentiation and division.

A multistep genetic model for colorectal cancer has been proposed in which specific genetic alterations of oncogenes and tumor-suppressor genes occur in an identifiable sequence, leading to the development of cancer. A study by Vogelstein and colleagues provided strong support for this model by demonstrating that as adenomas increased in size they were more likely to acquire specific mutations that are commonly found in colorectal cancer, including K-*ras* mutations and deletions on chromosomes 5, 17, and 18.

Further support for the adenoma to carcinoma sequence is seen in studies of the natural history of untreated polyps. A retrospective review was done at the Mayo Clinic of 226 patients with large (>1 cm) polyps found on barium enema between 1965 and 1970 who elected to not have the polyps removed. With a mean follow-up of 68 months, the cumulative risk of diagnosis of cancer at the polyp site at 5, 10, and 20 years was 2.5%, 8%, and 24%, respectively. In addition, 11 colorectal cancers were found at sites remote from the index polyp, and the risk of colorectal cancer at any site among this group of patients known to have large polyps was 35% at 20 years.

RISK FACTORS

Individuals vary in their susceptibility to the development of adenomas and carcinoma, with both genetic and environmental factors having clear significance (Table 72.1). In comparison with the general population, patients who have had colorectal adenomas found and resected have twice the risk of subsequent colon cancer. This risk increases with greater polyp number, size, or villous histology. Patients with a personal history of colorectal cancer are also at increased risk for a metachronous large bowel malignancy. In a National Cancer Institute study of 3,278 patients with resected stage II and III colon cancer, the incidence of a second primary was 1.5% at 5 years.

The presence of a family history of colorectal cancer is a well-recognized risk factor, and up to 30% of patients diagnosed with colon cancer in the United States have a family member with the disease. Among 87,031 American women participating in the Nurses' Health Study, those with a parent or sibling with colorectal cancer had nearly twice the risk of developing colorectal cancer themselves. The risk increased substantially if multiple family members were affected. First-degree relatives of patients with adenomas are at a similarly increased risk, particularly if the adenomas were found before the age of 60. The colon cancer risk is four times that of the general population if first-degree family members were diagnosed with colon cancer before age 45.

TABLE 72.1. Risk Factors for Colorectal Cancer

Personal
Advancing age
History of prior colorectal cancer or adenomas
History of endometrial or breast cancer
Long-standing ulcerative or Crohn colitis
Hereditary
First-degree relative with colorectal cancer or adenomas
Familial colorectal cancer syndromes (FAP/HNPCC)
Environmental
High-fat diet
Obesity
Lack of regular exercise
Alcohol intake
Cigarette smoking
Protective factors
Supplemental calcium
Supplemental folate
ASA/NSAIDs
Hormone replacement therapy

ASA, aspirin; FAP, familial adenomatous polyposis; HNPCC, hereditary nonpolyposis colorectal cancer.

Several familial colon cancer syndromes have been recognized that are inherited in an autosomal-dominant fashion and are associated with a very high risk of developing colon cancer. Although patients with these syndromes account for only a few colorectal cancers diagnosed each year, they provide great insight into the molecular pathogenesis of colon cancer and the relationship between colorectal cancer and other malignancies.

Familial adenomatous polyposis occurs as a result of a germline mutation in the adenomatous polyposis coli (APC) tumor-suppressor gene located on the long arm of chromosome 5 and represents less than 1% of colorectal cancer prevalence. Affected individuals begin developing adenomas in childhood and have hundreds to thousands of polyps throughout their colon by middle age, with an almost 100% chance of developing colorectal cancer by age 50. Variants of familial adenomatous polyposis that were initially thought to be distinct clinical entities have now been recognized as variable phenotypic expressions of APC gene mutations. These include Gardner syndrome, associated with osteomas and soft tissue tumors, and Turcot syndrome, associated with malignant central nervous system tumors.

Hereditary nonpolyposis colorectal cancer accounts for approximately 5% of colorectal cancer cases and is associated with a lifetime risk of colorectal cancer of 70% to 80%. A germline mutation in one of five genes responsible for repairing DNA nucleotide errors causes hereditary nonpolyposis colorectal cancer, which is phenotypically divided into two clinical syndromes, Lynch I and II. Although the malignancy risk in Lynch I patients is limited to the colon and rectum, Lynch II patients are at increased risk for extracolonic tumors, including endometrial, ovarian, gastric, small bowel, hepatobiliary, and urinary tract neoplasia. Endometrial cancer is most common, with a lifetime risk of 43% in Lynch II patients.

The incidence of colorectal cancer is also markedly increased in patients with inflammatory bowel disease. The degree of risk corresponds directly to the extent and duration of disease. Ulcerative colitis patients with proctitis alone have colon cancer rates comparable with the general population, whereas those with pancolitis may have up to a 15-fold greater risk. The incidence of colorectal cancer begins to increase 7 to 10 years after the onset of symptoms and rises by approximately 0.5% to 1% per year thereafter. Patients diagnosed with ulcerative colitis in childhood appear to be at the greatest risk. A Swedish study found that among patients diagnosed with ulcerative colitis before age 15, 40% had developed colorectal cancer by the age of 50. Patients with Crohn disease are at increased risk if they have significant colonic involvement.

Despite the importance of family history and underlying colitis, most colorectal cancers occur in individuals not known to be at increased risk for the disease. The incidence of colorectal cancer varies considerably throughout the world, and when individuals emigrate from areas of low incidence to high incidence areas, their risk soon rises. Environmental factors play a significant role in the development of colorectal cancer, and a number of factors have been studied.

High-fiber diets have long been thought to be protective against colon cancer. There are a number of different mechanisms by which fiber may act, including diluting carcinogens, binding with bile acids, or altering colonic microflora. Although animal studies and metaanalyses of observational studies have shown some benefit with increased fiber intake, recent prospective studies have been less encouraging. Data from the 88,757 women in the Nurses' Health Study did not find any association between fiber intake and colon cancer risk in women, and a prospective study of 1,303 men with adenomas failed to show any benefit in reducing recurrent adenomas with supplemental wheat bran fiber. Based on currently available data, fiber has no proven benefit for colorectal cancer prevention.

A number of studies have demonstrated a link between colon cancer and high-fat diets, particularly saturated fats and red meat. In a study of 2,079 patients with adenomas, however, adopting a low-fat and high-fiber diet did not influence the risk of recurrent adenomas. Another recent prospective study of almost 10,000 people in Finland failed to find any relationship between fat intake and colorectal cancer risk, although high cholesterol intake was associated with significantly higher rates of colon cancer.

Supplemental calcium and folate have both been shown to be protective against colorectal cancer in women. Although their mechanisms of action are unclear, each is thought to have a preventive role early in colon carcinogenesis. Dietary supplementation with antioxidant vitamins A, C, and E has been evaluated in several studies but has not been shown to be beneficial.

Although recent data are inconclusive, the American Cancer Society and the National Cancer Institute recommend limiting total fat intake to 30% of total calories and ingesting at least 20 to 30 g of fiber per diet with five servings of fruit or vegetables per day. Given that obesity, lack of regular exercise, cigarette smoking, and excessive alcohol intake have all been linked to an increased risk of colorectal cancer, the maintenance of a balanced diet and healthy lifestyle is likely to be beneficial through a number of different mechanisms.

In addition to dietary factors, a number of medications have been studied as potentially protective against colon cancer. Several large trials have supported the benefit of aspirin and other nonsteroidal antiinflammatory agents in lowering rates of colorectal cancer, although these benefits are primarily seen in patients who have taken the medications regularly over many years. In the Nurses' Health Study, the risk reduction from aspirin use was statistically significant only in women who had taken the drug consistently for 20 years or more.

Hormone replacement therapy in postmenopausal women may also be protective. In the Women's Health Study of 16,608 women, colorectal cancer rates were reduced by 37% in individuals receiving hormone replacement therapy. Unfortunately, it is unclear whether these benefits persist after hormone replacement is discontinued, and the potential for increased mortality from heart disease and breast cancer may outweigh the benefits of hormone replacement therapy for some patients.

CLINICAL PRESENTATION

The clinical presentation of patients with colorectal cancer varies depending on the extent of the disease. Most patients with early cancers found on screening are asymptomatic. More advanced lesions often result in a change in bowel habits, overt or occult gastrointestinal bleeding, or abdominal discomfort. In a retrospective study of 246 patients with colorectal cancer, 66% had symptoms referable to the lower gastrointestinal tract, most commonly hematochezia or abdominal pain.

Hematochezia is seen most often with rectal cancers, whereas iron deficiency anemia is frequently caused by malignancy in the cecum or ascending colon. Tumors of the left colon are more likely to result in a narrowed lumen and difficulty passing solid stool resulting in a complaint of constipation, a change in stool caliber, or tenesmus. Significant abdominal pain may represent bowel obstruction or perforation. Nonspecific symptoms such as malaise, weight loss, and anorexia usually occur in patients with advanced disease.

To recognize colorectal cancer at its earliest stage, a prompt evaluation of all patients with symptoms referable to the lower gastrointestinal tract is warranted. Physical examination may reveal lymphadenopathy, ascites, or a palpable mass, which may suggest metastatic disease. Stool should be tested for occult blood, although it may be negative in as many as 30% of patients with colorectal cancer. Women with suspected colorectal cancer should have breast and pelvic examinations to evaluate for associated gynecologic malignancies. Although iron deficiency anemia may be attributable to heavy menses in some young women, a study of 186 premenopausal women with iron deficiency found a clinically significant gastrointestinal lesion in 12% of patients. When iron deficiency occurs in postmenopausal women, however, colonoscopy and upper endoscopy are warranted. Although it may not be necessary in all younger patients, a colonoscopy to exclude malignancy should be done in any symptomatic individual over the age of 40.

LABORATORY AND IMAGING STUDIES

Patients diagnosed with a colorectal malignancy should have a thorough workup at presentation to determine the anatomic stage of the cancer and to rule out any synchronous cancers or polyps. A complete colonoscopy done at the time of diagnosis will reveal synchronous cancers in up to 5% of cases and synchronous adenomas in 20% to 40%. If a colonoscopy cannot be completed before surgery, it should be done within 3 to 6 months postoperatively. Chest x-rays are routinely done preoperatively. Liver function tests should be performed but are normal in a large number of patients with small hepatic metastases and cannot be used to rule out liver involvement.

The routine use of preoperative abdominal and pelvic computed tomography (CT) is controversial. CTs may demonstrate extension of tumor beyond the intestinal wall, regional lymphadenopathy, or distant metastases. Up to 25% of patients have liver lesions at the time of diagnosis, and these may be amenable to surgical resection. Synchronous ovarian malignancies are found in up to 8% of women with colorectal cancer, particularly premenopausal patients, and may be seen on a pelvic CT. The sensitivity of CT, however, is limited. In a study of 67 patients who underwent surgical resections for colon cancer, preoperative CTs detected only 75% of hepatic metastases and only 19% of patients with lymph node involvement were correctly staged.

Recent studies have suggested that positron emission tomography may be more sensitive than CT in detecting occult metastatic disease, although the role of preoperative positron emission tomography is still evolving. In patients with rectal cancer, endoscopic ultrasound provides the best means of staging and often determines the surgical approach. Carcinoembryonic antigen (CEA) levels are often elevated in patients with advanced colorectal cancer and have some prognostic value. Unfortunately, the sensitivity of CEA levels is poor in early disease, and they may be elevated with other malignancies or benign disease, so its use as a screening test for colorectal cancer is not recommended.

SCREENING

Colorectal cancer is a common disease resulting from an identifiable precancerous lesion, an adenoma, which in most patients takes many years to progress to malignancy. Screening tests designed to identify asymptomatic patients with adenomas or early stage colorectal cancers have the potential to reduce colorectal cancer mortality. In the National Polyp Study of 1,418 patients who underwent colonoscopic resection of adenomas, the incidence of colorectal cancer was reduced by over 75%. Several screening tests are available for colorectal cancer, including fecal occult blood testing (FOBT), sigmoidoscopy, double-contrast barium enema, and colonoscopy (Table 72.2).

FOBT is an easy and inexpensive means of identifying a group of patients at higher risk for having occult colon cancer. In a study of over 45,000 patients with an 18-year follow-up period, annual or biennial FOBT testing reduced the incidence of colorectal cancer by approximately 20%. False-positive tests are common, however, particularly if patients do not abstain from red meats, nonsteroidal antiinflammatory drugs, or peroxidase-containing vegetables while obtaining stool samples. In addition, small adenomas often will not bleed and thus will not be detected on FOBT.

TABLE 72.2. Colorectal Cancer Screening Recommendations

Average risk at age > 50
FOBT annually
Flexible sigmoidoscopy every 5 yr
FOBT annually and flexible sigmoidoscopy every 5 yr
Double-contrast barium enema every 5–10 yr
Colonoscopy every 10 yr
Family history of colorectal cancer or adenomas
Screening beginning at age 40 or 10 yr younger than youngest affected relative (colonoscopy preferred)
Personal history of colorectal cancer or adenomas
Colonoscopy every 3–5 yr (more often if multiple or large polyps, villous histology, or rectal cancer)
Familial adenomatous polyposis
Sigmoidoscopy beginning at ages 10–12
Hereditary nonpolyposis colorectal cancer
Colonoscopy beginning at age 25 then every 2 yr
Long-standing ulcerative colitis or Crohn colitis
Colonoscopy every 1–3 yr after 8–10 yr of disease
Colonoscopy annually after 20 yr of disease

FOBT, focal occult blood testing.

Sigmoidoscopy has been shown to reduce mortality from colorectal cancer by 60% to 85% Because sedation is not used, this test can be done in a doctor's office and is performed by many primary care physicians and nurse practitioners. Sigmoidoscopy to the splenic flexure will visualize approximately 50% of occult colorectal malignancies. Patients with distal adenomatous polyps, particularly adenomas greater than 1 cm in size, are at increased risk for proximal colonic cancers and should have a full colonoscopy.

Several recent studies suggested that a screening program with sigmoidoscopy will fail to detect a significant percentage of patients with proximal colonic lesions. Two studies with a total of 5,115 asymptomatic patients who underwent colonoscopic screening found that over 50% of patients with advanced proximal neoplasia did not have distal polyps. When a combination of FOBT and sigmoidoscopy was used for screening in a study of 2,885 patients, 24% advanced colonic neoplasias were not detected. Based on these studies, colonoscopy is now advocated as an initial screening test for colorectal cancer. It has the advantage of visualizing the entire colon and allows for removal of polyps at the time of initial testing. A colonoscopy is more expensive than flexible sigmoidoscopy, requires sedation with hemodynamic monitoring, and is associated with complications, including bleeding or perforation, in about 0.1% of procedures. However, recent studies suggest that colonoscopy is more cost effective overall than sigmoidoscopy for colon cancer screening in average risk individuals.

A recent cost-effectiveness analysis for the U.S. Preventive Services Task Force compared data on several different screening strategies, including annual FOBT, sigmoidoscopy every 5 years with or without annual FOBT, double-contrast barium enema every 5 years, and colonoscopy every 10 years. Although available evidence clearly supports screening in average risk patients over 50, no single method of screening was clearly found to be superior to the others. Current guidelines endorsed by multiple organizations including the American Cancer Society recommend screening for average risk patients begin at age 50 but allow physicians and patients to choose among the screening tests discussed above. Tests such as virtual colonoscopy and stool testing for genetic colorectal cancer mutations may soon provide additional screening options. At the present time, most surveys have found that less than 40% of eligible patients have been offered any screening test, and further efforts clearly need to be made to improve screening rates, whatever method is being used.

Patients known to be at higher risk for colorectal cancer need to be screened more frequently than those at average risk. If a parent or sibling is known to have colonic adenomas or colorectal cancer, screening should begin at age 40, and colonoscopy is generally the test of choice. In patients with higher familial risk (i.e., two first-degree relatives or a first-degree relative diagnosed at less than 60 years of age), a colonoscopy should be done either at age 40 or 10 years younger than the youngest affected relative. Patients who have had adenomas found and resected are at increased risk for recurrent polyps or cancer and need to have regular colonoscopic surveillance. Although the frequency of surveillance depends on the number, size, and histology of the polyps found, data from the National Polyp Study supports initial surveillance intervals of 3 years for most patients.

The risk of colorectal cancer in familial adenomatous polyposis patients is exceedingly high, and screening sigmoidoscopies should begin around age 10 with plans for colectomy when polyps begin to develop. In hereditary nonpolyposis colorectal cancer patients, colonoscopic screening is recommended beginning at age 25 and is usually repeated every 2 years. Individuals with chronic ulcerative colitis or Crohn colitis for over 8 years should have surveillance colonoscopies every 1 to 3 years, with multiple random biopsies taken from throughout the colon to detect dysplasia.

TREATMENT

The mainstay of curative therapy for colorectal cancer is surgical resection. The surgical approach varies with the location and extent of disease. In surgeries with curative intent, a wide resection of involved bowel and its lymph node–bearing mesentery is required. The abdomen is thoroughly explored at the time of surgery to allow for staging, often expressed in terms of the modified Dukes system. In this system, the designations are as follows:

A, a tumor limited to the mucosa.
B1, tumors extending into the muscularis propria that do not breach the serosa.
B2, tumors that penetrate the bowel wall without lymph node or distant metastases.
C, tumors with regional lymph node involvement without distant metastases.
D, tumors with distant metastases.

For patients with Dukes A and B1 lesions, surgery alone is frequently curative. In more advanced disease, adjuvant chemotherapy is often given postoperatively in an attempt to eradicate undetected microscopic disease. The best results have been obtained with 5-fluorouracil administered along with either leucovorin or levamisole. In a clinical trial with 929 Dukes C patients, 5-fluorouracil and levamisole given daily for 5 days and then weekly for 48 weeks reduced the recurrence rate by 40% and the death rate by 33% at a mean follow-up of 6.5 years. Similar results have been obtained using only 6 months of therapy with 5-fluorouracil and leucovorin in a variety of different regimens.

Rectal cancer can be particularly difficult to treat. From a surgical standpoint, a distal margin of at least 2 cm of normal bowel is required to perform a sphincter-sparing low-anterior resection. Patients with Dukes B and C rectal cancers have a high risk of local recurrence, and postoperative radiation therapy reduces this risk. Improvements in survival have been shown to occur when chemotherapy with 5-fluorouracil and leucovorin is combined with radiation therapy.

Colon cancer metastasizes most often to the liver, lung, and peritoneum, and the prognosis with distant metastases is very poor. Long-term survival has been reported after resection of isolated hepatic or lung metastases but occurs only rarely. Surgery, radiation, or chemotherapy may all be used for palliation, although the duration of response is generally brief.

FOLLOW-UP AFTER COLORECTAL CANCER

After curative resection for colorectal cancer, patients are at risk for both for local recurrence and the development of new adenomas or cancers. After a complete perioperative colonoscopy with resection of any adenomas, a surveillance colonoscopy should be performed in 3 years and every 3 to 5 years thereafter. The presence of multiple polyps, a poor preparation, and/or large sessile polyps with villous histology necessitates earlier follow-up colonoscopy (6–12 months). Patients with proximal rectal cancer who undergo sphincter-sparing low-anterior resections need to be more closely followed for local recurrence and should have flexible sigmoidoscopy every 3 to 6 months for the first 2 years after surgery. Women should also undergo age-appropriate screening for occult breast or gynecologic malignancies.

A rising CEA level may indicate the development or progression of metastatic disease before symptoms develop. In patients treated for Dukes B2 or C disease, CEA levels are usually obtained every 2 to 3 months postoperatively for up to 5 years. If an elevated CEA level is confirmed by retesting, an evaluation for metastatic disease is warranted. More aggressive surveillance regimens including annual colonoscopies, liver CTs, and chest radiography have not been shown to improve survival in patients with prior colorectal cancer.

CONSIDERATIONS IN PREGNANCY

Most cases of colorectal cancer occur in women over the age of 50, and therefore it is a malignancy rarely seen in pregnant patients. Unfortunately, the mortality from colorectal cancer in pregnancy is high because most cases are not diagnosed until the disease is at an advanced stage. Many of the presenting symptoms of colorectal cancer, including abdominal pain, altered bowel habits, fatigue, anorexia, and nausea, are common in pregnancy. Rectal bleeding is usually attributed to hemorrhoids, and a workup is frequently deferred. Colorectal cancer in pregnant patients is seen primarily in young patients and therefore often occurs in the setting of strong hereditary or environmental risk factors.

Prompt investigation of any concerning symptoms is warranted, particularly in high-risk individuals. Rectal cancers are seen more commonly than colon cancers in pregnant patients, and a digital rectal examination may be helpful. Flexible sigmoidoscopy can be safely performed and should be followed by colonoscopy if indicated, although the maternal and fetal risks of colonoscopy are not well defined and an obstetric consultation may be warranted. Abdominal CTs and barium studies are generally avoided during pregnancy, although transrectal ultrasonography is safe and often obtained.

Treatment of colorectal cancer in pregnancy depends on both the stage of disease and the gestational period in which diagnosis is made. For patients with localized disease diagnosed before 20 weeks' gestation, curative surgery is usually recommended at the time of diagnosis. After 20 weeks' gestation, surgery may be delayed until fetal viability, at which time delivery can be induced before surgery. Colorectal cancer in pregnancy has a high incidence of ovarian metastases, and oophorectomy is often performed. Adjuvant chemotherapy with 5-fluorouracil and levamisole or leucovorin is contraindicated in the first trimester but has been used in selected patients with Dukes C disease in whom the fetal risks were believed to be outweighed by maternal benefits. Radiation therapy is absolutely contraindicated during pregnancy.

As with colorectal cancer in general, improving mortality in pregnant women with colorectal cancer depends on making the diagnosis at an early stage. With greater numbers of women having children later in life, the number of pregnancies complicated by colorectal cancer will likely increase. Appropriate screening of high-risk individuals and prompt evaluations of symptomatic patients may improve the significant mortality now seen with colorectal cancers diagnosed in pregnancy.

CONCLUSION

Colorectal cancer is an important cause of morbidity and mortality in women. With an increased awareness of the risk factors for colorectal cancer and the need for appropriate screening and follow-up, health care providers have the opportunity to significantly improve the lives of the women in their care.

BIBLIOGRAPHY

Alberts DS, Martinez ME, Roe DJ, et al. Lack of effect of high fiber cereal supplementation on the recurrence of colorectal adenomas. *N Engl J Med* 2000;342: 1156–1162.

Atkin WS, Morson BC, Cuzik J. Long-term risk of colorectal cancer after excision of rectosigmoid adenomas. *N Engl J Med* 1992;326:658–662.

Bast RC, Ravdin P, Hayes DF, et al. 2000 update of recommendations for the use of tumor markers in breast and colorectal cancer: clinical practice guidelines of the American Society for Clinical Oncology. *J Clin Oncol* 2001;19:1865–1878.

Bini EJ, Micale PL, Weinshel EH. Evaluation of the gastrointestinal tract in premenopausal women with iron deficiency anemia. *Am J Med* 1998;105:281–286.

Bond JH. Colorectal cancer update: prevention, screening, treatment and surveillance for high-risk groups. *Med Clin North Am* 2000;84:1163–1182.

Cappell MS. Colon cancer during pregnancy: the gastroenterologist's perspective. *Gastrointest Clin North Am* 1998;27:225–256.

Eaden JA, Mayberry JF. Colorectal cancer complicating ulcerative colitis: a review. *Am J Gastroenterol* 2000;95:2710–2719.

Ekborn A, Hemick C, Zack M, et al. Ulcerative colitis and colorectal cancer: a population-based study. *N Engl J Med* 1990;323:1228–1233.

Friedman S, Rubin PH, Bodian C, et al. Screening and surveillance colonoscopy in chronic Crohn's colitis. *Gastroenterology* 2001;120:820–826.

Fuchs CS, Giovannucci EL, Colditz GA, et al. A prospective study of family history and the risk of colorectal cancer. *N Engl J Med* 1994;331:1669–1674.

Fuchs CS, Giovannucci EL, Colditz GA, et al. Dietary fiber and the risk of colorectal cancer and adenoma in women. *N Engl J Med* 1999;340:169–176.

Giovannucci E, Egan KM, Hunter DJ, et al. Aspirin and the risk of colorectal cancer in women. *N Engl J Med* 1995;333:609–614.

Green RJ, Metlay JP, Propert K, et al. Surveillance for second primary colorectal cancer after adjuvant chemotherapy: an analysis of intergroup 0089. *Ann Intern Med* 2002;136:261–269.

Greenlee RT, Murray T, Bolden S, et al. Cancer statistics 2000. *CA Cancer J Clin* 2000;50:7–33.

Imperiale TF, Wagner DR, Lin CY, et al. Risk of advanced proximal neoplasms in asymptomatic adults according to distal colorectal findings. *N Engl J Med* 2000;343:196.

Janne PA, Mayer RT. Chemoprevention of colorectal cancer. *N Engl J Med* 2000;342: 1960–1968.

Jarvinen R, Knekt P, Hakulinen T, et al. Dietary fat, cholesterol, and colorectal cancer in a prospective study. *Br J Cancer* 2001;85:357–361.

Jemal A, Thomas A, Murray T, et al. Cancer statistics 2002. *CA Cancer J Clin* 2002; 52:23–247.

Lieberman D. Colon cancer screening: role of endoscopy. *ASGE Clin Update* 2000; 8:1–3.

Lieberman DA, Weiss DG. One-time screening for colorectal cancer with combined fecal occult blood testing and examination of the distal colon. *N Engl J Med* 2001;354:555–560.

Lieberman DA, Weiss DG, Bond JH, et al. Use of colonoscopy to screen asymptomatic adults for colorectal cancer. *N Engl J Med* 2000;343:162–168.

Mandel JS, Church TR, Bond JH, et al. The effect of fecal occult blood screening on the incidence of colorectal cancer. *N Engl J Med* 2000;343:1603–1607.

McAndrew MR, Saba AK. Efficacy of routine preoperative computed tomography scans in colon cancer. *Ann Surg* 1999;65:205–208.

Moeretel CG, Fleming TR, MacDonald JS, et al. Fluorouracil plus levamisole as an effective adjuvant therapy after resection for stage III colon carcinoma: a final report. *Ann Intern Med* 1995;122:321–326.

Niederhuber JE. Colon and rectum cancer: patterns of spread and implications for work-up. *Cancer* 1993;71:4187–4192.

Pignone M, Saha S, Hoerger T, et al. Cost-effectiveness of colorectal cancer screening: a systemic review for the United States Preventive Health Services Task Force. *Ann Intern Med* 2002;137:E96–E106.

Rex DK. Sigmoidoscopy or colonoscopy: which way are we headed? *Am J Gastroenterol* 2000;95:1116–1118.

Rossow JE, et al. Risks and benefits of estrogen plus progestin in healthy postmenopausal women: principal results from the Women's Health Initiative randomized control trial. *JAMA* 2002;288:321–333.

Sander RS. Epidemiology and risk factors for colorectal cancer. *Gastrointest Clin North Am* 1996;25:717–735.

Schatzkin A, Lanza E, Corle D, et al. Lack of effect of low-fat, high-fiber diet on the recurrence of colorectal adenomas. *N Engl J Med* 2000;342:1149–1155.

Shoemaker D, Black R, Giles L, et al. Yearly colonoscopy, liver CT and chest radiography do not influence 5-year survival of colorectal cancer patients. *Gastroenterology* 1998;114:7–12.

Skilling JS. Colorectal cancer complicating pregnancy. *Obstet Gynecol Clin* 1998;25: 417–421.

Sonnenberg A, Delco F, Inadomi, JM. The cost-effectiveness of colonoscopy in screening for colorectal cancer. *Ann Intern Med* 2000;133:573–584.

Speights VO, Johnson MW, Stoltenberg PH, et al. Colorectal cancer: current trends in initial clinical manifestations. *South J Med* 1991;84:575–578.

Stryker SJ, Wolff BG, Culp CE, et al. Natural history of untreated colonic polyps. *Gastroenterology* 1987;93:1009–1013.

Van Stolk R. Familial and inherited colorectal cancer: endoscopic screening and surveillance. *Gastrointest Endocrinol Clin North Am* 2002;12:111–133.

Vogelstein B, Fearon ER, Hamilton SR, et al. Genetic alterations during colorectal-tumor development. *N Engl J Med* 1988;319:525–532.

Whiteford MH, Whiteford HM, Yee LF, et al. Usefulness of FDG-PET scan in the assessment of suspected metastatic or recurrent adenocarcinoma of the colon and rectum. *Dis Colon Rectum* 2000;53:759–770.

Winawer SJ, Fletcher RH, Miller L, et al. Colorectal cancer screening: clinical guidelines and rationale. *Gastroenterology* 1997;112:594–642.

Winawer SJ, Zauber AG, Gerdes H, et al. Risk of colorectal cancer in the families of patients with adenomatous polyps. *N Engl J Med* 1996;334:82–87.

Winawer SJ, Zauber AG, Ho MN, et al. Prevention of colorectal cancer by colonoscopic polypectomy. *N Engl J Med* 1993;329:1977–1981.

Winawer SJ, Zauber AG, O'Brien MJ, et al. Randomized comparison of surveillance intervals after colonoscopic removal of newly diagnosed adenomatous polyps. *N Engl J Med* 1993;328:901–906.

CHAPTER 73
Fecal Incontinence

Jeffrey L. Clemons

The ability to store feces and voluntarily empty at a socially desired time is a basic physiologic process that is taken for granted. Fecal incontinence can have a profound psychological impact, causing loss of self-esteem, anxiety, social isolation, frustration, anger, and reduced quality of life. Moreover, patients suffering from this condition frequently do not report it to their health care providers because of embarrassment.

Fecal incontinence is defined as any involuntary loss of gas, liquid, or solid stool. Many patients also have fecal urgency, with a need to defecate almost immediately. Fecal incontinence can be classified as either major or minor based on the severity of symptoms. Major incontinence is the loss of solid stool, whereas minor incontinence is the loss of flatus or occasional loss of liquid stool.

The prevalence of fecal incontinence varies between studies because of variations in patient populations and definitions (frequency and severity of incontinence). Fecal incontinence occurs in 2% to 7% of people in community-based studies, in up to 50% of nursing home residents, and in 20% to 50% of women after primary repair of an anal sphincter laceration. In a study of 881 patients aged 18 or older presenting to their primary care physician, the prevalence of fecal incontinence was 13%, and only one third of individuals had discussed the problem with a physician. Fecal incontinence is a common reason for institutionalization, and a 1992 Canadian nursing home study showed that 52 minutes daily were spent by staff dealing with fecal incontinence, at a total annual cost of almost $10,000 per patient.

PHYSIOLOGY

The rectum is normally compliant, storing up to 300 mL of feces without any increase in pressure. Beyond 300 mL, the rectal pressure increases and leads to a feeling of urgency. The anal sphincter is 3 to 4 cm long and consists of two concentric rings of muscle. The internal anal sphincter (IAS) consists of smooth muscle that extends upward to continue as a circular layer of smooth muscle of the rectum. The IAS maintains fecal continence at rest by providing 80% of the resting anal tone via sympathetic innervation. The IAS is inhibited by parasympathetic stimulation. The external anal sphincter (EAS) consists of skeletal muscle that surrounds the IAS and extends upward to continue with the levator ani. The EAS provides 20% of resting anal tone through innervation by the pudendal nerves (S2-4). The EAS maintains fecal continence by providing voluntary and reflex increases in anal squeeze pressure in response to increased rectal or abdominal pressure. The puborectalis muscle, although contiguous with the EAS, has separate innervation by the levator ani nerve (S3-4). The puborectalis maintains fecal continence by providing the resting anorectal angle (80–100 degrees), which becomes more acute (70 degrees) during voluntary squeeze in response to increased rectal or abdominal pressure.

Rectal distension occurs as stool or gas enters the rectum, and intact rectal sensation initiates the rectoanal inhibitory reflex. During the rectoanal inhibitory reflex, the IAS relaxes (parasympathetic), rectal contents enter the anal canal, and the EAS reflexively contracts. Anal sampling then occurs, as the sensitive anoderm of the anal canal samples the rectal contents to discriminate solid, liquid, and gas; sensory feedback is provided. If social conditions do not warrant passage of the rectal contents, a strong voluntary contraction of the EAS and puborectalis muscle will push the rectal bolus back up into the rectum, until the IAS is able to contract again (sympathetic). A maximal voluntary contraction of the EAS, however, lasts only 60 seconds and fatigues within 3 minutes. If the patient decides to defecate, the puborectalis and external sphincter are relaxed. This causes descent of the pelvic floor, a more obtuse anorectal angle (110 to 130 degrees), and a decrease in the anal squeeze pressure. Defecation then occurs.

ETIOLOGY AND DIFFERENTIAL DIAGNOSIS

Fecal continence depends on a complex process that involves anal sphincter and puborectalis muscle function, anorectal sensation and reflexes, rectal capacity and compliance, stool volume and consistency, and physical mobility and mental status. Disruption of any individual step in the continence process can usually be compensated for. However, multiple or severe insults will cause fecal incontinence.

Dysfunction of the anal sphincter (EAS and/or IAS) is a common cause of fecal incontinence, usually due to denervation, obstetric trauma, anal surgery, or primary degeneration of the IAS. Injury to the EAS causes urge-related or diarrhea-associated fecal incontinence, whereas injury to the IAS may cause passive incontinence, impaired sampling, or fecal seepage.

Before the advent of endoanal ultrasound, fecal incontinence in women was attributed to denervation, with subsequent atrophy and weakness of the anal sphincter and pelvic floor. Evidence of pelvic floor neuropathy is found in 80% of women with idiopathic (neurogenic) fecal incontinence. Additionally, denervation occurs with aging, and most women do not manifest incontinence symptoms until later in life. Pudendal neuropathy due to perineal descent and traction may occur with vaginal delivery, cesarean delivery after a long labor (>8 cm dilation), and chronic constipation with excessive straining. Several studies have shown occult pudendal nerve damage in up to 80% of primiparous women, often with recovery within 6 to 12 months.

Obstetric trauma is now recognized as a leading cause of anal sphincter dysfunction, due to mechanical injury to the IAS, the EAS, or the pudendal nerve. In a landmark study, Sultan and colleagues demonstrated *occult* anal sphincter defects with endoanal ultrasound in 35% and 44% of primiparous and multiparous women, respectively, despite clinically recognized anal sphincter lacerations (third-degree tears) occurring in only 2% and 0, respectively, of each group. Primiparous women were at greatest risk, because only 4% of multiparous women had developed new defects. No new sphincter defects were seen in women with a cesarean delivery. Occult sphincter injuries have been found in 30% to 40% of primiparous women in other studies and in 80% after forceps delivery. Only 15% to 40% of occult sphincter injuries are symptomatic, and most women have flatus incontinence or urgency. These women have decreased maximum resting and squeeze anal pressures, and they may develop more severe symptoms with aging. Clinically *diagnosed* sphincter injuries occur in 0.5% to 6% of vaginal deliveries. Risk factors for anal sphincter injury have been confirmed by many studies and include nulliparity, forceps delivery, episiotomy (midline more than mediolateral), macrosomia, prolonged second stage of labor, and occiput posterior position. Several studies have shown that 20% to 50% of women continue to suffer from fecal incontinence despite primary sphincter repair.

Prior anal surgery is associated with fecal incontinence, due to disruption of the IAS. With anal sphincterotomy, an excessively tonic IAS is intentionally incised, allowing relaxation, so that an anal fissure may heal. Other anal procedures that may injure the sphincter include hemorrhoidectomy, anal dilation and treatment of fistula-in-ano.

Primary degeneration of the IAS smooth muscle is a distinct disorder found in approximately 4% of patients. The symptoms are passive fecal incontinence without urgency, and the characteristic findings are a low anal resting pressure on manometry and a thin and hyperechogenic internal sphincter on ultrasound, consistent with fibrosis. Similar findings can occur after radiation therapy to the pelvis.

Abnormal anorectal sensation and reflexes can impair discrimination of rectal contents during sampling, causing incontinence, or lead to accumulation of stool, causing fecal impaction. Neurologic disorders associated with decreased sensation include dementia, cerebrovascular accidents, multiple sclerosis, Parkinson disease, spinal cord injury, neoplasm, and sensory neuropathy with diabetes mellitus. Fecal impaction occurs often in the elderly and may also be caused by antimotility drugs, anticholinergics, and opiates. Liquid stool flows around the impacted mass. The rectoanal inhibitory reflex may be chronically stimulated by rectal prolapse, causing relaxation of the IAS and fecal incontinence.

Rectal compliance is decreased by age, pelvic radiation, inflammatory bowel disease, scleroderma, amyloidosis, neoplasm, and scarring after surgery, resulting in rectal urgency at lower rectal volumes. Irritable bowel syndrome may cause high bowel pressures and loose stool, overwhelming a normal sphincter. Sphincter-sparing rectal excision for cancer or ulcerative colitis will cause a loss of rectal capacity, although a coloanal pouch will improve capacity and incontinence.

Altered stool volume and diarrheal states caused by infection, inflammatory bowel disease, irritable bowel syndrome, laxative abuse, malabsorption syndrome, short gut syndrome, or radiation enteritis can result in fecal incontinence, despite a mechanically and neurologically intact anal sphincter and rectum. Similarly, colonic transit with bile salt malabsorption or lactose intolerance may be so rapid that incontinence occurs.

Decreased physical mobility and mental status are associated with aging and are common in the institutionalized patient. Common causes include dementia, cerebrovascular accidents, spinal cord injury, multiple sclerosis, and meningomyelocele. In nursing home residents, risk factors for fecal incontinence are (in decreasing order) urinary incontinence, tube feeding, loss of ability to perform daily living activities, diarrhea, truncal restraints, pressure ulcers, dementia, impaired vision, fecal impaction, constipation, male gender, age, and increasing body mass index.

CLINICAL SYMPTOMS AND HISTORY

Because patients often do not volunteer their problem, the first step in making the diagnosis is to screen for it by simply asking if the patient experiences uncontrolled loss of solid or liquid stool or gas and how frequently incontinence occurs. Incontinence scoring questionnaires such as the Wexner Fecal Incontinence Scale (Table 73.1), are useful tools to screen for fecal incontinence and to monitor therapy. A Wexner Fecal Incontinence Scale score of 9 or more was associated with a significant decrease in the quality of life and correlated with loss of stool more than once a week, diaper use, and feeling restricted in daily functioning.

If fecal incontinence is elicited, the history should include the onset, duration, frequency, severity, use of pads, whether stool loss is insensible, and any prior therapy. Regarding bowel function, the frequency of bowel movements, fecal urgency, straining to defecate, manual manipulation to assist emptying, use of fiber, and use of stool softeners should be identified. Passive incontinence suggests IAS dysfunction, whereas urgency reflects EAS dysfunction. The clinician should inquire about the presence of hemorrhoids and should ask about symptoms associated with rectal and vaginal prolapse. Anal incontinence must be differentiated from pseudoincontinence, which is soiling due to a variety of anorectal conditions such as hemorrhoids, skin tags, fistula-in-ano, or poor hygiene.

The past medical and surgical history should identify any of the associated medical conditions listed above, especially urinary incontinence and irritable bowel syndrome. Medications such as anticholinergics, iron, antidepressants, calcium channel blockers, and antacids that contain aluminum or calcium can all cause constipation. An obstetric history should identify the method of delivery, whether forceps or vacuum was used, episiotomy, degree of lacerations, weight of the infant, length of second stage of labor, and any other delivery complications.

CLINICAL FINDINGS AND PHYSICAL EXAMINATION

The three key components are inspection, rectal examination, and pelvic examination. The anus, perineum, and vagina should be inspected. There may be prolapse of tissue from either the anus (hemorrhoid or rectal prolapse) or the vagina. The anus should have circumferential perianal creases; absence of these creases anteriorly is the dovetail sign and correlates with anterior anal sphincter defects. There may be dermatitis, a small or large perineal body (normal is 2–3 cm), or old episiotomy or laceration scars. A small or absent perineal body is consistent with an anal sphincter defect. A large perineal body is seen with perineal descent, which can be observed by asking the patient to bear down. Note any soiling of the skin or underwear.

Before the rectal examination, pudendal nerve function should be assessed by eliciting the anocutaneous reflex (anal wink) by stroking the perianal skin with a cotton swab and observing contraction of the EAS. Digital examination can detect anal pathology such as a mass or impaction and assess the resting sphincter tone. Decreased or absent anal sphincter tone may be due to a weak or injured IAS. The patient should next be instructed to squeeze. Decreased or absent squeeze may be due to an injured EAS. With aging, however, patients may squeeze poorly or use the wrong muscles. The clinician should attempt to identify the extent of anal sphincter defects with a finger and thumb. Anoscopy may reveal hemorrhoids, inflammation, or neoplasm.

On pelvic examination, two fingers are inserted to assess the pelvic floor. A gaping introitus is consistent with levator atrophy. Assess levator muscle strength by having the woman perform a Kegel squeeze. Any rectocele or other concurrent vaginal prolapse should be identified and a rectovaginal fistula sought along the posterior vaginal wall. Additionally, the patient's mobility and mental status should be noted, because this will have an impact on workup and treatment. An abdominal examination should be performed to rule out a mass or tenderness.

LABORATORY AND IMAGING STUDIES

Anal manometry provides an objective assessment of anorectal function. Water-perfused or microtransducer catheters are placed into the rectum. Information obtained includes resting anal pressure (a low value suggests an impaired IAS), squeeze anal pressure (a low value suggests an impaired EAS), and anal functional length. A balloon attachment to the catheter is then filled to assess rectal sensation, compliance, and the rectoanal inhibitory reflex. Surface electromyography (EMG) can be done with skin pads or an anal plug to evaluate the EAS.

Pudendal nerve terminal motor latency is a nerve conduction study that measures the time required for an electrical stimulus to travel from the pudendal nerve to the EAS. A St. Mark's glove with a stimulating electrode at the end of the index finger is inserted through the rectum to the ischial spine to stimulate the pudendal nerve, and a recording electrode at the proximal portion of the finger measures surface EMG of the EAS. Prolonged pudendal nerve terminal motor latencies are found in 80% of women with neurogenic fecal incontinence but inconsistently predict poor outcomes from anal sphincteroplasty.

TABLE 73.1. Wexner Fecal Incontinence Scale

Incontinence symptom	Frequency of incontinence				
	Never	<1 per mo	<1 per wk– ≥1 per mo	<1 per day– ≥1 per wk	≥1 per day
Gas	0	1	2	3	4
Liquid	0	1	2	3	4
Solid	0	1	2	3	4
Requires pad	0	1	2	3	4
Lifestyle alteration	0	1	2	3	4

Minimum score = 0, maximum score = 20.
Source: Jorge JM, Wexner SD. Etiology and management of fecal incontinence. *Dis Colon Rectum* 1993;36:77–97.

Endoanal ultrasound has become the gold standard for the evaluation of patients with fecal incontinence. It provides accurate and reproducible images of the puborectalis, IAS, and EAS. The integrity, thickness, and length of each can be measured. An endoprobe with a high frequency (7 or 10 MHz) transducer that allows a 360-degree image of the anal canal musculature is inserted. Images are recorded at the upper (puborectalis), mid (IAS), and lower (EAS) anal canal to map the sphincters. The IAS appears as a hypoechoic circle and the EAS as a hyperechoic circle. Anal sphincter defects usually occur anteriorly (from 10 to 2 o'clock in the lithotomy position), consistent with the location of obstetric trauma at delivery, and correlate well with manometric findings.

Other studies performed less often include needle EMG, defecography, colonic transit time (constipation), sigmoidoscopy or colonoscopy (intussusception and inflammatory or neoplastic conditions), and magnetic resonance imaging (pelvic floor anatomy). Needle EMG can identify abnormalities of the EAS such as denervation, reinnervation, and increased muscle fiber density. With contrast in the bladder, vagina, and rectum and the patient seated on a commode, defecography can evaluate the anorectal angle, pelvic floor descent, pelvic organ prolapse, intussusception, and paradoxical contraction of the puborectalis muscle (a defecation disorder).

TREATMENT

Most of the diarrheal causes of fecal incontinence are improved by treatment of the underlying medical condition. Current medications may need to be changed or the dose adjusted. Dietary modifications and the addition of fiber will help most patients, because formed stool is easier to control than liquid stool. Additional therapy may be used to reduce stool frequency and to increase stool bulk. Loperamide will reduce stool frequency, reduce urgency, and increase IAS tone. Hyoscyamine and amitriptyline have anticholinergic properties that increase stool transit time. Topical phenylephrine gel, which has been shown to increase anal resting pressure, is being investigated as treatment of fecal incontinence due to a weak IAS.

Management of constipation is important to avoid fecal impaction. Increased physical activity, fiber, and fluid intake are beneficial in most patients, although fiber can exacerbate fecal impaction. Stimulant laxatives may be used occasionally, but overuse can have significant side effects. Lactulose, docusate, and sorbitol are more effective and will take effect in 1 to 2 days.

In a nursing home study, residents with overflow incontinence due to fecal impaction and impaired rectal sensation were treated initially with daily enemas and then maintained with lactulose twice daily and a weekly enema (rectal sensation improves with time). Conversely, residents with neurogenic (passive) incontinence were treated with codeine to produce constipation and then two enemas weekly to produce predictable bowel movements. With treatment, 66% were continent, reaching 87% with full compliance.

Pelvic floor muscle (Kegel) exercises can improve incontinence symptoms, are easy to do, and can be done at any time or in any position. Patients are instructed to squeeze and hold (as if trying to stop a bowel movement) for 10 to 40 seconds, 10 times per set, three to four sets per day. Biofeedback can assist those unable to do these exercises by teaching patients how to properly contract the EAS and levator muscles. A systematic review of 46 studies and 1,364 patients found that 50% were cured and 70% were improved. There is no morbidity with biofeedback, and it is performed in an outpatient setting. Biofeedback may be used as a conservative treatment instead of surgery (especially with mild to moderate symptoms) or as an adjunct to improve results in patients with persistent symptoms after surgery.

Women with severe fecal incontinence due to anal sphincter defects are usually treated with an overlapping sphincteroplasty. The detached ends of the anal sphincter are each dissected completely and the scarred ends are overlapped in the midline and sutured together. A review of several large series has shown good to excellent results in 66%, fair results in 22%, and poor results in 12%. Whether preoperative pudendal nerve terminal motor latency studies predict postoperative success is controversial, because there are several conflicting studies.

Surgical treatments for patients who fail anal sphincteroplasty or who do not have anal sphincter defects are effective in relieving symptoms but have high complication rates. Gracilis transposition is a muscle transfer procedure that provides a passive neosphincter. Electrical stimulation from an external pulse generator provides continuous contraction without voluntary effort and can be turned off for defecation. Success rates range from 55% to 75%, but complications occur in half of the patients. The artificial anal sphincter is an inflatable plastic ring-shaped device that is implanted around the anus and deflated for defecation with a manual pump implanted in the labia majora. A successful outcome was achieved in 85% of patients with a functioning device, but intention to treat success was only 53%, because 37% had their devices explanted due to complications. Postanal repair is used less often due to decreased success (30%–40%) but may have a limited role in patients with intact sphincters. Colostomy may be useful in selected patients and can improve quality of life.

Sacral nerve stimulation (Interstim) was initially developed for urinary dysfunction and now is being investigated for fecal incontinence. Several short series have shown excellent success (80%–100%), but up to 25% have required revision or removal due to infection or lead dislodgement. The mechanism of action remains undetermined, although anal resting and squeeze pressures are improved.

CONSIDERATIONS IN PREGNANCY

What can be done to prevent pregnancy-related fecal incontinence? There are many preventive steps that can be taken, because known risk factors for anal sphincter laceration exist (listed above). Use of forceps and episiotomy should be minimized, especially if there is suspected macrosomia or occiput posterior position, to prevent anal sphincter lacerations. Forceps use is associated with greater sphincter damage than vacuum-assisted or spontaneous delivery. A mediolateral incision should be made when an episiotomy is needed. Perineal massage in nulliparas starting at 34 weeks is associated with a 5% to 10% absolute decrease in the risk of lacerated perineums. After primary repair of anal sphincter lacerations, 40% to 80% of women have persistent anal sphincter defects and 20% to 50% are symptomatic. Therefore, when anal sphincter lacerations occur, primary surgical repair could be improved by having the most experienced clinician complete the repair and by moving the patient from a birthing room to a delivery or operating room to provide better lighting, exposure, anesthesia, and assistance. Outcomes after primary repair of anal sphincter lacerations at delivery are similar between overlapping and approximation techniques.

How should women with prior pelvic floor trauma or fecal incontinence symptoms be managed in subsequent pregnancies? As noted above, 40% to 80% of women with primary repair have persistent anal sphincter defects, and occult defects can be found in 30% to 40% of women. In women without anal sphincter lacerations, the risk of permanent flatus incontinence was increased after the third vaginal delivery compared with the risk after the first and second delivery (8.3% vs. 1.2% and 1.5%, respectively). The effect of a second vaginal delivery on preexisting fecal incontinence symptoms has been investigated in three studies. Overall, among women without fecal incontinence after the first delivery, only 9% developed incontinence after the second delivery. Of women with transient incontinence after the first delivery, 41% became incontinent after the second delivery. For women with permanent fecal incontinence symptoms, 59% became worse. The effect of a second vaginal delivery on preexisting anal sphincter defects was similar: 38% of women with an anal sphincter defect (from their first delivery) reported fecal incontinence, compared with 10% of women without an anal sphincter defect. Minor incontinence symptoms such as flatus incontinence and urgency should be regarded as markers of anal sphincter trauma. Therefore, women with incontinence symptoms or a known prior anal sphincter laceration should be told that their symptoms may progress or recur with repeated vaginal deliveries and offered anorectal evaluation.

Women that have had a successful anal sphincteroplasty for fecal incontinence should be given the option of an elective cesarean delivery in subsequent pregnancies. However, there are no randomized trials to provide evidence that fecal incontinence will be prevented with elective cesarean delivery. Further research is needed to determine risk factors that identify which women would benefit from elective cesarean section.

DISCLAIMER

The opinions or assertions contained herein are the private views of the author and are not to be construed as official or as reflecting the views of the Department of the Army or the Department of Defense.

BIBLIOGRAPHY

Bannister JJ, Timms JM, Barfield LJ, et al. Physiological studies in young women with chronic constipation. *Int J Colorectal Dis* 1986;1:175–182.

Bek KM, Laurberg S. Risks of anal incontinence from subsequent vaginal delivery after a complete obstetric anal sphincter tear. *Br J Obstet Gynaecol* 1992;99: 724–726.

Borrie MJ, Davidson HA. Incontinence in institutions: costs and contributing factors. *CMAJ* 1992;147:322–328.

Buie WD, Lowry AC, Rothenber DA, et al. Clinical rather than laboratory assessment predicts continence after anterior sphincteroplasty. *Dis Colon Rectum* 2001;44:1255–1260.

Chapman AE, Geerdes B, Hewett P, et al. Systematic review of dynamic graciloplasty in the treatment of faecal incontinence. *Br J Surg* 2002;89:138–153.

Clemons JL, Aguilar VC, Myers DL, et al. Recommendations for delivery in pregnancy following pelvic reconstructive surgery. *Obstet Gynecol* 2002;99:108S.

Eason E, Labrecque M, Wells G, et al. Preventing perineal trauma during childbirth: a systematic review. *Obstet Gynecol* 2000;95:464–471.

Faltin DL, Sangalli MR, Roche B, et al. Does a second delivery increase the risk of anal incontinence? *Br J Obstet Gynaecol* 2001;108:684–688.

Fynes M, Donnelly V, Behan M, et al. Effect of second vaginal delivery on anorectal physiology and faecal continence: a prospective study. *Lancet* 1999;354:983–986.

Fynes M, Donnelly VS, O'Connell PR, et al. Cesarean delivery and anal sphincter injury. *Obstet Gynecol* 1998;92:496–500.

Johanson JF, Lafferty J. Epidemiology of fecal incontinence: the silent affliction. *Am J Gastroenterol* 1996;91:33–36.

Jorge JM, Wexner SD. Etiology and management of fecal incontinence. *Dis Colon Rectum* 1993;36:77–97.

Nelson R, Furner S, Jesudason V. Fecal incontinence in Wisconsin nursing homes: prevalence and associations. *Dis Colon Rectum* 1998;41:1226–12269.

Nelson R, Norton N, Cautley E, et al. Community-based prevalence of anal incontinence. *JAMA* 1995;274:559–561.

Norton C, Kamm MA. Anal sphincter biofeedback and pelvic floor exercises for faecal incontinence in adults—a systematic review. *Aliment Pharmacol Ther* 2001;15:1147–1154.

Rothbarth J, Bemelman WA, Maijerink WJ, et al. What is the impact of fecal incontinence on quality of life? *Dis Colon Rectum* 2001;44:67–71.

Ryhammer AM, Bek KM, Laurberg S. Multiple vaginal deliveries increase the risk of permanent incontinence of flatus and urine in normal premenopausal women. *Dis Colon Rectum* 1995;38:1206–1209.

Shiono P, Klebanoff MA, Carey JC. Midline episiotomies: more harm than good? *Obstet Gynecol* 1990;75:765–770.

Snooks SJ, Swash M, Henry MM, et al. Risk factors in childbirth causing damage to the pelvic floor innervation. *Int J Colorectal Dis* 1986;1:20–24.

Snooks SJ, Swash M, Setchell M, et al. Injury to innervation of pelvic floor musculature in childbirth. *Lancet* 1984;2:546–550.

Sultan AH, Kamm MA, Hudson CN, et al. Anal-sphincter disruption during vaginal delivery. *N Engl J Med* 1993;329:1905–1911.

Sultan AH, Kamm MA, Hudson CN, et al. Third degree obstetric anal sphincter tears: risk factors and outcome of primary repair. *BMJ* 1994;308:887–891.

Tetzschner T, Sorensen M, Lose G, et al. Anal and urinary incontinence in women with obstetric anal sphincter rupture. *Br J Obstet Gynaecol* 1996;103:1034–1040.

Tobin GW, Brocklehurst JC. Faecal incontinence in residential homes for the elderly: prevalence, aetiology and management. *Age Ageing* 1986;15:41–46.

Wong WD, Congliosi SM, Spencer MP, et al. The safety and efficacy of the artificial bowel sphincter for fecal incontinence: results from a multicenter cohort study. *Dis Colon Rectum* 2002;45:1139–1153.

CHAPTER 74
Hemorrhoids

Victor E. Pricolo and Matthew Vrees

Hemorrhoids affect approximately 5% of the general population in the United States, and close to 50% of people over the age of 50 are eventually affected. Despite a relatively high prevalence in the United States, hemorrhoids are often most misunderstood and poorly managed by patients and primary care providers.

Patients with perianal complaints often attribute them to hemorrhoids, but the differential diagnosis includes fissures, perianal warts, hypertrophied anal papillae, rectal prolapse, prolapsing rectal polyp, abscess, and, most importantly, anorectal neoplasms. Primary care clinicians must keep these conditions in mind as they evaluate women for perianal concerns.

ANATOMY AND CLASSIFICATION

Hemorrhoids are submucosal vascular cushions that lie both above and below the dentate line of the anal canal. They most commonly receive their blood supply from the superior rectal artery, the middle rectal arteries, and the inferior rectal arteries, allowing for natural portosystemic shunts. Hemorrhoids are typically located in the right anterior, right posterior, and left lateral positions of the anal canal. These cushions of tissue are made up not only of arterial and venous plexuses but also a rich supply of nerves, connective tissue, and smooth muscle.

An understanding of the classification system for hemorrhoids is essential to proper diagnosis and treatment and to differentiate from other common anorectal conditions. Hemorrhoids can be divided into two categories: internal and external. Internal hemorrhoids arise above the dentate line, are covered by transitional or columnar epithelium, and are classified on the basis of their degree of prolapse (Table 74.1). External hemorrhoids are distal to the dentate line and are covered by anoderm. They should be distinguished from simple skin tags, which are covered by true squamous epithelium.

ETIOLOGY

Major contributing factors to the development of hemorrhoids are believed to be chronic straining and a low-fiber diet. The

TABLE 74.1. Classification of Internal Hemorrhoids

Degree	Description	Symptoms	Treatment
First	Prolapse of hemorrhoid cushion into the lumen of the rectum and anal canal	Bleeding	Conservative Rubber band[a]
Second	Prolapse out of the anal canal with pressure and reduce spontaneously	Discomfort, swelling, and bleeding	Conservative Rubber band[a] Hemorrhoidectomy Excision/stapled
Third	Prolapse out of the anal canal with pressure and require manual reduction	Pain when prolapsed Thrombosis Bleeding	Conservative Hemorrhoidectomy Excision/stapled
Fourth	Prolapsed out of the anal canal and unable to be reduced	Severe pain Thrombosis/infarction	Hemorrhoidectomy

[a]*When conservative management fails.*

theory is that small caliber stools fail to activate the rectoanal inhibitory reflex. If the internal sphincter fails to relax, the intraluminal pressure in the anal canal is bound to rise, leading to mucosal injury. Other authors have demonstrated that patients with hemorrhoids have increased activity of the internal anal sphincter, although it has not been shown whether such changes are a cause or a consequence of the hemorrhoids.

EVALUATION

When evaluating a patient who complains of hemorrhoids, one must keep in mind that patients brand all pathology in the perianal region as " hemorrhoids." In other words, hemorrhoids are obviously not a complaint but a diagnosis. A clinician must be careful not to misdiagnose the problem, missing less common and potentially more dangerous pathology. An accurate diagnosis can be made in most cases by the history of symptoms and a properly performed examination.

Symptoms

INTERNAL HEMORRHOIDS

Bleeding is the most common symptom associated with internal hemorrhoids. The bleeding is typically episodic and described as bright red blood seen in the toilet bowl after a bowel movement. The blood may or may not be mixed with the stool, found just on the toilet paper, or can be more significant. Patients with chronic symptoms can present with any degree of anemia. In the evaluation of rectal bleeding we must always consider other causes of hematochezia and perform colonoscopy when indicated. Prolapse or protrusion of hemorrhoids may produce a feeling of pressure or a mass in the anal area. Patients may also complain of moisture or itching of the perianal skin from the production of mucus by the irritated epithelium of the hemorrhoidal mucosa. Prolapsed internal hemorrhoids may become thrombosed and potentially infarcted with associated severe throbbing pain. These symptoms are not relieved unless manual reduction or excision of the hemorrhoid is performed.

EXTERNAL HEMORRHOIDS

Complaints from external hemorrhoids range from acute to chronic symptoms. Unlike internal hemorrhoids, bleeding is not a symptom associated with external hemorrhoids in the acute phase. Patients almost exclusively complain of severe pain in the event of thrombosis. Symptoms may improve with time when the overlying anoderm sloughs, at which time some bleeding might be observed. With healing, redundant skin may develop and create anal skin tags, which become the complaint of patients in the later phase. Except in rare cases of associated dermatitis, the significance of skin tags is limited to perianal cosmesis and hygiene.

Examination

The examination of the perianal area, the anus, and rectum are best performed and most comfortable to the patient on a proctologic examination table with the patient in a prone or lateral decubitus position. The first part of every examination of this area is a complete inspection of the perianal region. This part of the examination is often overlooked but is crucial to appropriate diagnosis. Part of the inspection includes spreading of the buttocks, which allows good exposure to the distal anus, most fissures, external hemorrhoids, perianal skin tags, fistulae, and perianal dermatologic conditions. After inspection, the patient should be made aware that the next portion of the examination is the digital rectal examination. Because many patients present with a complaint of pain in the area of the anus, reassurance is imperative. It is important to remember that internal hemorrhoids are not typically palpable. The digital examination allows the estimation of sphincter tone and the presence of low rectal or anal cancer. The clinician may choose to omit the digital examination if there is severe anal pain from a visible thrombosed hemorrhoid, an abscess, or an acute fissure. After the digital examination, anoscopy should be performed. Anoscopy is the best maneuver for visualization of internal hemorrhoids. Carcinoma of the anus can also be observed during anoscopy. Other tests such as rigid or flexible sigmoidoscopy, colonoscopy, barium enema, or defecogram may be performed if indicated.

TREATMENT

Conservative

The initial treatment for all nonthrombosed hemorrhoids should be the addition of fiber to the patient's diet. In addition, patient's water intake should be increased to 8 to 10 glasses a day. Sitz baths help with pain and local hygiene. They consist of soaking the perianal region in warm water. No other topical remedy has ever been shown to significantly reduce the pain or duration of symptoms produced by hemorrhoidal disease. Internal hemorrhoids are not helped by any of the innumerable over-the-counter creams or ointments. In addition, the prolonged use of products that contain steroids may contribute to the risk of fungal infection and skin atrophy.

Ablative

RUBBER BAND LIGATION

Rubber band ligation is one of the most frequently used methods of hemorrhoidectomy in the United States. This procedure is best used in patients with symptomatic first- and second-degree hemorrhoids in the office setting. Care must be taken to place the band high above the dentate line to minimize any pain associated with the procedure. Over a 5- to 7-day period, the rubber band strangulates the tissue at which time the banded hemorrhoid will slough. Possible complications associated with rubber band ligation are uncommon but may include pain, bleeding, and urinary retention. To minimize the risk of bleeding, patients should be advised not to take antiplatelet medication (aspirin, Plavix, etc.) for at least 1 week after ligation. This procedure is contraindicated in patients requiring anticoagulation. Pelvic sepsis has rarely been reported and should be considered when pain and urinary retention are associated with fever.

INFRARED PHOTOCOAGULATION AND SCLEROTHERAPY

Infrared photocoagulation and sclerotherapy are two methods that create obliteration of the hemorrhoid and scarring of the tissue by using heat or a sclerosing agent, respectively. Infrared photocoagulation has never been shown to be superior to banding, whereas the cost is greater. Sclerotherapy may be safer in patients who are anticoagulated but can cause oleomas and abscesses.

HEMORRHOIDECTOMY

Surgical hemorrhoidectomy should be reserved for patients with third- and fourth-degree hemorrhoids. Although the surgical therapy for acutely thrombosed hemorrhoids has not changed over the last 30 years, there has been an evolution or perhaps a revolution in the treatment of nonthrombosed third- and fourth-degree hemorrhoids in recent years.

ACUTELY THROMBOSED HEMORRHOIDS

Conservative nonsurgical methods for the management of acutely thrombosed hemorrhoids have never been shown to be advantageous, when compared with surgical excision. Ice packs and analgesics may reduce the pain temporarily, but the time to complete symptom resolution is greatly prolonged. For acutely thrombosed external hemorrhoids, excision in the office with local anesthesia is the preferred treatment because it will alleviate the pain immediately and eliminate recurrence. Simple incision and drainage of the hemorrhoid may lead to persistent pain, drainage, superinfection of retained clot, and likely development of a skin tag. The treatment of acutely prolapsed and thrombosed internal hemorrhoids is best achieved by operative hemorrhoidectomy with regional or general anesthesia. Care to maintain sufficient intact anoderm between hemorrhoid columns is paramount to avoid an anal stricture.

CHRONIC SYMPTOMATIC HEMORRHOIDS

Hemorrhoidectomy is indicated if the patient has failed all previously described conservative treatments. Hemorrhoidectomy can be performed under local, epidural/saddle block, or general anesthesia. It is important to minimize the amount of intravenous fluids administered during the procedure to reduce the incidence of urinary retention associated with hemorrhoidectomy. It is crucial to preserve the internal sphincter fibers while excising the hemorrhoids. None of the different tools for cutting, including laser, harmonic scalpel, or cautery, has proven to be superior to scissors.

MANAGEMENT OF THE PATIENT AFTER HEMORRHOIDECTOMY

Complications of hemorrhoidal surgery include severe pain, bleeding, urinary retention, constipation, infection, fecal incontinence, and anal stenosis. All patients should be kept on fiber and perform sitz baths and should be immediately examined if fever or urinary retention is observed.

Restorative Surgery

STAPLED HEMORRHOIDECTOMY

Stapled hemorrhoidectomy is a novel approach in treating third- and fourth-degree hemorrhoids. Although referred to as a hemorrhoidectomy, it is really an anopexy with division of the vessels supplying the hemorrhoids. The hemorrhoids are not excised but are restored to their normal physiologic position using a circular stapling device. Randomized trials have demonstrated that stapled hemorrhoidectomy may offer advantages to the standard hemorrhoidectomy, including less postoperative pain and a quicker return to normal activities. Opponents to this technique criticize the added expense of the equipment and the lack of long-term follow-up.

CONSIDERATIONS IN PREGNANCY

The incidence of hemorrhoidal disease during pregnancy has been reported to be as high as 40%, nearly 10 times that of the general population. Certain physiologic and hormonal changes in pregnancy, which lead to increased abdominal pressure, constipation, and venous engorgement, theoretically explain the relatively high incidence. The symptoms are no different during pregnancy, and rigorous conservative management with increased fiber and water intake should not only be used as a treatment but as a preventive strategy. Importantly, if all conservative measures fail, hemorrhoid surgery during all trimesters can be performed safely under local anesthesia. After delivery, most cases of hemorrhoidal disease resolve, with the incidence no higher than the general population.

BIBLIOGRAPHY

Barwell J, Watkins RM, Lloyd-Davies E, et al. Life-threatening retroperitoneal sepsis after hemorrhoid injection sclerotherapy: report of a case. *Dis Colon Rectum* 1999;42:421–423.

Boccasanta P, Capretti PG, Venturi M, et al. Randomised controlled trial between stapled circumferential mucosectomy and conventional circular hemorrhoidectomy in advanced hemorrhoids with external mucosal prolapse. *Am J Surg* 2001;182:64–68.

Brodsky JB, Cohen EN, Brown BW Jr, et al. Surgery during pregnancy and fetal outcome. *Am J Obstet Gynecol* 1980;138:1165–1167.

Burkitt DP. Varicose veins, deep vein thrombosis, and haemorrhoids: epidemiology and suggested aetiology. *Br Med J* 1972;2:556–561.

Dennison AR, Wherry DC, Morris DL. Hemorrhoids: nonoperative management. *Surg Clin North Am* 1988;68:1401–1409.

Ferguson JA, Mazier WP, Ganchrow MI, et al. The closed technique of hemorrhoidectomy. *Surgery* 1971;70:480–484.

Haas PA, Fox TA Jr, Haas GP. The pathogenesis of hemorrhoids. *Dis Colon Rectum* 1984;27:442–450.

Hancock BD. Internal sphincter and the nature of haemorrhoids. *Gut* 1977;18: 651–655.

Johanson JF, Sonnenberg A. The prevalence of hemorrhoids and chronic constipation: an epidemiologic study. *Gastroenterology* 1990;98:380–386.

Johanson JF, Sonnenberg A. Temporal changes in the occurrence of hemorrhoids in the United States and England. *Dis Colon Rectum* 1991;34:585–591; discussion 591–593.

Kaman L, Aggarwal S, Kumar R, et al. Necrotizing fascitis after injection sclerotherapy for hemorrhoids: report of a case. *Dis Colon Rectum* 1999;42:419–420.

Kort B, Katz VL, Watson WJ. The effect of nonobstetric operation during pregnancy. *Surg Gynecol Obstet* 1993;177:371–376.

Leicester RJ, Nicholls RJ, Mann CV. Infrared coagulation: a new treatment for hemorrhoids. *Dis Colon Rectum* 1981;24:602–605.

Medich DS, Fazio VW. Hemorrhoids, anal fissure, and carcinoma of the colon, rectum, and anus during pregnancy. *Surg Clin North Am* 1995;75:77–88.

Moesgaard F, Nielsen ML, Hansen JB, et al. High-fiber diet reduces bleeding and pain in patients with hemorrhoids: a double-blind trial of Vi-Siblin. *Dis Colon Rectum* 1982;25:454–456.

Orrom W, Hayashi A, Rusnak C, et al. Initial experience with stapled anoplasty in the operative management of prolapsing hemorrhoids and mucosal rectal prolapse. *Am J Surg* 2002;183:519–524.

Randall GM, Jensen DM, Machicado GA, et al. Prospective randomized comparative study of bipolar versus direct current electrocoagulation for treatment of bleeding internal hemorrhoids. *Gastrointest Endosc* 1994;40:403–410.

Saleeby RG Jr, Rosen L, Stasik JJ, et al. Hemorrhoidectomy during pregnancy: risk or relief? *Dis Colon Rectum* 1991;34:260–261.

Thomson WH. The nature and cause of haemorrhoids. *Proc R Soc Med* 1975;68: 574–575.

Thomson WH. The nature of haemorrhoids. *Br J Surg* 1975;62:542–552.

PART

8

Urinary Tract Problems

CHAPTER 75
Urinary Tract Infections

Neil D. Jackson

Urinary tract infections (UTIs) in women are one of the most common types of infection seen by primary care providers. According to the National Ambulatory and Hospital Medical Care Survey, UTIs accounted for 7 million office visits, resulting in 100,000 hospital admissions. Nearly one in three women will have had a UTI by the age of 24. Almost half of all women will have had at least one UTI at some time in their life. Subgroups at increased risk for UTI include the elderly, infants, patients with spinal cord injuries, patients with indwelling Foley catheters, diabetics, patients with demyelinization disease, immunodeficient patients (e.g., human immunodeficiency virus), and patients with underlying urologic abnormalities. In noninstitutionalized elder patients, UTIs are the second most common form of infection, contributing to 25% of all infections.

Simple acute UTI in a nonpregnant female patient is considered a benign disease. Sequelae may be significant in the pregnant patient and in the pediatric population. The cost of UTI management in the United States is approximately $1.6 billion yearly.

UTIs encompass a wide spectrum of clinical and pathologic conditions ranging from asymptomatic bacteriuria to perinephric abscesses. UTIs are usually classified by the site of infection and are divided into lower and upper infections. Cystitis (lower UTI) is the clinical syndrome caused by pathogenic bacteria and is accompanied by lower urinary tract symptoms (e.g., dysuria, frequency, urgency, and suprapubic pain). Upper UTIs (e.g., pyelonephritis) are more ominous with respect to systemic disease and long-term morbidity and mortality. Acute pyelonephritis is often manifests with dysuria, urgency, frequency, flank pain, and significant bacteriuria ($\geq 10^5$ bacteria/mL). The symptoms of lower tract and upper tract infections may overlap, especially when both processes are occurring concomitantly, but the clinical picture is usually clear.

"Uncomplicated" infections are diagnosed in the urinary tract with no history of instrumentation. "Complicated infection" are diagnosed in the urinary tract where there is a structural or functional abnormality or instrumentation such as a Foley catheter. On many occasions these patients may be asymptomatic.

PATHOGENESIS

Lower genital tract bacteria colonize the lower urinary tract through various mechanisms, including adhesion to the uroepithelium mediated by papillae on the bacterial cell wall. The most common pathway of infection in the urinary tract is the ascending route. Hematogenous and lymphatic pathways also have been implicated as routes of UTI, but both are uncommon. Initiation of the ascent of bacteria occurs in the urethra. The short length of the female urethra, together with the tendency to periurethral contamination with pathogenic bacteria, may explain why UTIs are more common in females than in males. The urethra is a sterile organ except for the distal portion. The female urethra appears particularly susceptible to colonization with colonic Gram-negative bacilli because of its proximity to the anus, its short length (about 4 cm), and its termination beneath the labia. Migration of organisms from the urethra to the bladder is facilitated by sexual intercourse and diaphragm and spermicidal jelly utilization. Estrogen deficiency in postmenopausal women and nonsecretory status of ABO blood-group antigens are also considered risk factors for infection.

The incidence of UTI in ambulatory patients requiring intermittent straight catheterization of the bladder is about 1%. Patients with indwelling catheters and open drainage systems may develop UTIs within 3 or 4 days of initiation. Cultures of the periurethral and rectal areas have revealed an excellent correlation with the organisms subsequently found to be the cause of the UTI in catheterized patients. This evidence supports the suggestion that the ascending route is the most common pathway of infection in the urinary tract.

Although young women are susceptible to UTIs, the urinary tract is actually highly resistant to infection. Bacteria placed in the bladder, under normal circumstances, are cleared rapidly by the flushing and dilutional effects of voiding and the direct antibacterial properties of urine and the bladder mucosa. Bacterial growth is also inhibited by the high urea concentration, acidity, and high osmolality of the urine. Mucosal cells producing organic acids, along with local antibody responses and polymorphonuclear leukocytes in the bladder wall, appear to destroy bacteria that remain in the bladder mucosa after urination. When bacteria enter the urinary tract, UTI results only if inappropriate interaction occurs between the bacterial virulence factors, inoculum size, and adequacy of the host defense mechanism. The anatomic level of the UTI is also determined by these factors. Recurrent UTI is primarily a failure of normal host defense mechanisms rather than microbial characteristics.

The three major elements determining virulence of pathogenic bacteria are adhesions, hemolysis, and aerobactin. Most commonly, these characteristics are found in *Escherichia coli* strains. Adhesion was documented in 50% of patients with cystitis and 70% of patients with pyelonephritis. *E. coli* isolates from patients with pyelonephritis usually have virulence factors not usually present in ordinary fecal isolates. These factors include papillae (adhesions), which are surface organelles that mediate attachment to specific receptors on the epithelial cells of the vagina. At least four different types of adhesions have been described: type I papillae, type II papillae, the P adhesion, and diffuse adhesion. *E. coli's* avidity for iron constitutes the other two major elements believed to determine the virulence of pathogenic bacteria: the presence of hemolysins, which degrade red cells, and aerobactin, a siderophore that enhances iron uptake.

The most effective host defense mechanisms are the turnover of epithelial cells and the flushing effect of voiding. Researchers have reviewed tissue factors secreted from the lower urinary tract that should prevent bacteria from adhering to its mucosal membranes. These factors include oligosaccharides, uromucoids (Tamm-Horsfall proteins), immunoglobulins (IgG, IgA, and secretory IgA), and bladder mucopolysaccharides, which have the potential to inhibit or prevent attachment or to actively detach bacteria from the mucosal surface. The urothelial mucosal cells that produce these factors are deficient in women prone to UTIs, especially recurrent infections.

URINARY PATHOGENS AND URINARY TRACT INFECTIONS

As mentioned above, several endogenous factors help inhibit bacterial growth: high urine osmolality, urea concentration, organic acid concentration, and a low pH. The etiology of acute uncomplicated UTI rarely implicates more than one bacterial species. The presence of multiple organisms in a urine sample often reflects a contaminated specimen, unless the patient is at risk for a complicated UTI. Isolation of organisms usually residing as normal flora on the distal urethra and skin suggests contamination (e.g., *Staphylococcus epidermidis*, diphtheroids, lactobacilli, *Gardnerella vaginalis*, and anaerobes).

Pathogenic Gram-negative bacilli normally present in the gut are the source of organisms causing UTIs by the ascending route. The most common urinary pathogen, *E. coli*, accounts for about 80% to 85% of infections. *Staphylococcus saprophyticus* is the second most common cause of UTIs, particularly in young women. Other organisms found in uncomplicated infections include *Klebsiella, Proteus*, and *Enterobacter*.

E. coli accounts for half the UTIs in hospitalized patients. Other urinary pathogens in hospitalized patients include *Klebsiella, Enterobacter, Citrobacter, Serratia, Pseudomonas aeruginosa, Providencia*, enterococci, and *S. epidermidis*. Fungal infections are almost exclusively incurred by hospitalized patients. Diabetes and immunocompromised status are important risk factors. Fungi, especially *Candida* spp., may infect the urinary tract of patients with indwelling catheters receiving antimicrobial therapy. Other urinary pathogens associated with UTIs in the hospital in association with instrumentation and catheterization are *G. vaginalis*; lactobacilli; *Mycoplasma* spp., including *Ureaplasma urealyticum*; and *S. epidermidis*. Group B streptococcal infections are found predominantly in diabetic patients. Noninstrumented patients usually incur *Streptococcus faecalis*.

Sexually transmitted urethritis may involve pathogens such as *Chlamydia trachomatis, Neisseria gonorrhoeae*, and herpes simplex virus. Vaginitis caused by *Trichomonas vaginalis* and *Candida* spp. may mimic acute urethritis or urinary tract infection. *T. vaginalis* can also invade and infect the bladder (cystitis).

In the elderly, unlike in younger women, the pathogenesis of UTI is related to abnormal bladder function, bladder outlet obstruction, vaginal and urethral atrophy, use of long-term indwelling catheters, and puddling related to bed rest. The organisms causing infection in the elderly relate to the ecology of the patient's environment. Many have a greater variety of pathogenic organisms, especially women living in nursing homes and in particular those with permanent indwelling catheters. Many of these organisms may be antibiotic resistant.

The development of an infection and its outcome are determined by the interactions of the virulence of the bacteria and the host defense mechanisms. Some urinary pathogens are relatively opportunistic and avirulent and thus can induce UTI only when natural host defense mechanisms are compromised. Other organisms can cause infection and invade the lower or upper urinary tract in the absence of obstruction, other structural abnormalities, or urinary tract catheterization.

CLINICAL FINDINGS

There is a broad spectrum of symptoms accompanying UTI, ranging from irritative voiding to bacteremia, sepsis, or even death. Depending on the patient's age, the location of the infection, and concomitant urologic disease, symptomatology varies. Clinical signs and symptoms in adults with UTI include frequency, dysuria, small amounts of urine, urgency, hematuria, low back pain, or suprapubic pain. Low-grade fever may accompany lower tract infection. Lower tract infections in the elderly are often asymptomatic. The usual symptoms of lower tract infections (e.g., frequency, dysuria, hesitancy, and incontinence) are present in many noninfected elderly patients and therefore are nonspecific.

Classically, upper tract infections present with flank pain, nausea, vomiting, fever (38°C, often with chills and rigors), and costovertebral angle tenderness. Symptoms of cystitis may not be present. In moderate to severe cases of acute pyelonephritis, the temperature may be high (40°C), with intermittent spikes. If vomiting and insensible water loss have caused significant dehydration, the patient may be weak and may appear debilitated. Clinical hypotension may ensue and rarely progresses to overt septic shock. Lower tract symptoms are the only presentation in 10% to 50% of patients with concurrent upper tract infections. The elderly and neurologically impaired often have atypical clinical presentations. Symptoms may include appetite reduction, decreased social interaction and personal hygiene, changes in mentation, abdominal pain, incontinence, urgency, and nocturia.

Patients may present without symptoms but still have a lower or upper tract infection. Asymptomatic bacteria has been observed in up to 50% of catheterized hospitalized patients. The most common source of bacteremia produced by Gram-negative bacilli is UTI. In the presence of an indwelling catheter, bacteremia may occur with no urinary symptoms.

DIAGNOSIS

The initial step in the laboratory diagnosis of UTI is microscopic examination of the urine to look for pyuria and hematuria. Pyuria is present in almost all women with an acutely symptomatic UTI and in most women with urethritis. Pyuria without significant bacteriuria in a sexually active woman with dysuria suggests the diagnosis of urethritis, usually caused by either *N. gonorrhoeae* or *C. trachomatis.* The most accurate way to assess pyuria is to examine an unspun, voided midstream, urine specimen. In symptomatic women, urinalysis is the most accurate method for predicting bacteriuria. The periurethral and urethral areas are difficult to sterilize; therefore, frequent contamination of the urine specimen occurs. As a result, the presence of bacteria on urinalysis is not used as a single criterion for the diagnosis of UTI. The method of urine collection affects the results; the three acceptable methods for urine collection include midstream clean-catch, catheterization, and suprapubic aspiration. Catheterization avoids heavy vaginal contamination. However, a single catheterization carries a 4% to 6% risk of introducing an infection and is not justified merely to obtain a urine specimen for diagnosis. To decrease the chance of contamination, the patient must be properly instructed in how to obtain the specimen. A drop of unspun urine is examined, as well as the sediment from a specimen subjected to centrifugation for 5 minutes at 2,000 rpm. In an unspun urine, 10 or more leukocytes per cubic millimeter is considered abnormal, and most women with urinary tract infection have hundreds of leukocytes per cubic millimeter. In a centrifuged specimen, more than 8 to 10 white blood cells per high power field correlates with an excess of 400,000 cells shed per hour, which is the standard for the presence of infection.

Another useful test in the presumptive diagnosis of UTI is the microscopic examination of a specimen for bacteria. The presence of at least one bacterium per oil-immersion field in a midstream clean-catch, uncentrifuged, urine specimen correlates with 10^5 bacteria/mL of urine or more. In a stained sedimented specimen, the absence of bacteria in several fields indicates the probability of less than 10^4 bacteria/mL. Gram stain of urine smears is a rapid, accurate, and inexpensive way to detect greater than 10^5 bacteria/mL, with a 94% sensitivity, greater than 70% specificity, and a negative predictive value of 99%. However, low-count bacterial infection of the lower tract may be associated with a negative Gram stain.

Occasionally, microscopic or sometimes gross hematuria is seen in a patient with UTI. Red blood cells may reflect other disorders such as calculi, tumor, vasculitis, glomerulonephritis, or renal tuberculosis. White cell casts in the presence of an acute infectious process are strong evidence for pyelonephritis, but the absence of white cell casts does not rule out upper tract infection. White cells can also be seen in renal disease in the absence of infection.

A common but not universal finding in UTI is proteinuria. Patients with UTI usually excrete less than 2 g of protein in 24 hours; excretion of 3 g or more suggests glomerular disease.

Dipstick urine examination for leukocyte esterase or nitrite reductase is commonly used tests in ambulatory primary care. Leukocyte esterase is an indicator of pyuria, and nitrite is an indicator of bacteriuria. Dipsticks have a lower sensitivity and specificity when compared with a urine Gram stain. However, the dipstick method is a fraction of the cost of a Gram stain and is readily available in the office setting. A published metaanalysis of 51 studies concluded that a positive test for leukocyte esterase or nitrites reductase should be interpreted as a positive screen. However, a negative dipstick cannot exclude the diagnosis of UTI in a patient with a high likelihood of infection. Up to one half of UTIs in women with acute dysuria are characterized by growth of 10^2 to 10^4 bacteria/mL, and all rapid tests are relatively insensitive to detecting these lower levels of bacteriuria.

Microbiologic Criteria for Confirming Infection

Quantitative culture helps distinguish significant bacteriuria from contamination. Infection is usually present when at least 10^5 bacteria/mL are present in culture. Counts less than 10^4 bacteria/mL have traditionally been thought to reflect contamination. However, studies have shown that the criterion of 10^5 bacteria/mL has high specificity but low sensitivity. Up to one third of women with UTI symptoms have 10^2 to 10^4 colonies of *E. coli, S. saprophyticus,* or other pathogens per milliliter on culture. In women with acute dysuria, frequency, urgency, and pyuria on urinalysis, cultures with 100 or more colonies of a uropathogen per milliliter of urine have the highest sensitivity and specificity for identifying acute urinary tract infection. However, asymptomatic patients continue to be evaluated by the standard of 10^5 bacteria/mL.

Although urine culture results and quantitative assessment of bacterial colonization of the urine have been the gold standard in the diagnosis of urinary tract infection, they have limitations. Several studies have found that 29% to 32% of urine cultures were contaminated.

Most experts agree that urine cultures are not necessary in all patients with a suspected UTI. Patients with clear symptoms and a positive screening test do not need to incur the expense of a pretreatment culture, because the probability that the diagnosis is correct is high (80%–90%). In addition, posttreatment cultures are not necessary unless symptoms persist. Women with complicating factors should have cultures done. Indications for obtaining a culture include inability to distinguish UTI from vaginitis and sexually transmitted infections, suspected pyelonephritis, recurrent or relapsing infection, failure of short-course therapy, pregnant women with covert bacteriuria, patients about to undergo urologic surgery, and symptomatic patients with catheter- or instrument-associated nosocomial infection.

Under routine testing conditions, up to 15% of uncomplicated UTIs yield negative culture results. Organisms such as *C. trachomatis, U. urealyticum,* or *Mycoplasma hominis* should be considered when cultures are negative. Because pathogenic etiologies of UTI in the elderly are less predictable, urine cultures should guide antibiotic therapy in this population.

TREATMENT

The initial approach to the management of UTIs in women includes antibiotic therapy, administration of a high fluid volume to flush the system, and, if needed, the administration of urinary tract analgesics. The foundation of treatment for UTIs is antibiotic therapy. Antibiotic therapy usually produces symptomatic relief (clinical cure), but bacteriuria may persist. Appropriately chosen antibiotics relieve the symptoms shortly after therapy commences. Frequently, phenazopyridine hydrochloride is prescribed to relieve the symptom of burning. However, it should not be used more than 2 days because it may mask the symptoms of UTI progression. Patients with renal dysfunction should not use phenazopyridine because the incidence of adverse effects is greater in this population.

Infection severity and epidemiologic factors (e.g., age, institutionalization, underlying disease, and history of UTI) influence the choice of drug and the duration of treatment. The optimal antibiotic is one that achieves high urinary concentrations (above the infecting organism's minimum inhibitory concentration), has both Gram-positive and Gram-negative antimicrobial activity, has little potential for promoting bacterial resistance, has minimal effect on the anaerobic flora and microaerophilic normal flora but eradicates aerobic Gram-negative rods from the fecal and vaginal flora, has a long half-life (which facilitates long dosing intervals), has acceptable patient tolerance and adverse effect profile, and is inexpensive.

Antimicrobial Therapy

The characteristics of the antimicrobial agent and the location and etiology of the infection must be considered when selecting a therapeutic agent. Previously, sulfonamides and aminopenicillins were used to treat initial episodes of UTI in young women. However, more recently the relatively frequent resistance to these agents has lessened their use. Resistance rates vary from region to region. For example, resistance to trimethoprim/sulfamethoxazole (TMP-SMX) is present in up to 32% of recovered cultures in the western part of the United States but comprises only 11% to 12% in the northeastern parts of the United States. Resistance rates to ampicillin of 25% have been reported in studies evaluating the susceptibility patterns of uropathogens cultured from patients with nosocomial UTIs.

β-Lactamase resistance has been addressed with the development of clavulanate potassium, an irreversible competitive inhibitor of this enzyme. Clavulanate protects the β-lactam ring of amoxicillin. When used in combination with amoxicillin, a synergistic bactericidal effect results that expands the spectrum of activity of amoxicillin against many strains of β-lactamase–producing bacteria resistant to amoxicillin alone. UTIs caused by some resistant stains of *E. coli*, *Klebsiella* spp., *Enterobacter* spp., or *Proteus mirabilis* have been treated effectively with this combination.

Three generations of oral cephalosporins have been used in the treatment of UTIs. Cephalexin, cefuroxime, axetil, and cefixime can be used for the management of UTI but are always given as a 7-day regimen. These agents are relatively expensive, and their broad spectrum of activity may lead to an increased frequency of vulvovaginal candidiasis. The spectrum of activity of these agents varies. First-generation cephalosporins are more active against Gram-positive organisms; third-generation cephalosporins are more active against Gram-negative organisms. There is no oral cephalosporin with significant activity against enterococci and *Pseudomonas* spp. Cefixime has poor activity in vitro against *S. saprophyticus*. The long half-life of ceftriaxone, a parenteral third-generation cephalosporin with an extended spectrum of activity, allows once-a-day dosing.

The fluoroquinolones are a group of antibacterial agents that are structurally related to the prototype quinolone, nalidixic acid. The antibacterial spectrum and potency of this class of drugs have been broadened by the fluorination of the quinolone ring. Fluoroquinolones are effective in vitro against both Gram-positive and Gram-negative organisms, including *S. saprophyticus* and, in the case of ciprofloxacin, *P. aeruginosa*. Dosing on a once- or twice-daily basis is sufficient. They have been shown to be effective in both complicated and uncomplicated UTIs. Ambulatory care physicians are increasing their use of fluoroquinolones and nitrofurantoin, even though they are not recommended as first-line therapy and clearly are not the least expensive. Choices of antibiotic treatment for UTIs are influenced by clinical factors (e.g., drug allergies, pregnancy). However, nonclinical factors may come into play, such as tradition, habit, and subspecialty culture.

Nitrofurantoin, a nitrofuran-derivative antibacterial agent, has been an option for treatment of UTI for more than 50 years. It is active against most *E. coli*, *Staphylococcus aureus*, enterococci, and some strains of *Klebsiella* and *Enterobacter* but is relatively inactive against *Proteus* and *Pseudomonas* spp. Nitrofurantoin achieves high concentrations in the urine rapidly because it is readily absorbed in the gastrointestinal tract. It does not promote the emergence of resistant bacteria in fecal flora and therefore is effective as a chronic prophylactic agent in recurrent infections. It can be used during pregnancy and in pediatric populations. Because it does not achieve high serum levels and parenchymal penetration, it is not recommended for treatment of pyelonephritis. It is absolutely contraindicated for patients with renal failure.

Fosfomycin, the most recent addition to the antibiotic management of uncomplicated UTI, is a phosphonic acid bactericidal agent with activity against many common uropathogens (i.e., *E. coli*, *Citrobacter* spp., *Enterobacter* spp., *Serratia* spp., and *Enterococcus* spp.). The oral tromethamine salt has 40% bioavailability and is primarily excreted in the bladder essentially unchanged. A comparative study showed a 1-day course of fosfomycin tromethamine (one single dose of 3 g) to be as successful as a 5-day course of TMP.

UNCOMPLICATED URINARY TRACT INFECTIONS

Recommended therapy for uncomplicated UTIs has not changed in the past decade. However, there has been a divergence from these recommendations by prescribing physicians. The recommendation for initial therapy has been for a 3-day regimen of TMP-SMX (160/800 mg twice per day) or TMP (200 mg twice per day) for patients who are allergic to sulfa. The recommended second-line choice is for selected fluoroquinolones. Both drugs are effective in treating UTI, but there is a substantial cost differential. In a publication of the Archives of Internal Medicine, a comment was made that in 1999 a 10-day course of TMP-SMX was $1.79, whereas a course of ciprofloxacin cost $70.98.

Table 75.1 lists the dosage, side effects, and precautions for common antibiotics used in UTIs. Tetracycline is generally not prescribed because of the possibility of developing plasmid-mediated resistance in Gram-negative organisms. Doxycycline is occasionally used because less bacterial resistance develops and good urine concentrations are achieved; it is given twice daily. Resistance rates of 25% to 35% have been reported for *E. coli* with the use of ampicillin or sulfonamide. The high resistance rate reported for sulfonamide is overcome with the use of TMP-SMX. Other alternatives are the cephalosporins and amoxicillin/clavulanic acid.

Fluoroquinolones are impressive in the treatment of UTIs. Their greatest advantage is improved patient tolerance compared with TMP-SMX. However, higher doses of amifloxacin and fleroxacin have resulted in some adverse experiences. They are useful in a range of clinical situations but should not be considered first-line treatment because of their cost and the emergence of resistant isolates. Quinolones should be considered in complicated UTIs, in a patient allergic to a conventional agent, or in a patient whose infection is caused by Gram-negative bacilli with multiple resistance or if the toxicity of alternate therapy is greater.

TABLE 75.1. Dosage and Side Effects of Oral Antibiotics Commonly Used in the Treatment of Urinary Tract Infections in Young Women

Drug	Dosage: Treatment	Dosage: Prophylaxis	Side effects and precautions
Amoxicillin/clavulanate potassium	250 mg/125 mg every 8 h		Gastrointestinal, rash, *Candida* vaginitis
Cephalosporins			
Cefaclor	250–500 mg every 8 h		Cross-reactivity in 20% of patients with a history of anaphylactic reactions to penicillin, *Candida* vaginitis
Cefixime	400 mg once a day		
Cefuroxime	250–500 mg every 12 h		
Ceftriaxone	1–2 g daily IM		
Cephalexin	250 mg every 6 h or 500 mg every 12 h		
Fluoroquinolones			
Ciprofloxacin	250–500 mg every 12 h		Gastrointestinal, dizziness, headache; contraindicated in children and in pregnancy because induces cartilage erosion in young animals; *Candida* vaginitis
Norfloxacin	400 mg every 12 h		
Ofloxacin	400 mg every 12 h		
Lomefloxacin	400 mg once a day		
Nitrofurantoin	50–100 mg every 6 h	50–100 mg daily	Nausea, vomiting, neuropathy, pulmonary hypersensitivity reactions
Trimethoprim	100 mg every 12 h or 200 mg every day	100 mg at bedtime	Rash occurring 7–14 days after initiation of therapy; gastrointestinal
Trimethoprim/ sulfamethoxazole	160 mg/800 mg twice a day	40–80 mg/200–400 mg every day or three times a week	Rash, gastrointestinal, fatal hypersensitivity reactions (i.e., Stevens-Johnson syndrome)

IM, intramuscularly.
Source: Sravani A. Treatment of urinary tract infections in young women. American Urology Association Update Series, Lesson 6. 1993;12: 42, with permission.

SHORT-COURSE THERAPY

Because of its effectiveness, improved compliance, lower cost, reduced emergence of resistant bacteria, and fewer adverse reactions, short-course therapy has become the treatment of choice for uncomplicated lower tract infections. The regimens range from a single dose to multiple doses for up to 3 to 5 days. These regimens should be limited to young nonpregnant women presenting with symptoms of less than 7 days in duration who have insignificant urinary infection histories. Patients must be willing and able to come for follow-up. Longer treatment regimens should be prescribed for postmenopausal women. Relapse after a short or full course of therapy should be treated with a 2-week course of therapy.

The use of single-dose therapy for uncomplicated lower urinary tract infections has been advocated by some investigators and questioned by others (Table 75.2). This treatment regimen is less expensive and is associated with significantly fewer side effects than longer regimens. However, in clinical trials single-dose therapy has been found to be less efficacious than 3 or more days of therapy. Failure rates of approximately 20% have been observed, even with the use of the new quinolones as single-dose therapy. Thus, single-dose regimens are no longer the preferred therapy for women with acute cystitis.

In contrast, a 3-day course of therapy appears to be sufficient in most women with uncomplicated UTIs. Studies have shown that a 3-day course of TMP-SMX or the newer quinolones predictably cure approximately 95% of women clinically and microbiologically. Longer durations of therapy do not achieve significantly higher cure rates. Although quinolones are effective, they are expensive and there is concern about the emergence of bacterial resistance. β-Lactams are more effective when given for 5 days or more, compared with TMP-SMX, which is given for 3 days. Unfortunately, increasing numbers of uropathogens are resistant to ampicillin/amoxicillin. When treatment is given for more than 3 days, adverse reactions increase markedly overall. A 3- to 5-day course of therapy serves as a reasonable alternative to single-dose therapy for acute lower tract infection. If relapse occurs or if symptoms and bacteriuria persist after treatment, renal parenchymal involvement, bacterial resistance, or underlying urologic anomalies may be present.

TABLE 75.2. Single-Dose Oral Antibiotic Treatment Options for Urinary Tract Infections in Women

Drug	Dose
Amoxicillin	3 g
Cefaclor	2 g
Cefadroxil	1 g
Cefuroxime	1,000 mg
Cephalexin	3 g
Ciprofloxacin	250 mg, 500 mg
Enoxacin	600 mg
Fleroxacin	200 mg, 400 mg
Nitrofurantoin	400 mg
Norfloxacin	400 mg, 800 mg
Ofloxacin	200 mg, 400 mg
Sulfisoxazole	2 g
TMP-SMX	Two double-strength tablets
Trimethoprim	400 mg

TMP-SMX, trimethoprim/sulfamethoxazole in a 1:5 ratio by weight.
Source: Hatton J, Hughes M, Raymond C. Management of bacterial urinary infections in adults. *Ann Pharmacother* 1994;28:1264, with permission.

FOLLOW-UP CULTURE

The need for a follow-up culture after treatment of an uncomplicated lower tract infection is controversial. If done, the post-treatment urine culture should be collected 1 to 2 weeks after discontinuing therapy, primarily to detect relapses. In young nonpregnant women presenting with symptoms highly suggestive of UTI, empiric therapy without a urinalysis and culture is certainly acceptable. With recurrence or nonimmediate response to therapy, culture investigation and drug sensitivity will guide further therapy.

Treatment of Uncomplicated Upper Urinary Tract Infections or Pyelonephritis

Because pyelonephritis may result in serious complications such as renal scarring, immediate treatment with a broad-spectrum antibiotic should be initiated. Some believe that intravenous antibiotic therapy and hospitalization are necessary, but the more general consensus is that not all patients need intravenous antibiotic therapy, especially those who are minimally symptomatic. The goal is to achieve high urinary, serum, and tissue levels of antibiotic. Because more than 30% of strains causing acute pyelonephritis are ampicillin resistant, an oral quinolone antibiotic (e.g., ciprofloxacin, ofloxacin, levofloxacin, or gatifloxacin) is the recommended first-line agent. If the organism is known to be susceptible, oral TMP-SMX is an alternative. Many clinicians administer a single parenteral dose of antimicrobial (e.g., ceftriaxone, gentamicin, or a fluoroquinolone) before instituting oral therapy.

In patients who are sufficiently ill and require intravenous therapy, options include a parenteral fluoroquinolone, an aminoglycoside with or without ampicillin, or an extended-spectrum cephalosporin with or without an aminoglycoside. Treatment may be guided by the results of the urine Gram stain. Because very few *E. coli* are resistant to aminoglycosides, these agents can be administered as a once a day regimen, facilitating outpatient parenteral therapy. Aminoglycosides should be continued for 48 to 72 hours, at which time an appropriate switch is made to an oral agent indicated by the culture and sensitivity reports. With short-term therapy ototoxicity and nephrotoxicity of aminoglycosides are usually not a concern. After clinical improvement with parenteral therapy, as measured by resolution of fever (usually at 48–72 hours), it is appropriate to change to an oral regimen with agents active against the infecting organism. The fluoroquinolones and TMP-SMX are optimal broad-spectrum agents. Oral therapy should last 10 to 14 days. To diagnose a relapse, follow-up cultures are recommended. Evaluation of the upper tract for suppurative foci, calculi, or urologic disease should ensue if the patient remains febrile after 72 hours of treatment or if relapse occurs. With a relapse, treatment should continue for 6 weeks if no complicating factors are discovered.

Treatment of Complicated Urinary Tract Infections

Host factors such as a structural or functional abnormality of the urinary tract can complicate a UTI. The choice of antibiotic and the duration of treatment are affected when a UTI ascends to the kidney. Therapy may include parenteral antibiotics until the patient is afebrile for 12 to 24 hours; therapy is usually required for at least 14 days. Empiric therapy must consider the setting and medical history of the patient, as well as coverage for suspected Gram-negative organisms. Catheterization is an independent risk factor for UTI. Patients who develop bacteriuria from temporary catheterization (e.g., postoperatively) should receive antibiotic therapy before and for 24 hours after the catheter is removed. Others recommend antibiotic therapy only before and once or twice postoperatively. Asymptomatic patients less than 65 years old may be given a single dose of two double-strength TMP-SMX tablets to prevent UTI after catheterization. Cultures at 1 week and 1 month after catheter removal are recommended. When *P. mirabilis* is isolated, a full course of antibiotic therapy is prescribed; *P. mirabilis* can cause renal calculi and catheter encrustations, thus establishing a nidus of infection. With permanent catheter placement, bacteriuria is prevented by intermittent use of antibiotics but with eventual isolation of resistant organisms. When long-term catheterization cannot be avoided, the catheter must be changed every 3 to 4 weeks and cultures taken at that time Thus, treatment of bacteriuria in patients with permanent catheters is indicated if the patient is immunocompromised or if the threat of sepsis is evident.

In hospitalized patients, enterococci account for about 15% of UTIs. Aminopenicillins alone (ampicillin or amoxicillin) may be sufficient if the infection is confined to the bladder. However, if there is renal tissue involvement (and this may be difficult to diagnose), the combination of gentamicin and ampicillin may be required. The goal is a high urine concentration of aminoglycosides; therefore, serum concentrations may be kept low (40–50 μg/mL and 3–5 μg/mL, respectively). Vancomycin should be used in patients allergic to penicillin.

Patients who are debilitated, such as those in hospitals or nursing homes or those with spinal cord injuries, often acquire infections with more resistant Gram-negative rods. The isolates from the urine of these patients are usually *Enterobacter cloacae* and *P. aeruginosa*, microorganisms with a propensity to acquire resistance rapidly to many antibiotics. Broad-spectrum antibiotics are indicated if risk factors are present. Until the organism is identified and susceptibilities are known, reasonable empiric choices include antipseudomonal β-lactams (mezlocillin, piperacillin, ticarcillin, ceftazidime, ceftriaxone, cefotaxime), imipenem/cilastatin, aztreonam, aminoglycosides, and quinolones.

Often, atypical symptoms lead to delayed diagnosis and increase the risk of urosepsis. Broad-spectrum antibiotics should be included in the initial regimens. In high-risk populations, it is challenging to dose aminoglycosides empirically: Reduced muscle mass interferes with the interpretation of serum creatinine, and aminoglycoside concentrations are often higher than predicted. These patients have recurrent complicated UTIs, and thus repeated exposure to aminoglycosides may increase the risk for toxicity. Most studies reveal good to excellent cure rates with the quinolones, which were consistently more effective than the comparison drugs in complicated UTIs.

Complicated UTIs require aggressive management. Prolonged treatment for up to 6 weeks may be indicated in some cases.

Treatment of Urinary Tract Infections in the Elderly

With increasing age, the prevalence of UTI increases, reaching over 50% for institutionalized patients of either sex. Asymptomatic and symptomatic bacteriuria present a risk factor for bacteremia, sepsis, and increased mortality (especially for elderly women). Bacteriuria in the elderly is a complex problem. UTI is more difficult to treat, and its pathogenesis is related to abnormal bladder function, bladder outlet obstruction, vaginal and urethral atrophy, use of long-term indwelling catheters, and puddling related to bed rest. Bacteriuria is usually asymptomatic, and there is no indication for the treatment of asymptomatic bacteriuria except before invasive genitourinary procedures. Antimicrobial adverse effects and the emergence of resistant organisms, as well as the inability to prevent subsequent symptomatic episodes, form the rationale for not treating asymptomatic bacteriuria in elderly patients.

The most appropriate management in the elderly patient is controversial. There are no guidelines to identify patients likely to benefit from therapy. It must be borne in mind that an elderly patient who is incontinent of urine must not be considered asymptomatic. Bacteriuria in combination with urinary incontinence may be cause and effect related. As a first step in evaluating the mechanism of incontinence, treatment for the bacteriuria is preferred. Prevention of subsequent infections with treatment of bacteriuria has not been established. Commonly, there are increased adverse reactions, the development of resistance, and early recurrence. Patients with spinal cord injuries also experience early recurrence and therefore are treated if bacteria counts of 100 colony-forming units (cfu)/mL or more are associated with symptoms.

Recurrent bacterial infection in the elderly may be related to poor hygiene, particularly associated with fecal and urinary incontinence. Admission of elderly patients for Gram-negative bacteremia secondary to acute pyelonephritis is common. These patients can be treated effectively, resulting in a 97% survival rate.

Definition of Response to Therapy

The response of UTIs to antibiotic therapy can be assessed clinically and microbiologically. The clinical goal is the resolution of symptoms. There are four patterns of microbiologic response of bacteriuria to antimicrobial therapy: cure, persistence, relapse, and reinfection. Within 48 hours after initiation of an antimicrobial agent, the quantitative bacterial counts in urine should decrease, provided the microorganism is sensitive in vivo. It is unlikely that continued therapy will be successful if titers do not decrease within this time. Cure is defined as negative urine cultures achieved while the patient is on the therapy and during the 1- to 2-week follow-up period. Persistence means either significant bacteriuria after 48 hours of treatment or the presence of low numbers of the infecting organism in the urine after 48 hours. Drug resistance, subtherapeutic urinary antibiotic concentrations, or the presence of a bacterial nidus within the soft tissue or calculi may cause persistence. A relapse of UTI with symptoms can be the result of persistence.

Therapy is considered to have failed if the asymptomatic patient has 10^5 cfu/mL of uropathogen or if the symptomatic patient has 10^3 cfu/mL and pyuria occurring 5 to 9 days or 4 to 6 weeks after therapy.

Relapses and reinfections are differentiated on the basis of the second isolate identified. Relapse results when the original infecting organism persists in the urinary tract. Within 1 to 2 weeks after antibiotic treatment, a relapse can occur. Relapse may be associated with renal infection and structural abnormalities of the urinary tract. Women with acute UTIs experience frequent recurrences (about 20%) within the first 6 weeks after treatment, accounting for a great deal of morbidity, increased health care costs, and time lost from work. Reinfection, sometimes called superinfection, usually occurs after initial sterilization of the urine. It involves either a different bacterial species or a different serotype of the same species (usually *E. coli*) or the same serotype. It is attributed to contamination by fecal flora and occurs in 2% to 10% of patients. Superinfection can also occur during the treatment of a UTI. This is sometimes defined as the presence of a new organism resistant to the antibiotic.

RECURRENT URINARY TRACT INFECTIONS

UTIs recur in about 20% of the patients. The three primary causes of recurrent UTI are persistence of the organism in the urine during therapy, relapse caused by reemergence of the original infecting organism because of a failure to eradicate it from renal tissue, and reinfection caused by the entry of new organisms into the bladder from the fecal/perineal reservoir. In these patients, there is usually no anatomic or functional cause of infection. Women who use spermicidal contraceptives or diaphragms for contraception often have recurrent UTIs and should be advised to seek another means of contraception. Relapses occur whether single-dose or longer courses of therapy are prescribed. Most women who have had a 10- to 14-day regimen of antibiotic treatment without successful eradication of the infection are cured by 6 weeks of treatment, unless a pathologic condition of the upper urinary tract underlies the infection.

Therapeutic options shown to be effective in the management of recurrent UTIs include continuous low-dose oral antimicrobial prophylaxis, intermittent self-treatment, and postcoital prophylaxis. Women who experience two or more symptomatic UTIs over a 6-month period or three or more episodes over a 12-month period should begin prophylaxis, after any existing infection has been eradicated. In estrogen-deficient women, application of intravaginal estrogen cream has shown excellent benefits in preventing recurrent UTIs, whereas oral estrogen alone has not.

In patients with chronic or recurrent infections, continuous long-term therapy is useful. Continuous prophylaxis with daily or thrice-weekly doses of TMP-SMX, nitrofurantoin, or trimethoprim have been effective in controlling more than 90% of recurrences. Most authorities recommend a 6-month trial, after which the patient is recultured. Some patients require 2 or more years of antibiotic therapy. Postcoital prophylaxis with TMP-SMX (40 mg/200 mg), nitrofurantoin, or cephalexin should be used in women whose infections are temporally related to sexual intercourse. Reliable women who are uncomfortable taking antimicrobials over an extended period may self-treat with single-dose or 3-day antimicrobial therapy when they experience symptoms.

Often patients with recurrent UTIs are referred to the urologist or urogynecologist for evaluation. From 20 to 40 years of age in otherwise healthy women, the likelihood of finding a structural defect in the genitourinary system is very low. Such patients do not warrant cystoscopy or radiographic evaluation as long as there are no coexisting signs and symptoms of upper tract disease. Over the age of 40, and especially if there has been significant hematuria, cystoscopy and urography are indicated.

CONSIDERATIONS IN PREGNANCY

There are important physiologic and anatomic changes in pregnancy that contribute significantly to the persistence of bacteriuria in pregnancy. The presence of bacteriuria in pregnancy increases the possibility of symptomatic upper tract infection in untreated women, especially in the third trimester. Dilation of the ureters and renal pelves begins in the first trimester and progresses to term, allowing bacteria in the bladder to reach the upper tract. Dilatation of the upper collecting system occurs in most pregnancies and extends down to the level of the pelvic brim. These changes are more pronounced on the right side than on the left. Over 200 mL of urine may be contained in the dilated ureters and may contribute to the persistence of bacteriuria in pregnancy. Hormonal changes also contribute to hydroureter by decreasing peristalsis. After delivery, the dilated ureter rapidly returns to normal and is almost completely normal by the second month postpartum.

Asymptomatic Bacteriuria

Asymptomatic bacteriuria, present in 4% to 10% of pregnant women, develops into acute pyelonephritis in an estimated 20% to 40% of cases. Bacteriuria during pregnancy is associated with an increased incidence of adverse effects for the mother (persistent bacteriuria, symptomatic UTI, acute and chronic pyelonephritis, and probably anemia) and fetus (increased frequency of premature delivery, low birth weight, fetal infection, and risk of perinatal death). The fetal adverse effects are reported to be up to three times more common in the bacteriuric woman than in a nonbacteriuric woman. Pyelonephritis develops as an ascending infection from the lower urinary tract. Structural changes in the ureters due to high progesterone levels and ureteral compression by the gravid uterus are factors in the development of upper urinary tract infection. The time of greatest risk for pyelonephritis is in the second and third trimesters.

The bacteria responsible for most cases of pyelonephritis are primarily the aerobic inhabitants of the lower female genital tract. Members of the Enterobacteriaceae, such as *E. coli, Klebsiella pneumoniae,* and *P. mirabilis,* are the most commonly recovered, as well as other Gram-negative bacteria such as *Enterobacter, Citrobacter,* and Gram-positive organisms (e.g., group B streptococcus).

It is highly recommended that all pregnant patients be screened for asymptomatic bacteriuria early in the pregnancy. If found, bacteriuria should be treated because the 30% incidence of pyelonephritis that may occur later in pregnancy falls to 1% to 2% if bacteriuria is treated. Screening cultures are recommended for all women early in pregnancy; some experts suggest that the 16th week of gestation is the optimal time for screening. Urine cultures are the only satisfactory method for establishing the diagnosis of asymptomatic bacteriuria. The most efficient and cost-effective means of collecting and culturing the urine should be used. Women with negative initial cultures do not need further testing unless there is a history of recurrent UTIs. Women with positive screening cultures should have quantitative cultures and antimicrobial sensitivities performed. Treatment should be guided by sensitivities.

Urinary Tract Infections

UTIs are the most common bacterial infection in pregnant women. Pyelonephritis is the most common severe bacterial complication of pregnancy. Pyelonephritis occurs in 20% to 40% of pregnant women with untreated bacteriuria. The risk of developing pyelonephritis later in pregnancy falls from 30% to 1% to 2% if the asymptomatic bacteriuria is treated. One in 3,000 pregnant women with pyelonephritis develops end-stage renal disease if untreated. *E. coli* is responsible for about 80% of all community-acquired UTIs in pregnancy. Other pathogens, such as *K. pneumoniae, P. mirabilis,* and *Enterococcus faecalis,* are also common.

Treatment of Bacteriuria in Pregnancy

The duration of therapy for bacteriuria in pregnancy has received much attention. Short-course therapy (3 days) is more effective for bacteriuria than single-dose therapy. Short-course therapy minimizes potential toxicity; however, many experts still recommend 7-day regimens. Amoxicillin 250 mg three times a day for 3 or 7 days is one option; however, resistance to ampicillin/amoxicillin seems to be increasing. Nitrofurantoin is effective and nontoxic. There is more experience with the 7-day regimens of nitrofurantoin in pregnancy than the 3-day courses. One gram of sulfisoxazole followed by 500 mg every 6 hours for 7 days is a traditional regimen. However, sulfisoxazole should be avoided near term because of its association with neonatal hyperbilirubinemia. Both nitrofurantoin and sulfisoxazole have been associated with hemolytic anemia caused by glucose-6-phosphate dehydrogenase deficiency. Other options for therapy include amoxicillin/clavulanic acid and TMP-SMX. These agents are not usually recommended as first-line agents because of lack of clinical experience in pregnancy and the potential for toxicity. Quinolones are not used in pregnancy, because studies in immature animals report cartilage erosion. Follow-up cultures should be done approximately 1 week after treatment is completed. Treatment failure after a 3-day course should be treated with an additional 7- to 10-day course of therapy with a different agent based on antimicrobial sensitivities.

In the symptomatic pregnant patient with UTI, if the organism is susceptible, options include amoxicillin, TMP-SMX, nitrofurantoin, or cephalexin. If there is no improvement, even though the organism is susceptible to the agent, the patient should be retreated for 14 days. If resistant pathogens do not allow improvement, the pregnant patient should be retreated for 3 days with an antibiotic to which the organism is susceptible.

Acute Pyelonephritis

The clinical presentation of pyelonephritis in pregnancy is similar to that in nonpregnant women. Therapeutic approaches are also similar to nonpregnant patients. Quinolones, however, should not be used to treat upper urinary tract infections in pregnant women. Acute pyelonephritis in the pregnant patient is usually treated by hospitalization and parenteral antibiotics. Ampicillin and an aminoglycoside are typical first-line agents. More than 95% of patients will respond within 72 hours of intravenous therapy. A 14-day course of therapy should be completed and should be followed by suppressive therapy until delivery. Alternative diagnoses should be considered when there is nonresponse to therapy. Ultrasound imaging of the kidneys is indicated when pregnant women do not respond to antibiotic therapy.

BIBLIOGRAPHY

Andriole VT. Urinary tract infections in the '90s: pathogenesis and management. *Infection* 1992;20[Suppl 4]:S251.
Bailey RR. Management of lower urinary tract infections. *Drugs* 1993;[Suppl 3]:139.
Bent SA, et al. Does this women have an acute uncomplicated urinary tract infection? *JAMA* 2002;287:2701.
Bergman A. Urinary tract infections in women. *Curr Opin Obstet Gynecol* 1991;3:541.
Brown JS, et al. Urinary tract infections in postmenopausal women: effect of hormone therapy and risk factors. *Obstet Gynecol* 2001;98:1045.
Bump RC. Urinary tract infection in women: current role of single-dose therapy. *J Reprod Med* 1990;35:785.
Cunningham FG, Lucas MJ. Urinary tract infections complicating pregnancy. *Bailliere's Clin Obstet Gynecol* 1994;8:353.
Elder NC. Acute urinary tract infection in women: what kind of antibiotic therapy is optimal? *Postgrad Med* 1992;92:159.
Faro S. New considerations in treatment of urinary tract infections in adults. *Urology* 1992;39:1.
Fihn SD. Lower urinary tract infections in women. *Curr Opin Obstet Gynecol* 1992;4:571.
Foxman B. Epidemiology of urinary tract infections: incidence, morbidity, and economic costs. *Am J Med* 2002;113[Suppl 1A]:5S.
Gleckman RA. Urinary tract infection. *Clin Geriatr Med* 1992;8:793.

Hatton J, Hughes M, Raymond CH. Management of bacterial urinary tract infection in adults. *Ann Pharmacother* 1994;28:1274.
Hay A, et al. Clinical diagnosis of urinary tract infection. *JAMA* 2002;288:1229.
Hillebrand L, et al. Urinary tract infection in pregnant women with bacterial vaginosis. *Am J Obstet Gynecol* 2002;186:916.
Huang ES, Stafford RS. National patterns in the treatment of urinary tract infections in women by ambulatory care physicians. *Arch Intern Med* 2002;162:41.
Kiningham RB. Asymptomatic bacteriuria in pregnancy. *Am Fam Phys* 1993;47:1232.
Lawrenson RA, Logie JW. Antibiotic failure in the treatment of urinary tract infections in young women. *J Antimicrob Chemother* 2001;48:895.
Manges AR, et al. Widespread distribution of urinary tract infections caused by a multidrug-resistant *Escherichia coli* clonal group. *N Engl J Med* 2001;345:1007.
Neu HC. Urinary tract infections. *Am J Med* 1992;92:63S.
Nicolle LE. Prophylaxis: recurrent urinary tract infection in women. *Infection* 1992;20[Suppl 3]:5203.
Nicolle LE. Urinary tract infection: traditional pharmacologic therapies. *Am J Med* 2002;113[Suppl 1A]:35S.
Norrby SR. Evaluation of antibiotics for treatment of urinary tract infections. *J Antimicrob Chemother* 1994;33[Suppl A]:43.
Petrof EO, et al. Urinary tract infections and a multidrug-resistant *Escherichia coli* clonal group [letter, comment]. *N Engl J Med* 2002;346:535.
Sable CA, Scheld WM. Fluoroquinolones: how to use (but not overuse) these antibiotics. *Geriatrics* 1993;48:41.
Schaeffer AJ. New concepts in the pathogenesis of urinary tract infections. *Urol Clin North Am* 2002;29:241.
Sobel JD, Kaye D. Urinary tract infections. In: Mandell GL, Douglass RG, Bennett JE, eds. *Principles and practice of infectious diseases,* 2nd ed. New York: John Wiley & Sons, 1990:582.
Sravani A. Advances in the understanding and treatment of urinary tract infections in young women. *Urology* 1991;36:503.
Sravani A. Treatment of urinary tract infections in young women. *Am Urol Assoc Update Ser* 1993;12:42.
Sravani A, Bischoff W. Antibiotic therapy for urinary tract infections. *Am J Med* 1992;92:955.
Stamm WE. Criteria for the diagnosis of urinary tract infection and for the assessment of therapeutic effectiveness. *Infection* 1992;20[Suppl 3]:5151; discussion 5160.
Sultana RV, et al. Dipstick urinalysis and the accuracy of the clinical diagnosis of urinary tract 13 infection. *J Emerg Med* 2001;20(1).
Van Haarst EP, et al. Evaluation of the diagnostic workup in young women referred for recurrent lower urinary tract infections. *Urology* 2001;57:1068.
Vercaigne LM, Zhanel GG. Recommended treatment for urinary tract infection in pregnancy. *Ann Pharmacother* 1994;28:248.
Weissenbacher ER, Reisenberger K. Uncomplicated urinary tract infections in pregnant and non-pregnant women. *Curr Opin Obstet Gynecol* 1993;5:513.
Young JL, Soper DE. Urinalysis and urinary tract infection: update for clinicians. *Infect Dis Obstet Gynecol* 2001;9:249.

CHAPTER 76
Urethral Syndrome

Paul J. Russinko and Richard Caesar

Acute urethral syndrome (AUS) refers to dysuria and frequent urination, with a voided urine culture that is sterile or demonstrates low count bacteriuria. Chronic urethral syndrome (CUS) is similarly defined by dysuria and urinary frequency, which persists, but may have associated pelvic pain, suprapubic pain, dyspareunia, or urinary urgency. Symptoms of CUS are persistent or recurrent rather than acute. A specific infectious etiology for AUS can generally be determined and cure effected with antibiotic therapy. It should be viewed as a complex of symptoms for which specific etiologies exist and most of which are infectious and often related to vaginitis, urethritis, or cystitis. Urine cultures are sterile with CUS, and symptoms are more variable and can have multiple etiologies. Despite many recommended therapies, cure is often difficult to obtain.

Dysuria and frequency account for more than 5 million office visits per year in the United States. Fifty percent of women have an attack of urinary symptoms during their lives, and at least 25% experience at least one episode each year. About 40% of women with acute dysuria and frequency have AUS, whereas 60% have cystitis (defined as bacteriuria of ≥100,000 bacteria/mL of urine). The prevalence of CUS is unknown.

ETIOLOGY

The urethra plays an important role in the prevention of ascending bacterial infection. May and Hinman demonstrated that dogs display a high-pressure zone along the mid-urethra that can prevent bacterial ascent and implied that the mid-urethral segment performs a similar role in women. The female urethra functions more than a tubular conduit for urine. Kunnin et al. demonstrated various antibacterial mechanisms. Cells lining the urethra can bind bacteria, exfoliate, and thereby prohibit bacteria ascending the urethra. The paraurethral glands secrete mucus, which can also entrap pathogens along the urethra. A lower pH and recurrent washout by urine minimize the ascent and population of bacteria. Other potential antibacterial mechanisms are IgG production, cytokine mobilization, and leukocyte response.

Acute Urethral Syndrome

The cause of AUS is usually infectious. Stamm et al. reviewed 59 women with AUS and compared them with 35 asymptomatic women. Forty-two cases had pyuria, and 37 of these women demonstrated infected urine by catheterization or suprapubic aspiration. The majority of these women were infected with coliforms and the remaining demonstrated *Staphylococcus saprophyticus* or *Chlamydia trachomatis. Neisseria gonorrhoeae* and *C. trachomatis* may account for dysuria in 20% or more of cases.

Chronic Urethral Syndrome

The etiology of CUS is unknown and comprises a large list of differential diagnoses. Latham and Stamm extensively evaluated patients with this syndrome without identification of an infectious source, and all patients had an absence of pyuria.

Evidence of chronic inflammation or infection is suggested by the progressive structural and inflammatory changes that are sometimes found histologically in the periurethral glands. Splatt and Weedon performed histologic examination of patients with CUS that underwent urethroplasty. Their study implied patients with this syndrome had a noncompliant urethra replaced by collagen. However, these histologic structural changes have not been reproducible.

In many cases of CUS, urethral spasm and irritability of the external urethral sphincter have been urodynamically demonstrated. Barbalias and Meares performed video urodynamics on patients diagnosed with urethral syndrome. Ten of 18 patients demonstrated a narrowing localized to the middle urethra and extending to the lower third of the urethra, implying this was secondary to increased urethral musculature, periurethral muscles, or both. Both the smooth and skeletal muscles of the urethra are involved in this spasticity. Concomitant pelvic floor spasm or tension may also occur, including high resting urethral tone, increased mean and maximal urethral closure pressures, inability to relax the urethra voluntarily, incomplete funneling of the bladder neck, distal urethral narrowing, and intermittent urinary flow patterns. These changes may account for many of the symptoms of CUS, particularly dysuria, frequency, and postcoital voiding dysfunction. These voiding patterns may result in dysfunctional voiding. Pain may occur due to urethral spasticity and coincident stimulation of the pelvic muscle spindles with increased pelvic floor tension. Increased pelvic floor tension may result in pelvic muscular dysfunction and dyspareunia. Prolonged spasticity and increased tone may produce periurethral, urethral, or levator ani muscle fatigue, with resultant chronic pelvic pain. As suggested above, it may be due to inflammation or chronic infection in some cases. Biopsychosocial factors may influence the course of the disease and could have an etiologic role. Many clinical studies that assess personality profiles and screen for underlying psychopathology have failed to consistently demonstrate psychiatric illness as an etiologic role. Another hypothesis is that due to anatomic, physiologic, or psychological factors, some women are susceptible to repetitive urethral trauma with intercourse, and this plays the causative role in establishing urethral syndrome and producing its symptoms. It has become more apparent that interstitial cystitis is the underlying problem, and CUS and interstitial cystitis have many overlapping symptoms.

DIFFERENTIAL DIAGNOSIS

Acute Urethral Syndrome

The most common causes of acute dysuria or frequency are vaginitis, urethritis, and cystitis (Table 76.1). Vaginitis may also cause dysuria and dyspareunia, but a careful history usually identifies some differences. Dysuria associated with vaginitis is caused by urine leaving the urethra and then contacting the inflamed vulvar and vaginal tissues. Dyspareunia due to vaginitis is generalized in a vulvovaginal location rather than localized anteriorly at the vagina underlying the urethra and bladder base, as it is with urethral syndrome. Finally, with vaginitis the patient may have vulvovaginal pruritus, a symptom not present with urethral syndrome.

Urinary tract infection accounts for 50% of cases. Conventionally, a urine culture that grows one organism at a concentration of 100,000 bacterial colonies/mL confirms the diagnosis of cystitis. This definition of cystitis is based on the work of Kass; however, that work used the criteria of 100,000 bacteria/mL to distinguish women with pyelonephritis from women who were asymptomatic or had contaminated urine cultures and did not study women with only lower tract symptoms. There is evidence that the presence of 100 or more bacteria/mL in midstream urine is the most sensitive and specific diagnostic criterion of cystitis. Thus, many women diagnosed with dysuria and urinary frequency due to low bacterial counts actually have cystitis.

Chlamydia has been associated with urethritis 15% to 55%. *Neisseriae gonorrhea, Mycoplasma genitalia,* and *Ureaplasma urealyticum* have also been identified causes of urethritis. The initial genital infection with herpes produces dysuria in 80% of women.

TABLE 76.1. Differential Diagnoses of Acute and Chronic Urethral Syndromes

Acute urethral syndrome
Cystitis
Vaginitis
Urethreitis
Herpes genitalis
Chronic urethral syndrome
Chronic or recurrent cystitis
Interstitial cystitis
Dysfunctional voiding
Detrusor hyperreflexia
Detrusor hyperactivity
Urethral diverticulum

TABLE 76.2. Symptoms of Patients with Chronic Urethral Syndrome

Dominant symptoms	Percent
Frequency	65
Dysuria	60
Urgency	60
Dyspareunia	45
Postcoital voiding dysfunction	45
Postvoiding fullness	40
Nocturia	40
Abdominal pain	35
Suprapubic pain	25
Incontinence	25
Vulvodynia	25

Chronic Urethral Syndrome

CUS is generally a diagnosis of exclusion, requiring a high index of suspicion in women with suggestive symptoms (Table 76.2). Because it is often misdiagnosed as chronic or recurrent urinary tract infection, it is important that urine cultures be obtained before repeated antibiotic therapy. Urine cultures demonstrating at least 100 colonies/mL of a bacteria are negative in CUS. Repeated empiric antibiotic treatment of women with CUS may delay accurate diagnosis and make subsequent therapy difficult.

Interstitial cystitis presents with chronic irritative urinary tract symptoms similar to those of CUS. Patients with interstitial cystitis may complain of bladder or pelvic pain, pain on bladder filling, and nocturia. The reader is referred to the National of Institute of Arthritis, Diabetes, Digestive and Kidney Diseases consensus criteria for a complete definition of interstitial cystitis. Nocturia, when present with urethral syndrome (or cystitis), is usually early nighttime frequency related to sensory dysfunction of the urethra or bladder. In contrast, in interstitial cystitis the nocturia is due to limited bladder capacity and results with small volume voiding throughout the night. Pain with interstitial cystitis is usually suprapubic, may radiate to the low back or groin, and is associated with voiding. Dyspareunia is common with interstitial cystitis and CUS. Tenderness of the urethra and bladder base is usually found with urethral syndrome but is infrequent with interstitial cystitis. Cystoscopic findings are normal with urethral syndrome, and glomerulations or Hunner's ulcer is a classic finding associated with interstitial cystitis.

Urethral diverticula may present with similar symptoms to urethral syndrome, commonly urgency, frequency, and dysuria. Usually, urethral diverticula can be diagnosed by the presence of a midline mass along the urethra in the anterior vaginal wall. When fluctuant, they may present as a tender mass. Urethroscopy or positive pressure urethrography may be required to demonstrate the diverticulum.

CLINICAL PRESENTATION

The classic symptoms of AUS and CUS are urinary urgency, frequency, and dysuria. The symptoms may vary depending on the specific cause. Patients with AUS may also complain of low back pain, suprapubic pain, dyspareunia, or gross hematuria. Symptoms are usually of sudden onset when the syndrome is due to uropathogens but less so when due to chlamydia or gonorrhea.

Symptoms of CUS are similar to interstitial cystitis and may include incomplete voiding, urge or stress incontinence, voiding difficulties (especially postcoitally), suprapubic pain, low back pain, pelvic pain, or vaginal pain and urgency (Table 76.2). Dyspareunia is common with CUS and generally localizes to the anterior vagina. Coitus also often causes voiding dysfunction, burning dysuria, or urgency. A history of treatment of recurrent urinary tract infections without documentation of positive cultures is typical with CUS. Nocturia may be present with either AUS or CUS but is usually limited to the early nighttime.

PHYSICAL EXAMINATION

A pelvic examination is essential in the evaluation of both acute and chronic urethritis. In distinction to findings in males, women with AUS due to *N. gonorrhoeae* or *C. trachomatis* rarely have a frank urethral discharge. However, gentle massage of the urethra may yield a discharge, suggesting gonococcal or chlamydial infection. Inspection of the cervix for mucopurulent cervicitis may also suggest a chlamydial or gonococcal infection. Wet mount preparation and KOH preparation of vaginal secretions may be a useful adjunct to the physical examination.

Palpation should start with a gentle single-finger evaluation of the vulva and vagina, including palpation of the urethra, trigone, and bladder base. The tenderness elicited classically mimics the patient's pain with coitus. Pubococcygeal muscle tenderness is often present. Suprapubic tenderness can be associated with an inflammatory or infectious disease of the bladder. Visual inspection of the urethral meatus, decent of the bladder neck, vaginal vault, and labia is essential. The rest of the pelvic examination is usually normal, with absence of uterine or adnexal tenderness.

Cystoscopic and urodynamics can be helpful in these patients but should be used discriminantly. Either examination can help exclude an alternate etiology for their symptoms. In many of these patients, urethroscopy shows erythema, exudate, cystic dilation of the periurethral glands, and inflammatory fronds throughout the urethra during active urethritis. In women with pelvic pain as part of their symptom complex, urethroscopy invariably reproduces the pain symptoms. Passing a urethral catheter may often produce similar excessive pain in patients unable to relax the genitourinary diaphragm. Cystoscopic examination of the bladder and urethra will be variable pending the specific cause for their symptoms. When evaluating a patient for CUS, cystoscopic criteria for interstitial cystitis should be sought.

Urodynamic or video urodynamic evaluations can be useful in women with suspected CUS to examine or exclude voiding dysfunction detrusor instability or hyperactivity. It may also demonstrate incomplete funneling of the bladder neck and distal urethral narrowing. Urodynamic evaluations may show voiding abnormalities, including a high resting urethral tone, increased mean and maximal urethral closure pressures, inability to relax the urethra voluntarily, and intermittent urinary flow patterns. However, these findings likely represent an alternate underlying factor with impaired relaxation of the pelvic floor and genitourinary diaphragm.

LABORATORY STUDIES

Kass established 10,000 bacteria/mL as significant bacteriuria. It has been demonstrated that 100 bacteria/mL with symptoms of dysuria, frequency, and pyuria is accurate for cystitis. Stamm et al. defined women with more than 8 white blood cells per high power field as having significant pyuria in 42 of 59 symptomatic women. Thirty-seven of the 42 women demonstrated either coliforms, *S. saprophyticus*, or *C. trachomatis*, whereas women with less than 8 white blood cells per high power field did not demonstrate any bacteriuria.

A microscopic examination of a midstream urine sample for leukocytes and bacteria is essential. In uncentrifuged urine, a finding of one or more bacteria per oil-immersion field correlates with 100,000 or more bacteria/mL, whereas the absence of bacteria in several oil-immersion fields suggests a bacterial count of 10,000 or less bacteria/mL. Pyuria may be evaluated by direct hemocytometer counts of leukocytes in uncentrifuged urine. If centrifuged urine is to be examined, it is prepared by centrifuging 10 mL of urine, with resuspension of the resultant sediment in 1 mL of urine. In centrifuged urine, a finding of 5 to 10 leukocytes per high power field (×400) suggests pyuria; a finding of 100 or more bacteria per high power field is consistent with 100,000 or more bacteria/mL.

Urine cultures are indicated, as well as tests of the urethra and cervix for gonorrhea and chlamydia. Traditional midstream urine specimen cultures, however, may have limited usefulness in diagnosing AUS. For example, in patients with AUS, when cultures are directly taken of bladder urine via transurethral catheterization or suprapubic aspiration, more than 50% are positive for uropathogens but at concentrations of less than 100,000 bacteria/mL. When a single bacterial species is isolated from the bladder urine at less than 1,000 organisms/mL, the corresponding midstream voided specimens are positive for the same organism in less than half of cases. Furthermore, even when the organism is present in the midstream urine culture, it is mixed with one to four other bacterial species. Thus, in cases of AUS due to common uropathogens, midstream urine cultures are often nondiagnostic when the criterion of 10,000 bacteria/mL is used; however, one should consider 100 bacteria/mL as significant bacteriuria.

Biochemical urine tests are useful for diagnosing cystitis but are not well studied for usefulness in diagnosing AUS. A positive nitrite test correlates with bacteriuria of 100,000 or more/mL. A positive leukocyte esterase test implies pyuria of 8 or more leukocytes/mm^3. Pyuria strongly correlates with recovery of uropathogens from the bladder (but, as discussed above, not necessarily from a midstream specimen). Women with bacteria cultured from the bladder, even at low concentrations, usually have pyuria. Seventy percent of women with AUS show pyuria, and 90% of those with pyuria have cultures positive for uropathogens in the bladder (<100,000 organisms/mL) or for chlamydia or gonorrhea from the urethra or cervix.

Because women with chlamydial or gonococcal urethral infections tend to have pyuria, evaluations for chlamydia and gonorrhea should be done in patients with sterile pyuria. Chlamydia appears to cause AUS more often than does gonorrhea. More than two thirds of women with pyuria and sterile urine have chlamydia. Only 5% of women with symptoms of AUS without pyuria have chlamydia. Thus, the practitioner should sample the cervix and urethra for gonorrhea and chlamydia in women with pyuria without bacteriuria who are considered at risk for sexually transmitted diseases. Testing for gonorrhea and chlamydia is also indicated when mucopurulent cervical or urethral discharge is present. Gram stain of any cervical discharge may be useful, particularly if Gram-negative intracellular diplococci suggestive of gonorrhea are seen.

Urodynamic studies may be useful in patients with CUS again to exclude voiding dysfunction, detrusor hyperreflexia, or detrusor hyperactivity. Barabalias and Meares performed a

TABLE 76.3. Urodynamic Findings with Chronic Urethral Syndrome

Test	Chronic urethral syndrome	Normal
Mean urinary flow rate	<15 mL/s	>15 mL/s
Mean flow time	35–80 s	<30 s
Maximum urethral closure pressure	105 cm H_2O	50 cm H_2O
Residual volume	<50 mL	<50 mL

study on women diagnosed with urethral syndrome and evaluated these patients with video urodynamics. A summary of their findings is listed in Table 76.3. Their results imply that a structural abnormality exists, but this is misleading. A functional abnormality exists, impaired pelvic floor relaxation, which accounts for their findings. Despite the common symptom of incomplete emptying, women with CUS do not have increased residual volume. Not all patients with clinical evidence of CUS have urodynamic abnormalities (limited sensitivity).

Radiographic studies are not generally indicated in the evaluation of AUS or CUS. However, to rule out urethral diverticula in the differential diagnosis of CUS, a retrograde urethrogram may be useful.

TREATMENT

Acute Urethral Syndrome

For cystitis, single-dose and 3-day antibiotic regimens are effective (Table 76.4). Schultz et al. illustrated that single-dose therapy is reasonable, but multidose therapy resulted in fewer relapses in women with uncomplicated cystitis. Common short-therapy regimens for cystitis are listed in Table 76.4.

These regimens are not effective when AUS, caused by urethritis, is due to gonorrhea or chlamydia (Table 76.4). Chlamydia and gonorrhea may be treated with the regimens shown in Table 76.4. The Centers for Disease Control and Prevention has also recommended that all patients with gonorrhea be given treatment with a regimen effective against chlamydia (if chlamydia was not ruled out with testing), because up to 10% to 30% of patients with gonorrhea have concurrent chlamydia infection.

TABLE 76.4. Treatment Regimens for Acute Urethral Syndrome

Uropathogens
- Trimethoprim/sulfamethoxazole double strength, two tablets
- Trimethoprim/sulfamethoxazole double strength, one tablet twice a day for 3 days
- Amoxicillin/clavulanic acid, 250 mg three times a day for 3 days
- Norfloxacin, 400 mg twice a day for 3 days
- Ciprofloxacin, 500 mg twice a day for 3 days

Chlamydia
- Azithromycin, 1 g orally in a single dose
- Doxycycline, 100 mg twice a day for 7 days
- Erythromycin base, 500 mg orally four times a day for 7 days, or erythromycin ethylsuccinate, 800 mg four times a day for 7 days
- Ofloxacin, 300 mg orally twice a day for 7 days
- Levofloxacin, 500 mg orally daily for 7 days

Gonorrhea
- Cefixime, 400 mg orally once
- Ceftriaxone, 125 mg intramuscularly
- Ciprofloxacin, 500 mg orally once
- Ofloxacin, 400 mg orally once
- Levofloxacin, 250 mg orally once
- Plus one of the above regimens for chlamydia, if not ruled out.

TABLE 76.5. Results of a Randomized Placebo-Controlled Trial of Treatment of Acute Urethral Syndrome with Doxycycline

	Doxycycline (n = 32)	Placebo (n = 30)	P
Clinical cure			
Bladder bacteria	11/12	4/10	.016
Sterile pyuria	10/10	3/9	.003
No pyuria	7/10	8/11	.63
All cases	28/32	15/30	.002
Microbiologic cure			
Enterococcus coli/ S. saprophyticus	11/12	3/10	.005
Chlamydia trachomatis	4/4	0/3	.03
Resolution of pyuria			
Bacteria in urine	8/12	3/10	.09
Sterile urine	9/10	2/9	.005

Doxycycline is a good choice for empiric treatment pending cultures, because it has been well studied in a randomized, placebo-controlled, blinded study and showed efficacy for AUS due to either uropathogens or chlamydia (Table 76.5). Doxycycline should not be used in pregnancy.

Women with acute dysuria and frequency but without bacteriuria, positive cultures, or pyuria do not benefit from antibiotic therapy. Resolution of symptoms occurs in more than 70% of such women, and recovery is not hastened by antibiotic therapy. Half of the women with AUS treated with placebo show a clinical response, with resolution of symptoms (Table 76.5). Stamm et al. demonstrated that empiric antimicrobial therapy in the absence of any uropathogens or chlamydia did not reduce the duration of their symptoms.

Chronic Urethral Syndrome

Numerous treatments are used for CUS, including antibiotics, bladder neck opening, internal urethrotomy, urethral dilation, local steroid injections, estrogens, anxiolytics, and psychiatric therapy. Often the choice of treatment is based on tradition or empiric trial and error. Specific treatment should be based on a defined potential etiology and the desire to minimize adverse reactions. Procedures designed to increase the urethral diameter and reduce outlet obstruction (i.e., urethral dilation or urethrotomy) have not shown consistent reproducible improvement for patients and should be avoided.

A common and reasonable initial treatment for women with CUS is suppression with antibiotics (e.g., nitrofurantoin or tetracycline). In cases of CUS with urodynamic studies showing evidence of external urethral sphincter spasm, agents designed to relax the periurethral muscles and pelvic floor may be beneficial. Systemic therapy with anticholinergics, α-adrenergic blockers, and muscle relaxants has been advocated. Smooth muscle relaxants used alone or combined with a skeletal muscle relaxant such as diazepam can also be used in patients with urethral muscle spasm. Because the pudendal nerve innervates the external urethral sphincter, pudendal nerve block has also been used with some success.

Behavioral modification may also be helpful in patients with urethral sphincter spasm. Monitored relaxation and contraction of the pelvic floor (levator muscles) may lead to reestablishment of voluntary control of the urethral sphincter and cessation of involuntary spasm. Establishing a regular voiding schedule and implementation of a voiding diary are also helpful in this approach.

Surgical treatments for CUS have not been adequately evaluated. Surgical therapies are best done in research protocols and are not advised for widespread use. Many women with CUS are misdiagnosed and undergo unnecessary surgical and gynecologic evaluation or treatment. For example, in one case series 25% of patients had undergone total abdominal hysterectomy and bilateral salpingo-oophorectomy, 25% diagnostic laparoscopy, and about 12% ovarian cystectomy before the diagnosis of CUS was established.

CONSIDERATIONS IN PREGNANCY

Pregnancy symptoms themselves are unlikely to lead to a misdiagnosis of AUS or CUS. Pregnancy causes frequency of urination but not the other symptoms of either syndrome. Conversely, pregnancy has little effect on the symptoms of AUS or CUS. Pregnant women with symptoms suggestive of either should be evaluated as previously described.

Treatment options are affected by pregnancy. In particular, doxycycline, tetracycline, and quinolones are contraindicated. Erythromycin, amoxicillin (500 mg three times a day for 7 days), or azithromycin (1-g single dose) is recommended for treatment of chlamydial infections, and treatment with a cephalosporin or spectinomycin 2 g is indicated for gonorrhea. The use of trimethoprim/sulfamethoxazole is debatable during pregnancy, so alternatives are preferable when available. Nitrofurantoin appears to be safe, except for concerns about fetal hemolytic anemia if used near delivery.

BIBLIOGRAPHY

Barbalias GA, Meares EM. Female urethral syndrome: clinical and urodynamic perspectives. *Urology* 1984;23:208.

Hanno P, et al. Interstitial cystitis and related disease. In: Walsh P et al., eds. *Campbell's urology*, 7th ed. Philadelphia: WB Saunders, 1998:652.

Kunin CM, Evans C, Bartholomew D, et al. The antimicrobial defense mechanism of the female urethra: a reassessment. *J Urol* 2002;168:413–419.

Latham RH, Stamm WE. Urethral syndrome in women. *Urol Clin North Am* 1984;11:95–101.

Schultz HJ, McCaffrey LA, Keys TF, et al. Acute cystitis: a prospective study of laboratory tests and duration of therapy. *Mayo Clin Proc* 1984;59:391–397.

Splatt J, Weedon D. The urethral syndrome: morphologic studies. *Br J Urol* 1981; 53:263–265.

Stamm WE, Running K, McKevitt M, et al. Treatment of the AUS. *N Engl J Med* 1981;304:956.

Stamm WE, Wagner KF, Amsel R, et al. Causes of the AUS in women. *N Engl J Med* 1980;303:409.

Wesselmann U, Burnett AL, Heinberg LJ. The urogenital and rectal pain syndromes. *Pain* 1997;73:269–294.

Wilkins EGL, Payne SR, Pead PJ, et al. Interstitial cystitis and the urethral syndrome: a possible answer. *Br J Urol* 1989;64:39–44.

Workowski KA, Levine WC. Sexually transmitted disease treatment guidelines 2002. *MMWR Morb Mortal Wkly Rep* 2002;51(RR-6):1–77.

CHAPTER 77
Nephrolithiasis

Saurabh Agarwal and Richard Caesar

Urolithiasis is a significant worldwide health problem. It has afflicted humankind since the beginning of time. Egyptian mummies dating back to 4800 BC were found to have urinary calculi. The incidence has been estimated to be 2% to 3%. The cost of urolithiasis to the American economy in 1993 was approximately $1.7 billion. Calculi and their treatments have important implications on patients' quality of life and future renal function. In recent years there has been a trend toward less invasive surgical procedures, thereby minimizing patient morbidity. The metabolic evaluation popularized by Pak and directed medical therapy have led to significantly decreased rates of stone formation. Such therapy requires a dedicated effort by the patient and the primary care physician.

EPIDEMIOLOGY

Men are twice as likely to have a kidney stone in their lifetime than women (10% vs. 5%). Several studies have attributed this to lower testosterone levels in women and higher estrogen levels, which may be protective. Others have postulated that women have increased levels of citrate and other stone inhibitors in their urine.

ETIOLOGY OF STONE FORMATION

Kidney stones form when there is supersaturation of the urine with "salts." The most common type of stone is calcium oxalate. As the concentration of these salts rise, they can no longer be sustained in solution and thus precipitation occurs. The saturation point is dependent on the temperature, pH, and the solubility product (K_{sp}) specific to each crystal. Inhibitors of stone formation, including magnesium, citrate, and pyrophosphate, prevent nucleation of crystals by forming "complexes" that reduce their free ionic concentration. Promoters such as glycosaminoglycans and Tamm-Horsfall proteins provide a framework that facilitates crystalline formation. Stones enlarge by either homogeneous or heterogeneous nucleation once precipitation has occurred. Homogeneous nucleation occurs when the nucleus of the stone has formed in a pure solution. Crystal nuclei can form on red blood cells, debris, urine casts, or other crystals, called heterogeneous nucleation. Aggregation is the process by which these nuclei attach to one another, thus preventing them from being carried by the urinary stream. Knowledge of the physiology of stone formation is important in identifying risk factors and genetic predisposition to stone formation. This has come to the forefront of treatment in recent years because of the well-known recurrence rates of untreated stone disease and the significant reduction when proper therapy is initiated. Table 77.1 summarizes the incidence of the most common causes of nephrolithiasis.

Calcium Stones

Calcium stones represent about 75% to 85% of kidney stones in the United States. Approximately 90% of these are composed of calcium oxalate, whereas 10% are calcium phosphate. The pres-

TABLE 77.1 Major Causes of Nephrolithiasis

Stone type and etiology (% of all stones)	Occurrence of specific etiology (alone or with other causes) (%)	Female-to-male ratio
Calcium stones (80%)		1:2
Primary		
Hypercalciuria	60	1:2
Hyperuricemia	20	1:4
Hyperoxaluria	20	1:1
Hypocitraturia	20	1:1
Idiopathic	10	1:2
Secondary		
Medullary sponge kidney	20	1:2
Hyperparathyroidism	5	10:3
Distal renal tubular acidosis	1	1:1
Enteric hyperoxaluria	1	1:1
Primary hyperoxaluria	<1	
Other hypercalciuric states	<1	
Milk alkali syndrome		
Immobilization		
Sarcoid		
Vitamin D intoxication		
Malignancy		
Hyperthyroidism		
Uric acid stones (5%–10%)		
Gout	50	1:3
Idiopathic	50	1:1
Other	<1	
Myeloproliferative disorders		
Enzyme defect		
Enteric		
Cystine (1%)		1:1
Struvite (10%–15%)		5:1

ence of pure calcium phosphate stones mandates testing for rare causes of stone formation, such as distal renal tubule acidosis (type 1) and hyperparathyroidism.

Hypercalciuria is defined as calcium excretion exceeding 4 mg/kg a day. It has been found in 60% of patients with calcium oxalate stones. Paik and associates separated hypercalciuria into three categories: absorptive, attributed to increased intestinal absorption of calcium; renal, caused by increased excretion of calcium by the kidneys; and resorptive hypercalciuria, caused by increased bone resorption due to elevated levels of parathyroid hormone (PTH). This system is relevant because specific category-based therapy has yielded high success rates in prevention of stone recurrences.

Hyperoxaluria is found in up to 20% of patients who form calcium oxalate stones. Hyperoxaluria can be due to the deficiency of enzymes involved in protein metabolism. Malabsorption can lead to an increase in colonic permeability to oxalate and decreased free calcium to complex with oxalate in the intestinal lumen. Multiple studies have demonstrated that stone formation correlates better with oxalate excretion than with calcium excretion. Increases in oxalate excretion have a larger impact on the solubility product of calcium oxalate than do increases in calcium excretion. Patients with hyperoxaluria actually have increased stone formation when placed on a calcium-restricted diet. These patients need intestinal calcium to bind to free oxalate and form insoluble and nonabsorbable salts.

RENAL TUBULAR ACIDOSIS

Calcium nephrolithiasis often complicates distal (type I) renal tubular acidosis (RTA), which is characterized by a non-anion gap acidosis and a persistently elevated urine pH (>5.3 in a morning urine). Causes of RTA in adults include autoimmune disorders (particularly Sjögren syndrome), myeloma, or drugs such as lithium. A high urine pH in the presence of hypercalciuria promotes calcium phosphate precipitation. The excretion of citrate, which inhibits crystallization, is characteristically low (<150 mg/d) in distal RTA, contributing to nephrolithiasis. Patients with an "incomplete" form of distal RTA are not systemically acidotic but have defective urinary acidification and low urinary citrate excretion; like patients with "complete" RTA, they commonly present with calcium phosphate stones or nephrocalcinosis. Urinary citrate excretion should be measured if RTA is suspected.

MEDULLARY SPONGE KIDNEY

Medullary sponge kidney is a common condition present in up to 30% of women with calcium stones. It is characterized by obstruction and small cystic dilation of the collecting ducts at the papillary tips. The diagnosis is made by intravenous pyelogram, which demonstrates characteristic linear densities extending from the papillary tips. Medullary sponge kidney, in contrast to polycystic kidney disease and medullary cystic disease, is benign and does not result in proteinuria or renal insufficiency. The clinical manifestations include calcium stones, hematuria, and urinary tract infection. The stones (usually calcium oxalate or calcium phosphate) form within the cysts and commonly appear radiographically as nephrocalcinosis. It should not be assumed that the anatomic abnormalities are the sole cause of the stones. Hypercalciuria, for unknown reasons, is frequently present and should be treated.

HYPERURICOSURIA

Uric acid is a product from purine metabolism. Hyperuricosuria may be seen in patients with high purine diets and excessive cell turnover (i.e., neoplastic states). It was previously believed that elevated uric acid levels are associated with uric acid calculi. However, 20% of patients with calcium oxalate stones have elevated urinary uric acid levels. Uric acid crystals act as a nucleus for calcium oxalate precipitation. There is some evidence that uric acid may bind to inhibitors of stone formation, rendering them inactive.

HYPOCITRATURIA

Citrate is a product of the Krebs cycle and thus important in adenosine triphosphate generation. When excreted into the urine, it forms highly soluble complexes with calcium. It inhibits homogeneous nucleation of calcium oxalate and hinders aggregation of small nuclei. Hypocitraturia is one of the most common treatable causes of calcium stones. Up to 20% of those who form calcium stones have decreased urinary citrate levels. Hypocitraturia is defined as citrate excretion less than 115 mg/d in men and less than 200 mg/d in women. Acidosis and hypokalemia decrease citrate excretion. The intestinal absorption of citrate is unchanged; however, decreased urinary citrate levels are due to increase reabsorption of citrate within the distal nephron. Urinary citrate levels are higher in premenopausal women than in men, contributing to the decreased incidence of kidney stones in women. During pregnancy, urinary citrate excretion increases and offsets the concomitant increase in urinary calcium.

HYPERCALCEMIC NEPHROLITHIASIS

For the most part, the previously discussed states are all associated with low or normal serum calcium levels. Serum calcium levels in the following conditions is in the high-normal or high range.

Primary hyperparathyroidism is the most common cause of nephrolithiasis in the presence of hypercalcemia. Only 1% to 2% with hyperparathyroidism present with kidney stones. PTH acts on the distal nephron to increase calcium reabsorption and cyclic adenosine monophosphate excretion. It can be difficult to make the diagnoses; thus, unexplained high or high normal serum calcium should raise the index of suspicion and prompt an evaluation. Serum calcium levels are known to fluctuate, and so multiple samples must be taken. Primary hyperparathyroidism should be suspected in young patients, especially women, who present with bilateral renal calculi or recurrent stones. Typically, these stones are composed of calcium phosphate. Several different PTH assays are commercially available. The most sensitive are those that measure either the intact hormone or those that measure the carboxyl region.

Malignancy is the most common cause of hypercalcemia in the hospitalized population. Stone formation resulting from this hypercalcemia is exceedingly rare. Lung and breast cancer comprises 65% of this group. It was previously believed that destruction of bone by tumor invasion was the cause of the hypercalcemia. However, modern assays have detected a parathyroid-related peptide, which can bind to the same receptor as PTH and is responsible for bone resorption.

Another rare cause of hypercalcemic nephrolithiasis is sarcoidosis. Granulomatous disease such as sarcoidosis causes the production of 1,25-dihdroxyvitamin D, which is the activated form. Vitamin D acts directly in the small intestine to increase calcium absorption. The hypercalcemia causes suppression of PTH secretion.

Uric Acid Lithiasis

Uric acid is an end product of purine metabolism. It accounts for 5% to 8% of all stones in the United States. Humans do not have the ability to convert uric acid to allantoin, which is readily soluble in water. Uric acid is freely filtered and secreted into the urine. The solubility of uric acid is intimately related to the pH. It is 10 times more soluble in a pH of 6.5 than it is in a pH of 5.5. Therefore, the precipitation of uric acid crystals occurs with dehydration, acidosis, and hyperuricosuria. Approximately 20% of patients with clinically active gout will have uric acid stones. Disease states that result in increased cell turnover, such as acute leukemia and tumor lysis, can also lead to hyperuricosuria.

Infection Stones

Infection stones are called struvite, triple phosphate, or magnesium ammonium phosphate stones. Infection stones comprise 15% of all renal calculi. They are more common in women than in men. Urinary tract infections with urease-producing bacteria cause the production of ammonia and carbon dioxide. These products are converted to ammonium and bicarbonate in solution. An alkaline urine pH promotes struvite crystallization. Numerous bacteria produce urease, including *Proteus, Klebsiella, Pseudomonas*, and, rarely, *Escherichia coli*. The bacteria responsible for stone formation inhabit the interstices of the stones. Antibiotics cannot penetrate into all of these places to eradicate the infection; however, they are still important in keeping the infection contained and minimizing complications from intervention. Other than recurrent urinary tract infections, there are multiple other predisposing factors. Foreign bodies such as indwelling ureteral stents may serve as a nidus for infection. Neurogenic bladder or structural abnormalities of the urinary tract may cause urine stasis and promote urinary tract infections. Patients with urinary diversions frequently have their urinary tracts colonized with bacteria. People with struvite stones often present with staghorn calculi, which by definition is a stone that extends from the renal pelvis into one or multiple calyces. These stones are too large to pass spontaneously and often cause bleeding or obstruction, requiring urologic intervention.

Cystine Stones

Cystine is composed of two cysteine molecules connected by a disulfide bond. Cystine stones account for 1% to 2% of all nephrolithiasis in the United States. Cystinuria is an autosomal-recessive disorder characterized be the excretion of large amounts of cystine, ornithine, lysine, and arginine. The defective transport mechanisms are located in the proximal tubules and the small intestine. It is defined as excretion of greater than 250 mg of cystine per 24 hours. Of the four compounds excreted, cystine is the least soluble. Like uric acid, its solubility increases with an alkaline pH. The solubility is significantly higher at urine pHs above 7.5, whereas a pH of 6.5 is sufficient for uric acid lithiasis. The presence of hexagonal-shaped crystals in the first morning urine specimen is pathognomonic for cystinuria. These stones tend to be large on presentation and may even be staghorn calculi just like struvite stones.

CLINICAL MANIFESTATIONS

The clinical presentation of nephrolithiasis depends primarily on the size and the location of the stone. The type of stone can also affect symptomatology. The bacteria residing in struvite stone may enter the bloodstream and cause urosepsis. Many calculi are incidentally discovered on radiographic studies performed for other reasons. Nephrocalcinosis, which refers to calcifications within the renal parenchyma, are also often asymptomatic. These are often due to RTA, medullary sponge kidney, and hyperparathyroidism. Many calculi remain unchanged and asymptomatic over years of follow-up. However, about 50% of them will require urologic intervention within 5 years.

Larger stones are more likely to cause obstruction of urinary flow and thus distension of the renal capsule, resulting in visceral pain. Renal colic is intermittent and may last several minutes to hours. Patients are usually restless and writhing in pain. Free-floating stones within the renal pelvis usually do not cause symptoms unless they obstruct urine flow from a calyx or at the ureteropelvic junction. Smaller stones cause pain as they proceed from the kidney into the ureter. The location of the pain can provide clues to the location of the stone. Costovertebral or flank pain often indicates the stone is in the kidney or at the ureteropelvic junction. Pain radiating to the lower quadrant and into the inguinal region suggests the stone has progressed to the mid or distal ureter. Typically, pain in the urethra or labia occurs when the stone is in the distal ureter or at the ureterovesical junction. This can be mistaken for cystitis or urethritis.

Urinary calculi are the most common cause of microscopic hematuria. A thorough workup is required to exclude other causes, such as neoplasm and infection. Laboratory evaluation typically includes urinalysis, serum electrolytes, blood urea nitrogen, creatinine, and a complete blood count. Approximately 15% to 20% of patients with kidney stones will not have microhematuria. Pain associated with hematuria is typical.

RADIOGRAPHIC EXAMINATION

The first study that should be ordered is a plain abdominal x-ray. However, plain x-rays alone have a relatively low sensitivity and specificity. Calcium phosphate and oxalate stones are the most radiopaque, followed by struvite stones. Cystine stones are only slightly radiopaque, and pure uric acid stones are radiolucent. Stones must be differentiated from phleboliths or other extrarenal calcifications, which is sometimes difficult on a plain radiograph.

The intravenous pyelogram was the traditional study for the evaluation of nephrolithiasis. It helps to distinguish between intra- and extrarenal calcifications because the kidneys and collecting system are visualized. It can also assess the degree of obstruction of the system.

The noncontrast computed tomography is now the most frequently obtained imaging study for stones. It can be used in patients with renal insufficiency because no contrast is required. The incidence of contrast-induced nephropathy is estimated at 4% to 11% in patients with serum creatinine between 1.5 and 4.0. Additionally, a computed tomography does not require a bowel preparation or does not take as long as an intravenous pyelogram. A computed tomography can be used to diagnose extrarenal causes of flank pain such as acute appendicitis, making very useful in an emergency room setting.

Ultrasound can be used to detect hydronephrosis or kidney stones without radiation exposure. Ureteral stones are difficult to visualize, but hydronephrosis accompanied by the classic signs and symptoms of nephrolithiasis is diagnostic. This is the imaging modality of choice in pregnancy to minimize radiation to the fetus. The retrograde pyelogram is an excellent way to visualize stones and confirm their location within the urinary system. With the patient in the lithotomy position, a small catheter is inserted into the ureteral orifice cystoscopically. Radiopaque contrast medium is then injected through the catheter to visualize the collecting system. It is an invasive procedure that requires anesthesia and so it is often performed at the time of surgical intervention.

MANAGEMENT OF ACUTE NEPHROLITHIASIS

Most patients with symptomatic nephrolithiasis do not require immediate surgical management. Most can even be treated in an outpatient setting. Stones less than 5 mm have a 75% chance of passing spontaneously. Pain that is refractory to oral analgesics or intractable nausea and vomiting requires hospital admission. Fever or other signs of sepsis require immediate intravenous antibiotics and prompt surgical decompression. Infected urine within an obstructed system can progress to septic shock very rapidly. Diabetic patients should also be managed cautiously because of their decreased ability to fight infections. Bilateral ureteral calculi or stones in a solitary system require immediate treatment.

Ureteral Stent Insertion

This procedure involves placing a double J stent from the kidney to the bladder cystoscopically. The stent allows immediate drainage of the obstructed system and pain relief. This is an excellent procedure in the acute setting to provide symptom relief, but the stone must be addressed at a later date. In the setting of infection, manipulation of the upper urinary tract should be avoided. The system should be drained with a stent or percutaneous nephrostomy tube and the stone left in place. The stone may pass spontaneously after the ureteral dilation from the stent. Ureteral stents can cause flank discomfort, urinary urgency, and bladder spasms because of urothelial irritation.

Extracorporal Shock Wave Lithotripsy

In extracorporal shock wave lithotripsy (ESWL), shock waves are generated from an external source and directed into the body. Fluoroscopy or ultrasound on two axes localizes the stone. The focus of the shock wave is centered on the stone and its energy is concentrated there. The waves pass easily through the soft tissues of the body without losing energy or disrupting the surrounding structures. This procedure is performed under intravenous sedation and rarely requires general anesthesia.

Currently, ESWL is first-line treatment for stones less than 2.5 cm in the renal pelvis and less than 1.0 cm in the lower pole of the kidney or ureter. Stone-free rates range from 74% to 90%. Larger stones may be treated with ESWL, but stone-free rates drop to less than 60%. These stones are generally treated with percutaneous techniques. Cystine stones respond poorly to ESWL because they are much harder than calcium, uric acid, and struvite stones. Struvite stones are usually not treated with ESWL because they are often very large staghorns and the fragments harboring the bacteria must be removed to prevent rapid stone regrowth.

The absolute contraindications to ESWL are pregnancy, coagulopathy, and untreated urinary tract infection. Severe obesity and orthopedic deformities may cause difficulty in patent positioning and stone localization. Flank bruising and transient gross hematuria are not uncommon after the procedure. Patients require oral analgesics after ESWL because passage of the stone fragments may cause discomfort. Impaction of the stone fragments in the ureter is often caused by the large lead fragment and is called steinstrasse. The incidence of steinstrasse is 6.3% and requires ureteral stent placement or ureteroscopic stone extraction.

Ureteroscopy

Stones can be accessed endoscopically in a retrograde fashion using rigid or flexible ureteroscopes. The refinements in fiberoptic technology have lead to the development of smaller scopes, making this procedure safer for patients. These scopes are gently passed through the urethra, into the bladder, and then up into the ureter. Regional or general anesthesia is required, yet it can be performed on an outpatient basis. Recently, 3.5 and 4 French pediatric ureteroscopes have been developed for use in specialized pediatric urology centers. Thin laser fibers can be used through the ureteroscope to fragment large stones in the ureter and kidney. Specialized stone baskets are used to retrieve the stone fragments. Whether it is essential to remove the small stone fragments after ureteroscopy is currently controversial. Stone fragment retrieval may cause unnecessary trauma to the ureter because people often pass them spontaneously. Traditionally, a ureteral stent was always placed after ureteroscopy. This was done to minimize postoperative discomfort due to ureteral edema. Recently, more procedures are being performed without leaving stents. This eliminates future stent removal and the stent discomfort.

Percutaneous Nephrolithotomy

Percutaneous nephrolithotomy is reserved for large (greater than 2.5 cm) renal calculi or stones that have failed ESWL or ureteroscopic procedures. A percutaneous nephrostomy tube is placed into the collecting system under fluoroscopy. Rigid and flexible scopes are passed through the tract to fragment and extract the stone. Sometimes multiple nephrostomy tubes are necessary to access the entire stone. This procedure requires general anesthesia and several days of hospitalization. The procedure has success rates of 90% to 100%, even for very large stone burdens.

Open Nephrolithotomy

Open nephrolithotomy, once a very common procedure, is rarely performed today because of the refinements of ESWL, ureteroscopy, and percutaneous techniques. An incision is made in the kidney through the avascular plane between the anterior and posterior circulation. The collecting system is entered and the stone is extracted. The collecting system and the parenchyma are then sutured. This procedure is reserved for complex calculi, anatomic abnormalities of the collecting system, and failure of less invasive procedures. Success rates are 95% to 100%.

PREVENTION OF NEPHROLITHIASIS

All patients with a history of nephrolithiasis should undergo a full history and physical examination and limited laboratory and radiologic examination (Table 77.2). Initial evaluation is simplified if a stone has been retrieved: Uric acid, struvite, and cystine stones suggest specific diagnoses, and stones that are primarily calcium phosphate suggest RTA, primary hyperparathyroidism, or infection. The costs and potential side effects of a metabolic evaluation and medical therapy must be weighed against that of a recurrent stone. The recurrence rate is relatively low: 7% per year and 50% at 10 years. Most authorities recommend a full metabolic evaluation after a second stone episode. Simple dietary modifications can still be made, as described later.

Indications for a full metabolic evaluation are listed in Table 77.3. This is performed several weeks after the stone has been removed or has passed and the patient is back to their usual routines. The full evaluation was described by Paik et al. and requires three office visits. Two 24-hour urine collections on a random diet are analyzed for total volume, calcium, phosphate, uric acid, urea nitrogen, sodium, potassium, magnesium, citrate, oxalate, and creatinine. Table 77.4 lists the values for excretion of some of these metabolites. The third urine sample is collected after calcium, oxalate, and sodium restriction for 1 week followed by a calcium load. A urine calcium to creatinine ratio is determined after restriction but before the calcium load. Simpler versions of this test have been published; however, they yield less information. Whether this is clinically relevant or not is a matter of much debate.

TABLE 77.2. Evaluation and Prevention After the First Stone

History
Stone history
Previous radiologic evaluation
Calculi passed or removed
Stone analysis
Family history
Symptoms: pain, dysuria, grossly bloody urine
Associated conditions
Urinary tract infection and instrumentation
Gout
Inflammatory bowel disease
Sarcoidosis
Renal tubular acidosis
Malignancy
Medications associated with renal stones
Triamterene
Acyclovir
Acetazolamide
Vitamins C, A, D
Sulfonamides
Diet
Dairy products, meat/protein, soft drinks, alcohol, calcium supplementation
Oxalate-containing foods: spinach, nuts, chocolate, rhubarb
Water intake: amount and pattern
Laboratory
Urinalysis: for pH, crystals, evidence of infection
Calcium concentration (×2), renal function, electrolytes, phosphate, uric acid
Intravenous pyelogram and flat plate of abdomen
Stone analysis
General preventive measures
2–2.5 L urine output/d (6–8 glasses of water/d)
0.8–1 g/kg lean body weight protein (vegetable > animal)
< 3 g sodium, low oxalate diet

TABLE 77.3. Indications for Full Metabolic Evaluation of Nephrolithiasis

Recurrent stone formation
Women aged less than 30 y
Pediatric population
Osteoporosis, pathologic fracture
Urate stones or gout
Struvite stones
Cystine stones
Medullary sponge kidney
Positive family history
Intestinal disease

TABLE 77.4. 24-Hour Urinary Excretion of Several Metabolites

Solute	Men	Women
Calcium (upper limits of normal)		
mg/24 h	300	250
mg/g creatinine	140	140
mg/kg body wt	4	4
Uric acid (upper limits of normal)		
mg/24 h	800	750
Citrate (mg/24 h)		
Average excretion	600	700
Lower limits of normal	280	320
Renal tubular acidosis	<150	<150
Oxalate (range of normal)		
mg/24 h	20–40	20–40
Cystine (upper limits of normal)		
mg/24 h	400	400
Creatinine		
mg/kg body wt/d	20–25	15–20

Dietary Modifications

The primary therapy for the prevention of recurrent stone formation remains dietary modifications. These can be instituted without a metabolic evaluation. The success of therapy requires a team approach with close cooperation between the physician, patient, and nutritionist.

Fluid Intake

Increased fluid intake is the most effective therapy for prevention of kidney stones. Paik et al. demonstrated that a high fluid intake decreases the concentration of calcium, oxalate, phosphate, and uric acid. This reduces crystal formation. The incidence of kidney stones is much higher in hot climates where dehydration is prevalent. Patients should drink enough water to maintain a urine output of 2 to 3 L/d.

Protein

Studies have shown that the incidence of kidney stones is higher in countries in which the population has higher protein intake. Protein increases the urinary excretion of calcium, oxalate, and uric acid. The acid load generated from protein metabolism decreases urinary citrate levels and so predisposes to stone formation. A diet containing 60 g (0.8 g/kg lean body weight) of predominantly vegetable protein is recommended because it generates less acid than animal protein.

Sodium

Sodium and calcium are reabsorbed along the nephron at common sites. Increased dietary sodium causes increased sodium excretion and thus decreases calcium reabsorption. Patients who form recurrent stones are more apt to develop hypercalciuria with a high sodium diet. Most authors recommend a sodium intake of 3 g or less per day.

Oxalate

High urinary oxalate levels affect calcium oxalate supersaturation. Only 10% of urinary oxalate originates from dietary sources. It is reasonable to avoid oxalate-rich foods such as rhubarb, peanuts, tea, and spinach; however, strict oxalate restriction is unwarranted.

Calcium

Increased intestinal absorption of calcium occurs in many patients with recurrent nephrolithiasis. It would appear that limiting calcium intake would decrease stone formation. A study by Curhan found this was not the case. The mean calcium intake was actually lower in patients who formed stones than in those who did not. A high calcium diet was associated with a decreased risk of stone disease. Calcium binds with oxalate in the gastrointestinal tract, forming a compound that is not well absorbed. Free calcium and oxalate are readily absorbed. Furthermore, limiting calcium intake leads to a negative calcium balance and predisposes patients to osteoporosis. The optimal daily intake of calcium in not known, but certainly calcium restriction should be discouraged.

MEDICAL THERAPY FOR STONE DISEASE

Medical therapy for kidney stones is instituted after dietary modifications have failed to prevent stone recurrence. It is important to remind patients that they must continue to follow the dietary recommendations even after medical therapy is started. The type of stone a patient forms and any metabolic disorder that may be present must be determined by an appropriate stone analysis and metabolic workup before medical therapy.

Thiazides

Thiazides stimulate calcium reabsorption in the distal nephron and sodium excretion. They also increase PTH secretion. The usual dose is 25 to 50 mg twice daily. The effects of thiazides can be nullified by excess sodium intake. Bone mineral density may increase during therapy; however, the hypocalciuric affect is attenuated after maximal calcium saturation. The side effects of therapy include hypokalemia, hyperuricemia, and glucose intolerance.

Orthophosphates

Orthophosphates decrease the production of the activated form of vitamin D. This decreases the intestinal absorption of calcium. The renal excretion of phosphates is also increased, contributing to the inhibitor activity of urine. The side effects include gastrointestinal disturbance and diarrhea.

Sodium Cellulose Phosphate

Sodium cellulose phosphate is a nonabsorbable resin that binds intestinal calcium. It leads to a 50% to 75% decrease in urinary calcium excretion. It can be used in cases of increased intestinal calcium absorption. Severe nausea and diarrhea make it poorly tolerated in some patients. Oxalate absorption is increased by the reduction in calcium bioavailability; therefore, judicious oxalate restriction must be instituted.

Citrate

There are two options for citrate replacement: sodium citrate and potassium citrate. Citrate is a potent inhibitor of crystal formation. Both agents also alkalinize the urine, which is important in the dissolution of urate stones. Patients can be taught to measure their urine pH and titrate the citrate dose accordingly. Many patients with documented hypocitraturia, such as those with type 1 RTA, can be treated with oral citrates.

Allopurinol

Allopurinol is a potent xanthine oxidase inhibitor that reduces uric acid production. It can be used for the prevention of uric acid calculi and calcium stones associated with hyperuricemia. The usual dose is 100 mg three times per day.

Acetohydroxamic Acid

Acetohydroxamic acid is a urease inhibitor. It can be used to prevent the growth of struvite calculi. Side effects include gastrointestinal intolerance and deep vein thrombosis. Appropriate antibiotics must be instituted when treating infection stones.

D-Penicillamine and Mercaptopropionylglycine

Both agents are used for treatment of cystine stones. They form soluble salts with cystine and prevent the formation and growth of cystine stones. D-Penicillamine is an older agent with severe gastrointestinal toxicity. Mercaptopropionylglycine is much better tolerated by patients. It is important to remember that urine alkalinization and increased fluid intake are important adjuncts to this therapy.

SPECIAL CONSIDERATIONS IN PREGNANCY

During gestation, urinary calcium excretion increases two- to threefold and uric acid excretion also increases slightly. However, possibly because of a concurrent increase in citrate excretion, nephrolithiasis is no more common in pregnancy than in nonpregnant women. Complications of stone disease during pregnancy can be severe and are associated with a high incidence of preterm births. Most stones are diagnosed during the second or third trimester. The diagnosis should be considered in pregnant women with abdominal or flank pain or hematuria. It should also be considered if bacteriuria and urinary tract infections have not resolved after treatment with an appropriate antibiotic.

Establishing a firm diagnosis of nephrolithiasis is important, in part because empirical treatment for stones may be disastrous if another abdominal process is missed. Ultrasonography, although not as reliable as in the nonpregnant state, may be diagnostic in one half to two thirds of cases and should always be attempted initially. Modified excretory urography (0.4–1 rad) is then indicated if significant management decisions hinge on the results, but even this low level of radiation late in gestation may increase the risk of childhood malignancy. Promising diagnostic techniques that may decrease the need for exposure to radiation include use of Doppler ultrasound and vaginal ultrasound probe.

About 50% to 80% of stones in pregnancy pass spontaneously with supportive care that includes hydration and analgesia. Epidural anesthesia has been reported to augment the passage of calculi, possibly by decreasing ureteral spasm. Indications for invasive intervention include declining renal function, intractable pain, obstruction of a solitary kidney, infection proximal to an obstructing stone, and colic that precipitates premature labor.

Percutaneous nephrostomy, internal ureteral stent placement, and ureteroscopy are the major alternatives for definitive treatment of renal stone disease in pregnancy. Cystoscopic placement of an internal stent is generally recommended as the initial approach. X-ray guidance, which is relatively contraindicated early in pregnancy, generally is used in placement. However, avoidance of x-ray exposure by ultrasound placement of stents has been well described. If a stent cannot be placed or an abscess is present that cannot be drained by a stent, a percutaneous nephrostomy is inserted. This can be performed with local anesthesia and ultrasound guidance. In a septic patient, percutaneous nephrostomy may be preferable to stent placement to ensure drainage. The use of ureteroscopic stone removal as an alternative to percutaneous nephrostomy is controversial. Definitive treatment with ESWL or percutaneous stone removal should be deferred until after pregnancy. Crust tends to form on both internal stents and percutaneous nephrostomy tubes, mandating their replacement every 6 to 8 weeks; adequate hydration is essential to maintain patency.

BIBLIOGRAPHY

Coe FL, Parks JH, Asplin JR. The pathogenesis and treatment of kidney stones. *N Engl J Med* 1992;327:1141.

Consensus Development Panel, National Institutes of Health. Prevention and treatment of kidney stones. *JAMA* 1988;260:977.

Curhan GC, Willett WC, Rimm EB, et al. A prospective study of dietary calcium and other nutrients and the risk of symptomatic kidney stones. *N Engl J Med* 1993;328:833.

Hosking DH, McColm SE, Smith WB. Is stenting following ureteroscopy for removal of distal ureteral calculi necessary? *J Urol* 1999;161:48.

Kim SC, Nadler RB. ESWL: quo vadis? AUA Update Series, 2001:130.

Kurtzman NA, ed. Medical and surgical management of nephrolithiasis. *Semin Nephrol* 1990;10(1).

Levy FL, Adams-Huet B, Pak CYC. Ambulatory evaluation of nephrolithiasis: an update of a 1980 protocol. *Am J Med* 1995;98:50.

Loughlin KR. Management of urologic problems during pregnancy. *Urology* 1994; 44:159.

Mueller S, Wilbert D, Thueroff JW, et al. Extracorporal shock wave lithotripsy of ureteral stones: clinical experience and experimental findings. *J Urol* 1986;135: 831.

Paik ML, Wainstein MA, Spirnak JP, et al. Current indications for open stone surgery in the treatment of renal and ureteral calculi. *J Urol* 1998;159:374.

Pak CYC. Etiology and treatment of urolithiasis. *Am J Kidney Dis* 1991;18:624.

Parks JH, Coe FL. A urinary calcium-citrate index for the evaluation of nephrolithiasis. *Kidney Int* 1986;30:85.

Sulaiman MN, Buchholz NP, Clark PB. The role of ureteral stent placement in the prevention of steinstrasse. *J Endourol* 1999;13:151.

Uribarri J, Oh MS, Carroll HJ. The first kidney stone. *Ann Intern Med* 1989;111: 1006.

Yagisawa T, Chandhoke PS, Fan J. Comparison of comprehensive and limited metabolic evaluations in the treatment of patients with recurrent calcium urolithiasis. *J Urol* 1999;161:1449.

CHAPTER 78

Chronic Renal Disease

Seetharaman Ashok

Chronic renal disease results from a variety of pathologic entities, all of which are characterized by an irreversible reduction in glomerular filtration rate. *End-stage renal disease* (ESRD) refers to a total or near-total loss of renal function necessitating renal replacement therapy; *chronic renal insufficiency* refers to lesser degrees of irreversible renal injury. As of 2002, 350,000 people in the United States were being treated for ESRD. The incidence of ESRD has been increasing at approximately 8.8% per year since 1982. It seems likely that there are considerably more patients with lesser degrees of renal insufficiency. Differences in the incidence of ESRD exist between racial groups and the sexes, with

TABLE 78.1. Age, Gender, and Race Distribution of Major Causes of ESRD

			Each race's total ESRD (%)			
Disease	**Median age (y)**	**% Female**	**White**	**African-American**	**Asian**	**Native-America**
Diabetes mellitus	61	52.6	34	32.5	36.8	63.9
Hypertension	68	42	25.2	37.9	23.0	11.9
Glomerulonephritis	54	38.1	13.6	10.2	20.0	9.7
Collagen vascular disease	41	73.3	2.0	2.2	3.0	1.4
Cystic kidney disease	54	46.6	3.9	1.1	2.3	1.8
Interstitial nephritis	63	53.7	3.7	1.5	3.0	1.9
Obstructive nephropathy	68	27.5	2.5	1.1	1.4	1.3

Source: United States Renal Data System 1994 Annual Data Report. Publication No. PB95105003. Bethesda, MD: The National Institutes of Health, National Institute of Diabetes and Digestive and Kidney Diseases, with permission.

African-Americans and Native-Americans having an approximately fourfold higher incidence of ESRD than whites (Table 78.1). Overall, males with ESRD slightly outnumber females; however, this is primarily due to a predominance of males in the white population with ESRD. Among Native-Americans females predominate, whereas in African-Americans ESRD is evenly distributed between sexes. The etiology of ESRD also demonstrates some racial differences. Overall, diabetes mellitus is the most common cause of ESRD, particularly among Native-Americans. Hypertensive nephrosclerosis is the most common etiology among African-Americans.

The primary care physician plays a central role in the identification of chronic renal disease and, when possible, determination of a specific etiology. Long-term management of the multisystem complications of chronic renal insufficiency is also frequently overseen by the primary care physician. Referral to a nephrologist is appropriate when there is uncertainty regarding the etiology and appropriate therapy of chronic renal disease or when renal replacement therapy is indicated.

ETIOLOGY

Etiologies of ESRD are categorized as either systemic diseases with renal involvement or primary renal diseases (Table 78.2). The most common etiologies of chronic renal disease in the United States are discussed in the following sections.

Diabetes Mellitus

In the United States, end-stage diabetic nephropathy is steadily increasing in incidence and currently represents one third of all patients with ESRD. Considerably more data exist regarding the natural history and clinical course for insulin-dependent diabetes mellitus (IDDM) than are available for non–insulin-dependent diabetes mellitus (NIDDM). In IDDM, about 30% to 40% of patients ultimately develop nephropathy. This usually occurs after 10 or more years of diabetes and is manifest as persistent proteinuria, hypertension, and declining renal function. Microalbuminuria, defined as urinary albumin excretion at a rate below what is detectable by conventional laboratory tests, predicts eventual progression to overt diabetic nephropathy. Once persistent proteinuria is present, renal function slowly and inexorably declines, resulting in ESRD in approximately 7 to 10 years. The degree of proteinuria can vary significantly, ranging from 0.5 to 20 g/d. In those with overt nephropathy, associated diabetic complications such as retinopathy, neuropathy, and cardiovascular disease are very common.

The cumulative incidence of nephropathy in NIDDM is in the range of 10% to 20% for whites, but is somewhat higher for African-Americans and some Native-American tribes. The reasons underlying these racial differences are not well understood. As in IDDM, overt nephropathy is heralded by the development of persistent proteinuria, hypertension, and renal

TABLE 78.2. Etiology of ESRD

Disease	Total ESRD (%)
Systemic disease with renal involvement	
Diabetes mellitus	33.8
Hypertension	28.3
Autoimmune/collagen vascular disease	
Systemic lupus erythematosus	1.3
Goodpasture syndrome	0.3
Wegener granulomatosis	0.2
Scleroderma	0.2
Hemolytic uremic syndrome/TTP	0.2
Polyarteritis	<0.1
Henoch-Schönlein purpura	<0.1
Hereditary disease	
Autosomal-dominant polycystic kidney disease	3.0
Autosomal-recessive polycystic kidney disease	<0.1
Sickle cell disease	<0.1
Alport syndrome	0.3
Fabry disease	<0.1
Cystinosis	<0.1
Hyperoxaluria	<0.1
Dysproteinemia	
Multiple myeloma/light chain nephropathy	0.8
Amyloidosis	0.3
HIV-related nephropathy	0.3
Primary renal disease	
Glomerulonephritis	
Membranous nephropathy	0.4
Membranoproliferative glomerulonephritis	0.3
Focal glomerulosclerosis	1.4
IgA nephropathy	10.0
Interstitial renal disease	
Analgesic nephropathy	0.8
All other interstitial disease	2.2
Obstructive nephropathy	2.0
ESRD of unknown cause	11.8

TTP, thrombotic thrombocytopenic purpura.
Source: United States Renal Data System 1994 Annual Data Report. Publication No. PB95105003. Bethesda, MD: The National Institutes of Health, National Institute of Diabetes and Digestive and Kidney Diseases, with permission.

insufficiency. Progression to ESRD follows a time course roughly similar to that of IDDM. Evaluation of renal disease in patients with NIDDM is more complicated than with IDDM because these patients tend to be older with more complex medical problems.

Studies of the pathogenic mechanisms underlying the development of diabetic nephropathy have focused on the role of functional changes such as hyperfiltration and renal hypertrophy and ultrastructural changes such as thickening of the glomerular basement membrane and mesangial expansion. Whether sustained hyperglycemia alone or other aspects of the diabetic milieu are responsible for these changes is not yet known.

Hypertension

Arterial hypertension is both a common etiology and a consequence of chronic renal disease. About 25% of all patients with ESRD carry a diagnosis of hypertensive nephrosclerosis. This group of patients includes those with nephrosclerosis due to essential hypertension, those with malignant-phase essential hypertension, and those with renovascular disease. Hypertensive nephrosclerosis is predominantly a disease of African-Americans, perhaps due to the greater incidence of malignant-phase hypertension in this group.

ESSENTIAL HYPERTENSION

Patients in whom no specific or reversible etiology of hypertension can be determined are categorized as having primary or essential hypertension. Impaired pressure-induced sodium excretion and abnormally increased vasopressor tone have been proposed as pathophysiologic factors causing essential hypertension. Epidemiologic data further suggest an important role for both genetic and environmental factors. Hypertensive nephrosclerosis in patients with essential hypertension is usually seen in those with inadequately controlled diastolic hypertension or recurrent episodes of accelerated hypertension. The clinical course of hypertensive nephrosclerosis is variable, related to the severity of hypertension and effectiveness of control.

ACCELERATED MALIGNANT HYPERTENSION

Accelerated malignant hypertension is a hypertensive emergency. It is usually seen with diastolic blood pressures more than 140 mm Hg and is associated with evidence of rapidly progressing end-organ injury. Organ pathology seen in this setting may include rapidly worsening renal insufficiency, grade III or IV hypertensive retinopathy, encephalopathy, intracranial hemorrhage, acute myocardial infarction or left ventricular failure, and acute aortic dissection. End-organ injury in this syndrome results from an autoregulatory failure of resistance vessels, which allows transmission of the markedly elevated arterial pressure to the microvasculature. Before effective antihypertensive therapy became available, prognosis in malignant hypertension was dismal, with a 1-year mortality higher than 90%. Prompt recognition and effective treatment of malignant hypertension has greatly improved the outcome in these patients. Control of blood pressure in this setting may initially be associated with worsening of renal function. However, with sustained blood pressure control, renal function tends to improve over a period of weeks. Over the long term, however, many of these patients ultimately develop ESRD. Accelerated malignant hypertension most commonly represents an aggressive phase of underlying essential hypertension; it can also be seen, however, as a consequence of renovascular disease, acute glomerulonephritis, primary aldosteronism, pheochromocytoma, primary intracranial hemorrhage, or intoxication with a drug such as cocaine.

Renovascular Disease

Hemodynamically significant stenosis of one or both renal arteries results in renin-mediated hypertension. Chronic renal insufficiency develops when there is significant narrowing of both renal arteries, resulting in ischemic renal injury or the development of hypertensive nephrosclerosis in the non-stenotic kidney. The exact incidence of renovascular disease and its contribution to ESRD is not known, but it appears to be increasing. About two thirds of renovascular disease is atherosclerotic in origin; the remaining one third is due to fibromuscular dysplasia. Atherosclerotic disease is most commonly seen in men over the age of 55 years, whereas fibromuscular disease is predominantly a disease of younger women aged 15 to 40 years. Clinical clues suggesting the presence of renovascular disease include the presence of a systolic and diastolic abdominal bruit, the development of hypertension before the age of 30 years or over the age of 60 years, acceleration of previously well-controlled hypertension, and hypertension with associated renal insufficiency. A variety of screening procedures have been evaluated for the detection of renovascular disease, including captopril nuclear renography, Doppler ultrasonography of the renal arteries, magnetic resonance angiography, and intravenous digital subtraction angiography. The sensitivity and specificity of these tests vary from center to center and may be operator dependent (e.g., Doppler ultrasonography). Most experts consider hypertensive or rapid sequence intravenous pyelography an outmoded and insensitive screening study.

A form of renovascular disease seen with increasing frequency is cholesterol embolization. This is typically seen in patients with severe atherosclerotic disease after invasive vascular procedures such as arteriography, coronary artery bypass grafting, or repair of an abdominal aortic aneurysm. It is caused by the disruption of cholesterol plaque with subsequent showering of the microvasculature with cholesterol particles. Clinically, this may be manifest as livido reticularis seen primarily in the lower extremities, abdominal pain due to ischemic bowel or pancreatitis, stroke, or a sudden decrease in renal function. Less commonly, cholesterol embolization can occur spontaneously without vascular manipulation.

Glomerulonephritis

Glomerulonephritis may be seen as a primary renal disease limited to the kidney or as the renal manifestation of a variety of systemic diseases. When all forms of glomerulonephritis are grouped together, they constitute the third most common cause of ESRD (Table 78.1). Injury to the glomerulus and in particular the glomerular basement membrane by inflammatory and hemodynamic factors results in the characteristic clinical and histologic findings in glomerulonephritis. These include proteinuria and hematuria, both of which are consequences of a disrupted glomerular filtration barrier.

The nephrotic syndrome is characterized by heavy proteinuria (>3.5 g/d), hypoproteinemia, hyperlipidemia, and edema. The presence of oval fat bodies in the urine sediment is diagnostic of the nephrotic syndrome. In the nephritic syndrome, the urine sediment is more typically characterized by hematuria, often with red cell casts, but more modest degrees of proteinuria. Because of their transit through the glomerular basement membrane and renal tubules, red cells of glomerular origin are frequently dysmorphic in appearance. It is important to remember, however, that hematuria is overall more commonly the result of lower urinary tract pathology, which, in most cases, must first be excluded. Strong clues that hematuria is of glomerular origin are the presence of dysmorphic red cells, cellular casts, and proteinuria. The most commonly encountered types of primary and secondary glomerulonephritis are reviewed in the following sections.

PRIMARY GLOMERULOPATHIES

Membranous Glomerulonephritis

Membranous glomerulonephritis is the most common etiology of the nephrotic syndrome in adults, typically presenting as the gradual onset of proteinuria and edema. Urinary protein losses can be quite variable in this disorder, exceeding 20 g/d in some patients but less than 1 g/d in others. Membranous glomerulonephritis is most commonly idiopathic but may also result from a variety of infections (e.g., hepatitis B, *Plasmodium malariae*, syphilis), drugs (e.g., gold, captopril, penicillamine), or autoimmune disorders such as systemic lupus erythematosus (SLE). Primarily in patients over the age of 50, there is an association between membranous glomerulonephritis and the presence of malignancy. Screening examinations for occult malignancy are indicated in such patients. The urine sediment in membranous glomerulonephritis is typically bland, only rarely containing gross hematuria or red cell casts. On renal biopsy, the characteristic histologic findings are the presence of thickening of the glomerular basement membrane on light microscopy and the presence of subepithelial electron-dense deposits seen on electron microscopy.

The variable clinical course of this disorder complicates treatment. Spontaneous remission of proteinuria may occur in as many as 25% of patients, with 10-year renal survival rates varying between 50% and 90%. Clinical characteristics associated with a more favorable prognosis include female gender, normotension, younger age, and proteinuria below the nephrotic range.

Minimal Change Disease

Minimal change disease, also known as lipoid nephrosis and nil lesion, derives its name from the absence of any identifiable glomerular abnormality on light microscopy. Electron microscopy reveals fusion of epithelial cell foot processes—a nonspecific finding seen in all forms of nephrotic syndrome. Diagnosis is therefore one of exclusion. Minimal change disease is the most common cause of nephrotic syndrome in children, accounting for 90% of nephrotic syndrome in children under the age of 4 and 50% in those under the age of 10. In adults, however, the incidence is much lower, causing approximately 15% of all cases of the nephrotic syndrome. Onset of proteinuria is typically sudden and may follow a viral illness. Proteinuria can be massive, occasionally in excess of 20 g/d with associated anasarca. The urine sediment is typically bland, with heavy albuminuria, oval fat bodies, and occasionally microscopic hematuria. Gross hematuria and red cell casts are rare.

As with membranous glomerulonephritis, minimal change disease is most commonly idiopathic; however, it can be associated with malignancies, such as Hodgkin disease or T-cell lymphomas, and drugs, most commonly nonsteroidal antiinflammatory agents. As discussed below, response to corticosteroid therapy is very good in children but in adults is less dramatic and may take more prolonged courses of therapy.

Focal and Segmental Glomerulosclerosis

Focal and segmental glomerulosclerosis (FSGS) is a pathologic entity that derives its name from the presence of sclerotic lesions involving some glomeruli but leaving others uninvolved (focal) and affecting only portions of a given glomerulus (segmental). As with minimal change nephropathy, FSGS comprises approximately 15% of nephrotic syndrome in adults. FSGS is most commonly an idiopathic disease but can be seen in association with a variety of other disorders, including reflux nephropathy, human immunodeficiency virus (HIV) infection, sickle cell disease, morbid obesity, cyanotic heart disease, and heroin nephropathy. Some authors postulate that FSGS in certain patients may be a progressive form of minimal change disease seen in those patients who failed to achieve a long-term response to corticosteroid therapy. FSGS is seen more commonly in African-Americans than in whites and is the predominant cause of nephrotic syndrome in obese patients. The clinical course of FSGS is unfavorable, with most patients progressing to ESRD. This, however, may take up to 20 years from the time of initial presentation. In a subset of patients with FSGS, the clinical course is very rapid, with progression to ESRD in 2 to 3 years. This form of FSGS, called malignant focal sclerosis, tends to recur rapidly in transplanted kidneys.

Membranoproliferative Glomerulonephritis

Membranoproliferative glomerulonephritis (MPGN) is characterized histologically by the combination of thickening of glomerular capillary walls and mesangial hypercellularity. Pathologists identify two varieties. Type I, thought to be due to immune complex deposition, is characterized by immunofluorescence staining for complement fragments and immunoglobulins in capillary walls and mesangial areas. In type II MPGN, also known as dense deposit disease, continuous electron-dense deposits are seen in the glomerular basement membrane by electron microscopy. Of these two varieties, type I is much more common, accounting for approximately 10% of nephrotic syndrome in children and adults. Clinical manifestations are variable, with either a nephrotic or nephritic urine sediment being possible. At presentation, many patients have hypertension and renal insufficiency. MPGN usually follows a slow unremitting course, with approximately half of patients progressing to ESRD in 10 years. Characteristic laboratory findings include hypocomplementemia, which in some instances is due to the presence of circulating nephritic factors. These factors are autoantibodies that bind to convertases of the complement pathways, thereby preventing their degradation and promoting continued complement activation. Although usually idiopathic, MPGN may result from hepatitis B or C viral infection, cryoglobulinemia, chronic bacterial infection, SLE, or complement deficiency states. MPGN has a propensity to recur in transplanted kidneys.

IgA Nephropathy

Both in the United States and worldwide, IgA nephropathy is the most common cause of glomerulonephritis. It can be seen in association with Henoch-Schönlein purpura or chronic liver disease or as an isolated glomerulonephritis. Diagnostic histologic findings are immunofluorescent staining for IgA, predominantly in the mesangial areas. Electron microscopy usually demonstrates electron-dense deposits correlating to areas of IgA immunostaining. The clinical presentation is extremely variable, including isolated microscopic hematuria with or without proteinuria, chronic glomerulonephritis, rapidly progressive glomerulonephritis, or the nephrotic syndrome.

Both the initial presentation with hematuria and subsequent exacerbations often occur after upper respiratory tract infection. IgA nephropathy was previously considered a benign entity; it has become clear, however, that some patients do develop progressive renal insufficiency. In those who develop chronic renal insufficiency, it tends to be a very slow process, with approximately 20% of patients reaching ESRD after 40 years. Factors associated with a less favorable prognosis are the nephrotic syndrome, glomerular crescents on biopsy, and sustained hypertension. IgA nephropathy often recurs in transplanted allografts, but this should not prevent renal transplantation because it does not usually cause progressive loss of allograft function.

GLOMERULOPATHIES ASSOCIATED WITH SYSTEMIC DISEASE

Postinfectious Glomerulonephritis

Although most commonly seen after streptococcal infection, postinfectious glomerulonephritis can also be seen in association with a variety of other infections, such as visceral abscesses, osteomyelitis, bacterial endocarditis, or infection of ventriculovascular shunts. The most common postinfectious glomerulonephritis is an immune complex-mediated disease resulting from pharyngitis or impetigo due to group A streptococci. The risk of developing glomerulonephritis is slightly greater after impetigo than with pharyngitis. This is a disease primarily of children, but it does occur in adults.

Typically, patients with poststreptococcal glomerulonephritis present with hematuria, edema, flank pain, and sometimes with hypertension and signs of volume overload. A renal biopsy during the acute phase of the illness usually demonstrates an acute diffuse glomerulonephritis with neutrophils visible within glomerular capillary lumens. In most patients, these glomerular lesions slowly resolve, although occasionally with some focal residual scarring. Persistent microscopic hematuria or low-grade proteinuria may be present for many months. The long-term prognosis in children is excellent, with chronic renal insufficiency only rarely encountered. In adults, however, the prognosis may be less benign.

Systemic Lupus Erythematosus

SLE is a disorder predominantly affecting women, with a female-to-male ratio of 2:1. It is seen most commonly in younger patients, with the peak incidence between 15 and 40 years of age. Approximately half of all patients have clinical evidence of glomerulonephritis at the time of diagnosis with SLE, and an additional 25% have clinically apparent renal involvement at some point during their course. Even if clinical signs of renal involvement are absent, histologic evidence of lupus nephritis can be seen in 95% of all patients who meet the diagnostic clinical criteria for SLE. The presenting manifestations of lupus nephritis are variable and include microscopic or gross hematuria, low-grade proteinuria, nephrotic syndrome, and rapidly progressive glomerulonephritis. Hypertension is present in roughly half of all patients.

Lupus nephritis results from glomerular deposition of circulating immune complexes thought to be composed of DNA, anti-DNA, and complement fragments. The various histologic patterns seen with lupus nephritis have been categorized by the World Health Organization as follows:

- Class I—no identifiable lesion
- Class II—mesangial glomerulonephritis
- Class III—focal proliferative glomerulonephritis
- Class IV—diffuse proliferative glomerulonephritis
- Class V—membranous glomerulopathy
- Class VI—sclerosing nephropathy.

Histologic classification is of significant prognostic and therapeutic value. Patients with diffuse proliferative glomerulonephritis (class IV) have a less favorable prognosis, whereas a more benign course is seen in patients with class I and II disease. The prognosis in class V disease is less clear.

Antiglomerular Basement Membrane-Mediated Glomerulonephritis

Antiglomerular basement membrane-mediated glomerulonephritis is characterized by rapidly progressive glomerulonephritis and the demonstration of circulating autoantibodies to constituents of the glomerular basement membrane. Immunofluorescent microscopy shows linear deposition of IgG along the glomerular basement membrane, and light microscopy usually reveals glomerular crescents and variable degrees of segmental glomerular necrosis. In Goodpasture disease, anti- glomerular basement membrane–associated glomerulonephritis is seen in conjunction with alveolar hemorrhage. This syndrome affects predominantly men. There is a bimodal age distribution, with peaks in the third and sixth decades of life. Before glomerulonephritis is diagnosed, many patients complain of nonspecific symptoms such as weight loss or malaise for up to several months. Glomerulonephritis in this syndrome generally follows a rapidly progressive course to ESRD. Up to 75% of patients may have associated pulmonary involvement. Alveolar hemorrhage is most common in patients with an associated pulmonary insult such as respiratory tract infection, toxin exposure, or cigarette smoking.

Antineutrophil Cytoplasmic Antibody–Associated Diseases

Over recent years, several pathologic entities previously thought to be distinct have been shown to be associated with autoantibodies directed against components of neutrophil cytoplasm—termed antineutrophil cytoplasmic antibodies (ANCA). These pathologic entities include Wegener granulomatosis, microscopic polyarteritis nodosa, leukocytoclastic angiitis, and the pauci-immune variety of rapidly progressive glomerulonephritis. Two general classes of ANCA have been identified. These are *c-ANCA* and *p-ANCA*, correlating to the *cytoplas mic* or *perinuclear* immunostaining pattern of neutrophils by these autoantibodies. In general, p-ANCA is more commonly seen in those with disease limited to the kidney, whereas those with more systemic disease tend to have c-ANCA. It has recently been established that most c-ANCA are directed against proteinase 3, whereas p-ANCA are specific for myeloperoxidase. Most patients present with a prodrome of constitutional symptoms including fever, arthralgias, weight loss, or anorexia. Renal involvement is manifest by hypertension, renal insufficiency, proteinuria, and hematuria, frequently with red cell casts. Roughly half of patients with ANCA-associated glomerulonephritis have respiratory tract involvement. This may be manifest as pulmonary hemorrhage, sinusitis, or otitis media. Histologic examination of the kidney in these patients is notable for segmental necrotizing glomerulonephritis with crescent formation. Immunofluorescent studies are typically negative; thus the term *pauci-immune glomerulonephritis* has been applied to this entity. Most patients tend to be older, with a peak incidence in the fifth and sixth decades of life. Before the availability of more effective supportive and immunosuppressive therapy, these patients followed a rapidly progressive course resulting in a very high incidence of ESRD or death.

Dysproteinemia-Associated Renal Disease

A variety of renal lesions may result from the pathologic production of monoclonal proteins by plasma cells. In many patients, overt multiple myeloma is present, whereas in others there is an apparent plasma cell proliferative process as indicated by the production of monoclonal proteins but no pathologically identifiable neoplasia. Primary amyloidosis is the result of deposition within the glomerulus of immunoglobulin light chains that form amyloid fibrils. These deposits stain positively with Congo red. With primary amyloidosis, there is frequently cardiac involvement manifest as a restrictive cardiomyopathy and neural involvement characterized by peripheral neuropathy or carpal tunnel syndrome. The prognosis in primary amyloidosis is poor, with most patients succumbing to cardiac disease. Light chain deposition disease, which is characterized histologically by nodular nephrosclerosis similar to that seen in diabetic nephropathy, is also caused by deposition of light chains within the glomerulus. Patients with both of these entities typically present with the nephrotic syndrome. Other renal lesions associated with multiple myeloma include acute renal failure due to tubular obstruction from paraprotein casts and hypercalcemic nephropathy. Secondary amyloidosis is seen in chronic inflammatory diseases such as rheumatoid arthritis, inflammatory bowel disease, chronic cutaneous abscesses due to parenteral drug abuse, and familial Mediterranean fever. Amyloid fibrils in this disorder deposit in the kidney and other organs and result from production of serum amyloid A, a protein produced by the liver as an acute phase reactant in inflammatory states.

Human Immunodeficiency Virus–Associated Nephropathy

As our experience with HIV infection increases, renal complications of this infection are seen with greater frequency. The exact incidence of renal complications of HIV infection is not well known; however, approximately 1% of military recruits who test seropositive for HIV infection have urinary abnormalities. A variety of glomerular lesions has been reported in association with HIV infection, including membranous nephropathy, minimal change disease, focal and segmental glomerulosclerosis, membranoproliferative glomerulonephritis, and mesangial proliferative glomerulonephritis. The clinical presentation most frequently encountered is rapid onset of the nephrotic syndrome, frequently with very heavy proteinuria, large echogenic kidneys by ultrasonography, and the rapid progression to ESRD, usually within 6 months from the onset of proteinuria. African-American heterosexual males with a history of intravenous drug abuse make up most of these patients. This disorder therefore bears some demographic similarity to heroin nephropathy; it differs markedly, however, in that it progresses much more rapidly to ESRD. Pathologically, HIV nephropathy is most commonly characterized by focal and segmental glomerulosclerosis with the presence of tubuloreticular inclusions in vascular endothelium.

Indanivir, an antiviral agent in HIV management, is a well known cause of crystal-induced acute renal failure, dysuria, flank pain, and nephrolithiasis. Tubulointerstitial injury characterized by progressive rise in serum creatinine is another manifestation of toxicity. New onset hypertension, pyuria, and eosinophiluria indicates toxicity. Discontinuation of the drug reverses the condition.

Congenital or Inherited Renal Disease

AUTOSOMAL-DOMINANT POLYCYSTIC KIDNEY DISEASE

Autosomal-dominant polycystic kidney disease (ADPKD), affecting approximately 500,000 Americans, is one of the most common inherited disorders in the United States. As its name indicates, it is inherited in an autosomal-dominant fashion and therefore affects males and females equally. It is characterized by the presence of numerous and progressively enlarging cysts in both kidneys (Fig. 78.1). The exact incidence and prevalence of this disorder are not known, however, because only approximately one half of all affected patients progress to ESRD. Many affected persons therefore never manifest clinical signs or symptoms of ADPKD. Their disease is discovered incidentally during evaluation for some other problem or at postmortem examination. Cysts apparently arise from renal tubules, but the mechanism by which this happens remains unknown. The mechanism by which these cysts produce renal insufficiency is not clear either, but it may be related to compression of adjacent nephronal structures by enlarging cysts. Those who progress to ESRD generally do so in the fifth through seventh decades of life. Two varieties of this disorder, ADPKD-1 and ADPKD-2, have been differentiated based on the chromosomal location of the genetic defect. Approximately 10% of affected patients have no known family history of ADPKD, perhaps representing spontaneous mutations. Renal insufficiency develops very

A

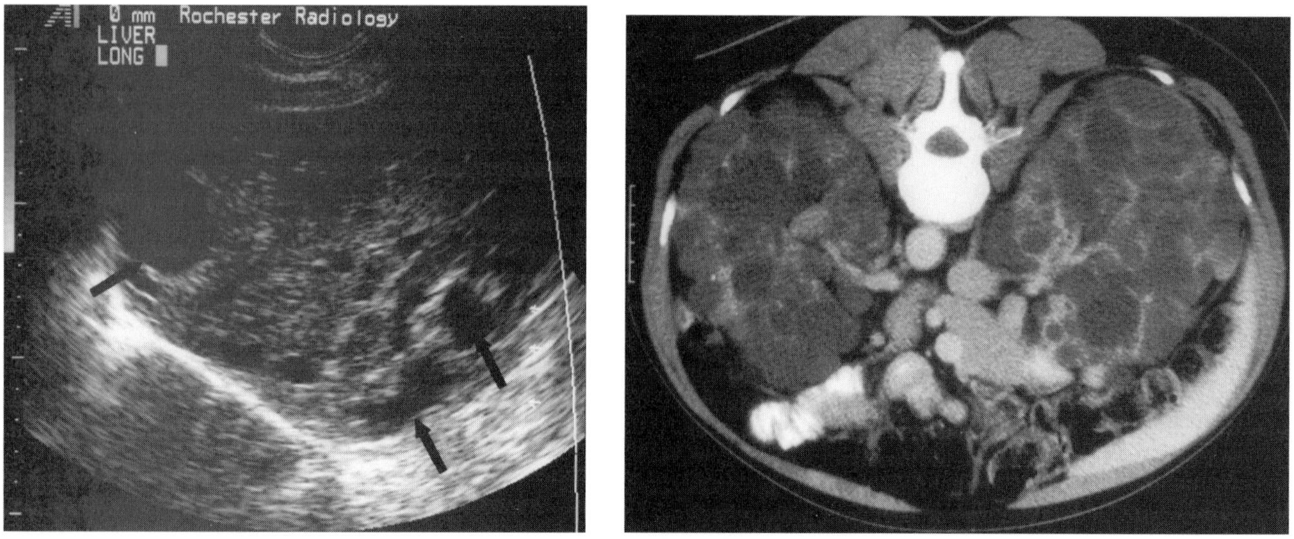

B

FIG. 78.1. A: Abdominal ultrasound of an asymptomatic 37-year-old woman with autosomal-dominant polycystic kidney disease. The *arrow* to the left indicates a large hepatic cyst, and the two *arrows* to the right identify two renal cortical cysts. The patient's blood pressure, urinalysis, and renal function were normal. **B:** Abdominal computed tomography of a 58-year-old man with massive renal enlargement and advanced renal insufficiency from autosomal-dominant polycystic kidney disease.

slowly in these patients and correlates with increasing cyst and kidney size. Hypertension often accompanies the development of renal insufficiency. The rate at which renal insufficiency develops in patients with ADPKD, however, is extremely variable, and, as noted earlier, approximately half of all patients never progress to ESRD.

Pathologically, ADPKD is characterized by the progressive enlargement of numerous cysts throughout both kidneys (Fig. 78.1). Roughly 90% of all affected patients have ultrasonically identifiable cysts by age 30 years. In many patients, however, cysts can be identified by ultrasonography or computed tomography at a much younger age and have even been visualized in utero.

In addition to hypertension and renal insufficiency, there are several other renal complications of ADPKD. These include bleeding into cysts, cyst infection, and urinary calculi. These episodes present with abdominal pain and can present a significant management problem. ADPKD is also associated with a number of extrarenal manifestations, including colonic diverticulosis, cardiac valvular abnormalities, hepatic cysts (Fig. 78.1), inguinal hernias, and, most importantly, intracranial aneurysms.

OTHER CYSTIC DISEASES

Autosomal-recessive polycystic kidney disease is rarer than ADPKD and usually progresses to ESRD in childhood. Medullary cystic disease, also quite rare, is divided into recessive and dominant forms. Both present early in life, with the usual clinical course being eventual progression to ESRD. Medullary cystic disease should not be confused with medullary sponge kidney, a disorder characterized by dilated intramedullary collecting ducts. Medullary sponge kidney is often complicated by urolithiasis and hypercalciuria but otherwise follows a benign course.

SICKLE CELL NEPHROPATHY

In the United States, approximately 4% of all patients with sickle cell anemia eventually develop ESRD. These patients usually present with hypertension and proteinuria, with focal and segmental glomerulosclerosis seen histologically. In patients with sickle cell trait, medullary ischemia can result in hematuria and impaired urinary concentration but rarely leads to ESRD.

HEREDITARY NEPHRITIS (ALPORT SYNDROME)

Hereditary nephritis (Alport syndrome) is an inherited renal disease with a gene frequency of approximately 1 in 5,000. In most affected families it has an X-linked transmission. Underlying this disorder is the absence of a component of type IV collagen from the glomerular basement membrane. This molecular defect is likely responsible for the frayed appearance and segmental thinning of the glomerular basement membrane as seen by electron microscopy. Patients typically present with microscopic or gross hematuria and modest degrees of proteinuria. Women with hereditary nephritis follow a more benign course, perhaps due to inactivation of one X chromosome per cell (the Lyon hypothesis). Approximately 20% of affected women develop ESRD but usually after age 50 years. Affected males invariably progress to ESRD. Extrarenal manifestations of hereditary nephritis include sensorineural hearing loss, ocular abnormalities, and leiomyomata of the gastrointestinal or genitourinary tract.

VESICOURETERAL REFLUX

Vesicoureteral reflux (VUR) usually presents in childhood in association with urinary tract infection. Progressive renal insufficiency from severe VUR represents a serious problem in children and accounts for approximately 10% of ESRD in the pediatric population. The mechanism by which VUR results in progressive renal insufficiency remains unknown. Also controversial is the role of coexisting bacterial infection in causing renal injury in this disorder. The severity of VUR is graded 1 through 5 based on findings on voiding cystourethrography. In grade 1, urine reflux is into the distal ureter but with no dilatation of the urinary tract, whereas in grade 5, urine reflux is into the renal calices, with marked dilatation of the entire urinary tract. Progressive renal insufficiency is usually associated with hypertension and proteinuria.

ANALGESIC NEPHROPATHY

Chronic use of a variety of analgesic preparations, including salicylates, acetaminophen, and nonsteroidal antiinflammatory drugs, results in chronic interstitial nephritis. In some countries, this is a significant problem, responsible for as much as 10% to 20% of all cases of ESRD. In the United States, it is seen less commonly and accounts for approximately 1% of all patients with ESRD. Cumulative intake of approximately 1 to 2 kg of analgesics over several years is usually required before this syndrome develops. It is seen more commonly in women and frequently is associated with some chronic pain syndrome such as headaches or rheumatoid or degenerative arthritis. Histologically, chronic interstitial nephritis, interstitial fibrosis, and papillary necrosis are seen. Progression to ESRD usually follows a very slow course over several decades. Transitional cell carcinomas of the urinary tract are associated with analgesic nephropathy.

CLINICAL SYMPTOMS AND SIGNS

Renal disease may manifest itself in a variety of ways. In many patients, renal disease is identified only incidentally after the performance of a routine urinalysis, blood chemistries, or blood pressure monitoring. Many other patients present in the advanced stages of chronic renal disease with nonspecific complaints such as fatigue, anorexia, and lethargy. Still others do not seek medical attention until overt uremia is present, manifest by anorexia, nausea, vomiting, slowed mentation, neuromuscular irritability, and serositis such as pericarditis or pleuritis.

When attempting to elicit a history suggestive of chronic renal disease, the physician should focus questioning on the presence of a previous history of renal disease, a family history of renal disease (e.g., ADPKD, hereditary nephritis), and the presence of any systemic illness that may have associated renal involvement (e.g., diabetes mellitus, SLE, vasculitis). Questions identifying specific symptoms and signs directly related to kidney disease should also be pursued. For example, patients with glomerular disease often present with complaints of edema or hematuria. A comprehensive past medical history is also very important in the evaluation of chronic renal disease. This should include any previous surgical or angiographic procedures and a medication history, with particular reference to nonsteroidal antiinflammatory agents. The etiology of chronic renal disease can often be determined from a careful history. In patients with long-standing diabetes mellitus complicated by retinopathy, proteinuric renal disease is most likely diabetic in origin. Long-standing essential hypertension, particularly if poorly controlled and in African-Americans, suggests hypertensive nephrosclerosis. Renal insufficiency associated with new onset or accelerated hypertension in a patient with known atherosclerotic vascular disease suggests the diagnosis of renovascular disease. Constitutional or rheumatologic symptoms such as fever, arthritis, arthralgias, skin rashes, or weight loss may point to a diagnosis of systemic lupus, vasculitis, or malignancy-associated glomerulopathy. Nocturia due to impaired urinary concentrating ability is also a common but nonspecific presenting complaint. History of recurrent urinary tract infections may suggest underlying VUR, whereas urinary hesitancy and frequency may indicate bladder neck obstruction. A detailed social history is also important, with specific reference to risk factors for transmission of HIV and exposure to environmental nephrotoxins such as lead.

A careful physical examination also plays a crucial role in the evaluation of patients with chronic renal disease. Blood pressure should be measured. An assessment of volume status is made by examining orthostatic blood pressures and jugular venous pressure. Peripheral edema and pulmonary congestion can reveal the presence of chronic renal disease. Depending on the nature of their renal disease, patients may present volume overloaded, euvolemic, or volume depleted. In patients presenting with advanced renal failure, the uremic syndrome may be present. On physical examination, this may be characterized by slowed mentation or confusion; neuromuscular irritability manifest by clonus, asterixis, or hyperreflexia; and the presence of uremic pleuritis or pericarditis with friction rubs. Uremic pericarditis may be associated with signs and symptoms of pericardial tamponade. Abdominal bruits or an abdominal aortic aneurysm raise the possibility of renovascular disease, whereas the presence of palpably enlarged kidneys might suggest ADPKD.

LABORATORY AND IMAGING EVALUATION

Laboratory studies and imaging procedures play an important role in the evaluation of patients with chronic renal disease. An overall scheme to the workup of renal insufficiency is given in Fig. 78.2. The goal of these studies is to identify in a minimally invasive manner the etiology of the patient's renal disease. In this attempt, special emphasis is given to treatable and potentially reversible forms of chronic renal disease. Once renal disease is identified, the first task of the clinician is to determine its duration. This information can best be obtained from the patient's medical history and previous laboratory studies revealing azotemia or urinary abnormalities. Imaging studies also play an important role in assessing the chronicity of renal disease.

The initial laboratory diagnosis of chronic renal disease is made by the elevation in serum creatinine and blood urea nitrogen, indicating a decrease in glomerular filtration rate, or the presence of urinary abnormalities such as hematuria, proteinuria, or pyuria. The measurement of glomerular filtration rate is an important step in assessing the severity of chronic renal disease. In the clinical setting, glomerular filtration rate is usually estimated by the clearance of creatinine calculated from the 24-hour urinary excretion of creatinine and the serum creatinine, according to the formula in Fig. 78.3A. The utility of creatinine as a filtration marker can be improved by the administration of cimetidine during the period of urine collection and blood sampling. Cimetidine blocks the tubular secretion of creatinine, thereby causing its clearance to be due almost completely to glomerular filtration. Radioisotopic methods for measuring glomerular filtration rate with a single injection of ^{125}I iothalamate have also been standardized. This method, however, is not available in all centers. In patients with a stable serum creatinine, the formula of Cockroft and Gault, given in Fig. 78.3B, can be used to estimate creatinine clearance.

Careful examination of the urine sediment by dipstick and microscopy also plays a major role in the initial evaluation of chronic renal disease. The presence of proteinuria, hematuria, pyuria, or cellular casts can significantly narrow the diagnosis of chronic renal disease. The presence of proteinuria should be assessed both by dipstick, which measures albuminuria, and sulfosalicylic acid, which identifies any form of urinary protein. Classification of renal disease based on urinary findings is given in Table 78.3.

Serum Chemistries and Serologic Evaluation

Depending on the type and severity of chronic renal disease present, abnormalities in a variety of serum chemistries may be present. With mild to moderate renal insufficiency (serum creatinine < 2.5 mg/dL), serum electrolytes and other chemistries may remain normal. With advanced renal insufficiency, abnormalities most commonly encountered include hyperkalemia, metabolic acidosis, anemia, and secondary hyperparathyroidism with hypocalcemia, hyperphosphatemia, and an elevated alkaline phosphatase. Diabetics in particular are prone to

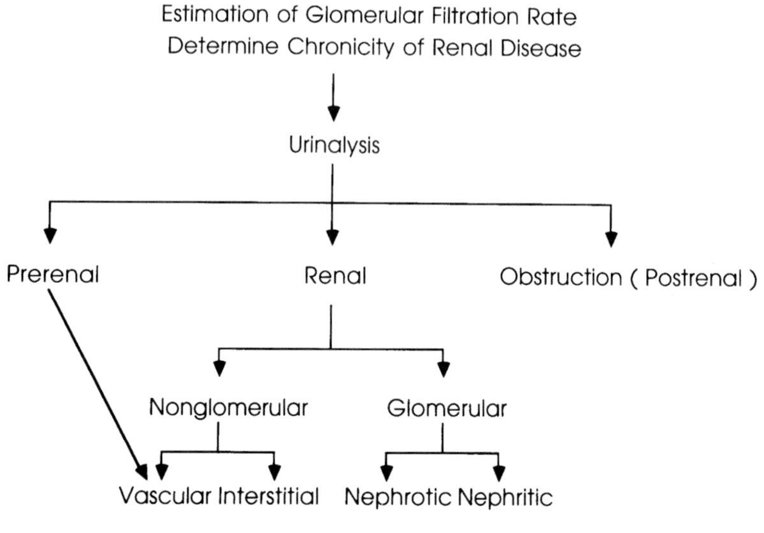

FIG. 78.2. Systematic approach to diagnosing the etiology of chronic renal disease. (From Rose BD. *Pathophysiology of renal disease,* 2nd ed. New York: McGraw-Hill, 1987, with permission.)

A

$$C_{Cr}\ (\text{ml/min}) = \frac{U_{Cr}\ (\text{mg/ml}) \times U_{Volume}\ (\text{ml/1440 min})}{P_{Cr}\ (\text{mg/ml})}$$

B

$$C_{Cr}\ (\text{ml/min}) = \frac{[140 - \text{age (years)}] \times \text{weight (kg)}}{P_{Cr}\ (\text{mg/dl}) \times 72} \times 0.85\ (\text{for women})$$

FIG. 78.3. A: Formula for determination of creatinine clearance from plasma creatinine and 24-hour urinary excretion of creatinine. **B:** Cockroft and Gault's formula for estimation of creatinine clearance.

hyperkalemia because of relative insulin deficiency and the presence in some of type IV renal tubular acidosis. Hypoalbuminemia and hypogammaglobulinemia may be present in heavily nephrotic patients. Serologic studies also play an important role in the evaluation of glomerular disease. The use of these studies should be tailored to the diagnostic possibility suggested by the patient's clinical presentation and urinary findings. Table 78.4 correlates laboratory findings with diagnostic possibilities.

TABLE 78.4. Laboratory Diagnosis of Renal Disease

Serologic finding	Diagnostic possibilities
Hypocomplementemia	SLE, MPGN (C3 nephritic factor), postinfectious glomerulonephritis, cryoglobulinemia
Antinuclear antibodies	SLE
Elevated anti-streptococcal antibodies	Poststreptococcal glomerulonephritis
Elevated IgA level (IgA-fibronectin aggregates)	IgA nephropathy
Hepatitis B surface antigen	MGN, MPGN, systemic vasculitis
Hepatitis C antibody	MPGN
HIV antibody	HIV-associated nephropathy
Cryoglobulinemia	MPGN
ANCA	ANCA-associated glomerulonephritis
Anti-GBM antibodies	Goodpasture syndrome, anti-GBM glomerulonephritis
Monoclonal paraproteinemia	Multiple myeloma, amyloidosis

ANCA, antineutrophil cytoplasmic antibodies; anti-GBM, antiglomerular basement antibodies; MGN, membraneous glomerulonephritis; MPGN, membrane proliferative glomerulonephritis; SLE, systemic lupus erythematosus.

Imaging Studies

A variety of imaging techniques that assess both renal structure and function is available. These greatly assist in diagnosing chronic renal disease and identifying its etiology. The most commonly used imaging studies are discussed, with a review of each procedure's utility, in the following sections. General goals in imaging evaluation of patients with renal disease are to use as noninvasive a test as possible, to avoid intravenous contrast where possible, and to avoid radiation exposure in pregnancy and to the gonads in younger patients.

PLAIN ABDOMINAL X-RAY

Plain abdominal x-ray provides limited information but can be helpful in identifying nephrocalcinosis and urolithiasis. Occasionally, it gives a gross estimate of renal size. Tomography improves the sensitivity of this study.

INTRAVENOUS PYELOGRAPHY

Intravenous pyelography provides a great deal of information about both urinary tract structure and function. It visualizes the entire urinary tract and also provides qualitative information regarding renal function. It was the initial study of choice in patients with suspected urolithiasis, renal trauma, or urinary tract tumors. In patients with advanced renal disease, however, renal concentration and contrast clearance may be significantly delayed, thereby preventing adequate visualization of the urinary tract. Rapid sequence or hypertensive intravenous pyelograms are relatively insensitive screening tests for renovascular disease.

TABLE 78.3. Classification of Renal Disease Based on Urinary Findings

Urinary finding	Etiology
Heavy proteinuria (>3.5 g/d), lipiduria	Nephrotic syndrome
Hematuria, red blood cell casts, proteinuria	Nephritic syndrome
Pyuria, low-grade proteinuria (<1.5 g/d), granular or waxy casts	Tubulointerstitial disease, obstruction
Normal or near normal: low-grade proteinuria, hyaline casts	Prerenal disease, renovascular disease, obstruction

Source: Rose BD. *Pathophysiology of renal disease,* 2nd ed. New York: McGraw-Hill, 1987, with permission.

ULTRASONOGRAPHY

Renal ultrasonography has numerous advantages. It provides good visualization of renal parenchyma, is noninvasive, requires no preparation, and does not use intravenous contrast. It is particularly useful during pregnancy, when avoiding radiation exposure is obviously of major concern. Ultrasonography, however, has the disadvantage of not providing information about renal function, and the quality of images can be affected by the skill of the operator and patient factors such as cooperation or obesity. This procedure is particularly helpful in evaluating suspected urinary tract obstruction, renal cysts, renal tumors, and stones. It also plays an important role in assessing the chronicity of renal disease. Indices of chronicity by ultrasound examination include small kidney size (<9 cm in an adult), cortical thinning, and increased parenchymal echogenicity. The safety and reliability of percutaneous renal biopsy has been improved when performed under ultrasound guidance.

Doppler renal flow study of the renal arteries is an important addition to renal ultrasound examinations. In skilled hands, the sensitivity of this technique in detecting renal artery stenosis has been reported to be 90% or greater. This technique has also been used to study renal venous flow when renal vein thrombosis is suspected clinically. As with routine ultrasonography, patient obesity can significantly impair the quality of this study.

RETROGRADE URETEROPYELOGRAPHY

Retrograde ureteropyelography is an invasive cystoscopic procedure performed by the urologist. It is the definitive study in ruling out urinary tract obstruction. When there is a strong clinical suspicion of obstruction and other imaging studies fail to demonstrate any obstruction, retrograde pyelography may be necessary. Other indications include better evaluation of urinary tract tumors, particularly ureteral tumors, urinary tract bleeding with a normal intravenous pyelogram, and ureteral strictures. This technique can also be used in patients who require visualization of the entire urinary tract but are allergic to intravenous contrast.

COMPUTED TOMOGRAPHY

Computed tomography is increasingly used for evaluating renal structure and function. Its main advantages are its high resolution and detailed cross-sectional views of the kidney. Its primary utility is in the evaluation of urolithiasis, renal trauma, renal tumors and cysts, but it is also helpful in identifying urinary tract obstruction and abscess formation. It is sensitive and specific for urolithiasis and important for the classification of renal trauma and its management. Use of intravenous contrast is frequently necessary to fully evaluate the possibility of renal cell carcinoma. Intravenous contrast also provides a qualitative assessment of renal function and can diagnose vascular disorders such as segmental renal infarction. Computed tomography guidance is also used in fine-needle aspiration of renal masses for diagnostic purposes.

MAGNETIC RESONANCE IMAGING

Magnetic resonance imaging is used primarily to further evaluate renal neoplasms or in patients who are allergic to radiocontrast material. Magnetic resonance angiography is an evolving technique that shows significant promise in evaluating renal artery stenosis.

ANGIOGRAPHY

Visualization of the renal arterial system is best achieved by an arterial approach using digital subtraction techniques. This procedure uses smaller catheters and a smaller quantity of contrast media than conventional arteriography and therefore reduces complications. Images produced by digital subtraction after the intravenous bolus administration of radiocontrast are frequently of inadequate quality. Indications for renal angiography include suspected renal artery stenosis, renal vasculitis, and, less commonly, evaluation of a renal mass. Complications of angiography include hematoma at the arterial puncture site, cholesterol embolization, contrast nephropathy, and radiocontrast allergy. Angiography has been utilized for therapeutic embolization for bleeding resulting from trauma and tumors in the urinary tract.

NUCLEAR RENOGRAPHY

A variety of radiopharmaceuticals that allow assessment of renal function is available. Because of poor imaging resolution, these are usually poor studies of renal anatomy, however. [^{99}TC] DTPA (diethylenetriamine pentaacetic acid) is most commonly used as a measure of glomerular filtration, whereas [^{131}I] iodohippuran is used to estimate renal perfusion. The principal utility of these studies is to measure right versus left kidney function to evaluate suspected renovascular disease. ^{99}m MAG3 [mercapto acetyl triglycine is excreted by tubular secretion and some glomerular filtration and is used for evaluation of renal transplants. There is good renal delineation in the presence of renal failure. ^{99}m DMSA [di mercapto succinic acid] is a cortical agent with scant renal excretion and can assess cortical damage from pyelonephritis or VUR. The sensitivity of the nuclear renogram in detecting unilateral renal artery stenosis can be improved to approximately 85% if it is performed after administration of captopril. Gallium 67 citrate or indium 111–labeled leukocytes may be helpful in the evaluation of renal inflammatory disorders, such as perinephric abscess and acute interstitial nephritis.

VOIDING CYSTOURETHROGRAM

Voiding cystourethrogram involves urethral or suprapubic catheterization of the bladder and instillation of radiocontrast material. Images are then taken during voiding to determine the presence and severity of VUR. In some centers, a voiding cystourethrogram can be performed using radioisotopes, thereby minimizing gonadal radiation exposure.

Approach to Urinary Abnormalities

PROTEINURIA

Once proteinuria is identified, the clinician must determine the quantity of proteinuria present and the type of protein excreted. Most commonly, the quantity of proteinuria is determined by the amount of protein present in a 24-hour urine collection. This procedure allows separation of those patients with significant proteinuria from glomerular disease from those with benign or transient proteinuria due to exercise, postural change, or fever. In an adult, protein excretion exceeding 150 mg/d is considered abnormal. An alternative method of quantitating protein excretion is to use the urinary protein-to-creatinine ratio. The ratio of protein concentration in mg/dL divided by the urinary creatinine concentration in mg/dL closely approximates the 24-hour protein excretion in grams. This method can be particularly useful in children and elderly patients for whom 24-hour collections are impractical. Protein excretion in excess of 1 g/d strongly suggests glomerular disease and in excess of 3.5 g/d indicates that the nephrotic syndrome is present. Benign orthostatic proteinuria can be assessed by performing two separate urine collections—one covering 16 hours during normal daytime activities and the second after 8-hour overnight recumbency. Total 24-hour excretion in this condition is less than 150 mg/d.

The initial step in determining the type of protein excreted is examination of the urine with sulfosalicylic acid. The presence of a positive reaction to sulfosalicylic acid with a negative dipstick suggests the presence of nonalbumin proteins. This is most commonly seen in multiple myeloma and is the result of excretion of large quantities of immunoglobulin light chains. To definitively identify the type of protein excreted, urine immunoelectrophoresis identifies any monoclonal protein present.

HEMATURIA

The discovery of hematuria on urinalysis is relatively common. The initial step in its evaluation is to search for other urinary findings suggestive of glomerular disease such as proteinuria or casts. Hematuria in the setting of proteinuria and red blood cell casts constitutes a nephritic urine sediment and is seen in a variety of glomerulonephritides. Urinary tract infection is also an important initial consideration and should be assessed by examination of the urine for pyuria and bacteriuria, along with a urine culture. If there is no evidence for glomerular disease in the urine sediment, the hematuria is most likely of urologic origin; overall, hematuria is most commonly of urologic origin. The list of diagnostic possibilities is sizable and includes carcinoma of the bladder, ureters, or kidney; urolithiasis; prostatitis; cystic renal disease; trauma; vascular malformations; and interstitial cystitis. Benign hematuria of glomerular origin is also a possibility and is seen after strenuous exercise and in thin basement membrane disease. Evaluation of persistent hematuria in the absence of evidence for glomerular disease should include intravenous pyelography and referral to a urologist for cystoscopy.

TREATMENT

Numerous advances have been made in our ability to treat chronic renal disease and its complications, thereby greatly improving the quality of life of these patients. As discussed in the following sections, treatment of these patients addresses the following issues: (a) treatment of the primary renal disease, (b) treatment aimed at slowing the progression of chronic renal disease, (c) treatment of extrarenal complications of chronic renal disease, and (d) renal replacement therapy in patients with ESRD.

Progression of Chronic Renal Disease

In many patients with established chronic renal disease, renal function slowly and inexorably declines to ESRD. This can occur regardless of the initial renal disease and even if the initial disease has become quiescent. The pathophysiologic mechanisms responsible for this progressive loss of renal function are summarized in Fig. 78.4. With reduced renal functional mass, the remaining nephrons undergo a variety of hemodynamic and metabolic adaptations. Although these adaptations serve the purpose of maintaining glomerular filtration in the short term, they may prove maladaptive in the long term by promoting further renal injury. Glomerular adaptations include increased plasma flow and filtration rates per remaining nephron with resultant glomerular hypertension. Altered permeability of the glomerular basement membrane leads to increased traffic of plasma proteins into the mesangium and activation of immune cells. Compensatory hypertrophy of nephrons is also associated with progressive renal injury. Tubular adaptations include accelerated rates of amniogenesis per nephron, increased production of reactive oxygen species, and interstitial deposition of calcium phosphate resulting from hyperphosphatemia. All these factors promote progressive glomerulosclerosis and tubulointerstitial fibrosis, thereby perpetuating a cycle of progressive injury.

Although no treatments exist that arrest progression of chronic renal disease, it is possible to slow it. This is best achieved with rigid control of hypertension and, to a lesser extent, with dietary protein restriction. Treatment of hypertension with angiotensin-converting enzyme inhibitors may offer additional benefit in slowing progression over conventional antihypertensive medications. This appears to be particularly true in diabetic patients and may be related to the ability of these agents to more effectively lower glomerular pressures. The efficacy of dietary protein restriction in slowing progression is more controversial. A recent large multicenter study, the Modification of Diet in Renal Disease Trial, did not show significant benefit of a low protein (0.58 g protein/kg body weight/day) in patients with an initial glomerular filtration rate below 25 mL/min. Use of very low protein diets (0.28 g/kg body weight/day) with ketoacid supplements also failed to demonstrate any clear-cut benefit. Smaller earlier studies, however, did seem to demonstrate some benefit from very low protein diets and ketoacid supplementation. This remains a controversial area among nephrologists, and definitive recommendations are therefore difficult to make.

Treatment of Initial Renal Disease

DIABETIC NEPHROPATHY

In addition to slowing progression of disease as noted earlier, several other interventions are worth considering in diabetics. Most studies of the treatment of diabetic nephropathy deal with IDDM, with less known about NIDDM. It is increasingly clear that strict metabolic control may at least delay the development of complications such as microalbuminuria, nephropathy, and retinopathy. Preliminary evidence indicates that pancreas transplantation also may delay the onset of nephropathy. Use of angiotensin-converting enzyme inhibitors has also been found to be beneficial even in normotensive diabetics with proteinuria. Diabetics with renal insufficiency who are treated with angiotensin-converting enzyme inhibitors must be followed closely for the development of hyperkalemia. This can frequently be prevented by concomitant use of a loop diuretic. Other diabetic complications that may impair renal function are the development of renovascular disease and functional urinary tract obstruction resulting from autonomic neuropathy involving the bladder.

GLOMERULONEPHRITIS

The decision of whether to treat primary or secondary glomerulonephritides is frequently complicated and in most cases merits referral to a nephrologist. Potential toxicities of immunosuppressive therapy coupled with the marginal response to therapy of many of these disorders warrant referral in most cases.

HYPERTENSIVE NEPHROSCLEROSIS

Little can be done for hypertensive nephrosclerosis other than control of hypertension and possibly dietary protein restriction. The possibility of underlying renovascular or glomerular disease should be excluded.

RENOVASCULAR DISEASE

Once a hemodynamically significant lesion has been identified angiographically, revascularization can be achieved by either balloon angioplasty or surgical bypass. Balloon angioplasty is most effective in the fibromuscular lesions and in non-ostial atherosclerotic lesions. Roughly one third of patients who respond to angioplasty will eventually restenose. Angioplasty is ineffective and carries a risk of atheroembolic complications when it is attempted for ostial lesions in patients with significant aortic atherosclerotic plaque. Deployment of vascular stents to maintain patency of a stenotic renal artery is a procedure increasingly used in many centers. The most commonly used surgical techniques are hepatorenal, splenorenal, or aortorenal bypass procedures.

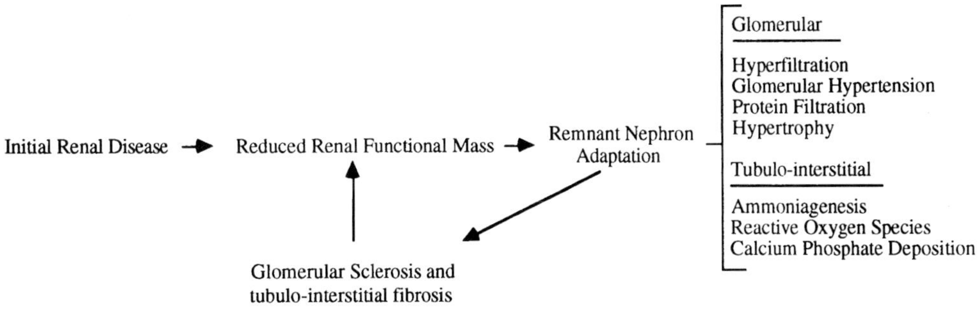

FIG. 78.4. Proposed pathophysiologic mechanisms responsible for progression of chronic renal failure.

AUTOSOMAL-DOMINANT POLYCYSTIC KIDNEY DISEASE

Treatment of ADPKD is geared toward slowing progressive renal insufficiency by blood pressure control and dietary protein restriction.

VESICOURETERAL REFLUX

Uncertainty exists among nephrologists, urologists, and pediatricians regarding the appropriate management of VUR. Infants and children should be screened for VUR with their first urinary tract infection. Preadolescent siblings of affected children also should be screened because up to 50% of them will have abnormalities on a voiding cystourethrogram. Bacteriuria should be treated aggressively with antibiotics, and some patients may require long-term suppressive therapy. A point of controversy in managing this problem is the appropriate role of antireflux surgery. It does not benefit patients with established renal insufficiency, hypertension, or persistent proteinuria. If surgery is to be effective, therefore, it must be instituted early. The issue is complicated by the fact that VUR resolves in many children as their urinary tracts mature. Referral for a urologic opinion is appropriate.

Extrarenal Complications of Chronic Renal Disease and End-Stage Renal Disease

Chronic renal disease and ESRD produce numerous derangements in the function of many other organ systems. The more prominent complications and their treatment are reviewed in the following paragraphs.

FLUID AND ELECTROLYTE DISTURBANCES

Volume overload caused by impaired salt and water excretion is best treated with loop diuretics, frequently in high dosages. Addition of metolazone significantly augments the diuretic response to a loop diuretic. Dietary sodium restriction also plays an important role in controlling volume overload in these patients. Hyperkalemia can also be managed with loop diuretics. Administration of sodium bicarbonate (2–4 g/d) also assists in the management of hyperkalemia by treating metabolic acidosis, which is frequently present, and also helps to prevent diuretic-induced volume depletion. Metabolic acidosis may alternatively be treated with sodium citrate solution (Bicitra) 10 to 30 mL four times daily.

HEMATOLOGIC ABNORMALITIES

Progressive anemia due to diminished renal production of erythropoietin is an almost universal finding in patients with advanced renal disease. Anemia frequently accompanies chronic renal insufficiency (<11 g/dL in dialysis patients, <12 g/dL in undialyzed patients). It can complicate the clinical picture by producing left ventricular hypertrophy and congestive heart failure. Correction of anemia by transfusions leads to associated complications such as iron overload, blood-borne infections, and development of cytotoxic antibodies that could preclude kidney transplantation. Correction of anemia, however, leads to regression of left ventricular hypertrophy. The introduction of recombinant human erythropoietin in 1988 has provided effective management of anemia in chronic renal insufficiency. Iron deficiency is the most common cause of poor response to recombinant human erythropoietin. Other causes of anemia include deficiency of vitamin B_{12}, folate, ascorbic acid, and nutritional causes. In predialysis patients, erythropoietin administration is usually started once the hematocrit is below 30 and the serum creatinine is greater than 3.0 mg/dL. Initial dosing is approximately 50 U/kg subcutaneously twice per week. Once the patient is on dialysis, it can be given intravenously with each dialysis treatment.

Coagulopathy due to abnormal platelet function is a frequent finding in advanced ESRD. This is best treated emergently with desmopressin acetate (0.3 μg/kg by slow intravenous infusion) or administration of a cryoprecipitate. More effective dialysis and conjugated estrogens have also been shown to improve platelet function in this setting.

RENAL OSTEODYSTROPHY

A variety of metabolic bone disorders is associated with chronic renal disease, including (a) secondary hyperparathyroidism and osteitis fibrosa, (b) aluminum-induced osteomalacia, (c) adynamic bone disease, and (d) dialysis-related amyloidosis. Secondary hyperparathyroidism results from diminished renal production of 1,25-dihydroxyvitamin D_3 coupled with phosphate retention. This is best treated by lowering the serum phosphorus with a phosphate-restricted diet and orally administered phosphate binders. Calcium-containing phosphate binders such as calcium carbonate and calcium acetate are most effective and should be administered with meals. Administration of exogenous calcitriol also plays an important role in treating secondary hyperparathyroidism by elevating serum calcium and suppressing parathyroid hormone secretion. Patients treated with calcitriol must be followed closely for the development of hypercalcemia. Dialysis patients with severe secondary hyperparathyroidism refractory to medical therapy may require parathyroidectomy.

Aluminum bone disease results from aluminum ingestion, usually in the form of aluminum-containing phosphate binders. If present, this can be treated by chelation with deferoxamine.

Adynamic bone disease is a poorly understood form of osteomalacia seen in dialysis patients. It may be the result of aluminum intoxication or of long-standing suppression of parathyroid hormone secretion by calcitriol administration.

Bone disease resulting from dialysis-related amyloid is due to bone deposition of β_2-microglobulin. β_2-Microglobulin is a low-molecular-weight protein that is poorly cleared by dialysis and therefore accumulates to high levels in these patients. Carpal tunnel syndrome is a common complication of this disorder.

ENDOCRINE ABNORMALITIES

Approximately 50% of premenopausal women with ESRD are amenorrheic, and an even greater percentage are anovulatory. Infertility, therefore, is a common problem among premenopausal women maintained on dialysis. This appears to be the result of a combination of factors, including hyperprolactinemia and impaired positive feedback of estrogens on pituitary gonadotropin release. Prolactin levels are rarely in excess of 100 ng/mL, and elevations of greater magnitude should prompt evaluation for pituitary adenoma.

Other endocrinopathies encountered with ESRD include insulin resistance, which may be the result of secondary hyperparathyroidism. Total serum levels of thyroxine and triiodothyronine may be low in ESRD due to displacement from protein binding sites. Free levels of triiodothyronine and thyroxine are normal. An elevation in serum thyroid-stimulating hormone is a reliable indication of hypothyroidism in these patients.

CARDIOVASCULAR DISEASES

Cardiovascular diseases contribute importantly to the morbidity and mortality of chronic renal insufficiency. Complications include left ventricular hypertrophy, ischemic heart disease, and peripheral vascular diseases. Exacerbating factors are hypertension, anemia, hyperparathyroidism, and dyslipidemias. Management of these factors can effectively reduce the burden of cardiovascular illnesses in the renal population through appropriate medical intervention.

CUTANEOUS MANIFESTATIONS

Nonspecific skin changes like pallor due to anemia and yellowish cast are due to urochrome and carotenoid deposition. Elastosis manifests as yellowish plaques in the sun-exposed areas. Lindsay's nails in which the proximal half of the nail is white and the distal half brown are seen in chronic renal insufficiency.

Specific skin changes include pruritus (58%–90%), perforating disorders, calcifying disorders, and bullous dermatoses. Calciphylaxis is a life-threatening manifestation due to progressive necrosis secondary to small vessel calcification, with a mortality of 60% to 80%. Porphyria cutanea tarda (bullous manifestation) is characterized by tense vesicles and bullae distributed on the dorsum hands, face, and occasionally feet.

Treatment Options and Renal Replacement Therapy

Patients with advanced renal insufficiency should be referred to a nephrologist for renal replacement therapy well in advance of their developing uremic symptoms. This allows adequate time for patient counseling, decision making, and planning for the modality of renal replacement therapy best suited for each patient. Twelve billion dollars are incurred annually as medicare expense for management of chronic renal insufficiency. In general, younger more active patients who wish to take a more active role in their own care do better with peritoneal dialysis or renal transplantation. Chronic hemodialysis is attractive to some patients because it requires less active participation on their part. One key disadvantage is the need to maintain long-term vascular access.

The most common treatment of ERSD is hemodialysis (60%), followed by kidney transplantation (30%) and peritoneal dialysis (10%). Kidney transplantation offers a longer life, improved quality of life, and lower health care costs. The limitation is the scarcity of donors.

On average, hemodialysis patients face two hospital admissions each year and a 23% mortality. Thirty-five percent of peritoneal dialysis patients switch to hemodialysis in the first 2 years.

Malnourishment, cardiovascular disorders, vascular access complications (infection, thrombosis), and peritoneal dialysis complications (peritonitis, exit site infection) are some of the common problems faced by patients with chronic renal insufficiency.

CONSIDERATIONS IN PREGNANCY

Physiologic Changes with Pregnancy

Renal function undergoes dramatic changes during normal pregnancy. These include an increase of approximately 30% to 40% increase in plasma volume with roughly 50% increases in renal plasma flow and glomerular filtration rate. As a result of this increased glomerular filtration rate, serum creatinine falls to an average value of 0.7 mg/dL and blood urea nitrogen to 9 mg/dL. Blood pressure also normally falls early in pregnancy and during the second trimester averages 105/60 mm Hg. Kidney size increases by 1 to 1.5 cm due to hyperperfusion. Under the influence of very high plasma levels of progesterone, ureters and renal calices dilate, producing the so-called hydronephrosis of pregnancy. Although this does not result in urinary tract obstruction, sluggish urine flow through the dilated collecting system may promote the development of bacteriuria. Electrolyte changes during pregnancy include a mild respiratory alkalosis due to the effect of progesterone and a reduction in plasma sodium concentration by approximately 5 mEq/L due to resetting of the hypothalamic osmostat.

Identifying renal disease in pregnancy must take into account the above physiologic changes. For example, a blood pressure of 140/90 might be considered normal in many adults but is clearly an elevated value in the pregnant patient. Serum creatinine and blood urea nitrogen values must also be judged against what should normally be found during pregnancy.

Chronic Renal Disease in Pregnancy

Pregnancy in women with chronic renal disease poses a difficult management problem, most appropriately referred to centers specializing in high-risk obstetric care. The two basic problems encountered are the role of chronic renal disease in affecting maternal and fetal outcome and the role of pregnancy in accelerating underlying chronic renal disease. Maternal morbidity is primarily affected by the increased risk of preeclampsia in women with underlying chronic renal disease, hypertension, or both. Fetal outcome is also adversely affected, with increased risks of preterm delivery and intrauterine growth retardation seen even with mild chronic renal disease (serum creatinine $<$ 1.4 mg/dL). Overall, fetal survival in these patients is approximately 95%. In women with more advanced renal disease, the clinical course of pregnancy is frequently complicated, with fetal survival as low as 50% to 75%. Pregnancy in women with ESRD on dialysis is rare, occurring in approximately 1% of all female dialysis patients of childbearing age. Management of these patients is complicated by worsening hypertension and anemia, and children are usually born prematurely and small for gestational age. The overall success rate of pregnancies in dialysis patients averages 50%.

The effect of pregnancy on the course of underlying chronic renal disease remains somewhat controversial. In patients with only mild renal insufficiency (serum creatinine < 1.4 mg/dL), there may be a transient increase in serum creatinine and worsening hypertension during pregnancy. After delivery, however, renal function generally returns to baseline levels. In those with proteinuric renal disease, the quantity of urine protein excretion commonly increases over the course of pregnancy. In patients with more advanced renal disease (serum creatinine > 1.4 mg/dL) the course is less clear. There may be an acceleration in the progressive loss of renal function induced by pregnancy in these patients. Inadequate control of hypertension may play an important role in the acceleration of renal disease in these patients. Protein-restricted diets should be avoided in pregnancy. Particular problems are presented by pregnant patients with underlying renal insufficiency due to IDDM and SLE. Difficulty with metabolic control in the diabetic and flares of lupus activity in the patient with lupus can significantly complicate the course of these pregnancies.

After successful renal transplantation, fertility is restored. Pregnancy in these patients may be complicated by accelerated hypertension, worsening renal disease, or graft rejection. In pregnancies that survive past the first trimester, the overall pregnancy success rate is 92%. Azathioprine and cyclosporine are generally well tolerated but may be associated with growth retardation.

A particularly difficult problem in managing pregnant patients with renal disease is accurately diagnosing preeclampsia in the setting of underlying renal disease. Many clinical and biochemical markers of preeclampsia, such as hypertension, proteinuria, renal insufficiency, and hyperuricemia, can all be seen with chronic renal disease alone. These patients therefore merit very close monitoring. The development of hyperreflexia strongly suggests preeclampsia, because this is only seen in chronic renal disease when the uremic syndrome is present. Other biochemical features of preeclampsia, such as elevation in liver enzymes, coagulopathy, thrombocytopenia, or microangiopathy, are relatively late signs.

Management

Prompt recognition and treatment of hypertension plays a vital role in the management of these patients. Blood pressure values higher than 140/85 mm Hg are clearly abnormal, and adverse fetal outcomes are associated with blood pressures above 125/75 mm Hg. Conservative management of hypertension consists of bed rest and avoidance of tobacco and alcohol. Dietary salt restriction should be avoided. In patients who are hypercoagulable from the nephrotic syndrome, prolonged bed rest increases their risk of venous thromboembolism. A variety of antihypertensive agents has proven effective and safe in managing hypertension in pregnancy when pharmacologic therapy is necessary. First-line agents include α-methyldopa, hydralazine, or beta-blockers. Experience with calcium channel blockers is limited. α-Methyldopa, which remains the first-line drug of choice, may be started at 250 mg three to four times daily and increased to a maximum daily dose of 2 g. In hypertensive emergencies, intravenous labetalol is the drug of choice. Antihypertensive agents to be avoided include all angiotensin-converting enzyme inhibitors, reserpine, sodium nitroprusside, ganglion blocking agents, and clonidine. Judicious use of diuretics may be necessary in the volume-expanded hypertensive patient with chronic renal disease. In patients with renal insufficiency, magnesium sulfate must be used cautiously in the treatment of preeclampsia. Impaired renal excretion of magnesium can lead to dangerous hypermagnesemia and respiratory muscle paralysis in these patients. Alternative antiseizure medications such as benzodiazepines should be considered in this situation.

Both peritoneal dialysis and hemodialysis have been used successfully in pregnant patients with ESRD. A special attempt should be made to provide efficient dialysis, keeping the blood urea nitrogen below 50 mg/dL. In those patients who progress to ESRD while pregnant, dialysis is generally initiated earlier than for the nonpregnant patient in an attempt to avoid any complications of the uremic syndrome.

BIBLIOGRAPHY

Bostom LR, Digiovanna JJ. Cutaneous manifestation of end-stage renal disease. *J Am Acad Dermatol* 2000;43:6.

Daugirdas JT, Ing TS. *Handbook of dialysis,* 2nd ed. Boston: Little, Brown, 1994.

Davison JM. Dialysis, transplantation, and pregnancy. *Am J Kidney Dis* 1992;17:127.

Gabow PA. Polycystic kidney disease: clues to pathogenesis. *Kidney Int* 1991;40:989.

Greenberg A, Cheung AK, Coffman TM, et al. *Primer on kidney diseases.* San Diego: Academic Press, 1994.

Hayslett JP. Maternal and fetal complications in pregnant women with systemic lupus erythematosus. *Am J Kidney Dis* 1991;17:123.

Henderson LW. Future developments in the treatment of ESRD: a North American perspective. *Am J Kidney Dis* 2000;35:4.

Jungers P, Houillier P, Forget D, et al. Specific controversies concerning the natural history of renal disease in pregnancy. *Am J Kidney Dis* 1991;17:116.

Kaplan NM. *Clinical hypertension,* 5th ed. Baltimore: Williams & Wilkins, 1990.

Kasiske BL, Kalil RSN, Ma JZ, et al. Effect of antihypertensive therapy on the kidney in patients with diabetes: a meta-regression analysis. *Ann Intern Med* 1993;118:129.

Kauz AT, et al. Anemia management in patients with chronic renal insufficiency. *Am J Kidney Dis* 2000;36:6.

Klahr S, Schreiner G, Ichikawa I. The progression of renal disease. *N Engl J Med* 1988;318:1657.

Knochel JP, Breyer JA, Cronin RE, et al. *Medical knowledge self-assessment program in the subspecialty of nephrology and hypertension.* Philadelphia: American College of Physicians, 1994.

Levin A. Cardiovascular disease in chronic renal failure. *Am J Kidney Dis* 2000;36[6 Suppl]:S24–S30.

Lindberg J. Research directions: new clinical frontiers. *Am J Kidney Dis* 2000;36[6 Suppl 3]:S52–S61.

Reece EA, Coustan DR, Hayslett JP, et al. Diabetic nephropathy: pregnancy performance and fetomaternal outcome. *Am J Obstet Gynecol* 1988;159:56.

Reilly RF, Tray K, Perazella MA. Indinavir nephropathy revisited: a pattern of insidious renal failure with identifiable risk factors. *Am J Kidney Dis* 2001;38:4.

Rose BD. *Pathophysiology of renal disease,* 2nd ed. New York: McGraw-Hill, 1987.

Schrier RW, Gottschalk CW. *Diseases of the kidney,* 5th ed. Vol. 1. Boston: Little, Brown, 1993.

Sehgal AR. What is the best treatment for end stage renal disease? *Am J Med* 2002;112:9.

Renal Data System. USRDS 1994 annual data report. Publication PB 95105003. Bethesda, MD: The National Institutes of Health, National Institute of Diabetes and Digestive and Kidney Diseases, July 1994.

Woodward JR, Rushton HG. Reflux nephropathy. *Pediatr Clin North Am* 1987;34:1349.

CHAPTER 79
Acute Renal Failure

Douglas Shemin

ETIOLOGY

Although renal function includes a wide variety of different components, including excretion of water-soluble solutes, prevention of urinary protein excretion, and regulation of total body water, sodium, acid-base, and potassium balance, renal failure is conventionally more narrowly defined as a decrease in glomerular filtration of solutes or as a decline in the glomerular filtration rate (GFR). Acute renal failure is defined as a sudden potentially reversible decrease in the GFR. It occurs relatively uncommonly in the general population—in population studies the incidence is less than 0.1% per year. However, it becomes more common in older individuals and in those with greater comorbidity: It is present in 1% of patients admitted to a general hospital, but because it frequently accompanies the progression of illness or its treatment, it may occur in over 5% of patients during their hospital course. Acute renal failure is even more common in critically ill patients and may develop in over 15% of patients in a medical intensive care unit or in a patients after cardiopulmonary bypass operation. No matter what the setting or the cause, a decrease in the GFR causes a decrease in filtration and renal excretion of nitrogenous waste products, sodium, water, hydrogen ion, phosphorus, and potassium, and acute renal failure therefore can potentially lead to serious systemic fluid and electrolyte disorders, including azotemia, volume overload, hyponatremia, metabolic acidosis, hyperphosphatemia, and hyperkalemia. These abnormalities in turn, if severe enough, may lead to dysfunction of many different organ systems and result in significant morbidity. When acute renal failure is severe enough to require the most aggressive therapy, renal replacement, the mortality rate can rise to above 30% in affected patients.

The development of acute renal failure is typically brought to the physician's attention by an increase in the serum levels of blood urea nitrogen (BUN) or creatinine concentration; both BUN and creatinine are small-molecular-weight water-soluble substances that are constantly produced and then filtered by normal glomeruli. Although the levels of both substances increase in acute renal failure, a rising serum creatinine concentration, by greater than 0.5 mg/dL per day, is the more reliable indicator of declining renal function. Creatinine is derived from muscle creatine and is removed from the blood primarily by glomerular filtration; a smaller proportion is excreted into the urine by tubular secretion. Because creatinine is produced at a fairly constant rate proportional to muscle mass, acute changes in its serum level usually reflect changes in GFR, with a rise in creatinine concentration indicating a fall in GFR (Fig. 79.1). Rare exceptions may occur when the normally small amount of tubular creatinine secretion is inhibited by pharmacologic agents such as trimethoprim or cimetidine. In such cases, there may be a small increase in the serum creatinine without a fall in the GFR.

Creatinine is released from skeletal muscle at a rate of 10 to 20 mg/kg/d (700–2,000 mg/d), depending on muscle mass. In a 70-kg individual containing 40 L of body water, the creatinine should theoretically increase by between 2.0 and 3.0 mg/dL for each day of acute renal failure. In clinical practice, the rate of increase is usually lower than this, because acutely ill, malnourished, and bedridden patients have a decrease in the muscular release of creatinine, and because many patients with acute renal failure have a decrement, but not a complete cessation, in the GFR. In general, the more rapid the increase in serum creatinine, the more severe the decrease in GFR. However, it may still take some time for an elevation in the GFR to be manifested as an elevated serum creatinine. For example, if the GFR drops to zero in a malnourished individual with a small muscle mass, the serum creatinine may increase by 0.5 mg/dL/d and rise from a baseline low level of 0.2 mg/dL to a still normal value of 1.2 mg/dL over the course of 2 days of acute renal failure.

A BUN level of greater than 25 mg/dL is abnormal and usually reflects a decrease in the GFR, but it is a less reliable marker of acute renal failure than the creatinine level. BUN is the end product of nitrogen metabolism, and the blood level may be elevated in the settings of excess catabolism of protein, in acute illness, or inhibition of anabolism (e.g., as in use of glucocorticoids) and in increased gastrointestinal absorption of protein,

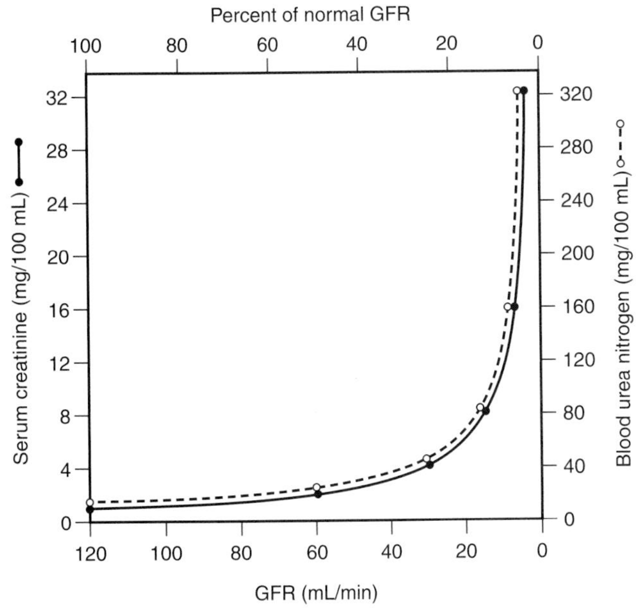

FIG. 79.1. Relationship of the serum creatinine and blood urea nitrogen to the glomerular filtration rate. (From Kassirer JP. Current concepts: clinical evaluation of kidney function/glomerular function. *N Engl J Med* 1971;285:385, with permission.)

such as in high protein diets and in gastrointestinal bleeding. Moreover, unlike creatinine, it is reabsorbed in the renal tubules; renal tubular reabsorption of urea increases in the settings of volume depletion (vomiting, diarrhea, dehydration) or effective volume depletion (left ventricular dysfunction and congestive heart failure). Elevation of the BUN can therefore occur in any of these settings in the absence of a marked decrease in the GFR.

Urine volume is not a reliable marker of renal function. Whereas oliguria (<500 mL of urine per day) does indicate that renal function is impaired, *the absence of oliguria does not mean that renal function is normal.* In fact, some estimates suggest that most cases of acute renal failure are nonoliguric, with the urine output remaining in the normal range.

DIFFERENTIAL DIAGNOSIS

There are hundreds of causes of acute renal failure. When it occurs, it is critical to identify the etiology, because prognosis and, more importantly, treatment will vary with the cause. In many cases, however, particularly in acutely ill and complicated patients with multiple organ system abnormalities receiving aggressive medical therapy, one single major cause of acute renal failure may be difficult to determine. Nevertheless, it is operationally useful to divide acute renal failure into three major etiologic categories (Table 79.1): prerenal failure, intrinsic renal failure, and postrenal failure.

Prerenal Failure

Prerenal failure is, in most large studies, the most common form of acute renal failure. It is defined as renal failure that develops as a consequence of reduced arterial perfusion to the kidneys. This may result from absolute volume depletion (hemorrhage, urinary or gastrointestinal fluid loss), effective volume depletion (congestive heart failure or pericardial tamponade), renal vasoconstriction despite systemic vasodilation (hepatic cirrhosis leading to the hepatorenal syndrome), or obstruction of the renal arteries (bilateral renal artery stenosis or dissection of the thoracic or abdominal aorta). Prerenal failure is reversible, with restoration of normal renal perfusion.

Although the hydrostatic pressure in the glomerular capillary is a critical determinant of GFR, a major reduction in renal perfusion pressure is required before the GFR falls in healthy people. This is because autoregulation maintains a relatively constant GFR and renal blood flow (RBF) over a wide range of perfusion pressures, until the mean arterial pressure falls below about 80 mm Hg; at this point RBF and GFR decline precipitously, with further decreases in blood pressure (Fig. 79.2). However, in patients with hypertensive, diabetic, or atherosclerotic vascular disease, the ability to autoregulate may be markedly impaired, predisposing such individuals to prerenal azotemia, even during small reductions in perfusion pressure.

When cardiac output is low, either because of hypovolemia or heart disease, blood pressure is maintained by high levels of systemically active vasoconstricting substances (e.g., angiotensin II and catecholamines). These vasoconstrictors also increase the resistance to blood flow in the kidney. If unopposed, this effect decreases RBF and GFR. Because renal vasoconstriction is mitigated by vasodilatory prostaglandins, the administration of nonsteroidal antiinflammatory drugs or cyclooxygenase-2 inhibitors, which block prostaglandin synthesis, can dramatically reduce RBF and GFR in patients with impaired renal perfusion.

Angiotensin-converting enzyme (ACE) inhibitors and angiotensin receptor blockers (ARBs) also can reduce the GFR

TABLE 79.1. Differential Diagnosis of Acute Renal Failure

- **Prerenal failure**
  - Absolute volume depletion
    - Hemorrhage
    - GI losses
      - Vomiting
      - Diarrhea
      - Anorexia
    - Renal losses
      - Diuretic drugs
      - Osmotic diuresis
      - Adrenal insufficiency
    - Third spacing
  - Effective volume depletion
    - Cardiac dysfunction
      - Heart failure
      - Arrhythmias
      - Valvular dysfunction
      - Pericardial tamponade
      - Pulmonary embolism
    - Peripheral vasodilatation
      - Sepsis
      - Liver failure/hepatorenal syndrome
      - Antihypertensive drugs
    - Renal vascular obstruction
      - Renal artery stenosis, thrombosis
      - Renal artery embolism
      - Dissecting aortic aneurysm
    - Impaired autoregulation
      - NSAIDs
      - ACE inhibitors
      - Angiotensin receptor blockers
- **Postrenal azotemia**
  - See Table 79.2
- **Intrinsic renal failure**
  - Glomerular Diseases
    - RPGN
    - Lupus nephritis
    - Goodpasture syndrome
    - Poststreptococcal GN
    - Endocarditis
  - Vascular disorders
    - Vasculitis
    - TTP
    - Scleroderma
    - Malignant hypertension
    - Cholesterol emboli
  - Tubular disorders
    - ATN
      - Ischemia
      - Nephrotoxins
        - Aminoglycosides
        - Radiocontrast agents
        - Heavy metals
        - Amphotericin
        - Cisplatin
        - Pentamidine
      - Intratubular obstruction
        - Myoglobinuria
        - Hemoglobinuria
        - Myeloma kidney
        - Ethylene glycol intoxication
        - Drugs: methotrexate
        - Drugs: acyclovir
        - Tumor lysis syndrome
  - Interstitial disorders
    - Hypersensitivity reactions
    - Sarcoidosis
    - Sjögren syndrome
    - Lymphomatous renal involvement

ACE, angiotensin-converting enzyme; ATN, acute tubular necrosis; GI, gastrointestinal; RPGN, rapidly progressive glomerulonephritis; TTP, thrombotic thrombocytopenic purpura.

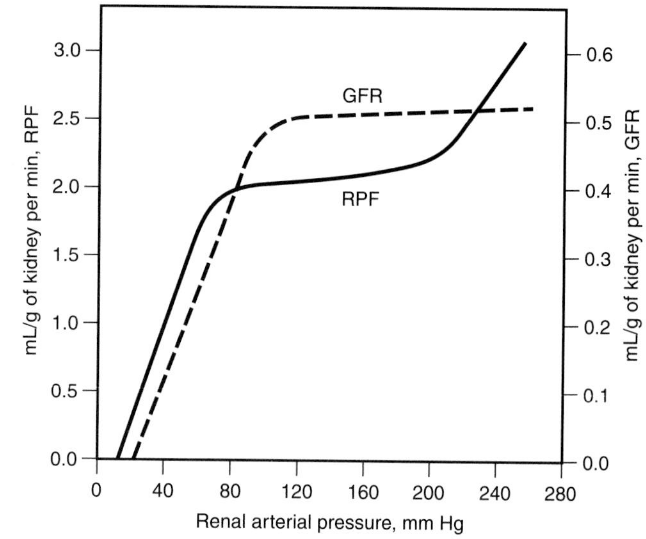

FIG. 79.2. Autoregulation of glomerular filtration rate and renal blood flow in the dog. (From Rose BD. Renal circulation and glomerular filtration rate. In: Rose BD, ed. *Clinical physiology of acid-base and electrolyte disorders.* New York: McGraw-Hill, 1984, with permission.)

when renal perfusion is compromised, as in bilateral renal artery stenosis, severe congestive heart failure, or volume depletion. In these conditions, maintenance of the GFR becomes dependent on angiotensin II, which constricts glomerular efferent arterioles and thereby preserves glomerular capillary hydrostatic pressure. The use of ACE inhibitors or ARBs in the setting of real or effective volume depletion prevents efferent arteriolar vasoconstriction and markedly decreases glomerular capillary hydrostatic pressure, decreasing the GFR.

Postrenal Failure

Postrenal failure refers to renal failure that develops as a consequence of obstruction to urine flow. Obstruction in the renal pelvis, ureters, bladder, or urethra increases the hydrostatic pressure in the renal tubules and Bowman space, thereby opposing glomerular filtration; when the tubular hydrostatic pressure exceeds transcapillary hydrostatic pressure, GFR declines. Like prerenal azotemia, if recognized and treated promptly, postrenal azotemia is completely reversible.

Postrenal failure may occur because of obstruction anywhere along the urinary tract (Table 79.2). However, because most people have two kidneys and because a healthy kidney can compensate in large part for the loss of its mate, obstruction must involve both renal collecting systems and both kidneys to cause a marked change in overall renal function. Therefore, when the serum creatinine is more than mildly elevated due to upper tract obstruction (i.e., above the bladder), this necessarily implies that either both ureters or both renal pelves are involved or that the patient had only one healthy kidney. On the other hand, lower urinary tract obstruction (e.g., of the urethra or bladder) requires only one localized anatomic process to interrupt the entire flow of urine, thereby causing renal failure in both kidneys.

It is a common misconception that when acute renal failure is caused by obstruction, the urine flow is always low. This is only true when urinary obstruction is complete. With partial obstruction, the patient usually is not oliguric. Therefore, postrenal azotemia may present with virtually any urine volume, including anuria (i.e., no urine), oliguria, and normal or

TABLE 79.2. Causes of Postrenal Azotemia in Women

Ureteral
Intraluminal
Stones
Sloughed papillae
Diabetes mellitus
Sickle cell disease
Analgesic nephropathy
Blood clots
Fungus balls
Ureteral malignancy
Extraluminal
Retroperitoneal or pelvic malignancy
Lymphoma
Colonic
Cervical
Ovarian
Retroperitoneal abscess, hematoma, or fibrosis
Pelvic abscess
Surgical injury
Endometriosis
Pregnancy
Uterine prolapse
Aneurysm
Bladder
Carcinoma
Neurogenic bladder
Diabetes mellitus
Spinal cord injury and disease
Anticholinergic drugs
Narcotics
Ganglionic blockers
Urethra
Carcinoma
Stones
Obstructed urethral catheter

even high urine flow. Rarely, when obstruction is intermittent, there may even be alternating polyuria and anuria.

Intrinsic Renal Failure

Intrinsic renal failure refers to an acute decline in the GFR secondary to one or more pathologic processes developing within the kidney itself. It is operationally useful to further subdivide these processes according to the primary structure affected: (a) the glomeruli themselves, (b) the renal arterial vasculature, (c) the renal interstitium, and (d) the renal tubules.

Glomerular diseases manifesting as acute renal failure may be limited to the kidney and idiopathic, such as idiopathic rapidly progressive glomerulonephritis; limited to the kidney and due to a known pathogenesis, such as antiglomerular basement membrane disease; or due to systemic disorders, with multiple organ system involvement, such as systemic lupus erythematosus or glomerulonephritis due to bacterial endocarditis. Vascular diseases may feature glomerular involvement (the glomerulus is, after all, a blood vessel); examples are Wegener granulomatosis or polyarteritis nodosa. They may also be due to obstruction of renal arterioles (as in thrombotic thrombocytopenic purpura or the cholesterol emboli syndrome) or intrinsic arteriolar damage (as in scleroderma or malignant hypertension). Interstitial diseases are usually hypersensitivity reactions to pharmacologic agents but can occur with connective tissue diseases or infiltrative diseases, such as Sjögren syndrome or sarcoidosis. Tubular diseases include acute tubular necrosis (ATN) due to ischemia, ATN due to nephrotoxins, and intratubular obstruction. Intratubular obstruction may develop from the precipitation of exogenously administered agents (acyclovir, methotrexate, oxalate in ethylene glycol overdoses) or overproduction and tubular obstruction of endogenous substances (uric acid in the tumor lysis syndrome, light chains in myeloma kidney, myoglobin in rhabdomyolysis). Intratubular obstruction differs from postrenal failure because in the former case thousands of tubules are obstructed, rather than the renal pelves and urologic structures. These categories are not mutually exclusive, and often several structures (the glomeruli and the vasculature, the tubules and interstitium) may be involved simultaneously. Furthermore, prerenal or postrenal failure can accompany and complicate intrinsic renal disease.

As discussed above, of all causes of intrinsic acute renal failure in hospitalized patients, ATN is by far the most common. The term ATN is to some extent a misnomer because histologic evidence of tubular necrosis is sparse and limited primarily to the late proximal tubule and loop of Henle. These parts of the nephron are located in the medulla, where the partial pressure of oxygen is normally low. The thick ascending limb of the loop of Henle is particularly susceptible to hypoxic or ischemic injury because its cells have the highest metabolic rate of any tubular cells; this explains the remarkable predisposition to the disproportionately hyperperfused kidney to ischemic injury during hypoxia, hypotension, or decreased intravascular volume.

ATN usually develops in the setting of serious illness or injury or postoperatively and, as outlined above, is caused by ischemia, nephrotoxins, or intratubular obstruction. Ischemic ATN is probably the most common form of severe hospital-acquired acute renal failure. It usually develops within 24 hours of a readily identifiable event that severely compromises renal perfusion, such as a hypotensive episode or sepsis and endotoxemia.

Multiple pharmacologic and medicinal agents may cause nephrotoxic ATN. Radiocontrast-induced acute renal failure is probably the leading cause in recent studies; it presents as a rising serum creatinine beginning within 24 to 48 hours of injection of the contrast agent, and the risk of its development is directly related to the dose of the contrast agent. Diabetics with baseline renal insufficiency are at greatest risk, but even in these patients, only some develop clinically important renal failure. Aminoglycoside nephrotoxicity has been an important cause of nephrotoxic tubular necrosis in the past and historically developed in about 10% of patients receiving a full course of therapy; its prevalence is less now that alternative antibiotics are used for treatment of Gram-negative infections. Other important causes of nephrotoxic ATN include heavy metals, such as the platinums, amphotericin B, and pentamidine.

Why the GFR falls in ATN is not certain. Theories include tubular obstruction secondary to cellular debris, back-leak of filtrate through damaged tubules, reduced RBF secondary to vasoconstriction (perhaps mediated by tubuloglomerular feedback), and a reduction in the permeability of the glomerular filtration barrier. In contrast to prerenal and postrenal azotemia, there is no established intervention that rapidly reverses ATN. Nevertheless, it is important to eliminate causative factors, because if the patient does not die from the underlying disease or its complications and if further renal insults are avoided, renal function usually returns to normal.

CLINICAL SYMPTOMS: HISTORY AND PHYSICAL EXAMINATION

When approaching a patient with an elevated serum creatinine concentration, the first step in the history and physical examination is to rapidly exclude life-threatening complications that require urgent treatment, such as hyperkalemia and pulmonary edema. Once this is accomplished, the first diagnostic issue to address is whether the elevation in creatinine is acute or chronic. The most reliable way to answer this question is to review previous laboratory data, if available. When previous creatinine values are unavailable, the serum creatinine should be checked daily for several days, because the resulting picture indicates whether renal function is stable or changing. Whenever the duration of renal failure remains in doubt, one should always assume that the process is new because acute renal failure may be treatable and reversible, whereas chronic renal failure is not. Furthermore, when a patient with known chronic renal disease develops a rising serum creatinine, one should not automatically assume that this is secondary to progression of the underlying disease; such patients are more susceptible to additional renal insults than are healthy individuals, and therefore the physician must exclude a superimposed new process.

After concluding that acute renal failure is present, the next step is to try to determine the cause. In general, patients should be evaluated in the hospital because of the danger of complications, unless renal failure is mild and easily correctable (e.g., worsening prerenal failure secondary to excessive gastrointestinal fluid losses in a patient with diarrhea). This evaluation should begin with a complete history and physical examination, as an attempt to diagnose the cause of acute renal failure, and to determine the severity of complications. In patients with acute renal failure, a variety of signs and symptoms may be encountered. These usually result from either the underlying pathologic process causing renal dysfunction or from the complications of renal failure.

Clinical Signs and Symptoms of the Causative Process

Although rarely diagnostic, historical data, signs, and symptoms may suggest the pathologic process causing acute renal failure. For example, symptoms of volume depletion are frequently detectable by history and physical examination; these include orthostatic dizziness, hypotension, and tachycardia, weight loss, vomiting, diarrhea, poor oral intake, and, on physical examination, orthostatic hypotension, dry mucous membranes, and skin tenting. Histories of uses of diuretics; antihypertensive agents, especially ACE inhibitors; ARBs; or nonsteroidal antiinflammatory drugs in the setting of clinical volume depletion support the diagnosis of prerenal failure. A clinical physical examination pearl is that, due to Starling forces, hypoalbuminemia frequently causes edema. The absence of edema in a hypoalbuminemic individual may then be a sign of volume depletion and prerenal failure. Similarly, symptoms of voiding difficulty and flank pain may accompany urinary tract obstruction, but this is not a specific sign; flank pain also may be seen with renal infarction, renal vein thrombosis, or inflammatory processes affecting the kidneys, such as glomerulonephritis or interstitial nephritis. Gross hematuria may suggest the postrenal failure diagnoses nephrolithiasis, papillary necrosis, or an obstructing malignancy. Complete anuria may be seen in acute total urinary obstruction, but it is not a sensitive or specific sign.

Processes causing intrinsic renal failure manifest a multiplicity of historical and physical examination findings, reflecting the multiplicity of renal diagnoses. A primary glomerular disease such as rapidly progressive glomerulonephritis may not manifest any symptoms other than general symptoms of the complications of renal failure, listed below. When glomerular or vascular disease is due to a systemic process, the manifestations of that process may dominate the clinical picture. For example, joint pain and skin rashes are common in patients with lupus nephritis; fever, anemia, and heart murmurs point to glomerulonephritis due to endocarditis (which can cause glomerulonephritis); focal digital ischemia and livedo reticularis (semipermanent bluish mottling of the skin of the legs and hands) are typical of cholesterol embolization; general malaise, joint pain, palpable purpura, and sinusitis suggest vasculitis; hemoptysis is frequent in Goodpasture syndrome; and thrombocytopenic nonpalpable purpura is characteristic of patients with thrombotic thrombocytopenic purpura. Fever, skin rash, and eosinophilia are typical of drug-induced acute interstitial nephritis, especially in the context of administration of a potentially offending drug, such as a cephalosporin or penicillin. Ischemic or toxic tubular disease is strongly suggested by the appropriate clinical context; for example, acute renal failure in a septic hypotensive patient in the intensive care unit implies ischemic ATN, and acute renal failure after a large dose of radiocontrast suggests nephrotoxic ATN.

Clinical Symptoms of the Complications of Acute Renal Failure

Numerous complications may punctuate the course of acute renal failure and result in a variety of signs and symptoms (Table 79.3). Because many of these complications accompany all causes of renal failure, they are not unique to prerenal, postrenal, or the various intrinsic renal etiologies. Continued intake of sodium and water in the face of impaired excretory capacity in postrenal and in intrinsic renal diseases causes volume overload, which may result in peripheral and pulmonary edema. In hemodynamically stable patients, however, the earliest and most common manifestation of volume overload, by far,

TABLE 79.3. Potential Complications of Acute Renal Failure

Electrolyte
Hyperkalemia
Hyponatremia
Metabolic acidosis
Hypocalcemia
Hyperphosphatemia
Hypermagnesemia
Cardiopulmonary
Pulmonary edema
Pericarditis
Hypertension
Gastrointestinal
Nausea
Vomiting
Anorexia
Hemorrhage
Hematologic
Anemia
Platelet dysfunction
Neurologic
Confusion
Obtundation
Asterixis
Myoclonus
Seizures
Dialytic
Infections
Urinary
Pulmonary
Wound
Bacteremia
Drug toxicity

is hypertension. If more free water is taken in orally or intravenously than is lost through renal and nonrenal routes, hyponatremia ensues. Hyperkalemia is an ever-present danger, particularly in oliguric patients, and may be precipitated by endogenous (e.g., secondary to tissue injury, as may occur in rhabdomyolysis or bowel ischemia) or exogenous sources of potassium; hyperkalemia may cause serious cardiac arrhythmias and, when severe, even cardiac arrest. High anion gap metabolic acidosis is common and results from an impaired ability to excrete the daily acid load and generate the bicarbonate buffer; compensatory hyperventilation may be manifested by Kussmaul respirations and dyspnea. Hypocalcemia and hyperphosphatemia, due to impaired renal hydroxylation of vitamin D and decreased glomerular filtration of phosphorus, are also frequently seen.

Neurologic complications of severe azotemia include altered personality, confusion, asterixis, neuromuscular irritability, seizures, and coma. Anorexia, nausea, and vomiting are classic gastrointestinal symptoms of renal failure, and gastrointestinal hemorrhage also may occur. Uremic pericarditis, increased susceptibility to infection, anemia, and a bleeding diathesis (secondary to platelet dysfunction) are other common complications.

LABORATORY AND IMAGING STUDIES

All patients should have a standard biochemical profile and a complete blood cell count because these may help pinpoint the etiology of acute renal failure and identify complications. For example, an increase in the BUN-to-creatinine ratio in the serum suggests prerenal failure, reflecting aggressive renal tubular urea nitrogen reabsorption in volume depletion. A low platelet count associated with hemolytic anemia raises the question of thrombotic thrombocytopenic purpura. Leukocytosis and eosinophilia suggest acute interstitial nephritis or cholesterol embolization. Other laboratory tests may also be helpful to rule in or to rule out specific diagnoses (Table 79.4). An isolated elevation of lactate dehydrogenase may be due to renal infarction or hemolysis (as seen in thrombotic thrombocytopenic purpura), whereas an elevated creatinine phosphokinase points to rhabdomyolysis and myoglobinuric renal failure. An extremely high uric acid level in a patient with a hematologic malignancy suggests uric acid nephropathy. Hypercalcemia, or even an inappropriately normal serum calcium, may be a clue to the presence of malignancy, especially multiple myeloma.

Blood cultures should be obtained in febrile patients to exclude endocarditis and sepsis. A serologic screen (including antinuclear antibody, complement, and antineutrophil cytoplasmic antibody levels) is indicated when renal involvement secondary to systemic lupus erythematosus or vasculitis is suspected. In elderly patients with unexplained acute renal failure, urine and serum protein electrophoresis should be obtained to exclude unsuspected multiple myeloma.

Urinalysis

A careful urinalysis, with examination of the sediment by the treating physician, can be of enormous help in determining the cause of acute renal failure (Fig. 79.3). A normal urinalysis suggests prerenal or postrenal azotemia, although hyaline casts are common in the former and hematuria or crystalluria may be seen in the latter, especially when postrenal failure is due to nephrolithiasis. When acute renal failure is due to intrinsic renal disease, the urine sediment is typically abnormal. Hematuria and proteinuria suggest either glomerular or vascular disease. In the absence of a urinary tract infection, white blood cells (especially eosinophils) and white blood cell casts suggest acute interstitial nephritis. Renal tubular cells and brown granular casts suggest ischemic or nephrotoxic ATN. Crystals, although seen in normal renal function, may raise the possibility of intratubular obstruction: Calcium oxalate crystals are seen in ethylene glycol intoxication, whereas uric acid crystals may be seen in acute uric acid nephropathy and in uric acid nephrolithiasis. Urine that is dipstick positive for blood but contains few or no red blood cells suggests myoglobinuria, from rhabdomyolysis, or hemoglobinuria.

TABLE 79.4 Diagnostic Studies in the Evaluation of Acute Renal Failure

Routine blood tests
BUN, creatinine
Glucose
Electrolytes
Calcium, phosphorus
Protein, albumin
Uric acid
LDH, bilirubin
CBC, differential
Selected blood tests
Arterial blood gases
Blood cultures
ANA
ANCA
ASLO titer, streptozyme test
Anti-GBM antibody
Cryoglobulins
Complement
Protein electrophoresis
CPK
Osmolality
Magnesium
Routine urine tests
Urinalysis
Selected urine tests
Hansel stain (eosinophils)
Sodium, osmolality, creatinine
Protein electrophoresis
Uric acid
Renal ultrasonography
Renal scan/MRA of kidneys/renal angiogram
Chest x-ray
Electrocardiogram

ANA, antinuclear antibody; ANCA, antineutrophil cytoplasmic antibody; anti-GBM, anti-glomerular basement membrane; ASLO, antistreptolysin-O; BUN, blood urea nitrogen; CBC, complete blood cell count; CPK, creatine phosphokinase; LDH, lactate dehydrogenase.

Urinary Indices

On occasion, it may be difficult to distinguish prerenal azotemia from ischemic or nephrotoxic ATN. In such cases, urinary indices measured on a "spot" urine specimen may be helpful (Table 79.5). Prerenal azotemia is characterized by a concentrated sodium-free urine, whereas in ATN the urine is isosmotic and contains sodium. However, there is overlap between these groups, especially when other factors affecting urinary concentrating ability and sodium excretion are at play (e.g., recent diuretic use). Overlap may be reduced, although not eliminated, by calculating the fractional excretion of filtered sodium (FeNa):

$$FeNa = \frac{(U/P)_{Na}}{(U/P)_{Cr}} \times 100\%$$

where U and P are the urine and plasma concentrations, respectively, of sodium (Na) and creatinine (Cr).

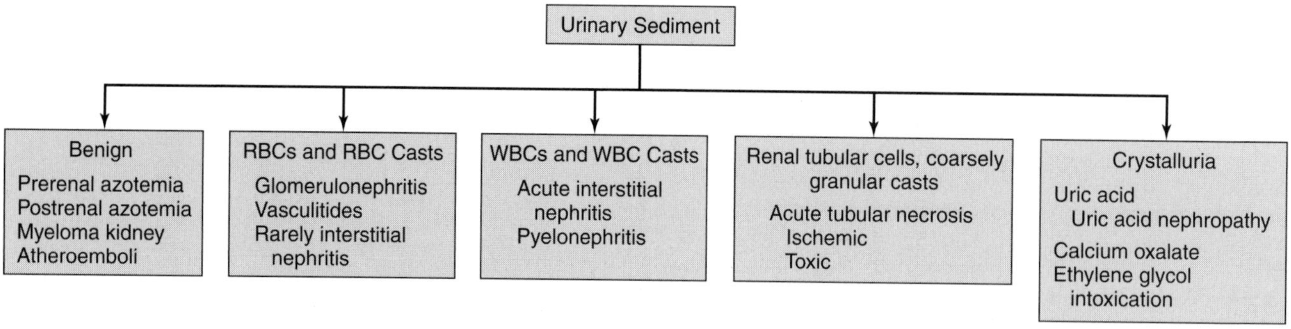

FIG. 79.3. Use of the urinary sediment to help localize the cause of acute renal failure. RBC, red blood cell; WBC, white blood cell.

Renal Imaging

In all patients with otherwise unexplained acute renal failure, urinary tract obstruction must be excluded, because this is a treatable reversible condition. Renal ultrasonography has emerged as the screening procedure of choice because it is both safe and has been shown to be highly sensitive and specific for the detection of obstruction. However, this technique does not detect obstruction directly but rather its usual consequence: dilatation of the collecting system. Rarely, urinary tract obstruction may not cause dilatation (e.g., when the ureters are encased by fibrosis or malignancy). In these unusual cases, renal ultrasonography may give false-negative results. Therefore, when the index of suspicion is high, despite normal findings on ultrasonography, other diagnostic approaches must be considered, including retrograde and antegrade pyelography.

Renal ultrasonography also provides a reliable estimate of renal size. This may be helpful when the duration of renal failure is uncertain. Small kidneys, with thin cortices, are indicative of chronic disease, and normal sized kidneys, with normal, thick, renal cortices, strongly suggest an acute process. Marked asymmetry of the kidneys on ultrasound suggests a unilateral obstruction or renovascular disease. A radionuclide renal scan provides an estimate of RBF and shows whether perfusion is homogeneous. This study may be useful to screen for suspected renal infarction or bilateral renal artery thrombosis. Magnetic resonance angiography and intraarterial contrast angiography can be helpful in evaluating renal arterial obstruction as a cause of acute renal failure. Magnetic resonance angiography avoids the risks of worsening renal failure by injection of contrast but is slightly less sensitive and specific in diagnosing renal infarction.

Renal Biopsy

Renal biopsy should be considered when the origin of acute renal failure remains unclear after a thorough history and physical examination and noninvasive laboratory and radiologic investigation. Renal biopsy also should be considered in patients with a presentation suggestive of rapidly progressive glomerulonephritis, which may occur as an idiopathic process or secondary to a variety of systemic diseases, because this disorder may be reversible with appropriate treatment.

TABLE 79.5. Urinary Indices in Acute Renal Failure

Index	Prerenal	ATN
U_{osm} (mOsm/kg H_2O)	>500	<350
U_{Na} (mEq/L)	<20	>40
FeNa (%)	<1	>1

ATN, acute tubular necrosis; FeNa, fractional excretion of filtered sodium; U_{Na}, urinary sodium concentration; U_{osm}, urinary osmolality.

TREATMENT

The goals of treatment of acute renal failure include facilitation of recovery of renal function, correction of established complications, and prevention of new complications.

Facilitation of renal recovery can be readily achieved when acute renal failure is caused by reversible factors that are identified and appropriately treated. For example, prerenal failure can be repaired by restoring renal perfusion. This involves administration of volume expanders (isotonic fluid) intravenously; discontinuation of agents that decrease intravascular volume or intracapillary hydrostatic pressure, such as diuretics, ACE inhibitors, ARBs, and cathartics; and increasing dietary sodium intake. Postrenal failure is improved by relieving urinary obstruction. This may be as simple as placing a bladder catheter in a patient with a urethral obstruction or bladder outlet obstruction; if urinary obstruction is higher, placement of antegrade or retrograde nephrostomy drains is necessary.

Certain types of intrinsic renal diseases, especially those due to a nephrotoxic agent, may reverse with removal of the offending agent. Renal involvement in some systemic diseases also may be treatable. Even when dealing with established ischemic ATN, renal hypoperfusion and nephrotoxic insults should be avoided because these may interfere with recovery. Good general supportive care, including prevention and eradication of infection and provision of adequate nutrition, also is extremely important.

Pharmacologic therapy for acute renal failure is generally reserved for acute glomerular, vascular, or interstitial diseases. In these cases specific and directed pharmacologic therapy—for example, use of glucocorticoids and cyclophosphamide in acute renal failure due to Wegener granulomatosis, a form of vasculitis—is given after a diagnosis is obtained, usually by a renal biopsy or other definitive evaluation.

For tubular diseases, especially ischemic ATN, there is no evidence to date that any general pharmacologic agent to improve renal function is beneficial. The agents that have most commonly been studied and prescribed in this setting are diuretics, and when administered early in the course, high doses of loop diuretics (furosemide, torsemide, bumetanide) theoretically may lead to an increase in urine flow and may convert oliguric acute renal failure to nonoliguric renal failure, which has a better prognosis. A recent observational study actually shows a poorer outcome in patients with ATN given diuretics, but that finding is complicated by the fact that patients who received diuretics tended to have a greater comorbidity. A scattering of clinical, experimental, and observational studies do show that other agents, such as low dose dopamine, the dopamine agonist fenoldopam, and atrial natriuretic peptide, all may improve urine output in patients with ischemic ATN. However, no large prospective trial supports the use of any of these agents, and many responders to any of these agents may simply be patients with less severe disease and a better overall prognosis. Nevertheless, because it is easier to manage nonoliguric patients, it is reasonable to try a single large dose of a loop diuretic such as furosemide (160–240 mg over 40–60 minutes), alone or in combination with low dose dopamine, early in the course of ATN. If there is no response within a 12- to 24-hour period, these agents should be discontinued.

Potential complications of acute renal failure have been discussed earlier. Perhaps the most lethal is hyperkalemia. To avoid this, plasma potassium (and other electrolytes) should be monitored at least daily and potassium intake should be restricted to below 40 mEq/d. However, severe hyperkalemia may develop despite exogenous potassium restriction because of cellular potassium release from injured tissue and hypercatabolism. Life-threatening hyperkalemia, defined as a plasma potassium concentration greater than 6.5 mEq/L or electrocardiographic changes beyond peaked T waves (e.g., loss of P waves, widened QRS complexes), requires immediate treatment with intravenous calcium gluconate, glucose, and insulin, and sometimes bicarbonate (Table 79.6). Inhaled β-agonists also can rapidly lower the plasma potassium in some patients. However, these treatments do not eliminate excess potassium from the body. Potassium removal is vital and can be accomplished in patients with some renal function and nonoliguria with high dose loop diuretics (160–240 mg furosemide intravenously) and with most patients with oral or rectal sodium polystyrene sulfonate (Kayexalate). Thirty grams of this cation exchange resin given orally (in sorbitol) every 2 to 3 hours is usually highly effective. In the unusual cases where this approach is unsuccessful, hemodialysis is required, which rapidly removes potassium from the body.

Volume overload and hyponatremia should be avoided by limiting sodium and water intake to match output. Large amounts of fluid often are given during the administration of drugs and must be taken into account. When volume overload occurs in oliguric patients or when large volumes of fluid are required to provide nutrition, fluid removal by dialysis or other renal replacement techniques is required. Daily weights are extremely helpful in assessing changes in volume status.

TABLE 79.6. Therapy for Hyperkalemia

Drug	Dose	Onset of action
Calcium gluconate	10–30 mL of 10% solution	Few minutes
$NaHCO_3$	44–132 mEq	15–30 min
Glucose and insulin	Glucose: 25–50 g/h by continuous IV drip Regular insulin: 5 U IV every 15 min	15–30 min
Sodium polystyrene sulfonate (Kayexalate)	Enema (50–100 g)	60 min
	Oral (40 g)	120 min

$NaHCO_3$, sodium bicarbonate.
Source: Tannen RL. Potassium disorders. In: Kokko JP, Tannen RL, eds. *Fluids and electrolytes*. Philadelphia: WB Saunders, 1986:197, with permission.

Acid-base status and calcium and phosphate levels also should be monitored regularly. Metabolic acidosis, although common, is usually not severe enough to require specific therapy. Indeed, aggressive correction of acidemia in hypocalcemic patients may precipitate tetany by decreasing the ionized calcium concentration. Furthermore, administration of sodium bicarbonate or potassium bicarbonate in patients with metabolic acidosis can worsen volume overload or hyperkalemia. Hypocalcemia and hyperphosphatemia can usually be controlled with oral calcium carbonate; this agent limits phosphorus absorption in the intestine while providing supplemental calcium. Magnesium or aluminum-containing antacids, although effective in decreasing gastrointestinal phosphorus absorption, should be avoided because magnesium and aluminum excretion is impaired in renal failure.

The dosage of medications that are excreted by the kidneys must be adjusted appropriately in acute renal failure. As previously discussed, when the serum creatinine is rapidly increasing, it cannot be used to estimate the GFR. In such cases, it is best to assume that the GFR is less than 10 mL/min and dose medications accordingly, following drug levels when possible. If the serum creatinine (S_{Cr}) stabilizes, the GFR for women can be estimated from the following formula:

$$140 - \text{age}/S_{Cr} \times \text{wt}/72 \times 0.85$$

Because infection remains the leading cause of death in acute renal failure, unnecessary instrumentation is to be avoided. Foley catheters are not useful in nonobstructed oligoanuric patients and also should be avoided in nonoliguric patients who are awake and able to void normally.

Patients with acute renal failure may have a prolonged bleeding time due to uremic-induced platelet dysfunction. If prolonged, the bleeding time may be shortened by intravenous deamino-D-arginine vasopressin (DDAVP) (0.3 μg/kg given over 30 minutes in 50 mL of normal saline). Blood transfusions, erythropoietin, and oral or intravenous estrogens may also improve the bleeding time. Erythropoietin is highly effective in treating anemia in chronic renal failure; a recent study supports its use in decreasing transfusion requirements in acutely ill patients in general, but its onset of action is probably too slow to effectively and acutely treat anemia in acute renal failure.

Finally, when acute renal failure is severe and prolonged, hemodialysis, peritoneal dialysis, or an alternative extracorporeal renal replacement therapy (slow continuous ultrafiltration, continuous venovenous hemofiltration, continuous venovenous hemodiafiltration, or continuous venovenous hemodialysis) is indicated. Dialysis and other renal replacement therapies use the physiologic principle of diffusion to promote the clearance of small-molecular-weight solutes down a concentration gradient across a semipermeable membrane, from blood to an extracorporeal fluid compartment, and the principle of convection to ultrafilter excess water and dissolved solutes from the blood to an extracorporeal fluid compartment. These therapies therefore effectively decrease intravascular concentrations of BUN, creatinine, potassium, hydrogen ion, and phosphate and decrease total body sodium and water. They are highly effective in improving the fluid and electrolyte status of patients with refractory volume overload, hyperkalemia, metabolic acidosis, and uremic complications, such as bleeding, neurologic impairment, or severe vomiting or malnutrition. Dialysis or other extracorporeal renal replacement therapy is also indicated when volume overload due to acute renal failure makes it impossible to administer necessary therapies, such as parenteral nutrition, antibiotics, or blood products. The effectiveness of these various therapies has begun to be studied in prospective randomized trials and studies. Based on preliminary evidence, hemodialysis is probably more effective and leads to a better outcome than peritoneal dialysis in ischemic ATN, and there is probably no significant difference in outcome between hemodialysis and continuous renal replacement therapies. Although studies are scarce, in both hemodialysis and in continuous venovenous hemofiltration, there seems to be a direct relationship between increased solute clearance, increased volume removal, and outcome, and that more aggressive therapy, including daily hemodialysis, leads to more rapid recovery of renal failure and a lower mortality rate.

ACUTE RENAL FAILURE IN PREGNANCY

Acute renal failure is distinctly uncommon in pregnant women, who are generally young and healthy and without systemic vascular diseases (diabetes, atherosclerosis, hypertension), which tend to predispose to prerenal failure and ischemic ATN. Nevertheless, to facilitate recognition of the rare cases that do occur, the physician should be aware of normal renal physiologic changes that take place during pregnancy and of the unique and rare conditions that may cause renal failure in this setting.

TABLE 79.7. Causes of Acute Renal Failure in Pregnancy

Prerenal azotemia
Hyperemesis gravidarum
Uterine hemorrhage
? Acute fatty liver
Postrenal azotemia
Ureteral compression by the gravid uterus
Renal azotemia
Cortical necrosis
Abruptio placenta
Puerperal sepsis
Septic abortion
Severe preeclampsia
Intrauterine death
Acute tubular necrosis
Uterine hemorrhage
Sepsis
Amniotic fluid embolism
Preeclampsia
HELLP syndrome
Postpartum HUS

HELLP, hemolysis, elevated liver function test results, and low platelet count; HUS, hemolytic-uremic syndrome.

Physiologic Changes in Renal Function and Blood Pressure during Pregnancy

During normal pregnancy, a reduction in systemic vascular resistance leads to a rise in cardiac output and a fall in diastolic blood pressure of about 10 to 15 mm Hg. Near term, the blood pressure rises again toward prepregnancy levels. In pregnant women, hypertension is defined as a systolic blood pressure level of 140 mm Hg or higher or a diastolic blood pressure level of 90 mm Hg or higher that occurs after 20 weeks of gestation in a woman with previously normal blood pressure. This condition is called gestational hypertension (previously pregnancy-induced hypertension). The renal plasma flow and GFR gradually increase to about 50% above prepregnancy levels by the second trimester, and these increases are sustained until delivery. As a result, the BUN and serum creatinine concentrations are diluted and fall to mean values of 9 and 0.5 mg/dL, respectively, with 15 and 0.8 mg/dL being the upper limits of normal. Urinary protein excretion also increases in pregnancy, so that 250 to 300 mg/d (rather than 150 mg) is the upper limit of normal. In response to hormonal changes and perhaps uterine compression, the urinary collecting system dilates during pregnancy and remains so for up to 12 weeks postpartum. This physiologic response may complicate noninvasive radiologic evaluation of possible urinary tract obstruction.

Causes of Renal Failure in Pregnancy

Acute renal failure is rare in pregnancy, with a recently reported incidence of 2 per 10,000 pregnancies. There are no large series of acute renal failure in pregnancy, as there are in the general and hospitalized populations, to quantify the most common causes of acute renal failure in pregnancy. Although pregnant women may develop any of the forms of acute renal failure previously discussed, there seems to be a few unique causes that comprise most cases of pregnancy-associated acute renal failure. This is based on the few series that do exist, general clinical experience, and case reports, which admittedly overemphasize unusual diseases. Table 79.7 lists these and other less common causes of acute renal failure unique to gestation.

Prerenal failure is uncommon in pregnancy, because pregnant women tend to be volume expanded, to have a baseline high GFR, and to lack systemic atherosclerotic and vascular disease; all these features protect against decreases in RBF. One important, though rare, cause of prerenal failure in pregnancy is hyperemesis gravidarum; this is a condition characterized by idiopathic intractable vomiting occurring during the first trimester of pregnancy. Classic volume depletion may result and induce prerenal azotemia. Treatment usually includes hospitalization; antiemetics; fluid, electrolyte, and vitamin replacement; and, in some cases, parenteral nutrition.

Postrenal failure is also rare, despite the appearance of urinary collecting system dilatation on radiographic studies. The gravid uterus, particularly when overdistended by polyhydramnios or multiple gestations, may obstruct the ureters and cause postrenal azotemia. This is quite rare but has been reported. Treatment options include delivery, drainage of polyhydramnios, bypassing the obstruction with ureteral catheters, or placing a percutaneous nephrostomy tube.

Of all intrinsic renal causes of renal failure, the preeclampsia–eclampsia continuum is probably the most common cause. Preeclampsia is a syndrome unique to pregnancy characterized by the development of hypertension, edema, and proteinuria occurring after the 20th week of gestation. The mechanism is not fully elaborated, but it does feature an increase in peripheral vascular resistance, which then causes decreased RBF and subsequent endothelial dysfunction. Renal insufficiency with a mild increase in serum creatinine is common and accompanies other systemic symptoms, including right upper quadrant pain and neuromuscular irritability, which may progress to seizures. Hyperuricemia and abnormal liver function tests are common. Preeclampsia is a vascular renal lesion; the characteristic pathologic finding in the kidneys is swelling of glomerular endothelial cells. In general, the serum creatinine rarely exceeds 1.3 mg/dL in the absence of other complications, but more severe renal failure, occasionally requiring dialysis therapy, may occur. Treatment begins with bed rest and antihypertensive therapy, but delivery is the ultimate therapy and is the treatment of choice if the fetus is viable. The syndrome of hemolysis, elevated liver function test results, and a *low* platelet count

(HELLP syndrome) is a severe variant of preeclampsia. It can cause acute renal failure, usually in association with other severe complications such as abruptio placenta and convulsions. HELLP syndrome can be differentiated from pregnancy-related hemolytic-uremic syndrome, discussed below, because it usually follows complicated preeclampsia.

Postpartum hemolytic-uremic syndrome is a vascular cause of intrinsic renal disease that, similarly to diarrhea-related hemolytic-uremic syndrome or thrombotic thrombocytopenic purpura, is characterized by microangiopathic hemolytic anemia and thrombocytopenia, along with varying degrees of acute renal failure. Histologically, platelet fibrin thrombi occlude small arterioles and capillaries; renal dysfunction is due to occlusion of these small blood vessels. It typically occurs 1 day to several weeks after delivery, although some cases may occur immediately antepartum. Patients are usually critically ill, with platelet counts that may be below 10,000, disseminated bleeding, and hemoglobins that are critically low due to bleeding and hemolysis. Therapy is similar to that for other thrombotic microangiopathies, with daily plasma exchange until hematologic remission. Corticosteroids are usually administered, although no good evidence-based data support their use. IgG, splenectomy, and vincristine can also be given in refractory cases. The mortality rate has historically been very high, and even now many patients who survive have persistent renal failure.

Although not, of course, unique to pregnancy, lupus nephritis is an important cause of primary glomerular disease in pregnancy, probably because lupus commonly occurs in young women. In a substantial number of patients, lupus nephritis may present during pregnancy. All histologic classes of lupus nephritis may be seen in pregnancy, but the more aggressive diffuse proliferative lesions have a worse prognosis for maternal and fetal outcome. Thrombotic complications related to lupus anticoagulants in lupus nephritis also increase morbidity risks.

Ischemic ATN, although rare in pregnancy, may develop after severe hypotension or during the course of sepsis. Thus, pregnant women with puerperal sepsis, septic abortion, amniotic fluid embolism, abruptio placenta, or other causes of uterine hemorrhage are at risk. Another complication of severe hypotension and sepsis, renal cortical necrosis, is caused by thrombosis of the small arteries, afferent arterioles, and glomerular capillaries in the cortex; the medulla is spared. Years ago the most common settings for cortical necrosis were complications of pregnancy, including abruptio placenta or other uterine hemorrhage; puerperal sepsis; septic abortion; preeclampsia; or prolonged intrauterine death. Extensive cortical necrosis is one of the few conditions that cause anuria; prolonged oliguria and bloody urine also may be seen. Fortunately, in more recent years this disorder has become unusual in developed countries with modern obstetric care; the decrease in number of illegally performed abortions may also account for its declining frequency.

Evaluation of Acute Renal Failure in Pregnancy

The approach to acute renal failure in the gravid woman follows the same general guidelines outlined earlier. Because mild hydronephrosis is normal in pregnancy, a renal ultrasound, commonly done in the general population to exclude postrenal failure, may not be as helpful; urinary obstruction can be detected by ultrasonography only when the collecting system is more dilated than anticipated for the stage of gestation. In questionable cases, a trial of urinary drainage may be necessary to see if renal function improves. When renal failure occurs in the third trimester or puerperium, liver function tests, a complete blood cell count and platelet count, red cell morphologic study, and coagulation tests should be obtained to rule out the potentially fatal postpartum hemolytic-uremic syndrome. A serum uric acid level that is elevated out of proportion to the degree of renal failure can be a clue to preeclampsia, because it features increased renal tubular reabsorption of uric acid. Renal biopsy is rarely indicated during pregnancy; if absolutely necessary it may be performed safely under ultrasound guidance.

Management and Prognosis

The same principles of general treatment outlined earlier apply to pregnant women. Additional caution must be used when prescribing medications, because the safety of many drugs has not been established in pregnancy and some are known to be dangerous. For example, the antihypertensive agents of the ACE inhibitor and ARB classes are absolutely contraindicated in pregnancy because they involve a high risk of fetal maldevelopment and neonatal renal failure.

General indications for dialysis also apply to pregnant women. Either peritoneal dialysis or hemodialysis may be used; there may be a theoretical advantage to peritoneal dialysis because continuous anticoagulation is not necessary. In pregnant women with chronic renal failure, recommendations are for early initiation of and more aggressive dialysis because of the assumption that minimizing the uremic environment reduces the risk of adverse events for both the mother and fetus and enhances fetal growth. Many authorities suggest starting dialysis when the BUN rises above 60 mg/dL and that dialysis be performed as needed to maintain the BUN at or below 50 to 60 mg/dL, regardless of the development of subjective uremic symptoms. These recommendations arise out of outcome data in women with chronic rather than acute renal failure but are probably still applicable. During dialysis, the growth and well-being of the fetus must be monitored closely, and even with aggressive treatment, there is a high rate of miscarriage, intrauterine fetal growth retardation, and low-birth-weight infants.

The prognosis of acute renal failure in pregnancy depends more on the precipitating process than on the severity of azotemia. Prerenal and postrenal azotemia is completely reversible with appropriate therapy. Renal dysfunction caused by preeclampsia and the HELLP syndrome usually improves after delivery. Renal failure may still persist up to 6 weeks postpartum. On the other hand, renal cortical necrosis often causes permanent renal injury, but because the process is frequently patchy, there may be some improvement over time. There is a substantial risk in postpartum hemolytic-uremic syndrome for irreversible renal failure even with appropriate and aggressive treatment.

BIBLIOGRAPHY

Abuelo JG. Diagnosing vascular causes of acute renal failure. *Ann Intern Med* 1995;123:601–614.

Allgren RL, Marbury TC, Rahman SN, et al. Anaritide in acute tubular necrosis. *N Engl J Med* 1997;336:828–834.

American College of Obstetricians and Gynecologists. Diagnosis and management of preeclampsia and eclampsia. ACOG Practice Bulletin No. 33. *Obstet Gynecol* 2002;99:159–167.

Badr KF, Ichikawa I. Prerenal failure: a deleterious shift from renal compensation to decompensation. *N Engl J Med* 1988;319:623–628.

Bagon JA, Vernaeve H, De Muylder X. Pregnancy and dialysis. *Am J Kidney Dis* 1998;31:756–765.

Brady HR, Singer GG. Acute renal failure. *Lancet* 1995;346:1533.

Brezis M, Rosen S. Hypoxia of the renal medulla-its implications for disease. *N Engl J Med* 1995;338:647–655.

DuBose TD, Molony DA, Verani R, et al. Nephrotoxicity of nonsteroidal anti-inflammatory drugs. *Lancet* 1994;344:515.

Epstein M. Hepatorenal syndrome: emerging perspectives of pathophysiology and therapy. *J Am Soc Nephrol* 1994;4:1735–1753.
Esson ML, Schrier, RW. Diagnosis and treatment of acute tubular necrosis. *Ann Intern Med* 2002;137:744–752.
Kaufman J, Dhakal M, Patel B, et al. Community-acquired acute renal failure. *Am J Kidney Dis* 1991;17:191–200.
Kellum JA, Decker JM. Use of dopamine in acute renal failure: a meta-analysis. *Crit Care Med* 2001;29:1526–1531.
Klahr S. Pathophysiology of obstructive uropathy: an update. *Semin Nephrol* 1991; 11:156–168.
Klahr S, Miller SB. Acute oliguria. *N Engl J Med* 1998;383:671–675.
Komers R, Anderson S, Epstein M. Renal and cardiovascular effects of selective cyclooxygenase-2 inhibitors. *Am J Kidney Dis* 2001;38:1145–1157.
Levy EM, Viscoli CM, Horwitz RI. The effect of acute renal failure on mortality. *JAMA* 1996;275:1489–1494.
Liano F, Pascual J. Epidemiology of acute renal failure: a prospective, multicenter, community based study. *Kidney Int* 1996;50:811–818.
McCrae KR, Cines DB. Thrombotic micrangiopathy during pregnancy. *Semin Hematol* 1997;34:148–158.
Mehta RL, Pascual MT, Soroko S, et al. Diuretics, mortality, and nonrecovery of renal function in acute renal failure. *JAMA* 2002;288:2547–2553.
Michel DM, Kelly CJ. Acute interstitial nephritis. *J Am Soc Nephrol* 1998; 9:506–514.
Moake JL. Thrombotic microangiopathies. *N Engl J Med* 2002;347:589–600.
Moroni G, Quaglini S, Banfi G, et al. Pregnancy in lupus nephritis. *Am J Kidney Dis* 2002;40:713–720.
Murphy SW, Barrett B, Parfrey PS. Contrast nephropathy. *J Am Soc Nephrol* 2000; 11:177–182.
Nash K, Hafeez A, Hou S. Hospital acquired renal insufficiency. *Am J Kidney Dis* 2002;39:930–936.
Nolan CR, Anderson RJ. Hospital acquired renal failure. *J Am Soc Nephrol* 1998;9: 710–718.
Nzerue CM, Hewan-Lowe K, Nwawka K. Acute renal failure in pregnancy: a review of clinical outcomes in an inner city hospital from 1986–1996. *J Natl Med Assoc* 1998;90:486–490.
Okunyande I, Abrinko P, Hou S. Registry of pregnancy in dialysis patients. *Am J Kidney Dis* 1998;31:766–773.
Phu NH, Hien TT, Mai NT. Hemofiltration and peritoneal dialysis in infection associated acute renal failure in Vietnam. *N Engl J Med* 2002;347:895–902.
Ronco C, Bellomo R, Homel P, et al. Effects of two different doses in continuous venovenous hemofiltration on outcomes in acute renal failure: a randomized prospective trial. *Lancet* 2000;356:26–30.
Schiffl H, Lang S, Fischer R. Daily hemodialysis and the outcome of acute renal failure. *N Engl J Med* 2002;346:305–310.
Selcuk NY, Tonbul HZ, San A, et al. Changes in frequency and etiology of acute renal failure in pregnancy. *Renal Fail* 1998;20:513–517.
Sibai BM, Ramadan MK, Usta I, et al. Maternal morbidity and mortality in 442 pregnancies with hemolysis, elevated liver enzymes, and low platelets (HELLP syndrome). *Am J Obstet Gynecol* 1993;169:1000–1006.
Thadhani R, Pascual M, Bonventre JV. Acute renal failure. *N Engl J Med* 1996;334: 1448–1553.
Vanholder R, Sever MS, Erek E, et al. Rhabdomyolysis. *J Am Soc Nephrol* 2000;11: 1553–1561.
Walker JJ. Preeclampsia. *Lancet* 2000;356:1260–1265.

CHAPTER 80
Interstitial Cystitis

Vivian C. Aguilar

Interstitial cystitis (IC) is a bladder syndrome characterized by irritative voiding symptoms, such as urinary urgency, frequency, and nocturia, and pelvic pain. The symptoms of IC can be debilitating and fluctuate in severity over time. In 1988 the National Institutes of Health-National Institute of Diabetes and Digestive and Kidney Diseases developed criteria for the diagnosis of IC for patient inclusion into clinical and drug trials (Table 80.1). Limitations of these criteria have been found when applied to clinical practice that can result in patient under-diagnosis as demonstrated by the National Institutes of Health Interstitial Database Study. In this study 60% of the patients judged to have IC by experienced clinicians failed to meet the National Institutes of Health-National Institute of Diabetes and Digestive and Kidney Diseases criteria.

TABLE 80.1. NIH-NIDDK Diagnostic Criteria of Interstitial Cystitis

Category A: At least one of the following findings on cystoscopy:
- Diffuse glomerulations (at least 10 per quadrant) in at least three quadrants of the bladder
- A classic Hunner ulcer

Category B: At least one of the following symptoms:
- Pain associated with the bladder
- Urinary urgency

Exclusion criteria:
- Age < 18 y[a]
- Urinary frequency while awake < 8 times per day
- Nocturia fewer than two times per night
- Maximal bladder capacity > 350 mL while the patient is awake
- Absence of an intense urge to void with the bladder filled to 150 mL of water with medium filling rate (30–100 mL/min) during cystometry
- Involuntary bladder contraction on cystometry using medium filling rate
- Duration of symptoms < 9 mo[a]
- Symptoms relieved by antimicrobial agents (antibiotics, urinary antiseptics), anticholinergics, or antispasmodics[a]
- Urinary tract or prostatic infection in the last 3 months[a]
- Active genital herpes
- Vaginitis[a]
- Uterine, cervical, vaginal, or urethral cancer within the past 5 years[a]
- Bladder or ureteral calculi[a]
- Urethral diverticulum[a]
- History of cyclophosphamide or chemical cystitis or tuberculous or radiation cystitis
- Benign or malignant bladder tumors

[a]Relative exclusion criteria.
Source: Walters MD, Karram MM. *Urogynecology and reconstructive pelvic surgery*, 2nd ed. St. Louis: Mosby, 1999:316, with permission.

IC has been diagnosed in children and adolescents as well as women of reproductive age and beyond. The disease seems to be unrelated to menopausal status, occurring both premenopausally and postmenopausally. The prevalence of IC is not known but is estimated at 30 cases per 100,000 in the United States and affects more women than men (ratio of 9:1).

ETIOLOGY AND PATHOGENESIS

The etiology of IC is unknown. Current thinking suggests that patients with IC have defects in the glycosaminoglycan layer of the bladder wall, although there is no evidence that the glycosaminoglycan is intrinsically defective or abnormal. The glycosaminoglycans of the bladder surface are hydrophilic polysaccharides that form a layer of micelles of water on the bladder epithelium. This micellar layer acts as a barrier between the transitional epithelial cells and urine. It is hypothesized that a defect in this layer allows "leaking" of the epithelium, resulting in a dysfunctional epithelium with excessive permeability. This causes exposure of the transitional epithelium and muscularis to noxious substances in the urine, which ultimately results in bladder inflammation and pain. However, this is only a partial explanation, possibly explaining the end-effect mechanism. It does not address the mechanism by which the permeability or leakiness of the glycosaminoglycan layer initially occurs.

The features of IC are similar to those seen in patients with chronic autoimmune processes. The pattern of disease is characterized by chronic symptoms with exacerbations and remissions. Several researchers demonstrated an increased number of mast cells in the bladder wall of patients with IC, which is consistent with a potential autoimmune process. Other proposed mechanisms include occult infection, toxin exposure, or other inflammatory mediators.

The physiologic causes of pain with IC also are not clear. Inflammatory mediators released by the sensory nerves cause nociceptor stimulation of visceral neural pathways, leading to pain. Substance P, a nociceptor transmitter, is integral in this pathway. When released, substance P leads to an inflammatory cascade, leading to mast cell activation and degranulation. Increased levels of substance P have been found in the urine of IC patients. In some patients, chronic inflammation results in a contracted bladder of limited capacity that may cause pain, urgency, and frequency. Such chronic visceral pain may result in inflammation and spasm of the pelvic floor muscles (levator ani syndrome) with resultant pelvic pain.

PRESENTATION AND DIFFERENTIAL DIAGNOSIS

Common clinical manifestations of IC may include severe suprapubic and bladder pain, frequency, urgency, nocturia, and dyspareunia. The suprapubic pain may be relieved for a short period of time after voiding. By the time IC is diagnosed, most patient have had symptoms for 2 to 4 years or more. Acute initial symptoms are commonly misdiagnosed as a urinary tract infection.

Frequency, urgency, nocturia, and pelvic pain may be associated with several other diagnoses. Acute, recurrent, or chronic infections of the urinary tract especially must be considered. A urine culture showing 100,000 or more bacterial colonies of one organism confirms cystitis. Infections of the urethra may show similar culture results but more commonly show either lower colony counts or negative bacterial culture results. Bladder tumors, including carcinoma in situ, may present with similar symptoms. Because of this possibility, urine cytologic studies and cystoscopically directed bladder biopsies generally should be performed as part of the diagnostic workup. A bladder tumor also may be suggested by the presence of microscopic hematuria.

The symptoms of IC can also mimic many symptoms of gynecologic disorders. These gynecologic diseases include pelvic tumors, vaginal atrophy, vaginal infections, vulvodynia, vestibulitis, pelvic relaxation, endometriosis, endometritis, pelvic adhesive disease, levator ani myalgia, and undiagnosed chronic pelvic pain. Disorders of the gastrointestinal system must be considered when evaluating pelvic pain, because IC patients will often complain of increased urinary symptoms associated with constipation and/or abdominal bloating. Irritable bowel syndrome, colitis, and diverticulitis can also cause irritative urinary symptoms. Thus, it is the task of the caregiver to consider all these organ systems in evaluating a woman who presents with pelvic pain, urgency, and frequency.

IC is most frequently diagnosed clinically on the basis of the symptoms of urinary urgency, frequency (more than eight voids during the day), nocturia (more than two voids during sleep), suprapubic pressure, and pelvic pain without the presence of infection or neoplasm. Pelvic examination in the female with IC may reveal anterior vaginal wall, bladder, or urethral tenderness. Cystoscopy under anesthesia with hydrodistention has been integral in the diagnosis of IC. The bladder is inspected initially and then hydrodistention is performed by filling the bladder under gravity at 800 cm of sterile water for 5 to 7 minutes. Glomerulations, petechiae, and submucosal hemorrhages may be visualized, and determination of reduced bladder capacity can be confirmed. Linear cracking and Hunner ulcer, first described by Hunner in 1914, may also be noted but are not always present. In addition, hydrodistention has been demonstrated to reduce symptoms in 20% to 30% of patients for up to 6 months. Biopsies obtained during cystoscopy may also aid in the diagnosis of IC by demonstrating the presence of inflammatory mast cells. Patients with mastocytosis may benefit from treatment with antihistamines.

In 1996, Parsons introduced the potassium sensitivity test as a method of diagnosing IC. A dilute solution of potassium (40 mEq in 100 mL of water) is infused into the bladder and left in for 5 minutes. The patient then rates the severity of provocation of urgency and frequency on a scale of 0 (no provocation) to 5 (severe provocation). A positive test is a change of score ≥ 2 from baseline. The test is based on the etiologic theory that damaged epithelium leads to increased permeability of toxic substances into the bladder wall, causing inflammation and pain. Although the potassium sensitivity test is relatively simple to perform in the office, it can be significantly painful to some patients. In addition, only 75% of patients with IC will have a positive test (sensitivity = 75%), and the test is also falsely positive in patients with cystitis, radiation damage, or detrusor instability.

In summary, the differential diagnosis of IC is not always easy. In a sense, it is a diagnosis of exclusion, being a disease of variable symptoms, of unknown etiology, possibly of heterogeneous causation, and with inadequate markers.

LABORATORY STUDIES

Urinalysis and urine culture should be part of the initial laboratory evaluation for IC to rule out urinary tract infection. In the presence of hematuria or microhematuria, urine cytology should be performed as well. A 48-hour voiding diary is obtained to reveal the severity of frequency, volume of voids during the day, and type of incontinence episodes, if any (Fig. 80.1). The diary can also reveal ingestion of bladder irritants such as caffeine and the total amount of fluid intake during the day. The number of voids during the day can be tallied and the average diurnal volume calculated. The number of voids during the night and the average nocturnal volume is also calculated in a similar fashion. It is helpful to obtain baseline voiding diaries not only to aid in diagnosis, but also to use as comparison later on to measure improvement with treatment. A postvoid residual is helpful to evaluate bladder emptying but may cause significant discomfort in patients with IC.

Radiologic studies such as renal ultrasound or intravenous pyelogram should be performed if the patient has a history of hematuria, prior pelvic surgery, renal calculi, or recurrent urinary tract infections. However, most laboratory studies in these patients are negative.

TREATMENT

Treatment can be a frustrating experience for both the patient and her physician, because none of the currently available therapies is curative. Significant biopsychosocial consequences are not surprising, considering the patient is told she has a disease of unknown cause with no known cure and with potentially incapacitating consequences. In addition, IC patients scored worse on quality of life questionnaires than patients on dialysis or age-matched healthy control subjects. Because of such issues, it is crucial that the physician educates and involves the patient fully, as well as the patient's family when possible or appropriate. A multidisciplinary approach is most successful in the treatment of IC with the primary goal of symptom reduction.

Time	Amount Voided	Activity	Urge Present	Leakage	Symptoms	Amount/Type Fluid Intake
6:15 am	*150*	*Waking up*	*Yes*			
7:00	*25*		*Yes*			
7:45	*50*		*Yes*			
8:30 am		*Sneezed*	*No*	*1-drops*		*1 cup of coffee*

FIG. 80.1. Example of a voiding diary.

Behavioral Modifications

Dietary change is an initial conservative approach to managing symptoms of IC. Urinary metabolites of certain foods excreted into the urine may exacerbate bladder irritation. Elimination of certain foods and beverages appears to improve symptoms of frequency and urgency in some patients. However, not every patient responds to the same diet. It is recommended that the patient eliminate all the possible foods causing flares for a week or two and then slowly add each food one by one. If a particular food is going to cause symptoms, it will usually do so within 6 to 12 hours of ingestion (Table 80.2). Food additives may be helpful in reducing the acidity of the food and the urine as well. Prelief, available over the counter, is a tasteless deacidifier sprinkled directly onto the food. Baking soda can also be used to neutralize the acidity of the urine; the recommended dose is ½ teaspoon of baking soda in a glass of water three times a day. Potassium citrate has also been used to decrease the acidity of the urine.

Increasing fluid intake is another important dietary change that further dilutes the acidic concentration of urine. Patients with IC tend to decrease their fluid intake to limit the frequency of voids; however, this concentrates the urine further, leading to increased irritation. By increasing fluid intake and urinary voided volumes, the urine becomes less toxic to a sensitive bladder.

Another useful treatment, as long as the patient does not have severe pain, is autodilation. This is a behavioral modification modality whereby the patient increases her bladder capacity through gradually increasing the intervals between voids. With this technique, the patient keeps a diary of times and volumes of urination, of fluid intake, of pain intensity, and of any suspected factors that might affect symptoms (e.g., menses, sex-

TABLE 80.2. Foods that May Cause a Worsening of Interstitial Cystitis Symptoms

Citrus fruits (oranges, grapefruits, lemons), apples, apricots, avocados, bananas, cantaloupes, cranberries, grapes, nectarines, peaches, plums, rhubarb, strawberries
Caffeinated beverages
Chocolate
Alcoholic beverages (particularly red wine)
Tomatoes and tomato sauces
Spicy foods
Carbonated beverages
Other foods, food additives, or beverages that might worsen symptoms include the following:
- Aspartame (Nutrasweet), saccharine, foods with artificial colors, monosodium glutamate (MSG), citric acid
- Cheeses (except American, cottage, cream, ricotta)
- Sour cream
- Yogurt
- Chicken livers
- Corned beef and other smoked meats
- Pickled herring
- Vinegar
- Salad dressing
- Mayonnaise
- Lentils, lima beans, fava beans, soy beans
- Nuts (almonds, pine nuts, and peanuts are okay)
- Onions
- Raisins, cranberries, prunes
- Rye and sourdough bread
- Soy sauce
- Tea (some herbal teas are okay, others are a problem—it is hard to tell which will have a negative effect).

Source: Moldwin R. *The interstital cystitis survival guide*. Oakland, CA: New Harbinger Publications, 2002:176–177, with permission.

ual activity, or stress). The patient and physician review the initial diary to establish baseline severity of symptoms and set concrete treatment goals. Specific goals need to be set and followed. The goals must be aimed toward a slow gradual progression. If the patient attempts to progress too rapidly, failure is inevitable. An initial increase of voiding intervals of no more than 15 minutes should be attempted. After about a month of successfully increasing the minimum voiding interval by 15 minutes, the minimum interval should be increased again. Generally, it is reasonable to try to increase the voiding interval by 15 minutes each month until a minimum interval of 3 to 4 hours is attained. The patient should continue to keep her diary throughout this treatment. This assists with compliance, adherence, motivation, and monitoring of her progress. Monthly physician visits are also helpful for the same reasons. Remission rates of 80% to 85% have been obtained with this treatment. However, relapse of symptoms is likely if the patient is not vigilant with the training. Success with autodilation is limited to patients with mild or controllable pain.

Hydrodistension of the Bladder

The mainstay of urologic treatment of IC for more than 50 years has been hydrodistention of the bladder. This procedure can be performed at the time of diagnostic cystoscopy if general or spinal anesthesia is used. After diagnostic evaluation is completed, the bladder is filled to maximal capacity under gravity at 80 cm H_2O for 2 to 7 minutes. The risk of bladder rupture with this procedure is rare; however, patients with a small-capacity scarred bladder are at an increased risk for rupture. Patients may complain of increased pain immediately postoperatively, and it is generally 2 to 3 weeks until they notice a remission of symptoms. About 30% to 50% of patients have a successful response to hydrodistention. Remission generally lasts for 6 months, with a gradual recurrence of symptoms in most patients. After recurrence, retreatment with hydrodistention has a greatly diminished success rate. The mechanism of action of hydrodistention is not known. Speculation is that one or both of the following mechanisms may apply: The dysfunctional epithelium is damaged and regeneration of normal epithelium is stimulated, or there is significant nerve damage with resultant denervation. Regardless of the actual mechanism, hydrodistention is a reasonable initial therapy. It has a good (albeit temporary) response rate, it is fairly easy and safe to perform, and it can be done at the time of the diagnostic cystoscopy.

Oral Therapy

Sodium pentosan polysulfate is the only oral medication approved by the U.S. Food and Drug Administration for the treatment of IC. Sodium pentosan polysulfate is a synthetic polyanionic analogue of heparin that is thought to augment the lining of the bladder and "repair" leaky epithelium. The medication is administered orally, 100 mg three times a day, and has 1⁄15 of heparin's anticoagulant effects. Reported results of its effectiveness have been mixed, but at least one placebo-controlled double-blinded study showed a 28% to 32% response rate compared with the placebo response rate of 13% to 16%. It is generally well tolerated, with the most common side effect of dyspepsia. Reversible alopecia, increased bruising, bloating, and diarrhea have also been reported. One drawback to this therapy is that a prolonged duration of treatment is needed before significant improvement is noted by the patient.

Hydroxyzine, a histamine-1 receptor antagonist, has been shown to improve IC symptoms by 40% in 95 of 140 patients who took the drug. In addition, those patients with a history of allergic problems or mastocytosis on biopsy had an increased response to 55% improvement in symptoms. The efficacy of hydroxyzine in the relief of IC symptoms may be due to mast cell stabilization. The sedating effects of hydroxyzine may be improved after 1 week of daily use and dosing at bedtime. The recommended starting dose is 25 mg at bedtime, which can be titrated up to 50 mg after 1 to 2 weeks.

TABLE 80.3. Medications for Irritable Bladder Syndrome

Medication	Dose
Anticholinergics/antispasmodics	
Flavoxate hydrochloride	100–200 mg q 6–8 h
Hyoscyamine sulfate	0.125–0.30 mg q 6–8 h
Oxybutynin chloride	5 mg q 6–12 h
Smooth muscle relaxants	
Phenoxybenzamine hydrochloride	10–20 mg q 8–12 h
Prazosin hydrochloride	1–5 mg q 8–12 h
Terazosin hydrochloride	1–5 mg qd
Skeletal muscle relaxants	
Carisoprodol	350 mg q 6–8 h
Cyclobenzeprine	10 mg q 8–12 h
Methocarbamol	500–1,000 mg q 6–8 h
Diazepam	2–10 mg q 6–12 h
Analgesics/others	
Phenazopyridine	200 mg q 8 h
Ketorulac tromethamine	10 mg q 6 h
Naproxen sodium	275–550 mg q 6–12 h
Ibuprofen	200–800 mg q 6–8 h
Amitryptilline	25–75 mg qd

The tricyclic antidepressant, amitriptyline, has many qualities that make it a common first-line agent in the treatment of IC (Table 80.3). The drug has the ability to down-regulate pain sensation by its effect on decreasing serotonin and norepinephrine reuptake in the central nervous system. Amitriptyline also appears to have a cholinergic effect on the bladder and the ability to stabilize mast cells. The sedative effect of the medication enables patients to have deeper and longer periods of sleep as well as improve mood. Uncontrolled studies of amitriptyline have shown 64% to 90% improvement in IC patients. The recommended starting dose is 10 to 25 mg at dinnertime and titration to effect with 75 to 100 mg/d. Adverse effects include fatigue, decrease in libido, anorgasmia, weight gain, urinary retention, dry mouth, thyroid dysfunction, and constipation.

Antiseizure medications, in particular gabapentin and carbamazapine, have been used in the treatment of neuropathic pain and IC. In a double-blind placebo-controlled trial, gabapentin was more effective than placebo in reducing postherpetic neuralgia. These agents are usually reserved as second-line therapy. Analgesics, such as nonsteroidal antiinflammatory drugs and opioids, have been used to treat the somatic pain component of IC. Narcotics are used in the treatment of IC for symptom flares and management of chronic pain refractory to other modalities.

Intravesical Therapy

Dimethyl sulfoxide (DMSO, Rimso-50) is the only drug with a U.S. Federal Drug Administration–approved indication for IC (Table 80.4). DMSO is a product of the wood pulp industry, a derivative of lignin. It is a superb solvent, being miscible with water, lipids, and organic agents. DMSO has several pharmacologic properties that led to interest in its use for IC: (a) membrane penetration without membrane damage, (b) enhance-

TABLE 80.4. Therapy of Interstitial Cystitis

Method	Success rate
Hydrodistention of bladder	6–10 mo
Autodilation	80%–85% (selected patients)
Dimethylsulfoxide, 50%, intravesical	40%–50%
Heparin, intravesical	40%–50%
Heparin, subcutaneous	30%–35%
Pentosanpolysulfate, oral	40%–50%
Nonsteroidal antiinflammatory drugs	—
Oxychlorosene, 0.4%, intravesical	—
TENS unit	—
Nd:YAG laser	—
Cystectomy and diversion	—

TENS, transcutaneous electrical nerve stimulation.

ment of drug absorption (e.g., steroids), (c) antiinflammatory activity, (d) topical analgesic activity via interruption of conduction in peripheral nerves, (e) promotion of collagen breakdown or dissolution via weakening of cross-linking, (f) muscle relaxation, (g) bacteriostasis, (h) vasodilation, and (i) enhancement of mast cell histamine release. All but the last of these pharmacologic properties are potential mechanisms by which DMSO might decrease symptoms in IC. In contrast, the DMSO effect on mast cells could account for the initial transient worsening of symptoms in some patients with IC undergoing DMSO treatment.

DMSO has low systemic toxicity. It is primarily excreted via the renal system as unchanged DMSO and dimethyl sulfone. A small percentage is excreted via the respiratory system as dimethyl sulfide. Dimethyl sulfide accounts for the garlic-like taste and breath odor after DMSO treatment. Some early animal studies raised concerns of lenticular opacities, but this has never been reported with therapeutic doses or human use. DMSO has been reported to be teratogenic in animal studies, so its use in pregnancy is contraindicated.

Intravesical treatment can be done as an office procedure. It is best to perform a urinalysis before treatments to exclude bacteriuria. Additionally, DMSO treatment should not be done in the 3 to 4 weeks after bladder biopsies to avoid excessive absorption via the unhealed biopsy sites. The urethra may be anesthetized with 2% lidocaine topically. Sometimes the treatment is painful, so analgesics before the procedure may be beneficial. A small urethral catheter (8–12 French) is inserted and the bladder emptied. A 50-mL volume of 50% DMSO (Rimso-50) is instilled and the catheter removed. The patient waits 15 to 30 minutes before voiding. Treatments are usually repeated four to eight times at 1- to 2-week intervals. As mentioned earlier, some patients find this treatment painful, so in these patients a pretreatment dose of ibuprofen, naproxen sodium, or ketorolac tromethamine might be considered. Some patients complain of significant irritation and burning of the urethra with DMSO treatment. This can be diminished by leaving the catheter in and clamped for the 15 to 30 minutes of treatment and then emptying the DMSO via the catheter before removal. Painful bladder spasms occur in about 10% of patients, and these may be treated with anticholinergics or belladonna and opium suppositories. All patients notice a garlic-like odor of breath and taste in the mouth for 24 to 48 hours after DMSO treatment. This can be personally and socially unpleasant for the patient, so each patient needs to be counseled about this side effect. Commonly, symptoms worsen transiently after the first treatment, so success cannot be determined until more than two treatments are done. In addition to subjective evidence of decreased symptoms, objective evidence of significantly increased bladder capacity (>100-mL increase) has been demonstrated. Unfortunately, DMSO treatments result only in remission of disease, not cure. At least 30% to 60% of patients relapse within the first year after successful treatment. Compounding this, retreatment with DMSO after relapse of symptoms is less effective, and many patients ultimately become resistant to DMSO treatment.

Heparin has been used intravesically to repair the glycosaminoglycan layer of the bladder. This modality has the advantage that the patient can be taught self-administration. Approximately 40% to 50% of patients respond to intravesical heparin therapy. Ten thousand units of heparin in 10 mL of sterile water are instilled into the bladder via a small urethral catheter (8–12 French) three to five times per week. The patient needs to retain the heparin without voiding for at least 1 hour. Four to 12 months of heparin therapy is necessary to achieve a clinical response. Heparin is not significantly absorbed into the circulation from the bladder, so partial thromboplastin time assays are not needed.

Intravesical instillations with anesthetic agents to directly anesthetize the painful bladder have been used with some success. One "anesthetic cocktail" as reported by Moldwin includes 30 mL of a 1:1 0.5% bupivacaine and 2% lidocaine jelly solution. Twenty-thousand units of heparin, 40 mg triamcinolone, and 80 mg gentamicin are added to the solution. The solution is instilled into the bladder, and the patient is instructed to hold the solution for 30 minutes before voiding. Instillations are repeated weekly for 8 to 12 weeks and patients describe significant pain relief.

Hyaluronic acid is a natural proteoglycan found in connective tissue and in human mast cell secretory granules. Instillation into patients with refractory IC showed a 70% improvement rate in symptoms after 14 weeks. Installation of other agents has shown symptom improvement as well (silver nitrate, bacillus Calmette-Guérin, capsaicin, and Resiniferatoxin), although these are not as widely available or commonly used.

Neuromodulation

Percutaneous sacral nerve root neuromodulation has been approved by the U.S. Food and Drug Administration for the treatment of IC. In a trial of neuromodulation, symptoms of urinary frequency, urgency, and pain were all improved in 15 women with refractory IC. Mean voided volumes increased, daytime frequency and nocturia decreased, and pain scores decreased as well in these patients. The procedure is performed in two stages. The first stage involves percutaneous placement of a test electrode in the S3 foramen that is attached to a small portable stimulator unit. During this test phase of stimulation, the patient keeps a voiding diary and monitors for symptomatic improvement. If the trial is successful, then a permanent electrode lead and stimulator unit is implanted. Although the exact mechanism of action for neuromodulation is unknown, success rates of up to 73% have been reported. Long-term outcomes and follow-up are necessary.

Surgical Intervention

Approximately 5% of patients have unresponsive, intractable, incapacitating symptoms that warrant surgical treatment as a last resort. Such patients usually have small fibrotic bladders and diminished capacity (<400 mL), void 18 to 20 times per day, and have severe uncontrolled pain. Cystectomy, urethrectomy, and continent diversion with a Koch or Indiana pouch have been the most successful and acceptable surgical treatment. However, in one series of such patients, 2 of 15 developed subsequent pouch pain.

A less aggressive surgical approach, with some degree of success, is neodymium:YAG laser ablation of the bladder lining. Of 24 patients with IC and Hunner ulcers who underwent treatment with the neodymium:YAG laser, all had symptom improvement within 2 to 3 days. However, relapse occurred in 11 patients, requiring one to four additional treatments. Although minimally invasive, treatment complications may include bowel injury with prolonged ablation at the dome.

In summary, the mainstays of current treatment for IC are a combination of behavioral changes, oral therapies, and hydrodistention followed by intravesical therapy. The effectiveness of combining these modalities has not been well studied. More research on the effectiveness of treatment for IC is needed, but such research is difficult to perform. Because the major clinical characteristics of IC are subjective symptoms, it is crucial that measurements such as visual or verbal analogue pain ratings, voiding intervals, voided volumes, and visual or verbal analogue ratings of urgency be used. Also, placebo-controlled studies are needed because studies show placebo response rates of 10% to 25% in IC patients. Given the poor quality of life scores reported by patients with IC, psychological, behavioral, and chronic pain counseling is an important adjunct to therapy.

BIBLIOGRAPHY

Baskin LS, Tanagho EA. Pelvic pain without pelvic organs. *J Urol* 1992;147:683–686.

Cannon TW, Chancellor MB. Pharmacotherapy of the overactive bladder and advances in drug delivery. *Clin Obstet Gynecol* 2002;45:205–217.

Chai TC. Diagnosis of the painful bladder syndrome: current approaches to diagnosis. *Clin Obstet Gynecol* 2002;45:250–258.

Gillenwater JY, Wein AJ. Summary of the National Institute of Arthritis, Diabetes, Digestive and Kidney Diseases Workshop on Interstitial Cystitis, National Institutes of Health, Bethesda, MD, August 28–29, 1987. *J Urol* 1988;140:203–206.

Maher CF, Carey MP, Dwyer PL, et al. Percutaneous sacral nerve root neuromodulation for intractable interstitial cystitis. *Urology* 2001;165:884–886.

Moldwin R. *The interstitial cystitis survival guide.* Oakland, CA: New Harbinger Publications, 2002.

Moldwin RP, Sant GR. Interstitial cystitis: a pathophysiology and treatment update. *Clin Obstet Gynecol* 2002;45:259–272.

Morales A, Emerson L, Nickel JC, et al. Intravesical hyaluronic acid in the treatment of refractory interstitial cystitis. *J Urol* 1996;156:45–48.

Myers DL, Aguilar VC. Gynecologic manifestations of interstitial cystitis. *Clin Obstet Gynecol* 2002;45:233–241.

Oberpenning F, van Ophoven A, Hertle L. Interstitial cystitis: an update. *Curr Opin Urol* 2002;12:321–332.

Parsons CL, Koprowski PE. Interstitial cystitis: successful management by increasing urinary voiding intervals. *Urology* 1991;38:207.

Parsons L. Interstitial cystitis: epidemiology and clinical presentation. *Clin Obstet Gynecol* 2002;45:242–249.

Peters KM. The diagnosis and treatment of intersitial cystitis. *Urol Nurs* 2000;20:101–107, 131.

Rofeim O, Hom D, Freid RM, et al. Use of the neodymium:YAG laser for interstitial cystitis: a prospective study. *J Urol* 2001;166:134–136.

Rothrock NE, Lutgendorf SK, Kreder KJ, et al. Stress and symptoms in patients with interstitial cystitis: a life stress model. *Urology* 2001;57:422–427.

Sant GR. Intravesical 50% dimethyl sulfoxide (RIMSO-50) in the treatment of interstitial cystitis. *Urology* 1987;29[Suppl]:17.

Sant GR, Hanno PM. Interstitial cystitis: current issues and controversies in diagnosis. *Urology* 2001;57[Suppl 6A]:82–88.

Theoharides TC, Kempuraj D, Sant GR. Mast cell involvement in interstitial cystitis: a review of human and experimental evidence. *Urology* 2001;57[Suppl 6A]:47–55.

Theoharides TC, Sant GR. New agents for the medical treatment of interstitial cystitis. *Exp Opin Invest Drugs* 2001;10:521–546.

Wein AJ, Hanno PM. Targets for therapy of the painful bladder. *Urology* 2002;59[Suppl 5A]:68–73.

Wesselmann U. Interstitial cystitis: a chronic visceral pain syndrome. *Urology* 2001;57[Suppl 6A]:32–39.

CHAPTER 81
Urinary Incontinence

Eric Sokol and Sarah Fox

Urinary incontinence (UI) affects approximately 13 million Americans with an estimated annual cost of more than $15 billion. It is estimated that 50% of patients who suffer from incontinence do not report the problem to a health care provider. Patients may not report symptoms because of the social stigma attached to UI, because they believe incontinence is an inevitable part of the aging process, or because of the lack of knowledge of available treatments. In addition, when UI is reported, many physicians and nurses are hesitant or ill prepared to manage the problem. As a result, this medical problem is vastly underdiagnosed and underreported. With a growing elderly population, it can be expected that even more people will be affected by UI in the future.

UI impacts the patient and her family in a number of ways. Patients are embarrassed by the leakage and odor. They may isolate themselves from friends and family and avoid intimacy due to the leakage of urine. A loss of self-esteem and even depression can result from their isolation. UI is a major cause of institutionalization of the elderly. Among nursing facility residents, the prevalence of UI is greater than 50%. UI is also a major cause of hip fractures in the elderly, which occur due to a fall while rushing to the toilet. Finally, the cost of incontinence pads, laundry, and medications for UI can be a hardship for patients on a fixed income.

Such a common and important medical problem deserves to be incorporated into routine health maintenance. This chapter addresses patient identification, prevention strategies, basic diagnostic techniques, and noninvasive, medical, and surgical management techniques.

ANATOMY

This section reviews anatomic topics related to UI. Female continence is maintained by the interaction of muscle, connective tissue, and nerves in the pelvic floor. The three layers of the pelvic floor function as a sheet of musculofascial tissue that spans the bony pelvis and provides critical support to the pelvic viscera. The first and deepest layer of the pelvic floor is the endopelvic fascia, which connects the vagina, urethra, and rectum to the side walls of the pelvis. The fascia is associated intimately with the pelvic viscera and the second layer of the pelvic floor, the levator ani.

The levator ani is a muscle complex consisting of several smaller muscles that function as a group (Fig. 81.1). It attaches anteriorly to the bony pelvis at the pubic bones, laterally to the ischial spines and arcus tendineus levator ani, and passes posteriorly behind the rectum to the sacrum and coccyx. The levator ani muscle group includes the iliococcygeus muscle and the puborectalis and pubococcygeus muscles, which are referred to together as the pubovisceral muscle. The iliococcygeus muscle arises from the pelvic side wall, specifically from the arcus tendineus levator ani. It inserts into a midline raphe, which forms a sheetlike layer over the midplane of the pelvis. The pubovisceral muscle extends in a U-shape around the rectum, attaching to the vagina and urethra as it passes by them. On contraction, the pubovisceral muscle lifts the rectum, vagina,

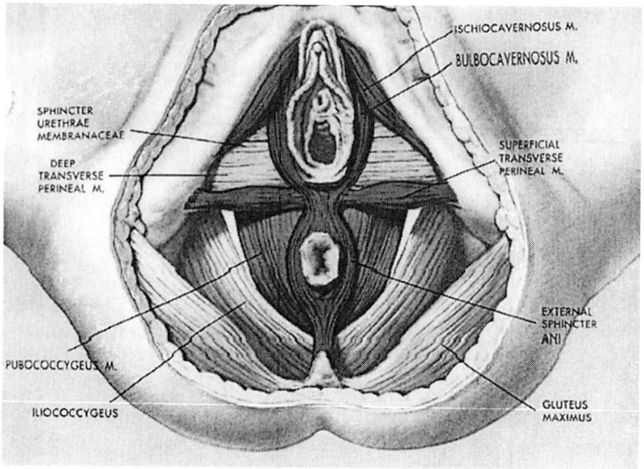

FIG. 81.1. Pelvic floor muscles as seen from below.

and urethra anteriorly, compressing the lumens of each structure. The close approximation of the endopelvic fascia and the levator ani form a pelvic diaphragm with tremendous strength, flexibility, and resiliency.

The third and most superficial layer of the pelvic floor is made up of the external urethral and anal sphincters and the perineal membrane. The perineal membrane is a triangular fibrous layer that attaches the perineal body and vaginal side walls to the pubis and limits descent of the pelvic viscera. The perineal membrane does not provide primary support to the pelvic viscera. Instead, it functions as a back-up support that prevents excessive downward movement of the perineal body and pelvic organs when the levator ani are relaxed, as during urination, defecation, and childbirth.

The striated urogenital muscle, or external urethral sphincter, is located just cranial to the perineal membrane and is made up of the bilateral compressor urethrae, the urethrovaginal sphincter, and the sphincter urethrae muscles. These muscles surround the central portion of the urethra and play a minor role in maintaining resting urethral pressures and a major role in increasing urethral pressures in response to a sudden increase in intra-abdominal pressures.

The internal sphincter is located at the vesical neck, where the urethra transverses the vesical wall. It is made up of the trigonal ring and detrusor loop muscles, which are smooth involuntary muscle extensions of the detrusor muscle of the bladder. The internal sphincter is the primary contributor to resting pressures in the urethra. The urethral mucosa, which is rich in estrogen receptors and mucosal and submucosal vessels, provides additional resting pressure and aids in coaptation of the urethra at rest.

The female continence mechanism relies on the levator ani muscular and arcus tendineus fascial attachments to urethral supports, internal and external sphincteric mechanisms, and mucosal and submucosal vasculature.

When abdominal pressure increases, such as with a cough, the urethra must maintain closure by maintaining a pressure that is higher than the intravesical pressure. Intact connective tissue attachments of the suburethral fascia to the fascia of the arcus tendineus and to the levator ani muscles result in a firm platform that remains relatively stable in the face of the force generated by a cough. As the downward force is halted, the urethra is compressed and continence is maintained. If damage occurs to the endopelvic fascia or the levator ani muscles, downward pressure will displace the urethra caudally and there will not be enough compression to increase urethral pressures above the vesical pressures, resulting in leakage of urine. In addition, if the internal sphincter is damaged and resting pressures are low, leakage can occur with sudden increases in intraabdominal pressure, even if the external urethral sphincter and levator ani muscles are functioning properly.

NEUROUROLOGY

Bladder function cannot be fully understood without basic knowledge of neurophysiology. The bladder is unique because it is an "involuntary" organ that is under voluntary control. During the filling phase of the storage and emptying cycle, the bladder relaxes and maintains a low resting pressure as it accommodates increasing urine volumes. There is a gradual increase in urethral resistance to prevent urine loss during the filling phase. When the bladder has filled to a specific volume, tension receptors in the bladder sense fullness, and when an appropriate time presents, a voluntary micturition reflex is initiated.

The lower urinary tract receives innervation from three sources. The sympathetic division of the autonomic nervous system controls urine storage, the parasympathetic division of the autonomic nervous system controls bladder emptying, and somatic innervation controls voluntary function of the pelvic floor musculature and the striated external urethral sphincter. Efferent sympathetic nerves arise from spinal cord segments T11 through L2 or L3 run through the hypogastric nerve plexus and innervate the pelvic organs, including the lower urinary tract, the rectum, and internal genital organs. Parasympathetic neurons arises from spinal levels S2-4 and run through the pelvic nerve and the hypogastric nerve plexus, meet with the sympathetic nerve fibers in Frankenhäuser's plexus, and then continue to the bladder and other pelvic organs. Spinal levels S2-4 also give rise to the pudendal nerve, which is responsible for somatic and sensory innervation to the pelvic floor and urethral and anal sphincters.

In the autonomic system, the preganglionic neurotransmitter is acetylcholine. Likewise, in the parasympathetic system, the postganglionic neurotransmitter is acetylcholine. The detrusor muscle is filled with muscarinic cholinergic receptors that, when stimulated, result in detrusor contraction and bladder emptying. This explains why anticholinergic medications are the mainstay of treatment for patients with detrusor overactivity. The postganglionic neurotransmitter for the sympathetic autonomic system is norepinephrine, which stimulates adrenergic receptors. α-Adrenergic receptors, found in the urethra and bladder neck, regulate vasoconstriction and smooth muscle contraction. When stimulated, the tone of the urethra will increase, maintaining continence. β-Adrenergic receptors are found in the bladder wall and function to relax the smooth muscle of the bladder and allow storage of urine.

Multiple complex facilitative and inhibitory pathways interact at the level of the spinal cord, which function under the control of higher centers. Above the level of the spinal cord, the most important facilitative motor center for micturition is the pontine micturition center located in the brainstem. The cerebellum is the major center for controlling pelvic floor relaxation and the rate and force of detrusor contractions. The basal ganglia are involved in inhibition of detrusor contractions. The cerebral cortex, primarily the frontal lobes, is important in inhibition of the pontine micturition reflex.

A promising area of neurourology involves the role of the external urethral sphincter in preventing stress UI. It has been noted that most patients with stress UI have reduced but measurable levels of sphincteric function. New research is addressing ways to improve sphincter function. Onuf's nucleus in the sacral spinal cord is the site of origin of somatic nerves to the external urethral sphincter. The neurons in Onuf's nucleus are of a unique size and are densely packed. Onuf's nucleus also has a high density of serotonin-2 (5-HT_2) receptors that, when stimulated, increase sphincter tone. These factors will allow researchers to develop medications that specifically target the neurons of Onuf's nucleus, thereby increasing external urethral sphincter tone and decreasing incontinence episodes.

CLASSIFICATION

Current classifications of UI are based on the 2002 recommendations from the International Continence Society.

Stress Urinary Incontinence

Stress incontinence is the loss of urine in the presence of increased abdominal pressure. Patients will describe leakage, often in small amounts, that occurs at the exact moment of coughing, sneezing, or any exertion that raises intra-abdominal pressure. The diagnosis of *urodynamic stress incontinence* (previously referred to as genuine stress incontinence) is made by urodynamic testing, confirming the presence of leakage of urine with increased intra-abdominal pressure without evidence of detrusor contractions. *Intrinsic sphincter deficiency* is a subtype of stress incontinence associated with very low urethral pressures due to a weakened urethral sphincter. The diagnosis of intrinsic sphincter deficiency is made by urodynamic testing and is discussed later in the chapter. It is important to identify patients with intrinsic sphincter deficiency before surgical interventions because they may require special surgical procedures.

Urge Urinary Incontinence

Hallmarks of urge incontinence include the loss of urine accompanied by the strong urge to void, *increased daytime frequency* (defined as more than eight voids in a 24-hour period), and *nocturia* (defined as waking more than once at night to void). Patients may report small amounts of leakage of urine or complete bladder emptying associated with triggers such as rushing to the bathroom, running water, cold weather, and hearty laughter. *Detrusor overactivity incontinence* is an urodynamic diagnosis of leakage accompanied by detrusor muscle contractions. *Neurogenic detrusor overactivity* is when detrusor contractions are caused by a neurologic cause such as a spinal cord injury. *Overactive bladder*, *detrusor instability*, and *sensory urgency* all are older terms for urge UI.

Mixed Incontinence

Mixed incontinence occurs when both stress and urge symptoms are present. The patient may note that either stress or urge symptoms are more prominent. It is very important to determine which symptoms bother the patient more and address them accordingly. These patients may present with a complex array of symptoms and may require further diagnostic testing before treatment.

Chronic Retention of Urine

When the bladder is unable to empty properly and becomes overdistended, urinary leakage may occur. In women, chronic retention may be due to a large uterine or vaginal wall prolapse partially obstructing the urethra, poor detrusor tone due to advanced age, or postsurgical complications. Patients with chronic retention may present with symptoms consistent with stress or urge incontinence, but if the underlying retention is treated, symptoms will usually resolve.

Extraurethral Incontinence

This category includes less common causes of UI, such as a fistula or an ectopic ureter. These patients will usually describe constant leakage, even during the night and without exertion. If incontinence is present since birth, an ectopic ureter should be suspected. A fistula is usually associated with previous surgery or radiation.

Uncategorized Incontinence

Some patients with a normally functioning bladder and urethra are unable to make it to the toilet because of physical constraints such as limited mobility or because of impaired mental status due to dementia or oversedation from medications.

PREDISPOSING FACTORS

Specific risk factors for incontinence should be identified and corrected with targeted interventions whenever possible. The incidence of incontinence is sufficiently high that the development of a prevention program addressing modifiable risk factors could reduce new cases of incontinence in community-dwelling women alone by approximately 50,000 cases annually. Age and female gender are major risk factors for UI. Modifiable risk factors include damage to the pelvic floor and bladder irritants.

The pelvic floor may become damaged by a number of mechanisms that can contribute to the development of UI. Trauma to the pelvic floor can weaken the collagen fibers that provide fascial support to the pelvic organs. These fibers can also be congenitally weak, contributing to UI and pelvic organ prolapse. Damage and stretch to the pudendal nerve, such as may occur in childbirth, weakens the levator ani muscles, which are crucial in the continence mechanism. Childbirth increases the risk of UI, particularly in patients who have difficult deliveries, operative deliveries, or large infants. However, a recent study by Buchsbaum et al. showed the incidence of UI to be almost 50% in a group of 149 nulliparous nuns. This study highlights the fact that the relationship between childbirth and UI is not straightforward, and that it is important to ask all women about UI, regardless of parity. Activities other than childbirth that can damage the pelvic floor include repetitive heavy lifting, smoking and chronic cough, asthma, and chronic constipation. Constipation, in addition to damaging the pelvic floor by repeated Valsalva maneuvers, can also cause worsening urge symptoms when the bladder is irritated by the chronically distended rectosigmoid colon. Foreign bodies such as bladder calculi and bladder tumors, urinary tract infections, and bladder irritants such caffeine, alcohol, and cigarette smoke increase the risk for urge incontinence.

The tissues of the pelvic floor, bladder, urethra, and vagina are rich in estrogen receptors. The reduced levels of estrogen during menopause result in atrophy and thinning of these tissues, thereby compromising their function. Urethral pressures may decrease with atrophy, accounting for more stress incontinence symptoms. The reduction in endogenous estrogens may help to explain why many women note the onset of UI in the perimenopausal period.

TABLE 81.1. Medications that Affect Bladder Function

Medications	Effect on the bladder
Diuretics	Polyuria, frequency, and urgency
Caffeine	Aggravation or precipitation of urge symptoms
Anticholinergic agents, including antihistamines, opiates, antispasmodics, anti-Parkinson agents	Urinary retention, overflow incontinence, fecal impaction
Psychotropics	
Antidepressants	Anticholinergic actions, sedation
Antipsychotics	Anticholinergic actions, sedation, rigidity, and immobility causing sedation, delirium, immobility, muscle relaxation
Sedatives/hypnotics/ CNS depressants	
Narcotic analgesics	Urinary retention, fecal impaction, sedation, delirium
α-Adrenergic blockers	Urethral relaxation
α-Adrenergic agonists	Urinary retention (present in many cold and diet over-the-counter preparations)
β-Adrenergic agonists	Urinary retention
Calcium channel blockers	Urinary retention

Neurologic diseases such as diabetes mellitus, multiple sclerosis, stroke, and spinal cord injury are often associated with UI. Initially, patients will note urge incontinence and neurogenic detrusor overactivity. As the nerve damage progresses, patients will have a large atonic bladder with poor detrusor function, which leads to chronic urinary retention.

The elderly are especially at risk for transient causes of incontinence, including delirium, infection, severe depression, restricted mobility, and stool impaction. Medications may affect bladder function (Table 81.1) or may be so sedating to the patient that she is not aware of her need to void.

The risk of worsening urinary function can be minimized by helping patients to control constipation, manage fluids and medications, lose weight, stop smoking, control asthma, and practice Kegel exercises, which are discussed later.

PATIENT INTERVIEW

The interview is an important aspect of the evaluation of a patient with UI. The clinician should screen all women, regardless of age, by asking if they have trouble holding their urine or have problems with urinary frequency or urgency. The patient may be ashamed of her symptoms and reluctant to offer information without direct questioning.

A thorough urogynecologic review of symptoms is long and can be time consuming (Fig. 81.2). Allowing the patient to fill out a questionnaire at home gives her the chance to think about her symptoms and provide more accurate information. The questionnaire should be reviewed with the patient at a subsequent visit. Although the patient history can help with diagnosis, it should be remembered that it is not a perfect predictor of the underlying disease process. Studies of the use of history to predict stress or urge UI have shown sensitivities of 70% to 90% and specificities of 50% to 55% when compared with the gold standard of urodynamic testing. History and physical examination may provide enough information to manage patients with nonsurgical interventions. For those with a complex history or those who wish to have surgical management of UI, further testing, including urodynamics testing, may be indicated. The most important part of the initial interview is to determine the patient's goals for the consultation. It may be that she believes her leakage is due to a cancer and simply wants reassurance, she may be worried that her symptoms will worsen over time, or she may find her current symptoms unacceptable and wish to have more aggressive treatment. The diagnostic and treatment plans should be tailored to the individual patient.

It is important to distinguish whether the patient experiences stress or urge symptoms and, if she has mixed incontinence, which symptoms are most bothersome. Patients with urge UI often find that symptoms may be stimulated by the sound or site of running water or by placing a key in the lock on returning home.

Women with incontinence may restrict their fluid intake in an attempt to minimize their incontinent episodes. This worsens symptoms because concentrated urine irritates the bladder and dehydration causes constipation. To get a better picture of daily intake, urine output, frequency, and number of incontinent episodes, a voiding diary is invaluable (Fig. 81.3). The patient is asked to keep such a diary for 24 to 48 hours and bring it with her on her next visit. This helps the clinician assess whether excessive fluid intake is part of the problem and can help to gauge the severity of the incontinence. The diary also helps follow progress as different therapeutic modalities are applied.

Systems related to the bladder should be reviewed as well. Does the patient note a vaginal bulge and is it necessary for her to manually replace the bulge to void or defecate? Does she have trouble with fecal incontinence or constipation? Is she sexually active and, if not, is the abstinence due to incontinence? Patients with hematuria, especially those who are heavy smokers or have a history of exposure to aniline dyes, should be screened for renal and bladder cancer with urine cytology and cystoscopy. If evaluation of the lower urinary tract is negative, intravenous pyelogram or computed tomography can be used to evaluate the upper urinary tract.

A full medical, neurologic, surgical, obstetric, and gynecologic history must be obtained. Pertinent aspects of the medical history include a history of asthma, renal disease, diabetes mellitus, poliomyelitis, stroke, arthritis, radiculopathies, sciatica, multiple sclerosis, syphilis, and vitamin B_{12} deficiency. Pertinent previous surgery includes hysterectomy (especially if done for previous prolapse), bladder repair, and urethral dilatation. Obstetric history should include any history of prolonged labor or complicated delivery and the weight of the largest infant. Careful examination of the medication list will determine

Urogynecology History Questionnaire

	Circle
1. Do you leak urine when you cough, sneeze, or laugh?	Y N
1A. If yes, does it come out in a spurt, dribble or constant stream?	Y N
2. Did you have bedwetting problems beyond age 5?	Y N
3. Have you wet the bed in the past year?	Y N
4. Do you ever have such an uncomfortably strong need to urinate that if you don't reach the toilet you will leak?	Y N
4A. If yes, do you ever leak before you reach the toilet?	Y N
5. How many times during the day do you urinate? ______________	
6. How many times at night do you get up to void? ______________	
7. Do you develop an urgent need to void when you are nervous, under stress, or in a hurry?	Y N
8. Do you develop a urgent need to void when you hear water running, prepare to bathe, or in cold weather?	Y N
9. Do you leak urine for no apparent reason at all?	Y N
10. Do you leak urine with intercourse?	Y N
11. Do you drink coffee, tea, or cola drinks, or eat chocolate? (Circle all that apply)	Y N
12. Do you find it hard to begin urinating?	Y N
13. Do you have a slow urinary stream?	Y N
14. Do you strain to pass urine?	Y N
15. After urination, do you have dribbling or a sense that your bladder is still full?	Y N
16. When passing urine, can you usually stop the flow?	Y N
17. Have you ever had a bladder infection?	Y N
17A. If yes, how many?__________ Any in past year?	Y N
18. Is your urine ever bloody?	Y N
19. Are you troubled by pain or discomfort when you urinate?	Y N
20. Have you ever had bladder/pelvic surgery?	Y N
21. Have you ever been treated with urethral dilatation?	Y N
21A. If yes, did it help?	Y N

(continued)

FIG. 81.2. Urogynecology history questionnaire. ***(continued on next page)***

Urogynecology History Questionnaire *(Continued)*

		Circle	
22. Did your urine problem start during or just after pregnancy?		Y	N
23. Did your urine problem start after an operation?		Y	N
Which type? ______________________________			
24. List all your medications (including vitamins, aspirin): ______________________________ ______________________________			
25. Did your urine problems start after radiation therapy?		Y	N
26. Have you ever been treated for:	kidney or bladder disease	Y	N
	kidney stones	Y	N
	kidney or bladder tumors	Y	N
	kidney or bladder injuries	Y	N
27. Did menopause make urine loss worse?		Y	N
28. Do you have problems with constipation or irregular bowel movements?		Y	N
29. Have you ever had brain, spinal, or back surgery?		Y	N
(Circle all that apply)			
30. Have you ever been treated for:	Paralysis	Y	N
	Polio	Y	N
	Multiple sclerosis	Y	N
	Stroke	Y	N
	Diabetes mellitus	Y	N
	Back pain	Y	N
	Syphilis	Y	N
31. Do you need to wear a pad because of leaking?		Y	N
31A. If yes, during the day only?		Y	N
all the time?		Y	N
32. How often do you leak in 24 hours? ______________________			
33. How long have you had a problem with leaking? ______________________			
34. Does anyone else in the family have a similar problem with leaking?		Y	N
35. Did/does anyone in your family have problems with bedwetting?		Y	N

FIG. 81.2. *(continued)*

NAME:					
DATE:					
INSTRUCTIONS: Place a check in the appropriate column next to the time you urinated in the toilet or when an incontinence episode occurred. Note the reason for the incontinence and describe your liquid intake (for example, coffee, water) and estimate the amount (for example, one cup).					
Time interval	Urinated in toilet	Had a small incontinence episode	Had a large incontinence episode	Reason for incontinence episode	Type/amount of liquid intake
6-8 a.m.					
8-10 a.m.					
10-noon					
Noon-2 p.m.					
2-4 p.m.					
4-6 p.m.					
6-8 p.m.					
8-10 p.m.					
10-midnight					
Overnight					
No. of pads used today:			No. of episodes:		
Comments:					

FIG. 81.3. Sample voiding diary.

whether there may be an iatrogenic component to the incontinence.

PHYSICAL EXAMINATION

Observation of the patient walking into the examination room reveals mobility problems that may make it difficult for the patient to reach the bathroom in time. Lower extremity edema, if present, should be noted. Patients with congestive heart failure may have third-spaced fluid in their lower extremities during the day and mobilize the fluid at night, leading to nocturia. Any pelvic or abdominal masses should be diagnosed and treated appropriately. A neurologic examination should include sensory and motor strength of the lower extremities. During the pelvic examination, further neurologic evaluation will include testing the bulbocavernosus reflex, which confirms proper function of the sacral reflex arcs. This reflex can be elicited by gently touching lateral to the clitoris with a cotton-tipped applicator and observing contraction of the external anal sphincter. Alternatively, an "anal wink" can be elicited by gently touching lateral to the external anal sphincter and observing the contraction of the anal sphincter. Bulbocavernosus or anal wink testing should be done at the beginning of the pelvic examination, because these reflexes accommodate to touch and are less likely to be elicited later in the examination. These reflexes are absent in about 15% of normal patients.

The pelvic examination continues with examination of the external genitalia, noting evidence of genital atrophy or excoriation and irritation, which may be due to contact with wet pads or undergarments. If the vulva is irritated, use of a petroleum-based barrier products (such as those used for diaper rash) and frequent pad changes should be encouraged. Vaginal and uterine support and the presence of pelvic organ prolapse should be documented, as discussed in Chapter 32. The urethra and bladder base should be palpated for tenderness and masses, which may lead one to suspect the presence of a diverticulum. At this point the patient should have a full bladder and the clinician can stand to the side, spread the labia, and ask the patient to perform a Valsalva maneuver or cough and observe for urine loss. If no urine loss is documented in the lithotomy position, the patient should be asked to stand and again to cough.

To perform an adequate bimanual examination, the patient's bladder must be empty, because a full bladder can interfere with the evaluation of the pelvic organs. After the patient empties her bladder, the clinician can measure a postvoid residual volume using either a sterile bladder catheter or by ultrasound measurement. If there is any evidence that the patient may not be able to empty her bladder completely, a postvoid residual volume should be performed. Although there is no defined normal value for a postvoid residual volume, those less than 50 mL are generally considered to be normal and those consistently over 100 mL are considered to have chronic retention of urine. Postvoid residual volume measurements should be repeated on at least two separate occasions for greater accuracy.

The Q-tip test was traditionally used to document urethral hypermobility in patients with UI. A cotton swab, lubricated with Xylocaine jelly, is placed into the urethra to the level of the urethrovesical junction. An orthopedic goniometer is used to measure the angle of excursion during a Valsalva maneuver. If the angle of excursion is greater than 30 degrees, the diagnosis of urethral hypermobility is made. Recent evidence has shown that in patients with stage 2 or greater cystocele, there is always hypermobility and the Q-tip test is unnecessary. The Q-tip test is most useful for patients without a large cystocele who are planning to have a surgical repair.

After examination of the cervix, uterus, and adnexa, the patient's ability to contract her levator ani muscles can be evaluated by asking her to squeeze the clinician's fingers with her vagina. The levator muscles can be palpated at the 5 and 7 o'clock position approximately 5 cm inside the vaginal introitus. The muscle response is graded on a 0 to 5 muscle strength scale, with 0 being no response and 5 being a strong contraction with the ability to hold for more than 5 seconds. This measurement can be used to monitor the patient's progress with pelvic floor exercises. If the patient's muscle strength is 0/5, they will be unable to perform Kegel exercises adequately and should look at other treatment modalities, such as electrical stimulation. It is also important to assess the external anal sphincter tone during the rectovaginal examination. Finally, a clean-catch urine specimen should be sent for urinalysis and culture to rule out infection and hematuria.

URODYNAMIC TESTING

Although outcome studies of urodynamic testing are lacking, most urogynecologists agree that any office evaluation of UI should include an assessment of bladder filling, voiding, and the urethral sphincter mechanism. One way of evaluating bladder and urethral function is by performing multichannel urodynamics, including cystometry, uroflowmetry, and urethral pressure profilometry. However, in this era of cost containment, the issue of which patients should undergo multichannel urodynamics is a contentious one. Although many urogynecologists have strong opinions about when these tests should be performed, appropriate indications for urodynamics remain unclear.

Clearly, urodynamic testing has a role in elucidating the etiology of UI. Most would agree that multichannel urodynamic testing is indicated if a surgical intervention is planned, if the patient has failed previous surgery, if the clinical picture is unclear, or if the patient has failed a medical therapeutic trial. Test results, however, are dependent on the skill of the clinician performing the studies. This is especially true when studying a patient with significant prolapse, where potential stress incontinence may be masked by urethral "kinking." The key to performing accurate studies is to reproduce the patient's symptoms in the laboratory.

The urodynamic examination allows identification and quantification of the in vivo process of urine storage and micturition. Figure 81.4 shows a typical urodynamic laboratory set up with a birthing chair and urodynamic software used in data processing. Though details about urodynamic testing are beyond the interest of most primary care physicians, it is helpful to know what information to expect when a patient is sent for such testing. The evaluation typically consists of a uroflow, cystometrogram, urethral pressure profile, and pressure-voiding study.

The uroflow is a screening tool for voiding dysfunction in which the patient voids into a special commode that can electronically measure time versus volume and thereby assess urine flow patterns (Fig. 81.5). A normal uroflow pattern is shown in Fig. 81.6. An intermittent or prolonged uroflow pattern suggests a voiding disorder such as an underactive detrusor muscle or outlet obstruction that should be further evaluated by pressure-flow studies.

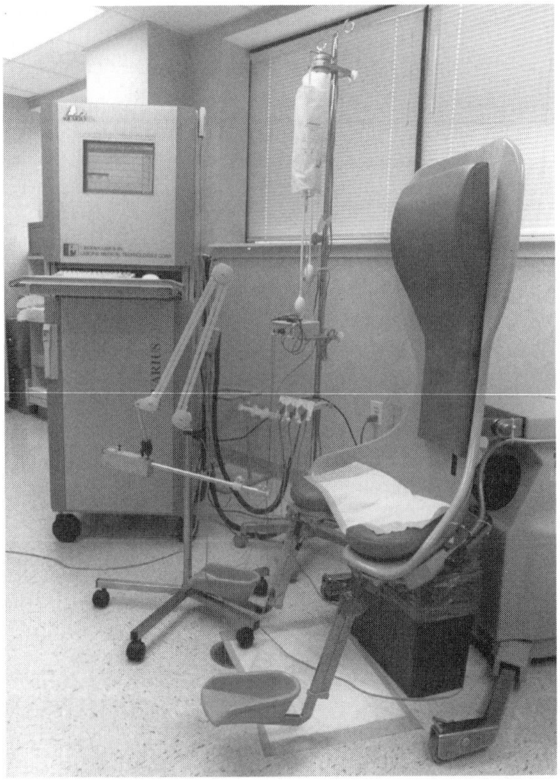

FIG. 81.4. Typical urodynamic laboratory.

The complex cystometrogram is performed by placing a pressure catheter into the vagina or rectum to measure abdominal pressure and a double-sensor catheter in the urethra and bladder. By subtracting the abdominal pressure from the vesical pressure, the true bladder (i.e., detrusor) pressure can be measured while filling the bladder with sterile saline or water.

The cystometrogram is performed with the catheters in place, with the goal of differentiating urodynamic stress incontinence from detrusor overactivity. The patient is asked to cough or perform Valsalva maneuvers at different times during bladder filling, and any leakage caused by these provocative maneuvers is noted. If the patient leaks at the exact moment of

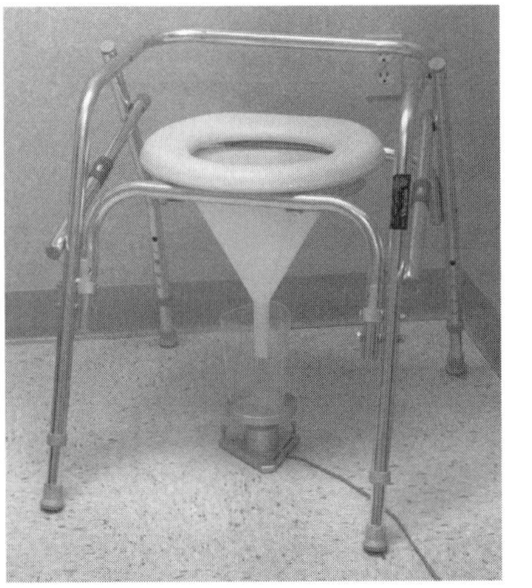

FIG. 81.5. Commode linked to electrical device to perform uroflow.

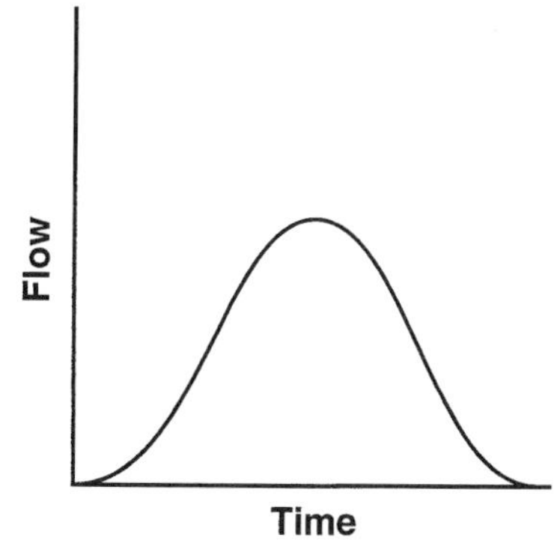

FIG. 81.6. Normal uroflow pattern.

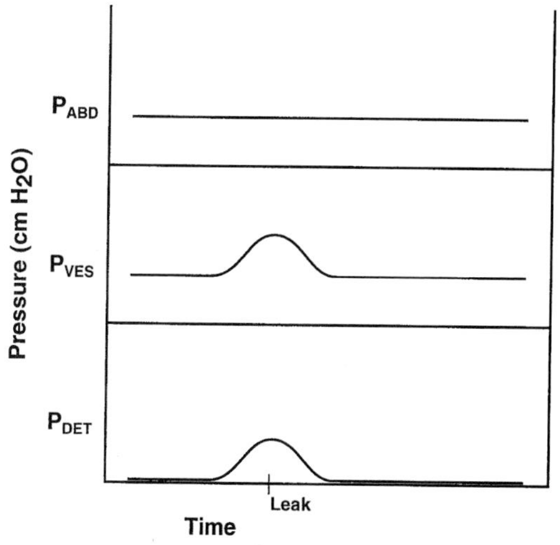

Abdominal Pressure = P_{ABD}

Bladder Pressure = P_{VES}

Detrusor Pressure = P_{DET}

FIG. 81.8. Detrusor overactivity.

increased abdominal pressure without a concomitant rise in detrusor pressure, then she has urodynamic stress incontinence (Fig. 81.7). If, on the other hand, any significant rise occurs in the true detrusor pressure during filling or provocation, detrusor overactivity is demonstrated (Fig. 81.8).

During the bladder filling phase, the patient is asked to state when she first becomes aware of bladder fullness (first sensation of bladder filling; normal is 100–150 mL), when she would definitely be looking for a bathroom (functional bladder capacity; normal is 350–500 mL), and when she can no longer tolerate any more fluid (maximal cystometric capacity; normal is 500–600 mL). These estimates of normal are general guidelines but may vary between patients. In addition, bladder compliance can also be assessed. As the bladder fills, the change in vesical pressure should be minimal. Low compliance or high vesical pressures may be associated with urge symptoms.

Two tests may be used to assess intrinsic urethral sphincter function. Abdominal leak point pressures are performed by recording pressures with a Valsalva at the time of leakage. Pressures less than 60 cm H_2O are associated with a diagnosis of intrinsic sphincter deficiency. The second test is the urethral pressure profile, which is performed by pulling the urethral catheter along the length of the urethra while measuring closure pressures (Fig. 81.9). A maximum urethral closure pressure of

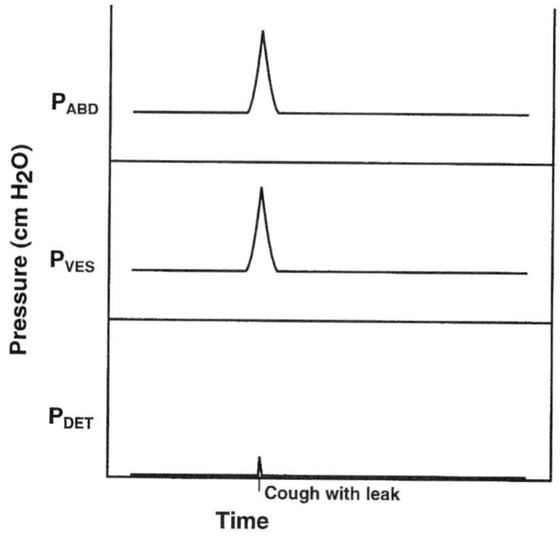

Abdominal Pressure = P_{ABD}

Bladder Pressure = P_{VES}

Detrusor Pressure = $P_{DET} = (P_{VES} - P_{ABD})$

FIG. 81.7. Urodynamic stress incontinence.

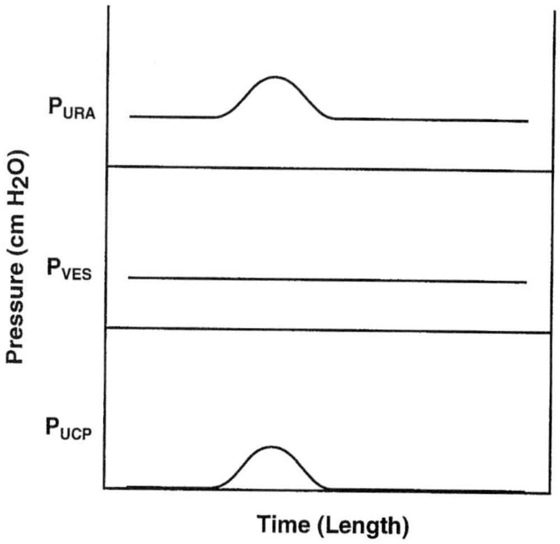

Urethral Pressure = P_{URA}

Vesical Pressure = P_{VES}

Urethral Closure Pressure = $P_{UCP} = (P_{URA} - P_{VES})$

FIG. 81.9. Urethral pressure profile.

less than 20 cm H_2O is another parameter that suggests intrinsic sphincter deficiency. This test can also measure the functional urethral length, that is, the length of the urethra that maintains a pressure above that of the bladder (normal, >2.5 cm).

Finally, the patient is instructed to void with the catheters in place, and a pressure-void study is performed to assess the voiding mechanism. A normal voiding mechanism involves urethral relaxation with detrusor pressure elevation (Fig. 81.10). Especially in the elderly, a prolonged uroflow pattern can sometimes be found in the absence of a functional outlet obstruction. Usually, these patients are found to have poor detrusor contractions, which can be documented during this examination.

Given the cost constraints of multichannel urodynamics, there are some simple, inexpensive tests that can be performed in a primary care office setting before moving on to more complex studies. The first simple test is to check a postvoid residual after the patient urinates. In general, postvoid residuals of less than 50 mL are considered adequate bladder emptying. Repetitive postvoid residuals ranging from 100 to 200 or higher are considered inadequate emptying and may be indicative of chronic urinary retention (i.e., detrusor failure), leading to overflow incontinence.

In place of a cystometrogram, simple cystometry can be performed by filling the bladder in a retrograde fashion with a 60-mL syringe (without its plunger) connected to a catheter. Water is poured into the syringe in 60-mL aliquots, and the patient's first bladder sensation and bladder capacity are noted. If the water level in the syringe begins to rise or overflow during filling, an uninhibited bladder contraction may be occurring. A standing cough stress test and supine empty bladder cough stress test can be performed at this time. These simple tests can help differentiate detrusor overactivity from stress UI and can give information about a patient's bladder sensation and bladder capacity.

A simple "uroflow" test can be performed by listening to the patient voiding in the bathroom. An astute clinician can obtain much valuable information from this simple test, such as the time to complete the void, the sound of the urine stream, and any sounds of straining or grunting, suggesting the need to Valsalva to complete voiding. Sounds of straining or a prolonged time to complete voiding may be suggestive of outlet obstruction or poor detrusor function.

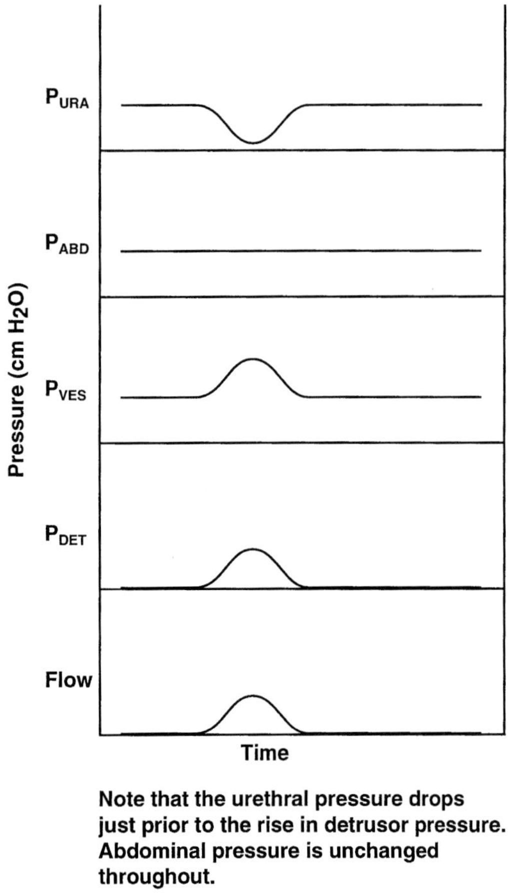
Pressure (cm H2O)
PURA
PABD
PVES
PDET
Flow
Time
Note that the urethral pressure drops just prior to the rise in detrusor pressure. Abdominal pressure is unchanged throughout.

FIG. 81.10. Pressure void study—normal.

MEDICAL MANAGEMENT

Stress Urinary Incontinence

Nonsurgical interventions can be instituted in patients who appear to have simple stress UI before referral for more advanced urodynamic testing. Some simple behavioral modifications can have a large impact on a patient's incontinence. For example, patients who admit to excessive caffeine use should be instructed to decrease intake or switch to noncaffeinated beverages because caffeine acts as a diuretic and bladder irritant. Also, overweight patients may benefit from an exercise and weight loss regimen. In addition to the obvious health benefits associated with weight loss, decreasing weight can reduce episodes of UI.

In the menopausal patient, an initial intervention is vaginal estrogen replacement, assuming no contraindications exist. Because the vagina and urethra are of similar embryologic origin, estrogen supplementation in postmenopausal women may restore urethral mucosal coaptation and increase vascularity, tone, and the α-adrenergic responsiveness of urethral muscle, which in turn may increase bladder outlet resistance and decrease stress incontinence. However, the exact role of estrogen, as well as its mechanism of action, are still unknown and deserve further research.

Another simple intervention that has been shown to improve outcomes is Kegel exercises. First described in 1938 by Dr. Arnold Kegel and later touted as a way to improve the sexual response, physicians quickly realized that patients performing these exercises suffered less from UI. Since that time, Kegel exercises have been popularized as a panacea for all types of UI. Although this view is certainly overly optimistic, Kegel exercises have been shown to reduce the frequency of urine loss in patients suffering from stress UI and can also improve the symptoms of urge incontinence.

To properly teach a patient to perform Kegel exercises, she should be instructed to squeeze her pelvic muscles around the examiner's fingers during a pelvic examination as if she were trying to stop the flow of urine or hold back gas. The clinician can explain that the levator ani muscles act as a hammock to hold up the bladder, vagina, and rectum. Once the patient has figured out the proper muscles to flex, she should be instructed to perform 10 repetitions of these exercises from three to eight times a day (between 30 and 80 repetitions). While doing the exercises, the patient should perform both short and long holds (up to 10 seconds). Typically, she should do up to four sets of each hold, remembering to completely relax her levator ani muscles between contractions. The short hold exercises work the fast-twitch muscle fibers, which account for approximately 30% of the levator muscle, whereas the long hold exercises will exercise the remaining 70% of slow-twitch muscle fibers. Patients should be discouraged from performing Kegel exercises by stopping urine flow because long-term performance of these exercises during voiding may worsen voiding function. These exercises should be performed daily for 3 months to see the best results.

For a patient with a large prolapse, performing Kegel exercises does not cure the prolapse but helps strengthen the pelvic floor and may forestall worsening of the condition. In addition, if the patient learns to perform these exercises efficiently, she may be able to prevent leakage by doing a Kegel squeeze when she is in a leak-type situation (e.g., coughing). In conjunction with medications, poor muscle tone may be improved with pelvic floor rehabilitation and electrical stimulation.

Other treatment modalities include pessaries, such as the incontinence dish and the incontinence ring. These devices can create a physical obstruction to the urethra and can stabilize the proximal urethra and bladder neck, reducing episodes of leakage caused by urethral hypermobility. Some patients with mild symptoms may find that a diaphragm or a tampon, used during exercise, can prevent leakage.

In addition to nonpharmacologic approaches, medicine can be tried in appropriate candidates. α-Agonists such as pseudoephedrine help stimulate closure of the bladder neck. Imipramine also has α-adrenergic effects and improves symptoms from stress UI in some patients. Duloxetine is a selective serotonin reuptake inhibitor that has some α-adrenergic properties and holds particular promise as a medical treatment for stress UI.

The rationale of pharmacologic therapy for stress UI caused by urethral sphincter insufficiency is based on selection of agents targeted toward the high concentration of α-adrenergic receptors in the bladder neck, bladder base, and proximal urethra. Sympathomimetic drugs with α-adrenergic agonist activity presumably cause muscle contraction in these areas and thereby increase bladder outlet resistance. Pharmacotherapeutic strategies that are designed to increase bladder outlet resistance include the use of drugs with direct α-adrenergic agonist activity, estrogen supplementation both for direct effect on urethral mucosal and periurethral tissues and for enhancement of α-adrenergic response, and β-adrenergic–blocking drugs that may allow unopposed stimulation of α-receptor–mediated contractile muscle responses.

If conservative measures do not improve a patient's symptoms, she should be referred for more extensive testing and possibly surgery. The ultimate surgical procedure chosen depends, to a large extent, on the underlying cause of the incontinence. Various surgical options include urethral fixation procedures, suburethral slings, or periurethral injections of bulking agents to improve urethral closure.

Detrusor Overactivity

Anticholinergic agents are effective as treatment for UI because they block contraction of the normal bladder and probably the unstable bladder as well. All anticholinergic drugs are contraindicated in patients with documented narrow-angle, but not wide-angle, glaucoma.

Oxybutynin has both anticholinergic and direct smooth muscle relaxant properties. Several randomized controlled studies have shown oxybutynin to be superior to placebo for the treatment of UI due to detrusor overactivity. Oxybutynin proved superior to placebo in six studies of middle-aged outpatients, reducing urge incontinence frequency by 15% to 58% over the response to placebo. In two of these studies, 43% and 67% of subjects became subjectively continent, a much better result than occurred with placebo. Oxybutynin has also been effective and well tolerated when instilled into the bladder of study patients, primarily those with neuropathic bladder.

Side effects from oxybutynin have been noted in all studies and include dry skin, blurred vision, change in mental status, nausea, constipation, and marked xerostomia (dry mouth). Severity of the side effects increased with dosage, with severe xerostomia occurring in 84% of subjects receiving 5 mg of oxybutynin four times per day. A newer extended-release formulation of oxybutynin has decreased the rate of intolerable side effects and is given 5 to 30 mg once daily.

Tolterodine is a newer anticholinergic agent that has similar effectiveness to oxybutynin and a similar side-effect profile. The immediate release formulation is taken as a 1- to 2-mg tablet twice a day. The long-acting formulation can be taken as a 2- or 4-mg tablet once daily and is well tolerated by most patients. Patients that have undesirable side effects from oxybutynin can be switched to tolterodine and vice versa, because patients may tolerate one medication more than the other.

Tricyclic antidepressants such as imipramine can be tried as a second-line therapy for detrusor overactivity in patients who fail to improve with oxybutynin or tolterodine. Imipramine acts to decrease bladder overactivity through its anticholinergic effects and can increase closing pressures in the proximal urethra through its α-adrenergic effects. Although a subset of patients will respond favorably to imipramine, there is a higher rate of side effects. The most common side effects are nausea and insomnia. Imipramine should be used with caution in the elderly because of risks of cardiac side effects.

Estrogen therapy can again be an important adjunctive therapy for patients with overactive bladder, particularly in the setting of mixed incontinence. It is imperative that patients curtail their caffeine intake and quit smoking, because both of these substances act as bladder irritants.

Patients with detrusor overactivity complain of urinary frequency, which can often be improved with a behavioral modification technique called bladder drill training. The patient is instructed to determine the longest interval she can wait between voids without risking an urge incontinence episode. She is then instructed to void on this initial schedule, increasing the interval by 15 to 30 minutes every week or two. For example, if a patient voids every hour during the day, then this is the interval that is initiated. She then progressively increases this interval, with a goal interval being every 3 to 4 hours. If the patient feels the urge to void sooner, she is instructed to attempt to dismiss the urge by performing three quick Kegel squeezes. By flexing the levator ani muscles, it is theorized that a reflex arc is interrupted, allowing the bladder to relax.

PHYSIOTHERAPY OF THE PELVIC FLOOR

When treating UI, pelvic muscle exercises may be used alone or augmented with bladder inhibition biofeedback therapy or vaginal weight training. Pelvic floor electrical stimulation is another method of pelvic muscle rehabilitation. Health care providers must teach patients the correct method of distinguishing and contracting the pelvic muscles through digital vaginal examination to verify appropriate muscle use, verbal feedback, or use of vaginal weights and biofeedback therapy to ensure accurate performance.

Biofeedback is performed by placing a sensor in the vagina and having the patient isolate her levator ani muscle by visual cues from a computer screen. Biofeedback strengthens the leva-

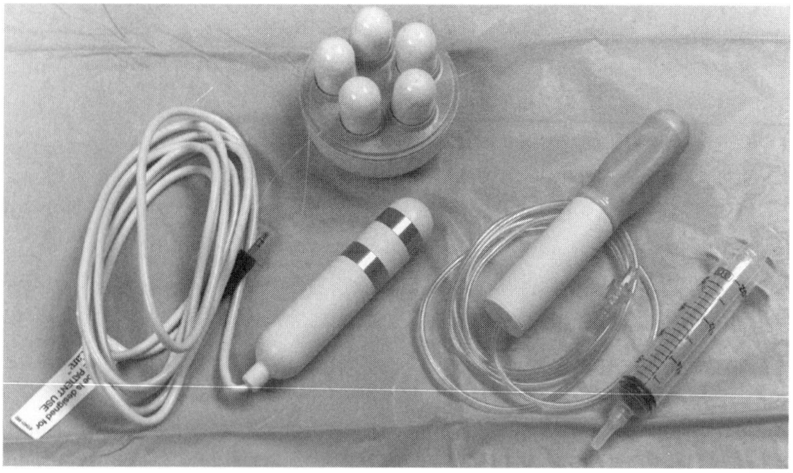

FIG. 81.11. Vaginal cones, vaginal sensors for electrical stimulation and biofeedback.

tor ani, thereby maintaining the bladder neck in a favorable position during stress, as well as strengthening the periurethral striated muscle, assisting in luminal coaptation.

Pelvic floor electrical stimulation (nonimplantable) produces a contraction of the levator ani, external urethral, and anal sphincters, accompanied by a reflex inhibition of the detrusor muscle; this activity depends on a preserved reflex arc through the sacral micturition center. Nonimplantable pelvic floor electrical stimulation uses vaginal or anal sensors or surface electrodes. Adverse reactions are minimal and include discomfort. Electrical stimulation (Fig. 81.11) is theorized to work in several ways. It may improve reinnervation of partly denervated pelvic floor muscles by promoting growth of the surviving motor axons. It also stimulates reflex inhibition of the detrusor muscle. Some suggest that it may restore normal urethral and bladder reflexes, although this is unproved.

Numerous studies show the efficacy of electrical stimulation. A 1994 study reviewed 52 patients in a prospective randomized fashion and found that electrical stimulation cured or improved 62% of them. A 1993 study showed this treatment to be effective in 71% of patients with stress urinary incontinence and 70% of patients with detrusor overactivity. When compared with the cumulative 5-year surgery success rate of 75%, these numbers are respectable. Another author found that biofeedback improved 66% of stress incontinence patients and 33% of those with detrusor overactivity. Remembering that the fundamental issue is one of quality of life, these modalities clearly are beneficial. Figure 81.12 shows a typical set-up, with screens to allow feedback to the patient as she is undergoing this therapy.

Specially designed vaginal weights for strengthening the pelvic muscles can augment pelvic muscle exercises. The patient receives a set of vaginal weights of identical shape and volume but of increasing weight (20–100 g). As part of a structured progressive resistive exercise program, women insert the weight intravaginally, with the tapered portion resting on the superior surface of the perineal muscle, and attempt to retain it by contracting the pelvic muscles up to 15 minutes. The weight is worn while the patient is ambulatory, and the exercise is done twice daily. The hypothesized mechanism of action is that the sustained contraction required to retain the weight increases the strength of the pelvic muscles, and the weight is assumed to provide heightened proprioceptive feedback to desired pelvic muscle contraction. A patient who cannot volitionally stop her urine flow by performing a Kegel exercise or one who has no

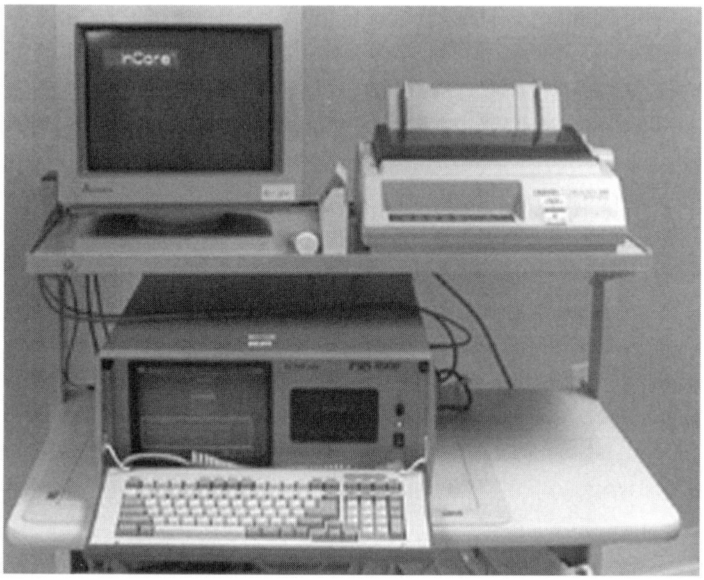

FIG. 81.12. Biofeedback monitor to enhance pelvic floor function.

palpable Kegel ability is probably not a good candidate for this therapy. Vaginal cones are shown in Fig. 81.11. Kegel exercises, biofeedback, electrical stimulation, and vaginal cones are all methods used to strengthen the pelvic floor muscles, and each can have a profound effect on the symptoms of UI when performed correctly.

SUMMARY

Due to an ever-aging population, UI is increasingly becoming a major public health problem. Though the consequences of incontinence are not generally life threatening, they can be socially isolating and devastating to patients. Primary care physicians are in a unique position on the "front line" of health care and therefore owe it to their patients to become familiar with the identification, prevention, treatment, and referral sources for UI.

BIBLIOGRAPHY

Abrams P, Cardozo L, Fall M, et al. The standardization of terminology of lower urinary tract function: report from the standardization sub-committee of the International Continence Society. *Neurourol Urodyn* 2002;21:167–178.

Buchsbaum GM, Chin M, Glantz C, et al. Prevalence of urinary incontinence and associated risk factors in a cohort of nuns. *Obstet Gynecol* 2002;100:226–229.

Cogan SL, Weber AM, Hammel JP. Is urethral mobility really being assessed by the pelvic organ prolapse quantification (POP-Q) system? *Obstet Gynecol* 2002;99: 473–476.

DeLancey JOL. Structural aspects of the extrinsic continence mechanism. *Obstet Gynecol* 1988;72:296–301.

Fantl JA, Newman DK, Colling J, et al. Urinary incontinence in adults: acute and chronic management. Clinical Practice Guidelines No. 2, 1996 Update. Rockville, MD: U.S. Department of Health and Human Services. Public Health Service, Agency for Health Care Policy and Research. AHCPR Publication No. 96-0682. March 1996.

Glazener CMA, Lapitan, MC. Urodynamic investigations for management of urinary incontinence in adults. Cochrane Incontinence Group. *Cochrane Database of Systematic Reviews* Issue 4, 2002.

Holmes DM, Montz FJ, Stanton SL. Oxybutynin versus propantheline in the management of detrusor instability: a patient-regulated variable dose trial. *Br J Obstet Gynaecol* 1989;96:607–612.

Mizunaga M, Miyata M, Kaneko S, et al. Intravesical instillation of oxybutynin hydrochloride therapy for patients with neuropathic bladder. *Paraplegia* 1994;32:25–29.

Moore KH, Hay DM, Imrie AE, et al. Oxybutynin hydrochloride (3 mg) in the treatment of women with idiopathic detrusor instability. *Br J Urol* 1990;66:479–485.

Riva D, Casolati E. Oxybutynin chloride in the treatment of female idiopathic bladder instability. *Clin Exp Obstet Gynecol* 1984;11:37–42.

Siu AL, Beers MH, Morgenstern H. The geriatric "medical and public health" imperative revisited. *J Am Geriatr Soc* 1993;41:78–84.

Tapp AJ, Cardozo LD, Versi E, et al. The treatment of detrusor instability in postmenopausal women with oxybutynin chloride: a double-blind placebo controlled study. *Br J Obstet Gynaecol* 1990;97:521–526.

Thor KB. Neurourology: exploring new horizons. *Johns Hopkins Adv Stud Med* 2002;2:677–680.

Thuroff JW, Bunke B, Ebner A, et al. Randomized, double-blind, multicenter trial on treatment of frequency, urgency and incontinence related to detrusor hyperactivity: oxybutynin versus propantheline versus placebo. *J Urol* 1991;145:813–817.

Vodusek DB, Plevnik S, Vrtacnik P, et al. Detrusor inhibition on selective pudendal nerve stimulation in the perineum. *Neurourol Urodyn* 1988;6:389–393.

Zeegers AGM, Kiesswetter H, Kramer AEJL, et al. Conservative therapy of frequency, urgency and urge incontinence: a double-blind clinical trial of flavoxate hydrochloride, oxybutynin chloride, emperonium bromide and placebo. *World J Urol* 1987;5:57–61.

PART 9

Immunologic and Infectious Diseases

CHAPTER 82
Allergies

Alison Ehrlich

The prevalence of allergic disease in the United States and many industrialized countries is increasing. The cost of allergic rhinitis (AR) alone in Europe is 1.0 to 1.5 billion Euros each year. AR has a prevalence of 3% to 19% in various countries and affects 20 to 40 million people in the United States. Although the reason for this increase in prevalence is unknown, some have hypothesized that increased awareness and improved diagnostic testing may attribute to this rise in reported allergic diseases. In addition, increased pollution, allergen exposure, and decreased challenge to the immune system may contribute to the rising prevalence.

The spectrum of allergic disease is broad, and therefore this chapter focuses on several of the most common allergic conditions. Specifically, atopic dermatitis (AD), allergic rhinitis (AR), urticaria, allergic contact dermatitis (ACD), and drug reactions are discussed. Allergies can be classified according to the Gell and Coombs classification of hypersensitivity: type I, IgE mediated; type II, cytotoxic; type III, immune complex; and type IV, cellular immune mediated. The main allergic reactions discussed in this chapter involve type I and type IV allergic reactions.

ETIOLOGY

Allergic disorders occur as a result of immune dysregulation. The immune system recognizes small molecules, called haptens, that trigger an immune cascade. The resulting clinical symptoms could be asthma, AD, AR, drug reaction, urticaria, and/or ACD.

Atopic Dermatitis and Allergic Rhinitis

Genetic susceptibility has been established for atopy and several related allergic disorders. Specifically, there is a genetic predisposition to the development of an IgE/mast cell/Th2 immune response. The triad of atopy—AD, asthma, and AR—is characterized by IgE reactiveness to various allergens, including dust mites, pollen, and animal dander. In the early phases of allergic reactions, the T cells are predominately $CD4^+$ helper type 2 (Th2) cells. Th2 cells produce interleukin (IL)-3, IL-4, IL-5, and IL-13 cytokines in response to allergen presentation by antigen-presenting cells. These cytokines mediate expansion of the immune response by regulation of IgE synthesis, eosinophil differentiation, and induction of vascular endothelial adhesion molecules. Although acute AD is associated with Th2 predominance, chronic AD is associated with interferon-γ and IL-5 expression. In addition, antigen-presenting cells from atopic skin lesions express CD1b, CD36, and a slightly increased amount of CD40. This atypical expression enhances recognition of self-T cells. In AR, the immune response represents a cascade of events, including release of inflammatory mediators and mobilization of cells to the nasal mucosa. IgE-coated mast cells degranulate upon recognition of allergens on nasal mucosa. Mucosal edema and rhinorrhea results from mast cell degranulation of inflammatory mediators: prostaglandin D_2, histamine, and leukotrienes. Also, late phase symptoms of AR such as fatigue and irritability may result from Th2 cytokines traveling to and exerting their effects on the hypothalamus.

Urticaria

The pathophysiology of urticaria can be IgE dependent (type I), complement mediated, nonimmunologic, or idiopathic. Some patients with chronic urticaria have IgG autoantibodies that cross-link with high affinity IgE receptors, which results in release of histamine from basophils and mast cells. These IgE receptors are found on basophils and mast cells in high concentrations. In type I hypersensitivity urticarial reactions (e.g., insect bites, food ingestion, or drug administration), specific IgE molecules are synthesized and, on repeat exposure, bind to the allergens. Then, the IgE molecules bind to their receptors on mast cells and basophils. Regardless of the mechanism, urticaria is characterized by mast cell degranulation and release of histamine and other inflammatory mediators. The IgE-dependent reactions are thought to be the mechanism responsible for physical, contact, or chemical urticaria. Complement-mediated reactions are associated with connective tissue disorders, angioedema, and transfusion reactions.

Drug Reactions

Drug reactions can be nonimmunologic or immunologic in nature. Characteristics of drug reactions are quite varied and include maculopapular eruptions, urticaria, angioedema, eczematous dermatitis, fixed drug eruptions, wheezing, and anaphylaxis. Severe drug reactions include Stevens-Johnson syndrome, toxic epidermal necrolysis, hypersensitivity syndromes, serum sickness, and vasculitis. The reactions discussed in this chapter focus on the most common eruptions.

The precise events, which occur in many drug allergies, are still unclear. Drug-specific T cells have been isolated in the blood of patients with allergy to penicillin, sulfamethoxazole, carbamazepine, and phenytoin. Activated $CD4^+$ and $CD8^+$ T cells (expressing HLA-DR) are evident in circulation during the acute phase of drug allergy. Hari et al. found that subjects with a predominance of activated $CD8^+$ T cells had more severe skin eruptions and were more likely to have liver involvement that subjects with a predominance of $CD4^+$ T cells. Subjects with a predominance of $CD4^+$ T cells are more likely to have maculopapular skin eruptions.

Allergic Contact Dermatitis

ACD is a delayed type allergic reaction (type IV). It is a T-cell–mediated process in which a genetically susceptible host has an exposure to a sufficient quantity of allergen. Most, but not all, allergens are haptens (small proteins < 500 Da) that must bind to carrier molecules in the skin. Allergens bind to major histocompatibility complex molecules on Langerhans cells. The Langerhans cells migrate to the lymph nodes and present the allergen to the T cells. This interaction results in production of accessory molecules on both the Langerhans cells and on the T cells. The interaction of B7 (on Langerhans cells) and CD28 (on T cells) is key for antigen sensitization, because tolerance will occur without this interaction. Upon repeated contact with allergen, memory T cells are activated and migrate with other inflammatory cells to the skin. This leads to the histologic changes seen in ACD: increased intercellular edema and a dermal infiltrate.

CLINICAL PICTURE

Atopic Dermatitis

The atopy triad consists of AD, AR, and asthma. (Asthma is discussed in Chapter 55.) There is considerable overlap between these three conditions, but all three conditions do not always occur together.

The onset of AD is frequently seen before age 2, and 30% to 40% of those affected will continue to have active disease as adults. Potential triggers for AD include bacterial proteins, superantigens, fungal and yeast antigens, viruses, contact allergens, food antigens, mite antigens, and self-antigens. Specific

TABLE 82.1. Clinical Features of Atopic Dermatitis

Major features
Pruritus
Facial/extensor involvement—infants and children
Flexural lichenification—adults
Chronic or relapsing dermatitis
Personal or family history of atopy
Minor features
Early age at onset
Food intolerance
Environmental or emotional factors
Xerosis
Ichthyosis, planter hyperlinearity, keratosis pilaris
Dennie-Morgan infraorbital folds
Nonspecific dermatitis of hands or feets
White dermatographism and delayed blanch
Cutaneous infections
Facial pallor or erythema
Nipple eczema
Pityriasis alba
Keratoconus
Anterior subcapsular cataracts

Source: Hanifin JM, Rajka G. Diagnostic features of atopic dermatitis. *Acta Dermatol Venereol (Stockh)* 1980;92:44, with permission.

criteria for the diagnosis of AD have been developed using clinical manifestations of AD (Table 82.1).

The distribution of skin lesions in AD changes throughout an individual's lifetime. Early in life, lesions are located primarily on the extensor surfaces of the body. In older children and adults, the flexural areas are more commonly involved.

Allergic Rhinitis

Watery nasal discharge, sneezing, pruritus, and nasal congestion characterize AR. Pruritus may involve the nose, ears, eyes, and/or throat. Other symptoms include ocular discharge, conjunctival injection, altered sense of smell, and headaches. Most cases of seasonal AR are attributable to tree and grass pollen allergens that vary by geographic region. Perennial AR is associated with a reaction to animal dander (especially domestic pets) and dust mites. Overlap exists between seasonal and perennial AR in many individuals.

The differential for AR includes nonallergic conditions such as infectious rhinitis, nasal polyps, nonallergic vasomotor rhinopathy, aspirin sensitivity, rhinitis medicamentosa (due to topical decongestants), and nonallergic inflammatory rhinitis with eosinophils.

Urticaria

Urticaria is characterized by erythematous pruritic wheals, which generally last less than 24 hours. The lesions of angioedema tend to be larger and more subcutaneous than classic urticarial lesions. Urticaria can be acute (duration of less than 6 weeks) or chronic (duration of greater than 6 weeks). The etiology of acute urticaria includes infections, foods, insect bites, contact and/or chemical exposure, and drugs. Chronic urticaria can be associated with connective tissue diseases, thyroid antibodies, infections, malignancy, and food additives. It can also be triggered by physical exposures: heat, cold, exercise, ultraviolet radiation, water, and vibration. It is important to note that most cases of chronic urticaria are idiopathic. If the lesions persist for greater than 24 hours and resolve with pigmentation, urticarial vasculitis should be considered in the differential. Systemic lupus erythematosus and Sjögren syndrome have been associated urticarial vasculitis.

Drug Reactions

Cutaneous drug reactions represent most allergic adverse reactions to medications. Immune-mediated drug reactions may present as urticaria, laryngeal edema, hypotension, fever, arthralgias, lymphadenopathy, and dermatitis.

Penicillin and its derivatives are responsible for most IgE-mediated drug reactions. Other classes of drugs associated with anaphylaxis include aminoglycosides, fluorinated quinolones, and several chemotherapy agents. Acute anaphylaxis may involve the skin, cardiovascular, pulmonary, and gastrointestinal organ systems. Skin findings include pruritus, flushing, urticaria, and angioedema. Cardiovascular symptoms include hypotension, rapid heart rate, syncope, and shock. Pulmonary complications include bronchospasm, laryngeal edema, and dyspnea. Gastrointestinal symptoms may include nausea, vomiting, diarrhea, and cramping.

Type IV cell-mediated hypersensitivity reactions occur with both topically applied medications and medications affixed to the skin in a patch preparation. Delayed type hypersensitivity reactions begin as localized eruptions and may develop into generalized skin eruptions.

Frequently, cutaneous drug reactions are not easily categorized using the Gell-Coombs classification system. Skin eruptions occurring in association with drug reactions include morbilliform, eczematous, exfoliative, targetoid, and blistering. Maculopapular or morbilliform eruptions are less likely to be IgE mediated than a urticarial reaction and are considered the most frequent types of drug-related skin eruptions. Annular or targetoid lesions are characteristic of erythema multiforme. When targetoid lesions occur in association with oral and ocular lesions, the major form of erythema multiforme is likely. Stevens-Johnson syndrome is characterized by widespread exfoliation and mucous membrane involvement. Sulfonamides and anticonvulsant medications have been associated with both erythema multiforme and Stevens-Johnson syndrome.

Allergic Contact Dermatitis

ACD is characterized by erythematous, scaly patches, and plaques in areas exposed to the culprit allergen. In the acute phase, affected areas may develop vesicles, crusts, and/or edema. The pattern of the dermatitis is frequently suggestive of the inciting allergen. For example, rubber ACD may present as dermatitis involving the hand and wrist. Textile ACD generally spares the axillary vault but involves the periaxillary region. Hair dye ACD will frequently spare the scalp but affect the anterior and posterior hairline. Fragrance ACD may present as a generalized eruption or patchy involvement of the face. Nickel ACD characteristically involves pierced ears, wrists (site of watch), and the periumbilicus (site of belt or pants button).

The differential diagnosis for ACD is somewhat dependent on location of the lesions. Conditions to consider in the differential include irritant contact dermatitis, AD, psoriasis, and seborrheic dermatitis.

HISTORY AND PHYSICAL EXAMINATION

Atopic Dermatitis

The history should include information on potential triggers, atopy, and the current skin care regime. The degree to which subjects are affected by pruritus should be ascertained. Frequently, severe AD patients are unable to sleep through the night due to severe pruritus. Physical examination should include inspection of the entire body for lesions and evaluation for evidence of superinfection. Any signs of topical steroid overuse, striae, and thinning of the skin should be documented.

Allergic Rhinitis

The history should include a detailed family and personal history for atopy. A complete social history should be taken, especially with regard to pets, floor covering, and recent geographic relocation. Information regarding nasal and ocular pruritus, repetitive clearing of throat, sneezing, and clear nasal discharge are useful in making the diagnosis of AR. Additionally, changes in taste, smell, ear fullness, and pressure over the sinuses may occur during peak pollination periods. Physical examination should include examination of the nasal mucosa and ocular conjunctiva.

Urticaria

It is important to ascertain whether the urticarial lesions have been occurring for greater than 6 weeks and therefore would be considered chronic. Also, triggers for physical urticaria should be elicited from the patient. Acute urticaria (occurring for less than 6 weeks) is likely to be related to drug reactions, insects, contact, or foods. History may assist in determining the etiology, but in 60% of cases there is no known cause. Physical examination should focus on evaluating the patient for causes of urticaria, such as thyroid disease or other connective tissue disease.

Drug Reactions

Accuracy and detail are key to successfully determining the culprit agent involved in causing a drug reaction. Even a vague history of penicillin allergy has been associated with a rate of positive skin testing of greater than 50%. It is important to establish the timing and duration of drug administration and development of skin eruption. Previous drug reactions and knowledge regarding frequency of drug eruptions with specific medications are helpful in determining the "culprit" medication. Furthermore, the duration and characteristics of drug reaction symptoms are useful to obtain. A complete list of all medications, including over-the-counter drugs, should be recorded. A thorough physical examination should be performed because drug reactions may involve more than one organ system.

LABORATORY TESTING

Allergic Rhinitis

Skin prick testing is the best diagnostic method for evaluating AR. This should be performed with standardized allergens. If skin prick testing is negative and the allergy is highly suspicious, intradermal testing may be useful. Antihistamines should be discontinued for at least 36 hours before skin prick testing. In addition, allergen-specific IgE can be measured in serum for specific allergens and/or groups of allergens. In vitro serum testing shows the presence of IgE specific for antigen, which may or may not be relevant to the clinical picture (e.g., RAST [radio-allergosorbent test], ELISA [enzyme-linked immunosorbent assay], EAST [enzyme allergosorbent test], CAP [Pharmacia ImmunoCap system]).

Urticaria

Laboratory testing for urticaria should be dictated by history and physical examination findings. A complete blood count, urinalysis, and chemistry panel are usually unremarkable. Further evaluation for connective tissue disease and/or thyroid disease should be pursued if indicated, and radiographic evaluation for sinus infections and dental infections may be warranted in some patients.

Allergic Contact Dermatitis

Patch testing is considered the most reliable method for diagnosis of ACD and so is indicated for patients with skin eruptions suggestive of ACD. Referral to a patch test specialist who performs both standard and custom patch testing is recommended. After patch testing, patients are educated about commercial products they should avoid using in the future and those products they can safely use.

Drug Reactions

The extent of laboratory investigation required for a drug reaction should be determined by the findings during the history and physical examination. Relevant studies may include complete blood count with differential, liver function tests, renal function tests, sedimentation rate, autoantibody tests, chest x-ray, and an electrocardiogram. Reactions caused by oral medications, especially penicillin, are best tested for by immediate hypersensitivity skin testing. Topical preparations should be tested by patch testing the agent and components of the agent (i.e., vehicle) if the reaction was consistent with a type IV delayed hypersensitivity reaction.

Drug skin testing (prick, scratch, or patch) should not be performed in patients who have had severe life-threatening reactions, such as vasculitic syndromes, Stevens-Johnson syndrome, or toxic epidermal necrosis. Additionally, these tests must be performed in clinics prepared for anaphylactic reactions in patients.

TREATMENT

Atopic Dermatitis

Food hypersensitivity rarely correlates with AD severity in adults, and food restriction diets are not thought to be useful for most individuals with AD. Teaching proper skin care to AD patients is very important for the success of their treatment. Patients should be instructed to use fragrance-free gentle cleansers and daily emollients. Oral antihistamines should be prescribed to control itching and topical steroids for flared areas. Patients should be educated about the side effects of topical steroids and warned about using potent steroids on areas of thinner skin such as the face, axilla, and groin. Oral antibiotics may be necessary because AD is prone to impetiginization.

Several new agents have recently become available for the treatment of AD. Tacrolimus and picrolimus have been shown to decrease cytokine expression of both Th1 and Th2 patterns. Both agents are steroid sparing and associated with mild burning or stinging when applied to affected skin. Recently, studies using recombinant humanized monoclonal anti-IgE antibody has shown clinical improvement in patients with seasonal AR.

Allergic Rhinitis

Treatment for AR consists of symptomatic therapy with oral antihistamines and/or nasal steroids. Oral decongestants may be used in conjunction with oral antihistamines to reduce nasal congestion, and topical antihistamines are available as eyedrops and nasal spray. Topical corticosteroids are efficacious for reducing nasal symptoms, and some consider them first-line therapy for moderate to severe AR. These intranasal sprays do not cause mucosal atrophy with long-term use. Environmental modification has proven to be rather effective in many cases of perennial AR. This is supported by studies showing that allergen concentration in an environment correlates with severity of AR. These modifications include removing wall-to-wall carpet, encasing mattresses and pillows, and washing bedclothes at 60° Celcius. More severe AR may require subcutaneous immunotherapy.

TABLE 82.2. Acute Anaphylactic Reaction Treatment

Oxygen
Maintain airway
IM or SC epinephrine (adults = 0.2–0.5 mL of 1:1,000 (1 mg/kg) every 15 min for two doses, then every 4 h as needed
Parenteral diphenhydramine (1–2 mg/kg or 25 to 50 mg)
Intravenous hydrocortisone
Intravenous fluids and vasopressors for hypotension
CPR as needed

Source: Executive Summary of Disease Management of Drug Hypersensitivity: a practice parameter. *Ann Allerg Asthma Immunol* 1999;83:665, with permission.

Urticaria

Nonsedating antihistamines are the first choice of treatment for urticaria and are helpful in reducing symptoms of pruritus and decreasing the number and frequency of wheals. Symptomatic control of hives, however, frequently requires higher doses of antihistamines than those generally recommended. The addition of H_2-receptor blockers in the management of chronic urticaria is helpful in some patients.

Drug Reactions

The treatment of drug reactions is specific to the type of hypersensitivity reaction. Anaphylactic reactions require emergency treatment with a standardized algorithm (Table 82.2). Less severe reactions can be treated with drug withdrawal and symptomatic care. Urticarial reactions and maculopapular drug reactions respond to oral antihistamines, topical anti-itch preparations, topical steroids, and, if necessary, oral steroids.

Allergic Contact Dermatitis

The most effective therapy for ACD is avoidance of the inciting allergen. In situations where avoidance is impossible or contact does occur, symptomatic therapy is required. Localized eruptions can be treated with topical steroids, oral antihistamines, and anti-itch preparations. Generalized eruptions may require a short course of oral steroids and/or ultraviolet-B phototherapy.

CONSIDERATIONS IN PREGNANCY

Allergies may worsen or improve during a pregnancy. Generally, allergies can be controlled during pregnancy, but poorly controlled asthma is considered a threat to the fetus. Many of the medications used to treat allergies have product labels stating they should be avoided during pregnancy. This is due to the paucity of fetal safety data for many medications. Intranasal steroids and sodium cromoglycate are considered safe in pregnancy. First-generation antihistamines are preferred over second generation due to longer safety experience with this class of medications. Specifically, chlorpheniramine has been recommended as the antihistamine of choice for pregnant women.

Women who have a history of atopy are more likely to have children who develop atopy. Maternal dietary antigen avoidance has not proven to have a protective effect on the development of atopic eczema and AR. Interestingly, Kramer et al. found that maternal dietary restriction is associated with a lower mean gestational weight.

BIBLIOGRAPHY

Alexander E, Provost T. Cutaneous manifestations of primary Sjögren's syndrome: a reflection of vasculitis and association with anti-Ro (SSA) antibodies. *J Invest Dermatol* 1983;80:386–391.

Bisaccia E, Adamo V, Rozan S. Urticarial vasculitis progressing to systemic lupus erythematosus. *Arch Dermatol* 1988;124:1088–1090.

Budd M, Parker C, Norden C. Evaluation of intradermal skin tests in penicillin hypersensitivity. *JAMA* 1964;190:203–205.

Casale T, Condemi J, LaForce C, et al. Effect of omalizumab on symptoms of seasonal allergic rhinitis. *JAMA* 2001;286:2956–2967.

Cauwenberge P, Bachert C, Passalacqua G, et al. Consensus statement on the treatment of allergic rhinitis. *Allergy* 2000;55:116–134.

Cooper K, Stevens S. T cells in atopic dermatitis. *J Am Acad Dermatol* 2001;45: S10–S12.

European allergy white paper. Brussels: UCB Institute of Allergy. 1997.

Graham-Brown R. Atopic dermatitis: predictions, expectations, and outcomes. *J Am Acad Dermatol* 2001;45:S61–S63.

Greaves M. Chronic urticaria. *N Engl J Med* 1995;332:1767–1772.

Hari Y, Frutig-Schnyder M, Hurni N, et al. T cell involvement in cutaneous drug eruptions. *Clin Exp Allergy* 2000;31:1398–1408.

Holm A, Fokkens W, Godthelp T, et al. A 1-year placebo-controlled study of intranasal spray in patients with perennial allergic rhinitis: a safety and biopsy study. *Clin Otolaryngol* 1998;23:69–73.

Kalish R, Wood J. Introduction of hapten-specific tolerance of human CD8+ urushiol (poison ivy) reactive T lymphocytes. *J Invest Dermatol* 1997;108: 253–257.

Kaplan A. Chronic urticaria and angioedema. *N Engl J Med* 2002;346:175–179.

Koponen M, Pichler W, de Weck A. Phenotypic analysis of in vitro activated cell subsets. *J Allergy Clin Immunol* 1986;78:645–652.

Korsgaard J. Mite asthma and residency. A case control study of the impact of exposure to house dust mites. *Am Rev Respir Dis* 1983;128:231–235.

Kramer M. Maternal antigen avoidance during pregnancy for preventing atopic disease in infants of women at high risk. *Cochrane Database Syst Rev* 2000;2: CD000133.

Leape L, Brennan T, Laird N, et al. The nature of adverse events in hospitalized patients: results of the Harvard Medical Practice Study II. *N Engl J Med* 1991; 324:377–384.

Leung DYM, Soter NA. Cellular and immunologic mechanisms in atopic dermatitis. *J Am Acad Dermatol* 2001;44:S1–S12.

Mauri-Hellweg D, Bettens F, Mauri D, et al. Activation of drug-specific CD4+ and CD8+ T cells in individuals allergic to sulfamethoxazole, phenytoin and carbamazepine. *J Immunol* 1995;155:462–472.

Meltzer E. The prevalence and medical and economic impact of allergic rhinitis in the United States. *J Allergy Clin Immunol* 1997;99:S805–S828.

Nalefski E, Rao A. Nature of the ligand recognized by a hapten and carrier-specific, MHC-restricted T cell receptor. *J Immunol* 1993;150:3806–3816.

National Asthma Education Program Report of the Working Group on Asthma and Pregnancy. Management of asthma during pregnancy. Bethesda, MD. NIH Publication No. 93-3279A. September 1993.

Neild V, Marsden R, Bailes J, et al. Egg and milk exclusion diets in atopic eczema. *Br J Dermatol* 1986;114:117–123.

Ring J, Kramer U, Schafer T. Why are allergies increasing? *Curr Opin Immunol* 2001;13:701–708.

Skoner D. Allergic rhinitis: definition, epidemiology, pathophysiology, detection, and diagnosis. *J Allergy Clin Immunol* 2001;108:S2–S8.

CHAPTER 83
Systemic Lupus Erythematosus

Christopher T. Ritchlin

Systemic lupus erythematosus (SLE) is a chronic autoimmune disorder characterized by wide diversity in clinical presentation and course. The disease is cyclic, with unpredictable flares and remissions, and disease severity ranges from fatigue, arthralgia, and a photosensitive rash to life-threatening major organ involvement. The diagnosis usually is based on information obtained from the history and physical findings combined with results from a number of serologic tests. Criteria have been developed to identify patients for clinical studies, but they also are useful to the practicing physician (Table 83.1). It is important that the primary physician caring for women be familiar with the cardinal signs and symptoms of SLE because it occurs primarily in female patients and is associated with a number of complications in the pregnant patient.

SLE has been described in all age groups but is most common between ages 13 and 40 years. Approximately 90% of the patients are female. In the older age groups, the female predominance lessens considerably. The disease is three times more common in Asians and African-Americans, with an annual incidence that varies from 6 per 100,000 in whites to 35 per 100,000 cases in African-Americans. The concordance rate for SLE in identical twins is approximately 30%, and the likelihood that first-degree relatives of an affected patient will develop SLE is about 5%.

ETIOLOGY AND DIFFERENTIAL DIAGNOSIS

The cause of SLE is unknown, but the epidemiologic and scientific data suggest a complex interplay between genetic and environmental factors, with the weight of each of these varying from patient to patient. The fundamental defects seem to include a loss of tolerance to self-antigens and excessive B-cell activity. This results in the overproduction of autoantibodies that alter cell function and formation of immune complexes that deposit in various tissues and stimulate an inflammatory response. SLE has been associated with the human leukocyte antigens (HLA) DR2 and DR3 and with deficiencies in complement proteins, particularly C2 and C4. Environmental agents associated with the onset of SLE include various drugs, ultraviolet light, and infections.

SLE mimics several other disorders. Prominent among these are subacute bacterial endocarditis, septicemia, sarcoidosis, tuberculosis, fibromyalgia, thyroid disease, and the acquired immunodeficiency syndrome. Other inflammatory joint disorders including rheumatoid, psoriatic, Lyme and viral arthritis must be considered. Differentiation from other autoimmune disorders, such as scleroderma, Sjögren syndrome, polymyositis-dermatomyositis, and mixed connective tissue disease, is based on characteristic clinical features and distinctive serologic tests.

HISTORY

The clinical manifestations of SLE are varied and often subtle, so the physician must take a complete history and maintain a high index of suspicion. Table 83.2 lists a series of questions that aid in making the diagnosis. Constitutional complaints are com-

TABLE 83.1. The 1982 Revised Criteria for Classification of Systemic Lupus Erythematosus[a]

Criterion	Definition
1. Malar rash	Fixed erythema, flat or raised, over the malar eminences, tending to spare the nasolabial folds
2. Discoid rash	Erythematous raised patches with adherent keratolic scaling and follicular plugging; atrophied scarring may occur in older lesions
3. Photosensitivity	Skin rash as a result of unusual reaction to sunlight, by patient history or physician observation
4. Oral ulcers	Oral or nasopharyngeal ulceration, usually painless, observed by a physician
5. Arthritis	Nonerosive arthritis involving two or more peripheral joints, characterized by tenderness, swelling, or effusion
6. Serositis	a. Pleuritis—convincing history of pleuritic pain or rub or heard by a physician or evidence of pleural effusion, or
	b. Pericarditis—documented by electrocardiogram or rub or evidence of pericardial effusion
7. Renal disorder	a. Persistent proteinuria 0.5 g/d or 3+ if quantitation not performed, or
	b. Cellular casts—may be red blood cell, hemoglobin, granular, tubular, or mixed
8. Neurologic disorder	a. Seizures—in the absence of offending drugs or known metabolic derangements, e.g., uremia, ketoacidosis, or electrolyte imbalance, or
	b. Psychosis—in the absence of offending drugs or known metabolic derangements, e.g., uremic ketoacidosis or electrolyte imbalance
9. Hematologic disorder	a. Hemolytic anemia—with reticulocytosis, or
	b. Leukopenia—$<4.0 \times 10^9$/L (4,000/mm^3) total on occasions, or
	c. Lymphopenia—$<1.5 \times 10^9$/L (1,500/mm^3) on at least two occasions, or
	d. Thrombocytopenia—$<100 \times 10^9$/L (x10^3/mm^3) in the absence of offending drugs
10. Immunologic disorder	a. Positive lupus erythematosus cell preparation, or
	b. Anti-DNA antibody to native DNA in abnormal titer, or
	c. Anti-Sm—presence of antibody to Sm nuclear antigen, or
	d. False-positive serologic test for syphilis known to be positive for at least 6 mo and confirmed by negative *Treponema pallidum* immobilization or fluorescent treponemal antibody absorption test
11. Antinuclear antibody	An abnormal titer of antinuclear antibody by immunofluorescence or an equivalent assay at a point in the absence of drugs known to be associated with drug-induced lupus erythematosus syndrome

[a]The proposed classification is based on 11 criteria. To identify patients in clinical studies, a person shall be said to have systemic lupus erythematosus if any 4 or more of the 11 criteria are present serially or simultaneously, during any interval observation.
Sm, Smith antigen.
Source: Condemi JJ. The autoimmune diseases. *JAMA* 1992;286:2882, with permission.

mon and include fatigue, fevers (usually less than 39°C [102°F]), and weight loss. Fatigue often is extreme, resembling that seen in fibromyalgia or chronic fatigue syndrome.

Nearly all patients complain of arthralgia or arthritis. The small joints of the hands, wrists, and knees are often painful, stiff, and swollen, particularly in the morning, resulting in an initial diagnosis of rheumatoid arthritis in many patients. Muscle aches and weakness also are frequent complaints. Skin involvement often presents as a malar blush or peripheral rash that is variable in appearance, generally nonscarring, and often induced by sunlight. Most patients complain of photosensitivity described as either a rash or an overall sense of not feeling well after sun exposure. Mouth ulcers tend to be painless, which differentiates them from canker sores. Transient hair loss is common during active disease.

It is essential to determine from the history whether major organs such as the lung, heart, or central nervous system (CNS) are affected in patients believed to have SLE. Pleuritic chest pain may represent pleural or pericardial inflammation. Dyspnea may be the result of pneumonitis, pleural or pericardial effusion, congestive heart failure, or pulmonary emboli. Neuropsychiatric symptoms range from mild, including mood lability, poorly localized headaches, and difficulty concentrating; to more severe, arising from psychosis, depression, seizures, strokes, peripheral neuropathy or transverse myelitis.

TABLE 83.2. Key Questions in Evaluating Patients for Systemic Lupus Erythematosus

1. Are your joints painful, swollen, or stiff?
2. Are you sensitive to the sun (not sunburn)?
3. Have you noticed painless sores in your mouth?
4. Have you ever been told that you have low blood counts?
5. Have you ever had protein or cells in your urine?
6. Have you ever had pleurisy or pain in deep breathing lasting more than a few days?
7. Do you have frequent headaches, difficulty concentrating, or memory loss?
8. Have you ever had a persistent facial rash?
9. Have you had periods of rapid hair loss?
10. Do your hands change colors or become uncomfortable in the cold?

Source: Shur PH. Clinical features of SLE. In: Kelly WN Jr, Harris ED Jr, Ruddy S, et al., eds. *Textbook of rheumatology,* 4th ed. Philadelphia: WB Saunders, 1993:1017, with permission.

PHYSICAL EXAMINATION

Low-grade fever often is associated with a lupus flare, and tachycardia may be the result of increased temperature, hyperthyroidism, anxiety, anemia, or volume depletion. Tachypnea may reflect pulmonary or cardiac involvement. Elevated blood pressure may be idiopathic in origin but often is related to underlying inflammatory kidney disease.

Acute skin lesions are variable in appearance and location. The typical butterfly rash is a nonpapular raised erythema over the cheeks and nose with sparing of the nasolabial folds. This is distinguished from rosacea which is more pustular in appearance. Maculopapular erythematous eruptions are frequently observed, and these can be triggered by sunlight or medications, especially sulfa drugs and penicillin derivatives. Urticaria and angioedema, bullae, palpable purpura, and livedo reticularis are less common skin eruptions. Painless mucosal ulcerations arise on the hard and soft palate but also are seen in the upper respiratory tract, nasal septum, and the vagina. Alopecia usually is diffuse, and hair loss is transient if scarring discoid lesions are not present.

CONSIDERATIONS IN PREGNANCY

Most patients with SLE can become pregnant and have successful outcomes, however, up to 70% of patients experience a flare. In patients who do flare during pregnancy, renal and hematologic involvement tends to be more common than arthritis. Moreover, pregnant SLE patients also are more likely to have problems with preeclampsia, hypertension, diabetes mellitus, and urinary tract infections than controls. Less common manifestations in the pre and postpartum period include stroke, uterine rupture, bilateral retinal detachments, deep venous thrombosis in patients with antiphospholipid antibodies, and the maternal syndrome of hemolysis, elevated liver enzymes, and low platelet count (HELLP syndrome).

The major events responsible for adverse fetal outcomes are fetal loss and preterm labor. Fetal loss occurs in both the first and second trimesters, but those in the second trimester are more strongly associated with elevated levels of anticardiolipin antibodies. Preterm birth can result from early labor, fetal distress, premature rupture of membranes, preeclamptic toxemia, and oligohydramnios. These complications are more common in patients with active lupus.

Neonatal SLE is a syndrome mediated by transplacental passage of maternal antibodies to Ro/La antigens that can manifest in utero or at birth. Infants with neonatal SLE can have thrombocytopenia, leukopenia, hepatosplenomegaly, and cutaneous lesions that typically resolve by 6 months of age without therapy. More serious complications include myocarditis, endocardial fibrosis, and congenital complete heart block. Congenital complete heart block can occur after the 16th week of gestation and is detected by a drop in fetal heart rate. Permanent pacemakers are often required in these newborns soon after birth. Interestingly, mothers of affected infants are frequently asymptomatic before and during the pregnancy, so autoimmune disease is not suspected. A significant percentage develop SLE (usually mild) or Sjögren syndrome later in life.

It is advisable that patients with SLE not conceive at a time when the disease is active. Mothers who develop active SLE during pregnancy or are in the midst of a flare when they become pregnant often require prednisone. Prednisone is metabolized by the placenta and does not pose a major risk to the fetus, but the drug increases the risk of diabetes, hypertension, and preeclampsia in the mother. It is recommended that women who have recurrent fetal loss and elevated antiphospholipid antibodies receive treatment with subcutaneous heparin (5,000–10,000 U twice daily) and low-dose aspirin throughout the pregnancy. Some physicians continue this therapy for 6 weeks postpartum. This therapy has improved pregnancy outcome. Hydroxychloroquine and azathioprine can be continued in the pregnant patient if they are required to control lupus activity, but methotrexate, cyclophosphamide, and NSAIDs should be discontinued because of possible adverse effects on the fetus. Low dose aspirin is well tolerated and may prevent preeclampsia.

Pregnant patients with SLE should be considered high risk, and close cooperation between the obstetrician and rheumatologist maximizes the possibility of a positive outcome. Generally, patients are followed monthly during the first two trimesters by both physicians and more frequently thereafter. Some groups start biophysical profiles and umbilical artery analysis after the 26th week of gestation. Mothers who have anti-Ro antibodies should have serial four-chamber echocardiograms beginning in the 18th week of pregnancy. If fetal heart block or myocarditis is detected early, plasmapheresis combined with high dose dexamethasone (or any steroid that crosses the placenta) can be effective in some cases if initiated early. Differentiating preeclampsia from a flare can be difficult, but falling complement levels, the absence of hypertension and improvement with prednisone are more strongly associated with active SLE.

PROGNOSIS

Patients with SLE have an excellent prognosis, with a 10-year survival rate of 90%, and most patients live a normal life span; however, recent data indicate that death rates have increased approximately 70% from 1979-1998 in African-American women aged 45 to 64 years. The factors responsible for the race-specific disparities in SLE are not well understood but possibilities include a higher incidence in black patients, delay in diagnosis, barriers to access of care or poor treatment response resulting from biologic factors or poor compliance. Patients with major organ disease, particularly involving the CNS and kidney, have a poorer prognosis, with infection, CNS lupus, and coronary artery disease responsible for most deaths.

BIBLIOGRAPHY

Askanase AD, Buyon JP. Reproductive health in SLE. *Baillieres Clin Rheum* 2002 (in press).

Chan TM, Li FK, Tang CSO, et al. Efficacy of mycophenolate mofetil in patients with diffuse proliferative lupus nephritis. *N Engl J Med* 2000;343:1156–1162.

Davidson A, Diamond B. Autoimmune diseases. *N Engl J Med* 2001;345:340.

Edworthy SM. Clinical manifestations of SLE. In Kelley WN Jr, Harris ED Jr, Ruddy S, et al., eds. *Textbook of rheumatology*, 6th ed. Philadelphia: WB Saunders, 2001:1105.

Ginzler EM, Diamond HS, Weiner M, et al. A multicenter study of outcome in systemic lupus erythematosus. I. Entry variables as predictors of prognosis. *Arthritis Rheum* 1982;25:601.

Levine JS, Branch DW, Rauch J. The antiphospholipid syndrome. *N Engl J Med* 2002;346:752–763.

Petri M. Pregnancy in SLE. *Baillieres Clin Rheum* 1998;12:449.

Ruiz-Irastorza G, Khamashta MA, Hughes GRV. Systemic lupus erythematosus. *Lancet* 2001;357:1027.

Sacks JJ, Helmick CG, Langmaid G, et al. Trends in death from systemic lupus erythematosus—United States 1979–1998. *MMWR* 2002;51:371–374.

Steinberg AD, Goarley AF, Austin HA, et al. Methylprednisone and cyclophosphamide, alone or in combination, in patients with lupus nephritis: a randomized, controlled trial. *Ann Intern Med* 1996;125:549–557.

Waltuck J, Buyon JP Autoantibody-associated congenital heart block: outcome in mothers and children. *Ann Intern Med* 1994;120:554.

CHAPTER 84

Sarcoidosis

Gary W. Wahl

Sarcoidosis is a multisystem disorder of unknown cause, pathologically characterized by nonnecrotizing granuloma. Although any organ system can be involved, the lung and mediastinal lymph nodes are the most prominent sites of involvement. Young adults are most frequently affected, but sarcoidosis has also been diagnosed in small children and in octogenarians. The incidence of sarcoidosis varies significantly among ethnic and geographic groups. In the United States, approximately 11 per 100,000 individuals are affected, but African-Americans (particularly women) have a rate of 20 per 100,000, almost 10 times that of whites. African blacks have incidence rates estimated at 2 to 4 per 100,000. Most patients have an uneventful spontaneous remission. However, many patients have significant symptoms while the condition is active that require careful monitoring to determine need for therapy.

ETIOLOGY

Sarcoidosis is characterized by nonnecrotizing granulomas that can involve any organ. The best current evidence suggests that still-unknown antigens stimulate circulating macrophages and lymphocytes to release cytokines. In the lung, a lymphocytic alveolitis that is composed of "killer" (CD4) lymphocytes results. This inflammatory process usually abates spontaneously within 6 to 24 months. In some individuals the process results in the proliferation of fibroblasts with extensive formation of fibrosis in the involved organ.

The causative antigen is unknown, and it is possible that sarcoidosis is a common injury response to several different triggers. Stimuli considered in the past have included infection with tuberculosis, fungi, viruses, and retroviruses; exposure to pine pollens, a variety of chemicals, and drugs; and autoimmune or genetic factors. In some studies, nearly one third of lymph nodes involved with sarcoid have DNA sequences in common with *Mycobacterium tuberculosis*, but other investigators have observed much lower rates.

DIFFERENTIAL DIAGNOSIS

Although noncaseating granuloma are the pathologic hallmark of sarcoidosis, they are not specific. Nearly identical lesions can be seen with beryllium exposure, tuberculosis, leprosy, hypersensitivity pneumonitis, Crohn disease, primary biliary cirrhosis, fungal infection, and local sarcoid reaction, which occur in lymph nodes draining neoplastic or chronically inflamed regions. Because the symptoms of sarcoidosis are also nonspecific, the diagnosis is often one of exclusion.

HISTORY

Sarcoidosis can present asymptomatically, with systemic symptoms of fever, malaise, and weight loss or with a history reflecting dysfunction of the organ system involved. In Japan, where the incidence of sarcoidosis is only about 1 in 100,000, 60% of patients are discovered on routine chest x-ray. In contrast, over 90% of African-American women with sarcoid present with symptoms. Table 84.1 reviews the most common complaints, by organ system, at initial presentation.

Pulmonary involvement occurs pathologically in 90% of all patients and is the most frequent cause of symptoms. Dyspnea with exertion, dry cough, and vague substernal chest pain is seen alone or in combination with other symptoms in over one third of patients. Occasionally, the chest pain is severe and mimics cardiac pain. Severe cough associated with wheezing can occur when there is extensive airway involvement. This presentation is often first mistakenly diagnosed as asthma. Hemoptysis (sometimes with cavitation of lung on x-ray), pleural effusion, and pneumothorax have all been described but are rare and prompt a careful investigation for an alternative diagnosis.

TABLE 84.1. Presenting Symptoms in Sarcoidosis

Presenting symptom	African-Americans (%)	White Americans (%)
Respiratory	30–50	30–50
Asymptomatic	5–15	10–25
Skin involvement	20–30	3–10
Constitutional signs	5–30	10–40
Erythema nodosum	2–5	7–10
Ocular	5–15	2–5

Presentation with nonspecific constitutional symptoms such as fever, weight loss, fatigue, anorexia, and even chills and night sweats occurs in about one third of patients. The association of constitutional symptoms, particularly fever, with erythema nodosum, migratory arthralgias (particularly the ankles), and bilateral hilar adenopathy syndrome (Löfgren syndrome) in young women is a common presentation with an excellent prognosis.

In over 20% of American patients, sarcoidosis is discovered when a routine chest x-ray is performed. Most commonly these patients have only bilateral hilar adenopathy, but some show evidence of pulmonary fibrosis.

One fourth of patients present with dermatologic complaints. Waxy maculopapular lesions and nodules on the extremities are the most common skin findings. Erythema nodosum (as part of Löfgren syndrome) is particularly common in white and Hispanic populations, particularly in young women. Lupus pernio is a violaceous lesion that occurs on the nose, cheeks, ears, and lips. It is a relatively specific finding for sarcoidosis.

Ocular findings occur in 20% of patients at some point in the course of sarcoidosis but only in a small percentage at presentation. Granulomatous uveitis is the most common finding. The acute inflammation results in a red frequently painful eye. This often clears spontaneously, but chronic uveitis (which may be painless) may lead to glaucoma, cataract formation, adhesion between the iris and lens, and even blindness. Conjunctival follicles, lacrimal gland enlargement, and keratoconjunctivitis sicca are also seen in this population. Most patients diagnosed with sarcoidosis should have formal ophthalmologic evaluation with slit-lamp examination.

Although 25% of patients have granuloma in the heart, symptomatic presentation with cardiac disease is rare. Abnormal conduction is the most common finding. It is occasionally associated with palpitations. Complete heart block with syncope and even sudden death has been described. Rarely, fibrotic replacement of myocardium can result in congestive heart failure.

Fewer than 5% of patients develop symptomatic neurologic involvement, but identification is important. Cranial nerve involvement, particularly cranial nerve VII (Bell palsy), is the most common abnormality. A predilection of the inflammatory process toward involving the base of the brain probably explains the development of these palsies as well as rarely seen episodes of aseptic meningitis, hydrocephalus, hypophyseal replacement, and pituitary dysfunction. Peripheral neuropathy and symptoms of space-occupying lesions may result from granulomatous inflammation in strategic locations.

Enlargement of cervical, supraclavicular, epitrochlear, or axillary nodes is fairly common, occurring in 10% to 50% of patients. The spleen is rarely enlarged. Granulomatous involvement of the liver is common but only rarely causes tenderness, cirrhosis, or jaundice. Among the 10% to 15% of patients with hypercalcemia, a small percentage develops kidney stones as a manifestation of the disease. One fifth of patients may develop arthralgia as a result of involvement of the joint capsule. Upper airway involvement has been reported to result in nasal obstruction and sinusitis.

LABORATORY AND IMAGING STUDIES

The diagnosis of sarcoidosis is based on clinical presentation, observation over time, and exclusion of other causes for the findings. Several laboratory and x-ray findings support the diagnosis, but none is specific. Biopsy demonstrating noncaseating granuloma is required an alternative diagnoses cannot be excluded with less invasive methods.

The chest x-ray is central to diagnosis and management in most patients. A staging system describes findings that correlate with lung function and prognosis. About 10% of patients have normal x-rays, which is stage 0 sarcoidosis. Stage I disease, bilateral hilar and mediastinal adenopathy with no evidence of lung parenchyma involvement, is seen in 35% to 45% of patients at presentation. Stage II sarcoidosis consists of bilateral hilar and mediastinal adenopathy along with parenchymal lung disease. The pulmonary involvement usually appears as a reticular pattern diffusely in the lung but occasionally is seen as multiple small nodules. Twenty percent of patients have stage III disease, which is diffuse lung involvement without adenopathy. There may be cystic changes associated with this more advanced involvement. Most stage I patients regress or remain stable, but longitudinal studies have shown that about 10% to 20% evolve from stage I to stage III. The risk of progression from stage II or III may be as high as 40%. Computed tomography can be helpful both to exclude other conditions and to support the diagnosis. The presence of widespread small nodules along vessels and subpleurally and thickened intralobular septae are particularly suggestive of sarcoidosis.

In stage I disease, lung function is usually normal, and over 80% of patients resolve completely or remain permanently stable. Stage II patients have mild lung dysfunction, and 60% to 80% remain stable or resolve. In stage III disease, lung function is much more disturbed, and 40% to 50% of patients have progressive disease.

Although often normal, pulmonary function studies frequently demonstrate a restrictive pattern. Patients with extensive airway involvement may demonstrate an obstructive pattern but generally have no response to inhaled bronchodilators like that seen in asthma patients. The diffusion capacity for carbon monoxide tends to be reduced, but not usually to extreme levels. Exercise-induced hypoxemia may occur when pulmonary involvement is severe.

There is no specific blood test to identify sarcoidosis. Anemia, leukopenia, lymphocytopenia, eosinophilia, thrombocytopenia, hypergammaglobulinemia, an increased erythrocyte sedimentation rate, hypercalcemia, and hypercalcuria may all be seen. Serologies for collagen vascular diseases show no abnormalities. Gallium scan and analysis of bronchoalveolar lavage fluid have been of some research interest but have not proved specific enough to be helpful in diagnostic or management decisions. The Kveim-Sitzbach test—injection of carefully processed splenic material followed by biopsy of the injection site—is only of historic interest because the reagent is no longer available.

The circulating level of angiotensin-converting enzyme is elevated in two thirds of patients with sarcoidosis. However, numerous conditions, including several in the differential diagnosis, also increase the angiotensin-converting enzyme level (Table 84.2). Although the role of angiotensin-converting enzyme as a diagnostic tool is limited, some believe the angiotensin-converting enzyme level is useful in following disease activity.

When alternative diagnoses cannot be excluded, confirmatory biopsy is often required. Transbronchial biopsy of the lung through a fiberoptic bronchoscope is the most commonly performed procedure. It carries a low morbidity and is diagnostic in 60% of patients when there is no lung abnormality on chest x-ray and in nearly 90% of patients when interstitial infiltrates are present (stages II and III). When there are visible skin lesions, palpable lymph nodes, or granular abnormalities of the conjunctiva, biopsy of these areas has a very high yield. Liver biopsy results are positive in most patients, particularly in those with abnormal liver function, but the procedure carries significant risk. Scalene lymph node biopsy or mediastinoscopy has very high yields but at significant expense and some risk. Open lung biopsy is rarely required to diagnose sarcoid.

TABLE 84.2. Conditions Associated with Elevation of Angiotension-Converting Enzyme Level

Likely alternative diagnoses	Unlikely alternative diagnoses
Asbestosis	Diabetes mellitus
Berylliosis	Gaucher disease
Coccidioidomycosis	Hyperthyroidism
Granulomatous hepatitis	Adult respiratory distress syndrome
Hypersensitivity pneumonitis	Inflammatory bowel disease
Lymphoma	Leprosy
Miliary tuberculosis	Liver cirrhosis
Pulmonary neoplasm	
Silicosis	

Some authorities believe biopsy should be performed on all patients before treatment is instituted, but this is controversial. Asymptotic patients with bilateral hilar adenopathy or those with erythema nodosum, arthralgias, and symmetric hilar adenopathy virtually always have sarcoidosis. In a large series of patients with bilateral hilar adenopathy, nearly 20% had lymphoma. All lymphoma patients have significant symptoms. The small percentage of patients with lung cancer were also symptomatic. Those with fungal or tuberculous causes had fever or purulent sputum. All patients in these series who were asymptomatic had sarcoidosis.

TREATMENT

The decision to treat sarcoidosis generally involves consultation. Corticosteroids are effective in treating sarcoidosis but are indicated in only some patients. Most patients remain stable or resolve spontaneously, and although steroids clearly accelerate recovery, there is no strong evidence that they affect long-term outcome. Obviously, the benefits of treatment must be balanced against the potentially serious side effects that 3 to 12 months' use of systemic steroids may cause.

The most important factor affecting the decision to treat with systemic steroids is the presence of symptoms. Asymptomatic patients with normal lung function and stage I radiographic changes should not be treated. If they have constitutional symptoms, arthralgias, or erythema nodosum, nonsteroidal antiinflammatory medications are usually effective. Sometimes short courses (5–10 days) of prednisone are needed to "carry" a patient through a difficult period. Stable patients are typically monitored with pulmonary function at 3 months, 1 year, and usually with pulmonary function 6 to 12 months after presentation.

Respiratory symptoms, particularly if progressive (cough, dyspnea, significant chest pain), usually are treated. Asymptomatic patients with involvement of the lung (stages II and III) observed on x-rays are frequently treated; if they are not treated, they are very closely followed for evidence of progressive pulmonary fibrosis. Patients with moderate or severe abnormalities of lung function, even if asymptomatic, should be treated.

Ocular, neurologic, cardiac, and upper airway involvement are indications for systemic treatment. Patients with asymptomatic hepatic involvement with normal liver function do not need to receive therapy but must be monitored frequently for deterioration.

The optimal dose and duration of therapy is not known. Most patients respond to 30 to 40 mg/d of prednisone, and this dose is usually reduced to 10 to 15 mg/d after 4 to 8 weeks. Alternate-day steroids are probably effective in the maintenance phase, although there are concerns about decreased compliance with these regimens. Therapy is generally continued for 3 to 6 months. Perhaps one fifth of patients with a good response to steroids have recurrence when therapy is tapered or discontinued, and in these patients long-term treatment may be required. Inhaled steroids are sometimes effective in patients with airway symptoms (i.e., cough, wheeze) but no other indication for therapy. Plaquenil has been anecdotally reported to benefit skin lesions of sarcoidosis. There are no good data studying steroid-sparing drugs such as methotrexate, cyclophosphamide, or azathioprine, which have had limited success in other forms of interstitial lung disease. They are, however, used by some in diabetic patients. Recurrence after complete resolution and successful withdrawal of steroids (if used in treatment) is unusual.

In stable or resolved patients, follow-up is usually performed 3 to 6 months after diagnosis with pulmonary function testing and chest radiographs. Patients are then tested annually for a total of 3 years.

CONSIDERATIONS IN PREGNANCY

Sarcoidosis does not affect fertility or pregnancy. The placenta has not been observed to be involved with sarcoid granulomas. Several studies of over 100 pregnancies in patients with sarcoidosis demonstrated no increase in cesarean section rates or in maternal or fetal difficulties, and pregnancy does not appear to affect disease activity in the mother. About 10% to 20% of patients have progression of their sarcoidosis during pregnancy, similar to the rate expected in a nonpregnant population. There are case reports of acceleration of sarcoid after delivery, so some suggest close follow-up in the first 6 months postpartum. Indications for treatment are said to be unchanged during pregnancy, although realistically there is a tendency to wait until delivery if symptoms are not severe.

BIBLIOGRAPHY

American Thoracic Society guidelines: Statement on sarcoidosis. *Am J Respir Crit Care Med* 1999;160:736.

Chesnutt AN. Enigmas in sarcoidosis. *West J Med* 1995;162:519.

Izumi T. *Sarcoidosis: pulmonary and critical care medicine.* Vol. 2. St Louis: Mosby-Year Book, 1992.

Johns CJ. *Sarcoidosis: pulmonary diseases and disorders,* 2nd ed. Vol. 1. New York: McGraw-Hill, 1988.

King TE. Restrictive lung disease in pregnancy. *Clin Chest Med* 1992;13:607.

Sharma OP. Pulmonary sarcoidosis and corticosteroids. *Am Rev Respir Dis* 1993; 147:1598.

Weissler JC. Southwestern Internal Medicine Conference: sarcoidosis-immunology and clinical management. *Am J Med Sci* 1994;307:233.

Winterbauer RH, Moores KD. A clinical interpretation of bilateral hilar adenopathy. *Ann Intern Med* 1973;78:65.

CHAPTER 85
Human Immunodeficiency Virus and Acquired Immunodeficiency Syndrome in Women

Jane Hitti and Susan E. Cohn

An estimated 40 million people in the world have been infected with human immunodeficiency virus type 1 (HIV), the virus that causes acquired immunodeficiency syndrome (AIDS). In the United States there has been a substantial increase in the proportion of women infected with HIV in recent years. As of 2001, an estimated 30% to 35% of all persons with HIV in the United States are female. Unfortunately, women have been less likely than men to enroll in clinical trials, so we know less about the pathogenesis, effective treatment, and complications of HIV among women than among men. Knowledge about HIV/AIDS continues to evolve rapidly, and HIV treatment guidelines are revised frequently and gaps in our knowledge do exist. The reader is advised to obtain the most current information about HIV treatment from up-to-date sources available on line. The HIV/AIDS Treatment Information Service is one excellent source of information (www.aidsinfo.nih.gov). Optimal HIV care must be individualized and must also account for rapidly changing knowledge in this field. For these reasons, we strongly recommend consultation with an HIV/AIDS expert when formulating a plan of care.

ETIOLOGY

HIV-1 is a retrovirus with an RNA genome and an outer lipid envelope. The term retrovirus describes a virus that contains reverse transcriptase, a viral enzyme that permits DNA to be copied from RNA. The copying direction is the reverse of cellular transcriptase, which copies RNA from DNA. HIV-2 is another human retrovirus found primarily in West Africa and is similar to HIV-1 but appears to be less destructive to the immune system and has slower disease progression. In this chapter, we limit discussion to HIV-1 infection and use the term "HIV" to refer to HIV-1.

HIV enters cells by means of attachment to a CD4 (or T4) receptor found on the surface of many cell populations. Several different cells in the body contain this receptor, including monocytes, macrophages, neuronal cells, glial cells, Langerhans-dendritic cells, follicular dendritic cells, colorectal cells, and the circulating lymphocyte (the CD4/T4 cell), also known as the helper-inducer T lymphocyte. Thus, many cells may be infected by HIV, not just the circulating CD4 lymphocyte cells.

Transmission of Human Immunodeficiency Virus

HIV can be transmitted by sexual contact, blood exposure through sharing needles, blood transfusion or organ transplantation, and from mother to infant during pregnancy, delivery, or breast-feeding. Heterosexual and male homosexual transmission of HIV is more likely in the setting of receptive anal intercourse, bleeding during sex, and the presence of another sexually transmitted disease (STD) in either the HIV-infected or susceptible partner. Sexual transmission is also more likely if the HIV-infected partner has advanced HIV disease and/or a high HIV viral load. HIV transmission occurs at a higher rate in a new sexual partnership than in an established partnership of 6 months or longer. As with other STDs, male-to-female HIV transmission occurs at a much higher rate compared with female-to-male transmission. This may be because susceptible endocervical cells are exposed to seminal fluid for a relatively long period of time after intercourse. In addition, the concentration of HIV is also higher in semen than in female genital secretions. Not all persons exposed to HIV become infected. This may be due to a difference in the virulence of HIV isolates, the amount of virus, the host immune response, or some combination of these factors. Although sexual HIV transmission is theoretically possible between women who have sex with women, to date, lesbians who are infected with HIV have been found to have other risk factors for HIV acquisition, such as sex with men, injection drug use, or transfusion.

Like other blood-borne viruses, HIV may be transmitted by injection drug use with sharing of contaminated needles or other equipment. HIV acquisition has also been associated with noninjection drug use, particularly the use of crack cocaine. The association between crack cocaine or other substance use and HIV acquisition is probably mediated by other behavioral risk factors, such as having a high-risk sexual partner, multiple partners, or the exchange of sex for drugs.

In the United States, blood products and other tissues have been screened for HIV since 1985. This process has virtually eliminated HIV transmission from transfusions or transplantation in this country. However, transfusion-associated HIV transmission still occurs in countries that do not yet have the resources to screen blood products for HIV.

Vertical HIV transmission can occur during pregnancy, at delivery, or postnatally during breast-feeding. It is estimated that breast-feeding increases risk for perinatal HIV transmission by approximately 40%. Excluding breast-feeding, approximately one third of perinatal transmissions occur during pregnancy and two thirds occur during labor and delivery. The management of HIV in pregnancy is described in more detail later in this chapter.

EPIDEMIOLOGY

The World Health Organization estimates that in 2001, 1% of the world's population between ages 15 and 49 were HIV infected, 5 million people became newly infected with HIV, and 3 million people died from HIV/AIDS. More than 95% of persons with HIV/AIDS live in developing countries. Worldwide, 80% of adults with HIV acquired the virus through heterosexual transmission, and over 90% of all HIV infections among infants and children occur through perinatal transmission. These alarming numbers underscore the urgent need for interventions that will limit further sexual and perinatal transmission of HIV. In particular, we need better prevention strategies that can be implemented in resource-limited settings. Upcoming international research should also focus on strategies to provide effective antiretroviral therapy to persons with HIV in developing countries.

In the United States, there has been a steady increase in the proportion of women with HIV/AIDS. By the end of 2001, women made up over 25% of all newly reported AIDS cases. HIV seroprevalence surveys estimate that women now make up approximately 30% to 35% of persons with HIV in the United States. Over 60% of women with AIDS acquired HIV through heterosexual transmission, often from a partner without recognized risk factors. Other risk factors for HIV among women include injection drug use and history of transfusion between 1978 and 1985. African-Americans, American Indian/Alaskan Natives, and Hispanics continue to be disproportionately infected with HIV.

Other STDs act as cofactors to increase likelihood of sexual HIV transmission. Herpes, syphilis, and chancroid all facilitate HIV transmission. These genital syndromes increase direct access of HIV to mucosal tissues, lymphatic drainage, and systemic leukocytes. Nonulcerative STDs such as *Chlamydia trachomatis, Neisseria gonorrhoeae,* and *Trichomonas vaginalis* probably also recruit inflammatory cells into the genital tract, resulting in enhanced HIV transmission. Recently, bacterial vaginosis (BV) has been associated with HIV acquisition. Lactobacilli, particularly the strains that produce hydrogen peroxide, play a critical role in maintaining an acidic vaginal pH and normal vaginal microflora and inhibiting HIV replication. Because women with BV have decreased or absent lactobacillus, an elevated vaginal pH, and no hydrogen peroxide production, the association between BV and HIV acquisition is scientifically plausible. Further, the anaerobic vaginal flora associated with BV may produce factors that stimulate HIV replication.

As yet, little is known about the effect of either endogenous hormonal variability (menstrual cycle, pregnancy, menopause) or exogenous hormones (contraception, hormone replacement therapy) on HIV acquisition and shedding. Although the amount of HIV in cervical secretions appears to increase in the late luteal phase of the menstrual cycle, as yet there are no data to suggest that endogenous hormonal variability modulates the risk of HIV acquisition. Several cross-sectional studies in developing countries have suggested that oral contraceptive use may be associated with HIV infection. However, it is not clear whether oral contraceptive use directly increases the risk of HIV acquisition or whether this association is mediated by increased cervical ectopy, risk behaviors, or other factors. In developing countries, male circumcision appears to decrease risk for HIV transmission. Again, it is not clear whether other behavioral or infectious risk factors mediate the association between male circumcision status and HIV transmission.

NATURAL HISTORY OF HUMAN IMMUNODEFICIENCY VIRUS INFECTION

Symptomatic primary HIV infection has been reported to occur in 30% to 70% of cases. The time of symptoms from exposure is typically 2 to 4 weeks but may be longer. Typical symptoms found in acute HIV infection include fever, myalgia, lymphadenopathy, pharyngitis, and an erythematous maculopapular rash. Less common symptoms include mucocutaneous ulcerations, diarrhea, nausea and vomiting, hepatosplenomegaly, and oral candidiasis, occurring in 10% to 30%. Neurologic features can include peripheral neuropathy, meningoencephalitis, facial palsy, cognitive impairment, and psychosis. Acute infection and seroconversion can also occur without symptoms.

After seroconversion, it may take a decade or longer for HIV infection to become symptomatic. During this asymptomatic period, there is a progressive decrease in the number of CD4 lymphocytes. The CD4 cells are central to the normal function of the immune system. They stimulate the maturation of B cells to plasma cells, which then secrete antibodies. They stimulate the maturation of CD8 cells (suppressor-cytotoxic lymphocytes), which kill cells infected with HIV and other pathogens. They suppress further growth of CD4 and CD8 cells when infection is controlled. They also proliferate into memory clones, which recognize and destroy pathogens to which the clones have previously been exposed. Thus, the decrease in

CD4 lymphocytes with progressive HIV infection results in disruption of both humoral and cell-mediated immunity. These defects in the immune system eventually increase susceptibility to a number of infections that can ultimately result in serious morbidity and mortality, in the absence of antiretroviral therapy. Fortunately, advances in antiretroviral therapy since the mid-1990s have substantially altered the course of HIV disease for persons with access to treatment.

Early symptomatic HIV infection includes complications that are more common and more severe because of the coexistence of HIV infection. Examples include oral candidiasis, persistent or recurrent vaginal candidiasis, cervical dysplasia, herpes zoster, and constitutional symptoms.

The most recent AIDS surveillance case definition includes the presence of an AIDS indicator condition or a CD4 cell count less than 200/mm^3. Examples of AIDS indicator conditions include *Pneumocystis carinii* pneumonia (PCP), recurrent bacterial pneumonia, *Candida* esophagitis, invasive cervical cancer, and pulmonary tuberculosis (TB). Patients with CD4 cell counts less than 50/mm^3 have a median survival of 1 to 1.5 years without prophylaxis and treatment for opportunistic infections (OIs) and/or antiretroviral therapy.

The median rate of progression from infection to the development of an AIDS-defining diagnosis, in the absence of treatment, is approximately 10 years. However, some HIV-infected individuals have remained clinically asymptomatic for more than 20 years, without antiretroviral therapy. These individuals have been referred to as "long-term nonprogressors" and may represent as many as 5% to 10% of all those infected with HIV. Whether this phenomenon is related to the host immune system or the infecting virus, or some combination of these factors, is not clear.

Manifestations of Human Immunodeficiency Virus/ Acquired Immunodeficiency Syndrome Specific to Women

Early clinical manifestations of HIV are generally similar among women and men. HIV-associated conditions specific to women include cervical and vulvar dysplasia and neoplasia, recurrent vulvovaginal candidiasis, and pelvic inflammatory disease (PID).

Compared with HIV-negative women, HIV-infected women are significantly more likely to have human papillomavirus (HPV) infection of the cervix, vulva, and anus. HPV infection may be asymptomatic or may manifest as genital warts. HPV is also a major cofactor in the pathogenesis of intraepithelial dysplasia and neoplasia at all these anatomic sites. The prevalence of genital dysplasia is approximately five times higher among HIV-infected women than HIV-negative women. Among HIV-infected women, the extent of HPV-associated genital dysplasia increases with advanced immunosuppression. Invasive cervical cancer has been designated as an AIDS-defining condition. HIV-infected women with cervical cancer are more likely to present with an advanced cancer stage, to have a shorter time to recurrence, and to die from cervical cancer compared with HIV-negative women.

Present guidelines for cervical cancer screening among HIV-infected women recommend performing a Pap smear at baseline and, if normal, a second Pap smear 6 months after the baseline evaluation. If both results are normal, Pap smears may then be done annually. The 2001 Bethesda consensus guidelines state that HIV-infected women with atypical squamous cells of uncertain significance or any grade of cervical dysplasia on Pap smear should be referred for colposcopy. Studies are underway to evaluate the role of HPV viral subtyping in the management of cervical dysplasia, both among HIV-infected and HIV-negative women. Intravaginal 5-fluorouracil cream has been shown to reduce the frequency of recurrence of high-grade cervical dysplasia after treatment among HIV-infected women. However, this treatment has not yet become the standard of care. Because the management of cervical dysplasia among HIV-infected women is beyond the scope of this chapter, expert consultation is recommended.

Symptomatic vulvovaginal *Candida* infection is a common gynecologic problem among HIV-negative and HIV-infected women. There is considerable variability between women in the frequency and severity of candida vulvovaginitis, independent of degree of immunosuppression. Some studies suggest that there does not appear to be a significant increase in the frequency of candida vulvovaginitis until the CD4 count is less than 100/mm^3. *Candida* species colonizing the genital tract appear to be distinct from those found in the oropharynx, suggesting that these conditions may arise independently. For women with severe persistent or recurrent candidiasis, prophylaxis with oral fluconazole (200 mg weekly) is an alternative to treatment limited to symptomatic episodes. However, it is not known if weekly fluconazole prophylaxis will increase the risk of developing azole-resistant fungal infections.

PID occurs more than four times more frequently among HIV-infected women compared with HIV-negative women. Several epidemiologic studies have suggested that HIV-infected women with PID may be more likely to present with fever and to have persistent fever for more than 48 hours, compared with HIV-negative women. HIV-infected women may also be more likely to develop tuboovarian abscesses and possibly more likely to require surgical intervention. The microbiologic findings among HIV-infected and HIV-negative women are similar. Although the clinical course of PID may be more severe among HIV-infected women than among HIV-negative women, the recommended antibiotic regimen is the same.

CLINICAL SYMPTOMS AND HISTORY

The goals of the initial HIV medical evaluation should be to assess the patient's level of immunosuppression, to identify any HIV-related infections or malignancies, and to identify any other medical conditions, particularly those associated with HIV risk behaviors. The evaluation should also include an assessment of the patient's understanding of HIV disease and her readiness for antiretroviral therapy. The ultimate goals should be to develop a partnership between the patient and her care provider, to develop strategies to prevent or delay the progression of HIV and its associated complications, to prevent the development of resistance to antiretroviral medications, and to prevent additional HIV transmission.

The provider should review prior HIV testing history and any prior HIV care, including past antiretroviral medication use, if applicable. The patient should be asked if she knows when and where she was first exposed to HIV, because approximately 50% of individuals progress to AIDS within 10 years of seroconversion in the absence of antiretroviral therapy. Also, the likelihood of infection with a resistant HIV strain is higher if infection occurred recently or in a geographic area with high prevalence of HIV drug resistance.

A complete medical history should be obtained, including current symptoms and prior HIV-related illnesses. The provider should ask specifically about the following symptoms: constitutional symptoms such as fever, weight loss, fatigue, and night sweats; pulmonary symptoms, including cough and shortness of breath; gastrointestinal symptoms such as diarrhea, difficulty swallowing, and sore throat; neurologic symptoms, including headaches, seizure disorders, and visual disturbances; and dermatologic and oral manifestations. The gynecologic history should include assessment of menstrual patterns, contraceptive use, history of STD, PID, and abnormal Pap smear, and obstetric history. Assessment of risk behaviors for HIV should include a sexual history, assessment of alcohol and drug use, past transfusion (particularly before 1985), and travel history. The social history is useful for assessment of available social support in general, as well as her degree of openness and available support in relation to her HIV status. Finally, during the interview it is particularly important to assess the patient's general coping style, degree of acceptance and/or understanding of HIV, and readiness for antiretroviral therapy if indicated.

CLINICAL FINDINGS AND PHYSICAL EXAMINATION

A baseline physical examination for an HIV-infected patient should emphasize careful assessment of the skin to look for abnormalities such as seborrheic dermatitis, psoriasis, molluscum contagiosum, folliculitis, herpes zoster, and Kaposi sarcoma. Retinal examination includes evaluation for exudates and hemorrhage suggestive of HIV retinopathy or cytomegalovirus (CMV) retinitis. The mouth and tongue should be examined carefully for evidence of oral hairy leukoplakia, candidiasis, aphthous ulcers, herpes simplex virus lesions, and other abnormalities. Lymphadenopathy should be assessed as well as the size of the liver and spleen.

Women with HIV infection should have a gynecologic evaluation, including Pap smear and testing for STD, at baseline. The external genitalia and perianal region should be carefully inspected for warts, ulcers, and other abnormalities. If genital or perianal ulcers or fissures suggestive of herpes simplex virus are noted, a swab from the base of the lesion can be sent for viral culture. If genital or perianal warts are seen, consider colposcopy and directed biopsies to evaluate for HPV-associated dysplasia, even if the cervical Pap smear is normal. Simple warts may be treated topically by a variety of methods, including cryotherapy. Bulky lesions may be better approached surgically, and expert consultation is recommended.

The vagina and cervix should be carefully inspected with a speculum. Any vaginal discharge should be evaluated for *Candida*, *T. vaginalis*, and BV. The cervix should be visualized and a Pap smear obtained using a technique to adequately sample the endocervix and transformation zone as well as the ectocervix. A bimanual examination of the cervix, uterus, and adnexal regions should be performed to rule out uterine or adnexal tenderness suggestive of PID. Finally, a rectovaginal examination is helpful to examine the adnexal regions adequately and rule out an adnexal mass such as a tuboovarian abscess or ovarian cyst.

Sexually Transmitted Disease Testing

Initial STD testing should include tests of cervical secretions for *C. trachomatis* and *N. gonorrhoeae* by immunofluorescence, culture, or nucleic acid-based methods. Of these techniques, nucleic acid testing is the most sensitive and may be performed with a "dirty catch" voided urine specimen as an alternative to testing cervical secretions. Women should also be assessed for vaginal candidiasis, *T. vaginalis*, and BV. Syphilis serology should be obtained, and a positive nontreponemal syphilis test (venereal disease research laboratory or rapid plasma reagin) should be quantified and also confirmed with a specific treponemal antibody test. STD testing should be performed annually for sexually active women or more frequently if indicated.

STD control is a vital component of HIV prevention. HIV-infected women with concomitant STDs probably have increased HIV in genital secretions and thus are more likely to transmit HIV to others. All HIV-infected women should be strongly urged to use condoms to decrease the risk of STD acquisition as well as the risk of HIV transmission to her partner. Condoms will also help to protect women from reinfection with HIV from an infected partner. Even when two HIV-infected persons are mutually monogamous, condom use is still recommended.

LABORATORY STUDIES

Table 85.1 summarizes the current laboratory monitoring recommended for HIV-infected women. Because recommendations may change over time, review of the most recent guidelines is suggested, and consultation with an HIV expert is strongly recommended.

Serologic Testing to Diagnose or Confirm Human Immunodeficiency Virus Infection

HIV serologic testing should be voluntary, with the informed consent of the patient obtained before HIV testing in accordance with local laws. Patient confidentiality must be ensured, and the possibility of discrimination toward those who test positive must be prevented if at all possible. In some cases, patients may prefer to obtain anonymous HIV serologic testing so as to completely avoid the possibility of inadvertent disclosure of their HIV serostatus.

The enzyme-linked immunosorbent assay (ELISA) antibody test screens for antibodies to HIV in the serum of infected individuals. The ELISA has high sensitivity but lacks specificity. A repeatedly reactive ELISA must be confirmed with a second confirmatory test (usually a Western blot) before diagnosing HIV infection. The Western blot is more time consuming and labor intensive than the ELISA but is extremely sensitive and specific for the detection of HIV infection. HIV antibodies are almost always detectable by ELISA and Western blot within 3 months of infection. However, because antibody tests do not screen directly for HIV, these tests may give false-negative results in persons with acute or recently acquired HIV infection who have not yet developed antibodies (the "window" period). Because patients with primary HIV infection may not have mounted an antibody response, the ELISA and Western blot may be negative or indeterminate at the time of initial serologic testing. The most sensitive assay for the detection of HIV infection is a quantitative plasma HIV RNA test by polymerase chain reaction (PCR), although this test is not currently licensed for diagnosing HIV. Of note, patients with acute HIV infection may have high levels of viremia (10^5 to 10^6 copies/mL). The diagnosis of acute HIV infection should be questioned if the plasma HIV RNA concentration is less than 2,000 copies/mL (potentially a false-positive result). All patients with suspected primary HIV infection should have a follow-up ELISA and Western blot in 3 to 6 months to confirm the diagnosis. In addition, many experts advocate aggressive antiretroviral therapy for primary HIV infection, and expert consultation is strongly advised.

Rapid tests for HIV antibodies are becoming available and are presently under investigation. It is likely that these tests will prove useful in settings where rapid diagnosis is desirable. For instance, a rapid HIV antibody test for a woman in labor may lead to maternal and/or neonatal antiretroviral therapy, and

TABLE 85.1. Laboratory Monitoring for HIV-Infected Women

Assessment	Frequency
T-lymphocyte subsets	3–4 mo[a]
Viral load quantification (HIV-RNA PCR)	3–4 mo[b]
CBC with differential and platelets	3–6 mo
Electrolytes, urea nitrogen, creatinine, liver function tests, glucose, lipid panel	3–6 mo[c]
Viral resistance testing	Virologic failure, suboptimal response to treatment, or suspected acute HIV infection
VDRL or RPR with quantitation and treponemal antibody test if positive	Annually and as indicated
Glucose-6-phosphate dehydrogenase test	Baseline
Hepatitis A antibody	Baseline
Hepatitis B surface antigen, surface antibody, core antibody	Baseline, repeat as indicated
Hepatitis C antibody	Baseline
Cytomegalovirus IgG	Baseline
Toxoplasma IgG	Baseline
Tuberculin skin test (PPD)	Baseline[d]
Neisseria gonorrhoeae and *Chlamydia trachomatis*	Annually, more often as indicated
Papanicolaou smear	Every 6 mo × 2, then annually if negative
Assessment for *Trichomonas vaginalis, Candida, bacterial vaginosis*	Annually, more often as indicated

[a]Perform CD4 counts with a CBC and differential to determine absolute CD4 count in addition to percent CD4.
[b]Obtain viral load immediately before initiation or change in antiretroviral therapy and every 4–8 weeks after initiation or change of therapy to monitor virologic response, until maximal viral suppression is reached. Thereafter, viral load should be monitored every 3–4 months. If the viral load increases more than three-fold without a clear explanation, obtain a repeat viral load to confirm virologic failure. Virologic failure should prompt the practitioner to assess the patient's adherence and to check for the presence of viral resistance. If infection with non-B clade HIV is suspected, a branched-chain DNA assay should be used to measure the viral load.
[c]Follow liver function tests closely, as recommended by the manufacturer, with initiation of nevirapine.
[d]Repeat tuberculin skin testing annually if negative.
CBC, complete blood count; IgG, immunoglobulin G; PCR, polymerase chain reaction; PPD, purified protein derivative; RPR, rapid plasma regain; VDRL, venereal disease reference laboratory.

possibly other interventions, to decrease the risk of perinatal HIV transmission. The current rapid HIV tests have about the same specificity as the ELISA, and positive results must be confirmed with a Western blot or other supplemental test.

Infants of HIV-infected women will have persistent maternal antibodies to HIV until at least 6 to 12 months of age. Accordingly, infant HIV diagnosis depends on serial HIV RNA or DNA PCR testing or peripheral blood mononuclear cell culture for HIV, not HIV serology. The Centers for Disease Control and Prevention has published guidelines for the diagnosis of pediatric HIV infection for perinatally exposed infants, and these can be found at the HIV/AIDS Treatment Information Service Web site.

Lymphocyte Markers

The absolute CD4 cell count and the percentage of CD4 cells are highly predictive of immune function, susceptibility to OI, and HIV disease progression. CD4 counts are used to guide the initiation of antiretroviral therapy and antibiotic prophylaxis for OIs. A CD4 count over 500/mm^3 implies relatively normal immune function, whereas a CD4 count less than 200/mm^3 indicates deteriorating immune function and increased susceptibility to PCP and other OIs. Lymphocyte counts should be monitored at a minimum of every 6 months and more frequently with declining CD4 counts and after initiation of therapy. In addition to antiretroviral therapy, factors that influence CD4 counts include laboratory variation, seasonal and diurnal variation, certain intercurrent illnesses, and corticosteroids. Thus, ideally lymphocyte markers should be measured at a consistent time of day and not during an acute illness. Lymphocyte markers should be ordered with a complete blood count with differential (CBC) to measure the absolute CD4 count and the percentage of CD4 cells. Current treatment guidelines as of 2002 recommend the initiation of antiretroviral therapy at a CD4 count in the range of 200 to 350/mm^3.

Viral Load Quantification

The amount of HIV RNA present in plasma or other body fluids may be quantified using PCR. Viral load quantification has become an extremely useful tool for monitoring response to antiretroviral therapy. Current ultrasensitive viral load tests have a lower limit of detection of 20 to 50 copies/mL. Prolonged suppression of HIV RNA to below this threshold is strongly associated with immune reconstitution and improvement in clinical status. In contrast, virologic rebound above 200 to 500 copies/mL after previously undetectable levels of HIV RNA may suggest the evolution of drug-resistant virus or nonadherence to antiretroviral therapy. The viral load should be followed closely after initiation of antiretroviral therapy (at 2–4 weeks after starting therapy and then every 4–8 weeks or more frequently if there are concerns about adherence or drug resistance). Once a patient has reached undetectable HIV RNA levels and appears to be stable with regard to adherence, the viral load can be followed less intensively (i.e., every 3–4 months). In the past, a high viral load (>55,000 copies/mL) was considered an indication to start antiretroviral therapy regardless of CD4 count. However, present antiretroviral treatment guidelines emphasize the role of the CD4 count over the absolute viral load.

Human Immunodeficiency Virus Antiretroviral Resistance Testing

HIV has the capacity to mutate rapidly in vivo. In general, nonmutated "wild-type" HIV is more fit than viral strains that carry mutations. However, certain viral mutations can confer survival advantages for the mutated virus in response to selection pressure from antiretroviral drugs. HIV strains carrying resistance mutations have become increasingly prevalent in recent years, in parallel with the increase in antiretroviral drug use.

Tests for antiretroviral resistance have been developed to attempt to optimize antiretroviral therapy. There are two main strategies for HIV testing: genotypic viral sequencing to detect resistance mutations and phenotypic assessment of the activity of selected antiretroviral agents against a viral isolate. Currently, both types of resistance testing require highly specialized laboratory resources and expert interpretation of the results. At present it appears that the main utility of antiretroviral resistance testing is to guide antiretroviral therapy in the setting of early virologic failure or for tailoring salvage therapy for antiretroviral-experienced persons. Current antiretroviral resistance testing methods are generally not sensitive enough to detect resistance mutations among persons who have not taken the drug of interest for several months. This is because wild-type virus usually becomes the predominant HIV strain in persons who stop antiretroviral therapy, even if there is a reservoir of resistant virus present.

Pharmacogenomic Testing

It is apparent that genetics plays a critical role in a person's response to drug therapy. Genetic polymorphisms can influence the rate of drug metabolism, the efficacy of a drug, and the potential for toxicity. The relationship between gene polymorphisms and antiretroviral pharmacokinetics, efficacy, and toxicity is presently under intense investigation. Pharmacogenomic testing is not presently available clinically and is only available in the context of clinical research. However, in the future, testing for specific gene polymorphisms may play an important role in the management of antiretroviral therapy. As an example, persons with a specific human leukocyte antigen subtype appear to be at increased risk for a hypersensitivity reaction to abacavir. Human leukocyte antigen typing before starting antiretroviral therapy could allow clinicians to avoid prescribing abacavir to persons at high risk for a hypersensitivity reaction while still using this drug in persons of lower risk.

Hematology and Blood Chemistry Assays

A CBC with differential is necessary for the interpretation of lymphocyte markers. Additionally, anemia and thrombocytopenia are common complications of untreated HIV. Anemia may also occur as a complication of antiretroviral therapy. Accordingly, the CBC should be monitored every 3 to 4 months or more frequently if indicated.

Baseline liver function tests are necessary to assess the patient's ability to tolerate treatment with potentially hepatotoxic agents. Liver function tests should be obtained at least every 3 to 6 months for persons on antiretroviral therapy and in some instances must be followed much more intensely (e.g., with nevirapine). A general chemistry panel should be obtained every 3 to 6 months, or more frequently as indicated, to monitor serum glucose, electrolytes, renal function, and nutritional parameters.

Given the frequency of lipid abnormalities in HIV-infected persons, many experts also obtain a baseline fasting lipid profile and subsequent measurements every 3 to 4 months, depending on the initial results and other risk factors for cardiovascular disease. Many HIV experts also recommend screening for glucose-6-phosphate dehydrogenase deficiency at baseline, in case medications such as dapsone and primaquine may be indicated.

Serologic Testing for Coinfections

Many HIV-infected persons have other viral and bacterial coinfections. It is important to screen for these coinfections to understand the full spectrum of the person's illness and to devise appropriate prevention and treatment strategies.

At baseline, HIV-infected patients should be screened for immunity to hepatitis A and B and current infection with hepatitis C virus (HCV). Persons who are susceptible to hepatitis A or B should be offered immunization. Persons with antibody (IgG) to hepatitis C are coinfected, and the extent of HCV infection can be assessed using a quantitative HCV RNA PCR. The management and indications for treatment of HCV in HIV-infected persons is an area of active investigation. Anti-HCV therapy is probably less suppressive among persons coinfected with HIV. Because the management of HCV is complex in the setting of HIV, expert consultation is recommended.

At baseline, it is helpful to test for latent CMV and toxoplasmosis infections. Many HIV-infected patients are coinfected with CMV as shown by a positive CMV IgG antibody test. Fortunately, primary CMV infection and reactivation do not usually cause systemic illness except in the setting of advanced immunosuppression (CD4 < 100 cells/mm^3). Similarly, toxoplasmosis serologic testing (IgG) demonstrates previous exposure to this organism. Persons with IgG to toxoplasmosis and advanced immunosuppression are susceptible to reactivation in the central nervous system.

Tuberculosis Testing

The Centers for Disease Control and Prevention recommends annual tuberculin skin testing with a purified protein derivative (PPD; Mantoux, 5TU units) if the result is not already known to be positive. The criterion for a positive PPD test in HIV-infected patients is 5 mm of induration, versus 10 to 15 mm in HIV-negative patients. Annual screening with the PPD is recommended if the initial test result is negative. Also, if the initial negative PPD test was obtained at a CD4 count less than 200/mm^3 and the patient subsequently has immune reconstitution on antiretroviral therapy such that the CD4 count is sustained above 200/mm^3, tuberculin skin testing should be repeated.

Persons with a positive PPD test should have a chest radiograph and clinical evaluation to look for active TB. Also, all HIV-infected persons with symptoms consistent with TB should have a thorough evaluation, including chest radiograph, even if the PPD is negative.

For current recommendations for the prophylaxis and treatment of TB, please consult current guidelines for the prevention and treatment of OIs associated with HIV infection, available on line.

TREATMENT

Principles of Antiretroviral Therapy

The philosophical approach to treating HIV infection has shifted in recent years from a "hit hard, hit early" strategy to a more conservative stance. The reasons for this shift include the recognition of the potential metabolic and other complications associated with long-term antiretroviral use. In addition, it has become increasingly clear that the decision to start antiretroviral therapy must be seen as a significant commitment on the part of the patient and that lack of adequate preparation to start antiretroviral therapy can lead to adherence difficulties that may have life-long consequences.

Because new information continues to become available at a rapid pace, HIV treatment guidelines are updated annually or more frequently. The most current treatment guidelines are available at the U.S. Department of Health and Human Services

AIDS information Web site (www.aidsinfo.nih.gov). The critical questions to be explored with a patient considering antiretroviral therapy include the following:

- When to start? Consideration of when to start therapy must go beyond the current CD4 and viral load criteria. The patient must be ready to commit to taking a potentially complex regimen exactly as prescribed for an indefinite period. This may mean changing her eating schedule; disclosing that she is on medications to friends, family, and coworkers; and coping with adverse effects.
- What drugs to use? Current guidelines recommend initiation of therapy with at least three potent, synergistic, antiretroviral drugs. The choice of initial regimen will depend on the patient's lifestyle and preferences and possibly her baseline liver function, past medical history, and likelihood of infection with a drug-resistant viral strain. For example, if the patient is pregnant or considering pregnancy, there are additional considerations regarding choice of antiretroviral therapy. Please see the section on pregnancy below for additional details.
- When to switch drugs or consider stopping treatment? Treatment may need to be modified or stopped because of patient intolerance or toxicity or because of virologic failure on the current regimen. If stopping treatment because of drug intolerance or toxicity, it is extremely important to stop all antiretroviral drugs simultaneously to minimize the risk of developing antiretroviral resistance. The definition of virologic failure requiring treatment switch or intensification is controversial, and the reader should consult current treatment guidelines on line. Antiretroviral resistance testing may be useful in the setting of possible virologic failure.

Specific Antiretroviral Medications

As the armamentarium of antiretroviral drugs continues to expand, we are learning more about the relative efficacy, complex interactions, and potential for toxicity with these agents. Following is a brief description of the antiretroviral drugs licensed by the U.S. Food and Dug Administration and available as of 2002. Because of the complexity involved with choosing and monitoring antiretroviral therapy, expert consultation is strongly recommended.

The nucleoside reverse transcriptase inhibitors (NRTI) are the oldest class of antiretroviral drugs. Zidovudine, lamivudine, didanosine, stavudine, zalcitabine, and abacavir are all nucleoside analogues in this class, and tenofovir is a nucleotide analogue. The major toxicity of the NRTI class is related to effects on mitochondrial DNA synthesis, and long-term use may lead to mitochondrial toxicity. This toxicity may be subtle (mild peripheral neuropathy) or fulminant (hepatic steatosis and liver failure). Abacavir can cause a rare, but potentially fatal, hypersensitivity reaction. Patients who start abacavir must be thoroughly counseled about symptoms of hypersensitivity, and those who stop abacavir because of suspected hypersensitivity should never be rechallenged with this drug.

The three approved nonnucleoside reverse transcriptase inhibitor (NNRTI) drugs are nevirapine, efavirenz, and delavirdine, with the latter being less commonly prescribed. Nevirapine is dosed at 200 mg once daily for the first 2 weeks during hepatic enzyme induction and is then increased to 200 mg twice daily, to decrease the likelihood of developing a rash. Skin reactions are the most common side effect of nevirapine, and in most cases the rash is mild and resolves spontaneously. However, rare cases of severe hypersensitivity reactions and fulminant hepatitis have been reported. Patients must be cautioned to report any symptoms suggestive of hepatotoxicity or systemic hypersensitivity reaction. Liver function tests should be monitored at baseline, 2 weeks after starting treatment before dose escalation, and frequently thereafter in accordance with the manufacturer's recommendations. Efavirenz is typically dosed once daily and is generally well tolerated. The most common side effects are mood alterations and sleep disturbance. Efavirenz has been shown to have teratogenic effects in primates, and so its use must be avoided in pregnancy. High-level resistance to all of the approved NNRTIs can occur with a single gene mutation of the reverse transcriptase enzyme, underscoring the need for excellent adherence when these medications are prescribed.

The protease inhibitor (PI) class includes the drugs nelfinavir, indinavir, saquinavir, ritonavir, amprenavir, lopinavir, and atazanavir. These drugs tend to require more capsules to be swallowed at one time (larger pill burden) compared with the NRTI and NNRTI drug classes. Ritonavir is often prescribed together with indinavir, saquinavir, amprenavir, and lopinavir to boost the levels of the second PI agent, enabling the PIs to be taken once or twice daily instead of more frequently. Most of the PIs have gastrointestinal side effects, including nausea, vomiting, bloating, gas, and diarrhea. Indinavir has been associated with renal stones and hyperbilirubinemia. Long-term use of PI-containing antiretroviral regimens has been associated with metabolic abnormalities, including hyperglycemia, hyperlipidemia, fat redistribution syndromes, and possibly also osteopenia and atherosclerotic cardiovascular disease. Atazanavir is the most recent PI to receive FDA approval. This drug can be taken once daily and may have less effect on lipid levels than other PIs.

There are new members of all these drug classes in development. Fusion inhibitors (such as enfuvirtide) and integrase inhibitors will provide additional strategies for the treatment of HIV infection. New antiretroviral drugs may be better tolerated, have improved side-effect profiles, and perhaps less complexity in terms of pill burden. These drugs will also provide some hope for treatment of HIV with multiple resistance mutations. Therapeutic vaccines and other immune-based therapies are also in development. However, all these strategies only limit or suppress HIV, converting what was once considered a terminal infection into a chronic disease. As yet there is nothing on the horizon that promises to be able to eradicate HIV once infection is established.

Prevention and Treatment of Opportunistic Infections

With the advent of highly active antiretroviral therapy, the incidence of PCP and most other OIs has dropped dramatically. Prophylaxis for OIs continues to be an important component of HIV care. In particular, persons with CD4 counts of less than $200/mm^3$ should receive antibiotic prophylaxis for PCP. Recent studies have demonstrated that it is probably safe to stop antibiotic prophylaxis for PCP in persons on antiretroviral therapy who have experienced a sustained rise in CD4 count over $200/mm^3$ for over 3 months. Current recommendations for the prevention and treatment of PCP and other AIDS-related OIs can be found at www.aidsinfo.nih.gov.

REPRODUCTIVE ISSUES

Preconceptual Counseling

As the clinical outlook for HIV has improved, more women with established HIV infection are contemplating pregnancy. Preconceptual counseling should include a thorough discussion of the woman's HIV status at present, including her most recent CD4 count and viral load; present and past antiretroviral medications; indications for antiretroviral treatment if not already on therapy; and whether the potential father is also HIV infected. Other factors to consider are summarized in Table 85.2.

The couple should be counseled that optimizing maternal health is the best strategy to have a healthy pregnancy and uninfected infant. If the woman is already on antiretroviral therapy, efforts should be made to ensure that she has maximal viral suppression and excellent adherence. If she has detectable virus on antiretroviral medications, resistance testing should be performed. Her antiretroviral regimen may need to be altered to minimize the risk of perinatal HIV transmission, optimize maternal health, and avoid the use of potentially teratogenic agents. In particular, efavirenz should be avoided before and during pregnancy. The patient should be counseled about the potential risks and benefits of antiretroviral therapy in the first trimester. Unless there is a clear maternal indication to start antiretroviral therapy before pregnancy, many clinicians wait until after 10 to 14 weeks' gestation to initiate treatment. Expert consultation is recommended.

If the potential father is also HIV infected, his antiretroviral therapy should also be optimized. The choice of antiretroviral drugs for the father will not have a teratogenic effect on the fetus. When both partners are HIV infected, one approach to conception is to have unprotected intercourse timed for the periovulatory phase of the menstrual cycle as documented by basal body temperature charting and/or urine luteinizing hormone testing. Partners should be encouraged to use condoms except when they are trying to conceive, so as to limit the possibility of reinfection. If the potential father is HIV negative, the safest approach to conception is to perform intravaginal or intrauterine inseminations during the periovulatory phase of the menstrual cycle. For couples without documented infertility, intravaginal inseminations are as effective as intrauterine inseminations.

Couples in which the woman is HIV negative and her male partner is HIV infected have limited alternatives for conception without putting the woman at risk for HIV acquisition. Published series demonstrate that intrauterine insemination after sperm washing appears to have a low risk for HIV transmission from an infected man to an HIV-negative woman. Intracytoplasmic sperm injection is another assisted reproductive technology that has been used to help HIV-discordant couples conceive with lower risk of infection to the woman. Although these techniques appear to be promising, they are not presently available in the United States outside of an academic setting, and they require an andrology laboratory capable of handling HIV-infected specimens and performing PCR testing on specimens in a timely manner before insemination. In addition, the high costs of reproductive technology are often not covered by insurance and are therefore not accessible to many couples.

Couples attempting to conceive should be advised that the likelihood of conception in any given cycle is less than 20%, that 50% of healthy couples attempting conception will become pregnant in 6 months, and that 80% to 90% will become pregnant in a year. Couples who have not conceived after a year may wish to consider infertility evaluation. Couples with clear risk factors for infertility (advanced maternal age, prior ectopic pregnancy, or documented tubal disease) may be referred for infertility evaluation sooner. The American Society for Reproductive Medicine has stated that it is ethical to provide infertility evaluation and services for HIV-infected women, just as for women with other chronic illnesses.

Preconceptual counseling for HIV-infected women should also include information about optimizing maternal health through adequate nutrition, including folic acid supplementation (at least 0.8 mg daily). The immunization history should be reviewed and immunizations updated as needed. Both partners should avoid alcohol, cigarettes, and other recreational drug use. In addition to the well-documented effects of alcohol and cigarettes on fetal development and placental function, both alcohol and marijuana can affect sperm production and motility.

Contraception

Condoms are an effective means of pregnancy prevention only if used consistently and correctly. Clinicians should offer HIV-infected women a second, female-controlled, contraceptive method. A second barrier method, such as the diaphragm, female condom, or cervical cap, is an excellent alternative. Some experts discourage the use of the intrauterine device among HIV-infected women because of the potential increased risk for upper genital tract infection. However, at least one study has demonstrated that the copper T intrauterine device (Paragard) is a safe and well-tolerated alternative for HIV-infected women who do not have other contraindications to its use. The levonorgestrel intrauterine device (Mirena) has not been investigated among HIV-infected women.

TABLE 85.2. Management of Other Pregnancy Risks for HIV-Infected Women

Risk factor	Comments
Diabetes	Women on protease inhibitors may have an increased risk of gestational diabetes. Evaluate family history, maternal age, and obesity as other risk factors for gestational diabetes. Consider early glucose tolerance testing in pregnancy, particularly for women on protease inhibitors.
Hepatitis C	HIV-infected women have approximately a 10% risk of transmitting hepatitis C to their infants. No interventions are available to decrease this risk.
Cervical dysplasia	Women who have had a prior cervical cone biopsy, including loop electrosurgical excision procedures, may have an increased risk of cervical incompetence, leading to late miscarriage or premature birth. Consider transvaginal cervical length monitoring in the late second and early third trimester.
Advanced maternal age	Women over age 35 have an increased risk of having a chromosomally abnormal pregnancy. Genetic amniocentesis may increase the risk of perinatal HIV and hepatitis C transmission, particularly through an anterior placenta. Targeted second-trimester ultrasound, first-trimester nuchal translucency measurement, and maternal serum biochemical screening are noninvasive alternatives to genetic amniocentesis. However, all these methods have diagnostic limitations. Genetic counseling should be performed by persons knowledgeable about HIV. The patient should make the final decision about genetic amniocentesis.

The interactions between hormonal contraceptive methods and various antiretroviral drugs are under investigation. It appears that some antiretrovirals, including nelfinavir and ritonavir, may increase hepatic metabolism of ethinyl estradiol, making oral contraceptives less effective when coadministered. Therefore, oral contraceptives should not be relied on as a sole means of contraception among women on antiretroviral therapy. Data will be available in the near future regarding interactions between antiretroviral agents and depot-medroxyprogesterone acetate (Depo-Provera).

Pregnancy

Many HIV-infected women in the United States have a planned or unintentional pregnancy after the diagnosis of HIV has been established. Other women learn of their HIV diagnosis as a result of serologic testing during pregnancy. Pregnant HIV-infected women should be presented with the range of alternatives available to them in a nonjudgmental manner, including pregnancy termination and pregnancy continuation. HIV-infected women are no more likely than HIV-negative women to choose pregnancy termination, and the choice to terminate a pregnancy usually hinges on life circumstances and not on the woman's HIV status.

Initial pregnancy counseling should include information about the effect of continuing a pregnancy on maternal health. Several large cohort studies in the United States and Europe have established that pregnancy does not accelerate the course of HIV infection. HIV-infected women do not appear to be at increased risk for pregnancy complications compared with HIV-negative women of comparable social and demographic backgrounds. There are conflicting data regarding whether combination antiretroviral therapy with a PI increases the rate of premature birth. Because these data are from observational studies, it unclear whether a possible association between maternal PI use and preterm birth might be mediated by some other factor, such as maternal medical status. Women should be informed of the possible association between PI use and preterm birth. However, the data are not convincing enough to recommend avoiding the use of PIs in pregnancy.

Advances in antiretroviral therapy have greatly reduced the risk of perinatal HIV transmission. Results from a randomized controlled trial (ACTG 076) found that zidovudine reduced the rate of HIV transmission from mothers to infants from 25.5% to 8.3%. In this study, HIV-infected pregnant women with CD4 counts over 200/mm^3 were randomized to receive placebo or maternal oral zidovudine after 14 weeks' gestation, intravenous zidovudine in labor, and infant oral zidovudine for the first 6 weeks of life. Subsequent trials have confirmed that zidovudine confers a significant reduction in perinatal HIV transmission even among women with advanced HIV disease, CD4 counts less than 200/mm^3, and women with prior zidovudine treatment. The mechanism by which zidovudine reduces perinatal HIV transmission is unclear and cannot be explained solely by its effect on maternal viral load. Zidovudine is converted to its active triphosphate metabolite by the placenta, and this may inhibit transplacental viral passage. When given intravenously, zidovudine reaches equivalent concentrations in maternal and fetal blood and reaches very high concentrations in the amniotic fluid (five times that of maternal blood). Thus, intravenous zidovudine in labor probably provides significant preexposure prophylaxis to the fetus.

More recent studies have shown that the single most important determinant of perinatal HIV transmission is maternal viral load. If the viral load is less than 1,000 copies/mL in pregnancy, the HIV perinatal transmission rate is estimated to be 2% or less. Among women with a viral load less than 1,000 copies/mL, antiretroviral therapy provides additional protection (1% perinatal transmission risk among women on treatment and up to 10% transmission among women on no antiretroviral therapy).

The goals of antiretroviral therapy in pregnancy are to optimize maternal health, to maximally suppress the viral load, and to avoid potential maternal or fetal toxicity. Given the data on maternal viral load and perinatal HIV transmission, current guidelines recommend consideration of potent combination therapy (at least three drugs) for pregnant women with a viral load greater than 1,000 copies/mL, regardless of CD4 count. Ideally, the woman's antiretroviral regimen should include zidovudine unless she is intolerant or resistant to this drug. If she is on stavudine, the option of replacing stavudine with zidovudine should be considered. Stavudine and zidovudine are competitive antagonists and should not be given together. Women with a viral load less than 1,000 copies/mL and a CD4 count in the normal range may be offered the alternative of zidovudine monotherapy because antiretroviral medication would be indicated primarily to prevent perinatal transmission. Table 85.3 summarizes the recommended zidovudine regimen, which may be prescribed as monotherapy or as part of a potent antiretroviral regimen. Dual combination nucleoside therapy (i.e., zidovudine plus lamivudine) should be avoided, because this combination is less likely to suppress HIV replication and may lead to development of resistance to lamivudine. The choice of additional antiretroviral drugs in pregnancy will depend on maternal health and previous antiretroviral experience. The combination of didanosine and stavudine should be avoided if possible, because of rare case reports of fulminant hepatitis and lactic acidosis in late pregnancy among women on these drugs. Efavirenz should be avoided in pregnancy, particularly in the first trimester, because of teratogenic effects in primate studies. The Antiretroviral Pregnancy Registry is a prospective database that compiles data on pregnancy out-

TABLE 85.3. Zidovudine Regimen[a] for the Prevention of Perinatal HIV Transmission

Phase	Timing	Dose
Antepartum	Begin at 10–14 weeks' gestation	300 mg orally twice daily throughout pregnancy
Intrapartum	With active labor or membrane rupture, or at least 3 h before planned cesarean	2 mg/kg intravenous loading dose, then 1 mg/kg/h intravenous infusion until delivery
Neonatal	Begin at 8–12 h age	2 mg/kg oral syrup every 6 h for 6 weeks

[a]Zidovudine should be included in the antiretroviral drug regimen in pregnancy, if at all possible. Under certain circumstances, zidovudine monotherapy may be considered.
ZDV, zidovudine.

comes after antiretroviral exposure. All cases of antiretroviral use in pregnancy should be reported prospectively to this database (www.apregistry.com).

HIV-infected pregnant women should also be counseled about other pregnancy risk factors as outlined in Table 85.3. Early glucose tolerance testing may be indicated for women on PIs, as well as those with other risk factors for diabetes. HIV-infected women who also have HCV have an increased risk of transmitting HCV to their infants, and there are no available interventions to decrease this risk. Women who have had a prior cervical cone biopsy or loop electrosurgical excision procedure (LEEP) may be at risk for cervical incompetence and early preterm birth, and they may benefit from transvaginal measurement of cervical length.

Amniocentesis for genetic testing or fetal lung maturity testing should be avoided if possible, especially sampling through an anterior placenta, given the theoretical increased risk of HIV transmission. Chorionic villus sampling and percutaneous umbilical blood sampling should also be avoided. A targeted second-trimester ultrasound has a 50% to 70% sensitivity for the detection of ultrasound markers associated with trisomy 21 and other karyotypic abnormalities. Some women may also wish to consider first-trimester fetal nuchal translucency measurements and/or first- or second-trimester maternal serum biochemical screening for chromosomal abnormalities. However, an abnormal maternal serum screening test may increase anxiety for women who might prefer to avoid an amniocentesis because of concerns related to HIV transmission risk. In these situations, genetic counseling with personnel who are familiar with HIV can be helpful.

There has been considerable controversy about mode of delivery for HIV-infected women. A metaanalysis of European and North American cohorts showed that in the context of zidovudine monotherapy, cesarean delivery before the onset of labor or ruptured membranes decreased the perinatal transmission rate to 2%. However, it is not clear whether scheduled cesarean delivery would further reduce the risk of perinatal HIV transmission among women with viral loads less than 1,000 copies/mL beyond the expected rate of 1% to 2%. The American College of Obstetricians and Gynecologists recommends that HIV-infected women have thorough counseling about the alternatives of vaginal and cesarean delivery and participate actively in the decision about mode of delivery. For women who choose to have a cesarean delivery, this may be scheduled at 38 weeks' gestation without requiring an amniocentesis for fetal lung maturity testing.

For women who plan a vaginal delivery, every effort must be made to avoid instrumentation that could increase fetal exposure to maternal blood and secretions. The membranes should be left intact for as long as possible, because perinatal HIV transmission has been correlated with duration of ruptured membranes. Fetal scalp electrodes should be avoided. Episiotomy should be avoided if possible. Vacuum extraction may be preferable to forceps if operative vaginal delivery is indicated.

In industrialized countries, where adequate infant nutrition can be achieved safely through the use of infant formulas, breast-feeding by HIV-infected women is strongly discouraged. There are no data on whether maternal antiretroviral therapy could decrease the risk of breast-feeding–related HIV transmission. Because breast milk is rich in lymphocytes, there may be considerable cell-associated HIV in breast milk.

It is important to discuss with women whether to continue antiretroviral treatment after delivery, particularly for those women who do not meet current treatment thresholds for nonpregnant adults. Even women who plan to continue antiretroviral treatment postpartum might consider a brief (4–12 week) break from antiretrovirals immediately after delivery, when adherence can be particularly challenging. Any decision about antiretroviral treatment interruption must be tailored to the individual and must consider the patient's present level of viral suppression and degree of immunosuppression, past antiretroviral history, adherence, and other factors.

IMPLICATIONS OF HUMAN IMMUNODEFICIENCY VIRUS FOR WOMEN AT DIFFERENT LIFE STAGES

Adolescents and Young Adults

Worldwide, adolescent girls and young adult women are the fastest growing age group of women with HIV. A new diagnosis of HIV infection presents unique challenges in this age group, because girls and young women have many other physical, social, emotional, and sexual transitions to negotiate. In addition, most girls and many young adult women are economically dependent on their parents or partners, and this may limit their access to HIV care because of confidentiality concerns. HIV-infected adolescents in the United States also appear to have high rates of physical and sexual abuse history, substance abuse, and psychiatric comorbidity. Although most HIV-infected adolescents have acquired HIV through adult behaviors, there is a growing population of perinatally infected girls who are now reaching young adulthood. This subset of HIV-infected young women has unique concerns related to chronic illness and prior substantial antiretroviral exposure.

Young women under age 25 have disproportionately high rates of acquisition of other STDs. This may be partly explained by behavioral risk factors and also by the increased prevalence of cervical ectopy in this age group. Accordingly, STD prevention, screening, and treatment must be emphasized. Young women are also at high risk for unintended pregnancy. Contraceptive counseling should follow the principles outlined previously.

Older Women

There is a paucity of information about HIV-infected women during and after menopause. It is difficult to estimate the proportion of HIV-infected women who have gone through menopause because of underdiagnosis in this age group. However, the trend to improved survival rates with potent antiretroviral therapy suggests that increasing numbers of HIV-infected women will be in this age group in the future. One retrospective study suggested that older HIV-infected women who were on hormone replacement therapy had improved survival compared with women not on hormonal therapy, and this difference persisted after adjustment for CD4 count and antiretroviral therapy. Because this was a retrospective analysis, it is possible that hormone use was a marker for improved access to health care, adherence to medication, or other factors.

As the population of HIV-infected women ages, we expect that osteoporosis, cardiovascular disease, and cognitive deficits will become increasingly important health concerns. Osteoporosis and cardiovascular disease are recognized complications of HIV antiretroviral therapy, and cognitive and other neurologic disorders are associated with HIV progression. It will be important to address the interactions between these common disorders of aging and HIV to optimize the health of older women with HIV.

INTERNET REFERENCES

Antiretroviral Pregnancy Registry. Access at www.apregistry.com.
Centers for Disease Control and Prevention, National Center for HIV, STD, and TB Prevention. HIV/AIDS surveillance in women (L264 slide series). Updated January 10, 2003. Access at www.cdc.gov/hiv/graphics/women.htm.
HIV/AIDS Bureau, Health Resources and Services Administration (Andersen J, ed.) A guide to the clinical care of women with HIV: 2001, 1st ed. Access at http://hab.hrsa.gov/womencare.htm.
Panel on Clinical Practices for the Treatment of HIV Infection. Guidelines for the use of antiretroviral agents in HIV-infected adults and adolescents. Updated February 4, 2002. Access at www.aidsinfo.nih.gov.
Perinatal HIV Guidelines Working Group. U.S. Public Health Service Task Force recommendations for the use of antiretroviral drugs in pregnant HIV-1 infected women for maternal health and interventions to reduce perinatal HIV-1 transmission in the United States. Updated June 16, 2003. Access at www.aidsinfo.nih.gov.
Perinatal HIV Guidelines Working Group. Safety and toxicity of individual antiretroviral agents in pregnancy. Updated May 23, 2003. Access at www.aidsinfo.nih.gov.
U.S. Public Health Service/Infectious Diseases Society of America. 2001 USPHS/IDSA guidelines for the prevention of OIs in persons infected with human immunodeficiency virus. Updated November 28, 2001. Access at www.aidsinfo.nih.gov.

BIBLIOGRAPHY

American College of Obstetricians and Gynecologists. Committee on Obstetric Practice. Scheduled cesarean delivery and the prevention of vertical transmission of HIV infection (number 234). Washington, DC. May 2000.
Barbosa C, Macasaet M, Brockmann S, et al. Pelvic inflammatory disease and human immunodeficiency virus infection. *Obstet Gynecol* 1997;89:65–70.
Clark RA, Bessinger R. Clinical manifestations and predictors of survival in older women infected with HIV. *J Acquir Immune Defic Syndr Hum Retrovirol* 1997; 15:341–345.
Cohn SE, Clark RA. Human immunodeficiency virus infection in women. In: Mandell GL, Bennett JE, Dolin R, eds. *Principles and practice of infectious diseases,* 5th ed. Philadelphia: Churchill Livingstone, 2000:1452–1467.
Connor EM, Sperling RS, Gelber R, et al. Reduction of maternal-infant transmission of human immunodeficiency virus type 1 with zidovudine treatment. Pediatric AIDS Clinical Trials Group Protocol 076 Study Group. *N Engl J Med* 1994;331:1173–1180.
Cu-Uvin S, Hogan JW, Warren D, et al. Prevalence of lower genital tract infections among human immunodeficiency virus (HIV) seropositive and high-risk seronegative women. *Clin Infect Dis* 1999;29:1145–1150.
Demeter L, Haubrich R. International perspectives on antiretroviral resistance: phenotypic and genotypic resistance assays—methodology, reliability, and interpretations. *J Acquir Immune Defic Syndr* 2001;26[Suppl 1]:S3–S9.
Edlin BR, Irwin KL, Faruque S, et al. Intersecting epidemics—crack cocaine use and HIV infection among inner-city young adults. Multicenter Crack Cocaine and HIV Infection Study Team. *N Engl J Med* 1994;331:1422–1427.
Ethics committee of the American Society for Reproductive Medicine. Human immunodeficiency virus and infertility treatment. *Fertil Steril* 2002;77:218–222.
Garcia PM, Kalish LA, Pitt J, et al. Maternal levels of plasma human immunodeficiency virus type 1 RNA and the risk of perinatal transmission. *N Engl J Med* 1999;341:394–402.
Gilling-Smith C, Smith JR, Semprini AE. HIV and infertility: time to treat—there's no justification for denying treatment to parents who are HIV positive. *BMJ* 2001;322:566–567.
Grosskurth H, Mosha F, Todd J, et al. Impact of improved treatment of sexually transmitted diseases on HIV infection in rural Tanzania: randomised controlled trial. *Lancet* 1995;346:530–536.
Haddow JE, Palomaki GE, Knight GJ, et al. Reducing the need for amniocentesis in women 35 years of age or older with serum markers for screening. *N Engl J Med* 1994;330:1114–1118.
Hader SL, Smith DK, Moore JS, et al. HIV infection in women in the United States: status at the Millennium. *JAMA* 2001;285:1186–1192.
Haubrich RH, Currier JS, Forthal DN, et al. A randomized study of the utility of human immunodeficiency virus RNA measurement for the management of antiretroviral therapy. *Clin Infect Dis* 2001;33:1060–1068.
Hetherington S, Hughes AR, Mosteller M, et al. Genetic variations in HLA-B region and hypersensitivity reactions to abacavir. *Lancet* 2002;359:1121–1122.
Iams JD, Goldenberg RL, Meis PJ, et al. The length of the cervix and the risk of spontaneous premature delivery. National Institute of Child Health and Human Development Maternal Fetal Medicine Unit Network. *N Engl J Med* 1996;334:567–572.
International Perinatal HIV Group. The mode of delivery and the risk of vertical transmission of human immunodeficiency virus type 1: a meta-analysis of 15 prospective cohort studies. *N Engl J Med* 1999;340:977–987.
Klebanoff SJ, Coombs RW. Viricidal effects of *Lactobacillus acidophilus* in human immunodeficiency virus type 1: possible role in heterosexual transmission. *J Exp Med* 1991;174:282–292.
Maiman M, Watts DH, Andersen J, et al. Vaginal 5-fluorouracil for high grade cervical dysplasia in HIV-infection: a randomized clinical trial. *Obstet Gynecol* 1999;94:954–961.
Mofenson LM, Lambert JS, Stiehm ER, et al. Risk factors for perinatal transmission of human immunodeficiency virus type 1 in women treated with zidovudine. *N Engl J Med* 1999;341:385–393.
Nicolaides KH, Heath V, Cicero S. Increased fetal nuchal translucency at 11–14 weeks. *Prenat Diagn* 2002;22:308–315.
Nduati R, John G, Mbori-Ngacha D, et al. Effect of breastfeeding and formula feeding on transmission of HIV-1: a randomized clinical trial. *JAMA* 2000;283: 1167–1174.
Reichelderfer PS, Coombs RW, Wright DJ, et al. Effect of menstrual cycle on HIV-1 levels in the peripheral blood and genital tract. WHS 001 Study Team. *AIDS* 2000;14:2101–2107.
Richardson BA, Morrison CS, Sekadde-Kigondu C, et al. Effect of intrauterine device use on cervical shedding of HIV-1 DNA. *AIDS* 1999;13:2091–2097.
Schuman P, Capps L, Peng G, et al. Weekly fluconazole for the prevention of mucosal candidiasis in women with HIV infection. *Ann Intern Med* 1997;126: 689–696.
Tuomala RE, Shapiro DE, Mofenson LM, et al. Antiretroviral therapy during pregnancy and the risk of adverse outcome. *N Engl J Med* 2002;346:1863–1870.
Watts DH. Management of human immunodeficiency virus infection in pregnancy. *N Engl J Med* 2002;346:1879–1891.
Wright TC, et al. 2001 consensus guidelines for the management of women with cervical cytological abnormalities. *JAMA* 2002;287:2120–2129.

CHAPTER 86
Sexually Transmitted Diseases

Patricia A. Coury-Doniger

EPIDEMIOLOGY

Sexually transmitted infections (STIs) are epidemic in the United States, more so than in any other developed country in the world. In the past 10 years, the annual incidence of STIs in the United States increased from 12 million to 15 million. Most of these infections occur in persons aged 15 to 35 years. The epidemiology of STIs is also changing. In the past, most known STIs were bacterial, including gonorrhea, syphilis, and chlamydia. Public health control programs were implemented to provide widespread testing and treatment, and the incidence of these infections decreased dramatically. In recent years, a new group of chronic viral STIs has been recognized, including herpes simplex virus (HSV), human papillomavirus (HPV), hepatitis B virus, hepatitis C virus, and human immunodeficiency virus (HIV). These newly recognized STIs have shown significant increases in incidence and morbidity over the past two decades. There is currently no curative treatment for these viral infections such that more than 65 million people in the United States are living with an incurable viral STI. Although most people with STIs are asymptomatic, these infections can cause serious diseases (sexually transmitted diseases [STDs]), disability, and death.

MEDICAL SEQUELAE

Women and children suffer disproportionate risks of morbidity and mortality related to STIs, including HIV. Women, especially teenagers, are more easily infected with STIs and are much more likely to develop complications of these infections. STIs in women can lead to pelvic infections, chronic pelvic pain, ectopic pregnancy, infertility, poor pregnancy outcomes, and cervical cancer. Each year, approximately 5,000 women in the

United States die as the result of invasive cervical cancer that is now known to be caused by infection with some types of HPV. HIV, which is often sexually transmitted to women, is now a leading cause of death of young women in the United States, particularly among African-Americans. An estimated 45,000 women have died of HIV/acquired immunodeficiency syndrome. Many STIs can be perinatally transmitted, resulting in birth defects, mental retardation, and fetal and infant death. Urban poor populations of women with high representation of racial and ethnic minorities experience an even higher disproportionate risk of STDs, including HIV.

INTERRELATIONSHIPS OF SEXUALLY TRANSMITTED DISEASES AND HUMAN IMMUNODEFICIENCY SYNDROME

It is now well known that the presence of an STD increases the risk of acquisition and transmission of HIV. That is, women without HIV are more readily infected with HIV if they have an STD. Likewise, women with HIV are more likely to transmit HIV to a sexual partner if they acquire a new STD. The interrelationships between STDs and HIV are behavioral, biologic, and epidemiologic.

Behavioral

STDs and HIV transmission occur as the result of sexual and substance use risk behaviors. Many risk factors and behaviors that lead to infection with various STDs are also responsible for the heterosexual transmission of HIV in women. For example, the exchange of sex for drugs, including crack/cocaine, increases a woman's risk of STDs and HIV.

Immunologic

HIV infects specific types of white blood cells, known as target cells. These include monocyte/macrophage and Langerhans cells, which are found in the genital submucosa. Inflammation of the mucosal surfaces causes these target cells to be recruited in large numbers to the surface where they are more readily infected with HIV. Therefore, women with genital ulcer diseases such as syphilis and herpes and inflammation of the cervix due to gonorrhea or chlamydia are more likely to be infected with HIV. It is increasingly common for women to be coinfected with various STDs and HIV. The natural history of HIV produces immunologic responses that can affect the clinical course of STDs, resulting in greater difficulty in diagnosis and treatment.

Epidemiologic

Populations with high STD rates are also at disproportionate risk of HIV, and the highest rate of heterosexual transmission of HIV is occurring within this population. STDs are now seen as modifiable risk factors for the heterosexual spread of HIV in women.

SEXUALLY TRANSMITTED DISEASE AND HUMAN IMMUNODEFICIENCY VIRUS SCREENING

Clinical Preventive Services for Women

Most STIs, including HIV, are asymptomatic in women yet are still transmissible. Therefore, from a patient care and public health perspective, the traditional approach of episodic STD/HIV diagnostic testing and treatment of symptomatic women is no longer adequate. To provide secondary prevention services, clinical providers must assume more responsibility for routine STD and HIV screening of sexually active young adolescents and young adults. Minimally, women at risk for or with STIs should be screened for HIV and women with HIV, for STIs. HIV counseling and testing should be routinely offered to all sexually active women seen in any primary care setting. It is also recommended that women with STIs be encouraged to consent to HIV testing to optimize the efficacy of their treatment. Primary care providers should realize that many women with STIs have multiple infections. All women presenting with any STI or STD should receive complete clinical evaluation and testing for other STIs, including HIV.

Sexually Transmitted Disease/Human Immunodeficiency Virus Behavioral Counseling for Women

Because there is no curative therapy for viral STIs (i.e., HPV, HSV, hepatitis B virus, and HIV), the primary prevention of these infections is now a priority. Primary prevention depends on reducing sexual and substance use risk behaviors and increasing health care seeking. In recent clinical trials of STD and HIV primary prevention interventions, the efficacy of social and behavioral science-based behavioral counseling was found superior compared with patient/client education. A consensus statement from the National Institutes of Health on effective HIV prevention interventions highlights brief interventions delivered by health care providers in clinical settings as effective in promoting behavior change. As a result, the Centers for Disease Control and Prevention now recommends prevention counseling models that are science based and incorporate essential elements for effectiveness, such as counseling that is (a) interactive, (b) focused on client's personal risks and circumstances, and (c) directed toward helping clients set and reach specific goals. Because STDs facilitate HIV acquisition and transmission, counseling models should be integrated. Most clinicians are experienced only in the more traditional patient education approach and need training in newer, more effective, behavioral counseling models.

SEXUALLY TRANSMITTED DISEASE SYNDROMES IN WOMEN

Vaginitis

ETIOLOGY

The three most common types of infectious vaginitis are *Trichomonas* vaginitis, candidal vulvovaginitis, and bacterial vaginosis. *Trichomonas* vaginitis is caused by a protozoal organism, *Trichomonas vaginalis.* Candidal vaginitis is the result of overgrowth of a fungal organism, *Candida albicans,* in the vaginal mucosa. Some nonalbicans yeast species such as *Candida tropicalis* and *Torulopsis glabrata* have been demonstrated to cause a small proportion of vaginal yeast infections. Bacterial vaginosis is the result of an overgrowth of a characteristic group of bacteria, including *Gardnerella vaginalis, Mycoplasma hominis,* and anaerobic species that replace the normal flora of the vagina, predominantly *Lactobacillus acidophilus.* The bacteria do not actually infect the squamous epithelial mucous membrane layer of the vagina but adhere to the surface of the squamous cells, resulting in a vaginosis as opposed to a vaginitis.

CLINICAL PRESENTATION

The histories of women with infectious vaginitis are highly variable; many are totally asymptomatic. Mild symptoms include increased vaginal discharge with abnormal color and odor. More severe symptoms usually result when a vulvitis component occurs and include itching, external dysuria, and dyspareunia. Predisposing factors for candidiasis include recent antibiotic therapy, oral contraceptive use, menstruation, diabetes mellitus, corticosteroid use, and, more recently, HIV infection. Because bacterial vaginosis does not result in an inflammatory response, women with this condition are often asymptomatic or mildly symptomatic with an increased vaginal discharge and a fishy odor that is often most noticed after sexual intercourse. The odor is the result of an increased amount of amines in the discharge that are the byproduct of the metabolism of the anaerobic bacteria characteristic of this condition. On examination, a thin, whitish, homogenous discharge is often seen adhering to the mucous membrane surfaces of the vagina and vulva. There is usually little erythema or edema.

T. vaginalis and *Candidal vaginalis* directly infect the squamous epithelial mucous membrane layer of the vagina and vulva. Thus, trichomoniasis and candidiasis can cause similar symptoms of severe itching, external dysuria, vulvar swelling, and dyspareunia. On examination, vulvar edema with excoriation may be seen along with marked erythema of the vaginal mucosa. The discharge of trichomoniasis, however, is often more profuse, frothy, greenish-yellow in color, and foul smelling, whereas candidiasis is characterized by a thick, white, curdlike vaginal discharge that can be seen adhering to the vaginal mucosal surfaces. Women with acute symptomatic trichomoniasis who remain untreated may become totally asymptomatic but have chronic infection.

CLINICAL CRITERIA FOR DIAGNOSIS

Because the symptoms of vaginitis are so wide ranging and nonspecific, the diagnosis rests mainly on physical examination, microscopic examination of the vaginal discharge (vaginal wet smear), and determination of its pH (normal range, 4.0–4.5). Because bacterial vaginosis is a polymicrobial syndrome rather than the result of a single etiologic microbe, clinical criteria have been established to aid in the diagnosis. These include the presence of characteristic "clue cells" on a vaginal wet smear, a positive "whiff" test, the observation of thin homogenous discharge on examination, and a pH greater than 5.0. Any three of these criteria establishes the diagnosis. Candidiasis and trichomoniasis are diagnosed primarily on the basis of the vaginal wet smear.

LABORATORY TESTING

A specimen is collected for the vaginal wet smear by swabbing the vaginal mucosal surfaces with a cotton-tipped swab that is then placed in a test tube containing a small amount of normal saline. In the office laboratory, a wet smear is made by placing a few drops of the saline mixture on one slide and placing a coverslip over the material. A second slide is prepared in the same manner with the addition of a few drops of 10% KOH (potassium hydroxide) to the mixture. The presence or absence of an amine (fishy) odor is noted immediately (whiff test) and then the slide is saved for later examination for yeast organisms. The wet smear is examined under the 40× objective of the microscope.

Normal findings on a wet smear include squamous epithelial cells with clear cytoplasm and linear borders, a few white blood cells, and a predominance of large rods, *L. acidophilus*. In bacterial vaginosis, characteristic clue cells can be seen along with a marked absence of *Lactobacillus* spp. and few white blood cells. Clue cells are squamous epithelial cells that have become covered with a variety of smaller coccobacilli bacteria that give the cytoplasm of the cells a stippled appearance and cause the cell borders to appear irregular. *T. vaginalis* can be seen as a single-celled protozoal organism approximately the same size as a white blood cell but with a flagellum. The flagellum can be seen undulating, producing a characteristic motility of the trichomonad. *C. vaginalis* can be seen either as budding yeast cells in the vaginal wet smear or in its pseudohyphae form on the KOH slide. The pseudohyphae are larger filamentous structures that enmesh and can be best seen using the 10× objective. In both conditions, there are an increased number of white blood cells in the smear.

T. vaginalis can be cultured using a selective Diamond medium. The culture has higher sensitivity than the wet smear but is generally not commercially available. A polymerase chain reaction test for *T. vaginalis* is available but not yet approved by the U.S. Food and Drug Administration. Yeast organisms can be cultured using Nickerson media. This is not generally helpful in detecting *C. albicans*, however, because this organism can be part of normal vaginal flora. However, if nonalbicans species are suspected, culture is often more reliable than wet smear. Newer tests for bacterial vaginosis include a DNA probe test for high concentrations of *G. vaginalis* and card tests for the detection of elevated pH and trimethylamine.

MANAGEMENT

Treatment of bacterial vaginosis, *Trichomonas* vaginitis, and candidal vulvovaginitis is provided in Table 86.1.

PATIENT EDUCATION AND COUNSELING

Sexual partners of women with trichomoniasis should be examined and screened for STDs and HIV. There is no reliable test to detect trichomonads in the male. Regular partners are presumed to be carriers and are treated presumptively and immediately with metronidazole 2 g. Recurrence of trichomoniasis should not occur unless there is reinfection from an untreated partner or a new sexual contact.

Although the characteristic group of bacteria that result in bacterial vaginosis are thought to be sexually transmitted, it is not the presence of these bacteria but their overgrowth that results in the clinical syndrome. Host factors that have not yet been identified play a role. Therefore, male sexual partners of women with bacterial vaginosis should be examined and screened for STDs and HIV but not routinely treated. Recurrence of bacterial vaginosis without reinfection frequently occurs.

Candidiasis results from overgrowth of the *C. albicans* organism. Again, host factors including decreased cellular immunity, inadequate *Lactobacillus* colonization, and increased glucose levels play a role in recurrence of this condition. *C. albicans* is not sexually transmitted, and treatment of the male sexual partner is not recommended. Recurrences are common, and suppressive antifungal regimens should be considered for some women.

Urethritis

ETIOLOGY

Although urethritis has been recognized as an STD in men for several decades, only recently have there been attempts to define this syndrome in women. The most common sexually transmitted organisms causing urethritis in women are *Chlamydia trachomatis, Neisseria gonorrhoeae,* and HSV. These organisms

TABLE 86.1. Treatment of Vaginosis and Vaginitis

Treatment of bacterial vaginosis
Recommended
Metronidazole 500 mg PO bid for 7 days
Metronidazole gel 0.75%, one applicator intravaginally once daily for 5 days
Clindamycin cream 2%, one applicator intravaginally once daily for 7 days
Alternative treatment
Metronidazole 2 g PO in a single dose
or
Clindamycin 300 mg PO bid for 7 days
or
Clindamycin ovules 100 g intravaginally once a day for 3 days
Treatment of trichomonas vaginitis
Recommended
Metronidazole 2 g PO in a single dose
Alternative treatment
Metronidazole 500 mg PO bid for 7 days
Treatment of candidal vulvovaginitis
Recommended
Butoconazole 2% cream intravaginally for 3 days
Butoconazole 2% cream (butaconazole 1—sustained release), single intravaginal application
Clotrimazole 1% cream intravaginally for 7–14 days
Clotrimazole 100 mg vaginal tablet for 7 days
Clotrimazole 100 mg vaginal tablet, two tablets for 3 days
Clotrimazole 500 mg vaginal tablet, one tablet in a single application
Miconazole 2% cream intravaginally for 7 days
Miconazole 200 mg vaginal suppository, one suppository for 3 days
Miconazole 100 mg vaginal suppository, one suppository for 7 days
Nystatin 100,000 unit vaginal tablet, one tablet for 14 days
Tioconazole 6.5% ointment intravaginally in a single application
Terconazole 0.4% cream intravaginally for 7 days
or
Terconazole 0.8% cream intravaginally for 3 days
or
Terconazole 80 mg suppository, 1 suppository for 3 days
Oral agent
Fluconazole 150-mg oral tablets. One tablet PO in a single dose

also cause cervicitis and urethritis, and both syndromes may be present simultaneously. *C. albicans* and *T. vaginalis* can cause a vulvitis with irritation of the urethral meatus but are not considered causes of urethritis. Cystitis is usually caused by *Escherichia coli, Proteus* spp., and *Staphylococcus saprophyticus*, which are not sexually transmitted agents.

CLINICAL PRESENTATION

The hallmark symptom of urethritis is dysuria, which is usually gradual in onset and intermittent. Women may complain of increased vaginal discharge if the cervix is also infected. Vulvitis usually results in a complaint of burning of the vulva that is exacerbated by the passage of urine over the inflamed tissue, referred to as external dysuria. Dysuria as the result of a cystitis usually has an abrupt onset and is more severe and continuous. Symptoms of gross hematuria, urgency, and bladder tenderness often help to distinguish cystitis from urethritis. All sexually active young women with dysuria or other urinary symptoms should receive a full genitourinary evaluation for urethritis, vaginitis, and cervicitis as well as cystitis. This includes a speculum examination with close examination for urethral discharge, vulvar lesions or inflammation, signs of vaginitis, and mucopurulent endocervical discharge.

CLINICAL CRITERIA FOR DIAGNOSIS

In men, the microscopic observation of more than four polymorphonuclear cells per high-powered field (1,000×) in a Gram-stained specimen of urethral discharge establishes the diagnosis of urethritis. At this time, no such simple criterion exist for women, and the diagnosis is made by consideration of the history, physical examination findings, and laboratory test results. Vulvovaginitis due to candidiasis or trichomoniasis should be ruled out. Clinical findings of herpetic lesions of the vulva or cervix and mucopurulent endocervical discharge support a diagnosis of urethritis. The condition of sterile pyuria, defined as increased numbers of white blood cells on urinalysis with a urine culture that shows no bacterial growth, is the best clinical criterion to support the diagnosis of urethritis in a woman.

LABORATORY TESTING

Laboratory studies should include urinalysis of a clean-catch urine specimen, a wet smear of vaginal discharge, a Gram stain of endocervical discharge, and specific testing for chlamydia and gonorrhea from urethral and cervical samples. A urine culture should be ordered if cystitis is suspected.

MANAGEMENT

Treatment for the presumptive diagnosis of acute urethral syndrome in women is doxycycline 100 mg by mouth twice a day for 7 to 10 days or azithromycin 1 g orally in a single dose. Additional treatment may be needed depending on test results.

PATIENT EDUCATION AND COUNSELING

It is most important for women to know that dysuria caused by urethritis is usually sexually transmitted. Sexual partners should receive a complete STD/HIV evaluation and testing. Testing should include a urethral Gram stain for urethritis and specific tests for gonorrhea and chlamydia. Treatment for chlamydia or gonorrhea should be provided empirically if tests in the woman are positive.

Cervicitis

ETIOLOGY

The most common recognized causes of infectious clinically recognizable cervicitis are *C. trachomatis, N. gonorrhoeae,* and HSV. These organisms can also cause urethritis, pelvic inflammatory disease (PID), and proctitis in women.

CLINICAL PRESENTATION

A familiarity with the normal anatomy and physiology of the cervix is necessary before an adequate assessment can be done. The cervix is composed of two main parts: the exocervix, which is contiguous with the vagina, and the endocervix, which is the lower part of the uterus. The exocervix is often covered by squamous epithelial cells, which are the same flat nonsecretory cells that line the vaginal walls. Squamous epithelial tissue appears clinically as pink smooth tissue. The endocervix includes the endocervical canal, which is lined with columnar epithelium. This tissue appears brick red in color, is more papillary, and secretes specific types of mucus in response to ovarian hormonal stimulation. The area where the squamous epithelium meets the columnar epithelium is called the transformation zone. A process called squamous metaplasia that occurs continuously at the transformation zone results in columnar epithelium being transformed into squamous epithelium over time.

In prepubescent girls, the endocervix, exocervix, and much of the vaginal walls are lined with columnar epithelial tissue.

For this reason, prepubescent girls can develop gonococcal vaginitis and chlamydial vaginitis. As the girl enters puberty, ovarian production of estrogen and progesterone supports a change of vaginal pH from alkaline to acidic. The acidic pH begins the squamous metaplastic process and the gradual replacement of the columnar tissue with squamous epithelium.

By the end of puberty, most women have only squamous epithelium lining the vagina but have areas of columnar epithelium still visible on the exocervix. This is clinically referred to as cervical ectopy and is evidence of an immature transformation zone. As women age reproductively, squamous metaplasia continues until the columnar tissue is located only in the endocervical canal and the entire exocervix is covered with squamous epithelium resulting in a mature transformation zone.

Cervical ectopy is not abnormal but does result in increased risk of certain STDs. *N. gonorrhoeae* and *C. trachomatis* infect columnar epithelium and not squamous epithelium. Women with an immature transformation zone are at higher risk for gonococcal and chlamydial infection because the ectopy on the exocervix provides more extensive exposure to potentially infectious semen in the vagina. Women with ectopy also experience an increased amount of normal discharge. Recent data suggest that women with cervical ectopy are at greater risk of HIV infection and cervical cancer.

Normal cervical discharge varies with the phases of the menstrual cycle. In the preovulatory phase, which is predominantly estrogenic, the cervical discharge is clear, stretchy, slippery, and lubricative. This is known as fertile mucus or Spinnbarkeit mucus. In the postovulatory phase, the progesterone hormone, which is produced by the corpus luteum of the ruptured ovarian follicle, dominates. Progesterone-influenced cervical discharge is white, thicker, more dense, and not stretchy. This is known as infertile or barrier mucus because it does not facilitate sperm transport. Cervical mucus mixed with squamous epithelial cells from the vaginal walls and *Lactobacillus* spp. of normal bacteria in the vagina creates the fluid that women experience as vaginal discharge.

This background understanding of vaginal and cervical anatomy and physiology serves as the basis for assessment of lower genital tract infections. After the speculum is inserted, the first step is to identify areas of squamous and columnar epithelium and assess each tissue for signs of infection. Clinical signs of infected epithelial tissue include erythema, hyperedema, friability, and abnormal discharge. Candidiasis and trichomoniasis of the vagina can extend to the squamous epithelium on the exocervix and result in an exocervicitis. In these cases, the clinical appearance of a red cervix is the result of erythematous changes of the squamous epithelium. The STD syndrome of cervicitis is an infection of the columnar epithelium that is really an endocervicitis in women with a mature transformation zone. In younger women with ectopy, the part of the exocervix containing columnar epithelium will also show signs of infection. In women with ectopy, the visual inspection of the exocervix is relevant to the diagnosis of cervicitis because the columnar epithelium can be directly assessed. In women without ectopy, the clinician has to rely on an assessment of the endocervical discharge rather than the appearance of the exocervix.

CLINICAL CRITERIA FOR DIAGNOSIS

Most women with cervicitis are asymptomatic. Some may notice an increase or a change in their vaginal discharge. Occasionally, spotting after intercourse may result from increased friability of cervical ectopy. Many women with cervicitis also have urethritis from coinfection with the same organism. The dysuria they experience from the urethritis may be their only symptom of cervical infection. Therefore, clinical criteria for the diagnosis of cervicitis do not rely on the presence of symptoms.

The following criteria can be used presumptively for the clinical diagnosis of mucopurulent cervicitis caused by gonorrhea or chlamydia:

- The observation of mucopurulent discharge from the endocervical os or areas of ectopy
- Observation of clinical signs of erythema, hyperedema, or friability in areas of ectopy on the exocervix or at the cervical os
- Demonstration of increased amounts of white blood cells in cervical discharge (this is less sensitive and specific).

Cervicitis due to genital herpes infection usually produces a number of shallow, ulcerative, necrotic lesions on the exocervix. Clear vesicles that are often highly diagnostic for genital herpes when seen on the external genitalia are not seen on the cervix. A profuse more watery cervical discharge can often be observed. This diagnosis must be confirmed by laboratory tests. It is estimated that up to 20% of women who develop genital herpes simplex infections have cervical involvement only without external lesions.

LABORATORY TESTING

A Gram stain of endocervical discharge can be used to confirm a clinical impression of mucopurulent endocervical discharge. An increased number of white blood cells is quantitated as 10 to 30 polymorphonuclear cells per high powered field using an oil-immersion lens with a magnification of 1,000×. Cervical tests for gonorrhea and chlamydia should also be performed. For gonorrhea, endocervical culture is still the gold standard, with 85% to 90% sensitivity, 100% specificity, and low cost. Tests for gonorrhea based on enzyme-linked immunosorbent assay and DNA probes are not as sensitive and specific and add cost. The chlamydial organism is more likely to lose viability during transport so that chlamydial cultures are impractical in many settings due to lower sensitivity and higher cost. Chlamydia tests based on enzyme-linked immunosorbent assay, direct fluorescent antibody, and DNA probes are currently widely used but have poor insensitivity (60%–80%). This means that women with mucopurulent endocervicitis should be presumptively treated for chlamydia even if the chlamydia test is negative. Recently, new tests have been approved by the U.S. Food and Drug Administration for the detection of both gonorrhea and chlamydia (urethra and cervix only). These tests are based on nucleic acid amplification and are known as polymerase chain reaction or LCR type tests. The sensitivity and specificity are both very high for both genital and urine specimens. Urine testing allows gas chromatography and computed tomography screening to be done in nonclinic settings that could be of benefit to women in criminal justice and other institutional settings.

If necrotic ulcerative areas are seen on the exocervix, a culture for HSV should be obtained directly from the lesions. Herpes simplex can be isolated from over 80% of cervical samples taken from women with primary genital herpes infections.

MANAGEMENT

Women who meet the criteria for mucopurulent cervicitis should be treated presumptively for *C. trachomatis* and *N. gonorrhoeae*, depending on the local prevalence of these STIs and the likelihood that a patient can be adequately followed (Table 86.2). If high sensitivity nucleic acid amplification tests are used and follow-up is ensured, treatment may be based on test results.

TABLE 86.2. Treatment of Cervicitis

Treatment of mucopurulent cervicitis
Empiric treatment should be considered if the prevalence of chlamydia or gonorrhea is high or the woman is unlikely to return for treatment.
Treatment of chlamydia
Recommended
Doxycycline 100 mg PO bid for 7 days
Azithromycin 1 g PO in a single dose
Alternative
Erythromycin base 500 mg PO qid for 7 days
Erythromycin ethyl succinate 800 mg PO qid for 7 days
Ofloxacin 300 mg PO bid for 7 days
Levofloxacin 500 mg PO for 7 days
For pregnant women
Recommended
Erythromycin base 500 mg PO qid for 7 days
Amoxicillin 300 mg PO bid for 7–10 days
Alternative
Erythromycin base 250 mg PO qid for 14 days
Erythromycin ethyl succinate 800 mg PO for 7 days
Erythromycin ethyl succinate 400 mg PO for 14 days
Azithromycin 1 g PO in a single dose
Treatment of gonorrhea
Cefixime 400 mg PO in a single dose
or
Ceftriaxone 125 mg IM in a single dose
or
Ciprofloxacin 500 mg PO in a single dose
Ofloxacin 400 mg PO in a single dose
or
Levofloxacin 250 mg PO in a single dose
plus
If chlamydia infection is not ruled out
Azithromycin 1 g PO in a single dose
Doxycycline 100 mg PO bid for 7 days
For pregnant women
Cefixime 400 mg PO stat
or
Ceftriaxone 125 mg IM stat
For pregnant women who are allergic to penicillin
Spectinomycin 2 g IM stat

PATIENT EDUCATION AND COUNSELING

Women with mucopurulent cervicitis must be advised that their infection may be due to gonorrhea or chlamydia even though approximately 40% of women with this syndrome do not have positive tests for gonorrhea or chlamydia. Lack of sensitivity of chlamydia testing may be partially responsible, but all the infectious causes of mucopurulent cervicitis are not known at this time. This condition, like urethritis, is only beginning to be understood and defined through research. Therefore, women with mucopurulent cervicitis should be advised to complete treatment even if their tests are negative. Women with herpetic cervicitis need extensive education and counseling (refer to the section on genital herpes, below).

TREATMENT OF THE SEXUAL PARTNER

Women who are treated for mucopurulent cervicitis should refer their partners for a complete STD/HIV evaluation and testing, even if they have no symptoms. Men should be specifically assessed for urethritis, tested for gonorrhea and chlamydia, and treated with a regimen effective against *C. trachomatis*, even if all test are negative.

Pelvic Inflammatory Disease

ETIOLOGY

PID describes any combination of upper genital tract infections, including endometritis (uterus), salpingitis (fallopian tubes), and oophoritis (ovaries). PID can be an acute first episode, recurrent, or chronic. These infections result from ascending organisms of the lower genital tract (i.e., vagina and cervix). The mechanism by which normal flora of the vagina and cervix are prevented from ascending is not known. However, certain bacterial pathogens, such as *N. gonorrhoeae, C. trachomatis,* and *Mycoplasma hominis* are known to circumvent these mechanisms and cause first-episode PID. Other bacteria, particularly anaerobic species such as *Bacteroides* spp. or *Peptostreptococcus* spp., also ascend from the lower genital tract, resulting in a polymicrobial infection. Once a woman has experienced an initial episode of PID, she is at increased risk of recurrent or chronic disease, even without reinfection with a sexually transmitted pathogen. This section addresses only acute first-episode PID, which is considered sexually transmitted unless there is a history of recent surgery or instrumentation.

CLINICAL PRESENTATION

Women with PID usually give a history of lower abdominal pain. The pain may be mild and intermittent, increasing slowly over a period of weeks, or severe and debilitating with an abrupt onset of a few hours or days. Women with endometritis may complain of increased vaginal discharge and intermenstrual bleeding and have uterine tenderness only on bimanual examination. Other symptoms of PID include dyspareunia, dysuria, and menometrorrhagia. In women with more severe pain, systemic symptoms such as fever, nausea, and vomiting may be present. All young sexually active women who present with lower abdominal pain must be tested for STDs and evaluated for PID with a thorough speculum and bimanual examination.

DIFFERENTIAL DIAGNOSIS

The clinical diagnosis of PID is challenging, partially because of the difficulties in adequately palpating upper reproductive tract structures in some women. Traditionally, the clinical diagnosis of PID has not correlated well with the results of microbiologic sampling of the endometrium and fallopian tubes. In Sweden, laparoscopic evaluations for PID are done routinely on an outpatient basis and increase the accuracy of the diagnosis. However, in the United States there is reliance on clinical criteria for the presumptive diagnosis and treatment of PID. The clinician should maintain a strong awareness of the likelihood of misdiagnosis and reexamine women with PID within 48 to 72 hours of initial treatment. Ovarian cysts, normal ovulation, ectopic pregnancy, appendicitis, and other intra-abdominal and pelvic conditions must be considered when making the diagnosis.

Diagnostic criteria for the presumptive diagnosis of PID include the following:

- Recent history of lower abdominal pain
- Pain reproduced by palpation of endometrium and/or fallopian tubes
- Cervical motion tenderness
- Evidence of lower genital tract infection.

Systemic signs such as elevated temperature, elevated erythrocyte sedimentation rate, and leukocytosis increase the specificity of the diagnosis but are not found in many cases of PID.

LABORATORY TESTING

Women with suspected PID should have a vaginal wet smear and an endocervical Gram stain to identify vaginitis or cervicitis. In addition, tests for chlamydia and gonorrhea should be taken from the cervix. Studies have demonstrated that correlations between the results of cervical sampling and fallopian tube sampling in cases of PID are poor. Therefore, a negative cervical test result for gonorrhea or chlamydia does not rule out the possibility of sexually transmitted PID. In addition, there is no commercially available test for *M. hominis*, another sexually transmitted pathogen.

MANAGEMENT

Because PID is a polymicrobial syndrome and the results of cervical sampling are not highly predictive of microbiologic etiology, all women with PID must be treated with a regimen that covers all the major STD pathogens as well as the facultative anaerobic bacteria. There is controversy over the use of outpatient versus inpatient treatment regimens. Some infertility experts believe that all women who desire future pregnancies should be hospitalized for PID management. Minimally, adolescents, patients with nausea and vomiting, and cases involving an adnexal mass should be hospitalized for treatment. In addition, women who do not show significant improvement within 48 to 72 hours should be hospitalized for further evaluation and treatment (Table 86.3).

Women treated for PID on an outpatient basis should be advised to rest for at least 2 to 3 days until the pain has subsided. Sexual intercourse should be avoided for at least 2 weeks. An IUD, if present, should be removed at the time of initial treatment.

PATIENT EDUCATION AND COUNSELING

Women with PID need to be educated about their potential risk of infertility even in cases with mild symptoms. Ways to reduce this risk, including full compliance with treatment and avoidance of reinfection, should be explained. Lack of laboratory proof of an STI can be frustrating and confusing for both patients and clinicians. Patients should be counseled about the presumptiveness of the diagnosis in relation to the serious medical sequelae of ectopic pregnancy or infertility if treatment is withheld.

TABLE 86.3. Treatment for Pelvic Inflammatory Disease

Outpatient treatment
Regimen A
Ceftriaxone 250 mg IM stat
followed by
Doxycycline 100 mg PO bid for 14 days
with or without
Metronidazole 500 mg bid for 14 days
Regimen B
Ofloxacin 400 mg PO bid for 14 days
or
Levofloxacin 500 mg PO once daily for 14 days
with or without
Metronidazole 500 mg bid for 14 days
Inpatient treatment
Regimen A
Cefoxitin 2 g IV every 6 h or cefotetan 2 g IV every 12 h
plus
Doxycycline 100 mg IV or orally every 12 h
Regimen B
Clindamycin 900 mg IV every 8 h
plus
Gentamicin loading dose IV or IM (2 mg/kg) followed by a maintenance dose (1.5 mg/kg) every 8 h

TREATMENT OF THE SEXUAL PARTNER

Multiple studies have shown that most male sexual partners of women with PID are asymptomatic. They are often carriers of gonorrhea or chlamydia or have asymptomatic urethritis. Therefore, all male sexual partners of women with PID must have a complete STD/HIV evaluation, including specific tests for gonorrhea, chlamydia, and urethritis. However, even if all the tests are negative, the male partner should still be treated with a regimen effective for uncomplicated gonorrhea and chlamydia.

SEXUALLY TRANSMITTED GENITAL AND DERMATOLOGIC LESIONS IN WOMEN

Syphilis

ETIOLOGY

Syphilis is a disease caused by the bacterial spirochete *Treponema pallidum*. This organism is sexually transmitted through intimate contact of mucous membrane surfaces. The latest heterosexual epidemic of syphilis in the United States began in 1986.

CLINICAL PRESENTATION

With much individual variation, most patients with untreated syphilis pass through distinct stages. Early syphilis, defined as syphilis of less than 1 year's duration, is further divided into four clinical stages—incubating, primary, secondary, and early latent.

Incubating syphilis is the stage between infection with *T. pallidum* and appearance of the first clinical symptom, which takes from 10 to 90 days. Primary syphilis is characterized by the appearance of one or more cutaneous or mucous membrane ulcers known as chancres. These lesions, which are relatively painless, heal without scarring within 2 to 3 weeks. Painless, unilateral, inguinal lymphadenopathy is usually also present. Secondary syphilis is a systemic infection resulting from the dissemination of replicated *T. pallidum* from the original chancre to the lymphatic system and bloodstream. This dissemination produces a significant antibody response resulting in a wide range of clinical signs and symptoms, from generalized lymphadenopathy and a rash to highly infectious condylomata lata and mucous membrane patches. Secondary manifestations typically persist for 2 to 12 weeks and then spontaneously resolve. Early latent stage occurs from the time of spontaneous resolution of secondary signs and symptoms until about 1 year after the original time of infection.

Late syphilis, also known as syphilis of greater than 1 year's duration, is divided into two additional stages—late latent stage and tertiary stage. Late latent stage occurs from the end of early latent stage until such time as symptoms reappear, usually after 15 to 20 years of untreated infection. At that time approximately 30% of patients develop tertiary stage syphilis, characterized by neurologic, cardiovascular, or bone deformation.

DIFFERENTIAL DIAGNOSIS

Staging is a clinical judgment made by considering the patient's medical and sexual history, physical examination, serologic tests, and epidemiologic investigation. Patients with primary and secondary syphilis have distinct clinical signs and symptoms that simplify staging. Distinguishing early latent from late latent disease is more challenging because such signs and symptoms are absent. Clinical staging must be completed before management decisions and accurate treatment can occur.

In general, patients with early syphilis are highly infectious through sexual or perinatal transmission and so are managed as priority cases by public health control programs. After 1 year, patients with untreated syphilis are no longer considered sexually communicable. However, perinatal transmission resulting in congenital syphilis can still occur. Epidemiologic investigation of sexual partners within the past year helps in differentiating early infectious syphilis from late noninfectious syphilis.

Syphilis has often been called the "great pretender" because the wide range of clinical signs and symptoms present during some stages can mimic so many other diseases. Primary stage chancres can be confused with genital herpes, chancroid, and Behçet lesions. The rash of secondary syphilis appears similar to pityriasis rosea; the condylomata lata lesions look like venereal warts. The clinician must maintain a high index of suspicion for syphilis in sexually active persons under the age of 40, especially if genital lesions, unexplained rash, lymphadenopathy, and alopecia are present.

LABORATORY TESTING

A successful culture system to isolate *T. pallidum* has not been developed, so clinicians must rely on direct microscopy and serologic antibody testing to aid in the diagnosis of syphilis. The sensitivity and specificity of each type of test varies with the stage of disease.

Microscopy tests include the dark-field examination and a newer DEN for *T. pallidum* test that is like a fluorescent dark field. These tests can be used only if mucous membrane lesions are present and are most helpful in primary syphilis when serology tests are not yet reliable. With adequate specimen collection, *T. pallidum* spirochetes can be seen, resulting in the most definitive diagnosis. Because most patients are seen in later stages, the clinical value of these tests is limited.

Serology testing for syphilis involves the use of two different types of antibody tests. Nontreponemal serology tests (non–T-STS) measure antilipid antibodies produced by the host and so are not specific for treponemal antibody. Non–T-STS are sensitive and inexpensive and so are effective for screening. In addition, the degree of reactivity is reported quantitatively, giving a numerical titer result. Non–T-STS titers correspond to the patient's clinical course and can be used to assist in clinical staging and to assess adequacy of response to treatment. All current direct T-STS use antigens of *T. pallidum* and detect specific antibody. For this reason, the T-STS have higher specificity and are used to confirm a diagnosis of syphilis.

MANAGEMENT

In general, patients with reactive screening non–T-STS and reactive T-STS, with no history of syphilis, are considered new cases to be staged and treated. If the patient has clinical signs of primary or secondary syphilis or can give a reliable history of symptoms consistent with primary or secondary stage within the past year, early syphilis can be diagnosed. If a patient has a negative serologic test for syphilis on record within the past year or is found to be the sexual partner of someone with an early case of syphilis, a presumptive diagnosis of early latent syphilis can be made. Patients who do not meet any of these criteria are diagnosed as cases of unknown duration and are treated for late latent syphilis.

For patients with reactive serology and a history of previous syphilis treatment, attempts should be made to contact the local health department in the area where the patient received treatment. Most county and state health departments maintain syphilis registries of all patients treated for syphilis. The syphilis registry can be used to verify treatment and thus avoid unnecessary retreatment in old cases of syphilis. This is particularly problematic for the many women treated in their early reproductive years, because the question of retreatment is raised at subsequent prenatal visits. They often are treated repeatedly and unnecessarily (Table 86.4).

TABLE 86.4. Treatment of Syphilis

Early syphilis (<1 y)
Penicillin G benzathine 2.4 million U IM × 1
Alternate treatment for penicillin allergy: doxycycline 100 mg bid for 14 days
Late syphilis (>1 y)
Penicillin G benzathine 2.4 million units IM × 3, at weekly intervals
Alternate treatment for penicillin allergy: doxycycline 100 mg bid for 28 days

PATIENT EDUCATION AND COUNSELING

Patients must be advised that the syphilis serology tests are antibody tests and so will remain positive even after treatment. Their serology titer should be explained at the time of treatment, as should the need to have repeat syphilis tests at specified intervals for 1 year to ensure adequate treatment. Successful treatment is usually defined as a fourfold or two-dilution decrease in titer within 3 to 6 months of treatment. Patients should be told their titers may remain at low levels (serofast) indefinitely after successful treatment. Many women with successfully treated syphilis continue to receive unnecessary treatment every time they have a positive antibody test. All patients with syphilis should be counseled and offered HIV testing. Persons coinfected with HIV and syphilis may follow a different clinical course and may need additional treatment.

TREATMENT OF THE SEXUAL PARTNER

All sexual partners of women with reactive syphilis serology should receive a complete STD/HIV evaluation and testing. Sexual partners exposed to a woman with early syphilis within the previous 90 days are offered prophylactic treatment for incubating syphilis, even if their serologic tests are negative. Because patients with late syphilis are not sexually communicable, male partners of women diagnosed with late latent infection do not need treatment if their own tests are negative.

Chancroid

ETIOLOGY

Chancroid is a disease caused by a bacterial bacillus named *Haemophilus ducreyi.* This organism is transmitted by direct intimate contact with infected mucous membrane surfaces. Usually, these bacteria colonize squamous epithelium in the genital region; however, female prostitutes have been found to maintain colonization in their pharynxes and to be able to transmit the disease through oral–genital sexual contact. Chancroid was very uncommon in the United States in recent years until 1986. Cases of chancroid have been linked to cocaine use and the exchange of sex for drugs. Since 1990, cases of chancroid have again decreased significantly.

CLINICAL PRESENTATION

The incubation time for chancroid is very short, usually 4 to 7 days. After that time, the patient usually notices a painful bump on the genitals that is often described as a pimple. The lesion quickly becomes larger and more painful and then ulcerates.

Unilateral, painful, inguinal lymphadenopathy develops in about 50% of cases.

Examination reveals a painful ulcer with a "dirty" necrotic-appearing base and sharp excavated edges. The exudate is yellowish and purulent, and secondary lesions due to autoinoculation from opposing mucous membrane surfaces are common in women. Ulcers are usually present around the introitus and on the surfaces of the labia minora. If unilateral lymphadenopathy is present, a characteristic inguinal bubo is formed that is pathognomonic for chancroid. The nodes become suppurative and a soft fluctuant mass that is exquisitely painful can develop. The skin overlying the bubo becomes erythematous and hot to the touch. If untreated, the bubo can spontaneously rupture through the surface of the skin and drain purulent material.

LABORATORY TESTING

A culture for *H. ducreyi* has been developed but requires a selective medium (i.e., New York City medium) that is not available in most areas. Culture results can also take more than 1 week and thus are not helpful in the initial management decisions. A Gram stain of exudate from the ulcers can demonstrate a predominance of small Gram-negative coccobacilli that are suggestive of *H. ducreyi*. However, the ulcers are often secondarily infected or contaminated with many other bacteria, resulting in difficulty in collecting an adequate specimen for Gram stain.

Other causes of genital ulcer disease must be ruled out. An HSV culture should be obtained, and a dark-field test, rapid plasma reagin, and FTA should be ordered to rule out syphilis.

DIFFERENTIAL DIAGNOSIS

Chancroid is often a diagnosis of exclusion. Women with a history of STD risk behavior who present with painful genital ulcer disease and demonstrate no laboratory evidence of syphilis or herpes should be presumptively treated for chancroid.

MANAGEMENT

The ulcers respond very quickly to antibiotic therapy and usually heal with no scarring. If an inguinal bubo is present, however, antibiotic therapy alone is not adequate treatment. An inguinal bubo should be aspirated by introducing a large-bore needle (14 gauge) through adjacent intact skin that has been locally anesthetized. Often, 15 to 20 mL of purulent exudate can be aspirated (Table 86.5).

PATIENT EDUCATION AND COUNSELING

Women should be told that this is an STD and the result of sexual contact within the previous 2 weeks. They should be counseled about the association between cocaine use and chancroid and the relationship between genital ulcer disease and HIV infection. They should be encouraged to refer their sexual partners for treatment.

TABLE 86.5. Treatment of Chancroid

Ceftriaxone 250 mg IM in a single dose
or
Azithromycin 1 g PO in a single dose
or
Erythromycin base 500 mg PO qid for 7 days
or
Ciprofloxacin 500 mg PO bid for 3 days

TREATMENT OF THE SEXUAL PARTNER

Sexual partners of women with chancroid should receive a full STD/HIV evaluation and testing. They should be treated empirically with a regimen effective for chancroid.

Genital Herpes

ETIOLOGY

HSV-1 and HSV-2 are the two recognized types of HSV. HSV-1 most often infects the mucous membranes of the mouth and is usually acquired nonsexually during childhood. This oral herpes infection is commonly known as cold sores or fever blisters. HSV-2 usually infects the genital mucous membranes and is acquired in adolescence or young adulthood as the result of sexual behavior. However, either type can infect either mucous membrane site. In recent years, oral–genital sexual techniques have become more common. This has resulted in up to 30% of cases of genital herpes being caused by HSV-1. Likewise, about 30% of new cases of oral herpes result from HSV-2 infection.

Young adults must be taught that cold sores are herpes simplex viral infections and oral–genital sex with a person with a cold sore can result in a genital herpes infection. Although HSV-1 can infect the genital area, it results in few recurrent outbreaks so that most recurrent genital herpes is due to HSV-2.

CLINICAL PRESENTATION

There is a wide range of clinical manifestations of genital herpes, from multiple painful ulcers to atypical minor lesions to asymptomatic shedding. An initial genital herpes infection in a woman who has never had oral herpes is called a primary outbreak.

Primary infections are usually the most severe. Women present complaining of severe vulvar pain and dysuria. On examination, multiple, small, clear vesicles and shallow ulcers can be seen covering the vulva and exocervix. The ulcers have a pink base, clear and watery exudate, and an erythematous border. In primary infection, painful, unilateral, inguinal lymphadenopathy is present and systemic signs and symptoms of viremia such as fever, headache, myalgias, photophobia, and meningismus may also be present. Women with primary genital herpes lesions of the cervix may also have signs and symptoms of PID. Without treatment, resolution of the infection takes about 3 weeks. During this time, all genital ulcers spontaneously heal and the HSV establishes latency in the sacral ganglia. At variable intervals, recurrences occur that result in a new outbreak of vesicular and ulcerative lesions.

An initial genital herpes infection of a woman with a previous history of oral herpes is called a first-episode genital infection. The clinical presentation of first-episode genital HSV and recurrent genital HSV is similar, with mild symptoms of genital pain and dysuria. On examination, a smaller number of vesicles and ulcers can be seen localized to a smaller area of the vulva. Inguinal lymphadenopathy or systemic signs or symptoms of viremia are absent. Lesions heal spontaneously in 3 to 7 days.

Sometimes genital herpes lesions are atypical and appear as a single erythematous papule or very shallow fissures with erythema in the perineal area. In addition, many women with genital herpes demonstrate asymptomatic shedding of HSV from the cervix or vulva with no visible lesions. Women who are asymptomatically shedding HSV represent a major potential source of transmission to infants and sexual partners. Men with genital HSV also demonstrate asymptomatic shedding and represent a major potential source of transmission to their sexual partners.

LABORATORY TESTING

The HSV culture has been the gold standard test for herpes. The sensitivity varies with the moistness of the lesions but is generally 90% within the first 3 to 5 days of an outbreak. A specimen is obtained by collecting cellular material from the base of the ulcers. This is best done using a small, sterile, urethral type, Dacron-tipped swab. Results usually take 7 days, so presumptive treatment may be initiated before culture results come back. The biggest limitation of the HSV culture is that it can be used only when there are visible lesions.

Newer rapid diagnostic tests for HSV have been developed using enzyme-linked immunosorbent assay or direct fluorescent antibody techniques. The sensitivities of these tests have been disappointingly low, however, in the range of 70% to 80% compared with culture. Therefore, these tests are being used only in areas where culture is not available. Sometimes the cytopathic effect of HSV can be seen as squamous epithelial giant cells on a Pap smear specimen. Cytologists report this as "evidence suggestive of HSV." The accuracy of this report depends largely on the experience of the cytologist but is considered presumptive and not definitive for genital herpes.

Type-specific HSV antibody serology tests have been developed based on the HSV-specific glycoprotein G2 for the diagnosis of infection with HSV-2 and glycoprotein G1 for the diagnosis of infection with HSV-1. These serology type–specific gG-based assays are sensitive and specific. These tests have been used by researchers to conduct large-scale seroprevalence surveys in various populations. Many studies have now shown that the prevalence of HSV-2 begins to increase in persons aged 15 to 19 years and then peaks at ages 30 to 35 years at approximately 30%. In studies of women with positive HSV-2 antibody, only about one third know they have genital herpes. Serology tests can be useful clinically, because many clients present with healing lesions that are likely to result in a false-negative HSV culture. Some are recommending the use of HSV serology tests for screening purposes to detect greater numbers of cases of genital herpes.

DIFFERENTIAL DIAGNOSIS

The history and physical examination are often sufficient to permit the clinical diagnosis of genital herpes. However, because of the psychological impact of a diagnosis of genital herpes and the future obstetric implications, women who present with painful vesicles or ulcers of the genitals should be cultured for HSV. Type-specific serology testing should also be considered. In addition, clinicians should maintain a high index of suspicion and culture all genital lesions with a pattern of recurrence, even if they appear atypical for genital herpes. Syphilis, chancroid, and candidiasis must be ruled out.

MANAGEMENT

Women with primary or first-episode genital herpes should be treated with oral antiviral therapy. Early treatment significantly reduces viral shedding and promotes healing so the infection usually resolves completely within 5 to 7 days of treatment. Systemic viremia symptoms and dysuria that result from HSV infection of the urethra also resolve quickly with treatment.

Women with recurrent outbreaks who desire oral therapy should be taught to self-administer the treatment within 24 hours of noticing a new lesion. This maximizes the clinical benefit of treatment of recurrences. Many recurrences do not require treatment because they are mild and resolve spontaneously in a few days.

Antiviral treatment can also be given daily to suppress recurrences. Although women taking suppressive therapy have significantly fewer recurrences, they may still demonstrate asymptomatic shedding and need to use barriers to prevent transmission. Suppressive therapy is best reserved for women whose pattern of recurrence is so frequent their lives and coping abilities are disrupted. Suppressive therapy has been proven safe and effective (Table 86.6).

TABLE 86.6. Treatment for Genital Herpes

First clinical episode
Acyclovir 400 mg PO tid for 7–10 days
Acyclovir 200 mg PO 5 times a day for 7–10 days
Famciclovir 250 mg PO tid for 7–10 days
Valacyclovir 1 g PO bid for 7–10 days
Recurrent genital herpes
Acyclovir 200 mg PO 5 times a day for 5 days
Acyclovir 400 mg PO tid for 5 days
Acyclovir 800 mg PO bid for 5 days
Famciclovir 125 mg PO bid for 5 days
Valacyclovir 500 mg PO bid for 3–5 days
Valacyclovir 1 g PO once daily for 5 days
Suppressive therapy
Acyclovir 400 mg PO bid
Famciclovir 250 mg PO bid
Valacyclovir 500 g PO once daily
Valacyclovir 1 g PO once daily

PATIENT EDUCATION AND COUNSELING

Women with genital herpes need extensive education and counseling about genital herpes to facilitate a healthy emotional adjustment. Women with this diagnosis experience the standard emotional stages of adjustment to any chronic illness—denial, anger, depression, and acceptance. Many women benefit from a short-term counseling program to enhance their acceptance of this chronic STD. Self-help support groups for women with genital herpes are available in many cities in the United States.

Most women newly diagnosed with genital herpes have numerous questions about transmission. Patients should be advised that even though they are most communicable to a sexual partner when they have active lesions, it is possible to transmit the virus even when no visible lesions are present. It is estimated that asymptomatic shedding is responsible for transmission in approximately 30% of new cases. Decisions about using barrier methods to prevent transmission resulting from asymptomatic shedding should be made by the woman and her sexual partner.

TREATMENT OF THE SEXUAL PARTNER

The sexual partner should be referred for a complete STD/HIV evaluation and testing. The absence of herpes lesions or any history of genital lesions does not rule out the diagnosis of genital herpes. Type-specific, HSV serology, gG-based assays should be used to screen sexual partners who are asymptomatic.

Genital Warts

ETIOLOGY

Genital warts are exophytic papules caused by specific subtypes of HPV. HPV subtypes 6 and 11 cause most exophytic warts and are benign. Other HPV subtypes that may infect the genital area are types 16, 18, 31, 33, and 35, which have been strongly associated with genital dysplasia and carcinoma. These types are often associated with subclinical infection or flat wart lesions but can be found in exophytic lesions. Genital warts are transmitted by direct sexual contact with infected skin or mucous membranes.

CLINICAL PRESENTATION

The average incubation period before lesions appear is 2 to 3 months. Many women with warts do not notice the lesions, resulting in long delays in diagnosis. Occasionally, women complain of symptoms of itching and tenderness of the tissue around the lesions. Genital warts usually appear as whitish, pinkish, or brownish solid papules with a characteristic verrucous cauliflower-like surface. The surface of the papules often feels firm and granular. Genital warts often appear at the fourchette and adjacent labial surfaces and may spread to other parts of the vulva and perineal areas. Lesions can also infect the exocervix and appear exophytic or as whitish flat lesions (flat condylomata).

DIFFERENTIAL DIAGNOSIS

The diagnosis is often made by visual inspection of the characteristic verrucous exophytic papules. These papules must be distinguished from molluscum lesions, skin tags, hymenal tags, moles, and prominent sebaceous glands. A clinical manifestation of secondary syphilis previously described as condylomata lata mimics the appearance of genital warts and should be considered in the differential diagnosis.

LABORATORY TESTING

Atypical papules or flat lesions may require a biopsy to identify the cytopathic effect of HPV in epithelial tissue. A Pap smear may be used to identify a typical halo appearance around the nuclei of squamous epithelial cells that is reported as "koilocytic atypia suggestive of HPV infection." Newer DNA probes have been developed to identify specific subtypes of HPV from cervical samples. These type-specific tests are beginning to be used to guide treatment and follow-up of women with abnormal pap tests. A screening serologic test for syphilis should be routinely done.

MANAGEMENT

The goal of treatment is removal of the exophytic lesions and is, in a sense, cosmetic. No therapy has been shown to eradicate HPV infection. Host immune factors are responsible for inactivation of this infection. Some experts believe that treating the wart lesions may reduce communicability and prevent new areas of squamous tissue from becoming infected, but this has not been proved. After successful treatment of the lesions, recurrences can occur, usually as the result of reactivation of the subclinical HPV infection. If left untreated, genital warts may spontaneously resolve, remain unchanged, or grow and spread to adjacent areas. For this reason, treatment of lesions is usually recommended (Table 86.7).

TABLE 86.7. Treatment of External Genital Warts

Provider applied
Cryotherapy with liquid nitrogen.
TCA or BCA 80%–90% applied to warts.
Patient applied
Podofilox 0.5% solution for self-treatment. Clients are advised to apply podofilox to warts twice a day for 3 days, followed by 4 days of no therapy. This cycle can be repeated as necessary for a total of four cycles. (This is not indicated for pregnant women.)
Imiquimod 5% cream. Patients should apply cream once daily at bedtime, 3 times a week for up to 16 weeks. Cream should be washed off with soap and water 6–10 h after each application.

PATIENT EDUCATION AND COUNSELING

Educating and counseling women about genital wart infections is particularly frustrating because of the lack of definitive research about many commonly asked questions about communicability, sexual transmission risks, and risks of subsequent carcinoma. It is most important to stress that treatment of the warts does not result in eradication of the HPV infection. For most women, their own immunologic response renders the virus inactive after approximately 6 months. Women with persistent HPV, however, are at increased risk of developing dysplasias and carcinoma in situ of the cervix.

The period of communicability after treatment of the lesions is unknown. Condom use is recommended at least until there is no evidence of active infection for 6 months in the woman or her sexual partner. At this time, it is assumed the host immune response has inhibited viral replication. However, the client must be advised that recurrences may occur throughout her life. Experts speculate that HPV infection may persist in a dormant state and recur if immunologic changes occur. Many women with genital warts can benefit from HPV support groups, which have formed in many cities around the country.

TREATMENT OF THE SEXUAL PARTNER

The sexual partner should be examined for genital warts and have a complete STD/HIV evaluation and testing. The partner may demonstrate exophytic warts, but many are subclinically infected with HPV and have no visible lesions. No practical screening tests for subclinical HPV are available for male partners. Condom use is recommended, but again the period of communicability is unknown.

Molluscum Contagiosum

ETIOLOGY

Molluscum contagiosum is a benign condition of the skin and mucous membranes characterized by multiple papular lesions. This condition is caused by infection with the molluscum contagiosum virus, which is a member of the poxvirus family. Molluscum contagiosum, like HSV, can be spread by both sexual and nonsexual routes of transmission. Children often develop this skin infection on the face, trunk, and extremities as the result of direct skin-to-skin contact of fomites. In adults, lower abdominal, thigh, groin, and genital lesions are common and are thought to result from direct skin-to-skin contact during sexual activity.

CLINICAL PRESENTATION

The incubation period for molluscum lesions to appear is approximately 2 to 3 months. Lesions develop as smooth pinkish papules that slowly enlarge over a period of weeks. At this time the papules are approximately 10 to 15 mm in diameter with a shiny pearly surface. At maturity, the papules demonstrate a highly characteristic central umbilication from which a caseous whitish "pearl" can be expressed. This pearl is the viral body, and its removal will result in resolution of the papule. Most women with molluscum papules are asymptomatic and unaware of the infection. Molluscum papules commonly occur in the groin areas frequently shaved by some women. Because of this distribution, many women who do notice the papules attribute them to shaving irritation.

Recently, atypical appearing and unusually large numbers of molluscum lesions have been described in persons infected with HIV, suggesting a role of host immunity in the control of molluscum contagiosum virus infection and its level of clinical expression.

DIFFERENTIAL DIAGNOSIS

Molluscum papules are often confused with venereal warts and diagnosed and treated inappropriately. The diagnosis is usually made by visual inspection and the identification of pink fleshy papules, often umbilicated, from which a pearl can be expressed. HPV lesions, as previously described, are solid papules with a verrucous surface.

LABORATORY TESTING

The only definitive diagnostic test for molluscum contagiosum is a biopsy of the papule. The material is histologically examined to identify enlarged epithelial cells with intracytoplasmic molluscum bodies that are pathognomonic. Biopsies are reserved for atypical lesions. Women with unusually large numbers or atypically appearing molluscum papules should be offered HIV counseling and testing.

MANAGEMENT

Molluscum infections are generally self-limited; individual lesions usually resolve spontaneously within 3 months and stop recurring in approximately 2 years. Decisions to use various treatments that may result in scarring must be made on an individualized basis. Treatment strategies are similar to those used for HPV lesions, that is, eradication of lesions by mechanical or chemical destruction techniques. Treatments do not eradicate molluscum contagiosum virus, however, and recurrences of lesions are common until there is an adequate host immune response.

Treatment of molluscum contagiosum includes removal of each papule by skin curettage, application of trichloracetic acid (TCA) and liquid nitrogen, and "coring" of lesions by expressing the pearl.

PATIENT EDUCATION AND COUNSELING

The female client should be told that molluscum papules are the result of a benign viral infection of the skin that may be the result of nonsexual or sexual contact. They should be clearly distinguished from venereal warts and HPV infection. The client should be aware that there are no known complications of this infection and that there is usually spontaneous resolution without treatment of the papules.

TREATMENT OF THE SEXUAL PARTNER

Sexual partners should be referred for inspection for molluscum lesions and a complete STD/HIV evaluation and testing.

Scabies

ETIOLOGY

Scabies is an infestation of the itch mite, *Sarcoptes scabiei*. This infestation can occur nonsexually through household contact and skin-to-skin contact or sexually as the result of prolonged skin-to-skin contact during sexual activity. The female mite burrows into the epidermal layer of the skin and, within hours, begins depositing eggs. The eggs hatch to form adult mites in 10 days.

CLINICAL PRESENTATION

The symptoms of scabies result from a sensitization reaction that develops in the human host over a period of several weeks. The most classic symptom of scabies is itching, particularly nocturnal itching. In addition, pruritic papules can be seen in a characteristic distribution in warm moist areas of the skin. Distribution sites include finger webs, wrists, elbows, axillary folds, the beltline of the trunk, gluteal folds, and the genital area. The papules have usually been scratched severely, resulting in crusted excoriations.

DIFFERENTIAL DIAGNOSIS

Diagnosis is usually made by the clinical history and visual inspection. A history of itching that is severe, worsens at night, and involves more than one household member or a sexual partner is highly suggestive of scabies. The clinical appearance of papules with excoriation and crusting appearing in classic distribution sites strengthens the diagnosis. Burrows may be seen on the skin, appearing as short, wavy, dirty-appearing fine lines formed by the burrowing and egg laying of the female mite. These burrows are pathognomic for scabies. Secondary infection or an eczematous reaction can complicate the clinical appearance.

LABORATORY TESTING

The most common test used is a skin scraping technique. The most recent unexcoriated papule is located. Mineral oil is placed on the skin, which is then scraped vigorously with a sterile scalpel blade to dislodge the papule or burrow. The material is then placed on a slide and examined for microscopic evidence of the mite or fecal pellets containing the eggs. A burrow ink test is sometimes used in which a fresh papule is rubbed with ink from a fountain pen. The ink is then wiped off the surface of the papule with an alcohol pad. In the burrow ink test positive lesion, the ink soaks down into the track of the mite burrow and forms a dark, zigzagging, fine line. In complicated cases, a skin punch biopsy may be needed.

MANAGEMENT

Treatment is directed at killing the mites. Signs and symptoms are caused by a sensitization reaction, however, and may persist for a few weeks after successful treatment. This results in overtreatment when clients are not properly educated and are self-treating. Treatment of scabies includes permethrin cream 5% applied to all areas of the body from the neck down and washed off after 8 to 14 hours or lindane 1%, 1 ounce of lotion or 30 g of cream, applied thinly to all areas of the body from the neck down and washed off after 8 hours. (Lindane is not recommended for pregnant women or children.) A newer treatment is Ivermectin 200 μg/kg orally, repeated in 2 weeks.

PATIENT EDUCATION AND COUNSELING

Clothing and bedding should be washed and dried on the hot cycles. All household members or a sexual partner should be treated at the same time. Clients especially need to understand that the itching and papules may persist for a week or two after treatment.

TREATMENT OF THE SEXUAL PARTNER

The regular sexual partner should be treated even if there are no signs or symptoms of scabies. The incubation period for an initial scabies infestation can be several weeks.

Pubic Lice

ETIOLOGY

Pubic lice, commonly called crabs, are caused by an infestation of *Phthirus pubis*. (This is a different species from those that cause head lice or body lice.)

CLINICAL PRESENTATION

The pubic louse is approximately 1 mm in length and wider at the abdomen, giving it the appearance of a crab. The pubic louse attaches itself to the base of a pubic hair follicle and buries its mouthparts under the skin where it feeds on the host's blood. Adult pubic lice can be seen as reddish brown spots at the base of the hair follicles. Eggs are deposited in cylindrical structures (nits) that are attached to the shaft of the pubic hair. The nits can be seen as whitish flakes that cannot be easily dislodged from the hair shaft. The eggs hatch within 5 to 10 days. Symptoms include itching of the skin in the pubic hair region and bluish or reddish spots on the affected skin.

DIFFERENTIAL DIAGNOSIS

The diagnosis is made by clinical history and careful inspection of the pubic region for adult lice and nits. Often, the adult louse may need to be dislodged from the base of the hair follicle with the blunt end of a wooden applicator. The legs can usually be seen moving.

LABORATORY TESTING

Confirmation of adult lice or nits can be made by microscopic assessment of samples using the 10× objective of a standard microscope.

MANAGEMENT

The ideal treatment kills both the adult lice and the eggs. All clothing and bedding should be washed and dried using the hot cycles. Recommended treatment is permethrin 1% creme rinse applied to affected area and washed off after 10 minutes or lindane 1% shampoo applied for 4 minutes and then washed off. (This treatment is not recommended for pregnant women or children).

PATIENT EDUCATION AND COUNSELING

The female client should be given proper treatment instructions and advised to wash her clothing and bedding at the same time as administering the treatment.

TREATMENT OF THE SEXUAL PARTNER

The regular sexual partner should be treated simultaneously even if asymptomatic to avoid reinfestation.

BIBLIOGRAPHY

Cates W Jr, Whittington WL. Checking out the new STD tests. *Contemp Obstet Gynecol* 1984;23:135.

Centers for Disease Control. Recommendations for the prevention and management of *Chlamydia trachomatis* infections. *MMWR Morb Mortal Wkly Rep* 1993; 42(RR–12).

Centers for Disease Control and Prevention, U.S. Dept. of Health and Human Services. *Tracking the hidden epidemic.* 2000:1–31.

Centers for Disease Control and Prevention, U.S. Dept. of Health and Human Services. HIV/AIDS surveillance report. 2001;13:1–43.

Centers for Disease Control and Prevention, U.S. Dept. of Health and Human Services. 1993 Sexually transmitted diseases treatment guidelines. *MMWR Morb Mortal Wkly Rep* 2002;51(RR-6):1–84.

Coury-Doniger PA. Syphilis: managing patients with reactive serologic tests. *STD Bull* 1993;12.

Coury-Doniger P, Levenkron JC, Knox K, et al. Use of stage of change (SOC) to develop an STD/HIV behavioral intervention: phase 1. A system to classify SOC for STD/HIV sexual risk behaviors—development and reliability in an STD clinic. *AIDS Patient Care STDs* 1999;13:493–502.

Coury-Doniger P, Levenkron JC, McGrath P, et al. From theory to practice: use of stage of change (SOC) to develop an STD/HIV behavioral intervention: phase 2. Stage based behavioral counseling strategies for sexual risk reduction. *Cogn Behav Pract* 2000;7.

De Vincenzi I. A longitudinal study of human immunodeficiency virus transmission by heterosexual partners. *N Engl J Med* 1994;331:341.

Edlin BR, Irwin KL, Faroque S, et al. Intersecting epidemics—crack cocaine use and HIV infection among inner-city young adults. *N Engl J Med* 1994;331:1422.

Gilchrist MIR, Rauh JL. Office microscopic examination for sexually transmitted diseases: a tool to lower costs. *J Adolesc Health Care* 1985;6:311.

Handsfield HH. *Color atlas and synopsis of sexually transmitted diseases.* New York: McGraw-Hill, 1992.

Holmes KK, Cates W, Lemon S, et al. *Sexually transmitted diseases,* 2nd ed. New York: McGraw-Hill, 1990.

Hook E III, Marra CM. Acquired syphilis in adults. *N Engl J Med* 1992;326:1060.

Koutsky LA. The frequency of unrecognized type 2 herpes simplex virus infection among women. *Sex Transm Dis* 1989;17:90.

Larsen SA. *A manual of tests for syphilis.* Washington, DC: American Public Health Association, 1990.

Martin DH, ed. Sexually transmitted diseases. *Med Clin North Am* 1990;74:1339.

McGrath PL, Levenkron JC, Knox KL, et al. The development, reliability, and validity of a rating scale of stage-based behavioral counseling skills for STD/HIV prevention. *J Public Health Practice* (submitted).

Mertz GJ. Frequency of acquisition of first-episode genital infection with herpes simplex virus from symptomatic and asymptomatic source contacts. *Sex Transm Dis* 1984;12:33.

Paavonen J, Stamm WE. Lower genital tract infections in women. *Infect Dis Clin North Am* 1987;1:179.

Stamm WE. *The practitioner's handbook for the management of STDs.* Seattle: HSCER Distribution, University of Washington, 1988.

Stamm WE. Dysuria: establishing a diagnostic protocol. *Contemp Obstet Gynecol* 1988:81.

Sweet RL, Gibbs RS. *Infectious diseases of the female genital tract,* 2nd ed. Baltimore: Williams & Wilkins, 1990.

Thomason JL, Gelbart SM, Broekhuizen FF. Advances in the understanding of bacterial vaginosis. *J Reprod Med* 1989;34:581.

Wasserheit JN. Pelvic inflammatory disease and infertility. *Maryland Med J* 1987;36:58.

Wasserheit JN. Epidemiological synergy: interrelationships between human immunodeficiency virus infection and other sexually transmitted diseases. *Sex Transm Dis* 1992;19:61.

Wasserheit JN, Aral AS, Holmes K, et al., eds. *Research issues in human behavior and sexually transmitted diseases in the AIDS era.* Washington, DC: American Society for Microbiology, 1991.

Wentworth B, Judson FN, eds. *Laboratory methods for the diagnosis of sexually transmitted diseases,* 2nd ed. Washington, DC: American Public Health Association, 1991.

Wisdom A. *Color atlas of sexually transmitted diseases.* Chicago: Year Book Medical Publishers, 1989.

CHAPTER 87
Chronic Fatigue Syndrome

Martin E. Olsen

Chronic fatigue syndrome is characterized by severe disabling fatigue associated with symptoms that predominately feature self-reported impairments in concentration and short term memory as well as sleep disturbance and musculoskeletal pain. Although many patients affected by chronic fatigue syndrome improve with time, most remain functionally impaired for several years. Twenty-three percent to 24% of the adult general population in the United States has had fatigue lasting 2 weeks or longer; in most patients, however, the source of the fatigue is a medical or pathologic condition other than chronic fatigue syndrome.

ETIOLOGY

The cause of chronic fatigue syndrome is undetermined. Various hypotheses have been suggested that involve immunologic, virologic, psychological, and neuroendocrine factors. No single definition is universally accepted. Frequently used definitions are the U.K. Oxford criteria and the U.S. Centers for Disease Control and Prevention definition. The fatigue may not be caused by other identifiable conditions. Fatigue must be debilitating and present for 6 months with some functional impairment.

Sixty percent of patients with fibromyalgia meet criteria for chronic fatigue syndrome. One issue in chronic fatigue syndrome research concerns a question of whether chronic fatigue syndrome is a pathologically discrete entity or a debilitating but nonspecific condition shared by other different entities. Somatoform disorder, anxiety disorder, major depression, and other affected disorders can manifest severe fatigue and psychological symptoms (Table 87.1).

TABLE 87.1. Diagnostic Criteria for Chronic Fatigue Syndrome

1. Self-reported persistent or relapsing fatigue lasting 6 or more consecutive months.
2. Four or more of the following symptoms are concurrently present for 6 or more months:
   A. Impaired memory or concentration
   B. Sore throat
   C. Tender cervical or axillary lymph nodes
   D. Muscle pain
   E. Multijoint pain
   F. Headache
   G. Unfreshed sleep
   H. Postexertional malaise

Source: Fukuda K, et al.

DIFFERENTIAL DIAGNOSIS

The following conditions exclude a patient from a diagnosis of chronic fatigue syndrome: (a) a chronic medical condition that may explain the presence of chronic fatigue, such as hypothyroidism, sleep apnea, narcolepsy, and side effects of medication; (b) a previously diagnosed medical condition whose resolution has been documented, such as malignancy or hepatitis B or C infection; (c) psychiatric conditions such as major depressive disorder, psychotic disorder, bipolar disorder, or schizophrenia; (d) dementias; (e) anorexia nervosa or bulimia nervosa; (f) alcohol or substance abuse; and (g) severe obesity (Table 87.2).

CLINICAL SYMPTOMS AND HISTORY

According to the Centers for Disease Control and Prevention criteria, at least 6 months of persistent or relapsing fatigue not relieved by bed rest and resulting at in at least 50% reduction in activity level must be present. In addition, four of eight specified symptoms on history must be present to make a diagnosis of chronic fatigue syndrome: (a) impaired memory, (b) sore throat, (c) lymph node pain, (d) muscle pain, (e) joint pain, (f) prolonged fatigue after previous tolerable levels of activity, (g) new headaches, and (h) sleep disturbance. History taking should assess medical and psychological circumstances of the onset of fatigue, depression, other psychiatric disorders, other episodes of medical unexplained symptoms, alcohol abuse, other substance abuse, prescription medication, over-the-counter medications, and food supplements.

TABLE 87.2. Exclusionary Criteria for Chronic Fatigue Syndrome

A. An active medical condition that may explain fatigue. Examples are untreated hypothyroidism, narcolepsy, sleep apnea, and medication side effects.
B. Unresolved previously diagnosed medical condition, such as malignancies or hepatitis B or C infection.
C. Current or previous diagnosis of major depression with psychotic or melancholic features, or bipolar affective disorders or schizophrenia or delusional disorders of any subtype or dementias or anorexia nervosa or bulimia nervosa.
D. Alcohol/substance abuse within 2 years before the onset of the fatigue.
E. Severe obesity.

Source: Fukuda K, et al.

CLINICAL FINDINGS AND PHYSICAL EXAMINATION

No definitive physical examination finding is linked to chronic fatigue syndrome. A recommendation has been made that a mental status examination is a minimal acceptable level of assessment for psychiatric evaluation. Such an assessment would include evaluation for abnormalities of mood, intellectual function, or personality. Attention should be directed toward the exclusion of neurologic or psychiatric disorders. Presence of psychomotor retardation would argue against a psychiatric or neurologic disorder.

LABORATORY AND IMAGING STUDIES

Diagnosis of chronic fatigue syndrome can be made only after other medical and psychiatric causes of chronic fatigue illness have been excluded. No pathognomic signs or diagnostic tests for this condition have been validated in scientific studies. Testing should be directed toward confirming or excluding other etiologic possibilities. Diagnosis can be made more difficult by the frequent finding of other clinical conditions that are commonly associated with chronic fatigue syndrome, such as (a) fibromyalgia, (b) irritable bowel syndrome, (c) multiple chemical sensitivity, (d) temporomandibular disorders, (e) interstitial cystitis, (f) postconcussion syndrome, (g) tension headache, (h) chronic low back pain, (i) chronic pelvic pain in women, and (j) chronic nonbacterial prostatitis in males. If appropriate, studies could be indicated to access the possibility of these commonly associated syndromes. These syndromes have in common an absence of objective findings on physical examination, disability out of proportion to the pathophysiology, and exacerbations associated with stress.

It was noted in a co-twin control study that identical twins with a diagnosis of chronic fatigue syndrome were more likely to experience one or more of the above-listed clinical conditions. Most commonly associated conditions in the twin study were fibromyalgia, irritable bowel syndrome, temporomandibular disorder, tension headache, and chronic low back pain.

Up to 70% of patients with chronic fatigue syndrome meet criteria for fibromyalgia. One group of authors suggested that fatigued persons often receive either inadequate or excessive medical evaluations. These authors suggested that a minimum battery of laboratory screening tests include complete blood count with leukocyte differential, erythrocyte sedimentation rate, serum levels of alanine aminotransferase, total protein, albumin, globulin, alkaline phosphatase, calcium, phosphorus, glucose, blood urea nitrogen, electrolytes, creatinine, determination of thyroid-stimulating hormone, and urinalysis. Examples of tests that would not be helpful are tests for Epstein-Barr virus, retroviruses, human herpes virus, enteroviruses, *Candida albicans*, immunologic function, magnetic resonance scans, radionuclide scans, computed tomography, and positron emission tomography.

Although hypocortisolism has been identified in chronic fatigue syndrome, it is unknown whether this is a primary feature or secondary to other factors. It may be one factor contributing to the symptoms of chronic fatigue, but at this point it is not diagnostic.

TREATMENT

Two thirds of patients have been described as dissatisfied with the quality of their medical care. Dissatisfied patients described delay, dispute, or confusion over diagnosis; a perception of doctors as demonstrating a lack of knowledge about chronic fatigue syndrome; or a feeling that the advice given was inadequate. Additionally, dissatisfied patients demonstrate a rejection of a psychiatric diagnosis. Satisfied patients perceive their doctors as caring, supportive, and interested in their illness. These satisfied patients indicated that they did not necessarily expect their doctors to cure chronic fatigue syndrome but perceived their physicians as a source of greatest help during their illness. These findings suggest that medical care was evaluated less on the ability of doctors to treat chronic fatigue syndrome and more on the physicians interpersonal skills. Diagnosis of chronic fatigue syndrome should not impede the treatment of coexisting disorders such as depression.

Whiting et al. accessed the effectiveness of all interventions by a systemic review of the literature. Three hundred fifty studies were accessed; only 44 met inclusion criteria. This review indicated that cognitive behavioral therapy demonstrated a positive overall effect, and the studies accessed were believed to be valid. Regimens that demonstrated insufficient evidence about treatment effectiveness are as follows: interferon, Ampligen, staphylococcus toxoid, terfenadine, oral NADH (reduced nicotinamide adenine dinucleotide), selegiline, acyclovir, moclobemide, fludrocortisone, antidepressants, sulbutiamine, growth hormone, galanthamine hydrobromide, magnesium supplements, general supplements, liver extract, homeopathy, massage therapy, osteopathy, combined programs, and buddy/mentor programs. Interventions that have shown promising results include cognitive behavioral therapy and graded exercise therapy.

All three studies evaluating graded exercise therapy found overall benefit of the intervention compared with control groups. No adverse effects were noted, although withdrawals from studies may have been related to the level of exercise. In one program, subjects were instructed to perform an aerobic activity such as walking/jogging, swimming, or cycling for 20 minutes at least three times per week. An exercise level that used 75% of the subjects' tested functional maximum ability was selected. Subjects monitored their exercise programs with pre- and postexercise heart rates and perceived exertion. Exercise intensity was increased when there was reduction of heart rate and reduction in perceived exertion. Cognitive behavior therapy would be best performed by those skilled in the therapeutic modality.

EFFECTS ON PREGNANCY

Pubmed, MD Consult, and DigiScript searches revealed no articles on chronic fatigue syndrome and pregnancy.

CONCLUSION

Concerns have been raised that no clear defining chronic fatigue syndrome community exists. The possibility has been expressed that several different communities exist; each is at risk of serving a particular constituency and may be united not so much in what they believe but in what they do not believe. Consumer patient activism is a force for change and can be a force for progress, but the two are not necessarily synonymous. Health providers must guard against potential disengagement. Abuse or intimidation of researchers for the production of unpopular research results has been reported.

BIBLIOGRAPHY

Aaron LA, Herrell R, Ashton S, et al. Comorbid clinical conditions in chronic fatigue: a co-twin control study. *J General Internal Medicine* 2001;16:24–30.

Buchwald D, Garrity D. Comparison of patients with chronic fatigue syndrome, fibromyalgia, and chemical sensitivities. *Arch Intern Med* 1994;154:2049–2053.

Cleare AJ, Blair D, Chambers S, et al. Urinary free cortisol in chronic fatigue syndrome. *Am J Psychiatry* 2001;158:641–643.

Deale A, Wessely S. Patients' perceptions of medical care in chronic fatigue syndrome. *Soc Sci Med* 2001;52:1859–1864.

Deyo RA, Psaty BM, Simon G, et al. The messenger under attack-intimidation of researchers by special-interest groups. *N Engl J Med* 1997;836:1176–1180.

Fukuda K, Straus SE, Hickie I, et al. The chronic fatigue syndrome: a comprehensive approach to its definition and study. *Ann Intern Med* 1994;121:953–959.

Fulcher KY, White PD. Randomised controlled trial of graded exercise in patients with the chronic fatigue syndrome. *BMJ* 1997;314:1647–1652.

Goldenberg DL, Simms RW, Geiger A, et al. High frequency of fibromyalgia in patients with chronic fatigue seen in a primary care practice. *Arthritis Rheum* 1990;33:381–387.

Klonoff DC. Chronic fatigue syndrome. *Clin Infect Dis* 1992;15:812–823.

Kruesi MJ, Dale J, Straus SE. Psychiatric diagnoses in patients who have chronic fatigue syndrome. *J Clin Psychiatry* 1989;50:53–56.

Powell P, Bentall RP, Nye FJ, et al. Randomised controlled trial of patients education to encourage graded exercise in chronic fatigue syndrome. *BMJ* 2001;322:387–392.

Price RK, North CS, Wessely S, et al. Estimating the prevalence of chronic fatigue syndrome and associated symptoms in the community. *Public Health Rep* 1992; 107:514–522.

Sharpe M, Archard L, Banatvala J. A report-chronic fatigue syndrome: guidelines for research. *J R Soc Med* 1991;84:118–121.

Walker EA, Katon WJ, Jemelka RP. Psychiatric disorders and medical care utilization among people in the general population who report fatigue. *J Gen Intern Med* 1993;8:436–440.

Wearden AJ, Morriss RK, Mullis R, et al. Randomised, double-blind, placebo-controlled treatment trial of fluoxetine and graded exercise for chronic fatigue syndrome. *Br J Psychiatry* 1998;172:485–492.

Wessely S. Chronic fatigue syndrome—trials and tribulations. *JAMA* 2001;286(11): 1378–1379.

Wessely S, Powell R. Fatigue syndromes: a comparison of chronic postviral fatigue with neuromuscular and affective disorders. *J Neurol Neurosurg Psychiatry* 1989;52:940–948.

White KP, Speechley M, Harth M, et al. Co-existence of chronic fatigue syndrome with fibromyalgia syndrome in the general population: a controlled study. *Scand J Rheumatol* 2000;29:44–51.

Whiting P, Bagnell AM, Sowden A, et al. Interventions for the treatment and management of chronic fatigue syndrome: a systemic review. *JAMA* 2001;286: 1360–1368.

Wilson A, Hickie I, Lloyd A, et al. Longitudinal study of outcome of chronic fatigue syndrome. *BMJ* 1994;308:756–759.

CHAPTER 88
Fibromyalgia

Martin E. Olsen

The source of fibromyalgia is unclear. Some discussion has occurred concerning the potential harm that could be dealt to patients by labeling them with fibromyalgia. Beliefs that communicating this diagnosis to patients might cause a disability or other changes in behavior have been the subject of speculation but little research. Some authors indicate fibromyalgia may be part of a spectrum of a chronic widespread pain syndrome or may be separate from a chronic widespread pain syndrome. Others regard fibromyalgia as a functional somatic disorder. Psychological abnormalities are significantly more common in patients with fibromyalgia than a control population.

Factors associated with fibromyalgia in the general population include female sex, divorce, failure to complete high school, low household income, decreased pain threshold, subjective joint swelling, parenthesis, morning stiffness, sleep disturbance, fatigue, irritable bowel syndrome, moderate or severe impairment demonstrated by the health assessment questionnaire, increased pain, fair or poor self-reported health status, and moderate dissatisfaction with health.

A prevalence of fibromyalgia in females of between 0.7% and 10.5% has been reported, but most studies reveal an incidence of 3% or less. Fibromyalgia is the second most common diagnosis in rheumatology clinics. Some authors, however, argue that fibromyalgia is not an autoimmune disease.

ETIOLOGY

Limited data exist with respect to risk factors; female sex and age are two consistent risk factors. A family history of fibromyalgia may also increase risk. Autonomic dysfunction has been recognized in fibromyalgia.

An elevation of prototypic pain transmitter (substance P) in the cerebrospinal fluid provides evidence that the pain of fibromyalgia is real. Some evidence exits that dysfunction of the hypothalamic-pituitary-adrenal axis is seen in patients with fibromyalgia.

Although in some studies patients with fibromyalgia have an increased history of emotional trauma more frequently than control subjects, these data suggest a subset of patients with fibromyalgia are more likely to have traumatic experiences, though not necessarily all patients. An increase in abuse has been noted in patients with fibromyalgia. It is believed, however, that evidence is insufficient at this time to make a statement concerning a causal relationship between abuse or trauma and fibromyalgia.

Other psychological factors associated with fibromyalgia include somatization, anxiety, depression, increased global severity of psychiatric illness, history of past or current depression, family depression, and increased application for disability benefits.

DIFFERENTIAL DIAGNOSIS

Differential diagnoses include the following rheumatologic conditions: osteoarthritis, rheumatoid arthritis, ankylosing spondylitis, polymyalgia rheumatica, systemic lupus erythematosus, Sjögren syndrome, chronic Lyme disease, osteomalacia, and polymyositis. Nonrheumatologic syndromes included in the list of differential diagnoses are as follows: chronic fatigue syndrome, hypothyroidism, hepatitis C infection, and anxiety or depression.

Other conditions may coexist with fibromyalgia. These conditions include primary systemic lupus erythematosus, rheumatoid arthritis, and osteoarthritis. Diseases such as human immunodeficiency virus and hyperprolactinemia may increase the risk of fibromyalgia. One third of patients with fibromyalgia may have a major depressive disorder.

Some experts suggest that chronic fatigue syndrome and fibromyalgia are two perspectives of the same disease process. Although both may demonstrate a subclinical inflammatory process, symptoms such as low-grade fever, lymph gland enlargement, and acute onset of the illness are not seen in fibromyalgia. Substance P is elevated in the cerebral fluid of fibromyalgia patients only.

CLINICAL SYMPTOMS AND HISTORY

In addition to pain, other central symptoms of fibromyalgia include sleep disturbance, fatigue, and stiffness. Some elements of these three symptoms are present in more than 75% of patients. The simultaneous presentation of all three symptoms is found in only 56% of patients.

CLINICAL FINDINGS AND PHYSICAL EXAMINATION

According the American College of Rheumatology, the criteria for fibromyalgia are as follows:

1. History of widespread pain. Pain is considered widespread when all the following are present: pain in the left side of the body, pain in the right side of the body, pain above the waist, and pain below the waist. In addition, axial skeletal pain (cervical spine or anterior chest or thoracic spine or low back) must be present. In this definition, shoulder and buttock pain is considered as pain for each involved side. "Low back" pain is considered lower segment pain.
2. Pain in 11 of 18 tender point sites on digital palpation (Fig. 88.1):
   Occiput: bilateral, at the suboccipital muscle insertions.
   Low cervical: bilateral, at the anterior aspects of the intertransverse spaces at C5-7.
   Trapezius: bilateral, at the midpoint of the upper border.
   Supraspinatus: bilateral, at origins above the scapula spine near the medical border.
   Second rib: bilateral, at the second costochondral junctions, just lateral to the junctions on upper surfaces.
   Lateral epicondyle: bilateral, 2 cm distal to the epicondyles.
   Gluteal: bilateral, in upper outer quadrants of buttocks in anterior fold of muscle.
   Greater trochanter: bilateral, posterior to the trochanteric prominence.
   Knee: bilateral, at the medial fat pad proximal to the joint line.

Digital palpation should be performed with an approximate force of 4 kg. For a tender point to be considered "positive," the subject must state that the palpation was painful. "Tender" is not considered "painful" (Fig. 88.1).

LABORATORY AND IMAGING STUDIES

Fibromyalgia is a clinical diagnosis. Studies are indicated to rule out those differential diagnoses not excluded on a patient's history and physical examination. Although elevated spinal fluid levels of prototypic pain transmitter (substance P) have been reported on fibromyalgia patients, it is not reasonable to routinely perform spinal taps.

TREATMENT

A successful fibromyalgia treatment program must address physical fitness, mental health, and environmental issues. Such environmental issues may include pain, sleep disturbances, mood disturbances, and fatigue. Other conditions commonly associated with fibromyalgia may require their own treatment; these conditions may include irritable bowel syndrome, interstitial cystitis, migraine headaches, temporomandibular joint dysfunction, disequilibrium, and sicca syndrome.

Many clinical trials have used only single-agent therapy. This may not be appropriate in that patients with fibromyalgia have a complex disease process that may benefit from more than one pharmacologic approach. An impressive placebo response is also evident in the treatment of fibromyalgia; this

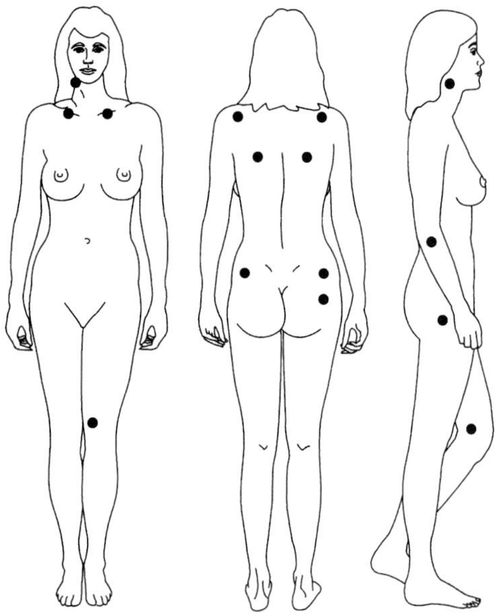

FIG. 88.1. Location of the major tender point sites in fibromyalgia.

increases the difficulty in evaluating response to therapy. A lack of consensus concerning optional and meaningful outcomes measures has also provided difficulty in analyzing successful treatment regimens. Antidepressants have received the most attention. Moderate improvement can be found with antidepressant therapy.

A multiple disciplinary treatment program may enhance a pharmacologic approach. Cognitive therapy and exercise therapy have been shown to improve outcome in a separate meta-analysis; this approach was found to be superior to pharmacologic therapy alone in this study.

The goal of treatment should be symptom improvement, not symptom extinction. This approach avoids patient disappointment and decreases the potential for overmedication. Medication should be prescribed after rank ordering the symptoms in terms of their importance to the patient and their impact on daily activities and quality of life. Pharmacologic therapy can then be symptom based. All medications should be periodically evaluated and tapered for justification of use. "Drug holidays" may assist in documentation of ongoing need for a medication. A technique to avoid habituation may include the cyclic use of agents with different modes of action.

Pain relief regimens frequently include the use of acetaminophen or nonsteroidal agents. The use of narcotic analgesia is controversial, but no randomized clinical control trials of opioid use in the treatment of fibromyalgia exist. Therefore, such treatment cannot be recommended. Input from a comprehensive pain management team would be preferable to the use of narcotics.

The use of tricyclic antidepressants with documented analgesic effects may be an important therapeutic mechanism. Selective serotonin reuptake inhibitors have less of an analgesic effect compared with other agents, but they do improve the emotional component of pain and could treat underlying mood disorder. In one study, a combination of fluoxetine and amitriptyline was more effective than either agent alone or as compared with placebo. Numerous publications indicate that both tri-cycle antidepressants and selective serotonin reuptake inhibitors are effective for symptoms of fibromyalgia.

Unrefreshed sleep with difficulty falling asleep and frequent awakening is a very common complaint in fibromyalgia. Sleep hygiene measures such as limiting caffeine beverages 4 to 6 hours before sleeping, avoiding intense exercise a few hours before retiring, and using the bedroom only for sleep and sexual activities (not for watching television, working, or arguing) may be important. Relaxation techniques such as stretching, yoga, and progressive relaxation using a sleep tape or the use of soothing music maybe helpful in promoting sleep. Pharmacologic agents may include sedatives, sedating antihistamines, and sedating antidepressants, such as amitriptyline. Significant caution must be exercised with benzodiazepines due to the risk of habituation; this author does not recommend continuous use. Trazodone is sometimes used in fibromyalgia due to its sedative effects.

Fatigue is a difficult symptom to treat. Selective serotonin reuptake inhibitors may improve fatigue. The clinician must be aware that patients may attempt to self-treat fatigue by ingesting large quantities of caffeine, which could result in rebound headaches, palpitation, bowel or bladder dysfunction, and insomnia.

The treatment of irritable bowel syndrome or migraine headaches may improve the patient's quality of life. One third of patients with fibromyalgia experience sicca symptoms that require individual treatment. Massage or physical therapy may be helpful in the treatment of fibromyalgia. The patient must be warned that a massage may be painful. Future research may include the use of growth hormone supplementation.

EFFECTS ON PREGNANCY

The effects of fibromyalgia on pregnancy were reviewed by Ostensen et al. in a retrospective patient recall study involving low numbers of patients. The condition of fibromyalgia was not believed to have any effect on neonatal outcome. Aggravation of fibromyalgia symptoms was reported in most patients. The aggravation of symptoms was reported as a gradual increase from the first trimester to the third trimester. Miscarriage was found to be significantly more prevalent as compared with rheumatoid arthritis, but the fibromyalgia patients did have an increase in smoking, a lower educational level, and a higher workload that may have been confounding variables. Worsening of symptoms after delivery was reported by greater than 80% of patients. Patients expressed the need for assistance with childcare and housekeeping significantly more often than control patients.

CONCLUSION

Fibromyalgia has been classified as a rheumatologic disease, but its exact etiology is unclear. Successful treatment programs may involve a multidisciplinary approach, with emphasis on symptom improvement, not necessarily symptom extinction.

BIBLIOGRAPHY

Alarcon GS, Bradley LA. Advances in the treatment of fibromyalgia: current status and future directions. *Am J Med Sci* 1998;315:397–404.

Arnold LM, Keck PE, Welge JA. Antidepressant treatment of fibromyalgia: a meta-analysis and review. *Psychosomatic* 2000;41:104–113.

Barkhuizen A. Pharmacologic treatment of fibromyalgia. *Curr Pain Head Rep* 2001;5:351–358.

Barsky AJ, Borus JF. Functional somatic syndromes. *Ann Intern Med* 1999;130: 910–921.

Bennett RM, Burckhardt CS, Clark SR, et al. Group treatment of fibromyalgia: a 6 month outpatient program. *J Rheumatol* 1996;23:521–528.

Brattberg G. Connective tissue massage in the treatment of fibromyalgia. *Eur J Pain* 1999;3:235–244.

Cote KA, Moldofsky H. Sleep, daytime symptoms, and cognitive performance in patients with fibromyalgia. *J Rheumatol* 1997;24:2014–2023.

Dessein PH, Shipton EA, Stanwix AE, et al. Neuroendocrine deficiency-medicated development and persistence of pain in fibromyalgia: a promising paradigm? *Pain* 2000;86:213–215.

Goldenberg D, Mayskiy M, Mossey C, et al. A randomized, double-blind cross-over trial of fluoxetine and amitriptyline in the treatment of fibromyalgia. *Arthritis Rheum* 1996;39:1852–1859.

Jung AC, Staiger T, Sullivan M. The efficacy of selective serotonin reuptake inhibitors for the management of chronic pain. *J Gen Intern Med* 1997;12:384–389.

Lindell L, Bergman S, Petersson JF, et al. Prevalence of fibromyalgia and chronic widespread pain. *Scand J Prim Health Care* 2000;18:149–153.

Makela M, Heliovaara M. Prevalence of primary fibromyalgia in the Finnish population. *BMJ* 1991;303:216–219.

Martinez-Lavin M. Overlap of fibromyalgia with other medical conditions. *Curr Pain Head Rep* 2001;5:347–350.

Neilson WR, Merskey H. Psychosocial aspects of fibromyalgia. *Curr Pain Head Rep* 2001;5:330–337.

Offenbacher M, Stucki G. Physical therapy in the treatment of fibromyalgia. *Scand J Rheumatol Suppl* 2000;113:78–85.

Ostensen M, Rugelsioen A, Hovern-Wigers S. The effect of reproductive events and alternations of sex hormone levels on the symptoms of fibromyalgia. *Scand J Rheumatol* 1997;26:355–360.

Rossy LA, Buckelew SP, Dorr N, et al. A meta-analysis of fibromyalgia treatment interventions. *Ann Behav Med* 1999;21:180–191.

Russell IJ. Fibromyalgia syndrome: approaches to management. *Bull Rheum Dis* 1996;45:1–4.

Russell IJ, Orr MD, Littman D, et al. Elevated cerebrospinal fluid levels of substance P in patients with fibromyalgia syndrome. *Arthritis Rheum* 1994;37:1593–1601.

Simms RW, Zerbini CAP, Ferrante N, et al. Fibromyalgia syndrome in patients infected with human immunodeficiency virus. *Am J Med* 1992;92:368–374.

Stahl S. Fibromyalgia: the enigma and the stigma. *J Clin Psychiatry* 2001;62: 501–502.

Walker EA, Keegan D, Gardner G, et al. Psychosocial factors in fibromyalgia compared with rheumatoid arthritis. II. Sexual, physical, and emotional abuse and neglect. *Psychosom Med* 1997;59:572–577.

White H. Classification, epidemiology, and natural history of fibromyalgia. *Curr Pain Head Rep* 2001;5:320–329.

Wolfe F, Anderson J, Harkness D, et al. A prospective, longitudinal, multicenter study of service utilization and costs in fibromyalgia. *Arthritis Rheum* 1997;40: 1560–1570.

Wolfe F, Symthe H, Yunus M, et al. The Americal College of Rheumatology 1990 criteria for the classification of fibromyalgia: report of the Multicenter Criteria Committee. *Arthritis Rheum* 1990;33:160–168.

PART

10

Hematologic and Oncologic Problems

CHAPTER 89
Anemia

Peter A. Kouides

Anemia is not a disease in itself—it is the end-laboratory abnormality of numerous disease processes. Informing a patient only that she is anemic is not sufficient. It is incumbent on the physician to then logically proceed with additional laboratory testing to determine the underlying disease. This, of course, enables the physician to go beyond measures such as a red blood cell (RBC) transfusion or iron replacement in the hope of permanently correcting the anemic state. Consequently, this chapter focuses more on diagnosis than on therapy.

What is the extent of the clinical problem of anemia? To answer this question, anemia must first be defined. In general terms, anemia is a reduction in the circulating red cell mass. In practical terms, anemia is defined by a reduction in the hematocrit, which is the percentage of red cells that make up the circulating blood volume or a reduction in the hemoglobin measured in g/dL. Obviously, the hematocrit goes hand in hand with the hemoglobin concentration, and both are spuriously elevated in the case of dehydration. The hematocrit (as well as the hemoglobin) is a continuous laboratory variable, and the normal range depends on several factors, including age, gender, and altitude:

- *Gender.* The World Health Organization criteria for anemia based on hemoglobin concentration are a cutoff of less than 13 g/dL for adult men, less than 12 g/dL for menstruating women, and less than 11 g/dL for pregnant women. The difference in gender has been explained in part because of higher androgen levels in men, which stimulate RBC production.
- *Age.* The definition of anemia should be adjusted downward by roughly 1 g/dL in elderly men (i.e., <12 g/dL) and probably also in elderly women (i.e., <11 g/dL). The difference related to age may be due to both normal senescence of hematopoietic cells and, in the case of men, decreased androgen secretion. There is also the possibility of a higher incidence of underlying occult illnesses in the older population.
- *Altitude.* A higher altitude is associated with a higher normal range.

These variables aside, the prevalence of anemia in the United States is up to 33% in the hospital setting. Two laboratory values other than hemoglobin and hematocrit that are indispensable in the evaluation of anemia are the mean cell volume (MCV) and the reticulocyte count. The MCV is the average size of the red cell, which is derived from the automated complete blood cell count (CBC). The normal range is from 80 to 100 fL. Disorders deficient in hemoglobin understandably result in a decreased MCV (<80 fL; i.e., microcytosis), whereas disorders with an elevated MCV (>100 fL; i.e., macrocytosis) often reflect an inability of the red cell to fully mature because of a block in DNA synthesis secondary to depletion of vitamin B_{12} or folate. Anemia associated with a normal MCV (normocytic RBCs) can reflect a systemic or marrow process that is inhibiting all phases of red cell development (erythropoiesis), thus resulting in decreased production with a normal RBC size. Occasionally, a normocytic or macrocytic anemia is due to normal red cell production in the setting of acute blood loss or red cell destruction (hemolysis). This can be determined by the reticulocyte count. The reticulocyte count is the percentage of RBCs that stain as reticulated (having cytoplasmic inclusions of ribosomal and protein aggregates) cells by a supravital stain. An additional stain must be requested for this, that is, a specific test for the reticulocyte count apart from the automated CBC. These young cells are larger than the older red cells. Consequently, their increase in the peripheral blood can increase the MCV from its baseline. The reticulocyte percentage must be corrected for the presence of anemia because it is spuriously elevated when the absolute number of RBCs is reduced and because reticulocytes released under clinical stress conditions have a longer life span than normal reticulocytes. The laboratory typically reports the reticulocyte count corrected for those reasons. Alternatively, the uncorrected percentage of reticulocytes can be multiplied by the RBC count—a value exceeding $100 \times 10^9/L$ is consistent with acute blood loss or a hemolytic process.

ETIOLOGY AND DIFFERENTIAL DIAGNOSIS

A very important point to remember about the pathophysiology of anemia is that a reduced red cell mass can be from essentially only two mechanisms—one "central" in terms of decreased production of the red cell mass and the other "peripheral" in terms of increased destruction of the red cell mass or acute blood loss. The initial step in evaluating an anemic patient is to check the reticulocyte count. If the anemia is from decreased production, the reticulocyte count is normal or decreased. It is increased if the anemia is due to destruction or acute blood loss, that is, the response of a normal marrow to peripheral destruction or loss of the red cell mass wherein more of the "young" larger red cells are released—those red cells that still have ongoing protein synthesis and thus stain as reticulocytes. Fig. 89.1 outlines the differential diagnosis of anemia, placing 25 to 30 conditions under the category of a decreased reticulocyte count (decreased production) and another 25 conditions under the category of an increased reticulocyte count (increased destruction).

Anemias of Decreased Production

THE MICROCYTIC ANEMIAS

Statistically, there are only a handful of anemias to consider that can be associated with a reduced MCV (wherein the reticulocyte count is reduced). The common pathway leading to decreased red cell production with small (i.e., microcytic) red cells is a decrease in hemoglobin production:

Indirectly in terms of a decrease in iron

- Iron deficiency anemia, wherein there is an absolute decrease in iron, typically from gastrointestinal (GI) or menstrual blood loss. Regarding the latter, at least two thirds of women with menorrhagia (>80 mL menstrual blood loss) have iron deficiency.
- Anemia of "chronic disease," wherein there is a decrease in free iron available for red cell production, one explanation being that the activated white cells of inflammation release a protein, lactoferrin, that binds to the iron. This reduces the iron available for hemoglobin synthesis and may be a mechanism for the anemia. An additional mechanism is that the cytokines liberated in the setting of inflammation suppress erythropoiesis and also impair iron utilization.

Directly in terms of a decrease in hemoglobin production despite available iron

- Thalassemia, an inherited defect in the gene coding for the α- or β-hemoglobin chains leads to decreased hemoglobin production.
- Heavy metal poisoning such as lead poisoning, aluminum toxicity, or zinc excess with subsequent copper deficiency. These metals probably affect heme biosynthesis, thereby leading to decreased hemoglobin production.
- Sideroblastic anemia, the congenital form in particular, is characterized by a genetic defect in one of the enzymes involved in heme biosynthesis. The acquired form (often normocytic or macrocytic) can be secondary to alcohol or to antituberculosis drugs.

THE NORMOCYTIC ANEMIAS

The peripheral blood smear can be very helpful in patients with a reduced reticulocyte count and a normal MCV. One reason may be that the anemia has more than one etiology, that is, it is a mixed anemia with one etiology, a microcytic process such as iron deficiency, and another etiology, a macrocytic process such as B_{12} deficiency that, in terms of the MCV, would then average out to a normal MCV. Some hematology textbooks mention the relative distribution width index as a helpful parameter in ruling out a "mixed" anemia. However, I have not found it more helpful than examining the peripheral blood smear.

A mixed anemia aside, the causes of a normocytic anemia can be broken down into either diseases within the bone marrow or diseases outside of the bone marrow such as inflammation or failure of the kidney, liver, or the endocrine organs. These disorders secondarily suppress red cell production of normal-sized red cells. It is worth making the distinction between a disease of the bone marrow and a disease outside of the bone marrow because once diseases outside the bone marrow are ruled out, a bone marrow examination is usually the next step.

Anemias secondary to diseases outside the bone marrow suppressing red cell production include the following:

- Anemia of renal failure, which is a major cause of a normocytic anemia. The kidney produces a growth hormone, erythropoietin, that is essential for normal red cell production. When the creatinine clearance decreases below approximately 40 mL/min, production of this hormone by the kidney begins to decrease, leading to the development of anemia.
- Anemia of chronic liver disease from multiple causes such as hypersplenism, variceal bleeding, and suppression of erythropoiesis from accumulating metabolites
- Anemia of endocrine failure (Addison disease, hypopituitarism, thyroid disease—usually hypothyroidism) can also lead to anemia because these various hormones (e.g., androgens) usually have a stimulatory role in RBC production.
- Anemia of chronic disease can be microcytic, as previously mentioned, but is often normocytic. Although anemia of chronic disease is the historic term for this condition, it is probably more helpful to refer to this as the "anemia of inflammation." This reminds the reader that it is not any disease that can cause anemia (certainly we do not see anemia attributable just to diabetes or chronic obstructive pulmonary disease) but the inflammatory component of the disease (as with chronic infection, collagen vascular disease, or malignancy) that accounts for the anemia by suppressing red cell production. This occurs in part from inflammatory cytokines such as interleukin-1, γ-interferon, and tumor necrosis factor and in part by impairing iron utilization as previously mentioned. On the other hand, the patient with chronic obstructive pulmonary disease or the diabetic who has developed a concurrent inflammatory state such as pneumonia or a foot ulcer, respectively, may become anemic.

The diseases that can cause a normocytic anemia that necessitate a bone marrow examination can be characterized further on the basis of the cellularity of the bone marrow specimen. If the bone marrow specimen shows more than the normal number of cells present in the marrow (i.e., if it is hypercellular), then invariably the disease is a malignant process (though occasionally it can be a granulomatous infection), either a solid tumor metastasis to the bone marrow (termed "myelophthisic" anemia) or a malignant process of the hematopoietic or lymphatic system—acute or chronic lymphocytic or myelogenous leukemia, myelodysplastic syndrome (MDS) (preleukemia), lymphoma, myeloma, or myeloid metaplasia with myelofibrosis. These infiltrating diseases crowd out normal red cell production and usually white cell and

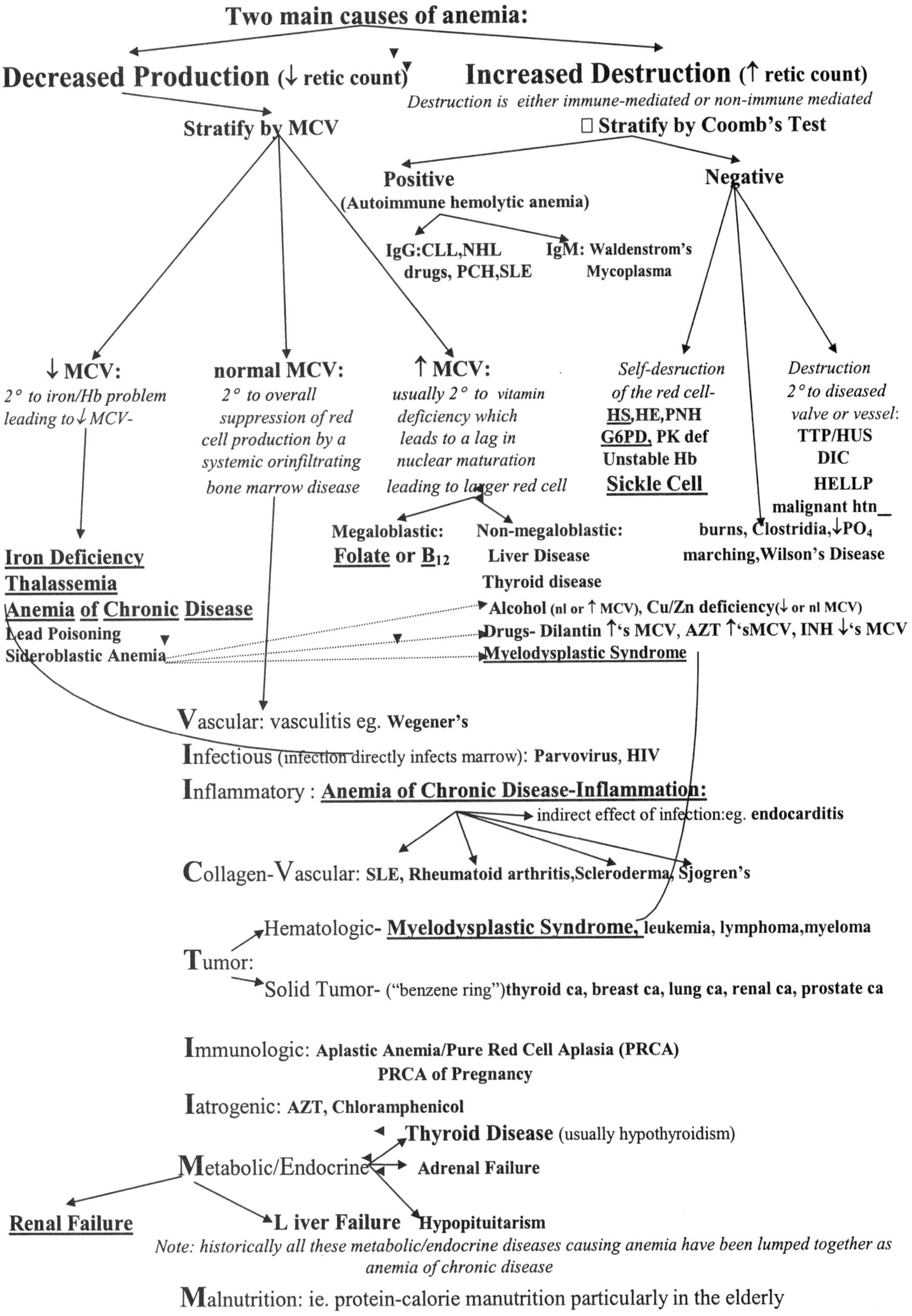

FIG. 89.1. Differential diagnosis of anemia—"physiology leads to pathology approach to anemia." One anemia can be in more than one category, as shown with dotted lines.

platelet production as well. One exception that may not present initially with associated platelet or white cell aberrations is MDS; it can present as an isolated anemia. Furthermore, in several studies of hospitalized patients, after iron deficiency anemia, anemia from acute blood loss, anemia from renal failure, and anemia of chronic disease are ruled out, MDS is the next most likely diagnosis, particularly in the elderly patient. Thus, this condition deserves consideration in any anemic elderly patient, but often such consideration is not made because MDS is a very difficult condition to understand, let alone diagnose. Part of the difficulty is that it is not a benign dysplastic disorder but a neoplastic disorder. It is a clonal disorder of hematopoiesis as in the case of the other primary hematologic malignant diseases previously mentioned, such as acute or chronic leukemia, lymphoma, and myeloma. In MDS, a clone at the level of the normal developing stem cell is present within the marrow. Over time it slowly expands, crowding out normal red cell and platelet production. In itself it does produce red cells, white cells, and platelets but not as effectively, hence the term "ineffective hematopoiesis." The morphologic manifestation is abnormal-appearing cells termed "dysplastic." Two implications are that (a) the initial laboratory manifestation will be a cytopenia, which typically involves the red cell series first (i.e., as an isolated anemia) and that (b) the red cells, white cells, and platelets produced are not entirely normal because they arise from an abnormal clone. Hence, these patients may be prone in part to infection and bleeding because of respective white cell and platelet dysfunction. Infection is a major cause of death from MDS, as is transformation to leukemia because the low-grade clonal expansion of the abnormal stem cell can lead in time to further genetic mutations and ultimately be clinically manifest as acute leukemia.

A hypocellular marrow that is associated only with a decrease in the cells of the erythroid lineage and not with the white cell- or platelet-producing lineage is termed pure RBC aplasia. If it is associated with the absence of cells in all three lineages, it is termed "aplastic anemia," a very serious condition that can be either idiopathic (though typically thought to be immunologic) or secondary. Secondary causes of pure RBC aplasia include collagen vascular disease, drug-induced (azathioprine, chloramphenicol, phenytoin, procainamide) disorders, lymphoproliferative disorders (particularly chronic lymphocytic leukemia or large granular lymphocyte leukemia), pregnancy, thymoma, and viral infections (parvovirus B19, hepatitis). Collagen vascular diseases, drugs, chemicals such as benzene, and viral infections have also been associated with aplastic anemia.

Anemias of Decreased Production with Increased Mean Cell Volume: the Macrocytic Anemias

The six or seven causes of a macrocytic anemia can be easily subdivided into those causes secondary to vitamin B_{12} or folate deficiency (pathologically termed "megaloblastic") versus the other causes (nonmegaloblastic). Typically, the MCV is markedly increased in vitamin deficiency (>115 fL), whereas the macrocytosis of the non–vitamin-deficiency states (alcohol use, chronic liver disease, drugs, familial, hypothyroidism, MDS) typically is milder—in the 100- to 110-fL range.

The usual cause of folate deficiency is dietary. In the case of B_{12} deficiency, several causes can be remembered best by understanding the physiology of B_{12} metabolism. The initial step is the dietary intake of B_{12}; thus, strict vegetarianism over a 10- to 15-year period can be a cause. The B_{12} then is liberated into a free form in the stomach by its acidic environment; hence, H_2 blocker use can be a cause. The stomach also produces a protein called "intrinsic factor," which is responsible for the absorption of B_{12}. Major loss of stomach tissue as in the case of a total or partial gastrectomy can be causative, as can be pernicious anemia, the specific autoimmune-mediated destruction of the intrinsic factor-producing parietal cells. Whereas B_{12} is liberated by the acidic environment in the stomach and then passes through the jejunum, further release of its bound form by pancreatic enzymes occur; therefore, chronic pancreatic insufficiency can be a cause of deficiency. Also, bacterial overgrowth from blind loops or diverticula or fish tapeworm in the jejunum compete with the host for the B_{12}. Absorption takes place in the presence of intrinsic factor in the terminal ileum. Malabsorption (that can also cause folate deficiency) can be from numerous causes such as Crohn disease, Whipple disease, tropical sprue, celiac disease, radiation ileitis, and infiltrative diseases such as lymphoma or scleroderma.

The non–vitamin-deficiency macrocytic anemias often are misdiagnosed initially as B_{12} or folate deficiency. A patient with a macrocytic anemia with a borderline low vitamin level may be started on folate or B_{12} injections without any further consideration for confirming the underlying cause of either folate or B_{12} deficiency. The clinician may observe after several months that the anemia is not responding to the vitamin supplementation.

Finally, certain drugs, particularly chemotherapy drugs and the antiretroviral drug, azidothymidine, can cause a macrocytic anemia, typically a macrocytosis without much of an anemia. Chemotherapy drugs can increase the MCV significantly in the range of B_{12} or folate deficiency. Two other drugs to mention under the heading of macrocytic anemia are phenytoin and sulfasalazine, which can interfere with folate absorption.

Anemia of Increased Destruction: the Hemolytic Anemias

The anemias of increased destruction do not occur as frequently as those of decreased production, although they include several that necessitate long-term primary care, such as sickle cell anemia and hereditary spherocytosis (HS). The two major categories of hemolytic anemias are immune-mediated and non–immune-mediated hemolytic anemias.

IMMUNE-MEDIATED HEMOLYTIC ANEMIAS: AUTOIMMUNE HEMOLYTIC ANEMIAS

The autoantibody causing the hemolysis can be either an IgG ("warm") or, less commonly, an IgM (cold). IgG-mediated hemolysis occurs via phagocytosis by splenic macrophages (extravascular hemolysis) engulfing part of the IgG-coated red cell membrane with each successive pass through the spleen, wherein the red cell may reseal after each pass, resulting in a spherical-shaped cell—a spherocyte. On the other hand, IgM-mediated hemolysis occurs in the intravascular compartment because this antibody is capable of fixing complement at a temperature less than 37°C and lysing the red cell without the help of the splenic macrophages. Making the distinction between extravascular and intravascular hemolysis has implications in terms of diagnosis and therapy. The indices of hemolysis (the red cell breakdown products lactate dehydrogenase, serum glutamic-oxaloacetic transaminase, hemoglobin) are more pronounced for the same degree of hemolysis in cold autoimmune hemolytic anemias (AIHA) compared with warm AIHA. In the latter, these products are absorbed within the spleen without much spillover into the plasma. Splenectomy would also have a therapeutic role in warm AIHA in contrast to cold AIHA.

In about 50% of cases of IgG- or IgM-mediated AIHA, an underlying cause is observed such as a lymphoproliferative disorder (chronic lymphocytic leukemia, lymphoma, Waldenström [IgM] macroglobulinemia), infection (usually the antibody is an IgM as in *Mycoplasma pneumoniae* or Epstein-Barr virus infection, rarely it is IgG and termed "paroxysmal cold hemoglobinuria," related to syphilis or certain viral infections), collagen vascular disease (lupus), delayed transfusion reaction, or drugs (IgG autoantibodies secondary to drugs such as quinidine, procainamide, penicillin, or Aldomet).

NON–IMMUNE-MEDIATED HEMOLYTIC ANEMIAS

Non–immune-mediated hemolytic anemias can be further subdivided into intrinsic red cell defects or processes extrinsic to the red cell that is responsible for red cell destruction. In the case of non–immune-mediated hemolysis secondary to an intrinsic red cell defect (i.e., the red cell is fragile), these conditions can be thought of in terms of their localization in relation to the various components of the red cell.

Disorders involving the Red Cell Membrane. These include congenital disorders characterized by certain red cell shape changes. HS is more common than hereditary elliptocytosis or hereditary stomatocytosis. HS is usually an autosomal-dominant disorder. The explanation for the change in the red cell from its normal discoid appearance to a spherical shape is usually because of a deficiency in spectrin. This protein is like a girder holding up a canopy. In HS, there is a genetic deficiency in the production of this protein or the proteins that maintain this girder (e.g., ankyrin, band 3 protein) and so in turn the canopy collapses, leading to a decrease in the surface-to-volume ratio. This spherical property (morphologically expressed as a spherocyte) confers a susceptibility to sequestration and destruction in the spleen. An acquired membrane disorder is paroxysmal nocturnal hemoglobinuria. This hemolytic disorder is secondary to a deficiency in a glycolipid anchor of the membrane that leads to a loss of several proteins on the red cell membrane, including a group of proteins that inhibits complement-mediated lysis of the red cell. This lysis is favored by an acidic environment; hence, the classic description of red urine upon morning awakening because of the relative acidosis that ensues during sleep from hypoventilation.

Disorders of the Cytoplasm. Disorders of the cytoplasm, for example, congenital deficiency of the glucose-6-phosphate dehydrogenase enzyme (which is an X-linked disorder) or one of the approximately 15 other red cell enzymes can lead to a decrease in the normal reducing power (i.e., the level of nicotinamide dehydrogenase/nicotinamide dehydrogenase phosphate [NADH/NADPH] is depleted) of the red cell and subsequent increased susceptibility to hemolysis in the setting of oxidative stress.

Disorders of Hemoglobin Structure. Sickle cell anemia is the classic example of a disorder of hemoglobin structure. Its genetic basis is a one-nucleotide mutation, which then codes for a different amino acid in the β-chain of the hemoglobin molecule. It is that one amino acid alone that changes the structural nature of the hemoglobin protein into one that can polymerize under hypoxic or acidic conditions with subsequent hemolysis or entrapment of the irreversibly sickled red cell. The latter leads to vaso-occlusion and ischemic pain. Far less common hemoglobin disorders that can be associated with hemolytic anemia are the unstable hemoglobins and the toxic hemoglobinopathies. The unstable hemoglobins are congenital disorders in which the hemoglobin molecules are susceptible to oxidative denaturation, leading to the conversion of hemoglobin to methemoglobin. Hemoglobin is also susceptible to oxidative denaturation if an agent (e.g., dapsone, sulfasalazine, chloroquine) is ingested that can directly oxidize it or if a congenital deficiency of the enzyme methemoglobin reductase is present.

Disorders outside the Red Cell. The last group of non–immune-mediated hemolytic anemias are those from a process extrinsic to the red cell. In these disorders, the red cell is normal but becomes an innocent bystander. Red cell destruction can be either from an infectious agent (*Bartonella*, babesiosis, or clostridia as in the classic setting of sepsis after an illegal abortion), trauma (marathon running—march hemoglobinuria or foot-strike hemolysis), metabolic perturbation (hypophosphatemia), or an abnormal heart valve or vessel (microangiopathic hemolysis) causing red cell fragmentation. In the case of a fragmentation-hemolysis anemia, patients with prosthetic valves, particularly mechanical valves in the aortic position, are at greatest risk for hemolysis. Hemolysis secondary to abnormal vessels occurs in the setting of any process that can decrease the lumen of the vessel in the microcirculation. The red cell must be able to bend through the microcirculation where the capillary diameter can be less than the diameter of the red cell. If the lumen is further narrowed by an inflammatory process, as in the case of vasculitis, eclampsia, or malignant hypertension, or if the narrowing is because of the development of intravascular thrombi, as seen in hemolytic uremic syndrome, thrombotic thrombocytopenic purpura, or disseminated intravascular coagulation, red cell fragmentation and hemolytic anemia may ensue. Examination of the peripheral blood shows red cells that have been injured because the passage through this narrow lumen leads to the appearance of fragmented red cells (schistocytes).

HISTORY

A history of the present illness should be taken. The classic common symptoms are fatigue; shortness of breath, particularly with exertion; lightheadedness or dizziness; tinnitus; and palpitations. Less common complaints include a whirring or humming sensation in the head (probably from rapid blood flow through the cranial arteries), loss of libido, inability to concentrate, change in mood, and change in sleep pattern. The onset of symptoms is acute if the cause is acute blood loss or hemolysis, although mild hemolytic disorders like HS can be associated with a gradual onset of symptoms. History that can suggest a specific diagnosis should also be sought:

- Craving (pica) for substances such as ice (pagophagia) or substances not usually ingested, such as venetian blind dust (coniophagia) or toothpicks (xylophagia) should suggest iron deficiency. Over 50 substances have been cataloged in the medical literature.
- History of changing the tampon/pad every 30 to 120 minutes, frequently staining underclothes, and loss of time from school or work because of heavy menstrual flow suggests iron deficiency anemia due to menorrhagia. Up to 20% of these patients may have additional mucocutaneous bleeding symptoms (epistaxis, history of dental or surgical related bleeding, easy bruising) consistent with the underlying congenital bleeding disorder, von Willebrand disease
- History of acute blood loss or recent blood donation.
- History of scleral icterus would suggest a hemolytic disorder such as HS.
- History of vegetarianism, paresthesia, ataxia, or cognitive changes suggests B_{12} deficiency.
- History of GI complaints suggests blood loss and iron deficiency; a history of GI disease such as sprue or Crohn disease suggests folate or B_{12} deficiency.

A past medical history should also be taken. Particularly if the patient has a normocytic anemia, a history for an inflammatory condition (collagen vascular disease, malignancy, or chronic infection) or organ failure (renal, liver, adrenal, pituitary, thyroid) should be sought. A history of gallstones suggests a chronic hemolytic disorder such as HS.

The patient should also be asked about family members with any of the congenital anemias, such as thalassemia, sideroblastic anemia, HS, sickle cell anemia, or glucose-6-phosphate dehydrogenase deficiency. Alcohol use can be associated with anemia of liver disease, sideroblastic anemia, or GI blood loss. And finally, certain drugs are associated with certain subsets of anemia (primarily hemolytic anemia or production defects) as mentioned earlier in the section on etiology and differential diagnosis. Iron deficiency anemia can be secondary to nonsteroidal drug-induced gastritis.

PHYSICAL EXAMINATION

The physical examination covers the following areas:

- *Vital signs.* Tachycardia and bounding pulse pressure are nonspecific findings.
- *HEENT (head-eyes-ears-nose-throat).* The word anemia is derived from a Greek word meaning "without blood," so obviously a pale appearance is typical. In people with dark pigmentation, this often is not readily apparent, so an additional helpful laboratory finding is obtained by examining the conjunctivae, which should appear pale. The sclera should also be examined for icterus, which suggests a hemolytic disorder. Retinal hemorrhages can be associated with severe anemia or anemia with thrombocytopenia as in acute leukemia.
- *Lymph nodes.* Palpable nodes should increase suspicion for lymphoma or chronic lymphocytic leukemia associated with AIHA or for a solid tumor malignancy associated with anemia of chronic disease or a myelophthisic anemia.
- *Cardiopulmonary.* A systolic ejection murmur may be present, and an S_3 can be noted if the anemia has led to cardiac failure.
- *Abdomen.* Splenomegaly suggests HS, lymphoma, hypersplenism, or warm AIHA.
- *Rectal.* Stool testing for occult blood should be a mandatory part of the physical examination given the fact that iron deficiency caused by blood loss is the most common cause of anemia.
- *Extremities.* Peripheral edema may be a nonspecific finding.
- *Skin and integument.* Progressive iron deficiency or B_{12} anemia also leads to deficiency of iron or B_{12} in the normal epithelial tissues. Iron and B_{12} are needed as cofactors for certain enzymes that maintain normal cellular functions, and their deficiency can account for spooning of the nails (koilonychia) seen occasionally in long-standing iron deficiency, breakdown of the epithelium at the juncture of the lips (cheilosis), and loss of the normal fissura of the tongue (glossitis) seen primarily in B_{12} deficiency. B_{12} deficiency can also be associated with vitiligo if the cause of the deficiency is pernicious anemia.
- *Neurologic.* Testing for position sense, vibration, and ataxia should be done because B_{12} deficiency can lead demyelination as well as anemia. It has been reported that patients with B_{12} deficiency can first present with such neurologic signs and symptoms before the development of a macrocytic anemia.

LABORATORY STUDIES

A hemogram should be obtained and whether the hematocrit is decreased noted. If it is decreased, the MCV should then be examined, because statistically the most common causes of anemia are those that decrease the MCV by reducing the amount of hemoglobin directly, as in thalassemia, or indirectly, as in iron deficiency.

A peripheral blood smear should be examined (laboratory technicians are usually helpful and willing to assist) and a reticulocyte count obtained in further consideration of anemias of decreased production or increased destruction. The associated morphologic abnormalities noted in the peripheral blood smear are shown in Table 89.1. They are often recorded as part of the CBC and differential. Fig. 89.2 outlines additional laboratory

TABLE 89.1. Peripheral Blood Cell Abnormalities in Relation to Categories of Anemia

Microcytic anemia	Normocytic anemia	Macrocytic anemia	Coombs negative hemolytic anemia	Coombs positive hemolytic anemia
Hypochromia in Fe deficiency, thalassemia	Burr cells (echinocytes) in renal failure	Macroovalocytes, hypersegmented WBCs, B_{12} or folate deficiency	Spherocytes in HS	Spherocytes in warm AIHA
Target cells in thalassemia	Spur cells (acanthocytes) and/or target cells in liver disease		Elliptocytes in HE Bite cells in G6PD deficiency	Rouleaux in AIHA secondary to cold-reacting antibodies, e.g., mycoplasma, Waldenström
Basophilic stippling in lead toxicity	Basophilic stippling, Pelger-Huet–like cells, (hypolobulated WBC), giant or agranular platelets all dysplastic features that are occasionally seen in MDS Tear drop cells in myeloid metaplasia with myelofibrosis		Red-cell fragments (schistocytes) in TTP/HUS, DIC, preeclampsia, malignant hypertension, prosthetic valve–related hemolysis, sickled cells, as in sickle cell anemia	

AIHA, autoimmune hemolytic anemia; DIC, disseminated intravascular coagulation; Fe, iron; G6PD, glucose-6-phosphate dehydrogenase; HE, hereditary elliptocytosis; HS, hereditary spherocytosis; MDS, myelodysplastic syndrome; TTP/HUS, thrombotic thrombocytopenic purpura/hemolytic uremic syndrome.

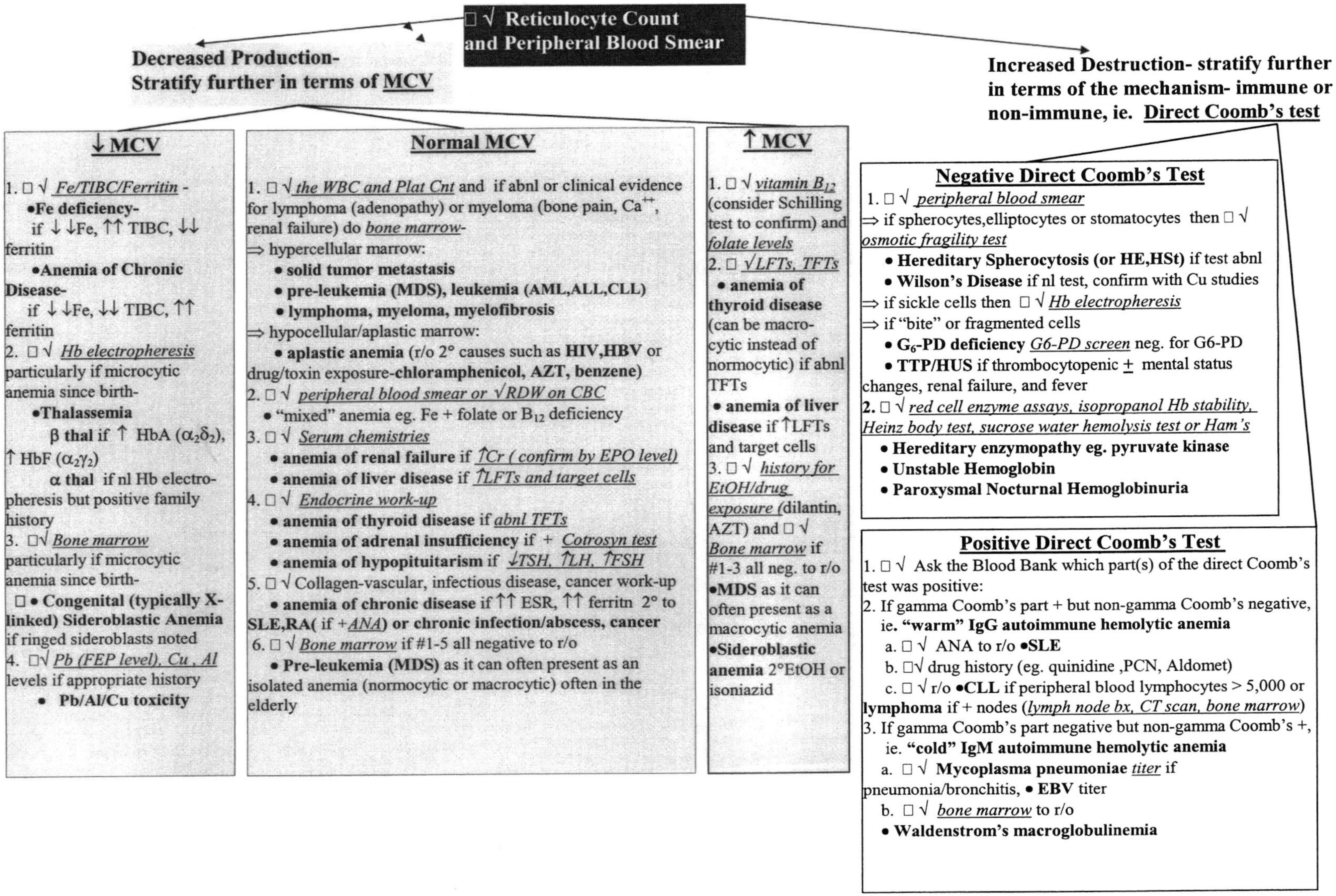

□ √ Reticulocyte Count and Peripheral Blood Smear
Decreased Production- Stratify further in terms of MCV
Increased Destruction- stratify further in terms of the mechanism- immune or non-immune, ie. Direct Coomb's test
↓MCV
1. □ √ Fe/TIBC/Ferritin -
•Fe deficiency-
if ↓ ↓Fe, ↑↑ TIBC, ↓↓ ferritin
•Anemia of Chronic Disease-
if ↓ ↓Fe, ↓↓ TIBC, ↑↑ ferritin
2. □ √ Hb electropheresis particularly if microcytic anemia since birth-
•Thalassemia
β thal if ↑ HbA ($\alpha_2\delta_2$), ↑ HbF ($\alpha_2\gamma_2$)
α thal if nl Hb electropheresis but positive family history
3. □√ Bone marrow particularly if microcytic anemia since birth-
□ • Congenital (typically X-linked) Sideroblastic Anemia if ringed sideroblasts noted
4. □√ Pb (FEP level), Cu, Al levels if appropriate history
• Pb/Al/Cu toxicity
Normal MCV
1. □ √ the WBC and Plat Cnt and if abnl or clinical evidence for lymphoma (adenopathy) or myeloma (bone pain, Ca^{++}, renal failure) do bone marrow-
⇒ hypercellular marrow:
• solid tumor metastasis
• pre-leukemia (MDS), leukemia (AML,ALL,CLL)
• lymphoma, myeloma, myelofibrosis
⇒ hypocellular/aplastic marrow:
• aplastic anemia (r/o 2° causes such as HIV,HBV or drug/toxin exposure-chloramphenicol, AZT, benzene)
2. □ √ peripheral blood smear or √RDW on CBC
• "mixed" anemia eg. Fe + folate or B_{12} deficiency
3. □ √ Serum chemistries
• anemia of renal failure if ↑Cr (confirm by EPO level)
• anemia of liver disease if ↑LFTs and target cells
4. □ √ Endocrine work-up
• anemia of thyroid disease if abnl TFTs
• anemia of adrenal insufficiency if + Cotrosyn test
• anemia of hypopituitarism if ↓TSH, ↑LH, ↑FSH
5. □ √ Collagen-vascular, infectious disease, cancer work-up
• anemia of chronic disease if ↑↑ ESR, ↑↑ ferritn 2° to SLE,RA(if +ANA) or chronic infection/abscess, cancer
6. □ √ Bone marrow if #1-5 all negative to r/o
• Pre-leukemia (MDS) as it can often present as an isolated anemia (normocytic or macrocytic) often in the elderly
↑MCV
1. □ √ vitamin B_{12} (consider Schilling test to confirm) and folate levels
2. □ √LFTs, TFTs
• anemia of thyroid disease (can be macrocytic instead of normocytic) if abnl TFTs
• anemia of liver disease if ↑LFTs and target cells
3. □ √ history for EtOH/drug exposure (dilantin, AZT) and □ √ Bone marrow if #1-3 all neg. to r/o
•MDS as it can often present as a macrocytic anemia
•Sideroblastic anemia 2°EtOH or isoniazid
Negative Direct Coomb's Test
1. □ √ peripheral blood smear
⇒ if spherocytes,elliptocytes or stomatocytes then □ √ osmotic fragility test
• Hereditary Spherocytosis (or HE,HSt) if test abnl
• Wilson's Disease if nl test, confirm with Cu studies
⇒ if sickle cells then □ √ Hb electropheresis
⇒ if "bite" or fragmented cells
• G_6-PD deficiency G6-PD screen neg. for G6-PD
• TTP/HUS if thrombocytopenic ± mental status changes, renal failure, and fever
2. □ √ red cell enzyme assays, isopropanol Hb stability, Heinz body test, sucrose water hemolysis test or Ham's
• Hereditary enzymopathy eg. pyruvate kinase
• Unstable Hemoglobin
• Paroxysmal Nocturnal Hemoglobinuria
Positive Direct Coomb's Test
1. □ √ Ask the Blood Bank which part(s) of the direct Coomb's test was positive:
2. If gamma Coomb's part + but non-gamma Coomb's negative, ie. "warm" IgG autoimmune hemolytic anemia
a. □ √ ANA to r/o •SLE
b. □√ drug history (eg. quinidine ,PCN, Aldomet)
c. □ √ r/o •CLL if peripheral blood lymphocytes > 5,000 or lymphoma if + nodes (lymph node bx, CT scan, bone marrow)
3. If gamma Coomb's part negative but non-gamma Coomb's +, ie. "cold" IgM autoimmune hemolytic anemia
a. □ √ Mycoplasma pneumoniae titer if pneumonia/bronchitis, • EBV titer
b. □ √ bone marrow to r/o
• Waldenstrom's macroglobulinemia

FIG. 89.2. Laboratory evaluation of anemia starting from the mean cell volume and reticulocyte count.

tests that allow the cause to be precisely pinpointed from about 50 conditions capable of causing anemia.

Laboratory Evaluation of the Microcytic Anemias

Tests for iron deficiency should be done first in this subset. If old records can be located and long-standing microcytosis is noted for more than 1 year or from childhood, a hemoglobin electrophoresis could be obtained to look for the β-thalassemia trait and the characteristic pattern of an increase in the minor adult hemoglobin (HbA_2) and the fetal hemoglobin (HbF). α-Thalassemia, however, cannot be diagnosed by electrophoresis. That diagnosis depends on finding other family members with a similar microcytic anemia or on studies of globin synthesis in peripheral blood reticulocytes or gene-mapping techniques. If both iron studies and hemoglobin electrophoresis and family history for α-thalassemia are nonrevealing, then the anemia of chronic disease should be considered. There should be adequate clinical or laboratory evidence for inflammation, and the serum ferritin must be elevated (although coincidental iron deficiency can lower the level to 20–100 ng/mL). Next, a free erythrocyte protoporphyrin level should be measured for consideration of lead poisoning if there is an appropriate clinical setting. If the diagnosis remains in doubt, a bone marrow examination should be done. The diagnosis of sideroblastic anemia may be established if red cell precursors in the bone marrow stain for deposits of iron in a perinuclear pattern.

The iron tests usually done to diagnose iron deficiency anemia include serum iron, total iron binding capacity, percentage of transferrin saturation (serum iron divided by total iron binding capacity), and serum ferritin. The typical pattern is a reduced serum iron, increased total iron binding capacity, decreased transferrin saturation, and reduced serum ferritin. Hematologists are often asked by general practitioners whether they need to do all these tests or whether they can just order one test, such as a serum iron or a serum ferritin. If the patient does not have any other ongoing medical condition—particularly one that can be inflammatory, such as malignancy, infection, or collagen vascular disease—it is probably adequate just to check the serum ferritin. What is clearly insufficient is to draw the serum iron. It can vary widely over a day, based on a recent meal, for example. It can be low in anemia of chronic disease despite normal or increased body iron. It is also insufficient for the clinician to begin iron replacement therapy without further studies to find the actual cause of the iron deficiency. Again, the common theme that arises here is that anemia, in this case iron deficiency anemia, is not a disease in itself. In women with microcytic anemia seemingly out of proportion to menses and/or age over 40 and/or abdominal symptoms and/or a fetal occult blood test, a GI lesion must be considered. But if the history is of very heavy menses in a female younger than age 40 and without abdominal symptoms, it might be reasonable to first give iron and determine if the hematocrit normalizes and remains stable before embarking on a GI workup.

LABORATORY EVALUATION OF THE NORMOCYTIC ANEMIAS

The first step that should be taken in this category is to look at the white blood cell count and platelet count recorded with the hematocrit on the CBC. If the white blood cell, platelet count, or both are abnormal, a bone marrow examination probably should be done next. If only anemia is present, the peripheral blood should be reviewed to rule out a mixed anemia, iron deficiency plus folate, or B_{12} deficiency wherein the MCV averages out. Before the peripheral blood smear is looked at for evidence of the elliptical or hypochromic cells of iron deficiency mixed with the large oval red cells and hypersegmented neutrophils of B_{12} or folate deficiency, a clue can be found in the red cell distribution width that is reported on the CBC. In such a mixed anemia, it should be increased. After ruling out a mixed anemia, the next step should be obtaining serum chemistries (liver function tests, serum creatinine with an erythropoietin level to confirm anemia of renal failure if the creatinine is increased) followed by endocrine testing (such as thyroid-stimulating hormone) as well as iron studies because anemia of chronic disease can present with normocytic indices. Finally, a bone marrow examination should be done if all the previous serum studies are within normal limits. Even if the white blood cell and platelet count are within normal limits, an MDS can present as an isolated anemia as previously mentioned. A bone marrow aspirate in consideration of MDS

- Has more cells than a peripheral blood sample to examine for the characteristic morphologic abnormalities (dysplasia) of this disorder
- Could be sent also for cytogenetic analysis because up to half of the cases have a confirmatory cytogenetic abnormality
- Can be examined for the percent of blasts for purposes of prognosis. Marrows with an increased percent of blasts portend a worse prognosis as the percentage reflects a higher probability of progression to acute leukemia.

LABORATORY EVALUATION OF A MACROCYTIC ANEMIA

A serum vitamin B_{12} and serum folate level should be drawn. In the case of folate, the RBC folate level is more sensitive than the serum levels, but for practical reasons most laboratories first do a serum folate level. A hemolytic anemia or GI bleed should be considered because the associated increased reticulocyte count also increases the MCV, albeit mildly. The clinician should at the very least ask the hematology laboratory to review the peripheral blood smear for the characteristic macroovalocytes and hypersegmented polymorphonuclear leukocytes. It is often said that the presence of just one six-lobed polymorphonuclear leukocyte or 5% of five-lobed polymorphonuclear leukocytes is consistent with the diagnosis of B_{12} or folate deficiency. If these findings are absent, the causes of a falsely low B_{12} level must be considered: multiple myeloma, oral contraceptive intake, folate deficiency, and pregnancy. If these causes are absent, then serology supportive for pernicious anemia can be drawn (an antiintrinsic factor antibody, antiparietal cell antibody). Historically, a Schilling test was first done, but this is done less frequently, although a recent study showed an alarmingly poor positive predictive value of 20% for a low B_{12} value.

If both folate and B_{12} levels are normal, a thyroid-stimulating hormone level evaluates for hypothyroidism and serum chemistries assess liver disease, either of which can be the cause of macrocytic anemia. Again, it is emphasized that non–vitamin-deficiency related microcytic anemias have only a mild macrocytosis (100–110 fL) compared with the marked macrocytosis (>115 fL) of B_{12} or folate deficiency. MDS can present as a macrocytic anemia; therefore, a bone marrow examination should be done after ruling out the above causes of a macrocytic anemia.

Laboratory Evaluation of a Hemolytic Anemia

If the anemic patient's reticulocyte count, as mentioned previously, is increased, a hemolytic workup should commence, starting with a direct Coombs test. Its sensitivity is approximately 90%. Reviewing the peripheral blood smear for spherocytes is helpful. They are still seen in that approximately 10% subset of AIHA with a negative direct Coombs test. The direct Coombs test involves adding a mixture of antibodies—IgG (gamma Coombs reagent) and complement (non-gamma reagent)—that react to the red cell suspension. In AIHA, reaction with a mixture of these reagents leads to agglutination of the red cells, which is viewed as a positive test. The gamma and non-gamma reagents are then reacted with the patient's red cells separately. If it is an AIHA from the production of IgG (warm-acting) antibody, the gamma reagent and usually the non-gamma reagent as well give a positive test for agglutination. Less commonly, the patient has a hemolytic anemia not because of the production of an IgG antibody but because of the production of an IgM (cold-reacting) antibody. In such a case, the gamma Coombs test is negative but the non-gamma Coombs test is positive.

Because of the frequent association of AIHA with a lymphoproliferative disorder, particularly in the older patient, some hematologists often proceed with a bone marrow examination to rule out a lymphoproliferative disorder. Serologies for Epstein-Barr virus or *Mycoplasma* infection are reasonable in the setting of cold AIHA if there is a consistent history.

If the Coombs test is negative, it is imperative to review the peripheral blood smear. The presence of spherocytes suggests HS (besides a false-negative direct Coombs test). An osmotic fragility test would be the confirmatory test in HS. If there are no spherocytes, paroxysmal nocturnal hemoglobinuria should be another membrane disorder to consider. A sucrose water hemolysis or acidified Ham test may be diagnostic, particularly if the patient has pancytopenia, unexplained thrombosis, or recurrent abdominal pain. If there are sickled cells, a hemoglobin electrophoresis should be done. If there are "bite" cells or if the previous tests are negative, a Heinz body test should be done. This would be positive in the setting of oxidative denaturation leading to hemolysis either from an RBC enzyme deficiency such as glucose-6-phosphate dehydrogenase deficiency (glucose-6-phosphate dehydrogenase screen should be done to confirm), an unstable hemoglobin, or methemoglobin reductase deficiency. An isopropanol instability test or the heat instability test establishes the presence of an unstable hemoglobin.

If fragmented or torn red cells are noted, the various causes of a microangiopathic anemia should be considered, including the hemolytic uremic syndrome or thrombotic thrombocytopenic purpura. The presence of fragmented red cells in a patient with a prosthetic valve should prompt a transesophageal echocardiogram to rule out valve dysfunction.

In either a Coombs-positive or Coombs-negative hemolytic anemia, serum chemistries to gauge the severity of the hemolysis should also be drawn, as outlined in Table 89.2. In intravascular hemolysis (i.e., the Coombs-negative hemolytic anemias), lactate dehydrogenase, SGOT [serum glutamate oxalate transferase], and indirect bilirubin are higher and the serum haptoglobin lower than in the extravascular hemolysis (i.e., Coombs-positive hemolytic anemias).

MANAGEMENT AND TREATMENT

Treatment of anemia involves treating the underlying cause. Table 82.3 outlines a pharmacologic classification of anemia.

Iron Deficiency Anemia

For iron deficiency anemia, 50 mg of elemental iron (325 mg in the sulfate form) is prescribed three to four times per day with a maximal absorption occurring 2 hours after a meal when there is a less acidic environment. An adequate response is a rise in the hemoglobin by more than 2 g/dL in 2 to 3 weeks. A common clinical problem related to iron therapy is GI symptoms, including constipation. An attempt can be made to switch to the ferrous gluconate formula 300 mg orally three times per day, although unfortunately it is not associated with as much free elemental iron. Also, trying iron sulfate in the elixir form may help the intolerance if the main problem is swallowing pills. Finally, a polysaccharide preparation can be tried, Niferex 150 mg orally twice a day, but it is costly. Despite these modifications, there will be an occasional patient who cannot tolerate any oral formulation of iron and therefore is a candidate for weekly intramuscular iron. A maximum of 100 mg at one time can be given once a week. Often the iron deficit is about 1,000 mg or more, so there is the inconvenience of numerous visits and the discomfort of the injection. Alternatively, the total iron deficit can be calculated and given as intravenous iron dextran over 4 to 6 hours. The total deficit is calculated as follows:

Iron deficit = {([the normal hemoglobin of 12 gm/dL in females] – [the patient's present hemoglobin]) × (their body weight in pounds)} + a correction factor of 600 mg

The risk of anaphylaxis is approximately 1 in 1,000 patients, so a test dose is advised. We premedicate the test dose of 25 mg

TABLE 89.2. Laboratory Features of Extra- and Intravascular Hemolysis

	Extravascular hemolysis	Intravascular hemolysis	
	Warm AIHA (e.g., autoantibody is IgG)	Cold ANA (e.g., autoantibody is IgM)	Nonimmune hemolytic anemia e.g., HS, PNH, G6PD deficiency, sickle cell disease, TTP/HUS)
Direct Coombs test	⊕ Gamma Coombs/ ± non-gamma Coombs	– Gamma Coombs/ ⊕ non-gamma Coombs	—
LDH	N or ↑	↑↑↑	↑↑↑
Haptoglobin	N or ↓	↓↓	↓↓
Urine hemosiderin	—	Occasionally	Occasionally

AIHA, autoimmune hemolytic anemia; ANA, anti-nuclear antibody; G6PD, glucose-6-phosphate dehydrogenase; HS, hereditary spherocytosis; IgG, immunoglobulin G; IgM, immunoglobulin M; LDH, lactate dehydrogenase; PNH, paroxysmal nocturnal hemoglobinuria; TTP/HUS, thrombotic thrombocytopenic purpura/hemolytic uremic syndrome.

TABLE 89.3. Pharmacologic Classification of Anemia

Pharmacologically responsive anemias	Pharmacologically unresponsive ("refractory") anemias
Nutrient responsive	**With cellular marrow**
Iron-deficiency anemia	Anemia of chronic disease (inflammation)
B_{12} deficiency	MDS
Folate deficiency	Metastatic tumor
Pyridoxine-responsive sideroblastic anemia	Thalassemia trait
Erythropoietin responsive	**With hypocellular marrow**
Renal failure anemia	Aplastic anemia
Synthroid responsive	Hypoplastic AML
Hypothyroidism	
Prednisone responsive	
Autoimmune hemolytic anemia	

AML, acute myeloid leukemia; MDS, myelo displastic syndrome.

iron dextran (0.5 mL of a 50-mg/mL vial) with Benadryl 25 mg orally, Tylenol 650 mg orally, and Solu-Medrol 40 mg IVSS (intravenous Solu-set). If there is no reaction after 60 minutes of observation, we proceed with the total dose over 4 to 6 hours as tolerated. We inform the patient that commonly 5 to 14 days after the infusion intense bone pain can develop, although typically it resolves with a nonsteroidal antiinflammatory drug.

Thalassemia

Management of thalassemia requires regular red cell transfusions for thalassemia major to maintain normal growth and development. This is at the price of iron overload, which develops after 10 to 20 units of RBCs. Such patients invariably need iron chelation with the subcutaneous iron chelator desferrioxamine. There has been expanding use of allogeneic bone marrow transplantation for thalassemia major primarily in Europe. No specific therapy is needed for thalassemia trait, because the diagnosis of α-thalassemia trait is one of exclusion. The reader is reminded that thalassemia can masquerade as iron deficiency, and iron should not be empirically prescribed for a microcytic anemia.

Anemia of Renal Failure

The successful use of erythropoietin in the correction of the anemia of renal failure has heralded a major advance—the use of the recombinant hematopoietic growth factors for hematologic disorders. Erythropoietin is given subcutaneously one to three times a week. The anemia of renal failure is corrected in most dialysis-dependent patients. In those not yet requiring dialysis and who still have some endogenous erythropoietin production, lower and/or less frequent dosing may be sufficient, such as 10,000 to 20,000 units subcutaneously every 1 to 4 weeks. Iron supplementation should be done concurrently so that erythropoietin augmented erythropoiesis does not "out-strip" the iron supply.

Myelodysplastic Syndrome

Because MDS is a clonal bone marrow disorder that originates in the stem cell, no chemotherapy can permanently eradicate the clone with restoration of normal hematopoiesis. Furthermore, because this is a condition primarily of older patients, the emphasis is on supportive care: transfusing red cells as necessary and treating infections with antibiotics. If there are recurrent infections, a trial with granulocyte colony-stimulating factor or granulocyte-macrophage colony-stimulating factor can be effective in increasing the number of white blood cells. At least one fifth of patients will respond to subcutaneous erythropoietin; an additional proportion of patients will respond to the addition of granulocyte or granulocyte-macrophage colony-stimulating factor subcutaneously one to three times a week.

Pure Red Cell Aplasia or Aplastic Anemia

Pure red cell aplasia or aplastic anemia is a presumed immunologic disorder that may respond to treatment with steroids and cyclosporine plus antithymocyte globulin. If there is a sibling who is histocompatible and the patient is under 40 years of age, then an allogeneic bone marrow transplant is preferable.

Anemias of Decreased Production: Macrocytic Anemia

Vitamin B_{12} deficiency requires lifelong repletion unless the patient has B_{12} deficiency from decreased gastric secretion secondary to H_2 blockers. The route is usually intramuscularly, but the subcutaneous route is just as effective. Some clinicians have even tried oral vitamin B_{12}. This is not as efficacious as the parenteral route because the majority of B_{12}-deficient patients have impaired absorption either directly because of bowel disease or indirectly through the lack of intrinsic factor though 3% of B_{12} is absorbed independently of intrinsic factor. Initially, treatment is given at 1 mg/d intramuscularly or subcutaneously for 1 week, then twice a week for 1 week, then weekly for a month, and then monthly indefinitely. In the case of folate deficiency, 1 to 5 mg of oral folate per day is advised. It is important to note the potential dangers of administering folate if vitamin B_{12} deficiency has not been ruled out. The folate replacement may correct the hematologic abnormality as the folate bypasses the B_{12} deficiency within the bone marrow, but it does not correct the neurologic deficit, which typically gets worse on folate.

Autoimmune Hemolytic Anemia

In the case of AIHA, the mainstay of therapy is corticosteroids at a dose of 1 to 2 mg/kg/d of prednisone. One third of patients do not achieve a durable remission, and so the next step is splenectomy. If that fails, trials of immunosuppressive agents such as azathioprine, cyclosporine, or intravenous IgG have met with varying success. In cases of severe anemia, plasmapheresis may be tried. Generally it works poorly for an IgG-mediated AIHA as opposed to an IgM because much of the IgG antibody is in the extravascular space.

Sickle Cell Anemia

Management of patients with sickle cell anemia could warrant a whole book in itself. The mainstay of treatment for vaso-occlusive crisis has been supportive and includes a combination of hydration, oxygenation, and pain management. Partial exchange transfusion (e.g., phlebotomize 500 mL whole blood, then infuse 300 mL normal saline, then phlebotomize another 500 mL whole blood followed by two to three units packed RBC transfusion) to reduce the HbS to less than 30% is indicated in the approximately 25% of patients who develop stroke and the approximately 30% who develop vaso-occlusion in the lungs ("acute chest syndrome") and occasionally preoperatively. Unfortunately, generally there has been no benefit in exchange transfusion for the most common complication of sickle cell disease—vaso-occlusive pain crisis. Painful crisis that necessitates a hospitalization is best managed with continuous-infusion morphine with dose adjustment by the patient (patient-controlled analgesia) as opposed to the historic practice of administering either morphine or meperidine (Demerol) intramuscularly on an as-needed basis.

Recently, prospective studies have shown benefit from the use of agents to reduce the frequency of vaso-occlusion by raising the level of fetal hemoglobin. An example is hydroxyurea, which actually is a chemotherapy drug. Based on an approximately 50% reduction in vaso-occlusive episodes in a double-blind, placebo-controlled, randomized trial of hydroxyurea, hydroxyurea may have a considerable beneficial impact. However, the potential long-term toxicity is not known. Because this is a drug that inhibits enzymes in the bone marrow cells, there has been some concern, mostly theoretical, that it could lead to stem cell injury and the development of secondary leukemia. At this point, without long-term toxicity follow-up, it is difficult to advocate hydroxyurea for all patients with sickle cell anemia, but certainly it appears to be indicated for patients whose quality of life has been significantly impaired because of recurrent vaso-occlusive crises.

Theoretically, sickle cell anemia could be prevented through the use of genetic screening. In the United States, the gene frequency for sickle cell anemia among African-Americans is quite high, roughly 8%. As such, statistically there is a 1 in 12 chance that an African-American will have a single gene defect (i.e., sickle cell trait) and, in turn, there is 1 in 640 chance that two such patients who marry and have a child with sickle cell anemia. Prenatal screening can be done by chorionic villus sampling or amniocentesis.

Patients with sickle cell trait are not anemic. Furthermore, they rarely have any complication of vaso-occlusion except for three relatively unusual situations: (a) strenuous exercise at high altitudes, which has been associated with sudden death; (b) acute papillary necrosis, which can be associated with sickle cell trait because the acidic hypoxic environment of the renal collection system can favor sickling; and (c) pain from vaso-occlusion, which can develop in joints with underlying inflammation such as rheumatoid arthritis.

Toxic Hemoglobinopathy

The use of methylene blue, 1 to 2 mg/kg intravenously, is effective in reducing methemoglobin to hemoglobin.

Anemia Secondary to Valve or Microangiopathic Hemolysis

The therapy for thrombotic thrombocytopenic purpura or hemolytic uremic syndrome involves plasmapheresis. In the case of thrombotic thrombocytopenic purpura, it has reduced mortality from more than 80% to approximately 20%.

CONSIDERATIONS IN PREGNANCY

In general terms, RBC transfusions are advised if the hematocrit is less than approximately 25% in the third trimester.

Iron Deficiency Anemia

Iron deficiency is very common in pregnancy. In socioeconomically disadvantaged patients, the prevalence reaches 50%; it is up to 80% in developing countries. The standard of care has been to prescribe 30 to 60 mg of elemental iron daily.

Folate Deficiency

Folate deficiency can be an endemic cause of anemia in certain areas in the world where folate supplements are not prescribed routinely. Its presence can also obscure the diagnosis of associated iron deficiency because the combination of these two could lead to normal MCV.

Pure Red Cell Aplasia and Aplastic Anemia

There are about 30 reports of pure red cell aplasia and aplastic anemia in pregnancy. In a laboratory model, ferrets that are in estrus can develop aplastic anemia, which suggests that excess estrogen can inhibit red cell production.

Autoimmune Hemolytic Anemia

AIHA can present during pregnancy because autoimmune diseases are relatively common among young women. Management is the same as in nonpregnant patients, initially with corticosteroids.

Sickle Cell Anemia

The management of sickle cell disease in pregnancy is controversial. Specifically, it is not clear whether all patients should undergo prophylactic red cell exchange transfusion to reduce the percentage of HbS. Close supportive care is mandatory because of the increased incidence of sickling complications in pregnancy, such as acute chest syndrome and stroke, and other complications, such as preeclampsia and urinary tract infections with sepsis. Even with close management, fetal outcome is impaired with increased rates of prematurity, decreased birth weight, and 30% risk of fetal wastage. High-dose folate supplementation (5 mg/d) is indicated to prevent megaloblastic arrest of maternal red cell production, because folate requirements increase further due to the needs of the fetus.

BIBLIOGRAPHY

Atweh GF, Schechter AN. Pharmacologic induction of fetal hemoglobin: raising the therapeutic bar in sickle cell disease [Review]. *Curr Opin Hematol* 2001;8:123–130.

Barton JC, Barton EH, Bertoli LF, et al. Intravenous iron dextran therapy in patients with iron deficiency and normal renal function who failed to respond to or did not tolerate oral iron supplementation. *Am J Med* 2000;109:27–32.

Farrell RJ, LaMont JT. Rational approach to iron-deficiency anaemia in premenopausal women. *Lancet* 1998;352:1953–1954.

Fitzsimons EJ, Brock JH. The anaemia of chronic disease [Editorial]. *BMJ* 2001;322:811–812.

Macdougall IC. Optimizing erythropoietin therapy [Review]. *Curr Opin Hematol* 1999;6:121–126.

CHAPTER 90

Bleeding Disorders in Women

Ronald Lewis Sham

The diagnostic approach to women with easy bruising or a suspected bleeding disorder includes a careful history, physical examination, and laboratory investigation. The history should elucidate whether or not a bleeding disorder exists and help to determine possible causes. The physical examination should be comprehensive to identify systemic illness yet also focused to evaluate clinical evidence of bleeding. The laboratory investigation should initially include only screening blood work; more specific diagnostic tests should be considered once the screening tests, clinical findings, and family history are reviewed. This chapter provides a framework for evaluating patients with suspected bleeding disorders or bruising and is organized in two sections: (a) a general approach to bleeding disorders discussed as abnormalities of coagulation factors, platelets, and disorders related to blood vessels and supporting tissues, and (b) bleeding disorders associated with pregnancy. Because many disorders are discussed, therapies are mentioned with the description of the disorder as opposed to a separate section. Emphasis is placed on bleeding problems seen in an ambulatory setting, and the complex coagulopathies seen in hospitalized patients are mentioned only briefly.

DIFFERENTIAL DIAGNOSIS AND APPROACH TO BLEEDING DISORDERS

Women with easy bruising, menorrhagia, mild bleeding symptoms, or abnormal coagulation or platelet studies are frequently seen by their primary care physician for evaluation of a possible bleeding disorder. These patients are distinct from patients with severe hemostatic abnormalities such as advanced liver disease or severe thrombocytopenia, and they do not require aggressive treatment or hospitalization. With the exception of specific bleeding disorders seen in pregnancy, the focus here is on patients who are otherwise well clinically and are seen in an outpatient setting. Women with clinically recognized bleeding generally have either hereditary hemostatic defects, acquired abnormalities due to medications or coexisting medical problems, or bleeding related to vascular abnormalities. There is often a subgroup in whom no diagnosis can be firmly established. Occasionally this is due to limitations of the laboratory evaluation. The more common bleeding disorders are discussed in this chapter; disorders that are uncommon or rare are listed in the summary tables.

Disorders of Plasma Coagulation Factors

Disorders of blood coagulation are either hereditary or acquired and may result in clinically significant bleeding or occasionally only abnormalities in laboratory studies (Table 90.1). Hereditary deficiencies are usually caused by a deficiency of a single coagulation factor. Hemophilia A (factor VIII deficiency) and B (factor IX deficiency) are extremely rare in women, although daughters of men with hemophilia are obligate carriers and may be clinically affected. A history of bleeding in male relatives is common, and specific assays for factor VIII and IX are needed and may reveal borderline low values in carrier women and a normal activated partial thromboplastin time (aPTT). Occasionally, more sophisticated genetic testing is necessary to determine carrier status. This becomes an issue when women in families with hemophilia are contemplating childbirth, because their sons have a 50% chance of being affected. Factor XI deficiency is a less common deficiency overall than factors VIII and IX but because of its autosomal inheritance will be seen equally in women and may present with mild bleeding. Bleeding due to hereditary deficiency of other coagulation factors is extremely rare.

TABLE 90.1. Coagulation Disorders

Hereditary disorders
Mild hemophilia (factor VIII, IX, XI deficiency)
von Willebrand disease
Dysfibrinogenemia
Factor XIII deficiency
α_2-Plasmin deficiency
Plasminogen activator inhibitor-1 deficiency
Acquired disorders
Circulating anticoagulants
Vitamin K deficiency
Liver disease
Amyloid (factor X deficiency)
Dysproteinemia
Myeloproliferative disorders
Warfarin therapy
Pregnancy-associated disorders
Disseminated intravascular coagulation
Acute fatty liver

von Willebrand disease (vWD) is one of the most common hereditary bleeding disorders, estimated to be present in 1% of the population. Affected patients often have easy bruising or mucosal bleeding and commonly present with heavy menstrual bleeding at menarche. This may be an unrecognized and underdiagnosed cause of menorrhagia in women. In women with menorrhagia, vWD may be present in up to 20% of such individuals. The screening laboratory data often show a prolonged bleeding time and aPTT. The diagnosis can be confirmed with specific assays for ristocetin cofactor activity, von Willebrand antigen, and factor VIII coagulant activity. A significant day-to-day variability is well recognized in these factor levels, affecting both screening tests and specific assays; therefore, the evaluation for vWD often needs to be performed on more than one occasion if the clinical suspicion is high. There may also be variation of factor levels with the menstrual cycle, further complicating the diagnostic evaluation. Patients with vWD usually have affected family members with similar degrees of hemostatic impairment. Affected patients usually have their bleeding complications managed by a hematologist and, depending on their clinical history, receive either desmopressin (1-desamino-8-D-arginine vasopressin) (DDAVP) or, in more severe cases, clotting factor concentrates. An intranasal form of DDAVP, Stimate, is useful in menorrhagia, and oral contraceptives may improve menorrhagia due to the beneficial effects of estrogen on the von Willebrand factor levels.

The most frequent acquired disorders of blood coagulation include vitamin K deficiency, warfarin therapy, liver disease, and coagulation inhibitors. The acquired inhibitors are due to antibodies that are reactive with specific coagulation factors, most commonly factor VIII. They usually cause severe bleeding, leading the patient to seek medical care, but can cause mild symptoms if residual factor levels are greater than 5%. Many cases are idiopathic, but inhibitors are often associated with autoimmune disease, medications, the peripartum state, and malignancy. The association of acquired inhibitors with pregnancy and autoimmune diseases makes this a notable problem in women despite the relative rarity of inhibitors seen in clinical practice. These inhibitors must be distinguished clinically and in the laboratory from the "lupus anticoagulant," which does not cause bleeding. Factor inhibitors almost always cause a prolongation of the aPTT or prothrombin time (PT), may cause severe bleeding, and often require hospitalization for management.

Vitamin K is a necessary cofactor for synthesis of functional factors II, VII, IX, and X. Deficiency can be seen based on diet but is often secondary to intrinsic gastrointestinal tract disease and malabsorption or can be seen in association with the use of antibiotics, which decrease the production of vitamin K by intestinal bacteria. Vitamin K deficiency can occur within a few weeks and should be suspected in the appropriate clinical setting in the presence of a prolonged PT. Vitamin K deficiency can usually be corrected with either oral or subcutaneous vitamin K.

Liver disease is a frequent cause of an acquired bleeding disorder with a complex pathogenesis, including decreased synthesis of coagulation factors, decreased clearance of activated coagulation factors, accelerated fibrinolysis, and abnormal platelet function. Patients with coagulopathy secondary to liver disease often have clinical manifestations of portal hypertension to support the diagnosis, although this may not be the case in acute severe liver dysfunction. Both PT and aPTT may be prolonged, and there are often decreases in fibrinogen, increased fibrin(ogen) degradation products, a prolonged bleeding time, and decreased platelets, particularly in patients with splenomegaly.

The last acquired disorder of coagulation to be discussed is that associated with amyloidosis. Amyloid fibrils can cause increased vascular fragility, which results in easy bruising. In addition, the amyloid protein can absorb factor X, resulting in an acquired coagulopathy that may further contribute to the bleeding disorder seen with amyloidosis.

TABLE 90.2. Platelet Abnormalities

Qualitative hereditary abnormalities
Receptor abnormalities (various defects described)
Bernard-Soulier syndrome
Glanzmann thrombasthenia
Signal transduction abnormalities (various defects described)
Granule abnormalities (various defects described)
Storage pool disease (α and dense granules)
Hermansky-Pudlak syndrome
Chediak-Higashi syndrome
Wiskott-Aldrich syndrome
Quantitative hereditary abnormalities
May-Hegglin anomaly
Mediterranean macrothrombocytopenia
Thrombocytopenia with absent radii
Qualitative acquired abnormalities
Medications (desired effect or side effect)
Uremia
Liver disease
Myeloproliferative diseases
Dysproteinemia
Acquired storage pool disease
Food/food additives (e.g., Szechwan purpura)
Attention deficit disorder
Cardiopulmonary bypass
Quantitative acquired abnormalities
Thrombocytopenia
Immune mediated
Nonimmune (marrow infiltration, aplasia)
Nutritional (vitamin B_{12} or folate deficiency)
Thrombocytosis with myeloproliferative disease
Pregnancy-associated abnormalities
Gestational thrombocytopenia
Immune thrombocytopenia
HELLP syndrome (hemolysis, elevated liver enzymes, and low platelets)
Thrombotic thrombocytopenia purpura/hemolytic uremic syndrome
Eclampsia
Disseminated intravascular coagulation

Disorders of Platelets

Disorders of platelets may be quantitative or qualitative and hereditary or acquired (Table 90.2). Thrombocytopenia and thrombocytosis can be associated with bleeding and are diagnosed easily by obtaining a platelet count. Thrombocytopenia is much more common, but patients with thrombocytosis due to myeloproliferative diseases such as essential thrombocythemia can have bleeding in the setting of an elevated platelet count. Bleeding either may be a presenting feature or may develop during the course of the illness. A variety of abnormalities in platelet function has been identified in these patients that contribute to bleeding and, in some patients, contribute to thrombotic complications. However, some patients have a normal bleeding time and normal platelet function tests and still show evidence of a hemostatic defect. Secondary thrombocytosis, such as that seen with inflammation, malignancy, or iron deficiency, is not associated with bleeding and needs to be distinguished from essential thrombocythemia. Because iron deficiency is common in women and can result in secondary thrombocytosis, this distinction is particularly notable in them.

Thrombocytopenia is a relatively common problem in women. The severity of bleeding due to thrombocytopenia is inversely correlated with the platelet count, with severe bleeding below 20,000/mL. Mild thrombocytopenia with a platelet count over 100,000/mL is typically asymptomatic, but mild bleeding and bruising is often seen with intermediate degrees of thrombocytopenia. The differential diagnosis of thrombocytopenia includes disorders due to decreased production and increased destruction of platelets. Disorders associated with decreased platelet production include hereditary abnormalities, drug toxicity, thrombocytopenia due to infiltrative marrow replacement (malignancy or infectious processes), and aplastic anemia. The hereditary abnormalities are rare and include Wiskott-Aldrich syndrome, thrombocytopenia with absent radii, and the May-Hegglin anomaly. Drugs that are frequently associated with decreased platelet production include alcohol, thiazide diuretics, and estrogens, but a large number of drugs have been associated with thrombocytopenia occasionally. Lists of these drugs can be found in many hematology textbooks. Finally, deficiency of vitamin B_{12} or folate may also cause decreased platelet production.

Thrombocytopenia caused by accelerated platelet destruction is often immune mediated (idiopathic thrombocytopenia purpura [ITP]) and is either idiopathic or secondary to a drug or medical disorder. There are many disorders associated with immune dysregulation, and there are a number of conditions associated with pregnancy that result in thrombocytopenia, which are discussed later. The evaluation of thrombocytopenia is dictated by the severity and by the presence of other clinical findings. The history should include a thorough review of both prescription and over-the-counter medications because of their frequent association with thrombocytopenia. Quinine, which is frequently taken for leg cramps, can cause immune thrombocytopenia. The evaluation should also focus on identifying autoimmune or collagen vascular disease, lymphoma, and human immunodeficiency virus (HIV) infection, which may be associated with immune thrombocytopenia. Many collagen vascular diseases such as lupus are relatively common in women, and HIV infection is being recognized more frequently in women and therefore should be considered when evaluating women with thrombocytopenia. Thrombocytopenia may be the first clinical sign of HIV infection; early in the infection it may be immune mediated and in more advanced disease is often due to marrow suppression. Treatment with antiretroviral drugs may improve HIV-associated thrombocytopenia. In many cases of thrombocytopenia in which no etiology is identified, it is presumed to be immune mediated and deemed "idiopathic." A number of treatment options for ITP exist, including glucocorticoids, intravenous gamma globulin, Rh immune globulin, splenectomy, danazol, and cytotoxic drugs. Whenever appropriate, therapy of any associated disorder should be undertaken. These patients should be managed with the assistance of a hematologist.

Qualitative platelet disorders include both common and rare diseases. The hereditary disorders are a heterogeneous group, often detected during childhood, and generally require specialized laboratory tests and a hematologist for diagnosis. They are caused by intrinsic abnormalities in platelet biology resulting in abnormal function and present with bleeding patterns similar to that seen in patients with thrombocytopenia. These disorders are discussed only briefly. Bernard-Soulier syndrome is associated with mild thrombocytopenia, giant platelets, and a prolonged bleeding time. Platelet aggregation studies show an impaired response to ristocetin due to an abnormality in the glycoprotein Ib-IX complex. Patients with Glanzmann thrombasthenia may have mild or severe bleeding, and platelet aggregation is impaired in response to epinephrine, adenosine diphosphate (ADP), and collagen due to an abnormality in glycoprotein IIb-IIIa, the primary platelet fibrinogen receptor. Platelet storage pool disorders result in abnormal platelet function and mild-to-moderate bleeding due to abnormalities in alpha granules, dense granules, or both. Defects in platelet membrane receptors or in specific enzymes required for intracellular signal transduction constitute a heterogeneous group of hereditary disorders of platelet function in patients with bleeding disorders.

In contrast to the rare hereditary disorders, acquired disorders of platelet function are commonly seen in medical practice. Drugs are the most common cause of qualitative platelet dysfunction. Aspirin acetylates the enzyme cyclooxygenase, thereby inhibiting the platelet release reaction and resulting in a prolonged bleeding time and abnormal *in vitro* platelet aggregation. The effect is irreversible, and all circulating platelets are affected by the single administration of aspirin in low dose, resulting in abnormal platelet function and a hemostatic defect that persists until sufficient new platelets are released into the circulation, typically 4 to 7 days. The hemostatic defect is mild but may be important in the presence of an additional abnormality such as vWD. The use of aspirin in prevention of arterial thrombotic disease has increased during the last two decades, making aspirin a common cause of acquired platelet dysfunction. Thienopyridines (ticlopidine and clopidogrel) are antiplatelet agents used either alone or with aspirin for patients with cardiac and vascular disease; their effect may last 4 to 7 days. Other common medications that may result in platelet dysfunction include penicillin antibiotics and nonsteroidal anti-inflammatory drugs. These medications differ from aspirin because the effects of these drugs on platelet function are reversible, last only as long as the drug is present, and improve with discontinuation of the medication.

A variety of medical illnesses is associated with acquired platelet disorders, the most common being uremia and severe liver disease. The exact pathogenesis of the platelet dysfunction in uremia is unknown, but it is postulated that abnormal interactions of von Willebrand factor and the subendothelium play an important role. Although there is no direct correlation with blood urea nitrogen or creatinine, bleeding tends to worsen as renal failure worsens and is commonly present in patients on dialysis. Patients with liver disease may have qualitative platelet abnormalities and coexisting acquired coagulation abnormalities that complicate the hemostatic defect. Abnormal platelet function can occur in myeloproliferative disorders and acute myelogenous leukemia and is associated with multiple functional defects. Patients with dysproteinemia such as multiple myeloma may manifest mild bleeding on the basis of paraprotein interference with platelet function. The platelet dysfunction improves with treatment of the underlying disorder.

Disorders of Blood Vessels

A number of vascular and connective tissue disorders have abnormalities in platelet function, coagulation, or fibrinolysis and are associated with mild bleeding and easy bruising (Table 90.3). Bleeding may be caused by increased transmural pressure, decreased mechanical integrity, or direct damage to the vessel wall. Bleeding associated with increased transmural pressure is typically petechial and mild. It occurs acutely on the upper body with childbirth, severe coughing, or vomiting or more chronically with chronic venous stasis of the lower extremities. Decreased integrity of the supporting tissue of blood vessels is seen in a variety of disorders causing purpura. Elderly women may develop senile purpura characterized by reddish purple lesions on the extensor surface of the forearms and hands, which are due to progressive decreases in collagen, elastin, and other proteins that occur with aging. Because this minor bleeding does not elicit an inflammatory response, senile purpura can persist chronically without reabsorption-induced color change. Patients with either exogenous or endogenous corticosteroid excess develop purpura, which appear similar to senile purpura. Steroid purpura is caused by loss of connective tissue and thinning of the epidermis making cutaneous vessels more fragile.

TABLE 90.3. Disorders of Blood Vessels (Vascular Purpuras)

Palpable
Vasculitis (including allergic purpura)
Dysproteinemia (including cryoglobulinemia)
Nonpalpable
Trauma, physical abuse
Senile purpura
Steroid purpura (endogenous and exogenous)
Solar purpura
Pseudoxanthoma elasticum
Ehlers-Danlos syndrome
Marfan syndrome
Osteogenesis imperfecta
Purpura simplex
Hereditary hemorrhagic telangiectasia
Psychogenic purpura (autoerythrocyte and DNA sensitivity)
Factitious
Pigmented purpuric eruptions (Schamberg disease)
Vitamin C deficiency (scurvy)
Amyloidosis
Purpura associated with infection
Purpura associated with disorders of hemostasis/thrombosis
Purpura associated with increased transmural pressure (valsalva delivery)

Vitamin C deficiency (scurvy) causes perifollicular purpura with corkscrew hairs; although rare, more extensive bleeding with severe deficiency or with trauma can be manifest in patients. Bleeding results from weakened skin connective tissue caused by defects in collagen synthesis, which is dependent on ascorbic acid for the conversion of proline to hydroxyproline. Patients with collagen disorders such as Ehlers-Danlos syndrome may have easy bruising and are recognized by clinical manifestations such as increased elasticity of the skin, joint hyperextension, pectus excavatum, and high arched palate. Other collagen disorders such as Marfan syndrome, pseudoxanthoma elasticum, and osteogenesis imperfecta may also be associated with easy bruising and are recognized by clinical features. Hemorrhagic skin lesions, termed "pinch purpura," can occur in patients with amyloid. These lesions are caused by increased vascular fragility due to amyloid infiltration of vessel walls. Patients with amyloid may also develop petechiae due to increased transmural pressure as seen with the Valsalva maneuver or after sigmoidoscopy.

Easy bruising is reported considerably more often in women than in men. Probably the most common diagnosis in women with easy bruising is purpura simplex. Its pathophysiology is poorly understood, but a hormonal sensitivity is likely because bruising often varies with the menstrual cycle. Patients with purpura simplex develop bruises that are often primarily a cosmetic concern, and these patients are not at risk for more significant bleeding. They occasionally have an extensive workup that is unrevealing. Hemorrhagic manifestations may occur with vasculitis of diverse causes, including hypersensitivity (anaphylactoid purpura) vasculitis, cryoglobulinemia, and the vasculitis associated with immunologic diseases such as systemic lupus or rheumatoid arthritis. These disorders should be considered in the appropriate clinical setting. Hereditary hemorrhagic telangiectasia (Osler-Weber-Rendu disease) causes mucocutaneous telangiectasia and bleeding, which often worsens with age and may be associated with abnormalities in von Willebrand factor levels that may contribute to the hemorrhagic diathesis. Other causes of easy bruising include psychogenic purpura (autoerythrocyte and DNA sensitivity), factitious purpura, and purpura associated with trauma. Purpura associated with trauma may be a manifestation of physical abuse and warrant more detailed questioning. Questions regarding possible physical abuse should be asked in a supportive environment. This evaluation may require repeat visits until a level of comfort is established.

TABLE 90.4. Approach to Patients with a Suspected Bleeding Disorder

Initial evaluation
History
Is there evidence for a bleeding disorder?
Bleeding that is always abnormal—hemarthrosis, gastrointestinal, genitourinary bleeding
Abnormal bleeding in a normal patient—epistaxis, bruising, gingival bleeding
Expected bleeding—may be abnormal quantity—menses, childbirth, surgery
What are the possible causes of bleeding?
Lifelong and family history—suspect congenital, need childhood history
Recent onset-suspect acquired bleeding, review medication, systemic diseases
Physical
Comprehensive search for systemic disease
Renal, hepatic, collagen vascular disease
Focused for signs of bleeding, bruising
Petechiae, purpura, ecchymosis size, location
Laboratory tests
Complete blood count with differential—blood smear review
PT, aPTT, bleeding time
Serum chemistries—liver and kidney function, serum globulins
Further evaluation
Abnormal screening test present
Evaluate for systemic disease, platelet or coagulation disorder
Normal screening tests
Low clinical suspicion
Evaluate for von Willebrand disease
High clinical suspicion
Evaluate for von Willebrand disease and other rare disorders

PT, prothrombin time; aPTT, activated partial thromboplastin time.

DIAGNOSTIC APPROACH TO SUSPECTED BLEEDING DISORDERS

History

A careful history is the most important element in the initial evaluation of a patient with a possible bleeding disorder. It serves to both establish the degree of clinical suspicion for a bleeding disorder and to provide clues to a specific diagnosis (Table 90.4). The history should establish the duration of the suspected bleeding disorder and also identify the sites and severity of bleeding and any inciting circumstances. It is often difficult to determine if the bleeding described is beyond the normal range, particularly when evaluating easy bruising. Some types of bleeding, such as hemoptysis, hematemesis, hematuria, hematochezia, and melena, are clearly pathologic but usually have anatomic causes, and the adequacy of prior diagnostic evaluation including endoscopy and imaging studies should be evaluated. Hemarthrosis is always abnormal and indicates a severe hemorrhagic disorder in the absence of trauma. It is often difficult to determine whether or not a bleeding disorder exists when evaluating what may be normal bleeding, such as that occurring with menses or childbirth, surgical bleeding, or bleeding with trauma. Because some blood loss is normal in these circumstances and because many patients consider themselves to be easy bleeders, it is often difficult to evaluate the seriousness of this bleeding. It is important to have an appreciation of the range of normal bleeding and to recognize the considerable reporting differences between patients. Objective assessment regarding the severity of bleeding can be obtained from information regarding the need for transfusions, reoperation, and development of iron deficiency anemia. Pictorial charts developed to quantitate menstrual bleeding have been useful for reproducibly diagnosing menorrhagia. Abnormal bleeding that is frequently seen in normal individuals without a bleeding disorder includes gingival bleeding, epistaxis, and skin bruising. It is important to determine the frequency and circumstances of such bleeding and its association with local problems such as gingivitis, nasal infection, allergy, and trauma.

The history may provide clues to a specific diagnosis. A history of lifelong bleeding suggests a hereditary disorder, and if the parents are available to interview, they may be able to provide information regarding childhood bleeding with dental eruptions, falls, minor injuries, and tonsillectomy. The family history is of critical importance and should be reviewed in detail. This sometimes requires more than one visit because the patient may need to discuss the family history further with relatives. If bleeding is of recent onset, questions regarding concurrent pregnancy, medical illnesses, and medications become important. A thorough medication history should include specific questions regarding aspirin and other medications that cause qualitative platelet dysfunction as well as drugs that could result in thrombocytopenia, such as quinine and other over-the-counter medications and herbal remedies that are frequently overlooked by patients. It is useful to review prior hemostatic challenges such as childbirth, menses, dental extractions, lacerations, fractures, and minor surgery. This information may allow the physician to date the onset of an acquired bleeding disorder.

Physical

A complete physical examination should be performed when evaluating a patient for a suspected bleeding disorder. The physical examination is useful in uncovering evidence of a systemic disease. The examination should also carefully evaluate any evidence of bleeding or bruising, examining the skin for petechiae and purpura and noting the location and distribution of lesions. The pattern and physical characteristics of the bruises may also be important, particularly in cases of suspected physical abuse. The nose and mouth should be examined in patients complaining of epistaxis or gingival bleeding. More severe gastrointestinal or genitourinary bleeding requires diagnostic imaging tests in addition to the physical examination.

Laboratory Evaluation

Laboratory tests that are required in nearly all patients include a complete blood count with differential, platelet count, a review of the peripheral blood smear, PT, aPTT, and bleeding time. The role of the bleeding time remains controversial, and new techniques such as platelet function analyzers may supplant the bleeding time in the future. Serum chemistries should be checked and may provide evidence of hepatic disease, renal dysfunction, or dysproteinemia. The extent of the further evaluation depends on the results of the initial findings. If the history and physical examination suggest the presence of a specific systemic disorder, this possibility should be pursued. In pregnant patients, there is a different spectrum of potential hemostatic disorders that needs to be pursued. These disorders are discussed later. Similarly, abnormal screening laboratory tests dictate further evaluation of specific coagulation or platelet disorders or systemic illness. Patients with a significant bleeding disorder usually have abnormal findings noted on the initial evaluation, which lead to a specific diagnosis. There are, however, patients in whom no abnormalities are identified in the initial evaluation. The evaluation of these patients, with normal screening studies, poses a diagnostic challenge and raises the question, How far should I go? This is difficult to answer; clinical guidelines follow.

Patients who are not on medication and who have no coexisting medical conditions may have a primary bleeding disorder. vWD has a relatively high frequency in the population and shows temporal variability in clinical severity and laboratory findings. Consequently, a normal aPTT and bleeding time may be found in mildly affected individuals. In many cases, it is necessary to repeat these tests and to obtain specialized tests such as assays for ristocetin cofactor activity, factor VIII coagulant activity, and von Willebrand antigen. These assays may need to be checked on more than one occasion if the clinical suspicion is high. The other causes of mild bleeding disorders are rare in the absence of clear abnormalities on the initial history, physical examination, and screening laboratory tests. It is inappropriate to pursue extensive laboratory evaluations in all patients who complain of easy bruising or have an equivocal history of mild bleeding. It is at this juncture that clinical judgment governs the decision regarding more extensive evaluation. If the clinical suspicion of a bleeding disorder is low initially and the screening studies are unremarkable, the patient should be reassured that it is very unlikely there is a significant bleeding disorder and advised that further evaluation would be required only in the presence of significant symptoms in the future. Women with a negative laboratory evaluation who have bruises in areas suggestive of physical abuse should be questioned further about this possibility.

If the initial clinical suspicion of a bleeding disorder is high, based on the history and physical examination, a more extensive laboratory evaluation is indicated. Rare disorders do occur, and in these individuals where a high clinical suspicion exists, the full range of possibilities should be systematically pursued. Many of these rare disorders are listed in Tables 90.1 through 90.3, and if such a disorder is suspected, hematology consultation would be appropriate. Mild coagulation factor deficiencies can occur with a normal aPTT or PT, and specific factor assays may be required. This is particularly notable in vWD where mildly affected patients may have a normal aPTT and bleeding time. Deficiencies of the fibrinolytic inhibitors, α_2-plasmin inhibitor, and plasminogen activator inhibitor type 1 do not affect screening coagulation tests, and specific assays are needed to detect these deficiencies. Severe factor XIII deficiency can be identified using a qualitative screening test. Most cases of dysfibrinogenemia result in a prolongation of the thrombin time. Specialized assays used to determine the presence of platelet functional abnormalities are also available. Finally, laboratory evaluation of family members is often useful, particularly if there is a suggestive family history.

BLEEDING DISORDERS ASSOCIATED WITH PREGNANCY

Many of the bleeding disorders already discussed may occur in pregnant women, may require treatment during pregnancy, or may be altered by pregnancy. In addition, a number of bleeding disorders develop in women only during pregnancy. Some of these disorders are clinically mild and diagnosed in the outpatient setting, whereas others have a more abrupt clinical presentation and often require hospitalization for management. Bleeding disorders that arise during pregnancy are, by definition, acquired processes and can be categorized as platelet abnormalities, coagulation abnormalities, or disorders in which both are present.

Platelet abnormalities that arise during pregnancy often require the same initial diagnostic approach as those in the nonpregnant patient. Management, however, has the additional concerns about the successful completion of the pregnancy and the health of the fetus. Pregnancy is not associated with acquired qualitative platelet disorders; however, preexisting disorders may pose management problems, but in general they are approached as discussed previously. An acquired quantitative platelet abnormality (i.e., thrombocytopenia) is a more common problem during pregnancy. The platelet count should not be altered by pregnancy *per se*; therefore, low values warrant further evaluation. Thrombocytopenia in the range of 100,000 to 150,000 that is new during the course of the pregnancy is most likely due to gestational thrombocytopenia. This is often a diagnosis of exclusion because platelet counts before the pregnancy may not be available. This is believed to occur in approximately 5% of pregnancies. Distinguishing gestational thrombocytopenia from chronic ITP may be difficult due to the frequent occurrence of ITP in women of childbearing age. Hematology consultation may be advisable. Gestational thrombocytopenia is usually self-limiting and not harmful to the mother or fetus, does not require treatment or alter the course of the pregnancy, and usually resolves postpartum.

ITP differs from gestational thrombocytopenia because it may require therapy during pregnancy and occasionally results in maternal or fetal complications. If the thrombocytopenia is severe, ITP is a more likely diagnosis and can be treated with steroids or intravenous immunoglobulin; splenectomy can be performed during pregnancy if necessary. The fetus may be at risk for thrombocytopenia due to transplacental passage of maternal antibody, and in certain cases, fetal scalp vein sampling or percutaneous umbilical blood sampling can be performed to determine fetal platelet counts. This is rarely required. Mothers with severe thrombocytopenia are more likely to have an affected child. Controversy regarding which pregnant patients with ITP require cesarean section persists, and therefore decisions about vaginal delivery must be individualized.

A number of acute disorders result in thrombocytopenia in pregnant women, usually in the setting of other clinical and laboratory evidence of a systemic illness. These include disseminated intravascular coagulation (DIC), thrombotic thrombocytopenic purpura and hemolytic uremic syndrome, coagulopathy associated with preeclampsia and eclampsia, acute fatty liver of pregnancy, and the HELLP syndrome (hemolysis, elevated liver enzymes, and low platelets). Women with these problems cannot be managed in an outpatient setting and should be hospitalized by their obstetricians and managed with the assistance of a hematologist. These disorders are discussed briefly.

Pregnancy results in a multitude of hemostatic changes, including hypercoagulability and decreased fibrinolysis. DIC that occurs during pregnancy is usually secondary to intrauterine fetal death or associated with another complication of delivery or abortion. Tissue factor derived from the deceased fetus may result in DIC, which usually resolves with delivery of the fetus and placenta. Placental abruption and amniotic fluid embolism may result in DIC in the peripartum period and are managed with delivery of the fetus and placenta and other supportive measures used for managing DIC in nonpregnant patients. Finally, DIC may be a factor in the coagulopathy associated with eclampsia and may be involved in the pathogenesis of eclampsia.

The pathogenesis of eclampsia is unknown but is believed to involve aberrant interactions between platelets and endothelial cells. Patients may develop a consumptive coagulopathy with greater effects on platelets than on coagulation factors. Three additional syndromes share some clinical features with the hemostatic defects associated with eclampsia: acute fatty liver of pregnancy, the HELLP syndrome, and thrombotic thrombocytopenic purpura/hemolytic uremic syndrome. These disorders can result in potentially devastating complications for the mother and fetus, including death, but usually improve with the delivery of the fetus. In summary, a number of hemostatic disorders may affect women during pregnancy. Mild disorders such as gestational thrombocytopenia and ITP require careful observation and occasional intervention. Severe hemostatic defects may be life threatening and require hospitalization and hematology consultation.

BIBLIOGRAPHY

Bick RL. Platelet function defects: a clinical review. *Semin Thromb Hemost* 1992; 18:167.

Burrows RF, Kelton JG. Fetal thrombocytopenia and its relation to maternal thrombocytopenia. *N Engl J Med* 1993;329:1463.

Burrows RF, Kelton JG. Thrombocytopenia at delivery: a prospective survey of 6,715 deliveries. *Am J Obst Gynecol* 1990;162:731.

Crowther MA, Burrows RF, Ginsberg J, et al. Thrombocytopenia in pregnancy: diagnosis, pathogenesis and management. *Blood Rev* 1996;10:8.

Kouides PA. Evaluation of abnormal bleeding in women. *Curr Hematol Rep* 2002;1:11.

Kouides PA, Phatak PD, Burkart P, et al. Gynecological and obstetrical morbidity in women with type I von Willebrand disease: results of a patient survey. *Hemophilia* 2000;6:643.

Lackner H, Karpatkin S. On the "easy bruising" syndrome with normal platelet count: a study of 75 patients. *Ann Intern Med* 1975;83:190.

Mammen EF. Coagulation defects in liver disease. *Med Clin North Am* 1994;78:545.

Mannucci PM. Desmopressin (DDAVP) in the treatment of bleeding disorders: the first 20 years. *Blood* 1997;90:2515.

Mannucci PM. How I treat von Willebrand disease. *Blood* 2001;97:1915.

Mannucci PM, Tuddenham EDG. The hemophilias-from royal genes to gene therapy. *N Engl J Med* 2001;344:1773.

McCrae KR, Cines DB. Thrombotic microangiopathy during pregnancy. *Semin Hematol* 1997;34:148.

McCrae KR, Samuels P, Schreiber AD. Pregnancy-associated thrombocytopenia: pathogenesis and management. *Blood* 1992;80:2697.

Rao AK. Congenital disorders of platelet function. *Hematol Oncol Clin North Am* 1990;4:65.

Sadler JE, Mannucci PM, Berntorp E, et al. Impact, diagnosis and treatment of von Willebrand disease. *Thromb Haemost* 2000;84:160.

Sham RL, Francis CW. Evaluation of mild bleeding disorders and easy bruising. *Blood Rev* 1994;8:98.

Weigert AL, Schafer AI. Uremic bleeding: pathogenesis and therapy. *Am J Med Sci* 1998;316:94.

CHAPTER 91
Venous Thromboembolic Disease in Women

Catherine Blackburn and Lucia Larson

Venous thromboembolic disease (VTE) is a major problem in the United States because of its high incidence and serious health consequences. Symptomatic deep vein thrombosis (DVT) and pulmonary embolism (PE) result in over 250,000 acute hospital admissions per year, and the total incidence is much higher if asymptomatic or undiagnosed cases are included. PE is the principal or a major contributing cause of mortality in 15% to 30% of all hospital deaths. It contributes significantly to the mortality and morbidity of chronically ill or bedridden patients and also affects otherwise healthy individuals, especially at times of increased risk, such as after surgery or trauma. PE also occurs more frequently during pregnancy and at parturition and is the most common cause of nonobstetric maternal mortality associated with live births. Anticoagulant treatment of venous thrombosis requires frequent laboratory monitoring and results in bleeding complications in 5% to 10% of patients, contributing to the high cost of care. Acute venous thrombosis can also lead to permanent vein damage and the postphlebitic syndrome, resulting in the chronic pain, swelling, and leg ulceration that affect approximately 500,000 individuals nationally. The annual cost of treating DVT in the United States has recently been estimated at $6 billion.

The clinical approach to VTE has undergone rapid evolution as a result of major advances in understanding its pathophysiologic mechanisms and improved clinical management. Increased understanding of hemostatic control mechanisms has led to definition of inherited abnormalities that contribute to a large proportion of cases of idiopathic venous thrombosis. The importance of an accurate objective diagnosis has been documented and new noninvasive diagnostic approaches introduced. Clinical studies have refined the therapeutic approach, improved anticoagulant therapy, and further defined the roles for thrombolytic and surgical management.

ETIOLOGY

In nearly all patients, venous thromboembolism begins in the deep veins of the calf as small thrombi. These thrombi may extend into larger and more proximal veins, causing leg symptoms, and they may also break free and embolize to the pulmonary arteries. Although most pulmonary emboli originate from thrombi in the leg veins, other sources include pelvic, renal, and upper extremity veins as well as the right heart. Abnormalities in any of the components in Virchow's triad (blood hypercoagulability, vessel wall damage, stasis of blood flow) contribute to the development of venous thromboembolism.

In the normal individual there is a fine balance between clot development for hemostasis and the limitation of excessive clot formation through the antithrombin III–heparin and protein C systems. Both inherited and acquired abnormalities within these pathways are described that cause a predisposition to coagulation. The inherited abnormalities, factor V Leiden mutation (which causes a resistance to activated protein C) and the prothrombin gene mutation (which increases the prothrombin antigen and activity), are the most common causes of the inherited thrombophilias and account for 18.8% and 7.1% of thrombophilias found in unselected patients with DVT. Deficiencies in protein S, protein C, and antithrombin (formally known as antithrombin III) and some cases of hyperhomocystinemia account for most of the other cases. Rarer thrombophilias are also described, as well as conditions that may be inherited (Table 91.1). Of these, elevated factor VIII levels in particular are associated with an increased rate of thrombosis. Persons with factor VIII coagulant activity levels greater than 150% of normal have been shown to have a 4.8-fold increased risk for venous thrombosis compared with persons whose levels of factor VIII coagulant activity were under 100% of normal.

Among the acquired abnormalities is the lupus anticoagulant-antiphospholipid antibody syndrome. This acquired hypercoagulable condition is caused by the presence of an autoantibody with phospholipid specificity, which often prolongs *in vitro* coagulation tests but results in an increased risk of both arterial and venous thrombosis and recurrent abortion. Such antibodies may occur in otherwise healthy individuals but are increased in frequency in patients with systemic lupus erythematosus and in the elderly. Other acquired causes of hypercoagulability are shown in Table 91.1.

TABLE 91.1. Risk Factors for Venous Thromboembolic Disease

Inherited hypercoagulable states
Common
Functional resistance to activated protein C, including factor V Leiden mutation
Prothrombin G20210A gene mutation
Homozygous mutation in methylenetetrahydrofolate reductase gene causing hyperhomocysteinemia
Less common
Antithrombin deficiency
Protein C deficiency
Protein S deficiency
Dysfibrinogenemia
Heparin cofactor II deficiency
Factor XII deficiency
Increased factor VIII
Congential venous abnormalities
Acquired hypercoagulable states
Antiphospholipid syndromes, including lupus anticoagulant and lupus-like inhibitor
Hyperhomocysteinemia
Functional resistance to activated protein C
Acquired conditions
Surgery, especially orthopedic, including presence of casts, splints
Trauma
Malignancy
Immobility
Obesity
Advanced age
Neurologic: stroke, paralysis
Prior deep vein thrombosis or pulmonary embolism
Myocardial infarction
Congestive heart failure
Myeloproliferative disorders—polycythemia vera, essential thrombocytopenia
Hyperviscosity: Waldenström macroglobulinemia, multiple myeloma, polycythemia vera, marked leukocytosis in acute leukemia, sickle cell anemia, paroxysmal nocturnal hemoglobinuria
Inflammatory bowel disease
Nephrotic syndrome
Pregnancy and puerperium
Medications: combined oral contraceptive and hormone replacement therapy, tamoxifen

Vessel wall injury is another contributor to thrombosis, and trauma or surgery that damages the vascular lining can initiate DVT. Whereas the normal venous endothelial lining is thromboresistant, deeper components are prothrombotic. After endothelial cell removal, platelets adhere rapidly to exposed subendothelial proteins, become activated, and promote thrombus formation. Fibroblasts and smooth muscle cells in the vessel wall also express tissue factor, a potent activator of the coagulation system. Endothelial thromboresistance also can be reduced by inflammatory cytokines, hypoxia, or exposure to endotoxin during sepsis.

Stasis plays yet another important role in thrombosis. It allows local accumulation of procoagulants that may become sufficient to generate fibrin and activate platelets, and it also contributes to endothelial cell hypoxia, which can stimulate secretion of activators of coagulation. Venous stasis is frequent in hospitalized or injured patients who are often immobilized with little effective calf muscle contraction, resulting in vasodilatation and blood pooling. Factors contributing to venous stasis include neurologic disease with paralysis, anesthesia, leg injuries, orthopedic procedures on the legs, casting, and splints. Slow venous flow also results from proximal obstruction occurring with tumors, pregnancy, congestive heart failure, and venous scarring from prior episodes of leg vein thrombosis. The risk for thrombosis is increased in these patient populations.

Other clinical conditions that may alter one or more of the components of Virchow's triad are associated with increased thrombotic risk (Table 91.1). These include surgery, trauma, malignancy, immobility, some medical conditions, and pregnancy and the postpartum state. These risk factors seem to act in an additive way, and multiple factors are often present in patients with VTE.

NATURAL HISTORY OF DEEP VEIN THROMBOSIS AND PULMONARY EMBOLISM

DVT usually occurs in the veins of the lower extremities. Distal calf DVT may resolve spontaneously or develop complications such as proximal extension and PE. Calf vein DVT are often asymptomatic, but symptoms occur with extensive thrombosis limited to calf veins or with proximal extension of thrombus into the popliteal or superficial femoral veins. Anticoagulant therapy modifies this natural history by preventing extension of calf vein thrombi, thereby permitting natural resolution through the processes of fibrinolysis and cellular organization. Untreated calf DVT has a low frequency of recurrence if proximal extension does not occur. This is unlike proximal DVT, which has a significant risk of recurrence. A frequent complication of DVT is chronic venous insufficiency, which results from vein scarring, chronic obstruction, and venous valve damage. With valve damage, the venous system is exposed to higher hydrostatic pressures and muscle contraction forces flow into superficial veins, resulting in dilatation, edema, collateral flow, and ultimately skin ulceration.

PE can occur as a single event or as successive emboli and is usually a complication of lower extremity deep venous thrombosis. Though a first event may be asymptomatic or may cause only minor symptoms, pulmonary emboli may have major clinical consequences, including death. The mortality of untreated PE is 25% to 30%, but with adequate anticoagulation the incidence of fatal and nonfatal recurrent PE is reduced to less that 8%. Factors associated with higher mortality are increased right ventricular afterload stress as detected by echocardiography, inadequate clot resolution, and revascularization of the pulmonary arterial and deep venous systems, advanced age, cancer, stroke, and cardiopulmonary disease. In a small number of patients, emboli do not resolve normally, and repeated embolization leads to chronic changes in the vasculature and pulmonary hypertension.

CLINICAL SYMPTOMS, SIGNS, AND DIFFERENTIAL DIAGNOSIS

Deep Vein Thrombosis

The clinical hallmarks of DVT are leg pain and swelling that usually have an acute onset but can be progressive over several days. Patients often complain of tightness or aching in calf muscles and the development of distal edema. Extensive proximal thrombosis can cause symptoms in the thigh, and dramatic swelling may result in bluish discoloration with compromise of arterial flow due to tense edema. Thrombosis confined only to a superficial vein usually presents with localized pain and redness, and a thrombosed vein can often be palpated as a superficial cord. These signs and symptoms should heighten clinical suspicion and lead to further investigation, but they are not sensitive or specific. The differential diagnosis is broad and includes cellulitis, muscle strain, arthritis, ligamentous injury to the ankle or knee, ruptured Baker cyst, muscle hematoma, and congestive heart failure.

Pulmonary Embolism

Symptoms of PE result from the respiratory and hemodynamic effects of pulmonary artery obstruction, and the severity is proportional to the degree of vascular obstruction. Large emboli cause acute pulmonary hypertension with right heart strain and decreased cardiac output, resulting in chest discomfort, weakness, collapse, or sudden death. Respiratory symptoms often include shortness of breath, wheezing, and cough. Pleuritic chest pain and hemoptysis result from pulmonary infarction and are less common. The most frequent physical findings are tachypnea and tachycardia. Major PE may present with hypotension, shock, and cyanosis. There may be evidence of right heart strain, including a right ventricular lift, gallop, and increased intensity of the pulmonary component of the second heart sound. Pulmonary findings include evidence of atelectasis, and infarction may result in findings of consolidation and a pleural friction rub. As is the case for DVT, the clinical findings of PE are neither sensitive nor specific, because small emboli may be asymptomatic. At least half of patients in whom embolus is suspected on the basis of clinical findings do not have the diagnosis confirmed with objective tests.

The differential diagnosis for PE is broad and includes lung disease, such as pneumonia, pleurisy, bronchitis, asthma, exacerbation of chronic obstructive pulmonary disease, lung cancer, pneumothorax, and atelectasis; cardiovascular disease, such as acute myocardial infarction, congestive heart failure, pulmonary edema, pericarditis, dissection of the aorta, pericardial tamponade, and primary pulmonary hypertension; and musculoskeletal pain; rib fracture; costochondritis; and anxiety.

LABORATORY TESTS AND IMAGING

Deep Vein Thrombosis

Because of the lack of specificity and sensitivity of clinical findings, objective tests are required to definitively diagnose DVT. Contrast venography remains the gold standard technique for the diagnosis of symptomatic DVT, but it is rarely performed now, because accurate noninvasive tests are available. It may be considered when other noninvasive tests are not diagnostic. The most commonly used noninvasive test for confirmation of diagnosis in symptomatic patients is compression ultrasound, which can both assess flow and image leg veins. Duplex ultrasound refers to a combination of compression ultrasound with venous imaging (real-time B-mode imaging) and Doppler venous flow detection in gray scale of color. Deep veins should be imaged from the common femoral vein to at least the level of the trifurcation of the popliteal vein. Inability to collapse the vein is a sensitive and specific indication of the presence of thrombus. The presence of intraluminal echoes from thrombus and abnormalities in venous flow patterns also provides confirmatory information. False-positive results can occur if venous compressibility is limited by leg obesity, edema, and tenderness or if there is extrinsic compression of a vein (e.g., by a pelvic mass). False-negative studies occur with calf DVT and with proximal DVT in asymptomatic patients. It is also unreliable in detecting iliac vein thrombosis. When compression ultrasound is negative in patients with suspected DVT, serial studies have proved to be a sensitive means by which to detect proximal extension of calf DVT in symptomatic outpatients. An advantage of compression ultrasound is that it can often provide an alternative diagnosis such as Baker's cysts, hematomas, lymphadenopathy, femoral artery aneurysm, superficial thrombophlebitis, and abscesses.

Impedance plethysmography is another noninvasive approach to DVT diagnosis based on changes in electrical resistance across the leg in response to compression with a venous tourniquet. The test has reasonable diagnostic accuracy in acute symptomatic proximal leg vein obstruction, but it is insensitive to calf DVT, often fails to detect partially obstructed clots, and can be difficult to interpret. Magnetic resonance imaging (MRI) is now emerging for the diagnosis of acute symptomatic DVT and may become more useful than other techniques for asymptomatic DVT because it directly images thrombi and can image nonocclusive clots. It appears useful for pelvic vein and thigh DVT but may be less sensitive than contrast venography for calf DVT. It is an expensive test, and accurate interpretation requires an experienced radiologist.

Pulmonary Embolism

Objective testing is required for diagnosis of PE. Initially, a chest x-ray is indicated to identify possible alternative diagnoses and to serve as a basis for interpreting lung scan findings. The findings of PE are highly variable on chest x-ray but may include atelectasis, infarction, or effusion if any abnormality is present at all. Vascular abnormalities are seen occasionally, including an abrupt cutoff of large vessels and areas of increased lucency due to hypoperfusion. Arterial blood gases may have clinical importance but are of limited diagnostic value. Patients frequently are hypoxic, but normal blood gas values do not rule out the diagnosis of PE. The electrocardiographic findings also are nonspecific, but evidence of right heart strain may be seen with large emboli. Echocardiography can be useful if thrombi are identified in right-sided chambers or in the pulmonary artery, and evidence of right ventricular overload also may be present.

If chest x-ray and electrocardiogram do not reveal an alternative diagnosis, a ventilation-perfusion scan is a useful initial screening test. The results are reported as normal, low probability, intermediate probability, and high probability for PE, but the most useful results are normal, which essentially excludes the diagnosis of PE, and high probability, which is considered diagnostic. A high probability scan result has a positive predictive value of 88% to 92% for the presence of PE and is considered sufficient evidence for the institution of treatment. Low and intermediate probability scan results are considered nondiagnostic and generally require further diagnostic evaluation, particularly if the clinical suspicion for PE is high.

Pulmonary angiography is regarded as the gold standard for the diagnosis of PE and is frequently used if the ventilation-perfusion scan is nondiagnostic. The sensitivity is in the region of 98% and specificity between 95% and 98%. Prospective studies have confirmed that it is safe to withhold anticoagulation in patients with a normal pulmonary angiogram. An invasive technique, it requires a properly equipped and experienced laboratory and is associated with a small risk of allergic reaction and induction of cardiac arrhythmias. With improved techniques, however, morbidity is now estimated at 1.5% to 2% and mortality at 0.1% to 0.5%. Relative contraindications are allergy to iodine containing contrast agents, impaired renal function, left bundle branch block, severe congestive heart failure, and severe thrombocytopenia. Severe pulmonary hypertension further increases the risk of complications.

Two other modalities are under active investigation and may soon be found to have a more clear role in the diagnosis of PE. These include computed tomography (CT) pulmonary angiography and MRI. CT pulmonary angiography refers to either contrast-enhanced electron-beam tomography or spiral (also known as helical) CT. Both techniques allow the direct visualization of pulmonary emboli within the pulmonary arteries. An advantage to CT is its ability to identify other pathology, such as lymphadenopathy, lung tumors, emphysemas, and other parenchymal abnormalities as well as pleural and pericardial disease. However, the diagnostic accuracy of spiral CT for PE is still under debate because its reported overall sensitivity is 53% to 89% and specificity is 78% to 100%. Investigators agree that spiral CT provides excellent results for the detection of emboli in the main, lobar, and segmental arteries with sensitivity and specificity estimated at 95%. However, sensitivities are less for isolated subsegmental emboli, which may be missed by this technique. Spiral CT still requires prospective management studies evaluating the safety of withholding anticoagulant therapy in patients with normal scan findings. A large prospective multicenter trial is currently underway that is designed to evaluate the role of spiral CT further and will evaluate whether spiral CT can be used as a definitive test in conjunction with or in place of other techniques. MRI is also now beginning to be used to evaluate for clinically suspected PE, but more studies are needed to determine how it will be best used. Interpretation is dependent on reader expertise, and larger studies are currently required to assess its accuracy.

Plasma D-dimers may be used as adjunct with other diagnostic tests for the diagnosis of VTE. D-dimers are produced by plasmin during fibrinolysis and are released into the circulation within 1 hour of thrombus formation. Levels can stay elevated for at least 7 days after thrombus formation. A positive D-dimer test supports the diagnosis of VTE, but a negative test does not exclude it, especially if the pretest probability is high. If used with other noninvasive diagnostic tests, such as leg ultrasound, a negative D-dimer may obviate the need for repeated investigations. For D-dimer results to be accurate, a validated assay must be used that includes the classic microplate enzyme-linked immunosorbent assay technique; a newer enzyme-linked immunosorbent assay test, the VIDAS (bioMerieux SA, Marcy-Etoile, France); and a second-generation latex agglutination test, the SimpliRED test (AGEN Biomedical Ltd, Brisbane, Australia). Certain other clinical conditions may also raise D-dimer levels, and the test cannot be reliably used in these circumstances. These include infection, cancer, surgery, cardiac or renal failure, acute coronary syndromes, acute nonlacunar stroke, pregnancy, and sickle cell crisis.

PREVENTION

Hospitalized patients are at increased risk for venous thromboembolic events. In one study, the incidence of VTE was over 130 times greater in hospitalized patients than among residents in the community. Further, PE is a leading preventable cause of hospital death in the United States. Fortunately, data establish that prophylactic measures cannot only decrease mortality and morbidity related to thrombosis but are also cost effective. Risk factors for thrombosis include increased age, immobility, stroke, paralysis, malignancy, previous thrombosis, surgery, trauma, obesity, congestive heart failure, indwelling central venous catheters, nephrotic syndrome, inflammatory bowel disease, pregnancy, and estrogen use. The exact risk associated with the thrombophilias is as yet unclear, but some are likely to have stronger associations than others. The presence of more than one risk factor increases the likelihood of a thrombotic event even further.

Determining the patient's risk for thrombosis based on these risk factors and the nature of the procedure to be performed is useful so that the risks of prophylactic measures can be balanced against the risk of not instituting such measures. The Sixth American College of Chest Physician Guidelines for Antithrombotic Therapy for Prevention and Treatment of Thrombosis stratify patients into low, moderate, high, and highest risk groups, which are summarized in Table 91.2. Patients who are at low risk (i.e., who are younger than 40 years of age, undergo a surgery lasting less than 30 minutes, and have no additional risk factors) have a less than 1% risk of developing proximal DVT or clinical PE without prophylactic measures. Patients at moderate risk have an overall incidence rate of calf DVT of 10% to 20%, proximal DVT of 2% to 4%, and PE of 1% to 4% if prophylactic measures are not administered. High-risk patients have a risk of calf DVT of 20% to 40%, proximal DVT of 4% to 8%, and PE of 2% to 4% without preventative measures. The highest risk patients include those over age 40 undergoing major surgery who have a history of previous VTE, cancer, or known thrombophilia, as well as orthopedic patients undergoing hip or knee arthroplasty, hip fracture surgery, or patients with major trauma or spinal cord injury. These patients have a risk of calf DVT of 40% to 80%, proximal DVT of 10% to 20%, and clinical PE of 4% to 10%. Surgery for gynecologic

TABLE 91.2. Recommended Preventative Strategies for Thromboembolism

Level of risk	Preventative strategy
Low risk Patients less than 40 years old without additional risk factors undergoing minor surgery	No specific measures Early ambulation
Moderate risk Nonmajor surgery in patients aged 40–60 years who have no additional risk factors Minor surgery in patients with additional risk factors Major surgery in patients less than 40 years old with no additional risk factors	Low dose unfractionated heparin q 12 h or low-molecular-weight heparin or elastic stockings or intermittent pneumatic compression stockings
High risk Nonmajor surgery in patients over age 60 Nonmajor surgery in patients with additional risk factors Major surgery in patients over age 40 Major surgery in patients with additional risk factors	Low dose unfractionated heparin q 8 h or low-molecular-weight heparin or intermittent pneumatic compression stockings
Highest risk Patients over age 40 undergoing major surgery who have a history of previous VTE, cancer, or a thrombophilia Hip or knee arthroplasty or hip fracture surgery Major trauma Spinal cord injury	Low-molecular-weight heparin or oral anticoagulants or intermittent pneumatic compression stockings/ elastic stocking plus low dose unfractionated heparin/low-molecular-weight heparin or Adjusted dose heparin

VTE, venous thromboembolic disease.

malignancies also represents a high-risk procedure. For nearly all moderate- and higher risk patients, safe and effective prophylaxis is available, including both pharmacologic and nonpharmacologic approaches.

Venous stasis is common in hospitalized patients, particularly after surgery when the effects of anesthesia, operative pain, and bed rest combine to decrease calf muscle activity. Simple measures to counteract venous stasis can be used in nearly all patients and include leg exercises for bed-bound patients and early ambulation for surgical and postpartum patients. Graded compression stockings exert maximal pressure at the ankle and gradually less pressure toward the thigh, decreasing venous capacitance and preventing blood pooling in leg veins. They are of value in low- to moderate-risk patients. External pneumatic compression uses boots or cuffs that rhythmically inflate to compress the leg; this action results in increased venous blood flow and also activates blood fibrinolytic activity. The absence of side effects makes this approach an attractive prophylactic modality, particularly in patients at high risk of bleeding in whom anticoagulant use is unacceptable. Used in combination with an anticoagulant, the prophylactic effect may be increased without additional risk.

The greatest experience with prophylaxis has been with low doses of heparin, and this is based on the rationale that lower concentrations of anticoagulant are needed to prevent than to treat venous thrombosis. Heparin is administered subcutaneously in a fixed dose of 5,000 units every 8 or 12 hours, beginning 2 hours before surgery and continuing until the patient is fully ambulatory. This regimen results in only slight prolongation of the partial thromboplastin time (PTT), and routine monitoring is not required. Its effectiveness in general surgery patients has been documented in many studies, and it results in an overall risk reduction of 67% for DVT and 47% for PE. The main side effect of heparin use is occasional bruising at the injection site and a 2% increase in wound hematomas, most of which are minor. Heparin-induced thrombocytopenia is rare but is life threatening if it occurs.

Low-molecular-weight heparin recently has been introduced and approved for use in prevention of DVT after orthopedic and high-risk surgery. It has a lower mean molecular weight than unfractionated heparin and improved pharmacologic properties. Data are conflicting regarding the relative effectiveness of low-molecular-weight heparin in comparison with unfractionated heparin in preventing venous thrombosis in general surgical patients, but both agents are considered acceptable. Warfarin is highly effective in preventing venous thrombosis, but its use is restricted primarily to high-risk patients, because low-dose subcutaneous heparin is effective and simpler to use in patients at moderate risk. Other pharmacologic agents include the heparin pentasaccharide, fondaparinux, which was approved by the U.S. Food and Drug Administration for prophylaxis in patients undergoing surgery for hip fracture and hip or knee replacement, but it is more expensive than low-molecular-weight heparin. Dextran is effective but has a limited use. Aspirin has a lower efficacy and appears to be associated with more bleeding than other agents, so that it is not generally recommended for prophylaxis for venous thromboembolism.

Recommendations for VTE prophylaxis are summarized in Table 91.3. Most hospitalized medical and surgical patients are in the moderate-risk category and require serious consideration for prophylaxis. Low-dose subcutaneous heparin is appropriate for most patients, whereas external pneumatic compression is an alternative for those with increased bleeding risk. The higher risk categories include those in whom frequent and serious venous thromboembolic complications occur in the absence of effective prophylaxis. Low-dose subcutaneous heparin is generally insufficient in these patient groups, and either warfarin,

TABLE 91.3. Sample Regimens to Prevent Venous Thromboembolic Disease

Low dose unfractionated heparin—heparin 5,000 units SC q 8–12 starting 1–2 h before surgery
Adjusted dose heparin—heparin SC adjusted to maintain a midinterval aPTT at high normal values
Low-molecular-weight heparin
Moderate risk, general surgery—dalteparin, 2,500 U SC 1–2 h before surgery and once daily postop, enoxaparin 20 mg SC 1–2 h before surgery and once daily postop
High risk, general surgery—daltparin 5,000, U SC 8–12 h before surgery and once daily postop, enoxaparin 40 mg SC 1–2 h before surgery and once daily postop
Orthopedic surgery—dalteparin 5,000 U SC 8–12 h before surgery and once daily starting 12–24 h postop

aPTT (activated partial thromboplastin time)

adjusted-dose heparin, external pneumatic compression, or low-molecular-weight heparin are appropriate choices.

TREATMENT

The goals of treatment of VTE are to provide symptomatic relief, to prevent disease extension or recurrence, and to minimize structural damage to deep leg veins and thereby prevent the long-term development of chronic venous insufficiency. Management requires a choice between several effective forms of anticoagulant, fibrinolytic, and surgical therapy to maximize patient benefit. The benefit-to-risk ratio is of central importance in making therapeutic choices, and this always involves difficult issues of clinical judgment focused on individual considerations of disease extent, risk of bleeding, patient ability to comply with long-term therapy, and coexisting medical illnesses that contribute to thrombotic risks or influence drug response. Careful assessment of bleeding risk is particularly important, because both anticoagulant and fibrinolytic therapies are associated with bleeding complications that compromise therapy and result in significant morbidity and occasional mortality.

Anticoagulation

PE and DVT most often are treated with heparin followed by a period of outpatient oral anticoagulation, usually with warfarin. For initial therapy, intravenous unfractionated heparin should be administered by a bolus followed immediately by a constant infusion in a dose adapted to body weight according to existing nomograms. Substantial evidence indicates that an important determinant of the efficacy of initial anticoagulation is the administration of sufficient heparin to prolong the activated PTT to within the therapeutic range of 1.5 to 2.5 times control.

Low-molecular-weight heparin can also be used for initial treatment. Its safety and efficacy has been established in trials for the treatment of DVT and nonmassive PE. Several forms are available, and the dose used is specific for each type but is usually as a subcutaneous injection once or twice daily. Laboratory monitoring is not required, except for platelet counts, unless prolonged treatment is planned. In this situation anti-Xa levels (heparin levels) are measured. Low-molecular-weight heparin may shorten hospital stay and improve quality of life for patients by allowing more outpatient treatment, at least of DVT, but outpatient treatment of PE cannot be recommended currently. Renal clearance of low-molecular-weight heparin is important, so some authors advocate the use of anti-Xa levels in the elderly and those with chronic renal failure. In addition, the proper dose of low-molecular-weight heparin in obese patients is unclear, so use in this patient population should be carefully considered.

The platelet count should be monitored frequently when heparin is begun because of the risk of heparin-induced thrombocytopenia, a rare but life-threatening side effect. Two forms exist: an early benign form reversible during treatment, due to a nonimmune mechanism, and a more serious form paradoxically associated with venous and arterial thrombosis. This form is immune mediated and usually occurs between 5 and 15 days of treatment. Heparin should be discontinued if there is a sudden unexplained decrease in platelet count less than 100/μL or a decrease of more than 50%. Cessation results in an increase in platelets over 10 days. The frequency of heparin-induced thrombocytopenia is greater with unfractionated heparin than with low-molecular-weight heparin. Other agents for anticoagulation are available for use in this situation if heparin needs to be discontinued. They include danaparoid sodium, r-hirudin, and argatroban.

Warfarin is the most frequently used oral anticoagulant and inhibits the synthesis of vitamin K–dependent clotting factors in the liver (factors II, VII, IX, X) and limits the carboxylation of the anticoagulant proteins protein C and S (carboxylation decreases their activity). Warfarin can be started during the first hospital day in a dose of 5 mg/d. No benefit has been found with using higher "loading" doses of warfarin. The prothrombin time should be checked daily and the dose adjusted to prolong the prothrombin time to an international normalized ratio (INR) of 2 to 3. Heparin can be discontinued after a minimum of 5 days, after the INR has reached the desired range on 2 consecutive days. The INR should be checked as an outpatient twice weekly until stable and then weekly or biweekly as needed. Patients should be advised to avoid aspirin-containing medications and to report any medication change to their physician, because it may impact on warfarin dosage.

Important side effects of warfarin are bleeding, which is more common when the INR is greater than 3.0, and skin necrosis. Bleeding can be reversed by withholding warfarin, oral or parenteral administration of vitamin K 1 to 2 mg, or, if severe, the concomitant administration of fresh frozen plasma. Warfarin-induced skin necrosis may occur within the first week of treatment and is associated with protein C deficiency. Subcutaneous unfractionated heparin or low-molecular-weight heparin is an alternative for both the initial and long-term treatment of venous thrombosis if oral anticoagulation cannot be taken. In addition to thrombocytopenia, osteoporosis is a potential risk of long-term heparin therapy.

Anticoagulation should be continued, in both patients with DVT and PE, for 3 to 6 months in patients with temporary risk factors. Six months should be considered for patients without predisposing risk factors after a first episode. Twelve months or an indefinite duration of anticoagulation should be considered if patients have recurrent episodes of VTE or active malignancy. Other indications for long-term anticoagulation include two or more spontaneous thromboses (one spontaneous thrombosis in the case of antithrombin deficiency or the antiphospholipid antibody syndrome), one spontaneous life-threatening thrombosis, one spontaneous thrombosis at an unusual site (mesenteric or cerebral vein), or one spontaneous thrombosis in the presence of more than a single genetic defect predisposing to a thromboembolic event.

Thrombolysis

Fibrinolytic therapy offers the potential for rapid clot dissolution, providing rapid relief of vascular obstruction, improving the hemodynamics, and preventing permanent vein damage. The results of thrombolytic therapy are best if treatment is given to patients most likely to respond and benefit. The use of thrombolysis in patients with DVT is controversial because most patients will have an uncomplicated course if treated with standard anticoagulation. However, because the risk of developing postphlebitic syndrome is highest in patients with extensive proximal DVT, thrombolytic therapy could be considered in this group. The greatest benefit of thrombolytic therapy for PE is expected in patients with large emboli and hemodynamic compromise, in whom the accelerated early clot lysis results in significant rapid clinical improvement. The risk of bleeding is minimized by careful patient selection. Intracranial bleeding is the most serious complication, and patients with recent head trauma, central nervous system surgery, or history of stroke, subarachnoid bleed, or intracranial metastatic disease should not be treated. Thrombolytic therapy also should be avoided in patients with a major risk of bleeding, such as those with active or recent gastrointestinal or genitourinary bleeding or major surgery or trauma within 7 days. Minimizing invasive vascular procedures also lowers the bleeding risk. Anticoagulation should be instituted when fibrinolytic therapy is discontinued to prevent recurrence.

Vena Cava Filters

Inferior vena cava filters can be inserted under local anesthesia through the jugular or femoral veins. In experienced hands, filters may be effective in preventing embolization of a DVT. Complications include development of venous stasis and occasional proximal migration of the device. The principal indication for placement of an inferior vena cava filter is DVT or PE in patients with severe bleeding in whom anticoagulation is contraindicated. A filter also should be considered in patients who have recurrent emboli while on optimal anticoagulation. Because the presence of a filter is thrombogenic and can obstruct or increase the rate of recurrent DVT, long-term anticoagulation treatment, if not contraindicated, should be considered.

Surgical Embolectomy

Surgical approaches to management of DVT are limited, but interruption of the venous system proximal to thrombus can prevent an embolus from reaching the lungs and may be useful in some patients. Acute pulmonary thrombectomy has a limited role in massive life-threatening PE. Operative mortality ranges from 20% to 50% and is determined by resuscitation before surgery, age, duration of symptoms, and number of episodes of PE. Long-term survival rate is acceptable with 71% surviving after 8 years, and major improvement in functional status is also seen.

CONSIDERATIONS IN PREGNANCY

Managing thromboembolic disease in pregnancy can be challenging, but as the leading cause of nonobstetric mortality in pregnant women, it is an entity that cannot be ignored. The risk for thromboembolism during pregnancy is increased five- to sixfold with an incidence estimated to be 0.5 to 3 in 1,000 pregnancies. A number of factors contribute to this increased risk, including an increase in clotting factors (such as fibrinogen, factors VII, VIII, IX, and X) and decreased fibrinolysis that are normal physiologic changes of pregnancy. Additional factors include progesterone-related venodilation and compression of the pelvic and lower extremity veins by the gravid uterus. At the time of labor and delivery there is vascular disruption so that all criteria of Virchow's triad (hypercoagulability, stasis, and vascular damage) are met during pregnancy. Further risk factors for thrombosis during pregnancy are the same as those in nonpregnant patients but also includes conditions specific to pregnancy such as hyperemesis, cesarean delivery, and ovarian hyperstimulation syndrome in women undergoing infertility treatment. The number of thromboembolic events that occur in association with pregnancy are evenly distributed through each trimester and the postpartum period, although relatively more DVT occur in the first and second trimesters and pulmonary emboli occur later and in the postpartum period. It is interesting to speculate that the thrombotic tendency of pregnancy may have been protective against obstetric hemorrhage in the past, but in the modern era it is a major cause of maternal morbidity and mortality.

Diagnosis of Venous Thromboembolic Disease in Pregnancy

When approaching a pregnant woman who may have had a thromboembolic event, one should remember that fetal health is dependent on maternal health so that an appropriate diagnostic evaluation and institution of treatment is not only to the mother's advantage but is of benefit to the fetus as well. Pregnant women should undergo evaluation and diagnosis of VTE in a manner similar to that in nonpregnant patients. However, a few caveats should be considered. PE is more likely to present with subtle signs and symptoms in pregnant women who generally do not have other cardiopulmonary pathology as compared with the general medical population. For example, in a study of pregnant women with documented PE, 58% had normal A-a gradients at initial presentation. Although lower extremity swelling is nearly universal in pregnancy, making this sign difficult to interpret, unilateral swelling should be considered especially suspicious for DVT. Left-sided swelling may be of greater significance because 90% of DVT in pregnancy occurs on the left. It should also be remembered that thrombosis may occur in the pelvic veins, particularly after a cesarean delivery. Therefore, a search for pelvic vein thrombosis is indicated when the clinical picture suggests DVT but lower extremity studies are negative.

The diagnosis of DVT and PE in pregnancy may be safely done in a manner similar to that of nonpregnant patients. Compression ultrasounds are safe even if serial studies are required. MRI and magnetic resonance venography (MRV) may be done safely and can be useful if ultrasound studies are inconclusive. Impedence plethysmography and venogram may also be done safely but can be difficult to interpret in pregnancy. Investigation for PE will require fetal exposure to radiation, but only to levels much lower than the 5 rads of total exposure during pregnancy deemed acceptable by the National Counsel on Radiation Protection. Initial evaluation with chest x-ray is associated with fetal exposures of less than 0.001 rods (comparable with the exposure of a transatlantic flight) and ventilation-perfusion scanning is associated with approximately 0.01 to 0.03 rads of fetal exposure. Likewise, a pulmonary angiogram can be safely performed with acceptable radiation exposures of less than 0.05 rads by a brachial route. The role of CT angiogram for the diagnosis of PE is evolving in nonpregnant patients. Though the radiation exposure is considered acceptable for pregnancy, it is not the gold standard for diagnosis, and the decision to use this test should be carefully considered. Unfortunately, D-dimers are not reliable for use in pregnancy because they are elevated by normal pregnancy and cesarean section.

Treatment of Venous Thromboembolic Disease in Pregnancy

Anticoagulation is required in women diagnosed with venous thromboembolism. Because warfarin crosses the placenta, is teratogenic, and may cause fetal bleeding associated with central nervous system abnormalities, it should be avoided except in rare circumstances. Neither unfractionated nor low-molecular-weight heparin cross the placenta and are considered the anticoagulants of choice in pregnancy. Important pharmacologic changes in pregnancy affecting heparin dosing include increased renal clearance and clearance secondary to placental production of heparinase. Unfractionated heparin may be monitored by the PTT in a manner similar to that in nonpregnant patients. However, the usual doses of low-molecular-weight heparin in nonpregnant patients cannot be reliably used in pregnant women. Twice daily dosing and heparin levels (anti-Xa levels) should be monitored to ensure adequate dosing when low-molecular-weight heparin is used in pregnancy. Though the advantages of less bleeding, thrombocytopenia, and bone loss with low-molecular-weight heparin are attractive, additional factors to consider are cost, the need to avoid epidural anesthesia within 24 to 48 hours of administration, and the inability to completely reverse it with protamine sulfate.

There is concern about the safety of outpatient management of pregnant women with acute DVT. Though the use of low-molecular-heparin in this situation been described, it may be prudent to treat acute DVT as an inpatient because of the physiologic changes of pregnancy causing hypercoagulability and venodilatation. When used for the treatment of an acute thromboembolic event in pregnancy, unfractionated heparin should initially be given intravenously followed 3 to 5 days later with subcutaneous unfractionated heparin in twice daily or three times daily doses. Dosing of subcutaneously administered heparin is adjusted by following the "mid-interval PTT" (PTT drawn midway between doses), which should be kept within the therapeutic range (1.5–2 times normal). Alternatively, enoxaparin 1 mg/kg twice daily may be administered with close follow-up of anti-Xa levels. Switching to unfractionated heparin at 36 weeks will ensure that epidural anesthesia is an option at delivery.

Pregnant Women with History of Venous Thromboembolic Disease

Pregnant women who have had a previous thromboembolic event or have other risk factors for thrombosis are at increased risk for recurrence. Those treated with lifelong anticoagulation on warfarin should be changed to therapeutic subcutaneous heparin in the manner described above. However, the optimal management of women who have had a single previous VTE and are not on long-term anticoagulation is not clear. One observational study attempting to define the magnitude of this risk included 125 women who were not known to have had a thrombophilia but who had had a previous thrombosis. These women were not treated with anticoagulation during pregnancy but were given heparin followed by coumadin for 4 to 6 weeks postpartum. A recurrence rate of 4.8% was observed with half of the events occurring antepartum. Though women with known thrombophilia were excluded from the study, a subgroup of study participants did have a thrombophilia workup. Patients were stratified by the presence or absence of a transient risk factor at the time of their index clot and by the results of thrombophilia testing. The recurrence rate for women who had a thrombophilia was from 13% to 20% depending on the presence or absence of a prior transient risk factor at the time of the initial thrombosis. Women who had no thrombophilia and prior idiopathic clot had a recurrence rate of 8%.

Many would advocate the use of heparin prophylaxis during pregnancy followed by a form of anticoagulation for 6 to 8 weeks postpartum in women who have had a previous thrombosis because of this risk of recurrence. Escalating doses of heparin are generally required throughout pregnancy because of the pharmacologic changes. A dose of 5,000 units of unfractionated heparin administered twice daily in the first trimester, 7,500 units twice daily in the second trimester, and 10,000 units twice daily in the third trimester is often used. Low-molecular-weight heparin can also be safely used (e.g., enoxaparin 30 mg twice daily), and the monitoring of heparin levels is recommended. In addition, changing to unfractionated heparin at 36 weeks will ensure that regional anesthesia is an option at labor and delivery.

Management during Labor and Delivery

Women who are treated with prophylactic doses of heparin should be instructed to discontinue their heparin injections when they develop contractions but otherwise do not require special management at labor and delivery. However, pregnant women treated with therapeutic heparin benefit from planning an induction so that their heparin may be discontinued on the evening before a morning induction. Prophylactic doses of unfractionated heparin and/or compression stockings may be used during this time in patients believed to be at particularly high risk for thrombosis. Heparin can be restarted 6 to 24 hours postpartum depending on the obstetricians judgment regarding the adequacy of hemostasis and the concern for recurrent thrombosis. When women on heparin present for labor and delivery, it is appropriate to check the PTT or anti-Xa level and complete blood count, including a platelet count.

Postpartum Management

It is not until 6 to 12 weeks postpartum that the physiologic changes in pregnancy resulting in a hypercoagulable state return to baseline. Therefore, thrombophilic women should be treated with anticoagulation for at least 6 weeks after delivery. For women who require therapeutic anticoagulation, warfarin (compatible with breast-feeding) is the best choice. Overlap with heparin is advised when warfarin is begun in postpartum women because protein S is known to decrease in pregnancy, and there is concern with precipitating warfarin skin necrosis otherwise. For those women who require prophylactic doses of anticoagulation, heparin or warfarin may be administered for 6 weeks postpartum. A reasonable regimen for unfractionated heparin is to give either 7,500 units twice daily for 2 weeks postpartum and then decrease to 5,000 units twice daily until 6 weeks postpartum or to simply administer 5,000 units twice daily for 6 weeks postpartum. Enoxaparin 30 mg twice daily may be continued as an alternative.

Obstetric Complications in Women with Thrombophilias

There is an increased risk for obstetric complications, such as recurrent miscarriage, fetal loss, and early severe preeclampsia, in women with antiphospholipid antibody syndrome. Placental thrombosis is thought to be the basis for these complications. Treatment with 81 mg aspirin in combination with prophylactic doses of heparin or 81 mg aspirin and prednisone throughout pregnancy has been shown to improve pregnancy outcome in women with antiphospholipid antibodies. Though women with other thrombophilias may also have increased obstetric risk, the optimal treatment of such women requires further research.

Hormones

Estrogen in the form of oral contraceptives or hormone replacement therapy carries a well-established risk for thrombosis. Women taking oral contraceptives have a risk of venous thromboembolism that is three to six times that of nonusers, although the absolute risk is quite low at 3 to 4 per 10,000 person-years during oral contraceptive use. The risk of thromboembolism is higher in the first year of use, and it is thought that women who develop clots during the first year of use may be more likely to have an underlying thrombophilia. In addition, it appears that the third-generation oral contraceptives have a higher risk of venous thrombosis than second-generation oral contraceptives. Likewise, hormone replacement therapy increases the rate of venous thromboembolism from 16 to 34 per 10,000 person-years. The American Heart Association recommends that women on hormone replacement therapy who become immobilized be taken off of hormone replacement therapy and consideration be given to instituting thromboprophylaxis.

BIBLIOGRAPHY

Atrash HK, Doonin LM, Lawson HW, et al. Maternal mortality in the United States, 1979–1986. *Obstet Gynecol* 1990;76:1050–1060.

Barritt DW, Jordan SC. Clinical features of pulmonary embolism. *Lancet* 1961;1: 729–732.

Bauer KA. The thrombophilias: well-defined risk factors with uncertain therapeutic implications. *Ann Intern Med* 2001;135:367–373.

Brill-Edwards P, Ginsberg GS, Gent M, et al. Safety of withholding heparin in pregnant women with a history of venous thromboembolism. *N Engl J Med* 2000;343:1439–1444.

Department of Health, Welsh Office, Scottish Home and Health Department and Department of Health and Social Services Northern Ireland. Confidential Enquiries into Maternal Deaths in the United Kingdom 1994–1996. London: TSO, 1998.

De Stefano V, Martinelli I, Mannucci PM, et al. The risk of recurrent deep venous thrombosis among heterozygous carriers of both factor V Leiden and the G20210A prothrombin mutation. *N Engl J Med* 1999;341:801–806.

Geerts WH, Heit JA, Clagett GP, et al. Prevention of venous thromboembolism. *Chest* 2001;119:132S–175S.

Gottschalk A, Stein PD, Goodman LR, et al. Overview of prospective investigation of pulmonary embolism diagnosis II. *Semin Nuclear Med* 2002;32:173–182.

Guidelines on diagnosis and management of acute pulmonary embolism. Task Force on Pulmonary Embolism, European Society of Cardiology. *Eur Heart J* 2000;21:1301–1336.

Heit JA, Melton LF, Lohse CM, et al. Incidence of venous thromboembolism in hospitalized patients vs. community residents. *Mayo Clin Proc* 2001;76:1002.

Hull RD, Raskob GE, Rosenbloom D, et al. Optimal therapeutic level of heparin therapy in patients with venous thrombosis. *Arch Intern Med* 1992;152: 1589–1595.

Hyers TM, Agnelli G, Hull R, et al. Antithrombotic therapy for venous thromboembolic disease. *Chest* 2001;119:176S–193S.

Kelly J, Rudd A, Lewis R, et al. Plasma D-dimers in the diagnosis of venous thrombolism. *Arch Intern Med* 2002;162:747–756.

Koster T, Rosendaal FR, de Ronde H, et al. Venous thrombosis due to poor anticoagulant response to activated protein C: Leiden thrombophilia study. *Lancet* 1993;342:1503.

Kupferminc MJ, Eldor A, Steinman N, et al. Increased frequency of genetic thrombophilia in women with complications of pregnancy. *N Engl J Med* 1999;340: 9–13.

Kupferminc MJ, Fait G, Many A, et al. Severe preeclampsia and high frequency of genetic thrombophilic mutations. *Obstet Gynecol* 2000;96:45–49.

Laskin CA, Bombardier C, Hannah ME, et al. Prednisone and aspirin in women with autoantibodies and unexplained recurrent fetal loss. *N Engl J Med* 1997; 337:148–153.

Lee RV, Rosene-Montella K, Barbour L, et al., eds. *Medical care of the pregnant woman.* Philadelphia: American College of Physicians-American Society of Internal Medicine, 2000.

National Counsel on Radiation Protection Report no. 91. Recommendations on Units for Exposure to Ionizing Radiation. Washington, DC: National Counsel on Radiation Protection, 1997.

Powrie RO, Larson L, Rosene-Montella K, et al. Alveolar-arterial oxygen gradient in acute pulmonary embolism in pregnancy. *Am J Obstet Gynecol* 1998;178:394–396.

Rai R, Cohen H, Dave M, et al. Randomised controlled trial of aspirin and aspirin plus heparin in pregnant women with recurrent miscarriage associated with phospholipid antibodies (or antiphospholipid antibodies). *Br Med J* 1997;314: 253–257.

Raschke RA, Reilly BM, Guidry JR, et al. The weight-based heparin dosing nomogram compared with a "standard care" nomogram: a randomized controlled trial. *Ann Intern Med* 1993;119:874–881.

Risks and benefits of estrogen plus progestin in healthy postmenopausal women: principal results from the Women's Health Initiative randomized controlled trial. *JAMA* 2002;288:321.

Salomon O, Steinberg DM, Zivelin A, et al. Single and combined prothrombotic factors in patients with idiopathic venous thromboembolism: prevalence and risk assessment. *Arterioscl Thromb Vasc Biol* 1999;19:511–518.

Stein PD, Henry JW. Prevalence of acute pulmonary embolism among patients in a general hospital and at autopsy. *Chest* 1995;108:78–81.

Tapson VF, Carroll BA, Davidson BL, et al. The diagnostic approach to acute venous thromboembolism: clinical practice guideline. American Thoracic Society. *Am J Respir Crit Care Med* 1999;160:1043–1066.

Thomson AJ, Walker ID, Greer IA. Low molecular weight heparin for the immediate management of thromboembolic disease in pregnancy. *Lancet* 1998;352:1904.

Vandenbroucke JP, Rosing J, et al. Oral Contraceptives and the risk of venous thrombosis. *N Engl J Med* 2001;344:1527–1535.

CHAPTER 92

Hematologic Malignancies: Leukemias and Lymphoma

Pradyumna D. Phatak

The hematologic malignancies are a heterogenous group of disorders that arise from malignant transformation of hematopoietic cells. The malignant cells proliferate in the bone marrow or lymphoid tissues or both, where they eventually result in impairment of normal hematopoiesis, immune dysfunction, or lymph node enlargement. Disorders in which the neoplastic cells originate in the bone marrow and often circulate in the peripheral blood are termed *leukemias.* Disorders that arise in lymphoid tissue and primarily cause lymph node enlargement and hepatosplenomegaly are termed *lymphomas.* Although the broad topic of hematologic malignancies also includes the plasma cell dyscrasias, the discussion in this chapter is restricted to the common forms of leukemia and lymphoma. As a group, these disorders tend to be quite widespread at presentation and are generally responsive to chemotherapeutic agents and radiation therapy. In general, the management of these disorders is best left to individuals accustomed to dealing with the intricacies of their treatment. Referral to a subspecialist is probably appropriate when one of these conditions is suspected or diagnosed.

CLASSIFICATION

Leukemias

The leukemias can be classified based on their cell of origin and clinical course.

MYELOID

The myeloid leukemias can be acute or chronic:

- *Acute.* Acute myelogenous leukemia (AML) results in a proliferation of primitive myeloid cells (myeloblasts). Particularly in elderly patients, this malignancy can sometimes evolve from another clonal hematopoietic disorder, most commonly myelodysplastic syndrome. Several subtypes of AML have been described, based largely on the presumed lineage of the myeloblast. Table 92.1 lists the commonly used classification of AML.

TABLE 92.1. Subtypes of Acute Myelogenous Leukemia

FAB type	Common name	Unique features
M1	Myeloid without maturation	
M2	Myeloid with maturation	t(8,21) in 10%
M3	Acute promyelocytic	DIC is common; response to retinoic acid
M4	Myelomonocytic	
M5	Monocytic	Gum and skin infiltrates
M6	Erythroleukemia	
M7	Megakaryoblastic leukemia	

DIC, disseminated intravascular coagulopathy.

- *Chronic.* Chronic myelogenous leukemia (CML) belongs to the myeloproliferative group of disorders in which both proliferation and maturation of myeloid cells occur. Thus, intermediate myeloid cells such as myelocytes and metamyelocytes predominate in the blood of patients with CML.

LYMPHOID

Proliferation of lymphoid cells in the bone marrow and lymphoid tissues with malignant cells appearing in the blood results in the lymphoid leukemias.

- *Acute.* In acute lymphoblastic leukemia (ALL) the predominant neoplastic cell is a primitive lymphoid cell (lymphoblast). Three subtypes (L1–L3) have been described based on the morphology of the lymphoblast. ALL may be derived from B- or T-lymphocyte precursors.
- *Chronic.* In chronic lymphocytic leukemia (CLL), mature lymphocytes predominate. This neoplasm is usually derived from B lymphocytes but sometimes can be from T lymphocytes as well.

Lymphomas

The lymphomas were recently reclassified at a consensus conference as outlined in Table 92.2.

TABLE 92.2. Clinical Classification of Lymphoproliferative Disorders (Prescreening Development Questionnaire Modification of REAL Classification of Lymphoproliferative Diseases)

Plasma cell disorders
- Monoclonal gammopathies of undetermined significance (MGU)
- Plasmacytoma (bone, extramedullary)
- Multiple myeloma
- Amyloidosis

Hodgkin lymphomas

Indolent lymphomas/leukemias
- Follicular lymphomas
  - Follicular small cleaved cell
  - Follicular mixed small cleaved and large cell
  - Diffuse small cleaved cell
- Diffuse small lymphocytic lymphoma/CLL—distinguish prolymphocytic leukemia (aggressive), T-cell granular lymphocytic leukemia
- Lymphoplasmacytic lymphoma/Waldenström macroglobulinemia
- Marginal zone lymphomas
  - MALT (extranodal B-cell lymphoma)
  - Monocytoid B-cell lymphoma (nodal B-cell lymphoma)
  - Splenic lymphoma with villous lymphocytes (splenic lymphoma)
- Hairy cell leukemia
- Mycosis fungoides/Sézary syndrome

Aggressive lymphomas/leukemias
- Diffuse large cell lymphomas—distinguish primary mediastinal large B-cell lymphoma, follicular large cell lymphoma, anaplastic large cell lymphoma (nodal versus cutaneous only), extranodal NK-cell/T-cell lymphoma (nasal type), lymphomatoid granulomatosis (angiocentric pulmonary B-cell lymphoma), angioimmunoblastic T-cell lymphoma, peripheral T-cell lymphoma (distinguish rare subtypes subcutaneous panniculitic and hepatosplenic gamma/delta T-cell lymphomas), enteropathy-type intestinal T-cell lymphoma, intravascular lymphomatosis
  - Diffuse mixed cell lymphoma
  - Diffuse large cell lymphoma
  - Immunoblastic lymphoma
- Burkitt lymphoma/diffuse small noncleaved cell lymphoma
- Lymphoblastic lymphoma
- Central nervous system lymphoma
- Adult T-cell leukemia/lymphoma (with HTLV-1)
- Mantle cell lymphoma
- Posttransplantation lymphoproliferative disorder
- Acquired immunodeficiency syndrome–related lymphoma
- True histiocytic lymphoma
- Primary effusion lymphoma
- Aggressive NK-cell leukemia

NK, natural killer.

ETIOLOGY

The etiology of leukemia is not known, but both genetic and environmental factors have been implicated. A familial tendency to develop leukemia has occasionally been noted, and some congenital disorders such as Down syndrome are associated with an increased risk of leukemia. Exposure to radiation has been associated with an increased risk of developing both AML and CML and possibly ALL as well.

Hodgkin disease occurs in a bimodal age distribution, and causative environmental factors have been strongly implicated, particularly in younger patients. Non-Hodgkin lymphomas occur with increased frequency in immunosuppressed individuals, including those with acquired immunodeficiency syndrome. Viruses have also been implicated in the pathogenesis of certain types of non-Hodgkin lymphoma, such as Epstein-Barr virus and Burkitt lymphoma.

HISTORY

Acute Leukemias

The acute leukemias, AML and ALL, share many clinical features. Characteristically, the initial presentation is acute with symptoms for weeks to a few months. About one fourth of patients with AML, particularly elderly patients, may have underlying myelodysplastic syndromes with associated cytopenia for many months before the diagnosis. The presenting symptoms of the acute leukemias usually relate to the ensuing cytopenia with weakness, fatigue, and shortness of breath due to anemia, bleeding at various sites due to thrombocytopenia, and infections due to neutropenia. Occasionally, patients with marked leukocytosis can present with symptoms of leukostasis such as visual blurring and shortness of breath. Rarely, pressure symptoms due to soft tissue masses of leukemia cells (chloroma), symptoms due to meningeal infiltration, or metabolic derangements due to tumor lysis syndrome can be presenting features.

Chronic Leukemias

The chronic leukemias have a more indolent presentation. CML may present with systemic symptoms such as fever and night sweats or may be incidentally detected as splenomegaly or leukocytosis. CLL is most often detected as an incidental lymphocytosis.

Lymphomas

Patients with lymphoma usually present with painless lymphadenopathy that may or may not be accompanied by systemic symptoms, including fevers, night sweats, weight loss, malaise, and pruritus. In Hodgkin disease, adenopathy most often involves cervical and mediastinal lymph node groups with occasional contiguous involvement of paraaortic and inguinal nodes. Only some patients have liver, spleen, bone marrow, or lung involvement at the time of diagnosis. Extralymphatic and noncontiguous involvement is more common in non-Hodgkin lymphomas. Patients with low grade lymphoma tend to have a more indolent presentation, whereas aggressive lymphomas can present with rapidly enlarging masses, systemic symptoms, or central nervous system involvement.

CLINICAL FINDINGS

The clinical findings in the acute leukemias usually relate to the accompanying cytopenia. Pallor is common, and petechiae and ecchymoses often occur. Occasionally, splenomegaly is palpable. The monocytic variant is more likely to present with signs of tissue infiltration, such as gum hypertrophy.

CML usually presents with splenomegaly. In CLL, both splenomegaly and lymphadenopathy can occur. Hodgkin disease and non-Hodgkin lymphoma often result in palpable lymphadenopathy or organomegaly.

A common dilemma facing the primary care provider is the approach to the workup of an enlarged lymph node. Most experts agree that biopsy should be performed on a firm lymph node that measures more than 1 cm, is not associated with an apparent infection, and persists more than 4 to 6 weeks. In an asymptomatic patient in whom enlarged lymph nodes are incidentally found, a period of observation is often reasonable. When the patient detects the enlarged lymph node, more urgent biopsy is usually required. Factors to consider in making the decision to biopsy include size and number of the enlarged lymph nodes, age of the patient, and the coexistence of symptoms.

LABORATORY AND IMAGING STUDIES

Acute Leukemias

Diagnosis of the acute leukemias requires examination of the bone marrow. Usually, involvement is extensive by the time clinical presentation occurs. The distinction between the various types of acute leukemia can be made on morphologic grounds and with the appropriate use of cytochemical stains. Immunofluorescent staining followed by flow cytometric analysis is now a standard part of the workup to assist with the differential diagnosis. From a management standpoint, it is very important to distinguish myeloid from lymphoid forms of acute leukemia, whereas distinction of various subtypes is less important. The one exception is acute promyelocytic leukemia for which there is a specific treatment modality (all-*trans* retinoic acid). In addition to tests required to make the diagnosis, the initial evaluation of patients with acute leukemia should include a chemistry profile to look for hyperuricemia, renal dysfunction, and other metabolic signs of tumor lysis because these may require urgent attention. A complete blood count is required to assess the presence of cytopenia and the need for transfusions.

Chronic Myelogenous Leukemia

The diagnosis of CML can often be suspected upon the examination of the peripheral blood smear. A moderate to marked leukocytosis is usually seen with the whole range of myeloid precursors being present, often referred to as a *garden party appearance.* There is a predominance of intermediate myeloid cells, including myelocytes and metamyelocytes. This type of blood morphology is sometimes seen in reactive states and is referred to as a leukemoid reaction. Features that distinguish CML from a leukemoid reaction include degree of leukocytosis (usually $<50{,}000/mm^3$ in leukemoid reactions), leukocyte alkaline phosphatase score (usually very low in CML), and the presence in most cases of CML of a unique cytogenetic abnormality, t(9,22), called the *Philadelphia chromosome.* The bone marrow in CML is usually hypercellular with predominance of myeloid precursors.

Chronic Lymphocytic Leukemia

CLL can often be diagnosed by the presence of lymphocytosis in the absence of an apparent infection. Morphologically, the peripheral blood lymphocytes are well differentiated and normal appearing. They tend to be fragile, leading to the frequent occurrence of "smudge cells" on the peripheral blood smear. Immunofluorescence staining with flow cytometric analysis can reveal the diagnostic predominance of B cells that often have a surface antigen called CD5 and have either kappa or lambda light chains, but not both, reflecting clonality. The bone marrow examination can reveal varying degrees of diffuse or nodular lymphocytosis. Physical examination and x-ray evaluation may reveal varying degrees of lymphadenopathy or hepatosplenomegaly. A complete blood count may reveal varying degrees of cytopenia.

Patients with CLL can develop immune hemolytic anemia or immune thrombocytopenia at any stage of the disease. The occurrence of immune cytopenia does not influence staging.

Lymphoma

The diagnosis of Hodgkin disease or non-Hodgkin lymphoma is usually based on the pathologic examination of an enlarged lymph node. After a pathologic diagnosis is established, further clinical, radiologic, and laboratory evaluation is directed toward defining the extent of the disease. Accurate clinical staging and is essential for selection of the most appropriate therapy.

The initial evaluation includes a careful history and physical examination with particular attention to lymph node–bearing areas, complete blood count, screening blood chemistries, and chest x-ray. Abnormal blood studies are common but not helpful in indicating stage or prognosis. If the chest x-ray is suspicious for mediastinal node involvement, computed tomography of the chest is indicated. An iliac crest bone marrow biopsy may reveal bone marrow involvement.

An abdominal computed tomography is performed to assess retroperitoneal and iliac lymph node involvement and to image the liver and spleen. Positron emission tomography can be of value in detecting areas of minimal involvement and in looking for minimal residual disease after treatment.

The commonly used staging system for lymphomas is as follows:

Stage I. Involvement of a single lymph node region (I) or localized involvement of a single extralymphatic organ or site (IE).

Stage II. Involvement of two or more lymph node regions on the same side of the diaphragm (II) or localized involvement of a single associated extralymphatic organ or site and its regional lymph nodes on the same side of the diaphragm (IIE).

Stage III. Involvement of lymph node regions on both sides of the diaphragm (III), which may also be accompanied by localized involvement of an associated extralymphatic organ or site (IIIE), or by involvement of the spleen (IIIS) or both (IIISE). Stage III1 indicates involvement of upper abdominal lymphatic structures: spleen, porta hepatis nodes, celiac nodes, or splenic hilar nodes. Stage III2 includes involved nodes in the paraaortic, iliac, mesenteric, or inguinal areas with or without involvement of the upper abdominal lymphatic structures.

Stage IV. Disseminated (multifocal) involvement of one or more extralymphatic organs with or without associated lymph node involvement or isolated extralymphatic organ involvement with distant (nonregional) nodal involvement.

If systemic symptoms of unexplained weight loss in excess of 10% of body weight, fever, or night sweats are present, the letter B is added to the stage. The letter A denotes absence of systemic symptoms.

TREATMENT

When the diagnosis of a hematologic malignancy is made, it is important to evaluate the patient for other underlying medical conditions. A therapeutic decision needs to be individualized weighing the intensity of the planned treatment regimen against the age and general condition of the patient. Older patients or those with significant underlying disease processes might not be appropriate candidates for intensive chemotherapy.

Acute Leukemias

The management of acute leukemias involves the use of intense myeloablative chemotherapy with intent to cure. The initial phase of treatment called *remission induction chemotherapy* is the most important phase. Intensive systemic chemotherapy is administered with the goal of reducing the leukemic cell burden below the level of detection. Because the chemotherapy drugs used have little selectivity for leukemic cells over their normal bone marrow counterparts, therapy is usually accompanied by the development of severe myelosuppression before achieving a complete remission. The two most active drugs used in AML are cytosine arabinoside and daunorubicin. The combination of these agents results in a complete remission rate of 60% to 80%. In the case of the promyelocytic variant, all-*trans* retinoic acid is a also a very effective treatment, and its use during induction improves cure rates. The therapy in ALL may be less intense, particularly in children. Prednisone and vincristine are an important component of the chemotherapy used for ALL (particularly in children). In adults with ALL, additional intense chemotherapy that includes an anthracycline is also typically used. Induction therapy usually results in myeloablation over the course of 5 to 7 days. This is followed in 3 to 4 weeks by recovery of the normal marrow components. Supportive care during this time is a critical part of the management and usually involves long-term hospitalization. Blood product support is usually needed, as is the appropriate management of intercurrent infections. It is generally advisable to use platelet transfusions to maintain the count over 15,000 to 20,000/mL. During the neutropenic phase, patients are at risk of developing potentially life-threatening infections. A fever in this setting requires prompt evaluation and often empiric therapy. Fungal infections are a common cause of morbidity and mortality in this setting, and the appropriate institution of empiric antifungal therapy is crucial to achieving a favorable outcome.

Involvement of the central nervous system requires special attention because most chemotherapy regimens do not cross the blood–brain barrier. Prophylactic central nervous system therapy is usually indicated in ALL because occult involvement of the central nervous system is common. Certain subtypes of AML such as the monocytic variants have an increased tendency for central nervous system involvement as well.

If remission induction therapy does not result in a complete remission, the prognosis is grave. Once a complete remission is achieved, it should be immediately followed by consolidation chemotherapy to achieve the best possible chance of a long-term remission. This therapy is also usually as intense as the initial induction treatment. In addition, the management of ALL typically involves lower dose maintenance therapy for several months.

Since the early 1980s, these forms of consolidation and maintenance chemotherapy have been replaced in part by bone marrow transplantation. Unfortunately, allogeneic bone marrow transplantation is a relatively risky procedure with high mortality and morbidity rates, particularly in older individuals. Most centers exclude patients over 55 years of age from their allogeneic bone marrow transplant programs. Moreover, only about 30% of individuals have an human leukocyte antigen–matched sibling donor available. There is some controversy in the literature as to whether every patient under age 55 years who has an human leukocyte antigen–matched sibling donor should automatically receive an allogeneic bone marrow transplant in first remission. Some centers reserve this technique for individuals who have disease relapses.

Modern-day intensive induction chemotherapy regimens followed by consolidation chemotherapy or bone marrow transplantation result in long-term cure rates in the order of 20% to 30% in patients with AML. Children with ALL have a better prognosis, with about 90% cure rates with chemotherapy alone. Adults with ALL have a prognosis similar to that of adults with AML.

Chronic Myelogenous Leukemia

The management of CML differs considerably from that of the acute leukemias. The disease course is characterized by an initial chronic phase in which most patients initially present. During this phase, mild oral chemotherapy using agents such as hydroxyurea and busulfan is usually sufficient to control the leukocytosis and associated symptoms. Unfortunately, these patients almost universally transform, in a median of 3.5 to 4 years, to an accelerated phase followed by blastic transformation.

Recently, a treatment targeted at the molecular defect in CML cells, called imatinib mesylate (trade name "Gleevec"), has become available and results in cytogenetic remissions in a high proportion of CML cases. The long-term outcome with this therapy is unknown because it has been use for only a few years.

The only proven curative therapy available is allogeneic bone marrow transplantation. This procedure is much more effective when performed in the chronic phase rather than after blastic transformation. Patients under 55 to 60 years of age who have human leukocyte antigen–matched sibling donors should be considered for bone marrow transplantation early in the course of their disease. Individuals who do not have matched sibling donors should be offered the possibility of a matched unrelated bone marrow transplant. Because this procedure involves considerable risk of morbidity and mortality, the decision to proceed is a more difficult one, particularly in older patients.

Chronic Lymphocytic Leukemia

CLL is a slowly progressive neoplasm, and the goals of therapy differ considerably from those noted previously. No curative therapy is currently available. On the other hand, patients with this disorder can enjoy long survival rates often with few symptoms. Therapy is indicated when symptoms occur or the disease is associated with significant cytopenia. Immune cytopenia are managed using steroids or splenectomy in a manner analogous to that used in these disorders when they occur in the absence of CLL. Cytoreductive therapy usually consists of oral alkylating agents, chlorambucil being most commonly used. The goal is to reduce the leukemic cell burden enough to relieve symptoms, shrink symptomatic lymphadenopathy and organomegaly, and relieve cytopenia.

Hodgkin Disease

The treatment of Hodgkin disease has improved dramatically in the past 30 years; most patients with localized disease are cured with radiation therapy, and most of those with disseminated disease are cured with combination chemotherapy or combined modality treatment. Current investigational efforts are directed toward finding treatment programs that maximize remission rates and durations and at the same time minimizing immediate and long-term complications.

Over the years, several effective chemotherapy regimens have evolved for the treatment of Hodgkin disease. The most widely used regimen is ABVD (adriamycin, bleomycin, vinblastine, and dacarbazine), which has supplanted earlier alkylating agent based combinations.

Non-Hodgkin Lymphomas

The management of non-Hodgkin lymphoma starts with accurate pathologic classification, discussed earlier, and staging. As in the case of the other hematologic malignancies, assessment of the general health of the patient and coexistent illnesses is necessary to determine potential complications from therapy.

In general terms, the indolent lymphomas have a relatively benign clinical course, and therapy is unlikely to be curative. The prototype pathologic subtype is the nodular, poorly differentiated, lymphocytic lymphoma. The goal of treatment in the indolent lymphomas is to achieve palliation of symptoms. If the patient is asymptomatic, observation without therapeutic intervention may be appropriate. If symptoms are due to regional lymph node enlargement, local radiation therapy may provide relief. For more generalized disease, systemic chemotherapy is often useful. Alkylating agents such as chlorambucil and cyclophosphamide are often used, sometimes in combination with prednisone and, occasionally, vincristine. More recently, nucleoside analogues, particularly fludarabine, have been used successfully in these neoplasms. A monoclonal anti-CD20 antibody called rituximab is effective in relapsed and refractory cases.

The intermediate to aggressive non-Hodgkin lymphomas are more likely to be symptomatic at presentation and have a rapidly fatal course if left untreated. On the other hand, a substantial proportion of these patients can be cured using combination chemotherapy. The prototype intermediate-grade lymphoma is diffuse large cell lymphoma. Standard chemotherapy for this disease includes a combination of cyclophosphamide, doxorubicin, vincristine, and prednisone (CHOP). Recently, the combination of CHOP with rituximab has been found to increase response rates and cure rates in these patients. Of these patients, about 60% achieve complete remission and about half of the remissions are sustained long term. The more aggressive lymphomas, such as Burkitt lymphoma and lymphoblastic lymphoma, are treated with aggressive chemotherapy regimens similar to that used in ALL.

In patients with intermediate to aggressive non-Hodgkin lymphomas that fail to respond or relapse after initial combination chemotherapy, salvage chemotherapy regimens have been used with limited success and little chance of sustained remission. Autologous and allogeneic bone marrow transplantation offer the only realistic chance of long-term disease control in this situation and are being increasingly used for this indication, particularly in younger patients.

Long-Term Sequelae of Therapy

Long-term survivors after chemotherapy or radiation therapy or both are prone to certain complications that primary care practitioners should be aware of. These complications have been best studied in Hodgkin disease survivors. Potential complications of radiotherapy include hypothyroidism, pericarditis, pneumonitis, spinal cord injury, infertility, and, rarely, damage to bone, liver, or kidney. Radiation to the mediastinum increases future risk of coronary atherosclerosis. Chemotherapy with older alkylating agent based combination regimens (e.g., mechlorethamine, vincristine, procarbazine, and prednisone [MOPP]) produces permanent sterility in almost all men and many young women. ABVD has a lower likelihood of leading to sterility, but the use of doxorubicin and radiation to the heart may cause cardiomyopathy, and increased risk of pulmonary damage occurs in patients treated with both bleomycin and chest irradiation. Greater myelotoxicity is observed in patients receiving combined modality therapy also. Second malignancies, especially AML and non-Hodgkin lymphomas, pose a substantial risk for patients treated with combined modality therapy or chemotherapy alone.

CONSIDERATIONS IN PREGNANCY

The occurrence of hematologic malignancies during pregnancy poses a particularly challenging therapeutic decision. Staging x-ray is contraindicated, at least relatively. The administration of chemotherapeutic agents during the first trimester is known to be teratogenic. A recent review of acute leukemia during pregnancy revealed a higher incidence of spontaneous abortion and premature delivery when leukemia was diagnosed and treated during the first or second trimester.

Factors to be considered when making therapeutic decisions during pregnancy include the following:

- The nature of the hematologic malignancy. In the aggressive neoplasms such as the acute leukemias, treatment is urgently needed. In the more indolent disorders such as the indolent lymphomas, treatment can sometimes be deferred until after delivery.
- The stage of pregnancy. In the first trimester, the teratogenic risk of chemotherapy is high, and it may be appropriate to terminate the pregnancy. In the second and third trimester, teratogenic effects are less likely and it may also be more feasible to delay therapy until after delivery.
- Patient preference. A detailed discussion with the patient about the prognosis of the malignancy is necessary to enable her to make an informed decision regarding the risks and benefits of chemotherapy, postponement of therapy, and continuation of the pregnancy.

The ultimate decision should involve close collaboration between hematologist/oncologist, radiation oncologist, obstetrician, primary care physician, and the patient.

BIBLIOGRAPHY

Aisenberg AC. Problems in Hodgkin's disease management. *Blood* 1999;93:761–779.
Allen HH, Nisker JA. *Cancer in pregnancy: therapeutic guidelines.* New York: Futura, 1986.
Armitage JO. Bone marrow transplantation in the treatment of patients with lymphoma. *Blood* 1989;73:1749.
Champlin R, Gale RP. Acute lymphoblastic leukemia: recent advances in biology and therapy. *Blood* 1989;73:2051.
Coltman CA Jr, ed. Introduction: Hodgkin's disease 1990. *Semin Oncol* 1990;17:641.
Foon KA, Gale RP. Therapy of acute myelogenous leukemia. *Blood Rev* 1992;6:15.
Foon KA, Rai KR, Gale RP. Chronic lymphocytic leukemia: new insights into biology and therapy. *Ann Intern Med* 1990;113:525.
Harris NL, Jaffe ES, Armitage JO. Lymphoma classification: from REAL to WHO and beyond. In: DeVita, VT, Hellman S, Rosenberg SA, eds. *Cancer: principles and practice of oncology updates.* Philadelphia: Lippincott Williams & Wilkins, 1999;13:1–14.
Hehlmann R. Chronic myelogenous leukemia: recent developments in prognostic evaluation and chemotherapy. *Leukemia* 1992;6[Suppl 3]:1105.
Mandelli F, ed. Therapy of acute leukemias. *Leukemia* 1992;6:1.
Stone RM, Mayer RJ. Treatment of the newly diagnosed adult with de novo acute myeloid leukemia. *Hematol Oncol Clin North Am* 1993;7:47.

PART

11

Musculoskeletal Problems

CHAPTER 93

Evaluation of the Patient with Musculoskeletal Symptoms

Yousaf Ali

HISTORY

Musculoskeletal diseases are the leading cause of disability in the United States. In the 1990s, an estimated 43 million Americans were affected, and this number is set to reach at least 60 million by 2020. In addition to the economic burden, the intangible costs include pain, limitation of activities, psychological stress, and change in appearance as a consequence of deformity. The ability to determine the origin of pain or inflammation depends on a thorough initial history and examination. An inadequate history and examination often lead to inappropriate testing and treatment.

The nature of the pain varies according to which tissue is involved. Neuropathic pain has a burning or lancinating quality and often a radicular pattern, whereas muscle pain is frequently described as a diffuse aching sensation. Determining whether extraarticular complaints are localized or systemic helps in the formulation of a differential diagnosis. Focal conditions include tennis elbow, trochanteric bursitis, muscle strain, and nerve entrapment syndromes. Generalized nonarticular pain suggests fibromyalgia, polymyositis, polymyalgia rheumatica, or a peripheral neuropathy.

Articular symptoms can arise from one joint (monarthritis) or more than one joint (polyarthritis) and may be secondary to inflammatory or noninflammatory processes. Inflammatory arthritis is associated with erythema, warmth, pain, and swelling in the joint. Systemic features such as morning stiffness, fatigue, low-grade fever, and generalized weakness are frequently present. A reasonable differential diagnosis can be determined based on the anatomic site of origin, number of joints involved, and the presence or absence of inflammation (Tables 93.1, 93.2). The possibilities can be narrowed further by considering the patient's age, sex, race, and family history. Systemic connective tissue diseases such as polymyositis, systemic lupus erythematosus (SLE), and Reiter syndrome are observed in younger patients, whereas osteoarthritis and polymyalgia rheumatica are more prevalent in patients older than 50 years of age. SLE and sarcoidosis are more common in blacks, whereas polymyalgia rheumatica and giant cell arteritis are rare in these patients. Women make up a much higher percentage of patients with SLE, rheumatoid arthritis, and fibromyalgia, but the spondylarthropathies and gout are more common in men. Disorders that tend to aggregate in families include rheumatoid arthritis (RA), ankylosing spondylitis, psoriatic arthritis, and some forms of osteoarthritis.

The pattern of joint involvement and mode of onset can provide valuable clues. Migratory arthritis is seen in subacute bacterial endocarditis, disseminated gonorrhea, early Lyme disease, and acute rheumatic fever. Progressive involvement of the small joints of the hands and feet over time is typical of RA, psoriatic arthritis, and SLE, whereas intermittent symptoms are suggestive of crystalline arthritis (gout or pseudogout), erosive osteoarthritis, or a foreign body in the joint. RA, SLE, and the spondylarthropathies tend to be insidious in onset. A sudden onset of inflammatory arthritis is more consistent with infection, crystalline arthritis, or a hypersensitivity reaction.

The presence of extraarticular symptoms in the skin, eyes, mucous membranes, and major organs suggests an under-

TABLE 93.1. Causes of Monarthritis

Inflammatory	
Infection	Bacterial and fungal infection, Lyme disease, viral infection (hepatitis B and C, HIV, parvovirus)
Crystals	Gout, pseudogout
Noninflammatory	
Osteoarthritis	
Ischemic necrosis	
Trauma	

TABLE 93.2. Causes of Polyarthritis

Inflammatory
Peripheral with axial involvement
Ankylosing spondylitis, Reiter syndrome, enteropathic arthritis, psoriatic arthritis
Peripheral asymmetric
Psoriatic arthritis, polyarticular gout, acute rheumatic fever, bacterial endocarditis, sarcoidosis
Peripheral symmetric
Rheumatoid arthritis, SLE, hepatitis B, serum sickness
Noninflammatory
Osteoarthritis
Hemochromatosis
Acromegaly
Amyloidosis

SLE, systemic lupus erythematosus.

lying inflammatory arthropathy or autoimmune disorder. Characteristic skin eruptions are observed in SLE, psoriatic arthritis, sarcoidosis, Reiter syndrome, and vasculitis. Ocular involvement is a frequent occurrence in Reiter syndrome, Sjögren syndrome, and sarcoidosis. A significant number of patients with Sjögren syndrome who present with xerostomia, vague arthralgias, and fatigue are misdiagnosed because of poor history taking. Vaginal dryness is also common and should be addressed if Sjögren syndrome is suspected. Painless oral ulcers are seen in patients with SLE; in persons with Behçet disease or inflammatory bowel disease, the ulcers are usually painful. Serositis is not uncommon in SLE but quite rare in RA. Interstitial lung disease, occasionally resulting in pulmonary hypertension, appears more commonly in mixed connective tissue disease, sarcoidosis, and scleroderma. Cold-induced vasospasm or Raynaud phenomenon also suggests SLE, scleroderma, or mixed connective tissue disease. Disorders of cognition can occur in SLE or Lyme disease, whereas peripheral neuropathies can be associated with a number of disorders, including RA, SLE, Lyme disease, vasculitis, and sarcoidosis.

Questions regarding functional losses are vital for determining the impact of disease on a patient. The ability to dress, groom, and perform the activities of daily living should be assessed. Patients with painful tender joints often have difficulty with simple tasks such as cutting meat, opening faucets, ascending stairs, and turning the ignition key. The ability to perform these tasks is often taken for granted or not inquired about in a short interview, and as a result, the patient may be left feeling isolated and helpless.

PHYSICAL EXAMINATION

The physical examination is an extension of the history and is guided by the same principal questions:

- Is the involvement articular or nonarticular?
- Is the process inflammatory or noninflammatory, diffuse or focal?
- What is the pattern of involvement, and is evidence of extraarticular disease observed?

The examination should be performed in an orderly sequence of inspection, palpation, and evaluation of range of motion. The cardinal findings of articular inflammation are joint margin tenderness, pain with motion, and swelling.

Inspection of the joints and periarticular structures for swelling, erythema, or deformities should help to localize the anatomic site of pain. Deformities can arise as a result of subluxation, ankylosis, synovitis, contracture, bony enlargement, or ligamentous inflammation. Close scrutiny of extraarticular sites can also provide important information. Characteristic skin lesions, including the malar rash of SLE, papulosquamous lesions in psoriasis and Reiter syndrome, and erythema nodosum associated with sarcoidosis and inflammatory bowel disease, are important clues. Ocular findings such as iritis and conjunctivitis may be indicators of an underlying spondylarthropathy, and dry eyes and mucous membranes are important features of Sjögren syndrome. Aphthous ulcers occur in Behçet disease and inflammatory bowel disease, in contrast to the erythematous lesions seen in SLE. Extensor nodules usually indicate RA but may also be seen in SLE and acute rheumatic fever.

Palpation of the joint reveals the presence or absence of synovial thickening, crepitus, tenderness, and warmth. Determining specific areas of tenderness can help to distinguish bursal inflammation from synovitis or tendinitis. Special attention should be focused on the extent and distribution of synovial swelling, tenderness, and warmth.

The active and passive movement of a joint through the range of motion can be very useful to the clinician. The patient is asked to imitate the examiner by moving the joint through the entire range of motion (active motion). If the complete range cannot be attained, the examiner moves the joint (passive motion). Normal passive but abnormal active range of motion is observed in patients with muscle, ligament, or tendon abnormalities. When the range of motion is equally diminished actively and passively, a block in the joint should be suspected, such as frozen shoulder or synovitis. Reproduction of a distinctive pattern of pain and limitation in a joint subjected to resisted movement helps to identify focal areas of tissue inflammation. For example, pain in the shoulder induced by resisted abduction of this joint arises from the supraspinatus muscle, whereas the pain of biceps tendinitis is increased following resisted supination of the forearm.

The distribution of objective joint findings helps in identifying the underlying cause. The axial skeleton (spine, hips, and shoulders) is involved in the spondylarthropathies (ankylosing spondylitis, Reiter syndrome, psoriatic arthritis, and enteropathic arthritis). A useful maneuver to assess lumbar mobility is the Schober test. A mark is made on the mid back at the level of the posterior iliac spine while the patient is standing. A second mark is placed 10 cm above the first, and the patient bends forward maximally. The two marks should be separated by at least 15 cm. Expansion to less than this amount is suggestive of a spondylarthropathy.

When the peripheral skeleton is examined, the small joints of the hands and feet deserve special attention. Symmetric swelling of the metacarpophalangeal and proximal interphalangeal joints suggests RA or SLE. Distal interphalangeal pain and swelling are associated with osteoarthritis or psoriatic arthritis. Diffuse swelling of a finger or toe ("sausage digit," or dactylitis) is commonly observed in the spondylarthropathies, particularly psoriatic arthritis and Reiter syndrome. A careful examination of the knees for signs of inflammation, decreased range of motion, locking, and crepitus should be carried out. Detection of a knee effusion can be very helpful because this joint is readily aspirated.

A complete neurologic examination, including tests of motor and sensory function in the peripheral extremities, is essential. Neuropathic and myopathic processes can mimic joint pain and also frequently accompany the different forms of inflammatory arthritis.

LABORATORY AND IMAGING STUDIES

In most circumstances, the diagnosis is clear by the end of the history and physical examination. Nevertheless, laboratory studies help to confirm clinical impressions and can provide measures of disease extent and severity. It is vital to be able to interpret the results of these tests to prevent unnecessary patient anxiety and further expensive testing. Patients who have an acute onset of inflammatory joint pain with symptoms lasting more than 6 weeks or systemic symptoms often require more extensive evaluation.

Routine blood cell counts, a urinalysis, and blood chemistries should be performed in all patients in whom a systemic inflammatory or infectious disease is suspected. The erythrocyte sedimentation rate (ESR) can help to differentiate inflammatory from noninflammatory musculoskeletal disorders, but the test is nonspecific and has not proved useful for screening. A Westergren ESR of more than 100 mm/h is generally seen only in systemic inflammatory, infectious, or neoplastic disease. The C-reactive protein level rises and falls quickly in response to inflammation and, unlike the ESR, is not influenced by anemia or elevated γ-globulins. The uric acid levels are usually elevated in patients with gout but may also be normal because they often fall during an acute attack (see Chapter 95). Tests for antinuclear antibodies and rheumatoid factor should be ordered for patients suspected of having SLE, RA, or a connective tissue disease (scleroderma, polymyositis, mixed connective tissue disease), but the specificity of these tests is poor, and the results can lead to an improper diagnosis if not placed in clinical context.

Synovial fluid analysis is mandatory in patients who present with acute monarticular arthritis or polyarthritis with fever. A white blood cell count, Gram stain, culture, and sensitivity and crystal analysis of the fluid help to differentiate noninflammatory from inflammatory effusions and confirm the presence of crystalline or infectious arthritis (Table 93.3). If only a few drops of synovial fluid are withdrawn, preference should be given to Gram stain and culture to exclude an infectious condition.

The findings on plain x-ray films are frequently normal in early inflammatory arthritis, although joint effusions and soft tissue swelling are often present. Roentgenography is important to exclude a fracture or foreign body. Special views of the sacroiliac joints can confirm the diagnosis of a spondylarthropathy, and calcification of joint cartilage seen on plain x-ray films of the knees, wrists, and symphysis pubis is a characteristic feature of calcium pyrophosphate deposition disease. It is important to point out that degenerative changes of sclerosis, joint space narrowing, and osteophytes are seen on the roentgenograms of most patients older than 60 years of age, and these findings frequently do not correlate with symptoms. Therefore, degenerative changes on an x-ray film may not explain the cause of a particular musculoskeletal complaint in an older patient.

Radionuclide scintigraphy (bone scan) provides information about distribution and extent of an arthropathy but is nonspecific, thereby providing little information regarding the underlying cause. In a patient with refractory pain, a bone scan can be useful to exclude a stress fracture missed on a radiograph. Magnetic resonance imaging (MRI) provides clear images of the cervical and lumbar spine and is useful in defining the architecture of peripheral joints, especially when a mechanical problem such as a rotator cuff tear or a torn meniscus in the knee is sought. Computed tomography can also be used to assess the axial spine, but imaging of the peripheral joints is limited by its relatively poor contrast resolution in comparison with that of MRI. Open MRI is now available for patients with claustrophobia, which makes the procedure more tolerable.

CONSIDERATIONS IN PREGNANCY

Most women experience musculoskeletal symptoms at some point during pregnancy. Generally, the problems are transient, but in some cases, short-term and even permanent disability can develop. The clinician needs to be aware of these conditions because simple interventions often provide dramatic relief. Patients presenting with hip pain in the third trimester require a prompt and thorough evaluation because two conditions affecting this joint, osteonecrosis of the femoral head and transient osteoporosis of the hip, can result in joint destruction, pain, and immobility.

Hormonal and mechanical alterations occurring during pregnancy can have profound effects on musculoskeletal structures. The release of the hormone relaxin causes increased

TABLE 93.3. Synovial Fluid Analysis

Type	Appearance	Cell count (WBCs/μL)	Etiology
Normal	Clear	<200	Physiologic
Noninflammatory	Clear yellow	200–5,000	Osteoarthritis, trauma
Inflammatory	Cloudy yellow	5,000–50,000	Crystalline arthritis, rheumatoid arthritis, SLE, seronegative arthritis[a]
Septic	Purulent	>60% PMNs >50,000	Infection (occasionally crystalline arthritis)
Hemorrhagic	Bloody	>85% PMNs RBCs predominant	Trauma, coagulopathy, sickle cell anemia

[a]Seronegative arthritis: psoriatic and enteropathic arthritis, ankylosing spondylitis, enteropathic arthritis.
PMNs, polymorphonuclear leukocytes; SLE, systemic lupus erythematosus; WBC, white blood cell.

mobility and widening of the sacroiliac joints and symphysis pubis at the same time that the enlarging uterus is placing a greater strain on the lumbar spine and sacroiliac region. Progressive edema of the upper extremities can compress adjacent joint structures, including nerves and tendons, and changes in nutritional requirements can result in deficiencies of important vitamins and minerals. Knowledge of these changes, combined with attention to anatomy and disturbed function, helps in making the proper diagnosis.

Low back pain is a common complaint, and the frequency of this problem increases with parity and maternal age. Initially, the pain and tenderness are usually localized to the sacroiliac joints, but they often progress to involve the lower lumbar region, with radiation to the back of the thigh. In one study, pelvic girdle pain developed in up to 20% of pregnant outpatients during gestation as a consequence of pelvic girdle syndrome, symphysiolysis, or sacroiliac dysfunction. Fibromyalgia and a herniated disc can also cause low back pain, but these entities should be readily diagnosed by history and physical examination.

Fibromyalgia is often described as diffuse muscle aching and fatigue with diagnostic tender points on examination. The pain from a herniated disc is referred to the lower extremities and may be associated with focal weakness and a loss of deep tendon reflexes in a radicular distribution.

Generalized edema can compress nerves and tendons in the wrist, resulting in carpal tunnel syndrome and de Quervain tenosynovitis. Carpal tunnel syndrome most often presents as nocturnal numbness, tingling, and pain in the hand during the second and third trimesters of pregnancy. These symptoms can be induced by having the patient flex both wrists (Phalen sign) or by tapping over the median nerve with a reflex hammer (Tinel sign). The symptoms are relieved by wearing nocturnal wrist splints and almost always resolve completely after delivery. The presentation of de Quervain tenosynovitis is pain at the base of the thumb that migrates to the hand or forearm. The extensor pollicis brevis and abductor pollicis longus tendons run in a common sheath adjacent to the styloid process. Synovitis is caused by friction (presumably triggered by edema) between the tendon sheath and styloid process. On examination, tenderness is noted over the radial styloid, frequently accompanied by crepitus. In the Finkelstein test, passive ulnar deviation of the wrist while the thumb is flexed over the palm usually reproduces the pain. Unlike carpal tunnel syndrome, de Quervain tenosynovitis tends to manifest postpartum and is often exacerbated by carrying the newborn baby.

Hip pain in a pregnant patient requires careful evaluation. Frequently, the pain emanates from the outer aspect of the hip over the greater trochanter and radiates down the outer aspect of the thigh. This pattern of discomfort is most commonly caused by trochanteric bursitis, not by any problems intrinsic to the hip joint. The pain can be induced by palpating over the site of the bursa and is not increased by passive or active movement of the hip. True hip pain is often located in the groin and radiates into the thigh. Hip pain in the third trimester may be secondary to osteonecrosis or transient osteoporosis of the femoral head. In both conditions, internal rotation of the hip and weight bearing elicit pain.

In most patients, musculoskeletal problems can be diagnosed by the history and physical examination. Patients with persistent severe low back pain, progressive neurologic symptoms in a radicular pattern, or hip pain may require imaging studies. Plain roentgenography should be avoided in the first trimester because of possible adverse fetal effects, and the findings are often normal in the early phases of osteonecrosis and lumbar disc disease. MRI provides detailed anatomic images of the spine and presumably does not pose a threat to the fetus, although long-term follow-up studies are not available.

BIBLIOGRAPHY

Albert HB, Godskesen M, Westergaard JG. Incidence of four syndromes of pregnancy-related pelvic joint pain. *Spine* 2002;27:2831–2834.

Colletti PM, Sylvestre PB. Magnetic resonance imaging in pregnancy. *Magn Reson Imaging Clin N Am* 1994;2:291–307.

Kanal E. Pregnancy and the safety of magnetic resonance imaging. *Magn Reson Imaging Clin N Am* 1994;2:309–317.

Kim EA, Lee KS, Johkoh T, et al. Interstitial lung diseases associated with collagen vascular diseases: radiologic and histopathologic findings. *Radiographics* 2002;22[Spec No]:S151–S165.

Lawrence RC, Helmick CG, Arnett FC, et al. Estimates of the prevalence of arthritis and selected musculoskeletal disorders in the United States. *Arthritis Rheum* 1998;41:778–799.

Noren L, Ostgaard S, Johansson G, et al. Lumbar back and posterior pelvic pain during pregnancy: a 3-year follow-up. *Eur Spine J* 2002;11:267–271.

Pozderac RV. Longitudinal tibial fatigue fracture: an uncommon stress fracture with characteristic features. *Clin Nucl Med* 2002;27:475–478.

Von Muhlen CA, Tan EM. Autoantibodies in the diagnosis of systemic rheumatic diseases. *Semin Arthritis Rheum* 1995;24:323–358.

Yelin E, Callahan LF. The economic cost and social and psychological impact of musculoskeletal conditions. National Arthritis Data Work Groups. *Arthritis Rheum* 1995;38:1351–1362.

CHAPTER 94
Inflammatory Arthritis

Charlene B. Varnis

Chronic inflammatory arthritis occurs in a number of rheumatologic diseases, of which rheumatoid arthritis (RA) is the most common. RA is a polyarticular and systemic disease that affects women two to three times more often than men; the peak incidence is in women in the fourth through sixth decades. Chronic inflammatory arthritis is also a manifestation of psoriatic arthritis, one of the seronegative spondylarthropathies, which can be distinguished from RA by the absence of rheumatoid factor, variable involvement of the sacroiliac joints (sacroiliitis) and spine (spondylitis), enthesitis (inflammation of tendons and ligament insertions on bone), and dactylitis (inflammation of joints and soft tissues of a digit that results in a "sausage" appearance).

RHEUMATOID ARTHRITIS

RA occurs in a worldwide distribution, affecting all races and ethnic groups. In the United States, the incidence of RA is 0.3% to 1.5%, with women more frequently affected. Familial clusters of cases are seen, suggesting genetic susceptibility to development of the disorder. The existence of a genetic component is further supported by a concordance rate of 15.2% in monozygotic twins, versus a rate of 3.6% in dizygotic twins. The rather low rate of concordance in monozygotic twins suggests that environmental factors play a major role in the development of RA. Genetic susceptibility is associated with the class II histocompatibility gene product HLA-DR4. The HLA-DR4 antigen confers a fourfold risk for the development of RA in Caucasians, with some variation seen in certain ethnic groups. In some populations, an additional HLA antigen, HLA-DR1, may be associated with a risk for development of the disease.

The cause of RA is unknown, although a potential role for infectious agents has long been of interest. No organism has been identified as the etiologic agent. The primary site of involvement in RA is the synovial lining of diarthrodial joints, usually a thin layer of tissue only one to three cell layers thick with no basement membrane; this becomes chronically inflamed and thickened. It is likely that in the initial stage of RA, the inflammatory response is triggered by an unknown antigen that reaches the synovial tissue via the circulation and is mediated by $CD4^+$ T lymphocytes. Cells at the site of inflammation release cytokines, such as interleukin-1 (IL-1) and tumor necrosis factor-α (TNF-α), which are important in driving both acute and chronic inflammation in RA.

The inflammatory response progresses with synovial proliferation, edema, and the formation of new blood vessels. The resulting proliferative synovium, or pannus, releases damaging enzymes into the joint that degrade the structural components of cartilage and bone. Damage occurs at bare areas of bone located at the margins of joints, where the synovium directly attaches. Microscopically, the pannus can be seen invading these parts of the joint, which correspond to areas of erosion visible on radiographs.

Clinical Features

RA is a systemic disease that initially presents with articular involvement. Often, the onset of arthritis is accompanied by constitutional symptoms, such as fatigue and malaise, reflecting the systemic nature of the disorder. In 55% to 70% of patients, joint pain and stiffness develop insidiously over weeks to months. The typical pattern is symmetric polyarticular involvement of the small joints of the hands, wrists, and feet. Stiffness lasting more than 30 minutes is significant for inflammatory involvement. Such stiffness is most marked after prolonged inactivity, particularly on awakening. Stiffness lessens with movement and use of the affected joints. In 8% to 15% of patients, RA presents with the acute development of pain and swelling within a few days. An intermediate onset of symptoms over days to weeks occurs in 15% to 20% of patients.

The metacarpophalangeal (MCP) and proximal interphalangeal (PIP) joints of the hands may be involved, but the distal interphalangeal (DIP) joints are almost always spared. Stiffness and pain often precede observable swelling. In the feet, metatarsophalangeal (MTP) joint involvement results in pain in the forefoot, particularly when the patient walks without shoes. The consequences of persistent synovitis include muscular atrophy, contractures, and a decreased range of motion of the affected joints. Deformities of the hands, such as ulnar deviation at the MCP joints, can progress to ulnar subluxation, which limits the ability to grasp and to extend the fingers. Similarly, palmar subluxation of the fingers at the MCP joints causes functional limitation, as do swan neck (DIP flexion with PIP hyperextension) and boutonnière (DIP hyperextension with PIP flexion) deformities of the fingers. Pannus involving the extensor tendons of the fingers can lead to extensor tendon rupture, which causes a loss of active extension of the affected fingers. Surgical intervention is required to correct the abnormality. Inflammation of the extensor carpi ulnaris tendon leads to pain and swelling at the ulnar styloid of the wrist. Foot deformities lead to abnormal mechanics, with loss of the metatarsal arch, severe hallux valgus, and plantar subluxation of the MTP joints leading to cock-up toe deformities.

Large joints of the extremities can be involved, including the knees, talar and subtalar joints, shoulders, and elbows. When the knee joint is involved, an accumulation of fluid in the gastrocnemius-semitendinosus bursa (Baker cyst) can produce the symptom of popliteal fullness. Rupture of the cyst leads to calf pain and swelling that mimic a deep venous thrombosis.

In the cervical spine, the junction of the first and second cervical vertebrae (C1-C2 articulation) or the apophyseal joints of the lower cervical levels can be involved. Synovial destruction at the C1-2 articulation can lead to instability of the joint and a risk for subluxation and spinal cord compression. Whenever a patient with RA requires intubation for general anesthesia, cervical spine radiographs should be obtained that include flexion and extension views to document possible instability of C1-2 before the neck is manipulated in any way, such as during oral intubation.

The clinician should be aware that hoarseness in a patient with RA may signify involvement of the cricoarytenoid joint. If movement of the cricoarytenoid is impaired as a result of rheumatoid inflammation, lung aspiration can occur.

A number of extraarticular manifestations in RA reinforce the systemic nature of the disease. Involvement at extraarticular sites can be clinically significant. It is important to perform a systems review to identify possible extraarticular involvement.

Rheumatoid nodules are seen in 30% to 40% of patients with classic RA, almost always in association with positive serum rheumatoid factor. They most commonly develop in subcutaneous locations, such as the extensor surface of the elbow, or at pressure sites, such as the occipital scalp, sacrum, and heels. The nodules are rarely painful, but depending on their location, they can mechanically interfere with function.

Nervous system involvement often presents as an entrapment syndrome when synovitis causes a median, ulnar, or posterior tibial neuropathy. The simultaneous occurrence of several isolated mononeuropathies (mononeuritis multiplex) may be a manifestation of rheumatoid vasculitis.

Pulmonary involvement includes pleural effusions, parenchymal rheumatoid nodules, and diffuse interstitial pulmonary fibrosis. Pericarditis is the most common cardiac manifestation. Occasionally, nodular disease or nonspecific myocarditis leads to conduction abnormalities.

The eyes can be affected by keratoconjunctivitis sicca, with symptoms of dryness, foreign body sensation, burning, and thick discharge. Inflammatory lesions of the eye may also occur, including episcleritis, scleritis, keratitis, and corneal ulceration. A painful eye should alert the physician to obtain a prompt ophthalmologic evaluation because scleritis or corneal inflammation with or without ulceration can progress rapidly and lead to complications, including perforation.

Clinically apparent vasculitis is a rare complication, usually seen in patients with long-standing seropositive disease. Cutaneous lesions are the most common manifestation of rheumatoid vasculitis and include periungual infarcts and vasculitic ulcers. Constitutional symptoms such as weight loss occur. Mononeuritis multiplex is the classic neurologic manifestation. The heart, lungs, and rarely the gastrointestinal tract can be involved.

Felty syndrome develops in patients with long-standing deforming RA who have seropositive nodular disease. Leukopenia and splenomegaly complete the syndrome. Neutropenia ($<100/mm^3$) correlates with increased bacterial infections in these patients. They may also have skin ulcerations and thrombocytopenia, and the syndrome can be present without active synovitis.

Laboratory and Imaging Studies

In the evaluation of a patient suspected of having RA, several laboratory studies help in the diagnosis, although none of these tests alone is considered diagnostic. Rheumatoid factor is present in 75% of patients. However, it must be recognized that rheumatoid factor is found not only in RA but also in other autoimmune diseases, such as primary Sjögren syndrome, certain chronic bacterial infections, a number of viral diseases, and several other idiopathic inflammatory diseases, such as sarcoidosis. The presence of rheumatoid factor in the sera of patients with RA is associated with more aggressive joint disease and a greater frequency of extraarticular manifestations.

The erythrocyte sedimentation rate (ESR) reflects inflammatory activity and can be elevated in a large variety of disorders, including other inflammatory arthritides, chronic and acute infections, chronic renal failure and end-stage renal disease, chronic hepatic disease, and malignancy, and after surgery. The ESR is mildly elevated during pregnancy. It is usually elevated in active RA, and elevation often correlates with disease activity.

Antinuclear antibody (ANA) may be present in patients with RA. Studies report a wide range in the frequency of ANA positivity (14%–60%). Patients with RA are more likely to be positive for ANA when they are also positive for rheumatoid factor, and ANA positivity is more likely in the setting of Sjögren syndrome. Rheumatoid factor and ANA can be present in a number of arthritides, and to reach a correct diagnosis, the results of these tests must be considered in the context of a carefully obtained history and the physical examination findings.

Radiographs, particularly of the hands, wrists, and feet, can be characteristic. In early disease, the findings may be normal. Later in the course, osteopenia develops in bone adjacent to the joints (juxtaarticular osteopenia), the joint spaces narrow diffusely, and erosions starting at the joint margins may be present.

The diagnosis of RA is based on the clinical history and presentation, laboratory evaluation, and radiographic findings. The American Rheumatism Association 1987 revised criteria may be helpful in guiding the diagnosis but are most applicable to defining populations for scientific studies (Table 94.1).

Treatment

Evidence suggests that in patients with RA, most of the damage occurs and disability progresses most rapidly during the first 2 years of disease. As a result, the approach to the treatment of RA has evolved to be more aggressive earlier in the course. The therapeutic goal is to administer medications that control inflammation and symptoms as soon as possible, in addition to other medications, disease-modifying antirheumatic drugs (DMARDs), that have the potential to reduce the destructive progression of the disease.

Nonsteroidal antiinflammatory drugs (NSAIDs) are used to reduce the symptoms and signs of inflammation and relieve pain. They have no major effect on the underlying RA disease process. The major pharmacologic action of this class of drugs is to inhibit cyclooxygenase, the enzyme that transforms arachidonic acid to prostaglandins, prostacyclins, and thromboxane. These products of the arachidonic pathway have homeostatic and cytoprotective effects in addition to proinflammatory actions. Thus, the NSAIDs are effective antiinflammatory agents but also have a wide array of potentially toxic effects, including gastric irritation, peptic ulcer formation, antiplatelet actions, reversible hepatocellular injury, reduced creatinine clearance, and acute interstitial nephritis. More recently, drugs such as rofecoxib and celecoxib have been developed that are selective for the COX-2 isoenzyme of cyclooxygenase; these inhibit the production of proinflammatory prostaglandins but have less effect on the products of the arachidonic acid pathway with cytoprotective properties. It has been shown that the COX-2 inhibitors are less likely to cause gastric irritation, ulcers, and antiplatelet effects.

Corticosteroids have potent antiinflammatory effects, and when given in low doses equivalent to 10 mg of prednisone or less daily, they can be a helpful adjunct in the treatment of RA, particularly to control inflammation while a DMARD is started. Even at low doses, corticosteroids may be associated with an accelerated loss of bone density, adrenal suppression, hypertension, hyperglycemia, mild fluid retention, and a redistribution of body fat. Other side effects that are probably rare at the lower-dose regimens are avascular necrosis, increased risk for infection, and cataracts. When corticosteroids are used to treat synovitis, they should be tapered because very gradual dose reductions are better tolerated. Intraarticular corticosteroids are often effective when inflammation is limited to one or two joints. It must be emphasized, however, that joint aspiration should be performed with Gram stain analysis and cultures to exclude the possibility of septic arthritis, particularly in a patient with no other sites of joint flare or symptoms of disease.

A DMARD should be considered for any patient with active inflammation or with factors indicating a poor prognosis, including female gender, positivity for rheumatoid factor, early erosions, nodules, and other extraarticular involvement. The DMARDs have diverse mechanisms of action that reduce inflammatory disease activity, damage, and the progression of RA. Drugs in this category include hydroxychloroquine, methotrexate, auranofin (oral gold), injectable gold, sulfasalazine, D-penicillamine, azathioprine, leflunomide, TNF-α inhibitors, and IL-1 inhibitor therapies.

Hydroxychloroquine is generally well tolerated but has a delayed onset of action at 3 to 6 months and is often reserved for mild RA. Potential side effects include dermatitis, nausea, headache, blurred vision, myopathy, and hemolytic anemia. Retinopathy may occur with an incidence of no more than 0.5%. The earliest changes in the retina are asymptomatic but can be detected by a careful ophthalmologic examination performed every 6 to 12 months. If any signs of retinal toxicity are seen, hydroxychloroquine should be discontinued.

Sulfasalazine has been approved by the Food and Drug Administration for the treatment of RA and is sometimes chosen for mild disease; its onset of action is at 6 to 12 weeks. Side effects include gastrointestinal upset, rash, drug-induced hepatitis, bone marrow suppression, idiopathic agranulocytosis, hemolytic anemia, reversible depression of sperm count in men, and rare instances of a lupus-like illness.

Methotrexate has become an important treatment for RA, favored by many as the DMARD of choice for patients with active, aggressive inflammation early in the course of the disease. It has a significant antiinflammatory effect, and a response is usually seen within 3 to 4 weeks after the initiation of therapy. Methotrexate is given as a single dose *once a week*. Stomatitis, nausea,

TABLE 94.1. Classification Criteria for Rheumatoid Arthritis

Morning stiffness lasting at least 1 hour
Arthritis involving at least three joint locations
Arthritis of hand joints (wrist, MCP, or PIP)
Symmetric arthritis
Rheumatoid nodules
Elevated serum rheumatoid factor
Roentgenographic abnormalities (well-defined juxtaarticular osteopenia or bony erosions)

Note: The first four criteria must be present at least 6 weeks. A diagnosis of rheumatoid arthritis is made if four of the seven criteria are present.
MCP, metacarpophalangeal; PIP, proximal interphalangeal.
Source: Adapted from Arnett FC, Edworthy SM, Block DA, et al. The American Rheumatism Association 1987 revised criteria for the classification of rheumatoid arthritis. *Arthritis Rheum* 1988;31:315, with permission.

vomiting, bone marrow suppression, hepatotoxicity with fibrosis and cirrhosis, lung hypersensitivity reactions, and teratogenesis are potential toxic effects of the drug. Supplementation with 1 mg of folic acid daily is helpful in preventing stomatitis and nausea without affecting efficacy. The risk for methotrexate-related hepatotoxicity is increased by alcohol intake, and patients should abstain from alcohol while on this medication. Fatty liver, as in obese or diabetic patients, may also increase the risk for hepatotoxicity. Trimethoprim/sulfamethoxazole antibiotics can cause synergistic toxic effects, including severe bone marrow suppression. Laboratory monitoring with complete blood cell counts and liver function tests should be performed regularly while a patient is taking methotrexate.

Gold compounds were used extensively to treat RA before methotrexate became the mainstay of therapy in the 1980s. Metaanalysis of past studies has shown that although the efficacy of parenteral gold was similar to that of methotrexate and sulfasalazine, its greater toxicity frequently led to discontinuation of the drug, and it is not commonly prescribed now. Rash and stomatitis are the most common side effects. Other serious side effects include immune complex-mediated membranous glomerulonephritis, leukopenia, thrombocytopenia, and rare instances of aplastic anemia. Oral gold (auranofin) is less efficacious than the other DMARDs and is used infrequently.

Azathioprine is an immunosuppressive drug that has been shown to be an effective treatment for RA. It is usually reserved for patients who have not responded to other therapies. A risk for lymphoreticular neoplasm may be associated with long-term use. Immunosuppression, myelosuppression, hepatotoxicity, nausea, gastrointestinal intolerance, and macrocytic anemia are side effects of the drug. The concomitant use of allopurinol or angiotensin-converting enzyme inhibitors and renal insufficiency are risk factors for myelosuppression. A response may begin after 12 weeks of treatment. Monitoring with complete blood cell counts is necessary.

The efficacy of D-penicillamine has been shown to be similar to that of intramuscular gold and azathioprine, but a significant number of side effects, including leukopenia, thrombocytopenia, rash, proteinuria, lupus-like disease, polymyositis, myasthenia gravis, and Goodpasture syndrome, have limited it use in the treatment of RA.

Leflunomide is a recent addition to the disease-modifying treatments for RA. Its efficacy is similar to that of methotrexate and sulfasalazine, with a response occurring by 2 to 3 months. In clinical trials, it has been shown to decrease the rate of radiographic progression of RA in comparison with placebo. Leflunomide can cause diarrhea, skin rash, hair thinning, and liver function abnormalities. The drug has a long half-life of about 16 days. The administration of cholestyramine increases the rate of drug excretion and quickly lowers the serum level and is recommended if serious side effects occur.

Drugs that work by inhibiting the proinflammatory cytokine TNF-α have been shown to decrease the inflammatory symptoms of RA and reduce the radiographic progression of disease, and they have become very important in the treatment of RA. Three TNF-α inhibitors are currently approved for the treatment of RA. Etanercept is a recombinant fusion protein consisting of soluble TNF-α receptor linked to the Fc portion of human immunoglobulin G1 (IgG1). It is administered by subcutaneous injection twice weekly. Infliximab is a chimeric IgG1 monoclonal antibody directed against TNF-α that is given to persons on methotrexate as an intravenous infusion at weeks 0, 2, and 6 and then every 8 weeks. Adalimumab is a recombinant human IgG1 monoclonal antibody against TNF-α that is administered as a subcutaneous injection every other week. Patients treated with these drugs often experience robust relief of inflammatory symptoms. For example, of patients treated with etanercept, 70% achieve 20% or greater improvement, 40% are 50% better, and 15% achieve 70% or greater improvement. A response often occurs within the first 2 weeks. The most common side effects are reactions at the local injection site for the subcutaneously administered drugs and occasional infusion reactions with infliximab. These drugs, by inhibiting TNF-α, may reduce natural defenses against certain infections. Reactivation of tuberculosis has been reported, and purified protein derivative (PPD) placement is recommended before therapy is initiated. Other serious infections have been reported, and patients should be advised to discontinue the drug while undergoing treatment for infection. Cases of multiple sclerosis, lupus-like illness, and lymphoma have been reported in persons treated with this class of drugs.

A drug that targets the proinflammatory cytokine IL-1 is available for the treatment of RA. Anakinra is a human recombinant IL-1 receptor antagonist that is administered by daily subcutaneous injection. It has been shown to reduce inflammatory disease activity and the radiologic progression of RA. Reactions at the injection site are the most common side effect. Immunosuppression and an increased risk for infection or malignancy were not identified in initial controlled trials.

An important aspect in the treatment of RA is patient education about the fluctuating nature of the disease and its systemic features, including fatigue. Advice regarding structuring rest periods during the course of the day can be helpful. Physical and occupational therapists can teach the patient proper techniques of joint protection and exercises that maintain range of motion and strength. Joint protection techniques enable the patient to continue performing daily activities while minimizing stress on affected joints. Occupational therapists can fabricate splints that are useful in resting actively inflamed joints and also provide patients with adaptive equipment.

Considerations in Pregnancy

RA generally remits during pregnancy, but it is common to see the arthritis flare postpartum, particularly in lactating women. High levels of prolactin may play a role in the inflammatory response.

Very few studies have examined the effects of inflammatory arthritis on pregnancy. Two studies have demonstrated that lower-birth-weight infants are born to mothers with inflammatory arthritis. One of these also found a higher incidence of preeclampsia and prematurity in mothers with inflammatory arthritis. The reasons for the findings are unknown.

Pregnancy in a patient undergoing treatment for RA raises concerns regarding the safety of the medications during gestation. Aspirin and NSAIDs cross the placenta and have been associated with prolongation of gestation and labor, more pronounced maternal anemia, greater intrapartum blood loss, and possible premature closure of the ductus arteriosus. Maternal use of indomethacin has been associated with reduced fetal urine production and oligohydramnios. Maternal use of aspirin is associated with increased cutaneous and intracranial bleeding in preterm and low-birth-weight infants, and aspirin should be discontinued at least 2 weeks before delivery. The American Academy of Pediatrics considers indomethacin, ibuprofen, naproxen, tolmetin, diclofenac, and piroxicam to be compatible with breast-feeding. Only trace levels of ibuprofen are detected in breast milk, and ibuprofen is the favored drug for lactating women. Daily and repeated doses of aspirin of 3 g or more can produce variable amounts of salicylate in breast milk, which may be sufficient to cause metabolic acidosis, altered pulmonary circulation, and bleeding in the nursing infant. Aspirin should be avoided by lactating women.

Experience with the use of DMARDs during pregnancy is variable. Although hydroxychloroquine can cross the placenta, it has not been associated with any fetal effect and can be continued during pregnancy if necessary. Sulfasalazine has been used to treat inflammatory bowel disease during pregnancy and has been found safe during both pregnancy and lactation. Folic acid supplementation should be given when a patient is treated with this medication. The literature describes a small series of patients with organ transplants who have had successful pregnancies while taking azathioprine. However, low levels of the drug and its metabolites are found in breast milk, and therefore its use is not advised in nursing mothers. Gold salts have been shown to be teratogenic in animal studies and are best avoided during pregnancy and lactation. Methotrexate is teratogenic and associated with increased spontaneous abortion. It is contraindicated during pregnancy, and sexually active women of reproductive age should be practicing effective contraception while on this drug. Methotrexate should be discontinued at least 3 months before conception is attempted. Only trace amounts of the drug are found in breast milk, but adequate data are lacking regarding the effect of even trace amounts on infant health; thus, methotrexate is best avoided during lactation. Leflunomide is teratogenic and contraindicated in pregnancy. If a woman who has been taking the drug is planning to conceive, the administration of cholestyramine (8 g three times a day for 11 days) will accelerate elimination of the drug; otherwise, complete elimination can take up to 2 years. Pregnancy should be avoided until the plasma level of drug is below 0.03 mg/L. Experience with the anticytokine therapies is early, and information regarding safety in pregnancy is lacking. TNF-α and other cytokines are important for both establishing and maintaining a successful gestation. Theoretically, inhibitors of TNF-α can interfere with its effects. However, when etanercept was administered to pregnant rats or rabbits in doses 60- to 100- fold greater than that used in RA, it had no apparent harmful effects on the fetus.

Corticosteroids in low to moderate doses (up to 20 mg of prednisone or the equivalent) are generally safe during pregnancy. They have not been found to cause a significant increase in miscarriages, fetal mortality, prematurity, or congenital anomalies. The maternal use of prednisone has been associated with gestational hypertension and diabetes, although this is probably of greater concern in patients with other rheumatic disorders that require treatment with high doses of steroids. Adrenal suppression in the neonate is rare but can occur with high maternal doses of corticosteroids, and the neonate should be monitored for this possibility. The various forms of corticosteroids differ in regard to placental passage. Prednisone and prednisolone are metabolized in the placenta, have the lowest passage rate, and are the preferred choice for maternal treatment. Minimal excretion of prednisone in breast milk is found at maternal doses of 20 mg or less, and prednisone appears safe in lactating women at these doses. Intraarticular steroids are an excellent choice for treating a patient with RA who experiences a flare in one or two joints while pregnant. Systemic absorption is relatively low, and intraarticular administration can be very effective in relieving the joint flare.

PSORIATIC ARTHRITIS

Psoriatic arthritis is an inflammatory arthropathy that occurs in approximately 5% to 10% of persons with psoriasis; men and women are equally affected. Although joint disease usually follows the onset of skin involvement, it precedes the appearance of psoriasis in up to 21% of cases; joint involvement presents concurrently with the onset of skin disease in up to 11% of cases. The skin involvement may be subtle, with only isolated nail findings of onychodystrophy or pitting, or small plaques in areas of skin that are difficult to observe, such as the scalp, intergluteal fold, and umbilicus.

The cause is unknown, but studies of families and twins suggest a genetic predisposition, with a high concordance rate seen in monozygotic twins. The development of skin or joint disease is much more likely in the first-degree relatives of persons with psoriasis or psoriatic arthritis than in the general population. Class I major histocompatibility antigens are associated with psoriatic arthritis, including HLA-B7, HLA-Cw6, and HLA-B17, whereas the class II antigen HLA-DR4 is associated with RA. The association with the class I major histocompatibility complex suggests that $CD4^+$ T lymphocytes are not mediators of the disease. This suggestion is further supported by the observation that in HIV infection, psoriatic skin and joint disease become very aggressive as the $CD4^+$ T-cell count declines. Guttate psoriasis, consisting of widespread small lesions, can be precipitated by streptococcal upper airway infection, indicating a possible role of bacteria or bacterial antigens in the pathogenesis.

Several patterns of joint involvement are seen. The most common, observed in 40% to 60% of patients, is a polyarticular pattern that is sometimes difficult to distinguish from RA, although the radiographic appearance may provide clues. An oligoarticular pattern (five or fewer affected joints in an asymmetric distribution), often with DIP or flexor tendon involvement and dactylitis, is observed slightly less frequently. Sacroiliitis with or without spondylitis occurs in 20% to 40% of patients, with a predominance in men. Extraarticular manifestations other than skin disease are occasionally seen, with a higher reported incidence of uveitis than that expected in the normal population.

Psoriatic arthritis was once thought to be a mild disease, but this concept has now been challenged. The peripheral arthritis of psoriatic arthritis can be as severe as that of RA, with severe, destructive, and deforming joint disease developing in 20% of patients.

Laboratory and Imaging Studies

No specific laboratory tests are available for psoriatic arthritis. Patients are usually negative for rheumatoid factor. An elevated ESR and mild anemia may be present, but the ESR and blood counts are often normal.

In early disease, radiographs may show no abnormalities. The juxtaarticular osteopenia observed in RA is not typical of psoriatic arthritis. The interphalangeal joints, including the DIP joints, which are usually spared in RA, may fuse or undergo destructive changes, such as erosion of the distal aspect of the phalanx proximal to the joint space and bony proliferation of the adjacent phalanx located distal to the joint. When this change is very advanced, it is described as a "pencil-in-cup" deformity. Resorption of the distal tufts of the fingers is sometimes observed. In the spine, ligamentous ossification results in the formation of syndesmophytes, which are often very large and asymmetric. Bony fusion of the apophyseal joints of the spine may occur. Sacroiliitis may be observed on x-ray films that is often asymmetric; erosions within the sacroiliac joint lead to a widened appearance of the joint, and increased sclerosis eventually progresses to ankylosis.

Treatment

NSAIDs are the initial treatment for psoriatic arthritis, but if the patient does not respond, treatment with DMARDs is begun. Sulfasalazine may be of benefit in the treatment of peripheral arthritis, and methotrexate has been effective in treating both psoriasis and psoriatic arthritis. The TNF-α inhibitors have shown great promise in the treatment of psoriasis and psoriatic arthritis, and etanercept is now approved by the Food and Drug Administration for the treatment of psoriatic arthritis. Intraarticular corticosteroids remain a treatment option when only one or two joints are actively inflamed, provided infection has been ruled out.

Patient education is an important part of treatment, particularly when spondylitis is prominent. The patient must be informed about the disease and the importance of proper posture and exercise. Physical therapy is an essential adjunct to train the patient in flexibility and spine extension. Proper posture encourages a position of function if the spinal disease progresses to fusion.

Considerations in Pregnancy

Relatively few data are available regarding psoriatic arthritis in pregnancy. Generally, women with psoriatic arthritis experience relief during gestation and a reappearance of symptoms during the first 10 weeks postpartum. Psoriatic arthritis does not appear to affect the outcome of pregnancy, including mode of delivery. Please refer to "Considerations in Pregnancy" in the "Rheumatoid Arthritis" section above for a discussion regarding the medications used to treat psoriatic arthritis, particularly the NSAIDs, sulfazaline, methotrexate, and TNF-α inhibitors.

BIBLIOGRAPHY

American College of Rheumatology Ad Hoc Committee on Clinical Guidelines. Guidelines for monitoring drug therapy in rheumatoid arthritis. *Arthritis Rheum* 1996;39:723.

American College of Rheumatology Ad Hoc Committee on Clinical Guidelines. Guidelines for rheumatoid arthritis management. *Arthritis Rheum* 1996;39:713.

Anderson RJ. Rheumatoid arthritis B: clinical and laboratory features. In: Klippel JH, ed. *Primer on the rheumatic diseases*, 12th ed. Atlanta, GA: Arthritis Foundation, 2001:218.

Arend WP, Dayer JM. Inhibition of the production and effects of interleukin-1 and tumor necrosis factor-alpha in rheumatoid arthritis. *Arthritis Rheum* 1995;38:151.

Arnett FC, Edworthy SM, Block DA, et al. The American Rheumatism Association 1987 revised criteria for the classification of rheumatoid arthritis. *Arthritis Rheum* 1988;31:315.

Barrett JH, Brennan P, Fiddler M, et al. Breast-feeding and postpartum relapse in women with rheumatoid arthritis and inflammatory arthritis. *Arthritis Rheum* 2000;43:1010.

Borigini MJ, Paulus HE. Rheumatoid arthritis. In: Weisman MH, Weinblatt ME, Louie JS, eds. *Treatment of the rheumatic diseases*. Philadelphia: WB Saunders, 2001:19.

Bowden AP, Barrett JH, Fallow W, et al. Women with inflammatory polyarthritis have babies of lower birth weight. *J Rheumatol* 2001;28:355.

Buckley LM, Bullaboy CA, Leichtman L, et al. Multiple congenital anomalies associated with weekly low-dose methotrexate treatment of the mother. *Arthritis Rheum* 1997;40:971.

Caldwell JR, Furst DE. The efficacy and safety of low-dose corticosteroids for rheumatoid arthritis. *Semin Arthritis Rheum* 1991;21:1.

Dayer JM, Feige U, et al. Anti-interleukin 1 therapy in rheumatic diseases. *Curr Opin Rheumatol* 2000;13:170.

Furst DE, et al. Consensus Statement. Updated consensus statement on tumour necrosis factor blocking agents for the treatment of rheumatoid arthritis and other rheumatic diseases. *Ann Rheum Dis* 2001;60:iii2.

Gladman DD. Current concepts in psoriatic arthritis. *Curr Opin Rheumatol* 2002;14:361.

Gran JT, Ostensen M. Spondyloarthritides in females. *Baillieres Clin Rheumatol* 1998;12:695.

Harris ED Jr. Clinical features of rheumatoid arthritis. In: Kelley WN Jr, Harris ED Jr, Ruddy S, et al., eds. *Textbook of rheumatology*, 4th ed. Philadelphia: WB Saunders, 1993:874.

Khan MA. Update on spondylarthropathies. *Ann Intern Med* 2002;136:896.

Maini RN, Zvaifler NJ. Rheumatoid arthritis and other synovial disorders. In: Klippel JH, Dieppe PA, eds. *Rheumatology*, 2nd ed. London: Mosby, 1998:5.1.1.

Nelso JL, Ostensen M. Pregnancy and rheumatoid arthritis. *Rheum Dis Clin North Am* 1997;23:195.

Ostensen M. The effect of pregnancy on ankylosing spondylitis, psoriatic arthritis and juvenile rheumatoid arthritis. *Am J Reprod Immunol* 1992;28:235.

Ostensen M. Treatment with immunosuppressive and disease-modifying drugs during pregnancy and lactation. *Am J Reprod Immunol* 1992;28:148.

Ramsey-Goldman R, Schilling E. Immunosuppressive drug use during pregnancy. *Rheum Dis Clin North Am* 1997;23:149.

Silman AJ. Epidemiology of rheumatoid arthritis. *APMIS* 1994;102:721.

Skomsvoll JF, Ostensen M, Irgens LM, et al. Obstetrical and neonatal outcome in pregnant patients with rheumatic disease. *Scand J Rheumatol* 1998;27[Suppl 107]:109.

CHAPTER 95

Crystal-Induced Arthritis: Gout and Pseudogout

Yousaf Ali

GOUT

Definition and Classification

Gout is a syndrome characterized by intermittent, acute swelling of the joints caused by an inflammatory response to monosodium urate (MSU) crystals. Although the host response to MSU crystals is variable, the disease manifests in only a limited number of ways:

- Acute gouty arthritis
- Accumulation of crystalline-rich aggregates (tophi)
- Renal dysfunction (gouty nephropathy).

Etiology

The development of hyperuricemia resulting in clinical events is multifaceted and occurs via two discrete mechanisms. Underexcretion of uric acid is the most common metabolic defect, and although not fully understood, this occurs secondary to a genetic abnormality, at least in certain patients. Approximately 85% of patients with gout are underexcretors of uric acid, with a urate clearance rate of less than 6 mL/min. This is important to know from a therapeutic standpoint because drugs can be used to accelerate the loss of uric acid if the daily tubular excretion is diminished. Occasionally, uric acid is overproduced; overproduction is associated with an excess of purine precursors, either from dietary sources or an abnormal handling of urate. In a very small minority of patients, inherited dysregulation of purine metabolism accounts for the hyperuricemia. In 1964, a familial disorder of urate overproduction combined with neurologic dysfunction and self-mutilation was described that was traced to a deficiency of hypoxanthine-guanine phosphoribosyltransferase (HGPRT). In this rare disease, the Lesch-Nyhan syndrome, the excessive production of uric acid is associated with the juvenile onset of gout.

The renal handling of uric acid remains the key factor in the development of hyperuricemia. Hence, hyperuricemia can be classified according to the underlying mechanism—overproduction or underexcretion of uric acid. This scheme is useful for the clinician attempting to correct the underlying cause of gout and direct therapy (Table 95.1).

The response of cells (usually polymorphonuclear leukocytes) to the presence of MSU crystals is pivotal in the pathophysiology of acute gouty arthritis. During an attack, the activation of signal transduction pathways leads to a rapid influx of neutrophils. Chemotactic factors such as interleukin-1, interleukin-6, and tumor necrosis factor perpetuate this process,

TABLE 95.1. Acquired Causes of Hyperuricemia

Urate overproduction	Urate underexcretion
HGPRT deficiency	Idiopathic
PRPP synthetase superactivity	Enhanced tubular reabsorption
Fructose administration	Lead nephropathy (saturnine gout)
Myeloproliferative disorders	Acidosis
Lymphoproliferative disorders	Hyperparathyroidism, hypothyroidism
Alcohol abuse	Drugs: diuretics, cyclosporine, nicotinic acid, pyrazinamide, low-dose aspirin, ethambutol
Psoriasis	

HGPRT, hypoxanthine-guanine phosphoribosyltransferase; PRPP, phosphoribosyl pyrophosphate.

which results in the systemic features commonly observed (e.g., fever, swelling, leukocytosis).

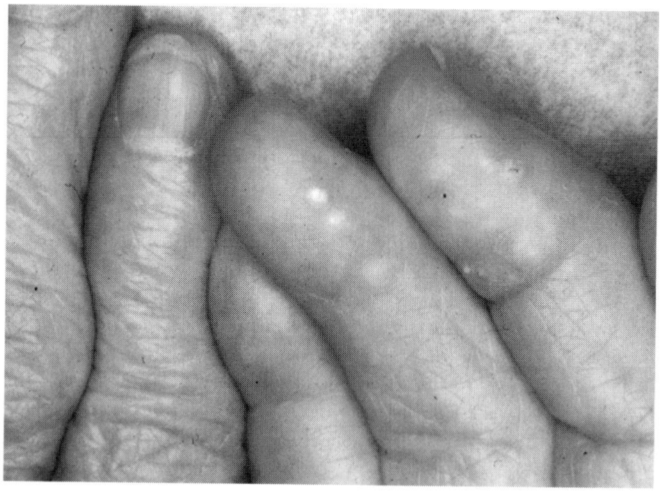

FIG. 95.1. Tophaceous gout affecting the digital pulp. (Photograph courtesy of John Conte, M.D.)

Epidemiology

Gout is predominantly a disease of middle-aged men. It is rare in children and premenopausal women. The peak incidence is in men between 40 and 50 years of age and in women older than 60 years. Estimates of the prevalence of gout vary widely. The prevalence of disease varies with age and increasing serum urate levels. In men, it is estimated to be between 5 and 28 per 1,000, and in women, between 1 and 6 per 1,000. The annual incidence is estimated at between 1 and 3 per 1,000 in men and at 0.2 per 1,000 in women.

Gout evolves in three distinct stages: asymptomatic hyperuricemia, acute intermittent disease, and chronic tophaceous disease. The latter stage usually develops after 10 to 15 years of intermittent gout. Although gout does not develop in most people with hyperuricemia, data from the Normative Aging Study showed a cumulative incidence of gouty arthritis of 3% in persons with levels of uric acid between 7.0 and 8.0 mg/dL. In subjects with levels above 9 mg/dL, the 5-year incidence rose to 22%. Both the age of the subject and the degree of hyperuricemia appear to be important predictors of the clinical outcome.

The risk for damage beyond the musculoskeletal system is not insignificant. Stones containing uric acid develop in approximately 10% of patients with gout, and possibly in as many as 50% of patients with a serum urate level above 13 g/dL. Obesity, hypertension, and hypertriglyceridemia are common in patients with gout.

If gout is untreated, subcutaneous tophi may develop, usually in the fingers, wrists, olecranon bursae, and Achilles tendons, and occasionally require surgical removal (Fig. 95.1).

Clinical Findings and Differential Diagnosis

> "The victim goes to bed and sleeps in good health. About two o'clock in the morning he is awakened by pain in the great toe.... The night is passed in torture, sleeplessness, turning of the part affected and perpetual change of posture."

Sydenham's classic description depicts the clinical scenario typical of gout. Severe pain usually develops in the affected joint, which becomes warm, red, and swollen. The attacks are usually monarticular and begin abruptly. Occasionally, nonarticular structures, such as the olecranon bursa and Achilles tendon, are involved. Most attacks are self-limited and resolve within 7 to 10 days.

Because MSU crystals are less soluble at lower temperatures, gout tends to affect acral areas. The joints most commonly involved include the first metatarsophalangeal joint (podagra), the insteps, ankles, heels, knees, wrists, and elbows (Fig. 95.2). An attack is often preceded by the ingestion of alcohol, trauma, or an acute medical illness. The admitting intern should learn to suspect gout in a febrile postoperative patient in whom a swollen, painful joint develops. The differential diagnosis for any swollen, warm joint includes infection, gout, and pseudogout. Because the clinical picture may be identical in all these conditions, a diagnostic tap should be performed in most, if not all, patients. Leukocytosis and fever may also be seen in any inflammatory arthritis and thus are not helpful in excluding infection.

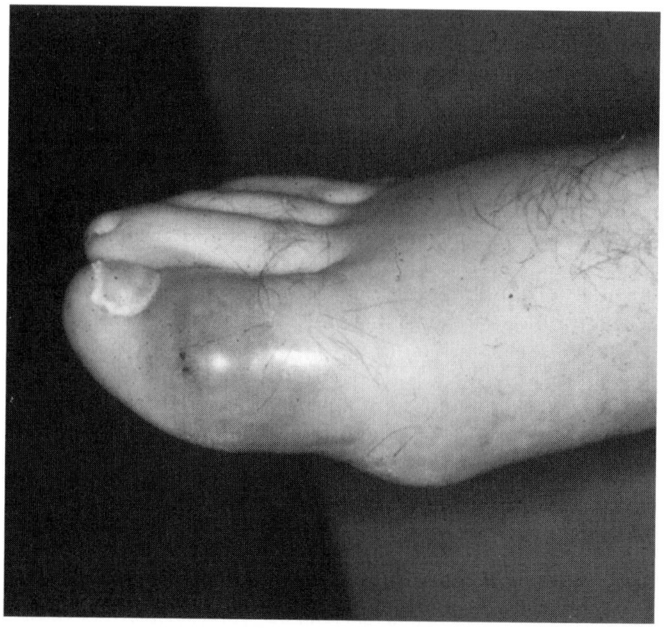

FIG. 95.2. A patient with acute podagra. (Photograph courtesy of John Conte, M.D.)

Laboratory Features and Diagnosis

The preferred method for confirming acute gout is arthrocentesis of fresh synovial fluid. Because sepsis and acute gouty arthritis are often difficult to differentiate, aspiration is essential. The presence of negatively birefringent, needle-shaped intracellular crystals is diagnostic for gout. Occasionally, extracellular uric acid crystals are innocent bystanders. Therefore, whenever septic arthritis is suspected, a culture should always be obtained.

The synovial fluid in acute gout is usually inflammatory, with a predominance of neutrophils (leukocyte count, 20,000–100,000/mm^3). The serum uric acid level is generally unhelpful during an attack because it is often normal. The hematologic indices often confirm acute inflammation, and acute phase reactants (erythrocyte sedimentation rate and platelets) are frequently elevated. If uricosuric therapy is being considered, a 24-hour urinary uric acid determination can be obtained to confirm urinary underexcretion. Provided the patient's diet is regular, the excretion rate of uric acid should not exceed 800 mg/24 h.

Imaging Studies

The radiographic studies of patients with gout are typically unremarkable early in the course of the disease. During an attack, soft tissue swelling is observed. After several years of exposure to uric acid crystals, both tophi and erosions are seen. Tophi appear as soft tissue densities overlying the joint that may become calcified. The erosions typically have sclerotic margins with overhanging edges. Because of their appearance, they are occasionally referred to as "rat bite" erosions. In comparison with rheumatoid arthritis, gout is characterized by the preservation of joint space and the absence of osteopenia.

Treatment

ACUTE GOUT

Patients in the midst of an acute attack experience excruciating pain. Therapy should have a rapid onset of action and be safe and effective. The three available choices are colchicine, nonsteroidal antiinflammatory drugs (NSAIDs), and corticosteroids. The NSAIDs are most widely used; they have a rapid onset of action but are unfortunately contraindicated in many patients. Indomethacin is frequently prescribed, but other NSAIDs may be equally effective.

Colchicine, an alkaloid derived from the plant *Colchicum autumnale*, has been used to treat gout for more than two centuries. It acts by inhibiting the polymerization of microtubules and prevents neutrophil chemotaxis and phagocytosis. When administered early in an attack, it can be extremely effective. Unfortunately, gastrointestinal upset is common, and side effects include increased peristalsis, nausea, abdominal pain, and cramping. Colchicine is usually given orally at a dosage of 0.6 mg/h until significant side effects develop or the symptoms subside. Generally, no more than 6 mg should be given at any one time, and further doses should be avoided for at least 7 days. To avoid the gastrointestinal side effects, colchicine may also be administered intravenously. One milligram should be diluted in normal saline solution, and dosing can be repeated up to 3 mg. Because the toxicity of colchicine is potentially irreversible and fatal, it should be administered intravenously only to patients with normal renal and hepatic function. Care should be taken not to allow extravasation of the drug because a local chemical thrombophlebitis can also occur.

When colchicine and NSAIDs are contraindicated, systemic corticosteroids may be used. Typically, 20 to 40 mg of prednisone or its equivalent can be given daily for the initial attack and then tapered during the next few days. Another option is 40 to 80 IU of adrenocorticotropic hormone given intramuscularly every 6 to 12 hours, although few data are available to demonstrate its superiority over traditional therapy. Urate-lowering drugs such as allopurinol should be avoided in the acute setting because fluctuations in the urate levels can prolong or precipitate an attack.

INTERMITTENT GOUT

Because many patients are asymptomatic between attacks, the decision to intervene should be balanced against the daily requirement for urate-lowering medication and lifestyle change. Treatment can be initiated once reversible risk factors, such as alcohol intake and dehydration, are corrected. Most rheumatologists start hypouricemic therapy if the patient has more than three attacks per year or asymptomatic hyperuricemia with levels above 12 mg/dL. If attacks occur despite a urate-lowering drug, the addition of once-daily colchicine should be considered because it can reduce the frequency of attacks by 75%.

CHRONIC TOPHACEOUS GOUT

The goal of therapy in tophaceous gout is the resorption of tophi such that erosive or compressive complications are avoided. Urate becomes soluble at levels below 5 mg/dL, which can usually be achieved with allopurinol or uricosuric drugs such as probenecid. Allopurinol is preferred because it is effective in both overproducers and underexcretors of uric acid. Doses of 300 mg daily are usually adequate. However, the dose should be adjusted for patients with renal insufficiency or who are elderly. Probenecid is an effective uricosuric drug but should be limited to patients who have a glomerular filtration exceeding 50 to 60 mL/min, are willing to drink at least 2 L of fluid daily, and have no history of nephrolithiasis.

CALCIUM PYROPHOSPHATE DIHYDRATE DEPOSITION

Definition and Classification

Calcium pyrophosphate dihydrate (CPPD) is a calcium-containing crystal. CPPD deposition in joints can result in an acute inflammatory arthritis, also termed *pseudogout*. Most patients with CPPD arthritis are elderly, although certain metabolic disorders appear to predispose to the condition. Strong associations with hyperparathyroidism, hemochromatosis, amyloidosis, hypomagnesemia, and hypophosphatasia have been shown.

Etiology

Acute pseudogout is caused by the release of CPPD crystals into a joint. Phagocytosis of the crystals by polymorphonuclear leukocytes ensues rapidly, and cytokine release activates the inflammatory cascade. Stimulated cells lining the joints secrete proteolytic enzymes such as collagenase, which damage the articular cartilage. Elevated levels of inorganic phosphate are found in the synovial fluid of most patients with CPPD crystals. It has therefore been postulated that interaction with calcium-containing crystals results in CPPD deposition.

Data on the calcification of articular cartilage (chondrocalcinosis) are derived mostly from radiographic surveys of the knee. Most studies suggest that the disease occurs predominantly in women between the ages of 65 and 75 years. The Framingham study showed an overall prevalence of 8% in people older than 63 years and a prevalence of up to 27% in patients older than 85 years.

Three presentations are commonly encountered: acute pseudogout, asymptomatic radiographic disease, and chronic arthritis. Acute attacks result in rapid inflammation of the joint and usually respond to aspiration alone. Generally, the pain subsides within 1 to 3 weeks. Polyarticular involvement may occur and usually requires longer therapy. In patients with relapsing disease, joint lavage may be required. When a more chronic form of the disease develops, the knee is generally involved, and patients experience chronic stiffness and restricted movement in this joint with or without superimposed acute attacks. The pattern of joint involvement typically results in severe degenerative changes at the metacarpophalangeal joints, wrists, elbows, and shoulders in addition to the knees. Unfortunately, a progressive, destructive arthropathy develops in a small percentage of elderly women that may resemble Charcot joints.

Clinical Findings and Differential Diagnosis

In acute pseudogout, swelling, pain, and warmth develop rapidly in the affected joint. The areas most often involved in descending order are the knees, wrists, metacarpophalangeal joints, hips, shoulders, elbows, and ankles. In comparison with gout, the attacks tend to be less severe but are also precipitated by trauma and acute illness. The presence of early morning stiffness, fatigue, and synovitis in a small minority of patients may cause confusion with rheumatoid arthritis. In these cases, it is vital to review all serologic and radiologic data to avoid the unnecessary administration of potentially toxic immunosuppressive agents.

Laboratory Features and Imaging Studies

The diagnosis of pseudogout is confirmed by arthrocentesis. An excess of polymorphonuclear leukocytes with weakly positively birefringent, rod-shaped intracellular crystals is characteristic. Other frequent laboratory values include a peripheral leukocytosis and elevated acute phase reactants. As in gout, septic arthritis may coexist. Therefore, a Gram stain and culture should be obtained, particularly in a hospitalized patient.

Chondrocalcinosis is a condition in which CPPD crystals deposit in cartilage. On radiographs, they are most commonly visualized in the triangular fibrocartilage of the wrist, the knee menisci, and the symphysis pubis. CPPD deposition differs from osteoarthritis in that isolated patellofemoral or wrist disease is quite common. Calcific deposits are also seen in ligaments, tendons, and the articular capsule. The distribution is usually punctate or linear and frequently parallel to the subchondral endplate of the bone.

Treatment

In most cases, arthrocentesis of the affected joint is adequate to abort an acute attack. Provided the synovial fluid cultures are sterile, I prefer a local corticosteroid injection (e.g., 20–40 mg of triamcinolone), which offers additional and more rapid relief of symptoms. Because patients are often hospitalized at the time of an attack, the affected limb should be rested, and topical ice may be helpful. Colchicine and NSAIDs may also be used but are often contraindicated in elderly patients with compromised renal and gastrointestinal function.

Unfortunately, no current therapies are available to reverse or retard the deposition of CPPD crystals, as they are for gout. Oral daily colchicine can be used as prophylaxis in patients with more frequent attacks. In patients younger than 55 years, secondary associated diseases such as hyperparathyroidism and hemochromatosis should be excluded.

CONSIDERATIONS IN PREGNANCY

During a normal pregnancy, the maternal serum level of uric acid decreases until about 24 weeks; between that time and 12 weeks postpartum, the serum urate level increases. If the pregnancy is complicated by preeclampsia or toxemia as a consequence of reduced renal urate clearance, the serum uric acid level is further elevated. Perinatal mortality is highest when the serum urate is significantly elevated (>6.0 mg/dL) and associated with diastolic hypertension above 110 mm Hg.

The transient increase in the serum uric acid level during normal labor is probably caused by a decrease in renal urate clearance and perhaps increased urate production. This increase persists for only a day or two postpartum.

The occurrence of the acute arthritis of gout or CPDD is extremely rare in pregnancy, although it has been reported. Oral prednisone, adrenocorticotropic hormone, or intraarticular steroid injection is the preferred method of treatment.

BIBLIOGRAPHY

Arnold MH, Preston SJ, Buchanon WW. Comparison of the natural history of untreated acute gouty arthritis vs. acute gouty arthritis treated with NSAIDS. *Br J Clin Pharmacol* 1988;26:488–489.
Axelrod D, Preston S. Comparison of parenteral ACTH with oral indomethacin in the treatment of acute gout. *Arthritis Rheum* 1988;31:803–805.
Bird HA, Ring EFJ. Therapeutic value of arthroscopy. *Ann Rheum Dis* 1978;37:78–79.
Campion EW, Glynn RV, DeLabry LO. Asymptomatic hyperuricemia: risks and consequences in the Normative Aging Study. *Am J Med* 1987;82:421–426.
Cheung HS, Ryan LM. Role of crystal deposition in matrix degradation. In: Woessner FJ, Howell DS, eds. *Joint cartilage degradation: basic and clinical aspects*. New York: Marcel Dekker Inc, 1995:209.
Cohen MG, Emmerson BT. Crystal arthropathies: gout. In: Klippel JH, Dieppe PA, eds. *Rheumatology*. London: Mosby, 1998:8.14.2.
Doherty M, Dieppe P. Clinical aspects of calcium pyrophosphate dihydrate crystal deposition. *Rheum Dis Clin North Am* 1988;14:395–414.
Emmerson BT, Nagal SL, Duffy DL, et al. Genetic control of the renal clearance of urate: a study of twins. *Ann Rheum Dis* 1992;51:375–377.
Felson DT, Anderson JJ, Naimark K, et al. The prevalence of chondrocalcinosis in the elderly and its association with knee osteoarthritis: the Framingham study. *J Rheumatol* 1989;16:1241–1245.
Hartung EF. History of the use of colchicine and related medications in gout. *Ann Rheum Dis* 1954;13:190–201.
Kelsall JT, O'Hanlon DP. Gout during pregnancy. *J Rheumatol* 1994;21:1365–1366.
Paulus HE, Schlosstein LH, Godfrey RC, et al. Prophylactic colchicine therapy of intercritical gout: a placebo-controlled study of probenecid-treated patients. *Arthritis Rheum* 1987;17:609–614.
Scott JT, Pollard AC. Uric acid excretion in the relatives of patients with gout. *Ann Rheum Dis* 1970;29:397–400.
Terkeltaub RA, Ginsburg MH. The inflammatory reaction to crystals. *Rheum Dis Clin North Am* 1988;14:353–364.
Wallace SL, Singer JZ. Systemic toxicity associated with intravenous administration of colchicine—guidelines for use. *J Rheumatol* 1988;15:495–499.
Wilson JM, Stout JT, Palella TD, et al. A molecular survey of hypoxanthine-guanine phosphoribosyl transferase deficiency in man. *J Clin Invest* 1986;77:188–195.
Wyngaarden JB, Kelley WN. *Gout and hyperuricemia*. New York: Grune & Stratton, 1976.

CHAPTER 96
Osteoarthritis

Elise M. Coletta

Osteoarthritis (OA), also known as *degenerative joint disease* or *osteoarthrosis*, is a noninflammatory type of arthritis. OA is the most frequent form of arthritis, and the most common cause of disability, in the United States. The prevalence of OA increases with age. The medical care sought by patients makes OA a significant factor in overall health care costs.

Epidemiologically, OA of the knee is twice as likely to develop in women as in men, and twice as likely in black women as in white women. The prevalence of OA of the hip is lower in Chinese, South African blacks, East Indians, and Native Americans than in Caucasians. It is uncommon for OA to be a problem during pregnancy because it generally affects women after their reproductive years.

ETIOLOGY

OA is classified as primary (idiopathic) or secondary depending on the absence or presence of an etiologic factor (Table 96.1.). Both the idiopathic and secondary forms are probably multifactorial in origin; the causes of the idiopathic form are unidentified.

The leading risk factor for primary OA is increasing age. Although the radiographic changes of OA are highly prevalent in older people, fewer than half of them are symptomatic. Genetic factors probably play a role in the development of OA because having a relative with OA does increase the risk.

Obesity increases the risk for OA of the knee, whereas arthritis of the hip is not as strongly associated with obesity. It is thought that the density of subchondral bone is increased in obese persons in response to greater stress on bone. The denser subchondral bone absorbs shock less effectively than normal or osteoporotic bone, so that wear on the cartilage is increased and OA develops. A weight loss of 5 kg can halve the risk for the development of symptomatic OA of the knee.

Joint trauma is a well-recognized risk factor for OA. Displaced intraarticular fractures often lead to arthritis. Injuries that result in malalignment of a joint or alter the mechanical function of a joint can generate an uneven distribution of forces in the joint, with a resultant increase in articular wear in areas of greater stress. Direct injury to the articular cartilage also can lead to OA, particularly because the ability of articular cartilage to repair itself is poor.

TABLE 96.1. Classification of Osteoarthritis

Primary (idiopathic)
Localized (single joint)
Generalized (multiple joints)
Sporadic
Familial (e.g., osteoarthritis of the hands)
Secondary
Trauma
Acute (e.g., intraarticular fractures)
Chronic (e.g., slipped capital femoral epiphysis)
Occupational (i.e., repetitive use)
Congenital/developmental
Developmental dysplasia of the hip
Legg-Perthes disease
Bone dysplasias (e.g., multiple epiphyseal dysplasia)
Metabolic
Alkaptonuria
Wilson disease
Hemochromatosis
Crystalline arthropathy (gout, calcium pyrophosphate dihydrate)
Septic arthritis
Other
Neuropathic arthropathy
Osteonecrosis
Hemophilia
Acromegaly
Paget disease

It is debatable whether the long-term repetitive use of joints (e.g., long-distance running) can lead to OA. The repetitive use of joints in athletics is generally not associated with OA unless other predisposing factors are present. Sports involving high-intensity direct impact on joints (e.g., football) may increase the likelihood of OA. The occupational repetitive activities of laborers or assembly line workers can increase the risk for OA in susceptible people.

PATHOPHYSIOLOGY

The primary damage in OA occurs at the weight-bearing portions of the joint. Initially, the articular cartilage swells as the water content increases secondary to damage to the collagen framework. Proteoglycan synthesis increases in an attempt to repair the damaged cartilage, but degeneration persists and overwhelms such attempts at repair. As the disease progresses, the joint cartilage thins and becomes soft, resulting in fibrillation and fissuring of the cartilage surface. The damaged cartilage can ultimately wear through to expose the underlying bone. Fibrocartilaginous repair tissue forms, but its ability to function as an articular surface is inferior to that of the native hyaline cartilage.

In addition to cartilage loss, bone changes occur, including the growth of subchondral appositional bone, eburnation of bone exposed by worn cartilage, microfractures, and the formation of bone cysts secondary to localized osteonecrosis. One of the hallmark changes of OA is the growth of cartilage and bone at the joint margins to form osteophytes. As a result of the cartilage and bone damage, joint deformity and malalignment may develop. Mild synovitis may also be seen in OA.

DIFFERENTIAL DIAGNOSIS

The diagnosis of OA is based on the entire clinical picture, including the history, physical examination findings, and radiographic evidence. OA is distinguished from other arthritides in the following ways: it generally affects older persons; a history of prior joint injury or deformity may be elicited; the larger weight-bearing joints, spine, and fingers are often affected; and classic radiographic signs of diminished joint space are present with associated bone sclerosis and osteophyte formation. Laboratory tests are not needed to make the diagnosis but are useful in atypical cases to rule out inflammatory types of arthritis.

Table 96.2 summarizes the criteria for the differential diagnosis of OA, rheumatoid arthritis, and soft tissue rheumatism (e.g., multifocal bursitis, fibromyalgia). Generally, the differential diagnosis includes other forms of arthritis and other types of musculoskeletal problems, but the possibility of a referred source of pain (e.g., bone metastases from cancer) should be considered, especially in elderly women.

CLINICAL SYMPTOMS/HISTORY

OA may involve one or multiple joints on presentation. Joint pain, the usual presenting symptom, is described as worse during activity and relieved by rest. The pain may be poorly localized to the joint; OA of the hip may present with groin or knee pain. In advanced OA of the hip, pain at night may interfere with sleep. Joint stiffness may occur in patients with OA, particularly after immobility or sleep. The duration of stiffness is usually no more than 30 minutes.

TABLE 96.2. Criteria for the Differential Diagnosis of Osteoarthritis

	Osteoarthritis	Rheumatoid arthritis	Soft tissue rheumatism
History	• More common in persons older than 50 years • Morning stiffness lasts <30 minutes • Rarely painful at rest	• More common in young and middle-aged women • Morning stiffness lasts >30 minutes • Pain at rest and with activity	• Affects adults of all ages • Morning stiffness atypical • Symptoms usually activity-related
Physical examination findings	• Rarely inflammatory • Asymmetric joint involvement • Affects an average of fewer than four joints • Common in the hands (first carpometacarpal, proximal interphalangeal [Bouchard nodes], distal interphalangeal [Heberden nodes] joints), spine, hips, knees, and first metatarsophalangeal joints of the foot	• Inflammatory • Symmetric joint involvement • Affects an average of more than eight joints • Common in shoulders, elbows, wrists, hands (metacarpophalangeal, proximal interphalangeal joints), knees, ankles, and metatarsophalangeal joints of the foot • Associated with systemic symptoms and extraarticular findings (e.g., rheumatoid nodules)	• Local tenderness may be present • Affects periarticular tissues
Laboratory findings	• Blood test results usually normal • Radiographic findings may be helpful	• Rheumatoid factor typically positive; sedimentation rate elevated • Radiographic findings helpful	• Blood test results usually normal • Radiographic findings not helpful

Source: Modified from Coletta EM, Lally EV. *Osteoarthritis reference guide*, 8th ed. Lexington, KY: American Board of Family Practice, 2002, with permission.

In advanced OA of the spine, compression of an isolated nerve root may cause radiculopathy, or stenosis of the spinal canal may lead to spinal cord impingement in the cervical spine or diffuse nerve root compression in the lumbar spine. Symptoms of neurogenic claudication and cauda equina syndrome can result from lumbar spinal stenosis. Symptoms of spinal stenosis may include diffuse pain, numbness, and tingling in the lower back, buttocks, or one or both legs. Symptoms are relieved by spinal flexion; characteristically, the patient notes less pain when sitting or pushing a shopping cart. Typically, the patient is elderly.

Systemic symptoms such as fatigue, rash, and recent weight change should be sought in the history; these are not associated with OA but may be present with an inflammatory type of arthritis. Elucidation of the risk factors listed in Table 96.1 may suggest possible causes of the arthritis.

The elderly patient in particular should also be questioned about any change in functional status resulting from the joint symptoms. A complete history of all prescribed and over-the-counter medications is essential. An assessment of comorbidity is relevant, especially a history of gastritis, peptic ulcer disease, congestive heart failure, or hypertension because the medications prescribed for OA may exacerbate these conditions.

CLINICAL FINDINGS/PHYSICAL EXAMINATION

Initially, the joints affected by OA may appear normal, with pain noted only at the extremes of joint range of motion. However, as the disease progresses with time, the joint range of motion may become limited. Because OA is an articular process, pain is present during both active and passive joint motion, a feature that differentiates OA from a periarticular process such as tendonitis or bursitis. Mild to moderate swelling of the joint, a result of low-grade synovitis, and a joint effusion may be detected, but frank inflammatory signs will be absent. In the later stages of OA, joint enlargement secondary to osteophytes, angular deformity, and at times joint instability may develop. The muscles controlling the affected joint may atrophy. The strength of the surrounding muscles should be assessed, as should gait and stance when the symptoms involve a joint of a lower extremity. Any body asymmetry should be noted. A general physical examination is important to detect signs that may indicate other diagnoses, including other forms of arthritis and other conditions that may affect the management of OA.

LABORATORY AND IMAGING STUDIES

Plain radiographs are usually the only imaging studies needed to diagnose OA. However, plain radiographs do not detect mild to moderate thinning of the articular cartilage; therefore, the results of these studies may appear normal during the early stages of disease. The sensitivity of knee radiographs can be improved by obtaining weight-bearing anteroposterior views, particularly with the knees partially flexed. Hallmark radiographic changes include a narrowed joint space secondary to progressive loss of cartilage, subchondral sclerosis of the bone, and the presence of osteophytes at the periphery of joints.

Computed tomography and magnetic resonance imaging (MRI) are generally not used to image osteoarthritic joints. However, there are a few exceptions. MRI of the hip is useful to rule out osteonecrosis of the femoral head. Early treatment of this disease can prevent the development of secondary OA. MRI may also be used to evaluate a patient for meniscal damage in the knees, the symptoms of which may mimic those of early OA.

The results of laboratory tests are usually normal in OA. Additional diagnostic tests may be necessary to rule out other diseases, as suggested by the history and physical examination findings. For example, a complete blood cell count, measurement of the erythrocyte sedimentation rate, and a determination of rheumatoid factor, antinuclear antibody, serum uric acid, and creatinine phosphokinase levels may be helpful, depending on the clinical presentation.

TREATMENT

The treatment of OA includes analgesia and appropriate joint rest to relieve pain, occasional intraarticular injection of corticosteroids to relieve inflammatory flares, physical therapy, and, for more severe disease, surgery.

Pharmacologic Therapy

Acetaminophen should be used initially to treat mild symptoms of OA because of its lower cost and reduced side effect profile in comparison with nonsteroidal antiinflammatory drugs (NSAIDs). If acetaminophen is ineffective, the patient's presenting symptoms are relatively severe, or the patient is experiencing an acute flare of symptoms, NSAIDs may be required. Because OA is generally not an inflammatory disease, NSAIDs may be therapeutic in less than the full antiinflammatory doses. The potential for gastrointestinal side effects with NSAIDs is significant, especially in elderly patients. In this population, 20% to 30% of all peptic ulcer disease-related deaths are related to treatment with NSAIDs. In addition, NSAIDs may affect renal and cognitive function in the elderly. In a patient of any age, kidney or heart disease increases the risk for NSAID-related gastrointestinal complications. NSAIDs that selectively inhibit the cyclooxygenase-2 (COX-2) isoenzyme are now available. Short-term studies have shown a reduction in gastrointestinal side effects and bleeding and endoscopically detected ulcers when these agents are used rather than traditional NSAIDs. It is unclear whether this benefit extends to patients with a history of peptic ulcer disease. The lack of long-term studies, the potential adverse cardiovascular and renal effects of COX-2 inhibitors, and possible drug interactions (e.g., with aspirin) prevent these agents from becoming first-line therapy for OA at this time. COX-2 medications should be used for patients who are at high risk for gastrointestinal side effects with traditional NSAIDs. Narcotic-containing analgesics may be needed when pain interferes with sleep. Counterirritant linaments (e.g., methyl salicylate) may help some patients, as may topical capsaicin.

The intraarticular injection of corticosteroids is often a second-line tool for the treatment of OA. The total number of injections should be limited because too many can accelerate the deterioration of articular cartilage, and inadvertent injection into adjacent tendons or ligaments can lead to atrophy and failure of these structures. The intraarticular injection of hyaluronic acid is a treatment option for OA of the knee. A trial would encompass three weekly injections. This treatment may be considered for patients with moderate to severe OA of the knee who do not respond to more standard therapy.

Physical Therapy

Physical therapy is important for maintaining joint range of motion and reducing loss of strength in supporting muscles. The application of moist heat with pads or baths can increase joint range of motion, and ice therapy may help during acute flares. Reducing stress on affected joints decreases joint pain. Weight loss and assistive devices, such as a cane, can be used to reduce the stress on affected weight-bearing joints of the lower extremities. The patient should be instructed to carry the cane in the hand contralateral to the affected joint.

An individualized exercise program tailored to the patient's specific needs is the best therapy plan. Non–weight-bearing exercises, such as bicycling or swimming, are preferable to running or aerobics. Available research supports the efficacy of exercise therapy for OA of the hip or knee. Improvement is seen in multiple areas, including level of pain, subjective and objective difficulty in walking, and global patient self-assessment of effect.

Other Therapies

Questionable treatments for OA abound. These include copper bracelets, dimethyl sulfoxide, bee venom, magnet therapy, and a variety of vitamins and herbs. None of them are likely to be effective. Glucosamine sulfate and chondroitin sulfate, marketed as dietary supplements, may relieve the arthritic symptoms of some patients, but it has not been proved that they affect the course of OA. Given the absence of significant adverse effects, many clinicians favor a trial of glucosamine. However, long-term safety and efficacy data are currently lacking for these two products.

Referral to Specialist

Referral to a specialist is appropriate when the diagnosis of OA is uncertain or the disease has not responded well to NSAID treatment and the patient is significantly impaired by her symptoms. The primary care physician can administer intraarticular injections of the knee, but injections of smaller joints (e.g., those of the hand) are better left to specialists.

Surgery

Surgery in OA is both preventive and therapeutic. For example, the early treatment of developmental dysplasia of the hip can prevent the long-term complication of arthritis of the hip. The preservation of torn menisci is important in preventing future arthritis. The appropriate management of fractures can prevent posttraumatic OA.

More surgical options are becoming available to patients with OA. Arthroscopic irrigation and debridement of damaged articular surfaces in the knee provides up to 5 years of relief in as many as 80% of patients with OA. Arthroscopy also allows direct visualization of the articular cartilage, making it possible to determine the stage and course of disease and obtain information that can be used to plan future surgical options.

In middle-aged patients with angular deformity of the knee, realignment osteotomies of the proximal tibia or distal femur can redistribute stresses in the knee joint to healthier areas of articular cartilage; satisfactory results beyond 10 years have been achieved. Intertrochanteric osteotomies of the hip may alleviate arthritic symptoms in the hip by unclear mechanisms.

Joint replacement has become the mainstay of treatment for patients with advanced OA. Replacement of the articular surfaces of the hip, knee, and shoulder with metal and polyethylene components has been tremendously successful. Satisfactory results beyond 20 years of follow-up for hips and 15 years for knees have been reported. More conservative replacement of only the affected portions of the knee joint is also possible with the use of unicompartmental components. Excellent results have also been achieved in the basal joint of the thumb with ligament reconstruction and joint replacement with interposition of a rolled-up tendon.

Fusion of affected joints is another surgical alternative, particularly in the distal interphalangeal joints and affected levels of the spine. Fusion is a more durable alternative in hips and knees than replacement and is often favored for younger, high-demand patients.

BIBLIOGRAPHY

American College of Rheumatology Subcommittee on Osteoarthritis Guidelines. Recommendations for the medical management of osteoarthritis of the hip and knee: 2000 update. *Arthritis Rheum* 2000;43:1905–1915.

Deal CL, Moskowitz RW. Nutraceuticals as therapeutic agents in osteoarthritis: the role of glucosamine, chondroitin sulfate, and collagen hydrolysate. *Rheum Dis Clin North Am* 1999;25:379–395.

Felson DT, Lawrence RC, Dieppe PA, et al. Osteoarthritis: new insights. Part I: The disease and its risk factors. *Ann Intern Med* 2000;133:635–646.

Felson DT, Lawrence RC, Hochberg MCC, et al. Osteoarthritis: new insights. Part 2: Treatment approaches. *Ann Intern Med* 2000;133:726–737.

Van Baar ME, Assendelft WJJ, Dekker J, et al. Effectiveness of exercise therapy in patients with osteoarthritis of the hip or knee: a systematic review of randomized clinical trials. *Arthritis Rheum* 1999;42:1361–1369.

CHAPTER 97

Osteoporosis and Complications

John M. Conte

Osteoporosis is a disease of epidemic proportions, with major public health significance. Its prevention and treatment must be carefully considered in women of all ages, especially in view of the increasing number of effective treatment options now available to the clinician. Osteoporosis, much like high blood pressure, is most often a silent disease that progresses slowly and imperceptibly over time until its secondary effects become manifest in the form of fractures, deformity, and pain. It is not possible to make a diagnosis in the early stages because clinical warning signs are lacking. Early diagnosis must therefore be based on a knowledge of predictive risk factors and a low threshold for initiating appropriate confirmatory imaging studies.

The term *osteoporosis* is defined as a decrease in bone mass resulting from microarchitectural deterioration that increases susceptibility to fracture. Although the composition of the bone mineral and matrix is normal, trabecular thinning leads to fragility. Thus, it is both the absolute amount of bone present and the quality of the bone that influence fracture risk. Osteoporosis is a systemic condition affecting the entire skeleton, but it may develop earlier and progress more rapidly in different areas of the skeleton, such as the spine or hip, based on genetic and other unknown factors. Osteopenia is the condition of bone mass reduction before fracture; of note, radiographic evidence of osteopenia indicates at least a 30% loss of bone mineral. The term *osteopenia* is defined more narrowly when used in the context of bone mineral density (BMD) measurement, as is discussed in further detail later. The term *osteomalacia* refers to abnormal mineralization of bone with normal matrix (often caused by vitamin D deficiency).

Osteoporosis can be characterized as primary (basic cause unknown, no underlying disease) or secondary (attributable to an inherited or acquired abnormality or disease state) (Table 97.1). In turn, primary osteoporosis is classified as type I, which results from estrogen loss during the 8 to 10 years after menopause, or type II, which results from altered calcium and vitamin D metabolism in persons of either sex after age 70. Other lifestyle and genetic factors also play a role in the pathogenesis of primary osteoporosis. As an aside, gonadal failure in men with a resultant decrease in circulating testosterone can also precipitate a period of more rapid bone loss.

TABLE 97.1. Common Causes of Secondary Osteoporosis

Hyperparathyroidism
Cushing disease
Hyperthyroidism
Multiple myeloma
Anorexia nervosa
Athletic amenorrhea
Chronic renal failure
Chronic liver failure
Immobility
Alcoholism
Medications (Table 97.3)

EPIDEMIOLOGY

Age-related bone loss occurs in all persons once they have passed the third decade, when bone mass peaks. Multiple factors, including hormonal, genetic, nutritional, and lifestyle influences, affect the development of primary osteoporosis. The disease is found throughout the world, although the incidence of fracture varies markedly, with the highest rates in developed countries such as the United States, Scandinavia, and New Zealand, and the lowest in rural Africa. The incidence is greater in urban than in rural populations and greater in Caucasian and Asian ethnic groups than in persons of African heritage.

The morbidity, mortality, and costs associated with osteoporotic fractures are significant. In the United States, osteoporosis affects more than 25 million persons and 25% of women older than 65 years of age. About 10% of women currently 35 years old will have a hip fracture later in life. Underlying osteoporosis contributes to more than 1.3 million fractures annually, including at least 250,000 hip fractures, 500,000 spinal fractures, and 240,000 wrist fractures. Costs, including those attributable to lost productivity, hospital care, and nursing care, are in excess of $10 billion each year. Hip fracture in particular is associated with a high rate of morbidity, in that half of those who sustain a hip fracture require short- or long-term nursing home care and half subsequently require assistive devices for mobility. A striking 5% to 20% excess mortality is also observed in the year after a hip fracture.

With demographic shifts leading to the "graying" of the U.S. population, some authors have projected that the direct and indirect costs of osteoporotic fractures may reach $60 billion annually by the year 2020.

CALCIUM AND BONE PHYSIOLOGY

Before a complete discussion of etiologic factors is presented, calcium and bone metabolism should be reviewed briefly. Changes that occur with aging should also be understood.

The major organs involved in calcium balance are the small intestine, kidney, and bone (Fig. 97.1). Optimal calcium intake in premenopausal women is about 1,000 mg/d, of which 20% to 40% is absorbed in the gut. Vitamin D is a major factor influencing the rate of calcium absorption through calcium-binding protein in the small intestine. With aging, the efficiency of both active and passive intestinal calcium absorption diminishes, as does the production and level of active vitamin D (calcitriol). As the efficiency of calcium absorption decreases, in part because of lower circulating levels of vitamin D, the resultant mild hypocalcemia triggers an increase in nocturnal parathyroid hor-

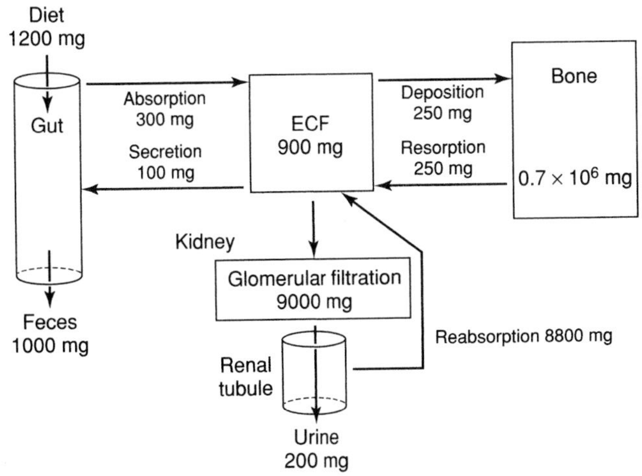

FIG. 97.1. Model of calcium metabolism. The principal organs (small intestine, kidney, and bone) involved in mass calcium transport and the approximate daily flux rates of calcium between the compartments in young normal women. The sizes of the compartments are given in milligrams, and the daily flux rates are indicated next to the corresponding *arrows*. (From Baylink DJ, Jennings JC. Calcium and bone homeostasis and changes with aging. In: Hazzard WR, Bierman EL, Blass JP, et al., eds. *Principles of geriatric medicine*. New York: McGraw-Hill, 1994:879, with permission.)

mone (PTH) levels and subsequent bone resorption—the "age-related" (type II, or non–estrogen-dependent) osteoporosis syndrome (Fig. 97.2).

Other factors that reduce calcium absorption include inadequate intake, lactase deficiency, sprue, pancreatic deficiency, and other malabsorptive states. Gastric acid, which is required to solubilize calcium and facilitate its absorption, also decreases with age. Any agents that diminish the production of gastric acid, such as histamine H_2 blockers and proton pump inhibitors, and disease states such as pernicious anemia also negatively influence calcium absorption. This is particularly true of calcium carbonate. Notably, calcium citrate is absorbed equally well in both acidic and alkaline environments and should be the supplement of choice in persons with relative achlorhydria, whether medication-induced, secondary to disease or surgery, or age-related.

The kidney filters and reabsorbs calcium and is not normally a major site of calcium excretion at any age. Calcium resorption is coupled to sodium transport and regulated by PTH levels. Primary hyperparathyroidism can induce a renal wasting of calcium. Proximal tubular disorders and syndromes of primary hypercalcuria are less common causes of negative calcium balance.

Bone is a unique organ in that it has a structural function in addition to being the major calcium repository of the body. Cortical bone, located in long bone diaphyses, is the major source of structural support. In cancellous bone, located in long bone metaphyses, vertebrae, and flat bones, the surface-to-volume ratio is higher, and cancellous bone is the primary site of calcium mobilization. Bone is a dynamic tissue comprised of a variety of cells, including osteoblasts, which form bone, and osteoclasts, which reabsorb bone in response to local and systemic hormonal stimuli, cytokines, and electromechanical forces. At any point in time, roughly 10% of the normal skeleton is undergoing a physiologic remodeling process. This is a balanced process such that the osteoblasts lay down an amount of bone equal to that absorbed by the osteoclasts. Predictably, the osteoblasts become less efficient after age 40, so that with each cycle of bone absorption and formation, slightly less bone is made than lost. Estrogen deficiency accentuates this negative balance after menopause. Thus, although healthy women do not lose a significant amount of bone between the peak years of bone formation in the 30s and menopause, bone is lost at a rate of 0.6% to 4% per year after menopause. By the 10th year, the average woman has lost 12% of her skeletal mass. As both women and men age, multiple factors, including hormone deficiency, lack of exercise, decreased calcium absorption, and lower levels of vitamin D with a secondary increase in PTH, all conspire to effect a net loss of bone that can become significant over time.

Several hormones are important to maintain calcium balance. PTH, secreted by the parathyroid glands, plays a major role in increasing serum calcium levels in response to hypocalcemia. It acts by increasing renal calcium resorption, increasing the conversion of vitamin D to its active form, and stimulating osteoclasts to mobilize calcium from bone.

Vitamin D acts at multiple sites to influence calcium metabolism. The vitamin is produced in the skin on exposure to ultraviolet light; the other major source is dairy products supplemented with vitamin D. Standard multivitamins also contain vitamin D. Vitamin D is hydroxylated in the liver to its storage form, 25-hydroxyvitamin D, then hydroxylated again in the kidney to its active form, 1,25-dihydroxyvitamin D. Major target organs of the active vitamin are the small intestine, bone, and parathyroid glands. As discussed previously, vitamin D facilitates calcium absorption from the gut, which in turn promotes bone formation. However, when PTH is present, vitamin D may also enhance its action.

Vitamin D deficiency is common in older persons and may be caused by several factors, including lack of exposure to sunlight, poor dietary intake of vitamin D, and decreased formation of the active hormone in the kidney as renal function predictably declines with age. Vitamin D status is best ascertained by measuring plasma levels of 25-hydroxyvitamin D, the storage form of the vitamin, together with serum PTH levels, which predictably rise during deficiency states, much in the same way that levels of thyroid-stimulating hormone rise in the face of low triiodothyronine/thyroxine states.

The effect of estrogen on bone in women is complex. In general terms, it stimulates bone formation and prevents net bone loss. During the 8 to 10 years after menopause, estrogen deficiency causes an increase in bone resorption with mobilization of calcium, which is then excreted (Fig. 97.3). In the postmenopausal state, mild hypercalcemia leads to suppression of PTH and vitamin D levels. This contrasts with age-related osteoporosis, in which PTH is elevated, although vitamin D is not. After 7 to 10 years, the rate of bone loss slows. Although the administration of exogenous estrogen can eliminate this phase of rapid bone resorption, loss begins as soon as estrogen is stopped.

↓Vitamin D → Calcium malabsorption → Small ↓ serum Ca → ↑PTH → ↑Bone resorption

FIG. 97.2. Type II ("age-related") osteoporosis.

Type I Estrogen-dependent Osteoporosis

↓ Estrogen → ↓ Bone formation → Small ↑ serum Ca
↓ Bone resorption
↓ PTH
↓ Vitamin D
↑ Ca excretion in urine

FIG. 97.3. Type I ("estrogen-dependent") osteoporosis.

TABLE 97.3. Medications Associated with Bone Loss

Corticosteroids
Heparin (long-term use)
Excessive thyroid hormone
Diphenylhydantoin (Dilantin)
Barbiturates
Antimetabolites (e.g., methotrexate, cyclophosphamide)

RISK FACTORS FOR OSTEOPOROSIS

Hormonal, genetic, and "lifestyle" factors influence the risk for osteoporosis (Table 97.2). Estrogen deficiency of any cause plays a major role in the development of the disease. Age-related decreases in calcium absorption and vitamin D production are also important, as previously discussed (see section "Calcium and Bone Physiology").

Multiple lifestyle factors affect the likelihood of osteoporosis. Achieving a high peak bone mass in the third decade of life is important, and this depends on an optimal calcium intake throughout the preceding years in addition to genetic factors. Weight-bearing exercise is receiving increasing attention as a preventive strategy. Walking and exercise with light weights have been shown to raise BMD in several studies. Excessive alcohol use, particularly in the setting of pancreatitis and chronic liver disease, is associated with osteoporosis. Smoking, by a direct negative influence of nicotine on circulating estrogen levels in women, may promote bone loss. An excessive dietary intake of protein causes an obligate urinary calcium loss, but whether this has an actual clinical effect is uncertain. Multiple medications may cause bone loss; these include corticosteroids, antimetabolites such as cyclophosphamide and methotrexate, anticonvulsants, heparin, cyclosporine, and thyroid hormone supplements in excessive doses (Table 97.3).

Genetic factors influence the risk for osteoporosis primarily through effects on the development of peak bone density. Women who have a positive family history, especially of maternal hip fracture, or a slight stature and low body mass are at greater risk. As previously noted (see section "Epidemiology"), osteoporosis is most common in women of European or Asian descent.

CLINICAL EVALUATION

A clinical evaluation of the perimenopausal and postmenopausal woman should include the information summarized in Table 97.4. The history should include information about diet, lifestyle, and genetic factors influencing the development of osteoporosis in addition to information about visual acuity, previous fractures and falls, and any arthritis, clotting disorders, or malignancies.

The physical examination should focus on excluding secondary causes of osteoporosis; signs of hyperthyroidism, hyperparathyroidism, chronic liver or renal disease, malabsorption, endogenous or exogenous hypercortisolism, and the proximal muscle weakness and long bone tenderness of osteomalacia should be sought. Laboratory testing in osteoporotic women without fracture should include measurement of electrolytes, blood urea nitrogen, creatinine, calcium albumin, phosphorus, and thyroid-stimulating hormone. In those with established

TABLE 97.2. Risk Factors for Osteoporosis

Estrogen deficiency
Natural or surgical menopause
Anorexia nervosa
Athletic amenorrhea
Age-related calcium malabsorption
Inadequate calcium intake
Inactivity
Alcohol use
Tobacco use
Excessive dietary protein
Genetic factors

TABLE 97.4. Clinical Evaluation of the Perimenopausal and Postmenopausal Woman

History
Age at menopause
Menopausal symptoms?
Calcium intake
Exercise
Smoking
Alcohol use
Past medical history
Cardiovascular risk factors: hypertension, diabetes mellitus, hypercholesterolemia, hypertriglyceridemia
Secondary causes of osteoporosis
Malignancy of breast, uterus, ovary
Medication use
Previous fractures
Family history
Osteoporosis
Cardiovascular disease
Malignancy of breast, uterus, ovary
Physical examination
Height, weight
Blood pressure, heart rate
Thyroid
Presence of vertebral fracture
Presence of blue sclerae (osteogenesis imperfecta)
Evidence of other systemic disease
Laboratory data: women without fracture
?Calcium, phosphorus, alkaline phosphatase
?Thyroid-stimulating hormone
Laboratory data: women with fracture
Calcium, phosphorus, alkaline phosphatase
Parathyroid hormone
Thyroid-stimulating hormone, thyroxine
Serum protein immunoelectrophoresis
Complete blood cell count
Vitamin D level
Consider 24-hour urine for calcium and creatinine
Further testing
Bone densitometry

osteoporosis, a more thorough evaluation is recommended to include a search for other causes of secondary osteoporosis, such as primary or secondary hyperparathyroidism, sprue, and myeloma. A 24-hour urine collection may be helpful to assess the adequacy of calcium intake both before and after supplementation and to rule out excessive calcium loss in the urine, as in idiopathic hypercalciuria, sarcoid, hyperparathyroidism, and vitamin D overdose. The severity of the patient's bone loss in addition to the age at onset should dictate the thoroughness of the evaluation.

QUANTITATIVE MEASUREMENT OF BONE MINERAL DENSITY

The BMD, calculated primarily as the ash content of bone divided by the area of measured tissue, correlates well with the strength of bone and is as good or better a predictor of fracture as the blood pressure is of stroke and the cholesterol level is of coronary disease. Moreover, the BMD can now be assessed quantitatively with reasonable accuracy and precision and applied clinically.

The BMD, much the same as the cholesterol level and mean blood pressure, is a continuous variable; nevertheless, risk for fracture has been stratified by the World Health Organization according to four broad categories of normal, osteopenic, osteoporotic, and severely osteoporotic individuals. These are defined as follows:

Normal: BMD within 1 standard deviation (SD) of the young adult reference mean.

Osteopenia: BMD more than 1 SD below the young adult mean but less than 2.5 SD below the young adult mean.

Osteoporosis: BMD more than 2.5 SD below the young adult mean.

Severe osteoporosis: BMD more than 2.5 SD below the young adult mean in the presence of one or more fragility fractures.

These are practical definitions based on the epidemiologic observation of an exponential increase in risk for fracture at values more than 1 SD below the young adult mean value. The loss of 1 SD represents an approximately twofold increase in risk for spinal fracture and a 2.5-fold increase in risk for hip fracture. With the caveat that an overlap of individuals with normal and low BMD values can certainly be found in a population with a history of fractures, the correlation of risk for future fracture with current BMD is excellent.

A category not specifically defined by the World Health Organization is that of persons with unusually high BMD values. They are not typically among those who sustain fractures but are clearly a subset of individuals with conditions ranging from osteoarthritis to Paget disease and metastatic bone cancer. Because the latter two conditions can cause pathologic fractures, the astute clinician should be aware of this not uncommon deviation from normal.

Currently, several noninvasive techniques are available for quantifying bone mass (Table 97.5). The most frequently used are single photon and single x-ray absorptiometry (SPA and SXA), dual-energy x-ray absorptiometry (DEXA), quantitative ultrasonography (QUS), and quantitative computed tomography (QCT). The bone density at a peripheral skeletal site (wrist or forearm) or central site (lumbar spine or hip) is determined and compared with those of age-matched controls. DEXA is considered the gold standard because it remains the test most thoroughly validated against fracture outcomes. Of note, computed tomography delivers significantly more radiation exposure than other techniques. In general, the greater number of sites measured, the more likely it is to be able to diagnose osteoporosis, given the heterogeneity of bone mass across both peripheral and central sites in any one person. Furthermore, a measurement of a specific site of interest, such as the hip, is a better predictor of fracture risk at that site than a measurement of a different site, such as the wrist or spine. BMD may vary in the same person by up to 15% depending on the manufacturer of the DEXA machine used for the measurement, such as Lunar, Hologic, and Norland. Follow-up measurements over time should be performed on the same machine if possible for optimal precision.

The indications for bone mass measurement have been outlined in a position paper by the National Institutes of Health and are included in the Medicare guidelines for BMD testing (Table 97.6). The cost of these techniques can be significant (in the range of $100–$300) but is reimbursed by most insurers who follow the Medicare rules. Testing may also be useful in women with inflammatory bowel disease or sprue, anorexia nervosa, athletic amenorrhea, an organ transplant, rheumatoid arthritis, or exposure to antimetabolites. Bone densitometry may be useful to follow the response to therapy but should

TABLE 97.5. Methods of Bone Mineral Density Measurement

Technique	Site of measurement	Advantages	Disadvantages
SXA/SPA	Radius Calcaneus	Low level of radiation Low cost Good reproducibility	Measures peripheral sites only
DEXA	Lumbar spine Femur Radius Total body	Low level of radiation Moderate cost Directly measures site of frequent fracture	Less precision at femur
QCT	Spine Radius	Allows separate assessment of trabecular and cortical bone	Higher cost Higher level of radiation Less accurate
QUS	Calcaneus	No radiation Low cost Portable	Measures peripheral sites only

DEXA, dual-energy x-ray absorptiometry; QCT, quantitative computed tomography; QUS, quantitative ultrasonography; SXA/SPA, single x-ray and single photon absorptiometry.

TABLE 97.6. Diagnoses that Support the Medical Necessity of Bone Mass Measurement for Medicare Reimbursement

Hyperparathyroidism
Ovarian failure
Menopause
States associated with artificial menopause
Osteoporosis (radiologic)
Osteopenia (radiologic)
Pathologic vertebral fractures
Postmenopausal status
Premature menopause
Postmenopausal hormone replacement
Treatment with adrenal cortical steroids
Gonadal dysgenesis

Notes:
1. Medicare will generally not cover follow-up bone mineral density measurements any sooner than 23 months. One exception is treatment with corticosteroids, when more rapid bone loss can occur.
2. Medicare will not pay for diagnostic tests performed for screening purposes alone.

be repeated at intervals of no less than 2 years given the precision limitations of the DEXA techniques and the temporal effects of available therapies. An exception to this rule would be patients with corticosteroid excess, in whom bone loss can be more rapid. Future trends in the "risk stratification" of perimenopausal women may include the increased use of biochemical markers of bone turnover to supplement BMD and historical data.

PREVENTION AND TREATMENT

To date, no prospective studies have provided direct evidence that screening at-risk populations actually reduces fracture rates. Nevertheless, several large studies do substantiate the usefulness of specific risk factors in helping to identify osteoporosis in a population of postmenopausal women. One of the most comprehensive reports in the United States is the Study of Osteoporotic Fractures (SOF), which used multivariable models to analyze data from 9,516 women older than 65 years in a prospective survey to identify 14 clinical risk factors as significant predictors for hip fracture. These included the following: age; maternal hip fracture; lack of weight gain; slight stature; poor self-rated health; hyperthyroidism; current use of benzodiazepines, anticonvulsants, or caffeine; not walking for exercise; lack of ambulation; inability to rise from a chair; poor scores on two measures of vision; high resting pulse rate; and any fracture since 50 years of age. Increased rates of hip fracture were identified in women with five or more risk factors. Unfortunately, no similar large studies with discriminating performance have been carried out in premenopausal women.

The U.S. Preventive Services Task Force has completed a scientific evidence review of screening for osteoporosis in postmenopausal women and made recommendations for screening. The Task Force concluded the following: (a) Good evidence indicates that the risk for osteoporosis and fracture increases with age and other risk factors, (b) bone density measurements accurately predict the risk for fractures in the short term, and (c) treating asymptomatic women with osteoporosis reduces the risk for fracture. According to the Task Force recommendations, women ages 65 and older should be routinely screened for osteoporosis. However, the Task Force made no recommendations for or against screening in postmenopausal women younger than 60 years or in women ages 60 to 64 who are not at increased risk for fractures.

Lifestyle Factors

Although the diagnosis of severe osteoporosis is definitive only with the occurrence of a fragility fracture, women of any age should be concerned with preventing osteoporosis. Avoidance of smoking and heavy alcohol use, in addition to an ongoing exercise program, should be encouraged. The current recommendations for calcium intake are summarized in Table 97.7. Calcium may be obtained from the diet or supplements; some common preparations are listed in Table 97.8. For someone with a relatively alkaline gastric pH or suppressed gastric acid secretion, calcium citrate is preferable because it is equally absorbed in either an acidic or alkaline environment.

Vitamin D supplements of 800 IU/d are recommended for women after the age of 60 years.

Prevention of Falls

Although significant loss of bone mass is extremely common in older women, some affected persons never experience a fracture. Falls are an important immediate contributing factor to osteoporosis morbidity and mortality and are common in community-dwelling older persons. Although some falls are minor, more than 90% of hip fractures are the result of a fall. Counseling older women about preventing falls is as important as choosing the appropriate medical regimen for patients at risk.

Falls are caused by a combination of numerous factors. Some risk factors include sensory loss (visual and hearing), disorders of gait and balance, arthritis, and medication use. In particular, medications that cause volume depletion, orthostatic hypotension, or sedation should be used with caution or not at all. The use of four or more medications has been found to be an independent risk factor for falling.

An assessment of the home environment is also beneficial. Uneven floor surfaces (steps or throw rugs), poor lighting, and lack of bathroom safety devices (grab bars, non-skid mats) may all contribute to a risk for falling.

Estrogen Replacement Therapy

During the past 50 years, estrogen replacement was historically the mainstay of treatment to prevent rapid bone loss at menopause despite never having been put to the test in a large randomized, prospective, placebo-controlled trial. As a consequence, the epidemiologic data regarding both the beneficial and adverse effects of estrogen were weakened, and some of the

TABLE 97.7. Optimal Calcium Intake

Age (y)	Elemental calcium (mg/d)
11–24	1,200–1,500
25–50	1,000
>50 (postmenopausal)	
On estrogen	1,000
Not on estrogen	1,500
Pregnant or nursing	1,200–1,500

Source: National Institutes of Health Consensus Panel, 1994.

TABLE 97.8. Common Calcium Supplements

Preparation	Milligrams of elemental calcium per gram of calcium salt	Dose to provide 1,000 mg of elemental calcium per day
Calcium carbonate[a]	400 mg/g	Four 650-mg tablets per day
Calcium citrate[b]	211 mg/g	Five 950-mg tablets per day

[a]Needs low pH to dissolve; take with meals.
[b]Dissolves independently of pH; use in achlorhydric patients.

putative associations of estrogen (e.g., with breast cancer) were difficult to interpret.

The data on breast cancer risk and estrogen use have been conflicting. Some gaps include the small number of studies of estrogen plus progestin regimens and the lack of large randomized, controlled trials. Most studies concur that the short-term use of estrogen (<5–7 years) is not associated with an increase in breast cancer risk. Some data show that long-term therapy (>8 years) may be associated with a 20% to 30% increase in the incidence of breast cancer, but others have not reported this finding.

With the release of the principal results of the arm of the Women's Health Initiative examining combined estrogen and progestin treatment, some of these issues have been addressed. The study population consisted of more than 16,000 healthy postmenopausal women with an intact uterus. Subjects were randomized to either placebo or a combination of equine estrogens (0.625 mg) and progesterone (2.5 mg) and were assessed for the primary outcomes of coronary disease and/or death in addition to secondary parameters of stroke, hip fracture, pulmonary embolism, endometrial cancer, colorectal cancer, and death from other causes. After an average follow-up period of 5.2 years, the study was terminated because of an observed increase in invasive breast cancer and smaller but persistent increases in myocardial infarction, stroke, pulmonary embolism, and deep venous thrombosis. A slight benefit was observed in terms of hip fractures and colon cancer. The conclusion of the authors was that the risks outweighed the benefit for the study population as a whole. It is important to note that the increased risk for breast cancer was noted only with the combination of estrogen and progesterone and not with estrogen monotherapy. A parallel trial of estrogen monotherapy in women who have had a hysterectomy is being continued until 2005.

With regard to bone metabolism, estrogen receptors have been identified on osteocytes where estrogen acts primarily as an antiresorptive agent. Estrogen is most effective when started before significant bone loss has occurred. Estrogen use is clearly linked to a decreased risk for hip fracture, with an overall risk reduction of approximately 25%. However, duration of use is an important variable; the fracture rate is lower in women who have used estrogen for a prolonged period (≥7–10 years) and, conversely, returns to baseline 6 or more years after therapy has been discontinued. Some studies have suggested a leveling of benefit after 5 to 7 years of use.

Because estrogen favorably affects lipoproteins, decreases platelet adhesiveness, and also directly affects vascular tone, estrogen therapy was believed to decrease the incidence of coronary disease in women with and without coronary disease when evaluated in observational studies. However, the Heart and Estrogen/progestin Replacement Study (HERS), performed over 4.1 years, found no overall benefit of estrogen replacement in providing secondary protection from cardiovascular disease in a population of postmenopausal women with established heart disease. It is more worrisome that a 50% increase in cardiovascular events was seen in the first year of the study.

The use of unopposed estrogen is associated with an increased risk for endometrial cancer, which is eliminated by the addition of a progestin to the regimen. Gallbladder disease occurs about twice as often in women who receive estrogen, as does a proclivity to clotting disorders. Not surprisingly, smoking greatly increases the thrombotic risk in estrogen users.

Overall, decisions about estrogen use must be based on an individualized assessment of a woman's risk for osteoporosis, breast cancer, cardiovascular disease, thrombosis, and colon cancer, in addition to the severity of vasomotor and central nervous system manifestations of estrogen deficiency. Although estrogen replacement therapy should be considered for all hypogonadal women at risk for osteoporosis, it can no longer be regarded as the agent of first choice because of the caveats previously noted. In women with a personal or family history of breast cancer or in the presence of significant coronary or cerebrovascular atherosclerosis, estrogens should be avoided and alternative interventions for preserving bone mass entertained. For patients at low risk for breast cancer, thrombotic events, and coronary disease, hormone replacement therapy may still be considered.

Calcitonin

The hormone calcitonin is produced by the parafollicular C cells of the thyroid in response to increased levels of PTH. This endogenous peptide binds to osteoclast receptors, inhibiting bone resorption. Despite its mechanism of action, exogenously administered calcitonin appears to have a lesser effect on BMD and fracture risk than other treatment options. In the Prevent Recurrence of Osteoporotic Fractures (PROOF) Trial, the most recent prospective, placebo-controlled trial to be performed in postmenopausal women, only modest increases in BMD at the spine and small decreases in risk for vertebral fracture were documented. No significant effects on hip density or fracture were noted, and no measurable effect in perimenopausal women with higher baseline BMD scores. Despite its less robust therapeutic effects, calcitonin therapy can be considered for patients with vertebral osteoporosis who experience side effects of hormonal manipulation and bisphosphonates or in whom these agents are contraindicated. Calcitonin has also been noted to have an analgesic effect when administered during the first few weeks after acute vertebral fracture, and it can therefore be used as an adjunctive therapy with narcotics and splinting. Calcitonin can be given either subcutaneously or intranasally. Side effects include flushing and nasal irritation.

Selective Estrogen Receptor Modulators

Selective estrogen receptor modulators (SERMs) act as estrogen receptor agonists in bone while blocking the effects of estrogen in breast and endometrial tissue. Raloxifene, the first SERM approved for the prevention and treatment of osteoporosis in postmenopausal women, was studied in the Multiple Outcomes of Raloxifene Evaluation (MORE), a large multicenter, placebo-controlled study that enrolled 7,705 postmenopausal women. Women with osteoporosis by DEXA or radiographic vertebral fractures received either 60 mg or 120 mg of raloxifene per day or a placebo and were followed for 3 years for the primary outcomes of vertebral and nonvertebral fractures. All study participants were given vitamin D and calcium supplements. The risk for vertebral fracture was reduced by 30% to 50% in the actively treated women with and without baseline vertebral fractures. The reduction in vertebral fractures occurred despite the fact that only a modest increase of 2% to 3% in BMD was achieved, approximately half the increase seen with bisphosphonates. Pooled data for both doses of raloxifene showed no reduction in the risk for nonvertebral fractures overall or hip fractures specifically. Thromboembolic events were increased by a factor of 3, similar to the risk observed with estrogens. Hot flashes and leg cramps were the most common side effects. In a separate analysis, the risk for invasive breast cancer was decreased by 76% during the 3 years of study participation. Raloxifene therefore offers an interesting and unique treatment option for osteoporotic women concerned about the development of breast cancer when vertebral osteoporosis is the main focus of treatment.

Bisphosphonates

Bisphosphonates are antiresorptive agents that bind to the hydroxyapatite crystalline structure in bone and decrease bone resorption by several postulated mechanisms, including a direct effect on osteoclast formation and function. They have been used to treat Paget disease and hypercalcemia of malignancy for more than a decade. Oral preparations of alendronate and risedronate have been approved by the Food and Drug Administration for both the prevention and treatment of postmenopausal osteoporosis. These medications are more effective and have fewer side effects than etidronate and pamidronate, the other two bisphosphonates available in the United States.

The ability of alendronate, a second-generation bisphosphonate, to reduce fracture risk in postmenopausal women ages 55 to 80 years with a low BMD in the femoral neck was evaluated in the Fracture Intervention Trial (FIT), a double-blinded, randomized, placebo-controlled study of more than 6,000 patients. The study was divided into two arms; one included patients with a low BMD in the hip but no prevalent vertebral fracture, and the second was composed of patients with a low BMD and at least one prevalent vertebral fracture. Participants were randomized to receive either placebo or 5 mg of alendronate for 3 to 4 years. After 2 years, the dose of alendronate was increased to 10 mg based on the results of other studies favoring the higher dose. In the 4,432 patients without pretreatment vertebral fractures, new vertebral fractures were reduced by 44% while the BMD increased significantly by 4.6% to 6.6%. In the 2,027 patients with preexisting vertebral fractures, new vertebral fractures were reduced by 47% and hip fractures by 51%, and a significant increase in BMD was observed.

The ability of risedronate, a third-generation bisphosphonate, to reduce vertebral fractures in postmenopausal women was examined in the Vertebral Efficacy with Risedronate Therapy (VERT) Trial, which was conducted in two separate arms. One enrolled 2,458 patients from North America who had at least two vertebral fractures or a low lumbar BMD and at least one vertebral fracture. The other enrolled 1,226 patients from Europe and Australia who had at least two vertebral fractures at baseline. All patients were randomized to placebo, 2.5 mg of risedronate, or 5 mg of risedronate. The 2.5-mg dose was discontinued by protocol amendment. During 3 years of follow-up, the risk for new vertebral fractures was reduced by 41% to 49% while the BMD increased by 4.3% to 5.9% at the lumbar spine and by 2.8% to 3.1% at the femoral neck.

The Hip Intervention Program (HIP) evaluated 9,497 women for 3 years in a multicenter randomized trial of postmenopausal women older than 70 years. Participants were treated with 2.5 mg of risedronate, 5 mg of risedronate, or placebo and were divided into two study groups. The first group included patients ages 70 to 79 years with either femoral neck osteoporosis (BMD > 4 SD below normal) or a BMD in the femoral neck more than 3 SD below normal and at least one clinical risk factor for fracture. The second group included patients 80 years of age or older with at least one clinical risk factor but no predetermined BMD requirement or with a BMD in the femoral neck 4 SD or more below normal. Interestingly, hip fractures were reduced by 39% to 58% in the patients with confirmed osteoporosis by actual BMD measurement but not in the patients included only on the basis of historical risk factors despite their advanced age. These findings support the desirability of basing treatment decisions on known BMD readings or the presence of pretreatment fragility fractures. Thus, with both alendronate and risedronate, hip fracture reduction was most evident in those women with documented osteoporosis, a history of vertebral fractures, or both.

Smaller dosing studies that followed these larger efficacy trials demonstrated the equivalence of weekly dosing of alendronate (70 mg) and risedronate (35 mg) in accruing BMD at the hip and spine in comparison with the daily dosing protocols. No large fracture prevention trials have used the once-weekly doses.

Because of concerns about local irritation of the esophageal and gastric mucosa, which increases with the duration of contact with the pill, both alendronate and risedronate must be taken with at least 8 oz of water while the patient remains upright in a seated or standing position. Because even under optimal conditions only 1% of an orally dosed bisphosphonate is absorbed, it should be taken on an empty stomach, with only water, at least 30 minutes before eating or drinking. Food or milk or other medications will inhibit absorption. Both drugs bind avidly to calcium, so that it is important to dose vitamins and calcium supplements with lunch or dinner at another time of the day. Nevertheless, as with all antiresorptive agents, adequate calcium and vitamin D supplementation is essential. Because of their proven efficacy in preventing hip fractures, bisphosphonates should be the agents of first choice for a patient with a history of previous hip fractures or documented osteoporotic BMD of the femoral neck or entire hip region.

An exciting alternative approach to oral bisphosphonate therapy is intravenous dosing with potent, long-acting agents such as zoledronic acid. This drug was examined for 1 year in 351 postmenopausal women in a placebo-controlled, randomized, double-blinded trial. Several dose regimens were evaluated, including 1 mg given intravenously every 3 months, 2 mg given every 6 months, and 4 mg given once a year. No significant differences were observed between the doses in accretion of BMD, which ranged from 3.1% to 3.5% at the femoral neck and from 4.3% to 5.1% at the lumbar spine in comparison with placebo. The level of C-telopeptide, a marker of bone resorption, reached a nadir after 1 month of therapy with all regimens, mirroring the physiologic effect of the orally dosed bisphosphonates. The possibility of convenient, once-yearly treatment with zoledronic acid to increase BMD and decrease fractures is currently being evaluated in a prospective multicenter study across the United States.

Parathyroid Hormone

A biologically active synthetic preparation of the 1–34 N-terminal portion of the native 84-amino acid human PTH, teriparatide, has been approved by the Food and Drug Administration for the treatment of women with established osteoporosis who are at high risk for recurrent fracture. Patients considered at high risk include those with previous single or multiple osteoporotic fractures and those who have failed to respond to or cannot tolerate other established therapies. Teriparatide is given as a 20-pg dose subcutaneously into the thigh or abdomen; peak serum concentrations that exceed normal levels of endogenous PTH are reached 30 minutes after dosing and fall to undetectable levels within 3 hours. Thus, although the chronically elevated levels of endogenous PTH seen in primary hyperparathyroidism are associated with significant bone resorption and calcium excretion, intermittent dosing of PTH has the opposite effect of stimulating bone formation by triggering a robust osteoblastic reaction. A large prospective, placebo-controlled study of 1,637 postmenopausal women with prior vertebral fracture who were given either 20 or 40 pg of teriparatide demonstrated a reduction in vertebral fractures of more than 65% and in nonvertebral fractures of 50%. Large increases in BMD were noted in the spine and moderate increases at hip sites. A small reduction in BMD in the distal radius was noted. Overall, only relatively minor side effects of headache and nausea were reported, and mild hypercalcemia in a few patients. The dropout rate was similar to that for placebo at the 20-pg dose. In another study, which compared 40 pg of teriparatide with 10 mg of alendronate, 146 postmenopausal women were followed for an average of 14 months. This study demonstrated an increase in BMD in the lumbar spine of 12.2% in the PTH group and of 5.6% in the bisphosphonate-treated patients. The only serious concern raised during preclinical animal studies was an observed increase in osteosarcomas in rats given extremely high doses (3–60 times normal) of teriparatide during their lifetime. This was not observed in monkey models. Furthermore, the risk for osteosarcoma is not increased in humans with hyperparathyroidism. The Food and Drug Administration concluded that this finding was not likely germane to the approved dosing protocol in humans, but it does advise through a "black box" labeling to avoid treating patients with a history of Paget disease, unexplained elevations of alkaline phosphatase, or prior skeletal radiation. Teriparatide is usually given for 1 to 2 years, after which a bisphosphonate or other antiresorptive treatment is given to maintain the gains in BMD.

Other Agents

Supplementation with 1,25-dihydroxyvitamin D and calcium in institutionalized or community-dwelling groups of elderly women has been shown to reduce fractures in some studies, but not in others. This likely speaks to the presence of significant vitamin D deficiency in both chronically institutionalized patients and many independently living elderly persons with inadequate exposure to sunlight and dietary intake of vitamin D. Screening for osteomalacia is important in this setting. In a large double-blinded, placebo-controlled, prospective 18-month trial, 3,270 elderly women were randomized to receive 1.2 g of elemental calcium and 800 IU of vitamin D_3. Hip fractures were reduced by 43% in the arm with calcium and vitamin D. However, another trial, which included 3,910 elderly persons, failed to show significant fracture reduction with a combination of 25-hydroxyvitamin D and calcium. In general, vitamin D and calcium supplementation alone, although helping to maintain BMD, cannot be considered adequate fracture prevention therapy in ambulatory women with confirmed osteoporosis. Because of the obvious benefit of these supplements to bone health and metabolism, however, they have been universally included in all trials of the newer antiresorptive agents.

Sodium fluoride stimulates bone formation and is approved for use in osteoporosis in several European countries, but not in the United States. Previous trials of fluoride reported an increase in bone mass but no reduction in the fracture rate and a significant percentage of side effects. Much lower doses of slow-release fluoride plus calcium supplementation have been shown to increase bone mass and reduce vertebral compression fractures, with minimal side effects. Because of a lack of supporting data from trials assessing fracture reduction, this combination is unlikely to be approved as a treatment in the near future.

Anabolic steroids also increase bone formation but have adverse effects on serum lipids, elevate hepatic enzymes, and induce virilization. They are not recommended for general use.

Supplementation with growth hormone has yielded mixed results in terms of accruing bone mass. Furthermore, no fracture studies have been performed, and this method is not likely to be approved for osteoporotic adults who are not deficient in growth hormone.

Vertebroplasty/Kyphoplasty

Successful treatment of the acute osteoporotic vertebral compression fracture remains challenging in view of the desire to provide adequate analgesia but avoid side effects, especially in elderly patients, in whom adverse complications are most often seen. Some patients are severely compromised and bedridden for days and weeks. Two procedures that are currently available often provide almost instant relief and facilitate a return to ambulation and function in many patients in whom conservative treatment has failed. In vertebroplasty, a needle is passed percutaneously into the collapsed vertebral body under fluoroscopic guidance, and polymethylmethacrylate bone cement is injected through the needle. In kyphoplasty, the needle is passed into the collapsed vertebra, and a balloon that is inflated through the tip partially reestablishes the height of the vertebral body and creates a cavity into which the cement is subsequently injected. Because these techniques provide mechanical stabilization, pain is often remarkably and quickly reduced with a low complication rate and good success. A caveat, however, is that in some patients, the contiguous vertebral segments collapse with time. Whether the procedure itself predisposes to such fractures or they simply represent the inevitable complications of osteoporosis in a high-risk population is not known. Consequently, to prevent future fractures, aggressive medical treatment of osteoporosis in these patients should be the rule.

BIBLIOGRAPHY

Allen SH. Primary osteoporosis: methods to combat bone loss that accompanies aging. *Postgrad Med* 1993;93:43.

Aloia JF, Vaswani A, Yeh JK, et al. Calcium supplementation with and without hormone replacement therapy to prevent postmenopausal bone loss. *Ann Intern Med* 1994;120:97.

Baylink DJ, Jennings JC. Calcium and bone homeostasis and changes with aging. In: Hazzard WR, Bierman EL, Blass JP, et al., eds. *Principles of geriatric medicine and gerontology*, 3rd ed. New York: McGraw-Hill, 1994:879.

Black DM, Cummings SR, Karpf DB, et al. Randomised trial of effect of alendronate on risk of fracture in women with existing vertebral fractures. Fracture Intervention Trial Research Group. *Lancet* 1996;348:1535.

Chapuy MC, Arlot ME, Duboeuf F, et al. Vitamin D_3 and calcium to prevent hip fractures in elderly women. *N Engl J Med* 1992;327:1637.

Chapuy MC, Chapuy P, Meunier PJ. Calcium and vitamin D supplements: effects on calcium metabolism in elderly people. *Am J Clin Nutr* 1987;46:324.

Chesnut C, Silverman S, Andriano K, et al. A randomized trial of nasal spray salmon calcitonin in postmenopausal women with established osteoporosis: the Prevent Recurrence of Osteoporotic Fractures Study. *Am J Med* 2000;109:267.

Chesnut CH III. Osteoporosis. In: Hazzard WR, Bierman EL, Blass JP, et al., eds.

Principles of geriatric medicine and gerontology, 3rd ed. New York: McGraw-Hill, 1994:897.
Consensus Development Conference. Diagnosis, prophylaxis, and treatment of osteoporosis. *Am J Med* 1993;94:646.
Cummings S, Eckert S, Krueger K, et al. The effect of raloxifene on risk of breast cancer in postmenopausal women. Results from the MORE randomized trial. *JAMA* 1999;281:2189.
Ettinger B, Black DM, Mitlak BH, et al. Reduction of vertebral fracture risk in postmenopausal women with osteoporosis treated with raloxifene: results from a 3-year randomized clinical trial. Multiple Outcomes of Raloxifene Evaluation (MORE) Investigators. *JAMA* 1999;282:637.
Felson DT, Zhang Y, Hannan MT, et al. The effect of postmenopausal estrogen therapy on bone density in elderly women. *N Engl J Med* 1993;329:1141.
Garay L, Parreno J, Gonazalez Y. A prospective multicentric, randomized study to evaluate the effect of tricalcium phosphate versus tricalcium phosphate plus 25(OH)-vitamin D on the risk of fractures in older women. *Geriatrika* 1997;13:24.
Healy B. PEPI in perspective—good answers spawn pressing questions [Editorial]. *JAMA* 1995;273:240.
Harris ST, Watts NB, Genant HK, et al. Effects of risedronate treatment on vertebral and nonvertebral fractures in women with postmenopausal osteoporosis: a randomized controlled trial. Vertebral Efficacy with Risedronate Therapy (VERT) Study Group. *JAMA* 1999;282:1344.
Heaney RP. Fluoride and osteoporosis [Editorial]. *Ann Intern Med* 1994;120:689.
Henrich III. The postmenopausal estrogen/breast cancer controversy. *JAMA* 1992; 268:1900.
Hulley S, Grady D, Bush T, et al. Randomized trial of estrogen plus progestin for secondary prevention of coronary heart disease in postmenopausal women. Heart and Estrogen/progestin Replacement Study (HERS) Research Group. *JAMA* 1998;280:605.
McClung MR, Geusens P, Miller PD, et al. Effect of risedronate on the risk of hip fracture in elderly women. Hip Intervention Program Study Group. *N Engl J Med* 2001;344:333.
Neer RM, Arnaud CD, Zanchetta JR, et al. Effect of parathyroid hormone (1–34) on fractures and bone mineral density in post-menopausal women with osteoporosis. *N Engl J Med* 2001;344:1434.
Nelson H, Helfand M, Woolf S, et al. Screening for postmenopausal osteoporosis: a review of the evidence for the U.S. Preventive Services Task Force. *Ann Intern Med* 2002;137:529.
Nelson ME, Fiatarone MA, Morganti CM, et al. Effects of high-intensity strength training on multiple risk factors for osteoporotic fractures: a randomized control trial. *JAMA* 1994;272:1909.
NIH Consensus Conference. Optimal calcium intake. *JAMA* 1994;272:1942.
Pak CY, Sakhaee K, Piziak V, et al. Slow-release sodium fluoride in the management of postmenopausal osteoporosis: a randomized control trial. *Ann Intern Med* 1994;120:625.
Reginster J, Minne HW, Sorensen OH, et al. Randomized trial of the effects of risedronate on vertebral fractures in women with established postmenopausal osteoporosis. Vertebral Efficacy with Risedronate Therapy (VERT) Study Group. *Osteoporos Int* 2000;11:83.
Reid I, Brown J, Burckhardt P, et al. Intravenous zoledronic acid in postmenopausal women with low bone mineral density. *N Engl J Med* 2002;346:653.
Steinberg KK, Thacker SB, Smith J, et al. A meta-analysis of the effect of estrogen replacement therapy on the risk of breast cancer. *JAMA* 1991;265:1985.
Tilyard M, Spears GFS, Thomson J, et al. Treatment of postmenopausal osteoporosis with calcitriol or calcium. *N Engl J Med* 1992;326:357.
U.S. Preventive Services Task Force. Screening for osteoporosis in postmenopausal women. Rockville, MD: Agency for Healthcare Research and Quality, 2002. Available at *www.ahrq.gov/clinic/3rduspstf/osteoporosis/osteorr.htm*. Originally in *Ann Intern Med* 2002;137:526–528.
Watts NB, Harris ST, Genant HK. Treatment of painful osteoporotic vertebral fractures with percutaneous vertebroplasty or kyphoplasty. *Osteoporos Int* 2001;12: 429.
Writing Group for the PEPI Trial. Effects of estrogen or estrogen/progestin regimens on heart disease risk factors in postmenopausal women. *JAMA* 1995;273:199.
Writing Group for the Women's Health Initiative Investigators. Risks and benefits of estrogen plus progestin in healthy postmenopausal women: principal results from the Women's Health Initiative Randomized Controlled Trial. *JAMA* 2002;288:321.

CHAPTER 98
Neck and Back Pain

Phillip R. Lucas, Mark Palumbo,
Robert Campbell, and Mauricio A. Valdes

Back and neck pain are second only to upper respiratory complaints as a reason for visits to a physician. Men and women are equally affected, with the initial presentation most often between the ages of 30 and 50 years. Some studies estimate that 60% to 80% of adults have experienced low back pain, and 2% to 5% are affected on a yearly basis. Low back pain is the most common and expensive cause of chronic disability and therefore one of the most frequent reasons for early retirement in Western countries. Impairments related to back pain are among the leading causes of time lost from work and permanent disability.

Although most cases of back and neck pain resolve without invasive intervention, approximately 4% of the population will undergo a spinal procedure in their lifetime. Recent years have seen a dramatic rise in the overall rates of spinal surgery. From 1988 to 1997, rates of spinal surgery among U.S. Medicare enrollees increased 57%, to a rate of 3.4 per 1,000 members of the population.

ETIOLOGY

Pain is an unpleasant sensory and emotional experience associated with actual or potential tissue damage. Several structures have been implicated in the development of back or neck pain. These include the intervertebral discs, ligaments, overlying muscles, neural elements, and osseous spine. In addition, neck and back pain can be the result of pathologic processes involving the adjacent viscera and vascular structures. Therefore, the causes of neck and back pain are many. One way to organize the numerous causes is to categorize them as spondylogenic, neurogenic, vascular, visceral, or psychogenic (Table 98.1). These categories overlap significantly. Although it is thought that malingering patients are rare, an underlying psychological component may magnify the underlying symptoms and disability of many patients.

Often, in both acute and chronic situations, no significant structural abnormalities may be noted in the physical examination and diagnostic studies. In this case, biochemical substances probably play an important role. Metabolites involved in inflammation, such as substance P, prostaglandins, and bradykinins, may reach the dorsal ganglia and nociceptors and cause hyperactivity in cells located at this level, with implications for pain.

TABLE 98.1. Sources of Spinal Pain

Spondylogenic
Muscle
Ligament
Disc
Osseous structures
Neurogenic
Nerve root
Peripheral nerve
Spinal cord
Vascular
Aneurysm
Peripheral vascular disease
Visceral
Genitourinary system
Gynecologic
Gastrointestinal system
Psychogenic

HISTORY/PHYSICAL EXAMINATION

Because of the extensive differential diagnosis, a complete and accurate history is essential. All the standard parameters, such as the location, duration, and severity of symptoms and any positively or negatively modifying factors, must be clearly determined and documented. Diagnostic acumen is vital in identifying patients with an acute condition that requires rapid, high-level attention to prevent progression and permanent disability (Table 98.2).

Examination allows continued focusing of the clinical problem. As always, the examination begins with careful observation. Appreciating the way a patient moves or does not move provides early clues to pain and dysfunction. The patient should always be properly exposed. It is possible to maintain modesty and still expose the areas that must be examined. Inspection includes gait, spinal curvature, alignment, and pelvic tilt. Palpation should be performed and range of motion carefully assessed throughout the spinal column. The abdomen and distal pulses should also be evaluated. A genital and rectal examination must be included in accordance with the symptoms and presentation. Flexion, extension, lateral bend, and rotation are easily checked in the cervical and lumbar spine.

A very important part of the assessment is the neurologic examination. This includes an evaluation of muscle strength and sensation, including light touch, pinprick, propioception, and reflexes, with any asymmetric or pathologic changes noted.

The presence of certain historical, symptomatic, and physical examination "red flags" (Table 98.3) should alert the physician. These patients require further investigation to rule out underlying and potentially dangerous pathologic conditions.

DIAGNOSTIC STUDIES

Depending on the presenting symptoms and physical findings, many patients do not require diagnostic studies. The severity and duration of symptoms determine what tests should be ordered.

Except in the diagnosis of a variety of infectious problems, laboratory studies are not very helpful in the diagnosis of back pain. The white blood cell count, erythrocyte sedimentation rate, and level of C-reactive protein are all used to diagnose infection, but obviously, the results are often nonspecific, and the information must be applied in the context of the overall clinical presentation. Other nonspecific parameters, such as the alkaline phosphatase level, may be elevated in the event of spinal tumor or metabolic disease, but in general they play a minor adjunctive role. The levels of parathyroid hormone, ionized calcium, albumin, and inorganic phosphate are similarly used in the diagnosis of metabolic bone disease.

TABLE 98.2. Elements of the History

Age
Sex
Trauma Mechanism: seat belt, airbag, damage to vehicle
Symptoms
Location: pinpoint, diffuse, radiating
Duration
Alleviating factors
Aggravating factors
Nocturnal/diurnal variation
Radiating to where?
Onset
Sensory/motor deficits
Bowel/bladder dysfunction
Sexual dysfunction
Progression over time
Occupational activities
Leisure activities
Psychosocial factors
Smoking
Previous therapeutic modalities

TABLE 98.3. "Red Flags"

Age
Fever
Sudden neurologic changes
Immunosuppressive drugs
History of cancer
Weight loss
Drug abuse
Pain at rest

Radiologic studies are a mainstay of the assessment of neck and back pain. Many practitioners believe that radiology may be overused in a scattergun approach to diagnosis. However, there is no doubt that the following studies, when properly used, can augment the physician's diagnostic arsenal:

Plain films have long been a mainstay of diagnosis. Applications include fracture, scoliosis, vertebral alignment, flexion/extension views, spondylolisthesis, degenerative disease, destruction of bone secondary to infection or tumor, seronegative spondylarthropathies, and osteoporotic changes.

Ultrasonography is used mainly to evaluate collections of fluid, such as seromas, hematomas, infections, and possibly tumors.

Myelography was more important before the advent of magnetic resonance imaging (MRI). It is now used mostly to evaluate spinal stenosis with computed tomography as the imaging modality.

Scintigraphy offers the advantage of whole-body scanning, but its low specificity is a disadvantage. It is used mostly to evaluate tumors and infections.

Computed tomography allows a precise visualization of the bony anatomy. It is extremely useful to evaluate fracture, especially in complex anatomic areas, such as the spine and pelvis.

MRI is best for imaging soft tissues, such as ligaments, muscles, intervertebral discs, and neural elements. It is also useful for the evaluation of infections and tumors.

Bone densitometry is used to assess bone mineral content and risk for osteoporotic fracture.

CLINICAL PRESENTATION AND TREATMENT

Because the presentations and causes of neck and back pain share many features, they can be grouped into two main categories, acute and chronic.

Acute

After a thorough history and examination have ruled out visceral or vascular conditions and suggested that the origin of the pain is in spinal structures, the most common cause is a musculoskeletal imbalance, more commonly known as *mechanical pain*. Although trauma may be a precipitating event, acute pain may also be the result of day-to-day mechanical stresses superimposed on biochemical changes. Overuse of the neck and back can cause muscular strain. *Generally*, the evaluation of patients with this initial presentation reveals pain during movement and muscle tenderness without neurologic abnormalities. No diagnostic studies are necessary at this time unless a "red flag" is encountered (Table 98.3). Usually, such patients are treated with analgesics, nonsteroidal antiinflammatory drugs (NSAIDs), and mild muscle relaxants. If symptoms persist, diagnostic studies, beginning with radiographs, are indicated. Physical therapy may be of some benefit at this point.

A percentage of patients in this category have an underlying disc herniation. The initial presentation may be the same as in muscle strain, but the symptoms often do not resolve within a short time. In some cases, neurologic symptoms and signs may develop in the extremities secondary to a proximal nerve compression. Initial treatment includes a brief period of rest and analgesics, but if pain persists or the neurologic findings worsen, then MRI of the suspected region should be performed (Fig. 98.1). At this point, the use of oral or epidural steroids has been shown to have beneficial effects. Even with positive MRI findings, the symptoms of most patients resolve spontaneously within 4 to 6 weeks. Approximately 10% of patients presenting with acute neck and back pain and positive neurologic findings require surgical intervention.

Surgery may be required in certain cases, as when mass lesions within the spinal canal cause severe neurologic impairment. Mass lesions such as herniated discs, epidural abscesses, and metastases may occur at all levels of the spine.

Chronic

In about 7% of patients who present with acute back pain, longstanding or chronic symptoms develop that may severely interfere with day-to-day function.

Treatment of these patients requires a thorough diagnostic workup and most often a multidisciplinary approach including pain management, physical therapy, changes in lifestyle, and rarely surgical intervention, such as fusion.

The Elderly Patient

Elderly patients may experience neck and back pain as a result of degenerative arthritis or metabolic changes causing osteoporosis. In addition, the incidence of metastatic disease necessitates not only a complete history and examination but also an early diagnostic imaging evaluation, beginning with plain radiographs (Fig. 98.2). MRI and bone scan are often necessary. If the symptoms are of nonradiating pain without red flags, a diagnosis of degenerative arthritis may be made, and treatment should involve the use of NSAIDs, physical therapy, and possibly changes in lifestyle.

In a patient with symptoms that radiate to an upper or lower extremity or gait abnormalities, the spinal cord or cauda equina is often compressed. Such a patient may be treated symptomatically, but depending on the neurologic findings, degree of disability, and general health, surgical intervention may be required. Despite age and comorbid conditions, good to excellent results of surgical intervention may be achieved in 80% of these cases.

Metabolic changes as a result of endocrine abnormalities and changes in the nutritional state of an elderly patient may lay the

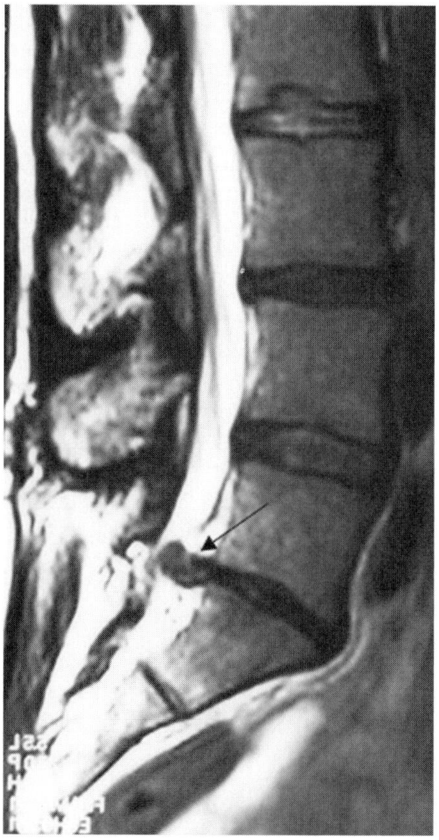

FIG. 98.1. Magnetic resonance image of the lumbar spine showing a herniated disc *(arrow)* at the L5-S1 level.

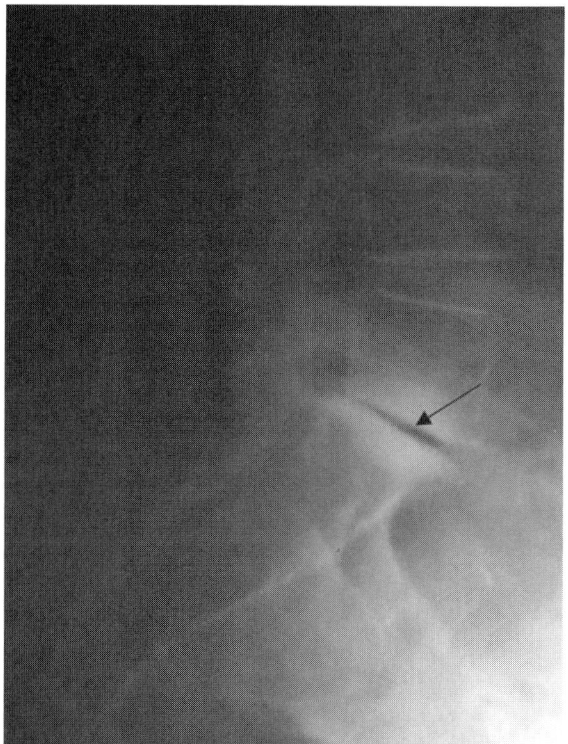

FIG. 98.2. Lateral plain x-ray film of the lumbar spine showing marked degenerative changes at the L5-S1 level. Loss of height of the intervertebral space *(arrow)* is associated with sclerotic changes of the adjacent vertebral bodies and osteophytes.

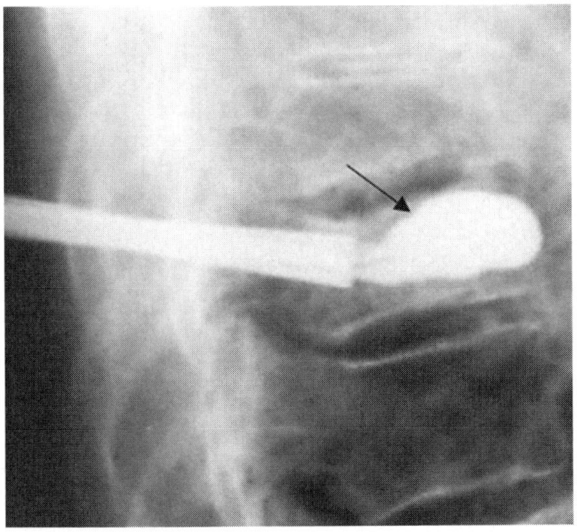

FIG. 98.3. Lateral plain x-ray film of the thoracolumbar junction. A kyphoplasty procedure (transpedicular cement injection) *(arrow)* has reestablished the vertebral body height.

groundwork for osteoporosis or osteomalacia. Compression fractures may occur in the thoracic or lumbar spine even without trauma. Management should include prevention with an adequate diet (calcium intake) and periodic evaluation with dual-energy x-ray absorptiometry (DEXA). If osteopenia is present, supplemental treatment with bisphosphonates, calcitonin, and vitamin D is required; in the case of postmenopausal women, hormonal supplementation with estrogens has shown benefit. An adequate exercise program with weight bearing is always advised.

When a fracture does occur, neurologic involvement is rare. Treatment in this case consists of symptomatic relief of pain with analgesics and the use of a back support. If the patient remains symptomatic for a period of weeks, then treatment with vertebroplasty or kyphoplasty may be indicated (Fig. 98.3). Surgical decompression with stabilization is generally reserved for the rare patient with neurologic compromise.

CONSIDERATIONS IN PREGNANCY

Because this is a textbook of primary care for women, a discussion of back pain in pregnancy is warranted. Back pain is especially common during pregnancy, experienced by 50% or more of pregnant women. Back pain is so frequent during pregnancy that it is often viewed as an expected part of the process.

Multiparity, Caucasian race, heavier weight, short stature, younger age, and psychological problems have all been related to a greater frequency of back pain during pregnancy. Back pain during pregnancy is also associated with a history of previous back pain, especially when the pain presents between the 12th and 28th weeks of gestation. Interestingly, the onset of back pain during pregnancy has also been associated with a greater frequency of spontaneous abortion. The intensity of pain correlates with the time required for resolution postpartum. Ten percent to 25% of women with persistent back pain report an onset during pregnancy, and about 7% still have serious residual pain at 18 months postpartum that affects their ability to carry out daily activities and work. The risk for recurrence of back pain during a second pregnancy is high.

Etiology

Changes occurring during pregnancy influence the onset of back pain. The mean total body content of water increases during pregnancy. As a consequence of fluid retention in and around connective tissues in the vertebral column and pelvis, they become more lax.

The weight gained can be as much as 25% of the body weight before pregnancy. Because of a shift in the center of gravity, changes in posture are required to maintain balance, and an increase in lumbar lordosis causes an imbalance that may lead to muscular fatigue. These alterations may play a role in disc herniation, but the literature fails to show a higher prevalence of disc disease during pregnancy.

Hormonal changes also influence the development of back pain. Relaxin increases ligamentous laxity around the pelvic joints, especially in the symphysis pubis and sacroiliac joints, which leads to instability and decreased joint support.

Engorgement of the epidural veins secondary to hypervolemia and obstruction of the inferior vena cava by the enlarged uterus in the supine position may result in hypoxia and metabolic disturbances of unmyelinated nerves, which cause positional and predominantly nocturnal back pain.

Evaluation

Radiographic examination is recommended only after the first trimester. Most patients with classic symptoms and signs limited to low back pain that is not severe and sacroiliac instability can be managed without radiographic evaluation.

Patients in whom severe and unusual symptoms develop may undergo a lumbar spinal x-ray series, and if needed, MRI can be performed.

Clinical Presentation

Some studies suggest that back pain in pregnancy is not a single syndrome and should be separated into lumbar back pain and posterior pelvic pain. Others include posterior pelvic pain within the diagnosis of low back pain.

Uncomplicated low back pain occurs over the area of the lumbar spine and may or may not radiate to the leg.

Posterior pelvic pain is four times as prevalent as low back pain. The pattern is similar to the one described for sacroiliac pain, the pain of ligamentous laxity, or pelvic insufficiency. Posterior pelvic pain is deep. It is usually felt distal to L5-S1 over the sacroiliac joint and posterior superior iliac spine and sometimes radiates to the posterior thigh or knee; it may also present as a typical "catching" of the leg during walking, worsening with certain postures and asymmetric loading of the pelvis. Pain at the pubic symphysis may be associated.

Low back pain and posterior pelvic pain can be differentiated by location and by the posterior pelvic provocation test, which consists of hip flexion on the affected side to 90 degrees while the opposite iliac crest is stabilized. Vertical pressure is applied through the flexed thigh, and a positive test result reproduces the patient's symptoms.

Management

Preventive measures for women planning a pregnancy can have definite positive effects. General care of the back, education, and fitness programs certainly diminish the incidence of back-related problems during pregnancy, especially for women with a history of previous back pain.

Management is generally conservative. Measures include limitation of physical activity, wearing low-heeled shoes, application of heat, and resting in bed with pillows under the knees if the pain is acute.

The analgesic of choice is acetaminophen. Severe muscle spasm can be managed with methocarbamol. Other drugs, such as codeine, aspirin, and NSAIDs, are relatively contraindicated and should be avoided as much as possible. They can be used on a case-to-case basis for a short time only. Long-term use should be avoided to lessen the possibility of intracranial bleeding and improper timing of closure of the fetal ductus arteriosus.

Other conservative measures include the use of devices that support the back, such as sacroiliac corsets and trochanteric belts. Individual education and physical training programs that include pelvic tilting exercises have effectively managed severe pain during this period.

The treatment of herniated disc and sciatica in pregnant women is similar to that for other patients with these conditions; surgery is reserved for those with severe unremitting pain and neurologic emergencies.

BIBLIOGRAPHY

Anderson GBJ. Epidemiological features of chronic low-back pain. *Lancet* 1999;354:581–585.
Advanced trauma life support course manual. Chicago: American College of Surgeons, 1997.
Berg G, Hammar M, Moller-Nielsen J, et al. Low back pain during pregnancy. *Obstet Gynecol* 1988;71:71–75.
Castro WHM, ed. *Examination and diagnosis of musculoskeletal disorders: clinical examination, imaging modalities.* New York: Thieme Medical Publishers, 2001.
Chan YL, Lam WWM, Lau TK, et al. Back pain in pregnancy—magnetic resonance imaging correlation. *Clin Radiol* 2002;57:1109–1112.
Damen L, Buyruk H, Guler-Uysal F, et al. Pelvic pain during pregnancy is associated with asymmetric laxity of the sacroiliac joints. *Acta Obstet Gynecol Scand* 2001;80:1019–1024.
Deyo RA, Weinstein JN. Low back pain. *N Engl J Med* 2001;344:363–370.
Farndon DF, Garfin SR, eds. *Orthopaedic knowledge update, spine 2.* Rosemont, IL: American Academy of Orthopaedic Surgeons, 2002.
Fast A, Shapiro D, Ducommun EJ, et al. Low back pain in pregnancy. *Spine* 1987; 12:368–371.
Greene WB, ed. *Essentials of musculoskeletal care,* 2nd ed. Rosemont, IL: American Academy of Orthopaedic Surgeons, 2001.
Heckmann JD, Sassard R. Musculoskeletal considerations in pregnancy. *J Bone Joint Surg Am* 1994;76:1720–1730.
Hoppenfeld S. *Orthopaedic neurology.* Philadelphia: Lippincott-Raven, 1997.
Kristiansson P, Svardsudd K, Von Schoultz B. Back pain during pregnancy. *Spine* 1996;21:702–709.
Kristiansson P, Svardsudd K, Von Schoultz B. Serum relaxin, symphyseal pain and back pain during pregnancy. *Am J Obstet Gynecol* 1996;175:1342–1347.
MacEvilly M, Buggy D. Back pain and pregnancy: a review. *Pain* 1996;64:405–414.
Miller MD, ed. *Review of orthopaedics,* 2nd ed. Philadelphia: WB Saunders, 1996.
Nirkmeyer NJO, Weinstein JN, et al. Design of the Spine Patient Outcomes Research Trial (SPORT). *Spine* 2002;27:1361–1372.
Noren L, Ostgaard S, Johansson G, et al. Lumbar back and posterior pelvic pain during pregnancy: a 3-year follow up. *Eur Spine J* 2002;11:267–271.
Ostgaard HC, Anderson GBJ, Karlsson K. Prevalence of back pain in pregnancy. *Spine* 1991;16:549–552.
Ostgaard HC, Andersson GBJ. Previous back pain and risk of developing back pain in a future pregnancy. *Spine* 1991;16:432–436.
Ostgaard HC, Zetherstrom G, Roos-Hansson E. Back pain in relation to pregnancy: a 6-year follow up. *Spine* 1997;24:2945–2950.
Perkins J, Hammer RL, Loubert PV. Identification and management of pregnancy-related low back pain. *J Nurse Midwifery* 1998;43:331–340.
Sturesson B, Uden G, Uden A. Pain pattern in pregnancy and catching of the leg in pregnant women with posterior pelvic pain. *Spine* 1997;22(16):1880–1883.
Sydsjo A, Sydsjo G, Alexanderson K. Influence of pregnancy-related diagnoses on sick-leave data in women aged 16–44. *J Womens Health Gender-Based Med* 2001; 10:707–714.
Weinstein JN, Rydevik BL, Volker KH. *Essentials of the spine.* New York: Raven Press, 1995:1–54.

CHAPTER 99
Hip and Knee Pain

Robert Shalvoy, Gary M. Ferguson, and Roy K. Aaron

HIP PAIN

Etiology

ANATOMIC CONSIDERATIONS

Articular or periarticular hip pain must be distinguished from pain originating in related anatomic areas. Because of the proximity of the hip to the lower abdominal quadrants, retroperitoneum, and iliopsoas muscle, which originates from the lumbar spinous processes and passes through the retroperitoneum to insert on the lesser trochanter, disease in these areas may present as hip pain. An example is the well-described retroperitoneal abscess that is associated with diverticulosis or inflammatory bowel disease and may present as hip irritability on range of motion. In women, femoral herniae present occasionally as hip pain. In addition, the fourth lumbar nerve root supplies sensation to the groin and anteromedial thigh, and conditions such as spinal stenosis and herniated lumbar disc with L4 nerve root entrapment may present as hip pain.

The blood supply to the femoral head, in particular the arterioles and venules, appears to be unusually sensitive to alterations in intraosseous pressure and microthrombosis, which has major implications in terms of osteonecrosis, described in more detail later. Several sources of periarticular pain have an anatomic basis. Two major bursae are close to the hip. Inflammation of the trochanteric bursa may present as tenderness directly over the greater trochanter, or scarring and fibrosis of the bursa may lead to symptoms of snapping hip. Inflammation of the psoas bursa presents as deep medial groin pain. A large number of muscles originate from the pelvis, notably hip flexors from the anterior pelvis, abductors from the lateral pelvis, and hamstrings from the ischial tuberosity, and avulsion or inflammation of these structures in athletically active women may present as acute and severe periarticular pain localized over the muscle origins.

DIFFERENTIAL DIAGNOSIS

Several distinct pathologic entities frequently involve the hip joint and present as hip pain.

Osteoarthritis. The female-to-male ratio in persons with osteoarthritis (OA) is 2:1. Two thirds of patients undergoing hip or knee arthroplasty are women. OA may be idiopathic or secondary. Some forms of idiopathic osteoarthritis may be genetic, and osteoarthritis-prone populations of patients are being studied. OA is often secondary to trauma, dysplasia, sepsis, inflammatory conditions, or, more rarely, metabolic disorders.

OA of the hip presents as groin or buttock pain that is often of significant severity and may radiate to the anterior and anteromedial thigh as far distally as the knee. Pain tends to develop at the end of the day and is accompanied by a reduction in gait capabilities, which may be experienced as fatigue. Patients present with an antalgic gait and may exhibit some true shortening of the affected limb as a consequence of loss of articular cartilage.

The radiographic characteristics of osteoarthritis are a patchy, nonconcentric loss of joint space, subchondral sclerosis, and cysts and reactive bone, including osteophytes and capsular calcification. Osteophytes at the medial hip joint and loss of cartilage on the weight-bearing portion of the femoral head may together result in a superolateral migration of the femoral head within the acetabulum.

Inflammatory Arthritis. The prototype of inflammatory arthritis is rheumatoid arthritis (RA), in which the female-to-male ratio is 3:1. Other inflammatory arthritides include systemic lupus erythematosus, scleroderma, and mixed connective tissue disease, also with a strong female predominance, and the inflammatory spondylarthropathies; in general, these conditions are less destructive to joints than RA. RA classically presents as a migratory, symmetric oligoarticular or polyarticular arthritis but at times is monarticular, especially early in the course. The presentation of pain in the hip is similar to that of OA.

The first radiographic finding in RA is periarticular osteopenia. The loss of cartilage is usually more uniform than in OA, resulting in concentric joint space narrowing on x-ray films. Reactive bone and sclerosis are unusual, but subchondral cysts and erosions are common. Acetabular protrusion may occur, and patients with RA of the hip who are not candidates for surgical intervention at one observation should be followed with periodic hip roentgenography to monitor for medial migration of the femoral head and acetabular protrusion.

Osteonecrosis. Osteonecrosis is a circulatory disorder of bone that prominently involves the femoral head. Concepts of pathophysiology leading to cell death have focused on the vulnerable microcirculation of the femoral head and the consequences of vascular occlusion and ischemia leading to osteocyte necrosis. The mechanical interruption of the circulation to the femoral head in hip dislocations or displaced hip fractures is the most obvious and best-understood pathogenic mechanism. The pathogenesis of alcohol- or corticosteroid-associated osteonecrosis is considerably less well understood. Current evidence suggests that intravascular coagulation with microcirculatory thrombotic occlusion is the most likely final common pathway for nontraumatic osteonecrosis with a variety of etiologic associations.

A number of medical conditions have been associated with osteonecrosis as presumed causes. However, it is difficult to assess the frequency of each of these because data have largely been derived from cross-sectional, rather than prospective, studies. The demographic composition of reporting centers varies widely and, in cross-sectional studies, may result in an over- or under-representation of presumed etiologic factors. The best-associated causes are dysbarism, corticosteroid intake, excessive alcohol use, and hemoglobinopathies, although the exact incidence and prevalence of these factors remain in some dispute. Other conditions that are more or less strongly associated include Gaucher disease, hyperlipidemias, pregnancy, and other states of thromboplastin release.

The clinical presentation of pain is often sudden, as in an infarct. It is important to realize, though, that osteonecrosis may occasionally present with an insidious onset of pain or even be silent. Osteonecrosis may be multifocal, but in such cases, the hip is always involved.

The findings on anteroposterior and "frog lateral" x-ray films are normal in stage I. Technetium bone scans or magnetic resonance imaging (MRI) makes the diagnosis in this pre-radiographic stage. In stage II, x-ray films of the femoral head show patchy sclerosis, representing areas of dead bone laminated with new bone, and lucency, representing resorption. The spherical shape of the femoral head is preserved, and the joint space is normal. In stage III, a subchondral fracture or "crescent sign" is seen, which represents true subchondral fracture and collapse of the subchondral trabeculae, resulting in incongruity of the hip joint.

The ability to preserve the femoral head with hip-sparing treatment depends on the stage at which the diagnosis is made. Therefore, it is critically important to maintain a high index of suspicion for osteonecrosis in high-risk populations and screen with MRI. Several rapid, inexpensive, screening MRI protocols are available.

The major differential diagnosis of osteonecrosis is bone marrow edema syndrome (transient osteoporosis) of the hip. The clinical presentation may be quite similar. Radiographs may show demineralization of the femoral head and neck, and technetium bone scans exhibit increased radionuclide uptake. The MRI provides an important diagnostic distinction. Whereas in osteonecrosis a low signal intensity is observed on both T1- and T2-weighted images, in bone marrow edema syndrome, a decreased signal intensity is noted on the T2 images.

Osteoporosis. Osteoporosis in itself does not usually cause spontaneous or resting bone pain. In contradistinction, other metabolic bone diseases, such as hyperparathyroidism and osteomalacia, may indeed cause bone pain. However, osteoporosis can be accompanied by stress fractures or fractures after minimal trauma to the hip, including, prominently, pubic or ischial ramus fractures. These heal spontaneously with supportive care. Fractures about the acetabulum, or those involving both anterior (ramus) and posterior portions of the pelvic ring, may be more problematic and may require surgical stabilization. Fractures of the hip commonly complicate osteoporosis. Fractures of the femoral neck that are intracapsular can interrupt the circulation to the femoral head and lead to nonunion or osteonecrosis. These require surgical stabilization in a young patient, or replacement with hemiarthroplasty in an older patient. Fractures at the intertrochanteric or subtrochanteric region are extracapsular and do not interfere with circulation in the femoral head. They are usually treated with surgical stabilization rather than arthroplasty.

Risk factors for osteoporosis are female gender, increasing age, Caucasian/northern European extraction, and a low body mass index. Other important associated clinical factors are early menopause without hormone replacement therapy, dietary calcium restrictions (e.g., lactose intolerance), smoking, excessive caffeine intake, and physical inactivity. Although plain x-ray films of the hip may show a diminished trabecular pattern in osteoporosis (Singh index), they are relatively insensitive to moderate losses of bone mass. The standard way of diagnosing osteoporosis is dual-energy x-ray absorptiometry (DEXA). Screening of bone mineral density by DEXA should be considered in women at risk for osteoporosis. In fact, the U.S. Preventive Services Task Force has concluded that women 65 years of age and older should be screened routinely for osteoporosis and that routine screening should begin at age 60 for women at increased risk for osteoporotic fractures.

History and Physical Examination

Descriptions of the pattern and location of pain are important in the diagnosis of hip and thigh pain. Pain or tenderness directly over the greater trochanter is usually characteristic of trochanteric bursitis. True articular hip pain usually presents as groin or buttock discomfort and may radiate to the anterior or anteromedial thigh as far distally as the knee. Radiation of true hip pain below the knee is distinctly unusual. Patients may describe "gelling," or tenderness on arising from a sitting to a standing position. Overuse because of workplace demands or dedication to a running exercise program and a tight or inflamed iliotibial band are perhaps among the most common causes of hip pain in women younger than 55 years. After age 55, hip complaints are more likely to result from early or established degenerative change, fatigue and deconditioning of the paraspinal muscles, or spinal stenosis. The mechanism by which paraspinal muscle strain and spinal stenosis present as hip pain are complex, but these conditions commonly respond to a dedicated formal physical therapy program.

On physical examination, the *posture* of the limb should be examined. A shortened, externally rotated limb that is acutely painful on log rolling is often indicative of hip fracture. A leg that is held with the hip flexed and externally rotated and that is painful on internal rotation may indicate acute inflammatory or other intraarticular pathology, such as infection or hemorrhage. *Stance* and *gait* may suggest intrinsic hip or spinal pathology, and the overall pelvic and spinal alignment should be observed. Limp may be caused by pain (antalgic), leg length discrepancy, or weakness. Leg length is best assessed by measurement from the anterior-superior iliac spine to the medial malleolus. This is the true leg length. Measurement of the apparent leg length from the umbilicus to the medial malleolus helps account for pelvic tilt and may have to be compared with the true leg length for a complete analysis. Scoliosis and pelvic tilt may be a reaction to muscle spasm, particularly of the paraspinal muscles. An antalgic gait is characterized by a shortened stance phase. *Range of motion* of the hip can be measured in extension (log rolling) or flexion. Internal rotation is usually the movement lost first in intrinsic hip disease, and patients with inflammatory synovitis, infection, or intraarticular hemorrhage describe groin pain on internal rotation in either flexion or extension. Descriptions of pain elsewhere, for example over the greater trochanter or pelvic brim, should direct the observer to periarticular disease. Active straight leg raising against resistance increases intraarticular pressure and causes pain in patients with hip disease. However, avulsion or strain of the hip flexor muscles attaching to the pelvic brim also cause discomfort on active straight leg raising, and the location of the pain should be observed.

In addition to intrinsic musculoskeletal disease, neurologic and vascular conditions may present as hip or thigh pain. A careful neurologic examination may be necessary to rule out an L4 nerve root lesion. Because the L4 nerve root supplies sensation to the anterior and anteromedial skin, hypesthesia often accompanies L4 nerve root irritability. Weakness of the quadriceps and depression of the knee reflex are signs of L4 motor involvement and may be useful diagnostically. However, an L4 radiculopathy may present with pain only and normal neurologic findings. Spinal or vascular claudication may rarely present as exercise-related thigh pain but usually presents symptomatically below the knee.

Diagnostic Imaging

Anteroposterior views of the pelvis with the hips in physiologic position and flexed, abducted, and externally rotated ("frog lateral" position) should be obtained routinely in all patients who have hip or pelvic pain. For patients with hip pain sufficiently severe that the frog lateral position is not possible, a shoot-through or true lateral x-ray film can be obtained. Other studies, including oblique and inlet and outlet views, are useful in special cases. Examination should be performed of the joint space, surrounding sclerosis, and cysts associated with arthritis; the trabecular texture of the femoral head for osteonecrosis and osteoporosis; the femoral neck and trochanteric cortical outlines for fracture; and periarticular calcifications and avulsions for muscle injury. Fairly trivial trauma may cause pubic or ischial ramus fractures in osteoporotic women.

Persistent or severe hip pain with or without trauma may present with normal radiographic findings. MRI is proving to be of great diagnostic value and cost-effectiveness in the diagnosis of occult hip pain. In the setting of falls or other trauma, MRI can diagnose occult fractures of the pelvis or proximal femur. In athletic or dance injuries, MRI often reveals stress fractures. Acute intraarticular disease (e.g., infection, hemorrhage) presents as acute joint effusions demonstrable on MRI. The bone marrow edema syndrome and osteonecrosis commonly present with normal radiographic findings but are demonstrated on MRI. MRI should be considered for any woman with persistent or severe hip pain and normal findings on x-ray films.

Treatment

Overall, the two most generally useful treatment modalities for hip pain are a formal physical therapy routine and modification of activity. Antiinflammatory agents are helpful but alone rarely effect meaningful improvement. Ibuprofen is typically a good initial choice because most patients have had experience with that drug. Often, simply increasing the dosage to 600 or even 800 mg three times a day orally provides prompt benefit. The drug should be discontinued after 4 weeks to avoid the increased potential for side effects. This decision, however, is always tempered by the response of the patient's condition overall. Injection therapy with steroid derivatives is also a useful adjunct, but only when a specific entity can be confirmed. With hip disease, this is usually trochanteric bursitis. Injection of the posterior-superior iliac spine is sometimes useful in treating the tendinitis that can cause pain at that location.

The goal of physical therapy is to improve muscle kinematics and flexibility, and the improved power can create a more mechanically stable hip that is less vulnerable to routine demands. OA, RA, a variety of overuse syndromes, paraspinal strain that radiates to the hip, iliotibial band pain and tightness, and iliopsoas tendinitis/bursitis would all be expected to respond favorably to such a program. This typically consists of two formal sessions per week for 4 weeks. The importance of the patient's taking over the program herself as a long-term maintenance and preventative effort should be strongly emphasized.

The effectiveness of activity modification to eradicate hip pain in a female patient is directly related to how much care is taken to understand the relationship between activity demands and the pain itself. The nature and frequency of a female athlete's running routine, the requirement for repetitive cycles of sitting and standing or prolonged positioning in the workplace, and the selected position of the driver's seat in an automobile can all have a significant effect on hip pain. In general, reducing repetitive cycles of activity and avoiding prolonged positions of strain are helpful. Often, with some discussion, the patient herself can provide suggestions for improvement.

Considerations in Pregnancy

Transient osteoporosis of the hip is a rare disorder seen in pregnant women. It presents during the third trimester and is characterized by pain and decreased range of motion. The pain is worse with weight bearing. Unilateral and bilateral osteopenia with a normal joint space is seen on x-ray films. An accurate diagnosis is essential because continued weight bearing can lead to fracture of the femoral neck and disastrous consequences—for example, avascular necrosis and degenerative joint disease. Treatment includes protective weight bearing until the symptoms resolve.

Widening of the symphysis pubis is another potentially painful condition during pregnancy. Hormonal changes, such as an increase in relaxin from the corpus luteum, lead to ligamentous laxity at the sacroiliac joints and pubic symphysis. Often, radiographic examination during the first trimester demonstrates widening of the pubic symphysis. This widening may gradually increase until term but almost always resolves postpartum and rarely requires surgical intervention.

KNEE PAIN

Etiology

ANATOMIC CONSIDERATIONS

The knee is a complex joint that moves in three planes. Reducing the knee to a simple hinge joint greatly limits one's ability to understand how it works and therefore the injuries, disorders, and forms of malfunction to which it is susceptible. The knee is capable of flexion and extension, angulation (varus/valgus), and rotation. All these are accomplished simultaneously to make possible the many intricate motions and positions of both everyday and athletic functioning. A thorough history, physical examination, and routine radiographs can diagnose most, if not all, disorders of the knee. The ease of diagnosis is directly related to one's understanding of its anatomy and function. In treating women, one should be especially aware of extensor mechanism disorders and anterior cruciate ligament injuries.

The knee is a perfect balance of mobility and stability, which means it can move the body smoothly across the environment by accommodating changes in terrain, direction, or speed while providing a stable base for the body and a base for power movements. This is accomplished in part by the surface anatomy of the knee, in which two cam-like condyles at the femur and concave/convex platforms on the tibia form the main articulation. The surfaces of these structures are covered with articular cartilage, which provides a low-friction gradient ideal for gliding. Stability is enhanced by ligaments—cord-like cruciate ligaments within the joint and capsular ligaments around the periphery—that limit the extent of motion and absorb stress. The wedge-like menisci (medial and lateral) set between the femur and tibia further enhance stability and neutralize stress across the joint, preserving the articular cartilage. Layered on top of the joint are the muscles and tendons that provide dynamic stability to the joint, initiating motion and controlling motion and forces across the joint.

In addition to the tibiofemoral joint, the knee comprises a patellofemoral joint. Less constrained than the tibiofemoral joint, the patella is contained within an expansion of the quadriceps musculature that continues distally to the tibia via the patellar tendon and is subject to forces for its ultimate alignment. The articular surface, however, is well contoured and also covered with cartilage for articulation with the femur.

DIFFERENTIAL DIAGNOSIS

Traumatic Lesions and Fractures. Fractures may involve the femur, tibia, or patella and may result from athletic trauma. Ligamentous injuries may present as avulsion fractures around the knee. Fractures present with pain, swelling (local or global), focal tenderness to palpation, and difficulty bearing weight. The diagnosis is usually confirmed by radiographs. Early treatment includes the application of ice, compression dressing, and protection with crutches or immobilization. Incongruity of the joint surface or mechanical instability may require surgical intervention.

Extensor Mechanism Injuries. Injuries to the patella and extensor mechanism can be either acute or chronic. Acute injuries include subluxations and dislocations of the patella in addition to fractures. Tenderness immediately around the patella may be accompanied by swelling or ecchymosis. A defect may be palpable in the extensor mechanism if a tear has occurred, and weakness in the quadriceps. The patella may be unstable to lateral displacement, or the patient may be apprehensive of such stress. If the patella is dislocated, the knee will be locked in flexion with an obvious deformity.

Chronic injuries include soft tissue inflammation around the patella, injury or softening (chondromalacia) of the cartilage of the patella, and tendinitis in the quadriceps or patellar tendons. This is caused by repeated trauma or stress from patellar malalignment or overly vigorous activity. Findings include tenderness in the affected tissues, tendons, or the patella itself. Quadriceps atrophy may be noted. Pain is typically localized to the anterior knee and noted during prolonged sitting and athletic activity. Jumping activities may be involved. Treatment includes the application of ice and antiinflammatory medication. Stretching of the soft tissues and tendons can be particularly helpful, along with strengthening of the quadriceps. A physical therapy referral is appropriate. The patella may be stabilized with taping or a specialized brace.

Meniscus Tears. Meniscus tears are often sustained during athletic activities if compression and twisting are applied across the knee joint. When this happens, the meniscus becomes a source of sharp focal pain centered on the joint line. A meniscus tear can also cause swelling and locking of the joint. On examination, in addition to joint line tenderness, sharp catching pain is present with full flexion of the knee and with flexion and rotation (McMurray test).

Plain x-ray films will not reveal a meniscus tear, and MRI may be indicated to confirm the diagnosis.

Symptoms typically persist because the healing capability of the meniscus is limited, and surgery to address the tear is recommended. A torn meniscus may be repaired or the torn portion removed arthroscopically, depending on the patient's age and the location and pattern of the tear. Meniscus tears are commonly seen in conjunction with anterior cruciate ligament injuries.

Articular Cartilage Injuries. The articular cartilage can be injured either by direct trauma to the knee surface or by continual wear and tear. Like the meniscus, articular cartilage does not heal readily, and damaged cartilage may present with symptoms. Pain is common, usually dull and achy in nature. The pain may be poorly localized and increased by weight-bearing activities. Swelling may be present. On examination, tenderness may be vague or focal. Swelling, joint line tenderness, and limited range of motion are common. Locking may occur if a cartilage fragment has broken loose within the joint.

Articular cartilage is poorly visualized with plain radiographs, and MRI may be indicated. Arthroscopy may be indicated to evaluate the nature and extent of the injury.

Conservative treatment includes application of ice, rest, and physical therapy to restore function. Lesions less than 2 cm in diameter are most likely to heal. If symptoms persist, arthroscopic surgery is indicated. At arthroscopy, damaged cartilage can be removed and the underlying bone drilled, or a "microfracture" created, in an attempt to stimulate healing. For larger lesions, transplantation of cartilage may be necessary to heal the defect, eliminate symptoms, and prevent further destruction of the articular surface.

Anterior Cruciate Ligament Injuries. An athlete stops and cuts or lands a jump, and her knee buckles or gives way. A "pop" can be heard, followed by rapid swelling within minutes to hours after the event. Such is the typical presentation of an anterior cruciate ligament tear. Pain develops after the swelling, along with difficulty in bearing weight. The knee may be locked if the meniscus has been torn at the same time. The physical examination is significant for a positive Lachman test result—the most reliable test for an anterior cruciate ligament tear—followed by a positive anterior drawer test result. The results of medial and lateral stress testing may be positive in the face of other ligament injuries and may indicate a more serious knee injury.

Acute management includes frequent icing, careful compression, and protected weight bearing. Once symptoms are controlled, further evaluation may include MRI of the knee. In most cases, physical therapy is indicated to eliminate swelling and stiffness in the knee before surgery is contemplated.

Surgery is recommended for persons with multiple ligament injuries or with anterior cruciate ligament and meniscus injuries, high-demand athletes, and those with symptoms of instability, including persistent pain, swelling, or functional giving way. Surgery consists of reconstructing the torn ligament with patellar tendon, hamstring tendons, or allograft tendon. Results with patellar tendon and hamstring tendons have been equally promising.

In groups of soccer and basketball players, it has been observed that the incidence of anterior cruciate ligament injuries is twofold to 10-fold higher in female athletes than in their male counterparts. Whether hormonal changes are related to this observation is controversial. Data linking injury and the menstrual cycle are inconsistent, and altering hormones or the play schedule is not indicated. Likewise, anatomic differences have not been found to be causative. The most promising data thus far suggest neuromuscular differences in jumping between male and female athletes, and preliminary results show a reduction in injuries after neuromuscular training.

Nontraumatic Conditions. The knee is subject to a number of inflammatory conditions, and effusion and synovitis are accessible to observation, as is sampling of joint fluid.

Osteoarthritis. The female-to-male ratio in persons with OA is 2:1. Two thirds of patients undergoing knee arthroplasty or arthroscopy for OA are women. In older women, OA may coexist with chondrocalcinosis of both the articular and meniscus cartilage. This is usually, but not exclusively, a consequence of the deposition of calcium pyrophosphate crystals. Occasionally, calcium hydroxyapatite or calcium urate crystals may present as chondrocalcinosis. However, in elderly women with OA, chondrocalcinosis is for the most part caused by the deposition of calcium pyrophosphate crystals. Gout is much less common in women than in men. Pseudogout is the clinical presentation of acute inflammation associated with warmth and effusion together with crystal-associated OA. Pseudogout can be confused with a true gouty attack or even sepsis. The diagnosis is usually made readily by synovial fluid analysis (see later discussion) and responds extremely well to the aspiration of joint fluid and instillation of corticosteroids. Although intimately related, chondrocalcinosis, calcium pyrophosphate deposition disease, and pseudogout are not identical clinical entities. They may exist separately but overlap considerably.

The radiographic characteristics of OA include a nonconcentric loss of articular cartilage leading to valgus or varus angular deformities, subchondral sclerosis, cysts, and osteophytes. In long-standing OA, the angular deformities may become fixed, requiring special ligament-balancing techniques at arthroplasty.

Inflammatory Arthritis. The inflammatory arthritides include RA, systemic lupus erythematosus, scleroderma, mixed connective tissue disease, and a number of inflammatory spondylarthropathies, including Reiter syndrome and psoriatic arthritis. The initial presentation of RA may be monarticular, but in its classic form, RA is a migratory polyarticular arthritis that is usually symmetric. The first radiographic finding in RA is periarticular osteopenia. The loss of the cartilage space is more uniform than in OA, resulting in concentric joint space narrowing involving all three compartments of the knee. Valgus angulations may be more common in RA than in OA. Subchondral cysts and erosions at the osteochondral junction are common, but reactive bone, osteophytes, and sclerosis are unusual.

Osteonecrosis. Osteonecrosis of the knee presents very characteristically in women. Although some patients may have a circulatory disorder of bone similar to that seen in the hip, spontaneous osteonecrosis of the knee involves the femoral condyles much more frequently in women than in men. This leads to damage of the overlying cartilage and compartmental joint destruction, and replacement arthroplasty is often required. No risk factors for this form of osteonecrosis are known other than advanced age and female gender. Other forms of osteonecrosis, caused by corticosteroids, alcohol, and the various risk factors typically associated with osteonecrosis in other joints, may develop in a metaphyseal or epiphyseal location about the knee. These cases should be distinguished from the distinct entity of spontaneous osteonecrosis of the knee.

Imaging studies in osteonecrosis of the knee are similar to those in osteonecrosis of the hip, although the staging system is less formal. Spontaneous osteonecrosis of the knee presents as a subchondral lucency at the femoral condyle, often surrounded by a halo of sclerotic bone. With time, subchondral fracture or chondrolysis of the articular cartilage develops, with secondary incongruity of the joint and OA.

History and Physical Examination

Much can be determined from the history. A history of a specific injury history versus a history of more insidious or progressive symptoms is an obvious but nonetheless critical element in making the correct diagnosis. Pain is common in knee injuries. The nature of the pain—sharp or dull, throbbing, aching or burning—is significant, as are its location and intensity and whether it is constant or intermittent.

Any swelling and signs of inflammation in the knee or surrounding areas should be noted. The presence of stiffness, weakness, and mechanical symptoms, such as instability, locking, and giving way, is routinely ascertained.

General features such as symmetry, gait, body alignment, and posture should be noted. Sometimes, these provide the only clues to what is happening during functional activity. Any examination of the knee must include an evaluation of the hip because hip disease often presents as medial knee pain radiating from the thigh. Log rolling of the hips and passive range of motion of the hip in flexion should be assessed, and a straight leg raise test should be performed. Any duplication of the patient's symptoms should cause the examiner to look more closely at the hip joint as a source of the problem.

Next, the quadriceps and extensor mechanism are evaluated. Check for muscle asymmetry, such as atrophy on the affected side, and defects in the musculature or areas of swelling. Check the patient's ability to raise the leg straight without the knee lagging into flexion. Palpate for tenderness at and around the patella and in the tendons above and below the patella. Patellar stability is best evaluated with the leg relaxed and the knee flexed at about 30 degrees. Direct the patella both medially and laterally in this position while checking for instability or pain. Comparison with the contralateral knee is best. Active range of motion of the knee is observed for malalignment of the patella; abnormal tracking or jumping of the patella should be sought.

The tibiofemoral joint is palpated along the joint line medially and laterally and across the front. Just off the joint line, the medial collateral ligament, hamstring tendons, and pes bursae can be palpated medially, and the lateral collateral ligament, iliotibial band, and biceps femoris can be palpated laterally. Also lateral and slightly posterior is the fibular head, which articulates just distal to the knee joint. The knee range of motion should be observed, with either deficient or excessive motion and painful motion during the arc documented. Stability is examined with medial and lateral stress in 0 and 30 degrees of flexion. A Lachman test is performed in 30 degrees of flexion. The leg is relaxed, and the thigh is stabilized with one hand while the examiner's other hand is placed on the tibia just below the joint. This hand is used to draw the tibia anteriorly toward the examiner, and the extent of forward excursion of the tibia relative to the fixed femur is noted. The anterior drawer test is performed with the knee flexed to 90 degrees. The leg is relaxed and the foot stabilized on an examination table. Both of the examiner's hands are placed on the tibia to draw the tibia forward relative to the femur. The patient's foot should be rotated internally and the test repeated. The foot is then externally rotated and the test performed again. Routine manual muscle testing for strength of the thigh and leg muscles is performed. Sensory testing and a reflex examination of the lower extremity completes the evaluation.

Diagnostic Imaging

A complete radiographic examination of the knee consists of an anteroposterior view taken in the standing position and lateral, tunnel, and sunrise views. The lateral view should be obtained with the knee in a flexed position; the tunnel view is useful for detecting lesions of osteochondritis dissecans or loose bodies in the intercondylar notch; the sunrise view is useful to determine the patellofemoral position and reveal arthritis. Occasionally, especially in conditions of trauma, oblique views may be useful to delineate small cortical infractions. Radiographs may be supplemented by MRI, which is useful for determining subtle fractures, circulatory disorders of bone including osteonecrosis, and soft tissue injuries, notably ligamentous disruptions and meniscus tears. MRI is particularly diagnostic in osteonecrosis and may offer supporting objective evidence, especially when ligamentous or meniscus tears are suspected.

Joint Fluid Analysis

The knee is a relatively large-volume joint, and because of its proximity to the surface and tendency to present with swelling, joint fluid analysis is commonly performed. The aspiration of fluid from an acutely inflamed knee often provides substantial symptomatic relief in addition to diagnostic information. Joint fluid is conveniently aspirated from the suprapatellar pouch, usually from a superolateral approach entering just beneath the patella. The presence of hemarthrosis strongly suggests an underlying ligamentous injury or fracture. Fat droplets are often seen in the aspirate in cases of bony fracture. Fluid obtained from a knee with OA is usually clear and yellow, and the white cell count may vary from very low to moderately high, occasionally as high as 20,000 to 25,000/mm^3, especially when calcium pyrophosphate crystal deposition is also present. Fluid from OA knees should be examined for the cell count and presence of crystals. Cloudy fluid often accompanies inflammatory conditions of the knee and reflects the relatively higher concentration of white blood cells. The viscosity is usually reduced. The synovial fluid should be examined for the cell count and presence of crystals, and culture and sensitivity and a Gram stain should be performed. In cases of inflammatory arthritis in which sepsis cannot be ruled out at the time of aspiration, instillation of corticosteroids is probably best deferred until a definite cytologic and bacteriologic diagnosis is made.

Treatment

The primary care physician should be aware of the general initial management of trauma, including ligamentous injuries, as previously outlined. Supportive splinting and the application of cold packs to minimize swelling and bleeding are particularly useful strategies until definitive diagnosis and treatment can be carried out. The frequent application of ice can control pain and swelling. The skin should be protected to prevent thermal injury. Compression should be applied to control swelling. Ace bandages, Jones dressings, or cold compression devices are acceptable. Frequent reapplications avoid injury from compression. Painful weight bearing can be managed with crutches or other assistive devices. Immobilization can be used for acute pain or instability. Nonsteroidal antiinflammatory medication is helpful in controlling pain and reducing swelling unless contraindicated by allergy, gastric intolerance, or drug interaction. In the nontraumatized knee, antiinflammatory strategies, both oral and intraarticular, are useful initial approaches. Synovial fluid is readily sampled and may facilitate the diagnosis, literally within hours. The removal of synovial fluid is especially indicated for treatment in cases of tense hemarthrosis or effusion, crystal-associated OA, including both gout and pseudogout, and septic arthritis.

Considerations in Pregnancy

The increased weight of pregnancy tends to aggravate preexisting conditions. Problems of patellar malalignment causing anterior knee pain about the patella are common in young women. Hence, if a pregnant patient has any history of prior knee pain of this nature, she should avoid squatting, kneeling, or excessive stair climbing while carrying extra weight.

BIBLIOGRAPHY

Aaron R. Osteonecrosis: etiology, pathophysiology, and diagnosis. In: Callaghan J, Rosenberg A, Rubash H, eds. *The adult hip*. New York: Lippincott-Raven, 1998:451–466.

Garvin K, McKillip T. History and physical examination. In: Callaghan J, Rosenberg A, Rubash H, eds. *The adult hip*. New York: Lippincott-Raven, 1998: 315–332.

Griffin L. *Prevention of noncontact anterior cruciate ligament injuries*. Rosemont, IL: American Academy of Orthopaedic Surgeons, 2001.

Snider R, et al. *Essentials of musculoskeletal care*. Rosemont, IL: American Academy of Orthopaedic Surgeons, 1997.

U.S. Preventive Services Task Force. *Screening: osteoporosis. Update, 2002 release*. (Available at *www.ahrq.gov/clinic/uspstf/uspsoste.htm*. Accessed May 24, 2003.)

CHAPTER 100

Principles of Fracture Diagnosis and Care

Eric M. Bluman and Trimble S. Augur

The primary care physician is often the first one to examine a patient with an acute fracture. It is common for primary care physicians to see patients with fractures that were initially undermanaged or improperly managed in the emergency department. Although many fractures require minimal care, some that appear relatively innocuous may heal in a way that is harmful to the biomechanics of the adjacent joints or soft tissues. The liberal and early use of orthopedic consultation is recommended.

The injury should be viewed as part of a whole, not just as a limb with a broken bone. It may be advantageous in some cases to think of fractures as soft tissue injuries that have a bony component. Awareness of the soft tissues means thoroughly assessing the neurovascular status of the limb as close to the time of injury as possible and repeating the evaluation at every follow-up visit, especially if a circumferential dressing is part of the treatment.

The primary care practitioner must also avoid thinking that a fracture of a small bone is a small problem. Undertreatment or improper treatment of a fracture may lead to late and often irreversible sequelae, such as posttraumatic arthritis, unacceptable deformity, and joint stiffness. This chapter seeks to present some of the principles of fracture care. Learning these simple principles allows the primary care physician to manage many fractures with an excellent outcome. A comprehensive survey of fracture care cannot be presented here, but many reference sources are available for the primary care physician.

ETIOLOGY AND DIFFERENTIAL DIAGNOSIS

The cause of most fractures is trauma in the form of outside energy. The bone and surrounding tissues receive an input of kinetic energy, which is then dissipated in the bone and surrounding soft tissue. The fracture and soft tissue injury are the result of the transmission of energy to the tissues. The magnitude of the energy relative to the toughness of the bone to which it is imparted determines whether a fracture will occur. Energy can be transmitted when an object strikes a person or a person strikes an object.

The severity of an injury is related to the amount of energy transmitted and absorbed by the anatomic site in question. At the same velocity, one is much less likely to survive a head-on encounter with a large truck (greater mass and therefore greater momentum) than with a motorcycle. In a fall, the velocity at the moment of impact, and thus the magnitude of the energy imparted, depends on the distance of the fall.

The same mechanism of injury and the same amount of energy dissipated in the tissues cause different injuries in persons of different ages because the relative strength and elasticity of the tissues change throughout life. For example, bone and ligamentous structures are much more compliant in a young woman than in one who is elderly. Therefore, much more energy is required to produce the same bone displacement in a Colle's wrist fracture in a 20-year-old woman than in a 70-year-old woman. Consequently, more energy is dissipated into the surrounding soft tissues, causing more damage and tissue destruction in the 20-year-old. In another example, a knee forcefully struck on the lateral aspect will be displaced into valgus (knock-knee position). This mechanism causes markedly different injuries depending on the age of the patient. In a youngster with open growth plates, a fracture may occur through the distal femoral growth plate. In a woman in her 20s, the medial collateral ligament may be torn. A lateral tibial plateau or distal femoral fracture may be caused by a mechanism of this type in a woman in the sixth decade of life or older because her bone is weaker than the ligaments. The age-related weakening of the skeleton is a major contributor to the high incidence of wrist, shoulder, and hip fractures resulting from mild falls in older women.

Patients with stress fractures or pathologic fractures have no antecedent history of acute kinetic loading. A stress fracture is a spontaneous fracture of normal bone that results from a summation of stresses, any of which in isolation would be harmless. In pathologic fractures, the weakened state of the abnormal bone allows fracture to occur within the range of physiologic loading.

Healthy bone can support loads because its design allows it to resist compressive forces and shear and tension stresses. Compression fractures occur when the bone fails in axial loading. Avulsion fractures are a form of failure in tension loading. Fractures associated with shear loading display simple or complex patterns, depending on the speed and direction of loading.

HISTORY

A thorough history is required not only to understand the cause of a fracture but also to gauge the accompanying soft tissue damage and detect clues of accompanying injuries that may be masked by acute pain. The history, physical examination, and roentgenography often provide all the information needed to understand the character of a fracture.

High-energy fractures are frequently accompanied by other injuries. These "secondary" injuries may be masked early in the evaluation and treatment of fractures because of the distracting pain of the "primary" injuries. A common example is the patient who sustains a lumbar vertebral compression fracture in addition to the calcaneal fracture caused by a fall from a height. It is essential to examine the entire injured extremity thoroughly before treatment is initiated. The physician should also consider whether the level of energy that caused the injury explains the findings. For instance, if mild trauma causes an arm to break, a pathologic process may have weakened the bone.

A complete history is also essential for medicolegal reasons. The history should not state merely that the patient fell on her outstretched wrist; it should include much more detail. The physician should try to obtain a complete history of how the fall occurred, in the patient's own words. If the events are unclear, a statement to that effect should be included in the documentation.

PHYSICAL EXAMINATION AND CLINICAL FINDINGS

The injured part should be examined before x-ray films are ordered. A complete neurovascular examination must be carried out. With a cooperative patient, the physician can start by performing a sensory examination of the limb distal to the injury. The sensory distribution of all the major nerves must be evaluated and any deficiencies recorded. Sensation to light touch or pinprick is the most useful test. Any deficiencies in sensation must be noted before the patient undergoes diagnostic imaging and before the fracture is reduced, in case changes develop after the initial examination.

As stated earlier, a fracture should not be thought of as a bony injury in isolation. For example, a fracture of the distal radius may be associated with damage to the articular cartilage and wrist ligaments and nerve compression in the form of an acute carpal tunnel syndrome. If the physician were to treat only the bony component of an injury with all these elements, posttraumatic arthritis, an unstable wrist, or permanent nerve damage might develop in the hand despite a normal appearance of the distal radius on follow-up radiographs.

The motor examination may be difficult because of the patient's pain, but integrity of motor function and the nerve supply can be verified. In the upper extremity, median, ulnar, and radial nerve function is easily verified by asking the patient to make an "OK" sign with the thumb and index finger (median nerve), spread the fingers widely (ulnar nerve), and extend the thumb (radial nerve). In the lower extremity, peroneal and posterior tibial nerve function is also easily verified. Resisted extension of the great toe confirms peroneal nerve function, and flexion confirms posterior tibial nerve function. These tests can be performed even in the presence of a severely fractured tibia. Knowing the status of nerves early is essential to diagnosing compartment syndrome in evolution.

Compartment syndrome should be considered, and the patient evaluated for it, in all but the most minor forms of musculoskeletal trauma. Pain on passive stretch of the deep compartment muscles is the first sign of compartment syndrome. Extreme pain with passive extension of the index finger is an early warning sign if forearm swelling is present. In the lower extremity, pain on passive flexion or extension of the great toe with a tense swollen leg is a "red flag" for compartment syndrome. An immediate consultation with an orthopedic surgeon is required for all suspected cases of compartment syndrome in an extremity.

After the preliminary neurosensory examination has been completed, the physician should carefully palpate the injured part, evaluating the areas of maximal swelling and ecchymosis and paying close attention to the skin status.

A superficial abrasion or laceration must be distinguished from skin penetration that communicates with the fracture site. In an open (compound) fracture, the fracture communicates with the outside environment through a break in the skin. Often, a puncture wound is found where a sharp fragment of bone has perforated the skin. No matter how small the opening, bacterial contamination is possible. These wounds often have a characteristic appearance, with frankly bloody, fat-filled drainage because of their communication with the marrow cavity. A fracture of a distal phalanx with bleeding around the nail bed is also likely to be an open fracture. Any fracture that the physician suspects is open should be evaluated in a timely manner by an orthopedic surgeon.

Open fractures should be treated by a specialist. Antibiotic and tetanus prophylaxis is prudent. Antibiotic coverage must be individualized and may include a first-generation cephalosporin, penicillin, an aminoglycoside, or a combination thereof, depending on the extent of the associated soft tissue injury and the environment in which the fracture occurred. Wounds considered tetanus-prone are those contaminated with soil, saliva, or fecal material, burns, frostbite, and crush injuries. Tetanus toxoid should be administered to patients who may be at risk for tetanus infection but who never completed a series of toxoid immunization or have not had a tetanus booster within the last 5 years. If the wound is severe, human tetanus immune globulin should be administered in addition to the tetanus toxoid. Patients who are immunodeficient should also receive human toxoid immune globulin for passive immunization soon after injury.

Pain and tenderness are always present in neurologically intact patients. The physician should palpate and identify the points of maximal tenderness. Bony crepitus—the sound and feel of edges of broken bone rubbing together—is sometimes noted. Often, deformity is observed. Ends of fractured bone bleed, and a fracture hematoma leads to swelling.

LABORATORY AND IMAGING STUDIES

After the physical examination, appropriate radiographs should be ordered. Two orthogonally opposed views of every bone fractured are a minimum for the most simple fracture patterns. Most fractures can be imaged adequately with only an anteroposterior and a lateral radiograph. Multiple fractures in close proximity may all be imaged adequately with a single set of radiographs oriented orthogonally to one another. Fractures involving comminution through multiple anatomic planes and those that are intraarticular may be characterized better with oblique views and computed tomography of the area.

The injured patient sent for imaging studies must be well protected in a temporary supportive splint that immobilizes the injured part. This provides comfort and protects the soft tissue structures as the patient is positioned for radiographs. Fiberglass splinting material is preferred over that made from plaster of paris because the former is more radiolucent and less likely to obscure fine detail.

Ordering and interpreting x-ray films can be difficult and inefficient if all involved parties are not using a standard nomenclature (Table 100.1, Fig. 100.1). Communications with

TABLE 100.1. Fracture Nomenclature

Diaphysis: The shaft of a long bone; made up primarily of compact cortical bone.
Metaphysis: The widened portion of a long bone at each end; made up of a high percentage of spongy trabecular bone.
Epiphysis: Each end of a long bone, from which growth occurs.
Torus or *greenstick fractures:* Fractures in which one cortex breaks and the opposite bends (like a "green stick"). These occur most frequently in children, whose bones are more elastic.
Displaced: Fracture fragments separated in the plane of the fracture. Measurement in terms of distance should be given.
Transverse: Pattern in which the fracture crosses the bone perpendicular to its long axis.
Oblique: Pattern in which the fracture line crosses the bone at an angle.
Spiral: Pattern in which the fracture line winds helically around the long axis of the bone.
Extraarticular: Fracture line that does not enter a joint.
Intraarticular: Fracture line that enters a joint.
Comminuted: Fracture pattern with multiple fragments and fracture lines.
Butterfly fragment: A generally triangular third fracture fragment separate from the proximal and distal fragments. This fragment results from a bending force perpendicular to the longitudinal axis of a bone.
Segmental fracture: Fracture pattern in which two distinct areas of fracture in one bone create three major fragments.
Apposition: Percentage of the cross-sectional area of the proximal and distal fracture fragments remaining in contact.
Angulated: Fracture in which the longitudinal axis of the distal fragment subtends at an angle to the longitudinal axis of the proximal fragment. This displacement should be measured accurately with a goniometer.
Varus angulation: Apex away from the midline.
Valgus angulation: Apex toward the midline.

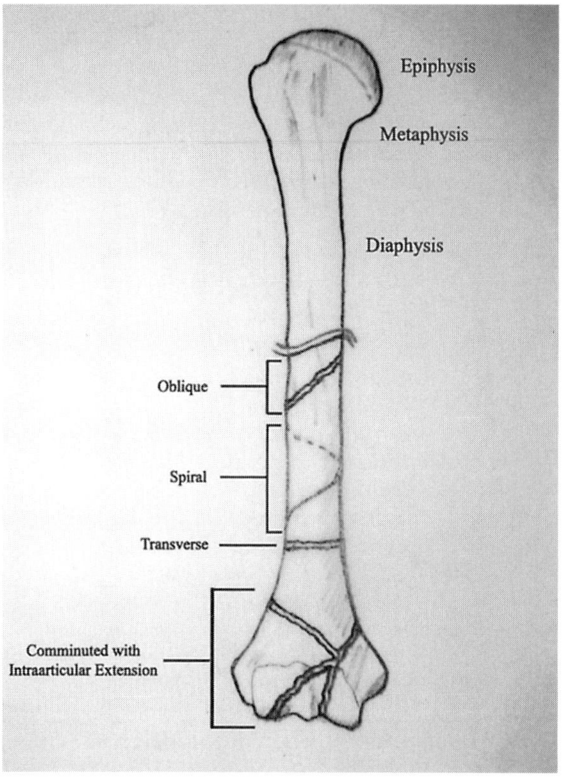

FIG. 100.1. Anatomic regions of long bones and types of fracture patterns. The three anatomic regions of the long bones are labeled on the right side of the illustration. Basic fracture patterns are demonstrated in the bottom half of the figure.

colleagues and consultants should include minimal components that provide a thorough and descriptive foundation on which to base treatment decisions (Table 100.2). Because the term "slightly displaced" means different things to different people, it is better to abandon this descriptor and quantify the amount of displacement in millimeters.

It is important to describe the appearance in two planes because the two views often differ. A short oblique tibia may appear to have 90% apposition and 5 degrees of varus on the anteroposterior view but 10% apposition and 40 degrees of apex anterior angulation on the lateral view.

TABLE 100.2. Important Points of the Fracture Evaluation to Communicate to Colleagues

Location of injury
Bones involved
Whether the fracture is open or closed
Associated neurologic or vascular compromise
Location of fracture within bone
Angulation
Displacement
Comminution
Whether or not fracture extends into joint
Presence of joint dislocation or subluxation with fracture
Condition of soft tissue envelope
Presence of associated injuries

TREATMENT

Once the initial evaluation has been completed, the patient should be made as comfortable as possible while alignment is restored and the limb protected, usually with a splint or cast. Heat should never be part of the treatment of an acute fracture. Cold and elevation are safe and reduce pain and the need for analgesics. Fracture pain is caused by swelling and motion, neither of which can be completely eliminated. However, a well-applied cast or splint helps reduce swelling and pain by means of mild circumferential compression. Molding by three-point fixation helps reduce fracture motion. Many patients with a fracture feel motion of the bone ends for several weeks, even in a well-fitting cast.

Many fractures can be managed by several equally effective means. A tibial fracture may be treated in a long leg cast, a short leg cast, or a plastic orthosis. Different types of surgical treatment may be equally correct. The optimal treatment considers and integrates the patient's age, occupation, bone quality, coincident injuries, and other medical problems. It also depends on the physician's experience and comfort with various treatment techniques. Treatment must be individualized because each fracture has a unique personality.

Patients who are known to smoke should be counseled to abstain from or at least minimize smoking tobacco while their fracture heals. Multiple studies have shown that complete fracture healing takes longer and that nonunion occurs in a greater percentage of fractures in smokers.

CONSIDERATIONS IN PREGNANCY

Fractures heal at the same rate in pregnant women as in those who are not pregnant. However, fracture healing may be impaired by deficiencies of vitamin D or calcium.

Fractures that are best treated operatively in a patient who is not pregnant should be treated similarly in a pregnant patient. Treatment with prolonged bed rest and immobilization can lead to complications. The goal of early mobilization, which is often realized by early surgical treatment, can be valuable in a pregnant patient. In most cases, anesthesia can be delivered effectively for both mother and fetus with minimal disturbance of physiology.

Motor vehicle accidents are the leading cause of death in pregnant women. Seat belts should be fastened properly, low across the anterior superior iliac spines, to protect mother and fetus.

In the peripartum period, a painful significant widening of the pubic symphysis may develop in the mother. Although most cases resolve spontaneously, some may result in continued debilitation and require consultation with an orthopedic surgeon.

CONSIDERATIONS IN LATER LIFE

Osteoporosis and Fractures

Just as osteoporosis is a risk factor for fractures, so too are fractures a risk factor for osteoporosis. Multiple studies have demonstrated that long-term and frequently permanent osteoporosis develops after a fracture. The primary care provider must ensure that all modalities to increase and preserve bone mass are being used appropriately. These may include physical and occupational therapy, bisphosphonate therapy, hormone replacement therapies, and calcium and vitamin D supplementation if the dietary intake of these nutrients is inadequate.

Elder Abuse

It is estimated that 1% to 2% of older persons living at home are abused in some way. Some risk factors for abuse of the elderly are cognitive impairment of the victim, dependence of the abuser on the victim, shared living arrangements, and social isolation.

CONCLUSION

Many fractures can be treated successfully by primary care physicians. A thorough and systematic history, physical examination, and radiographic examination are required. Orthopedic surgical consultation should be obtained for patients with multiple orthopedic injuries or open fractures and in cases of abuse. The soft tissue envelope must be evaluated and treated just as aggressively as the osseous component of the injury. Not only are patients with osteoporosis more likely to sustain fractures, but significant and irreversible osteoporosis may develop in patients with fractures.

ACKNOWLEDGMENTS

We thank Dr. Peter G. Trafton for his generosity and expertise in teaching orthopedic traumatology and Dr. Richard A. Lewis for the previous version on which this chapter is based.

BIBLIOGRAPHY

Browner BD, Jupiter JB, Levine AM, et al., eds. *Skeletal trauma*, 2nd ed. Philadelphia: WB Saunders, 1998.
Charnley J. The closed treatment of common fractures. In: Green DP, ed. *Operative hand surgery*, 3rd ed. New York: Churchill Livingstone, 1993.
Chen AL, Koval KJ. Elder abuse: the role of the orthopaedic surgeon in diagnosis and treatment. *J Am Acad Orthop Surg* 2002;10:25.
Deal DN, Tipton J, Rosencrance E, et al. Ice reduces edema: a study of microvascular permeability in rats. *J Bone Joint Surg Am* 2002;84:1573.
Fildes J, Reed L, Jones N, et al. Trauma: the leading cause of maternal death. *J Trauma* 1992;32:643.
Heckman JD, Sassard R. Musculoskeletal considerations in pregnancy. *J Bone Joint Surg Am* 1994;76:1720.
Järvinen M, Kannus P. Injury of an extremity as a risk factor for the development for osteoporosis. *J Bone Joint Surg Am* 1997;79:263.
Kocher MS, Kasser JR. Orthopaedic aspects of child abuse. *J Am Acad Orthop Surg* 2000;8:10.
Lane JM, Riley EH, Wirganowicz PZ. Osteoporosis: diagnosis and treatment. *J Bone Joint Surg Am* 1996;78:618.
Porter SE, Hanley EN. The musculoskeletal effects of smoking. *J Am Acad Orthop Surg* 2001;9:9.
Wolf ME, Alexander BH, Rivara FP, et al. A retrospective cohort study of seat belt use and pregnancy outcome after a motor vehicle crash. *J Trauma* 1993;34:116.

CHAPTER 101
Common Disorders of the Hand and Wrist

Scott D. Allen, Julia A. Katarincic, and Arnold-Peter C. Weiss

CARPAL TUNNEL SYNDROME

Etiology

Carpal tunnel syndrome, a common source of hand pain and numbness, is caused by compression of the median nerve at the wrist. The carpal tunnel consists of a bony floor and bony walls (the carpal bones) and a ligamentous roof formed by the transverse carpal ligament. This rigidly confined space contains nine flexor tendons in their investing sheaths and the median nerve. With constant use or repetitive activities and some systemic conditions, inflammation of the sheaths and swelling develop, increasing pressure within the carpal tunnel and compressing the median nerve at this site. Compression leads to nerve ischemia and the characteristic carpal tunnel symptoms of numbness and tingling in the sensory distribution of the median nerve, described later. Carpal tunnel syndrome is far more common in women, especially those who are pregnant, and in patients with diabetes mellitus or thyroid disease. Less common causes of carpal tunnel syndrome, all of which increase the volume within the carpal tunnel, include trauma, an anomalous flexor muscle belly, amyloidosis, collagen-vascular diseases, and rheumatoid arthritis. The prevalence of carpal tunnel syndrome may also be increased in women using oral contraceptives.

Differential Diagnosis

The differential diagnosis of carpal tunnel syndrome includes conditions causing compression of the median nerve at sites other than the wrist, ulnar neuropathy, and other systemic neuropathic conditions. Cervical spondylosis may cause compression at the nerve root. In addition, the median nerve may be compressed throughout its course in the arm and forearm by fascial and muscular structures. As a result, the "double crush" phenomenon may develop, in which sensitivity of the nerve is increased at the wrist because of compression at a more proximal site. Hand pain and numbness are also caused by ulnar neuropathy with compression at the elbow in the cubital tunnel or at the wrist in the canal of Guyon. Other conditions include peripheral neuropathy associated with diabetes, alcoholism, metabolic abnormalities, or drug reactions.

Clinical Findings/Physical Examination

A brief review of median nerve anatomy enhances the understanding of the clinical presentation of carpal tunnel syndrome. After passing through the carpal tunnel, the median nerve provides sensation to the thumb, index finger, middle finger, and radial half of the ring finger. The sensory distribution is over the volar surface of these structures and usually extends to the dorsal surface of the distal phalanges. Approximately 4 cm proximal to the carpal tunnel, the median nerve gives rise to the palmar sensory branch. Sensation in the palm is usually spared in carpal tunnel syndrome because this branch does not pass through the carpal tunnel, a fact that may help to distinguish carpal tunnel syndrome from more proximal causes of nerve compression. The distal motor branch of the median nerve innervates the thenar muscles and the radial two lumbricals. This branch usually exits distal to the carpal tunnel; however, in several anatomic variations, it passes through the transverse carpal ligament, which is important to remember during surgical release. Sensory nerve fibers are usually affected first when the nerve is compressed, and the motor fibers later after prolonged compression.

Patients usually describe numbness and tingling in the sensory distribution of the median nerve or in all five fingers, which may be accompanied by wrist pain. The symptoms are usually worse at night, and patients commonly report awakening with numb hands. Activities involving repetitive stress or prolonged wrist flexion or extension may exacerbate the symptoms. These include typing, repetitive manipulation of machinery, and constant fine manipulation. Activities involving more prolonged flexion include gripping a steering wheel, blow drying hair, holding a book or newspaper, and carrying household items. Symptoms may have been present for weeks or months. Earlier stages are characterized by symptom-free intervals. Later stages present with constant sensory symptoms and hand weakness or thenar atrophy.

On physical examination, inspection may reveal thenar muscle atrophy, which is a late feature. Comparison with the opposite hand is helpful. Thumb palmar abduction strength is tested by having the patient rest the dorsum of the hand on a table and lift the thumb off the table against resistance. Light touch is assessed in the median and ulnar nerve distributions, although this is not a very sensitive test. A more sensitive test of sensation is two-point discrimination. This determines the distance that must separate two fine objects touching the hand before the patient can distinguish between them. A space of approximately 5 mm or less is normal; a distance of 7 mm or more may indicate mild neuropathy, and a distance of more than 14 mm represents severe neuropathy.

Provocative testing is an integral part of the physical examination. In the Tinel test, the examiner taps the patient's wrist over the carpal tunnel (Fig. 101.1). A positive test result is a sensation of tingling ("pins and needles" or "electric shocks") radiating into the thumb and fingers in the median nerve distribution. Pain is not considered a positive test result. The carpal compression test, in which pressure is applied directly over the carpal tunnel, may also elicit these symptoms. The main provocative test is the Phalen wrist flexion test (Fig. 101.2). The wrist is flexed fully and held in this position for up to 60 seconds. Again, a positive test result is a sensation of tingling radiating into the thumb and fingers. It is likely that a faster elicitation of symptoms indicates more severe compression.

Laboratory Tests/Imaging Studies

The Semmes-Weinstein monofilament test is also useful in the diagnosis of carpal tunnel syndrome. This is a very accurate test for diagnosing early nerve compression. Plastic monofilaments of increasing diameter are pressed onto the skin until the filament bends. The smallest-diameter filament that the patient is able to feel is noted. When combined with the wrist flexion provocative test, monofilament testing increases the sensitivity of the diagnosis of carpal tunnel syndrome from 75% with the Phalen test alone to 82%, and increases the specificity of the diagnosis from 47% with the Phalen test alone to 86%.

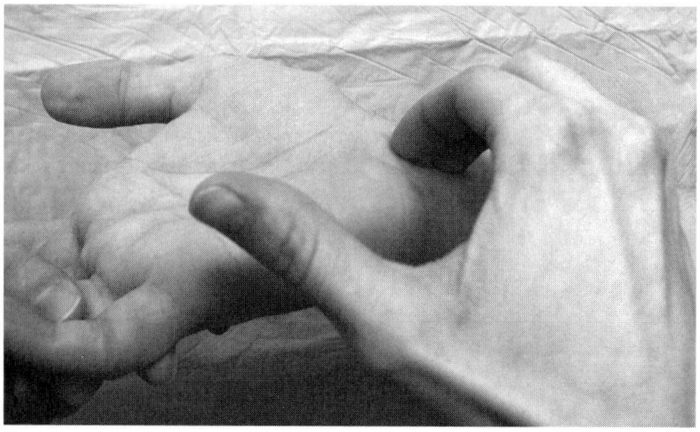

FIG. 101.1. Tinel test. The examiner taps over the median nerve where it enters the carpal tunnel. A positive result is distal radiation of tingling and numbness in the median nerve distribution.

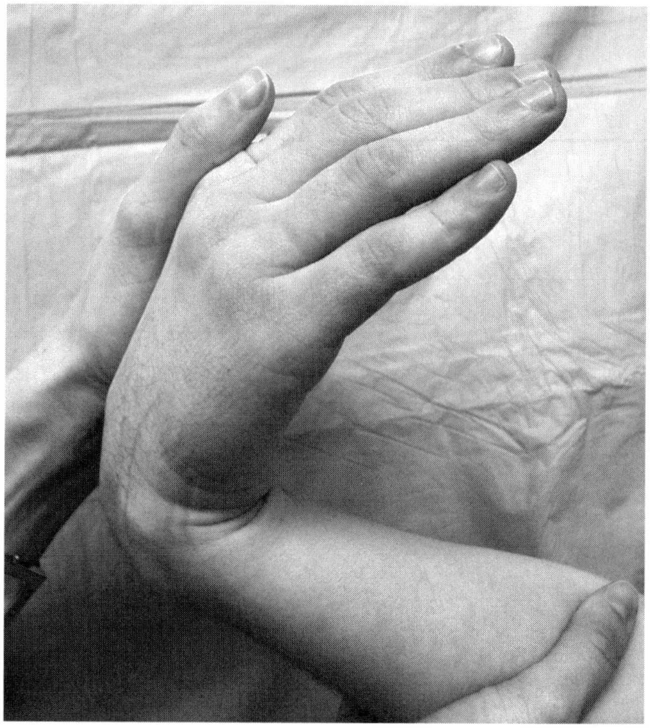

FIG. 101.2. Phalen test. The examiner holds the patient's affected wrist in a flexed position for up to 60 seconds. A positive result is distal radiation of tingling and numbness in the median nerve distribution.

Electrodiagnostic studies may also aid in the diagnosis and in monitoring the progression of carpal tunnel syndrome. Sensory and motor nerve responses are tested by passing an electric current through needle electrodes and observing the response. Sensory nerve conduction velocities and latencies are noted. Nerve conduction velocities may be decreased in early nerve compression. Electromyography of the hypothenar muscles innervated by the median nerve may also be performed. Denervation potentials with or without obvious atrophy indicate more prolonged nerve compression. The results of these tests may be either false-positive or false-negative; thus, a negative test result does not rule out carpal tunnel syndrome. Furthermore, it has been shown that electrodiagnostic testing does not correlate with a better final outcome after carpal tunnel release. One study showed similar high rates of symptomatic relief after surgical release in groups with positive preoperative test results, negative preoperative results, and no preoperative electrodiagnostic tests. Thus, the exact role of specific tests is unclear. They may be helpful in diagnosing carpal tunnel syndrome in patients without a classic presentation.

Treatment

Nonoperative management includes splinting the wrist in a neutral position, nonsteroidal antiinflammatory drugs (NSAIDs), and corticosteroid injection (Fig. 101.3). Soft splints may be used during the day. However, a firm wrist neutral splint should be worn at night to prevent wrist flexion during sleep. Modification of the workstation to support the wrists in a neutral position is also helpful. Corticosteroid injection may provide 20% to 25% of patients with long-term relief. However, even if relief is for a short period of time, a positive response to injection may predict a successful surgical outcome. It has been shown that splinting and corticosteroid injection are most suc-

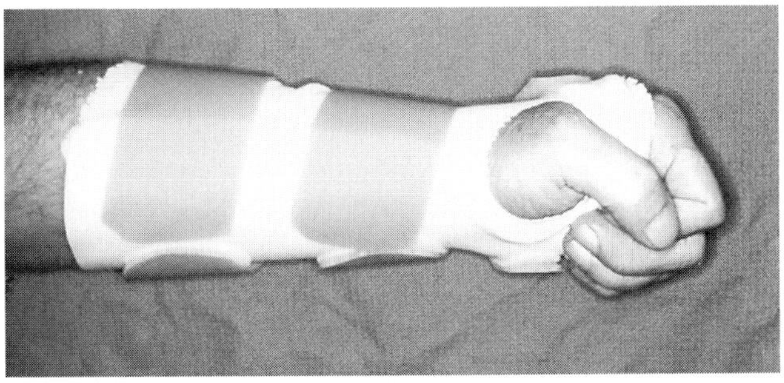

FIG. 101.3. Wrist neutral forearm-based resting splint. This is a typical custom-made night-time splint used in the conservative treatment of carpal tunnel syndrome. It prevents wrist flexion and subsequent compression of the median nerve during sleep.

cessful in patients with mild symptoms in whom carpal tunnel syndrome is diagnosed early. Relapse is more likely in patients with more severe symptoms and physical findings. Resolution of symptoms with conservative management appears to be least likely in young women. It has also been suggested that diuretics may reduce edema, although this treatment is not widely used. Any underlying systemic disease should also be addressed.

Operative management is surgical release of the transverse carpal ligament by a variety of techniques. In the traditional open carpal tunnel release, a 2- to 3-cm incision is created over the carpal tunnel, then the palmar fascia and transverse carpal ligament are divided under direct vision. Care is taken to avoid anomalous motor branches, the palmar sensory branch, and distal vascular structures. A larger open incision is typically used in patents with a prior fracture of the distal radius or rheumatoid arthritis requiring a synovectomy. A variation of this technique, the mini-open carpal tunnel release, is becoming popular (Fig. 101.4). Creation of a smaller, 1-cm incision over the distal extent of the carpal tunnel is followed by division of the palmar fascia and distal aspect of the transverse carpal ligament under direct vision. After this exposure has been achieved, a special knife is used to divide the proximal extent of the ligament (under the skin) while a protective skid prevents the knife from injuring the median nerve. In an alternative method, the endoscopic carpal tunnel release, the transverse carpal ligament is divided through one or two small portals under endoscopic visualization. The single-portal technique avoids a palmar incision altogether. After a small incision is made at the volar wrist crease, an endoscopic knife is inserted through the volar forearm fascia and into the carpal canal. While the deep surface of the ligament is visualized through the endoscope, the knife is used to divide the transverse carpal ligament. Complications include injury to the median nerve within the canal, the palmar cutaneous branch, and the recurrent motor branch. The superficial palmar vascular arch is also at risk at the distal extent of the transverse carpal ligament. A possible complication of the endoscopic technique is incomplete ligament release because of poor visualization of the ligament during surgery. The outcomes of all techniques are similar at 6 months postoperatively, with no significant difference noted in relief of symptoms. Although some palmar pain is still associated with the mini-open and endoscopic techniques, the smaller palmar incision in the mini-open technique and the lack of a palmar incision in the endoscopic technique may allow an earlier return to normal function.

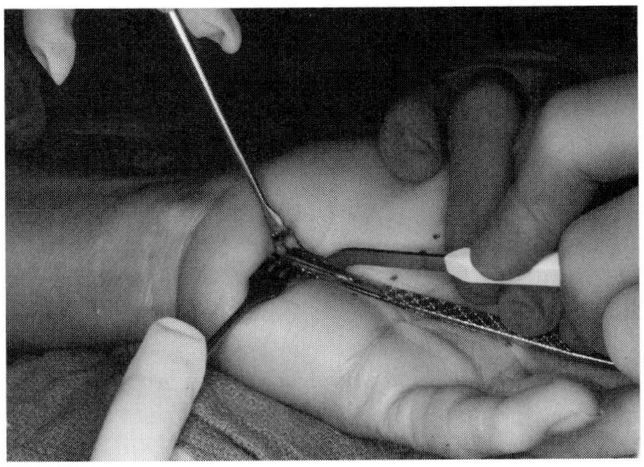

FIG. 101.4. Mini-open carpal tunnel release. The transverse carpal ligament is transected by the white-handled carpal tunnel knife as it is slid between the subcutaneous tissues and the protective skid, which is positioned superficial to the median nerve.

Overall, early disease responds better to both nonoperative and surgical management. A trial of splinting is appropriate when the diagnosis is made early. If the symptoms progress, the patient should be referred to a specialist. If the disease is diagnosed at a later stage—for example, when constant numbness or thenar atrophy has developed—referral should be made sooner. Thenar atrophy cannot be reversed by surgery. Operative release is likely to prevent progression and decrease pain at this late stage. Late-stage return of sensation is variable.

Effects of Pregnancy on Disease

Carpal tunnel syndrome is the second most frequent musculoskeletal problem developing in pregnancy, second only to low back pain. It is diagnosed most often in the third trimester, although symptoms may have been present earlier. Carpal tunnel syndrome that develops during pregnancy is usually bilateral and may be more common in older primiparas, women with preeclampsia, and those with generalized edema. Splinting and occasionally corticosteroid injection are the preferred treatments during pregnancy. The symptoms of up to 80% of patients in whom carpal tunnel syndrome develops during pregnancy resolve during the first month postpartum. In a smaller percentage of women, the symptoms are prolonged, and surgical release may be required as definitive treatment. Symptoms have also been associated with breast-feeding and fluid retention caused by prolactin. Subsequent relief of symptoms has been noted at the cessation of nursing.

DE QUERVAIN DISORDER

Etiology

De Quervain disorder, or stenosing tenosynovitis of the first dorsal compartment of the wrist, is a common painful condition of the hand and wrist. The first dorsal compartment is located at the radial border of the distal radius just proximal to the radial styloid. It consists of a bony floor (the distal radius) and a fibrous roof (the extensor retinaculum) and contains multiple slips of the abductor pollicis longus and extensor pollicis brevis tendons and the tenosynovium lining the tendons. Pain at the first dorsal compartment is caused by inflammation and ultimate narrowing of this fibro-osseous canal, which irritates the tendons traveling within. Pain is exacerbated by activities involving repeated abduction of the thumb and ulnar deviation of the wrist, as in highly repetitive manipulation in the workplace or continual lifting of small children. It usually occurs in patients ages 30 to 50 years and is more common in women, especially postpartum.

Differential Diagnosis

Other conditions that cause symptoms similar to those of de Quervain disorder (pain at the radial border of the wrist) should be kept in mind when this diagnosis is made. Arthritis of the thumb carpometacarpal joint may present with pain on the radial side of the wrist. However, point tenderness is usually localized to the base of the first metacarpal in this condition. A radiograph may demonstrate degenerative changes in this and other involved joints. Radiographs may also show a scaphoid fracture. In this case, the pain is usually localized over the scaphoid in the "anatomic snuffbox." In addition, de Quervain disorder may be confused with intersection syndrome, another condition caused by inflammation and tendon irritation. Intersection syndrome develops where muscles of the first dorsal compartment cross over the radial wrist extensors of the second dorsal compartment, which also may be involved. The location of the pain is usually more proximal and ulnar, over the tendons of the second dorsal compartment. These conditions may also occur in conjunction with de Quervain disorder.

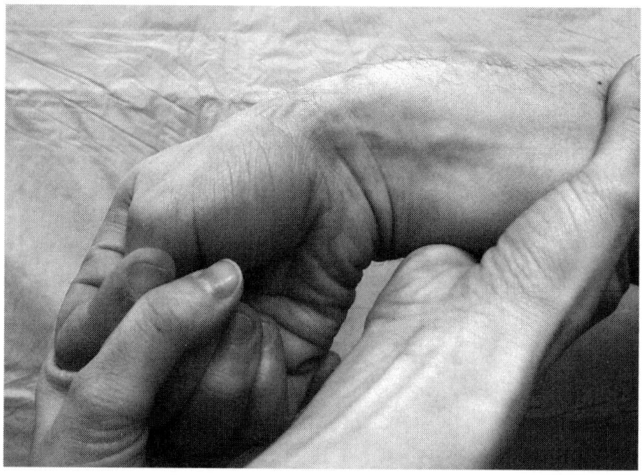

FIG. 101.6. Finkelstein test. The examiner has the patient grasp the flexed thumb and deviate the involved wrist to the ulnar side. The abductor pollicis longus and extensor pollicis brevis tendons and their investing inflamed sheath are stretched through the fibro-osseous canal of the first dorsal compartment. The elicitation of pain by this maneuver is a positive test result.

Clinical Findings/Physical Examination

Patients describe pain at the radial side of the wrist that is made worse by various activities involving characteristic motions of the thumb and wrist. Variable periods of relief with rest are common. On physical examination, tenderness to palpation is localized over the first dorsal compartment of the wrist, just proximal to the radial styloid at the radial border of the distal radius (Fig. 101.5). Pain in this area combined with a positive provocative test result (Finkelstein test) confirms the diagnosis (Fig. 101.6). In the Finkelstein test, pain is elicited over the first dorsal compartment by having the patient grasp the flexed thumb in the affected hand and deviating the wrist to the ulnar side.

Treatment

Nonoperative management includes splinting, modification of activity, NSAIDs, and corticosteroid injection. In a study comparing the results of splinting alone with corticosteroid injection alone and with splinting plus corticosteroid injection, splinting with the thumb abducted and wrist slightly extended provided complete relief of symptoms in only 20% of patients, which represents an 80% failure rate. In the same study, the symptoms of 67% of the patients in the steroid injection group resolved completely. When steroid injection was combined with splinting, the rate of symptom relief was not improved. It was suggested that splinting is unnecessary because the failure rate is high and patients are less restricted without a splint. A trial of NSAIDs and activity modification may also be warranted. Nonoperative treatment may be more successful in acute cases. Patients with tendons traveling in a tight fibro-osseous tunnel are more likely to fail conservative therapy. Complications include fat atrophy and loss of skin pigmentation with corticosteroid injection. Those who fail conservative management may benefit from operative intervention.

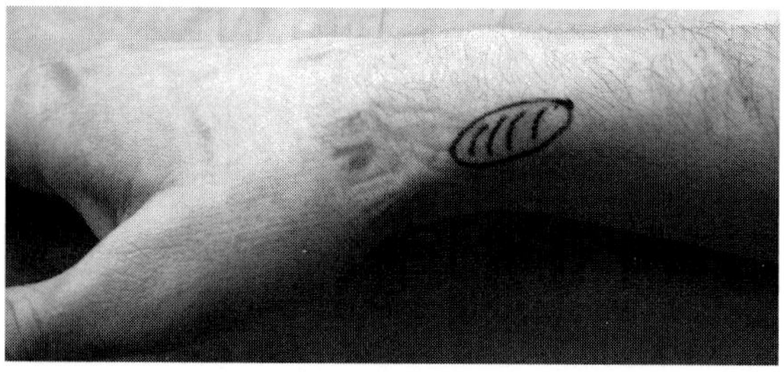

FIG. 101.5. De Quervain disorder point of maximal tenderness. Tenderness to palpation over the first dorsal compartment of the wrist *(circled area)* is usually elicited in the diagnosis of de Quervain disorder.

Surgical treatment involves making a small incision proximal to the radial styloid. Care is taken to avoid branches of the superficial sensory branches of the radial nerve. Next, the fibrous extensor retinaculum is incised, which is usually found to be inflamed. The tendons of the abductor pollicis longus and extensor pollicis brevis are identified. Exploration ensures identification and release of the multiple slips of the abductor pollicis longus tendon, which may travel in separate fibrous sheaths. Incomplete identification and release of these multiple tendon slips may lead to an early recurrence of symptoms. The encasement of the tendons slips in separate sheaths may explain the poor response to nonoperative management. Complications include injury to the superficial branches of the radial nerve and incomplete release. Most patents experience relief after this procedure. Incomplete relief appears most common in working women with occupations requiring repetitive activities.

Effects of Pregnancy on Disease

De Quervain disorder is another frequent cause of hand pain during and after pregnancy. It is thought to be a result of hormone-related swelling and occasionally starts during the second or third trimester. Symptoms may resolve postpartum or at the cessation of nursing. More commonly, women first notice symptoms in the immediate postpartum period, within 1 to 3 months after delivery, or a significant worsening of symptoms after delivery. The combination of hormonal imbalance, fluid retention, and lifting the newborn appears to be responsible for this condition in most cases.

THUMB CARPOMETACARPAL JOINT OSTEOARTHRITIS

Etiology

Osteoarthritis (OA) in the joint formed by the base of the thumb metacarpal and the saddle-shaped trapezium, known as the *thumb carpometacarpal (CMC)* or *trapeziometacarpal (TM) joint*, is another common source of hand pain. The thumb CMC joint is the foundation for the many movements and functions of the thumb. Motion at this joint is greater than at the other, more restrained CMC joints because the opposable thumb is involved in activities of pinch and grasp. Thus, once established, OA may be exacerbated by many activities, especially those that are repetitive. It usually develops in adults in the fifth or sixth decade. More than 50% of women older than 40 years are symptomatic. In addition, women are at a 5% to 10% greater risk for this condition than men, and radiographic evidence is found in 25% of older women, versus only 8% of men. Other risk factors besides female gender and older age include hand dominance and hereditary predisposition.

As for OA in general, no clear causes of thumb CMC arthritis have been identified. Suggested mechanisms include excessive joint laxity, traumatic ligament rupture, and inflammatory disease. Excessive joint laxity combined with repetitive axial loading may lead to synovitis, eventually articular degenerative change, and subluxation of the TM joint. The articular surface of the TM joint displays the same degenerative changes over time as other weight-bearing joints. The articular cartilage becomes soft and frayed. Eventually, cartilage fissures and wears off, and bone eburnation develops. Bony sclerosis is evident, in addition to outgrowths of bone, or osteophytes. These ultimately lead to metacarpal and trapezium bone-on-bone contact, which causes pain, inflammation, and loss of function. Pinch and grasp may be further compromised by compensatory thumb metacarpophalangeal joint hyperextension when subluxation of the TM joint develops.

Differential Diagnosis

The differential diagnosis for thumb CMC joint arthritis includes de Quervain disorder and carpal tunnel syndrome, as previously described. Trigger thumb, or stenosing tenosynovitis of the first annular flexor pulley, may also be confused with this disorder. An inflamed flexor pollicis longus tendon passing through a narrowed annular pulley causes a clicking or locking sensation when the thumb is extended from a flexed position. Tenderness is elicited just proximal to the metacarpophalangeal joint over the first annular pulley. This location is more distal than the typical location of thumb CMC arthritis. Finally, degenerative arthritis at the joint formed by the scaphoid, trapezium, and trapezoid (STT joint) is also in the differential. Tenderness is usually localized dorsally over this joint, which is proximal and ulnar to the base of the thumb metacarpal.

Clinical Findings/Physical Examination

The predominant clinical symptom is pain localized to the radial side of the hand and thumb. Pain may also be localized to the thenar eminence and radiate proximally. Symptoms have usually been present for months or years at the time of diagnosis. Cramping in the first web space or thenar eminence may be noted. Pain is usually exacerbated by activities that load the CMC joint, such as writing, using scissors, and turning keys. Pain is usually relieved by rest and NSAIDs. Functional limitations at work and during hobbies may be noted. In older adults, pain may interfere with the activities of daily living.

The physical findings include localized tenderness to palpation at the volar base of the thumb metacarpal and CMC joint. Active and passive range of motion may be decreased. Joint laxity may be demonstrated, as may weakness in grip and pinch.

As in the previously described conditions, provocative testing is an essential part of the physical examination. The axial grind test elicits pain in the diseased first CMC joint (Fig. 101.7). The metacarpal of the affected thumb is grasped in the hand of the examiner, and an axial load with rotation is applied across the CMC joint. Forceful pinch may also cause pain in the diseased joint.

Laboratory Tests/Imaging Studies

Plain radiographs are extremely helpful in the diagnosis of thumb CMC arthritis (Fig. 101.8). The Eaton classification was developed to characterize the different stages of disease and determine appropriate treatment strategies. Three views of the thumb and CMC joint, including a pronated posteroanterior view, and a CMC joint stress view are obtained. Based on the radiographic findings, disease is in one of four stages.

Stage I disease is characterized by normal findings on standard radiographs. Some joint widening may indicate synovitis. The stress view may show some degree of CMC joint subluxation with a normal scaphotrapezial joint.

Stage II disease is characterized by narrowing of the CMC joint, indicating loss of cartilage. Minimal sclerotic changes and small osteophytes or loose bodies may be present. The scaphotrapezial joint is normal.

Stage III disease is characterized by marked narrowing of the CMC joint, subchondral sclerosis, and larger osteophytes. Subluxation of the CMC joint has usually developed at this stage; however, the scaphotrapezial joint is still normal.

Finally, stage IV disease is characterized by advanced disease of both the CMC and scaphotrapezial joints.

Treatment

The goals of OA treatment are to reduce or eliminate pain and restore function. The nonoperative treatment of thumb CMC joint arthritis is similar to the management of OA at other locations. A course of splinting for 3 to 6 weeks in conjunction with NSAIDs may provide variable relief. Splinting is usually more successful at earlier stages of disease or after an acute exacerbation of symptoms. Occasionally, an intraarticular corticosteroid injection provides limited relief. Patients may also benefit from physical therapy and activity modification. For example, using a larger-diameter golf grip may relieve symptoms. The goal of conservative treatment is to decrease symptoms to a tolerable level. Many patients may have no or only mild pain between acute exacerbations. When conservative management fails and symptoms interfere with activities of daily living, it is appropriate to consider operative intervention.

Operative management is chosen when the patient experiences persistent pain and functional disability. Whether TM arthritis is present alone or in conjunction with scaphotrapezial arthritis determines the operative course. In the latter situation, both arthritic joints must be addressed at the time of surgery to ensure a successful outcome. Treatment for early stage I disease involves a reconstruction of the incompetent volar ligament, which adds stability to the CMC joint and allows normal loading of the joint. Several treatments are used for stages II through IV disease, including simple trapeziectomy alone, trapeziectomy

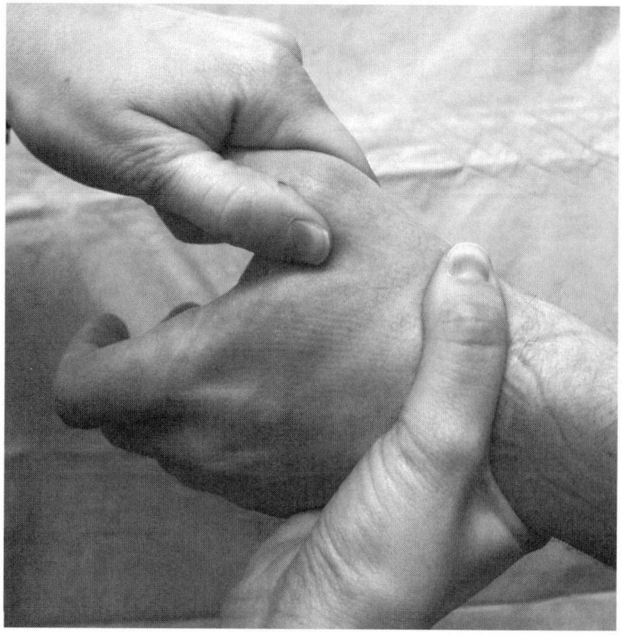

A

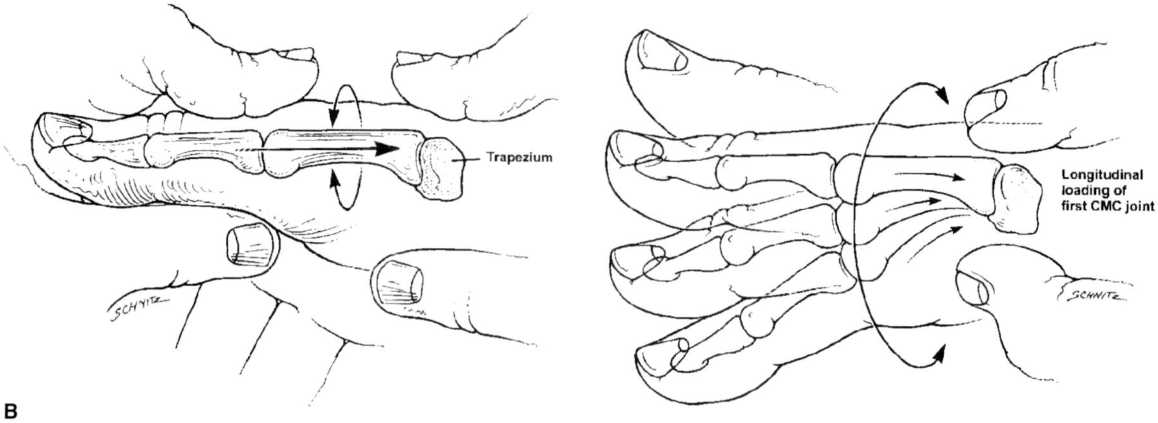

B

FIG. 101.7. First carpometacarpal joint grind test. The examiner grasps the metacarpal of the affected thumb and applies an axial load with rotation. The elicitation of pain by this maneuver is a positive test result.

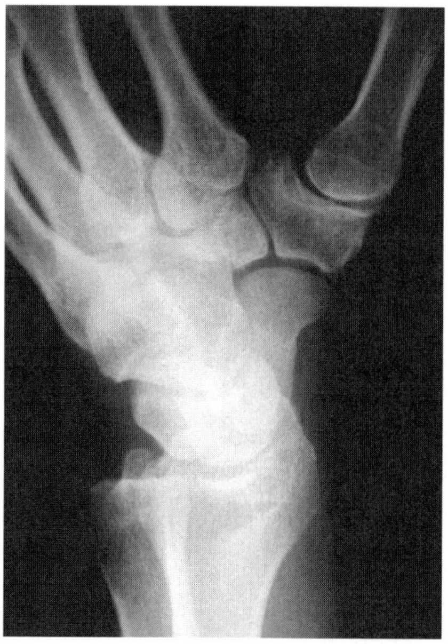

FIG. 101.8. This radiographic view of the pronated first carpometacarpal joint demonstrates Eaton stage II degenerative changes. Narrowing of the joint with sclerotic changes indicates a loss of articular cartilage. At this stage, the scaphotrapezial joint is preserved.

and placement of interpositional material into the space formerly occupied by the trapezium, and trapeziectomy with placement of interpositional material and volar ligament reconstruction. CMC joint arthrodesis may be considered for patients whose occupations require heavy labor, but only if the scaphotrapezial joint is preserved. The metacarpophalangeal joint must be evaluated before surgery. Patients with metacarpophalangeal joint hyperextension benefit from metacarpophalangeal fusion at the time of their other procedure. This improves pinch postoperatively.

Most outcome studies have shown that all these procedures relieve pain and improve range of motion (with the exception of arthrodesis) and strength. Comparisons of trapeziectomy alone, trapeziectomy with interposition, and trapeziectomy with interposition and volar ligament reconstruction have not shown significant differences in patient satisfaction.

It should be kept in mind that up to 40% of patients may present with carpal tunnel syndrome in addition to CMC arthritis. This should also be addressed to optimize functional outcome.

Effects of Pregnancy on Disease

We are unaware of any association between pregnancy and OA of the thumb CMC joint.

BIBLIOGRAPHY

Agee JM, Peimer CA, Pyrek JD, et al. Endoscopic carpal tunnel release: a prospective study of complications and surgical experience. *J Hand Surg [Am]* 1995;20:165–171; discussion 172.

Armstrong AL, Hunter JB, Davis TR. The prevalence of degenerative arthritis of the base of the thumb in post-menopausal women. *J Hand Surg [Br]* 1994;19:340–341.

Belcher HJ, Nicholl JE. A comparison of trapeziectomy with and without ligament reconstruction and tendon interposition. *J Hand Surg [Br]* 2000;25:350–356.

Brown RA, Gelberman RH, Seiler JG III, et al. Carpal tunnel release: a prospective, randomized assessment of open and endoscopic methods. *J Bone Joint Surg Am* 1993;75:1265–1275.

Courts RB. Splinting for symptoms of carpal tunnel syndrome during pregnancy. *J Hand Ther* 1995;8:31–34.

Davis TR, Brady O, Barton NJ, et al. Trapeziectomy alone, with tendon interposition or with ligament reconstruction? *J Hand Surg [Br]* 1997;22:689–694.

Downing ND, Davis TR. Trapezial space height after trapeziectomy: mechanism of formation and benefits. *J Hand Surg [Am]* 2001;26:862–868.

Eaton RG, Glickel SZ. Trapeziometacarpal osteoarthritis: staging as a rationale for treatment. *Hand Clin* 1987;3:455–471.

Eaton RG, Lane LB, Littler JW, et al. Ligament reconstruction for the painful thumb carpometacarpal joint: a long-term assessment. *J Hand Surg [Am]* 1984;9:692–699.

Gelberman RH, Aronson D, Weisman MH. Carpal-tunnel syndrome: results of a prospective trial of steroid injection and splinting. *J Bone Joint Surg Am* 1980;62:1181–1184.

Glowacki KA, Breen CJ, Sachar K, et al. Electrodiagnostic testing and carpal tunnel release outcome. *J Hand Surg [Am]* 1996;21:117–121.

Graeber MC, Lucas AB. Management of pregnancy-related carpal tunnel syndrome. *J Miss State Med Assoc* 2000;41:790–791.

Green DP. Diagnostic and therapeutic value of carpal tunnel injection. *J Hand Surg [Am]* 1984;9:850–854.

Heckman JD, Sassard R. Musculoskeletal considerations in pregnancy. *J Bone Joint Surg Am* 1994;76:1720–1730.

Imaeda T, An KN, Cooney WP, et al. Anatomy of trapeziometacarpal ligaments. *J Hand Surg [Am]* 1993;18:226–231.

Koris M, Gelberman RH, Duncan K, et al. Carpal tunnel syndrome: evaluation of a quantitative provocational diagnostic test. *Clin Orthop* 1990;251:157–161.

North ER, Rutledge WM. The trapezium-thumb metacarpal joint: the relationship of joint shape and degenerative joint disease. *Hand* 1983;15:201–206.

Schned ES. De Quervain tenosynovitis in pregnant and postpartum women. *Obstet Gynecol* 1986;68:411–414.

Schumacher HR Jr, Dorwart BB, Korzeniowski OM. Occurrence of de Quervain's tendinitis during pregnancy. *Arch Intern Med* 1985;145:2083–2084.

Stahl S, Blumenfeld Z, Yarnitsky D. Carpal tunnel syndrome in pregnancy: indications for early surgery. *J Neurol Sci* 1996;136:182–184.

Szabo RM. Entrapment and compression neuropathies. In: Green DP, Hotchkiss RH, Pederson WC, eds. *Green's operative hand surgery*. New York: Churchill Livingstone, 1999:1404–1417.

Tomaino MM, Pellegrini VD Jr, Burton RI. Arthroplasty of the basal joint of the thumb: long-term follow-up after ligament reconstruction with tendon interposition. *J Bone Joint Surg Am* 1995;77:346–355.

Turgut F, Cetinsahinahin M, Turgut M, et al. The management of carpal tunnel syndrome in pregnancy. *J Clin Neurosci* 2001;8:332–334.

Wand JS. Carpal tunnel syndrome in pregnancy and lactation. *J Hand Surg [Br]* 1990;15:93–95.

Weiss AP, Akelman E, Tabatabai M. Treatment of de Quervain's disease. *J Hand Surg [Am]* 1994;19:595–598.

Weiss AP, Sachar K, Gendreau M. Conservative management of carpal tunnel syndrome: a reexamination of steroid injection and splinting. *J Hand Surg [Am]* 1994;19:410–415.

Wolfe SW. Tenosynovitis. In: Green DP, Hotchkiss RH, Pederson WC, eds. *Green's operative hand surgery*. New York: Churchill Livingstone, 1999:2034–2038.

CHAPTER 102
Injuries of the Ankle and Foot

Christopher W. DiGiovanni and
Florian Nickisch

The foot and ankle complex represents our "end organ." It is our constant contact with the environment. We are so accustomed to our feet working well that when they fail, we are surprised by how much disability is incurred. The magnificent biomechanical design and durability of the human foot—which has taken 30 million years of evolution to produce—is continually taken for granted. Few members of the wild kingdom can walk on their heels the way we can, and this ability remains our most distinctly human trait. Our feet rely on the unique interdependence of 28 bones, 31 articulations, and their supporting soft tissue structures to fulfill daily functions requiring load bearing of up to three to seven times body weight. Despite its size, the foot and ankle complex remarkably tolerates these bodily stresses for many years, often with little sign of fatigue in the absence of injury.

Injury to the foot and ankle is important to recognize because of the drastic effect it can have on the delicate biomechanical balance of these structures. When the female foot and ankle complex is examined, however, two kinds of subtle, insidious trauma are less obvious to the clinician but nonetheless must always also be considered in the absence of the typical trauma we think of in an emergency room setting. The physiologic changes of pregnancy add weight across the female foot, which is concomitantly subjected to increased levels of hormones that relax the connective tissues supporting its architecture. Thus, heel pain, stress fractures, and progressive flatfoot deformity are not unusual in the third trimester of pregnancy. Women's fashionable shoes have also long been known to cause foot deformity through low-grade, continual pressure, and additionally they place the ankle at risk for injury. Shoes with pointed toes and high heels can result in an eightfold increase in debilitating toe maladies, such as hammertoes and bunions. They can also cause Achilles tendon contracture, which exacerbates plantar fasciitis. When such shoes are worn, the talus is plantarflexed into a more vulnerable and less stable position within its ankle mortise; combined with the intrinsic instability of the shoe on uneven surfaces, these changes are a setup for ankle sprains or falls. Both of these age-old problems can be at least partially circumvented with preventative care, such as gastrocnemius-soleus stretching exercises, weight control, and wearing appropriately supportive, low-heeled, accommodative toe box shoes.

Today, overt traumatic insults to the foot and ankle complex represent one of the most common reasons that a patient seeks the attention of a primary care physician or musculoskeletal specialist. The literature suggests that the incidence of delayed diagnosis of foot and ankle injuries can approach 30%.

ANKLE SPRAINS

The vast majority of ankle injuries seen in a primary care physician's office are sprains. The term *ankle sprain* is inclusive of any stretching, partial tear, or even complete tear of one or more of the stabilizing ligaments supporting the ankle, so long as the joint remains congruent (located). Because of a common misconception among caregivers and patients, more concern is still raised when ligaments are "torn" rather than stretched or "partially torn," but in reality, these injuries differ little in regard to treatment or clinical outcome except for time to recovery. Thus, although surgery was very popular for acute ankle ligament injuries many years ago, it is very rarely performed today because in 90% to 95% of patients presenting with acute ankle sprains, an excellent long-term outcome is achieved with appropriate conservative management.

Anatomically, ankle sprains can be classified as lateral, medial, or "high" (syndesmotic) sprains. The bony and ligamentous anatomy places the lateral side of the ankle at highest risk for ligamentous injury because the lateral malleolus extends significantly more distally than the medial malleolus and so provides a strong buttress against eversion. The medial side is further stabilized by an extremely strong, dense ligament complex collectively known as the *deltoid ligament*. Consequently, 85% of ankle sprains are *inversion sprains that affect the lateral side* of the ankle. Because the talar dome is wider anteriorly, maximal bony stability is provided with the ankle in dorsiflexion, when the talus is locked more securely in its mortise. As a result of the greater play in plantar flexion, the lateral ligament complex—the anterior talofibular ligament (ATFL), calcaneofibular ligament (CFL), and posterior talofibular ligament (PTFL)—become the primary stabilizers against inversion. In contradistinction, hyperdorsiflexion (often with external rotation) typically sprains the syndesmotic ligaments—the anterior inferior tibiofibular ligament (AITFL), interosseous membrane, and posterior inferior tibiofibular ligament (PITFL). Injuries to these structures are usually considered higher-energy injuries that result in greater soft tissue damage and require prolonged recovery. Such "high" sprains account for approximately 10% of ankle ligament injuries.

Because the great majority of ankle sprains occur laterally, this discussion focuses on their particular treatment. Various classification systems are used to grade the severity of lateral ankle sprains, but the most common and useful one is based on the clinical examination findings. In this system, grade 1 ankle sprains signify stretching of the ATFL. They are moderately painful, with mild swelling, no demonstrable instability, tenderness along the anterior distal fibular margin, and a generally low-energy twisting mechanism; patients with such injuries are able to advance to weight bearing within days or so after the injury. Grade 2 ankle sprains correlate anatomically with complete tearing of the ATFL and partial tearing (or stretching) of the CFL. Clinically, they are somewhat painful, with moderate swelling, often ecchymosis, no demonstrable instability, and tenderness along the entire distal fibular region; patients are frequently unable to advance to weight bearing for 1 to 2 weeks after injury. In grade 3 ankle sprains, both the ATFL and CFL are completely ruptured. These injuries are usually markedly painful, diffusely tender about the lateral ankle, and significantly swollen or ecchymotic (depending on the timing of the presentation), and they may exhibit some instability on examination; patients are usually unable to bear weight for 2 to 4 weeks after injury. In any patient with proximal tenderness or ecchymosis extending up the anterolateral leg, a syndesmotic injury should be considered to be superimposed, and the patient should be evaluated by a specialist. Also, because of discomfort and the patient's tendency to guard, a stability examination is generally not recommended in the acute setting; rather, it should be performed at follow-up within 4 to 6 weeks after injury, when it is better tolerated (and therefore interpreted).

The *mechanism of injury* is important to identify in patients with ankle sprains because the joint position at the time of injury and the direction of the applied force determine injury patterns. A good evaluation should also assess functional capacity; note the onset of the ability to bear weight, walk, and jump; and elicit a history of any locking, clicking, or popping and any previous ankle sprains or feelings of instability on the injured side. Repetitive sprains raise concern for chronic ankle instability or other more subtle problems, such as subtalar instability, tarsal coalition, osteochondritis dissecans, and peroneal tendon dislocation, all of which are best managed by a specialist.

On *physical examination*, the normal, uninjured ankle provides a baseline for assessing the anatomic landmarks and ligament stability. The amount and location of swelling and ecchymosis are noted. The anatomic landmarks palpated for points of maximal tenderness should include the lateral and medial malleoli, entire fibula, fifth metatarsal, and, in skeletally immature patients, distal tibial and fibular physes. Soft tissue palpation includes the ATFL, CFL, PTFL, peroneal tendons, deltoid ligament, and anterior joint line. Range of motion and stability can be tested gently to minimize guarding. The *anterior drawer test* assesses ATFL integrity. With the ankle slightly plantarflexed, the anterior shin is stabilized with one hand while the other hand is used to cup the heel and generate an anteriorly directed force to the foot. A poor endpoint or anterior translation of the talus of more than 10 mm or of more than 3 mm in comparison with the uninvolved side suggests ATFL rupture (grade 2 sprain). Additional injury to the CFL is tested with the *talar tilt test*. The tibia is braced with one hand while the other hand gently inverts the hindfoot and ankle. One finger should palpate the lateral aspect of the talus during this maneuver to ensure that motion occurs at the ankle and not at the subtalar joint. Again, a poor endpoint or talar tilt at least 10 degrees greater than that of the uninjured side suggests complete rupture of the ATFL and CFL (grade 3 ankle sprain). It is important to note that these tests are much more valuable in the subacute or chronic setting than acutely, when surrounding soft tissue swelling and patient guarding interfere. Furthermore, the limited interpretation of the results in the acute setting rarely changes initial management of the sprained ankle. To diagnose a syndesmotic sprain, the *squeeze test* and *external rotation test* can be used. With the patient's foot maximally dorsiflexed, the tibia and fibula are gently squeezed together in the proximal half of the leg. Pain over the space between the distal tibia and fibula suggests a high ankle sprain. In the *external rotation test*, the patient's knee is flexed over the end of the examining table, and while one hand stabilizes the tibia proximally, the other hand applies a gentle external rotation force to the foot; if this maneuver generates radiating discomfort along the anterolateral margin of the leg, the test result is positive. Results of strength and proprioception testing are likely to be abnormal in the acute setting.

Radiographs should usually be obtained by the physician who plans to manage the ankle sprain to resolution. The Ottawa clinical decision rules were proposed in an effort to reduce the number of unnecessary radiographic studies performed for ankle sprains without sacrificing sensitivity for detecting fractures. Accordingly, x-ray films should be obtained for patients who are unable to bear weight or walk four steps or who have tenderness over bony landmarks such as the malleoli or fifth metatarsal. Whenever the diagnosis is in doubt, films should also be obtained. When radiographs are indicated, the standard anteroposterior, lateral, and mortise views should be ordered. Contrary to popular belief, bone scan, computed tomography, and especially magnetic resonance imaging are of limited use in the initial evaluation of an ankle sprain, and the decision to order these tests should be left to the specialist in recalcitrant cases.

The treatment and outcome of lateral inversion ankle sprains depend largely on establishing an accurate diagnosis and ruling out associated injuries. Conservative therapy and rehabilitation for inversion sprains can be divided in four phases. The goal in phase 1 is to control pain, reduce swelling, protect any injured ligaments, and preserve or regain active range of motion. Rest, ice, compression, and elevation (RICE protocol) are the mainstays of this acute treatment. Depending on the severity of the injury, the ankle can be protected initially in either an ankle stirrup brace (grade 1), controlled ankle motion (CAM) walker (grades 2 and 3), or, in cases of severe discomfort, a short leg cast (grade 3) for the first few weeks. Weight bearing with crutch support as needed should be encouraged as soon as possible. Phase 2 begins once the swelling has subsided and the patient is ambulating without major discomfort. Active range of motion and muscle strengthening, especially of the peroneals (which stabilize the ankle against inversion), are emphasized provided they can be performed without pain or swelling. Once joint motion and strength return to normal, the patient is ready for phase 3. At this point, the proprioception that is predictably lost with ankle sprains is restored. Phase 4 consists of functional progression from rehabilitation exercises to the activities of daily living and athletics. When all activities can be performed without pain or limitation, rehabilitation is complete. Protection with taping or bracing is recommended during rehabilitation until strength returns to normal. This rehabilitation protocol is indicated and similar for all grades of inversion ankle sprains, although the duration depends on the severity of the injury (grade). Rehabilitation for *minor* medial and syndesmotic sprains is essentially the same, but progression is generally slower in these patients.

Immediate referral to a specialist for an ankle sprain is necessary whenever it is associated with a break in the skin, neurovascular compromise, severe soft tissue swelling, fracture, tendon rupture or subluxation, significant syndesmotic injury, or demonstrable joint instability. Many of these patients require surgery in the acute setting for optimal outcome. Delayed referral is indicated for any patient who begins to experience mechanical locking or catching, fails to progress with an appropriate physical therapy regimen, or feels pain out of proportion to what is normally expected based on the description of the injury. Complex regional pain syndrome is an unusual but reported sequela of ankle sprains. Another group of patients who warrant the attention of a specialist are those with a history of repetitive ankle sprains or mechanical malalignment because chronic instability is associated with significant disability and arthritic change if left untreated. Surgical treatment in the setting of an acute, isolated ankle sprain is *rarely* indicated and controversial, generally being reserved for elite level athletes with grade 3 inversion sprains.

ANKLE FRACTURES

The incidence of both low- and high-energy ankle fractures is steadily rising in Western countries. From long-term follow-up studies, we have learned that satisfactory alignment, early range of motion, and controlled weight bearing are paramount for restoration of optimal function. Thus, prompt diagnosis and treatment are important. Only small (<2 mm) avulsion-type fractures resulting from a low-energy injury should be treated by the primary care practitioner. Any fracture associated with large fragments, open wounds, neurovascular compromise, malalignment, or unusual or rapidly progressive swelling or in which the talus or additional bones of the foot are involved should be managed by a specialist. Obviously, this list also includes any injury that the physician does not feel competent to manage for whatever reason.

Beware the patient referred to you with "negative" radiographs and a diagnosis of "ankle sprain," particularly if (a) no films are available to look at, (b) a high-energy mechanism is involved, (c) the sprain is "chronic" (chronic sprains generally do not exist), or (d) pain, swelling, or ecchymosis is greater than expected. Maintaining a high index of suspicion is often half the battle. The physician should always inspect and palpate the entire length of the leg (tibia *and* fibula) and foot in any patient presenting with acute ankle trauma. The skin and neurovascular structures should always be inspected carefully, and joint stability and the location of any tenderness should be determined. No patient should be evaluated without accompanying radiographs (anteroposterior, lateral, and mortise) of the ankle. In the event that the traumatic mechanism traveled through the ankle and up the leg, injuries to other structures beyond the ankle are often present, such as a high fibular fracture or syndesmotic injury (Fig. 102.1). These

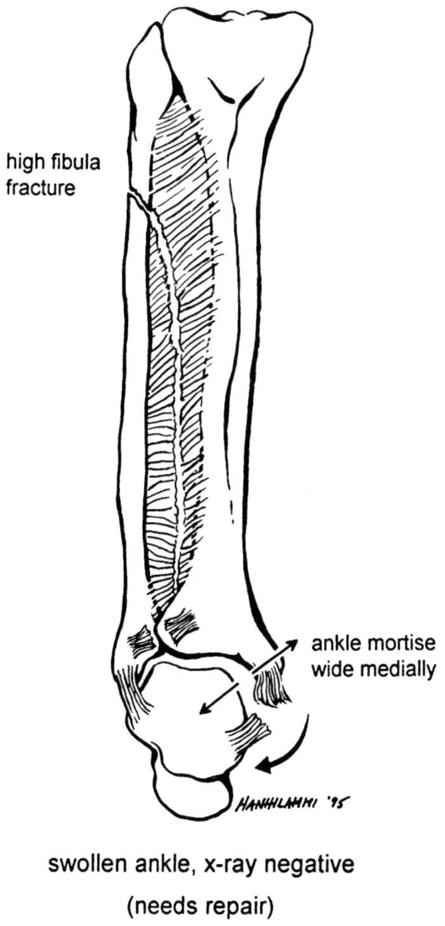

FIG. 102.1. Swollen ankle with severe ligamentous injury and high fibular fracture.

often require surgical intervention. The fracture of the fibula in such cases is not the problem; rather, the restoration of congruent ankle anatomy remains the focus. Whenever the mortise of the ankle appears widened, regardless of whether a fracture is present, referral to a specialist to consider operative repair is in order. When this decision is difficult, a comparison view of the opposite side is often a quick and easy way to compare normal with abnormal.

Stability is of prime importance in determining the right treatment plan for an ankle fracture. The assessment of stability requires a basic understanding of ankle biomechanics and fracture patterns. The components of the ankle joint can be thought of as a closed ring; the talus, the distal fibula and its lateral ligaments, the distal tibia and its medial ligaments, and the syndesmosis between tibia and fibula form a stable ring (Fig. 102.2A). The ring can be disrupted by any combination of ligamentous and bony damage. If the ring is disrupted in one spot, it is still quite stable, but if it is broken in two places, it becomes quite unstable (Fig. 102.2B). Instability is most frequent when disruption occurs on both the lateral and medial sides (Fig. 102.2 C,D). The best way to ensure that the ring is broken in only one place is by carefully examining the patient and the x-ray films. For example, in the event of a stable, isolated, undisplaced fibula fracture with lateral tenderness and swelling, the physician should carefully examine the medial side. If the medial skin and soft tissues appear unharmed on examination, this suggests that the deltoid (medial) ligament is intact (Fig. 102.2B). If the deltoid is intact and the radiograph suggests only a lateral and no medial malleolar fracture, then the ring is likely broken in only one spot and the pattern is considered stable. It is unlikely that the mortise will widen in this situation. Because a lack of medial tenderness sometimes correlates poorly with integrity of the deep deltoid ligament, however, careful examination of the medial clear space on x-ray films, in addition to close follow-up of the patient, is prudent. When clinical suspicion remains, sometimes stress x-ray films can be helpful in demonstrating subtle ligamentous instability. Whenever doubt arises, referral to a specialist should be made because posttraumatic instability or arthritis of the ankle is a problem that is highly likely to lead to disability.

Low-energy ankle injuries deemed stable in a proper evaluation can be successfully treated by short-term immobilization in a cast, walking boot, or stirrup, depending on the severity, followed by rapid mobilization with physical therapy, NSAIDS, and a RICE protocol. In the vast majority of such cases, an excellent functional outcome can be expected by 6 to 8 weeks of follow-up. Any divergence from this expected gradual improvement should also prompt rapid evaluation by a specialist.

RUPTURED ACHILLES TENDON

Patients who sustain an acute Achilles tendon rupture often describe feeling as if they had suddenly been struck with a bat in the back of the leg, or feeling a "pop" in the back of the leg. Typically, this occurs in "weekend warriors" between the ages of 35 and 55 years at the moment of a rapid change in direction or push off during a sporting event. Weak plantar flexion of the foot is still possible, and the patient may even be able to limp gingerly after complete Achilles tendon rupture. This is possible because of the action of the nearby toe flexors, peroneals, and posterior tibial tendon. The examiner must confirm whether the Achilles tendon is intact because this sequence of events sometimes results simply from a plantaris rupture or gastrocnemius-soleus muscle pull, both of which can be reliably treated with physical therapy and rapid progression to weight bearing. An Achilles tendon rupture, on the other hand, is often (but not always) best treated surgically. To test the integrity of the heel cord, the patient should lie prone on the examining table with the feet off the end of the table. If the Achilles tendon is ruptured, a defect is often visible and palpable, most commonly 4 to 6 cm above the calcaneus, with some surrounding ecchymosis. Moreover, the involved foot is in a neutral position or even slight dorsiflexion in comparison with the uninvolved side. When the patient is asked to bend the knee actively to 90 degrees, the foot drops further into dorsiflexion. The Thompson test is probably the best way to diagnose an Achilles tendon rupture; gentle manual compression of the mid calf should produce slight plantar flexion of the foot. If no foot motion is noted, the result of the Thompson test is positive, suggesting discontinuity of the Achilles tendon with the heel. Comparison with the uninvolved side is always helpful.

It is debated in orthopedic circles whether to treat these injuries by open or closed methods. Operative treatment has been shown to result in a greater (and sometimes faster) return to the preinjury functional level, greater gastrocnemius-soleus power, and lower rate of recurrent rupture. Surgery is generally recommended for active patients but does entail the usual associated risks. Conservative treatment with serial equinus casting is an alternative treatment that should probably be reserved for patients who are elderly, medically unstable or at high risk, or predominantly sedentary.

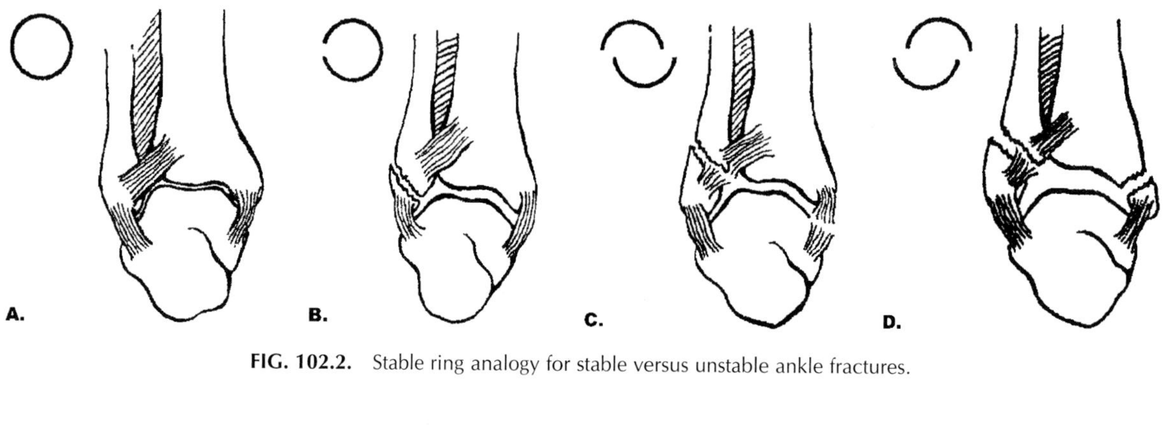

FIG. 102.2. Stable ring analogy for stable versus unstable ankle fractures.

TARSAL INJURIES

The evaluation of patients with a foot fracture includes documentation of the neurovascular status, condition of the soft tissue envelope, any deformity or swelling, and stability, and an examination of the presumably uninjured opposite foot. Routine radiographs (anteroposterior, lateral, and oblique) of the injured foot are always obtained. The ankle should also be quickly assessed in these patients. Because the foot is not a single structure but actually a multitude of bones and joints that act together, these are also often injured together. Thus, even if a patient's problem is in one particular area, the examiner should check the entire hindfoot, midfoot, and forefoot.

In general, fractures involving the major tarsal bones of the foot (calcaneus, talus, navicular, and cuboid) are typically caused by high-energy mechanisms and often indicate relatively severe and global injury patterns. With the exception of small, extraarticular avulsion fractures, which are most aptly treated by a RICE protocol and progressive weight bearing as tolerated in well-cushioned shoes, such injuries warrant special attention and are best treated by an experienced surgeon familiar with the myriad associated problems and complications. We often teach that tarsal injuries represent severe soft tissue trauma that happens to be associated with a break in the bone.

As in many cases of orthopedic trauma, the soft tissues usually dictate the urgency of care. Any acute, significant (>2 mm) talar fracture should be considered relatively urgent by the primary care physician, and the patient is most appropriately kept from weight bearing, splinted, and referred. The talus is the bone around which the entire foot moves and the single connection between the foot and ankle. Therefore, significant injury to the talus often has devastating consequences. This bone is covered mostly by articular cartilage, has a tenuous blood supply, and comprises a major portion of the ankle and subtalar joints. The calcaneus is also a complex bone that requires rapid evaluation and treatment by a specialist after injury; it is often fractured in high-speed vehicular crashes or falls from heights. Injury to the precariously thin soft tissue cover of the calcaneus bodes special problems, and every effort should be made to keep swelling to a minimum. The axial loading responsible for a fractured heel often simultaneously causes vertebral fractures or abdominal injuries, so the physician should always check for back tenderness or peritoneal signs in a patient with a broken heel. These injuries frequently result in surgical intervention. *Compartment syndrome* should always be ruled out when significant swelling or pain develops in a patient with a foot injury. This can be challenging even for an experienced examiner because signs of neurovascular compromise are usually late. Compartment syndrome is a leading cause of medicolegal action in the United States, and the foot is the most notoriously difficult area of the musculoskeletal system in which to make this diagnosis. The most reliable signs are pain out of proportion to the physical findings, extreme swelling, and pain on passive toe stretch. Any question about the existence of this problem should prompt rapid tertiary referral.

The tarsal navicular and cuboid are often injured together in a combination of either bony or ligamentous injury. Much like a round pretzel, it is difficult to break one side of the foot without damaging the other. Tiny avulsion fractures in this region not caused by a high-energy mechanism and without much swelling can usually be treated with a RICE protocol, early weight bearing, and sometimes short-term (2–3 weeks) casting for initial comfort. Patients with these injuries typically recover well without functional limitation, whereas avulsion injuries associated with major bony or soft tissue damage are telltale signs of significant underlying instability or degloving and warrant the attention of a specialist. A small ossicle (accessory navicular) is often found on the medial aspect of the navicular and mistaken for an acute fracture. It typically lacks the common cardinal signs of swelling, tenderness, and irregular radiographic contours found in acute fractures. The ossicle is the attachment site of the posterior tibial tendon and is present in many feet. True fractures of the tarsal navicular are other bad injuries that often require surgery and may result in avascular necrosis, nonunion, or chronic foot pain. The lesser tarsal bones (cuneiforms) are also seldom injured in isolation.

TARSOMETATARSAL FRACTURE AND FRACTURE DISLOCATION

Isolated dislocation of the bones or joints of the foot are actually rare. Disruption of joints in the foot occurs most frequently at the level of the tarsometatarsal (Lisfranc) joints. If left untreated, this usually results in chronic foot pain, progressive deformity, and disability. The Lisfranc joints are supposed to be rigid structures with very little movement, providing stability to the arch. Injury to the Lisfranc joints often results in symptomatic collapse of the arch and abduction of the foot. Such injuries are easily missed on x-ray films and clinical examination unless a physician with a high index of suspicion checks the intermetatarsal *and* tarsometatarsal (junction of forefoot and midfoot) alignment. Comparing the injured foot with the uninjured foot provides valuable clues to the patient's normal anatomy clinically and radiographically. These injuries are almost always caused by a high-energy mechanism, as in a motor vehicle accident or on football turf, and present with acute swelling, midfoot tenderness, and sometimes abduction deformity or instability. Subtle widening between the base of the first and second metatarsals is often noted on x-ray films, indicating a large ligamentous injury to the tarsometatarsal joints (Fig. 102.3). A tiny fracture (fleck sign) in this location may imply the same. Although this is often quite obvious on x-ray films, subtle anatomic relationships are sometimes the tip-off; on the oblique view, the medial aspect of the cuboid should line up exactly with the medial border of the fourth ray, and on the anteroposterior view, the medial border of the second metatarsal base should line up exactly with the medial base of the second cuneiform. Stress or comparison radiographs are often very helpful in this regard (Fig. 102.3). Typically, these fractures/dislocations are unstable and require operative fixation. Although it is clear that patients do best after operative anatomic restoration, it is difficult for them to regain normal foot function after a tarsometatarsal injury, and complete recovery (as in many hindfoot/midfoot injuries) often takes 1 to 2 years. When such injuries are suspected, evaluation by a consultant is always appropriate.

METATARSAL FRACTURES

In static loading, weight is evenly distributed between hindfoot and forefoot. Although their bases are uneven, each metatarsal head is level with the next and distributes weight relatively evenly in proportion to its size. The weight of the forefoot is distributed so that the great toe, with its two underlying sesamoid bones, takes one third, and each of the lesser

A,B
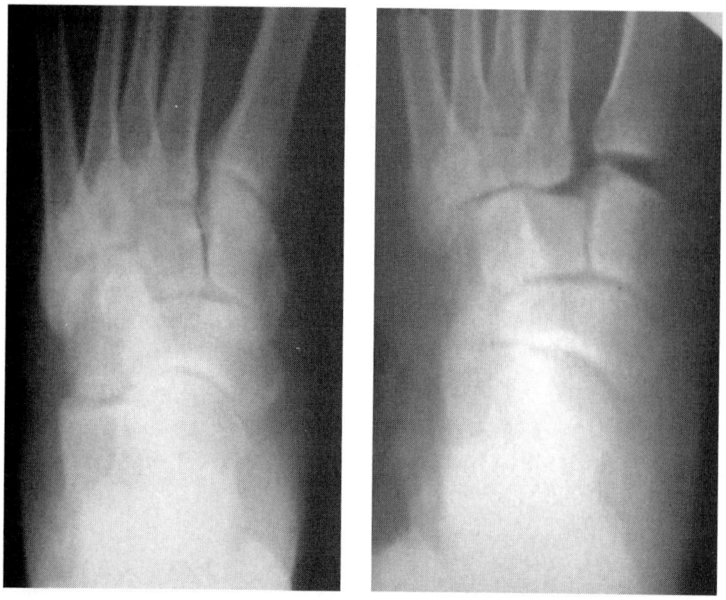

C,D
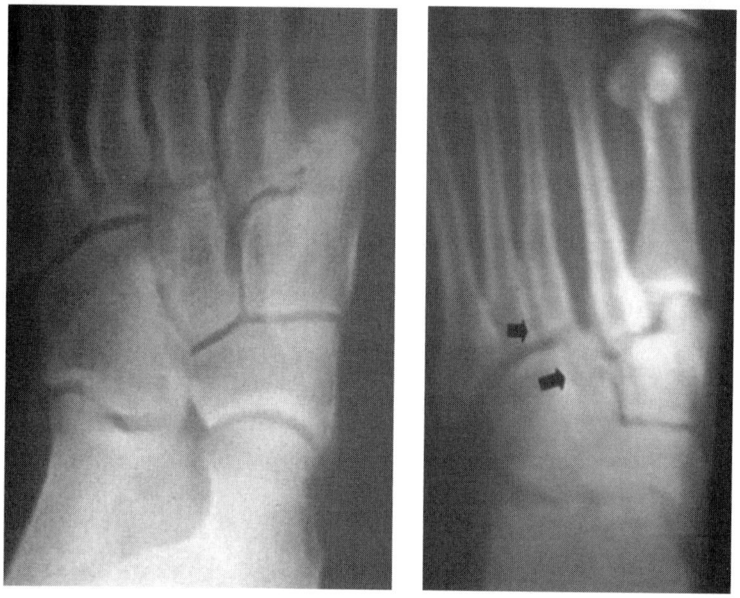

FIG. 102.3. Anteroposterior and medial oblique roentgenographic views of the tarsometatarsal joint. **A:** Normal joint alignment on anteroposterior view. **B:** Tarsometatarsal injury with lateral migration of first and second rays. **C:** Normal joint alignment on medial oblique view. **D:** Tarsometatarsal injury with lateral displacement of the fourth metatarsal in relation to the medial border of the cuboid *(arrows)*.

four toes takes about one sixth. In a metatarsal fracture, the physician must bear in mind the weight-bearing function of the bone. Single fractures of the metatarsal shaft are usually minimally displaced and well splinted by the strong and balanced intermetatarsal ligaments. As soon as the initial pain and swelling abate (usually within 2–3 weeks), protected weight bearing in a short leg cast or CAM walker boot can usually begin. Fractures of the metatarsal head and neck, which are typically angulated, can sometimes reduce into correct alignment with weight bearing. Fractures of the base of metatarsals I through IV should initially be evaluated to rule out tarsometatarsal joint injuries because of their anatomic proximity and subtle instability patterns. Although the vast majority of metatarsal fractures can be treated conservatively, the "border" fractures of metatarsals I and V require more attention because it is difficult to fit shoes in the event of displacement in the transverse plane. Consultation with a specialist should be reserved for patients with these injuries, multiple metatarsal or intraarticular fractures, high-energy or severely displaced fractures, or any fractures that threaten the overlying skin, make the clinician uncomfortable, or arouse suspicion of compartment syndrome. A fracture in the proximal diaphysis of the fifth metatarsal (Jones fracture) is often slow to heal and relatively unique in this array of injuries in that a non–weight-bearing cast is required for the first 6 weeks of treatment, or even early operative fixation in some cases. In contrast, the adjacent, more common avulsion fracture of the base of the fifth metatarsal is quick to heal and can easily be treated in a comfortable walking shoe (Fig. 102.4). With most of these fractures, 8 weeks or so is required until solid bony union is obtained, although some swelling or a dull "ache" is often present for months thereafter.

TOE FRACTURES

Most lesser toe (II–V) fractures respond well to conservative care. They are often sustained when a toe is stubbed or struck

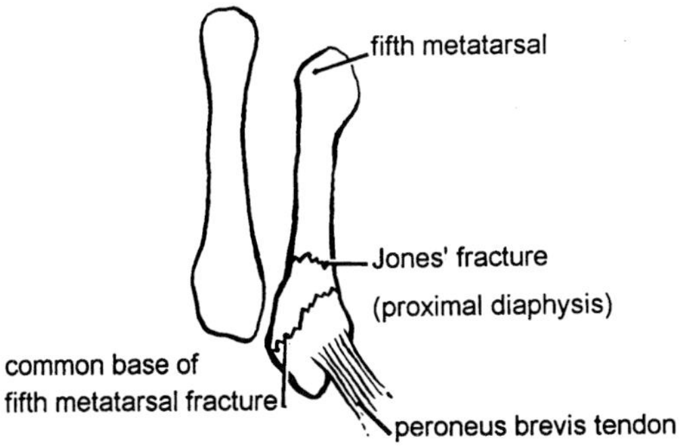

FIG. 102.4. Different types of fifth metatarsal fractures.

by a falling object. The treating physician must be sure that the fracture is a closed injury that does not enter (extraarticular) or disrupt (subluxation or dislocation) a joint. Alignment of the toes as a unit must also be (and usually is) appropriate. Even initially displaced fractures or deformed toes can usually be reduced and aligned with gentle traction or Chinese finger traps and then taped to adjacent toes with a wisp of lamb's wool in between. Casting is rarely needed. A supportive, semirigid, comfortable shoe can often used to allow weight bearing on the rest of the foot. On the other hand, intraarticular problems of the great toe (I) require careful attention, and this toe is less forgiving of small amounts of displacement than the lesser toes. Except for a tuft fracture of the end of the toe, anatomic reduction should be ensured in all fractures of the great toe for optimal outcome. Although deviations from this rule are occasionally acceptable, they should be the responsibility of the specialist, not the primary care physician.

FRACTURES OF THE SESAMOID BONES

The sesamoids are the two weight-bearing bones beneath the first metatarsal head. If they suddenly sustain too heavy a load or, more commonly, too much repetitive stress, they can fracture. However, they may also be congenitally bipartite structures that just appear to be fractured. Again, the tip-off here is discerning rounded, sclerotic edges from the jagged, abrupt ones seen in trauma. The foot should be examined carefully for tenderness and the radiograph scrutinized in search of cortical disruption. If a fracture is present, a prolonged period of protected weight bearing is usually required, first in a cast and later in an unloading orthotic. If these treatments are unsuccessful after 3 months, referral to a specialist and, rarely, surgery are necessary.

BIBLIOGRAPHY

DiGiovanni CW, Benirscke SK, Hansen ST. Foot injuries. In: Browner BD, Jupiter JB, Levine AM, Trafton PG, eds. *Skeletal trauma, basic science, management and reconstruction*, 3rd ed. Philadelphia: WB Saunders, 2003.

Judd DB, Kim DH. Foot fractures frequently misdiagnosed as ankle sprains. *Am Fam Physician* 2002;66:785–794.

Kannus P, Palvanen M. Increasing number and incidence of low-trauma ankle fractures in elderly people: Finnish statistics during 1970–2000 and projections for the future. *Bone* 2002;31:430–433.

Kerkhoffs GM, Handoll HH, De Bie R, et al. Surgical versus conservative treatment for acute injuries of the lateral ligament complex of the ankle in adults. *Cochrane Database Syst Rev* 2002;3:CD000380.

Kocher MS, Bishop J, Marshall R, et al. Operative versus nonoperative management of acute Achilles tendon rupture: expected-value decision analysis. *Am J Sports Med* 2002;30:783–790.

Luo RS, Tejwani NC, DiGiovanni CW, et al. Outcome after open reduction and internal fixation of Lisfranc joint injuries. *J Bone Joint Surg Am* 2000;82:1609–1618.

Rockwood CA, Green DP, Heckman JD, et al., eds. *Fractures in adults*, 5th ed. Philadelphia: Lippincott Williams & Wilkins, 2001.

PART

12

Neurologic Problems

CHAPTER 103
Headache

Joshua Hollander

Headache is a problem that most people encounter at some time. Headaches are generally infrequent and not excessively severe. Most people deal with an occasional headache by taking over-the-counter (OTC) drugs and do not consult a physician. In about a third of the population, headaches are more frequent and more severe. Some of these people suffer disabling symptoms without troubling their physician because of the common belief that a physician can do little for a headache anyway. A patient presenting to a physician because of headache is one of a few persons in the affected population who have reached the point of being unable to cope. The complaint of headache in a patient who is no longer able to cope should be dealt with in a serious and sustained fashion because major advances in management are now available. When a patient does seek medical help, a proper diagnosis requires the physician's time and interest, with careful attention to the symptoms, more than technology. A clear explanation of the cause of the problem is needed in addition to relief of pain. Patients with infrequent headaches may respond to abortive agents, but for those with frequent headaches, prophylaxis should be attempted. Chronicity implies a benign origin but also necessitates more care and support from the physician. Multiple agents may be tried, and the patient's understanding and cooperation are essential. Because the problem is not life-threatening, it is often dismissed all too casually by the treating physician.

ETIOLOGY AND DIFFERENTIAL DIAGNOSIS

Although brain tissue per se is not sensitive to pain, numerous intracranial structures are nociceptive. The scalp, dural sinuses, falx, and proximal larger arteries are innervated by the trigeminal nerve in the anterior and middle fossa and by the upper cervical roots and glossopharyngeal and vagus nerves in the posterior fossa. Traction on nociceptive structures distorts them and causes pain. It is generally referred to the frontotemporal region when it arises in the anterior and middle fossa and to the posterior cervical region, ear, or throat when structures of the posterior fossa are involved. Sinus headache does occur but manifests with frank purulent material. *Sinus headache* is the term popularized on television to denote migraine without an aura. The eyes may be a source of headache primarily when glaucoma or injection is present.

The overwhelming majority of patients with headache have a benign condition, but many insist that they must have a structural cause of their headache. The misconception that brain tumors commonly present with severe headaches contributes to the anxiety provoked by recurrent and resistant severe headaches. The first consideration for the caregiver is to distinguish common benign headaches from the infrequent headaches with an ominous presentation. The physician must always balance the need to recognize a life-threatening condition against the cost of imaging studies. The differential diagnosis for a first acute headache is quite different from that for chronic, recurrent headaches. A headache that stands out against a background of infrequent, deep aching or is described as the "worst headache of my life" is probably only a migraine but is worrisome, especially when sudden in onset. A change in the pattern of chronic headache is also disturbing and requires careful reevaluation. A first severe, explosive headache, especially if associated with a stiff neck, suggests meningeal irritation. It is important to remember that the full expression of meningeal signs may await breakdown of blood or progression of meningitis. An explosive onset of headache and stiff neck without fever suggests subarachnoid hemorrhage, and a more gradual development of headache and stiff neck with fever suggests meningitis. The detection of either pus or blood requires lumbar puncture. If the history or physical findings suggest lateralized masses, posterior fossa masses, or increased intracranial pressure, computed tomography (CT) may be required before lumbar puncture is performed.

The headache associated with increased intracranial pressure occurs in the morning or after naps and remits after the patient arises. Patients experience headaches on more than half of mornings that crescendo during weeks to months. The intensity varies. The headache associated with a local lesion is constant, nonpulsatile, and maximal in a small area determined by the location of the lesion.

The International Headache Society has developed a new classification of headache; a simplified version is presented in Table 103.1. Only some classes of headache are reviewed here.

TABLE 103.1. Classification of Headache

- Migraine
  - Migraine without aura
  - Migraine with aura
    - Typical aura with migraine headache
    - Typical aura with non-migraine headache
    - Typical aura without headache
    - Migraine with prolonged aura
    - Familial hemiplegic migraine
    - Sporadic hemiplegic migraine
    - Basilar-type migraine
  - Childhood periodic syndromes that commonly precede migraine
    - Cyclic vomiting
    - Abdominal migraine
    - Benign paroxysmal vertigo of childhood
  - Retinal migraine
  - Complications of migraine
    - Chronic migraine
    - Status migrainosus
    - Persistent aura without infarction
    - Migrainous infarction
    - Migraine-triggered seizures
- Tension-type headache
  - Episodic tension-type headache
  - Chronic tension-type headache
- Cluster headache and other trigeminal-autonomic cephalalgias
  - Cluster headache
    - Episodic cluster headache
    - Chronic cluster headache
  - Paroxysmal hemicrania
    - Episodic paroxysmal hemicrania
    - Chronic paroxysmal hemicrania
  - Short-lasting unilateral neuralgiform headache with conjunctival injection and tearing (SUNCT)
  - Hemicrania continua
- Other short-lasting head pains
  - Primary stabbing headache
  - Primary cough headache
  - Primary exertional headache
  - Primary headache associated with sexual activity
    - Dull type
    - Explosive type
  - Hypnic headache
- Headache attributed to head or neck trauma
- Headache attributed to cranial or cervical vascular disorders
- Headache attributed to nonvascular, noninfectious intracranial disorder
- Headache attributed to a substance or its withdrawal
- Headache attributed to infection
- Headache attributed to a disturbance of homeostasis
- Headache or facial pain associated with a disorder of the cranium, neck, eyes, nose, sinuses, teeth, mouth, or other facial or cranial structures
- Headache attributed to a psychiatric disorder
- Cranial neuralgias and central causes of facial pain

Note: Simplified after the International Headache Society draft.

Migraine

Migraine is the most common type of headache, affecting almost half of persons with significant headache. Migraine is a complex blend of head pain and neurologic and vegetative symptoms. The diagnosis is based on the history. In all persons with headache, the severity of the headaches varies. Mild migraine without an aura may blend into tension-type headache, but a severe headache tends to be of a type usually associated with migraine. Migraine most typically is unilateral, throbbing, aggravated by routine activity, severe enough to interfere with daily activities, and associated with photophobia and phonophobia. A person experiencing a migraine headache prefers to lie down in a quiet, dark place. The headache lasts 4 to 72 hours but may be terminated by sleep. The frequency of "ice pick" pains and "ice cream" headaches is increased in migraine.

Migraine is significantly more prevalent in women. The prevalence peaks at the age of 40 years, abates somewhat by age 55, and decreases significantly later in life. The incidence peaks somewhat earlier in teenagers who have migraine with aura. The female-to-male prevalence ratio begins to increase at puberty and peaks at 3.5:1 at age 40. Genetic factors have been noted in twin studies. An individual has a 40% chance of having migraine if one parent is affected, and a 70% chance when both parents have migraine. The migraine personality has not stood up to scrutiny, but psychogenic factors as triggers remain important. Depression is almost universal in people with daily headaches, but it is less clear whether depression or migraine is the primary condition. It may well be that each exacerbates the other.

Some migraineurs are unaware of any clear precipitants of headache, but most can identify some stimulus likely to provoke an attack. Psychosocial factors may manifest as a slump headache on days off rather than at times of peak stress. Emotional stress, too much or too little sleep, bright light, loud, blaring music, and olfactory stimulants all probably act on central mechanisms. Missed meals, foodstuffs, food additives, medications, and altered barometric pressure presumably act systemically. Many potentially precipitating agents, such as sharp cheddar cheese, chocolate, and nuts, contain vasoactive agents such as tyramine and phenylethyl amine. Vasodilators such as nitrates and nitrites may precipitate migraine in susceptible persons. Red wine and changes in the barometric pressure act by uncertain mechanisms. Excitatory amino acid transmitters, such as monosodium glutamate and aspartame, may be precipitants. Foodstuffs are important triggers for a small number of individuals, and it is not generally helpful to embark on massive dietary restrictions unless it is clearly relevant to the individual patient. Medications said to cause headache include antihypertensives, vasodilators, calcium channel blockers, histamine H_2 blockers, hormones, and antibiotics. Agents such as ergotamine and caffeine are associated with rebound headache. A factor in the conversion of migraine to chronic daily headache is the analgesic rebound headache. The effects of menses and pregnancy are discussed later in this chapter.

Premonitory symptoms or prodromes are warnings of impending headache but may precede the attack by hours or days. They include changes in mood, behavior, energy level, and appetite, or vague cervical and cephalic sensations. These may not always occur but can be sufficiently striking to alert family and friends to an impending attack.

The aura is a transient attack of neurologic dysfunction that develops gradually during 5 to 20 minutes and lasts for less than 60 minutes. It usually precedes head pain. The aura is most commonly a sensory disturbance, either visual or somatosensory. The most characteristic aura is a C-shaped, shimmering, prismatic, jagged scotoma best seen with the eyes closed. It is usually in one hemifield and slowly moves across the field to the periphery. As it moves away, either visual loss or a new scintillation may develop. A large variety of visual phenomena occur, including hemianopia, blindness, and photopsia. Monocular phenomena raise the specter of retinal or nerve disease but may be a retinal migraine in which a brightly colored light progresses to visual loss that clears with the onset of headache. Dysesthesias of the mouth and hands are the most common somatosensory phenomena. Other phenomena include motor abnormalities, vertiginous states, aphasia, and behavioral and perceptual states. The metamorphopsia and perceptual alterations have been referred to as the *"Alice in Wonderland" syndrome* .

Although migraine with aura is easy to recognize in its most typical form, patients with a prolonged aura or with aphasia and hemiplegia should provoke greater concern and require further evaluation. Patients who have migraine with aura may sometimes experience headache without aura or aura without headache. In persons who had headaches earlier in life that disappeared, transient neurologic dysfunction may develop that must be differentiated from transient ischemic attacks. Transient migrainous attacks spread slowly across the cortex, and the visual, motor, or sensory loss may take 5 to 20 minutes to spread fully, whereas the full distribution of transient ischemia is manifested almost immediately.

Despite great advances in clarifying the pathophysiology of migraine, major gaps remain. For many years, a vascular mechanism was hypothesized; intracranial vasospasm was thought to be the cause of the migrainous aura, with subsequent vasodilation and stretching of vessels causing pain. This hypothesis could not be confirmed experimentally and failed to reconcile major clinical findings in migraine. Experimental studies led to the neurogenic inflammation theory. The trigeminal nerve innervates the proximal portions of the large intracranial vessels and can transmit nociceptive stimuli centrally, but at branch points it can also conduct antidromically and release algesic substances that promote vascular inflammation and increase pain. Vomiting may develop secondary to the trigeminal activation of brainstem centers involved in vomiting. The migrainous aura is now believed to be related to the spreading cortical depression of Leao rather than vasospasm. Potassium is released in spreading depression, and a leading wave of depolarization, commencing in the calcarine cortex (aura of "classic migraine"), reaches the trigeminal fibers and initiates the nociceptive trigeminal vascular circuit. This theory fails to explain the initiation of spreading cortical depression in migraine with aura, the initiation of nociception in migraine without aura, and the role of precipitating perceptual or psychic factors. Important roles have been postulated for the mesencephalic periaqueductal gray matter and medullary raphe nuclei. These are pain-modulating centers, and a failure of negative feedback loops because of either hereditary instability or neural inputs could allow the trigeminal vascular system to spiral out of control. Alterations of serotonin function have been observed at many levels in migraine, but their role is uncertain. Positron emission tomography has revealed major activation of the raphe nuclei (serotoninergic) during an attack. Adrenergic transmitters, in addition to such peptides as calcitonin gene-related peptide, have also been implicated. The identification of genetic factors in familial hemiplegic migraine and its relationship to genes associated with P/Q-type calcium channels has opened a new window on the pathogenesis of migraine. Regrettably, a unified theory of migraine capable of explaining all the complex phenomenology characterizing this common disorder is lacking.

Tension-Type Headache

Recurrent, episodic, bilateral headaches of mild-to-moderate intensity that are not worsened by activity or accompanied by nausea and that last 30 minutes to 7 days are called *tension headaches*. The pain is of a pressing, tightening quality. These headaches do not occur daily (<15 per month); when they do occur more frequently for a prolonged time, they are referred to as *chronic tension-type headaches*. The incidence of both intermittent episodic and chronic tension headaches is higher in women. Psychosocial stress is a significant component of tension-type headaches. Analgesic abuse and withdrawal are important considerations in the chronic form, especially when it blends into chronic daily headache. Oromandibular dysfunction is also more prominent in chronic forms.

This disorder was formerly called *muscle contraction headache* when it was thought to be caused by cervical or fronto-occipital muscle spasm. Electromyography has failed to confirm such a mechanism. It is now postulated that an acute attack may occur in an otherwise normal person as the result of a complex interaction of pericranial muscle strain, myofascial pain sensitivity, and descending limbic effect on brainstem nociception. Chronicity may manifest with predominantly central mechanisms.

Cluster Headache and Chronic Paroxysmal Hemicrania

Cluster headache is a dramatic disorder (affecting 0.1% of the population) associated with a host of synonyms. The abrupt onset of a strictly unilateral headache characterized by severe orbital, supraorbital, and temporal pain may occur with a periodicity of weeks to months or more frequently (from several times a week to up to eight times a day). Individual attacks affect the same side and last 15 to 180 minutes. One or more of the following associated signs are seen on the painful side: conjunctival injection, lacrimation, nasal congestion, rhinorrhea, forehead and facial sweating, miosis, ptosis, and eyelid edema. The pain may be described as boring, burning, or throbbing. It elicits a local sensitivity, and persons with this type of headache tend to engage in intense physical activity for a short time, unlike those with migraine, who seek rest. Cluster headache is unusual in that it is more common in men. Unlike patients with migraine, those with cluster headache usually lack a family history. The headaches generally occur in periodic clusters, with many months between. During the cluster, small amounts of alcohol can precipitate a headache. Most commonly, the headaches awaken the subject from sleep. Chronic cluster headache lacks periodicity but is infrequent.

Chronic paroxysmal hemicrania is an uncommon (only 1% as frequent as cluster headache) related disorder that affects primarily women. The onset is in early adulthood. It differs from cluster primarily in the brevity and frequency of attacks, which are excruciatingly painful. They usually last only 2 to 24 minutes but may recur 2 to 30 times a day. Patients usually keep still during attacks, which may be mechanically triggered. An absolute responsiveness to indomethacin is a diagnostic feature.

Miscellaneous Headaches without an Associated Structural Lesion

IDIOPATHIC STABBING HEADACHE

Idiopathic stabbing headache (jabs and jolts, ice pick-like pains) manifests with fleeting stabs or a series of stabs confined to the head, most specifically in the distribution of the first division of the trigeminal nerve. The headaches occur at irregular intervals and are a common feature in migraineurs, usually on the side habitually affected by migraine. Structural disease must be excluded.

EXTERNAL COMPRESSION HEADACHE

External compression headache is a constant pain that results from the application of external pressure to the head (e.g., swim goggles, tight hat, tight wig). It is felt in the area of pressure and relieved by removal of the compression.

COLD STIMULUS HEADACHE

Cold stimulus headache can be elicited by external cold or, more commonly, the ingestion of a cold substance (ice cream headache). After rapid ingestion of a cold stimulus, pain rises to the middle of the forehead. It may be intense but subsides within 5 minutes. It is benign but associated with migraine.

BENIGN COUGH HEADACHE

Benign cough headache is a brief bilateral headache of sudden onset that is precipitated by coughing. The presentation is identical to that of a posterior fossa mass, and imaging is required. Straining or heavy lifting induces a similar phenomenon in patients with an intracranial mass, and this should be distinguished from a benign exertional headache, which is a bilateral throbbing headache brought on by exercise that lasts from 5 minutes to 24 hours.

HEADACHE ASSOCIATED WITH SEXUAL ACTIVITY

Headache associated with sexual activity (benign coital cephalalgia), precipitated by the sexual excitement of masturbation or coitus, is a bilateral headache that occurs in three forms: a dull ache increasing to orgasm, an explosive orgasmic headache to be distinguished from subarachnoid hemorrhage, and a postural headache like that associated with low cerebrospinal fluid pressure.

SPECIFIC CONSIDERATIONS WITH REGARD TO MENSES

Menstrual migraine has not been specifically defined in the new headache classification. Migraine worsens around the time of menses, but the term *menstrual migraine* refers specifically to migraine without aura that occurs primarily during or just before menses. The headache seems to be precipitated by a fall in plasma estradiol and manifests as a severe, 2- to 3-day attack associated with nausea and vomiting. Recurrent menstrual migraine can be delayed by estrogen but not progesterone. Headache still occurs when the estradiol level is allowed to fall. Estrogen levels distinctive to this population of women have not been observed. Although alterations in hypothalamic control systems have been said to occur, they still would not explain the headache associated with estradiol withdrawal. Numerous hormonal manipulations have been tried with dubious benefit.

The track record of oral contraceptive pills has been colored by the viewpoint of neurology or gynecology. All series tend to be weak, but neurologists claim a significant increase in the frequency and duration of headache, whereas gynecologists seem unconcerned. Both worsening of headache and the onset of menstrual migraine during oral contraceptive use are probably problems for some women. Headaches that worsened may become less severe 1 to 12 months after oral contraceptives are discontinued. The risk for stroke is probably increased in women who use oral contraceptives, especially those who have migraine with aura associated with smoking and hypertension.

Pregnancy has a beneficial effect on migraine in most women, particularly in the last two trimesters and in women with menstrual exacerbation. A few patients may have a first attack during pregnancy. Relapse is not uncommon in the first week postpartum.

Menopause is said to cause a transient worsening that is followed by improvement, but in large numbers of women, the headaches do not change or worsen. Hormone replacement is common. The daily administration of estrogens may lessen headache. Cyclic therapy reduces the risk for endometrial carcinoma but may worsen headache.

HISTORY

Patients often find it difficult to describe in detail all the headaches they have experienced, so it is simpler to focus on the current headache, the typical headache, and the worst headache. The frequency, duration, location, quality, and severity are determined. Is there more than one variety? Has the pattern changed? When did the headaches first appear? Are there typical times or modes of onset?

After the pain itself has been explored, associated phenomena, such as prodromal symptoms, aura, autonomic features, and residua, are sought. Precipitating, exacerbating, and mitigating factors may shed light. A careful history of any previous workups is necessary. What treatments have been used, at what dose, and for how long? Many useful agents are discarded prematurely. Toxicity should be clarified. OTC agents are frequently omitted by patients, who do not consider them real medicine. Many patients take herbal preparations (such as feverfew) and often do not mention them to physicians. The safety of these agents in pregnancy is unknown, and the composition of the preparations may be questionable. Recent imaging studies need not be repeated. Is there a family history of headache? What is the occupational or home life like? Does the patient have an exposure to precipitating foods, medicines, recreational drugs, or occupational agents? Marital discord may make management impossible. Does the patient already know what brings on or relieves the headaches? Patients with obstructive sleep apnea may experience headache. The interview frequently establishes a relationship, which is then furthered to ensure the patient's trust and compliance with the maneuvers needed to deal with a chronic illness.

PHYSICAL EXAMINATION

The physical examination is primarily of value in eliciting findings that signal structural causes of headache. High blood pressure is freely blamed for headache but should not be invoked unless an acute rise in the diastolic pressure of more than 25% has occurred. Careful examination of the head should include a visual field and a funduscopic examination. The tympanic membranes and temporomandibular joints should be observed. Any conjunctival injection, sinus tenderness, occipital nerve tenderness, carotid or superficial artery tenderness, or meningeal signs should be noted. In addition to nuchal rigidity (resistance to flexion but not rotation), one should test for the Kernig sign (with the hip and knee at 90 degrees, extending the leg on the thigh elicits pain), the more specific leg Brudzinski sign (on testing for the Kernig sign, the contralateral hip and knee flex), and the neck Brudzinski sign (neck flexion elicits flexion of the hips and knees). During a headache, patients with migraine look ill and may well have difficulty complying with a detailed physical and neurologic examination. The neurologic examination findings may be dismissed as nonfocal, without testing of the visual fields, a cortical sensory examination, or an evaluation of higher cortical function.

LABORATORY AND IMAGING STUDIES

Lumbar puncture may be required in subarachnoid hemorrhage, central nervous system inflammation, or benign intracranial hypertension. An abnormal erythrocyte sedimentation rate may alert the physician to temporal arteritis in older patients. Testing for lupus anticoagulant or antiphospholipid antibodies is useful in atypical migraine, especially if the patient has a history of spontaneous abortion or venous thrombosis. Usually, the patient with headache learns more about the toxic effects of the chronic use of medication than about headache from the laboratory test results.

Although some physicians advocate obtaining imaging studies for all patients with headache to avoid later problems of a medicolegal sort, the cost to the health care system of ordering 20 million CT or magnetic resonance imaging (MRI) studies for the 10% of the U.S. population who have migraine is prohibitive. The decision to order a study is based on a sense of disquiet about the headache or the associated symptom history. Imaging should not be necessary for a patient with a typical history in whom no abnormalities are detected during a physical or neurologic examination. A neurologic consultation is generally less expensive and more helpful. CT is usually more readily available in emergency situations to rule out intracranial hemorrhage (not subarachnoid hemorrhage), hydrocephalus, or a large mass lesion. MRI is generally a more definitive study in less acute situations, especially to exclude posterior fossa lesions or Arnold-Chiari lesions. Magnetic resonance angiography and careful CT angiography with volume rendering are the procedures of choice to exclude dural venous sinus thrombosis.

TREATMENT

In the management of any patient with recurrent headache, a relationship must be established, and the patient's major concerns about the possibility of a brain tumor and finding the cause of the pain must be addressed. Some discussion of the nature of the headache syndrome in addition to reassurance that others are experiencing similar phenomena may improve the outlook for some patients. A "headache log" is necessary to establish a baseline; pharmacotherapy may then be undertaken.

Migraine

Two major approaches to migraine therapy are available: abortive and prophylactic. Abortive therapy attempts to terminate an already established headache and is preferable when headaches are infrequent. Therapy should be optimized, and care should be taken to include all medications in the assessment. Patients frequently do not regard OTC nonsteroidal anti-inflammatory drugs (NSAIDs), aspirin, acetaminophen, or mixtures as true medications and may be ingesting large quantities without volunteering the information. Analgesic rebound headache and analgesic hepatic or renal toxicity must be considered when headaches occur weekly or more often. Specific problems associated with migraine include nausea and vomiting with gastric stasis, which may eliminate oral therapy. Migraine may respond to aspirin or NSAIDs, but the patients will usually have tried acetaminophen, aspirin, ibuprofen, or naproxen in OTC preparations before consulting a physician. A variety of OTC headache mixtures are also available. Caffeine appears to provide an added benefit. Many patients will have tried a variety of medications in a suboptimal dosage or for a suboptimal period of time. After a careful history to assess the headache type and medication history, a trial of naproxen (500–1,000 mg) or ibuprofen (600 mg) may be attempted. For patients unable to tolerate NSAIDs, acetaminophen (1,000 mg) or isometheptene (Midrin) may be tried. Caffeine is a useful adjuvant, as is rest in a quiet, dark place.

The abortive treatments fall into the categories of nonspecific or specific therapies. The analgesics, NSAIDs, and butalbital compounds fall into the nonspecific camp and are primarily for milder forms of headache. The patient with more severe attacks or who responds poorly to NSAIDs should get treated with more specific remedies. The triptans were the first agents designed to treat migraine and have revolutionized therapy because they not only relieve the pain but stop the entire syndrome. As with the nonspecific agents, triptans may induce rebound. Step therapy has been suggested with a nonspecific agent (cheaper) used first and only when this fails use the specific agent. Efficacy is maximal if treatment is given early and step therapy has maximized disability. Many patients have only severe headaches or are able to identify which of their attacks are going to develop into severe migraine. Stratified therapy has been suggested to maximize efficacy in these patients. This entails the use of analgesics for mild attacks and a triptan early for those attacks which will be severe. There are now multiple triptans available and all are effective. Differences are based on mode of administration, time of onset, duration of action, and side effect profile. The presence of early nausea and vomiting may restrict therapy to injectable sumatriptan which comes in a convenient fixed dose injector, intranasal sumatriptan, zolmatriptan, or dihydroergotamine (DHE 45). The nasal preparations are somewhat of a problem to use and the sumatriptan is distasteful. For patients who may be nauseated but are not yet vomiting the sublingual (absorbed through stomach) rizatriptan or zolmatriptan may be effective. The pill preparations take longer to work and are less suitable for patients with a steep onset profile. Sumatriptan injection has the fastest onset but wears off fast as well. Oral sumatriptan, rizatriptan, zolmatriptan, almotriptan, and eletriptan have the highest 2-hour efficacy. Naratriptan and frovatriptan have long duration efficacy but slow onset. Almotriptan, frovotriptan, and naratriptan may have fewer adverse effects. All of the triptans (almotriptan, eletriptan, frovatriptan, naratriptan, rizatriptan, sumatriptan, and zolmatriptan) are effective but all are arterial constrictors and should be avoided in patients with coronary artery disease or hypertension or are at risk for these problems. Sumatriptan injection may also cause a nonspecific chest tightness. In the emergency room when the patient has not taken a triptan the long acting intravenous dihydroergotamine (0.6 mg) can be given with high efficacy. Because nausea is a common accompaniment, metoclopramide (10 mg IM or IV) is given 10 min prior to the DHE. In the emergency department, one can also use a small dose of intravenous prochlorperazine (10 mg) or, less optimally, chlorpromazine (1 mg/kg). Hypotension may result, and intravenous fluids and careful observation are in order.

Prophylactic therapies are warranted to avoid analgesic toxicity or rebound headache. This approach may fail if the patient is having serious interpersonal problems (e.g., if the patient is having serious marital problems, prophylactic therapy is probably doomed to failure) or a chronic daily headache, perhaps from analgesic rebound or depression. Considerable time seems to be needed to achieve efficacy and avoid confusing minor fluctuations in the frequency or intensity of headache with true relief. It is probably best to not worry about how each agent is relieving the headache while so many headache mechanisms remain controversial. Each agent may not be acting in the manner implied by its classification in the therapeutic armamentarium. The effective dose varies with individuals and may require titration. The doses are frequently assumed to be very low, and potentially valuable agents are abandoned because of a lack of efficacy at inadequate doses. Major prophylactic agents include β-adrenoreceptor blockers, antidepressants, calcium channel blockers, methyl ergonovine, and valproate. Methysergide is less popular because of toxicity, and cyproheptadine is of limited efficacy.

The efficacy of β-adrenoreceptor blockers in migraine is variable. Effective agents include propranolol, nadolol, timolol, atenolol, and metoprolol. Ineffective β-blockers include alprenolol, oxprenolol, pindolol, and acebutolol. A lack of efficacy is not related to cardiac selectivity, penetration into the central nervous system, membrane-stabilizing activity, or affinity for serotonin-binding sites. Partial agonist activity correlates negatively with efficacy. The main effect is to reduce the frequency of headaches. Side effects include fatigue, sleep disturbances, depression, dizziness, and hypotension. The doses used for hypotension and bradycardia are probably equipotent in migraine prophylaxis.

The role of calcium channel blockers is also variable. The response to nifedipine and nimodipine is poor. The best-documented studies of efficacy show a strong benefit of flunarizine, an agent not available in the United States. The efficacy of verapamil in doses of 240 to more than 320 mg/d is less rigorously documented, but when maintained for 6 to 8 weeks, verapamil is probably quite effective. Side effects include constipation, nausea, edema, hypotension, and atrioventricular block. Verapamil should not be used in combination with a β-blocker, and it should not be given to patients with bradycardia, sick sinus syndrome, or atrioventricular block.

Antidepressant medications have been known to have benefits comparable with those of propranolol. The cyclic compounds documented in control trials are amitriptyline and doxepin. These drugs are tolerated relatively poorly by patients with migraine, and doses must be titrated up from between 10 and 25 mg to between 75 and 100 mg. The disturbing sedation usually wears off, but dry mouth, constipation, aggravation of glaucoma, and urinary retention can all be problems. Excessive sweating and altered myocardial depolarization can also develop. The other tricyclic antidepressants, in addition to the heterocyclic trazodone, may be better tolerated, but their efficacy is less clearly documented. Imipramine appears ineffective. Of the serotonin reuptake inhibitors, fluoxetine has proved effective. This is one of the few migraine prophylactic agents that does not cause weight gain. Sertraline has less of a stimulant effect and has been thought effective. Monamine oxidase inhibitors such as phenelzine have been shown to be helpful, but concerns about hypertension precipitated by the ingestion of certain foods, in addition to other toxicities, have caused most physicians to use these agents as a last resort.

The α-agonist clonidine showed some early promise but is ineffective.

The anticonvulsant valproate clearly is effective in the treatment of migraine, but phenytoin and carbamazepine are not. Valproate can be titrated by blood level. Care must be taken because of the possibility of teratogenicity (neural tube defects). Other toxic effects include hyperammonemia, hair loss, and weight gain. Serious hepatic toxicity is reported only in children. Topiramate is also effective. Resistant menstrual migraine may benefit from a short course of prophylactic NSAIDs. The antihistamine cyproheptadine is also a weak antiserotonin agent, but it provides only minimal benefit.

Tension Headaches

Tension headaches are not easily managed if they have progressed from episodic events that respond to OTC preparations to chronic intractable headaches. Most physicians have difficulty finding a suitable explanation for the pain in view of our current lack of understanding of the underlying process. One possible explanation is that spiraling headache and depression or anxiety feed on each other. After a strong dose of reassurance has been offered, aspirin, acetaminophen, or nonsteroidal anti-inflammatory agents may be used. For chronic tension-type headaches, amitriptyline appears highly beneficial. Some patients may benefit from nonpharmacologic therapy, such as relaxation exercises or biofeedback. The possibility of oromandibular dysfunction should be explored.

Cluster Headaches

Cluster headaches are relatively intense and brief. The administration of 100% oxygen by tight mask at a rate of 7 L/min can abort a headache in 5 to 10 minutes, even though cerebral oxygen consumption does not increase. Oxygen availability may be a problem. Sumatriptan has been very effective, but relapses may occur. Sumatriptan remains effective even after prolonged use. Ergotamine and dihydroergotamine are now less popular than formerly. Prophylactic therapy is obviously in order for patients whose cluster is prolonged or whose problem is chronic. Rectal ergotamine-caffeine is effective for nocturnal attacks. Verapamil is usually used before lithium is tried. Steroids have been widely used, but their efficacy has never been clearly demonstrated. Valproate is claimed to be effective, but further study is in order.

A group of headaches that respond to indomethacin includes chronic paroxysmal hemicrania, idiopathic stabbing headache, and benign exertional headache. Headaches associated with sexual activity are indomethacin-responsive when the patient also has benign exertional headaches. Propranolol can be helpful because exertional headaches may be associated with hypertensive surges. Diltiazem has been claimed to be effective. The main consideration here is concern about possible subarachnoid hemorrhage.

CONSIDERATIONS DURING PREGNANCY

Although many women experience some headaches early in pregnancy, they are usually a minor problem and respond to acetaminophen. Migraine, especially menstrually exacerbated migraine, remits in approximately 70% of pregnant women, most strikingly during the last trimester. Unfortunately, some women experience migraine throughout pregnancy, and in a small number, the onset of migraine occurs during pregnancy. Tension-type headaches continue throughout pregnancy.

The pharmacologic management of headache during pregnancy raises concern about the possibility of teratogenicity early in pregnancy and labor-related problems later. For abortive therapy, acetaminophen is generally used. The teratogenicity of the NSAIDs has not been adequately addressed. Aspirin (acetylsalicylic acid) is probably the best studied of these agents, but not much is known about its possible teratogenic effects. Aspirin causes primarily labor-related problems, but some other NSAIDs are teratogenic. Although ibuprofen is relatively safe, it is probably best to avoid all inhibitors of prostaglandin synthesis. β-Blockers such as propranolol and atenolol are thought safe but may cause neonatal bradycardia. All ergot derivatives are probably inappropriate because of their potential effects on the uterus. Acetaminophen for abortive therapy and amitriptyline for prophylaxis are the best options. Biofeedback, meditation, and other nonpharmacologic means can also be used. Triptans and dihydroergotamine are not used while nursing.

BIBLIOGRAPHY

Davidoff RA. *Migraine: manifestations, pathogenesis, and management,* 2nd ed. New York: Oxford University Press, 2002.

Ferrari M, Roon K, Lipton R, et al. Oral triptans (serotonin 5-HT 1B/1D agonists) in acute migraine treatment: a metaanalysis of 53 trials. *Lancet* 2001;358:1668.

Headache Classification Committee. Classification and diagnostic criteria for headache disorders, cranial neuralgia and facial pain. *Cephalalgia* 1988;8:1.

Kors EE, Van den Maagdenberg AMJM, Plomp JJ, et al. Calcium channel mutations and migraine. *Curr Opin Neurol* 2002;15:311.

Olesen J, Tfelt-Hansen P, Welch KMA. *The headaches.* Philadelphia: Lippincott Williams & Wilkins, 2000.

Raskin NH. *Headache,* 2nd ed. New York: Churchill Livingstone, 1988.

Silberstein SD, Lipton RB, Goadsby PJ. *Headache in clinical practice,* 2nd ed. London: Martin Dunitz, 2002.

CHAPTER 104
Dizziness

Joshua Hollander

Sensations of heat and cold are consistently learned experiences of childhood. No such uniformity exists for dizziness, and the physician must first understand what a patient means by that word. Most are relating a loss of spatial orientation. Correct sensory input, proper central integration, and an appropriate motor response are all required. Vision, vestibular input, proprioception, touch and pressure, and hearing all serve as orienting sensations. Attention and alertness are necessary for full spatial orientation. Vision contributes horizontal and vertical meridians and is a primary orienting sensation in humans. The labyrinth assesses angular acceleration in three perpendicular axes through the semicircular canals, and the otoliths measure linear acceleration in the vertical (gravity) and horizontal (fore-and-aft) planes.

Problems causing dizziness include spontaneous false sensations, such as acute vestibular dysfunction; sensory mismatch, experienced when printed matter is read in a rocking boat cabin; sensory distortion, experienced by patients with new cataract lenses; poor central integration, a feature of multiple sclerosis; impaired motor execution with cerebellar dysfunction; and servoloop failure, as in Parkinson disease. Most patients with true rotational vertigo have vestibular disease, but the range of problems referred to as *dizziness* is quite broad.

The vestibulo-ocular reflex is more important than the vestibulospinal reflex in humans. In this regard, some clarification of eye movement systems is required. Vergence systems (convergence and divergence) integrate independent eye movements to allow the binocular fusion of targets at varying distances. Saccadic eye movements are quick flicks that change the line of sight and include nystagmus fast phases. These bring the target to the high-acuity fovea. The moving image is stabilized on the retina by optokinetic and pursuit systems. The vestibulo-ocular reflex allows ocular stabilization despite head movements.

Voluntary saccades are ballistic eye movements initiated by signals from the frontal eye field to the paramedian pontine reticular formation, with the superior colliculus reorienting gaze to novel stimuli. A complex process produces signals via the median longitudinal fasciculus to the oculomotor and abducens nuclei, allowing both yoked eye movements and reciprocal inhibition. Smooth pursuit is triggered by retinal slip with low target speed.

The vestibular end organ comprises two interconnected subsystems, three perpendicularly oriented semicircular canals and the otoliths. The canals detect angular acceleration when endolymph motion bends a group of hair cells with nonmotile stereocilia. This motion is bidirectional and results in conjugate deviation of the eyes through the yoked medial and lateral recti. The eye movements should be equal in amplitude and opposite in direction to the head movement; this vestibulo-ocular reflex is much faster than the smooth pursuit system. Slow deviation of the eyes may be followed by a corrective saccade. The resultant alternating fast and slow eye movements in the plane of the stimulated semicircular canal are called *vestibular nystagmus*. In the utricle and saccule, the otoliths (calcium carbonate crystals) are attached to hair cells oriented to respond to linear acceleration in the vertical or horizontal plane. The vestibular system then adjusts the position of the eyes in the orbit to compensate for the position of the head in space.

Vestibulospinal reflexes contribute to posture and tone. Unilateral labyrinthectomy decreases ipsilateral extensor tone and increases contralateral tone. Bilateral lesions abolish decerebrate rigidity.

ETIOLOGY AND DIFFERENTIAL DIAGNOSIS

Among a large number of unselected patients presenting to Northwestern University with the complaint of dizziness, many were actually found to have low-level hyperventilation or multisensory impairments (Fig. 104.1). Symptoms of vertigo syndromes include the illusion of movement caused by the impaired perception of a stationary environment by central nervous system space-constancy mechanisms.

Multisensory impairments cause the additional loss of an outside stationary reference system, which is required for orientation and postural regulation, and thereby contribute to a sense that the self or the surroundings are moving. Such impairments include peripheral large fiber neuropathy with a diminished sense of position; visual disturbances, such as those associated with cataract removal without implant, major refractive change, or macular degeneration; cervical osteoarthritis that limits neck movement; and impairment of auditory or vestibular sensitivity.

Otolithic lesions cause static head tilts or ocular skew or torsion. Unilateral labyrinthine lesions cause an imbalance in the tonic vestibular firing rate as the ipsilateral vestibular nucleus loses spontaneous activity and becomes unresponsive to ipsilateral rotational signals. The symptoms usually reflect the problems in the horizontal semicircular canals because the vertical canals cancel each other out. Such patients, attempting fixation, experience visual blurring as an object appears to move away from the side of the lesion toward the fast phase of the vestibular nystagmus. Eye proprioception is lacking, and target displacement on the retina is perceived as motion. Eye closure eliminates visual correction, and the vestibular input imbalance is perceived as subjective rotation toward the affected labyrinth.

Dizziness reflects cortical spatial disorientation. Nystagmus is caused by direction-specific vestibulo-ocular reflex imbalance. Ataxia or imbalance is caused by impaired vestibulospinal signals. Nausea and vomiting are caused by activation of the adjacent medullary vomiting center. Compensation occurs as the normal vestibular nuclei reduce their firing rate and the commissural fibers induce new tonic firing. Compensation probably requires the participation of the cerebellum and reticular formation; this is why it is more difficult to compensate for central vertigo. The problem of the "double hit" develops in the face of both central and peripheral lesions with poor compensation. Compensation is poor for otolithic lesions, and chronic mild imbalance may be perceived. Compensation occurs most rapidly if vestibular exercises and stimulation are begun as soon as possible after injury. Patients with bilateral vestibular dysfunction experience visual blurring when walking or driving because they are left with only a slow smooth pursuit system and, lacking the vestibulo-ocular reflex, cannot maintain fixation.

Symptoms are thus influenced by laterality, chronicity, and severity. The clinical axioms are the following:

- Acute unilateral vestibular dysfunction causes vertigo.
- Compensated unilateral vestibular dysfunction does not cause vertigo.
- Uncompensated intermittent unilateral vestibular dysfunction causes vertigo.
- Recurrent dysfunction of the same or opposite labyrinth may cause vertigo.

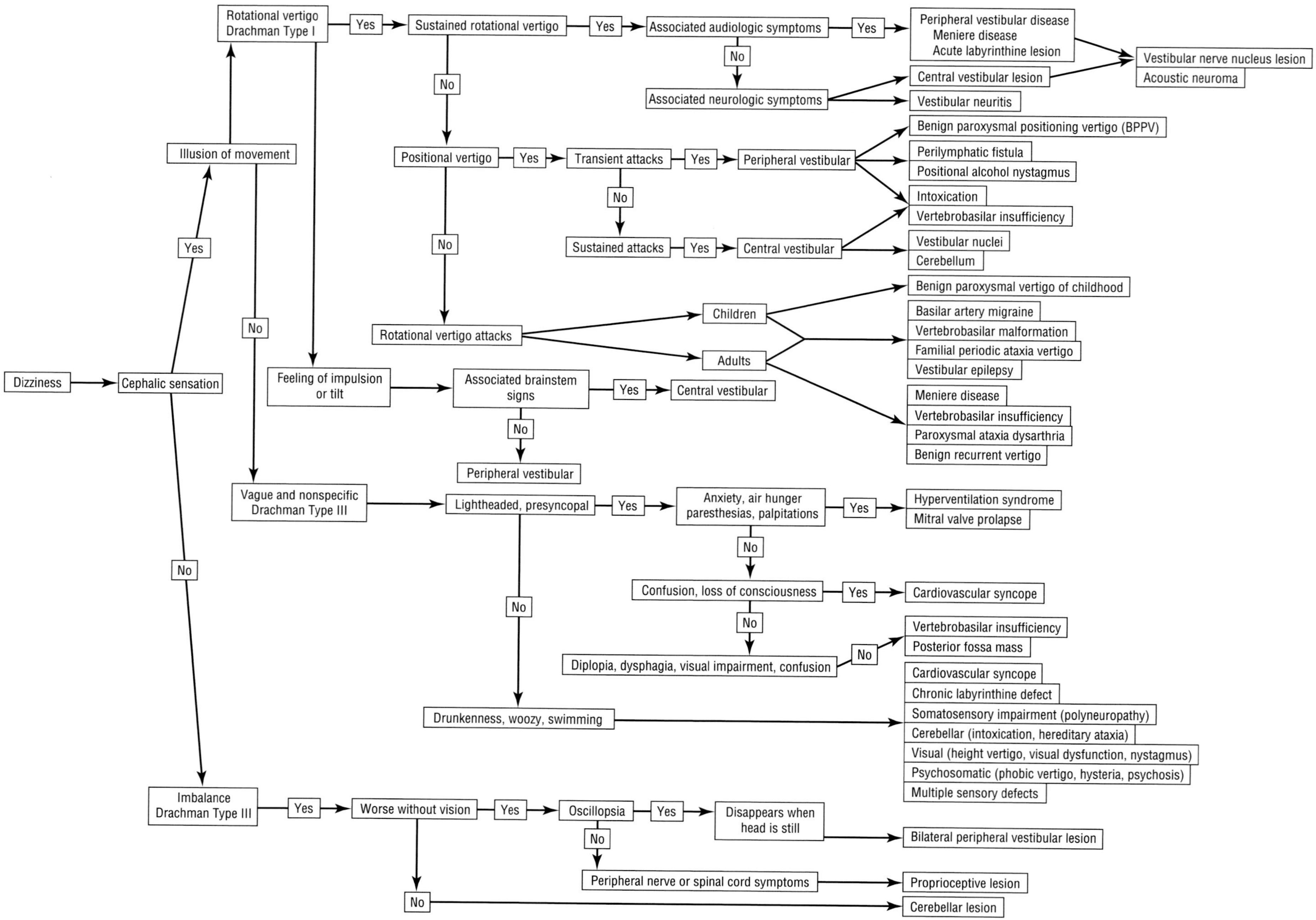

FIG. 104.1. Differential diagnosis of dizziness.

- Bilateral absent vestibular function may cause lifelong symptoms but not vertigo.

Physiologic vertigo develops when external stimuli act on a normally functioning sensory system. Motion sickness, the most common form, is elicited by unfamiliar body acceleration or intersensory mismatch and is exacerbated by fear or insecurity. Visual-vestibular conflict is important and is reduced by ample peripheral vision. A provocative activity might be reading a book in the back of a car traveling on a winding road. Symptoms include apathy, salivation, nausea and vomiting, pallor, perspiration, and prostration.

Height vertigo is a visually induced subjective instability in postural balance and locomotion, with fear of falling and vegetative symptoms. The response is subject to adaptation, but a phobic reaction may supervene.

Head extension vertigo is important because it is often confused with vertebrobasilar insufficiency. The otoliths are nonfunctional in head extension and flexion. Flexion is a more common position, and we accommodate. When we look up with no visual cues (darkness) or conflicting cues (moving clouds without a horizon line), we may fall when we lift a foot.

Space sickness, visual vertigo, somatosensory vertigo, auditory vertigo, alternobaric vertigo, and pilot's vertigo (spatial disorientation) are all manifestations of physiologic vertigo. They are important but are not discussed further here.

As previously discussed, visual and somatosensory problems may cause pathologic vertigo. A more detailed discussion of vestibularly mediated vertigo follows.

Peripheral Vestibular Vertigo

Acute unilateral peripheral vestibulopathy or vestibular dysfunction has been suggested in patients with poorly understood pathogenetic mechanisms. These patients are acutely vertiginous and experience vegetative distress. They lie with the affected ear up and avoid looking toward the good ear. Vestibular neuritis is a single episode of acute vertigo, nausea, and vomiting that tends to affect younger persons. Hearing is unaffected. Vertigo is severe, with commensurate spontaneous nystagmus.

Antecedent infection has been described, but the cause is unknown. This condition may be related to the epidemic vertigo seen in the spring and summer. Viral labyrinthitis is a similar disorder that follows a childhood exanthem and is usually associated with hearing loss. Ramsay Hunt syndrome (herpes zoster oticus) may be associated with facial paresis in addition to vertigo, hearing loss, and canalicular vesicles.

Patients with Ménière disease experience the classic tetrad of aural fullness, fluctuating sensorineural hearing loss, low-pitched tinnitus, and decrescendo attacks of nystagmus-vertigo. Recovery takes place during hours or days, with remissions of a month or longer. In most cases, the condition remits in 5 years. The pattern on electronystagmography may be normal but usually displays positional nystagmus or canal paresis. Ménière disease is usually unilateral. It is thought that impaired endolymphatic duct drainage results in endolymphatic hydrops. Periodic rupture decompresses the membranous labyrinth but releases high-potassium endolymph into the perilymph, causing vestibular nerve discharge and then paresis. End-stage Ménière disease may present with otolithic catastrophes of Tumarkin and abrupt alterations of postural tilt (and altered perception of the vertical) that cause the patient to fall to the floor.

Posttraumatic vertigo comprises a mixed group of disorders ranging from postconcussion syndrome to benign paroxysmal positional vertigo, labyrinthine concussion, perilymph fistula, and temporal bone fracture. Syphilis may present with labyrinthitis or hydrops. Vascular problems include internal auditory artery occlusions, small vessel infarcts from diabetes, and hemorrhage from bleeding diatheses. Acoustic schwannomas grow slowly, and vestibular compensation usually causes hearing loss without much vertigo.

Recurrent Unilateral Vestibular Dysfunction

Recurrent unilateral vestibular dysfunction may be caused by Ménière syndrome. Otosclerosis, a familial disorder associated with abnormal bone growth and resorption, results in hearing loss in the second or third decade. Some of these patients experience gait disturbances and episodic vertigo.

Paroxysmal Positional Vertigo

Benign paroxysmal positional vertigo is common and usually seen in women between the ages of 50 and 60 years. Rotational vertigo (vertical-torsional nystagmus) begins 10 to 15 seconds after the head is tilted toward the affected ear and subsides after 10 to 60 seconds, when the response becomes fatigued. The vertigo is usually worse in the morning but is triggered by lying down, rolling over in bed, or extending the head when upright. It is confirmed on examination by a classic Hallpike response. The mechanism is presumed to be a disruption of otoconia from the utricular macule, which then lodge in the posterior semicircular canal. As a result, the canal is converted from an angular acceleration receptor into a gravity receptor. Other types of lithiasis involving other semicircular canals have been reported but are uncommon.

Other forms of positional nystagmus have been divided into central and peripheral types, but this classification may not have merit. Failure of fixation suppression may be the best indicator of central pathology but has been noted in lithiasis of the horizontal canal, which may also show direction-changing nystagmus.

Bilateral Vestibular Dysfunction

Positional alcohol nystagmus is the most common form and results from overindulgence. Alcohol enters and leaves the cupula at a different rate than the endolymph, inducing a specific gravity differential that causes movement-induced vertigo during intoxication and 5 to 10 hours later, during recovery. A similar mechanism may be related to the vertigo of macroglobulinemia.

Ototoxicity is a symptom complex without vertigo. It is associated with impaired balance in darkness in addition to an impaired vestibulo-ocular reflex. Visual difficulty develops during head movement and unsteadiness during head turns. The patient actively seeks medical attention, or the condition may be detected when a patient is mobilized after a major illness or surgery. Aminoglycosides, which concentrate in endolymph, are common offenders. The diagnosis depends on the electronystagmographic demonstration of bilateral canal paresis and a history of ingestion of a potentially ototoxic drug or of a major illness or surgery. Prophylactic or therapeutic use in any patient, but especially one with impaired renal function, may be the only history obtained. Other ototoxic drugs include nonsteroidal antiinflammatory agents, loop diuretics, antiprotozoal agents, anticancer agents, and a host of less common offenders. These must be distinguished from the long list of agents causing nonvestibular dizziness, which clears after drug withdrawal.

Disequilibrium of aging comprises a complex of disorders. Degenerative cupulolithiasis causes benign paroxysmal positional vertigo. Loss of end-organ function (depressed vestibulo-ocular reflex) may cause vestibular ataxia of aging. These patients are asymptomatic when still but have trouble controlling their center of gravity when walking and trying to maintain a fixed head position for visual reference. Loss of central inhibition (hypersensitive vestibulo-ocular reflex) may result in vertigo with angular head movements. Vertigo develops when the position of the head is changed relative to gravity. The patient sits on the edge of the bed before walking. Orthostatic hypotension must be excluded.

Multiple sensory defects may also contribute to disequilibrium of aging. Age-associated changes develop in the vestibular system and in proprioception. These, in combination with hearing loss and visual loss caused by cataracts or senile macular degeneration, may result in disequilibrium, even though no one system alone is sufficiently involved.

Bilateral Ménière syndrome may occur, but the symptoms are no different from those of the unilateral form. Autoimmune sensorineural hearing loss manifests as progressive hearing loss, tinnitus, pressure, and reduced vestibular function. Bilateral relentless hydrops or an associated autoimmune disorder may suggest this rare entity.

Central Vestibular Vertigo

Central vestibular vertigo may be caused by lesions of the vestibular nuclei, vestibular cerebellum, or their connections. Pure nystagmus vectors tend to be central in origin, and a neurologic examination usually elicits associated findings.

Vascular disease tends to be invoked in older patients quite freely, with a disregard of other possibilities. Although vertebrobasilar insufficiency is commonly associated with vertigo (reduced supply to the vestibular nuclei and cerebellum), brainstem or cerebellar symptoms or signs may also occur, including vegetative signs, dysarthria, postural imbalance, visual loss, diplopia, paresis, and paresthesias of one or both sides. Occipital headache is common. The onset is abrupt, and the symptoms taper within 30 minutes or less. Vertebrobasilar insufficiency may be hemodynamic in origin, and Stokes-Adams attacks and subclavian steal must be considered. Vertebral artery occlusion may cause the lateral medullary syndrome (posterior inferior cerebellar artery syndrome) of ipsilateral ataxia, loss of ipsilateral facial pain and temperature sensibility, loss of contralateral pain and temperature sensibility, and Horner syndrome (ptosis, miosis, relative enophthalmos). The vestibular nuclear lesion causes vertigo and fall to the affected side; utricular involvement causes skew deviation (one eye slightly higher in orbit). Anterior inferior cerebellar artery syndrome is a lateral pontomedullary syndrome often associated with labyrinthine infarction and deafness. Cerebellar hemorrhage is a potentially lethal disorder easily seen by computed tomography in a patient with the sudden onset of headache, nausea, vomiting, vertigo, and ataxia.

Multiple sclerosis with brainstem or cerebellar involvement may cause dizziness, but associated brainstem signs should be present unless only the vestibular nerve root entry zone is affected.

Basilar artery migraine is an uncommon disorder seen primarily in adolescent girls or young women. The aura consists of vertigo, ataxia, and bilateral visual changes. This is followed by an occipital throbbing headache. Benign paroxysmal vertigo of childhood is thought to be a migraine variant. Various lesions of the foramen magnum and eye movement disorders may induce dizziness, usually as a consequence of oscillopsia (conscious perception of visual movement in nystagmus).

Psychogenic Vertigo

Psychogenic vertigo is common in anxiety neurosis, hysteria, depression, and schizophrenia. Low-grade hyperventilation is frequent. Panic attacks with vertigo as a major feature may occur with or without agoraphobia.

HISTORY

Four areas in the neurologic history must be explored: time course, precipitating factors, predisposing factors, and associated symptoms.

Time Course

Dizziness with a sudden onset and offset may suggest a cardiac or vascular cause. Psychogenic vertigo builds up gradually and ends abruptly. A single bout that tapers over days to weeks suggests acute peripheral vestibulopathy. Brief episodes of minutes to hours occur in Ménière disease. Brief paroxysms elicited by changes of head position suggest benign paroxysmal positional vertigo. New-onset nystagmus may cause an illusory environmental movement (oscillopsia).

Precipitating Factors

Orthostatic dizziness may also be seen in orthostatic hypotension, but dizziness elicited by lying down or rolling over in bed is characteristic of benign paroxysmal positional vertigo. Other movements are nonspecific. Carotid kinking can occur and is as common as vertebral kinking. The Tullio phenomenon of vertigo induced by loud noise is seen in perilymph fistula and Ménière disease.

Predisposing Factors

Alcohol may affect the relative specific gravity of the endolymph and macula. Phenytoin is a cerebellar toxin, and aminoglycosides are ototoxic. Anticoagulants may induce bleeding. Sedatives may cause nonvestibular dizziness.

Associated Symptoms

- Aural: hearing loss, tinnitus, fullness, otalgia, otorrhea
- Autonomic: nausea, vomiting, sweating
- Neurologic: facial motor or sensory loss, dysarthria, dysphagia, loss of coordination, visual problems, altered consciousness, weakness, paresthesias
- Psychogenic: phobias (particularly agoraphobia) suggested if fear of dizziness confines the patient to the home
- Visual: Oscillopsia secondary to nystagmus and the inability to focus on the macula during motion, reflecting bilateral vestibular impairment, must be distinguished during the history and explored during the physical examination.

PHYSICAL EXAMINATION

When performing the general neurologic examination, the physician must pay particular attention to the cranial nerves and cerebellum and to proprioception. The general physical examination must include an otoscopic inspection of the drum for vesicles (Ramsay Hunt syndrome), drainage, and inflammation. A blue drum suggests glomus tympanicum. The hearing can be grossly checked with a ticking watch or a 512 tuning fork. Rubbing the fingers may mask the other ear, and whispered words may reveal the impaired verbal discrimination of nerve deafness.

Vestibular imbalance may manifest as nystagmus that is fixation-suppressed. It may be detected by ophthalmoscopy and accentuated by covering the viewing eye to block fixation suppression. The head can be shaken while the subject reads, and visual blur or corrective saccades imply abnormal vestibular gain. A minimal caloric test can be performed with 1 mL of ice water in the ear and the erect head tipped back 60 degrees or the supine head elevated 30 degrees. Normally, the ensuing nystagmus is named for the fast component and is cold-opposite. A secretarial swivel chair can be used to perform an approximate Barany rotation; 10 rotations with the head tipped back 60 degrees usually suffices. Nystagmus and dizziness can be elicited. The patient should be able to suppress the nystagmus by fixing the gaze on an outstretched finger. Failure to do so (failure of fixation suppression) is a central sign. Abnormalities of the otolithic system may be revealed by head tilt or visual skew deviation.

The vestibulospinal system is tested by gait and station. In the Romberg maneuver, the cerebellar function must be intact to allow the patient to stand in place with the feet together. The eyes are then closed. Without visual cues, position sense and vestibular sense are necessary to maintain stance. If the position sense is significantly impaired, the patient falls in a random manner. If unilateral vestibular impairment is present, the fall is to the involved side or in the direction of the nystagmus slow phases. The patient is asked to march in place and slowly rotates in the direction of the Romberg fall. Past pointing is tested by having the outstretched arm come down on the examiner's finger with the eyes closed. The patient's finger deviates in the direction of the Romberg fall.

Saccades may be dysmetric in cerebellar dysfunction and are best tested by having the patient look from a lateral gaze to a medial target. Smooth pursuit can be tested by having the patient follow a slowly moving target. The eye movement should not consist of multiple jerky saccades. The patient is examined for nystagmus, which may be pendular (symmetric in both directions) or jerk (rapid in one direction and slow in reverse). The fast component of jerk nystagmus is a corrective saccade. Optokinetic nystagmus is elicited by moving a series of targets across the visual field; a nystagmus ensues with a fast component in the direction from which the target is coming (as though the eye followed the target until it passed by and then moved to find a new one at the edge of the field). Asymmetric optokinetic responses are seen in parietal lobe disease. End-point nystagmus is a physiologic nystagmus occurring in the direction of gaze. It should not be asymmetric and is not seen at less than 20 degrees of lateral gaze (when the limbus crosses the lachrymal puncta). Gaze-evoked nystagmus is the pathologic form and is associated with drugs, myasthenia, and multiple sclerosis. Limitation of the adducting eye and dissociated nystagmus in the abducting eye reflect a median longitudinal fasciculus lesion, common in multiple sclerosis. Positional nystagmus does not occur in the primary position (head and eyes facing forward) but manifests in any other position. Vestibular nystagmus is always conjugate and is more evident in the direction of gaze of the fast component (away from the nonfunctioning vestibular system). Peripheral vestibular nystagmus is common, always conjugate, never vertical, not usually purely horizontal, reduced by visual fixation (fixation suppression), sometimes marked, and often associated with tinnitus or deafness. Romberg fall, past pointing, and compass turn are in the direction of the slow phase, but subjective environmental spin is to the fast phase.

Provocative maneuvers are useful if a sensation is elicited that is comparable with the patient's subjective sensation. Both physician and patient are reassured by a mutual understanding of the patient's complaint. Orthostatic hypotension is sought by measuring pulse and blood pressure with the patient in the supine position and again after 3 minutes of standing. A potentiated Valsalva maneuver can be performed by having the patient squat, stand, and blow forcefully for 15 seconds. A limited Barany rotation in a swivel chair was described previously, as was the limited ice water caloric test. The Barany maneuver (also called the *Nylan-Barany* or *Dix-Hallpike maneuver*) can be performed before the patient is placed supine for examinations. The patient's head is turned 45 degrees to one side, and the patient is brought down to a 45-degree hanging head position and observed for 1 minute. Typical nystagmus may appear after 15 to 20 seconds, associated with vertigo and fatigue in about 1 minute. The patient is then returned to the sitting position; vertigo and reversed nystagmus appear after a similar delay. Fixation suppression may eliminate the nystagmus. The patient should avoid fixation, and Frenzel lenses should be used if available.

LABORATORY AND IMAGING STUDIES

Routine laboratory studies are not often helpful but should include the following: complete blood cell count; measurement of levothyroxine, thyroid-stimulating hormone, antinuclear antibody, and lipids; a fasting glucose test; serum protein electrophoresis; and a fluorescent treponemal antibody absorption test.

Audiometry is used if a vestibular mechanism is suspected. Routine pure-tone audiometry with air conduction, bone conduction, and masking is supplemented with impedance audiometry and tympanometry. The diagnostic audiologist should know that site-of-lesion testing is desired.

Short-latency brainstem auditory evoked potentials (auditory evoked responses) play a major role in site-of-lesion testing. Electrodes are placed on the head, and the far-field potentials are recorded. A repetitive click is the auditory stimulus, and time-locked signal averaging allows resolution of the potentials elicited by the auditory stimulus from the more random electric activity of the brain. The first five waves occur within less than 10 milliseconds and are little affected by drugs or level of awareness. Despite lack of certainty about the specific generators, prolonged interwave latencies or loss of later waves can localize the pathology. An increase in interwave latency in waves 1 to 3 is a sensitive test for acoustic neuroma; a prolongation of waves 3 to 5 indicates intrinsic brainstem pathology.

Electronystagmography makes it possible to observe nystagmus behind closed lids and record eye movements. A more leisurely and quantitative analysis becomes possible because a corneal-retinal potential difference makes the eye a dipole, and eye movements can be tracked electrically. Variability is present, and this test is really only semiquantitative. The tests usually performed include a search for pathologic nystagmus with changes in gaze position, head position, and fixation. Saccades, smooth pursuit, and optokinetic nystagmus are generally tested to assess central oculomotor control systems. The vestibulo-ocular reflex is studied with a bithermal caloric test. Major findings include unilateral canal paresis in unilateral vestibular dysfunction, as in vestibular neuritis or acoustic neuroma; bilateral canal paresis in ototoxicity; failure of fixation suppression in central pathology; and the classic Hallpike response in benign paroxysmal positional vertigo.

Rotational or sinusoidal testing is better tolerated than caloric stimulation. It effectively detects bilateral canal paresis and failure of fixation suppression but detects unilateral vestibular dysfunction poorly. It is expensive and of limited clinical use.

Posturography is a test of the vestibulospinal reflex. The patient stands on a force platform, and a computer analysis of Romberg sway is performed. Linear acceleration stimuli and shifts in platform angle and visual surround provoke compensatory force shifts that can be analyzed. This test is becoming more popular, but its usefulness has not been fully defined.

Thin-cut computed tomography through the internal auditory canal visualizes small intracanalicular acoustic neuromas but has been surpassed by magnetic resonance imaging, which does not have the problem of bone artifact. The cochlea and semicircular canals, in addition to the eighth nerve, can be seen on imaging studies, but these have little relevance in most cases of dizziness.

TREATMENT

Spatial disorientation and postural instability are frightening in themselves, and they also induce dread of an ominous cause. Despite the distressing lack of therapeutic accompaniments to the increasingly sophisticated research being performed in vestibular and oculomotor physiology, the physician can provide a careful explanation of the basis of the patient's complaint. An explanation of what the patient is experiencing and what is not happening can have a powerful therapeutic effect. Learning about vestibular compensation may sustain the patient through a trying time.

The acutely vertiginous patient must lie still and be given sedation, antiemetics, and fluids as needed. As soon as the nausea and vomiting have subsided sufficiently, the patient should be mobilized to promote early vestibular compensation. Excessive sedation or maintenance therapy should be avoided during recurrent attacks in favor of standby therapy. Medication is often given inappropriately for positional vertigo, even though the symptoms usually subside before the medication takes effect, and the medication may delay vestibular compensation. Physical therapy is probably preferable.

Pharmacologic Measures

The spontaneous firing rate of the vestibular primary afferent neurons and the transmission of firing through the vestibular nuclei are in equilibrium. Transmission from the primary to the secondary vestibular neurons is thought to be cholinergic. A cholinergic facilitatory reticulovestibular system is balanced by a monoaminergic inhibitory reticulospinal system. An imbalance in the spontaneous firing rate can be corrected by suppressing spontaneous firing on both sides with anticholinergic drugs, but their use is limited by mental status changes in addition to the more frequent dry mouth, constipation, prostatism, and glaucoma. Transdermal scopolamine (0.5 mg three times daily) is effective for motion sickness when instituted several hours before anticipated exposure. Inadvertent ophthalmic contamination because of lack of sufficient care in handling the disc can cause mydriasis, visual impairment, and anxiety.

Antihistamines are the most commonly prescribed agents, but their mode of action is unknown. Meclizine is usually given for vertigo and dimenhydrinate for motion sickness. Trimethobenzamide has antiemetic properties and may be more useful in acute vertigo. Adrenergic agents such as ephedrine may be adjunctive.

Phenothiazines have been used for their antiemetic properties. Chlorpromazine is a classic dopaminergic blocking agent with some antihistaminic and anticholinergic properties. It suppresses both the spontaneous vestibular and stimulation-induced firing rates and has sedative and antiemetic effects. The use of prochlorperazine should be avoided because it can induce severe dystonic reactions in addition to antiemetic effects. Butyrophenones are potent agents and can be used when others fail, provided the risk for extrapyramidal side effects is kept in mind. Benzodiazepines depress the spontaneous vestibular firing rate and interact with central pathways. Short courses of low-dose diazepam may be very helpful in younger patients.

Vestibular compensation requires exposure to the vertiginous stimulus, and suppressant medication should be discontinued as soon as possible after the most severe symptoms have subsided.

Ménière disease is usually treated with salt restriction and thiazides. Topical gentamicin may be applied to the tympanic membrane in patients with bilateral disease for several weeks in a fashion designed to reduce vestibular function without ablation.

Patients with central vertigo are difficult to treat. If they fail to respond to benzodiazepines, a trial of acetazolamide may be used. Carbamazepine may be useful in patients with quick spins who fail to respond to other approaches.

Vestibular Physical Therapy

Since it first became clear that vestibular compensation is facilitated by early exercise, Cooksey-Cawthorne exercises and the later Brandt modification have been used. Exposure to mismatch during eye, head, and body movements somehow restores the fragile balance in vestibular firing, presumably by restoring the depressed spontaneous firing rate. It is not surprising that centrally mediated vertigo is helped less by vestibular compensation, which requires a central recalibration of sensory mismatch. Compensation depends on cerebellar function and can be lost if a cerebellar stroke occurs later ("double hit"). Sedatives and alcohol can induce transient loss.

Positional vertigo can be managed by having the patient assume the appropriate ear-down supine position, maintain it until the response becomes fatigued, then sit up to reproduce the symptoms. This maneuver is repeated until the response does not occur. The exercise is performed several times a day until the symptoms abate. Patients are often so terrified of the symptoms that they will not hold the position, so sometimes a family member must assist. Whether the therapy helps by shaking an otoconium loose or by promoting vestibular compensation is unknown.

Patients with the very common benign paroxysmal positional vertigo of the posterior canal can usually achieve complete remission with a modified Epley maneuver, and patients with the less common canal variants can use similar maneuvers. These are not be described here for lack of space, but the practitioner should either learn these maneuvers or refer the patient to someone experienced in their use, who can thereby relieve a very distressing symptom.

Surgical Therapies

Ménière disease may remit spontaneously or respond to salt restriction or the administration of diuretics. When these treatments fail, various procedures have been undertaken. The efficacy of endolymphatic sac shunting is questionable. Vestibular nerve section may preserve hearing but can be complicated, and separating the vestibular from the auditory nerves is not always feasible. When residual hearing is minimal or absent in unilateral disease, destructive labyrinthectomy may be undertaken. Medical ablation with streptomycin may also be used. When cupulolithiasis is unremitting, deafferentation of the posterior semicircular canal may be achieved by singular nerve section, which preserves hearing. "Disabling positional vertigo" (not well defined) is reportedly caused by microvascular loops that compress the vestibular nerve; surgery has been performed to correct this condition.

CONSIDERATIONS DURING PREGNANCY

Considerations relate primarily to possible orthostasis and hypoglycemia associated with pregnancy. Vascular tumors and arteriovenous malformations enlarge during pregnancy. Posterior fossa meningiomas and acoustic schwannomas may be involved in such enlargement, but this is unlikely.

BIBLIOGRAPHY

Baloh RW, Honrubia V. *Clinical neurophysiology of the vestibular system,* 2nd ed. Philadelphia: FA Davis, 1990.

Brandt T, Daroff RB. The multisensory physiologic and pathologic vertigo syndromes. *Ann Neurol* 1980;7:195.

Brandt T, Steddin S, Daroff RB. Therapy for benign paroxysmal vertigo, revisited. *Neurology* 1994;44:796–800.

Drachman D. An approach to the dizzy patient. *Neurology* 1972;22:323–334.

Epley JM. The canalith repositioning procedure for treatment of benign paroxysmal positional vertigo. *Otolaryngol Head Neck Surg* 1992;107:399–404.

Lanska DJ, Remla B. Benign paroxysmal positioning vertigo: classic descriptions, origins of the provocative positioning technique, and conceptual developments. *Neurology* 1997;48:1167–1177.

CHAPTER 105
Seizures

Gerald W. Honch

Epilepsy is a chronic heterogeneous neurologic condition in which abnormal electric discharges in the brain are manifested clinically as two or more unprovoked seizures. It is clinically important to separate the observation of seizures from the diagnosis of epilepsy. Seizures arise from the abnormal, paroxysmal electric discharges of cerebral neurons. They are symptomatic of an underlying process affecting cortical electric excitability. Seizures are the manifestation of this electric excitability. Many conditions, such as infections, metabolic changes, or toxic states, may temporarily cause seizures. These are potentially treatable or reversible, and once they have been corrected, the patient is free of the risk for further seizures. Epilepsy is characterized by recurrent seizures that are not provoked by a metabolic or toxic disturbance. The causes of epilepsy are diverse, and many types of epilepsy have been described; these can be treated with an enlarging group of drugs at the clinician's disposal.

It is difficult to examine the scope of this medical problem accurately because of an inability to identify all persons with the disease. Reporting biases limit such data. The social stigma of the epileptic disorders makes affected individuals reluctant to report the condition. Those patients whose seizures are controlled with medication or who have not recently had a seizure may not report epilepsy as a medical problem in a survey. Epilepsy and seizures affect 2.3 million Americans of all ages. Approximately 181,000 new cases of seizures and epilepsy occur each year. About 10% of the American population will experience a seizure in their lifetime. Epilepsy will develop in 3% by the age of 75 years. In about 25% of the total epilepsy population, seizures persist despite treatment and are considered intractable.

TERMS

The terms or language of epilepsy and epileptologists are confusing, and some definitions are required:

Absence—a brief lapse of consciousness.

Antiepileptic—a drug or mechanism that prevents seizures.

Aura—the warning that precedes an epileptic seizure and is regarded as part of the seizure itself.

Clonic—characterized by rhythmic motor activity alternating with motor relaxation.

Cure—a term not freely used by epileptologists, who are somewhat reluctant to declare with absolute confidence that seizures will not recur. The clinical test lasts a lifetime.

Epileptogenic lesion—a structural disturbance (e.g., a tumor or a scar) that gives rise to seizures.

Focal—characterized by a single epileptic focus. May be bilateral or multifocal and independent. Contrast with diffuse or generalized (nonfocal).

Generalized seizures—bilateral involvement of the brain.

Grand mal—an unfortunate and outdated term. Usually taken to mean seizures with loss of both consciousness and postural tone, both tonic and clonic components, tongue biting, incontinence. It is what most witnesses mean when they refer to a seizure. This is a "usual" or "regular" seizure.

Ictus—the epileptic seizure itself.

Major motor seizure—this term has replaced *grand mal seizures.*

Partial seizures—seizures that begin in a part of the brain or are limited to one hemisphere. Simple partial seizures do not impair consciousness. Complex partial seizures impair consciousness.

Petit mal—an unfortunate and outdated term that refers to a specific, well-defined clinical event in children (absence) that is associated with characteristic electroencephalographic (EEG) features (3-per-second spike and wave). Does not mean "small" events.

Postictal—occurring when an ictal event has ended. Transient clinical or electrophysiologic abnormalities in brain function may appear postictally and last minutes to a day or two.

Pseudoseizure—any nonepileptic event that resembles an epileptic seizure. It is often a difficult and meddlesome task to clarify and treat pseudoseizures, which are also known as *psychogenic seizures.*

Secondary epileptogenesis—a process in which focal epileptogenic abnormalities give rise to distant epileptogenic zones. Also may be referred to as *kindling.*

Seizure-free—no longer afflicted with seizures. The term is not synonymous with *cured* but is used to denote a clinical state without detectable epileptic events.

Temporal lobe seizures—also known as *psychomotor seizures.* Another unfortunate and outdated set of terms. Modern terminology uses the term *complex partial seizures* with focal identification or limbic descriptors.

Tonic—characterized by sustained motor activity without rhythmic phenomena. A tonic seizure may result in a slow or sustained motor manifestation affecting posture or position.

CLASSIFICATION

A classification of the various seizure types serves many purposes. Most importantly, defining by type facilitates an understanding of the patient's symptoms. Proper identification clarifies communication regarding a specific seizure type. Treatment choices may be directed by the seizure type, and the success of treatment is closely linked to choosing an anticonvulsant appropriate for the seizure type.

The International League Against Epilepsy published the first International Classification of Epileptic Seizures in 1970. This was revised in 1981 (Table 105.1). The classification is based on distinctive behavioral and electrophysiologic features of the epileptic ictal events and does not specify pathophysiologic mechanisms or anatomic substrates. It uses impairment of consciousness as the sole means of distinguishing between simple and complex partial seizures. In addition, it takes into account the symptom progressions that characterize most epileptic seizures. Alternative classifications may be more useful clinically for those working in the field.

ETIOLOGY

Epilepsy can be classified by etiology or by clinical manifestations. Epilepsy with a known cause is referred to as *symptomatic* or *secondary epilepsy*. Epilepsy without an identifiable cause is referred to as *idiopathic epilepsy*. This distinction is clinically important because treating or relieving the cause of seizures may improve or favorably affect the ultimate result of treatment with anticonvulsants.

A seizure can be provoked in any normal person given the right combination of circumstances. People differ in their threshold for seizures, however. One can think of the threshold as a level that can be raised or lowered depending on various circumstances. The resting state of neuronal excitability and synchronization plus the rate of change in the basal state determine the point at which a seizure occurs. In addition, one can consider a number of inhibiting mechanisms that may exert a protective effect. The threshold is not a static phenomenon and changes with time and biochemical factors. The incidence of seizures is higher in the very young and the aged.

Some patients are genetically susceptible to seizures. This susceptibility is nonspecific (aside from inherited metabolic disorders). The susceptibility to epileptiform EEG patterns and epileptic seizures is increased in the first-degree relatives of persons with epilepsy. A genetic basis for nonspecific seizure susceptibility is now accepted. Hence, the manifestation of epileptiform EEG abnormalities or seizures requires the interplay of both genetic and environmental factors. Genetic traits may underlie specific epileptogenic disturbances (e.g., the 3-cycle-per-second spike-and-wave EEG discharge, photosensitivity). A number of genes inherited in a mendelian manner have been identified. The Epilepsy Foundation has established the Gene Discovery Project to identify families with epilepsy, facilitate linkage analysis, and find genetic markers that congregate within epilepsy families.

The threshold for seizures fluctuates with normal biologic rhythms. Circadian rhythms are related to diurnal cycles in hormone levels or to alterations in neuronal activity that accompany sleep and wakefulness. Some patients may have seizures predominantly while awake and others predominantly during sleep. A time of particular vulnerability to seizures is the twilight period of transition from wakefulness to sleep or vice versa. Cyclic fluctuations in the threshold may be longer. A common example is catamenial epilepsy. An increased occurrence of seizures in women around the time of menses is largely secondary to changes in estrogen and progesterone levels. Premenstrual and ovulatory exacerbations of seizures occur. Estrogen appears to lower the seizure threshold, and progesterone raises it. Epilepsy also affects hormone levels and function. An interplay between antiepileptic drugs, hepatic enzyme systems, and birth control medication may lead to a failure of birth control and the need for a higher dose of replacement hormone. Potentially persistent interictal effects of seizures lead to reproductive endocrine disorders. More than 50% of women with epilepsy have a menstrual disorder. Amenorrhea affects 14% to 20% of women with epilepsy (oligomenorrhea 20%). Prolonged or shortened menstrual cycles are noted in 20%. The incidence of polycystic ovarian syndrome is higher in women with epilepsy.

Environmental factors may alter the capacity of cerebral neurons to be excited or synchronized. The seizure threshold can be raised or lowered by various means. Nonspecific factors such as systemic illness, psychological stress, sleep deprivation, alcohol or sedative drug withdrawal, and fever may all lower the seizure threshold and precipitate an event. Certain drugs, such as the neuroleptics and antidepressants, are not likely to cause seizures in nonepileptic persons, but they can increase the risk for seizures in persons with specific epileptogenic factors. Other drugs, such as cocaine or amphetamines, may cause a seizure at the time of use in an otherwise healthy person who is not predisposed to epilepsy.

Acquired brain lesions may lower or raise the seizure threshold in certain cerebral areas. Often, focal seizures are the result of focal injuries to the cerebral cortex. Cortical scarring and irritation resulting from traumatic injury is the most common example. Other focal cortical injuries, such as those associated with cerebral infarction (10%–15% of patients with stroke), arteriovenous malformation (berry aneurysms, Sturge-Weber syndrome), multiple sclerosis, and other disorders, increase the risk

TABLE 105.1. International Classification of Epileptic Seizures

Partial (focal, local) seizures
- A. Simple partial seizures
  - 1. With motor signs
  - 2. With somatosensory or special sensory symptoms
  - 3. With autonomic symptoms or signs
  - 4. With psychic symptoms
- B. Complex partial seizures
  - 1. Simple partial onset followed by impairment of consciousness
  - 2. With impairment of consciousness at onset
- C. Partial seizures evolving to secondarily generalized seizures
  - 1. Simple partial seizures evolving to generalized seizures
  - 2. Complex partial seizures evolving to generalized seizures
  - 3. Simple partial seizures evolving to complex partial seizures evolving to generalized seizures

Generalized seizures (convulsive or nonconvulsive)
- A. Absence seizures
  - 1. Typical absences
  - 2. Atypical absences
- B. Myoclonic seizures
- C. Clonic seizures
- D. Tonic seizures
- E. Tonic-clonic seizures
- F. Atonic seizures (astatic seizures)

Unclassified epileptic seizures

Source: From the Commission on Classification and Terminology of the International League Against Epilepsy. *Epilepsia* 1981;22:489, with permission.

for epilepsy. Hypertensive encephalopathy is considered the cause of seizures in toxemia of pregnancy. Residual pathologic changes in the cerebral cortex can act as a focus for chronic epilepsy. Seizures can also occur in patients with blood dyscrasias (sickle cell anemia and coagulopathies), perivascular infiltrates secondary to leukemia, and cerebral disturbances induced by collagen-vascular diseases.

Seizures occur in 20% to 70% of patients with various types of intracranial tumors. It is possible that small, unrecognized tumors account for a relatively high percentage of focal epileptic disorders. Magnetic resonance imaging (MRI) has been particularly valuable in demonstrating small lesions in areas difficult to assess, such as the mesial temporal lobes. Meningiomas and arachnoid cysts cause seizures through irritation rather than destruction. Malignant tumors are more aggressive and associated with areas of increased vascularity and tumor necrosis, which may contribute to cortical irritability. Hamartomas and nonneoplastic masses consist of abnormal mixtures of vascular, glial, and neuronal tissue that may give rise to seizures. Hamartomas are occasionally encountered in temporal lobe tissue removed from patients with complex partial seizures. Tubers are disorganized collections of large pleomorphic astrocytes, often with calcification; these also are occasionally encountered in temporal lobe tissue removed from patients with partial complex seizures. Cortical dysgenesis accounts for 15% of patients with epilepsy.

The acute infections of meningitis, encephalitis, or abscess commonly precipitate seizures. Cortical irritation, local metabolic changes, reduced glucose levels, and cellular changes all contribute. Chronic or more indolent infections can cause seizures. The most common cause of focal seizures in Latin America is cysticercosis. Syphilis is once again becoming an important cause of seizures. Today, AIDS is an important cause of neurologic symptoms in adults and children. Opportunistic infections, lymphomas, and AIDS encephalopathy can manifest with epileptic seizures.

Acquired degenerative diseases are occasionally associated with epileptic seizures. Two percent of patients with multiple sclerosis have seizures. The incidence of seizures is increased 10-fold in patients with presenile and senile dementia of the Alzheimer type. Local degenerative changes may cause seizures.

Hippocampal sclerosis is the most common lesion encountered in patients with complex partial seizures. The cause of this change, which alone may lead to seizures, is debated. It has been postulated that hippocampal sclerosis results from epileptic activity. It has also been suggested that prolonged febrile convulsions (commonly reported in the history of patients with complex partial seizures) damage the hippocampus. Later in life, a structural abnormality of this type becomes an epileptogenic lesion.

HISTORY

The clinical story or history is absolutely essential in establishing the diagnosis of a seizure disorder. The history is usually obtained from an observer and may be retold by multiple other, well-meaning witnesses. There is no substitute for questioning the primary observer. Seizures are dramatic and frightening to witnesses. The records are often incomplete and include the emotional contributions of the observer. The patient may be able to provide valuable information regarding the prodrome or period before the event and may also be able to document the time in recovery from the postictal state. An eyewitness account is usually more reliable than the patient's account.

The course of events during a seizure must be recorded logically and concisely. It is never reasonable to accept a diagnosis of a seizure disorder without sifting through the events that took place, no matter how well qualified or well intentioned the historian. A video recording made by family members is particularly valuable and can be analyzed repeatedly by multiple persons. It is very easy to be misled by an incorrect diagnosis. The obvious consequences are multiple: The correct treatment is not given, various social and financial problems are invited, and the true diagnosis is missed.

It is best to start with the circumstances under which the event occurred: the time of day, activity of the patient, general health and condition of the patient, and any contributing circumstances. What was the effect of the episode on the patient's consciousness? How long did the event last? Has more than one type of event occurred? Stress, deprivation of sleep, fatigue, alcohol, drugs, hunger, or bizarre dietary changes may be important.

Did the patient experience an aura (warning) or prodrome before the event? Is this warning a recognizable phenomenon that might be useful in predicting or recognizing another event? The usual questions asked relate to olfactory sensations (usually unpleasant), odd tastes, abdominal discomfort, or a rising sensation (in the genital areas). Some visual disturbances occur, such as distortions of size, shape, color, or form. Did the patient experience formed or unformed hallucinations? Was any "forced thinking" noted (the patient may experience repeated or stereotyped thinking patterns or memories)? Some of these can be quite unusual, such as a fragment of music, a voice, or a familiar dialogue. Visual or auditory experiences are not usually volunteered by patients out of embarrassment or fear. Feelings of familiarity (*déjà vu*, *déjà entendu*, and *déjà vécu*) or strangeness (*jamais vu*, *jamais entendu*, *jamais vécu*) occur in partial complex seizures. Fear is the most common affective symptom.

The observer must record the duration of the event and note the evolution of activity within an event. Focal clonic or tonic movements or forced versive deviations of the limbs or eyes may be important clues to the origin of the epileptiform activity. Attention should be paid to the number and variety of seizure types. Is there some cycling or clustering of seizures?

The past history requires careful scrutiny. The birth history with gestational risks and the delivery should be explored. A history of past head trauma or surgical procedures performed on the central nervous system (CNS) may be relevant. Is there a relationship to other CNS disorders? Are there any known medical disorders (e.g., systemic lupus erythematosus) that might be causing seizures? Is there a family history of a seizure disorder?

PHYSICAL EXAMINATION

The general physical examination may provide clues to systemic illnesses predisposing the patient to seizures. In both the acute and nonacute settings, the general physical examination may yield useful signs of such disorders as infection, hypertension, drug intoxication, and metabolic disturbances. In addition, signs of trauma must be noted. The skin may indicate a phakomatosis (e.g., the port-wine stain of Sturge-Weber syndrome, the café au lait spots of neurofibromatosis, or the ash leaf spots and shagreen patches of tuberous sclerosis). Inspection of the scalp and palpation of the skull may reveal evidence of trauma or prior surgical procedures.

The neurologic examination findings are often normal in the patient with idiopathic epilepsy. Focal or lateralized features can help distinguish partial from generalized epileptic disorders.

Careful examination during the immediate postictal period may reveal diagnostically useful fleeting focal or lateralized dysfunction that would not be apparent later. Findings of minimal brain dysfunction, such as clumsiness, synkinesis, abnormal posturing of the hands, hyperreflexia, and mild mental retardation or dementia, may support a diagnosis of secondary rather than primary epilepsy. Memory disturbances can result from the epileptogenic lesion itself and are often exacerbated by the effects of antiepileptic drugs. It is important to remember that a postictal Todd paralysis or phenomenon (focal paralysis following a seizure) usually does not last longer than 24 to 48 hours.

LABORATORY AND IMAGING STUDIES

The laboratory studies should be tailored to the needs and presentation of the patient. In an acute setting with a first convulsive episode, the laboratory workup is generally more extensive. For the patient with an established seizure disorder, the laboratory workup is more specific.

In the acute setting, the following studies are helpful: complete blood cell count; measurement of electrolytes, calcium, and glucose; hepatic and renal screen; and urinalysis. A serum magnesium determination is generally not considered useful. A lumbar puncture is performed if the history and physical examination findings suggest that the cerebrospinal fluid may be helpful in establishing another diagnosis. A toxic screen of blood and urine is useful in selected patients. The serum prolactin level is elevated after complex partial and generalized seizures (blood should be drawn within 20 minutes after the episode). The serum levels of anticonvulsant drugs are very helpful in guiding the treatment of a patient with an established seizure disorder.

EEG is the single most informative laboratory test for the diagnosis of epilepsy and is noninvasive, benign, and relatively inexpensive. Every patient with suspected epilepsy should undergo EEG. There is no reason to decrease a patient's antiepileptic medication before EEG is performed. The routine repetition of EEG at specific intervals without asking specific questions is not justified. EEG can be useful in establishing the following:

Does the patient have epilepsy? EEG will help distinguish seizures from other conditions.

What kind of epilepsy does the patient have? Certain EEG patterns help to diagnose characteristic types of epilepsy, and this knowledge guides the selection of specific drugs.

EEG can detect signs of drug toxicity. In some instances, EEG is useful as a guide to therapy. For instance, EEG is indispensable in following the response to treatment of a patient with status epilepticus.

EEG is useful for establishing the location of interictal EEG spike discharges and the focal nature of the electric activity.

A variety of EEG protocols are used. In a routine study, the electrode placement, duration of the examination, and use of activation procedures such as hyperventilation and photic stimulation are well established. Sleep studies help activate interictal EEG spike activity. Special facilities for all-night recording or long-term monitoring are available in certain laboratories. Special monitoring facilities are equipped for simultaneous EEG and video recording. Additional recording electrodes may be used (e.g., nasopharyngeal, sphenoidal). Computed tomography (CT) and MRI are useful in demonstrating focal structural lesions of the CNS. CT is less expensive, more often available on an emergency basis, and generally superior to MRI in demonstrating hemorrhage or a meningioma. MRI is vastly superior for demonstrating subtle lesions of the mesial temporal lobe, vascular lesions (e.g., an arteriovenous malformation), and cortical dysplasias.

TREATMENT

Once epilepsy has been diagnosed, long-term treatment with antiepileptic drugs must be designed. The goal is to achieve complete seizure control with a minimum of adverse side effects. The price of medication is also an important consideration in the current era of cost containment. It is well to remember that the cost of antiepileptic medications ranges from relatively small to enormous when taken for a lifetime. The primary antiepileptic drugs in use today include phenytoin, carbamazepine, valproate, ethosuximide, phenobarbital, and primidone. Since 1993, eight new antiepileptic drugs have become available in the United States for the treatment of epilepsy (felbamate, gabapentin, lamotrigine, topiramate, tiagabine, levetiracetam, oxcarbazepine, and zonisamide). No drug is able to control all seizure types, and no drug is without the potential to cause adverse side effects. Careful selection of the initial antiepileptic drug is based on identification of the seizure type and the epilepsy syndrome, as discussed previously. Both symptoms and drug levels must be monitored in a patient with epilepsy. Any anticonvulsant used in subtherapeutic amounts cannot be expected to be effective. The fewer the number of agents used, the simpler the management scheme.

A thorough appreciation of the medication being used is mandatory. The importance of anticipating the problems that may be encountered and being familiar with the idiosyncrasies of each anticonvulsant in use cannot be emphasized strongly enough. Uncontrolled seizures and disabling side effects compromise the quality of life. Both patient and physician must be well informed.

Poor compliance, a major problem in treating this illness, is often linked to psychological issues. Loss of control over one's health, resentment about the need to take medication, and dependence on medication to be able to lead a normal life are all very real issues to the patient. Denial of illness is very common initially. The nature of epilepsy and the proper use of medication are educational issues that the physician must return to again and again. The social stigma of epilepsy alters the way these patients live and relate to the world in diverse ways; schooling, job and career selection, marriage, sports, driving, and the ability to live independently are all affected. Discrimination is still commonplace.

The vast majority of patients (50%–80%) are able to achieve adequate seizure control with a minimum of side effects by using a single drug effectively. Approximately 50% become seizure-free with the first antiepileptic drug tried (provided the drug selected is appropriate for the seizure type). These results are commonly attained with low or moderate doses. When a second drug is tried, the seizures of an additional 15% of patients are brought under control. Adding a third drug in combination or as monotherapy helps just another 5%. Hence, one can tell early in the course of treatment whether long-term success will be achieved. This is important for the selection of antiepileptic drugs early in the patient's course of treatment. Patients with mesial temporal lobe epilepsy are excellent candidates for epilepsy surgery. Polypharmacy has a role but should be the exception, not the rule. Selection of the most effective agent for the seizure type is the first step.

Partial seizures—primary and secondarily generalized: carbamazepine, phenytoin, gabapentin, tiagabine, oxcarbazepine, phenobarbital, primidone, levetiracetam.

Broad spectrum—all seizure types, including partial, absence, myoclonic, tonic, and generalized tonic-clonic: valproic acid, lamotrigine, topiramate, felbamate, zonisamide, and levetiracetam.

Absence only: ethosuximide.

Infantile spasms: valproic acid and zonisamide.

Knowledge of the pharmacokinetics of each drug is necessary to determine the dose and the timing of the doses. Table 105.2 notes the half-life of the frequently prescribed drugs. Drugs with a long half-life may be given once or twice per day. Drugs with a relatively short half-life must be taken multiple times per day to avoid wide differences between peak and trough concentrations. The same concept applies to the measurement of drug levels. It is generally best to obtain drug levels at the estimated trough time (in the morning); in this way, a consistent pattern of analysis is established.

Protein binding is more important for some drugs than others. Drugs that are highly protein-bound are affected by states that alter serum protein levels (e.g., renal failure, pregnancy). It may be necessary to obtain free levels in these special circumstances.

The therapeutic range is meant to be a guide, not absolutely rigid. The fixation of both patients and physicians on achieving the therapeutic range is often difficult to overcome. The pharmacokinetics of antiepileptic drugs is not always a straight line function (first-order kinetics). For most of them, zero-order kinetics prevail, in which the enzyme necessary for drug metabolism becomes saturated. The serum drug level then increases exponentially as the dose is increased. After a certain point, very small changes in the dose result in very large changes in the serum drug level. It is the physician's mission to control seizures with the smallest number of side effects; it is very easy to slip from a therapeutic to a toxic range with only a minor increase in the dose. Levels are most useful in sorting out questions of toxicity and compliance, and in planning and monitoring the effects of changes in dose. Steady-state levels are reached roughly once a period equal to five half-lives of the drug in question has elapsed. This is a very useful guide for monitoring drug levels after a dosage adjustment.

In the acute situation, the question of "loading" the patient must be considered. Loading a patient who has status epilepticus or frequent seizures with anticonvulsants is certainly a practical and necessary step. In most patients with a single seizure, loading is unnecessary. Loading is generally performed only with agents that have a relatively long half-life (phenytoin and phenobarbital). The antiepileptic drugs with a short half-life are not suitable for this use (carbamazepine). With a drug that has a short half-life, the threshold to toxicity is reached quickly. It is also important to remember that certain agents (e.g., carbamazepine) gradually induce the hepatic enzyme systems to higher levels over days to weeks. Hence, early doses of these agents must be smaller, with gradual titration to higher-dose regimens.

Drug interactions are complex, both between the various drugs used to control epilepsy and between antiepileptic drugs and any others administered concurrently. The effect may be to enhance or retard drug metabolism. Hence, the addition of

TABLE 105.2. Pharmacokinetics of Anticonvulsant Drugs

Drug	Usual adult dose (mg/d)	Half-life (h)	Metabolism	Usual effective plasma concentration (μg/mL)	Time to peak concentration fraction (h)	Protein-bound (%)
Phenytoin *(Dilantin)*	300–400	22	>90% hepatic with induction	10–20	3–8	90–95
Carbamazepine *(Tegretol, Carbatrol)*	800–1,600	8–22	>90% hepatic with induction	8–12	4–8	75
Phenobarbital	90–180	100	>90% hepatic with induction	15–40	2–8	45
Primidone *(Mysoline)*	750–2,000	Primidone 8–22	40%–60% renal >40% hepatic	Primidone 5–12	6–8	Primidone 20
Valproate *(Depakote, Depakene)*	1,000–3,000	15–20	>95% hepatic with inhibition	50–120	3–8	80–90
Ethosuximide *(Zarontin)*	750–1,500	60	65% hepatic, no induction	40–100	3–7	<5
Felbamate *(Felbatol)*	2,400–3,600	14–23	60% hepatic	20–140	2–6	25
Gabapentin *(Neurontin)*	1,800–3,600	5–7	>95% renal	4–16	2–3	<5
Lamotrigine *(Lamictal)*	100–500	12–60	>90% hepatic, no induction	2–16	2–5	55
Topiramate *(Topamax)*	200–400	19–25	30% hepatic, no induction	4–10	2–4	9–17
Tiagabine *(Gabitril)*	32–56	5–13	>90% hepatic, no induction	(not established)	1	95
Oxcarbazepine *(Trileptal)*	600–1,800	8–10	>90% hepatic, mild induction	10–35	3–13	40
Levetiracetam *(Keppra)*	1,000–3,000	6–8	>65% renal excretion	5–45	1	<10
Zonisamide *(Zonegran)*	100–400	63	70% hepatic, no induction	10–40	2–6	40

another agent may render the anticonvulsant levels subtherapeutic or toxic, depending on the drugs in question. In other situations, no apparent interaction occurs. The careful selection of antiepileptic drugs, and a consideration of how they interact with other antiepileptic drugs and other drugs in general, is essential. A safe practice should always include a referral to a source to address these possibilities.

Single seizures are an important and difficult area. The patient with a single unprovoked seizure does not have epilepsy by definition and does not warrant treatment with anticonvulsant drugs. The chance for recurrence of seizures in a patient who has had an isolated seizure is 16% to 61%. The likelihood of recurrence is increased in patients with:

- Recent or remote symptomatic neurologic disease
- A family history of epilepsy
- Partial complex seizures
- Abnormal findings on a neurologic examination
- An abnormal EEG.

If seizures are going to recur, they generally do so within 1 year. The longer a patient remains seizure-free (measured in years), the lower the likelihood of recurrence. After a patient has had a second unprovoked seizure, the risk for recurrence is high (79%–90%).

The question of when and how to discontinue antiepileptic drugs is never easily answered. There are no absolutes to address this question, and the "test" or trial period off antiepileptics lasts for the lifetime of the patient. However, some general guidelines are quite helpful. The longer the duration of seizure control with antiepileptic drugs, the better the prognosis. The chances for successful drug withdrawal are greatest in patients with:

- No seizures for 2 to 5 years while taking antiepileptic drugs
- A single type of seizure (either partial or generalized)
- Normal neurologic examination findings
- A normal intelligence quotient
- An EEG that normalizes during treatment.

Both patients and third party payers frequently ask about the feasibility of generic antiepileptic medication. Cost containment is the issue. The price of medication over the lifetime of a patient can be enormous.

Current Federal Drug Administration guidelines assume that bioavailability can vary safely by 20%. No scientific evidence indicates that this or any other range of variability can be tolerated safely by patients with epilepsy. The three pharmacologic risk factors to consider are a low level of water solubility, a narrow therapeutic range, and nonlinear pharmacokinetics. With generic preparations, the time to maximum blood level after each dose may vary. Variability in shelf life may be questioned.

When generic drugs are used, neither the patient nor the physician is kept informed about which manufacturer's generic formulation is actually dispensed at a particular time. Multiple manufacturers may offer a single drug, each version differing in regard to binding or coloring agents, dissolution and absorption times, bioavailability, and time to maximum serum concentration. Generic substitution can be approved only if safety and efficacy are not compromised.

Convulsive status epilepticus has been the subject of controversy and special study. Status epilepticus is defined as continuous seizure activity lasting more than 30 minutes, or the occurrence of two or more sequential seizures without full recovery of consciousness between them. The outcome is often linked to the cause. The setting is important. In patients with life-threatening illnesses such as anoxia and CNS infection, the outcome is less favorable. When status epilepticus is the first manifestation of a seizure disorder or when a dose of antiepileptic drugs has been reduced abruptly, the outcome is more favorable. More than half of patients with status epilepticus respond to therapy with a single agent. Status epilepticus associated with an acute or progressive neurologic disorder is more likely to be refractory.

Like the management of any unresponsive patient, the initial management of a patient with status epilepticus includes the ABCs of life support: supporting respiration (airway), maintaining the blood pressure, gaining access to the circulation, and, when possible, identifying and treating the probable cause. The patient's fluids, levels of electrolytes, blood urea nitrogen, creatinine, glucose, and antiepileptic drugs, and temperature must be evaluated and addressed. Simply correcting a fever may be helpful in stopping the seizure activity.

The goal of therapy is rapid termination of the clinical and electric seizure activity. The longer an episode of status epilepticus goes untreated, the more difficult it is to control with medication. There is no substitute for a clear plan of treatment, the prompt administration of effective drugs in adequate doses, and attention to the possibility of apnea or hypoventilation. Neuromuscular paralysis without the administration of antiepileptic drugs is inappropriate because sustained electric discharges in the brain can cause irreversible brain injury. Intramuscular therapy has no place in the treatment of status epilepticus or seizures in general. Drugs should be administered by the intravenous route only.

Table 105.3 compares the agents used to treat status epilepticus. These should be given only under conditions of close monitoring, such as in an intensive care unit or emergency department where ventilatory support is immediately available. Diazepam is probably the most popular agent and works extremely rapidly. Unfortunately, a single dose of diazepam no longer effectively prevents seizures 15 to 30 minutes after administration. Hence, breakthrough or a return to status epilepticus may occur. Lorazepam does not work as rapidly as diazepam but is nonetheless very fast. The major advantage of lorazepam is its duration of action; its anticonvulsant effect lasts several hours. As the seizure activity comes under control, a longer-acting agent such as phenytoin or fosphenytoin should be added promptly.

Treatment with midazolam and more recently propofol has been suggested for cases of refractory generalized status epilepticus. These agents have been reserved for patients in very special circumstances of prolonged convulsive status epilepticus unresponsive to standard doses of intravenous benzodiazepines, phenytoin, and phenobarbital. Midazolam and propofol are given as a slow bolus followed by a continuous infusion for several hours. EEG monitoring is recommended to follow the seizure activity. An adjustment of the maintenance dose to stop electrographic seizures is based on EEG monitoring. Phenytoin and phenobarbital are continued as maintenance medications. The midazolam or propofol is discontinued after about 12 hours while the patient is monitored clinically and the EEG is followed to detect further electrographic seizure activity.

CONSIDERATIONS IN PREGNANCY

Both the medical community and laypersons are aware of the teratogenic potential of antiepileptic drugs. It is estimated that 1 in 250 newborns are exposed to antiepileptic drugs in utero. The risks include major malformations, minor anomalies, failure of intrauterine or postnatal growth, and psychomotor retardation. The absolute risk is that 7% to 10% of children exposed

TABLE 105.3. Drugs for Status Epilepticus

	Diazepam	Lorazepam	Phenytoin	Phenobarbital	Midazolam	Propofol
Adult IV dose (mg/kg)	0.15–0.25	0.1	15–20	20	Bolus of 200 µg/kg followed by continuous infusion of 0.75–10 µg/kg/min	1–3 followed by continuous infusion of 1–15 mg/kg/h
Maximum rate of administration (mg/min)	5	2.1	50	100		
Time to stop status (min)	1–3	6–10	10–30	20–30	>5	>5
Effective duration of action (h)	0.25–0.5	>12–24	24	>48	Titrate	Titrate
Elimination half-life (h)	30	14	24	100	1.5–3.5	1.5–28
Side effects						
Depression of consciousness	10–30 min	Hours	None	Days	Yes	Yes
Respiratory depression	Yes	Yes	Rare	Yes	Yes	Yes
Hypotension	Rare	Rare	Yes	Rare	Rare	Yes
Cardiac arrhythmias	No	No	With history of heart disease	No	No	Brady

to antiepileptic drugs will have such defects. This risk is two times higher than that in the general population. The more serious effects include congenital heart malformations (phenytoin and phenobarbital) and neural tube defects (valproate and carbamazepine).

A possible genetic predisposition for some of these defects in certain families is a matter of concern. The anomalies in the children of mothers with epilepsy (treated or untreated with antiepileptic drugs) tend to be slightly higher than in the children of fathers with epilepsy or in control subjects. Teratogenicity is generally considered to be related to antiepileptic drugs, not to epilepsy. The effects of tonic-clonic seizures on the fetus during pregnancy are not well established. Physical injury to the mother, hypoxia, hypotension, and antiepileptic drugs may all contribute significantly to the risk for defects. No information is available regarding which of the four major antiepileptic drugs (phenytoin, carbamazepine, valproate, or phenobarbital) is the most teratogenic or which causes the most significant malformations. Table 105.4 lists the major antiepileptic drugs in use today and their associated potential teratogenic effects. The risk to the fetus is greatest during the first trimester.

The role of folic acid in birth defects is controversial. Some have suggested that antiepileptic drugs cause neural tube defects by interfering with folic acid metabolism. After one child has been born with a neural tube defect, supplementation with folic acid (4 mg/d for at least 1 month before conception) can reduce the risk for neural tube defects in subsequent children from 3.5% to 0.7%. It is safer to recommend that all women who may bear children consume a diet that contains adequate amounts of folic acid, that all women with epilepsy who are being treated with antiepileptic drugs receive folic acid daily, and that normal folic acid concentrations be ascertained in the serum and red blood cells pregnant women with epilepsy who are being treated with antiepileptic drugs.

The risk for teratogenicity is increased by the following:

- A high daily dose of an antiepileptic drug
- High serum levels of an antiepileptic drug
- Polypharmacy
- Low folate levels (neural tube defects).

It is important that adequate preconception and prenatal counseling be given. More than 90% of women with epilepsy who take antiepileptic drugs during pregnancy deliver a normal child free of birth defects. Some simple measures are suggested:

- Discussing and making the patient aware of the potential risk before conception
- Realistically and accurately weighing risk potential against alternatives to antiepileptic drugs
- Discussing diet and ensuring adequate folate
- Maintaining seizure control with monotherapy if possible
- In a patient seizure-free for at least 2 years, considering withdrawal of antiepileptic drugs

TABLE 105.4. Teratogenic Effects of Antiepileptic Agents

Drug	Teratogenicity	Secreted in breast milk
Carbamazepine	Spina bifida	Yes
Clonazepam	Unclear	Yes
Ethosuximide	High prevalence of severe birth defects, physical anomalies, growth and mental retardation	Yes
Phenobarbital	Cleft lip and palate, congenital heart and urogenital defects	Yes
Phenytoin	Cleft lip and palate, congenital heart and urogenital defects	Yes
Primidone	Adds to phenobarbital risk	Yes
Valproic acid	Spina bifida, cardiovascular and urogenital malformations	Yes
Gabapentin	Unknown	Unknown
Lamotrigine	Unknown	Yes
Felbamate	Unknown	Yes

- Administering the lowest antiepileptic drug dose and maintaining the lowest plasma level that protects against seizures.

During pregnancy, the serum levels of antiepileptic drug may vary. The dose should be altered after a consideration of the clinical issues, not simply the serum levels of antiepileptic drug. The reasons for fluctuating serum levels are increased hepatic and renal clearance rates, reduced albumin levels, plasma protein binding of increased levels of unbound drug, and increased plasma volume by the third trimester.

During labor and delivery, a tonic-clonic seizure occurs in 1% to 2% of women with epilepsy. It is important to maintain adequate antiepileptic drug levels at this time, when doses may be missed. The drug half-life (Table 105.2) guides the dosing frequency. After delivery, the doses of antiepileptic drug must be returned to those used before pregnancy to avoid toxicity during the first few weeks of the puerperium.

All antiepileptic drugs are secreted in breast milk (Table 105.4). The concentration depends on the level of protein binding in the mother's serum (the higher the rate of protein binding, the less the amount of drug available for secretion into breast milk) (Table 105.2). Sedation of the infant may be a problem with agents that have sedative potential. Breast-feeding is not recommended with clonazepam or the newer agents (felbamate, gabapentin, and lamotrigine). Reported concentrations of antiepileptic drugs in breast milk range from 10% to 80% of the maternal serum levels.

Antiepileptic drugs may induce hepatic microsomal enzymes sufficiently to alter the metabolism of oral contraceptive agents. Breakthrough bleeding is an early sign of such interference. The effectiveness of the oral contraceptive may be reduced, so that a higher dose of hormone in the oral contraceptive becomes necessary. In addition, a similar mechanism of enzyme induction by oral contraceptives may reduce the serum levels of antiepileptic drugs and increase the frequency of seizures. Antiepileptic drug levels may have to be adjusted when oral contraceptives are started or changed.

The long-term use of phenytoin, phenobarbital, carbamazepine, or primidone is associated with decreased bone density and an increased risk for fractures. Induction of the cytochrome P-450 system by these drugs leads to excessive enzymatic degradation of vitamin D and bone demineralization. Valproate causes an increase in bone resorption with a subsequent decrease in bone mass.

BIBLIOGRAPHY

Abramowicz M. Drugs for epilepsy. *Med Lett* 1995;37:37.

Cascino GD. Epilepsy: contemporary perspectives on evaluation and treatment. *Mayo Clin Proc* 1994;69:1199.

Commission on Classification and Terminology of the International League Against Epilepsy. Revised clinical and electroencephalographic classification of epileptic seizures. *Epilepsia* 1981;22:489.

Delgado-Escueta AV, Janz D. Consensus guidelines: preconception counseling, management and care of the pregnant woman with epilepsy. *Neurology* 1992; 42[Suppl 5]:149.

Devinsky O. Patients with refractory seizures. *N Engl J Med* 1999;340:1565–1570.

Devinsky O, Yerby M, eds. *Women with epilepsy: reproduction and effects of pregnancy on epilepsy.* Philadelphia: WB Saunders, 1994.

Dodson WE, Lorenzo RJ, Pedley TA, et al. Treatment of convulsive status epilepticus. *JAMA* 1993;270:854.

Donaldson JO. Epilepsy. In: Donaldson JO, ed. *Neurology of pregnancy.* Philadelphia: WB Saunders, 1989:229.

Engle J. *Seizures and epilepsy.* Philadelphia: FA Davis Co, 1989.

Epilepsy: a report to the nation. Landover, MD: Epilepsy Foundation of America, 1999. Available at *www.efa.org/news/nation/nation.html.* Accessed August 15, 2002.

Krumholz A. Epilepsy in pregnancy. In: Goldstein PJ, Stern BJ, eds. *Neurological disorders of pregnancy.* Mount Kisco, NY: Futura Publishing, 1992:25.

Kumar A, Bleck TP. Intravenous midazolam for the treatment of refractory status epilepticus. *Crit Care Med* 1992;20:483.

Kwan P, Brodie MJ. Early identification of refractory epilepsy. *N Engl J Med* 2000; 342:314–319.

Kwan P, Brodie MJ. Effectiveness of first anti-epileptic drug. *Epilepsia* 2001;42: 1255–1260.

Leis AA, Ross MA, Summers AK. Psychogenic seizures: ictal characteristics and diagnostic pitfalls. *Neurology* 1992;42:95.

Lindhout D, Omtzigt JGC. Pregnancy and the risk of teratogenicity. *Epilepsia* 1992; 33[Suppl 4]:S41.

Morrell MJ. Hormones and epilepsy through the lifetime. *Epilepsia* 1992;33[Suppl 4]:549.

Noort SVD. Assessment: generic substitution for antiepileptic medication. *Neurology* 1990;40:1641.

Parent JM, Lowenstein DH. Treatment of refractory generalized status epilepticus with continuous infusion of midazolam. *Neurology* 1994;44:1837.

Praxad A, Worrall BB, Bertram EB, et al. Propofol and midazolam in the treatment of refractory status epilepticus. *Epilepsia* 2001;42:380–386.

Prevalence of self-reported epilepsy—United States, 1986–1990. *JAMA* 1994:272: 1993.

Theodore WH, Porter RJ. *Epilepsy: 100 elementary principles.* Philadelphia: WB Saunders, 1995.

Treiman DM. Epileptic emergencies and status epilepticus. In: Grotta JC, ed. *Management of the acutely ill neurological patient.* New York: Churchill Livingstone, 1993:111.

CHAPTER 106

Parkinson Disease and Other Movement Disorders

Joshua Hollander

Parkinson disease and other movement disorders are manifested by difficulty in both initiating and sustaining movements and are therefore divided into *hypokinetic* (akinetic-rigid syndromes) and *hyperkinetic* (dyskinetic) disorders. Despite a rich terminology for describing movement disorders, a major advance in this field has been the use of videotaping, which makes it possible to analyze uncertain movements, consult with other physicians, and document therapeutic interventions. Because these problems are best visualized on videotape, such tapes have been made available for educational purposes. Some of the specific terms used to describe the phenomenology include *rigidity, bradykinesia, tremor, chorea, athetosis, ballism, dystonia, myoclonus, tics,* and *stereotypies. Rigidity* is stiffness or resistance throughout the range of passive movement. It is the same in both extensors and flexors and relatively independent of velocity. Rigidity is reinforced by contralateral movement, anxiety, and stress. When interrupted by tremor, it is called *cogwheel rigidity;* without tremor, it is referred to as *lead pipe* or *plastic rigidity. Bradykinesia* is a complex of delayed motor initiation, slow performance, inability to execute simultaneous or sequential movements, difficulty in reaching a target with a single movement, rapid fatigue with repetition, and defective kinetic automatisms (loss of associated movements, such as arm swinging during walking). *Akinesia* may be a synonym but implies greater severity.

Potentially overlapping terms are used to describe adventitious movements. *Dyskinesia* denotes excessive or abnormal involuntary movements. *Tremor* is a rhythmic oscillation about a point that varies in frequency and in relation to motion. *Chorea* ("dance") is a quick, irregular, and predominantly distal semipurposive movement. *Ballism* is a proximal, high-amplitude, wild, uncontrollable, and sustained flinging (ballistic) movement that evolves to chorea during recovery. *Athetosis* refers to continuous, slow, writhing (Balinese dancer) movement. A recent tendency has been to lump all these movements together in the category of chorea. *Myoclonus* is a sudden movement caused by contractions of one muscle or a group of muscles that may be single or repetitive in the same part of the body. It may be spontaneous or precipitated by movement. Negative myoclonus, induced by the inhibition of agonist and antagonist muscle group contractions, is called *asterixis* ("flap"). *Dystonia* is an involuntary, often twisting movement that ends in a sustained contraction. Muscle tone is normal between spasms. Dystonia may manifest only with action. *Akathisia* is a restlessness resulting in an inability to sit or stand still. *Tics* are sudden, transient, complex, coordinated movements. They tend to be repetitive and are subject to brief voluntary suppression. *Stereotypies* are involuntary, coordinated, repetitive, patterned, purposeless, ritualistic-appearing movements, postures, or utterances. With the exception of sleep myoclonus and seizures, abnormal involuntary movements cease during sleep.

Parkinson disease, essential tremor, and the drug-induced movement disorders are the most common problems encountered and are stressed in this discussion.

ETIOLOGY AND DIFFERENTIAL DIAGNOSIS

The complex connections of the basal ganglia can be reviewed only briefly here. The pars compacta of the substantia nigra contains dopaminergic cells that project to the putamen (striatonigral pathway). It is these cells that are depleted in Parkinson disease. Striatopallidal pathways are both direct and indirect. The direct γ-aminobutyric acid (GABAergic) inhibitory path to the internal pallidum (GPi) reduces GABAergic inhibition of the ventrolateral thalamic nucleus, which results in the release of stimulation of the supplementary motor cortex. The cortex has direct stimulatory connections to the striatum. A similar GABAergic inhibitory path to the external pallidum (GPe) inhibits a GABAergic output to the subthalamic nucleus that has glutamatergic facilitatory output to the GPi. Omitted are numerous other neurotransmitters, multiple receptor types, and loop pathways. In Parkinson disease, a loss of nigral cells results in the loss of GPi inhibition and hence the loss of thalamic activation of the supplementary motor cortex. This results in bradykinesia and rigidity. Huntington chorea is characterized by the loss of striatal inhibition of the GPe and resultant inhibition of the subthalamic nucleus. In hemiballismus, an infarct or tumor of the subthalamic nucleus reduces GPi activation, resulting in a lack of movement suppression.

Parkinson Disease

Parkinson disease is a progressive neurodegenerative disorder that usually begins in the sixth or seventh decade of life. The prevalence is about 1 per 1,000. Cardinal features are bradykinesia, rigidity, tremor, and impaired postural reflexes. Bradykinesia contributes to a masklike facies, a diminished arm swing and associated movements, slow movement, a gait characterized by small steps, difficulty in initiating movements, hypophonia, and micrographia. The characteristic tremor is a resting tremor of low frequency (4–5 Hz) and coarse amplitude, but a low-amplitude action tremor may also be seen. The appearance of the patient sitting at repose, with tremor clearing during movement, is striking. Cogwheel rigidity (primarily in the upper limbs) reflects the tremor detected during motion. A loss of postural reflexes results in a loss of balance and an inability to invoke righting reflexes. Manifestations of autonomic dysfunction include impotence, seborrhea, constipation, and orthostatic hypotension. The eye movements tend to be hypometric. Blepharospasm may be seen. Depression with associated psychomotor retardation may be erroneously diagnosed in a patient with Parkinson disease. It is not unusual for a patient with Parkinson disease to be depressed. Therapy, as in other types of depression, is appropriate. Subcortical dementia is seen in 20% of patients and may confound therapy. A wide variety of psychiatric disorders are associated with either Parkinson disease or its treatment.

Parkinson disease is caused by a loss of dopaminergic cells of the striatonigral path, but the reason for the loss is still uncertain. Studies of parkinsonism induced by the designer drug MPTP led to the thesis that chronic exposure to environmental oxidative toxins causes cell loss. Some cell loss occurs merely as a result of aging, but it may be compounded by oxidative toxicity in Parkinson disease. Symptoms develop after a critical threshold of cell loss has been passed. Some cases are familial, but most are sporadic. A cohort of persons with postencephalitic parkinsonism related to the world pandemic of von Economo encephalitis in 1919 has aged and essentially passed from the scene. Several other causes of atypical parkinsonism may have a similar pathogenesis.

A group of diseases is sometimes referred to as *Parkinson plus*. Lewy bodies, which are eosinophilic, hyaline, cytoplasmic inclusions, are seen in the nerve cells. (Diffuse Lewy body disease with extensive cortical involvement is discussed in Chapter 108.) In Parkinson disease, the Lewy bodies tend to be located in the basal ganglia, but in some cases of Parkinson disease, no Lewy bodies are seen at all. *Multiple system atrophy* comprises a group of disorders that account for about 10% of cases of parkinsonism, including *Shy-Drager syndrome, olivopontocerebellar atrophy,* and *striatonigral degeneration*. Oligodendroglial tubular inclusions are a characteristic feature of these disorders. The presence of severe autonomic dysfunction, absence of resting tremor, early postural instability and falls, early dementia, and poor response to levodopa should alert the clinician to the possibility of one of these conditions. Corticobasal ganglionic degeneration is an akinetic-rigid syndrome with severe cortical sensory impairments, apraxia, myoclonus, tremors, and other abnormal involuntary movements. Cognitive impairment and oculomotor impairments (gaze apraxia) are also seen. Disordered voluntary gaze characterizes *progressive supranuclear palsy*. The upward gaze is decreased in normal aging and more so in Parkinson disease. Patients with progressive supranuclear palsy show a striking early impairment of downward gaze. This results in an inability to use bifocals and a tendency to fall while descending steps. The diagnostic tetrad for progressive supranuclear palsy is supranuclear oculomotor palsy, axial rigidity, pseudobulbar palsy, and subcortical dementia.

The disorder most frequently confused with Parkinson disease, after the akinetic-rigid syndromes, is essential tremor, which is the most common of the movement disorders. When a positive family history (50%) is elicited, the condition is called *familial tremor*. When the onset is after the age of 65 years, it is called *senile tremor*. Subtetanic motor unit stimulation with intact stretch reflexes results in a low-amplitude oscillation with a frequency directly proportional to muscle stiffness and inversely proportional to the mass. This physiologic tremor is enhanced to visible levels by adrenergic excess secondary to anxiety, stage fright, hypoglycemia, hyperthyroidism, caffeine, levodopa, or adrenergic medication. Physiologic tremor is an action tremor and is not present at rest. Quite similar is essential-familial tremor. The tremor is quiet at rest, but movement, such as attempting to drink a glass of water or sign a check, causes a distressing and embarrassing tremor. It should be easily distinguished from parkinsonism because of the absence of a resting tremor, rigidity, bradykinesia, and postural instability.

The two continue to be confused, perhaps because the incidence of essential tremor is increased in patients with parkinsonism.

Drug-induced parkinsonism usually develops within months after the institution of antidopaminergic drug therapy. Although it may mimic Parkinson disease, it occurs at any age, usually resolves within days to months after drug withdrawal, is symmetric, and displays both a relatively rapid resting and an action-postural tremor. Bradykinesia is a major feature. The drugs with the highest capacity for dopaminergic blockade in the nigrostriatal system, such as the piperazine phenothiazines and butyrophenones, cause denervation hypersensitivity. These are also associated with a high incidence of both drug-induced parkinsonism and tardive dyskinesia. The dopamine (D_2) receptor antagonist metoclopramide can cause both parkinsonism and tardive dyskinesia. The concept of dopaminergic blockade causing drug-induced parkinsonism and subsequent denervation hypersensitivity causing tardive dyskinesia may be an oversimplification but is useful in considering these problems.

Choreiform Disorders

The *choreiform disorders* comprise both hereditary and sporadic types, but the clinician is often hampered by an inadequate history as a consequence of adoptions, unrecognized paternity, and lost or suppressed family data. *Huntington disease,* which has a prevalence in the United States of 5 to 10 per 100,000, is the best-known of these disorders. The mean age at onset is 40 years. Chorea or disordered motor control is the usual presentation, but bradykinetic and psychotic forms also occur. Chorea may resemble abnormally quick voluntary movements, especially if the patient incorporates them into seemingly purposeful movements or parakinesias. The movements are increased by stress and walking, and in Huntington disease, they are frequently associated with slower athetoid or later dystonic movements. More generalized motor disorders have features of impaired eye and tongue movements and repetitive movements, which ultimately make driving or even holding a knife unsafe. Dysarthria and dysphagia become end-stage problems. An emotional change near onset is common. Cognitive problems tend to involve attention, concentration, and executive planning. Visual memory is affected more than verbal memory. Huntington disease is an autosomal-dominant disorder characterized by an excessive number of trinucleotide CAG repeats (coding for glutamine) on chromosome 4. A direct correlation between the number of repeats and the age at onset has been found. A mutated form of the normal protein huntingtin is produced in excess. Other diseases have been found associated with abnormal CAG repeats, and many features of the pathogenesis are yet to be clarified. Pathologic studies have shown an extensive loss of caudate head and striatal GABAergic cells of the indirect path to the GPe. Senile chorea and essential chorea may well be late-life forms of Huntington disease.

The inheritance of *neuroacanthocytosis* can be either dominant or recessive. Less severe chorea may manifest as myoclonic jerks, tics, vocalizations, dystonia, and self-mutilation. More than 15% of the red blood cells on smear are acanthocytes. Less common hereditary choreas include *benign hereditary chorea* and *paroxysmal dystonic choreoathetosis*.

The most common *sporadic chorea* is *Sydenham chorea,* which is seen in post-streptococcal infection as part of the rheumatic fever complex. The frequency is decreasing as a consequence of aggressive antibiotic therapy of streptococcal infections. The movements are swifter than those of Huntington disease, and the patients are younger. In addition to the risk for cardiac problems, patients may have some residual chorea and an increased susceptibility to recurrent chorea caused by medications, birth control pills, and pregnancy. *Chorea gravidarum* is chorea during pregnancy. Many patients have a prior history of Sydenham chorea, but a hormonal factor may also be involved. Although vasculitis must be excluded, the pregnancy can proceed to term. Chorea associated with birth control pills is quite similar and ceases when the hormonal preparations are withdrawn. Other causes of sporadic chorea include hyperthyroidism, polycythemia vera, and vasculitis associated with lupus, dopa, or stroke. Neuroleptics may cause tardive dyskinesia (orobuccolingual dyskinesia or a pelvic thrusting form), which may be mistaken for chorea but tends to be more repetitive and stereotypic.

Hemiballismus most commonly occurs as the result of a stroke in a small penetrating artery in the subthalamic nucleus of Luys. The movements are continuous and more violent than in chorea and may result in injury. Hemiballismus tends to subside spontaneously and may evolve into a hemichorea phase.

Athetosis is most commonly associated with perinatal injury, as in prematurity or kernicterus. Later progression may occur. When athetosis develops in response to movements in other parts of the body, it is referred to as *overflow*.

Dystonias

A large group of disorders, referred to as *dystonias,* are the subject of multiple overlapping classifications. *Idiopathic torsion dystonia* begins in childhood and is more common among Ashkenazi Jews. A dominant inheritance pattern and chromosome have been identified, but these may not apply in persons who are not Jewish. Idiopathic torsion dystonia is a generalized process beginning as a localized phenomenon and displaying overflow. It can be a seriously disabling disorder. Affected persons frequently master sensory tricks to suppress abnormal movement. Although dystonia is generally thought of as a sustained posture, movements of varying speeds and types are associated. The sporadic and localized dystonias are 10 times more common, with a prevalence of 30 per 100,000. *Spasmodic torticollis* is the most common form of cervical dystonia; it is often interrupted by placing a finger on the chin. When combined with cranial dystonias, such as blepharospasm, it is referred to as *Meige syndrome*. Other common dystonias include spastic dysphonia and hand dystonias, such as writer's cramp and other occupational cramps. Blepharospasm may be sufficiently severe to cause functional blindness.

Wilson disease is a rare autosomal-recessive disorder (chromosome 13) that presents in childhood with rigidity, bradykinesia, dystonia, and liver dysfunction. Adults may have a psychiatric presentation with tremor (may be coarse) and dysarthria. A Kayser-Fleischer ring in the cornea may be detected as a brown deposit, but a slitlamp examination performed by an ophthalmologist is often required. This disorder is associated with the excessive deposition of copper in affected organs secondary to impaired biliary excretion. The myoclonic disorders are not discussed in this text. However, the presence of myoclonus should prompt consultation of more detailed sources.

HISTORY

The history must include a careful exploration of the birth history. Neurologic disease in the family, in addition to possible psychiatric illness, must be reviewed, with input from older members of the family to obtain information about persons who may have slipped out of family gatherings because of their chronic illness. It may prove necessary to see some family members directly. A history of carbon monoxide exposure must be specifically sought, as must the use of street or designer drugs.

Because of the wide range of movement disorders seen after the use of neuroleptics, including their use for nonpsychiatric purposes (e.g., nausea and vomiting), careful questioning and a high index of suspicion may be required. It is important to remember that tardive movement disorders develop after the reduction or withdrawal of neuroleptic medications, and the patient may be diffident about discussing a nervous breakdown.

The disturbances in posture or movement itself must be analyzed in regard to sudden versus insidiously progressive movement, sensory tricks, ameliorating factors such as alcohol, and exacerbating factors such as stress. Although the spectrum of psychogenic movement disorders is wide, it is important to remember that many tremors and hyperkinetic disorders are exacerbated by stress. A spouse may bitterly complain that the patient with Parkinson disease is more mobile and performs better in the physician's office than at home. Inquiries about time required to dress in the morning and difficulty adjusting clothing after toileting may be helpful.

Autonomic dysfunction should be sought, including orthostatic symptoms, urinary and sweating disturbances, and bowel problems, including constipation.

Because cognitive impairments are associated with many of these disorders, job performance or home responsibilities should be explored.

PHYSICAL EXAMINATION

It may be faster to have an assistant put the patient in a room, but watching the patient walk to the examining room, struggle with clothing, and get on and off the examining table may be more useful than the remainder of the examination. The stooped, small-stepped, shuffling gait of a patient with Parkinson disease immediately raises the diagnostic possibility. Is there any loss or reduction of associated movements? Can the patient rise freely from a sitting posture without having to make several attempts or requiring help from the arms? Are overflow movements elicited by walking or contralateral limb movements? Can the patient stay still or maintain a posture? Is the patient merely fidgety or is the movement abnormal and involuntary? Unfortunately, this group of disorders requires that the examiner look at the patient and reach a diagnostic conclusion both while the patient is aware that an examination is under way and when this is not suspected.

Tremor may be present at rest, while posture is held, and during action. What is the speed and amplitude of tremor? Associated cerebellar ataxia should be sought. Warm sweaty palms, tachycardia, or proptosis in a patient with tremor may direct attention to the thyroid. Resting tremor should always be present in Parkinson disease but can be fairly inconspicuous and asymmetric. Complete absence suggests Parkinson plus. Although postural tremor may be seen in Parkinson disease, it is critical to avoid making a diagnosis on tremor alone in the absence of rigidity and bradykinesia.

Tone should be checked in the distal and proximal muscles and in the axial musculature, such as that of the neck. This may be brought out by asking the patient to make an alternating movement with the other hand. Cogwheel rigidity may be the only indication of a subtle tremor when bradykinesia and rigidity are present. Diminished blinking, a bland and masked facies, micrographia, and a hypophonic voice that fades during a sentence may be seen in akinetic-rigid syndromes. Rigidity is an increase in tone throughout the range of movement that is unrelated to speed. Spasticity is velocity-dependent and is best characterized by the spastic catch. Spasticity is associated with corticospinal dysfunction. Paratonia increases with age and manifests as *gegenhalten* (involuntary intermittent resistance to passive movement) and *mitgehen* (a seeming effort to cooperate with the examiner); it is associated with dementia when marked.

The Babinski reflex is absent in Parkinson disease but present in some other disorders. It must be distinguished from the "striatal toe," which is really a dystonic dorsiflexion and is more prolonged and not related to the stimulus.

The eye movements must be examined for ocular dysmetria and hypometric or hypermetric saccades, in addition to impairments in vertical or horizontal gaze. Lost voluntary eye movements in progressive supranuclear palsy are surprisingly full with head turning (which elicits the oculocephalic reflex).

The patient should be checked for orthostatic hypotension and sweating. Early orthostasis, anhidrosis, bladder dysfunction, and impotence may reflect multiple system atrophy rather than Parkinson disease.

Retropulsion and postural instability can be checked by standing behind the patient and giving a quick backward pull. Parkinson disease may progress to the stage at which the postural reflexes are lost and the patient falls backward in the direction of the pull with no attempt to compensate. Patients with Parkinson disease fall, but when the falls occur early in the course, progressive supranuclear palsy should be considered.

Some interesting phenomena include the retained ability of patients with Parkinson disease to catch a ball of paper thrown to them despite considerable bradykinesia. Rocking the patient will facilitate walking, as will stripes on the floor.

Normal movements should be smooth without unexplained interruptions. Motor impersistence may characterize chorea, and the examiner should watch for parakinesias. The patient who holds a finger or hand to the chin may be demonstrating a sensory trick used to stabilize torticollis or to assist weak cervical muscles in myasthenia gravis.

The patient with involuntary movements should be observed long enough to determine whether the movements display a recurrent pattern and whether they are generalized or segmental. Videotaping may make it possible to analyze the patient's movements outside the office setting.

The neurologic examination must be sufficiently thorough to indicate whether the problem is really a multisystem atrophy. The mental status examination must determine the presence of either dementia or depression.

LABORATORY AND IMAGING STUDIES

In many of the movement disorders, the diagnosis is based completely on the clinical evidence, including the history and an analysis of the patient's motor function. Imaging studies may be needed to explain an unexpected finding, such as an extensor plantar response associated with an old stroke or myelopathy. The neurologic workup of all these disorders follows the neurologic examination. Exceptions include visualization of the ventricles when hydrocephalus is being considered and atrophy of the caudate head in possible Huntington disease, and genetic analysis in olivopontocerebellar atrophy and Huntington disease. Measurement of the serum ceruloplasmin and urinary copper levels or a liver biopsy to detect the effects of copper may help in the diagnosis of Wilson disease.

TREATMENT

The treatment of Parkinson disease is evolving as new agents are developed and our understanding of the pathogenesis improves. Early disease does not require treatment. The management generally involves a slow initiation of medications, preferably at low doses. When polypharmacy proves necessary, only one medication should be changed at a time. Selegiline is a monoamine oxidase (MAO) B inhibitor that prolongs the efficacy of levodopa. It can therefore be used to manage end-of-dose wearing off. It has a minimal effect in untreated patients, but evidence suggests that it may slow the progression of disease. Induction of hypertensive crises is not a problem unless doses above the recommended 10 mg/d are used, when MAO A activity can develop. Side effects include interactions with meperidine and fluoxetine, activation of peptic ulcers, orthostatic hypotension, and an increase in levodopa-induced confusion. Insomnia can be avoided by administering the drug early in the day.

The antiviral agent amantadine (100 mg twice daily) has a greater effect on rigidity and bradykinesia than anticholinergics and a smaller effect than levodopa. It may act at presynaptic and postsynaptic dopaminergic terminals, in addition to having an anticholinergic effect. The effect declines with time, but some can be sustained. Side effects include livedo reticularis, edema, dry mouth, and blurred vision. Confusional states may require reduction of the dose or withdrawal, especially in demented patients. Excretion is renal.

Anticholinergic drugs were the old standards. These reduce symptoms to a modest degree. They are used only minimally now for tremor and rigidity. Slow titration of trihexyphenidyl to 2 mg three times daily or benztropine to 0.5 mg four times daily can be used. Side effects of anticholinergics include aggravation of glaucoma, urinary retention, and constipation. Sialorrhea may be decreased by anticholinergics. The most significant problem is a relatively poor tolerance of these agents in the elderly, with associated delirium, hallucinations, memory loss, and sedation.

The most significant advance in the pharmacotherapy of Parkinson disease was the discovery of levodopa. Levodopa can pass the blood-brain barrier (unlike dopamine) and is decarboxylated in the brain to dopamine. Aromatic amino acid decarboxylase is diminished in Parkinson disease, but not as severely as the rate-limiting enzyme tyrosine hydroxylase. Extensive peripheral decarboxylation was a problem until a peripherally active decarboxylase inhibitor that does not cross the blood-brain barrier, carbidopa, was administered concurrently with levodopa (Sinemet). An unresolved issue is the possibility that dopamine increases oxidative toxicity and accelerates the progression of disease. Some physicians start with dopamine agonists and delay levodopa therapy for this reason. Most neurologists begin Sinemet therapy when bradykinesia and rigidity begin to impede job performance or interfere with the activities of daily living. The medication is usually introduced as half of a 25-100 pill three times daily, with a gradual increase to a 25-100 pill three times daily. Early side effects, which tend to subside, include anorexia, nausea and vomiting, orthostatic hypotension, and cardiac rhythm disturbances. When lower doses of Sinemet are used for a protracted period, it may be necessary to add supplemental carbidopa. Initially, gastrointestinal intolerance is avoided by giving the medication with meals. Supplemental carbidopa may be helpful, as may be domperidone. (Domperidone is not approved in the United States and must be obtained from Canada at significant expense to the patient.) Because other aromatic amino acids interfere with the absorption of levodopa, the doses are timed not to be taken concurrently with meals high in protein after initial therapy seems satisfactory. The effect is gradual, and weeks must be allowed to assess the maximum therapeutic benefit. Most patients with Parkinson disease show sustained improvement with therapy, and the absence of such improvement calls the diagnosis into question. Reasons for levodopa failure include inadequate dosing or the concurrent administration of a dopaminergic blocker, such as metoclopramide, a phenothiazine, or a butyrophenone. Patients and referring physicians are often disturbed by a lack of control of tremor or even an increase in tremor. This reflects a failure to use the correct index of rigidity or bradykinesia. Levodopa is a poor agent for controlling tremor. Reducing rigidity and bradykinesia, may allow tremor to be manifest. Patients can clearly benefit by increasing the dosage (Sinemet 25-250 three or four times daily) to titrate against side effects. A large minority of neurologists try to minimize the levodopa dosage by using dopamine agonists early if moderate doses of levodopa prove inadequate.

Levodopa therapy is complicated by a variety of intercurrent problems. Although the patient with Parkinson disease can respond to stress (jumping up from the porch rocker and running away when someone shouts "Fire," only to freeze subsequently), the bradykinetic state returns once the patient is safe. The number of these fluctuations increases as the severity of disease and duration of therapy increase. Freezing may occur during turning or when a doorway is reached. *Freezing* is the term used to describe the behavior of a patient who has been ambulating successfully and suddenly stops. Freezing is most distressing to both patient and caregivers, who may think freezing is a voluntary effort of the patient to be ornery. Initially, the episodes tend to be simple wearing-off phenomena that are relieved by more frequent dosing, use of the sustained-release form of levodopa or longer-acting dopamine agonists. When fluctuations occur, the patient must keep a log indicating the time of "off" periods. The patient may not distinguish between tremor and chorea unless this log is reviewed. Although the sustained-release preparation would appear to be an easy solution (with Sinemet CR 50-200 substituted for Sinemet 25-100), this is not the case. Retitration becomes necessary. The response in the morning may be inordinately delayed. As the central storage capability decreases, frequent small doses are helpful, but it may be difficult for patients to comply with this suggestion. Supplemental agonists may be helpful because of their lesser tendency to induce dyskinesias. These are discussed later. A wide variety of abnormal movements are induced by levodopa. High- and low-dose dopa dyskinesias are being clarified by dopamine receptor subtype analysis. Foot dystonia is often a low-dose phenomenon. High-dose chorea and low-dose dystonia often respond to lowering the levodopa dose at the price of decreased mobility. Levodopa holidays fail to produce lasting effects and can be life-threatening.

The dopamine agonists readily enter the brain and require no metabolic conversion. Those in current use have a long half-life and are highly potent. Because, unlike levodopa, they are not generators of free radicals, they have the theoretic advantage of not accelerating progression of the disease. Semisynthetic ergot alkaloids such as bromocriptine (D_2 receptor) and pergolide (D_1 and D_2 receptors) were the initial agents but were replaced by pramipexole and ropinirole, which are not ergots. These agents all are active at D_2 receptors but vary in their D_1, serotoninergic, and noradrenergic actions. Pramipexole may cause a profound urge to sleep. Bromocriptine is most familiar to gynecologists because it is used to prevent galactorrhea. The agonists have a long blood half-life, but their anti-Parkinson effect is significantly shorter. When they are used as initial monotherapy, levodopa supplementation may be required within a year. As supplements of levodopa, they may allow dose reduction, and their longer duration of action may reduce nocturnal or early morning immobility or dystonia. Some reduction in wearing off can be anticipated. Agonist side effects resemble those of levodopa. Except for the dyskinesias, the side effects tend to be more severe and last longer. The dosage varies: bromocriptine (15–60 mg/d), pergolide (2–4 mg/d), pramipexole (to 4.5 mg/d), ropinirole (up to 12 mg/d).

The problems of frequent dosing and motor fluctuations were addressed by the development of the catechol-O-methyl transferases entacapone and tolcapone. Although tolcapone has some attractive features, its potential to cause hepatotoxicity limits its appeal.

Depression affects almost half of patients with Parkinson disease and can be treated with a serotonin reuptake inhibitor or a tricyclic agent, but MAO A inhibitors must be avoided because of the risk for hypertensive crises when they are combined with Sinemet.

All the anti-Parkinson medications cause mental side effects, and too frequently these limit therapy. Dementia occurs in about 15% of patients with Parkinson disease, and the rate is higher in the Parkinson plus group. The caregiver should be alert to the possibility of delirium because this is probably a reversible process. Although it may be a sign of systemic illness, it may also be drug-induced. An early feature in levodopa therapy is visual hallucinosis. This may manifest as hallucinations of soft, fuzzy, nonfrightening "critters" in the patient's bed or figures standing in the room at night. Benign hallucinosis may progress so that these things are perceived as real, and paranoid ideation may develop. Reducing medications may resolve this problem, but at a loss of therapeutic benefit. Overt psychosis is more common in patients with incipient dementia and generally includes features of florid visual hallucinations and paranoia. Clozapine in very low doses may be effective and make it possible to continue anti-Parkinson medications. Clozapine is associated with agranulocytosis. Olanzapine has the potential to enhance parkinsonian symptoms, and the drug most often used now is quetiapine.

Sleep disturbances are common in the elderly and are increased by nocturia, sleep fragmentation secondary to the use of alcohol and other sedative drugs, the pain of arthritis, and many other factors. This chapter is concerned only with Parkinson-related factors. Sleep apnea is increased in Parkinson disease. Restless legs and nocturnal myoclonus may benefit from clonazepam or propoxyphene. Depression should be treated if present. Rigidity makes rolling over in bed a problem, and tremor may retard sleep. A trapeze can help the patient roll over and facilitates arising for toileting.

Pain may occur primarily in the shoulder girdle and respond to anti-Parkinson medications. Dystonia can be painful, and akathisia may be described as pain.

Constipation is almost the rule. High-fiber diets, bulk-forming agents, and stool softeners should be tried early. Cisapride seems to be well tolerated and is effective. Lactulose and other osmotic agents may induce a watery diarrhea that is difficult for a patient with reduced mobility to manage. Mineral oil predisposes to aspiration in this population.

Swallowing problems and aspiration are not unusual.

Urinary problems are multifactorial in this population. Nocturia may be relieved by oxybutynin or tolterodine. Detrusor hyperreflexia may be suppressed by anticholinergics, which may also cause retention. The risk for retention is less problematic in women because they do not have prostatism. One cannot assume that urinary problems are either disease- or drug-related without an evaluation. Sexual dysfunction is common and related to chronic illness, immobility, mental status changes, and autonomic dysfunction.

Falling is complex and does not respond to levodopa.

Surgical procedures decreased markedly after the advent of levodopa, but they have regained a significant role in this disorder. Ventrolateral thalamotomy reduces tremor and rigidity, but not bradykinesia. Posteroventral pallidotomy has relieved tremor, rigidity, and bradykinesia. The most exciting procedures are probably deep brain stimulation of the ventroposterolateral thalamus for tremor and of the subthalamic nucleus for rigidity and bradykinesia. Fetal cell transplantation remains experimental.

Treating early Parkinson disease is frequently a simple and very gratifying affair for the first few years. However, once wearing off, dyskinesias and other problems develop, treatment is best managed by a physician experienced in the subtle nuances that allow a patient to remain functional.

Neuroleptic malignant syndrome is a potentially lethal condition characterized by fever, muscle rigidity, autonomic instability, and altered consciousness that can be precipitated by dopaminergic withdrawal, lithium, and neuroleptics. Prompt dopaminergic restitution is in order.

Essential tremor is relieved by alcohol, but this therapy is problematic because of the potential for abuse. Primidone in low doses has proved the most effective agent for management, but because of side effects of nausea, unsteadiness, vertigo, and clouding of consciousness, very slow initiation of therapy is required. The use of more than 250 mg seems to add little to effectiveness. Blood levels are not helpful. If tolerated, propranolol in doses of up to 240 to 360 mg/d seems optimal. Propranolol may be tried if primidone is not tolerated.

Wilson disease is managed with copper chelators. A wide range of agents is used for Huntington disease, including dopamine receptor antagonists, dopamine-depleting agents, benzodiazepines, and anticonvulsants. Therapy for Huntington disease must be considered unsatisfactory and can best be managed by an experienced specialist in movement disorders.

Dystonias can be managed by local injections of botulinum toxin when the symptoms are sufficiently discrete, such as blepharospasm, spastic dysphonia, and cervical dystonia. The generalized dystonias have been variously treated with anticholinergics, dopaminergics, antidopaminergics, benzodiazepines, and baclofen. Surgical therapy includes thalamotomy, selective nerve root section, and myotomy. Myoclonus may be reduced by clonazepam. The therapy of dystonia, myoclonus, and tic disorders, including Tourette syndrome, is complex and best referred to experienced physicians. Tardive dyskinesias can be managed by titrating the neuroleptic to the lowest possible dose in unstable patients and then considering specific therapy with dopamine-depleting agents or benzodiazepines. The dose may be slowly tapered in a stable patient and the patient then observed off the drug to determine the degree of disability. The management is complex and fraught with medicolegal problems. Referral to experienced physicians is urged.

CONSIDERATIONS DURING PREGNANCY

Major issues to be considered in pregnancy include the teratogenicity of the specific agents used and the risks associated with drug withdrawal. Selegiline is best withdrawn several weeks before surgery and meperidine avoided. In patients with essential tremor, medication withdrawal seems best. Parkinson disease rarely affects women of childbearing age. Tardive dyskinesias have been reported in the offspring of patients treated with neuroleptics. Patients with the other movement disorders should be managed in concert with experts. Many of these disorders involve hereditary factors, which should be explored with the prospective mother before pregnancy.

A specific issue is chorea gravidarum, which is the development of chorea during pregnancy. A third of these patients have a history of Sydenham chorea. Although they should be checked for activation of streptococcal infection, this is infrequent. Thyrotoxicosis and connective tissue disease must be ruled out. There is no reason to terminate the pregnancy.

BIBLIOGRAPHY

Jankovic J, Tolosa E, eds. *Parkinson's disease and movement disorders,* 4th ed. Philadelphia: Lippincott Williams & Wilkins, 2002.

Jankovic J. Parkinson's disease therapy: tailoring choices for early and late disease, young and old patients. *Clin Neuropharmacol* 2000;23:252.

Joseph AB, Young RR, eds. *Movement disorders.* Boston: Blackwell Science, 1992.

Kurlan R. *Treatment of movement disorder.* Philadelphia: JB Lippincott, 1995.

Limousin P, Krack P, Pollak P, et al. Electrical stimulation of the subthalamic nucleus in advanced Parkinson's disease. *N Engl J Med* 1998;339:1105.

Marsden CD, Fahn S, eds. *Movement disorders 3.* Oxford: Butterworth-Heinemann,1994.

Nutt JG, Hammerstad JP, Gancher ST. *Parkinson's disease: 100 maxims.* St. Louis: Mosby, 1992.

Parker WD Jr, Boyson SJ, Parks JK. Abnormalities of the electron transport chain in idiopathic Parkinson's disease. *Ann Neurol* 1989;26:719

Sethi KD. Clinical aspects of Parkinson disease. *Curr Opin Neurol* 2002;15:457.

CHAPTER 107

Transient Cerebral Ischemia and Stroke

Joshua Hollander

Stroke remains the third leading cause of death in the United States and is also a major cause of disability. The management of stroke is far less effective than prevention, so it is gratifying that major inroads have been made in identifying stroke risk factors and interventions. Research into the mechanisms and management of acute stroke has dramatically advanced, and the large number of promising treatment trials in progress suggests that an array of therapeutic options for acute stroke may soon be available.

In an ischemic stroke, a core area of the cerebrum is subjected to profound ischemia, and necrosis is a consequence. An area of sublethal ischemia (ischemic penumbra) can be preserved if flow is restored promptly. The therapeutic window is not well defined but probably is measured in hours, not minutes. The tissue in the ischemic penumbra may recover or may progress to delayed programmed cell death through a series of complex changes not yet fully identified; changes related to increased intracellular calcium levels, calcium-activated cytotoxic enzymes, free radicals, excitatory amino acid toxicity, cytokines, intercellular adhesion molecules, and programmed cell death have all been explored. We are at the stage of excellent management of experimental stroke in rodents, but in humans, successful treatments are as yet unproven.

The older classification of stroke by temporal profile has fallen into disfavor because of the realization that transient ischemic attacks (TIAs) last no more than 1 hour, the frequent finding on neuroimaging studies of areas of minor infarction in patients with TIAs, and the absence of well-defined areas of infarction in many patients with clearly persistent deficits. Temporal classification and the TIA concept were of considerable early value but later served to retard stroke research. Treatment was withheld for 24 hours in trials to prevent confusing stroke with TIA. As a result, the therapeutic window (3–8 hours) was allowed to pass, and the failure of any treatment under consideration was almost guaranteed. Rational stroke therapy requires the treating physician to analyze the probable mechanism of stroke and select appropriate measures for treatment and prevention.

Many trials of the treatment of stroke will yield results within the next few years. We are faced with the need to enroll patients in trials of hyperacute (90–180 minutes) or acute (3–8 hours) management because we must remain within the therapeutic window. However, the public and many health care professionals have not yet accepted the concept of stroke as a "brain attack" worthy of care as serious and urgent as that given for a heart attack. Time may be muscle, but it is also brain. The more we delay in getting patients with stroke into the system, the fewer patients will be available for trials and the more years will elapse before a meaningful therapeutic intervention is discovered.

Predictors of stroke include factors that we cannot control, such as age and male sex. Race is a complex factor; blacks are excessively prone to hypertension, hemorrhagic and ischemic stroke, and intracranial vascular disease. Persons of Japanese ancestry exhibit different stroke profiles in Japan, Hawaii, and the mainland United States, presumably related to dietary factors. Hispanics (a mixed population) occupy an intermediate position. Genetic factors are not fully defined. Modifiable risk factors include hypertension for all types of stroke and heart disease for ischemic stroke. Nonvalvular atrial fibrillation becomes a progressively more important risk with increasing age. Coronary heart disease, left ventricular hypertrophy on electrocardiography, and congestive heart failure all increase the risk for stroke. Prior major stroke, minor stroke, transient hemispheric ischemia, transient monocular blindness, and asymptomatic carotid stenosis all increase the risk for stroke, in declining order. Diabetes increases the risk for all types of ischemic stroke, and cigarette smoking is associated with a lesser increase in all types of stroke. Hypercholesterolemia is a minor risk factor independent of heart disease. Alcohol is more of a risk factor for hemorrhagic stroke, and hypocholesterolemia may increase the risk for intracerebral hemorrhagic stroke.

The number of deaths caused by stroke has been declining gradually for many years. This trend has accelerated since effective, well-tolerated therapy for hypertension became available. The effective treatment of streptococcal infections has reduced the rate of rheumatic heart disease, and attention to lifestyle and serum lipid levels has reduced or delayed ischemic heart disease. Carotid endarterectomy markedly reduces the risk in patients with symptomatic stenoses occluding more than 70% of the lumen. The beneficial effect is much lower in asymptomatic patients and occurs primarily in men. Warfarin therapy markedly reduces cardioembolic events, including those secondary to nonvalvular atrial fibrillation.

ETIOLOGY AND DIFFERENTIAL DIAGNOSIS

The older classification of stroke based on the temporal profile is being replaced by one that emphasizes mechanism (Table 107.1). When the etiologic mechanisms of stroke are assessed, a large percentage of strokes are classified as cryptogenic, but newer diagnostic techniques are reducing the size of this group, which is thought to include many cases of embolism without an identifiable source.

Large vessel thrombosis is usually associated with atherosclerosis. Extracranial vascular disease is more common among whites, but the incidence of intracranial stenosis is higher in blacks. Atherosclerosis of the coronary arteries tends to develop 10 years earlier than carotid disease. The risk for carotid steno-

TABLE 107.1. Classification of Stroke by Mechanism

Ischemic
Thrombosis
Large vessel extracranial occlusion
Large vessel intracranial occlusion
Small vessel intracranial occlusion
Embolism
Cardiogenic
Paradoxical
Arterioarterial
Impaired systemic perfusion
Other known causes
Coagulopathies
Vasculitis
Cryptogenic
Hemorrhagic
Subarachnoid hemorrhage
Intracerebral hemorrhage

TABLE 107.2. Cardiac Diseases Causing Cerebral Embolism

Cardiac dysrhythmias
Nonvalvular atrial fibrillation
Chronic sinoatrial disorder
Ischemic heart disease
Acute myocardial infarction
Left ventricular aneurysm
Rheumatic valvular disease
Mitral stenosis
Mitral incompetence
Aortic valve disease
Prosthetic heart valves
Less common sources
Mitral annulus calcification
Mitral valve prolapse
Idiopathic hypertrophic subaortic stenosis
Cardiomyopathies
Nonbacterial thrombotic endocarditis
Infective endocarditis
Cardiac myxoma
Paradoxical embolism

sis is higher in patients with peripheral vascular disease. Carotid stenosis may present with major vascular territory symptoms or with tandem branch occlusions. Strokes in the anterior cerebral territory generally affect the lower limbs; strokes in the middle cerebral territory, which are far more common, tend to involve the face and hands. Dysphasia, acalculia, and apraxias tend to be associated with left perisylvian lesions (especially in right-handed patients); impaired prosody implicates the right temporal lobe, and spatial perceptual problems are associated with strokes in the right parietal area. Carotid occlusions may be asymptomatic or present with partial or complete middle cerebral territory infarcts, or even combined massive anterior and middle cerebral territory infarcts. Partial infarcts may be arterioarterial emboli or distal field ischemia. Distal field ischemia tends to favor watershed involvement; this is generally associated with proximal weakness rather than the typical distal weakness. Posterior cerebral territory infarcts are more commonly embolic and cause visual field loss and memory loss if bilateral. Basilar territory strokes present with crossed cranial nerve and long tract signs. The "top of the basilar" is the first narrow point in the posterior circulation; various syndromes develop if saddle emboli become fragmented and occlude the mesencephalic vessels, the vessels that penetrate the thalamus, or the superior cerebellar or posterior cerebral artery. Strokes in the territory of the posterior circulation may affect consciousness.

Small vessel intracranial disease is primarily associated with hypertension, but the rate is also increased among diabetics. Lacunar strokes, infarcts of about 5 mm, are caused by the occlusion of small deep penetrating arteries (primarily secondary to hypertension). Multiple clinical syndromes have been defined, such as pure motor hemiplegia, pure sensory stroke, ataxic hemiparesis, sensory-motor stroke, and clumsy hand-dysarthria syndrome.

Embolic stroke may be cardiogenic, paradoxical, or arterioarterial. Some cardiogenic mechanisms are listed in Table 107.2. The risk for recurrent embolization varies with the source; it is high in transmural anterior wall myocardial infarction and low in mitral valve prolapse. Some cardiac lesions, such as mitral annulus calcification, increase the risk for stroke but may be associated with intracranial pathology rather than embolization. Paradoxical emboli require a connection between the pulmonary and systemic circulations, such as an atrial septal defect or intrapulmonary shunt. The Valsalva maneuver or a pulmonary embolus may shift pressures and open a foramen ovale or induce right-to-left shunting. Older patients are also prone to aortic arch plaque and clot with secondary embolization. Ulcerated carotid plaque with stenosis may also be a source of arterioarterial embolization. Embolic lesions may cause branch occlusions and present with isolated hand weakness and numbness, isolated aphasia, or isolated hemianopia.

Impaired systemic perfusion results from prolonged hypotension below the limits of autoregulation. Inadequate cerebral blood flow is most marked in the watershed territory between the distribution areas of the major cerebral vessels and causes the previously described characteristic pattern of deficits.

Generally, thrombosis does not occur in small cortical branches because atherosclerosis does not usually develop there. Vasculitis and hypercoagulable states are exceptions, as is distal field ischemia resulting from a proximal occlusion and inadequate perfusion (with or without overly enthusiastic antihypertensive therapy).

Venous sinus thrombosis or cortical vein thrombosis occurs primarily in the context of hypercoagulable states and presents a less familiar pattern. When the venous sinuses are involved, hemorrhagic infarction is not unusual, and intracranial pressure may be increased because of impaired venous drainage.

Intracerebral hemorrhage is usually associated with vascular malformations in the young. These continue to be a problem later in life, but other factors, such as hypertensive ganglionic hemorrhage, also contribute. This used to be the most common cause of intracerebral hemorrhage, but as a result of more effective antihypertensive therapy, hypertensive ganglionic hemorrhage now occurs less frequently. Cerebral amyloid angiopathy is currently the major cause of intracerebral hemorrhage and is seen as lobar hemorrhage in elderly patients.

The frequency of subarachnoid hemorrhage has not decreased, and we have not succeeded in reducing the associated mortality. Many patients with aneurysmal subarachnoid hemorrhage die of the first bleed before an aneurysm is detected. Spontaneous subarachnoid bleeding in children is caused primarily by vascular malformations, but in teenagers and older persons, the primary consideration is aneurysm.

The full definition of a stroke requires attention to both the vascular and functional anatomy of the brain. The physician should be able to make a reasonable estimate of the location and mechanism of a stroke based on the history, neurologic and vascular examination findings, results of laboratory and imaging studies, and pattern of symptoms. No single test provides all the information required, but experienced physicians can classify most patients. The mechanism of a stroke may remain obscure, either because none is evident or because multiple factors may be responsible (e.g., atrial fibrillation, hypertension, diabetes, and carotid stenosis are all present). Not every neurologic event or deficit is vascular in origin.

HISTORY

Typically, the onset of a stroke syndrome is abrupt and apoplectic, but thrombotic strokes may present with a stuttering onset. Carotid strokes may evolve over a day; basilar occlusions may progress over several days. Newer therapies require a precise definition of the time of onset of ischemic strokes, and careful probing may be necessary to elicit subtle behavioral changes or mild degrees of unsteadiness or weakness. Patients who awaken with a deficit are more likely to have a thrombotic stroke; an abrupt onset in an awake, active patient favors embolic mechanisms. The onset of stroke is dated from the last time the patient was well; in a patient who awakens at 8 a.m., the onset of stroke is considered to be at bedtime. A history of recurrent stereotypic events such as transient visual loss or hemiparesis favors large vessel extracranial disease. Recurrent pure motor hemiparesis or pure hemisensory syndromes may be signs of lacunar stroke. The repertory of responses to injury of the nervous system is limited, and once the lesion is localized, the tempo of the lesion leads to the diagnosis.

A previous TIA favors thrombotic stroke and, depending on the clinical profile, suggests either large vessel or lacunar syndrome. Recurrent symptoms brought on by arm use may suggest subclavian steal, which is caused by proximal subclavian occlusion with secondary reversal of flow in the vertebral artery to deliver blood to the involved arm.

Transient neurologic dysfunction can have many causes. Nocturnal hand numbness and tingling, in addition to finger weakness, may reflect carpal tunnel syndrome or cervical radiculopathy secondary to cervical osteoarthritis. The deficit of a TIA of vascular origin is abrupt and changes little during the attack. The hand may drop limply to the bed, with diminished sensation. When the deficit begins in the fingertips and slowly moves up the hand and arm over a 15-minute period, a transient migrainous attack is more likely. Migraine subsides later in life, and if an isolated migrainous aura develops many years later, the patient may not recall the similarity to the old migrainous aura unless specifically questioned. Such questioning may obviate the need for an expensive workup.

The "worst headache of my life" suggests subarachnoid hemorrhage. Headache, nausea and vomiting, and a rapidly progressing stroke imply intracranial hemorrhage. Ischemic stroke cannot be fully distinguished from hemorrhagic stroke by the history alone.

PHYSICAL EXAMINATION

A patient having a stroke requires a careful neurologic examination to attempt to localize the lesion and its vascular pattern. The screening neurologic examination should assess the mental status (level of consciousness, attention, language, memory, gnosis, and praxis), cranial nerves, motor and sensory function (including at least one cortical sensory modality), coordination, and reflexes. Stance and gait must be evaluated. The general examination should include the vital signs. The peripheral pulses should be noted, including the carotid and vertebral pulses and bruits, in addition to the timing of the radial pulses to exclude subclavian steal. The possibility of aortic dissection should be considered during the pulse examination. The heart is checked for murmurs or rhythm disturbances and signs of congestive failure. A funduscopic examination may provide insight into the severity and duration of diabetes mellitus and hypertension. Subhyaloid hemorrhages are characteristic of subarachnoid hemorrhage. The skin, mucous membranes, and conjunctivae should be surveyed for embolic lesions. Fever may occur with time in subarachnoid or pontine hemorrhage but is otherwise unusual in stroke; if present, it suggests endocarditis as a cause of embolic stroke or intercurrent pulmonary or urinary tract infection.

Loss of consciousness is uncommon in stroke and should alert the examiner to the possibility of a subdural hematoma or other intracranial mass lesion. Brainstem or large hemispheric strokes or bleeds may alter consciousness, but the "sleepy stroke" warrants prompt imaging studies.

Patients with small sentinel bleeds of subarachnoid hemorrhage may not exhibit any focal neurologic signs; if subarachnoid hemorrhage is suspected because the patient has a thunderclap headache, meningeal signs should be sought (photophobia, nuchal rigidity [resistance to neck flexion but not rotation], Kernig and Brudzinski signs). The Kernig sign, which is relatively nonspecific, is pain in the back of the thigh in response to knee extension when the hip, knee, and ankle are flexed at 90 degrees. The leg Brudzinski sign is contralateral hip flexion elicited when the Kernig maneuver is performed. The neck Brudzinski sign is flexion of both hips when the neck is passively flexed. Meningeal signs may take time to develop; they are most striking when blood breakdown has already occurred.

Forced eye deviation away from the hemiplegic side occurs in supratentorial lesions; the reverse may be seen in brainstem stroke. Eyes beating to the side of the hemiparesis should alert the examiner to the likelihood of status epilepticus. A Horner syndrome, with or without neck and orbital pain, may suggest carotid dissection. Intracerebral hemorrhage may cause characteristic disturbances in eye movement. Putaminal hemorrhage may cause early transtentorial herniation, with the development of a nearly blown pupil on the side of the lesion as a consequence of third nerve compromise. Thalamic hemorrhage may cause downward pressure on the superior colliculi, with impairment of upward gaze and the so-called sunset sign, in which one or both eyes look toward the nose. Patients with cerebellar hemorrhage may display nystagmus and gaze palsy without hemiparesis early in the bleed. Pontine hemorrhage is associated with pinpoint pupils secondary to loss of descending sympathetics.

LABORATORY AND IMAGING STUDIES

Routine laboratory studies should include a complete blood cell count, platelet count, and measurement of the prothrombin time and partial thromboplastin time to screen for sepsis, blood dyscrasias, and coagulopathies. Urinalysis and the Westergren sedimentation rate may provide clues to concurrent vasculitis. Hyperglycemia is a poor prognostic sign. Screening chemistries should also be performed. A chest film and an electrocardiogram are obtained and may be followed by a Holter examination if intermittent atrial fibrillation is suspected but not seen on the initial electrocardiogram.

Patients younger than 60 years should undergo a more detailed battery of tests to exclude a procoagulant state before anticoagulants are administered. Appropriate studies might include screening for protein C, protein S, antithrombin III, resistance to activated protein C (factor V Leiden), prothrombin 20210, lupus anticoagulant, and anticardiolipin antibodies and a serologic test for syphilis. These studies are important mainly in patients with cryptogenic stroke or a history of recurrent thrombotic episodes and in young patients,.

It takes time for cerebral computed tomography (CT) to show a stroke, and the National Stroke Data Bank studies indicate that up to 40% of strokes are never apparent on CT. CT is usually performed early in the stroke because it is exquisitely sensitive to intracranial hemorrhage and can exclude mass lesions. Early changes may include subtle effacement of the sulci or a white vessel suggestive of an occlusion. CT is less sensitive to subarachnoid hemorrhage but detects more than 90% of cases on day 1, decreasing in sensitivity with time from the ictus. The thickness of the clot on CT is a good predictor of the delayed development of an ischemic neurologic deficit.

When the mechanism of stroke remains obscure despite studies, it sometimes helps to perform another imaging study after 3 to 5 days. Magnetic resonance imaging (MRI) can be used for this purpose. MRI is more sensitive than CT and can detect lesions in the posterior fossa. It also detects significantly smaller lesions than can be seen on CT. It was formerly less specific for acute hemorrhage than CT, but the use of echoplanar imaging has greatly enhanced this capability. When available readily, MRI is much more useful than CT. It visualizes a stroke within 15 minutes after the ictus by means of diffusion-weighted imaging. Discrepancy between the area of infarction delineated by diffusion-weighted imaging and the area of perfusion abnormality seen on perfusion MRI may display the ischemic penumbra (brain at risk). Fluid-attenuated inversion recovery (FLAIR) sequences are helpful in showing the extent of prior areas of infarction.

Selective angiography performed via the femoral route is the definitive method of visualizing the cerebral circulation. Digital subtraction techniques allow more rapid studies with less catheter time and a lower dose of contrast. This minimizes risk, but about 1% of patients still sustain a transient or permanent neurologic deficit. Arch aortography is associated with a comparable risk, creates images with overlapping shadows, and does not provide intracranial images. MRI can be combined with magnetic resonance angiography. This technique takes advantage of the lack of signal in blood moving rapidly perpendicular to the plane of examination to show vessels without contrast. Magnetic resonance angiography tends to overestimate stenoses, and other limitations do not allow it to serve as a gold standard, but nevertheless it often provides adequate information to obviate the need for more invasive studies.

In spiral CT, a slipped conduction ring (allowing the radiation source and detectors to make continuous circular movements) and a steadily moving table (thrusting the head through the gantry) allow ultrarapid filming. With a contrast injection, a reliable image of the carotid bifurcation can be obtained. CT angiography, especially with volume rendering, is an elegant technique that may show aneurysms and intracranial stenoses.

Carotid duplex examinations (B-mode image of the vessel combined with pulsed-wave Doppler measurement of velocity) have a sensitivity and specificity of more than 90% in detecting high-grade carotid stenoses and should especially be performed in patients with anterior circulation strokes. Transcranial Doppler sonography offers a picture of the collateral circulation, cerebrovascular reserve, and intracranial posterior circulation. A pattern of microembolic signals may provide evidence of cardiogenic or arterioarterial sources. Transcranial Doppler sonography makes use of temporal bone thinning (window) and the planar arrangement of the circle of Willis. Distal branches cannot be examined. Two-dimensional imaging has not added much to the usual blind technique.

Transthoracic echocardiography is performed when the patient does not have atrial fibrillation or another known source of embolic stroke. Left ventricular wall dysfunction or ventricular aneurysm may suggest an embolic source. A 3- to 4-mm clot is sufficient to obstruct the middle cerebral artery and is near the limit of resolution of transthoracic echocardiography, so that performing transthoracic echocardiography to detect clot is unrewarding.

When the mechanism of stroke remains cryptogenic, especially in a young patient, transesophageal echocardiography may be helpful. This tends to be avoided because the patient must swallow the probe catheter and often requires sedation. The view displays the left atrium and appendage and the interatrial septum; part of the thoracic aorta can also be seen. This is the best study for cardiac embolic disease, showing the mitral valve, interatrial septal aneurysm, interatrial septal defect, spontaneous echo contrast (smoke), and aortic wall clot. An injection of agitated saline solution provides microbubble contrast, which clarifies a right-to-left shunt. A Valsalva maneuver may be needed to open the flap of a patent foramen ovale. Transcranial Doppler ultrasonography can also be used to demonstrate a right-to-left shunt. It provides no direct evidence of the intracardiac defect but may detect intrapulmonary shunts. Almost 15% of normal persons have a patent foramen ovale, but young patients with cryptogenic stroke tend to have larger shunts, and the frequency is three times greater.

Lumbar puncture has become less important in patients with stroke since the advent of new technology but remains the definitive test for subarachnoid hemorrhage. If this is clinically suspected but the CT findings are negative, a careful lumbar puncture should be performed. The opening pressure should be recorded and three or four tubes collected. If the fluid is bloody, the first and fourth tube counts should be compared to assess clearing. The spun supernatant fluid should be examined for xanthochromia. When the peripheral blood cell counts are normal, the fluid usually contains 700 red cells for each white cell and 1 mg of extra protein (if the tap is traumatic). When the tap is performed several days after a subarachnoid hemorrhage, an excess of white cells is usually noted, and only a culture can definitively confirm infection.

TREATMENT

The prevention of stroke is far more effective than treatment. Control of hypertension, cessation of smoking, and reduction of cardiac disease by reduction of risk factors are all in order. Prophylactic aspirin is ineffective in healthy persons but offers a 20% relative risk reduction in patients at risk. Ticlopidine offers a 30% relative risk reduction in comparison with aspirin but is associated with infrequent neutropenia and frequent diarrhea. The addition of clopidogrel provides a choice for patients who cannot tolerate aspirin but is probably no more effective. Combining aspirin with clopidogrel because they have different sites of action on platelets seems appealing and is being studied. A combination of long-acting dipyridamole and a very low dose of aspirin may be more effective. Head-to-head comparison trials are in the planning stages. Patients with valvular atrial fibrillation are anticoagulated with warfarin (international normalized ratio, 2–3). Nonvalvular atrial fibrillation, especially in older patients with left ventricular dysfunction, is also treated with warfarin. Patients younger than 60 years with lone atrial fibrillation and no other evidence of heart disease are not anticoagulated. Aspirin offers a 20% relative risk reduction in patients at risk but does not prevent large cardiac embolic strokes in patients with atrial fibrillation.

TIA is followed fairly soon by stroke in patients with high-grade stenosis (North American Symptomatic Carotid Endarterectomy Trial [NASCET] index >70%). These patients should promptly undergo a workup and carotid surgery before stroke ensues.

When stroke occurs, the patient should be admitted promptly to a hospital. Controlled studies have demonstrated better results when patients are admitted to a dedicated stroke unit.

Airway support and ventilatory assistance are in order when consciousness is depressed. Oxygen is appropriate when hypoxia is present. Rapid drops in blood pressure are to be avoided, and hypertension is generally treated orally unless the mean arterial pressure exceeds 130 mm Hg. Treatment is cautious. Fever should be controlled to reduce the cerebral metabolic demands. The blood sugar should be normalized, but no data indicate a better outcome with this therapy.

Cerebral edema peaks at 3 to 5 days. Corticosteroids are ineffective, but osmotherapy may be used. Shunting or ventricular drainage for hydrocephalus may be helpful, but patients with large cerebellar infarctions or hematomas may require posterior fossa decompression. Anticonvulsants are used to control seizures.

Swallowing is assessed by observing the patient swallow from a cup of 50 mL of water. If this is followed by coughing or wet speech, a speech pathologist should be asked to help evaluate the safety of deglutition and request a program to reduce risk.

Deep vein thrombosis is common in plegic legs. Prophylactic heparin (5,000 U twice daily) is given to patients with thrombotic stroke. Patients with intracranial bleeding should wear pneumatic compression stockings.

Aspirin has never been shown to be of benefit acutely and can be anticipated to be of marginal benefit. The early use of antithrombotic therapy is nevertheless mandated as a quality measure. Heparin has never been properly studied. Hemorrhagic transformation of embolic stroke is commonly noted at postmortem examinations. Good data are not available, but it seems likely that patients with large embolic strokes are at higher risk for symptomatic hemorrhagic transformation. Early anticoagulation of embolic strokes is in order to prevent repeated embolization. The physician can wait 2 to 3 days and have another CT performed before heparinizing the patient. If hemorrhagic transformation has occurred, anticoagulation is delayed an additional week. However, this may be unduly cautious.

Secondary measures of stroke prevention include carotid endarterectomy in patients who have stenoses occluding more than 70% of the lumen (NASCET index), in patients whose life expectancy is a year or more, and in patients whose deficit leaves them with more function to lose. Patients with cardiac embolism who can be safely anticoagulated with warfarin should be so treated. Studies of low-molecular-weight-heparins and heparinoids have shown no benefit for the stroke. Warfarin versus aspirin in cryptogenic stroke has been studied, with no benefit for warfarin. A disturbing finding in this study was a higher recurrence rate in patients who had had a stroke while on aspirin regardless of the treatment choice. Ticlopidine has been touted as better than aspirin in African-Americans, but this claim was not borne out in a study. A study of the relative merits of aspirin versus warfarin in patients with symptomatic large vessel intracranial stenoses is under way. Retrospective data suggest that warfarin may be more effective than aspirin.

Clinical trials are evaluating the efficacy of many drugs as cerebral protective agents, but thus far, they offer hope only to rodents. Properly selected patients with middle cerebral occlusions seen within 180 minutes after the ictus can be safely treated with tissue plasminogen activator. This treatment has been approved by the Food and Drug Administration. Relatively few patients are treated because they tend to present too late, and emergency departments may not be ready for them. However, this is a potentially dangerous treatment (increased rate of intracerebral hemorrhage), and its safe use requires careful understanding. The standard is a door-to-needle time of 60 minutes, including CT to rule out hemorrhage. The rate of satisfactory opening of large vessels with this technique is not high. Studies of intraarterial prourokinase (not available) showed good results with a longer time window. This has led to the use of intraarterial tissue plasminogen activator (off label) in many centers where a team capable of catheterizing the middle cerebral artery is available. Some gratifying results have been obtained.

The medical complications of stroke include aspiration, pneumonia, malnutrition, deep vein thrombosis, pulmonary embolism, myocardial infarction, urinary tract infections, decubitus ulcers, contractures, and frozen shoulder.

Experienced physicians should manage patients with subarachnoid hemorrhage. Subarachnoid hemorrhage causes death by direct bleeding, rebleeding, and vasospasm. Little can be done about direct bleeding, but we must do better in recognizing small bleeds. Early angiography and surgery can be performed in patients in good condition (low Hunt-Hess grade), with clipping of the aneurysm and elimination of rebleeding. Aneurysms may be treated by such endovascular therapies as Guglielmi detachable coils. The use of endovascular procedures is growing. All patients should be treated with prophylactic nimodipine, which reduces death and disability caused by the delayed vasospasm that occurs after day 4 in patients with subarachnoid hemorrhage and thick clot. Nicardipine reduces vasospasm but fails to decrease either death or disability. Presumably, nimodipine acts as a cerebral protective agent. Blood pressure is controlled but perfusion is maintained. Hyposmolar agents should be avoided, and hyponatremia should not be casually treated with fluid restriction without a consideration of the need to maintain the intravascular volume.

The management of intracerebral hemorrhage is unsatisfactory and remains controversial. A large cerebellar hemorrhage should be decompressed before the patient becomes comatose.

CONSIDERATIONS DURING PREGNANCY

Pregnancy and the puerperium represent a special risk for stroke because of the procoagulant state. It was once thought that these strokes were usually venous, but recent data have shown that strokes in pregnancy and the first week postpartum are arterial. Venous infarction occurs in the succeeding month. The incidence of strokes is about 10 times greater during pregnancy and the puerperium. Equal numbers occur during pregnancy and the puerperium. A careful workup is necessary, and anticoagulation is given when appropriate. Warfarin crosses the placenta, so heparin is usually used. Care must be taken not to induce thrombocytopenia. The anticardiolipin antibody syndrome is associated with increased spontaneous abortion, but patients have carried to term with steroids and aspirin. These strokes are usually in the carotid territory. The low level anticardiolipin elevations seen in elderly patients with stroke probably do not require therapy.

Venous thrombosis may be suspected when the patient presents with headache, seizures, and obtundation later in the puerperium. Specific syndromes may point to specific dural venous sinuses. Cranial nerves III, IV, V, and VI suggest the cavernous sinus, aphasia the lateral sinus, and leg weakness the sagittal sinus. Although these lesions often are quite hemorrhagic, heparin therapy seems to be helpful.

Vascular lesions may grow during pregnancy. When a patient experiences subarachnoid hemorrhage during pregnancy, the abdomen should be shielded and prompt angiography performed. The risk for bleeding appears greatest during the second trimester, but rupture may occur during parturition. If the lesion cannot be readily managed, careful vaginal delivery can be allowed if the Valsalva maneuver can be avoided; Valsalva increases the venous pressure and the likelihood of rupture. Cesarean section may be needed to protect the mother. The risk drops after delivery but is still high enough to warrant prophylactic surgery, if feasible.

The risk for aneurysmal bleeding increases with each month of pregnancy. Aneurysmal bleeding is likely to recur severely and soon. Labor may be triggered by aneurysmal rupture. The risk for rebleeding during vaginal delivery is not prohibitive if the patient is multiparous or in good control. If the patient is late in pregnancy, delivery and aneurysmal surgery should be undertaken. If the patient is early in pregnancy, the aneurysm must be managed.

Stroke in pregnancy may create problems for the mother's ability to care for her offspring. The problem of subarachnoid hemorrhage is highly complex even without pregnancy, and a careful multispecialty effort is critical to a successful outcome. The death rate of patients treated conservatively is in the range of 60% to 70%, and delay should be avoided.

The increased risk for stroke with oral contraceptives seems to be associated with factors such as hypertension and smoking.

BIBLIOGRAPHY

Barnett HJM, Mohr JP, Stein BM, et al., eds. *Stroke: pathophysiology, diagnosis, and management,* 2nd ed. New York: Churchill Livingstone, 1992.

Bogousslavsky J, Caplan L, eds. *Stroke syndromes,* 2nd ed. New York: Cambridge University Press, 2001.

Caplan LR. *Stroke: a clinical approach,* 3rd ed. Boston: Butterworth-Heinemann, 2000.

Fisher M, ed. *Clinical atlas of cerebrovascular disorders.* London: Mosby–Year Book Europe, 1994.

Fisher M, ed. *Stroke therapy.* Boston: Butterworth-Heinemann, 1995.

Fisher M, Bogousslavsky J, eds. *Current review of cerebrovascular disease.* Philadelphia: Current Medicine, 1993.

Fisher M, Bogousslavsky J, eds. *Current review of cerebrovascular disease,* 4th ed. Philadelphia: Current Medicine, 2001.

Hankey GJ, Warlow CP, eds. *Transient ischaemic attacks of the brain and eye.* London: WB Saunders, 1994.

Norris JW, Hachinski VC, eds. *Prevention of stroke.* New York: Springer-Verlag, 1991.

Yatsu FM, Grotta JC, Pettigrew LC. *Stroke: 100 maxims.* St. Louis: Mosby, 1995.

CHAPTER 108
Dementia (Alzheimer Disease and Other Types)

Joshua Hollander

Dementia is a persistent decline in previous intellectual functioning. Cummings has defined dementia as an acquired persistent impairment of intellectual function with compromise in at least three of the following spheres of mental activity: language, memory, visuospatial skills, emotion or personality, and cognition (e.g., abstraction, calculation, judgment, executive functioning). The fourth edition of the *Diagnostic and Statistical Manual* of the American Psychiatric Association (DSM-IV) continues to require memory loss as a basic requirement while abandoning the need for demonstration of progression. Therefore, persons who have suffered a severe but not progressive brain insult (cardiac arrest) can be included. The requirement for memory impairment excludes some early dementing disorders. The decline in memory or other cognitive functions can be determined by a history of performance decline, the clinical examination, or neuropsychologic testing. The diagnosis cannot be made when consciousness is impaired by delirium, drowsiness, stupor, or coma, or when the mental status cannot be adequately evaluated because of other clinical problems (National Institute of Neurological Disorders and Stroke—Alzheimer's Disease and Related Disorders Association [NINDS-ADRDA]).

Dementia is a growing societal and health care problem because its frequency increases with aging and people are living longer. Most forms of dementia progress insidiously, and the physician or family members may not be aware of even serious deterioration if the patient is not challenged to provide an orderly detailed history. It is the presence of major gaps or inconsistencies that may alert the physician to a cognitive problem. New difficulty at work may bring these deficiencies to attention. Families tend to cover up problems and may gradually assume responsibility for household finances or cooking. Women make up a greater share of the elderly, and the incidence of the problem is higher in women. The prevalence rate of significant dementia may reach 20% in persons older than 80 years and almost 50% in those older than 85 years. Dementia has multiple causes, with only a small fraction amenable to therapy. Alzheimer disease is by far the most common form, affecting almost 50% of all demented people. The dementing illnesses are not homogeneous and are characterized by discrepancies between different forms of cognition.

ETIOLOGY AND DIFFERENTIAL DIAGNOSIS

Etiologic classifications exist but are not as useful as one might wish because of the large number of disorders placed in the unknown category. As research continues to evolve, the group of degenerative dementias will continue to shrink. A vast array of neurologic disorders can cause dementia because the repertoire of responses of the nervous system to injury is limited. The more common and the potentially treatable disorders are addressed here. No more than a few general categorizations about most of these disorders can be attempted in this context (Tables 108.1–108.3).

TABLE 108.1. A Brief Etiologic Classification of the Dementias

Degenerative
Cortical
Subcortical
Vascular
Infectious
Metabolic
Inherited disorders with dementia
Hydrocephalic
Pseudodementias
Miscellaneous

TABLE 108.2. Etiologic Classification of the Dementias

- **Degenerative dementias**
  - Cortical dementias
    - Dementia of the Alzheimer type
    - Pick disease
    - Focal cortical atrophies
      - Primary progressive aphasia
        - Nonfluent aphasia (anterior perisylvian)
        - Fluent aphasia (temporal and posterior perisylvian)
        - Anomic aphasia (anterior temporal)
        - Mixed aphasia (temporal and perisylvian)
      - Perceptual-motor syndromes
      - Progressive visual syndromes (parietooccipital/parietotemporal, posterior cerebral atrophy)
      - Progressive motor syndromes (parietofrontal)
      - Progressive frontal lobe syndromes (frontal lobe dementia)
        - Neuropsychiatric
        - Progressive spasticity/primary lateral sclerosis
        - Mixed
      - Bitemporal syndromes
        - Progressive amnesia
        - Progressive prosopagnosia
        - Progressive neuropsychiatric syndrome with anomia and amnesia
        - Posterior cerebral atrophy
  - Subcortical dementias with basal ganglia involvement
    - Huntington disease
    - Parkinson disease
    - Diffuse Lewy body disease
    - Progressive supranuclear palsy
    - Wilson disease
    - Hallervorden-Spatz syndrome
    - Spinocerebellar degeneration
    - Idiopathic calcification of the basal ganglia (Fahr disease)
    - Thalamic degeneration
    - Corticobasal degeneration
    - Progressive subcortical gliosis
    - Motor neuron disease with dementia
- **Vascular dementias**
  - Superficial infarctions
    - Multiple emboli, vasculitis
  - Deep infarctions
    - Lacunar state
    - Binswanger disease
  - Combined superficial and deep infarctions
    - Multi-infarct dementia
  - Hypoperfusion syndromes
- **Viral dementias**
  - Postencephalitic dementias
    - Arbovirus infection
    - Herpes simplex
  - Postinfectious encephalomyelitis
    - Exanthematous
    - Nonexanthematous
    - Postvaccination
  - Progressive dementia caused by conventional viruses
    - Human immunodeficiency virus 1
    - Progressive multifocal leukoencephalopathy
    - Subacute sclerosing panencephalitis
    - Progressive rubella panencephalitis
  - Prion diseases
    - Creutzfeldt-Jakob disease
    - Kuru
    - Gerstmann-Straeussler-Scheinker disease
    - Alper disease
    - Thalamic dementia
- **Bacterial, fungal, and parasitic dementias**
  - Chronic meningitis
    - Fungal
      - Cryptococcosis; coccidioidomycosis; histoplasmosis; candidiasis; blastomycosis; aspergillosis; paracoccidioidomycosis; dermatomycosis; infection with *Clodosporium, Allescheria, Cephalosporium, Sporotrix, Actinomyces, Nocardia*
    - Parasitic
      - Malaria
      - Cysticercosis
      - Coenurosis
      - Toxoplasmosis
      - Amebiasis
    - Chronic bacterial
      - *Mycobacterium tuberculosis*
      - Syphilis
        - General paresis
        - Meningovascular
        - Syphilitic meningitis
  - Neurobrucellosis
  - Lyme borreliosis
  - Whipple disease
  - African trypanosomiasis
- **Metabolic dementias**
  - Medications
  - Heavy metals
    - Lead
    - Mercury
    - Manganese
    - Arsenic
    - Thallium
    - Others: aluminum, gold, tin, bismuth, nickel
    - Industrial toxins
  - Endocrinopathies
    - Thyroid (myxedema, thyrotoxicosis)
    - Adrenal (Addison, Cushing)
    - Parathyroid (hyperparathyroidism with hypercalcemia, hypoparathyroidism)
    - Hypopituitarism
  - Nutritional deficiencies
    - Hypoglycemia
    - Thiamin
    - Niacin
    - Cyancobalamin
  - Anoxias
    - Transient severe anoxia with postanoxic dementia
    - Carbon monoxide
    - Chronic hypercapnic encephalopathy
    - Hyperviscosity syndromes
  - Chronic renal failure
    - Uremic encephalopathy
    - Dialysis dementia
  - Hepatic dysfunction
    - Portosystemic encephalopathy
    - Chronic non-Wilsonian hepatocerebral degeneration
  - Pancreatic disorders
- **Inherited disorders with dementia**
  - Leukodystrophies
    - Metachromatic leukodystrophy
    - Adrenoleukodystrophy
    - Cerebrotendinous xanthomatosis
  - Poliodystrophies
    - Adult G_{M1} gangliosidosis
    - Adult G_{M2} gangliosidosis
    - Adult Gaucher disease
    - Membranous lipodystrophy
    - Neuronal ceroid lipofuscinosis (Kufs disease)
    - Niemann-Pick disease, type C
  - Corencephalopathies
    - Subacute necrotizing encephalomyelitis (Leigh disease)
    - Hepatolenticular degeneration (Wilson disease)
    - Hallervorden-Spatz syndrome
    - Neuroacanthocytosis
  - Diffuse encephalopathies
    - Acute intermittent porphyria
    - Adult polyglycosan body disease/Fabry disease (multi-infarct dementia)
  - Mitochondrial encephalomyelopathies

(continued)

TABLE 108.2. (*continued*)

Kearns-Sayre syndrome	Superficial hemosiderosis of the central nervous system
Myoclonus epilepsy with ragged red fibers (MERRF)	Hydrocephalus ex vacuo
Mitochondrial myopathy, encephalopathy, lactic acidosis, and stroke-like episodes (MELAS)	**Pseudodementias**
Progressive myoclonus epilepsy (Unverricht-Lundborg)	Dementia syndrome of depression
With Lafora bodies	Ganser syndrome
Without Lafora bodies	Malingering
Spinocerebellar degeneration	Miscellaneous psychiatric disorders
Friedreich syndrome	**Miscellaneous dementias**
Olivopontocerebellar atrophy	Trauma
Dentatorubral-pallidoluysian atrophy	Dementia pugilistica
MAST syndrome	Closed head injury
Sensory radicular neuropathy	Chronic subdural hematoma
Myotonic dystrophy	Multiple sclerosis
Homocystinuria	Tumors
Hydrocephalic dementias	Direct
Spontaneously arrested hydrocephalus	Mass
Obstructive, noncommunicating hydrocephalus	Local
Obstructive, communicating hydrocephalus (normal pressure)	Neoplastic meningitis
Subarachnoid hemorrhage	Paraneoplastic limbic encephalitis

Degenerative Dementias

Clinically differentiated forms can be divided into cortical, subcortical, and mixed types. Not all dementias fit into this classification, but it allows the clinician to make some useful clinical distinctions at the bedside. Although the concept of "axial dementia" has been suggested to cover pure impairments of new memory formation (Korsakoff psychosis), it has not been generally accepted.

CORTICAL DEMENTIAS

Cortical dementias are characterized by a sparing of motor function until quite late in the course of the illness, when the patient finally may be reduced to lying curled in hypertonic flexion. The early onset of gait disturbance should not occur. The major features are the early involvement of mental status, with impairment of language, calculation, visuospatial perception, memory, judgment, and abstraction. The patient may become disinhibited or apathetic.

A prototype disorder is *Alzheimer disease,* which is the most common form of dementia, affecting almost half of demented persons. The duration of this disorder is 10 to 20 years. The incidence increases with age, from 10% in persons older than 65 years to 35% in those older than 85 years. It has been estimated that Alzheimer disease affects as many as 4 million Americans at an annual cost of $90 billion.

Initial features include memory deficits, which are more severe for new memories. Visuospatial skills decline, and mild language dysfunction develops. Indifference or irritability may be noted, and the patient may be sad. Later, the memory defects become more global (both recent and remote). Visuospatial skills further deteriorate so that even simple constructions cannot be performed. A fluent aphasia, acalculia, and apraxia are manifested. Restlessness and possibly delusions occur. Finally, a severely deteriorated intellect is combined with rigid, flexed posture and incontinence. Seizures may occur late. The disorder may unfold over 10 years, but the rate of progression is somewhat variable.

Risk factors include age, female sex, genetic predisposition, lack of education, and head trauma. Less clear is a potential role for late maternal age. Aluminum toxicity was touted but has not borne up in further study. Protective benefits of higher education and intellectual pursuits have been noted. Patients with typical Alzheimer pathology may be more profoundly affected if they have intercurrent cerebrovascular disease.

The cause of Alzheimer disease is unclear as yet, but some important clues are emerging. It is possible that multiple etiologic factors and pathogenetic mechanisms result in a converging pattern of neuronal dysfunction, synaptic impoverishment, and ultimate neuronal loss. Loss of synaptic function adversely affects signal transmission and correlates with intellectual decline. The involvement of the nucleus basalis results in a major loss of frontal subcortical to cortical cholinergic tone, which correlates with memory impairment. This system comprises nerve growth factor receptors. Other neurotransmitters are also involved, predominantly in younger patients. Excitatory amino acids have been implicated in excessive intracellular calcium influx and have been thought to be a possible mechanism of cell death. Although the role of glutamate transmission in ischemic cell death seems more clearly established, it is possible that injured neurons are more sensitive to excitatory amino acid toxicity. The role (or lack of it) of amyloid angiopathy in the pathogenesis of neuronal loss is not clear. Several kindreds of early-onset autosomal-dominant Alzheimer disease have led to the finding of multiple genetic loci (presenilin-1, presenilin-2, apolipoprotein E4 [apoE4], amyloid precursor protein) that may suggest multiple converging pathogenic mechanisms.

Alzheimer disease primarily damages association areas; parietal and temporal regions are more severely affected than frontal regions. The brain is atrophic, with neuronal loss and astrocytic gliosis. Intraneuronal neurofibrillary tangles, neuritic plaques, granular and vacuolar degeneration, and amyloid

TABLE 108.3. An Abbreviated Classification of the Dementias

Drug
Emotional
Metabolic
Eyes and ears
Nutritional
Tumor
Infection
Atherosclerosis

angiopathy are noted. Dendritic arborization is diminished. Each of these histologic findings is nonspecific

Two abnormal proteins have been identified. Microtubule-associated tau protein of normal brain is found in large amounts. Neurofibrillary tangles are paired helical intracellular filaments containing abnormally phosphorylated tau protein and ubiquitin. β-Amyloid is found in the neuritic plaques and degenerating nerve terminals. Senile or neuritic plaques contain neuronal and glial processes in addition to β-amyloid. Amyloid precursor protein, a cell adhesion peptide, is a constituent of brain across many species with many minor amino acid variants and a high turnover rate. This is a large, coiled glycoprotein with straightened ends, one of which is embedded in the neuronal membrane. It exhibits serine protease properties and may be involved in cell growth. Degradation of the amyloid precursor protein at the wrong site results in the formation of β-amyloid, an insoluble protein resistant to degradation.

The amyloid precursor protein gene is located on chromosome 21, and it is interesting that long-lived persons with Down syndrome (21 trisomy) exhibit changes of Alzheimer disease. The apoE gene codes for a serum lipoprotein and occurs in three forms. It is located on chromosome 19, and whereas apoE4 is seen in 14% of controls, it occurs in 30% to 40% of late-onset sporadic cases and 80% of late-onset familial cases. The chance for the development of Alzheimer disease by the age of 85 years in persons homozygous for apoE may be 90%. Estimates are that 25% to 40% of cases are attributable to apoE4. ApoE4 has a high affinity for β-amyloid, and patients with the gene have larger plaques. The continued rapid evolution in the understanding of the neurobiology and genetics of this common tragic disorder may lead to useful therapeutic manipulations.

The *frontotemporal dementias,* which are mostly tauopathies, include frontotemporal dementia, Pick disease, corticobasal degeneration, primary progressive aphasia, and the pathologically distinct progressive subcortical gliosis. *Pick disease* is a much less common disorder than Alzheimer disease; personality is affected early, with amnesia, visuospatial problems, and acalculia developing late. Linguistic disturbances also occur but tend to be anomia and stereotypic speech. Because of the selective atrophy of the frontal and temporal lobes, Klüver-Bucy syndrome, with hypersexuality, gluttony, hyperorality, and emotional blunting, may develop. The pathology includes argyrophilic intracytoplasmic Pick bodies or inflated cells with argyrophilic cytoplasm. Dendritic spines are lost, and white matter gliosis is seen.

SUBCORTICAL DEMENTIAS

Unlike the cortical dementias, the subcortical dementias manifest with early abnormalities of gait, stance, movement, and tone. Speech is more impaired than language, and both speech and cognition appear slowed. The mood is apathetic, and the memory exhibits retrieval problems. These patients may really have a loss of frontal-subcortical connections with resultant difficulty in switching sets, and the term *subcortical dementia* may be somewhat of a misnomer. An example might be Huntington disease or the lacunar state.

Huntington disease is an autosomal-dominant disorder with complete penetrance characterized by atrophy of the caudate head and a loss of cortical neurons. The gene is localized to the short arm of chromosome 4. The defect is known to be a polymorphic trinucleotide CAG repeat. A potential role for excitotoxic amino acids and depleted γ-aminobutyric acid has been presented. The onset is usually between 30 to 50 years of age, with a duration of about 15 years. The prevalence is about 5 per 100,000 people. Features include motor, cognitive, and emotional impairments. The motor disorder is not just chorea but includes athetosis, dystonia, and other movements. Rigidity occurs in juvenile-onset and late disease. The cognitive disorder may be preceded by impairment of frontal lobe "executive" functions, such as organization and judgment. The cortical features tend to be spared, with memory deficit, cognitive slowing, and apathy the rule. Loss of perception of shapes, impaired comprehension of prosody, and dysarthria are other features. Psychiatric problems include depression, impulsive behavior, intermittent explosive disorder, and, less commonly, schizophrenia and antisocial behavior. Suicide is excessive, as would be expected in a population with a 33% rate of major depression.

Parkinson disease is a common (prevalence of 1 per 1,000 people) disorder. The four cardinal features are rigidity, bradykinesia, tremor, and postural instability. The onset is at about 60 years, and the duration is about 10 years. A loss of pigmented neurons occurs that is most severe in the pars compacta of the substantia nigra. Neuronal loss and gliosis are associated with the more specific finding of cytoplasmic round eosinophilic hyaline bodies with halos called *Lewy bodies*. The movement disorder is related to the loss of nigral dopaminergic input to the striatum. Some mental impairment occurs in 20% to 30% of patients, especially at late stages of the disorder. The dementia in most cases is only mild to moderate, with bradyphrenia, impaired problem solving, slowed and impaired recall, decreased spontaneity, impaired visuospatial perception, impaired set shift, and depression. A strong association of limbic cortex Lewy bodies and large numbers in the mesencephalon has been noted, and the limbic Lewy body concentration is strongly associated with dementia. When severe cognitive deficits develop, changes of Alzheimer disease may be noted. One group of patients has moderate cortical Lewy body involvement and dementia without Parkinson disease. These patients are said to have *diffuse Lewy body disease* and present with a primarily cortical dementia. Diffuse Lewy body disease is probably a common cause of dementia. An additional complexity is the ability of anti-Parkinson medications to induce visual hallucinations and delirium.

Progressive supranuclear palsy is only 1% as common as Parkinson disease and may be confused with Parkinson disease early in its course. It presents with axial rigidity, pseudobulbar palsy, dysarthria, and supranuclear ophthalmoplegia. The posture tends to be in extension rather than in flexion as in Parkinson disease. An impairment of upward gaze develops in patients with Parkinson disease, but patients with progressive supranuclear palsy characteristically have a striking impairment of downward gaze. The eye movement problem is supranuclear, evidenced by the ability to induce reflex eye movements in response to head turning (oculocephalic reflex). The impairment of downward gaze causes severe reading problems for patients who must wear bifocals and, in combination with instability of posture, frequent falls. The dementia develops late and is typically frontal subcortical in type.

Other causes of subcortical dementia include Wilson hepatolenticular degeneration, Hallervorden-Spatz syndrome, amyotrophic lateral sclerosis-parkinsonism-dementia complex of Guam, and spinocerebellar degeneration.

MIXED DEMENTIA

Mixed cortical and subcortical dementias also exist and include some forms of vascular dementia and neurosyphilis.

Vascular Dementia

The term *vascular dementia* presents special problems because it harkens back to the days when cerebral arteriosclerosis was accepted by general physicians as *the* cause of dementia.

Although the term is now used more cautiously, a clear definition and an understanding of the relationship between the vascular lesion and the dementia are still lacking. It is recognized that some 25% of patients with stroke from the Stroke Data Bank have dementia. Of those with dementia, 56% are thought to have dementia as a consequence of the stroke, and an additional 36% are thought to have mixed vascular dementia and Alzheimer disease. The extent, location, laterality, and total volume of the vascular disease appear to determine the development of dementia, rather than the nature of the vascular disease itself. For each of the factors cited, no clear criteria exist. Evidence for a chronic ischemia of nerve cells rather than multiple infarctions has not been presented. Whether this diagnosis is overused or underused is the subject of controversy.

The classic clinical features that implicate a vascular cause are male sex, sudden onset, stepwise course, focal signs, relative preservation of personality, history of vascular disease, vascular risk factors, and hypertension. These were quantified into an ischemic scale by Hachinski, which evolved and was then simplified by Rosen. The scale does serve to distinguish patients likely to have stroke from those in whom stroke is unlikely (Table 108.4).

Patients with large areas of infarction are not controversial because they also present with obvious neurologic findings and so are not easily confused with other patients with dementia. In elderly persons with chronic nonvalvular atrial fibrillation, the embolic stroke burden is excessive. They are therefore subject to granular cerebral atrophy, which can cause a cortical dementia, but the frequency of this condition in the elderly is unclear.

Lacunes are small deep infarcts of gray and white matter resulting from hypertensive fibrinoid changes in the small penetrating arteries at the base of the brain. They are also caused by atherosclerosis in the mouth of these vessels. Less commonly, they may be caused by emboli or small bleeds. When the lesions are bilateral and multiple, the condition is referred to as the *lacunar state*.

The hemispheric white matter is supplied by long, fine penetrating vessels that arise from major cortical branches but are themselves end vessels subject to hypertension-induced changes similar to those that cause lacunar infarction. These changes may result in subcortical infarcts or incomplete lesions in which the tissue integrity is preserved but axons and myelin are lost, with subsequent disconnection from the overlying cortex. The subcortical dementia that ensues is characterized by apathetic behavior, memory disturbances, emotional lability, and preservation of insight. This is superimposed on a background of incontinence, pseudobulbar palsy, and pyramidal and extrapyramidal signs. This condition is known as *Binswanger disease*. In addition, these areas are in the watershed territory between major blood vessels and may be damaged if hypotension develops or antihypertensive regimens are used overzealously, especially if large vessel disease is also present. Binswanger disease shares many of the features of a lacunar state but may show more cortical features. Large vessel involvement may result in the *angular gyrus syndrome*, which can be confused with Alzheimer disease but spares topographic skills and memory on nonverbal testing.

TABLE 108.4. Rosen Modification of Hachinski Ischemic Scale

Abrupt onset	2
Stepwise deterioration	1
Somatic complaints	1
Emotional incontinence	1
History of hypertension	1
History of strokes	2
Focal neurologic symptoms	2
Focal neurologic signs	2

Note: Degenerative dementia is suggested by a score below 3, vascular dementia by a score above 3. A score of 3 is then indeterminate.

The term *leukoaraiosis* was coined to describe changes in the white matter seen by computed tomography (CT), to distinguish a radiographic appearance of uncertain nature from Binswanger disease. Magnetic resonance imaging (MRI), with finer resolution, better delineates these changes, which are very common. Leukoaraiosis correlates with age, stroke, and hypertension. Mild changes, seen as ventricular caps, are frequent, and some changes merely reflect the cribriform state, which is an increase in perivascular spaces in the atrophic brains of hypertensive patients. In other cases, larger confluent areas are associated with white matter pathology, similar to that described in Binswanger disease, that bears some relation to cognitive decline and focal neurologic findings. Increased leukoaraiosis in Alzheimer disease has been attributed to wallerian degeneration or hypotension and hypoperfusion. Leukoaraiosis is strongly correlated with dementia and, when severe, has been thought in itself to be a cause of dementia. An error that is too commonly made is attempting to define dementia or its cause in radiographic terms.

It is not possible to cover all the dementing illnesses, but several infectious causes are worthy of mention. Creutzfeldt-Jakob disease is a rare, rapidly progressive dementia with features of myoclonic jerks and characteristic electroencephalographic (EEG) findings. Several clinical varieties have been described. Of great importance was the discovery that it is caused by a transmissible agent. This and other spongiform encephalopathies have been shown to be transmitted by prions—small proteinaceous infectious particles that resist inactivation by procedures that modify nucleic acids. Creutzfeldt-Jakob disease occurs in sporadic, inherited, and iatrogenic forms. Human transmission has occurred through organ transplantation, and therefore dementia must be regarded as an absolute contraindication to such grafts. A recent description of the brain 14-3-3 protein in cerebrospinal fluid and an abnormal appearance of the basal ganglia or thalamus on MRI may be helpful. The variant Creutzfeldt-Jakob disease (mad cow disease) may present in an atypical fashion with anxiety, depression, early ataxia, and sensory disturbance and a lack of EEG findings. Mad cow disease may affect women of childbearing age.

A form of dementia that is increasing, especially among the young, is the AIDS dementia complex (HIV encephalopathy). Patients may present with dementia before they have full-blown AIDS. The disorder usually presents as a subcortical dementia but is ultimately expressed as a more generalized process. It has not been amenable to therapy thus far and leads to an early demise. A critical consideration for the physician is ruling out such opportunistic infections as toxoplasmosis, cryptococcal meningitis, cytomegalovirus infection, progressive multifocal leukoencephalopathy, and primary central nervous system lymphoma.

Neurosyphilis is a major cause of dementia, but the incidence has profoundly declined, with new cases now rare. Despite the problem of reemerging syphilis, it will be some years before new cases of tertiary syphilis are seen again.

A rare but much discussed syndrome is normal pressure hydrocephalus, which is most readily diagnosed after subarachnoid hemorrhage or meningitis. It manifests as a dementia in which slowed mental processing deteriorates to apathetic forgetfulness, suggestive of a subcortical type, but admixtures of cortical dysfunction may be seen. A gait disturbance is always associated, and the gait is usually an apraxic type rather than spastic. Urinary incontinence is a later feature of the diagnostic triad. In normal pressure hydrocephalus, a communicating hydrocephalus (no blockage in the flow of spinal fluid from the ventricles to the subarachnoid space) is associated with impaired absorption of spinal fluid into the pacchionian granulations and sagittal sinus. Because it is difficult to distinguish enlarged ventricles from atrophy (hydrocephalus ex vacuo), the diagnosis is frequently considered. The diagnosis is somewhat problematic because the condition is relieved in fewer than a third of patients after ventriculoperitoneal shunting. Improvement is more common when the syndrome is new, and the mental changes may be at least amenable to treatment.

Early in its course, a dementing illness must be distinguished from the normal cognitive changes of aging. As people age, they experience a normal increase in the difficulty of immediate recall and may assume that this is a manifestation of impending dementia. Reassurance from the physician is essential to their sense of well-being. Early in the illness, when the complaints may merely reflect a high achiever's loss of a subtle edge, the standard interview may prove quite inadequate. Patients may be brought back in follow-up when the distinction between normal aging and perhaps too many responsibilities, as opposed to incipient dementia, is not evident to the examiner. The family benefits not only from knowing about the presence of an illness but also from anticipating its possible course. The diagnosis currently is based primarily on clinical judgment and familiarity with the possibilities. Unfortunately, no simple blood or imaging tests are diagnostic, and a careful cognitive examination takes time. Detailed neuropsychologic testing is available and often quite helpful, but many insurance plans are reluctant to pay for it. The physician should be reluctant to accept a diagnosis as gloomy as this without a serious consideration of possible alternatives. A precise diagnosis will assume greater importance as more specific treatments become available.

Patients exhibiting memory deficits greater than those anticipated for their age but lacking sufficient cognitive impairment for a diagnosis of dementia are said to have *mild cognitive impairment*. Most of them become demented eventually, but sometimes not for years.

HISTORY

A general medical history must include questions about endocrine, hematologic, and infectious (including HIV) factors. Inquiries about possible causes of neurologic dysfunction, such as head injury, stroke, and seizure, should be made. A family history of dementing illness may not be volunteered and must be elicited. Early features, such as forgetting names, must be distinguished from normal age-associated memory impairment. In the case of a patient who is mismanaging work or financial affairs, an independent history from family or coworkers may be required. It is important to remember that the organ that gives the history is the organ that is ill. It is said that when a physician feels more and more frustrated or provoked by a patient's inability to provide a consistent and reasonable history, dementia should be considered as a possible diagnosis. Many families cover for patients, and answers to indirect questions about who handles the checkbook and whether the cooking has changed may yield clues. Difficulty with appointments or scheduled medications may follow. A loss of creativity or an inability to learn new skills or retain a topographic orientation usually precedes any loss of linguistic or perceptuomotor skills. The pattern of development of the disorder will vary both with the individual patient and with the type of dementia. Apathy must be distinguished from depression. Depression may also follow a loss of intellect. It is not usually a key etiologic factor unless the patient has a prior history of mood disturbance. The use of prescription, over-the-counter, or recreational drugs or alcohol should be queried. The family may have to check the medicine cabinet for such things as a dead spouse's medication, multiple out-of-date prescriptions, and prescriptions from multiple physicians.

The family or friends may contribute information about changes in the patient's personality and routines. Appetite, weight, sleep, dress, and toilet must all be assessed. The office situation can usually be manipulated to allow a private conversation with the caregiver except in the case of a patients who is extremely paranoid. Failure to do so will necessitate a specific arrangement so that the history can be obtained from the family or coworkers in the patient's absence.

Difficulties in learning and retaining information (being repetitive, forgetting conversations, misplacing objects), handling complex tasks (preparing meals, balancing checkbook), reasoning (planning and problem solving, observing the social amenities), spatial ability and orientation (driving, becoming lost in familiar surroundings), language (finding words, following a conversation), behavior (being passive, irritable, suspicious and misinterpreting stimuli) are all alerting symptoms that should prompt evaluation.

PHYSICAL EXAMINATION

A general physical examination is necessary because intercurrent illness can seriously compromise the results of mental status testing, particularly in the elderly. The so-called frontal signs are more reflective of diffuse disease. These include the glabellar response (inability to suppress forced eye closure in response to tapping the forehead), suck reflex, forced grasp response, impaired visual smooth pursuit, impaired upward gaze, and paratonia (resistance to passive movements intermingled with facilitation of such).

The patient's level of consciousness and attentiveness must be assessed. An *alert* person with the ability to attend to the task is needed before a mental status test can be performed reliably. *Attention* is gauged by having the patient spell *world* backward or perform serial subtractions. A demented patient may have delirium with clouding of consciousness, but one should not rush to diagnose dementia in a patient with delirium. The mental status examination should take cognizance of general behavior and mood. Language function must be evaluated early because the ability to comprehend a cognitive test may be compromised by aphasia. Aphasia with severe neologisms and paraphasia may be confused with the sudden onset of schizophrenia, an unlikely event in the elderly. Delusions, illusions, and hallucinations may have a paranoid flavor but tend to be more visual and simpler than in primary psychotic disorders. Insight may be lacking.

Cognition is tested by a series of questions directed at different aspects of higher function. The patient's prior level of intellect and education will have a major impact on performance. Most physicians do not have a set of testing materials available and make do with pencil and paper. The Folstein Mini-Mental Status Examination is well-known to many physicians and medical students. This 5-minute test can be quite helpful for screening provided it is recognized that the results are affected by illness and medication, and it also may be inadequate to evaluate early and late disease. For example, mild deficits do not serve to distinguish between age-associated memory impairment and Alzheimer disease. Many areas are covered in this scale, but the observation of deficits or a worrisome history should lead to further exploration.

Orientation to time, place, and person is assessed. A patient who has been hospitalized for a prolonged period is frequently uncertain about the day of the month.

Memory is frequently tested by immediate recall, but this is primarily a function of attention. *Fund of information* (old learning) can be measured by questions directed at age of children and schooling, occupational history, geography, politics, sports, or hobbies. The ability to retain new information and retrieve old information can be tested. A memory task, usually learning the names of three objects, is assigned, and the examination continues after the examiner is certain that the names have indeed been learned. Other aspects of the mental status are pursued, and the examiner returns to memory task later. Recognition may be better than recall in aged patients.

Comprehension, judgment, and *abstractions* can be tested with proverbs ("Rome wasn't built in a day"), similarities ("What do an orange and an apple have in common?"), and problems ("Why do we pay taxes? What would you do if you found a sealed, stamped, addressed envelope?").

Apraxia has been defined as an inability to carry out purposeful movements on oral command in the absence of comprehension or motor deficits. In *constructional tasks,* the patient may be asked to draw a daisy or the face of a clock, copy a design, or build with blocks or matches. Other forms of apraxia may be tested by asking the subject to demonstrate how to use a comb or scissors. The patient should be observed dressing.

Motor aspects of *speech* are tested, but dysarthria, as opposed to the more symbolic processing of language, is not usually seen early in cortical dementia. *Language* is evident during the history through *comprehension* of the questions and *spontaneous speech.* Abnormal language may be either nonfluent (sparse, slow, effortful, telegraphic) or fluent but devoid of nouns, verbs, and content. Letter or word substitutions (paraphasia) or nonwords (neologisms) may be interspersed, or the sentence may be directed around a word that will not be found. *Naming* is tested, as are reading, writing, and repetition.

Other cognitive abnormalities that may be noted include topographic disorientation, right-left confusion, finger agnosia, unilateral neglect, impaired motor sequences (rock, paper, scissors), and impaired calculation.

A formal neuropsychologic evaluation is quite helpful, but a physician with sufficient time to spend with a patient can obtain much useful information. The references should be consulted for more details of the technique of the mental status examination, if this is desired.

LABORATORY AND IMAGING STUDIES

Laboratory testing is usually not of great help in evaluating dementia because diagnostic testing is not available for the most frequent causes. The importance of laboratory testing lies in excluding potentially treatable disorders and in making a specific diagnosis in many of the rare cases. This type of bleak outlook deserves some effort at detecting the more treatable possibilities. Routine blood cell counts and serum chemistries, including glucose, renal, hepatic, and protein studies, are performed. Vitamin B_{12} determinations are necessary, even if the blood picture is unremarkable, to exclude combined degeneration. Thyroid studies, including measurement of thyroid-stimulating hormone, are indicated, in addition to measurement of calcium and perhaps cortisol. The sedimentation rate and perhaps antinuclear antibody testing may help exclude inflammatory diseases. The results of a serum venereal disease research laboratory (VDRL) test or similar test may be negative in 40% to 50% of cases of tertiary syphilis, and a fluorescent treponemal antibody absorption (FTA-ABS) test is needed. When anything arouses clinical suspicion, a toxic drug screen or heavy metal analysis may be in order. A lumbar puncture is not part of the routine diagnostic workup but is required when chronic fungal meningitis is considered. Specific tests may be ordered to rule out some of the more exotic causes.

An imaging study can be performed to exclude chronic subdural hematoma, which may present with more behavioral than motor signs. This will also be helpful in cases of chronic meningitis and other intracranial masses and will exclude normal pressure hydrocephalus. MRI provides more information and is usually performed in preference to CT. In normal pressure hydrocephalus, an acute angle between the frontal horns and a depressed third ventricular floor with ventriculomegaly and minimal sulcal enlargement are most easily seen in MRI, as is transependymal absorption of spinal fluid. In suspect cases, assessment of the spinal fluid flow pattern by indium cisternography may be helpful. Isotope injected into the lumbar cerebral spinal fluid should flow over the convexities and be absorbed normally. In normal pressure hydrocephalus, the isotope enters the ventricle and remains there for days without passing to the sagittal sinus. Plain roentgenography is seldom helpful, and the results of imaging and other studies lack sensitivity and specificity.

EEG is generally unrewarding but may show characteristic suppression bursts (sharp waves on a low-voltage slow background) in Creutzfeldt-Jakob disease and triphasic slow waves in some metabolic encephalopathies. Cerebral evoked potentials are specific forms of EEG activity seen in response to a stimulus. A signal averager or computer averages out variable EEG activity as background noise in response to hundreds of stimuli, leaving only EEG activity that is linked to a specific stimulus. It has been claimed that event-related potentials with long latency, in response to a novel stimulus, distinguish depression from true dementia. This is not fully established, and such testing is not performed routinely.

Positron emission tomography (PET) and single photon emission tomography (SPECT) provide functional brain imaging that is useful primarily in supplementing clinical and neuropsychological data. These studies, combined with CT or MRI, may yield only equivocal results. Although clearly positive, SPECT findings are more likely to be obtained in advanced disease, they are also less likely to be needed. SPECT may display a pattern of cerebral blood flow more suggestive of Alzheimer disease than other types of dementia, but no pattern is completely diagnostic.

TREATMENT

The first step in the management of dementia is deciding that a cognitive deficit is present; the second is deciding whether the disease is progressing and at what rate. Once treatable causes have been excluded, treatment is primarily supportive. The patient and family will require information about the process and expectations for the future. Considerable repetition and review are needed. The physician or nurse can be a significant source of support, but most families can also derive much benefit from contact with the Alzheimer's Association, especially if a local support group is available.

Little specific therapy is available for Alzheimer disease. A cholinergic deficit in this disorder is associated with involvement of the nucleus basalis of Meynert. Tacrine is a cholinergic agent (a reversible cholinesterase inhibitor) that has been shown to improve cognitive scores and results of global assessments. However, it is not well tolerated, and many patients cannot achieve an optimal dosage. The newer generation of cholinergic drugs (centrally acting acetylcholinesterase inhibitors) includes donepezil, rivastigmine, and galanthamine. Galanthamine may also stimulate nicotinic receptors. Although the experience is greatest with donepezil, these all have similar benefit as cognitive enhancers. The major toxicity is gastrointestinal, and women may experience serious weight loss with galanthamine. Because the effect is not expected to be sustained, some formal assessment of cognitive function should be made. If efficacy cannot be sustained, the drug should be withdrawn slowly. These agents do not affect the basic pathogenetic mechanism and do little to relieve behavioral problems, which may show some response to valproate or carbamazepine. If major antipsychotic agents are required, the atypical newer agents are preferred (risperidone, olanzapine, and quetiapine). Selective serotonin reuptake inhibitors are reasonably tolerated, but anticholinergics should be avoided. Vitamin E and selegiline have been reported to slow progression. Results with estrogens and cyclooxygenase-2 inhibitors have been disappointing.

In my experience, most families and patients will consider entry into clinical trials, and the physician should be aware of local trials. Participation in clinical trials offers additional support systems to care providers.

Patients with mild-to-moderate disease may still manifest disturbing behavior. Those with restless agitation may benefit from a calm routine, food, familiar surroundings, and quiet. Catastrophic reactions may have common triggers, which should be avoided. Feeding problems may be reduced by offering favorite foods that require little effort to eat; these can be left out for snacking if the patient likes to eat but cannot handle the structure of regular, infrequent meals. Bathing may cause conflict, especially if the patient is incontinent. The caregiver may execute a strategic withdrawal and try again another time. Urinary incontinence is not uncommon in moderate-to-severe disease, but it can also reflect problems of the prostate or pelvic floor. A workup is in order when this problem occurs to a degree inappropriate for the mental status. Evening fluids and diuretics should be minimized. Leaving lights on at night and scheduling toileting may be helpful. Protective garments are a last resort but may be needed to avoid decisions for institutional care. *Sundowning* is an evening exacerbation of deficits that may be severe. It is alleviated by adequate light and reorientation. Lower levels of activity and a companion may help.

Even more disruptive for the caregiver, who may have a day job, is an exaggeration of the patient's normally increased nocturnal awakening and loss of deep sleep. This may lead to caregiver burnout and must be addressed. Long, restful naps in the day should be avoided, and bedtime snacks and afternoon activity help. Avoidance of nocturnal diuretics, pain, and disorientation is desirable. Sleep medications are avoided but may be necessary briefly. The anticholinergic properties of Benadryl may cause confusion. A sedating antidepressant in small doses may be more beneficial over time than the more direct, intermediate-acting benzodiazepines.

Wandering may occur at any time but is more of a problem if the caregiver is asleep or if it takes the patient out of the house inappropriately attired and unable to find the way home. A double lock may restrict departure, and the patient should wear an identification bracelet with a phone number. A well-lighted path to the toilet may alleviate the problem. Having an enclosed space, such as a yard or garden, available where the patient can pace may also be helpful.

An additional stress on the caregiver is the need of the patient to shadow the caregiver, preventing any rest and personal time. If possible, a friend or relative can spend some time with the patient to allow the caregiver a chance for shopping or relaxation. An audiotape of the caregiver's voice may also be helpful. As previously discussed, agitation may be relieved by pharmacologic means if needed.

Fecal soiling may be reduced by avoiding cathartics and using bulk, bran, fluids, exercise, and planned evacuations or enemas. If fecal soiling is caused by an inability to remove clothing, simpler attire with elastic or Velcro straps may help. Feeding problems and refusal of food are usually an end-stage phenomenon.

It is important to remind the caregiver that the patient is not trying to be difficult. Instructions should be given simply and one step at a time. It is useful to capitalize on the patient's strengths and perhaps assign a simple repetitive task. The Alzheimer's Association has patient information sheets with clues on how to communicate and guidelines for caregivers. A major problem can be taking away the car keys. A face-saving excuse may be better accepted unless the patient has had many accidents or has repeatedly been lost. Not allowing the patient to drive is a serious issue in communities where the automobile is the major means of transportation. The widespread availability of guns also can be a problem.

As the disease becomes worse, institutionalization must be considered. Legal and financial questions should be explored well in advance. Early in the disease, while the patient retains insight, living wills or health care proxies should be discussed and prepared. Unless the patient is abusive or the caregiver has burned out, institutionalization should be delayed because deterioration frequently accelerates afterward.

CONSIDERATIONS DURING PREGNANCY

Dementia is not a common problem in pregnancy but is of great concern when it does occur because possible etiologic factors are disorders such as HIV infection and neurosyphilis, which can be transmitted to the fetus. Variant Creutzfeldt-Jakob disease (bovine spongiform encephalopathy, mad cow disease) has been reported in this country but probably is still restricted to people who have traveled abroad. Surveillance is actively under way because of the possible importation of contaminated animal feed. The physician should be alert to possible dementia and thoroughly explore treatable or transmissible disorders.

BIBLIOGRAPHY

American Psychiatric Association. *Diagnostic and statistical manual of mental disorders,* 4th ed. Washington, DC: American Psychiatric Association, 1994.

Appel SH, ed. *Current neurology,* vol 15. St. Louis: Mosby–Year Book, 1995.

Burns A, Levy R, eds. *Dementia.* London: Chapman & Hall, 1994.

Chertkow H. Mild cognitive impairment. *Curr Opin Neurol* 2002;15:401.

Cummings JL, ed. *Subcortical dementia.* New York: Oxford University Press, 1990.

Cummings JL. Dementia: the failing brain. *Ann Neurol* 1993;33:568.

Cummings JL, Benson DF, eds. *Dementia: a clinical approach,* 2nd ed. Boston: Butterworth-Heinemann, 1992.

Gruetzner HM, ed. *Alzheimer's: a caregiver's guide and sourcebook.* New York: John Wiley & Sons, 1988.

Heilman KM, Valenstein E, eds. *Clinical neuropsychology.* New York: Oxford University Press, 1993.

Meyer JS, Lechner H, Marshall J, et al., eds. *Vascular and multi-infarct dementia.* New York: Futura Publishing, 1988.

Tatemichi TK, Desmond DW, Paik M. Clinical determinants of dementia related to stroke. *Lancet* 1993;33:568.

Waldemar G. Functional brain imaging with SPECT in normal aging and dementia: methodological, pathophysiological, and diagnostic aspects. *Cerebrovasc Brain Metab Rev* 1995;7:89.

Whitehouse PJ, ed. *Dementia.* Philadelphia: FA Davis Co, 1993.

CHAPTER 109
Brain Tumors

Gerald W. Honch

Brain tumors are relatively common in both children and adults. About 17,000 new primary brain tumors occur in adults each year in the United States. About half of these are relatively benign and can be successfully treated with an excellent prognosis. The others are more aggressive, are less successfully treated, and carry a limited survival rate. The more common primary brain tumors are listed in Table 109.1. The mean age (in years) at diagnosis is included.

Although neurons are the most common cells in the brain, they cannot reproduce. The glial cells are the supporting cells of the brain. They are numerous and perform many structural and metabolic functions. Glial cells do reproduce and are the source of most of the primary tumors of the central nervous system (CNS). Cancer arises in association with the accumulation of specific structural molecular genetic alterations (mutations) within cells. These cells proliferate inappropriately, lose the differentiated characteristics of the cells of origin, and acquire the ability to invade surrounding normal tissues and resist antineoplastic therapies.

Two types of molecular alterations cause these changes. One is a loss of or decrease in cellular activities that operate physiologically to restrain growth (tumor suppressor genes). The other is an inappropriate activation of genes that enhance cellular proliferation (protooncogenes). Many malignant tumors induce the formation of new blood vessels, thereby increasing their own nutrient supply and enhancing their own growth. Both benign and malignant tumors may cause edema in the surrounding brain; some secrete factors that increase vascular permeability.

SYMPTOMS AND DIAGNOSIS

Brain tumors present with a variety of clinical signs and symptoms that depend largely on the type of tumor and its location. Seizures (partial or generalized), visual loss, hearing loss, focal motor or sensory phenomena, ataxia, double vision, and headache develop frequently. Increased intracranial pressure may cause nonspecific symptoms of headache, nausea, and vomiting. The headache secondary to increased intracranial pressure is more noticeable in the morning and dissipates within a few hours. Personality changes may be associated with increased intracranial pressure and with masses in the frontal region or posterior fossa. Changes in libido or menstrual cycles may occur. This mixture of protean and specific complaints is the reason medical attention is sought.

On physical examination, the focal signs may help direct the workup. The fundi may reveal papilledema. With slow-growing tumors, the findings are generally more subtle because the CNS may be more accommodating. A rapid evolution of signs and symptoms is generally cause for alarm.

In the past, lumbar puncture with cerebrospinal fluid (CSF) analysis, electroencephalography, nuclear scanning, pneumoencephalography, ventriculography, and angiography were the mainstays of the workup for brain tumors. These studies have been supplanted by computed tomography (CT) and magnetic resonance imaging (MRI). MRI may provide a better evaluation of the anatomy of the CNS, and a better definition of edema versus tumor mass. Angiography remains a useful modality, especially for vascular tumors. CSF analysis may be used for staging purposes, to demonstrate meningeal seeding, and to detect shedding of malignant cells into the CSF (i.e., primary CNS lymphoma).

TABLE 109.1. Distribution of Primary Brain Tumors by Tumor Type

Tumor	Percentage of cases (%)	Mean age at diagnosis (y)
Glioblastoma	40	54
Astrocytoma	16	37
Meningioma	18	55
Schwannoma	2	57
Pituitary adenoma	12	39
Lymphoma	2	46
Other	10	—

CLASSIFICATION

Neuropathology has played a major role in improving our understanding of tumor pathogenesis. The analysis of tissue obtained by biopsy or resection is the only method of exact diagnosis. Although the location and behavior of the mass and its character on CT or MRI may provide important clues to the diagnosis, there is no substitute for a microscopic examination with differential staining and other advanced pathologic techniques. Several different scales or classification protocols are followed. Glial tumors are graded pathologically on the basis of the most malignant area identified (World Heath Organization system or the St. Anne-Mayo system). These systems use the presence or absence of nuclear atypia, mitosis, microvascular proliferation, and necrosis to establish a specific grade. The Karnofsky performance score is an important clinical grading scale commonly used to evaluate the patient across various stages of treatment and follow-up. Patients are assigned a score of 10 to 100 according to their ability to perform daily tasks. Thus, simple survival scores have been expanded to include the quality of survival.

BENIGN TUMORS

Benign tumors of the nervous system (Table 109.2) generally grow slowly and do not invade surrounding structures. They are often subtle in their presentation. A tumor is benign on the basis of its cellular character and behavior. However, benign tumors may not be resectable if they adhere to adjacent tissues or surround essential structures.

Meningioma

Meningiomas arise from meningothelial cells and are technically not true brain tumors. Meningiomas occur twice as often in women as in men, usually in later life. They are more common after previous cranial radiation and in persons with neurofibromatosis type 2. The incidence of meningiomas is increased in patients with breast carcinoma. Meningiomas contain receptors for sex hormones and other ligands, including progesterone, estrogen, androgen, dopamine, and the β-receptor for platelet-derived growth factor; of these, the progesterone receptor is the

TABLE 109.2. Benign Tumors of the Central Nervous System

Tumor	Clinical presentation	Location	CT features	MRI features	Treatment issues
Meningioma	Subtle, slow growth and lack of invasion; seizures, headache, focal deficits	Arachnoid origin, along dural planes	Well-defined, enhances well with contrast	Similar to brain on T1 and T2, enhances with contrast	Not always curable; site, accessibility, and biologic aggressiveness; hormonal relation
Pituitary adenoma	Endocrine, visual symptoms; mass effect incidental	Sella turcica and suprasellar region	Use contrast; transaxial and coronal views (bone and tissue)	Best on T1; contrast; sagittal, coronal, and transaxial virus	Observation, hormone (bromocriptine), surgery
Acoustic neuroma	Sensorineural hearing loss, tinnitus, dizziness	Vestibular nerve in internal auditory meatus	Bony changes and mass	Best seen with MRI and contrast	Observation surgery, radiation
Craniopharyngioma	Growth failure in children; sexual dysfunction/visual loss in adults	Suprasellar	Low density with calcification	Low density with calcification	Observation, radiation, stereotactic and surgical resection; combination
Epidermoid	Seizures, cranial nerve abnormalities, hydrocephalus	Cisterns at base of brain	Low density, irregular rim that enhances	Low density, irregular rim that enhances	Surgery only
Colloid cyst	Headache or obtundation secondary to obstruction of foramen of Monro	Third ventricle	Low, isodense or enhancing; location is key	Low, isodense, or enhancing; location is key	Surgery, may need shunting; stereotactic aspiration
Hemangioblastoma	Posterior fossa obstruction, hydrocephalus	Cerebellum	Vascular nodule with surrounding cyst	Vascular nodule with surrounding cyst	Surgical resection

most robust. These may have important implications for pathophysiology and future therapies. The characteristic histologic features are whorls formed around central hyaline material. This eventually calcifies and forms psammoma bodies or interlacing bundles of elongated fibroblasts with narrow nuclei. Several pathologic classifications have been developed.

The classic primary treatment has been surgical, but size, location, and relation to neighboring structures may preclude total resection. External beam radiotherapy has been shown to slow regrowth in selected patients with inoperable, partially resected, or recurrent meningiomas. Chemotherapy for meningioma has been disappointing.

Pituitary Adenoma

Pituitary adenomas account for 10% to 15% of intracranial tumors. The four most frequent presentations of a pituitary adenoma are the following: a hypersecretory endocrine syndrome, visual symptoms, symptoms of a mass effect (e.g., headache), and an incidental finding on MRI or CT.

Of the hypersecretory syndromes caused by pituitary adenomas, the most common is hyperprolactinemia secondary to a prolactin-secreting tumor (40%). In women, galactorrhea, amenorrhea, or infertility develops. The serum prolactin levels can be measured and monitored. Growth hormone-secreting adenomas (15%) cause acromegaly in adults. Major changes in other organs (e.g., hypertension, cardiomyopathy, hepatosplenomegaly, arthritis) may occur. A third hypersecretion syndrome is Cushing syndrome, caused by excess secretion of cortisol or adrenocorticotropic hormone (10%). The clinical signs include moon facies, truncal obesity, abdominal striae, buffalo hump, facial hirsutism, diabetes mellitus, and hypertension. Follicle-stimulating hormone, luteinizing hormone, and thyroid-stimulating hormone may all be affected.

Pituitary adenomas typically cause a bitemporal hemianopia when they compress the fibers within the optic chiasm. Symptoms of a mass effect with headache are often nonspecific. Pituitary apoplexy with hemorrhage or infarction into the pituitary gland can cause collapse and symptoms similar to those of subarachnoid hemorrhage. Several other tumors can mimic a pituitary adenoma if they occupy the sellar and suprasellar regions. These include meningiomas, craniopharyngiomas, and rare primary and metastatic tumors (breast cancer and non–small cell lung cancer).

MRI is the modality of choice for imaging pituitary structures and provides excellent definition of the suprasellar extent of the tumor in addition to retrosellar and parasellar extension. CT is an excellent second choice. Both MRI and CT should be performed with and without contrast.

The management of these tumors depends on their size and type and the clinical syndrome. Often, neurology, neurosurgery, ophthalmology, and endocrine consultants are necessary. In the case of prolactin-secreting tumors, a dopamine agonist (e.g., bromocriptine) lowers the prolactin levels and shrinks the tumor mass. The other pituitary tumors are best treated by surgery. Transsphenoidal surgery is the procedure of choice, with a morbidity rate of 5% to 10% and a mortality rate of nearly zero. CSF leak is the most common postsurgical problem. Radiation therapy is used adjunctively.

Acoustic Neuroma

Acoustic neuromas are more correctly called *vestibular schwannomas* because they are composed of Schwann cells and arise from the vestibular nerve. These are benign neoplasms. The incidence is about 1 per 100,000. Ninety-five percent are unilateral and not associated with other entities. Five percent are bilateral and associated with neurofibromatosis type 2 (von Recklinghausen disease), an autosomal-dominant disorder. No sexual predilection is noted.

The most common presenting complaint is sensorineural hearing loss. Other symptoms include tinnitus, dizziness, and disequilibrium. As the tumor expands, it fills the internal auditory meatus, compressing the cochlear and facial nerves. Late signs include brainstem compression, ataxia, and hydrocephalus. Audiometry shows sensorineural hearing loss, usually for high frequencies. Brainstem auditory evoked potential testing demonstrates prolongation of waves I through III. CT shows an isodense enhancing mass originating at the internal auditory meatus (internal auditory canal erosion is often seen on bone windows) and a mass in the cerebellopontine angle. MRI with gadolinium is the imaging modality of choice. Other lesions of the cerebellopontine angle include meningiomas, gliomas, cholesteatomas, arachnoid cysts, metastatic tumors, lipomas, hemangiomas, and aneurysms.

The therapeutic options include observation, surgery, and radiation therapy. Acoustic neuromas tend to grow slowly; hence, a small tumor incidentally found in an elderly patient may warrant observation for an extended period. A young patient with progressive neurologic deficits or evidence of tumor growth requires definitive treatment. Surgery is the treatment of choice. CSF leakage is a potential postoperative problem. Newer microsurgical techniques preserve hearing and avoid facial nerve damage. Patients with large tumors or tumors that have enveloped cranial nerves or distorted the brainstem are at higher risk. Radiation therapy has had limited success.

Craniopharyngioma

Craniopharyngiomas are benign suprasellar tumors arising from epithelial remnants of the Rathke pouch. Children with a craniopharyngioma present with growth failure, and adults with sexual dysfunction. MRI and CT may be diagnostic because of the location and variable contents of these tumors, which range in appearance from areas of low density to areas of calcification. Treatment options include observation, various surgical approaches, and radiation. Postoperative problems include memory deficits, appetite and behavioral disturbances, and endocrine dysfunction.

Epidermoid

Epidermoids are collections of misplaced ectoderm (by implantation or sequestration). They generally develop at the cerebellopontine angle and base of the skull. Patients usually present with headache, signs of obstruction, or cranial nerve abnormalities. On CT, the tumors are of low attenuation and lobulated in the expected location. On MRI, the T1 and T2 values are prolonged. The treatment is surgical, although the tendency of the tumors to grow along cranial nerves may preclude removal. The cyst contents are notorious for inciting an aseptic meningitis (responsive to steroids).

Colloid Cyst

Colloid cysts are spherical cysts in the roof of the third ventricle. Patients present with headache and other signs of obstructive hydrocephalus. Sometimes, the cysts are found incidentally on a scan performed for other reasons. They are low or isodense spheres on CT and MRI; some enhance. The treatment is surgical, but their location can make removal difficult.

Hemangioblastoma

Hemangioblastomas are most commonly found in the cerebellum. About 10% of patients have polycythemia secondary to tumor production of erythropoietin. The tumors occur sporadically or as a component of autosomal-dominant von Hippel-Lindau disease. They are associated with retinal angiomatosis, renal cell carcinoma, visceral cysts, and adrenal pheochromocytomas. A cystic lesion with a nodule is seen on CT and MRI. Surgical resection is the preferred treatment.

MALIGNANT TUMORS

The term *malignant* generally refers to the ability of a tumor to metastasize. This has no relevance in the CNS, but seeding or spreading of tumor along surfaces is possible. Malignant CNS tumors infiltrate the parenchyma and are poorly circumscribed (Table 109.3). Metaplasia (a nonneoplastic conversion of one adult cell type to another) and anaplasia (change from a more differentiated to a less differentiated state) occur. Tumor necrosis develops when tumor growth outpaces blood supply. Other important signs of malignancy are grading by histologic differentiation, palisading and pseudopalisading, rosette formation, desmoplasia (proliferation of mesenchymal tissue), and endothelial proliferation (capillaries).

Astroglial Neoplasms

Tumors of the astrocytic series comprise the largest and most heterogeneous group of neuroepithelial tumors. Astrocytoma, anaplastic astrocytoma, and glioblastoma represent an evolution of the same process. Malignant changes may transform a well-differentiated astrocytoma over time. The astrocytoma is considered a mildly hypercellular tumor with pleomorphism but no vascular proliferation or necrosis. The anaplastic astrocytoma exhibits vascular proliferation, moderate pleomorphism, and moderate hypercellularity. The glioblastoma shows these characteristics plus necrosis. The absence of necrosis is the principal criterion for distinguishing anaplastic astrocytoma from glioblastoma.

The astroglial tumors are also described on the basis of their location: optic nerve glioma, hypothalamic glioma, brainstem (tectal, pontine, or medullary) glioma, cerebellar astrocytoma, corpus callosum glioma, cerebral hemisphere astrocytoma, and so forth. The location of the tumor may have important implications for treatment. Brainstem gliomas occur primarily in children. Widespread infiltration of the brain parenchyma is rare; when it occurs, it is termed *gliomatosis cerebri*.

The mean age of patients at the onset of anaplastic astrocytoma is 46 years. The tumors are usually located in the cerebral hemispheres. The average survival time from diagnosis is 2 years.

Glioblastoma multiforme is the most common primary brain tumor in adults, comprising about 50% of all gliomas. It is the most aggressive, malignant, and lethal primary tumor of the CNS parenchyma. The peak age at onset is 40 to 60 years; the average survival time from diagnosis is 10 months. The tumor occurs in the deep white matter, basal ganglia, or thalamus; rarely, it is found in the cerebellum or spinal cord. The affected portion of the brain is usually replaced by a single well-circumscribed lesion that infiltrates the cerebral cortex and spreads to the opposite hemisphere via the corpus callosum.

TABLE 109.3. Malignant Tumors of the Central Nervous System

Tumor	Clinical presentation	Location	CT features	MRI features	Treatment issues
Astroglial neoplasm	Headache, progressive neurologic deficit, seizures	Range from optic nerve to brainstem	Range from low density to contrast enhancing rim with variable edema	More sensitive than CT, better demarcation of tumor vs. edema	Surgical resection with radiation; chemotherapy options
Oligodendroglioma	Seizures and headache, rarely hemorrhage	Variable	Hypodense, often with calcification; no enhancement	Hypodense, often with calcification; no enhancement	Surgical resection, radiation questionable, chemotherapy an option
Ependymoma	Headache, obstructive hydrocephalus, seizures	Posterior fossa masses in children, supratentorial in adults	Isodense or hyperintense lesions that enhance with contrast	Variably enhancing, heterogeneous tumors lining the ventricles	Surgical resection with radiation
Ganglioglioma	Seizures	Temporal or frontal lobe	Hyperdense, no enhancement; calcification	Hyperdense, no enhancement; calcification	Surgical resection, radiation an option
Medulloblastoma	Headache, gait disturbance, diplopia, increased intracranial pressure	Cerebellar vermis in children, cerebellar hemisphere in adults	Nonspecific posterior fossa mass with hydrocephalus	Nonspecific posterior fossa mass with hydrocephalus	Surgical resection when possible, radiation therapy
Pineal region tumor	Headache, gait disturbance, Parinaud syndrome	In region of the pineal gland with obstruction and compression of adjacent structures	Variable: isodense, hyperdense, heterogeneous; contrast enhancing	Best study; variable: isodense, hyperdense, heterogeneous; contrast enhancing	Variable depending on type, size, and extension: surgery and radiation
Lymphoma	Focal symptoms and signs, headache, increased intracranial pressure, immunocompromise	Mass in periventricular region of deep white matter	Isodense or hyperdense in supratentorial periventricular regions, enhances, ring enhancing at times	Isodense or hyperdense in supratentorial periventricular regions, enhances, ring enhancing at times, little edema	Steroids oncolytic, surgery for biopsy only, radiation therapy the treatment of choice, chemotherapy in selected cases
Cerebral metastases	Occur in 30% with systemic cancer (melanoma, breast cancer, small cell lung cancer); progressive deficit, seizure, hemorrhage	Distal arterial fields	Enhancing lesions with edema	More sensitive than CT, enhancing lesions with edema	Biopsy if primary not known, surgical excision for single accessible lesion, radiation

Most patients with an astrocytoma present with headaches, a progressive neurologic deficit, or seizures. A seizure occurring for the first time in an adult (without evident cause) should alert the clinician to the possibility of a brain tumor. This should be investigated by CT or MRI. The appearance of the tumors is quite varied. Low-grade tumors are seen on CT as areas of low density (containing either tumor cells or edematous fluid). MRI is more sensitive than CT in distinguishing tumor from edema. The border of glioblastoma multiforme enhances with contrast medium on MRI (ringlike enhancement).

Surgical resection is the mainstay of treatment. The width of the resection should be as vigorous as possible with guidance and limitation by location. Radiation to the whole brain plus the tumor itself prolongs survival. Brachytherapy (stereotactic implantation of radiation) may be useful for recurrence. Various chemotherapeutic agents have been used; some have small but definite advantages over surgical resection and radiation therapy. Hence, the routine use of chemotherapy is controversial. No clinical feature can identify the patients who are likely to benefit from chemotherapy. The use of chemotherapy increases the proportion of long-term survivors from less than 5% to approximately 15% to 20%.

Oligodendroglioma

Oligodendroglial tumors comprise only 1% of brain tumors in children and fewer than 5% of brain tumors in all age groups. The frontal lobes are often the site of these tumors. Seizures are the presenting symptom in about two thirds of patients. Almost 25% are hemorrhagic. On occasion, they bleed sufficiently to manifest a stroke-like presentation, but headache and seizures are the usual presenting features.

These tumors do not enhance with contrast on CT or MRI. They characteristically are of low density and contain areas of calcification. Histologically, the cells have uniform nuclei surrounded by clear cytoplasm ("fried egg" appearance).

It may be elected to defer treatment until evidence of progression is noted. The accepted treatment is surgical. Radiation treatment is optional, with several studies demonstrating benefit; controversy exists regarding timing, dose, and response.

Chemotherapy has been shown to benefit some of these patients. Most oligodendrogliomas eventually progress by becoming malignant.

Ependymoma

Ependymomas arise from the cells that line the ventricles, and the tumors project from the ependymal surface to occupy the ventricle. Obstructive hydrocephalus is the usual mode of presentation. Ependymomas comprise 4% of all brain tumors and are the third most common CNS tumor in children. They occur most frequently in children younger than 10 years. Ninety percent are in the brain; the rest are in the spinal cord. Most are infratentorial.

Radiographically, they appear on CT as isodense or hyperintense lesions that enhance with contrast. Forty percent are calcified. MRI demonstrates the anatomic location well and may reveal spread. The tumors may seed the subarachnoid space and spinal canal. Histologically, they are characterized by sheets of cells interrupted by perivascular rosettes and canals (glandlike structures lined by cells resembling those that line the ventricles).

The treatment is surgical resection with radiation. If seeding is evident, full craniospinal radiation is performed. Chemotherapy for these tumors is not well established.

Ganglioglioma

Gangliogliomas occur in children and young adults; 80% of the patients are younger than 30 years. They may develop anywhere in the brain, but the temporal lobe is the most common site. Patients present with long-standing epilepsy. CT and MRI are often nonspecific. The lesions are nonenhancing and hyperdense, but occasionally a nodule enhances. Calcifications may occur.

Pathologically, gangliogliomas resemble low-grade astrocytomas with sheets or bundles of spindle cells. Some neurons may acquire a dysplastic appearance.

The treatment is surgical resection. Radiation therapy is added for unresectable recurrent tumors and for subtotally resected gangliogliomas with an anaplastic component.

Medulloblastoma

Medulloblastoma is the most common malignant brain tumor of childhood. Twenty-five percent occur in adults, but most of these patients are younger than 20 years. Medulloblastomas are rare after the fourth decade. Patients present with posterior fossa signs or signs of obstruction (headache, nausea, vomiting, diplopia, gait ataxia, nystagmus, papilledema). In children, the tumors arise in the cerebellar vermis; in adults, they arise in the cerebellar hemisphere.

Histologically, these are highly cellular tumors with abundant, dark-staining, round or oval nuclei, scant cytoplasm, and frequent mitoses. Pseudorosettes, characterized by carrot-shaped nuclei arranged radially around amorphous, eosinophilic centers, are present in 40% of the cases.

The CT and MRI appearance of medulloblastomas is nonspecific. They appear as isodense or hyperdense masses arising from either the cerebellar vermis or cerebellar hemisphere. Contrast enhancement is variable. Hydrocephalus is common.

Medulloblastomas tend to spread locally within the ventricles or seed the subarachnoid space and spine. Staging is helpful for planning treatment and establishing a prognosis.

The first line of treatment is surgical. The goal is to remove as much tumor as possible without neurologic compromise. Shunting for hydrocephalus may be necessary. Craniospinal radiation is the mainstay of postoperative treatment. Chemotherapy has been beneficial in patients who are poor candidates for surgery or radiation therapy.

Tumors of the Pineal Region

Tumors in this area comprise only 1% of adult brain tumors; they are more common in children. Various types of tumors develop in the pineal region, more than half of them of germ cell origin. Germinomas (which account for two thirds of the germ cell tumors), teratomas, dermoids, malignant choriocarcinomas, endodermal sinus tumors, and embryonal tumors comprise the germ cell tumor list, in descending order of frequency. Twenty percent are of pineal cell origin (pinealocytoma and pineoblastoma).

These tumors cause symptoms by obstructing CSF flow at the aqueduct or posterior third ventricle and by compressing adjacent brainstem structures. Hydrocephalus is common. Presenting symptoms include headache, lethargy, nausea, vomiting, and gait disturbance. Tectal compression causes Parinaud syndrome (impairment of upward gaze, loss of convergence, pupillary abnormalities, and retraction nystagmus).

The tumors are of variable cell type, and their appearance on CT and MRI also varies, from isodense to hyperdense to heterogeneous. Some are calcified. Contrast may enhance them.

Surgical treatment with attention to the hydrocephalus is the usual approach. Seeding along CSF pathways may be a concern. Radiation may be helpful.

Lymphoma

Primary CNS lymphomas occur in both immunocompetent and immunosuppressed populations, but the highest incidence is in patients with AIDS. They are also associated with other immunodeficiency states, both congenital (e.g., Wiskott-Aldrich syndrome) and acquired (e.g., after organ transplantation). The origin is unknown because no lymph nodes or lymphatics are found in the CNS. These are not likely to be metastases from an occult systemic lymphoma. The tumors arise within and are confined to the nervous system. The biologic basis of primary CNS lymphoma in immunocompetent patients is poorly understood. The Epstein-Barr virus genome is found in immunocompromised patients with primary CNS lymphoma.

The tumors typically occur as a mass lesion in the periventricular region of the deep white matter. Seventy-five percent are supratentorial. Primary CNS lymphoma is multifocal in about 50% of immunocompetent patients but in all AIDS patients (often with leptomeningeal spread). Hemorrhage into the tumor is uncommon in primary CNS lymphoma but frequent in patients with AIDS (especially after surgery). Tumor necrosis is characteristic of AIDS-related lymphomas. Lesions in identical locations in the two hemispheres (mirror images) are commonly encountered in AIDS patients.

Most tumors are of B-cell origin. The tumor cells are usually large, of high grade, pleomorphic, discohesive, and infiltrative. The tumors are often infiltrated by reactive T lymphocytes.

Primary CNS lymphoma occurs in all age groups. The peak incidence is in the sixth and seventh decades in immunocompetent patients, earlier in the immunosuppressed population. Patients present with focal symptoms and symptoms of increased intracranial pressure. Personality and cognitive changes are common. Seizures are uncommon. Symptoms progress over weeks to months.

Contrast-enhanced CT or MRI reveals periventricular masses with indistinct borders, homogeneous enhancement, and little surrounding edema. Before enhancement, the tumors are isodense or hyperdense. Multiple lesions are seen in 50% of patients.

CSF analysis may be helpful. The CSF protein level is elevated in 85% of patients. The CSF glucose level may be low in cases with leptomeningeal spread. Lymphocytic pleocytosis is present in 50% of the patients. Immunohistochemical staining may establish the malignant nature of the pleocytosis. Lymphomatous infiltration of the eye is found in 20% of the patients at presentation.

Corticosteroids are oncolytic agents in primary CNS lymphoma and should not be given until the disease is established by biopsy. Steroid responsiveness should not be used as a diagnostic test. Surgery is limited to biopsy only.

The radiographic appearance in patients with AIDS may mimic that of toxoplasmosis. In patients with AIDS and a CNS mass lesion, empiric antitoxoplasmosis therapy is usually given first. If the patient has primary CNS lymphoma, neurologic deterioration usually occurs during antibiotic treatment.

Whole-brain radiation therapy has been the mainstay of treatment in the past because of the widespread distribution of lymphoma within the brain. Primary CNS lymphoma can recur within the brain, but at a site distant from the original tumor. Radiation therapy induces a complete response in 90% of patients. The median survival is 12 to 18 months, with a 5-year survival rate of 3% to 4%. Chemotherapy has been shown to be of benefit. High-dose methotrexate is associated with a complete response rate of 50% to 80%. A better response is obtained with the combination of radiation and chemotherapy. Delayed neurotoxic effects may be seen in patients older than 60 years.

CEREBRAL METASTASIS

Neurologic symptoms occur in about 20% of patients with cancer. Metabolic encephalopathy is the most common neurologic sequela in patients with cancer, but it is usually a terminal complication representing organ failure. Metastatic lesions of the brain parenchyma are the most common nonterminal neurologic event in patients with cancer. Almost 25% of patients with cancer have brain metastases at autopsy, and about 10% have metastases confined to the brain parenchyma.

More than 25% of all autopsy-proven brain metastases have a pulmonary source; breast cancer and melanoma are second and third most common sources, respectively. Malignant melanoma (which represents only 1% of all cancers) is the most likely of all systemic malignant tumors to metastasize to the brain. Most brain metastases are spread hematogenously, arising from circulating tumor cells or from frank tumor emboli. They occur at the junction of gray and white, which is characteristic of an embolic event. Metastases are multiple in about 50% of patients and typically are well demarcated and solid. Occasionally, they are cystic, necrotic, or hemorrhagic. Tumors arising from the kidney, colon, breast, and thyroid and adenocarcinoma of the lung are most often associated with a single metastasis; metastases from melanoma, small cell carcinoma of the lung, and tumors of unknown origin tend to be multiple. Melanoma, renal cell carcinoma, and germ cell malignant tumors (especially choriocarcinomas) tend to be hemorrhagic. Brain metastases of lung origin are often identified early in the course of the disease; metastases from breast cancer typically develop late, usually after the disease has spread systemically.

Most patients with brain metastases present with a combination of focal and generalized symptoms and signs within a subacute, progressive time frame. Those with hemorrhage or seizures present acutely in a dramatic fashion. CT usually provides sufficient information. Contrast enhancement and the presence of white matter edema and multiple lesions are the compelling features of metastases. MRI can detect metastases occult on CT, identify associated leptomeningeal disease, and disclose early therapeutic complications.

Treatment options are tempered by the patient's neurologic condition and functional and overall performance status, extent of the primary tumor and other systemic disease, number and sites of the brain metastases, and radiosensitivity of the tumor type. The goal of treatment is to control the neurologic symptoms; cure is rarely possible. Corticosteroids produce a prompt improvement in most patients with brain metastases. The improvement may be seen in just a few hours, and 70% of patients show substantial improvement within 48 hours. Corticosteroids may have a specific oncolytic effect in lymphomas and breast cancer. The long-term use of corticosteroid medication is associated with substantial side effects and risks. Whole-brain radiation and other radiation techniques may extend the duration and quality of life. Chemotherapy for cerebral metastases remains uncertain.

Surgical options include the resection of solitary lesions, treatment of increased intracranial pressure, biopsy of tumors from an unknown primary cancer, and administration of stereotactic radiosurgical therapy. Up to 50% of patients have a solitary metastasis. About half of these are not surgical candidates because of tumor inaccessibility, extensive systemic metastases, or other medical problems. In patients who qualify, resection of an isolated metastasis followed by radiation therapy offers better survival than radiation therapy alone. The best survival rates are in patients younger than 65 years with a single brain metastasis, a score of at least 70 on the Karnofsky performance scale, and a controlled primary tumor.

CONSIDERATIONS DURING PREGNANCY

The incidence of intracranial tumors (except pituitary tumors) is not increased during pregnancy. Intracranial neoplasms may manifest initially during pregnancy because of three factors. First, tumors may enlarge during pregnancy as a result of retention of salt and water in the systemic vasculature. Vascular tumors such as meningiomas are most likely to manifest in this way. Second, mild immunologic suppression during pregnancy may decrease the patient's ability to tolerate a tumor. Third, some tumors may be hormonally dependent. Pregnancy does not appear to influence the growth of vestibular schwannomas.

The pituitary gland may enlarge up to 70% during pregnancy because of a proliferation of prolactin-secreting cells. When a woman with an unknown adenoma or other pituitary tumor becomes pregnant, the tumor may rapidly enlarge and become symptomatic. The most common symptoms include headache and a bitemporal hemianopic visual field defect. As previously stated, adenomas may be hypersecretory or hyposecretory for prolactin, growth hormone, or adrenocorticotropic hormone.

Management depends on the severity of symptoms. If vision is threatened, surgical management is unavoidable. In most instances, however, surgery may be delayed if the tumor can be controlled with steroids and bromocriptine (for prolactin-secreting tumors). These agents are safe to use during pregnancy. Bromocriptine suppresses lactation in the postpartum period. Abrupt blindness resulting from pituitary apoplexy mandates urgent surgical intervention.

It has been reported that meningiomas and vascular tumors frequently present during pregnancy, and that the symptoms of these tumors progress rapidly during pregnancy, then decrease after parturition. Progesterone and estrogen receptors are frequently detected in meningioma cells and are thought to have a direct hormonal effect on the tumor growth rate. Indeed, the symptoms of a meningioma may fluctuate with the menstrual cycle. Tamoxifen (a potent antiestrogen agent useful in breast cancer) does not clinically affect tumor size or symptoms in patients with inoperable meningiomas.

Choriocarcinoma is a malignant tumor that arises from fetal trophoblastic tissue. The trophoblastic tumor invades the maternal uterine blood vessels and metastasizes. The rate of cerebral metastases is high (up to 28%). These may manifest as an embolic stroke, subarachnoid hemorrhage, or intracerebral hematoma. Choriocarcinomas are highly vascular tumors that bleed at the site of metastatic involvement. A strong relationship has been found between cerebral metastatic lesions and mortality from choriocarcinoma. Chemotherapy and radiation therapy are the initial treatment modalities for the metastatic cerebral tumors. Surgery is reserved for acute hemorrhagic complications.

In the management of brain tumors diagnosed during pregnancy, several important considerations must be weighed: the suspected nature of the tumor, the stage of pregnancy during which the tumor is detected, the patient's neurologic stability, the anticipated maternal and fetal outcomes with medical versus surgical management, the efficacy of vaginal versus cesarean delivery, and fetal viability.

BIBLIOGRAPHY

Black PM. Brain tumors. *N Engl J Med* 1991;324:1471.

DeAngelis LM. Brain tumors. *N Engl J Med* 2001;344:114.

Donaldson JO. Neurology of pregnancy. In: Walton J, ed. *Major problems in neurology*. Philadelphia: WB Saunders, 1989.

Fox MW, Harms RW, Davis DH. Selected neurologic complications of pregnancy. *Mayo Clin Proc* 1990;65:1595.

Heffner RR. Pathology of nervous system tumors. In: Bradley WG, Daroff RB, Fenichel GM, et al., eds. *Neurology in clinical practice*. Boston: Butterworth-Heinemann, 1996.

Jaeckle KA, Cohen ME, Duffner PK. Clinical presentation and therapy of nervous system tumors. In: Bradley WG, Daroff RB, Fenichel GM, et al., eds. *Neurology in clinical practice*. Boston: Butterworth-Heinemann, 1996.

Laws ER, Thapar K. Brain tumors. *CA Cancer J Clin* 1993;43:263.

Olivi A, Brem RF, McPherson R, et al. Brain tumors in pregnancy. In: Goldstein PJ, Stern BJ, eds. *Neurological disorders of pregnancy*. New York: Futura Publishing, 1992.

O'Neill BP, Buckner JC, Coffey RJ, et al. Brain metastatic lesions. *Mayo Clin Proc* 1994;69:1062.

Weinreb HJ. Demyelinating and neoplastic diseases in pregnancy. In: Yerby M, Devinsky O, eds. *Neurologic complications of pregnancy*. Philadelphia: WB Saunders, 1994.

Wen PY, Black PM. Brain tumors in adults. *Neurol Clin* 1995;13:4.

CHAPTER 110

Spinal Cord Syndromes

Joshua Hollander

Spinal cord diseases can be confusing if the clinician is not familiar with the anatomy of the cord and its circulation, and the relationship of the cord to the spinal canal and its bony levels. The growth of the cord does not match that of the spinal column, and the cord slowly recedes in a rostral direction. In adulthood, the cord ends at the L1-2 vertebral level. The cervical region comprises seven vertebrae and eight roots. C1 through C7 emerge above the vertebral level; the C8 root emerges below the vertebra in the manner characteristic of the rest of the vertebral column. The clinician must remember the discrepancy between the cord and column levels in planning investigations. The dermatomal distribution is discussed in the section on radiculopathy.

In cross section, the white matter columns of the cord surround the interior gray. The posterior columns are involved in ipsilateral discriminative touch and limb proprioception, crossing in the brainstem. The ventrolateral spinothalamic and spinoreticular columns conduct pain, temperature, touch, and pressure. The cell bodies of the sensory neurons are in the dorsal root ganglia, and the sensory neurons may form synapses in the dorsal horn of the cord. Most spinothalamic fibers cross through the central cord. The lateral columns contain descending motor fibers. The anterior horns of the central gray contain the lower motor neurons, which exit through the anterior root. Many complex interneurons and multiple transmitters are found in the cord that are not dealt with here.

The circulation of the cord is complex. Two posterior spinal arteries course downward near the dorsal root entry zones with multiple radicular collaterals (Fig. 110.1). The anterior cord is less well endowed, with an anterior spinal artery arising from branches of each vertebral artery. Anterior collaterals are less frequent; small ones may be found at about C6 and some in the thoracic cord. A major lateralized collateral is the great radicular artery of Adamkiewicz in the lumbar area. The location of this vessel is somewhat variable but is usually at T11 on the left. Blood flow is such that the major watershed area is around T4, but another may be found at T12.

ETIOLOGY AND DIFFERENTIAL DIAGNOSIS

The approach of Young and Woolsey (1995) to disorders of the spinal cord is followed here, and their work can be consulted for a more complete discussion. They divided the disorders into five neurologic abnormalities and nine cord syndromes; their system allows a clinical classification before any expensive studies are performed.

The five neurologic abnormalities are pain, motor abnormalities, sensory abnormalities, abnormalities of reflex and motor tone, and bladder symptoms.

Pain may be local, radicular, or central. Local pain is related to the involvement of ligamentous and bony structures at the level of a lesion; the time course of the evolution of pain can indicate the type of process. Radicular pain in intrinsic disease usually occurs at the level of a lesion and tends to radiate only short distances. It is less useful in localization than paresthesias. Central pain has a diffuse burning, aching quality that is associated with sensory loss in the relevant area.

The most significant motor abnormality is weakness, which requires a loss of 50% of descending motor neurons or a similar loss of anterior horn cells. Weakness is most striking in lesions with an abrupt onset. Slowly progressive lesions are more likely to cause fatigability, clumsiness, and unsteadiness. Spasticity of the upper motor neuron type may be prominent but is usually less of a problem. Involvement of anterior horn cells may be associated with atrophy and fasciculations. Hand problems are more readily detected.

Sensory abnormalities include positive and negative features. Positive features, or paresthesias, are manifested in damaged sensory pathways. The presentation is of either the posterior column type ("pins and needles," tingling) or spinothalamic pathway type (thermal sensation or itching). The Lhermitte sign is an electric shocklike sensation radiating down the back or limbs that is elicited by cervical flexion in cases of cervical myelopathy. Negative symptoms of numbness or

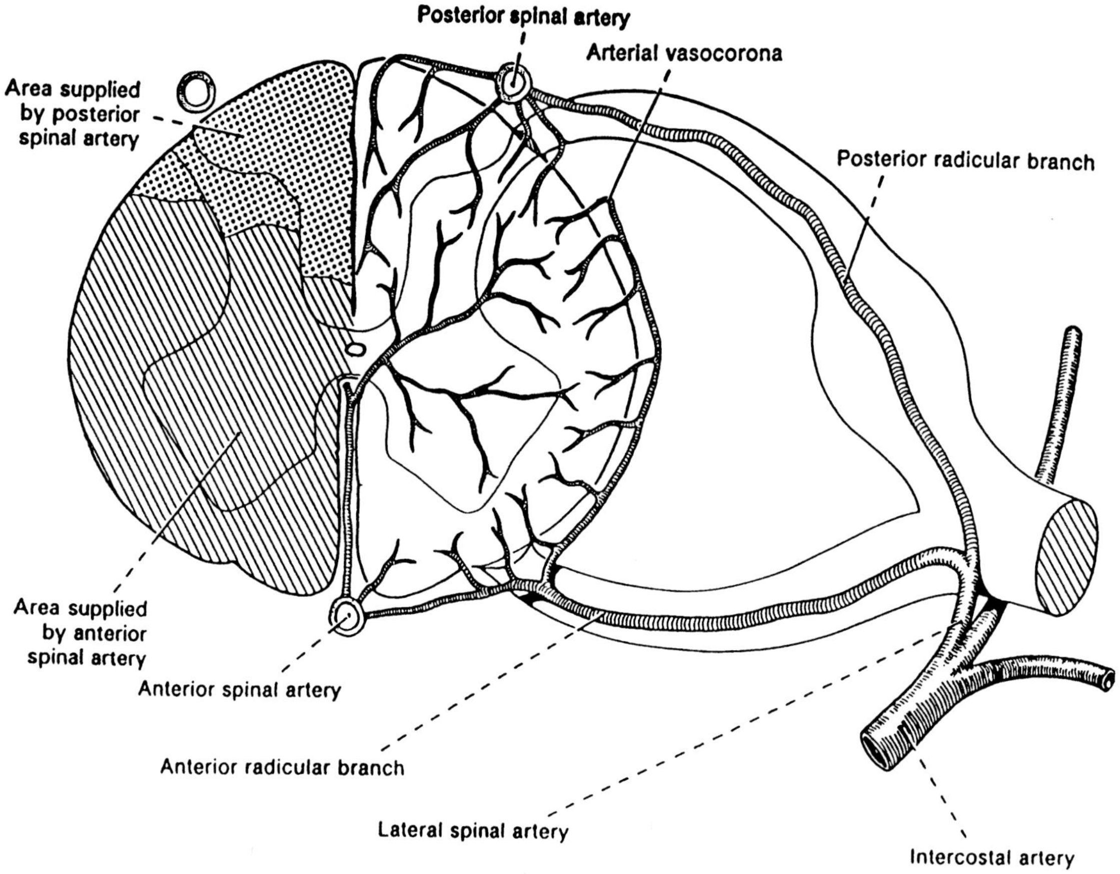

FIG. 110.1. Circulation of the spinal cord.

"deadness" reflect posterior column involvement. Spinothalamic loss may be noted only by an inability to gauge the temperature of shower water on one side. Characteristic patterns include loss of position and vibratory sense in the feet with spared reflexes (dorsal cord syndrome), loss of position and vibratory sense in the feet with a clear sensory level to pinprick on the trunk (thoracic cord lesion), bilateral segmental upper limb sensory loss sparing the lower limbs (central cord syndrome), loss of pinprick and contralateral position and vibration (Brown-Séquard syndrome), loss of pinprick on the trunk and lower limbs with a level but preserved perianal sensation (sacral sparing, intramedullary or anterior extramedullary cord lesion), loss of perianal and posterior thigh sensation (conus medullaris or high cauda lesion), and loss of pinprick on the trunk and lower limbs with a level (anterior cord syndrome).

Reflex changes include spinal shock (when acute lesions result in paralysis) and areflexia (from a loss of descending facilitative impulses). More slowly developing lesions manifest with hyperactive reflexes below the level of the lesion, and reflexes may be absent or hypoactive at the level of the lesion. Hyperactive limb reflexes with a hyperactive jaw jerk suggest an intracranial localization; a hypoactive jaw jerk suggests a high cervical localization. The extensor plantar response is a polysynaptic reflex that may be seen early in cord disease.

Bladder dysfunction varies with the level of the lesion and the rate of development. Urinary retention with overflow incontinence is seen with acute cord lesions and lesions of the conus medullaris and cauda equina. More slowly progressive myelopathies result in hyperactive detrusor reflexes that present as urgency, frequency, and incontinence. A more confusing problem is detrusor/sphincter dyssynergia, seen in disorders that cause lesions at multiple levels.

The nine cord syndromes of Woolsey and Young are as follows:

The complete cord syndromes (paraplegia or quadriplegia with local pain, altered reflexes, nonselective sensory loss, and loss of bladder function) occur as acute or subacute disorders. *Acute complete cord syndromes* are caused primarily by vascular or traumatic mechanisms. Trauma is usually associated with a history of injury and local pain. Infarction tends to occur in the more vulnerable anterior cord, sparing the posterior columns. Spontaneous epidural hemorrhage and acute cord compression from a herniated disc are rare. These conditions are associated with spinal shock. *Subacute complete cord syndromes* may evolve over hours or weeks. More rapid syndromes, such as transverse myelitis, may display areflexia; more slowly evolving syndromes are associated with hyperreflexia and extensor plantar responses. A spinal epidural tumor or abscess causes early radicular pain. The bladder is involved acutely and late in subacute processes.

Chronic spastic paraplegia with gait ataxia evolving over months or years is associated with three syndromes. The *pure motor syndromes* include motor neuron diseases, familial spastic paraplegia, and the myelopathy of cervical spondylosis. Bladder involvement is minor. The *dorsal cord syndromes* (paraplegia or quadriplegia with loss of position and vibratory sense) include multiple sclerosis, subacute combined degeneration of the spinal cord (vitamin B_{12} deficiency), myelopathy of cervical spondylosis, arteriovenous malformations, axial or extraaxial cord tumors, spinocerebellar degeneration, arachnoiditis, and spinal cord trauma. Bladder involvement is a late event. *Disorders with loss of pain sensation* include bilateral (anterior cord syndrome) and unilateral (Brown-Séquard syndrome) variants. Causes may be extrinsic cord tumors, spondylotic myelopathy, radiation myelopathy, cord trauma, and myelitis.

Chronic atrophic paralysis of the hands evolving over months or years can be classified according to the presence or absence of sensory loss. Features include a segmental loss of pain sensation *(central cord syndrome)* and involvement of multiple modalities. The loss begins in a cape or glove distribution. Associated conditions include syringomyelia, intrinsic cord tumors, and trauma. *Pure motor syndromes* include motor neuron disease, cervical spondylosis, and extrinsic high cervical tumors.

Cauda equina syndromes (paraplegia with low back pain, areflexia, saddle anesthesia, and loss of bladder function) can be grouped by time course. *Acute syndromes* can be precipitated by lumbar spine trauma with fracture, a central lumbar disc herniation, or AIDS lumbosacral polyradiculopathy. *Subacute or chronic syndromes* may be caused by lumbar disc protrusion, lumbar spinal stenosis, arachnoiditis, and tumor.

Acute transverse myelitis is a rare monophasic demyelinating disorder; although the name implies a segmental lesion, the pathology may extend more broadly. The typical scenario is an antecedent viral illness followed by back pain, weakness, sensory loss and paresthesias, and urinary retention. Acute transverse myelitis tends to affect the lower thoracic cord. A more acute onset leads to more severe necrosis and residua. An association with multiple sclerosis has been noted, but the frequency is controversial (perhaps 5%–10%). Specific infectious agents have rarely been associated with acute transverse myelitis, but the infectious forms more often present with a necrotizing myelopathy or a more subacute involvement. Antecedent infections include herpesvirus infection, toxoplasmosis, schistosomiasis, and Lyme borreliosis. Toxic myelopathy is seen with intrathecal methotrexate and cytosine arabinoside. Enthusiasm for chymopapain treatment for herniated disc waned when transverse myelitis became associated with this therapy. The acute transverse myelitis of systemic lupus erythematosus is similar to the other types but has features of rapid onset, clear sensory level, and back pain. The transverse myelitis of lupus has a subacute multiple sclerosis-like fluctuating course. No clear association with anticardiolipin antibodies has been noted.

Spinal cord ischemia is rare, possibly because of the rich collateral supply of the cord and its relative resistance to ischemia (in comparison with the brain). The most vulnerable areas are the central gray matter and the watershed area in the thoracic cord. Most cases are caused by a loss of the segmental radicular arteries of the aorta. The great radicular artery (Adamkiewicz) may be lost during spontaneous dissection of the descending thoracic or abdominal aorta or during surgery on this section of the aorta. The usual presentation is sudden tearing chest or abdominal pain, paraplegia, and a sensory level.

Atheromatous (aorta), myxomatous (heart), and fibrocartilaginous (disc) emboli usually spare the cord, but such cases have been reported. Aortic atherosclerosis has been implicated in some patients with spinal cord claudication (exercise-induced painless paraparesis and sphincter disturbance), but again, vascular disease of the cord is rare. Iatrogenic vascular lesions of the cord are more common than spontaneous lesions; causes include aortic surgery, intraaortic counterpulse balloons, radiographic catheters, and possibly spinal or epidural continuous anesthesia with vasoconstrictive potentiators. Systemic hypotension has also been implicated.

Spinal cord vascular malformations include true arteriovenous malformations of both intramedullary and extramedullary, intrathecal types and dural arteriovenous fistulae. The true malformations tend to be thoracic and dorsal to the cord. They may have multiple feeders but frequently a large one in the lumbar area. The onset may be caused by subarachnoid hemorrhage and is associated with stabbing pain in the back *(coup de poignard)* and perhaps paraparesis. Exertional or postprandial paraparesis has also been noted. The dural lesions may manifest as a progressive myelopathy later in life secondary to increased venous pressure.

Progressive necrotic myelitis (syndrome of Foix and Alajouanine) usually presents with sensory, motor, and sphincter loss that progresses to higher cord levels over years. Abnormal hypertrophic vessels and spastic paraparesis with ascending amyotrophy are features of this disorder.

Radiation myelopathy presents as a gradual symmetric loss of long tracts secondary to vascular changes. It is related to the dose and fractionation and may occur 6 to 48 months after exposure. A transient cord syndrome has been described, but this usually develops over weeks and is permanent.

The perivenous demyelinating diseases include acute disseminated encephalomyelitis and multiple sclerosis (see Chapter 111). The nervous system is affected more widely in these disorders, and the diagnosis is not based on the spinal findings alone because these are nonspecific. An uncommon variety of multiple sclerosis presents late in life as a chronic progressive or relapsing/progressive spinal degeneration, with or without a remote spinal or optic event. An asymmetric onset, asynchrony in the posterior column, and motor signs may help distinguish this condition from vitamin B_{12} deficiency. Because vitamin B_{12} deficiency tends to occur later in life, the concurrent presence of cervical spinal degeneration with osteophytic ridges may cause confusion.

Degeneration of the cervical spine is associated with osteophyte formation and the subluxation of joints; disc herniation may also occur. The spinal canal or neural foramina, or both, may be compromised. The usual presentation of cervical spondylosis is a painful stiff neck, pain and numbness in the arms and hands, and spastic (perhaps ataxic) paraparesis. The evolution is over months or years, with intermittent painful exacerbations. Bladder problems may include urgency incontinence. Purely radicular syndromes are more suggestive of a herniated disc. The vertebral spaces most often involved are C4-5 (C5), C5-6 (C6), and C6-7 (C8). The severity does not always correlate with the size of the osteophyte. Other determinants are the size of the cervical canal (cervical stenosis) and the presence of redundant ligaments, which can contribute to a myelopathy as repeated cord trauma is caused by flexion and extension. The diagnosis requires a good correlation of the location and severity of signs with the radiographic findings.

Motor neuron or motor system diseases include progressive muscular atrophy, progressive bulbar palsy, primary lateral sclerosis, and amyotrophic lateral sclerosis. The latter disorder is the most common one. The combination of upper and lower motor neuron features in the same muscle groups is important for the diagnosis. Lower motor neuron features are atrophy, weakness, and fasciculations at rest; upper motor neuron features are spasticity, hyperreflexia, and extensor plantar responses. The affected limb is atrophic and weak, but the reflexes are preserved. Cervical spondylosis may cause atrophy in the hands, but the only hyperreflexia is in the legs. The onset may be asymmetric, and the bulbar muscles may be involved. Intellect and sensation are spared. Either lower motor neuron or upper motor neuron signs may be prominent early. The predominantly lower motor neuron variant, progressive muscular atrophy, tends to follow an indolent course rather than causing death within 4 to 7 years. The onset of hereditary spinal muscular atrophies is in infancy or childhood.

Familial spastic paraplegia is a progressive syndrome beginning in childhood or adulthood that presents with progressive weakness and spasticity of the legs. It probably represents a mixture of disorders.

Spinocerebellar degenerations present with ataxia as a prominent sign. The best-known condition is Friedreich ataxia. The onset is in childhood or adolescence, with slow progression over decades. This autosomal-recessive disorder affects the dorsal root ganglia, posterior columns, and spinocerebellar and corticospinal tracts. Progressive ataxia and loss of touch, vibration, and position sense are combined with areflexia. Dysarthric speech, impaired swallowing, and nystagmus are present. Skeletal deformities such as pes cavus and kyphoscoliosis are secondary features. Death is usually from the associated cardiomyopathy.

Syringomyelia is a cavitation of the central cord, usually in the cervical region, and presents with a central cord syndrome. Pain and temperature sensation are usually lost in a glove or shawl distribution; painless injuries to the fingers are not unusual. Other sensory modalities are usually spared but may be affected below the lesion. Segmental muscle atrophy and weakness are features. The differential diagnosis includes intramedullary tumor, which may also be associated with a syrinx. The cavity may extend to involve the medulla, with resultant cranial nerve dysfunction. The medulla is also affected in the half of these patients who have an associated Chiari type I malformation (plugging of the foramen magnum and downward protrusion of a medullary tongue and cerebellum). A syrinx may also develop in response to trauma and arachnoiditis.

Subacute combined degeneration of the spinal cord (vitamin B_{12} deficiency) is becoming less common. Paresthesias and sensory ataxia are followed by spastic paraparesis. Neuropathy is also seen. The presentation is usually symmetric, with progression from paresthesias to sensory ataxia and then an ataxic paraparesis. The reflexes vary, depending on the stage of the disease. The involved tracts have a spongiform appearance. Primary nutritional deficiency of vitamin B_{12} is rare, and the classic syndromes result from malabsorption of vitamin B_{12} secondary to lack of intrinsic factor (addisonian pernicious anemia), gastrectomy, blind loops of bowel, or extensive bowel resection. Rarer forms are caused by defects of cobalamin or methyl group metabolism. A macrocytic anemia with hypersegmented polymorphonuclear leukocytes and a marrow picture of megaloblasts may provide the needed clues. The administration of folate may obscure these features, and this is important to remember in women of childbearing age, who require folate supplementation.

Infectious forms of myelopathy include tropical spastic paraparesis, which is caused by human T-lymphotropic virus (HTLV-1). A chronic meningoencephalitis leads to spastic leg weakness with variable sensory and sphincter problems. Tropical spastic paraparesis is usually seen in middle-aged persons who have lived in North Africa or the West Indies. It may be transmitted by transfusion. Infection with HTLV-1 is usually asymptomatic.

AIDS is associated with various infections, such as the herpes group, but a vacuolar myelopathy occurs in 10% to 30% of patients. This resembles subacute combined degeneration, but without vitamin B_{12} deficiency. The variable clinical picture tends to include a spastic ataxic gait, proprioceptive sensory loss, and sphincter disturbance. The cause is unclear.

The frequency of adhesive arachnoiditis is decreasing as greater care is taken about what is placed in the spinal fluid. This progressive fibrosis of the pia mater and arachnoid can manifest as chronic pain in the low back, thighs, and legs, with adhesions seen on myelography. Another picture is that of a progressive spastic ataxia.

Spinal tumors are only 25% as common as intracranial tumors. The most common spinal tumors are meningiomas and schwannomas, which account for more than half. Ependymomas and metastases represent an additional fourth, with astrocytomas and a miscellaneous group completing the list. Meningiomas are more common in women and ependymomas in men, so that spinal cord tumors are more common in women overall. The peak incidence is in the fifth decade. Tumors are classified as intramedullary, intradural extramedullary, or extradural. Neurofibromas may present as dumbbell lesions projecting through the neural foramen.

Intramedullary tumors include both primary and metastatic lesions. Intramedullary metastases usually occur in advanced disease, with additional lesions at other sites. Primary intramedullary tumors resemble extramedullary tumors if localized to a segment. If the root entry zone is affected, pain is prominent. Most commonly, multiple segments are involved, and the patient presents with a central cord syndrome resembling syringomyelia. If the lesion is thoracic and the expanding tumor affects the spinothalamic tracts, the sacral fibers are affected last, resulting in sacral sparing.

Extramedullary tumors tend to involve few segments and present with local and radicular pain and paresthesias. Radicular weakness and wasting follow, then cord compression. Cord compression affects the outer pathways first. The clinical syndrome of spinal cord compression is a neurologic emergency. Clinical features include spastic weakness below the lesion, a sensory level at the level of the lesion, reflex hyperactivity, loss of superficial reflexes and extensor plantar responses, and impaired bladder (ultimately rectal) control. If effective treatment is not promptly instituted, progression to complete cord transection follows. When epidural cord compression occurs in the context of advanced cancer, symptoms may be overlooked. An unsteady gait may be sensory ataxia; limb weakness or paresthesia or unrelenting pain may be bony metastases with incipient cord compression. Primary tumors include lung, breast, and gastrointestinal cancers, melanoma, and lymphoma. Intradural tumors are more likely to be neurofibromas, meningiomas, or schwannomas.

Foramen magnum tumors may affect posterior column sensation in addition to causing a spastic paraparesis. The lower cranial nerves (IX–XII) may be involved if the tumor extends rostrally. The C2 dermatome is on the occiput and may be missed. Cervical tumors present with features related to the specific level. Upper cervical lesions cause spastic tetraplegia. Lower lesions produce a level of flaccid atrophic muscle; spastic paresis is present below that level. The C4 dermatome involves sensation to the epaulet area and innervation of the diaphragm. The C5 dermatome provides sensation to the outer upper arm and motor innervation to the deltoid, biceps, supinator, supraspinatus, and infraspinatus muscles. The upper arm hangs limply, and the biceps reflex is lost. The C6 dermatome provides sensation to the radial forearm and the first two digits. Motor supply is to the triceps and wrist extensors. The triceps reflex is lost, and the partly flexed forearm exhibits a partial wrist drop. The C7 dermatome provides sensation to the middle finger and motor supply to the wrist flexors and finger flexors and extensors; attempted hand closure produces mild wrist extension and slight finger flexion ("preacher's hand"). The C8 dermatome provides sensation to the ulnar forearm and the fourth and fifth digits and motor supply to the intrinsic muscles of the hand. A claw hand *(main-en-griffe)* is seen. Horner syndrome (ptosis, miosis, hypohidrosis, and relative enophthalmos) can be subtle. Although Horner syndrome is caused by involvement of the C8 root, intramedullary tumors can involve the descending sympathetic fibers anywhere along their path.

The manifestations of thoracic tumors depend primarily on the sensory level. Lumbar tumors of L3-4 sparing the cauda equina cause weakness of the quadriceps with loss of reflex and preservation of ankle jerk. The cauda is usually involved, with lower limb flaccid areflexic paralysis or some combination of findings. Conus or cauda tumors cause pain in the low back, perirectal area, and both lower legs, with sensory loss in the saddle area and the remaining lumbosacral dermatomes. Bladder function is lost early. Flaccid lower limbs with atrophy and areflexia develop later.

HISTORY

The estimated incidence of spinal cord trauma is 900 per 1 million persons; almost 80% of victims are male. The causes include motor vehicle accidents, falls, recreational activities (diving), and assaults. Major sites of injury are the neck (especially C5 and C6) and thoracolumbar junction. Patients should be stabilized and transported to a suitable facility for specialized care after means are taken to ensure that no further cord injury occurs.

The history is of paramount importance. The temporal sequence and rate of progression are defined. Attention is directed toward the five features previously described. Pain (it may be absent) is localized, radicular, or diffuse. Weakness may manifest as fatigability or clumsiness. Gait may be unsteady. The patient may describe being unable to perform specific functions; this suggests a direction for the muscle examination. Paresthesias may define root involvement more specifically than associated pain or sensory loss. The Lhermitte sign, in which flexion of the neck elicits a fleeting electric shocklike sensation that radiates down the spine and perhaps into the limbs, indicates cervical cord pathology (posterior column involvement); it is nonspecific for multiple sclerosis..

Some patients are reluctant to discuss bladder or bowel function, but the examiner must specifically inquire about this, in addition to sexual function. An atonic bladder may present as urinary retention with overflow incontinence. Urgency, frequency, and incontinence reflect a spastic neurogenic bladder. The symptoms of detrusor/sphincter dyssynergia are more variable. Urinary tract infection may manifest as retention, urgency, or frequency and must be ruled out. Incontinence should suggest neurologic involvement.

The history should also explore features suggestive of other levels of nervous system involvement. Involvement of a cerebral hemisphere is more likely to cause a loss of position sense than loss of pinprick. Dementia may favor frontal lobe dysfunction. Cough or exertional headache may favor a concurrent Chiari malformation. Exposure to toxic or infectious agents should be explored. Antecedent optic neuritis can be overlooked if remote. The family history should not be overlooked.

PHYSICAL EXAMINATION

The physical examination should include an assessment of spinal curvature and mobility. Tenderness is elicited. Skin lesions may suggest neurofibromatosis, and axillary freckles should be sought. Pulses may indicate aortic involvement. The bladder can be palpated and percussed. A cutaneous angioma may be present in patients with arteriovenous malformations.

The cranial nerves are checked with a funduscopic examination and visual fields. The lower cranial nerves must be assessed. Horner syndrome is subtle because the bright lights usually used for the examination cause pupillary constriction in the normal eye, obscuring the pathology. A faint light from the side makes it possible to estimate the pupillary size in relative darkness.

The sensory examination is most quickly performed with a pin to ascertain the presence of a sensory level; the examiner proceeds from the area of decreased sensation to more normal areas. The sacral areas must be checked for clues to conus or cauda syndromes or for sacral sparing. It is useful to elicit clues to possible radicular sensory loss during the history. A mental dermatome map is needed to allow fluid sensory testing. The sensory examination is the most difficult for both patient and examiner and is best done briskly to avoid excessive fatigue. When patients are anxious about pins, the side of a tuning fork should feel cold and may well suffice. Posterior column sensation is less readily defined in terms of a sensory level, although vibratory sense on the spine may provide useful information about a level. The evaluation of both spinothalamic tracts and posterior columns is necessary to define the nature of the syndrome.

Motor strength and tone are evaluated. Weak muscles are carefully assessed for atrophy, and the presence of fasciculations is determined by examining exposed limbs at rest. These small subcutaneous ripples represent the spontaneous firing of large motor units. They should be noted in weak muscles and should not be restricted to a single muscle group. The tongue can be examined in the floor of the mouth and the "bag of worms" effect seen.

A level above which the reflexes are normal and below which they are increased must be determined. Landry-Guillain-Barré syndrome may exhibit areflexic weakness but usually does not show diminished pinprick. Weakness and atrophy in association with preserved or increased reflexes suggest amyotrophic lateral sclerosis.

LABORATORY AND IMAGING STUDIES

New technology has made evaluation of the spinal cord safer and more accurate; however, it cannot be used efficiently if the region and question are not adequately defined.

Evoked potentials are obtained by administering a repetitive stimulus and recording electric activity from the skin overlying the spine or skull. This activity is then averaged while time-yoked to the stimulus. Somatosensory potentials are elicited by administering repetitive electric stimuli to the area of the median, ulnar, posterior tibial, or peroneal nerve. Potentials can be elicited from the back, cervical spine, thalamus, and sensory cortex. A central conduction time can thus be determined. Because the large myelinated fibers of the posterior columns conduct most rapidly, this test reflects primarily posterior column function. Transcranial or transspinal magnetic stimulation allows painless activation of the corticospinal tracts; complex polyphasic electromyographic waveforms are then recorded, and a central motor conduction time can be determined. These electrophysiologic tests allow the noninvasive measurement of cord function.

In myelography, the spinal canal is filmed after the cerebrospinal fluid has been rendered radiodense with a water-soluble contrast medium. The contrast medium is introduced by lumbar arachnoid puncture or lateral C2 puncture and is excreted by the kidneys. The use of contrast makes it possible to visualize the cord shadow and anything impinging on it. Carcinomatous meningitis may manifest as multiple nodules on nerves. Because a study of the full spine requires the administration of intrathecal contrast and high doses may be toxic, lumbar myelography has been combined with cervical or thoracic computed tomography to image the cord.

Magnetic resonance imaging has replaced most other imaging modalities. T1-weighted images provide great anatomic detail, showing black cerebrospinal fluid and a gray-white cord. Sagittal images visualize syringes and vascular malformations. T2-weighted images are less crisp but tend to highlight pathology. Intravenously injected gadolinium enhances many pathologic lesions.

Lumbar puncture makes it possible to examine the cells for inflammation and malignancy. An elevated protein level may suggest tumor or other neoplasia. A low sugar level is consistent with infection or neoplasia. Cytology may be helpful. The need for and uses of lumbar puncture are decreasing.

TREATMENT

Treatment must be directed at the primary disease process. Meningiomas and schwannomas are benign tumors that can be removed without definite neurologic injury. Neurofibromas are benign but intermingled with nerve fibers, so removal entails loss of the nerve root. Ependymomas may take the form of a string of beads that can be shelled out of the central cord, but recurrence is possible. Astrocytomas require radiation, with potential cord injury. Epidural metastatic lesions are best managed by radiation without surgery. The tumor may have destroyed the anterior elements, and decompression by posterior laminectomy may render the spine unstable. Anterior procedures are more complex. The lesion must be approached surgically when a prior diagnosis of cancer has not been made.

Patients with spinal cord trauma may be helped by the urgent administration of very high doses of steroids, and surgery is indicated in some cases to decompress the cord and stabilize the vertebrae. As for all too many of these conditions, no therapeutic options are available for spinal cord ischemia.

Cervical spondylosis may benefit from anterior fusion or posterior laminectomy. Foraminotomy is less successful but may be required for intense pain. The problem is susceptibility of the root to traumatic injury. In many cases, short courses of steroids or nonsteroidal antiinflammatory agents provide relief. The usefulness of collar and traction is controversial, but some patients seem to benefit.

Patients with syringomyelia may experience periods of stabilization, so that it is difficult to evaluate the many surgical procedures available. Posterior fossa decompression is useful in patients with concurrent Chiari malformations. Drainage of the cyst itself may be necessary in others. The goal is to arrest the process, but some patients do improve.

Of these conditions, subacute combined degeneration of the spinal cord has the best prognosis. All but the most severely affected patients show some response to the intramuscular administration of vitamin B_{12}.

Advances in our understanding of amyotrophic lateral sclerosis have led to a new treatment, riluzole. It offers limited benefit, but more meaningful therapy is anticipated in the future.

CONSIDERATIONS DURING PREGNANCY

Meningiomas are vascular tumors that enlarge during pregnancy. Arteriovenous malformations also enlarge during pregnancy, as a consequence of increased estrogen and perhaps enhanced perfusion.

The delivery of high doses of radiation to the fetus in myelography can be avoided with magnetic resonance imaging, which may well be safe in pregnancy.

Because women are less often involved and their responses are less readily measurable, far fewer studies of female sexual dysfunction in spinal cord injury have been performed. Traumatic injury has been the best studied, and problems may include loss of psychogenic or reflex stimulation of vaginal lubrication, clitoral enlargement, and labial swelling. Bowel and bladder soiling, in addition to pelvic muscle spasticity, may be avoided by elimination before intercourse and the use of muscle relaxants to reduce spasticity. Once a seriously embarrassing event has occurred, sexual contact may be avoided. Pregnancy is possible, and contraception may be indicated. Women with higher cord lesions may have delivery problems as a consequence of autonomic instability and ineffectual contractions. Blood pressure control may be a problem, as may recurrent urinary tract infections. Before delivery, careful planning is necessary to allay the mother's anxiety about being able to care for her child.

BIBLIOGRAPHY

Barnett HJM, Foster JB, Hodgson P. *Syringomyelia.* London: WB Saunders, 1973.

Byrne TN, Benzel EC, Waxman SG. *Diseases of the spine and spinal cord.* New York: Oxford University Press, 2000.

Chiles III BW, Cooper PR. Current concepts: acute spinal injury. *N Engl J Med* 1996; 334:514.

Hoppenfeld S. *Orthopaedic neurology: a diagnostic guide to neurologic levels.* Philadelphia: JB Lippincott, 1977.

Ropper AH, Wijdicks EFM, Truax BT. *Guillain-Barré syndrome.* Philadelphia: FA Davis Co, 1991.

Young RR, Woolsey RM. *Diagnosis and management of disorders of the spinal cord.* Philadelphia: WB Saunders, 1995.

CHAPTER 111
Multiple Sclerosis

Lawrence M. Samkoff

Multiple sclerosis (MS) is an immune-mediated, inflammatory, demyelinating disease of the central nervous system (CNS) that is a major cause of disability in young adults. Although thought to be primarily a disease of CNS myelin, recent neuropathologic studies have convincingly demonstrated evidence of axonal injury in both the early and late stages of MS. In the United States, approximately 250,000 to 400,000 persons have MS, with a female-to-male ratio of 2:1. MS primarily affects persons between the ages of 15 and 50 years, with a peak onset between the ages of 28 and 30 years. Although the course of illness is variable, 50% of patients with MS will require an aid for ambulation 15 years after disease onset. The last decade of the 20th century was witness to the development of treatments for many neurologic diseases, but arguably for none more than MS. The development of pharmacologic agents for MS paralleled advances in our understanding of disease pathophysiology, neuroimmunology, and neuroimaging.

ETIOLOGY AND PATHOGENESIS

The cause of MS is unknown. The most commonly advanced hypothesis is that it is an immune-mediated disorder affecting genetically susceptible persons, possibly triggered by an aberrant immunologic response to a nonspecific infectious agent encountered early in life. Numerous viral and bacterial pathogens have been implicated, including human herpesvirus 6 (HHV-6), human T-lymphotrophic virus (HTLV), Epstein-Barr virus, and *Chlamydia pneumoniae,* each of which has been detected in the CNS and blood of patients with MS. However, none has been definitively linked to the pathogenesis of MS.

Evidence for a genetic influence in MS is compelling. The concordance rate is sixfold higher in monozygotic twins (30%) than in dizygotic twins (5%). The risk for the development of MS in first-degree relatives is 20 to 40 times higher than that in the general population. Although multiple genetic factors are undoubtedly involved, genes regulating immune function are of interest. One recognized susceptibility gene is the HLA-DR2 allele, which encodes major histocompatibility complex (MHC) proteins. Some evidence also indicates that the course of the disease may be affected by genes associated with the interleukin-1 cell receptor, immunoglobulin Fc receptor, and apolipoprotein E.

An immunologic basis for MS has been postulated because of its similarity to experimental autoimmune encephalitis, the animal model for MS. The pathologic hallmark of MS in the CNS is the MS plaque, which is a zone of demyelination, axonal transaction, and gliosis. MS plaques of all ages contain variable components of inflammatory cells (lymphocytes, macrophages, and microglia). They are found mostly in the perivenous white matter, corresponding to areas where activated T lymphocytes from the periphery may penetrate the CNS.

One widely accepted hypothesis of the pathogenesis of MS postulates a central role for activated T lymphocytes. It is theorized that circulating potentially myelin-reactive T cells become activated on interacting with antigen-presenting cells that express MHC class II molecules bound to myelin peptides. This trimolecular complex of T cell, T-cell receptor, and antigen-presenting cell in the periphery leads to the formation of myelin-sensitized activated $CD4^+$ T cells, which migrate across the blood-brain barrier. Activated T lymphocytes express adhesion molecules and produce matrix metalloproteases, promoting attachment to endothelial cells, disruption of the blood-brain barrier, and entry into perivenous areas of CNS white matter. Release of chemokines and proinflammatory cytokines (e.g., tumor necrosis factor, interferon-γ) by activated T lymphocytes in the CNS recruits additional inflammatory cells (B cells, macrophages) and stimulates CNS-based microglia and astrocytes, producing an enzymatic cascade that leads to inflammation, demyelination, and axonal damage. The extent of irreversible axonal injury, the biologic substrate for fixed disability in patients with MS, is proportional to the extent of inflammatory demyelination.

CLINICAL HISTORY

MS is classically described as a disorder of the CNS white matter that is disseminated in time and space. In 80% to 85% of patients, it presents in a relapsing-remitting pattern, in which episodes of neurologic dysfunction lasting several days to weeks are followed by variable intervals of clinical improvement. Complete or nearly complete recovery is the rule in the early stage of relapsing-remitting MS, but disability increases stepwise as relapses continue over time. In approximately one half of persons with relapsing-remitting MS, secondary progressive MS develops, causing insidiously burdensome disability independently of attack frequency within 10 years after presentation. In 15% to 20% of patients, the MS course is primary progressive, in which impairment advances slowly after disease onset without relapses. More rarely, occasional acute or subacute episodes of neurologic dysfunction develop in patients with primary progressive MS (progressive-relapsing MS). Patients with primary progressive MS and progressive-relapsing MS are typically older than 40 years at disease onset, and the female-to-male ratio is 1:1.

The clinical manifestations of MS are protean and correspond to the location of plaque; none are pathognomonic for MS. Symptomatic lesions are typically located in the optic nerves, brainstem, cerebellum, and spinal cord. Lesions of the subcortical white matter and corpus callosum may be clinically silent early in the course but can be associated with cognitive dysfunction as the disease progresses.

In relapsing-remitting MS, neurologic symptoms and signs of at least 24 hours' duration define attacks; discrete relapses are separated by at least 30 days. Approximately 30% of patients with relapsing-remitting MS present with unilateral optic neuritis, which is characterized by a progressive monocular loss of visual acuity over several days that is usually accompanied by pain during eye movement. Symptoms of brainstem-cerebellar origin are also common and include diplopia, dysarthria, dysphagia, trigeminal neuralgia, vertigo, gait unsteadiness, and tremor of the limbs. Spinal cord lesions cause sensory disturbances (paresthesias of the limbs and trunk), limb weakness and clumsiness, spasticity, bladder dysfunction (urinary urgency, hesitancy, and incontinence), constipation, and sexual dysfunction. The Lhermitte phenomenon (an electric shocklike sensation radiating along the spine and into the arms and legs when the neck is flexed) is also frequently encountered and is caused by plaque in the posterior columns of the cervical spinal cord. Acute transverse myelitis, with a rapidly progressive sensory-motor deficit, may be an initial presenting feature of MS. Additionally, many patients with relapsing-remitting MS experience disabling fatigue that usually occurs in the late afternoon and is disproportionate to the degree of physical disability. Uncommon features of relapsing-remitting MS include seizures, paroxysmal tonic limb spasms, and sensory useless hand syndrome. Seizures are fivefold more frequent in patients with MS than in the general population; lesions located at the junction between the white and gray matter are presumed to be causative. Paroxysmal tonic spasms are brief, painful dystonic movements that typically affect the extensor muscles of the arms. Patients with sensory useless hand syndrome usually have a severe tactile and proprioceptive deficit that impairs routine manual activities.

The clinical course of relapsing-remitting MS is variable and unpredictable in any one patient. Indicators of a poor prognosis include the early onset of motor or cerebellar symptoms, incomplete remissions, and an older age at onset. The frequency of attacks typically lessens over time, but the pattern in most patients then evolves into a secondary progressive phase.

Primary progressive and secondary progressive MS typically present as a slowly evolving myelopathy, with spastic paraparesis or quadriparesis, bladder disturbances, and sexual dysfunction. More infrequently, a progressive cerebellar syndrome may develop in patients with primary progressive MS, characterized by truncal ataxia, action tremor of the limbs, and scanning dysarthria.

Occasionally, patients with MS present initially with dementia, although cognitive impairment usually occurs later in the disease. Neuropsychiatric disturbances are present in more than half of patients with MS and can develop in either the relapsing or progressive phase of the disease. Depression is an important feature in both relapsing-remitting and primary progressive MS. The cognitive deficits associated with MS include problems with short-term memory, impaired information processing, visuospatial deficits, and poor attention and concentration.

PHYSICAL EXAMINATION

The neurologic examination should reveal evidence of lesions disseminated in space. Reduced visual acuity is the hallmark of acute retrobulbar optic neuritis and is associated with an afferent papillary defect (paradoxical pupillary dilation of the affected eye with the swinging flashlight); the optic disc may be swollen but typically appears normal. Optic atrophy may develop after recovery. Signs of brainstem involvement include internuclear ophthalmoplegia, horizontal or vertical nystagmus, impaired extraocular smooth pursuit, and pseudobulbar syndrome (dysarthria, hyperactive gag reflex). Cerebellar findings include intention tremor of the limbs, truncal ataxia, and scanning dysarthria. Spinal cord dysfunction causes spastic limb weakness (quadriparesis or paraparesis), decreased vibratory sensation and proprioception in the lower extremities, hyperreflexia, an absence of superficial abdominal reflexes, and Babinski signs. Clinical evidence of gray matter disease (e.g., aphasia, agnosia, apraxia, choreoathetosis), lower motor neuron involvement (muscle atrophy, fasciculations), or peripheral neuropathy is distinctly unusual and should prompt a search for an alternative diagnosis.

DIAGNOSIS AND DIFFERENTIAL DIAGNOSIS

No specific diagnostic test for MS is available. The diagnosis relies on the clinical history and examination, which reveal neurologic symptoms and signs disseminated in time and space. The clinical diagnosis of MS is supported by abnormalities of the brain and spinal cord seen on magnetic resonance imaging (MRI), delayed evoked potentials (visual, brainstem auditory, and somatosensory), and increased immunoglobulin (IgG) or oligoclonal bands in the cerebrospinal fluid (CSF). CSF lymphocytic pleocytosis (<50 cells) or elevated protein (>100 mg/dL) may occur in MS.

Cranial MRI is the most sensitive diagnostic tool for MS and is able to discriminate between active and inactive disease (MS plaques) in more than 90% of patients. Abnormalities include hyperintense white matter signals on T2-weighted and fluid-attenuated inversion recovery (FLAIR) images, gadolinium enhancement of active lesions, and hypointense "black holes" and brain atrophy on T1-weighted studies. On cranial MRI, MS lesions are commonly found in the periventricular white matter, corpus callosum, brainstem, and cerebellum. Activity on MRI serial studies is a much more sensitive indicator of disease progression and has become an important outcome measurement in therapeutic trials. Less consistently, spinal MRI may reveal hyperintense signals, contrast-enhancing lesions, and spinal cord atrophy. Spinal MRI is useful in patients with transverse myelitis and can easily exclude compressive lesions that mimic progressive MS.

Cranial MRI is particularly helpful in patients who present with isolated demyelinating syndromes (e.g., optic neuritis, transverse myelitis) typical of MS. The presence of MRI abnormalities consistent with MS significantly increases the 2-year risk for the development of clinically definite MS (i.e., a second clinical demyelinating episode); conversely, normal findings on the initial MRI reduce the long-term risk for clinically definite MS.

The differential diagnosis of MS is extensive and comprises entities that cause multifocal or progressive neurologic disease. These include systemic disorders, CNS infections, metabolic illnesses, and primary neurologic diseases that can usually be excluded by a careful history and physical examination and the appropriate laboratory tests. In many cases, neuroimaging and CSF analysis can help distinguish these diseases from MS.

Systemic illnesses with multifocal neurologic involvement that can mimic MS include systemic lupus erythematosus, Sjögren syndrome, Behçet disease, polyarteritis nodosa, sarcoidosis, anticardiolipin syndrome, and Wegener granulomatosis. Serum and CSF testing can usually exclude CNS infections such as neurosyphilis, Lyme disease, HTLV-1 myelopathy, and HIV-associated myelopathy. Metabolic diseases such as vitamin B_{12} deficiency (subacute combined degeneration) and adrenomyeloneurotrophy can produce myelopathy indistinguishable from that of primary progressive MS. Mitochondrial cytopathies with predominantly CNS or optic nerve features (e.g., Leber optic atrophy) can also be confused with MS.

Neurologic diseases that should be considered in the differential diagnosis of MS include neoplasms (spinal cord tumor, CNS lymphoma, gliomatosis cerebri); neurovascular disorders (primary CNS angiitis, cerebral autosomal-dominant angiopathy with subcortical infarcts and leukoencephalopathy [CADASIL]); posterior fossa disorders (Arnold-Chiari malformation, hereditary ataxia); and spinal cord disorders (spondylotic myelopathy, primary lateral sclerosis).

TREATMENT

The management of MS comprises three separate but parallel pathways: disease modification, symptomatic treatment, and rehabilitation. Disease-modifying agents affect the natural history of MS, symptomatic therapies target the clinical manifestations, and rehabilitation is aimed at designing adaptive strategies to mitigate the dysfunction and disability associated with MS. The appropriate interventions must be made on an individual basis.

Disease-Modifying Therapy

MS is a chronic disease. Natural history studies have demonstrated that secondary progressive MS develops in more than 50% of patients with relapsing-remitting MS after 10 years. One half of patients with relapsing-remitting MS require an aid for ambulation between 15 and 23 years after disease onset. As recently as the early 1990s, most physicians considered MS untreatable, and disease modification therapy was limited to episodic courses of corticosteroids for MS relapses. Since 1994, the Food and Drug Administration has approved four agents for patients with relapsing-remitting MS or secondary progressive MS: interferon-β-1a (IFN-β-1a), IFN-β-1b, glatiramer, and mitoxantrone (Table 111.1). These medications have revolutionized the approach to patients and have transformed MS into a treatable illness.

CORTICOSTEROIDS

Corticosteroids are widely used for the short-term treatment of acute exacerbations of MS, although their role in maintenance therapy in secondary progressive MS is under study. Steroids generally hasten the time to recovery after a clinically significant relapse. No consensus has been reached regarding the optimal formulation, dosage, route of administration, and duration of treatment. Many neurologists favor a 3- to 7-day course of intravenous methylprednisolone followed by an oral taper of prednisone for approximately 10 days. The results of the Optic Neuritis Treatment Trial indicate that clinically disabled patients with acute optic neuritis should receive intravenous corticosteroids rather than oral therapy alone.

TABLE 111.1. Current Disease-Modifying Therapies for Multiple Sclerosis

Agent	MS type	Dose	Adverse effects
IFN-b-1b (Betaseron)	RR ? SP with relapses	8 million IU SC qod	Flulike syndrome Injection site reaction Depression (?) Menstrual irregularities
IFN-b-1a (Avonex)	RR	30 mg IM weekly	Flulike syndrome
IFN-b-1a (Rebif)	RR	22 or 44 mg SC three times weekly	Flulike syndrome
Glatiramer acetate (Copaxone)	RR	20 mg SC qd	Post-injection syndrome[a] Injection site reaction
Mitoxantrone	Worsening RR, SP	12 mg/m^2 IV q 3 mos × 2–3 y (maximum: 140 mg/m^2)	Alopecia Nausea Menstrual disorders Leukopenia, rare leukemia Cardiomyopathy (at cumulative doses >100 mg/m^2

[a]Chest pain, palpitations, flushing, anxiety.
IFN, interferon; IM, intramuscular; IV, intravenous; RR, relapsing/remitting; SC, subcutaneous; SP, secondary progressive.

INTERFERON-β

Three IFN-β products have been approved for the treatment of MS in the United States and Europe. These recombinant agents differ in mode of production, chemical structure, route of administration, and dosage. Each has been shown to reduce the relapse rate, progression to disability, and MRI activity in relapsing-remitting MS; however, their benefit in secondary progressive MS has not been clearly established.

IFN-β-1b (Betaseron; Berlex Laboratories, Montville, New Jersey), a nonglycosylated recombinant product derived from *Escherichia coli,* was the first medication approved by the Food and Drug Administration for relapsing-remitting MS. It differs from natural IFN-β by a single amino acid substitution. In a 2-year multicenter, double-blinded, placebo-controlled study of 372 ambulatory patients with relapsing-remitting MS, the subcutaneous administration of 8 million IU of IFN-β-1b every other day was found to decrease the annual exacerbation rate by 32%. An intermediate dose of IFN-β-1b, 1.6 million IU, was also significantly effective in comparison with placebo, but less so than the higher dose. Cranial MRI disease activity was also significantly reduced in patients treated with 8 million IU of IFN-β-1b in comparison with placebo at the end of 3 years. Although progression of disability was confirmed in fewer patients on IFN-β-1b after 5 years, this difference did not reach statistical significance. IFN-β-1b has also been studied in patients with secondary progressive MS, but results have been conflicting. In a European controlled trial, a significant delay in time to confirmed disability progression was noted in patients treated with 8 million IU of subcutaneous IFN-β-1b every other day. Unfortunately, a second North American study of subcutaneous IFN-β-1b in secondary progressive MS failed to show clinical benefit. Thus, the role of IFN-β-1b in the treatment of secondary progressive MS remains controversial.

Two IFN-β-1a agents (Avonex; Biogen, Cambridge, Massachusetts, and Rebif; Serono, Boston, Massachusetts), both naturally sequenced glycosylated recombinant mammalian products, have also been approved for the treatment of remitting-relapsing MS. In a randomized, placebo-controlled, double-blinded study of 301 patients with remitting-relapsing MS, a weekly 30-μg dose of intramuscular IFN-β-1a (Avonex) brought about a 37% reduction in sustained disability over 104 weeks. Weekly intramuscular IFN-β-1a also significantly reduced the exacerbation rate (by 18%) and cranial MRI gadolinium enhancement. Subcutaneous IFN-β-1a (Rebif) at doses of 22 and 44 μg three times a week reduced relapse rates during 1 and 2 years by 27% and 33%, respectively. Accumulation of sustained disability was decreased in both IFN β-1a groups. The MRI burden of disease was also lower in both treatment arms. In a 2-year blinded extension study, patients initially given placebo were randomized to receive 22 or 44 μg of subcutaneous IFN-β-1a three times weekly (crossover groups) while patients on active treatment continued to be followed on their assigned doses. The results of the extended trial confirmed the ongoing efficacy of high-dose IFN-β-1a in reducing the relapse rate, progression of disability, and MRI activity in patients with remitting-relapsing MS. Furthermore, delaying treatment appeared to affect these same parameters adversely because patients in the crossover groups fared significantly worse on clinical and MRI measures of disease activity.

Intramuscular (30 μg) IFN-β-1a and subcutaneous (22 μg) IFN-β-1a given weekly were also demonstrated to be beneficial in patients with a first isolated demyelinating event (optic neuritis, partial transverse myelitis, or brainstem-cerebellar syndrome and MRI evidence of prior demyelination). Such patients are at high risk for the development of clinically definite MS within 3 years. Both intramuscular IFN-β-1a and subcutaneous IFN-β-1a given weekly were shown to delay the 3-year risk for a second demyelinating event significantly in this cohort of patients. The long-term significance of these findings is unknown.

IFN-β is associated with a number of adverse events, including flulike symptoms, depression, menstrual irregularities (breakthrough bleeding, spotting), reactions at the injection site, and increased spasticity. The flulike syndrome tends to abate after several months and usually responds to acetaminophen, ibuprofen, or prednisone. Alternatively, to reduce side effects, IFN-β may be initiated at one-fourth to one-half the recommended dose and then gradually titrated to the full dose. The most commonly reported laboratory abnormalities associated with IFN-β are leukopenia and elevated liver enzymes; these usually reverse with temporary cessation of therapy. Neutralizing antibodies to IFN-β develop in 12.5% to 38% of patients and may attenuate its therapeutic efficacy.

The mechanism of action of IFN-β in remitting-relapsing MS is not precisely known. IFN-β binds to surface receptors on lymphocytes, monocytes, and endothelial cells, resulting in a cascade of nuclear events that modulate proinflammatory and antiinflammatory cytokine production, antigen presentation, and T-cell trafficking across the blood-brain barrier. These cellular activities take place in the peripheral circulation.

The optimal dosage and route of administration of IFN-β in patients with remitting-relapsing MS are unknown. Multiple studies comparing IFN-β-1a and IFN-β-1b at weekly dosages ranging from 22 to 144 μg demonstrate a dose-response in both clinical and MRI parameters. The investigations performed to date all have limitations and have not generated enough long-term results that firm recommendations can be made. Nevertheless, it is possible that more frequent, higher-dose IFN-β is more beneficial than lower-dose, less frequent IFN-β in patients with more active clinical or radiologic disease. Patients with early MS treated with any of the IFN-β agents require close monitoring to evaluate treatment efficacy.

GLATIRAMER ACETATE

Glatiramer acetate (Copaxone; Teva Pharmaceuticals USA, North Wales, Pennsylvania), formally known as *copolymer-1,* is a mixture of synthetic polypeptide chains consisting of four amino acids: L-glutamate, L-lysine, L-alanine, and L-tyrosine. Glatiramer acetate was originally developed as an analogue to myelin basic protein and was found to modify or suppress experimental autoimmune encephalomyelitis, the animal model of MS. Subsequent studies confirmed its usefulness in the treatment of remitting-relapsing MS. In a randomized, multicenter, placebo-controlled trial, the daily subcutaneous administration of 20 mg of glatiramer acetate resulted in a 29% reduction in the relapse rate in comparison with placebo. The disability scores of patients in the treatment arm were significantly improved at the end of the study. In a 12-month extension study, glatiramer acetate continued to decrease the relapse rate and progression of disability. In separate studies, glatiramer acetate reduced MRI disease activity.

Glatiramer acetate is well tolerated. The most common adverse effect is a reaction at the injection site consisting of mild erythema and induration. More rarely, glatiramer acetate may be associated with a post-injection syndrome characterized by a variable combination of chest tightness, flushing, dyspnea, palpitations, and anxiety. This benign but troublesome systemic reaction is sporadic and unpredictable and was reported at least once in 15% of patients. It typically occurs within minutes after an injection and resolves spontaneously in 30 seconds to 30 minutes. It is not associated with any cardiac abnormality.

The mechanism of action of glatiramer acetate in MS is unknown. Proposed immunomodulatory activities include inhibition of myelin-reactive T cells by blocking HLA, T-cell receptor antagonism, and induction of antiinflammatory T helper subset 2 (Th2) cells.

MITOXANTRONE

Mitoxantrone is an anthracenedione used to treat numerous malignancies. It has demonstrated efficacy in patients with both remitting-relapsing and secondary progressive MS, although the results of a major study have been published only in abstract form. In a multicenter, double-blinded, placebo-controlled trial, 194 patients were randomized to receive quarterly intravenous infusions of 12 mg of mitoxantrone per square meter, 5 mg of mitoxantrone per square meter, or placebo for 2 years. Both doses of mitoxantrone reduced the relapse rate, progression of disability, and MRI activity and increased the time to first exacerbation. The treatment was generally well tolerated; alopecia, urinary tract infections, nausea, and vomiting were the most common adverse events reported. Because cumulative doses of mitoxantrone above 140 mg/m^2 are associated with cardiomyopathy, its long-term use in MS will likely be limited. Although mitoxantrone been approved by the Food and Drug Administration for treating worsening remitting-relapsing and secondary progressive MS, further recommendations regarding its use await the publication of peer-reviewed data.

OTHER AGENTS

Benefit has been reported for a variety of immunosuppressive agents in MS. In addition to the first-line therapies previously discussed, azathioprine, methotrexate, pulse intravenous methylprednisolone, intravenous immunoglobulin, plasmapheresis, and cyclophosphamide have shown some efficacy in both relapsing and progressive forms of MS. Although these treatments have been supplanted by newer medications, they continue to be used; their potential as adjunctive therapies in combination with the interferons or glatiramer awaits further study. Interestingly, oral estradiol was found to reduce MRI activity in nonpregnant women with MS; a large controlled trial is planned. Most recently, a phase II study of monthly intravenous natalizumab, a monoclonal antibody against α_4-integrin, a mediator of lymphocyte and monocyte migration across the endothelium-based blood-brain barrier, demonstrated reduced MRI and clinical activity in patients with remitting-relapsing MS.

SELECTING A DISEASE-MODIFYING AGENT

A consensus is growing that disease-modifying therapy should commence early in patients with remitting-relapsing MS. It is speculated that starting immunomodulatory treatment during the early inflammatory phase of the disease will delay the onset of irreversible axonal loss that predominates in the later stages of MS. Confirmation of this hypothesis awaits evidence-based long-term study.

Although IFN-β-1a, IFN-β-1b, and glatiramer acetate have each been shown to affect relapse rates, progression of disability, and MRI activity favorably, evidence is emerging that these agents are not equally efficacious. Several studies, some uncontrolled, comparing IFN-β-1a and IFN-β-1b at different doses and intervals of administration demonstrated a dose effect on both clinical and MRI measures. In one 12-month open label study comparing IFN-β-1a, IFN-β-1b, and glatiramer acetate, the reduction in relapse rate was statistically significant only in the IFN-β-1b and glatiramer acetate groups. It is plausible that patients with more active remitting-relapsing MS—that is, those with more frequent exacerbations or more incomplete remissions—may respond better to high-dose IFN-β-1a, IFN-β-1b, or glatiramer acetate than to low-dose IFN-β-1a. Low-dose IFN-β-1a or glatiramer acetate may be a reasonable option in patients with isolated demyelinating syndromes or less active remitting-relapsing MS.

Another factor influencing the choice of immunomodulatory treatment is tolerance of adverse drug effects. Both low-dose IFN-β-1a and glatiramer acetate are better tolerated than high-dose IFN-β-1b. IFN-β-1a and IFN-β-1b are both associated with the formation of neutralizing antibodies, but their clinical relevance remains uncertain.

Patients whose disease progresses while they are on a primary immunomodulatory agent pose a difficult dilemma. None of these drugs halt disease activity, and relapses are expected to continue, albeit less frequently. Some patients on an IFN-β may benefit from switching to glatiramer acetate. Alternatively, raising the weekly IFN-β dose may be helpful, although this may produce intolerable side effects. Institution of therapy with monthly pulses of intravenous methylprednisolone (1,000 mg) or an immunosuppressive agent such as mitoxantrone, either alone or in combination, may also be considered.

Symptomatic Therapy

Patients with MS experience a variety of secondary symptoms of neurologic dysfunction, including neuropathic pain, spasticity, fatigue, cerebellar tremor, and neurogenic bladder. Neuropathic pain, such as dysesthetic limb pain or trigeminal neuralgia, may be relieved with gabapentin, phenytoin, or carbamazepine. Spasticity may be reduced with an oral agent such as baclofen, tizanidine, or diazepam. Patients with refractory spasticity may benefit from intrathecal baclofen delivered by a surgically implantable programmable pump. Disabling fatigue may be managed with pemoline, amantadine, or modafinil. Although cerebellar tremor rarely responds to medication, carefully selected patients with MS may benefit from stereotactically targeted long-term thalamic stimulation. Finally, neurogenic bladder disturbances such as urinary frequency and incontinence can be treated with anticholinergic agents and intermittent catheterization. Vigilant monitoring for urinary tract infection is also essential because of the high incidence of bladder dysfunction in MS.

PREGNANCY ISSUES

Because MS is a disease that primarily affects women in their childbearing years, issues regarding the decision to become pregnant, the effects of pregnancy on MS, and the consequences of MS treatments on the pregnancy and developing fetus commonly arise. The decision to become pregnant is clearly an individual one and may be based partly on the degree of disability.

MS disease activity is influenced by pregnancy, possibly as a consequence of the fetal-placental down-regulation of cell-mediated immunity. Before 1998, several small reports suggested that the relapse rate decreased during pregnancy and then increased during the postpartum period. The Pregnancy in Multiple Sclerosis (PRIMS) Study, a European prospective, multicenter investigation, resolved this important issue. The PRIMS Study enrolled 254 women during 269 pregnancies who were followed for up to 12 months postpartum. The relapse rates during each trimester were compared with the rates 1 year before pregnancy. The relapse rates were found to decline progressively through the third trimester, with the greatest decline noted in the third trimester (0.2 ± 1.0, $P < 0.001$) in comparison with the rate before pregnancy (0.7 ± 0.9). The relapse rate then increased during the first 3 months postpartum (1.2 ± 2.0, $P < 0.001$) and then returned to the value noted before pregnancy. Epidural anesthesia and breast-feeding did not adversely affect either the postpartum relapse rate or the progression of disability.

It is generally recommended that pregnant and nursing women stop using disease-modifying agents during pregnancy and postpartum, and this advice is corroborated in part by the protective effects of pregnancy on clinical disease activity. IFN-β has been found to be abortifacient in animal studies, although no teratogenicity was detected in rhesus monkeys. The effects of IFN-β and glatiramer on the human fetus are unknown, and prospective data are not available.

BIBLIOGRAPHY

Confavreux C, Hutchinson M, Hours MM, et al., and the Pregnancy in Multiple Sclerosis Group. Rate of pregnancy-related relapse in multiple sclerosis. *N Engl J Med* 1998;339:285–291.

Coyle PK. Multiple sclerosis. In: Lahita RG, Chiorazzi N, Reeves WH, eds. *Textbook of autoimmune disease*. Philadelphia: Lippincott Williams & Wilkins, 2000: 595–609.

Miller DH, Khan OA, Sheremata WA, et al. A controlled trial of natalizumab for relapsing multiple sclerosis. *N Engl J Med* 2003;348:15–23.

Noseworthy JH, Lucchinetti C, Rodriguez M, et al. Multiple sclerosis. *N Engl J Med* 2000;343:938–952.

Sicotte NL, Liva SM, Klutch R, et al. Treatment of multiple sclerosis with the pregnancy hormone estradiol. *Ann Neurol* 2002;52:421–428.

Walther EU, Hohlfeld R. Multiple sclerosis: side effects of interferon beta therapy and their management. *Neurology* 1999;53:1623–1627.

CHAPTER 112
Mononeuropathies

Harold Lesser and Anne Moss

Isolated injuries to peripheral nerves are frequently seen in the primary care setting. The most common are injuries to the median nerve at the wrist, ulnar nerve at the elbow, and peroneal nerve at the fibular head. Whereas many mononeuropathies are isolated events, others develop in patients with underlying systemic illnesses or significant risk factors for nerve injury. Identifying underlying risk factors may help to limit recurrent trauma to an affected nerve, prevent future nerve injury, and determine the prognosis.

The clinical course and management of nerve injuries depend on the severity of the injury. Injuries that affect only the myelin sheath carry a better prognosis than those affecting the integrity of axons themselves. Neurapraxia, the mildest of nerve injures, is a temporary focal disruption of nerve function without disruption of the anatomic integrity of the nerve or its sustaining structures. The limb that "falls asleep" and recovers over minutes is a common example. Repeated or more severe neurapraxia injuries can produce symptoms lasting for days. When the myelin sheath surrounding the nerve sustains a significant injury, conduction block (focal nerve conduction failure) can develop at the site of injury. The acute functional consequences of severe conduction block are identical to those of nerve transection: loss of sensorimotor function distal to the site of injury.

Axonotmesis is a more severe form of nerve injury associated with some degree of axonal loss, but the integrity of the supporting structures of the nerve is preserved. Weakness, sensory loss, and loss of reflexes develop acutely. Over time, wallerian degeneration develops in the axons disconnected from their sustaining cell bodies. The most distal portions of the axons and their myelin coating degenerate first, then degeneration spreads proximally. When axonotmesis is mild by both clinical and electrodiagnostic measures, functional recovery is more likely because regenerating axons can regrow along intact nerve infrastructure.

Neurotmesis or transection is the most severe form of nerve injury. Immediate and potentially permanent loss of sensorimotor and autonomic function occurs distal to the transection site. Severe muscle atrophy develops during subsequent months. Surgical exploration should be attempted when neurotmesis is suspected because surgical reanastomosis provides the only hope for functional recovery. Unfortunately, despite surgical intervention, scarring and neuroma formation at the transection site often inhibit regeneration and may lead to chronic nerve irritation and pain.

Nerve conduction studies provide an accurate estimate of the degree of axonal loss if they are performed after sufficient time has elapsed for wallerian degeneration to develop. If performed too early (i.e., within the first few weeks after injury), the results underestimate the ultimate degree of axon injury. Needle electromyography is exquisitely sensitive to axon loss, but again, timing is critical. When motor axons are injured and die, trophic (nutritional) support to the muscle fibers that they previously innervated is lost. Denervated muscle fibers undergo degeneration, causing membrane instability, which leads to abnormal spontaneous discharges known as *p-waves* and *fibrillations*. Abnormal spontaneous activity (also known as *denervation*) can be detected after injury to as few as 3% of motor axons.

In cases of severe axonotmesis, the question often arises of whether *any* axons remain intact. When only a few motor axons survive, they often activate so few muscle fibers that no muscle contraction is visible. Electromyographic demonstration of volitional motor unit activation implies a greater chance for recovery than when no volitional motor units can be activated. Electromyographic evidence of ongoing axonal sprouting and reinnervation, when present, also is an encouraging sign.

ETIOLOGY AND DIFFERENTIAL DIAGNOSIS

The common compressive mononeuropathies (median at the wrist, ulnar at the elbow, and peroneal at the fibular head) are often associated with underlying disorders or risk factors that increase the probability that mononeuropathies will develop. Numerous medical conditions (e.g., malnutrition, alcoholism, diabetes, hypothyroidism, uremia) predispose to the compressive injury of individual nerves. Prolonged unconsciousness or immobility and severe weight loss are risk factors for compressive injuries to the ulnar nerve at the elbow, radial nerve at the spiral groove, and peroneal nerve at the fibular head. Carpal tunnel syndrome (CTS) or lateral femoral cutaneous neuropathy (meralgia paresthetica) often develops during pregnancy.

HISTORY

When mononeuropathies are evaluated, a patient's handedness, occupation, and hobbies should be ascertained. A history of trauma to the symptomatic limb, even in the distant past, may be relevant. The recent use of casts, orthotic devices, or crutches should be considered. If the patient has been hospitalized recently, the examiner should inquire about periods of immobility or unconsciousness and intravenous or phlebotomy sites.

A detailed medical history should be obtained, and the family history should be probed for diabetes, hypothyroidism, connective tissue disorders, and neuropathy. A family history of high arched feet, hammer toes, gait disorders late in life, or simply "funny feet" should suggest the possibility of an inherited neuropathy.

PHYSICAL EXAMINATION

Identifying a mononeuropathy requires a fairly detailed knowledge of peripheral nerve anatomy. The cutaneous distribution of the peripheral nerves in the limbs is shown in Figs. 112.1 through 112.3. This information must be compared and contrasted with the dermatomal patterns shown in Figs. 112.4 and 112.5 because the differential diagnosis of peripheral nerve lesions often includes nerve root compression (e.g., ulnar neuropathy vs. C8-T1 radiculopathy).

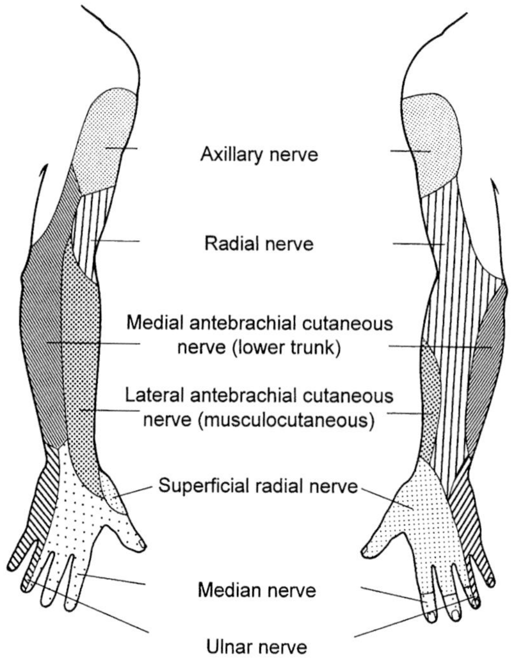

FIG. 112.1. Cutaneous innervation of the left arm. (Modified from Binney CD, Cooper R, Fowler CJ, et al. *Clinical neurophysiology: EMG, nerve conduction, and evoked potentials*. Oxford: Butterworth-Heinemann, 1995:114, with permission.)

CLINICAL FINDINGS

Upper Extremity Mononeuropathies

MEDIAN MONONEUROPATHIES

Compression of the median nerve at the wrist, or CTS, is the most common mononeuropathy. The carpal tunnel is a fibrous channel, bound by the transverse carpal ligament, through which the median nerve and nine finger flexor tendons enter the wrist. Overuse of the hands, particularly repetitive motions performed under stress, produces focal nerve injury. Other predisposing factors for CTS include diabetes, weight gain, pregnancy and lactation, hypothyroidism, and rheumatoid arthritis. CTS is more likely to develop in women than in men.

Classically, patients describe numbness and tingling involving the thumb and index and middle fingers. Difficulty holding a newspaper or steering wheel and clumsiness of the hand are often reported, as is nocturnal awakening with paresthesia. The discomfort of CTS may be poorly localized, involving the whole hand, forearm, shoulder, or even neck. Alternate diagnoses, such as a proximal median mononeuropathy at the elbow, brachial plexopathy, or cervical radiculopathy, must be considered when such complaints are evaluated.

In mild CTS, a paucity of findings may be noted on examination. The presence of a Tinel sign—paresthesias (abnormal sensation of pins and needles) provoked by percussion over the median nerve at the wrist—indicates local axonal injury and regeneration at the site of percussion. The Phalen sign—the reproduction of symptoms by forcible hyperflexion of the wrist for 30 to 60 seconds—also suggests local nerve injury. Decreased sensation on the median (lateral) half of the fourth digit with sparing of sensation on the ulnar half is characteristic. Sensory loss and thenar atrophy are seen in more advanced

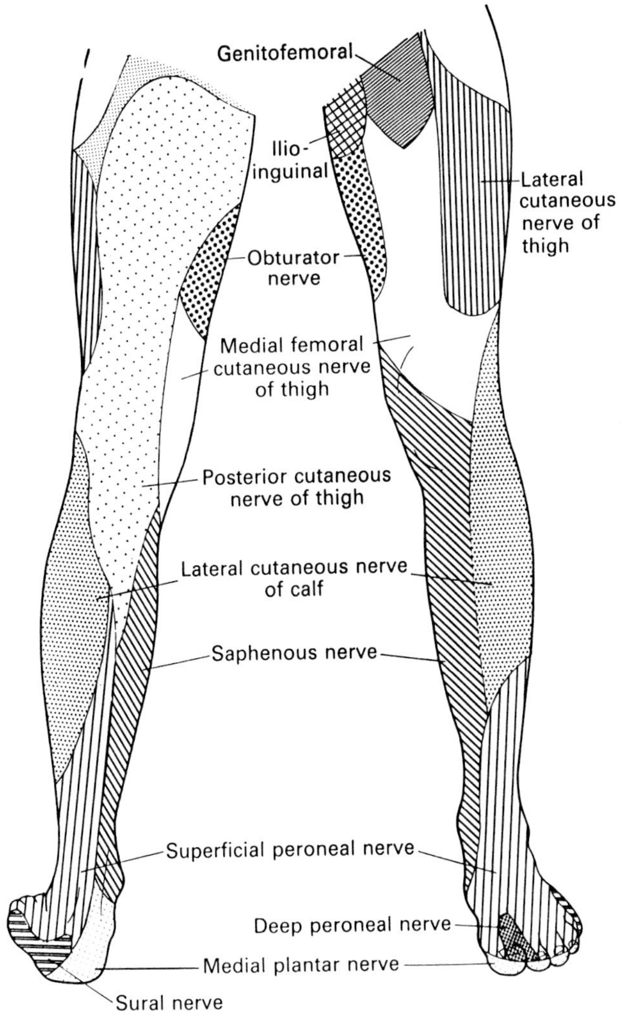

FIG. 112.2. Cutaneous innervation of the left leg. (Modified from Binney CD, Cooper R, Fowler CJ, et al. *Clinical neurophysiology: EMG, nerve conduction, and evoked potentials.* Oxford: Butterworth-Heinemann, 1995:127, with permission.)

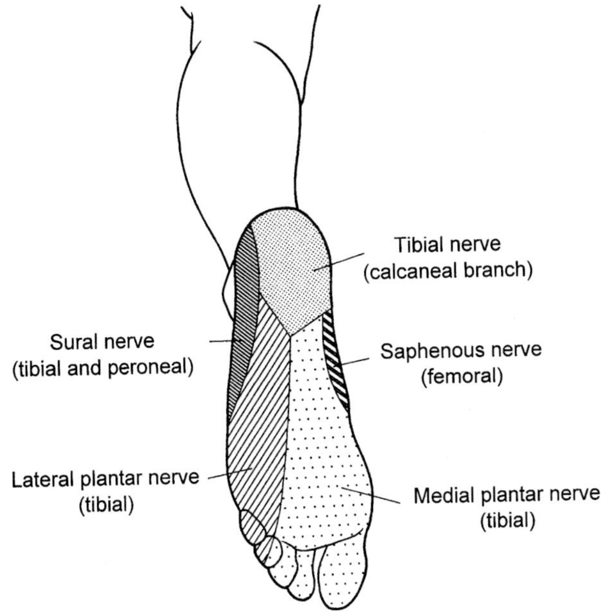

FIG. 112.3. Cutaneous innervation of the sole of the left foot. (Modified from Binney CD, Cooper R, Fowler CJ, et al. *Clinical neurophysiology: EMG, nerve conduction, and evoked potentials.* Oxford: Butterworth-Heinemann, 1995:135, with permission.)

cases. Both hands should always be evaluated for signs and symptoms because the syndrome is commonly bilateral. The differential diagnosis of CTS should include DeQuervain syndrome (tenosynovitis of the thumb extensor tendon), C6 radiculopathy, and proximal median mononeuropathy.

Mild CTS can be managed with nocturnal wrist splinting to prevent passive flexion of the wrist during sleep. Splints reduce both nocturnal awakening and the ongoing nerve injury that is associated with daytime symptoms. Reducing repetitive movements and strain at work and home may also be helpful. Symptoms often progress despite these interventions. Local injections of long-acting steroids into the carpal tunnel may be of use in patients without evidence of axonal injury. Injections can provide temporary or occasionally sustained relief in some patients; however, no controlled trial supports the efficacy of this treatment.

Electrodiagnostic testing can be used to confirm CTS, assess the need for surgical management, and rule out alternate diagnoses. Surgical intervention is generally warranted for injuries causing axon loss. Once significant atrophy develops, the recovery of function after surgery may be incomplete. A more conservative approach should be taken when symptoms arise during pregnancy.

ULNAR MONONEUROPATHY

Ulnar mononeuropathy at the elbow is the second most common compressive mononeuropathy. Leaning on the elbows is the most frequent cause. It also occurs commonly in unconscious and immobilized patients. Antecedent trauma can predispose some people to the development of ulnar mononeuropathy years or even decades later—so-called tardy ulnar palsy. Bony overgrowth from the original injury renders the nerve more susceptible to further injury. Specific inquiry about previous trauma is important because patients rarely associate their past injury with current difficulties. Because all muscles innervated by the ulnar nerve share a C8-T1 root supply via the lower trunk of the brachial plexus, both cervicothoracic radiculopathy and lower trunk plexopathy must be considered in the differential diagnosis.

Patients with ulnar nerve injury at the elbow should be instructed how to avoid nerve damage and to use an elbow pad. When clinical examination, electrodiagnostic testing, or both indicate significant axon loss at the elbow, surgical ulnar transposition should be considered. The nerve is typically relocated to a site anterior to the cubital tunnel, although alternative approaches can be used. Surgical intervention should be considered cautiously for patients with an underlying polyneuropathy (e.g., diabetes).

RADIAL MONONEUROPATHY

The radial nerve is vulnerable to injury in the axilla (crutch injury) and as it wraps behind the distal third of the humerus at the spiral groove. "Saturday night palsy" is radial neuropathy resulting from prolonged pressure on the nerve in the spiral groove, frequently after alcoholic stupor. Humeral fracture is another common cause of injury. Lead toxicity characteristically causes radial mononeuropathies.

A finding of wrist drop, finger drop, or both is the hallmark of most radial mononeuropathies; triceps weakness is seen only with the most proximal of radial injuries. Weakness of the brachioradialis suggests a lesion at or proximal to the spiral

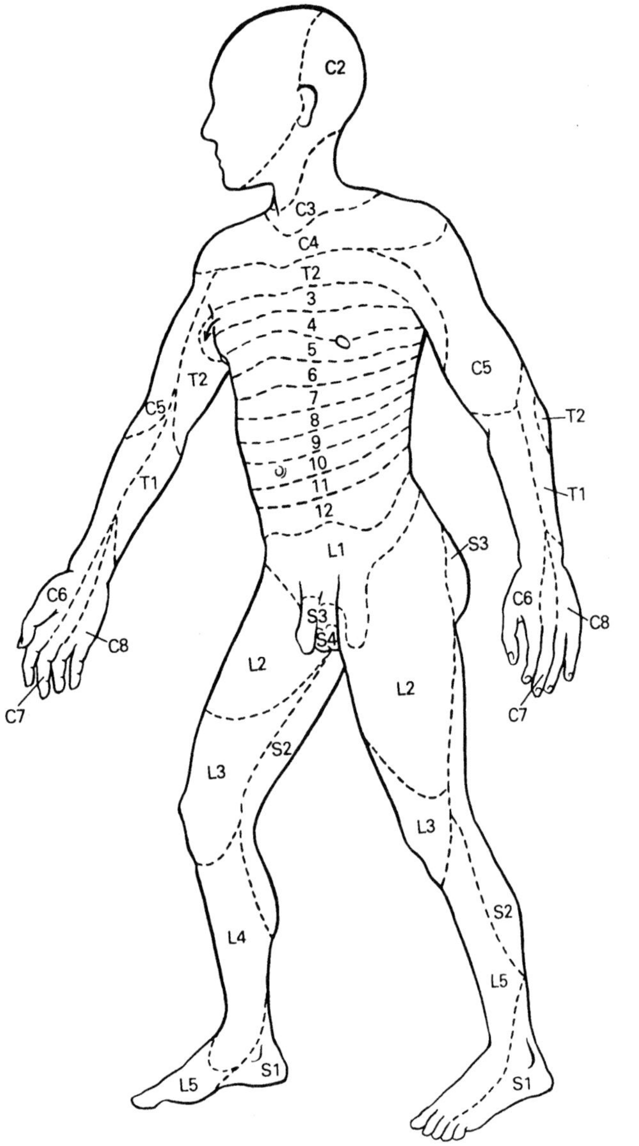

FIG. 112.4. Dermatomes in anterior oblique view. The arm is supplied by C5-T2, the leg by L2-S2. Common landmarks include the T4 dermatome at the level of the nipples and the T10 dermatome at the level of the umbilicus. (From Devinsky O, Feldmann E. *Examination of the cranial and peripheral nerves.* Oxford: Churchill Livingstone, 1988:37, with permission.)

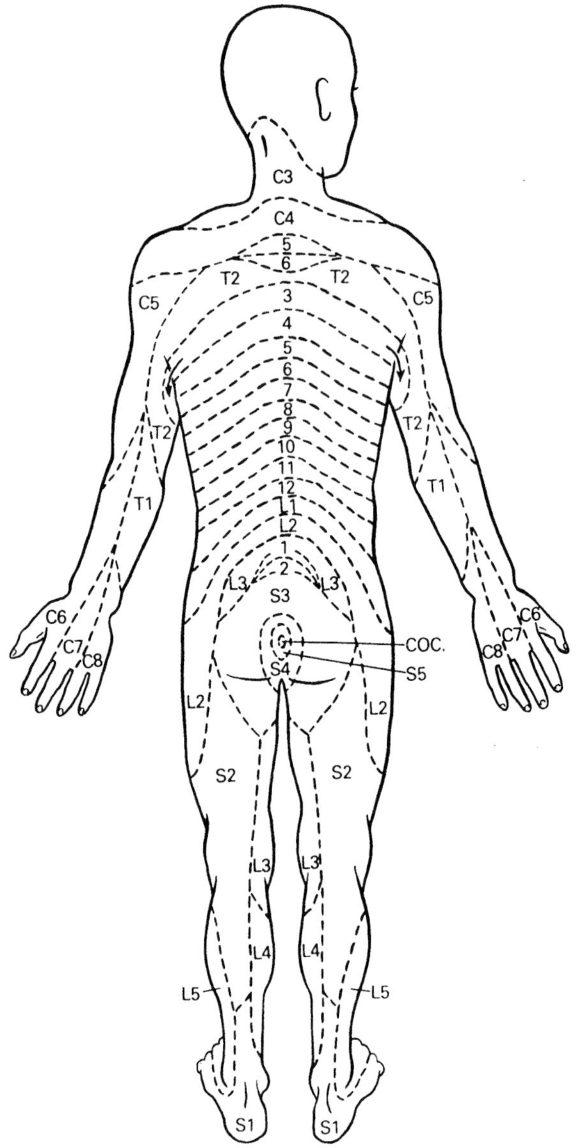

FIG. 112.5. Dermatomes in the posterior view. (From Devinsky O, Feldmann E. *Examination of the cranial and peripheral nerves.* Oxford: Churchill Livingstone, 1988:37, with permission.)

groove. To test this muscle, the examiner should place the patient's forearm midway between pronation and supination (as if ready to pound the fist on the table) and have the patient flex the arm at the elbow.

Weakness from radial mononeuropathy is often mistaken either for a stroke, which causes greater extensor than flexor weakness in the upper extremity, or for an ulnar mononeuropathy, which causes weakness of the hand intrinsic muscles. The hand intrinsics help to spread the fingers apart and work to mechanical advantage only when the fingers are fully extended. Without radial nerve-mediated finger extension, the fingers assume a flexed position in which they do not generate full power. Placing the hand flat on the examination table before testing restores the optimal mechanical advantage, and the normal strength of the ulnar nerve-innervated intrinsic muscles can be demonstrated.

OTHER UPPER EXTREMITY MONONEUROPATHIES

The long thoracic nerve supplies the serratus anterior, which helps to stabilize the scapula against the chest wall. Traction or blunt injuries lead to scapular winging with medial translocation of the scapula. Stretch injury or direct trauma to the nerve is an infrequent complication of mastectomy or thoracotomy. The suprascapular nerve can be compressed as it passes under the suprascapular notch on its way to supply the infraspinatus. A suprascapular mononeuropathy results in weakness of external rotation of the arm. The axillary nerve supplies the teres minor and deltoid muscles and provides sensory supply to a small patch of skin overlying the deltoid muscle. Humeral neck injuries, blunt trauma, and injection injuries account for most axillary mononeuropathies. The cutaneous territory of the axillary nerve is shown in Fig. 112.1.

Lower Extremity Mononeuropathies

Pelvic masses, pregnancy, vaginal delivery, and certain pelvic procedures are commonly complicated by focal nerve compression, so that women are at special risk for the development of mononeuropathies of the lower extremity. The evaluation of abnormalities of the lower extremity is complicated by the close anatomic interrelationships of its peripheral nerves. The sciatic nerve gives rise to both the peroneal and tibial nerves, and all three share a similar root supply. To complicate matters further, the sheer strength of the leg muscles makes it difficult to detect mild muscle weakness. Sensory findings are often most helpful in localizing a problem to a particular root level.

SCIATIC MONONEUROPATHY

The sciatic nerve innervates the hamstrings, and its branches supply all the muscles below the knee. It is composed of both peroneal and tibial fascicles, which remain anatomically distinct along the entire course of the nerve. The peroneal and tibial fascicles finally separate to form the common peroneal and tibial nerves in the distal third of the thigh. The sensory territory of the sciatic nerve includes portions of the lateral leg and the lower leg and foot. The fact that injuries to the sciatic nerve are often partial is a testament to its size and deep location.

Sciatica is a common presenting complaint in outpatients. The term *sciatica* is used loosely by patients and physicians to cover a wide range of symptoms referable to the low back and lower extremity. The history and physical examination should narrow the differential diagnosis of sciatica. The differential diagnosis includes spinal cord pathology (typically in the lower thoracic cord or conus medullaris), lumbosacral radiculopathy (particularly at the L5-S1 level), mononeuropathies (sciatic, posterior femoral cutaneous, peroneal, or tibial nerve), lumbosacral plexopathy, and simply nonspecific low back pain. Electrodiagnostic testing may be required to distinguish among these possibilities.

Trauma to the proximal sciatic nerve occurs with pelvic fractures and dislocations, fractures of the acetabulum, and penetrating wounds. Misplaced buttock injections (inferomedially instead of superolaterally near the ischial rim) are the most common iatrogenic cause, followed by hip arthroplasty and malpositioning during surgery. Hematomas can arise after trauma or surgery, or they can develop spontaneously in patients taking anticoagulant therapy. More unusual causes include prolonged sitting in the yoga position or sitting on a large wallet in the hip pocket. Pelvic tumors can directly compress the sciatic nerve. Endometriosis can cause catamenial sciatica, symptoms of sciatic compression that vary with the menstrual cycle, by compressing the nerve either at the sciatic notch or as it passes under the piriformis muscle.

In the piriformis syndrome, patients experience groin discomfort when internally rotating their flexed and adducted hip (i.e., sitting on the floor with legs crossed) and often report dyspareunia. The syndrome is said to result from compression of the sciatic nerve or its peroneal division as it passes under the piriformis muscle toward the greater sciatic foramen. Despite the anatomic plausibility of this syndrome, little firm electrodiagnostic evidence supports its existence.

PERONEAL MONONEUROPATHY

The common peroneal nerve separates from the sciatic nerve in the distal third of the thigh. It winds around the fibula relatively unprotected from external compression, so that common peroneal mononeuropathy at the fibular head is one of the most frequently seen compressive mononeuropathies. The common peroneal nerve gives off superficial and deep branches, each with their respective motor and sensory supplies. The deep peroneal nerve supplies the "anterior compartment" of the ankle and leg, including the ankle and toe dorsiflexors, and provides sensation to the web space between the great toe and second toe. The superficial peroneal nerve supplies the ankle evertors and provides sensation to the dorsum of the foot, except for the most lateral portions, which are supplied by the sural nerve (Figs. 112.2, 112.3). The lateral (external) hamstring jerk is mediated by the peroneal nerve; the medial (internal) hamstring jerk is mediated by the tibial nerve.

Compression at the fibular head produces painless footdrop, toe-drop, or both, often with little sensory loss. Eversion of the foot is also weak. The most common cause in healthy patients is habitual or prolonged leg crossing or squatting. Thin persons, those with significant recent weight loss (either intentional or in the setting of cachexia), and diabetic patients are all at increased risk. The peroneal nerves of patients who deliver in the lithotomy position may be compressed by the improper use of stirrups, or even by pressure exerted with the patients' own hands as they attempt to flex and externally rotate their hips forcefully.

Patients with footdrop have a characteristic gait. The inability to dorsiflex the foot makes it impossible to advance the affected leg without external (lateral) rotation or unnatural elevation of the hip. Patients report tripping over their toes, catching the edge of carpeting, or scuffing the tops of their shoes. An ankle-foot orthosis "cures" footdrop and permits a nearly normal gait, even when the ankle dorsiflexors are flaccid. When footdrop is mild, high-top sneakers may substitute for an ankle-foot orthosis.

Chronic footdrop places patients at risk for the development of shortening of the Achilles tendon and contractures. Once contractures develop, dorsiflexion of the foot becomes impossible, even with normal ankle dorsiflexor strength. The use of a foot board at night, appropriate supports (ankle-foot orthosis or high-top shoes) during the day, and passive lengthening exercises can help to preserve normal heel cord length.

The differential diagnosis of peroneal mononeuropathy includes L5 radiculopathy, sciatic mononeuropathy, lumbosacral plexopathy, and other conditions. Upper motor neuron injuries (i.e., stroke, spinal cord injury) can also cause footdrop. L5 radiculopathies are typically associated with back pain and weakness of both foot inversion *and* eversion, whereas peroneal mononeuropathies cause greater eversion weakness. The peroneal fascicles in the sciatic nerve are selectively vulnerable to compression, and compression of these fascicles often mimics more distal injuries to the common or deep peroneal nerve. Electromyographic evaluation should be sufficiently detailed to exclude this possibility.

TIBIAL MONONEUROPATHY

The tibial nerve arises from the medial portion of the sciatic nerve. It supplies the posterior calf muscles and foot intrinsic muscles. Tibial mononeuropathies cause weakness of ankle plantar flexion ("stepping on the gas") and inversion. The ankle jerk and medial hamstring jerk are both mediated by the tibial nerve. The sensory territory of the nerve includes the posterior leg, lateral border of the foot, and sole via the medial and lateral plantar nerves (Figs. 112.2, 112.3).

The tibial nerve and the medial sciatic nerve from which it arises are relatively immune to injury. Proximal injuries are rare, occurring with total knee replacement, severe knee trauma, Baker cysts, and aneurysms of the popliteal artery. Distal compressive injuries at or below the ankle are more common but still unusual. Tarsal tunnel syndrome is the most common of the tibial mononeuropathies. The syndrome results from entrapment of the tibial nerve under the flexor retinaculum (just behind the medial malleolus). Sensory loss is prominent on the plantar surface of the foot in the distribution of the median and lateral plantar nerves (Fig. 112.3). Sensation in the heel is spared because the calcaneal branch of the tibial nerve arises just proximal to the tarsal tunnel and is not compressed. Weakness of the lateral toe flexors develops. A Tinel sign may be elicited below the medial malleolus. Diabetic and hypothyroid patients are at increased risk for tarsal tunnel syndrome, as for other forms of entrapment.

FEMORAL MONONEUROPATHIES

The femoral nerve supplies the quadriceps (knee extensors), iliopsoas (hip flexor), and sartorius (external rotator of the knee) and provides sensory supply to the anteromedial thigh, knee, and medial calf via the saphenous nerve. The patellar jerk is mediated by fibers of the femoral nerve. Placing a patient in the lithotomy position, either for surgical procedures or delivery, can compress the femoral nerve under the inguinal ligament, and cephalopelvic disproportion can lead to direct compression of either the femoral nerve or the lumbosacral plexus from which it arises. Retroperitoneal hemorrhage can produce devastating proximal femoral mononeuropathies. Spontaneous retroperitoneal bleeding often develops in patients on anticoagulation therapy. Inguinal pain followed by weakness of the proximally innervated iliopsoas and quadriceps muscles strongly suggests the diagnosis, which can be confirmed by pelvic computed tomography. Timely surgical intervention may spare femoral nerve function.

In diabetic amyotrophy, severe subacute thigh pain is followed by pronounced quadriceps atrophy (see Chapter 114). Although the distribution of signs and symptoms is reminiscent of an ischemic femoral mononeuropathy, a more proximal injury at the level of the lumbosacral plexus is more likely.

OBTURATOR MONONEUROPATHY

The obturator nerve supplies the hip adductors. Mononeuropathies are uncommon but can occur in the setting of difficult vaginal deliveries or gynecologic surgery because the nerve lies in close approximation to the uterus. Endometriosis can cause nerve compression in rare instances. Weakness of hip adduction and flexion (a secondary action of the adductor muscles) is seen. An L2-3 radiculopathy can cause a similar picture, although hip flexion, mediated by the femoral nerve-innervated iliopsoas muscle, is more severely affected, and back pain is likely.

GLUTEAL MONONEUROPATHIES

The gluteal nerves supply the gluteal muscles (gluteus maximus, gluteus minimus, gluteus medius) and the tensor fasciae latae, a muscle that inserts into the iliotibial band of the fascia lata on the lateral thigh. Both nerves exit the sciatic foramen with the sciatic nerve and can be injured by misplaced injections into the buttock. The inferior gluteal nerve supplies the gluteus maximus, which primarily extends but also abducts and laterally rotates the thigh. The superior gluteal nerve supplies the gluteus medius and gluteus minimus and the tensor fasciae latae.

PUDENDAL MONONEUROPATHIES

The pudendal nerve exits the greater sciatic foramen along with the sciatic and both gluteal nerves. It reaches the perineum via the pudendal canal. The nerve can be injured by misplaced injections, bicycle riding, or trauma during vaginal delivery or surgery. Branches of the nerve subserve sexual function and bowel and bladder control, so that mononeuropathies are particularly devastating. More proximal injuries to either the lumbosacral plexus or the sacral roots in the cauda equina can produce a clinical and electrodiagnostic picture similar to that of a pudendal mononeuropathy and must be considered in the differential diagnosis.

The first branch of the pudendal nerve within the pudendal canal is the inferior rectal nerve, which provides motor supply to the levator ani and external anal sphincter and perirectal cutaneous sensation. The perineal nerve arises from the pudendal nerve shortly after the inferior rectal branch and supplies both the posterior labia and the external urethral sphincters. The dorsal nerve of the clitoris is the final pudendal branch.

Electrodiagnostic studies are useful in the evaluation of urinary and fecal incontinence. Pudendal motor conduction studies can be performed with a flexible St. Mark electrode attached to an examination glove. Needle electromyography of the urethral and anal sphincters also can be performed.

SENSORY MONONEUROPATHIES OF THE LOWER EXTREMITY

Several of the proximal mononeuropathies of the lower extremities produce sensory-only symptoms. The cutaneous distribution of these nerves is shown in Fig. 112.2. The most common proximal mononeuropathy is lateral femoral cutaneous neuropathy—the syndrome known as *meralgia paresthetica* ("painful thigh"). The lateral femoral cutaneous nerve of the thigh is typically injured by tight pants or seat belts, or it can be injured by leaning against the edge of a table or during pregnancy. Patients who are diabetic or obese are particularly prone to this condition. They report sensory loss or dysesthesia over the anterolateral thigh. The symptoms typically resolve spontaneously, so conservative management is generally appropriate. Nonsteroidal antiinflammatory agents may provide sufficient pain relief for some patients, but others may require local steroid injection or nerve block. The presence of motor signs or symptoms, back pain, or an atypical pattern of sensory loss should suggest an alternate diagnosis. The differential should include a high lumbar radiculopathy (L2-3 level) and lumbosacral plexopathy. Nerve conduction studies may be helpful, although they are often most difficult to perform in the very patients who are at risk—obese persons and those with diabetes.

The saphenous nerve is the terminal branch of the femoral nerve. It is a purely sensory nerve that supplies the medial calf and medial dorsum of the foot. Inadvertent injury during saphenous vein grafting, knee surgery, and varicose vein surgery are the most common causes of mononeuropathy. Improper stirrup use can result in isolated injury. Both a proximal femoral mononeuropathy and an L4 radiculopathy cause a similar pattern of sensory loss.

Cutaneous sensation in the perineum is mediated by nerves arising from the lumbar plexus (Fig. 112.6). Most mononeuropathies result from abdominal or pelvic surgery, although retroperitoneal malignancy must be considered. When bilateral abnormalities are present, spinal cord disease must be ruled out. The iliohypogastric nerve supplies the skin overlying the medial portion of the inguinal ligament. It is most commonly injured during procedures requiring transverse low abdominal or suprapubic incisions. The ilioinguinal and genitofemoral nerves traverse the inguinal canal and are therefore more at risk during herniorrhaphy, appendectomy, and pregnancy. Ilioinguinal nerve injuries produce sensory loss or pain over the extreme medial portion of the thigh and upper half of the labia majora. Thus, sensation to the labia majora is supplied by two anatomically distinct pathways—the upper half of the labia majora by the ilioinguinal nerve and L1 nerve roots and the lower half by the pudendal nerve and S2-3 nerve roots. Iatrogenic causes of genitofemoral neuropathy predominate. Sensory loss involves the femoral triangle—the anterior thigh below the inguinal ligament in the region of the femoral nerve, artery, and vein. Sensation to the clitoris is supplied by the dorsal nerve of the clitoris, a terminal branch of the pudendal nerve. The lower half of the labia majora and the labial minora share this root supply. The posterior femoral cutaneous nerve (S1-3) arises from the sacral plexus and traverses the greater sciatic foramen beside the sciatic nerve. It courses under the piriformis to supply the medial aspect of the buttock, posterior inner thigh, and upper portion of the posterior calf. Fractures of the hip or upper femur or misplaced buttock injections can

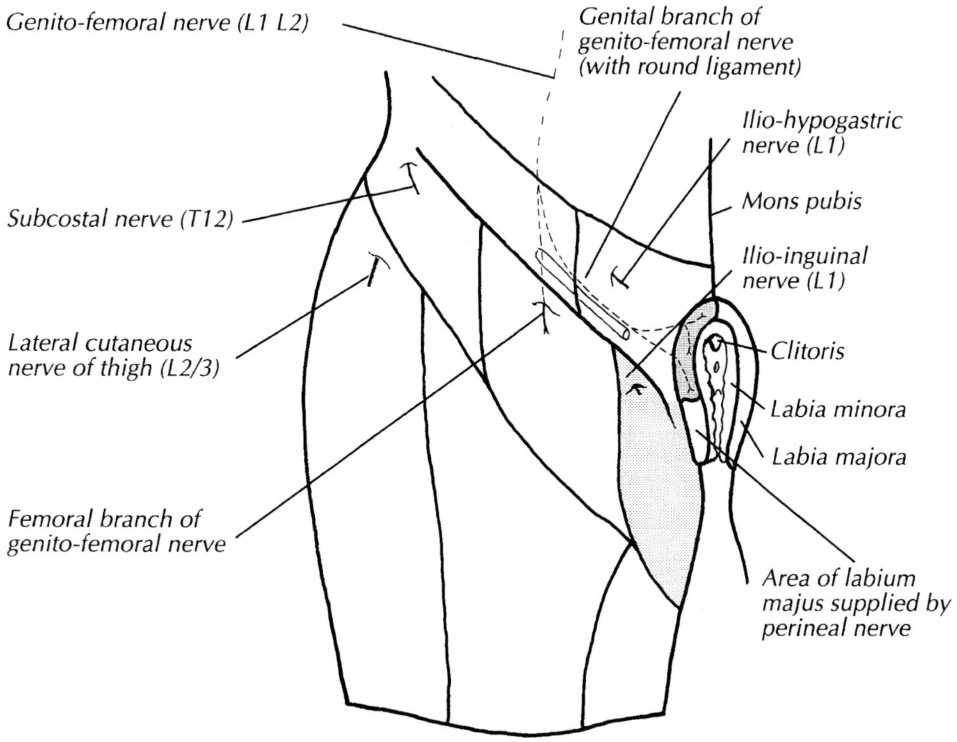

FIG. 112.6. Cutaneous nerve supply to the female perineum. The superior portion of the labia majora is supplied by both the ilioinguinal nerve and the genital branch of the genitofemoral nerve. The inferior portion of the labia majora is supplied by the perineal nerve. The ilioinguinal nerve supplies the superomedial thigh adjacent to the perineum. (Modified from Patten J. *Neurological differential diagnosis,* 2nd ed. Berlin: Springer-Verlag, 1996:313, with permission.)

injure this nerve. The inferior rectal nerves (see section "Pudendal Mononeuropathies") supply perirectal sensation.

The sural nerve receives contributions from both the tibial and common peroneal nerves. It supplies the medial third of the posterior calf and portions of the lateral calf and foot. The sural nerve can be injured when the posterior calf is pressed against a hard edge or when improperly fitting ski boots are worn. This nerve is commonly harvested for nerve biopsy because of its accessibility and the inconsequential nature of the subsequent sensory deficit. Unfortunately, in a small percentage of patients, a neuroma forms at the distal stump of the transected nerve and causes chronic pain.

Injury to the tibial nerve-derived interdigital nerves under the metatarsal heads of the lateral toes causes Morton metatarsalgia, in which chronic toe pain is exacerbated by weight bearing and walking. Deep interdigital palpation may reveal local tenderness or local nerve enlargement. Tight shoes and high heels are major risk factors for local nerve injury; hence, most patients with this condition are women. Conservative measures such as changing footwear should be attempted before surgical exploration is considered. At surgery, local nerve enlargement (neuroma) is detected in some patients. Resection of the neuroma or nerve transection more proximally can lead to symptomatic relief.

CONSIDERATIONS IN PREGNANCY

Table 112.1 lists the most common mononeuropathies associated with pregnancy, vaginal and cesarean delivery, and surgical positioning. Most are self-limiting conditions that can be

TABLE 112.1. Common Pregnancy-Associated Mononeuropathies

	Pregnancy	Vaginal delivery	Cesarean delivery	Surgical positioning
Sensorimotor	Median (CTS) Sciatic Obturator	Lumbosacral plexus Pudendal Obturator Peroneal Femoral	Lumbosacral plexus Pudendal Femoral	Ulnar Sciatic Obturator Femoral Peroneal
Sensory only	Median (CTS) Meralgia paresthetica	Saphenous	Genitofemoral Ilioinguinal Iliohypogastric Saphenous	Saphenous

CTS, carpal tunnel syndrome.

managed conservatively. The most frequent, CTS, occurs in up to 2% of patients and is often bilateral. Vaginal delivery can result in a mononeuropathy because the lumbosacral plexus or peripheral nerves may be directly compressed by the descending fetal head. The use of surgical instruments to assist the delivery can also result in injury. Cesarean section and other surgery can cause local injuries to the nerves of the lower abdominal wall and inguinal region or compressive injuries as a consequence of improper patient positioning.

BIBLIOGRAPHY

Abrams BM. Entrapment and compressive neuropathies: upper extremity progression. *Neurology* 2000;2:3.

Asbury AK, Thomas PK, eds. *Peripheral nerve disorders: blue books of practical neurology*. Oxford: Butterworth-Heinemann, 1995.

Cohen BS, Felsenthal G. Peripheral nervous system disorders and pregnancy. In: Goldstein PJ, ed. *Neurological disorders of pregnancy*. Mt. Kisco, NY: Futura Publishing, 1986:153.

Devinsky O, Feldmann E. *Examination of the cranial and peripheral nerves*. Oxford: Churchill Livingstone, 1988.

Donaldson JO. Neurology of pregnancy. In: Walton J, ed. *Major problems in neurology*, 2nd ed, vol 19. London: WB Saunders, 1989.

Editorial Committee for the Guarantors of Brain. *Aids to the examination of the nervous system*. East Sussex, UK: Bailliere Tindall, 1986.

Patten J. *Neurological differential diagnosis*, 2nd ed. Berlin: Springer-Verlag, 1996: 282.

Stewart JD. *Focal peripheral neuropathies*, 2nd ed. New York: Raven Press, 1993.

CHAPTER 113
Cranial Neuropathies

Gerald W. Honch

The cranial nerves are 12 paired sets of nerves named for their function. The first two cranial nerves do not originate in the brainstem, but the rest do. A knowledge of brainstem anatomy is essential for localizing a lesion at that level, as is an understanding of anatomic and functional relationships at the level of the brainstem. As the cranial nerves leave the brainstem and course toward an end organ or structure, they are vulnerable to injury. A knowledge of the course of these nerves and the anatomic pitfalls of entrapment or injury is helpful diagnostically.

DIFFERENTIAL DIAGNOSIS

If the clinician can discern from clinical clues at the presentation where an insult occurred, more than half the diagnostic challenge has been met. Diagnostic tools can be selected only after an insult has been localized by clinical examination. A judicious investigation is both logical and economical. Roentgenography is useful for evaluating bony structures. Computed tomography (CT) is ideal for evaluating bony structures and the sinuses, but its utility in the brainstem parenchyma is limited. Magnetic resonance imaging (MRI) is ideal for brainstem structures but not very helpful for bone. Angiography is useful for vascular anatomy and its anomalies but is invasive. Functional electric testing (electromyography and nerve conduction studies) requires experienced neurophysiologic personnel and a knowledge of the specific questions to be answered. Evoked response testing of vision and the brainstem can be helpful, but again, specific questions must be answered.

CLINICAL FINDINGS, IMAGING STUDIES, AND TREATMENT

An exhaustive review of neuroanatomy and functional anatomy within the skull is not intended here. Table 113.1 provides a quick guide to the 12 cranial nerves and their relationships within and outside the brainstem. Landmarks are given to help the clinician recognize valuable clues to localization. Only cranial nerves II through VIII are discussed in detail here; these have been chosen because of their importance and frequent involvement.

Cranial Nerve II: Optic

The optic nerve receives neural input from the rods and cones in the retina. Each optic nerve extends from the posterior orbit to the optic chiasm just in front of the pituitary stalk. The course of this nerve as it leaves the globe is extremely complex. Its relationship to the extraocular nerves, bones of the orbit, carotid artery, and pituitary gland may provide anatomic clues of great localizing value. The appearance of the retina and optic disc must be assessed. The size, shape, and extent of a visual field defect must be recorded. Whether a field defect and any changes noted on funduscopic examination are unilateral or bilateral is of great localizing significance (to define whether the problem is within the eye, supporting structures, or brain). Papilledema (swelling of the head of the optic nerve) may be difficult to appreciate in mild cases but is dramatic in others. Optic atrophy as a residuum of prior papilledema or optic neuritis manifests as a pale disc and a reduction in the fine retinal vasculature and disc size.

Optic neuritis is more common in women (77%) and associated with ocular pain and rapid (not sudden) visual loss of varying severity. Edema of the optic disc may occur. Color vision is impaired in 90% of patients. Most patients recover their visual acuity with time alone; treatment with high-dose steroids is controversial. Many patients with a history of optic neuritis are subject to future attacks. Multiple sclerosis later develops in some patients who have experienced an episode of optic neuritis. MRI reveals lesions of the brain white matter in 25% to 75% of patients with an episode of optic neuritis. It is unclear how to interpret an MR image that demonstrates white matter lesions in the absence of other symptoms. Most neurologists would be reluctant to diagnose multiple sclerosis on the basis of a single episode of optic neuritis and abnormal MRI findings without other supportive historical, laboratory, or physical changes; however, data strongly suggest that multiple sclerosis is more likely (ultimately) in a patient with abnormal MRI findings.

Anterior ischemic optic neuropathy is caused by impaired perfusion in the anterior portion of the optic nerve (supplied by the posterior ciliary arteries). Clinically, the patient experiences sudden painless visual loss in one eye. The cause may be systemic or local hypotension, glaucoma, vasculitides such as giant cell arteritis, hypertension, diabetes mellitus, or atherosclerosis. Recovery is poor. Temporal arteritis is the most important (only 5% of cases) disease to consider because it is treatable.

Tumors may develop in the optic nerve, chiasm, or tract. These tend to be more aggressive in children. Neurofibromas may also occur in this region. Many other neoplastic lesions develop in the optic nerve pathway, such as metastases, germinomas, dermoids, craniopharyngiomas, meningiomas, pituitary adenomas, hamartomas, and epidermoids. Mass effects from aneurysms, arachnoid cysts, sarcoidosis, or a craniopharyngioma may be a cause of symptoms referable to the optic nerve pathways. Attention to these areas by CT or MRI may be helpful.

TABLE 113.1. Summary of Cranial Nerves

Nerve						
Number	Name	Function	Brainstem anatomy	Landmarks	Related nerves	Issues/problems
I	Olfactory	Sensory	Not applicable	Upper nose, cribriform plate, olfactory bulb, olfactory tract	None	Odors to supplant basic taste Diseases within the nose or trauma
II	Optic	Sensory	Not applicable	Orbit, carotid artery, pituitary, chiasm	None	Vision; field defects Unilateral vs. bilateral Optic neuritis
III	Oculomotor	Motor	Midbrain near midline Relates to medial longitudinal fasciculus	Medial longitudinal fasciculus, tentorial edge, cavernous sinus, orbit	IV, V, VI	All extraocular muscles except superior oblique and lateral rectus Pupillary constrictor muscle
IV	Trochlear	Motor	Medial tegmentum of midbrain at inferior colliculus	Exits brainstem ventrally; petrous bone, cavernous sinus, orbit	III, V, VI	Motor to superior oblique
V	Trigeminal	Motor/sensory	Pons to the gasserian ganglion Three sensory divisions to face	Meckel's cave in petrous part of temporal bone Exits skull via foramen ovale	III, IV, VI	Motor to muscles of mastication Sensory from surface of head and neck, sinuses, meninges, and tympanic membrane
VI	Abducens	Motor	Dorsal medial pons near 4th ventricle	Petrous bone, cavernous sinus, orbit	III, IV, V	Motor to lateral rectus muscle
VII	Facial	Motor/sensory	Pontine tegmentum Winds around the 6th nerve nucleus	Enters the internal auditory canal via cerebellopontine angle Travels in facial canal Exits skull at stylomastoid foramen	Special relation to 6th nerve nucleus in brainstem Travels with 8th nerve in facial canal	Muscles of facial expression and stapedius Sensation from tympanic membrane Taste on anterior two thirds of tongue
VIII	Vestibulocochlear	Sensory	Enters medulla at junction with pons Lateral to 7th nerve	Travels with 7th nerve in the internal auditory canal	VII	Balance and hearing
IX	Glossopharyngeal	Motor/sensory	Series of rootlets between inferior olive and restiform body of lateral medulla	Travels the jugular fossa Exits skull via jugular foramen	X, XI	Motor to stylopharyngeal muscle, parotid gland Sensation around external ear and tympanic membrane Taste posterior third of tongue
X	Vagus	Motor/sensory	Dorsal motor nerve of vagus and nucleus ambiguus	Wanders from brainstem to splenic flexure Exits skull via jugular foramen; travels in carotid sheath Laryngeal, recurrent laryngeal, and cardiac branches	IX, XI	Motor/sensory to pharynx and larynx Parasympathetic to thoracic and abdominal viscera
XI	Accessory	Motor	Lower motor neuron cell bodies in spinal cord	Exits cranium via jugular foramen	IX, X	Motor to sternomastoid and trapezius muscles
XII	Hypoglossal	Motor	Medullary tegmentum near midline	Exits brainstem as rootlets between pyramid and inferior olive; exits skull via hypoglossal canal near foramen magnum	None	Motor to intrinsic and extrinsic muscles of the tongue

Cranial Nerves III, IV, and VI: Oculomotor, Trochlear, and Abducens

These three motor nerves move the eye within the orbit. Six extraocular muscles in each eye rotate the eye about three mutually orthogonal axes. The patient with a lesion presents with double vision (diplopia). An understanding of the function of these three nerves and their relationship to the muscles they serve will help the clinician describe the diplopia and decide whether referral to a neurologist or ophthalmologist is appropriate.

The lateral and medial rectus muscles abduct and adduct the eye, respectively. The superior rectus and inferior oblique muscles elevate the eye. The inferior rectus and superior oblique muscles depress the eye. The superior and inferior oblique muscles and the superior and inferior recti act in concert to provide torsion movements to the eye.

The central control of eye movement is divided among the supranuclear, internuclear, and nuclear areas. In supranuclear and internuclear lesions, premotor input to the nerve nucleus is disrupted; certain types of eye movements may be affected, but others are spared. The classic example is internuclear ophthalmoplegia, in which conjugate horizontal eye movements are affected but vergence eye movements are spared. In nuclear lesions or lesions beyond the nucleus in the nerve itself, all types of eye movements in which the affected nerve is involved are disrupted.

OCULOMOTOR NERVE

The oculomotor nucleus is located in the medial tegmentum of the midbrain near the periaqueductal gray matter at the level of the superior colliculus. This oculomotor complex of subnuclei innervates the ipsilateral medial rectus, inferior rectus, superior rectus, and inferior oblique muscles of each eye, in addition to the levator palpebrae muscles of the eyelid. Control of pupillary function also is mediated by related nuclear structures. The medial longitudinal fasciculus relates components of the third and sixth nerve nuclei on the opposite sides of the brainstem to coordinate horizontal eye movements.

The course of the third nerve, after it exits the brainstem, is complex. It passes between the posterior cerebral and superior cerebellar arteries and runs parallel to the posterior communicating artery (relationships to vascular structures may provide clues to the localization of berry aneurysms occurring in this area). It passes on the edge of the tentorium (providing localizing clues in uncal herniation). The third nerve passes along the superior region of the cavernous sinus and relates to other cranial nerves (IV, V, and VI) at this intimate crossroads. Finally, it enters the orbit through the superior orbital fissure (a bony landmark).

A complete oculomotor nerve palsy causes ptosis and a fixed, dilated pupil. The eye is abducted at rest as a result of unopposed tonic activity in the lateral rectus. Adduction, elevation, and depression of the eye are lost. In less severe palsies, all the features are less severe or even incomplete. If the pupil is spared, the physician must consider myasthenia gravis, hypertension, diabetes mellitus, restrictive orbit disease, or rarely an aneurysm. A tonic (Adie) pupil or a dorsal midbrain lesion (Parinaud syndrome) may produce light near dissociation. Local instillation of drugs that affect the pupil should be considered when a patient has a dilated pupil and no other findings. The anatomic localization of lesions damaging the oculomotor nerve depends on the associated neurologic and orbital signs. These clues may place the lesion at various locations within the brainstem, along the course of the third nerve and adjacent structures, or within the orbit. An accurate assessment of these findings simplifies and directs the workup.

TROCHLEAR NERVE

The trochlear nucleus is located in the medial tegmentum of the midbrain, ventral to the periaqueductal gray matter and at the level of the inferior colliculus. The fibers decussate before exiting the brainstem. This is the only cranial nerve to exit the brainstem dorsally. The trochlear nerve passes ventrally around the cerebral peduncle and then enters the cavernous sinus (lateral). It enters the orbit through the superior orbital fissure to innervate the superior oblique muscle (contralateral to the trochlear nerve nucleus of origin). The fourth cranial nerve has the longest intracranial course.

The superior oblique muscle depresses the eye when it is adducted and intorts the eye when it is abducted. Hence, trochlear nerve palsies cause vertical and torsional diplopia. The diplopia is most severe during downward gaze and when the head is tilted toward the side of the paretic muscle. Patients often maintain a typical head posture to minimize the diplopia (chin down and head tilted toward the normal eye). A trochlear nerve lesion is easy to identify when it coexists with an oculomotor nerve lesion (when the abnormal eye is examined during attempted downward gaze, subtle rotatory movement can be seen in the conjunctival vessels if the trochlear nerve is intact).

The trochlear nerve can be damaged by lesions in the brainstem, subarachnoid space, cavernous sinus, or orbit. Trauma is the most common cause of acquired trochlear nerve palsy.

ABDUCENS NERVE

The abducens nerve nucleus is located in the dorsal medial pons, under the floor of the fourth ventricle. The nerve exits the brainstem ventrally at the pontomedullary junction and then ascends in the prepontine cistern. It travels along the apex of the petrous bone, passes through the cavernous sinus, and enters the orbit through the superior orbital fissure. It innervates the lateral rectus muscle. The tortuous course of this nerve makes it vulnerable to various injuries in multiple anatomic locations.

Abducens nerve palsies present with horizontal diplopia. The distance between the images becomes more pronounced as the patient looks toward the paretic lateral rectus muscle. The diplopia worsens with distance vision and is less severe with near vision. On examination, reduced abduction of the involved eye is often grossly apparent. In primary position, esodeviation of the involved eye may occur because the medial rectus is unopposed. Restrictive orbital problems (as in Graves disease) and ocular myasthenia gravis may have to be considered.

Lesions that damage the abducens nucleus or nerve often involve adjacent neural structures. When a brainstem lesion affects the abducens nucleus, an ipsilateral nuclear facial palsy and a contralateral hemiparesis are common. Involvement of the medial longitudinal fasciculus may cause contralateral medial rectus dysfunction. The combination of a lesion of the abducens nucleus and involvement of the ipsilateral medial longitudinal fasciculus is referred to as the *one and one-half syndrome* (the only remaining horizontal eye movement is abduction of the contralateral eye). Pontine lesions involving the abducens nucleus or nerve can result from ischemic infarction, hemorrhage, abscess, neoplasm, Wernicke encephalopathy, or demyelination. Many disorders that involve the subarachnoid space (e.g., meningioma, carcinomatous meningitis, infection) can affect the abducens nerve. Lesions at the bony petrous apex (usually from complicated otitis media) can cause an abducens nerve palsy associated with ipsilateral facial (retro-orbital) pain and decreased facial and corneal sensation (Gradenigo syndrome). Neoplastic processes may also invade the petrous apex. Increased intracranial pressure may cause an abducens palsy (as a false localizing sign) solely on the basis of pressure on the very long subarachnoid course of the nerve. In the cavernous sinus and orbit, abducens nerve palsies occur in conjunction with losses in adjacent cranial nerves (III, IV, and V). Isolated abducens palsies can occur as the result of occlusion of the vasa nervorum secondary to hypertension or diabetes mellitus.

Cranial Nerve V: Trigeminal

The three sensory divisions of the trigeminal nerve are the ophthalmic (V1), maxillary (V2), and mandibular (V3). These cover the facial territory extending from the vertex of the scalp (but not the scalp posterior to the ear) to the lower margin of the mandible. The outer canthus of the eye separates V1 from V2, and the corner of the mouth separates V2 from V3. The three sensory divisions merge at the gasserian ganglion (in a depression of the petrous part of the temporal bone called *Meckel's cave*). The trigeminal nerve extends proximally from the gasserian ganglion and merges with the ventrolateral aspect of the pons. Within the pons, some sensory fibers remain in the main trigeminal nucleus; others extend caudally to the level of the second cervical segment, and still other sensory fibers terminate in the mesencephalic nuclei at the edge of the periaqueductal gray matter. The motor nucleus of the trigeminal nerve is in the lateral pontine tegmentum. Motor fibers pass forward along the inferior surface of the gasserian ganglion to become incorporated into the mandibular division. The motor component of the mandibular division leaves the skull through the foramen ovale and enters the anterior trunk of the mandibular division to innervate the muscles of mastication (masseter, temporalis, and medial and lateral pterygoid). Branches are sent to the tensor tympani, tensor veli palatini, mylohyoid, and anterior belly of the digastric muscles.

Primary vascular afferents contain neuropeptides that modulate pain. This trigeminal-vascular system is central to the pathogenesis of migraine headaches.

Injury to one or all of the divisions or branches of the trigeminal nerve results in loss of sensibility in the corresponding cutaneous area. The range of sensory losses include light touch, pain, and temperature. Dysesthesia or hyperpathia can occur. Interruption of the ophthalmic division can cause a diminution or loss of the corneal reflex. Lesions of the mandibular nerve lead to loss of the masseter or jaw reflex. Paralysis of the masseter or temporalis muscle may be seen.

Trigeminal neuralgia (tic douloureux) is intense, lightning-like pain that occurs in one or more divisions of the trigeminal nerve. It generally begins after the age of 40. The pathophysiology is unclear but is related to increased afferent activity and diminished inhibitory control, with paroxysmal discharges in the trigeminal nucleus in response to sensory input. The neurologic examination findings are usually normal. Trigeminal neuralgia is more common in women than men (ratio of 1.74:1); the incidence is 4.7 per 100,000. It is rarely familial. The patient experiences brief episodes of severe, focal pain described as electric, jabbing, or lancinating. The pain is usually within a single dermatome (most often V2 or V3). The painful paroxysms can occur repeatedly around the clock, often with a characteristic trigger point. The trigger point may be so sensitive that the patient avoids washing an affected area, brushing certain teeth, or even eating or talking in an effort to avoid pain. The trigger point is generally in the same division of the trigeminal nerve as the pain. These episodes have an extremely rapid onset and a slightly slower offset. Each paroxysm of pain lasts only a few seconds but is so intense that the patient may exaggerate its duration. Between attacks, the patient is free of pain and can carry on usual activities with caution to the trigger areas. Some patients have a prodromal pain syndrome that consists of continuous dull, achy discomfort. After a paroxysm of pain, a refractory period may occur during which stimulation of the trigger zone does not precipitate pain. Hence, immediately after experiencing a painful episode, the patient may be able to eat or wash her face without triggering another episode. The episodes of pain may remit spontaneously for months or years. The patient lives in dread of the next episode of pain.

The precise pathophysiology of trigeminal neuralgia is unclear, but vascular compression of the trigeminal nerve root entry zone is favored. Several studies have demonstrated compression of the nerve by an artery (less commonly by a vein). Trigeminal neuralgia is more common in patients with multiple sclerosis. Trigeminal neuralgia also occurs in conditions in which the nerve is stretched, as in mass lesions, syringobulbia, brainstem infarctions, aneurysms, and vascular malformations.

Most patients (90%) respond to carbamazepine. Other medical therapies include phenytoin, baclofen, gabapentin, sodium valproate, and lamotrigine, alone or in combination. Once the patient has obtained relief, the dosage should be tapered slowly to define a maintenance level. Once the symptoms have remitted, the medication should be tapered further and discontinued. Surgical procedures are best used when conservative approaches have failed. These include percutaneous radiofrequency neurolysis, glycerol or alcohol block, microvascular decompression, and peripheral neurectomy. Some neurosurgical procedures (radiofrequency) attempt to destroy pain-transmitting fibers and spare touch sensation. Complete anesthesia may cause a loss of the corneal reflex or a painful anesthesia of the face (anesthesia dolorosa). Some recommend microvascular decompression of the trigeminal nerve with a retromastoid craniectomy. The success rate is improved if vascular distortion of the nerve can be demonstrated.

Sensory trigeminal neuropathy is a sensory loss in the trigeminal nerve distribution. It may occur alone or as part of a more widespread neurologic constellation. The symptoms may be acute or subacute and unilateral or bilateral, and they may affect parts of or the entire trigeminal nerve distribution. Sensory trigeminal neuropathy may be painless or associated with constant pain or even paroxysmal symptoms of trigeminal neuralgia. Headache may also occur. Motor findings are absent. The causes or associated diseases cover a wide spectrum: inflammatory diseases, multiple sclerosis, neoplastic disease (primary or metastatic), trauma, and infections; the condition may also be idiopathic.

Mental neuropathy (numb chin syndrome) may be caused by a lesion of the mandibular division of the trigeminal nerve, the inferior alveolar nerve, or its terminal branch, the mental nerve. The condition has various causes, but the most common is cancer.

Cranial Nerve VII: Facial

The voluntary control of facial movement, including eyelid closure, originates in the cortex (lower third of the precentral gyrus). The fibers course downward in the genu of the internal capsule and decussate in the basis pontis to terminate in the facial nucleus. The nuclear component of the forehead receives cortical contributions bilaterally. The innervation of the lower facial muscles is predominantly contralateral. Hence, in an upper motor lesion (above the facial nucleus), sparing of the forehead is an important finding. In a lower motor lesion (at the facial nucleus or in the facial nerve), the forehead is involved.

The facial nerve originates from the facial nucleus at the level of the pontine tegmentum. Fibers from the nucleus wind around the sixth nerve nucleus and then exit the pons in the region of the cerebellopontine angle medial to the acoustic nerve. The nerve enters the internal auditory meatus (in the facial canal) accompanying the eighth nerve. The facial canal is 1 cm long and contains the geniculate ganglion. Within the facial canal, the chorda tympani and branches to the stapedius muscle are given off. After leaving the skull via the stylomastoid foramen, the facial nerve passes through the parotid gland, where it divides into a number of branches to supply the muscles of facial expression.

The parasympathetic component of the facial nerve originates from the lacrimal and superior salivatory nuclei. The fibers from these nuclei emerge from the pons as the nervus intermedius. This merges with the motor root of the facial nerve in the internal auditory canal, although its course may be separate from that of the seventh and eighth nerves. The parasympathetic fibers pass through the geniculate ganglion on their way to the lacrimal and nasopalatine glands and the sphenopalatine ganglion. The parasympathetic fibers destined for the submaxillary and sublingual glands also pass through the geniculate ganglion and proceed with the seventh nerve to the chorda tympani.

The taste chemoreceptor cells of the tongue reside in the anterior two thirds of the tongue. This sensory information travels through the lingual nerve to the chorda tympani and hence to the facial nerve. Stimuli are conveyed centrally via the nervus intermedius to the nucleus solitarius. Second-order fibers go to the thalamus through the medial lemniscus on their way to the sensory cortex.

Supranuclear lesions cause predominantly weakness of the lower half of the contralateral face. The greatest weakness is around the mouth, with drooping of the corner of the mouth and flattening of the nasolabial fold. Any weakness of the forehead is usually slight and transient. Closure of the eyelid may be compromised slightly. Emotional and associated movements of the face may be retained, but voluntary movement is compromised.

Most pontine lesions do not affect facial function without affecting neighboring structures such as the abducens nucleus. A proximal pontine facial nerve lesion may spare the parasympathetic and taste components of the facial nerve.

With complete peripheral facial nerve palsies, all movements of the affected side of the face are lost, both voluntary as well as associated and emotional. The weakness extends from the mouth and nasolabial fold to the eyelid and forehead. When eyelid closure is attempted, the eye rotates up and out (Bell phenomenon). Blinking is lost, and tears collect and overflow. Food tends to collect between the gum and cheek. Corneal sensation is intact, but the blink reflex is lost. If the nerve to the stapedius muscle is affected, auditory acuity may be increased (hyperacusis). Taste is lost or distorted over the anterior two thirds of the tongue with compromise of the chorda tympani nerve. Most patients who report a loss of taste have actually lost smell; taste on the tongue is limited to sweet, sour, bitter, and salty.

Peripheral facial nerve palsy has many causes. It can be part of a constellation of neurologic findings or occur in isolation. The onset may be acute or slowly progressive. The palsy can be unilateral or bilateral, recurrent, or congenital.

Idiopathic facial nerve palsy, or Bell palsy, is an inflammatory demyelinating neuropathy. It is rare in childhood, and the incidence increases with age. Bell palsy is more common in patients with diabetes mellitus. No sexual preference is noted, although it is three times more common during pregnancy, especially during the third trimester and the first 2 weeks postpartum. In some series, toxemia appears to be a risk factor, but in others, this is not significant. Bell palsy may be recurrent. Periauricular pain occurs in 60% of patients, dysgeusia in 57%, hyperacusis in 30%, and diminished tearing in 17%. Examination of the cerebrospinal fluid may reveal a mild mononuclear pleocytosis and mildly elevated protein. The facial nerve and muscles can be examined with nerve stimulation studies and electromyography. Within the first few days after paralysis, distal nerve degeneration is minimal, so the results of nerve conduction studies are normal distal to the stylomastoid foramen. If recovery has not occurred spontaneously in days to weeks, repeated studies may demonstrate abnormalities. These findings may be useful prognostically. About 85% of patients recover completely within 3 months. If the patient does not recover fully within 3 months, complete remission is unlikely. Older patients have a poorer recovery rate than younger ones. The more severe the facial weakness, the poorer the rate of recovery.

Protecting the eye from dryness and foreign material cannot be overemphasized. Closure of the eyelid with paper tape or an ophthalmologic consultation to stitch the eyelid closed (tarsorrhaphy) may be necessary. Artificial tears are often prescribed but are useful only briefly because they dry out. Protecting the eye during sleep must not be overlooked (ophthalmic ointment). Steroid treatment remains controversial because of the large proportion of patients who recover spontaneously. Those who advocate steroids give 1 mg of prednisone per kilogram per day as soon as possible after onset and continue it for 1 to 2 weeks. Herpes simplex virus (type 1) has been suggested as the cause of Bell palsy. Treatment with acyclovir has been advocated, but the results are mixed. No evidence has been found that surgical intervention to treat typical patients with idiopathic facial nerve palsy is helpful.

Ramsay Hunt syndrome is peripheral facial nerve palsy with herpes zoster oticus. The herpes zoster represents activation of the varicella-zoster virus residing in the geniculate ganglion. Recovery is less certain than with idiopathic or Bell palsy. Treatment with acyclovir alone or in combination with corticosteroids may lead to a better outcome.

Melkersson-Rosenthal syndrome is characterized by recurrent facial paralysis, a fissured tongue, and unilateral, recurrent, nonpitting facial and lip edema. Only part of the triad may be present. This may be a spectrum of orofacial granulomatous disorders.

Facial palsies may be caused by various infectious and inflammatory diseases, including Lyme disease, sarcoidosis, tuberculosis, syphilis, HIV infection, infectious mononucleosis, rubella, mumps, Guillain-Barré syndrome, Behçet syndrome, and Wegener granulomatosis. Various neoplasms, in addition to carcinomatous meningitis, may produce facial palsies. Facial palsies are more common in metabolic disorders, such as diabetes mellitus, uremia, hypothyroidism, and porphyria.

Surgical techniques to reinnervate facial muscles are considered within the context of serious traumatic injury to the facial nerve, surgical resection causing discontinuity of the facial nerve, and the rare patient with a poor recovery 1 year after the onset of facial neuropathy. In traumatic injury, efforts are directed at reapproximating the nerve and stump. Nerve grafts are sometimes used. A hypoglossal-facial nerve or spinal accessory-facial nerve anastomosis can be created.

Hemifacial spasm is characterized by paroxysmal involuntary tonic and clonic contractions of the muscles innervated by the facial nerve on one side. Women are affected twice as often as men. The orbicularis oculi is usually the first muscle affected. The orbicularis oris is the other most commonly affected muscle, but all the facial muscles can be involved. The spasms may continue during sleep and are worsened by stress, chewing, speaking, light, and cold. The most frequent cause is microvascular compression of the facial nerve at its root exit zone, although many other causes have been cited. Carbamazepine or clonazepam may be helpful. Botulinum toxin injections can be tried. Decompressive surgery may be helpful.

Facial myokymia is characterized by continuous involuntary mild facial muscle contractions (usually unilateral). It is associated with many conditions.

Möbius syndrome is characterized by the sporadic occurrence of congenital sixth and seventh nerve palsies and associated skeletal deformities (syndactyly, brachydactyly, and oligodactyly). Brainstem nuclei are hypoplastic or absent.

The facial nerve can be imaged with CT and MRI. High-resolution CT provides excellent detail of the bones of the internal auditory canal, the facial canal, and adjacent vestibular and auditory structures. MRI with contrast visualizes the brainstem, proximal facial nerve, and facial nerve within the facial canal. These two modalities should be used to complement each other, not as exclusive studies.

Cranial Nerve VIII: Vestibulocochlear

The vestibulocochlear nerve carries two kinds of sensation, vestibular (balance) and auditory (hearing), from special sensory receptors in the inner ear. The central processes of these neurons form the eighth nerve, which travels through the internal auditory meatus in the company of the seventh nerve. This complex enters the medulla at its junction with the pons, just lateral to the seventh nerve.

The end organ of the vestibular system is the vestibular labyrinth, which is divided into two components—the semicircular canals and the otolith organs. In each ear, three semicircular canals are arranged at right angles to one another in the three planes of the body. The semicircular canals sense head rotation. The otolith organs (utricle and saccule) sense linear acceleration, including that caused by gravity. These structures are constantly active, firing at a basal rate even when the subject is stationary. During movement, the baseline firing increases. The structures are physiologically paired with those on the opposite side such that rotation or movement activating a semicircular canal on one side inhibits the paired semicircular canal on the other side. Head rotation and eye movements are related. The vestibulo-ocular reflex is an opposite response of the eyes to rotational movement of the head (i.e., when the head turns to the right, the eyes turn to the left). Both the saccule and the utricle contain a patch of sensory receptors (macula) that consist of ciliated hair cells covered by a gelatinous mass. Tiny crystals of calcium carbonate (otoliths) are embedded in the gel. When the head changes position relative to gravity or accelerates linearly, the otoliths stimulate the hair cells by bending the cilia in different directions.

The vestibular ganglion in the periphery collects this sensory information regarding motion. Central processes of the ganglion cells form the vestibular portion of the eighth nerve. These axons run with the cochlear portion and with the seventh cranial nerve through the internal auditory meatus to terminate in the vestibular nuclear complex in the floor of the fourth ventricle. Secondary neurons travel to the cerebellum and to lower motor neurons in the brainstem and spinal cord (to maintain balance). All nuclei in the vestibular complex contribute fibers to the medial longitudinal fasciculus. This complex arrangement allows the eyes to maintain fixation on an object while the head is moving.

Damage to or dysfunction of the vestibular apparatus results in dizziness, falling, and abnormal eye movements. Nausea and vomiting may accompany these symptoms because of connections between the vestibular and vagal nuclei. The clinical clues to localization are related to the onset of symptoms (acute or chronic), whether they are constant or intermittent, hearing changes, effects of position, contribution of motion, disorders of eye movement (including nystagmus), and findings within other cranial nerves. More information is provided in Chapter 104.

The cochlear component of eighth nerve function serves to convert sound waves (which distort and move structures within the external ear) to mechanical vibrations in the middle ear. Essentially, the sound waves cause the tympanic membrane to vibrate. The vibrations are transmitted via the round window to move three small ossicles (malleus, incus, and stapes). Vibrations of the stapes create waves in the fluid within the cochlea. The cochlea contains a complex array of organized structures that receive, sort, and convert these mechanical changes, which are converted into an electric signal that is transmitted along the acoustic portion of the eighth nerve. The cochlear nuclei at the junction of the pons and medulla receive the primary sensory neurons. The pathway to the auditory cortex is complex and not well understood.

Damage to the auditory apparatus (tympanic membrane, ossicles, cochlea) or nerve is commonly the result of skull fractures or infections. These cause a loss of hearing in the affected ear. Mass lesions within the internal auditory meatus (meningioma or acoustic neuroma) may damage components of the eighth nerve and also the accompanying seventh nerve.

BIBLIOGRAPHY

Albers JW, Bromberg MB. Bell's palsy. In: Johnson RT, ed. *Current therapy in neurologic disease*. New York: BC Decker, 1990.

Bromberg MB. Bell's palsy and idiopathic cranial neuritis. In: Feldmann E, ed. *Current diagnosis in neurology*. St. Louis: Mosby, 1994.

Donaldson JO. *Neurology of pregnancy*. Philadelphia: WB Saunders, 1989.

Goldstein PJ, Stern BJ. *Neurologic disorders of pregnancy*. Mt. Kisco, NY: Futura Publishing, 1992.

Morrow MJ. Bell's palsy and herpes zoster oticus. *Curr Treatment Options Neurol* 2000;2:407–416.

Optic Neuritis Study Group. The 5-year risk of MS after optic neuritis: experience of the Optic Neuritis Treatment Trial. *Neurology* 1997;49:1404–1413.

Rosenbaum RB, Donaldson JO, eds. Neurologic complications of pregnancy. *Neurol Clin North Am* 1994;12:461–478.

Stern BJ, Wityk RJ, Lewis RE. Disorders of the cranial nerves and brain stem. In: Joynt RJ, ed. *Clinical neurology*. Philadelphia: JB Lippincott, 1993.

Wilson-Pauwels L, Akesson EJ, Stewart PA. *Cranial nerves: anatomy and clinical comments*. New York: BC Decker, 1988.

CHAPTER 114

Polyneuropathies

Harold Lesser and Anne Moss

Unlike mononeuropathies, which affect individual nerves, polyneuropathies affect all the peripheral nerves in varying degrees. They produce a wide range of pathology and symptomatology and are often associated with underlying systemic disorders. The differential diagnosis of neuropathy is so extensive that it becomes both daunting and confusing. The history and physical examination can determine the relative involvement of sensory, motor, and autonomic function and the temporal course of the illness. Once classified in this manner, the differential diagnosis becomes more focused and can help guide further workup. The distinction between axonal and demyelinating neuropathies can be difficult to make without electrodiagnostic testing or nerve biopsy and thus is less helpful in directing the early investigation of a neuropathy.

ETIOLOGY AND DIFFERENTIAL DIAGNOSIS

Sensorimotor polyneuropathies are the most common; conditions affecting predominantly sensory, motor, or autonomic function occur less frequently. The differential diagnosis of the polyneuropathies is summarized in Table 114.1. For simplicity, many rare inherited disorders and less common drug toxicities have been omitted.

Sensorimotor Polyneuropathy

ACQUIRED SENSORIMOTOR POLYNEUROPATHY

Sensorimotor polyneuropathy is the most common pattern of polyneuropathy. Diabetes, alcohol abuse, and hypothyroidism account for a large percentage of cases, so that these neuropathies are frequently encountered in the primary care setting.

Diabetic Polyneuropathy.The neuropathy of diabetes is the prototype of the sensorimotor polyneuropathies. Symptomatic neuropathy develops in 15% to 20% of diabetic patients, and neuropathy can be detected in twice as many. Neuropathic symptoms often lead to a previously unsuspected diagnosis of diabetes. Like many other neuropathies, the neuropathy of diabetes is characterized by length-dependent axonal injury. The longest axons, those subserving sensation to the toes, are affected earliest; the shorter axons supplying the fingers are typically not affected until lower extremity symptoms reach the knees. As the neuropathy progresses, a glove-and-stocking pattern of sensory loss (i.e., distal and symmetric) emerges. The deep tendon reflexes are reduced or absent, and vibratory sensation and position sense are impaired. Motor signs appear somewhat later and are manifested by symmetric distal weakness (e.g., footdrop or, somewhat later, wrist drop). Loss of trophic (nutritional) support may produce chronic skin and nail changes. Profound sensory loss can lead patients to traumatize their extremities repeatedly, with the subsequent bony destruction of digits in the hand or foot (Charcot joints). Nerve conduction studies show low-amplitude sensory and motor compound action potentials, reflecting the axonal nature of the neuropathy. Conduction velocities may be mildly decreased secondary to demyelination accompanying the axonal loss.

Other Diabetes-associated Conditions. Diabetics are at increased risk for the development of compressive mononeuropathies at sites frequently subjected to compression (median nerve at the wrist, ulnar nerve at the elbow, peroneal nerve at the fibular head). Patients presenting with multiple mononeuropathies, such as bilateral carpal tunnel syndrome, or cranial mononeuropathies, such as Bell palsy, should undergo screening for diabetes.

Diabetic autonomic neuropathy can develop when a significant number of small fibers are injured. Its effects on blood pressure regulation, gastrointestinal and bladder function, thermoregulation, sexual function, and the ability to detect hypoglycemia can be disabling.

Diabetic amyotrophy presents with the sudden onset of severe pain in one or both lower extremities, followed days to weeks later by atrophy. The condition may be caused either by an ischemic injury to the femoral nerve or, more likely, by a proximal process within the lumbosacral plexus. The pain of diabetic amyotrophy is intense, and patients require narcotics acutely and tricyclic antidepressants for chronic discomfort. The time needed to recover motor function can be prolonged when severe atrophy develops. The association between amyotrophy and diabetes is strong enough to warrant a careful screen for diabetes in all patients with this clinical picture.

Diabetic neuropathic cachexia is a frightening complication of diabetes that is often associated with attempts to bring severe diabetes under better control. Patients experience months of profoundly decreased appetite, severe weight loss, and depression that cause most to undergo an unrevealing workup for occult malignancy. The pathophysiology of the disorder is unknown. The treatment is supportive, with antidepressants and analgesics. The end of the illness is often heralded by a return of appetite sufficient to permit weight gain. Many patients ultimately make a good recovery after a year or more of debilitating illness.

Alcoholic Polyneuropathy. Chronic alcohol abuse, even heavy social drinking, can lead to alcoholic polyneuropathy. A symmetric, axonal sensorimotor polyneuropathy affecting distal more than proximal fibers results. Most patients with an alcoholic neuropathy exhibit other physical, neuropsychological, and social stigmata of alcohol abuse. Direct ethanol toxicity and nutritional depletion (especially of thiamin, vitamin B_{12}, and folate), the result of substituting alcohol for normal caloric intake, have been implicated as potential causes of neuropathy. A clinically indistinguishable polyneuropathy can develop secondary to vitamin B_{12} and folate deficiencies in strict vegetarians and in AIDS patients with intestinal malabsorption.

Lancinating foot pain is often the first sign of an alcoholic polyneuropathy. With continued alcohol use, similar symptoms ultimately appear in the upper extremities. A gait disorder often develops later. The causes of gait difficulties in alcoholics are multiple and include impaired sensory inflow to the cerebellum secondary to neuropathy and direct ethanol toxicity to the cerebellum itself.

Other Acquired Sensorimotor Polyneuropathies. As shown in Table 114.1, numerous other conditions can cause acquired sensorimotor polyneuropathy. Specific inquiries should be made about exposure to the medications and chemotherapeutic agents listed, possible toxic exposures, unusual dietary practices, recreational drug use, and other active illnesses. Critical illness polyneuropathy and chronic inflammatory demyelinating polyradiculoneuropathy and related disorders are discussed later in this chapter.

INHERITED SENSORIMOTOR NEUROPATHY

Dozens of neuropathies are inherited, including sensorimotor, sensory, motor, and autonomic types. Almost all are rare and within the province of the neuromuscular specialist. Two fairly common sensorimotor neuropathies deserve mention because they are likely to be encountered frequently in the primary care setting.

Charcot-Marie-Tooth disease (hereditary motor-sensory neuropathy type I [HMSN I], peroneal muscular atrophy) is the most common inherited neuropathy. The course of this autosomal-dominant disorder, which begins in the first or second decade, is extremely indolent. The disease often goes unrecognized, even in families with many affected members. Pathologically, the neuropathy shows a predilection for the largest myelinated fibers, in which it causes repeated bouts of demyelination and remyelination that lead to a microscopic appearance reminiscent of onion bulbs and to palpable nerve hypertrophy. Patients usually present with motor complaints. On examination, they often have high-arched feet (pes cavus), hammertoes, and “stork legs” (peroneal muscle atrophy). The deep tendon reflexes are diminished or lost, vibratory sensation is reduced, and nerve hypertrophy may be appreciated. Footdrop may be present. Despite these abnormalities, many patients with HMSN I are minimally disabled. Nerve conduction studies reveal conduction velocities far below the lower limits of nor-

TABLE 114.1. Polyneuropathy

	Sensorimotor	Sensory or sensory > motor	Motor or motor > sensory	Autonomic
Common	Diabetes^{M}, alcohol, hypothyroidism^{M}, uremia^{M}	Diabetes^{M}, alcohol, uremia, hypothyroidism^{M}	AIDP^{D} Diabetic amyotrophy, ALS^{N}	Diabetes^{M}, amyloid, alcohol, renal and hepatic failure
AIDS-associated	HIV infection^{AD} Medications: ddI/ddC	Distal symmetric polyneuropathy of AIDS Medications: ddI/ddC, thalidomide	AIDP/CIDP^{D} Cytomegalovirus-associated polyradiculoneuropathy, distal symmetric polyneuropathy, motor neuron disease	
Chemotherapy	Chlorambucil, vincristine, suramin^{M}	Cisplatin, docetaxel, paclitaxel, vincristine		Paclitaxel, vincristine
Connective tissue disorders	Rheumatoid arthritis^{D} Periarteritis nodosa, systemic lupus erythematosus^{M}	Sjögren syndrome^{N}	Systemic lupus erythematosus^{M}	Rheumatoid arthritis^{D}
Endocrine	Acromegaly^{D} Diabetes^{M}, hypothyroidism^{M}	Diabetes^{M}, hypothyroidism^{M}	Diabetic amyotrophy	Diabetes^{M}
Idiopathic	Critical illness polyneuropathy	Dorsal root ganglionitis^{N}	ALS^{N}	Shy-Drager syndrome, primary idiopathic orthostatic hypotension
Immune	COP^{D} Amyloid, cryoglobulinemia, multiple myeloma, osteosclerotic myeloma^{M}, sarcoid, Waldenström macroglobulinemia	anti-MAG^{D} Amyloid, Crohn disease, cryoglobulinemia, hepatitis C, paraproteinemia, primary biliary cirrhosis, Sjögren syndrome	AIDP^{D}, MMN/CB with anti-GMT antibodies^{D} Axonal AIDP, brachial neuritis	AIDP^{D} Amyloid
Infectious	Diphtheria^{D} Lyme disease	AIDS, Lyme disease,leprosy^{M}, syphilis (tabes dorsalis)	Diphtheria^{D} AIDS, botulism, leprosy^{M}, polio^{N}, tick paralysis	AIDS, leprosy^{M}, botulism
Inherited	HMSN I^{D}, HMSN II, hereditary neuropathy with tendency to pressure palsy (HNPP)^{D} Myotonic dystrophy	Friedreich ataxia, amyloid, rare hereditary sensory neuropathies	Porphyria^{D} Hereditary ALS^{N}, Werdnig-Hoffman syndrome^{N}	Amyloid, porphyria
Medications (other than chemotherapy)	Amiodarone Chlorpropamide, colchicine, ddI, ddC, disulfiram, ergots, gold, indomethacin, isoniazid, lithium, metronidazole, phenytoin, tolbutamide, tricyclic antidepressants	ddI, ddC, isoniazid (slow acetylators), metronidazole, phenytoin, thalidomide, vitamin B_6 overdose^{N}	Dapsone, tricylic antidepressants	
Metals	Arsenic, gold^{M}, mercury, thallium	Arsenic, gold^{M}, thallium, methyl mercury	Gold^{M}, lead	Arsenic, inorganic mercury
Neuronopathy		anti-Hu^{N} (see paraneoplastic), dorsal root ganglionitis^{N}, Sjögren syndrome^{N}	See paraneoplastic	
Nutritional	Vitamin B_{12}, folate, thiamin deficiencies, gestational	Vitamin B_{12} deficiency, vitamin E deficiency		Vitamin B_{12} deficiency
Paraneoplastic	Mild distal neuropathy of cancer	anti-Hu (lung > breast > ovary > lymphoma)	Lymphoma, Hodgkin motor neuron disease	Adenocarcinoma, anti-Hu, Lambert-Eaton syndrome
Toxic	Ethylene oxide, nitrous oxide, hexacarbons (glue sniffing)	Ethylene oxide, nitrous oxide	Acrylamide, hexacarbons, organophosphate poisoning	Acrylamide

Note: Unless noted, all neuropathies are axonal. Exceptions are indicated by a superscript, as in demyelinating^{D}, mixed^{M}, neuronopathy^{N}, axonal^{A}.
AIDP, acute inflammatory demyelinating polyradiculoneuropathy; ALS, amyotrophic lateral sclerosis; anti-GMT, anti-GMT gangliosides; anti-Hu, also called anti-ANNwA (antineuronal nuclear antibody); CIDP, chronic inflammatory demyelinating polyradiculoneuropathy; ddC, 2′,3′-dideoxycytidine (zalcitabine); ddI, 2′,3′-dideoxyinosine (didanosine); HMSN I, hereditary motor sensory neuropathy type I (Charcot-Marie-Tooth disease); MAG, myelin-associated glycoprotein; MMN/CB, multifocal motor neuropathy with conduction block.

mal. The diagnosis can also be established by DNA testing, which is available both prenatally and postnatally.

A similar clinical picture can arise from the axonal form of Charcot-Marie-Tooth disease (HMSN II), although the underlying pathology and electrophysiology are dominated by axon loss. The inheritance is also typically autosomal-dominant. Symptoms begin somewhat later, in the second decade. Nerve enlargement is absent, and arm involvement is less common. Electrodiagnostic studies show essentially normal conduction velocities and evidence of axon loss.

Sensory-Predominant Polyneuropathies

The differential diagnosis of the sensory neuropathies differs from that of the more common sensorimotor polyneuropathies, although several conditions can lead to either. The presence of a purely sensory neuropathy is often unsuspected early in the course because in the more common sensorimotor polyneuropathies, sensory symptoms develop first. The diagnosis is often first suggested when electrodiagnostic tests reveal the near-absence of motor involvement. The most common sensory neuropathies are caused by diabetes, alcohol abuse, and uremia. Of the nearly two dozen other causes listed in Table 114.1, a few deserve special mention.

Nutritional deficiency states, especially vitamin B_{12} and folate deficiencies, cause a selective injury of sensory fibers. Vitamin B_{12} and folate deficiencies are most common in alcoholics and less common in strict vegetarians, as previously noted. A macrocytic anemia is anticipated. Spasticity and extensor plantar responses, which indicate upper motor neuron damage, coexist with lower motor findings, such as areflexia. Vitamin E deficiency, typically associated with fat malabsorption syndromes, can produce both a sensory neuropathy and spinocerebellar degeneration.

Several chemotherapeutic agents commonly used to treat malignancies of the reproductive organs—vincristine, cisplatin, paclitaxel, and docetaxel—produce fairly predictable dose-dependent sensory neuropathies. A progressive loss of deep tendon reflexes is followed by distally predominant sensory loss. Vincristine can also cause significant autonomic problems, including orthostatic hypotension, impotence, and abdominal pain. Doses of paclitaxel larger than 200 mg/m^2 are likely to result in an acute distal sensory-predominant neuropathy. With doses of cisplatin smaller than 500 mg/m^2, the neuropathy may be reversible.

Leprosy (Hansen disease) is the most common cause of peripheral neuropathy worldwide, although it is uncommon in the United States (except for a few southern states). In the lepromatous form, local bacterial invasion and sensory loss are seen in cooler areas of the body. The tuberculoid form causes hypopigmented skin lesions with reduced pain and temperature sensation. Isolated or multiple mononeuropathies may develop. Chronic joint injury, leading to autoamputation, is common. Dapsone, a drug commonly used to treat leprosy, can produce a motor-predominant neuropathy.

Sensory Neuropathies

The most disabling sensory neuropathies develop when the cell bodies, which reside in the dorsal root ganglia, are damaged. The term *neuronopathy* is used to indicate a process that damages the cell body or neuron as a whole, in contrast to a *neuropathy,* in which damage is limited to the axon. Sensory neuronopathies are caused by toxic agents. Selective and severe damage to the sensory fibers mediating joint position sense leads to profound functional disability with little weakness and few sensory complaints. The inability to detect either movement or static position of the limbs may lead to apparent weakness that often resolves if the patient is retested while the limb being evaluated is watched. Patients often cannot sit or stand unsupported.

When a sensory neuronopathy develops within days, the cause is probably idiopathic. Subacute and chronic sensory neuropathies are more likely to be secondary to carcinoma or Sjögren syndrome, although idiopathic cases also occur. Among the carcinomas, small cell lung tumors are the most frequent causes, followed by breast, esophagus, kidney, and liver cancers. A careful history can help exclude prior toxic exposures to heavy metals, drugs, or toxins.

FRIEDREICH ATAXIA

Friedreich ataxia is an autosomal-recessive disorder in which sensory abnormalities are prominent. Patients present in the preteen years with the gait difficulties of lower extremity ataxia. With time, the arms become involved, and dysarthria develops. High-arched feet (pes cavus) and scoliosis are common. As in patients with vitamin B_{12} deficiency, the curious combination of areflexia and bilateral Babinski signs is seen. Large fiber sensory loss results in a loss of vibratory sensation and position sense. Motor weakness often appears later in the illness. Cardiomyopathy is common, and diabetes mellitus develops in many cases. Pathologic findings are noted in the dorsal root ganglia and posterior columns, accounting for the prominent large fiber sensory loss. Abnormalities in the corticospinal tracts explain the spasticity and extensor plantar responses.

Motor-Predominant Polyneuropathies

Several polyneuropathies affect motor fibers nearly exclusively. Acute causes include acute inflammatory demyelinating polyradiculoneuropathy (Guillain-Barré syndrome) and critical illness polyneuropathy; chronic disorders include chronic inflammatory demyelinating polyradiculoneuropathy. The remaining illnesses listed in Table 114.1 are uncommon.

ACUTE INFLAMMATORY DEMYELINATING POLYRADICULONEUROPATHY

Acute inflammatory demyelinating polyradiculoneuropathy (AIDP) is treatable but dangerous. In two thirds of patients, the disorder is preceded by a viral respiratory illness, diarrhea, vaccination, or surgery. Distally predominant weakness develops over hours or days. At initial presentation, patients may have vague symptoms of distal paresthesias, back pain, and subtle weakness. In many cases, a viral syndrome, anxiety, or hysteria is diagnosed initially. Subtle bilateral facial weakness or signs consistent with autonomic instability (tachycardia, excessive sweating, orthostatic hypotension) are easily overlooked. The persistence of reflexes, which are classically absent or depressed, can falsely reassure the unwary physician early in the clinical course. Ultimately, the constellation of symptoms becomes clearer, so that the proper diagnosis is more likely.

AIDP typically progresses within days to a month at most. Symptoms often stabilize during a plateau phase of 1 or 2 weeks; stabilization is followed by recovery over many months. The vast majority of patients with acute inflammatory demyelinating polyradiculoneuropathy make a substantial and often complete recovery, but up to 20% have residual motor deficits at 1 year. Progressive weakness for more than a month or exacerbations and remissions should suggest an alternate diagnosis.

As many as 10% to 20% of patients with AIDP require mechanical ventilation during the early phase of the illness. Failure to recognize impending respiratory distress can be a fatal mistake. When a physician is called about a patient with possible AIDP, the first question should be, "Can she cough?" Patients who can cough have a vital capacity well over 1 L, so that immediate respiratory failure is unlikely. If the cough is weak or absent, the patient should be transferred to an intensive care unit, regardless of how well she appears otherwise. Blood gas measurements are often falsely reassuring; elective intubation should be performed in patients who show signs of respiratory fatigue, including but not limited to a forced vital capacity below 12 to 15 mL/kg and a negative inspiratory force below –30 mm H_2O. When respiratory failure is properly managed, the mortality of AIDP drops to 2% to 4%, with most deaths caused by cardiac arrhythmias or hospital-acquired infections.

A particularly severe form of AIDP often follows a bout of bloody diarrhea secondary to infection with *Campylobacter jejuni*. Whereas the primary pathology is demyelinating in typical AIDP, axonal injury predominates in this form. The illness is often explosive, and profound weakness develops within hours to a day. Early electrodiagnostic testing reveals absent responses from both motor and sensory fibers. The prognosis for recovery is guarded because axonal regeneration is often incomplete.

CHRONIC INFLAMMATORY DEMYELINATING POLYRADICULONEUROPATHY

Chronic inflammatory demyelinating polyradiculoneuropathy (CIDP) is a cousin of AIDP. Many of the clinical features are the same, but the management is much different. CIDP presents as a progressive, symmetric sensorimotor polyneuropathy. Unlike AIDP, CIDP progresses over months to years, and exacerbations and remissions are common. CIDP accounts for nearly 20% of cases of chronic neuropathy. It often presages the development of another disorder; a paraproteinemia, lymphoma, granulomatous disease, an autoimmune disease (e.g., lupus, rheumatoid arthritis, Sjögren syndrome), or HIV infection develops later in up to a third of patients. Plasma cell dyscrasias from multiple myeloma are especially common. A few patients demonstrate antibodies directed against myelin (anti–myelin-associated glycoprotein [anti-MAG]).

Symptoms are often more prominent in the legs, and sensory symptoms are often more prominent than in AIDP. Tremor and nerve hypertrophy are fairly common in CIDP but not in AIDP. As in AIDP, a cell-albumin dissociation is noted in the cerebrospinal fluid (CSF). Electrodiagnostic criteria have been established for CIDP, although in some cases, nerve biopsy may be required to establish the diagnosis. Onion bulb pathology, the residua of bouts of demyelination and remyelination, strongly supports the diagnosis.

MULTIFOCAL MOTOR NEUROPATHY WITH CONDUCTION BLOCK

Multifocal motor neuropathy with conduction block is a treatable disorder. The presentation can mimic that of amyotrophic lateral sclerosis. Patients present with asymmetric, progressive weakness that is often worse in the arms. Anti-GM1 antibodies are present in the serum in most patients. Electrodiagnostic studies play a crucial role, demonstrating evidence of conduction block in affected limbs. Treatment with intravenous immunoglobulin or immunosuppression with cyclophosphamide is effective.

CRITICAL ILLNESS POLYNEUROPATHY

Critical illness polyneuropathy often develops in the setting of sepsis but has also been associated with the concomitant use of neuromuscular blocking agents and high-dose steroids. A generalized neuropathy ensues that causes diffuse weakness and diaphragmatic weakness or paralysis. This diagnosis should be considered in the acutely ill patient with unexplained ventilatory dependence or weakness. AIDP can also develop in this setting and must be considered.

Autonomic Neuropathies

Autonomic involvement is characteristic of a few neuropathies, in many of which sensorimotor fibers are affected concurrently. The most common associated conditions are diabetes, alcoholism, and amyloidosis. Autonomic instability is frequently observed in patients with AIDP; in some cases, bouts of severe hypotension and hypertension alternate within minutes. Autonomic instability and associated cardiac rhythm disturbances account for a large percentage of deaths in patients with AIDP. Severe autonomic involvement is also seen in Shy-Drager syndrome, a parkinsonian syndrome characterized by rigidity, gait disturbances, impotence, and relative unresponsiveness to L-dopa.

MONONEURITIS MULTIPLEX

The term *mononeuritis multiplex* is applied to a condition in which multiple peripheral nerves are injured in a haphazard pattern. At onset, it often appears to be a simple mononeuropathy, but as additional nerves are affected, it becomes evident that the process is multifocal. The inability to classify the neuropathy under one of the common schemas (i.e., distal, axonal, sensorimotor) should suggest this diagnosis. Mononeuritis multiplex follows no simple rules. In some cases, the distal nerve fibers are injured preferentially. Multiple nerve injuries may cause confluent sensory loss that replicates the glove-and-stocking pattern of distal symmetric polyneuropathies. Clues to the correct diagnosis are often obtained from a careful history revealing either abrupt, stepwise changes in sensorimotor function or events in the distant past that the patient thought insignificant (e.g., old carpal tunnel syndrome). A detailed physical or electrodiagnostic examination may uncover evidence of unsuspected neuropathies.

The conditions most frequently causing mononeuritis multiplex are diabetes, rheumatoid arthritis, sarcoid, polyarteritis nodosa, HIV infection, hepatitis, and leprosy. Although routine laboratory studies (fasting blood glucose and serum angiotensin-converting enzyme levels, rheumatoid factor and HIV titers) may be useful, a definitive diagnosis often requires nerve biopsy.

HISTORY

Sensory symptoms are usually the first to appear in sensorimotor polyneuropathy. Patients experience paresthesias or burning discomfort or state that they feel as if they are "walking on cardboard" or "wearing too many socks." They rarely report sensory loss itself. Gait instability, particularly in the dark, can be caused by the loss of joint position sense that accompanies the loss of large sensory axons. Distal hand numbness may cause clumsiness, or patients may have trouble identifying objects deep in their pockets. Injuries to the feet, such as blisters, puncture wounds, and infections, may go unnoticed. The motor component of neuropathy leads to distally predominant weakness and only much later to atrophy. Footdrop or toe-drop develops first. Patients may report catching their toes on the edge of carpeting, scuffing the tops of their shoes, or slapping their feet as they walk. Autonomic symptoms, such as feeling faint on standing, nausea, vomiting, diarrhea, and impotence, are often prominent but may be mistakenly attributed to non-neuropathic causes.

The clinical course of the neuropathies varies from acute (hours or days) to very indolent (decades). The symptoms of ischemic neuropathies begin abruptly. The course of chronic demyelinating neuropathies, both acquired and inherited, is slow and relentless.

PHYSICAL EXAMINATION AND CLINICAL FINDINGS

Early in the course of a neuropathy, symptoms may be unaccompanied by signs of nerve dysfunction on the examination. Later in the illness, the physical examination is more revealing. The goal of a peripheral nervous system examination is to describe the findings concisely—for example, "a distal, symmetric sensory greater than motor polyneuropathy with evidence of axonal features." While taking the history and examining the patient, the physician should consider several questions: When did the symptoms begin? What is the clinical course of the process (e.g., acute, subacute, chronic, relapsing, progressive)? Where did the symptoms start? Are they symmetric? Is a glove-and-stocking pattern of abnormalities apparent (suggestive of a distal-to-proximal dying-back neuropathy), or does the sensory loss suggest a radicular (dermatomal) pattern or the pattern of an individual mononeuropathy? Are small or large nerve fibers preferentially affected? Sometimes, these questions can be answered by a careful history; in other cases, even a detailed physical examination leaves many questions unanswered. An electrodiagnostic evaluation often helps to clarify the nature and degree of pathology, but sometimes only nerve biopsy can reveal the specific diagnosis.

The sensory examination is particularly helpful in assessing patients with polyneuropathy because distal sensory signs occur so early in the clinical course. When large sensory fibers are involved, a progressive loss of distal vibratory sensation and a decrease in joint position sense (the ability to detect passive movement of a joint or its position in space) are noted, and the deep tendon reflexes are diminished. Small sensory fibers, which mediate pain and temperature sensation, are spared in some neuropathies and preferentially involved in others. Diseases affecting the small fibers, such as amyloidosis, may also cause significant autonomic dysfunction, evidenced by decreased sweating and orthostatic hypotension.

The motor examination assesses large motor axon function. Muscle weakness and atrophy develop only after fairly significant axonal loss; thus, the physical examination often misses signs of early motor neuropathy. Needle electromyography, however, is exquisitely sensitive to axonal loss; the loss of just 3% of motor axons within a nerve increases membrane instability in muscle, detectable as p-waves and fibrillations (denervation). Denervation can be noted when strength, bulk, and reflexes are all normal.

LABORATORY EVALUATION

Polyneuropathy is not a diagnosis unto itself. The physician must establish a probable cause of the polyneuropathy, excluding the treatable (predominantly demyelinating) neuropathies and reducing or eliminating ongoing risks to the peripheral nervous system (e.g., medications, alcohol, toxins). The laboratory evaluation should begin by focusing on the most common conditions associated with each subtype of polyneuropathy. If screening laboratory studies for the relevant conditions fail to establish a diagnosis, the patient should be referred to a neuromuscular specialist for further evaluation. The cost of screening neuropathy panels, touted by some laboratories as a one-size-fits-all workup, far exceeds that of a neurologic consultation; furthermore, these panels are often unrevealing. Unfortunately, even exhaustive workups at major referral centers fail to identify the cause of a neuropathy in up to 30% of patients.

Nerve conduction studies are crucial in some patients; they help to classify the neuropathy and serve as a possible prelude to nerve biopsy. Biopsy specimens of clinically and electrically normal nerves are rarely abnormal. When severely affected nerves are sampled, end-stage pathologic changes may obscure the primary pathologic process. Nerve conduction studies can help determine whether a biopsy should be performed and which nerve should be selected.

In patients with a sensorimotor polyneuropathy, screening laboratory tests should include the following: random glucose study; determination of the hemoglobin A_{1c} level; thyroid function tests; measurement of the blood levels of blood urea nitrogen, creatinine, vitamin B_{12}, and folate; serum and urine protein electrophoresis; and serum immunofixation. If the history suggests heavy metal exposure, a 24-hour urine sample should be obtained.

In patients with sensory neuronopathy, laboratory studies should include measurement of the vitamin B_{12} level, determination of the vitamin E level in patients at risk for fat malabsorption, serum and urine protein electrophoresis, and immunofixation. A chest roentgenogram should be obtained for all patients, and an anti-Hu antibody titer for those at risk for lung malignancy by history or chest roentgenography. CSF should be obtained and examined for abnormal cytology or the anti-Hu antibody (although the latter can often be detected in serum). An AIDS test should be considered for patients with risk factors or an unrevealing laboratory workup. Laboratory screening for Sjögren syndrome should include anti-Ro (SS-A) and anti-La (SS-B) tests. An ophthalmologic evaluation, including a Schirmer test for tear production and rose bengal staining of the cornea, can establish the diagnosis. The gold standard for diagnosing Sjögren syndrome is a minor salivary gland biopsy.

Laboratory tests play a central role in diagnosing the acquired demyelinating polyneuropathies. In AIDP, the most useful confirmatory tests are CSF analysis and electrodiagnostic tests. Additional tests should be performed to exclude the most common AIDP look-alikes and search for possible causes. The CSF should be examined for the characteristic cell-albumin dissociation (protein elevation without elevation of white cells). The CSF may remain normal during the early days of the illness, and the CSF protein never rises in up to 10% of patients. A significant CSF leukocytosis should raise concern about the polyradiculopathies associated with carcinoma, AIDS, Lyme disease, or cytomegalovirus infection. Nerve conduction studies can demonstrate evidence of distal conduction block or temporal dispersion secondary to early demyelinating changes. Electromyography can detect denervation secondary to motor axon injury after 1 to 2 weeks. Ancillary testing should probably include an HIV test, a porphyria screen, *C. jejuni* titers, a hepatitis screen, and a mononucleosis spot. If clinically indicated, a urinary heavy metal screen should be performed or diphtheria titers measured.

In CIDP, the CSF should be evaluated as in AIDP. It is critical to look for evidence of plasma cell dyscrasia. Screening tests should include a serum and urine protein electrophoresis and immunofixation. A bone marrow analysis may be necessary to exclude an underlying hematologic malignancy. A skeletal survey should be performed to look for evidence of lytic lesions, which suggest multiple myeloma. Lifelong surveillance for myeloma is required. Worsening CIDP or the appearance of a new protein spike on serum protein electrophoresis warrants a repeated skeletal survey. Radiation or resection of a new lytic lesion relieves the neuropathy in some patients. AIDP and CIDP are more common in HIV-positive patients and can be the initial manifestation of HIV infection.

TREATMENT

No specific therapy is available for many of the polyneuropathies, although some interventions may be of benefit. When the neuropathy accompanies a systemic disorder, such as diabetes or hypothyroidism, treatment of the underlying condition may slow the progress of the neuropathy. Uremic patients may do especially well as their condition improves. The toxic effects of drugs, alcohol, heavy metals, or industrial solvents must be considered (Table 114.1) and all potential offending agents eliminated.

A few polyneuropathies require specific interventions. Diabetic neuropathy requires preventive and, when necessary, symptomatic treatment. Prevention consists of redoubling efforts to control blood sugar levels. The Diabetic Control and Complications Trial, completed in 1994, demonstrated that long-term tight control of blood sugar levels slows the progression of diabetic neuropathy in insulin-dependent patients. Symptomatic treatments can help reduce the chronic burning dysesthesias that bother many patients. Low nocturnal doses of a tricyclic antidepressant (e.g., 10–50 mg of amitriptyline orally at bedtime) are often helpful; carbamazepine and phenytoin are also effective. Some patients benefit from the local application of capsaicin cream (derived from pepper plants), although a 30-day trial of application four times daily may be necessary to establish efficacy.

Effective treatments are available for the acquired demyelinating polyneuropathies (AIDP and CIDP). Therapy for AIDP consists of total plasma exchange or infusions of intravenous immunoglobulin. Steroids, once the standard of care, are ineffective. Plasma exchange is most effective when begun during the first 2 weeks of the illness, but treatment during the first month is probably warranted if the patient is sufficiently weak. Typically, five or six plasma exchanges are performed on an alternate-day schedule. If the final exchange is completed during the second or third week of the illness, the patient may require one or two weekly "clean-up" exchanges to prevent relapse during the first month of the illness. Intravenous immunoglobulin is an equally effective treatment for AIDP. The standard dose is 0.4 g/kg daily for 5 days. Intravenous immunoglobulin is particularly useful in children and in patients with limited intravenous access or vascular instability.

Although steroids have no therapeutic role in AIDP, they are useful in CIDP. Many patients require long-term immunosuppression with steroids or steroid-sparing agents such as mycophenolate mofetil (CellCept) or azathioprine (Imuran), although some can be managed with intermittent plasma exchange or intravenous immunoglobulin. Patients with CIDP and gammopathy require lifelong screening for worsening gammopathy or lytic bony lesions. The detection and treatment of a previously occult malignancy can mitigate the neuropathy.

CONSIDERATIONS DURING PREGNANCY

Few of the polyneuropathies are specifically exacerbated in pregnancy; the two exceptions are the inflammatory demyelinating polyneuropathies (AIDP and CIDP). AIDP appears to be no more common during pregnancy than at other times. The primary treatment modalities, plasma exchanges and intravenous immunoglobulin therapy, can both be used safely during pregnancy. CIDP may present or relapse at a higher rate during pregnancy. Normally, CIDP is treated with prednisone, but this should be avoided during pregnancy if possible; plasma exchange is a safe alternative. Long-term immunosuppressive therapy is commonly used in CIDP. Women of childbearing age must be counseled about the considerable teratogenicity of these therapies, and a highly effective form of birth control should be used.

A gestational distally predominant sensorimotor polyneuropathy can develop in women with significant nutritional deficiency, but this is uncommon in developed countries. In rare families predisposed to brachial plexopathy or mononeuritis multiplex, pregnancy may provoke a new attack.

BIBLIOGRAPHY

Aminoff MJ, ed. *Neurology and general medicine.* London: Churchill Livingstone, 1995.

Asbury AK, Thomas PK, eds. *Peripheral nerve disorders: blue books of practical neurology.* Oxford: Butterworth-Heinemann, 1995.

Boonyapisit K, Katirji B. Severe exacerbation of hepatitis C-associated vasculitic neuropathy following treatment with interferon alpha: a case report and literature review. *Muscle Nerve* 2002;25:909.

Bosch EP, Mitsumoto H. Disorders of peripheral nerves. In: Bradley WG, Daroff RB, Fenichel GM, et al., eds. *Neurology in clinical practice,* 2nd ed. Oxford: Butterworth-Heinemann, 1996:1881.

Chaudhry V, Cornblath DR, Griffin JW, et al. Mycophenolate mofetil: a safe and promising immunosuppressant in neuromuscular diseases. *Neurology* 2001; 56:94.

Cohen BS, Felsenthal G. Peripheral nervous system disorders and pregnancy. In: Goldstein PJ, ed. *Neurological disorders of pregnancy.* Mt. Kisco, NY: Futura Publishing, 1992.

Donaldson JO. Neurology of pregnancy. In: Walton J, ed. *Major problems in neurology,* 2nd ed. Philadelphia: WB Saunders, 1989.

Dyck PJ, Thomas PK, Griffin JW, et al. *Peripheral neuropathy.* Philadelphia: WB Saunders, 1993.

Lindenbaum Y, Kissel JT, Mendell JR. Treatment approaches for Guillain-Barré syndrome and chronic inflammatory demyelinating polyradiculoneuropathy. *Neurol Clin* 2001;187–199.

Mowzoon N, Sussman A, Bradley WG. Mycophenolate (CellCept) treatment of myasthenia gravis, chronic inflammatory polyneuropathy and inclusion body myositis. *J Neurol Sci* 2001;185:119–122.

CHAPTER 115
Myasthenia Gravis

Harold Lesser and Anne Moss

Myasthenia gravis (MG) is the most common disorder of neuromuscular junction transmission and probably the best-understood autoimmune disease. Patients with MG experience fatigable weakness that may be restricted to the ocular muscles (ocular MG) or oculopharyngeal muscles (bulbar MG). In generalized MG, the skeletal and respiratory muscles are affected. MG was recognized more than 300 years ago, but effective treatments were not discovered until the early 1900s. As recently as the late 1950s, MG was a disabling disorder with a 30% mortality rate. Today, MG is manageable, most patients lead full lives, and fatalities are unusual. The disorder is sporadic, with an annual incidence of 2 to 5 per million and a prevalence of 5 to 12 per 100,000. There are 35,000 cases in the United States. MG tends to develop in women in their 20s and 30s, and in men in their 60s and 70s.

ETIOLOGY AND DIFFERENTIAL DIAGNOSIS

Weakness, the primary symptom of MG, results from disturbed transmission across the synapse that bridges the motor axon and muscle membrane. Neurotransmission is mediated by acetylcholine (ACh), which is released from synaptic vesicles in the axon terminal and crosses the synaptic cleft, where it binds to acetylcholine receptors (AChRs) embedded in the muscle endplate. ACh binding leads to the production of an action potential in the postsynaptic muscle membrane. Autoantibodies to the AChR reduce the number of available receptors, thereby decreasing the ability of ACh to generate an action potential. At rest or with minimal effort, the physiologic reserve is sufficient to make the generation of an action potential likely; with exertion, the probability of successful neurotransmission is reduced, and weakness results. In addition to decreasing the number of available postsynaptic receptors, autoantibody binding and complement activation result in a structural simplification of the muscle membrane and a shortened life of the AChR, both of which impair neuromuscular transmission.

The autoimmune basis of MG is well established. The passive transfer of patient sera to experimental animals produces disease, immunoglobulin G autoantibodies to the AChR have been isolated from sera, and the AChR and its autoantibodies have been characterized at the molecular level. The autoimmune nature of the disease is further supported by the increased risk for autoimmune disorders such as lupus, rheumatoid arthritis, and thyroiditis in patients and their first-degree relatives. As in most autoimmune diseases, the primary trigger for the disorder is not well understood; however, evidence suggests a pathophysiologic link to the thymus.

The differential diagnosis of MG is limited in patients who present with marked, clear diurnal variation. The differential is broader in patients with symptoms limited to the ocular or oculopharyngeal muscles, particularly when some degree of fixed weakness is present. Disorders to consider include thyroid eye disease, intracranial mass lesions in the region of the superior orbital fissure, multiple sclerosis, brainstem masses, multiple cranial mononeuropathies, and myopathy (oculopharyngeal dystrophy, progressive external ophthalmoplegia). In cases without definite laboratory evidence of MG, a brain imaging study may be necessary to exclude other conditions.

Weakness that involves both the bulbar and limb musculature suggests several other disorders, including amyotrophic lateral sclerosis, polio, botulism, and some myopathies. Patients with amyotrophic lateral sclerosis usually exhibit both upper motor neuron signs (spasticity, diffuse hyperreflexia, extensor plantar responses) and lower motor neuron signs (weakness, fasciculations, atrophy). In polio and botulism, the clinical course is fairly acute, and pupillary abnormalities are typical in botulism. Proximal muscle weakness is common in many myopathies, including polymyositis. Except for a few rare metabolic myopathies, the characteristic pattern of myopathy is fixed rather than variable weakness. Many myopathies are associated with an elevated level of creatine kinase, particularly in the acute phase. The creatine kinase level is not elevated in MG.

The Lambert-Eaton myasthenic syndrome (LEMS) is another disorder of neuromuscular transmission that is occasionally confused with MG. The unfortunate choice of the term *myasthenic syndrome* to refer to Lambert-Eaton syndrome makes confusion with *myasthenia* all too easy. Fortunately, the differential diagnosis is usually straightforward.

LEMS is rare in comparison with MG. An underlying malignancy is found in 50% to 60% of patients with LEMS. Like patients with MG, those with Lambert-Eaton syndrome experience variable weakness; however, their strength may improve with repeated effort. They often report dryness of the mouth and are frequently areflexic. The antibodies that cause Lambert-Eaton syndrome attack the voltage-gated calcium channels of the presynaptic axon terminal, thereby reducing ACh release. Positivity for voltage-gated calcium channel antibodies is noted in 85% to 90% of patients with LEMS.

Drug-induced MG can occur in patients who receive D-penicillamine for rheumatoid arthritis. These patients have otherwise typical MG, with positivity for antibodies and abnormal results of repetitive stimulation studies. The myasthenic symptoms typically disappear after the medication is discontinued.

HISTORY

The symptoms of MG develop insidiously. Patients with ocular MG may notice blurring of vision after prolonged reading or driving. Ptosis can also develop in this setting. Questions about new ptosis or facial weakness can often be settled by reviewing old photographs; a driver's license photo is often readily available. Patients with bulbar MG may report nasal speech, decreased speech volume, nasal regurgitation of fluids, and difficulty swallowing. Weakness of the facial muscles can make it difficult to drink from a straw. When a "myasthenic snarl" replaces a normal smile, family and friends often mistakenly believe the patient to be depressed or angry. In generalized MG, patients may have difficulty performing activities of daily living. They often subconsciously adjust their activities to accommodate their symptoms. The ability to perform activities of daily living requiring good proximal muscle strength should be assessed (e.g., washing one's hair, lifting heavy objects out of cupboards, climbing stairs, getting in and out of a car, arising from a low couch or a squatting position). A good history may reveal a significant decrease in strength either as the day goes on (i.e., diurnal variation) or following exertion.

PHYSICAL EXAMINATION AND CLINICAL FINDINGS

The physical examination should be directed at demonstrating either fatigable or fixed weakness. Fatigable weakness of the extraocular or limb muscles is the hallmark of MG. Ptosis or diplopia may be elicited by having the patient stare at the ceiling for 1 or 2 minutes. The palpebral fissures should be measured both before and after testing. The pattern of diplopia may be confusing because multiple muscles in both eyes are often affected. Limb weakness can be provoked by repetitive exertion of specific muscle groups. The patient is asked to exert a maximal effort five to 10 times against the examiner's resistance. Patients with significant MG may demonstrate decreasing strength with repeated efforts. After a few minutes of rest, strength returns to normal. Tests of upper extremity fatigability are usually performed on the deltoid; lower extremity strength can be evaluated by having the patient repeatedly stand from a squat.

Fixed weakness often develops in the neck extensors and facial muscles. In a normal person, the examiner should not be able to overcome forcefully closed eyes or lips or a forcefully extended neck. When profound weakness of the neck extensors develops, the patient's chin may be on her chest, or the patient may resort to propping her head up with her hands. This symptom is also seen in polymyositis and amyotrophic lateral sclerosis. MG is not associated with sensory deficits or reflex abnormalities. Strength in the distal muscles is typically well preserved.

LABORATORY EVALUATION

The laboratory evaluation of MG is important to confirm the diagnosis and aid treatment decisions. The major categories of testing are serology, electrodiagnostic studies, supplementary laboratory evaluation, and imaging studies.

Antibody testing should be performed whenever the diagnosis of MG is seriously considered. AChR antibodies are present in 85% of patients with generalized MG and 50% of those with ocular or bulbar MG. The absolute titer of AChR antibodies does not predict the severity of disease between patients, but a rising titer in an individual patient may indicate the progression of disease. Seronegative patients are clinically indistinguishable from those who are seropositive, and they respond to similar treatments. False-positive antibody test results are rare. False-negative results are occasionally obtained during the first year of disease, so repeating the AChR antibody test 1 year after an initially negative workup may be revealing.

Electrodiagnostic testing is helpful in evaluating MG. Repetitive motor conduction studies can demonstrate fatigue at the neuromuscular junction. At a normal neuromuscular junction, repetitive nerve stimulation at a low rate (2–5/s) evokes motor responses of equal amplitude. In MG, neuromuscular fatigue causes the amplitude of the responses to decline. The effect is most pronounced in proximal muscles (e.g., trapezius, facial muscles) and is absent in some patients. In contrast, in patients with Lambert-Eaton syndrome, the amplitude of the motor responses is low at rest and markedly increases after exercise or repetitive stimulation at a high rate (50/s).

In patients with a normal repetitive stimulation test result, single-fiber electromyography may be helpful. This test detects abnormally increased variability ("jitter") in the timing of activation of adjacent muscle fibers. The degree of jitter correlates well with the severity of the neuromuscular transmission defect. Abnormalities are often seen even in clinically normal muscles. Single-fiber electromyography has a sensitivity well above 95%, and the result of this test may be the only one that is abnormal in some patients with MG.

Supplementary laboratory testing is critical to rule out underlying conditions that can be confused with MG or complicate its management. Given the association of MG with autoimmune disorders, it is rational to order thyroid function tests, an antinuclear antibody (ANA) test, and a rheumatoid factor assay. If the diagnosis is in question, it is reasonable to obtain thyroid function tests, a creatine kinase measurement, and a determination of the vitamin B and folate levels. If the diagnosis is established, baseline laboratory studies may be appropriate before steroid treatment or immunosuppression is undertaken. Tuberculosis should be excluded in any patient in whom chronic immunosuppression is anticipated. In patients with newly diagnosed MG, computed tomography (CT) of the chest should be performed to look for an enlarged thymus in the mediastinum; chest roentgenography detects only the largest of masses and is therefore an inadequate screening test.

Malignant thymoma should be suspected in all patients with newly diagnosed MG. Chest roentgenography detects only the largest of thymomas; therefore, CT of the chest should be performed instead. If the result of an antistriated muscle antibody titer is positive, malignant thymoma is highly probable. Patients with suspected thymoma require more aggressive therapy (see section "Treatment").

In some centers, the edrophonium (Tensilon) test is routinely performed to evaluate patients with possible MG; however, since the advent of modern electrodiagnostic and serologic techniques, the use of this test has decreased. A definite abnormality must be noted on the examination, such as objective ptosis or diplopia, dysphonia, or weakness. The test should be performed by experienced practitioners in a facility where atropine and resuscitation equipment are available because anticholinergic agents can precipitate profound bradycardia or respiratory arrest. A positive test result is an improvement in muscle strength for up to 5 minutes after the injection. Some physicians perform the test in a blinded fashion to avoid observer bias. False-positive results are possible if the patient has another disease that causes weakness.

TREATMENT

MG should be managed by a specialist. All the treatments have serious potential side effects, and mismanagement can lead to unnecessary morbidity and mortality. The treatment comprises both symptomatic and immunosuppressive arms.

Symptomatic treatment is accomplished with anticholinesterase agents such as pyridostigmine (Mestinon). By inhibiting the action of acetylcholinesterase, pyridostigmine increases the availability of ACh in the neuromuscular junction, thereby facilitating neuromuscular transmission. Side effects of pyridostigmine include cramps, nausea, vomiting, and diarrhea. Excessive doses may lead to a cholinergic crisis, severe weakness that is clinically indistinguishable from MG itself. In addition to the oral form of pyridostigmine, parenteral and sustained-release (Mestinon Timespan) formulations are available.

Immunosuppressive treatments help, in part, by reducing the production of AChR antibodies. Prednisone and prednisone-sparing agents, in addition to immunomodulating therapies such as plasma exchange and immunoglobulin infusions, are used. Prednisone is the mainstay of therapy for many patients. This drug should be initiated on an inpatient basis because nearly half of patients experience an increase in weakness during the first week of treatment, and respiratory failure may develop rarely during this time. Initial doses of 60 to 100 mg of prednisone per day are often required to bring symptoms under control, but ultimately many patients can be managed on alternate-day therapy in doses as low as 2.5 to 5 mg.

Some patients fail to respond to prednisone or require such large doses that long-term side effects are inevitable. Prednisone-sparing agents are particularly helpful in such cases. Azathioprine (Imuran) is commonly used. Because it may take up to 6 months to work, it is often started concurrently with oral steroids. An intolerable flulike syndrome affects at least 10% of patients treated with azathioprine, and they must discontinue the drug. In others, severe neutropenia develops. Patients of childbearing age must be cautioned about the significant risk of this and other immunosuppressive agents to the fetus and should be offered highly effective contraceptives.

Mycophenolate mofetil (CellCept) has been shown to be effective in the treatment of immune-medicated neuromuscular diseases. Benefit is experienced with this agent sooner than with azathioprine, and in some cases of MG, mycophenolate mofetil precludes the need for steroids.

Cyclosporine is an alternate immunosuppressant that is effective in MG. Its primary side effects are nephrotoxicity and hypertension. It acts sooner than azathioprine, within 1 to 2 months after treatment is initiated.

Plasma exchange is a highly effective, rapidly acting immunotherapy for MG. It is particularly useful in acute crises. A series of four to six exchanges every other day removes circulating autoantibodies and improves neuromuscular transmission. Plasma exchange may also exert modulatory effects on antibody production by mechanisms that are not well understood. Intravenous immunoglobulin is effective in MG and may be suitable for children and patients with difficult vascular access.

Thymectomy may be the most powerful immunomodulating therapy. A controlled trial of thymectomy in MG is under way. Unlike any of the treatments previously mentioned, it can increase the remission rate up to 40%. The value of thymectomy was recognized in the 1930s, when malignant thymomas were first resected. Although patients with thymoma had more severe MG, a surprising number went into remission postoperatively. The observation that the remission rate improved even among patients whose preoperative "thymoma" was pathologically benign led to trials of thymectomy in patients without thymoma. Surgery is nonelective in patients with a thymoma, and radiation therapy is usually administered postoperatively. In patients without a thymoma, series have demonstrated increased remission rates during the 3 to 5 years after surgery. Surgery benefits even very young children, but the benefit is uncertain in patients older than 60 years. Before surgery, symptomatic patients should undergo a course of plasma exchange to maximize their ventilatory capacity and strength. Transsternal thymectomy should be performed because it better exposes the mediastinum and permits more complete resection of both the thymus and scattered ectopic rests of thymic tissue.

When the symptoms of MG worsen, several possibilities must be considered. Noncompliance with medication is always a possibility, but in its absence, an underlying infection is the most likely culprit. Severe respiratory compromise can develop in the setting of a "simple" urinary tract infection or pneumonia—the myasthenic crisis. An increased body temperature accelerates the rate at which acetylcholinesterase degrades ACh, thereby compromising neuromuscular transmission. Patients experiencing frank dysphagia or coughing after eating or drinking are at high risk for aspiration and respiratory failure and require close attention, often in an intensive care setting. A vital capacity below 15 mL/kg or a negative inspiratory force below –20 cm H_2O is an indication for intubation, even if the blood gas measurements are normal. A brief course of plasma exchange is often the best way to improve function at the neuromuscular junction rapidly in this setting.

Cholinergic crisis, a result of the excessive use of pyridostigmine, can also cause progressive weakness. Patients often have signs of cholinergic excess. Salivation can be misleading because it can just as easily reflect difficulty in handling secretions as a consequence of bulbar weakness. Profound bradycardia and diarrhea may be more helpful signs. Management involves the discontinuation of medications, respiratory support, and the slow reintroduction of low doses of anticholinesterases at a later time.

Concurrent medications are a potential concern because several different drugs can compromise the function of the neuromuscular junction. However, few, if any, are absolutely contraindicated. The aminoglycoside antibiotics such as gentamicin are commonly cited as a potential risk, but they should not be withheld in the setting of significant Gram-negative infection.

Thymic hyperplasia and thymoma can also cause MG to worsen. Chest CT should be repeated in patients who have undergone thymectomy to look for residual thymic rests that may have become hypertrophic after surgery. "Second-look" surgery may lead to substantial improvement in such cases.

CONSIDERATIONS IN PREGNANCY

Myasthenic patients require special attention during all phases of pregnancy, beginning before conception and continuing through the postpartum period. Women of childbearing age should use highly effective contraceptives if they are being treated with azathioprine or cyclosporine. Prednisone should be avoided but can be used during pregnancy if it is essential. Plasma exchange is safe throughout pregnancy and may be used in patients whose condition deteriorates. Treatment with pyridostigmine can be continued, but the parenteral form should be avoided because it can induce uterine contractions.

MG is not an indication for cesarean section. Spinal anesthesia should be used whenever possible. Nondepolarizing neuromuscular blocking agents should be avoided because the response to these medications may be prolonged in a myasthenic patient.

If preeclampsia develops in a myasthenic patient (a chance occurrence because the two conditions are not related), caution should be used in administering magnesium sulfate. Magnesium is a neuromuscular depressant, and its effect may be more pronounced in a patient with preexisting difficulties of neuromuscular transmission.

During the first few days postpartum, neonates born to myasthenic mothers must be monitored for signs of weakness. Evidence of transitory neonatal MG is detected in up to 15% of infants; difficulty in feeding or breathing or a weak cry is a common sign. The passive transfer of AChR antibodies from mother to fetus during gestation underlies this condition. Neonatal weakness can persist for weeks to months until the maternal antibodies are cleared. Although breast milk contains measurable amounts of maternal antibodies to AChR, no evidence has been found that it poses a significant threat, even to infants with transitory neonatal MG. Treating infants symptomatically with pyridostigmine is usually adequate, although intravenous immunoglobulin or plasma exchange is required in some. Affected infants are not at increased risk for the development of MG later in life, although like all first-degree relatives, they are at increased risk for the development of other autoimmune disorders.

BIBLIOGRAPHY

Chaudhry V, Cornblath DR, Griffin JW, et al. Mycophenolate mofetil: a safe and promising immunosuppressant in neuromuscular diseases. *Neurology* 2001;56: 94.

Drachman DB. Medical progress: myasthenia gravis. *N Engl J Med* 1994;330:1797.

Drug-induced myasthenia gravis. *Micromedex* 1996;87.

Gilchrist JM. Myasthenia gravis. In: Feldmann E, ed. *Current diagnosis in neurology*. St. Louis: Mosby, 1994:350.

Lopate G, Pestronk A. Autoimmune myasthenia gravis. *Hosp Pract* 1993;28:55.

Pascuzzi RM. Pearls and pitfalls in the diagnosis and management of neuromuscular disorders. *Semin Neurol* 2001;21:425.

Sanders DB, Howard JF Jr. Disorders of neuromuscular transmission. In: Bradley WG, Daroff RB, Fenichel GM, et al., eds. *Neurology in clinical practice*, 2nd ed. Oxford: Butterworth-Heinemann, 1996.

Seneviratne U, DeSilva R. Lambert-Eaton myasthenic syndrome. *Postgrad Med J* 1999;75:516–520.

Toyka KV. Myasthenia gravis. In: Johnson RT, ed. *Current therapy in neurologic disease*. Philadelphia: BC Decker, 1990:85.

CHAPTER 116

Low Back Pain and Sciatica

Joshua Hollander

Low back pain affecting the area between the rib cage and the gluteal folds is the most common complaint of patients heard by primary care physicians and the most frequent cause of disability among persons younger than 45 years of age. About 75% of the population experiences low back pain (lumbago). The annual prevalence is 15% to 20% in the United States. About 25% of patients with low back pain also have back-related pain that radiates along the course of the sciatic nerve to one or both legs distal to the knee (sciatica). Although low back pain affects persons of both sexes equally, men more often undergo surgery. Physically fit people recover more readily from back pain. Related physical factors include work that involves lifting heavy objects, static posture, bending, and twisting; muscle fatigue and deconditioning predispose to injury. Job dissatisfaction and monotony increase the likelihood of a complaint.

The lumbar spine comprises a series of vertebrae linked by anterior discs and posterior facet joints. The vertebral discs are fibrocartilaginous remnants of the notochord. The ovoid gelatinous nucleus pulposus is contained within the firm concentric collagenous fibrous rings of the annulus fibrosus. Discs have a minimal blood supply and are innervated by a branch of the posterior primary ramus. Their water content drops from 88% at birth to 66% at age 70. In a normally functioning disc, an incompressible cushion distributes forces. An isolated vertebra compresses before a disc does, but the spine in situ withstands forces far in excess of those tolerated ex vivo. The abdomen, its muscular wall, and the paraspinal muscles disseminate forces widely, protecting the spinal column. The typical weight lifter's trochanter belt serves a similar function.

The aging (early) spine loses both water and proteoglycans and its collagen content increases, resulting in a loss of gel behavior. Tears may develop in the annulus, causing lumbago. Disc herniation and fragment compression of a root cause sciatica. Thus, disc degeneration develops in three stages: a dysfunctional stage of nuclear degeneration and traumatic tears of the annulus leading to nuclear prolapse, an unstable stage of disc and facet degeneration and capsular laxity, and a restabilization stage of disc collapse and fibrosis and osteophyte formation resulting in a stiff joint. Goldthwait related lumbago and sciatica to the lumbar disc. Mixter and Barr demonstrated a clear relationship between herniated lumbar discs and lumbago and sciatica, in addition to therapy with lumbar disc excision. The role of muscle spasm and injury is controversial, and these may be only an epiphenomenon.

The clinical symptoms that signal a need for caution and early workup include the following: sciatica with an evolving neurologic deficit; unrelenting pain at rest, which suggests cancer or infection; and the writhing pain of intra-abdominal or vascular processes.

Musculoskeletal disorders of the lower back are discussed in Chapter 98.

NEURAL ROOT COMPRESSION SYNDROMES

A *herniated lumbar disc* may be easily recognized by the acute onset of lumbago and sciatica. In another presentation, a patient with chronic lumbago and segmental (hip and thigh) pain now experiences less back and proximal pain and primarily distal radicular discomfort instead. Specific symptoms relate to the root affected and whether the lesion is lateral and compressing a single root or central and compressing the conus. The presentation of *lumbar spinal stenosis* may be similar to that of a herniated disc. Central stenosis presents with neurogenic claudication and neurogenic bowel and bladder. It may be confused with vascular claudication when a patient experiences leg pain while walking that is relieved by rest. Patients with neurogenic claudication can comfortably ride a stationary bike, however, because the legs are flexed. The symptoms of lateral stenosis may be vague, with only segmental leg pain. The syndrome of neurogenic claudication with pain on walking that is relieved by rest may be related to nerve root ischemia induced by compression of the roots. Mechanical (instability) syndromes may be manifested by low back or segmental pain that is aggravated by weight bearing, bending, or twisting and relieved by recumbency.

HISTORY

Acute low back pain is pain of less than 6 weeks' duration and is only infrequently associated with a specific diagnosis. Subacute back pain is pain of 7 to 12 weeks' duration, and chronic low back pain is pain of longer duration. Sciatica is pain radiating along the course of the sciatic nerve to one or both legs distal to the knee. A damaged lumbar disc may cause pain to the knee, as may hip disease, but the pain does not radiate below the knee. The history should include questions about the onset, duration, distribution, course, and quality of the pain. Factors that aggravate or alleviate symptoms should be explored. Radiation in a radicular pattern, paresthesias, motor loss, and bowel or bladder dysfunction should alert the physician to potentially more serious problems. Other potentially serious problems can be signaled by fever (especially in drugs users, diabetics, or immunocompromised patients), abdominal symptoms, known cancer, unexplained weight loss, and osteoporosis. Lack of fitness, psychosocial problems, and marked scoliosis are risk factors. Patients must be asked about traumatic causes. Inflammatory spondylopathies may worsen pain after bed rest and cause morning stiffness. Tumor pain is usually increased by recumbency. Patients with disc disease have difficulty sitting, and those with lumbar spinal stenosis may have neurogenic claudication and require rest after walking modest distances. Patients who are unable to be at rest may have abdominal pathology with colic.

PHYSICAL EXAMINATION

The physical examination should include a general physical examination, especially of the abdomen. Motor and sensory skills, coordination, and reflexes are checked. An assessment of sphincter tone and the anal wink test may be required. The spine should be evaluated for normal curvature, tenderness, mobility (flexion, extension, later flexion), and paravertebral spasm. A shelf suggests spondylolisthesis. Tenderness should be sought 2 or 3 cm lateral to the spine for facet joint disease. A sciatic list is away from the irritated nerve root when the herniation is lateral to the root and toward the side of the irritated root when the herniation is medial. Sciatic notch tenderness is checked with the Valsalva maneuver. The jugular compression test reproduces the pain in the radicular distribution, as does coughing and straining. Gait testing includes toe and heel walking. The usual upper limb muscle is weaker than a lower limb

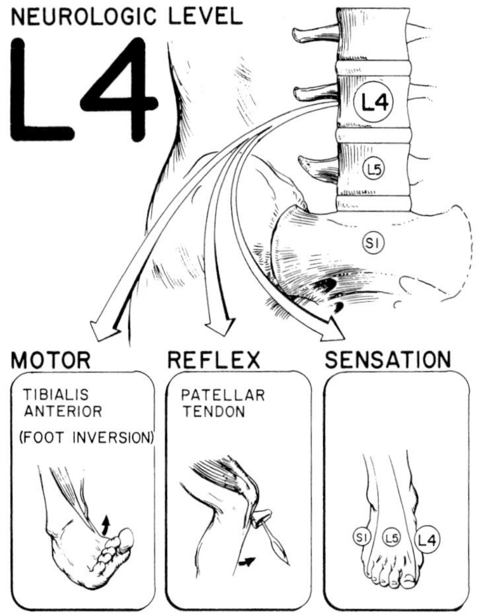

FIG. 116.1. Fourth lumbar root. (From Hoppenfeld S. *Orthopaedic neurology: a diagnostic guide to neurologic levels.* Philadelphia: JB Lippincott, 1977:52, with permission.)

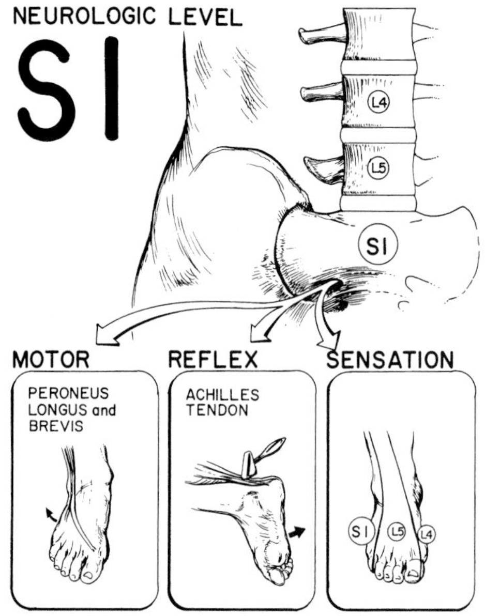

FIG. 116.3. First sacral root. (From Hoppenfeld S. *Orthopaedic neurology: a diagnostic guide to neurologic levels.* Philadelphia: JB Lippincott, 1977:58, with permission.)

muscle, and patients with questionable weakness on formal strength testing may display obvious weakness when tested functionally. The knee and ankle reflexes are most easily elicited with the hip, knee, and ankle flexed at 90 degrees and the foot pressing lightly down on a supporting hand. The straight leg-raising (Lasègue) test stretches a trapped nerve root at less than 50 degrees of hip flexion. This test can also be performed with the patient in the sitting position; the knee is extended in such a manner as to disguise the purpose if the examiner is suspicious of the patient's symptoms. Sensitivity is increased by the Bragard test, which involves lowering the leg after a positive straight leg-raising test result and then dorsiflexing the foot to reproduce the patient's pain. The well leg straight leg-raising test is highly specific, but its sensitivity is poor. The Hoover sign is elicited when the examiner's hand is placed under the heel of the good leg in a supine patient. The patient attempts to raise the weak leg, exerting a downward force on the examiner's hand with the good leg. If this force is not present, the patient is not really trying. Simplified schemas of dermatome features are presented in Figs. 116.1 through 116.3.

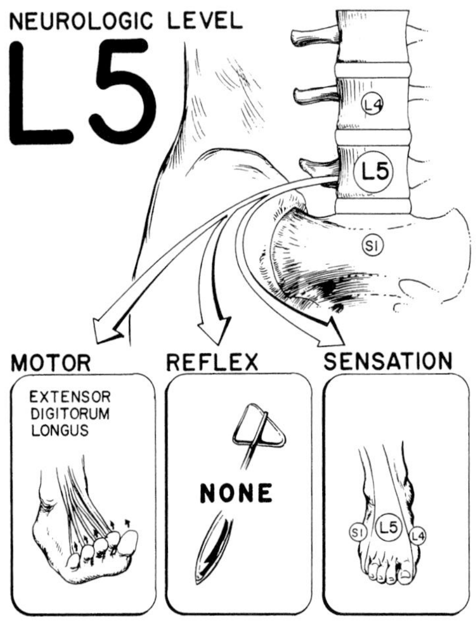

FIG. 116.2. Fifth lumbar root. (From Hoppenfeld S. *Orthopaedic neurology: a diagnostic guide to neurologic levels.* Philadelphia: JB Lippincott, 1977:54, with permission.)

LABORATORY AND IMAGING STUDIES

The investigation of uncomplicated acute low back pain requires only that a history be taken and a physical examination performed unless the examiner's impression after this evaluation is that the patient is at risk and requires early workup.

Acute low back pain with sciatica is more worrisome. If a cauda equina syndrome is suggested or a neurologic deficit progresses, workup must be considered. Multiple imaging techniques are available. Plain spine films are inexpensive, and they are useful in detecting the less common causes of back pain, such as tumor, congenital anomalies, and spondylolisthesis. They also have the advantage of not subjecting the patient to high doses of radiation. These films provide little information about the disc itself or the spinal canal, however. Magnetic resonance imaging (MRI) is expensive but visualizes the spine, disc spaces, and contents of the spinal canal. It has replaced most other lumbar imaging studies. MRI provides information about far lateral disc protrusion that does not disturb the canal. Computed tomography (CT) may be sufficient for straightforward disc disease but does not provide any information about the contents of the spinal canal. However, it does show the details of cortical bone and may be preferable to MRI for visualizing bony disorders because MRI visualizes marrow but not dense bone. Myelography may be performed with water-soluble contrast material and used in concert with CT to evaluate the contents of the spinal canal. In most cases, adequate images can be obtained with only one modality. If the findings are equivocal, however, or if inconsistencies are noted between the clinical and imaging findings, multiple investigations are in order. Isotope bone scanning is helpful in inflammatory disease of the bones or joints and in tumor. The use of discography has undergone a minor resurgence, but it has generally been abandoned. Epidural venography is no longer held in high esteem. Electromyography is unfortunately overly sensitive and less specific and therefore not as useful as it might be. It is valuable for (a) excluding a more distal lesion, (b) confirming evidence of root compression, and (c) localizing the compression to one or more roots.

In an evaluation of the results of any of these studies, it is important to remember that in one third of patients, disc herniation is not accompanied by sciatica. Weakness and paresthesias may occur without pain, or disc herniation may cause back pain without sciatica.

TREATMENT

In many cases, acute low back pain can be relieved by 2 days of bed rest (supine in a modified Fowler position) or by back mobilization exercises. Chiropractic treatment is controversial. Patients may experience satisfactory results. Acute low back pain with sciatica is of greater concern, but more than 50% of patients recover without surgery. Some clinicians have greater reservations about manipulation in the face of sciatica.

Subacute low back pain (a residual in 10% of patients with acute low back pain) requires more extensive treatment. A limited workup is in order. Limited bed rest may help. Lumbar traction probably exerts its benefit by confining the patient to bed. Heat and cold may be used, with variable effect. Injections of facet joints, epidural steroids, and peripheral nerve blocks are of questionable value. Many patients appear to benefit from the use of a lightweight flexible support with a molded plastic insert, which restricts lumbosacral motion and provides abdominal support and postural correction.

A patient with subacute low back pain and sciatica requires an attempt at a more specific diagnosis, with therapy then directed at the presumed underlying condition. In most cases, this kind of pain is caused by a herniated nucleus pulposus. Surgical removal of a disc fragment that has been visualized and correlated with symptoms and signs promotes recovery in the 10% of patients who appear to require surgery. Chymopapain injections have become less favored because of a high incidence of anaphylaxis and reports of transverse myelopathy. Lumbar fusion is performed infrequently. Newer procedures for disc removal are far less extensive and appear not to lead to an unstable back.

Many patients with severe neurogenic claudication secondary to lumbar spinal stenosis are elderly. They nevertheless tend to benefit from large-scale decompressive laminectomy. This procedure should not be withheld purely on the basis of age.

Patients with back pain that persists despite conservative measures and a serious effort at finding a treatable cause may require referral to a pain specialist. Such patients may have to learn to live with some pain. Concurrent depression should be treated.

CONSIDERATIONS DURING PREGNANCY

Although only half of pregnant women experience back pain, it is almost certainly more common during pregnancy. The need to maintain an erect posture while the enlarging uterus protrudes anterior to the center of gravity forces an increasingly lordotic posture. Periodic bed rest and the avoidance of high-heeled shoes are in order. Standing with one foot raised on a step may be helpful. When, infrequently, sudden severe pain with sciatica and features of herniated disc develops, bed rest is in order. Cauda equina syndrome requires surgical intervention even during pregnancy, but other deficits should be managed conservatively, if possible. MRI may be undertaken if either cauda equina syndrome or progression of a neurologic disability indicates that surgery may be appropriate.

BIBLIOGRAPHY

Acute low back problems in adults. *Clinical practice guidelines.* U.S. Department of Health and Human Services publication no 14, 1994.

Borenstein DG, Wiesel SW, Boden SD. *Low back pain: medical diagnosis and comprehensive management,* 2nd ed. Philadelphia: WB Saunders, 1995.

Devereaux M. *Acute low back pain.* San Francisco: American Academy of Neurology Annual Courses, 1996:423.

Empting LD. Ten questions about lower back pain. *Neurologist* 1996;2:2.

Frymoyer JW. Back pain and sciatica. *N Engl J Med* 1988;318:291.

Hoppenfeld S. *Orthopaedic neurology: a diagnostic guide to neurologic levels.* Philadelphia: JB Lippincott, 1977.

Malmivaara A, Hakkinen U, Aro T, et al. The treatment of acute low back pain—bed rest, exercises, or ordinary activity? *N Engl J Med* 1995;332:351.

PART

13

Ophthalmologic Problems

CHAPTER 117

Examination of the Eye

Gwen K. Sterns and James Frank

Taking a systematic approach to the examination of the eye helps the primary physician uncover pathology that threatens vision. A properly conducted, organized examination ensures appropriate intervention and timely referral.

OCULAR HISTORY

The basic eye examination begins with a thorough patient history of current symptoms and problems, including their onset, duration, and severity. Loss of vision should be noted and defined as monocular, binocular, episodic, complete, or partial. Other symptoms, including glare, photosensitivity, spontaneous pain, pain with motion, discharge, and crusting (especially in the morning on awakening), should also be included. A detailed past ocular history and medical history, including current medications, allergies to medications, social history, and family history, should be elicited.

The patient's age is an important part of the history and should be considered strongly in the differential diagnosis. For example, a 40-year-old patient's description of the gradual onset of blurred vision for near tasks may lead the clinician to a presumptive diagnosis of presbyopia. An 80-year-old patient with the same problem is more likely to have a cataract.

The past history can provide important information to aid in the diagnosis. A young woman with a long history of cold sores on her lip who now presents with a red, painful eye may have herpes simplex keratitis. A contact lens wearer with similar symptoms may have a vision-threatening corneal ulcer. A sudden loss of vision in the eye of a woman who has a prosthetic heart valve may suggest an embolus. Severe headaches in a woman with fluctuating vision should suggest the possibility of an intracranial process, such as pseudotumor cerebri or a pituitary mass.

ASSESSMENT OF VISUAL FUNCTION

Visual Acuity

Every eye examination should include testing for visual acuity, regardless of the presenting problems. A vision testing chart, such as a Snellen chart for distance acuity, is placed 20 feet from the patient under adequate diffuse illumination. Each eye is tested independently with and without the patient's most recent distance spectacle correction. Acuity is noted as cc (with correction) or sc (without correction). If the patient can see all letters on the 20/20 line at a distance of 20 feet from the chart, this is recorded as 20/20. If the patient missed two letters on the 20/20 line, then the vision should be recorded as 20/20–2. A patient who reads all the letters on the 20/40 line and two additional letters on the 20/30 line has an acuity of 20/30+2. Ophthalmologists use the Latin designation OD *(oculus dexter)* for the right eye and OS (oculus sinister) for the left eye.

Acuity is recorded as a ratio of the distance at which the patient can see an object divided by the distance at which the object can be seen by someone with normal vision. For most patients, the test objects are letters or numbers. For example, an acuity of 20/50 means that the patient can read at 20 feet an object that a person with normal vision can read at 50 feet. Alternatively, the testing distance can be moved closer to the patient, with the numerator adjusted accordingly. This can be helpful in evaluating patients with severely reduced vision who require standardized testing to monitor their progress. For example, the acuity of a patient with a retrobulbar neuritis may be reduced to 3/100. This means that the patient can read a test object at 3 feet that a person with normal vision can read at 100 feet.

If the patient cannot read the largest letter on the Snellen chart at any distance, then the distance at which the patient can perceive hand motion is noted and is recorded as HM at stated distance. If no hand motion is detected by the patient, then light perception is recorded as LP, or no light perception is recorded as NLP. If the patient's vision is limited to light perception, the light should be shone from each of the four field quadrants and the patient asked to identify the direction from which the light is shining. If the answers are consistently correct, the vision may be recorded as light perception with projection in four quadrants. Each eye must be tested independently.

The pinhole visual acuity test helps identify patients with uncorrected refractive errors and corneal irregularity. Patients with a visual acuity of less than 20/30 in either eye should undergo this test. The pinhole aperture is placed in front of each eye independently and the patient is asked to read the Snellen chart through one of the pinholes. The pinhole compensates for any uncorrected refractive error down to the 20/25 line. Therefore, a patient with a refractive error as the sole reason for diminished visual acuity should see the 20/25 Snellen acuity line. A patient who has 20/40 vision in the right eye without correction and 20/25 vision with the pinhole should be recorded as OD VA sc 20/40, PH 20/25. If vision is not improved with the pinhole aperture, the examiner should suspect a cause other than refractive error or corneal irregularity. Possible causes include media opacity (e.g., vitreous hemorrhage), cataract, diabetic retinopathy, and optic nerve disease. These patients should be referred to an ophthalmologist for further evaluation.

Near vision should be tested with the patient wearing reading glasses or bifocals. Near vision is tested with the Rosenbaum pocket vision screener or other equivalent near card. The patient holds the card about 14 inches away, and the smallest line discernible is read. The vision may be recorded in the Jaeger notation as J1; the testing distance and whether the test was performed with or without correction should be specified. Again, each eye is tested separately.

Confrontation Visual Fields

Many conditions are associated with loss of the peripheral visual field. Specialized visual field equipment is usually available only in a specialist's office. Confrontation visual field testing can be performed to screen for gross visual field defects and often is as accurate as formal perimetry testing. In addition, this may be the only method available for patients with physical disabilities that prevent them from sitting at a field analyzer.

In one technique of confrontation field testing, the examiner and the patient face each other about an arm's length apart. The patient is instructed to occlude the left eye with an occluder or hand and look at the examiner's left eye with her right eye. The field of the examiner's left eye is used as a standard for measuring the field in the patient's right eye and vice versa. The examiner asks the patient to count the number of fingers on the hand that the examiner presents to each of the four quadrants. Next, the examiner uses both hands and simultaneously presents fingers to both the nasal and temporal fields of the eye. The patient's responses are recorded and visual field loss noted. This examination can reveal visual field loss and help direct further examination and referral for more formalized testing.

Color Testing

Color defects are rare in women and may be associated with other vision problems. Color testing can be performed with standardized color test charts such as the pseudoisochromatic plates of Ishihara. Diminished color perception in conditions such as optic neuritis may help in the diagnosis. The patient with optic neuritis may perceive a red target as a dull brown in the affected eye.

ASSESSMENT OF INTRAOCULAR PRESSURE

Tonometry, the determination of intraocular pressure, is easily accomplished in the typical office setting and can be part of a general physical examination performed by the primary care physician. Tonometry should always be part of a formal eye examination. Patients with a positive family history of glaucoma should also undergo this test.

The intraocular pressure can be measured with the readily available Schiotz tonometer. A topical anesthetic is required. The patient must lay her head back or be supine. The eyelids are held open and the tonometer is held gently over the cornea. The degree to which a specific weight indents the cornea indicates the intraocular pressure. A tonopen can also be used to check the intraocular pressure. In this device, an electronic sensing of an applanation force is used to record the intraocular pressure. A topical anesthetic is required. The patient can be seated. The eyelids are held open and the tonopen is placed against the cornea with sufficient pressure to indent it. The intraocular pressure is recorded electronically.

EXTERNAL EXAMINATION

The examination of the ocular adnexa should proceed in an orderly fashion. With a penlight, the lids can be examined for evidence of infection, such as crusting, swelling, and erythema. Lid position should be noted, together with any ptosis, proptosis, or lid lag. Lesions on the lid margin should also be noted. Entropion, which is a turning inward of the lid, may cause tearing and irritation; ectropion, which is eversion of the lid margin, suggests a lid neoplasm in a young patient and lid laxity causing excessive tearing in an older patient.

PUPILS

The pupils should be inspected for size, shape, reaction to light and near stimuli, and the presence or absence of the consensual light response. An irregularly shaped iris may suggest synechiae (adhesions) between the iris and lens resulting from iritis, trauma, or acute glaucoma. An afferent pupillary defect can alert the examiner to an optic neuritis or retrobulbar neuritis.

MOTILITY

Eye movement is assessed in the cardinal positions of gaze: up and right, right, down and right, left and up, left, and left and down. The primary position of gaze should also be evaluated by having the patient fix her gaze on a distant target; the examiner observes the position of the corneal light reflex. Any gross asymmetry of the light reflex in one or both eyes indicates a deviation of that eye.

OPHTHALMOSCOPY

The technique of direct ophthalmoscopy should be a part of all ophthalmic and general physical examinations. The first step in ophthalmoscopy is to look for the red fundus reflection, which can easily be seen without magnification at a distance of 20 to 40 cm. A full red reflex quickly rules out gross corneal lesions, dense media opacities, and complete retinal detachments. Any opacities appear as black forms against the red background of the reflex. Next, the cornea is inspected with a strong plus lens of about +10.00 to +15.00 diopters. From a distance of 2 cm, one may easily see corneal scars, ulcers, and foreign bodies. In ocular herpes simplex keratitis, dendritic corneal lesions may also be seen by this technique.

Abnormalities of the anterior chamber aqueous, such as hyphema or hypopyon, can be seen. Adequate visualization of the detail of the iris architecture with a +15.00 diopter lens can be used to rule out tumor, nodules, and synechiae. With a slightly lower power of +4.00 to +8.00 diopters, the lens can be examined and cataracts sought.

By extending the focus into the vitreous cavity with +4.00 to +8.00 power, opacities in the vitreous can be seen. Blood in the vitreous appears bright red in recent hemorrhage or as dark brown clumping in more chronic hemorrhage.

The funduscopic examination should include an inspection of the optic nerve, vessels, macula, and mid periphery. The disc is normally round or oval, with the nasal edge less distinct than the temporal edge. The sclera may be seen surrounding the optic nerve in myopic patients. The disc, with a central white depression (cup), may be seen. Cup-to-disc ratios should be recorded; ratios larger than normal suggest glaucoma.

The macula is temporal to the disc. It may appear darker than the surrounding retina. The central reflex in the macula is the foveal reflex. Clumping or loss of pigment in this region, with resultant loss of central vision, suggests macular degeneration.

The retinal vessels should be examined for caliber, course, and crossing appearance. The ratio of the normal venous diameter to the arteriolar diameter is 3:2. Changes in this ratio, defects in the crossings, and increases in the light reflex of the arteriolar color suggest arteriolar sclerotic or hypertensive retinopathy.

SUMMARY

If the examination described yields an abnormal finding that requires additional evaluation, the patient should be referred to an ophthalmologist. Supplemental diagnostic testing such as indirect ophthalmoscopy, neuroimaging, gonioscopy, perimetry, ultrasonography, and fluorescein angiography may be performed.

BIBLIOGRAPHY

Berson FG, ed. *Ophthalmology study guide.* San Francisco: American Academy of Ophthalmology, 1987.

Tasman W, Jaeger EA, eds. *Duane's clinical ophthalmology.* Philadelphia: JB Lippincott, 1994.

CHAPTER 118

Red Eye

Ronald D. Plotnik and Gwen K. Sterns

The term *conjunctivitis* denotes inflammation of the conjunctiva associated with various disorders, usually manifested as a "red eye" or "pink eye." These conditions may range from inconsequential to severe. Causes include infection, trauma, allergy, and toxins. In addition, a variety of conditions unique to the eye (e.g., glaucoma, dry eye) may result in redness.

The eye appears red because the conjunctiva is inflamed. The conjunctiva is the outermost layer adjacent to the white sclera and normally is clear. Injection or dilation of the blood vessels results in the redness seen. The conjunctiva may be affected primarily, as in infection, or become red in a generalized reaction to other ocular conditions. In the primary care setting, the history often provides a clue to the cause, and the associated symptoms are often helpful in delineating the cause.

In most primary care settings, a biomicroscope ("slitlamp"), the device ophthalmologists use to examine the eye, is not available. A slitlamp magnifies the features of the eye, and examination with this instrument often reveals the cause of a red eye. It then becomes imperative to be able to decide who can be treated empirically and who requires urgent referral. Furthermore, the range of treatments available in a primary care setting should be broad enough to allow management of the most common conditions but narrow enough to preclude inappropriate therapy. In a practical sense, common bacterial and viral conjunctivitis can be treated by the primary care physician, whereas cases of conjunctivitis with other causes require referral. Certain warning signs ("red flags") indicate which patients should be referred and that topical antibiotics are not the appropriate treatment.

ETIOLOGY AND DIFFERENTIAL DIAGNOSIS

Table 118.1 provides a partial list of some of the more common causes of a red eye. Each has characteristic signs and symptoms and requires a specific treatment. The most common cause of a red eye is bacterial or viral conjunctivitis.

HISTORY

In the ophthalmologist's office, the history may be important, depending on what signs are noted on the slitlamp examination. In the primary care setting, however, the history is imperative because the only other information available is whatever is visible to the primary care provider's naked eye.

The history can be divided into two parts. In the first, the patient is questioned about onset, exposures, past medical history, course, and symptoms. In the second, all symptoms that require urgent referral are specifically excluded.

TABLE 118.1. Common Causes of Conjunctivitis

Infectious
Bacterial conjunctivitis
Viral conjunctivitis
Bacterial keratitis
Herpes simplex
Herpes zoster
Fungal keratitis
Orbital/preseptal cellulitis
Chlamydia infection
Traumatic
Subconjunctival hemorrhage
Traumatic iritis
Corneal abrasion
Conjunctival lacerations
Foreign bodies
Chemical injury
Ocular conditions
Contact lens overwear
Blepharoconjunctivitis
Acute glaucoma
Dry eye (Sjögren syndrome)
Iritis (intraocular inflammation)
Scleritis (inflammation of the sclera)
Allergic/toxic
Contact
Hayfever
Contact lens reactions
Atopy
Chemicals

The timing of the onset can be an important differentiating historical point. More severe conditions tend to develop relatively quickly. A history of exposure to other persons with a red eye is important. Close contact with another person with a red eye, especially a child, often antedates bacterial and viral forms of conjunctivitis. Certain sexually transmitted diseases affect the eye. Exposure to a "cold sore" may be important. A previous upper respiratory infection or fever may provide additional information. A history of connective tissue disease, shingles, chickenpox, atopy, rosacea, herpes simplex labialis, or previous red eye suggests the cause. A history of trauma, contact lens wear, use of eye drops, exposure to chemicals, certain occupations, or previous ocular surgery or conditions is also helpful.

Ocular symptoms include tearing, sensitivity to light (photophobia), reactive eyelid closure (blepharospasm), discharge, decreased vision, eye pain or irritation, foreign body sensation, itching, double vision, pain during eye movement, periocular swelling, pupils unequal in size, decreased or restricted eye movement, headache, proptosis (eye partially projecting out of the socket), and associated nausea and vomiting. Warning signs and symptoms that the condition is more than a simple case of conjunctivitis and that the patient requires urgent referral are the following:

- Decreased vision
- Unequal pupils
- Significant ocular or periocular swelling
- Significant photophobia
- Associated nausea or vomiting
- Significant ocular pain
- Double vision
- Proptosis
- History of contact lens wear.

Often, these symptoms indicate corneal involvement, significant ocular inflammation, infection, or elevated eye pressure (glaucoma). Such conditions must be treated by an ophthalmologist.

PHYSICAL EXAMINATION

In the primary care setting, the ocular examination should be directed to diagnosing conjunctivitis and excluding other ocular diseases. Certain signs can be evaluated, even without the use of specialized equipment. The examination should begin with a determination of visual acuity. A wall or hand-held chart is optimal. If the patient wears corrective glasses, they should be worn for this test. Conjunctivitis usually does not decrease visual acuity.

The penlight can be a very useful instrument. Pupil size and reactivity should be determined. The pupils should be equal in size, round, and reactive to the light. The corneal surface can be evaluated by shining the penlight directly on the eye. The corneal reflection of light, or "reflex," is usually smooth and bright. Irregularities of the corneal surface may dull or distort the reflex. A whitish opacity or spot, graying, or a foreign body on the cornea may be visualized in some conditions.

The periorbital skin should be inspected for signs such as vesicles, redness, thickening, swelling, purulence, scaling, and excoriation. The conjunctiva should be grossly inspected for injection (redness) and chemosis (swelling). Gross purulence is usually present in bacterial and sometimes in viral conjunctivitis.

The nature of the ocular redness also may be important. Redness primarily in a circle around the cornea, redness with a purple hue, redness that affects only one portion of the eye, intense redness, or marked enlargement of vessels should prompt referral.

Fluorescein dye can be instilled in the eye, after which the eye is viewed with a cobalt blue light filter. A blue filter is built into most direct ophthalmoscopes or may be available as a penlight attachment. Defects in the corneal surface cell layer (epithelium) show up as bright green in ordinary light and bright yellow in the cobalt blue light. Any uptake of dye by the cornea suggests corneal disease (as opposed to primary conjunctivitis), which requires referral. If a slitlamp biomicroscope is available (such as in some offices and emergency rooms), the eye should be examined to rule out other disease.

LABORATORY STUDIES

In the ophthalmologist's office, cultures are often helpful, especially if the symptoms and signs are nonspecific and infection is suspected. Certain bacteria are considered to be normal flora on the eye (such as coagulase-negative staphylococci), but even these can cause infection in certain situations. In suspected bacterial conjunctivitis, cultures are obtained only if the clinical response to treatment is poor. Most topical antibiotics effectively treat bacterial conjunctivitis, and therefore cultures are usually not helpful. Cultures must be obtained with antibiotic sensitivities for any corneal ulcer because this is a much more serious condition.

Typical lesions of herpes simplex or herpes zoster do not require cultures because the clinical picture is often sufficiently clear without them. Similarly, cultures in probable cases of viral conjunctivitis are usually not worthwhile when the diagnosis is strongly suspected clinically. Lesions of herpesvirus and adenovirus may affect the cornea in the form of an immune reaction, but results of cultures during this phase are usually negative. With certain slitlamp findings, testing for infection with *Chlamydia* can be helpful.

In the primary care setting, cultures usually are not warranted. If the clinician is sufficiently concerned—in terms of either the diagnosis or antibiotic sensitivity—to obtain a culture, the patient should be referred to an ophthalmologist for a slitlamp examination.

CLINICAL FINDINGS AND TREATMENT CONSIDERATIONS

The following discussion covers many of the more common causes of red eye. It is by no means exhaustive, and the patient's broader clinical situation must be taken into consideration.

Infectious Conjunctivitis

BACTERIAL CONJUNCTIVITIS

Bacterial conjunctivitis is common and may follow exposure to a child or adult with "pink eye." The infection causes tearing, occasional mild blurring of vision caused by pus on the eye (which can be "blinked away"), and redness. The discharge ranges from mucoid to frank yellow or green pus. The usual organisms isolated include *Staphylococcus aureus*, coagulase-negative *Staphylococcus*, *Streptococcus*, and, in children, *Haemophilus influenzae*. Although uncommon, gonococcal conjunctivitis produces a copious purulent discharge and requires systemic treatment. Infections with other organisms usually require only 7 days of topical antibiotic treatment. Most organisms are overwhelmed by the antibiotic, and specific sensitivity tests usually are not needed unless the patient does not respond to treatment.

An antibiotic-steroid combination or steroids alone should never be used because they may lead to significant complications, including potentiation of the herpes simplex virus and exacerbation of bacterial and viral infections. As a general rule, primary care physicians should not use steroids at all before a detailed slitlamp examination is performed, which usually requires a referral. Contagious precautions should be taken because patients may be infectious for several days. Additionally, topical anesthetics should never be dispensed because they are toxic to the ocular surface and prevent healing.

VIRAL CONJUNCTIVITIS

Viral conjunctivitis is usually caused by adenovirus. The incubation period can be as long as 2 weeks, and the patient often has a history of exposure. Viral conjunctivitis may follow an upper respiratory tract infection, and fever may be associated. The condition is typically bilateral, although one side is usually more severely affected. The eyes are red, and the discharge is watery to mucoid. The vision may be decreased later in the course of the disease. Mild photophobia may be present, and an enlarged, tender preauricular node is often noted. Viral conjunctivitis usually runs its course without major sequelae but may lead to corneal problems and decreased vision. Treatment consists of keeping the eye clear of accumulating discharge, using cool compresses, and taking contagious precautions. Viral conjunctivitis is extremely contagious and can be transmissible for approximately 2 weeks after the onset of symptoms. Patients should be advised to be prudent about hand washing and avoid sharing towels or pillows. Because of the infectious and often epidemic nature of adenovirus conjunctivitis, health care providers and others, including day care workers, must often be secluded for 2 weeks. The virus can live on dry surfaces for many hours.

BACTERIAL KERATITIS

Bacterial keratitis is an ophthalmic emergency requiring the frequent administration of fortified antibiotic drops. It is essential for the primary care provider to exclude this diagnosis. The vision is usually markedly decreased, but not always. The eye is typically extremely red, and discharge may be copious. Contact lens wear, especially extended wear, is a risk factor. Sometimes, a white opacity is seen on the cornea, or the corneal luster may be decreased. Cases in which this diagnosis is a possibility require urgent referral.

CHLAMYDIA INFECTION

Infection with *Chlamydia* is sexually transmitted and usually spreads to the eyes by way of the fingers. A history of urethral or vaginal discharge may be elicited. Infection with *Chlamydia* causes a red eye that is minimally responsive to topical antibiotics. The vision may be decreased slightly. Treatment should consist of systemic doxycycline or similar medication for 2 to 3 weeks. It is important also to treat the sexual partners of patients. Coinfection with *Chlamydia* should be considered when other sexually transmitted eye infections, such as gonococcal infections, are treated.

HERPES SIMPLEX

Herpes simplex may affect the eye primarily, but ocular herpes simplex more often represents a reactivation of latent infection in the trigeminal ganglion. The virus travels out of the nerve axons to cause infectious conjunctivitis or keratitis. Precipitating factors may include a fever, "flu," or trauma. Although used to treat the sequelae of herpes simplex, the administration of topical steroids during an acute infection may markedly worsen the condition and cause permanent visual loss. This is the main reason why a primary care physician should not treat a "red eye" with steroids or antibiotic-steroid combinations. Acute infection often takes the form of a "dendrite" or branch-like lesion on the cornea that stains with fluorescein dye. Treatment consists of the application of topical antiviral agents tapered during a course of 3 weeks. Oral antiviral agents may be of additional benefit.

HERPES ZOSTER

Herpes zoster may affect the eye in the form of "shingles" or, less often, after a case of chickenpox. In the more common form, an adult who had chickenpox as a child presents with right- or left-sided dermatomal involvement of the scalp, forehead, eye, nose, or cheek. Eye findings range from minimal conjunctivitis to severe ischemic ocular disease. The corneal sequelae of herpes zoster can last for many years, and topical steroids may be required to control inflammation. Topical antiviral agents are usually not given, but oral antiviral agents have been shown to decrease ocular complications of the disease significantly. Postherpetic neuralgia can often be controlled with topical capsaicin, an inhibitor of substance P.

FUNGAL KERATITIS

Fungal keratitis or corneal infection is more common in tropical climates and may be associated with contact lens wear. Treatment consists of topical and oral antifungal agents. The corneal surface usually displays a defect that stains with fluorescein dye, and an underlying white spot is usually noted.

ORBITAL AND PRESEPTAL CELLULITIS

The orbital septum divides the periorbital skin from the actual eye orbit or socket. Infection of the preseptal or skin region must be treated with oral antibiotics. Gram-positive organisms are usually the cause. Deeper infection of the orbit itself is an ocular emergency requiring intravenous antibiotics. Urgent computed tomography or magnetic resonance imaging is also indicated to rule out orbital abscess, which requires incision and drainage. Although preseptal cellulitis may manifest as a mild red eye, no other signs are noted in the eye or orbit. Orbital cellulitis presents as proptosis, restriction of eye movement, abnormal pupil responses, marked swelling, decreased vision, copious discharge, and abnormalities of the fifth cranial nerve (i.e., paresthesia).

Traumatic Causes of Conjunctivitis

SUBCONJUNCTIVAL HEMORRHAGE

In subconjunctival hemorrhage, mild bleeding develops in the space beneath the conjunctiva, over the white sclera. The blood appears vibrant red and is homogenous. Blood vessels are not engorged. Subconjunctival hemorrhage is usually sectorial; it is inconsequential and requires no treatment. Resolution may take as long as 2 weeks. Subconjunctival hemorrhage may be caused by minor trauma, significant coughing, systemic anticoagulation, or daily use of aspirin, or it may occur as an isolated event.

TRAUMATIC IRITIS

Any blunt trauma to the eye can cause intraocular inflammation. At the slitlamp examination, this is evidenced by the presence of white blood cells floating free in the anterior chamber of the eye. Photophobia, decreased vision, tearing, and pain are frequently associated. Topical steroids and dilating drops are usually prescribed. A slitlamp examination is required to make the diagnosis.

CORNEAL ABRASION

The surface layer of cells of the cornea, or epithelium, can be abraded in a variety of ways. Patients may report having been hit in the eye by a baby's finger, tree branch, or piece of paper. Topical antibiotic ointment, either with or without patching, is usually indicated. One type of abrasion warrants special mention. Contact lens wearers may present with what they believe is an abrasion. The clinical examination findings may also be consistent with this, but corneal infection must be ruled out. It is safer not to patch contact lens "abrasions" and to treat with topical antibiotic ointment. Patching may exacerbate infection, but this is not a concern in most abrasions of other causes.

CONJUNCTIVAL LACERATIONS

Trauma may cause a laceration of the conjunctiva that involves the underlying sclera. Referral is indicated if this is suspected.

FOREIGN BODIES

Conjunctival and corneal foreign bodies are relatively common. Many are metallic and occupationally related. Conjunctival and corneal foreign bodies can be removed easily with a needle or burr at the slitlamp examination. Sometimes, the foreign body can be seen with the naked eye, and a moistened cotton swab can be used to remove it. Conjunctival foreign bodies are more amenable to removal by this method than corneal foreign bodies. Antibiotic ointments are usually prescribed for several days as prophylaxis.

CHEMICAL INJURY

Chemical injuries vary from mild to catastrophic. Mild injuries cause a red eye with no decrease in vision. Topical antibiotic-steroid combinations may be used if other causes of red eye have been ruled out. Referral is usually indicated if the symptoms are severe or persistent. More severe injuries are caused by alkali or acid. Alkaline injuries are worse and may cause significant and permanent ocular damage. Immediate treatment for chemical injury consists of copious irrigation at the site of injury, which is continued into the emergency room. The pH level must be checked periodically to assess progress and then again after irrigation to make sure no residual alkaline or acidic particles remain. Urgent referral is indicated for most chemical injuries. Patients with minor injuries, a mild red eye, no fluorescein staining, and no other symptoms may be observed carefully.

Ocular Conditions Causing Red Eye

CONTACT LENS OVERWEAR

Contact lens overwear may cause a severe red eye that is often associated with tearing, photophobia, and decreased vision. The history often includes sleeping in daily wear lenses. Temporary cessation of lens wear is necessary. The frequency of infectious keratitis is significantly increased in these patients, and referral for a slitlamp examination is required to rule out signs of infection. Cultures may be taken. Patching is not indicated, nor is topical steroid use. Contact lens solution toxicity may be an additional factor. Often, topical antibiotics are used empirically.

BLEPHARITIS AND DRY EYE SYNDROME

The tear film is composed of water from the lacrimal glands and oil from the meibomian glands. With aging, a decrease in water from the lacrimal glands gives rise to dry eye syndrome. Sjögren syndrome is a form of dry eye syndrome. Blepharitis, or plugging of the oil glands in the eye lids, results in a decreased amount of lubricating oil in the tears. These conditions are associated with chronic irritation and redness that result from the poor quantity and quality of the tear film. A gradual onset and long-lasting symptoms in an adult, especially a woman, can be characteristic. Slitlamp examination and special testing can confirm the diagnosis.

ACUTE GLAUCOMA

In predisposed persons, dilation of the pupils in dim light can cause acute angle-closure glaucoma. *Angle closure* refers to the anatomic changes that cause this type of glaucoma. The extremely high ocular pressure causes severe pain, a red eye, a hazy cornea, and often nausea and vomiting. Urgent referral is required to prevent visual loss. Treatment consists of lowering the pressure with drops and oral medications; a laser procedure is then performed as the definitive treatment. The development of symptoms in an older adult in the dim light of a movie theater is the classic scenario. Dilation of the pupils as part of the eye examination can also precipitate this condition in some persons.

IRITIS (INTRAOCULAR INFLAMMATION)

Although iritis precipitated by trauma was described previously, iritis may also occur without precipitating factors as an intrinsic entity associated with intraocular inflammation. Iritis often develops in the setting of connective tissue diseases, in which its incidence is significantly increased. Treatment includes topical steroids and a dilating drop, which can prevent intraocular scarring. In an otherwise healthy person, a systemic workup may be indicated if the iritis is bilateral, recurrent, or severe. Visual loss, photophobia, tearing, and pain are usual accompanying symptoms.

SCLERITIS (INFLAMMATION OF THE SCLERA)

Inflammation of the sclera presents as a red eye. It can be severe and may be associated with visual loss, a small nodule on the eye, sectorial redness, corneal inflammation, and iritis. Although scleritis is not necessarily associated with systemic connective tissue disease, it often is, and a systemic workup is usually indicated. Although topical steroids and nonsteroidal antiinflammatory drugs may be helpful, systemic treatment is usually required. This consists of indomethacin (Indocin) or another nonsteroidal antiinflammatory agent, with prednisone or systemic immunosuppressants used in more severe cases.

Allergic Reactions: Hay Fever

Seasonal allergies may give rise to a red eye accompanied by prominent itching. Tearing and conjunctival swelling may be present. Allergic conjunctivitis can be treated with cool compresses and systemic antihistamines. Several topical products are available that may help, including antihistamines, mast cell stabilizers, and nonsteroidal antiinflammatory drugs.

CONSIDERATIONS IN PREGNANCY

A primary consideration in pregnancy is the use of diagnostic and therapeutic drops. Each small drop instilled is absorbed systemically. Two techniques can diminish absorption significantly. Normally, the excess drop is removed from the eye surface through the lacrimal drainage system, which consists of two small openings (puncta) on the medial side of the lids (one upper and one lower) connected to a lumen that empties into the nose. This is why crying results in clear rhinorrhea. Blinking helps to propel the excess drop into this system. Five minutes of lid closure, without blinking, after drops have been instilled decreases systemic absorption. In a second technique, pinching the bridge of the nose, including the medial corner of each eye, effectively closes the openings to the system. Combined lid closure and punctal occlusion may be even more effective.

The usual course of antibiotic treatment is dosing four times daily for 1 week. Treatment for 5 days may be effective. Eye drops are usually preferred to ointments. Antiviral drops may have to be used and are often continued, while the dose is tapered, for 3 weeks. The use of fluorescein dye and dilating drops, especially phenylephrine, should be avoided. Topical steroids should be used at the lowest possible dose. Antihistamines and other drops should be avoided unless symptoms necessitate their use. Lid closure and punctal occlusion should always be performed after dosing. Obstetric consultation should be obtained before any drops are used.

BIBLIOGRAPHY

Arffa RC. *Grayson's diseases of the cornea*, 3rd ed. St. Louis: Mosby–Year Book, 1991.
Fraunfelder FT, Roy FH. *Current ocular therapy*, 4th ed. Philadelphia: WB Saunders, 1995.
Smolin G, Thoft RA. *The cornea: scientific foundations and clinical practice*, 2nd ed. Boston: Little, Brown, 1987.

CHAPTER 119

Corneal Diseases and Treatment

Julie H. Tsai, Bryant Shin, and Steven S. T. Ching

ANATOMY OF THE EYE

The human eye is roughly spherical, averaging 24 mm in diameter. Posteriorly, 80% of the surface consists of *sclera*, a white, opaque layer composed of connective tissue and collagen fibrils that measures about 1 mm in thickness. The muscles that move the eye are attached to the sclera, and blood vessels and nerves penetrate the sclera to gain access to intraocular structures. The sclera meets the *cornea*, the anterior surface of the eye, at a transition zone called the *limbus*. The *conjunctiva* covers the anterior portion of the sclera and inside of the eyelids and ends at the limbus (Fig. 119.1).

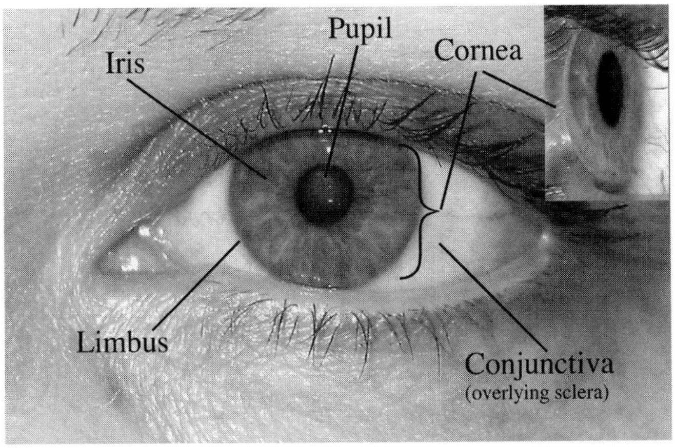

FIG. 119.1. External anatomy of the eye. (Photograph courtesy of Cathy Burkat, M.D.)

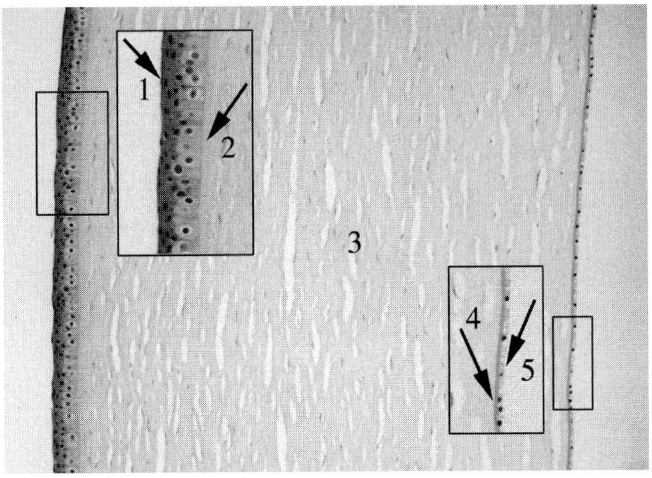

FIG. 119.2. **A:** Slitlamp photograph of a normal cornea. **B:** Light microscope photograph of normal corneal anatomy. From anterior to posterior: *1*, epithelium; *2*, Bowman membrane; *3*, stroma; *4*, Descemet membrane; *5*, endothelium. (Photographs courtesy of William Fischer, M.S.)

Cornea

The cornea is a clear, regularly curved structure that acts as the primary refractive lens of the eye. It is transparent because of its unique collagen structure, and its surface is smooth to provide maximal optical clarity. The cornea is avascular and devoid of lymphatic tissue but can stimulate immunologic responses via cytokines and other cellular signals.

The cornea is composed of five layers (Fig. 119.2). The outermost layer, the *epithelium*, is five to seven cells thick and the layer most often damaged in a corneal abrasion. The next layer is the *Bowman membrane*, which is composed of collagen and connective tissue. It serves as a supporting tissue for the overlying cells of the epithelium. Beneath the Bowman membrane is the *stroma*, which comprises the bulk of the corneal thickness. The stroma is composed of an orderly array of collagen fibrils, and this arrangement of lamellae is responsible for the transparency of the cornea. Beneath the stroma lies the *Descemet's membrane*, which is the basement membrane of the innermost layer, the *endothelium*. The endothelium is composed of a single layer of cells that do not divide and pumps fluid actively out of the cornea into the eye, so that a thin, clear cornea is maintained.

CLINICAL CONDITIONS

Ocular Inflammation and Infection

The hallmark of ocular inflammation is conjunctival injection. However, conjunctival injection may develop when structures adjacent to or contiguous with the conjunctiva become inflamed. These include the sclera, episclera, cornea, and iris. Depending on the structure involved, such inflammation is termed *scleritis*, *episcleritis*, *keratitis*, or *iritis*. Conjunctival inflammation ranges from mild to severe hyperemia, and the discharge may vary in character from clear to copious and purulent. The most common infectious causes of *conjunctivitis* are bacteria and viruses, with the latter responsible for most of the cases of conjunctivitis evaluated per year in offices and emergency rooms. The most serious form of infective conjunctivitis is caused by *Neisseria gonorrhoeae*; this entity can lead to corneal ulceration and perforation. Typically, gonococcal conjunctivitis is explosive in onset and characterized by severe injection and copious mucopurulent discharge.

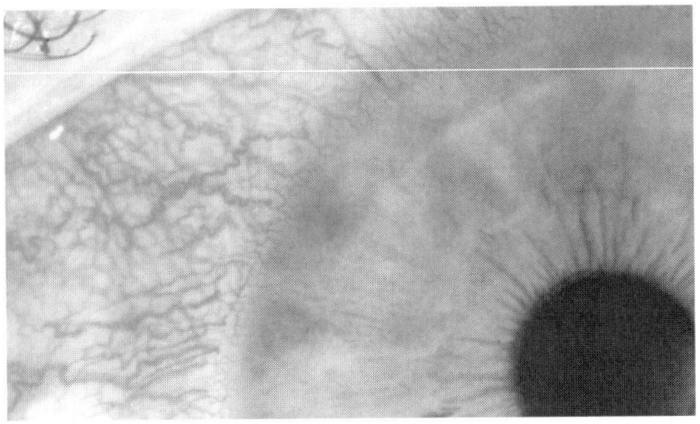

FIG. 119.3. Ciliary flush. Note that injection is more prominent near the limbus. (Photograph courtesy of Steven S. T. Ching, M.D.)

Other causes of conjunctivitis are immunologic, allergic, chemical, mechanical, and idiopathic.

Episcleritis, which is an inflammation of the thin layer of vascularized connective tissue overlying the sclera, is relatively uncommon. It is generally benign and self-limited and may be idiopathic or associated with systemic diseases, particularly autoimmune diseases. *Scleritis*, which is an inflammation of the sclera itself, is also uncommon. The red eye associated with scleritis is often accompanied by pain that is typically severe and tenderness of the globe.

Keratitis is an inflammation of the cornea. A keratitis can be infective, immunologic, or mechanical. Bacterial infective keratitis is oftentimes caused by the bacterial flora of the adjacent lids, most commonly *Staphylococcus* and *Streptococcus* species. Other causes of severe infective keratitis include *Pseudomonas* species or *Acanthamoeba* in contact lens wearers, acute and chronic ocular infection with herpes simplex virus, and rarely fungi. Examples of noninfective keratitis include the following: *keratitis sicca*, caused by a deficiency of tears; neurotrophic keratitis; marginal keratitis, caused by a hypersensitivity to staphylococcal breakdown products; and keratitis resulting from trauma. Because the cornea is the main lens of the eye, inflammation may result in ulceration and scarring with loss of vision. Therefore, once it is recognized that a red eye is secondary to a keratitis, the patient should be referred to eye care professionals for treatment.

Other causes of a red eye include *iritis*, which is an inflammation of the iris or the iris and ciliary body, and *acute angle-closure glaucoma*, which results from a sudden and complete occlusion of the anterior chamber angle by iris tissue.

In an isolated conjunctivitis, dilated conjunctival vessels do not usually involve the limbus, whereas in inflammation of the sclera, cornea, and iris, vascular injection surrounds the cornea at the limbus, a condition termed *limbal* or *ciliary flush* (Fig. 119.3). Conjunctivitis can be differentiated from other causes of a red eye by the presence of ciliary flush, visual loss, pain, changes in corneal clarity, and pupillary abnormalities (Table 119.1).

Neonatal and Perinatal Conditions

Neonatal conjunctivitis is rarely seen these days given the widespread empiric therapy of newborns after birth. However, it is important to note that chlamydial and gonococcal forms of conjunctivitis can be seen after birth and in young children. An appropriate diagnostic workup should be pursued in these particular instances and treatment instituted promptly.

Corneal abnormalities at birth may be classified as abnormalities of size or clarity. Abnormalities of size include *microcornea*, in which the cornea is smaller than 10 mm, and *megalocornea*, in which it is larger than 12 mm.

Abnormalities of corneal clarity include developmental abnormalities, neonatal corneal infection, trauma, and glaucoma. Examples of significant developmental abnormalities are *sclerocornea* and *Peter anomaly*, which describes a spectrum of malformations of the anterior chamber that may include central corneal clouding and adherence of the lens to the cornea. In *congenital hereditary endothelial dystrophy*, corneal clouding is present at birth or develops shortly after. The condition is bilateral, symmetric, and noninflammatory. Other conditions associated with corneal clouding include congenital glaucoma, congenital rubella, neonatal herpes simplex keratitis, and injury from forceps delivery. Congenital glaucoma is also characterized by high intraocular pressures and enlarged corneal diameters. Perinatal infections such as rubella are significantly associated with other malformations of the anterior segment of the eye. Neonatal herpes simplex keratitis is important because of the possibility of corneal scarring and neonatal viremia. Forceps injuries can cause a partial rupture of the cornea, with corneal edema and scarring. The severity of the corneal edema depends on the extent of the injury. Although the cornea may eventually clear after any of these insults, the visual deprivation may cause amblyopia.

Effects of Topical Medications during Pregnancy

Topical medications are the mainstay of medical treatment in ophthalmology. However, it is important to realize that common ophthalmic drops have side effects, especially during pregnancy. Ophthalmic medications are often absorbed systemically. For instance, topical ocular beta-blockers can decrease the forced expiratory volume in 1 second (FEV_1) and

TABLE 119.1. Common Causes of Red Eye, with Differential Diagnoses

	Ciliary flush	Visual loss	Pain	Corneal clarity	Pupillary abnormality
Conjunctivitis	Negative	None	Usually none	Clear	None
Episcleritis	Segmental +	None	Occasional	Clear	None
Scleritis	Yes	Usually none	Moderate to severe	Clear (unless associated with keratitis	None
Keratitis	Yes	Often	Mild to severe	Decreased	None
Iritis	Yes	Sometimes	Photophobia or pain with accommodation	Usually clear	Constricted or irregular shape
Angle-closure glaucoma	Yes	Yes	Severe	Decreased	Usually 5 mm and nonreactive

Source: Adapted from Bradford CA, ed. *Basic ophthalmology for medical students and primary care residents.* San Francisco: American Academy of Ophthalmology, 1999, with permission.

precipitate asthma in susceptible patients. Brimonidine (Alphagan), a glaucoma medication, has been shown to cause somnolence or coma when used in children, and secretion in breast milk is unknown. Also, patients taking psychiatric medications, such as monoamine oxidase inhibitors, are advised to avoid the medication because of possible drug interactions. Atropine sulfate and scopolamine are two anticholinergic agents used to dilate the pupil. Topical application of these drugs can occasionally result in depression of the respiratory drive, urinary retention, changes in mental status, and tachycardia. To minimize systemic absorption, digital pressure can be applied over the medial canthus for 5 minutes when the medication is applied. The use of these and other ophthalmic medications should be discussed with an eye care professional when a pregnancy is confirmed.

Disorders of Corneal Curvature

The curvature of the cornea provides the primary refractive power of the eye. Subtle changes in curvature associated with astigmatism can be easily corrected with glasses or contact lenses. However, in a few conditions, glasses or contact lenses alone cannot completely correct the refractive error, such as when the curvature of the cornea is excessively thinned or ectatic. Corneal ectasia may occur centrally or peripherally.

Keratoconus is the most common of these disorders; the name is derived from the conical shape of the cornea that develops during the course of the disease. The apex of the cone becomes fairly thin, and visual acuity decreases as the irregularity of the corneal curvature increases (Fig. 119.4). Pellucid marginal degeneration is a variant of keratoconus characterized by thinning of the peripheral cornea. Both forms of corneal ectasia result in abnormal curvature of the cornea and irregular refraction of light through the cornea. In severe cases, the thinning results in rupture of the Descemet membrane, which causes acute corneal edema (acute hydrops). In these changes of corneal curvature, glasses are first used to treat the decreased visual acuity. Eventually, the irregularity can be corrected only with rigid, gas-permeable contact lenses. When medical therapy with glasses or rigid contact lenses fails because of poor visual acuity or intolerance of contact lenses, a corneal transplantation may be performed.

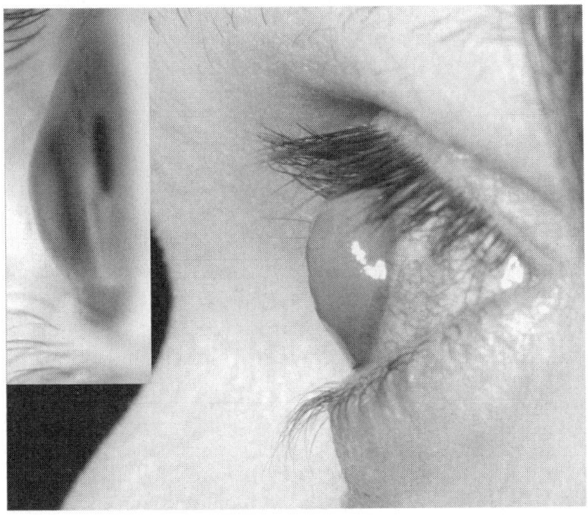

FIG. 119.4. Keratoconus with acute hydrops. **Inset:** Side view of a cornea with keratoconus. (Photographs courtesy of Steven S. T. Ching, M.D.)

Endothelial Dysfunction

The endothelium serves as a mechanical pump, actively removing fluid from the stroma of the cornea. Inadequate function of the pump leads to corneal edema, loss of corneal clarity, and reduced visual acuity. Endothelial dysfunction can result from hereditary conditions such as congenital hereditary endothelial dystrophy, Fuchs' endothelial dystrophy, and posterior polymorphous dystrophy. The endothelium may also be compromised after trauma (forceps injury or intraocular surgery) or chronic intraocular inflammation (uveitis).

Fuchs' endothelial dystrophy is an autosomal-dominant disorder that affects women 2.5 times more often than men. It is a bilateral process, although it may present asymmetrically, rarely in persons younger than 50 years. On the other hand, posterior polymorphous dystrophy, which is also bilateral and may present asymmetrically, affects younger patients, in their second to third decade. It is mostly asymptomatic and can be associated with glaucoma. As discussed previously, congenital hereditary endothelial dystrophy, a condition diagnosed in newborns, also presents with endothelial dysfunction. Definitive treatment for these conditions involves transplantation of a donor cornea to replace the affected tissue.

Dry Eye

The normal tear film consists of three layers: a superficial lipid layer, a middle aqueous layer, and lastly a basal mucin layer. The three act in conjunction to provide a stable tear film, which is distributed over the surface of the eye during a normal blink. Any disruption of the production of these components can lead to symptoms of a dry eye. Tear insufficiencies are usually caused by lipid or aqueous disorders. The meibomian glands, located in the eyelid margin, produce the lipid of the tear film. Dysfunction of these glands can result in an unstable tear film and dry eye secondary to evaporative causes. A decrease in the production of the aqueous component is another cause of dry eye.

Systemic diseases also contribute to dry eye syndromes. Autoimmune disorders such as Sjögren syndrome and Graves thyroid ophthalmopathy can contribute to a tear-deficient state. Lid abnormalities or changes resulting from injury can cause dry eye secondary to exposure of the ocular surface with incomplete closure or improper distribution of the tear film with poor blinking. Some medications affect the tear film, most notably oral contraceptives and antihistamines. Treatment for these conditions ranges from replacement with artificial tears to surgical intervention.

TREATMENT

Corneal Transplant Surgery

The clarity and regular surface of the cornea are paramount in maintaining good vision. After disease or injury, the cornea may become cloudy, irregular in shape, scarred, or irreparably damaged. If medicines are ineffective, the damaged cornea can in some cases be replaced with a healthy cornea from a deceased person. This replacement procedure is called *corneal transplantation*. Several types of corneal transplantation have been developed. Depending on the extent and nature of the disease, the surgeon may choose to perform an anterior partial transplant *(lamellar keratoplasty)* or full-thickness transplant *(penetrating keratoplasty)*.

Corneal transplantation was the first successful transplant surgery performed (Eduard Zinn in 1906). The success rate of the procedure varies depending on the disease of the host but approaches 90% in persons with noninflammatory disorders. Approximately 35,000 procedures are performed each year in the United States.

Corneal tissue for transplantation is received at an eye bank as part of an organ donation program, much like organs such as the heart or liver. The donor tissue is carefully inspected and tested to rule out any disease that might be transmitted to the recipient. The donor's medical history is also reviewed for any transmissible diseases; if positive, the tissue is not accepted. The cornea can be stored for several days in a nutrient fluid before use. When healthy tissue becomes available, the local eye bank enters the information into a nationwide computer network. The use of HLA matching or cross-matched tissue has been controversial, but in a large multicenter study, matching was not shown to reduce the chance of graft rejection.

INDICATIONS AND PROCEDURE

A replacement cornea is indicated when loss of vision is caused by a lack of corneal clarity, as in scarring or edema, or an abnormal corneal curvature, as in corneal ectasia.

The most frequently performed corneal transplant procedure is the full-thickness penetrating keratoplasty, in which a full-thickness circular piece of tissue is removed. Under a microscope, a circular knife (trephine) is used like a cookie cutter to remove the center of the diseased cornea. A "button" of similar size is cut from a donor cornea. The donor tissue is then sewn in place with multiple fine nylon sutures or one or two continuous sutures. If it has been determined before surgery that a cataract is present, it can be removed and an intraocular lens implanted during the corneal transplant operation.

After the surgery, topical antibiotics and topical steroids are used to prevent infection and rejection of the new graft. Very rarely, a patient is given systemic immunosuppressive medication.

The recovery period required to achieve good vision can be up to 1 year because of the slow healing rate of the avascular cornea. Patients should be informed that the corneal wound will be weak for the entire lifetime of the eye and that proper precautions must be taken. Possible complications include, but are not limited to, astigmatism, infection, bleeding, retinal detachment, glaucoma, and cataract. Occasionally, the donor cornea is rejected and becomes cloudy. Early rejection is indicated by symptoms of pain, conjunctival injection, ocular discharge, and decreased visual acuity. If detected early, 90% of rejection reactions can be reversed by increasing steroid administration. The risk for graft rejection is highest in the first year after transplantation but remains throughout the lifetime of the graft.

Contact Lenses

The most commonly used contact lens is the soft contact lens. It offers many advantages: comfort, quick adaptation, reduced incidence of lens dislodgement, ease of placement, and disposability. The selection of soft contact lenses is also greater, with various materials and designs available. With flexibility of function, such as daily wear, extended wear, and bifocal lenses, contact lenses can be customized to the patient's lifestyle.

Rigid, gas-permeable contact lenses have been slightly less popular because of the longer "breaking in" period required. They can be less comfortable than soft contact lenses, especially during the initial fitting period. Difficulty in stabilizing the lens may resulting in image movement or dislodgement. However, rigid lenses offer many advantages, including superior quality of vision, correction of astigmatism, durability, ease of handling and removal, and lower overall cost.

Complications of contact lens wear include abrasions, infection, sterile inflammation (keratitis), and irregular corneal shaping (warpage). The comfort and fit of contact lenses may change during pregnancy. Intolerance may develop during pregnancy as a result of a change in the corneal curvature, an increase in corneal thickness or edema, or a change in the tear film. Any of these may cause blurred vision, a change in the lens prescription, or a change in the fit of the contact lenses. It is recommended that one wait several weeks postpartum before a new refraction is prescribed.

Bacterial infections are an uncommon but devastating complication of contact lens use. Annually, an infection develops in 1 in 2,500 daily contact wearers and 1 in 500 overnight lens wearers. Because of this risk, contact lens wearers are advised to discontinue lens wear temporarily if pain, conjunctival injection, or ocular discharge develops.

Refractive Surgery

The refractive nature (ability to bend light) of the eye depends on the length of the eye, corneal curvature, and power of the internal crystalline lens. If the light is focused exactly on the retina, the patient is *emmetropic*. If light rays are focused in front of the retina, the person is *myopic*, or nearsighted. If the light rays are focused behind the retina, the person is *hyperopic*, or farsighted. The objective of refractive surgery is to refocus light onto the retina.

The cornea is a lens that accounts for two thirds of the refractive power of the eye. For this reason, small changes on the corneal surface can cause significant changes in refractive power. The corneal tissue is also readily accessible and can be modified without entering into the eye. Currently, the corneal curvature can be modified by photorefractive keratectomy (PRK), laser in situ keratomileusis (LASIK), or laser epithelial keratomileusis (LASEK).

PHOTOREFRACTIVE KERATECTOMY

In PRK, the epithelium of the eye is removed with a spatula or blade. Once the underlying corneal tissue is exposed, an excimer laser, which uses a cool ultraviolet light beam to precisely remove, or *ablate*, small amounts of tissue from the surface of the cornea, reshapes it. Often, a bandage contact lens is placed for comfort until the corneal epithelium heals.

In nearsighted persons, the laser is used to flatten the overly steep cornea and decrease its refractive power. In farsighted people, selective ablation in the mid peripheral cornea steepens the cornea and increases its refractive power. Also, excimer lasers can correct astigmatism by smoothing an irregular cornea into a more normal shape.

LASER IN SITU KERATOMILEUSIS

In LASIK, a corneal "flap" is created with an instrument called a *microkeratome*. This thin, circular flap in the cornea is folded back out of the way, and the tissue underneath is reshaped with an excimer laser. The flap is then laid back in place to cover the area where the corneal tissue was removed.

The advantages of LASIK over PRK include less perioperative pain and a more rapid return of vision because the surface layers of the eye are maintained.

LASER EPITHELIAL KERATOMILEUSIS

In LASEK, the epithelium is cut not with the microkeratome used in LASIK but with a finer circular blade called a *trephine*. The surgeon covers the area with an alcohol solution to loosen the edges of the epithelium. After removing the alcohol solution from the eye, the surgeon uses a tiny instrument to lift the edge of the epithelial flap and gently fold it back out of the way. An excimer laser is used to sculpt the corneal tissue underneath. Afterward, the epithelial flap is replaced carefully, and a bandage contact lens is placed over the eye.

COMPLICATIONS OF REFRACTIVE SURGERY

Although refractive surgery has been quite successful, it is not without complications. Undercorrection or overcorrection is possible and necessitates further treatment. The patient's vision may gradually revert to its preoperative prescription, a process called *regression*. Patients often temporarily experience dry eye, which is a consequence of interruption of the corneal nerves during the procedure. They may also be bothered by halos or glare or experience double vision, usually for a few days but sometimes for several months. This may be caused by infection, irregularly healing epithelium, or decentered areas of laser treatment. The development of scarring or haze in the area of treatment can result in clouding of vision. Rarely, sterile inflammation can occur underneath the flap after LASIK, a condition called *diffuse lamellar keratitis*.

SUMMARY

As refractive surgery has become more commonplace, it is important to remember that not every patient is a good candidate for the procedure. In-depth evaluation and measurements are required to determine which procedure is most likely to benefit the patient, or whether refractive surgery should be performed at all. It should be noted that the shape of the cornea can change during pregnancy, and refractive surgery should be deferred until after the postpartum period.

BIBLIOGRAPHY

Azar DM. Refractive surgery. In: Yanoff M, Duker J, eds. *Ophthalmology*. London: Mosby, 1999:1.1–7.16.

Berlin RJ, Lee UT, Samples JR, et al. Ophthalmic drops causing coma in an infant. *J Pediatr* 2001;138:441–443.

Bradford CA. The red eye. In: Bradford CA, ed. *Basic ophthalmology for medical students and primary care residents*. San Francisco: American Academy of Ophthalmology, 1999.

Davis EA, Dana MR. Pregnancy and the eye. In: Albert DM, Jakobiec FA, Azar DT, et al., eds. *Principles and practice of ophthalmology*, 2nd ed. Philadelphia: WB Saunders, 2000:4767–4783.

Feder RS. Noninflammatory ectatic disorders. In: Krachmer JH, Mannis MJ, Holland EJ, eds. *Cornea*. New York: Mosby, 1997:1091–1106.

Kim T, Palay DA. Developmental corneal anomalies of size and shape. In: Krachmer JH, Mannis MJ, Holland EJ, eds. *Cornea*. New York: Mosby, 1997:871–883.

Lindquist TD. Conjunctivitis—an overview and classification. In: Krachmer JH, Mannis MJ, Holland EJ, eds. *Cornea*. New York: Mosby, 1997:745–758.

O'Brien TP. Bacterial keratitis. In: Krachmer JH, Mannis MJ, Holland EJ, eds. *Cornea*. New York: Mosby, 1997:1139–1155.

Stein HA, Freeman MI, Stein RM, et al. *CLAO resident contact lens curriculum manual*, 2nd ed. New York: Kellner/McCaffery Associates, 1999.

Sugar J. Cornea and external disease. In: Yanoff M, Duker J, eds. *Ophthalmology*. London: Mosby, 1999:1.1–15.6.

CHAPTER 120
Retinal Diseases

Steven J. Rose

The retina is the specialized tissue that lines the back of the eye and is most commonly associated with the transformation of light energy into perceived visual images. The anatomic arrangement of the nine layers of the retina clearly identifies it as one of the most highly organized tissues of the body (Fig. 120.1). Light energy is received at the level of the photoreceptors; it is modified and reorganized as it travels through the retina to the optic nerve and then onto the occipital cortex of the brain, where visual imaging actually takes place.

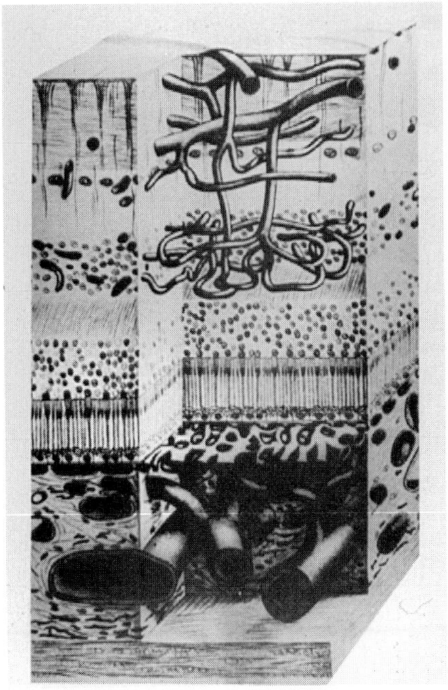

FIG. 120.1. Anatomic arrangement of the retina. The top of the figure represents the vitreous side, the bottom is choroidal.

The vitreous body, which constitutes most of the volume of the eye, is essentially an optically empty chamber. In normal, healthy persons, the various structural and physiologic roles of the vitreous maintain optical integrity. Abnormal vitreoretinal relationships can, however, lead to a number of disease states that ultimately affect vision.

This chapter presents the most common retinal diseases encountered in a primary care setting: retinal vascular diseases, diabetic retinopathy, age-related macular degeneration, inflammatory and infectious diseases, retinal tears, and retinal detachment. Recognition of these disease states and the need for referral to the appropriate ophthalmologist is stressed.

EXAMINATION OF THE FUNDUS

Before the retinal diseases likely to be encountered in practice are described, the practical aspects of the retinal examination are presented.

A thorough examination of the fundus requires excellent powers of observation, and clinical experience with ophthalmoscopy is necessary. Most clinicians have been introduced to the direct ophthalmoscope at the beginning of their clinical training in medical school, with emphasis placed on observation of the optic nerve head and, secondarily, the blood vessels. Unfortunately, the most helpful adjunct to examining the retina, pupillary dilation, has never been stressed consistently. Examination of the fundus, and especially the retinal periphery, is greatly facilitated by a well-dilated pupil. Suggested dilating medications include 1% tropicamide (Mydriacyl) and 2.5% phenylephrine drops (Mydfrin), one drop of each in both eyes. Most patients' eyes dilate adequately after 20 to 30 minutes; however, darkly pigmented irises dilate more slowly. The reluctance to dilate eyes originates from the fear that dilation will precipitate attacks of

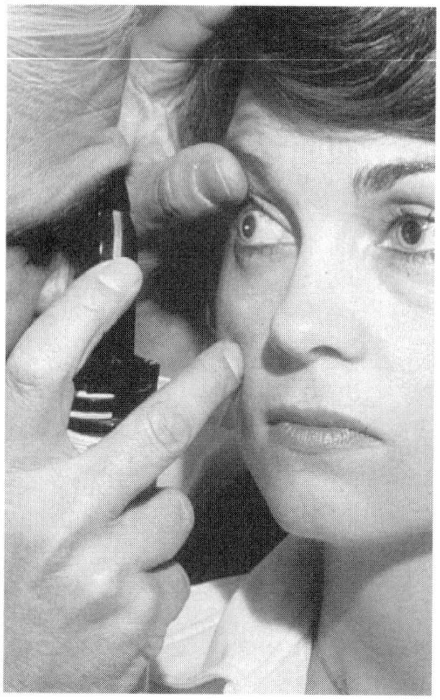

FIG. 120.2. Examination of the fundus with direct ophthalmoscope.

narrow-angle glaucoma. However, this is a concern for only a few patients, and the cases of disease missed through failure to dilate the pupils are, in my opinion, potentially more harmful than the glaucoma, which can be safely treated.

To examine the ocular fundus, specialized instruments are necessary. The simplest and most familiar to primary care practitioners is the direct ophthalmoscope, which is, in essence, a miniature flashlight held close to the examiner's and patient's eyes and shone through the pupil (Fig. 120.2). The fundus is viewed monocularly through a small aperture just above the source of illumination; an upright, virtual image is produced that magnifies the area being examined about 15 times. A set of neutralizing lenses built into the ophthalmoscope can be dialed to achieve the sharpest image for the examiner.

Although magnification and resolution are good with the direct ophthalmoscope, some disadvantages limit its effectiveness. The lack of stereopsis (depth perception), inadequate illumination in the presence of media opacities (corneal scars), visualization of only about 8% of the total retinal area, and considerable degradation of the image in patients with significant lens opacities all contribute to a suboptimal screening examination. Furthermore, the direct ophthalmoscope does not provide an undistorted view of the peripheral retina, so that its use is limited to the posterior retina. The use of other ophthalmoscopes, such as the binocular indirect ophthalmoscope, is beyond the scope of practice for the primary care provider and is not covered here.

In summary, the direct ophthalmoscope, in conjunction with pupillary dilation, serves the primary care practitioner well as a screening device for evaluating papilledema, macular degeneration, and diabetic and hypertensive retinopathy.

RETINAL VASCULAR DISEASES

Diabetic Retinopathy

Diabetic retinopathy is one of the four most frequent causes of new blindness in the United States and the leading cause in the 20- to 64-year-old age group. An estimated 14 million Americans have diabetes mellitus. Of these, 10% to 15% have insulin-dependent diabetes mellitus (type 1), which usually is diagnosed before 40 years of age. Most patients, however, have non–insulin-dependent diabetes mellitus (type 2), which is usually diagnosed in patients older than 40 years. Although the incidence of severe ocular complications is higher in patients with type 1 diabetes mellitus, the number of patients with type 2 diabetes mellitus is larger overall, so that they account for the majority of clinical cases.

The prevalence of all types of retinopathy in the diabetic population increases with the duration of diabetes and advancing age. The prevalence of any degree of retinopathy reaches 50% in persons with disease of 7 years' duration and approaches 90% after 17 to 25 years. Systemic hormonal changes occurring at puberty result in an increased prevalence of retinopathy after 13 years of age. Furthermore, associated health and medical conditions present a significant risk for the development and progression of diabetic retinopathy. These include pregnancy, hypertension, chronic hyperglycemia, renal disease, and hyperlipidemia.

The cause of diabetic microvascular disease is not known. It has been suggested that protracted hyperglycemia results in the glycosylation of tissue proteins and ultimate damage. Certain physiologic abnormalities have been identified to occur early in the course of diabetic retinopathy. These include impaired autoregulation of retinal blood vessels, alterations in blood flow, and breakdown of the blood-retinal barrier, a normally impermeable vascular entity.

Studies suggest that the speed of retinal blood flow in large vessels increases with progressive disease. Subsequent capillary closure causes retinal ischemia, which at some critical point results in the release of a vasoproliferative factor that stimulates the growth of new blood vessels from the retina, optic nerve, or iris.

The clinical features of diabetic retinopathy most likely are present before any visual symptoms occur; therefore, it is critical to screen for this disease in yearly examinations performed in the primary practitioner's office. Various retinal lesions identify the risk for progression of retinopathy and visual loss.

The first clinical signs of diabetic retinopathy are microaneurysms, which are saccular outpouchings of retinal capillaries (Fig. 120.3). Ruptured microaneurysms and decompensated capillaries result in intraretinal hemorrhages. The clinical appearance of these hemorrhages reflects the retinal level at which they occur. Hemorrhages at the nerve fiber layer tend to be flame-shaped, whereas those deeper in the retina look like

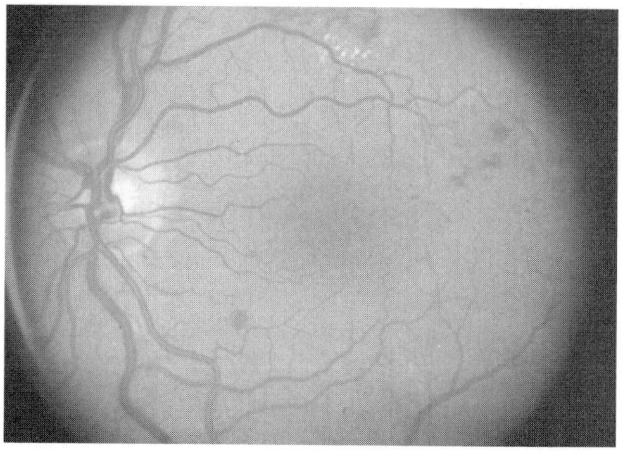

FIG. 120.3. Macular area of a diabetic patient with small hemorrhages from microaneurysms.

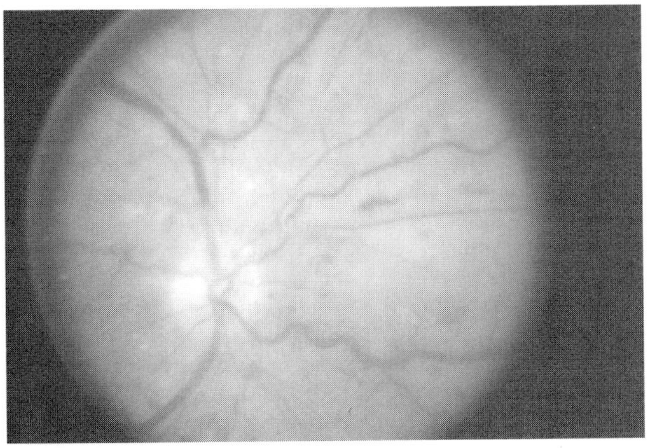

FIG. 120.4. Venous abnormalities in a patient with diabetic retinopathy. Note the sausage shape of the vasculature.

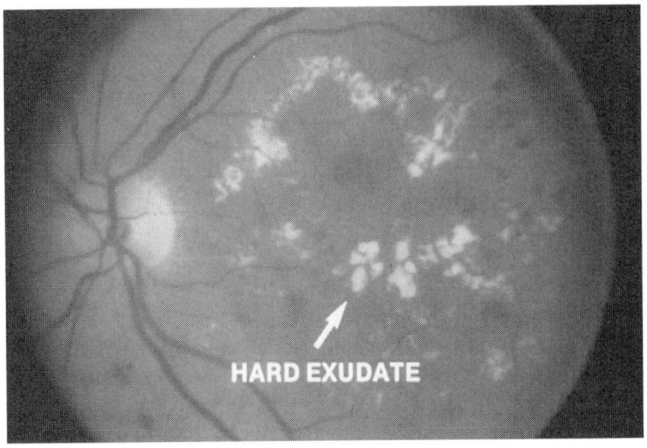

FIG. 120.6. Macular edema with significant hard exudates.

pinpoints or dots. Abnormalities of venous caliber indicate severe retinal hypoxia. These changes can be venous dilation, venous beading, or loop formation (Fig. 120.4).

Proliferative diabetic retinopathy (Fig. 120.5) is marked by proliferating endothelial cell tubules. They grow either at or near the optic disc (neovascularization of the disc) or elsewhere in the retina (neovascularization elsewhere). Fibrous tissue may appear to grow with these new vessels.

Diabetic retinopathy is classified in two main stages: nonproliferative and proliferative. The nonproliferative stage is characterized by focal intraretinal capillary closure and increased retinal vascular permeability. The hemorrhagic changes described previously are the clinical manifestations of this stage. In addition, exuded serum proteins, including lipoproteins, are seen as hard exudates (Fig. 120.6).

Retinal thickening is an important consequence of abnormal retinal vascular permeability. Edema involving the macula is probably the most common cause of decreased vision in diabetic retinopathy. Diabetic maculopathy may present as focal or diffuse retinal thickening with or without deposits of intraretinal lipoprotein exudates.

The diagnosis of diabetic retinopathy, although mainly based on clinical findings, is aided by an imaging technique known as *fluorescein angiography*. Sodium fluorescein, a dye, is injected into a peripheral vein. Up to 70% of the injected dye molecules are bound to serum albumin and other large protein molecules; an unbound portion is left that can diffuse through small intercellular spaces. As the dye enters the retinal circulation, fluorescence is documented with a special fundus camera and black and white film. Abnormal leakage (Fig. 120.7) is noted and can guide treatment. Although fluorescein angiography can be performed safely during pregnancy with little apparent risk to either mother or fetus, it is recommended that the test not be performed unless absolutely necessary. Similar precautions are advised during breast-feeding.

The treatment of diabetic retinopathy consists of medical control of retinopathy, laser therapy, and surgery.

The medical control of diabetic retinopathy has been a long-sought but elusive ideal. In the Diabetes Control and Complications Trial, a nationwide clinical trial that compared tight control of blood glucose levels with standard control, tight control significantly reduced the rate of progression and severity of diabetic retinopathy.

The association of hypertension with the development of diabetic retinopathy is well documented, but the degree to which it exacerbates retinopathy is uncertain. One study showed systolic blood pressure to be a predictor of the incidence of diabetic retinopathy, and diastolic blood pressure to be a predictor of the progression of retinopathy.

Laser photocoagulation remains the cornerstone of treatment for both nonproliferative and proliferative diabetic retinopathy. A collimated beam of light energy at certain wavelengths is used to create focal burns at the level of the retina.

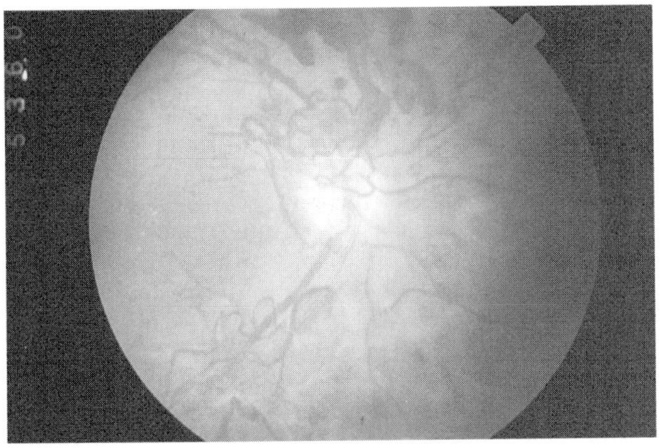

FIG. 120.5. Proliferative diabetic retinopathy with florid neovascularization of the optic nerve.

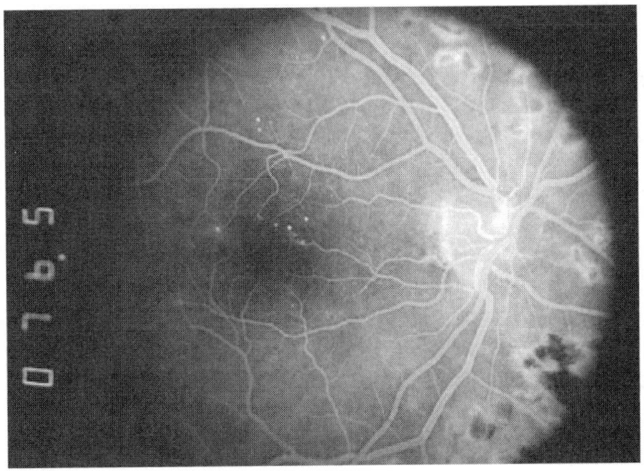

FIG. 120.7. Fluorescein angiogram of macula with pinpoint leaks near the fovea from diabetic microaneurysms.

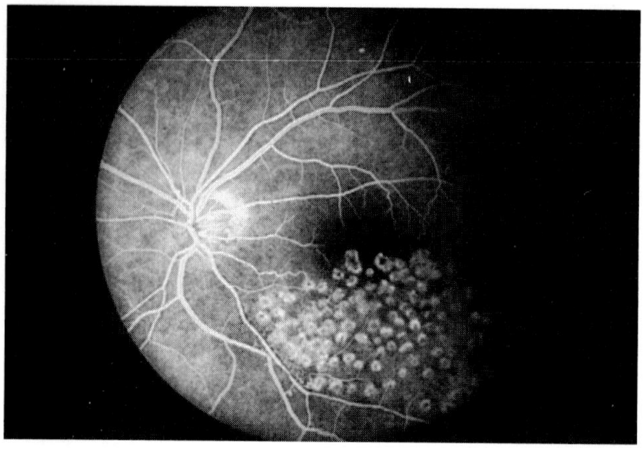

FIG. 120.8. Fluorescein angiogram depicting grid laser treatment pattern.

Focal macular edema is treated by direct focal closure of the leaking blood vessels, whereas diffuse macular edema is treated with an indirect grid pattern (Fig. 120.8). Scatter photocoagulation (Fig. 120.9) is used to treat proliferative diabetic retinopathy. Multiple laser burns (total of 1,500–2,500 burns) are placed in the mid peripheral retina during two or more sessions. The response to laser treatment varies, but since its introduction in the latter half of the 20th century, millions of diabetics have been saved from certain blindness.

If a patient fails to respond to laser treatment, surgical intervention in which the vitreous (vitrectomy) and abnormal fibroproliferative tissues are removed can also save many eyes from severe visual loss. These techniques require specialized training and experience and are performed by ophthalmologists who subspecialize in vitreoretinal diseases and surgery.

Pregnancy presents a unique situation with regard to diabetic retinopathy. The acceleration of proliferative retinopathy and poor control of hyperglycemia are well-known clinical phenomena in pregnant women with diabetes. Glucose metabolism is disturbed by the anabolic needs of the developing fetus and the hormonal state of pregnancy. Patients with advanced retinopathy formerly were cautioned against pregnancy because of retinopathy and maternal and neonatal complications. Currently, the efficacy of laser photocoagulation has eliminated retinopathy as a contraindication to pregnancy.

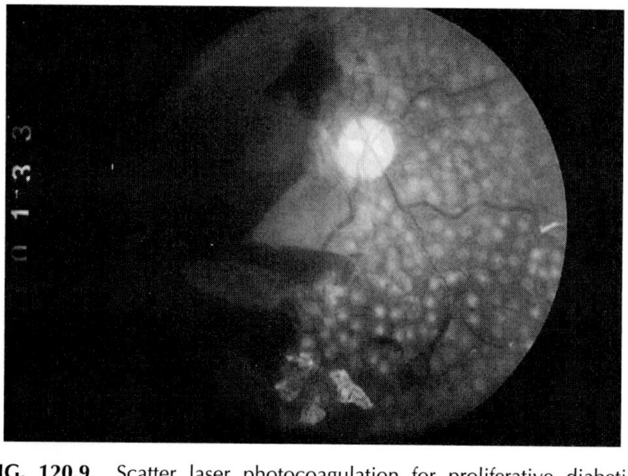

FIG. 120.9. Scatter laser photocoagulation for proliferative diabetic retinopathy.

The effect of pregnancy on the progression of retinopathy is controversial. Few randomized prospective studies have compared pregnant and nonpregnant diabetic women. Diabetic women with no or minimal nonproliferative retinopathy are at minimal risk for the development of vision-threatening complications during pregnancy. Macular edema can be marked during pregnancy, especially in women with hypertension or nephropathy, but is unlikely to lead to permanent visual loss.

Pregnant women with relatively severe nonproliferative retinopathy are at higher risk for progression to proliferative retinopathy. Without laser treatment, more than half progress to proliferative retinopathy during pregnancy. Increased intravascular volume and Valsalva maneuvers during delivery may increase the risk for vitreous hemorrhage. Prompt laser photocoagulation should be considered for pregnant women with severe nonproliferative diabetic retinopathy or early proliferative retinopathy. Macular edema can be treated at the same time. In patients who have undergone laser treatment for proliferative retinopathy with complete regression, progression has been noted during subsequent pregnancy, although this is rare.

Until a cure for diabetes is found, the emphasis must be on identification, careful follow-up, and timely laser intervention. Proper care results in a reduction of personal suffering in addition to a substantial cost savings for all involved. Table 120.1 provides guidelines for an eye examination schedule.

Hypertensive Retinopathy

Systemic hypertension initially causes a local or generalized vasoconstriction of the retinal arterioles. Prolonged acute systemic hypertension may disrupt the blood-retinal barrier, resulting in leakage of plasma and formed blood elements into the retina, similar to the diabetic changes previously described.

A consequence of prolonged systemic hypertension is thickening of the walls of the retinal arterioles. Clinically, the thickened arterioles have a broader and brighter reflex. Because the arteries and veins share an adventitial sheath where they cross, characteristic changes can be seen at the arteriovenous crossings, including nicking (Fig. 120.10). If arteriolar sclerosis advances significantly, several complications may occur, including macroaneurysm formation and occlusion of the central retinal artery or vein.

During pregnancy, hypertensive retinal changes may develop secondary to preeclampsia or toxemia of pregnancy. Visual loss ranging from mild to total blindness can occur. The pathologic changes are seen at the level of the choroid, or blood supply under the retina. The acute hypertensive crisis causes reversible damage to the network of small blood vessels (lamina choriocapillaris), which in turn damages the overlying retinal pigment epithelium. As a result of the breakdown in the pigment epithelial barrier, fluid collects under the retina. In extreme cases, a total exudative retinal detachment occurs, with total loss of vision.

Toxemia can also cause optic nerve swelling with or without concomitant retinal damage.

Treatment is directed at the underlying cause, and direct treatment of the retina is rarely required. In most cases, vision returns to normal. The primary care provider and the ophthalmologist should work closely together during these periods.

Arterial Occlusive Disease

The blood supply to the inner layers of the retina is entirely from the central retinal artery, a branch of the ophthalmic artery, which is in turn a branch of the internal carotid. Retinal ischemia develops when disease affects the afferent vessels, any-

TABLE 120.1. Eye Examination Schedule for Diabetic Patients

Type of diabetes	Recommended time of first examination	Routine minimal follow-up interval
Type 1 (IDDM) and Type 2 (NIDDM)	Five years after onset or at time of diagnosis	Yearly
During pregnancy	Before pregnancy for counseling Early in first trimester	Each trimester or more frequently as indicated 3–6 months postpartum

IDDM, insulin-dependent diabetes mellitus; NIDDM, non–insulin-dependent diabetes mellitus.

where from the common carotid artery to the retinal arterioles. The signs and symptoms of arteriolar obstruction depend on the vessel involved. Ophthalmic artery disease can cause total blindness, whereas occlusion of an extramacular arteriole may be asymptomatic. The loss of vision is usually abrupt, although symptoms of intermittent loss of vision (amaurosis fugax) may precede the final event.

The two major types of arterial occlusion are branch retinal artery occlusion (BRAO) and central retinal artery occlusion (CRAO). In BRAO, the patient usually notices a partial blind spot or scotoma near the central visual field. Clinically, acute BRAO manifests as an edematous, white retina caused by infarction of the affected vessel (Fig. 120.11). With time, the edema resolves, and the vessel reopens or recanalizes. A permanent field defect remains. Three main varieties of emboli are recognized: cholesterol emboli arising from the carotid artery, platelet-fibrin emboli associated with large vessel arteriosclerosis, and calcific emboli from diseased cardiac valves. Rare forms of emboli include fat emboli from long bone fractures, emboli from cardiac myxoma, septic emboli from infective endocarditis, and talc emboli in intravenous drug abusers.

Management is directed toward determining the systemic etiologic factors. No specific, proven ocular therapy is available.

CRAO is characterized by a sudden, painless loss of vision in one eye. The retina becomes opaque and edematous, particularly in the posterior pole, where the nerve fiber and ganglion cell layers are the thickest. An orange reflex, from the intact choroidal vasculature beneath the intact foveola, stands out in contrast to the surrounding opaque retina, producing a "cherry red" spot (Fig. 120.12). With time, the central retinal artery reopens and the retinal edema clears.

The effect on visual acuity is usually devastating, with most eyes ending up with vision of hand motions or less than 20/400. Loss of vision or no light perception usually results from concomitant choroidal vascular obstruction.

CRAO is usually caused by arteriosclerosis-related thrombosis at the level of the optic nerve. Emboli may be important in some cases. For any patient in the 60- to 80-year-old age range presenting with CRAO or BRAO, temporal arteritis should be high on the list of differential diagnoses, and a sedimentation rate should be obtained as a screening test.

CRAO is an ophthalmic emergency, and patients must be referred immediately. Therapeutic steps include reduction of the intraocular pressure by paracentesis, ocular massage, inhalation therapy with carbogen (95% oxygen and 5% carbon dioxide), and the use of aspirin. One study showed the prognosis to be poor with or without treatment; however, anecdotal cases of visual recovery are common.

Venous Occlusive Disease

The venous supply from the retina also is at risk for blockage, which causes disease associated with mild to severe visual loss. Like the arterial diseases, the venous diseases can be divided into branch retinal vein occlusion (BRVO) and central retinal vein occlusion (CRVO).

The ophthalmoscopic findings of acute BRVO include superficial hemorrhages, retinal edema, and often cotton wool spots in an affected sector of the retina (Fig. 120.13). The obstructed vein is dilated and tortuous, and the corresponding artery may become narrowed and sheathed. The superior temporal quadrant is most commonly affected, and the site of occlusion is usually an arteriovenous crossing point. Histologic studies suggest that the common adventitia at these points binds the artery and

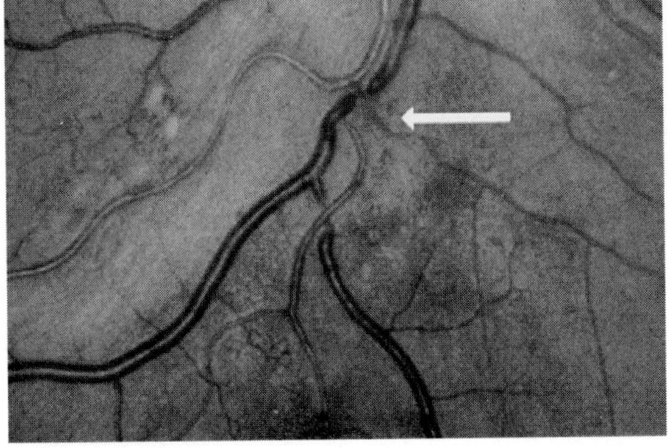

FIG. 120.10. Hypertensive retinal vascular changes illustrating arteriovenous nicking.

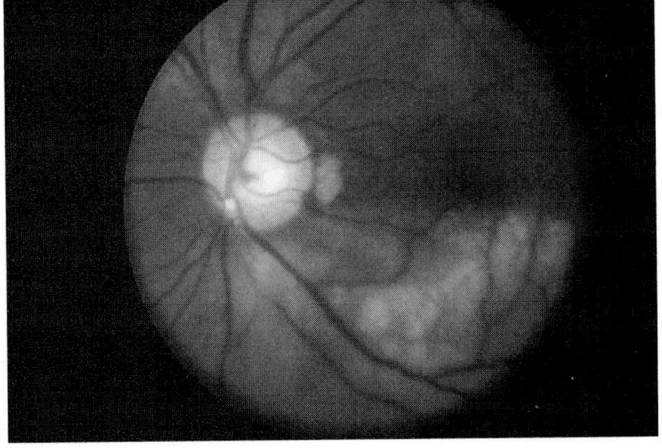

FIG. 120.11. Occlusion of the inferior macular branch artery. Note white, edematous retinal tissue.

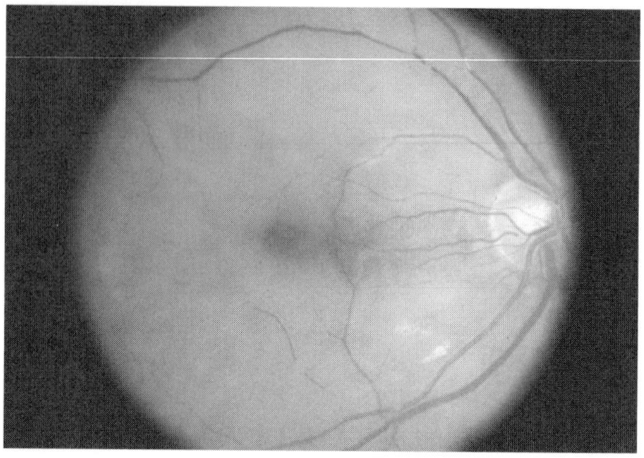

FIG. 120.12. Central retinal artery occlusion with cherry red spot.

vein together and that a diseased arterial wall impinges on the vein, causing turbulent flow, endothelial cell damage, and thrombotic occlusion. Arterial disease related to systemic hypertension, diabetes, or arteriosclerosis may predispose to BRVO.

The visual prognosis depends on the extent of capillary damage and retinal ischemia, and on whether macular edema is present. Fluorescein angiography is used to assess the extent and location of capillary damage. Acutely, vision may be reduced by macular edema, hemorrhage, or capillary occlusion. With time, capillary compensation and reperfusion may allow recovery of flow, with resolution of edema and improvement in visual acuity. In other eyes, progressive capillary occlusion may develop. Extensive retinal ischemia can result in the growth of new blood vessels on the retina or optic nerve, similar to the neovascularization of diabetes. In such cases, visual loss can be caused by vitreous hemorrhage.

Laser photocoagulation therapy is considered for the two major complications of BRVO: chronic macular edema and neovascularization. For eyes with macular edema, it is important to delay treatment for 4 months to allow maximum spontaneous resolution. Therapy has been shown to enhance resolution of the edema. Scatter photocoagulation in the diseased quadrant of the retina is an effective treatment for eyes with neovascularization, causing the new vessels to regress. For eyes in which persistent vitreous hemorrhage develops, vitrectomy surgery may be indicated.

CRVO is usually a much more dangerous and devastating disease. Several forms are recognized. Partial or venous stasis retinopathy, a milder form, has the early findings of a full CRVO, yet visual acuity is usually good. This fundus picture is commonly seen in younger women with no significant medical history. Histologic studies suggest a common mechanism in all forms of CRVO, which is thrombosis of the central retinal vein at the level of the optic nerve. The extent of the thrombosis appears to determine the severity of the retinal findings and the variable course.

Partial CRVO is characterized by mild swelling of the optic disc and mild dilation and tortuosity of all branches of the central retinal vein. Dot and flame hemorrhages are present in all quadrants of the retina. Macular edema with loss of visual acuity may be present. Complete resolution is seen in a significant percentage of patients, partial resolution in about one third, and progression to complete CRVO in about one third to one half.

Complete CRVO is characterized by extensive four-quadrant retinal edema and hemorrhage, with marked venous dilation and a variable number of cotton wool spots (Fig. 120.14). The visual prognosis is extremely poor for this group as a whole; only 10% achieve vision better than 20/400. In addition, the incidence rate of abnormal blood vessel growth in the front of the eye (iris neovascularization) is high (20%–60%); this results in a painful type of glaucoma that is difficult to treat.

Both types of CRVO are similar in regard to age at onset, associated local and systemic findings, and laboratory studies. Ninety percent of patients are older than 50 years at onset. CRVO may occur in younger persons and is not always benign. Frequent systemic associations include cardiovascular disease, hypertension, and diabetes. Unusual diseases that affect the blood vessel wall or cause clotting abnormalities or changes in blood viscosity may be associated with a CRVO, including blood dyscrasia, dysproteinemia, and causes of vasculitis (e.g., syphilis, sarcoidosis, lupus). Oral contraceptive use has also been implicated in CRVO.

Laboratory parameters that are often abnormal in patients with CRVO include glucose tolerance, serum cholesterol, lipoproteins, triglycerides, and gamma globulins. All patients presenting with CRVO should undergo a complete systemic evaluation with the appropriate laboratory studies to identify factors that may promote thrombus formation.

In eyes with partial CRVO, no treatment is useful unless an underlying systemic cause is found. In eyes with ischemic CRVO, full-scatter laser photocoagulation is effective therapy for preventing glaucoma.

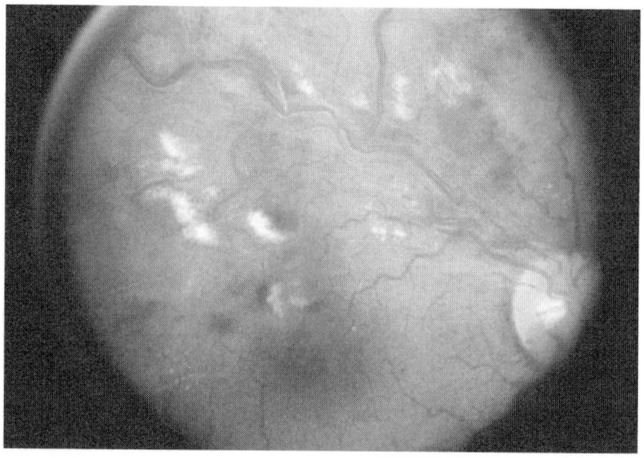

FIG. 120.13. Superior temporal branch vein occlusion with hemorrhages and cotton wool spots.

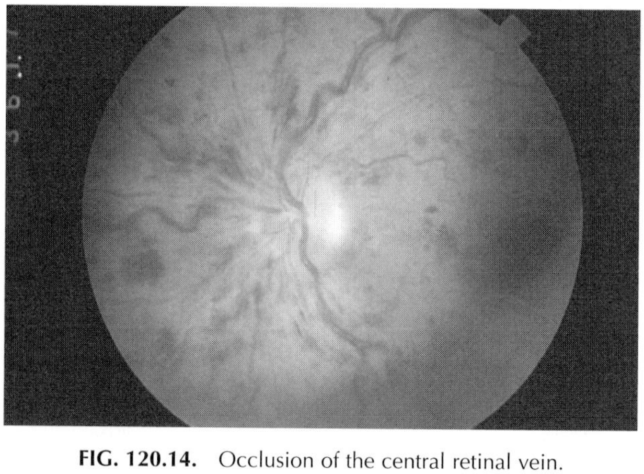

FIG. 120.14. Occlusion of the central retinal vein.

MACULAR DISEASES

The macula, or central area of the retina, is a highly specialized structure made up predominantly of cones. This area allows normal, healthy persons to achieve 20/20 vision or better. A variety of retinal diseases affect the macula preferentially, and those more frequently encountered in primary care are reviewed.

Age-Related Macular Degeneration

Age-related macular degeneration is extremely prevalent in the United States, affecting more than 20 million persons. Although it is most common in people older than 65 years, younger persons may also be affected, and early signs of the disease can be seen in the third and fourth decades. This disease affects primarily central vision, which is relied on for close work such as reading and writing. Macular degeneration can also affect the ability to drive if severe enough. Normal senescence results in a spectrum of clinical and histologic changes in all layers of the macula. The cell principally affected appears to be the retinal pigment epithelial cell.

The retinal pigment epithelium lies beneath the retina and is important in maintaining macular health. The anatomy of the retinal pigment epithelium is unique, and it promotes normal macular function in three ways: (a) formation of a barrier between the blood supply to the retina and the sensory retina, (b) phagocytosis of rod and cone segments, and (c) vitamin A metabolism.

Changes in the retinal pigment epithelium with age and disease include a loss of pigment granules and the formation of hyaline deposits on the supporting structure of the layer, the Bruch membrane. These deposits, called *drusen*, are the hallmark of age-related macular degeneration (Fig. 120.15). Thickening and weakening of the Bruch membrane allow vascular ingrowth from the blood vessel layer beneath the retina (lamina choriocapillaris).

As a result of the processes associated with drusen formation, complications may ensue that cause visual loss. The most frequent of these is loss of the retinal pigment epithelium, leading to atrophy. Visual loss is caused by the attendant loss of photoreceptors, a condition generally known as *dry macular degeneration*. A second complication of drusen formation, accounting for almost 90% of cases of severe visual loss from macular degeneration, is subretinal neovascularization, generally called *wet macular degeneration*; this develops when neovascular membranes enter through the Bruch membrane into the subretinal space, where they leak fluid, blood, or both, causing severe visual loss. The hemorrhage stimulates the proliferation of scar tissue, with loss of cone function.

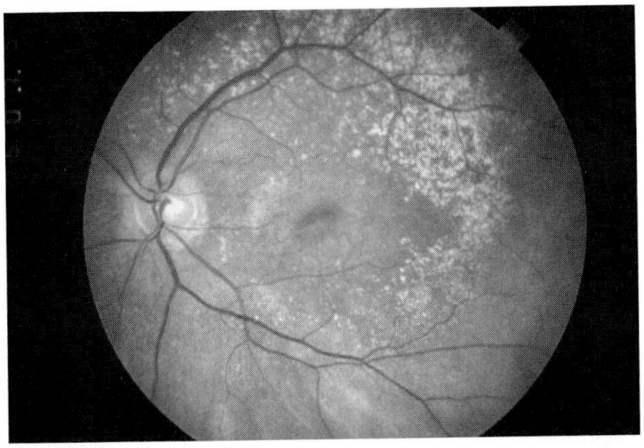

FIG. 120.15. Macular drusen are the hallmark of age-related macular degeneration.

The pathogenesis of macular degeneration is unclear. The primary abnormality appears to be degeneration or a metabolic disturbance of the retinal pigment epithelium and its biochemical relationship with the photoreceptor cells, resulting in a thickening of the Bruch membrane and drusen formation. Hereditary factors will most likely prove to be the most important determinant of the development of this disease.

No effective medical treatment is available for the dry form of macular degeneration. Patients with drusen, particularly if the fellow eye has a macular scar, should be instructed to monitor their central acuity with an Amsler grid, which is essentially a graph paper pattern with a central fixation point. Patients test each eye independently and look for blind spots or distortion of the lines. Any abnormal symptom should be reported to the ophthalmologist. Fluorescein angiography can be performed to detect evidence of treatable subretinal neovascular complexes.

Reports of the efficacy of zinc in the diet have spawned a host of dietary "eye vitamins," none of which has been proven to delay the onset or cure the damage of macular degeneration. In a randomized, masked, double-blinded study sponsored by the National Eye Institute, supplementation with high doses of vitamins A (as β-carotene), C, and E, in addition to zinc, significantly slowed progression of the disease in patients with high-risk drusen and other retinal pigment epithelial changes. Other studies have shown some stabilization of the disease when patients consumed a diet rich in green leafy vegetables such as spinach and collard greens.

The efficacy of laser treatment for the wet or exudative form of macular degeneration has been demonstrated in a national randomized, double-blinded study, the Macular Photocoagulation Study. Patients enrolled had angiographic evidence of a choroidal neovascular membrane at least 200 cm from the center of the fovea. After 18 months, severe visual loss had developed in 65% of the untreated eyes, compared with 25% of the treated eyes.

Many eyes cannot be treated effectively, and a patient can progress to legal blindness in each eye in a short period of time. Photodynamic therapy, which has been approved for the treatment of wet macular degeneration with abnormal blood vessel growth directly underneath the fovea, has been successful in slowing the progression of visual loss and in some cases has reversed it. In this therapy, pharmacologic treatment with verteporfin (Visudyne) is combined with low-level red laser. In another pharmacologic approach, anti-vascular endothelial growth factor (anti-VEGF) substances are used to destroy abnormal blood vessels. This approach avoids potential damage from the laser. Progression of disease in an otherwise healthy, independent adult can result in a dramatic change in lifestyle. Affected persons may no longer be able to drive or live by themselves. Both the ophthalmologist and primary care provider should watch for signs of depression during this period. Aids for people with low vision and support groups can be useful. Referral for evaluation by local state services for the visually handicapped may be appropriate.

Central Serous Choroidopathy

Central serous choroidopathy is characterized by the development of a serous detachment of the sensory retina caused by a focal leakage in the retinal pigment epithelium. It tends to occur in young men, who present with the sudden onset of blurred vision and distortion. Women are affected, although rarely.

The sensory retina is elevated, and the leakage point is sometimes identified as a small area of retinal pigment epithelial clumping or atrophy. Occasionally, an extensive serous detachment of the retina may develop from one or more leak points outside the macula and clinically may resemble a large retinal detachment.

In most eyes with central serous choroidopathy (80%–90%), spontaneous resorption of the subretinal fluid and recovery of vision are noted within 1 to 6 months after the onset of symptoms, although patients may continue to feel that their vision is not right. In some eyes, permanent visual loss develops, and many patients experience recurrent episodes.

Although central serous choroidopathy is less common in women, some studies of the effects of pregnancy on this disease have been performed. Subretinal fibrinous exudates were common in this population of women. No racial predilection was noted, and in all patients studied, the central serous choroidopathy resolved during the term of the pregnancy. One patient had a subsequent pregnancy without involvement.

Laser treatment of the site of leakage has been shown to shorten the duration of disease but does not affect final visual acuity in comparison with no treatment. Most ophthalmologists elect to observe the first episode of central serous choroidopathy and treat it only if it persists beyond 6 months. Recurrences are more likely to be treated, and a fellow eye with visual loss from central serous choroidopathy should also be treated.

Macular Hole

Macular hole occurs primarily in women in the sixth through eighth decades of life. The formation of a hole in the central macula causes a loss of reading vision (Fig. 120.16). The symptoms usually worsen with time; however, some patients report a sudden visual loss. Visual acuity can drop to the 20/400 level, with preservation of the peripheral visual field. Patients with developing macular holes that have not yet progressed to full thickness may present with less extreme changes in visual acuity.

The pathogenesis of macular hole formation is not known; however, the relationship between the macula and its overlying vitreous is implicated. Tractional or pulling forces exerted by a thin layer of vitreous seem to cause a hole to develop in susceptible persons.

Previously, no successful treatment was available for this condition, but within the last decade, surgery has made it possible to recover most of the visual loss. Removal of the vitreous gel with microsurgical techniques, in addition to peeling the thin layer of adherent vitreous over the macula, is the mainstay of treatment. The vitreous is replaced with a premeasured concentration of a long-acting gas bubble, and the patient is instructed to remain face down for 12 to 14 hours per day for up to 2 weeks postoperatively. The success rate of this procedure approaches 95%.

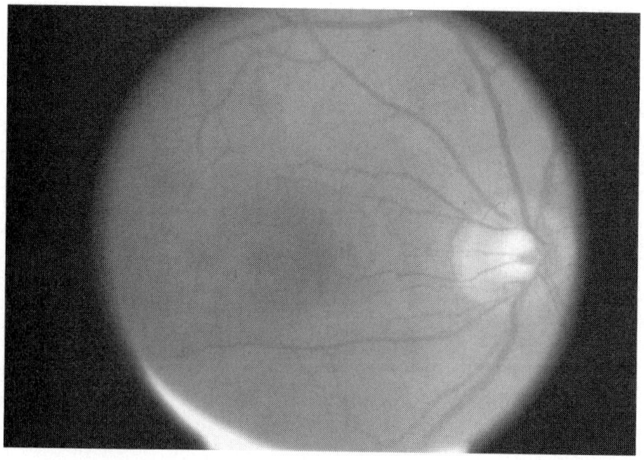

FIG. 120.16. Macular hole measuring approximately 300 μm.

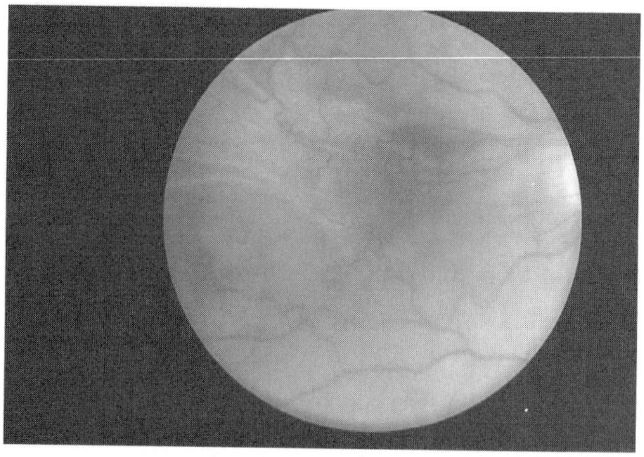

FIG. 120.17. Epiretinal membrane over the macula distorting the underlying retina.

The incidence of bilateral disease is reported to be up to 10%. Thus, the development of an effective surgical intervention has had a considerable impact on patients with macular holes. Patient selection remains crucial in the success of this procedure.

Epiretinal Membrane

Epiretinal membranes are extraretinal tissues that tend to form at or near the macula, blurring and distorting vision (Fig. 120.17). The membranes develop in patients in the sixth through eighth decades, and if they exert sufficient pull, they can cause a marked reduction in visual acuity in association with macular edema. The pathogenesis is unclear; however, histologic studies show that some of the cells of which the membranes are composed are retinal pigment epithelial and retinal glial cells.

The treatment is surgery if vision drops to a level at which reading or driving is difficult. Although most of the membranes are idiopathic, some are secondary to a variety of conditions, including retinal vascular occlusion, uveitis, trauma, and intraocular surgery.

INFLAMMATORY AND INFECTIOUS DISEASES

A variety of inflammatory and infectious diseases can affect the retina and vitreous. The degree of inflammation varies, and visual loss ranges from mild to severe. The importance of an accurate diagnosis cannot be overemphasized because appropriate and timely treatment considerably affects outcome. The major diseases reviewed here are toxoplasmosis and AIDS-related diseases of the eye.

Toxoplasmosis

Patients with ocular toxoplasmosis usually present with symptoms of floaters and blurred vision. The floaters are caused by inflammatory cells in the vitreous. The source of the cells is a focus of inflammation in the retina that can usually be seen oph-

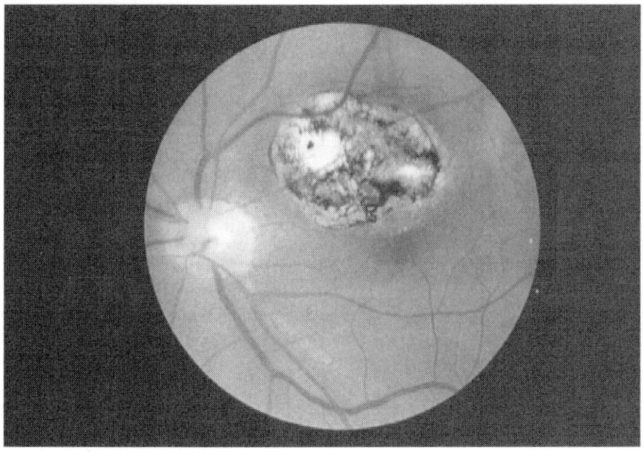

FIG. 120.18. Typical toxoplasmosis scar with heavy pigment.

thalmoscopically as a white, raised retinal lesion with indistinct borders. The causative organism is *Toxoplasma gondii*, which multiplies preferentially in the inner retinal layers.

The acute retinal lesions heal spontaneously within 6 months and leave a chorioretinal scar with variable pigmentation (Fig. 120.18). Usually, the vitreous clears, and vision returns as long as the retinitis has not involved the macula.

Repeated attacks are caused by recurrent foci of retinitis, most often at the edge of old atrophic lesions, thought to be caused by the breakdown of *Toxoplasma* cysts in the retina and the subsequent release of viable organisms. The encysted organism may remain latent in the retina for many years.

The congenital form of toxoplasmosis is transmitted from an infected pregnant woman across the placenta to the fetus and affects multiple organs. The eye and brain are especially susceptible, particularly if the fetus acquires the infection during the first trimester. Infants born with congenital toxoplasmosis often have a large macular scar, and recurrence of the disease may be lifelong.

Cats are the natural host of the organism and shed the cysts in their feces. These can contaminate foods or infect animals eaten by humans. Raw or undercooked meat is a major and avoidable source of infection.

The diagnosis of ocular toxoplasmosis is made by observing a focal, necrotizing retinitis in association with an old chorioretinal scar and by detecting any levels of anti-*Toxoplasma* antibodies in the sera. The enzyme-linked immunosorbent assay is most useful for this purpose.

It is generally recommended that active ocular toxoplasmosis be treated in patients with extensive involvement or with lesions that threaten the macula. Treatment consists of orally administered pyrimethamine and sulfonamide along with prednisone for 6 weeks. Clindamycin has also been found to be effective in place of sulfonamides.

AIDS: Retinal and Choroidal Infections

At least a dozen infectious agents have been identified in the retina or choroid of patients with AIDS. The prevalence of these varies, but all can lead to loss of vision or blindness. Because retinal biopsy and vitreous culture are difficult and serologic testing for ocular pathogens is inaccurate, clinical diagnosis remains the major method of differentiating the cause of an AIDS-related retinopathy.

The most common retinal manifestation of AIDS is a microangiopathy that manifests clinically as single or multiple cotton wool spots. The lesions are usually found in the macular area. Retinal hemorrhages, microaneurysms, or other microvascular changes may be associated.

No specific treatment is required; however, these changes probably indicate an advanced stage of the illness. HIV retinopathy has been shown to be related to a decreasing ratio of $CD4^+$ to $CD8^+$ cells.

Cytomegalovirus (CMV) retinitis is the most common retinal infection in AIDS. The exact prevalence is not known, but most investigators believe that CMV retinitis develops in at least 20% of patients with AIDS during the course of their disease. CMV retinopathy is usually a late manifestation of the AIDS syndrome, and its presence alone is sufficient for making a diagnosis of AIDS.

The diagnosis of CMV retinopathy is based on the clinical findings. The presence of anti-CMV antibodies or CMV from other body sites cannot be used to confirm the diagnosis of CMV retinopathy because most patients with AIDS have been infected with CMV.

CMV retinitis may be unilateral or bilateral. Clinically, two presentations are described. The first, or hemorrhagic type, is the classic form; it usually develops in or near the macula and has a "crumbled cheese and ketchup" appearance. Large areas of retinal hemorrhage are associated with regions of thick, whitish retinal necrosis along blood vessels (Fig. 120.19). The second form, most often seen in the peripheral retina, is the granular type. In this form, the lesions spread out from a central focus. The advancing border has a yellow-white granular appearance with little or no hemorrhage. The location of these changes is mostly impossible to see with the direct ophthalmoscope, so it is important for an ophthalmologist to screen patients at risk for the development of CMV retinitis every 90 days.

CMV retinitis is an indolent infection that spreads during many weeks and eventually involves the entire retina. Without treatment, vision is usually lost because of optic nerve involvement. Spontaneous remission is rare. Treatment was successfully undertaken in 1985 with ganciclovir, an analogue of the antiviral acyclovir. Ganciclovir stabilizes the retinitis, halting or delaying progression and visual loss and decreasing viral shedding. The drug is given intravenously for a 2- to 3-week induction period at a dosage of 5 mg/kg twice daily. After induction, patients continue on a maintenance dosage of 5 to 6 mg/kg per day given 5 to 7 days during the week. The patient must be monitored for renal dysfunction and the development of neutropenia while on this therapy. Therapy continues indefinitely

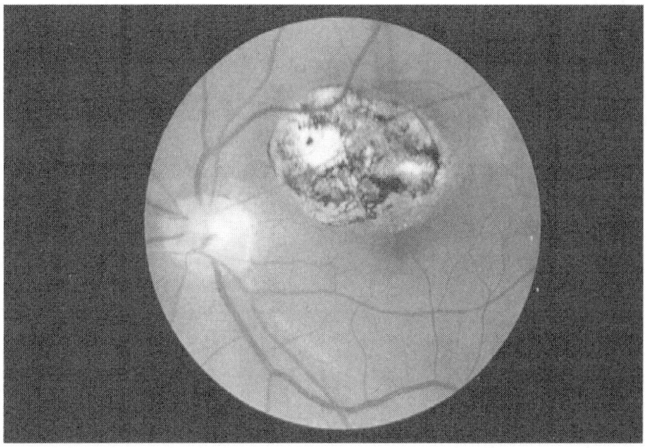

FIG. 120.19. Cytomegalovirus retinitis with hemorrhages and retinal necrosis.

unless a resistant CMV infection or life-threatening side effects develop.

Initially, 70% to 80% of patients with CMV retinitis respond to ganciclovir; however, CMV can recur in up to 40% of patients on maintenance therapy. Patients must be followed closely every 2 to 3 weeks while undergoing treatment.

The primary alternative to ganciclovir is foscarnet, which is a potent inhibitor of herpes simplex virus DNA polymerase and retrovirus reverse transcriptase. Foscarnet also is virustatic for CMV. Continuous therapy is required. The most problematic side effect is nephrotoxicity.

Other treatment modalities include direct injection of ganciclovir into the vitreous cavity in patients unable to tolerate the systemic side effects. A long-acting ganciclovir pellet that can be surgically inserted into the vitreous is now the initial treatment of choice for many patients. The pellet lasts about 8 months and obviates the need for systemic treatment.

CMV retinitis used to be associated with a mean survival of 4 to 6 months. With improved treatments of AIDS in general, survival has been lengthened to years. The ability to preserve vision becomes more important as survival time increases. Highly active antiretroviral therapy (HAART) has improved the survival rates of many of these patients with less morbidity.

Several other opportunistic infections affect the retina and underlying choroid. These are only mentioned here, and the interested reader is referred to sources cited at the end of the chapter for more detailed information. Infection with *Pneumocystis carinii* is usually seen in advanced cases of AIDS. Syphilis, herpes zoster, toxoplasmosis, and infections with *Mycobacterium* and *Cryptococcus* have all been described.

RETINAL TEARS AND RETINAL DETACHMENT

Retinal tears or retinal detachment can develop at any time during a person's life. A retinal break is a full-thickness discontinuity of the retinal tissue, usually in the peripheral retina. It is clinically significant in that it provides an access route for vitreous fluid to enter the subretinal space, causing a retinal detachment. Normally, the retina is kept in place by a variety of mechanical, physical, and metabolic forces. The strong pumping mechanism of the retinal pigment epithelium keeps the subretinal space relatively dry. When forces of fluid movement are strong enough to overcome the pump mechanism, the retina detaches.

The precursor of a retinal tear is the condition known as *posterior vitreous detachment*. The vitreous in persons uniformly fills the vitreous cavity. With senescence, the vitreous gel liquefies and can pull away from where it adheres at the back of the eye (Fig. 120.20). Adhesion in the peripheral retina is strongest near the insertion of the vitreous (vitreous base), which is where tears usually occur. In symptomatic posterior vitreous detachment, patients experience the sudden onset of floaters or flashing lights. The sensation of flashing lights (photopsia) indicates persistent pulling or traction on the retina and may be present with or without a retinal tear. Symptomatic posterior vitreous detachment requires immediate referral to an ophthalmologist and a careful retinal examination. If the collapsing vitreous pulls on the retinal blood vessels, a vitreous hemorrhage can occur, with a dramatic loss of vision.

If a retinal tear is identified, it is usually treated the same day. As long as large amounts of subretinal fluid have not developed in association with the tear, it can be treated with laser or freezing (cryopexy). These are office-based procedures with minimal morbidity and high rates of success.

If too much fluid has accumulated under the retina, then a retinal detachment has occurred, (Fig. 120.21) and major eye surgery is usually indicated. A retinal detachment is usually an ophthalmic emergency, and surgery is performed within 12 to 24 hours. If the detachment is limited to a peripheral part of the retina and does not involve the macula, then the surgery takes on added urgency. If the detached retina can be repaired before fluid accumulates under the macula, the chances of preserving 20/20 vision are much greater. Patients with a detachment threatening the macula usually undergo surgery within hours.

Surgery may involve outpatient or inpatient hospital services. The standard procedure is a scleral buckle. The tears all are identified under controlled conditions in the operating room suite and treated with cryopexy to induce retinal pigment epithelium adhesion. A silicone or sponge material is then sutured onto the wall of the eye under the tears to support the weakened areas of tear. The eye wall is indented effectively, relieving the pulling on the retinal tear (Fig. 120.22). Some retinal detachments require more involved surgery, such as vitrectomy. An office-based procedure used for certain selected retinal detachments is pneumatic retinopexy. A long-acting gas (2–4 weeks) is instilled into the vitreous cavity after the tear(s) have been treated with laser or cryopexy. The patient then is positioned so that the intraocular gas bubble remains in contact with the tear for 12 to 16 hours per day. This procedure is tolerable primarily for superior detachments.

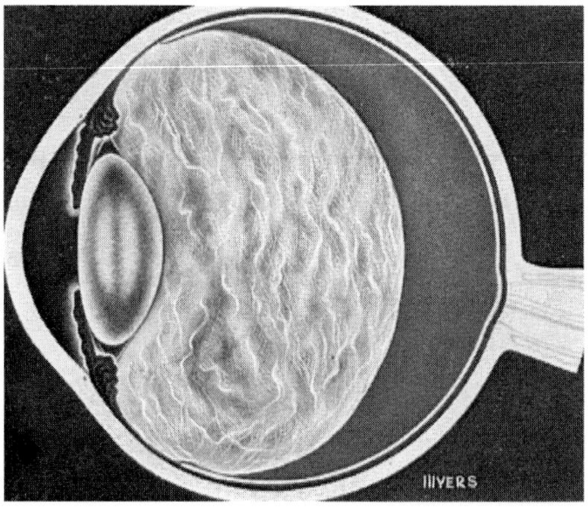

FIG. 120.20. Posterior vitreous detachment. Note the adhesions remaining anteriorly.

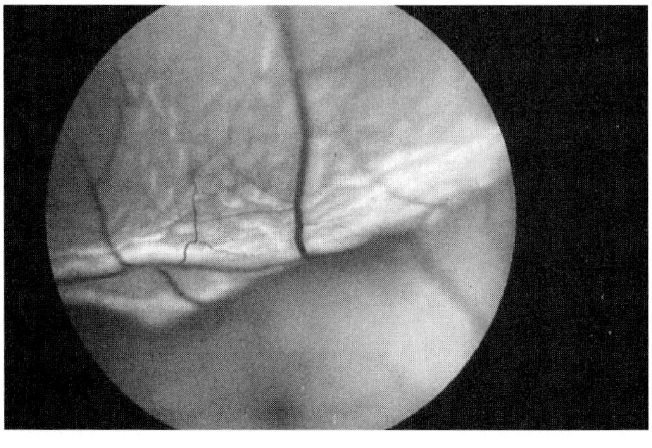

FIG. 120.21. Typical appearance of a retinal detachment.

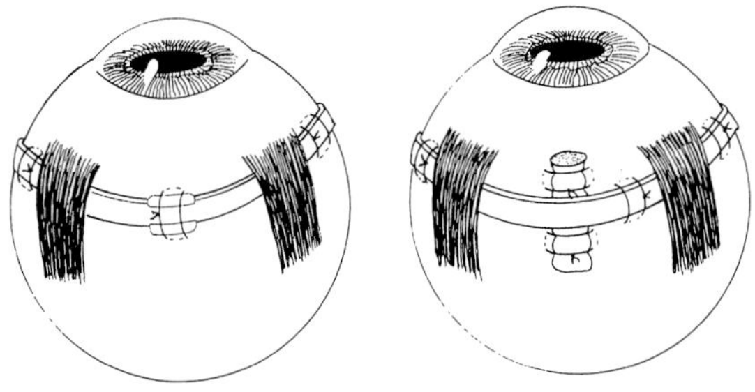

FIG. 120.22. Location of scleral buckle surgery.

Retinal detachment surgery is successful more than 90% of the time. Failure of the retina to reattach results from a variety of reasons, and reoperation may be necessary.

BIBLIOGRAPHY

Diabetes Control and Complications Trial Research Group. Progression of retinopathy with intensive versus conventional treatment in the Diabetes Control and Complications Trial. *Ophthalmology* 1995;102:647.

Duane T, ed. *Clinical ophthalmology*, vol 3. Philadelphia: Harper & Row, 1986.

Gass JDM. *Stereoscopic atlas of macular diseases*. St. Louis: Mosby, 1987.

Lewis H, Ryan SJ, eds. *Medical and surgical retina: advances, controversies and management*. St. Louis: Mosby, 1994.

Macular Photocoagulation Study Group. Argon laser photocoagulation for senile macular degeneration: results of a randomized clinical trial. *Arch Ophthalmol* 1982;100:912.

Ryan SJ, ed. *Retina*. St. Louis: Mosby, 1989.

Schepens C. *Retinal detachment and allied diseases*, vols 1 and 2. Philadelphia: WB Saunders, 1983.

Stenson S, Friedberg D. *AIDS and the eye*. Herndon, VA: Contact Lens Society of America, 1995.

CHAPTER 121
Cataracts

Steven S. T. Ching and Richard I. Chang

Cataracts are the major cause of visual disability worldwide. Approximately 2.7 million cataract surgeries were performed in the United States in 2002. A cataract is the result of a change in the clarity of the crystalline lens. Some form of lens change is present in 95% of people older than 65 years of age. Therefore, the term *cataract* should include a change in visual function with the noted anatomic change. Fifty percent of people between 65 and 74 years of age and 70% of those older than 75 years of age are visually impaired because of cataract.

FORMATION OF CATARACTS

The eye is a natural camera. It captures images of the world and transmits them to the brain. As in any camera, a lens system refracts or focuses light. The eye has an external lens, the cornea, and an internal lens, the crystalline lens. A condition in which the internal lens looses its clarity or abnormally focuses light is termed a *cataract*.

The crystalline lens grows throughout life as the lens cells proliferate and differentiate in layers. Analogous to growth rings of a tree, the external layers are the newest. The newly formed layers contain nuclei and with age eventually loose the nuclei. On slitlamp examination, the center of the lens is termed the *nucleus*, and the periphery is the *cortex*.

Cataracts that develop with age present in three forms: nuclear sclerosis, peripheral cortical opacification, and posterior subcapsular opacification (Fig. 121.1). After the age of 65 years, the nucleus begins to increase in density and change in color from clear crystalline to yellow-brown. This change, termed *nuclear sclerosis*, results from the formation of insoluble protein aggregates that alter the refractive index, scatter light rays, and reduce transparency. Initially, the increased index of refraction tends to increase the refracting power of the lens. Nearsightedness or myopia may be induced, and a person may be able to see without glasses at near. This phenomenon of regaining near vision with advancing age is termed *second sight*. As the nuclear sclerosis progresses, vision eventually becomes distorted, with loss of visual clarity.

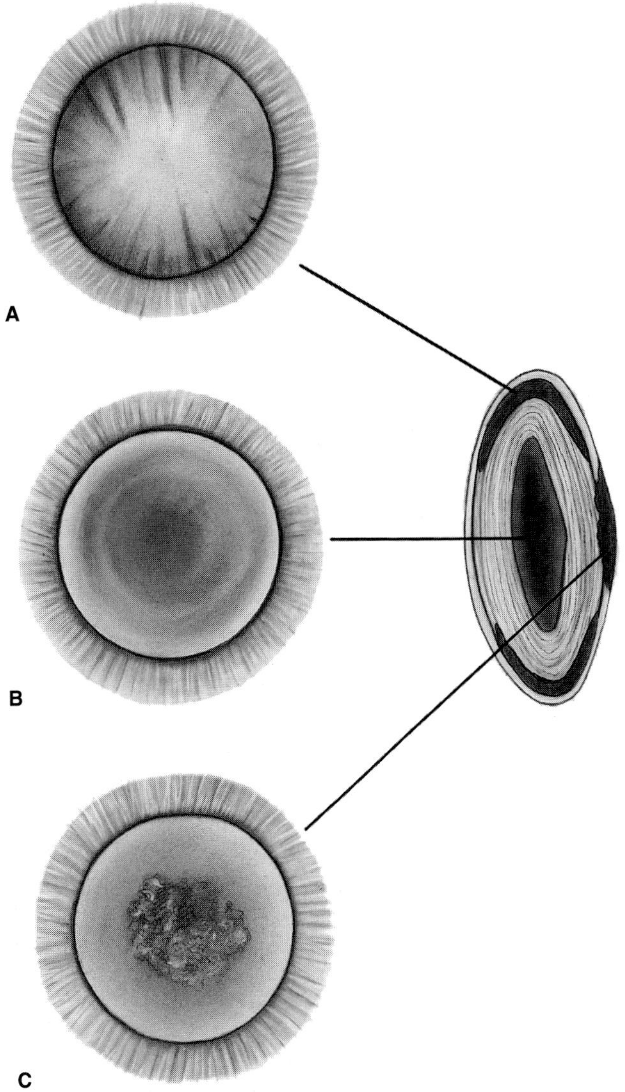

FIG. 121.1. **A:** Cortical cataract: peripheral lens fiber abnormalities look like the spokes of a wheel ("cortical spokes," or cuneiform cataract). **B:** Nuclear cataract: the nucleus of the lens is denser than the periphery. This causes a "bull's-eye" appearance. **C:** Posterior subcapsular cataract: posterior axial abnormal lens fibers cause focal opacification. The axial location of the opacity leads to early visual symptoms.

If the growth of the cortical lens fibers is disturbed, a focal opacity of the lens results. This phenomenon occurs with age and leads to the formation of peripheral lens opacities. On slit-lamp and ophthalmoscopic examination, these look like the spokes of a wheel and are termed *cortical spokes*. Because of the peripheral location of the opacities, cortical cataracts cause symptoms of glare and a mild decrease in visual acuity.

In the third form of cataract, lens fibers migrate posteriorly near the posterior capsule and fail to differentiate. This results in an opacity in the posterior lens termed a *posterior subcapsular cataract*. Because of its axial and posterior location, this form of cataract causes the greatest degree of visual disability. Patients usually experience sensitivity to light and decreased vision in bright light.

DIAGNOSIS

Patients experience decreased visual acuity, sensitivity to light, monocular multiple images, halos, loss of stereopsis, and the appearance of flaring around point sources of lights. They may regain reading vision, and the frequency of eyeglass changes may increase.

The examiner may notice discoloration of the pupil. Of note, the direct and indirect pupillary response to light should be normal. Cataracts, even when severe, do not alter the pupillary light response. An abnormal pupillary response indicates optic nerve dysfunction, retinal disease, or central nervous system disease. To view the lens and retina, the pupil should be dilated with 2.5% phenylephrine (Neo-Synephrine) and 1% tropicamide (Mydriacil). Before dilation, the examiner should estimate the depth of the anterior chamber to ensure that the patient is not at risk for an attack of angle-closure glaucoma (see Figure 122.4). The examiner should view the lens with a direct ophthalmoscope with a +10 diopter setting at 10 cm or a +3 diopter setting at 33 cm. The red reflex in nuclear sclerosis appears as a bull's-eye with a central dark reflex and peripheral lucency. In nuclear sclerosis, the indices of refraction of the central lens vary. When the fundus is viewed through the ophthalmoscope, optical distortion of the retinal structures may be noted. Cortical spokes appear as peripheral linear opacities, and the posterior subcapsular cataract appears as a central axial dark spot.

DIFFERENTIAL DIAGNOSIS

Cataract is the most common cause of visual disability in the elderly. However, it may coexist with another ocular disease, such as glaucoma or macular degeneration. Therefore, other causes of visual loss should be ruled out.

Optical aberrations viewed by the direct ophthalmoscope can be localized by parallax. Varying the observer's position makes it possible to discern the location of the opacity in relation to the lens. Anterior visual aberrations arise from the cornea, and posterior opacities are in the vitreous.

A late stage of cataract formation has the appearance of a white pupil, or leukocoria. In an adult, leukocoria can be secondary to cataract, retinal detachment, intraocular tumor, or vitreous membranes.

ETIOLOGY

In normal aging, it is thought that photooxidative stress is induced in lens proteins and lens cells by radiation of ultraviolet waves of A length (UVA) and B length (UVB). The effects of radiation may be mediated by a loss of intralenticular antioxidant activity or photosensitization of lens proteins. These processes eventually cause protein aggregation, areas with varying indices of refraction, and light scattering.

Ultraviolet light, alcohol, and smoking increase the risk for cataract. Two important causes of cataract are the use of systemic steroids and diabetes mellitus. Systemic steroids are associated with an increased incidence of cataract, seen in patients with rheumatoid arthritis. Cataracts develop in 30% to 40% of patients with rheumatoid arthritis when they take prednisone at doses of 10 mg/d for 2 years; the rate increases to 100% in those treated for 4 years. Diabetes mellitus is thought to accelerate the rate of cataract formation by 20 to 30 years through the damaging effects of sorbitol on lens cells. Hyperglycemia also decreases antioxidative activity of the lens and thereby potentiates other lens damage.

MEDICAL MANAGEMENT

No chemical agent effectively reduces the incidence or progression of cataract. Clinical trials of aspirin, aldose reductase inhibitors to lower sorbitol levels, and antioxidants are under investigation. Damage of the lens secondary to UV radiation comes from a lifetime of exposure, and short-term measures to reduce such exposure probably would have little effect.

Colored lenses, usually amber to brown, limit the spectra of incoming light and may limit glare and increase contrast. Optimizing lighting and using magnifiers may be beneficial. If the cataract is axial and of limited area, pupillary dilation may be helpful.

SURGERY

Indications

The decision to intervene surgically is based on the patient's visual disability as a consequence of the cataract, the patient's visual needs, the surgical risks, and the medical risks of the ocular disease. Cataracts can cause symptoms of glare and monocular diplopia. The blurred vision caused by a monocular cataract can interfere with the functioning of the opposite eye. If these symptoms are bothersome and interfere with the patient's lifestyle, cataract surgery can be considered.

The visual needs of patients vary considerably. For example, a machinist or pilot may require stereopsis and fine binocular acuity. Other persons may not require stereopsis and do not have to undertake the risks of surgery. Patients with nuclear sclerotic cataracts usually have limited distance vision but may have excellent near vision. If a patient's social situation is such that perfect distance vision is not crucial, surgery may not be necessary. Usually, a critical level of vision in the elderly is that necessary to maintain a driver's license. In most states, 20/40 vision in either eye is required to maintain an unrestricted driver's license. The requirements for a limited daytime license vary from 20/50 to 20/70, depending on the state. Patients may have to maintain other minimum visual standards as mandated by government or industry.

In some instances, cataracts must be removed for medical reasons. For example, in patients with diabetic retinopathy or glaucoma, visualization of the retina and optic nerve is necessary to monitor and treat the underlying disease. If a cataract is significantly advanced, inflammatory or angle-closure glaucoma can be precipitated.

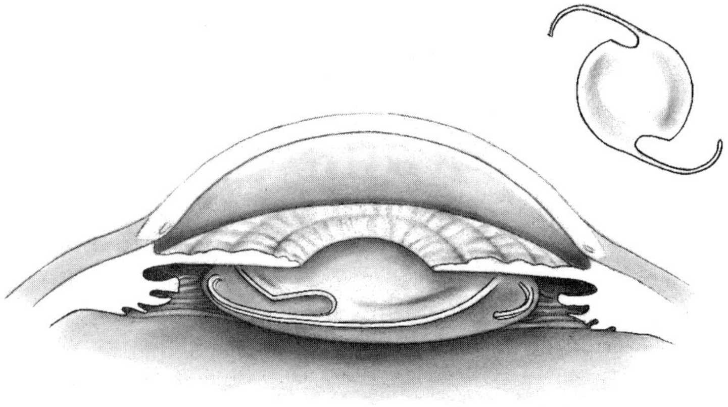

FIG. 121.2. The intraocular lens is a plastic prosthetic lens. This schematic shows a lens situated in the capsule of the original crystalline lens in the posterior chamber. The arms of the lens act as springs that stabilize it against the peripheral capsule.

The risk for an ocular complication of cataract surgery varies from 1% to 3%. The complications of cataract surgery are discussed in greater detail later in this chapter. To undergo surgery, a patient must be capable of lying flat and tolerating local or topical anesthesia.

Methods

Three major methods are used to remove cataracts surgically: intracapsular removal, extracapsular removal with a standard incision, and extracapsular removal by phacoemulsification with a small incision. In intracapsular cataract surgery, the entire lens is removed. This method was popular through the 1970s. It has the advantage of being relatively simple and does not require extensive technologic surgical instrumentation. This method is still used in third world countries because of its simplicity. However, it is performed infrequently in the United States today because it limits intraocular lens choices.

In extracapsular cataract surgery, the lens contents are removed without the external lens capsule. The capsular remnant serves to hold or anchor an artificial intraocular lens. At 4 months postoperatively, the visual results and complications of the standard technique and the small-incision phacoemulsification technique appear to be the same. The small-incision phacoemulsification technique has the advantage of quicker rehabilitation but may not be suitable for all types of cataract.

Visual Correction after Surgery

The internal crystalline lens accounts for 35% of the refracting power of the eye, loss of which must be compensated for after cataract surgery. This can be accomplished with high-power plus lenses (cataract spectacles), a contact lens, or an intraocular artificial lens. Cataract spectacles are safe but associated with significant optical disadvantages. They magnify images approximately 30%, thereby causing significant perceptual problems for patients. In addition, high-power plus lenses significantly limit peripheral vision and cause peripheral distortion. Contact lenses are difficult for most patients to manage. The incidence of dry eye is increased in elderly persons, who may not be candidates for contact lenses.

Intraocular lenses have been used since 1949. Lens designs and surgical techniques have evolved such that intraocular lenses are considered the standard of care in the United States. Ninety-eight percent of all cataract surgeries are performed with intraocular lens implants. Some types of intraocular lenses in the 1970s and early 1980s were associated with significant complications of intraocular inflammation, bleeding, glaucoma, and corneal edema. Today's implants are placed in either the posterior chamber (Fig. 121.2) or anterior chamber and carry a low risk for complications. Intraocular lenses in patients younger than 18 years are investigational.

Ocular Complications after Cataract Surgery

No surgical procedure is without risk. Usually, the risk of cataract surgery is low. Early severe complications include choroidal hemorrhage (0.3%) and intraocular infection, or endophthalmitis (0.08%–0.13%). Significant late complications include corneal edema (0.3%), clinically significant macular edema (1.4%), and retinal detachment (0.8%). Rarely, persistent intraocular inflammation (uveitis) and long-term raised intraocular pressure develop.

Laser after Cataract Surgery

After extracapsular cataract surgery, the capsular remnants may undergo opacification. This occurs in approximately 20% of patients in the first year after surgery. A neodymium:yttrium-aluminum garnet laser is used to create a pupil in the posterior capsule. This procedure is mistakenly interpreted by patients as removal of a cataract by laser.

CONCLUSION

Cataract formation is a natural consequence of aging. Not all cataracts require removal. Although the risks of surgery are relatively low and the results excellent, the decision to remove a cataract surgically is a complex one and should be individualized based on the patient's visual needs.

BIBLIOGRAPHY

Cataract symposium. San Francisco: American Academy of Ophthalmology, 1994.

Andley U. Photooxidative stress. In: Albert DM, Jakobiec FA, Azar DT, et al., eds. *Principles and practice of ophthalmology*, 2nd ed. Philadelphia: WB Saunders, 2000:1428–1449.

Bradford CA, ed. *Basic ophthalmology for medical students and primary care residents*, 7th ed. San Francisco, American Academy of Ophthalmology, 1999.
Floyd RP. History of cataract surgery. In: Albert DM, Jakobiec FA, Azar DT, et al., eds. *Principles and practice of ophthalmology*, 2nd ed. Philadelphia: WB Saunders, 2000:1463–1476.
Javitt JC, Street DA, Tielsch JM, et al. National outcomes of cataract extraction: retinal detachment and endophthalmitis after outpatient cataract surgery. *Ophthalmology* 1994;101(1):100–105.
Johns KJ, Feder RS, Hamill M, et al. *Basic and clinical science course. Section 11: Lens and cataract*. San Francisco, American Academy of Ophthalmology, 2002.
Powe NR, Schein OD, Gieser SC, et al. Synthesis of the literature on visual acuity and complications following cataract extraction with intraocular lens implantation. *Arch Ophthalmol* 1994;112(2):239–252.
Schein OD, Steinberg EP, Javitt JC, et al. Variation in cataract surgery practice and clinical outcomes. *Ophthalmology* 1994;101:1142–1152.
Streeten BW. Pathology of the lens. In: Albert DM, Jakobiec FA, Azar DT, et al., eds. *Principles and practice of ophthalmology*, 2nd ed. Philadelphia: WB Saunders, 2000:3685–3749.
West SK, Valmadrid CT. Epidemiology of risk factors for age-related cataract. *Surv Ophthalmol* 1995;39:4:323.

CHAPTER 122
Glaucoma

Steven S. T. Ching and Richard I. Chang

The term *glaucoma* refers to a group of ocular disorders associated with raised intraocular pressure (IOP), optic atrophy, and visual field changes. Anatomically, glaucoma can be classified according to the anatomy of the anterior chamber angle. In angle-closure glaucoma, the peripheral iris apposes and occludes the trabecular meshwork of the anterior chamber angle. In open-angle glaucoma, the iris is not in apposition to the trabecular meshwork. Glaucoma is primary if no secondary causes (e.g., inflammation, abnormal neovascularization, congenital anatomic abnormalities) can be identified.

Glaucoma causes 12% to 15% of cases of blindness in the United States. It is the leading cause of blindness in African-Americans and the third leading cause of blindness in white Americans. Two million Americans have glaucoma.

IDENTIFYING AND MONITORING GLAUCOMATOUS DAMAGE

Intraocular Pressure and Production of Aqueous Humor

A characteristic form of optic atrophy and visual field loss is observed in eyes with elevated IOPs. The level of IOP at which damage to the optic nerve occurs varies with individuals. This raises the question, What is normal IOP and what is a safe pressure?

The mean IOP, based on the results of pooled epidemiologic studies, is 15.5 mm Hg with a standard deviation of 2.5 mm Hg. Any IOP above 21 mm Hg is considered suspect. However, no level of IOP is clearly safe. Some eyes become damaged with IOPs of 18 mm Hg, whereas others tolerate IOPs above 30 mm Hg without damage. Major risk factors for glaucomatous damage include diabetes mellitus, cardiovascular disease, a history of central retinal vein occlusion in either eye, older age, and black race (the incidence of glaucoma is higher in blacks). In the presence of risk factors, treatment is more likely to be undertaken for borderline IOPs. The ophthalmologist must weigh the benefits of treatment to lower the IOP against its side effects and cost. The incidence of optic nerve damage is greater in eyes with higher IOPs, and therefore most ophthalmologists institute treatment if the IOP exceeds 30 mm Hg.

IOP measurements are subject to considerable variability. In normal persons, a diurnal variation of 6.5 mm Hg is noted. In patients with primary open-angle glaucoma, the average diurnal variation is 10 mm Hg. Other causes of transient alterations of IOP include exercise, changes in postural position, and the use of drugs such as alcohol and tobacco. These fluctuations in IOP make it difficult to judge when it is well controlled. In some instances, it is necessary to take multiple readings throughout the day and night to ensure that the peak IOPs are not excessive.

The IOP depends on the balance between aqueous humor production and aqueous outflow from the eye. Most cases of glaucoma result from some form of obstruction or increased resistance to aqueous outflow (Fig. 122.1). The aqueous humor maintains the IOP, provides metabolic substrates, and aids in the removal of metabolic products. It is formed in an area posterior to the iris, the ciliary body. It is secreted into the posterior chamber and then passes forward to the anterior chamber through the pupil. The major drainage of the aqueous is through the trabecular meshwork, an area located at the juncture of the cornea and the iris. Between 5% and 15% of aqueous drains from the eye via an alternative pathway, the uveoscleral pathway, which involves the ciliary muscle, supraciliary space, and suprachoroidal space.

Multiple methods are used to measure IOP. The Shiotz tonometer is inexpensive, durable, relatively easy to use, and well suited for use by primary care providers to screen for glaucoma.

Optic Nerve Head

The optic nerve contains 1.2 million fibers. The average area of the intraocular portion of the optic nerve is 1.5 mm^2. The normal intraocular nerve can be divided into three regions: the neural rim, a central depression termed the *optic cup*, and an area of central pallor. The optic cup is delineated by retinal vessels and usually corresponds to the area of pallor. The ratio of the area of the optic cup (C) to the total area of the nerve (D) is the cup-to-disc ratio (C/D). Similarly, one may define a pallor-to-disc ratio (P/D). In most eyes, the cup-to-disc ratio is less than 0.5, and this ratio is greater than 0.7 in only 5% of the population (Fig. 122.2). The average cup-to-disc ratio may be greater in blacks than in whites because of the greater average size of the optic nerve. The areas of the optic cup and pallor are significant because enlargement over time indicates optic nerve damage secondary to glaucoma.

The direct ophthalmoscope is an important tool with which to screen for and follow the progress of glaucoma. The following guidelines may be helpful in using the direct ophthalmoscope:

1. The examiner's right eye should be used to observe the patient's right eye, and the examiner's left eye to observe the patient's left eye; this prevents collision of the two noses and allows the patient to maintain fixation.
2. The observer's contralateral eye should be kept open to minimize observer accommodation.
3. One should view the nasal retina first to identify a retinal vessel and then follow this vessel back to the optic nerve head. Observation of the nasal retina causes less photophobia for the patient than observation of the temporal retina and thereby facilitates a better view.
4. The following parameters should be noted: optic nerve margins, course of the nerve vessels, delineation of the optic cup by the optic nerve vessels, area of central pallor, symmetry of

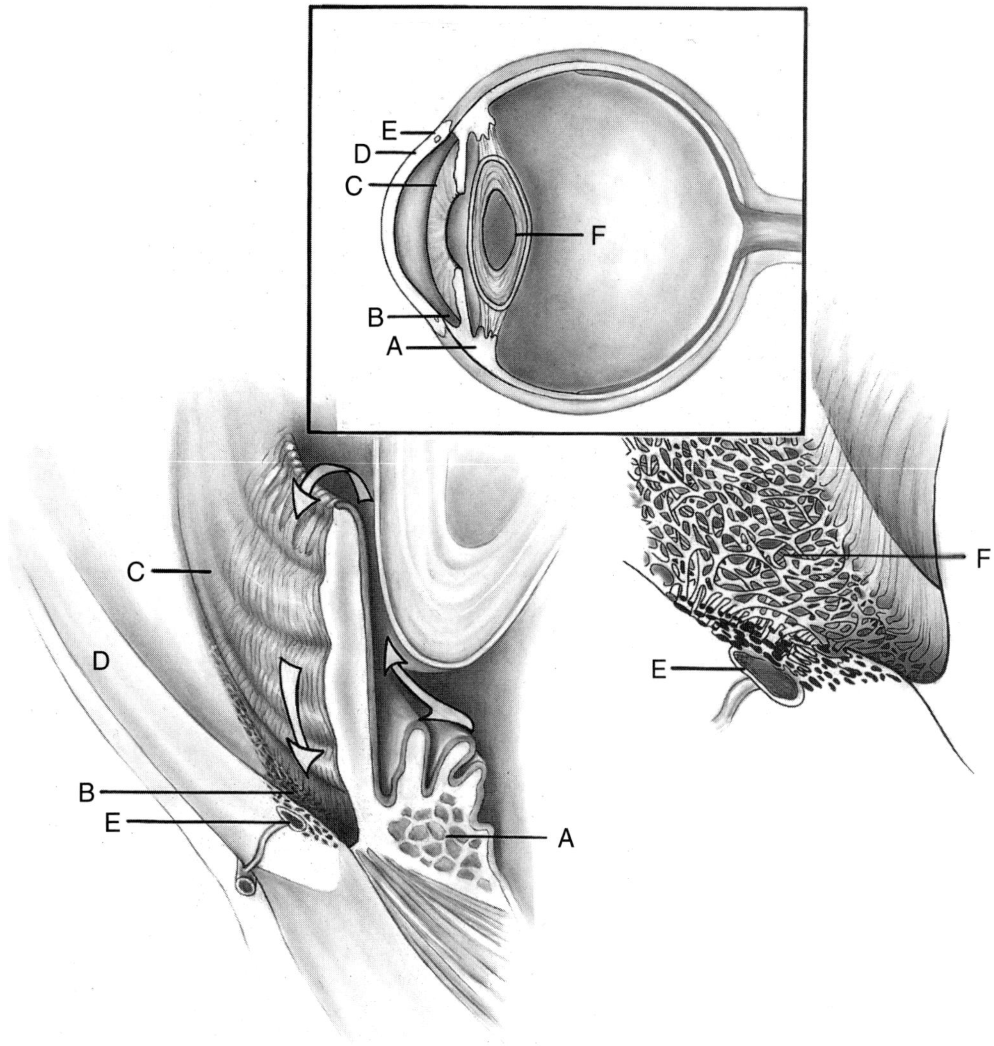

FIG. 122.1. **A:** Ciliary body. **B:** Trabecular meshwork. **C:** Iris. **D:** Cornea. **E:** Schlemm canal. **F:** Crystalline lens. Aqueous humor is formed in the ciliary body, flows through the pupil, exits the anterior chamber through the trabecular meshwork to the Schlemm canal, and subsequently drains to an episcleral venous network.

the cup in relation to the neural rim, presence of peripapillary hemorrhages, and equality of the cup-to-disc ratios in the two eyes.

5. The optic cup and pallor are usually best seen with lower levels of light from the direct ophthalmoscope. Also, directing the light to an area adjacent to the cup may retroilluminate the cup and allow a better study of subtle variations in color and vessel topography of the optic nerve head.

The optic cup and area of pallor are the key indicators of glaucomatous damage. Any cup-to-disc ratio greater than 0.5 should be suspect. In glaucoma, the cup and area of pallor seemingly enlarge as the neural rim diminishes. This enlargement is frequently asymmetric in a vertical direction or in a specific sector. The observer must note the relationship of the optic cup and area of pallor. Cup enlargement, demarcated by the optic nerve vessels, may precede enlargement of the area of pallor in glaucoma. The reverse, in which the area of pallor extends beyond the vessel surrounding the cup, may also indicate optic nerve damage. Glaucoma is frequently asymmetric. Any disparity of 20% or greater between the cup-to-disc ratios of the two eyes is significant. Hemorrhages on the neural rim are frequently seen in glaucoma; sectorial atrophy at the hemorrhage site on the neural rim develops subsequently.

Optic nerve damage in glaucoma is thought to occur in two ways. A raised IOP compresses the optic nerve fibers and decreases axoplasmic flow, with resultant optic nerve atrophy. An abnormal IOP can also cause damage by decreasing perfusion in the optic nerve.

Visual Fields

A visual field examination aids in identifying glaucomatous damage during initial screening and allows the practitioner to judge the effectiveness of therapy over time. The visual field

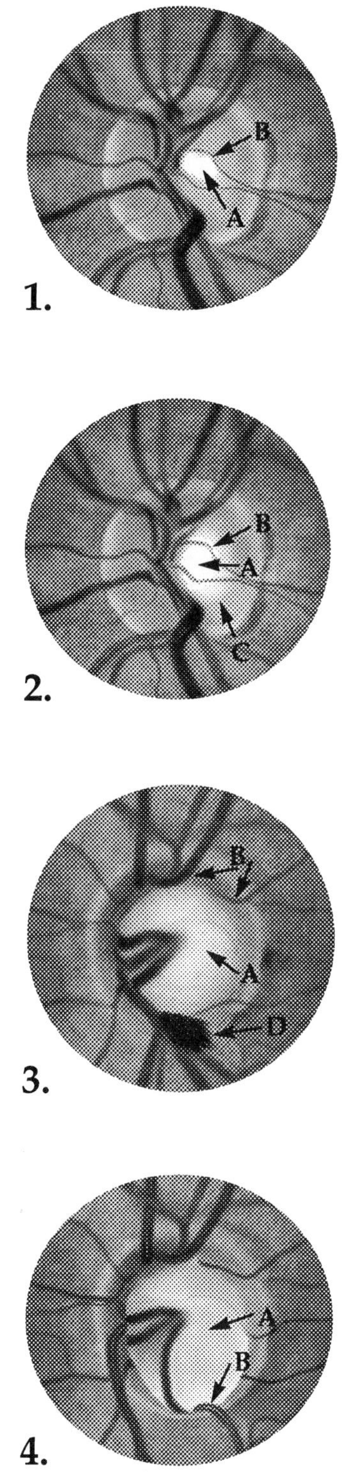

FIG. 122.2. *1.* Normal optic nerve head. Note the blood vessel **(B)** outlining the optic cup. The central pallor **(A)** usually occupies the same area as the optic cup. *2.* The area of pallor **(C)** is beginning to exceed that of the optic cup. *3.* The optic cup and area of pallor are markedly increased. A hemorrhage **(D)** is seen inferiorly on the neural rim. The borders of the cup are delineated by the surrounding vessels. *4.* Note the extensive cupping and pallor of this glaucomatous optic nerve head. The cup is asymmetric in a vertical direction. Very little neural rim remains at the inferior pole of the nerve head.

defects noted in glaucoma follow the distribution of the retinal nerve fiber layer. These fibers do not cross the horizontal midline. Usually, damage to the inferior and superior retinal fibers is not concurrent. Glaucomatous visual field defects therefore do not cross the horizontal midline unless both hemifields are damaged simultaneously. The site of nerve fiber damage determines the resultant visual field defect. Typical nerve fiber defects are shown in Fig. 122.3. The classic defect is the arcuate scotoma. Other defects may be thought of as partial arcuate defects. The nasal visual field (corresponding to the axons that enter the optic nerve temporally from the temporal retina) is the most susceptible to damage, which results in the classic nasal step visual defect. The retinal fibers from the fovea are the most resistant to glaucomatous damage. Thus, the central visual field is often the last area to be lost in glaucoma.

Visual field defects that respect the horizontal midline indicate pathology of the optic nerve and retinal nerve fibers. Typically, defects of this nature are caused by glaucoma or vascular insults to the retina. Visual field defects that respect the vertical midline typically arise from the optic tracts or further posteriorly in the optic radiations and visual cortex and therefore indicate neurologic disease.

Other Methods

Several newer technologic devices for detecting and monitoring the progression of glaucoma may be more sensitive than the visual field examination and human observation of the appearance of the optic nerve. These include the confocal scanning laser ophthalmoscope (Heidelberg Retina Tomograph), scanning laser polarimetry (GDx Nerve Fiber Analyzer), and optical coherence tomography. These computerized devices provide quantitative measurements describing the optic disc and retinal nerve fiber layer. Each machine uses a different feature of the retinal nerve fiber layer and different properties of light to quantify the topography of the optic nerve and thickness of the retinal nerve fiber layer. This information may help the ophthalmologist detect glaucoma earlier, because changes in the thickness of the retinal nerve fiber layer and damage to the optic nerve have been shown to precede visual field loss, and follow patients for progression of damage.

PRIMARY OPEN-ANGLE GLAUCOMA

Primary open-angle glaucoma affects more than 60% to 70% of the persons in whom glaucoma is diagnosed in the United States. As many as 1% of Americans older than 40 years of age have this disease; the incidence increases to 3% for persons older than 70 years of age. The disease is more severe and prevalent in Caribbean and African populations. In the United States, 4% of patients are blind; in Nigeria, 34% of patients with the disease are blind bilaterally and 91% are blind monocularly.

The prevalence of the disease is higher in the relatives of patients with glaucoma, in whom the risk for the development of glaucoma is five to six times greater than that in the general population. Genetically, glaucoma is thought to be polygenic.

Clinical Features

This entity is insidious, slowly progressive, and painless. Because the central vision is affected last, the disease may go unnoticed until damage has become severe. A raised IOP is the primary risk factor. However, 50% of patients have normal IOPs at initial screening. Not all patients with IOPs above 21 mm Hg have glau-

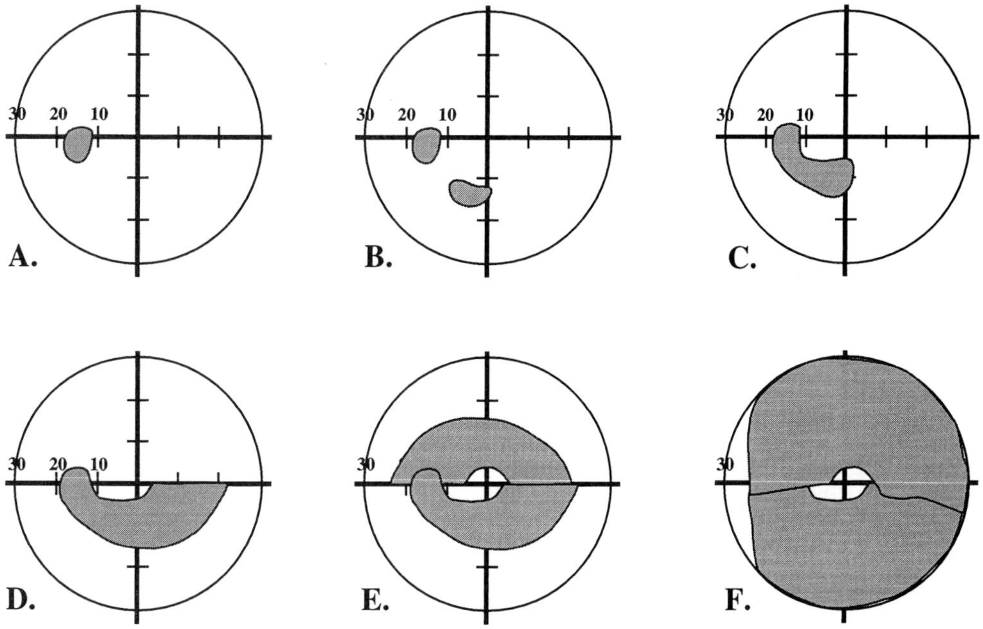

FIG. 122.3. **A:** Normal visual field. **B,C:** Partial lesions. **D:** Arcuate nerve fiber defect. **E:** Arcuate defect in the upper and lower hemifields. **F:** Late stage of glaucoma with sparing only of a central and temporal island of vision.

coma. Primary open-angle glaucoma may be diagnosed by a combination of raised IOP, optic nerve changes, visual field deficits, an open anterior chamber angle on gonioscopy, and the absence of other factors causing a raised IOP. The percentage of the population with a raised IOP increases with age. Table 122.1 illustrates the prevalence of raised IOP and glaucoma as a function of age.

As discussed previously, one of the greatest challenges for the ophthalmologist is to decide when a raised IOP poses a threat and consequently requires therapy. Practitioners have three choices: (a) Treat all patients with IOPs above 21 mm Hg. With this strategy, a large number of patients are treated who may not require therapy. (b) Treat only those with accompanying disc and visual field deficits. The problem is that significant loss of nerve fibers may occur before visual field loss is first detected. (c) Treat patients with risk factors (e.g., diabetes mellitus, cardiovascular disease, strong family history), excessively high IOPs, or suspect optic nerve changes. Most ophthalmologists choose the third option.

Medical Therapy

The topical agents used in ophthalmology have systemic side effects. These can be lessened by applying digital pressure to the medial canthal area for 5 minutes after the agent has been applied to the eye. This maneuver limits drainage through the lacrimal ducts and nasal mucosa and thereby minimizes systemic absorption.

β-ADRENERGIC ANTAGONISTS

These topical agents lower the IOP by decreasing the production of aqueous humor. Six topical β-adrenergic antagonists are available in the United States: betaxolol (Betoptic), carteolol (Ocupress), levobetaxolol (Betaxon), levobunolol (Betagan), metipranolol (OptiPranolol), and timolol (Timoptic). Betaxolol is a relatively selective β_1-adrenergic blocking agent, whereas the other agents have both β_1-adrenergic and β_2-adrenergic antagonist effects. Systemic side effects are infrequent but include bradycardia, heart block, bronchospasm, decreased

TABLE 122.1. Prevalence of Raised Intraocular Pressure as a Function of Age

Age (y)	Percentage of population with IOP >23 mm Hg (%)	Percentage of population with open-angle glaucoma (%)
Total population		0.50
>30	1.6	—
30–39	1.25	—
50–55	—	0.2
70–79	10.5	2

IOP, intraocular pressure.
Adapted from Ritch R, Shields MB, Krupin T. The glaucomas. St. Louis: CV Mosby, 1999:789–795.

libido, and mood changes. β-Adrenergic blockade in a neonate has been described when timolol was used during the period of delivery. Timolol is excreted in breast milk, but studies thus far indicate that the daily dose is below what would be expected to cause cardiac effects in an infant.

ADRENERGIC AGONISTS

Topical epinephrine (Epifrin) was used before the introduction of dipivefrin. Dipivefrin (Propine) is a prodrug of epinephrine with greater therapeutic effectiveness locally in the eye and fewer systemic side effects. This class of glaucoma agent is thought to enhance the outflow of aqueous through the uveoscleral pathway. Systemic side effects include hypertension, extrasystole, headache, and localized adrenochrome deposits in the conjunctiva. Apraclonidine hydrochloride (Iopidine) and brimonidine tartrate (Alphagan) are topical alpha$_2$-adrenergic agonists. Apraclonidine hydrochloride lowers IOP by reducing aqueous secretion and is used after neodymium:yttrium-aluminum garnet laser capsulotomies to prevent pressure spikes, but a high incidence of topical sensitivity has been noted with long-term use. Brimonidine tartrate lowers IOP by decreasing aqueous production and increasing uveoscleral outflow. Its side effects include hyperemia, fatigue, insomnia, depression, and anxiety.

CHOLINERGIC AGONISTS

These topical agents induce pupillary miosis and ciliary muscle contraction, which increase fluid outflow through the trabecular meshwork. Pilocarpine (Isopto Carpine) works directly on the motor endplates as a cholinergic agonist. Echothiophate (Phospholine Iodide) and demecarium bromide (Humorsol) act indirectly by inhibiting the effect of acetylcholinesterase and thus increasing the duration of action of acetylcholine. Carbachol (Isopto Carbachol) has both direct and indirect actions on the cholinergic system. The systemic side effects of this family of drugs, including diarrhea, abdominal cramps, increased salivation, and enuresis, are usually caused by the indirect agents. The indirect agents inhibit systemic anticholinesterase levels; therefore, agents used in general surgery, such as succinylcholine, should not be administered for at least 6 weeks after the topical medication has been discontinued.

CARBONIC ANHYDRASE INHIBITORS

This class of agents acts to decrease aqueous production. Systemic acetazolamide (Diamox) and methazolamide (Neptazane) are used often, and dichlorphenamide (Daranide) less frequently. Topical carbonic anhydrase inhibitors include brinzolamide (Azopt) and dorzolamide (Trusopt). The carbonic anhydrase inhibitors are often associated with systemic side effects, less so in their topical forms. Patients experience paresthesias of the fingers, toes, and lips. Weight loss, abdominal cramping, diarrhea, fatigue, and depression develop, as may aplastic anemia. Acetazolamide has been noted to cause congenital defects in rats, rabbits, and mice. However, despite widespread use, no reports link acetazolamide with human congenital defects.

Acetazolamide is secreted in breast milk, but signs and symptoms in lactating infants have not been reported. The American Academy of Pediatrics feels that this drug is compatible with breast-feeding.

PROSTAGLANDIN ANALOGUES

These topical agents enhance uveoscleral outflow to lower IOP. Three agents are currently available: latanoprost (Xalatan), travoprost (Travatan), and bimatoprost (Lumigan). Some unique side effects include increased pigmentation of the iris, hypertrichosis, cystoid macular edema, and uveitis. Unoprostone isopropyl (Rescula) is a docosanoid that is a structural analogue of an inactive biosynthetic cyclic derivative of arachidonic acid, prostaglandin $F_{2\alpha}$. It increases aqueous outflow by an unknown mechanism. It has side effects similar to those of the prostaglandin analogues.

HYPEROSMOTIC AGENTS

These agents dehydrate the vitreous humor and thereby lower IOP. They are usually used for a short course of treatment because they cause significant systemic effects and lose efficacy as the osmotic gradients equalize in the body. Reported side effects are headache, backache, and mental confusion. Glycerin can cause hyperglycemia in diabetics. Because they increase the intravascular volume, these agents can aggravate congestive heart failure. The agents most commonly used are oral glycerin, oral isosorbide, and intravenous mannitol.

Surgical Therapy

Argon laser therapy can be used in open-angle glaucoma. In this procedure, argon laser trabeculoplasty, laser burns are delivered to the trabecular meshwork. This therapy increases aqueous outflow through the trabecular meshwork and is indicated if medical therapy is inadequate.

If medical and laser therapy does not control IOP sufficiently to prevent the progression of optic nerve damage, surgical filtration surgery can be performed. A variety of surgical techniques are used to create an internal fistula that allows aqueous to drain to the episcleral space. The complications of these procedures are cataract formation in addition to all the complications of cataract surgery.

PRIMARY ANGLE-CLOSURE GLAUCOMA

Angle-closure glaucoma results from apposition of the iris to the trabecular meshwork, which blocks the exit of aqueous humor. The most common cause of angle-closure glaucoma is primary angle-closure glaucoma with pupillary block. Other causes of angle closure include neovascular glaucoma secondary to inflammation or diabetes mellitus, intraocular tumors, and associated ocular diseases.

Pathophysiology

The precipitating event may be mild pupillary dilation (iatrogenic or in normal situations, such as a darkened room or sympathetic stimulation). In angle-closure glaucoma, the peripupillary iris maintains contact with the crystalline lens; fluid formed by the ciliary body in the posterior chamber cannot travel forward through the pupil to the anterior chamber and is trapped. The peripheral iris bulges forward to appose the trabecular meshwork. The egress of aqueous fluid is blocked. Aqueous humor continues to be formed and the IOP builds.

Epidemiology

Angle-closure glaucoma with pupillary block has a hereditary component. The prevalence of this disease in the United States is much less than that of primary open-angle glaucoma. However, in Eskimos, Japanese, and Southeast Asians, this is a significant form of glaucoma. Hyperopic eyes, in which the anterior chambers tend to be shallow, are more susceptible to angle-closure glaucoma. With age, the lens continues to grow and displaces the iris anteriorly. Also with age, the pupil becomes more miotic. Therefore, angle-closure glaucoma tends to occur in people older than 60 years.

Significance

Angle-closure glaucoma occurs precipitously and is a true ocular emergency. Because the pressures rise precipitously and to very high levels, vision can be lost in a relatively short period of time. Patients may experience severe pain with nausea, vomiting, and dehydration. The patient may be obtunded secondary to dehydration at presentation. This form of glaucoma may be precipitated by pupillary dilation that develops when systemic drugs with atropinic effects are used.

Symptoms

Patients may experience mild to severe eye pain. The pain may be sufficiently severe to cause nausea and vomiting. Patients may describe seeing halos around light, blurred vision, or severe loss of vision.

Signs

The following are signs of angle-closure glaucoma: engorgement of the limbal blood vessels; decreased visual acuity; corneal edema manifested by an irregular corneal luster and light reflex; decreased corneal clarity; an irregular, nonreactive, mid position pupil; raised IOP; and poor view of the retina with ophthalmoscopy.

Diagnosis

The examiner should use a hand light and examine the conjunctiva. Note injection and the distribution of redness. In angle-closure glaucoma, the blood vessels around the cornea are engorged, and a red halo appears to surround the cornea.

By projecting light across the anterior chamber from the temporal to the nasal side, the examiner can estimate the anterior displacement of the iris. In a shallow anterior chamber, the iris bows forward and blocks the pathway of the light. Consequently, a shadow is seen on the nasal side of the iris (Fig. 122.4).

Examine the reflection of the light from the cornea. Normally, the corneal reflection of light is very uniform and smooth. If corneal edema is present, the light reflex is pebbly and irregular. Multiple light reflexes may be seen rather than one.

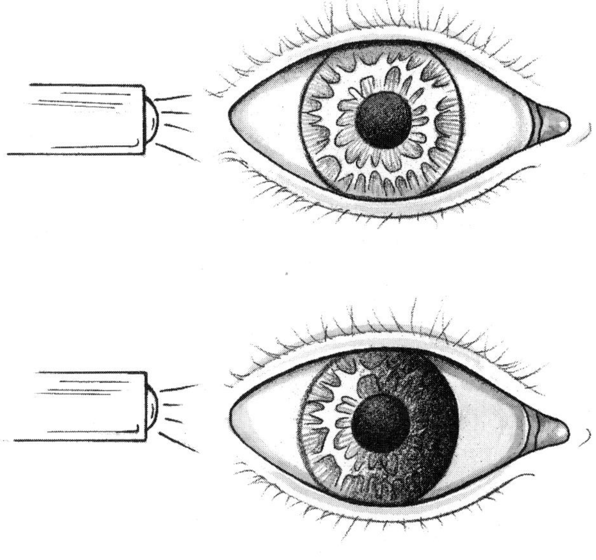

FIG. 122.4. A penlight is shone across the anterior chamber from the temporal to the nasal side. If the anterior chamber is shallow, the temporal side of the iris casts a shadow.

The clarity of the cornea should be compared with that of the contralateral eye. Through a normal cornea, one should be able to visualize the iris, lens, and retinal detail. If the cornea is edematous, it will appear hazy, and the view of the iris, lens, and retina is poor.

The pupil may be misshapen and react poorly to light in comparison with the contralateral eye.

The IOP is usually elevated. However, attacks of angle-closure glaucoma may abate spontaneously and recur episodically (subacute angle-closure glaucoma). Therefore, the IOP may be normal if the patient is seen during the recovery phase of the episode. In the subacute phase, the cornea may be clear. Varying degrees of optic atrophy or optic nerve pallor may be observed.

Treatment

Laser iridectomy is the treatment of choice. A hole created in the iris provides an alternate pathway from the posterior to the anterior chamber. The entrapment of aqueous humor and resultant anterior displacement of the iris are decreased.

If laser iridotomy is not possible, the attack can be treated medically with topical and systemic agents (see section "Medical Therapy" under "Primary Open-Angle Glaucoma").

Surgical iridectomy can be performed if previous therapies have been unsuccessful.

SUMMARY

Glaucoma affects more than 2 million Americans. The disease is frequently silent, but if treated early, visual loss can usually be prevented. The primary care physician may recognize early signs of the disease primarily by optic disc changes (cup-to-disc ratio greater than 0.5, unequal cup-to-disc ratios in the two eyes, and asymmetry of the optic cup relative to the neural rim). Other indications for referral include IOPs above 21 mm Hg, risk factors for glaucoma (family history of glaucoma, diabetes mellitus, or severe cardiovascular disease), and signs of acute angle-closure glaucoma.

BIBLIOGRAPHY

American Academy of Pediatrics Committee on Drugs. The transfer of drugs and other chemicals into human milk. *Pediatrics* 1994;93(1);137.

Berson FG, ed. *Ophthalmology study guide*, 5th ed. San Francisco: American Academy of Ophthalmology, 1993.

Bradford CA, ed. *Basic ophthalmology for medical students and primary care residents*, 7th ed. San Francisco: American Academy of Ophthalmology, 2000.

Briggs GG, Freeman RK, Sumner JY. *Drugs in pregnancy and lactation*, 6th ed. Philadelphia: Lippincott Williams & Wilkins, 2002.

Cantor L, Berlin MS, Fechtner A, et al. *Basic and clinical science course. Section 10: Glaucoma*. San Francisco: American Academy of Ophthalmology, 2002.

Glaucoma prescribing guide. In: *Physicians desk reference*, 4th ed. Montvale, NJ: Medical Economics, 2002.

Haley MJ, ed. *The field analyzer primer*. San Leandro, CA: Allergan Humphrey, 1987.

Newell FW. *Ophthalmology: principles and concepts*, 8th ed. St. Louis: Mosby, 1996.

Shields MB. *Textbook of glaucoma*, 4th ed. Baltimore: Williams & Wilkins, 1997.

Thomas JV. Primary open-angle glaucoma. In: Albert DM, Jakobiec FA, Azar DT, et al., eds. *Principles and practice of ophthalmology*, 2nd ed. Philadelphia: WB Saunders, 2000:2682–2707.

Trobe JD. *The physician's guide to eye care*, 2nd ed. San Francisco: American Academy of Ophthalmology, 2001.

Wilson MR, Martone JF. The epidemiology of primary open-angle glaucoma and ocular hypertension. In: Ritch R, Shields MB, Krupin T, eds. *The glaucomas*, 2nd ed. St. Louis: Mosby, 1996.

Zangwill LM, Bowd C, Berry CC, et al. Discriminating between normal and glaucomatous eyes using the Heidelberg retina tomograph, GDx nerve fiber analyzer, and optical coherence tomograph. *Arch Ophthalmol* 2001;119:985–993.

CHAPTER 123
Ophthalmic Emergencies

King To

The purpose of this chapter is to help you, the primary care physician, recognize an ocular emergency and initiate the appropriate care and referral. The management and visual prognosis of patients with these conditions are not discussed here. An ocular emergency is not always easy to recognize. The initial care provided by the primary care physician is sometimes crucial until the patient can be seen by an ophthalmologist. A good example is the patient with a chemical burn.

OCULAR BURNS

Ocular burns may be classified as chemical, thermal, electric, or caused by radiation. Chemical burns of the eye are by far the most common and most urgent of all ocular burns. Potent chemicals containing alkaline material, such as lye or ammonia in household cleaners, or acidic material, such as battery acid or bleach, can cause serious ocular injury and blindness. In general, alkaline injuries are more serious than acid burns. Acid burns denature the ocular tissue proteins, and the resultant precipitation of proteins sets up a barrier against further penetration of the chemical into the eye. Conversely, strong alkaline chemicals rapidly penetrate the ocular tissues and cause widespread damage. The severity of a chemical burn depends on the amount and nature of the chemical to which the eye has been exposed and the length of time it has been in the eye. Therefore, the single most important thing to do in case of a chemical burn is to irrigate the affected eye(s) immediately with copious amounts of water, saline solution, or any available bland fluid. Ideally, the irrigation is performed after a drop of topical anesthetic has been applied, and the eyelids are retracted with a lid speculum. If an anesthetic or eyelid speculum is not available, separate the eyelids as best you can and irrigate the eye until the pH paper readings are between 7.3 and 7.7. This can be difficult to do because the patient is already experiencing a great deal of discomfort and will likely have trouble keeping the eyes open during the irrigation. But irrigate you must.

The management of a chemical injury is best handled by an ophthalmologist. After you have irrigated the eye as best you can, refer the patient to an ophthalmologist. The medical and surgical therapy for serious chemical burns of the eye can be quite complex and is beyond the scope of this chapter.

OCULAR INFECTIONS

Infections of the eye and ocular adnexa in general are not ocular emergencies except in a few cases, one of which is orbital cellulitis. Orbital cellulitis is a true ocular emergency because when treatment is delayed, blindness secondary to optic nerve compression or even death can result. Orbital cellulitis must be distinguished from preseptal or periorbital cellulitis. In preseptal cellulitis, the infection and inflammation are limited to the skin and muscle of the eyelids and remain anterior to the orbital septum. In orbital cellulitis, the inflammation has spread behind the septum and into the orbital space. Clinical findings suggestive of orbital cellulitis include fever, decreased vision, afferent pupillary defect, proptosis (anterior displacement of the eye), and restricted eye movements. If one or more of these signs are present in a patient with cellulitis of the eyelids, prompt referral to an ophthalmologist is indicated. The key lies in the examination of the eye. An example of cellulitis of the eyelid is shown in Fig. 123.1. To determine whether this patient also has orbital cellulitis, the eyelid must be elevated and the eye examined for vision, pupillary response, proptosis, and extraocular motion. Preseptal cellulitis in adults can usually be managed with oral antibiotics in an outpatient setting. In children, preseptal cellulitis can quickly progress to orbital cellulitis; as a result, hospital admission with intravenous antibiotic therapy is often warranted for children with this condition.

External infections of the eye can usually be managed by the primary care physician. However, serious infections of the cornea, such as a corneal ulcer, and of the conjunctiva, such as hyperacute gonococcal conjunctivitis, require the immediate attention of an ophthalmologist. When a defect is present in the superficial epithelial layer of the cornea, the cornea is at risk for infection. If an infection develops, an inflammatory infiltrate (corneal ulcer) appears in the stroma of the cornea. Corneal ulcers can progress rapidly and result in a permanently scarred cornea and blindness. A predisposing factor for corneal ulcers is contact lens wear, especially in patients who do not care for their lenses meticulously and who sleep with the lenses in their eyes. Corneal ulcers, especially in the early stages, can be difficult to identify without the aid of a slitlamp. The primary care physician should refer any patient, particularly a contact lens wearer, who presents with a painful red eye, foreign body sensation, and decreased vision to an ophthalmologist to rule out a corneal ulcer. A corneal opacity, depending on the size of the corneal ulcer, may or may not be noted during a penlight examination in the primary care physician's office.

Infectious conjunctivitis is a very common condition and often does not require any treatment. However, gonococcal conjunctivitis is a rare but serious eye emergency. If not promptly treated, the infection can quickly advance to perforation of the cornea. The hallmark of gonococcal conjunctivitis is a tremendous amount of pus or discharge actively draining from the eye(s) (Fig. 123.2), unlike that seen in any other type of conjunctivitis. Rapid diagnosis with Gram stain of the conjunctival discharge reveals Gram-negative intracellular diplococci. Such patients require topical ocular antibiotic therapy in addition to systemic antibiotic therapy.

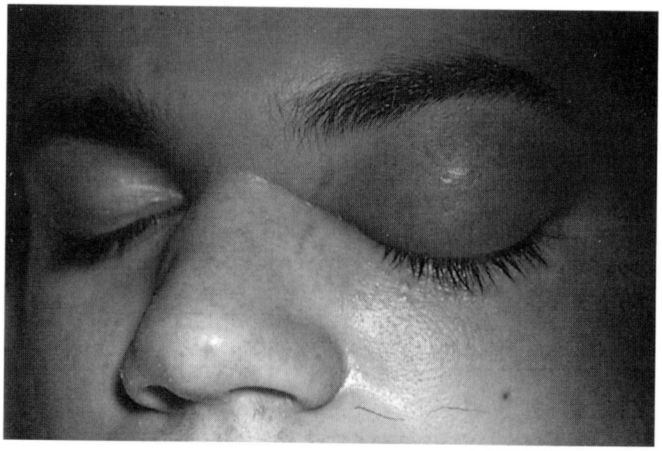

FIG. 123.1. Marked cellulitis of the upper lid in a patient with orbital cellulitis.

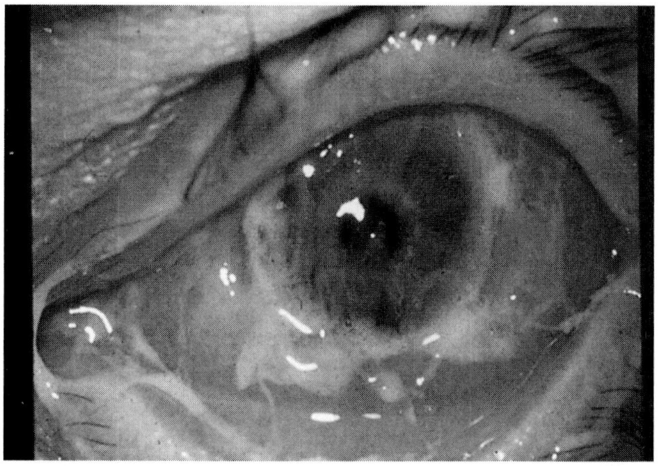

FIG. 123.2. Hyperacute purulent conjunctivitis secondary to *Neisseria gonorrhoeae* infection.

DIPLOPIA

Patients with diplopia, or double vision, may present initially to their primary care physician. Which patients with an acute onset of diplopia warrant immediate ophthalmologic or neurosurgical consultation? In general, any patient with diplopia should be evaluated by an ophthalmologist, but diplopia associated with a cranial nerve III palsy requires an immediate ophthalmologic consultation. The many causes of a cranial nerve III palsy include diabetes, hypertension, trauma, tumors, temporal arteritis, multiple sclerosis, and intracranial aneurysm. In a patient with a cranial nerve III palsy, the affected eye typically deviates outward and down, and the upper eyelid droops (ptosis). If the pupil is also dilated, an expanding posterior communicating artery aneurysm that may rupture should be ruled out immediately (Fig. 123.3). Palsies of two other cranial nerves can result in diplopia: those of cranial nerves IV and VI. Patients with cranial nerve IV palsy experience vertical diplopia, in which images from one eye are above or below images from the fellow eye. Causes include trauma, diabetes, temporal arteritis, tumor, and a congenital cranial nerve IV palsy that has decompensated over time. Patients with a cranial nerve VI palsy have horizontal diplopia, in which the double images are side by side. The involved eye is turned inward, and the ability to abduct the eye is decreased. Causes of cranial nerve VI palsy include diabetes, hypertension, inflammation, multiple sclerosis, brain tumor, and increased intracranial pressure. Cranial nerve VI is particularly susceptible to increased intracranial pressure. The pressure can cause a downward displacement of the brainstem that results in a cranial nerve VI palsy by stretching the subarachnoid segment between the point of exit of cranial nerve VI from the brainstem and its dural attachment on the clivus.

A

B

C

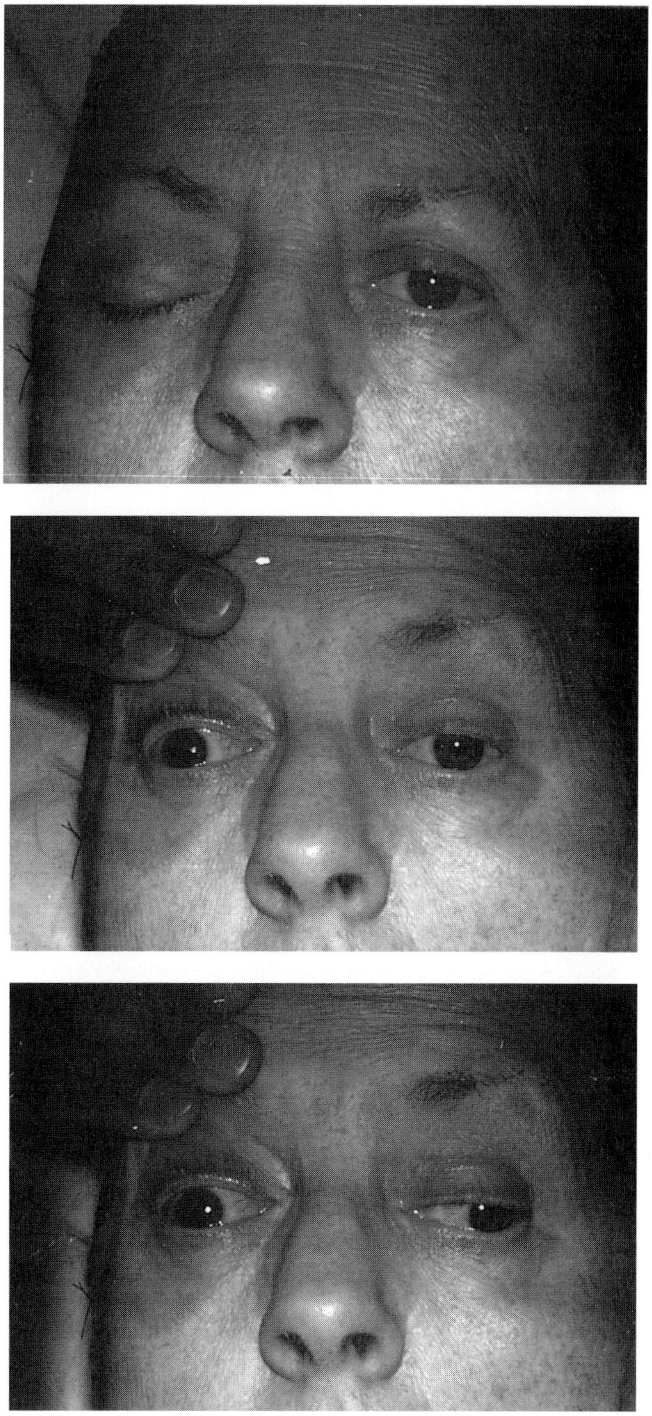

FIG. 123.3. **A:** Complete ptosis of the right side in a patient with a cranial nerve III palsy secondary to a life-threatening expanding posterior communicating artery aneurysm. **B:** With the lid elevated, the right eye is deviated outward and down. **C:** When instructed to look to the left, this patient is unable to do so with the right eye because the medial rectus muscle is controlled by cranial nerve III.

OCULAR TRAUMA

Trauma to the eye warrants an evaluation by an ophthalmologist because such patients may not be able to cooperate with an eye examination, so that a serious injury is left hidden and untreated. Most trauma cases do not require immediate attention, but the following are unique ocular injuries for which an immediate ophthalmologic consultation is necessary.

A ruptured globe is a true ocular emergency. Rupture of the eyeball may be the result of a serious contusion or penetrating trauma. Subconjunctival hemorrhage in the eye may mask the rupture. The site of a globe rupture can be very difficult to determine, and in some cases this author has had to take the patient to surgery to look for occult sites of rupture. If a perforation of the globe is discovered, immediate surgical repair is indicated. If a perforation is left untreated, infection and uveitis (intraocular inflammation) can and do often lead to a blind and painful eye.

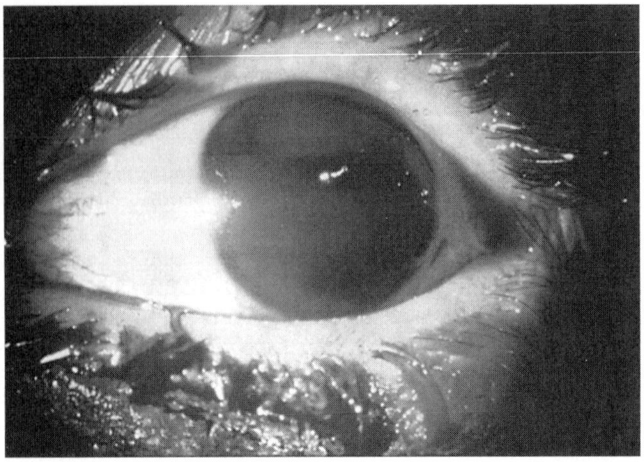

FIG. 123.4. Traumatic hyphema (blood in the anterior chamber).

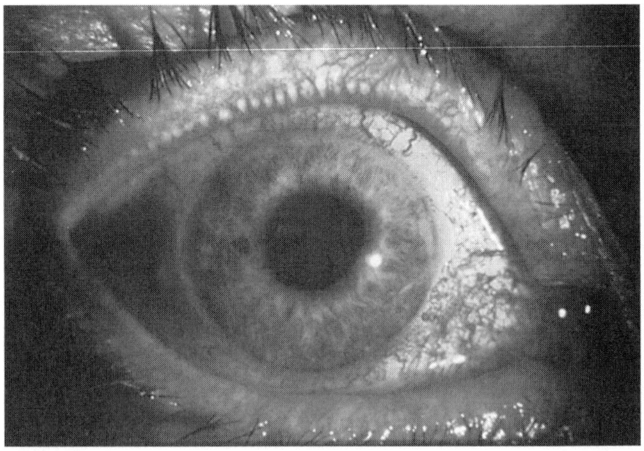

FIG. 123.5. Ocular appearance of acute glaucoma in a patient presenting with eye pain, tearing, halos, blurred vision, nausea, and vomiting.

Although one of the physical findings associated with a globe rupture is a soft eye, it is not a good idea to attempt to palpate the eyeball. In an effort to diagnose a ruptured globe, even gentle palpation can result in the extrusion of intraocular tissue and permanent ocular damage. When a ruptured eyeball is suspected, the primary care physician's examination is over. Everyone, including the patient, must be instructed not to touch the injured eye. Ideally, if an eye shield is available, it is taped over the eye to protect it from further injury. An urgent ophthalmic consultation is warranted.

When an intraocular hemorrhage such as a hyphema (blood in the anterior chamber) is suspected, it is reasonable to conclude that the eyeball may also be ruptured. Any injury severe enough to cause an intraocular hemorrhage may well perforate the globe. The vision of such a patient is typically reduced, and on penlight examination, the pupil may be obscured by the hemorrhage (Fig. 123.4). Immediate treatment by an ophthalmologist is necessary to prevent the development of glaucoma and further bleeding. Even without a ruptured globe, an intraocular hemorrhage is a true eye emergency. I should emphasize again that one must be mindful that unnecessary manipulation of the eye can cause additional ocular damage. The examination of such patients must be very gentle, and if the primary care physician is unable to assess the severity of the injury, an ophthalmologist should be contacted.

ACUTE GLAUCOMA

Acute angle-closure glaucoma is an ocular emergency. These patients present with the sudden onset of blurred vision, eye pain, and nausea and vomiting. On penlight examination, the eye is injected and the details of the iris are hazy because the cornea is edematous (Fig. 123.5). The pupil is usually fixed (poorly responsive to light) and slightly dilated. Measurement of the intraocular pressure and a gonioscopic examination by an ophthalmologist confirm the diagnosis. The vast majority of patients with glaucoma have the open-angle form and are not predisposed to acute angle-closure glaucoma.

ACUTE VISUAL LOSS

The patient who presents with acute painless visual loss requires an emergent evaluation by an ophthalmologist. The causes of profound acute loss of vision are numerous. The following are ocular emergencies: retinal detachment, central retinal artery or vein occlusion, exudative macular degeneration, and anterior ischemic optic neuropathy.

A retinal detachment can cause central visual loss if the macula is involved, or it can create a "shadow" or defect in a particular field of vision. Symptoms associated with central or peripheral field loss include floaters and photopsia (sensation of seeing flashes of light). On ophthalmoscopy, inward bulging of the retina toward the center of the eye creates folds in the retina. An associated retinal hole or tear is present where the detachment started, but this is very difficult to visualize unless the pupil is dilated and examined with an indirect ophthalmoscope or a three-mirror lens. Prompt laser or surgical repair of a retinal detachment often successfully restores vision.

Central retinal vein occlusion has a distinctive funduscopic appearance and is easier to identify on ophthalmoscopy than a retinal detachment. The extent of visual loss is quite variable. I have seen patients with asymptomatic mild central retinal vein occlusion and patients with severe central retinal vein occlusion who have become legally blind. Central retinal vein occlusion is more common in patients with diabetes, hypertension, collagen-vascular diseases, and hyperviscosity syndromes. Examination of the fundus reveals hemorrhages in all four quadrants of the retina, dilated and tortuous retinal veins, a swollen optic nerve, and an edematous macula.

Unlike central retinal vein occlusion, in which the degree of visual loss is quite variable, central retinal artery occlusion is typically associated with profound visual loss. In addition, the funduscopic appearance of a central retinal artery occlusion is rather unimpressive in comparison with that of a central retinal vein occlusion. No retinal hemorrhages are seen; instead, diffuse retinal ischemia and edema make the macula look like a "cherry red spot" (Fig. 123.6).

Exudative degeneration of the macula is one of the leading causes of blindness and the leading cause of blindness in patients older than 65 years of age in the United States. In exudative or wet macular degeneration, new abnormal blood vessels (choroidal neovascular membrane) invade the subretinal space. Vascular invasion is associated with development of hemorrhage, subsequent permanent scarring of the macula (disciform scar), and blindness. Exudative macular degeneration accounts for 90% of the cases of severe visual loss that occur in patients with age-related macular degeneration. Identification of the new blood vessels by fluorescein angiography allows prompt treatment with laser photocoagulation. This

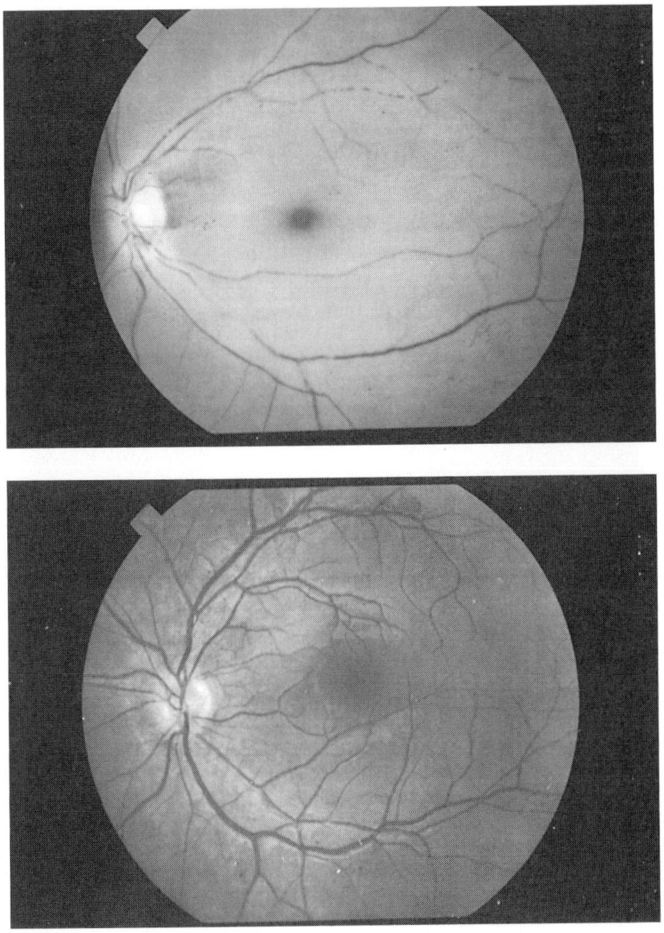

A

B

FIG. 123.6. **A:** Characteristic appearance of the "cherry red spot" seen in central retinal artery occlusion. Segmentation of the blood column ("boxcars") can be observed in the retinal vessels. **B:** For comparison with **A**, a healthy retina.

treatment should be administered as soon as possible before any significant hemorrhage or scarring develops.

Anterior ischemic optic neuropathy is an infarction of the prelaminar portion of the optic nerve. It may be caused by hemodynamic instability associated with severe blood loss, profound hypotension, emboli (as a complication of coronary artery bypass surgery), or arteriosclerosis (typically in a middle-aged patient with hypertension, diabetes, or both). However, only one form of anterior ischemic optic neuropathy can be considered a true ocular emergency: that associated with temporal arteritis, also known as *giant cell arteritis*. This condition is a disease of the elderly. The anterior ischemic optic neuropathy of temporal arteritis is rare before the age of 60 years and typically occurs in persons older than 70 years.

Little can be done for an eye with anterior ischemic optic neuropathy, and patients with temporal arteritis are at high risk for the development of anterior ischemic optic neuropathy in the fellow eye within hours to days. It has always amazed me, in my 17 years of practicing ophthalmology, how many of my patients adjust and lead happy and productive lives after the

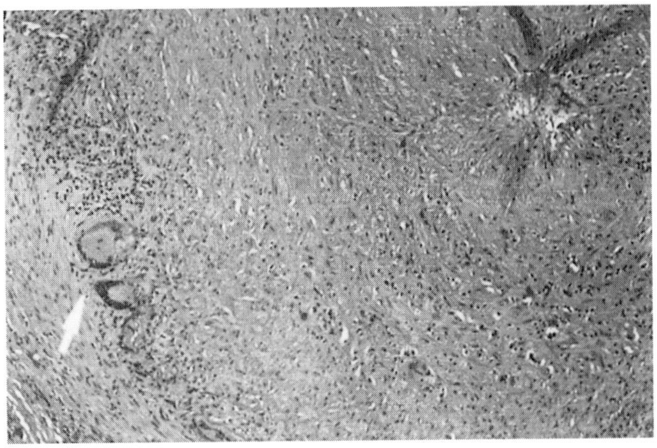

FIG. 123.7. Temporal artery biopsy specimen demonstrating vasculitis in all layers of the vessel. Note the prominent granulomatous giant cell reaction in the wall of the artery *(arrow)*.

loss of vision in one eye. Of course, in the truly disastrous scenario of bilateral blindness, as may occur in anterior ischemic optic neuropathy associated with temporal arteritis, these patients' lives are sadly changed forever. Therefore, it is of great importance to recognize anterior ischemic optic neuropathy promptly in a patient with temporal arteritis and refer the patient to an ophthalmologist so that treatment can be initiated to prevent involvement of the other eye.

The key to recognizing anterior ischemic optic neuropathy in association with temporal arteritis is in the patient's history. Temporal arteritis is a generalized inflammatory disease of large and medium-size arteries that occurs in the elderly. Consequently, these patients often have one or more of the following systemic symptoms: malaise, loss of appetite, weight loss, fever, scalp tenderness, muscle and joint stiffness and pain (polymyalgia rheumatica), headache, and jaw claudication. Therefore, if an elderly patient is encountered with acute vision loss and these systemic symptoms, a diagnosis of temporal arteritis should be considered and the following steps taken: A sedimentation rate should be obtained at once and the patient referred to an ophthalmologist immediately. Caution must be exercised, because although most patients with temporal arteritis have an elevated sedimentation rate (>50 mm/h), 5% of them actually have a normal rate. If an ophthalmologist is unable to evaluate the patient right away, the initiation of high doses of oral steroids (typically 60–80 mg of prednisone) should be considered. Biopsy of the temporal artery should be scheduled within 14 days after the start of therapy (Fig. 123.7). The results of biopsies performed after 2 weeks of steroid therapy may be false-negative, although not always.

BIBLIOGRAPHY

Albert DM, Jakobiec FA, Azar DT, et al., eds. *Principles and practice of ophthalmology*, 2nd ed. Philadelphia: WB Saunders, 2000.

Kanski JJ, ed. *Clincal ophthalmology*, 4th ed. Boston: Butterworth-Heinemann, 2000.

To KW, Enzer YR, Tsiaras WG. Positive temporal artery biopsy after corticosteroid therapy. *Am J Ophthalmol* 1994;117:265–267.

Yanoff M, Duker JS, eds. *Ophthalmology*, 2nd ed. Philadelphia: Mosby International, 1999.

PART

14

Ear, Nose, and Throat Problems

CHAPTER 124

Acute and Chronic Rhinosinusitis

James A. Hadley

HISTORY

Acute infectious rhinosinusitis is an extremely common medical problem, affecting more than 20% of the United States population each year and accounting for nearly 25 million office visits per year. It is an inflammatory and usually infectious process of the linings of the paranasal sinuses and the nasal cavity. The disease is responsible for the expenditure of millions of dollars for medications and antibiotics to alleviate the symptoms of pain, nasal congestion, and lethargy, which is characteristic of the process. Some experts believe that acute and chronic rhinosinusitis are becoming more prevalent, perhaps due to air pollution damage to the respiratory linings and increased exposure to upper respiratory infections in day care settings and "tight" buildings.

The symptoms of acute rhinosinusitis (nasal congestion, postnasal discharge, facial discomfort, and cough) are often confused with the common head cold, and this misunderstanding leads to prolonged inflammation due to lack of early treatment. Primary care physicians must be aware of the symptoms to render early effective treatment and to differentiate between other causes of sinonasal disorders. For example, pregnancy often renders the nose stuffy, primarily due to the estrogenic effects on the nasal mucosa; allergic rhinitis may affect up to 20% of the population and may be seasonal or perennial.

Treatment of infectious rhinosinusitis is necessary to prevent possible serious complications and is based on appropriate antibiotic therapy. The recent emergence of antibiotic-resistant bacteria, especially *Streptococcus pneumoniae,* has made selection of appropriate antibiotic regimens crucial.

In the past decade, technical advances in paranasal imaging and endoscopic examination have led to a new understanding of the physiology of the paranasal sinuses. These developed concepts have led to a better overall management of this common problem. Medical therapy should be effective for most patients with persistent rhinosinusitis, but surgery may be recommended for recalcitrant cases and specifically for patients with complications of acute or chronic rhinosinusitis.

ANATOMY AND PHYSIOLOGY

The paranasal sinuses, paired air-containing cavities in the anterior skull, include the maxillary, ethmoid, frontal, and sphenoid sinuses. Phylogenetically presumed to lighten the otherwise heavy skull, they are lined by the same respiratory pseudostratified ciliated squamous epithelium characteristic of the bronchial tree. They develop as outpouchings of respiratory epithelium within the facial bones, and their primary role is to provide aeration, humidification, and warming of inhaled air and protection from foreign objects inhaled through the nose. Ventilation and transport of mucus occur through the small ostia from the sinuses into the nose. These important mechanisms depend on the ability of the ciliated respiratory epithelium to move mucus through the narrow ostia.

Maxillary Sinus

The maxillary sinuses are the largest and develop first from pea-sized pouches extending into the cheeks from the nose. They begin to develop around the third month of gestation and change shape to a triangular cavity during the child's growth. The maxillary sinus ultimately develops into a pyramidal cavity, occupying most of the maxilla. The maxillary antrum communicates with the middle meatus via the infundibulum of the middle meatus through a natural ostium.

The natural ostium drains into the hiatus semilunaris, a slit-like ostium between the ethmoid cells, the uncinate process, and the orbit. Accessory ostia may develop as a result of chronic infection.

Ethmoid Sinus

The ethmoid sinuses develop during the third trimester into a labyrinth of small sinus cells medial and superior to the maxillary sinuses. They enlarge by pneumatization over the person's growth. The ethmoid cells vary in number (from 4 to 50 individual cells) and location. The most anterior cells are the frontal cells; next to them, the infundibular cells are anterior to the ethmoid bulla. These cells drain the frontal sinuses into the nose. The bullar cells may form a large cell and drain into the middle meatus just posterior to the agger nasi cells. Conchal cells of the ethmoids involve the anterior aspect of the middle turbinate and may cause obstruction of the middle meatus or give rise to pressure points. The posterior ethmoid cells lie behind the basal lamella of the middle turbinate and drain into the sphenoethmoidal recess.

Frontal Sinus

The frontal sinuses become pneumatized from the ethmoids directly into the frontal bone after about the third year of life. This pneumatization of the frontal bones is often asymmetric, and the sinuses are sometimes hypoplastic or nonexistent or large with several compartments. They drain into the nasofrontal recess directly into the middle meatus alongside the anterior ethmoid cells.

Sphenoid Sinus

The sphenoid sinus does not appear until about the third year of life, growing as an outpouching of the sphenoethmoidal recess. Pneumatization enlarges the sinus to the sella turcica, attaining maximal growth in mid-adolescence. It drains usually through a small ostium in the sphenoethmoidal recess that is superior to the floor of the sphenoid sinus.

Physiology of the Paranasal Sinuses

The sinuses are lined by a respiratory epithelium composed of a pseudostratified columnar layer of cells lying on a supporting layer of fibroelastic tissue associated with goblet cells. The function of this layer of respiratory epithelium is to provide the sinuses with a supporting blanket of mucus.

The nose is designed to protect the respiratory tract from a hostile environment, and the sinuses play a major role in this defense through the elaboration of a mucous blanket. This blanket functions to warm and humidify ambient air and clears debris and pathogens from the body.

A mucous lining consisting of a biphase inner sol layer and an outer thick layer coats the respiratory epithelium. It is made from seromucinous glands within the epithelium and provides both protective and barrier functions. Respiratory mucus, found in the nose, sinuses, and eustachian tube, can insulate, lubricate, waterproof, humidify, and provide a medium for ciliary action. The outer gel layer traps foreign material, which is then transported to the natural drainage ostia by means of the ciliary action of the cells beating in the inner thinner layer of mucus. Enzymatic proteins, including lysozyme, lactoferrin, and secretory IgA, are contained in the inner serous layer. These digest foreign bacteria and viruses and are the first line of defense. In the healthy state, the cilia propel the mucus to the natural ostia of the nose, from which it is eventually expelled.

Mucociliary clearance through the natural ostia may become impaired after a viral infection. Stasis of secretions occurs, and a secondary bacterial infection may result from this stagnation. The small size of the natural drainage pathways predisposes to obstruction of the natural ostia from even minor swelling of the mucous membranes after an upper respiratory inflammation, allergic inflammatory response, or infection (Fig. 124.1). These events set the stage for sinus infection.

The ventilation and drainage portals of the sinuses are small ostia that vary in size and position. The natural ostium of the maxillary sinus is located behind a lamella of bone, termed the uncinate process. The frontal sinus drains and ventilates through a recess superior to the ethmoid bullar cell (the largest of the many ethmoid cells) directly into the middle meatus, along with the ethmoid cells (Fig. 124.2). The sphenoid sinuses have their own ostia, which drain into the sphenoethmoidal recess posterior and medial to the middle turbinate (Fig. 124.3).

After a viral upper respiratory infection, the seromucinous glands secrete an increased amount of plasma proteins to help fight the infectious process. The increased vascular permeability that results creates the symptoms of nasal congestion and engorgement with increased rhinorrhea. These secretions thicken as the infection progresses, resulting in the symptoms of thick postnasal discharge.

Allergic reactions play a role in the development of inflammations within the paranasal sinuses. Type I hypersensitivity reactions involve the release of inflammatory mediators from the mast cell after sensitization. During the early stage of this reaction, histamine and other preformed kinins are released, causing increased capillary permeability, edema formation, and increased mucous production. This is followed by a late phase several hours later, characterized by the influx of cells into the inflammatory site. These cells include neutrophils, eosinophils, and lymphocytes that elaborate lymphokines and other mediators, prolonging the inflammation within the mucosa. This inflammatory state within the sinus mucous membranes may

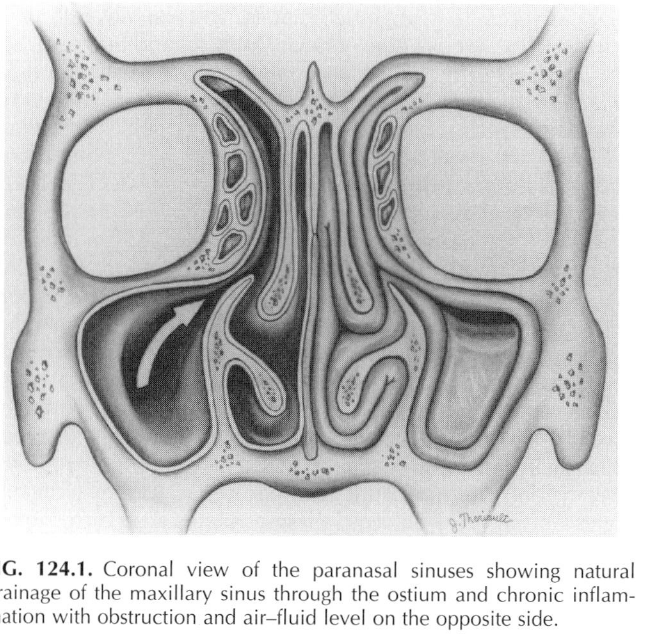

FIG. 124.1. Coronal view of the paranasal sinuses showing natural drainage of the maxillary sinus through the ostium and chronic inflammation with obstruction and air–fluid level on the opposite side.

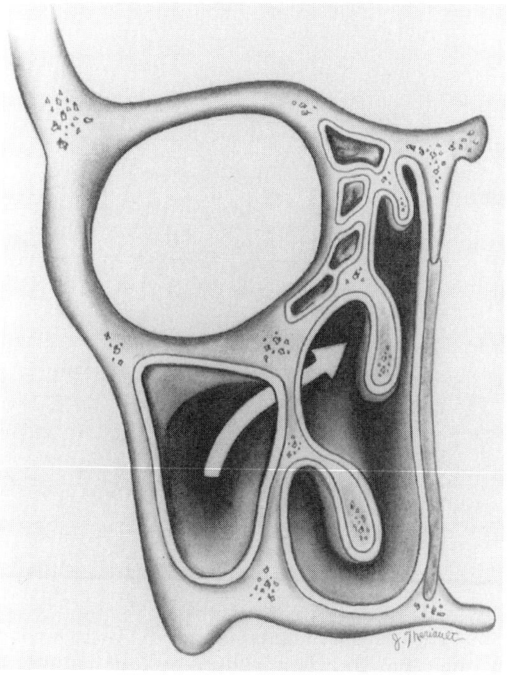

FIG. 124.2. Drainage pathway through the natural ostium located at the osteomeatal complex.

predispose the patient to secondary invasion of bacterial pathogens, giving rise to an episode of rhinosinusitis.

Histopathologic examination of paranasal sinus tissue from patients with chronic rhinosinusitis reveals an infiltration of the mucosa by eosinophils. These cells liberate major basic protein, eosinophil cationic protein, and other chemical mediators that affect the mucosa, stimulating the generation of polypoid mucous membranes.

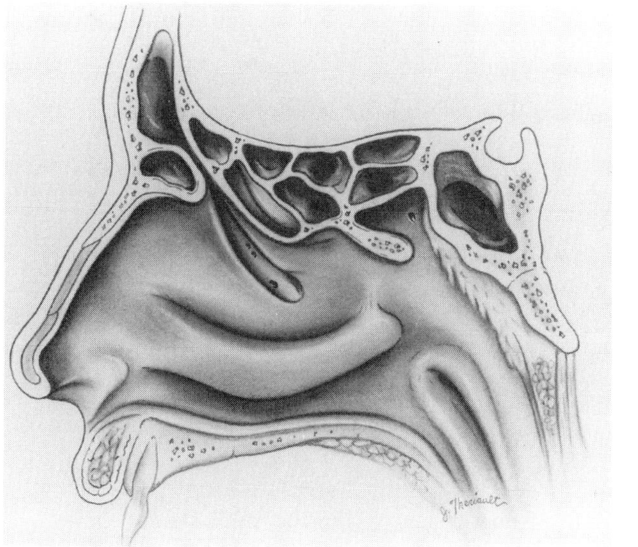

FIG. 124.3. Lateral view of the paranasal sinuses with the ethmoid labyrinth and frontal sinus recess draining into the hiatus semilunaris. The sphenoid sinus ostium is clearly seen in the sphenoethmoidal recess. The middle turbinate has been removed for clarification.

Cytokines released by the late phase of the inflammatory reaction attract eosinophils and other inflammatory cells to prolong the inflammatory state. These cytokines include histamine and the leukotrienes LTB_4, LTC_4, LTD_4, and LTE_4, which are potent bronchoconstrictors that induce symptoms of asthma with cough in many patients with inflammations of the paranasal sinuses. We now begin to comprehend the association of asthma and acute or chronic sinusitis due to the release of these inflammatory mediators during the late-phase reaction.

PREDISPOSING FACTORS FOR RHINOSINUSITIS

Certain patients have a predisposition to the development of acute or chronic rhinosinusitis. For example, this predisposition occurs in 15% to 20% of patients with allergic rhinitis. Other factors predisposing to infection include structural abnormalities (nasal septal deviations, concha bullosa formation of the middle turbinates, paradoxic middle turbinates) and nasal polyps or tumors that block the outflow tract of the osteomeatal complex (Table 124.1). Metabolic abnormalities include cystic fibrosis, ciliary dyskinesia, immune deficiencies, acquired immunodeficiency syndrome, and hyperreactive respiratory lining, especially in patients with asthma.

ETIOLOGY OF SINUS INFECTIONS

A primary respiratory event (either viral or allergic) leads to an inflammatory reaction and consequent edema of the respiratory epithelium. The inflammation of the mucosa at the narrow ostia eventually shuts down the ventilation and drainage of the sinus cavity. With the change in aeration, a vicious cycle develops that leads to continued inflammation and poor drainage (Fig. 124.4). A change in the pH occurs, and the mucosal gas metabolism is altered, with resultant damage to the cilia of the epithelium. Secretions stagnate, creating a culture medium for bacterial overgrowth within a closed cavity. Sneezing, nose blowing, or sniffling may allow bacteria to enter the sinus. A secondary infection, usually bacterial, decreases the mucociliary clearance and continues the inflammatory process.

The source of the inflammation is usually at the osteomeatal complex, the narrowest channel between the maxillary and the ethmoid sinuses. Experience with computed tomography (CT) and diagnostic nasal endoscopy has proved that the pathogenesis of sinus infections is within this narrow region.

TABLE 124.1. Predisposing Factors in Rhinosinusitis

Local problems	Systemic problems
Nasal septal abnormalities	Cystic fibrosis
Turbinate abnormalities	Allergic rhinitis
Rhinitis medicamentosa	Ciliary dyskinesia
Environmental aberrations	Immunodepression (acquired immunodeficiency syndrome)
Choanal atresia	Immunoglobulin deficiencies
Barotrauma	
Nasal polyps or tumors	
Foreign bodies	

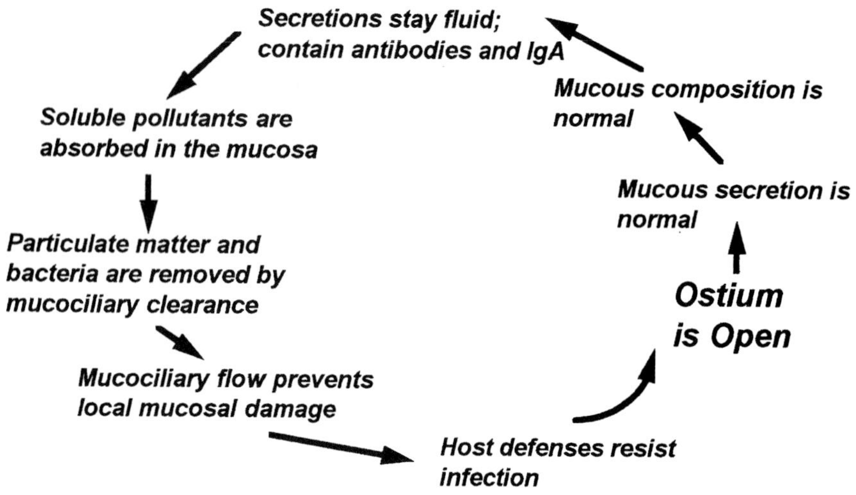

FIG. 124.4. Normal cycle of sinus secretions.

CLINICAL MANIFESTATIONS

The symptoms of rhinosinusitis are often confused with those of allergic disease or a common upper respiratory tract infection. The practitioner must be able to differentiate among these disorders to manage the acute manifestations before they become chronic.

Acute Rhinosinusitis

Acute rhinosinusitis presents with symptoms of thick purulent nasal discharge, facial pain, and severe nasal congestion, often accompanied by cough and fever. The facial pain may localize to the maxillary region, with associated dental pain, or to the periorbital and forehead regions, with associated severe headache. These acute headaches may be confused with migraine or temporal arteritis. Younger patients may not have as much pain, but they have purulent rhinorrhea and bad breath. Younger patients often present with cough, which may be confused with an asthma-like picture. Rhinosinusitis is considered acute if the symptoms persist no longer than 6 to 8 weeks or if there are fewer than four episodes per year of acute symptoms lasting 10 days or less and no mucosal damage remains.

Acute ethmoid sinusitis presents with symptoms of nasal congestion, purulent rhinorrhea, and pain localized to the inner canthal area or periorbital pain and pressure. The infection is often accompanied by infection in the maxillary sinus as well. Patients feel worse when supine or coughing and when wearing glasses. Minimal disease within this small cavity often leads to maximal symptoms.

Acute maxillary sinusitis tends to localize over the cheekbone or on one side of the face. The pain may resemble a toothache, and consequently the patient may present to the dentist. Thick purulent discharge comes primarily from the middle meatus on the involved side. The pain becomes more intense while walking or in an upright position and may improve when supine.

Acute frontal sinusitis presents with severe forehead discomfort. This may rapidly progress to an intracranial complication,

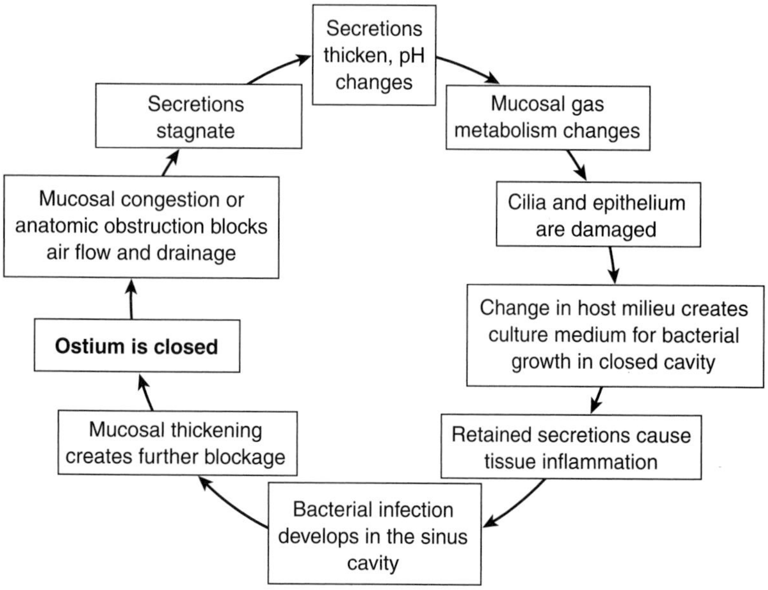

FIG. 124.5. Vicious cycle leading to chronic rhinosinusitis.

especially in younger patients. The headache is usually the worst the patient has experienced and may be confused with meningitis. Patients need early referral to an otolaryngologist to avoid the complications of intracranial spread, epidural abscess, subdural empyema, and brain abscess.

Acute sphenoid sinusitis is relatively rare and is a medical emergency for surgical drainage. Patients complain of a deep occipital-type headache with referral to the top of the head. Impending central nervous system complications include visual loss and cavernous sinus thrombosis.

Chronic Rhinosinusitis

The clinical manifestations of chronic rhinosinusitis present a diagnostic challenge because they are poorly localized to any one area and are usually more subtle and mild than those of acute rhinosinusitis. After a period of persistent inflammation, the ostia of the sinuses become blocked with an inflammatory reaction. This leads to stasis and thickened secretions, predisposing to an anaerobic environment. Symptoms include all the common complaints seen in the acute phase of the infection, including purulent yellow or green postnasal discharge and facial discomfort (not typically pain but a constant feeling of pressure). Fever may coexist but may be low grade or subclinical. Other symptoms include decreased sense of smell, chronic sore throat with or without hoarseness, and lethargy or generalized fatigue.

Chronic rhinosinusitis may precipitate a worsening of an underlying asthmatic condition. Patients who have asthma frequently have associated chronic rhinosinusitis, and the asthmatic inflammatory state is not resolved until the infection is cleared. Between 30% and 50% of patients with asthma have radiologic evidence of mucous membrane abnormalities of the paranasal sinuses. The lower respiratory tract inflammation may be due to several factors, including reflex increase of vagal tone from trigeminal stimulation within the sinuses and liberation of inflammatory mediators (leukotrienes), which are strong bronchoconstrictors.

COMPLICATIONS

Sinus infections, unless treated early and with proper antibiotics, can lead to severe complications, including blindness and intracranial abscess. Physicians must become familiar with the symptoms of acute sinus infection so they can prevent the spread of the disease into the orbit or brain.

Orbital Complications

Infection within the sinus can easily transgress the thin lamella of bone that separates the ethmoid and maxillary sinuses. Inflammation of the sinus mucosa creates a thrombophlebitis within the veins draining the ethmoid sinuses, and infection can spread easily through the valveless veins of the diploic bone of the skull. The development of vasculitis and early inflammation with cellulitis around the orbit can eventually lead to subperiosteal abscess, then orbital abscess, and finally cavernous sinus thrombosis.

The symptoms of periorbital cellulitis include edema and erythema of the ipsilateral eyelid. This may be confused with an eye infection, but the underlying cause is directly related to the ethmoid sinus infection. Severe headache and fever are common. If not treated aggressively, this process may progress to orbital subperiosteal abscess formation. At this stage, the patient may have decreased motion of the involved eye, chemosis of the eyelid, and proptosis. The CT shows a subperiosteal collection of purulence that requires immediate surgical drainage.

Progression of orbital involvement may lead to thrombophlebitis of the veins of the paranasal sinuses, which may progress to the development of cavernous sinus thrombosis. Signs of this potentially fatal infection include severe deep orbital pain, complete ophthalmoplegia, and spiking fevers. This is a medical and surgical emergency requiring intravenous antibiotics and surgical drainage.

Intracranial Complications

The spread of the infection from the paranasal sinus into the brain is rare with the use of broad-spectrum antibiotics. Usually, this infection occurs as a direct result of frontal sinus infection. The signs of intracranial infection include prostration, severe headache with nausea and vomiting, photophobia, and papilledema. CT confirms the diagnosis. Lumbar puncture may show infection but may be contraindicated in the presence of increased intracranial pressure.

DIAGNOSIS AND EVALUATION

Historically, physicians relied on the chief complaints and physical examination to diagnose rhinosinusitis. Modern diagnostic techniques involve direct examination of the nasal cavity and sinus ostia, which permits direct culture, and radiographic studies, including CT.

History

A comprehensive history is important to evaluate the patient's complaints and to rule out other causes of nasal complaints, including an evaluation for allergy. The history should include the type, consistency, and duration of nasal discharge; the location of facial pain (to determine the involved sinus cavity); and associated symptoms (e.g., loss of sense of smell, presence of cough or fever).

The past medical history should be reviewed with reference to asthma, allergies, chronic bronchitis, or possible immunologic disorders. A thorough review of prior medications, including over-the-counter medications, and drug reactions is necessary.

Physical Examination

FACE

The face is observed for evidence of swelling or erythema over an involved sinus. In frontal sinusitis, the physician may note significant edema and tenderness to palpation. Percussion over the cheeks or forehead may elicit tenderness.

NOSE

The nose is inspected using ample light via headlamp and nasal speculum (an otoscope may be used for a child), looking for mucosal edema and swelling within the middle meatal region between the middle and inferior turbinates. Direct cultures can be obtained from this region. Otolaryngologists may use a nasal endoscope, which provides superior illumination and visualization of the drainage pathways. The nose is inspected for obvious anatomic abnormalities, including nasal septal deformities and nasal polyps or tumors. The color, texture, and quality of any nasal discharge are assessed.

SINUSES
Transillumination of the paranasal sinuses is performed in a darkened room using a bright light source applied against the patient's cheek, looking into the open mouth, and applied under the eyebrow, looking at the forehead. Swollen infected sinuses block the transillumination of the light.

HEAD AND NECK
The examiner should evaluate the throat for discharge, swollen membranes, and foul breath. The ears may present with serous middle ear effusions or symptoms of eustachian tube dysfunction, with a retracted or reddened ear drum.

Laboratory Tests

Direct culture of sinus fluid is the best way to diagnose sinusitis. Maxillary sinus puncture is an invasive procedure that represents the gold standard. Direct nasal cultures have not correlated well with the results of the fluid within the involved sinus cavity and should not necessarily be relied on to direct antibiotic coverage (Table 124.2).

Radiography

X-ray evaluation of the paranasal sinuses has evolved with CT, and more precise images can be obtained that make plain views of the sinuses almost obsolete. Plain sinus radiography gives limited information but may be sufficient for the practitioner to justify therapy or referral. It is useful to document maxillary or frontal sinus disease and may have a role in following the progress of infection, but it cannot evaluate the ethmoid sinuses properly. CT is preferred because it provides the best images of the relation of the mucous membranes to the surrounding bony structures.

When nasal endoscopy fails to document the source of presumed infection, CT is indicated to search for inflammation or obstruction, primarily within the anterior ethmoid sinuses. This evaluation is also needed by the otolaryngologist when a patient is a candidate for surgery. CT may also confirm the presence of chronic sinusitis and the need for referral for definitive therapy.

Magnetic resonance imaging is generally not indicated: It does not address the bony confines but shows primarily mucosal disease or possible fungal invasion. This technique is helpful, however, for the differential diagnosis of tumors or the possibility of intracranial complications of acute or chronic sinusitis.

TABLE 124.2. Common Pathogens in Acute Rhinosinusitis

Species	Positive cultures (%)[a]
Streptococcus pneumoniae	41
Haemophilus influenzae	35
Anaerobes	7
Streptococcal spp.	7
Moraxella catarrhalis	3.5
Staphylococcus aureus	3
Others	3.5

[a]In 383 pretreatment sinus aspirates.
Source: Gwaltney JM Jr, Scheid WM, Sande MA, et al. The microbiology, etiology and antimicrobial therapy of adults with community-acquired sinusitis: a 15-year experience at the University of Virginia and review of other selected sites. *J Allerg Clin Immunol* 1992;90:457, with permission.

Ultrasonography, using either a-mode or b-mode scanning, reportedly has had some success in diagnosis, but the technique is not well established and requires considerable experience. For now, ultrasonography provides little diagnostic or therapeutic information.

DIFFERENTIAL DIAGNOSIS

Allergic Rhinitis

Allergic rhinitis presents with very similar symptoms of nasal congestion, facial pressure, and rhinorrhea, but the nasal discharge is primarily clear (Table 124.3). The patient also has a history of seasonal or year-round symptoms of an itchy and runny nose associated with sneezing. Other allergic symptoms may coexist, including red itchy eyes and dark circles under the eyes ("allergic shiners") due to vascular blush from nasal congestion. Usually, these and other symptoms of the allergic state tip the practitioner to this diagnosis. However, allergic patients may become acutely infected; treatment relies on reduction of infection first, with subsequent allergy control.

Nasal Polyposis

Nasal polyps are benign, frequently large, saclike appendages of nasal and sinus mucosa that arise primarily from the lateral wall of the nose, from the ethmoid sinuses and middle turbinate. They develop as a result of an inflammatory process that occurs after an infection or allergic process. Patients complain of constant nasal congestion, anosmia, and chronic nasal discharge. Secondary infection of the sinuses can occur as well. The inflammatory reactions that result from nasal polyps can progress to involve all the paranasal sinuses with a hyperplastic mucosa that fills all the sinuses. Earlier surgical treatments of nasal polypectomy led to recurrence, but current techniques usually avoid this problem.

Fungal Infection of the Sinuses

Fungal infections of the sinuses may occur after ineffective treatment of a sinusitis or de novo. These infections may be asymptomatic or present with symptoms of facial pressure or an infection that persists despite adequate antibiotic therapy. The discharge associated with allergic fungal sinusitis is characteristically thick, tenacious, and dark green or brown; patients may also present with nasal polyposis. CTs reveal an opacified sinus and areas of hyperdensity but usually no invasion into the bone. The most common fungus is *Aspergillus,* although other species are beginning to appear in case reports. Diagnosis is based on review of the CT and identification of allergic mucin

TABLE 124.3. Sinus Infection versus Allergy

Infection	Allergy
Nasal obstruction/congestion	Nasal obstruction/congestion
Pressure with pain	Itchy runny nose
Thick nasal discharge	Paroxysmal sneezing
Toothache	Thin watery nasal discharge
Fever	History of sinusitis during allergy season
Cough or irritability	Other allergic symptoms

by rhinoscopy or at the time of surgery. Treatment is primarily surgical debridement or removal of the fungus ball. Invasive fungal infections of the sinuses present as surgical emergencies.

Sampter Triad

These patients present with symptoms of recurrent rhinosinusitis, usually with nasal polyposis, asthma, and sensitivity to aspirin. Their asthma symptoms worsen after ingestion of aspirin products or other nonsteroidal antiinflammatory agents, due to a blockade of the cyclooxygenase pathway of arachidonic acid metabolism, favoring the production of leukotrienes. These mediators stimulate bronchial smooth muscle contraction. Patients depend on the combination of medical management and surgical removal of nasal polyps with sinus ventilation to improve their quality of life.

Cystic Fibrosis

This disease is due to an autosomal recessive gene affecting the exocrine glands, resulting in the combination of pancreatic insufficiency, pulmonary dysfunction due to excessive mucus, and abnormal sweat. These children present with rhinosinusitis due to nasal polyposis, an otherwise rare finding in children.

Cysts and Tumors

Mucous retention cysts, benign lesions within the maxillary sinuses, develop in patients with inflammation of the sinuses due to allergy or infection. They are found incidentally on radiographic evaluation. Mucoceles are more symptomatic and can cause expansile masses within the frontal sinus.

TREATMENT

The treatment of paranasal sinusitis centers around proper medical management in the acute stages and consideration of surgical drainage and ventilation in chronic sinusitis or refractory cases.

Acute Rhinosinusitis

The management goals in the treatment of acute rhinosinusitis include control of infection, reduction of mucosal edema, improvement of sinus drainage, restoration and maintenance of sinus ostia patency, and breakup of the vicious cycle leading to chronic rhinosinusitis (Table 124.4).

Antibiotics are the mainstay of management of acute rhinosinusitis. Once the diagnosis has been established, the decision to place the patient on appropriate antibacterial medications should be made. Antibiotic therapy should be directed against the primary pathogens in acute sinusitis (Table 124.2). The recent emergence of resistant bacteria has presented a problem in the choice of appropriate antibiotics. Strains of *S. pneumoniae* and especially *Haemophilus influenzae* have become resistant to ampicillin-like agents due to the production of β-lactamase. Current antibiotics recommended for the treatment of acute rhinosinusitis are listed in Table 124.5. The antibiotic selections listed in Table 124.5 are stratified by disease severity, age of the patient, and recent antibiotic exposure. The preferred agents are active against the common acute sinusitis pathogens—*S. pneumoniae, H. influenzae,* and *M. catarrhalis*. Switching to a second agent is suggested if after 72 hours the patient's condition does not clinically improve or worsens.

First-line therapy for adult patients with mild disease and no antibiotic therapy during the previous 4 to 6 weeks is limited to high-dose amoxicillin, amoxicillin/clavulanate, cefpodoxime proxetil, and cefuroxime axetil. The guidelines note that cefprozil may have a bacterial failure rate of up to 25%. Similarly, although clarithromycin, trimethoprim/sulfamethoxazole, doxycycline, or erythromycin may be considered for patients with β-lactam allergies, bacteriologic failure rates of 20% to 25% have been reported. The use of trimethoprim/sulfamethoxazole also has been associated with potentially fatal toxic epidermal necrolysis. For adults with mild disease who have had recent antibiotic therapy or for those with moderate disease with no recent antibiotic therapy, first-line treatment recommendations include amoxicillin/clavulanate, high-dose amoxicillin, cefpodoxime proxetil, and cefuroxime axetil. Appropriate agents for β-lactam–allergic or –intolerant patients include gatifloxacin, levofloxacin, and moxifloxacin. In adult patients with moderate disease and recent antibiotic use, the indicated agents are amoxicillin/clavulanate, gatifloxacin, levofloxacin, moxifloxacin, or combination therapy—amoxicillin or clindamycin for Gram-positive coverage plus cefixime or cefpodoxime proxetil for Gram-negative coverage.

The clinician must consider the efficacy of the medication, the side-effect profile, the convenience of administration, and the cost. Erythromycin and tetracycline are ineffective in acute rhinosinusitis. Certain second-generation cephalosporin antibiotics may not have activity against *H. influenzae* and should be avoided.

Adjunctive medical therapy is helpful to reduce tissue edema and promote drainage of the sinus cavity. Topical and systemic decongestants may be used to provide relief of tissue edema and subjective improvement of nasal congestion. Topical decongestants (oxymetazoline) act on adrenergic receptors in the nasal mucosa, shrink the swollen inflamed tissue, and promote oxygenation of the sinus. They should be used for no longer than 3 days to avoid rebound effects. Systemic decongestants (pseudoephedrine, phenylpropanolamine) also stimulate α-adrenergic receptors in the nose to provide subjective relief, and they may improve ostial patency by reducing nasal blood flow. Their use in the first trimester of pregnancy is con-

TABLE 124.4. Medical Therapy for Rhinosinusitis

Adequate medical therapy is the key to successful treatment.
Antibiotics help to control the infection in the closed sinus cavity.
Decongestants may help to maintain ostial patency.
Mucoevacuants may also help to maintain patency and thin secretions.
Topical or oral corticosteroids help in chronic rhinosinusitis but are not indicated in acute rhinosinusitis.

TABLE 124.5. Antibiotics for Acute and Recurrent Acute Rhinosinusitis

Doxycycline (100 mg bid)
Trimethoprim sulfamethoxazole (bid)
Clarithromycin (500 mg bid)
Amoxicillin clavulanate (875/125 mg bid)
Cefuroxime axetil (250 mg bid)
Cefdinir (250 mg bid)
Duration of therapy, 10–14 days

traindicated, and the use of over-the-counter medications should be discouraged.

Antihistamines are indicated solely for allergic rhinitis and are not useful in acute rhinosinusitis. They control type I hypersensitivity reactions by reducing the release of histamine and other chemical mediators and thus should be used only when allergy is a predisposing factor for infection. They are effective for reducing the symptoms of rhinorrhea, sneezing, and nasal itching, but the older classic antihistamines may cause too much drying, inhibiting clearance of nasal secretions.

Other adjunctive measures are important. The patient frequently complains of significant pain, so analgesics are important. Humidification of the nasal membranes is important and may be delivered by nasal saline spray, steam inhalation, or cool vapor humidifiers. Mucolytic agents have potential benefit, especially in patients with thick nasal secretions. Guaifenesin is the mucolytic of choice and may be combined with a systemic decongestant.

Maxillary sinus irrigation is occasionally indicated in acute rhinosinusitis. This office procedure is relatively benign and allows direct culture of the involved sinus cavity with the removal of the infected sinus material. Irrigation of the sinus cavity may help restore sinus ostial patency. It should be considered in patients who are immunocompromised, especially in patients with acquired immunodeficiency syndrome.

The role of topical nasal steroids in acute rhinosinusitis has not been established. These medications are indicated for the treatment of chronic sinusitis. Topical nasal steroids reduce the inflammation within the nasal mucosa but require several days before subjective improvement is obtained.

In summary, therapy for acute rhinosinusitis includes antibiotics, analgesics, decongestants (topical or systemic), mucolytic therapy (saline or systemic mucolytics), adjunctive therapy (topical saline or humidification), and sinus irrigation in refractory or immunocompromised cases.

Chronic Rhinosinusitis

Chronic rhinosinusitis is a direct result of persistent inflammation within the mucous membranes of the paranasal sinuses. This problem occurs after recurrent acute episodes or persistent infection lasting more than 3 months. At this stage, the sinus ostia are more or less irreversibly blocked by fibrous tissue or hyperplastic mucosa that prevents adequate ventilation and drainage of the involved sinus cavities. As the sinus cavity becomes depleted of oxygen, the bacterial species change and become anaerobic; treatment regimens must change accordingly.

Chronic rhinosinusitis in adults should be managed using the same therapies as for acute disease: antibiotics, analgesics if necessary, decongestants, mucolytics, and the addition of topical nasal and sometimes systemic steroids.

Antibiotics directed against anaerobic bacteria should be prescribed (e.g., amoxicillin/clavulanate, clindamycin, or the association of penicillin and metronidazole [Flagyl]). They should be prescribed for at least 3 weeks to achieve maximal effect. However, even intensive and prolonged antibiotic therapy may not affect a cure.

Medical therapy to reduce tissue edema is important. Topical nasal steroids are the primary medications used to help reduce tissue edema around the sinus ostia. Used appropriately, the risk of systemic side effects is very low; however, their use in pregnancy is controversial. Five topical steroids are available: dexamethasone, beclomethasone, budesonide, flunisolide, and triamcinolone acetonide. Dexamethasone is prescribed as a short-term, high-potency, topical nasal steroid. It is recommended when a rapid onset of action is desired and for cases of hyperplastic nasal polyposis. The other second-generation topical nasal steroids have a slower onset of action but are effective in the management of inflammation. Patients should be cautioned to use the topical corticosteroids at their recommended dosage; the risk of systemic absorption is small at appropriate dosages. Dosages should be adjusted according to the response and reduced to the lowest possible maintenance level. Side effects with the use of topical nasal steroids include nasal irritation, epistaxis, and minor headache (Table 124.6).

TABLE 124.6. Topical Steroids in Rhinosinusitis[a]

Beclomethasole dipropionate
Triamcinolone acetonide
Flunisolide
Budesonide
Fluticasone
Mometasone

[a]Topical corticosteroids reduce edema, inflammation, and mucous secretion in chronic rhinosinusitis but are not indicated in acute rhinosinusitis.

Consultation with an otolaryngologist should be considered when the patient does not respond to this regimen. Surgical procedures may afford greater success when the patient has had symptoms for more than 6 months or three or more episodes of acute sinusitis each year for 3 years in a row.

CONSIDERATIONS IN PREGNANCY

Rhinosinusitis may be confused with the symptoms of nasal congestion induced by estrogens during pregnancy. Patients often complain of a stuffy nose, which can be ameliorated with the use of a topical nasal steroid during the second trimester. Topical decongestants may also give relief, and they have less risk to the fetus than systemic medications.

Patients with infections of the sinuses require antibiotics. Penicillins (ampicillin, ampicillin/clavulanate) are the antibiotics of choice. Their risk to the fetus is small. Cephalosporins also have a low risk of teratogenicity, although they cross the placenta and are excreted into the amniotic fluid like the penicillins.

Sulfonamides and combinations with trimethoprim cause no risk to the fetus during the first trimester. They may be combined synergistically with erythromycin.

Antibiotics for chronic rhinosinusitis include clindamycin, which has not been associated with any congenital defects. It crosses the placenta and achieves serum cord levels 50% of those in maternal serum.

BIBLIOGRAPHY

File TM, Hadley JA. Rational use of antibiotics to treat respiratory tract infections. *Am J Manag Care* 2002;8:713–727.

Gwaltney JM, Scheld WM, Sande MA, et al. The microbiology, etiology and antimicrobial therapy of adults with community-acquired sinusitis: a 15-year experience at the University of Virginia and review of other selected sites. *J Allergy Clin Immunol* 1992;90:457.

Hadley JA. The microbiology and management of acute and chronic rhinosinusitis. *Curr Infect Dis Rep* 2001;3:209–216.

Hadley JA, Bakos R, Regenbogen V. Middle cranial fossa epidural abscess, an unusual complication of acute sinusitis: etiology, evaluation, and treatment. *Am J Rhinol* 1991;5:181.

Kaliner MA. Human nasal host defense. *J Allergy Clin Immunol* 1992;90[Suppl]:424.

Kennedy DW, Zinreich SJ, Rosenbaum AE. Functional endoscopic sinus surgery: theory and diagnostic evaluation. *Arch Otolaryngol Head Neck Surg* 1985;111:576.

Kennedy DW, Zinreich SJ, Rosenbaum AE. Functional endoscopic sinus surgery: technique. *Arch Otolaryngol Head Neck Surg* 1985;111:643.
Mabry RL. Corticosteroids in rhinology. *Otolaryngol Head Neck Surg* 1993;108:768.
Raphael GD, Baraniuk JN, Kaliner MA. How and why the nose runs. *J Allergy Clin Immunol* 1991;87:457.
Sinus and Allergy Health Partnership. Antimicrobial treatment guidelines for acute bacterial rhinosinusitis. *Otolaryngol Head Neck Surg* 2000;123[Suppl]: S1–S32.
Stammberger H. Endoscopic endonasal surgery—concepts in treatment of recurring rhinosinusitis. *Otolaryngol Head Neck Surg* 1986;94:143.

CHAPTER 125
Otitis

Wen Jiang

Otitis is divided into otitis externa, otitis media, and labyrinthitis. Each type represents a distinctly separate entity in terms of cause, treatment, and potential sequelae.

OTITIS EXTERNA

The ear canal inclusive of the tympanic membrane is covered with desquamating squamous epithelium. The canal is about 3 cm long and consists of a lateral cartilaginous portion and a medial bony portion. The bony part of the canal is covered by a thin layer of skin that adheres to the periosteum and contains no accessory structures. On the other hand, the epithelium in the cartilaginous portion of the canal is relatively thick with numerous hair follicles and apocrine glands, including the ceruminous glands that form cerumen. Cerumen provides lubrication to the epithelium as well as a protective coating. Otitis externa may be categorized as acute, subacute, and chronic depending on the time course of the infection.

Etiology

Approximately 10% of all people may be affected by otitis externa at one point in their lives, and 90% of the time the infection is unilateral. This disease occurs with a higher frequency in warm humid climates and is more common in swimmers because of local maceration of the canal skin, which facilitates the entry of pathogenic bacteria (e.g., swimmer's ear). Infection occurs with occlusion of the apopilosebaceous units and subsequent bacterial proliferation. Another common predisposing factor is trauma to the canal with removal of cerumen by cotton-tipped applicators or other instrumentation. This mechanical removal of cerumen causes maceration of the canal skin, atrophy of the ceruminous and sebaceous glands, and overall disturbance in the chemical balance of the external canal, which all contribute to the increased susceptibility to infection by bacteria and fungi.

The pH of the canal skin is a very important factor in the growth of bacteria, in addition to the temperature, moisture content, and aeration of the external auditory canal. A rise of pH above 6.0 is a prerequisite for the development of infection. Because of its relatively narrow diameter, any significant inflammation with the attendant edema or indurations may rapidly lead to obstruction, which favors the growth of Gram-negative and anaerobic bacteria. Finally, hearing aids, absence of cerumen, a narrow and long external canal with poor self-cleaning ability, foreign bodies, and allergy to medications may also be causative factors.

Physical Examination and Clinical Findings

In acute otitis externa, the patient typically presents with a 2- to 3-day history of unilateral otalgia, pruritus, and discharge not associated with an upper respiratory tract infection or fever. There may be a history of water exposure, from either swimming or showering. Physical examination reveals an acutely inflamed canal with erythema and edema. The cartilaginous portion of the canal is painful to the touch, and the canal is often filled with debris and foul-smelling discharge. The tympanic membrane is intact but may be difficult to assess because of otalgia, swelling, and obscuring debris. Impacted cerumen may be present; this requires removal. If the canal is open, tuning fork and hearing test should be normal, indicating that the middle ear is not involved. There may be a mild conductive hearing loss depending on the degree of obstruction of the canal.

The auricle and the cartilaginous canal have a very rich lymphatic drainage to an extensive regional network consisting of parotid, retroauricular, infraauricular, and superior deep cervical nodes. Infections of the external canal frequently present with significant swelling in these areas with variable cellulitis of the adjacent skin.

Recurrent acute infections may eventually lead to the atrophy of the epithelial lining, reduction of the protective film, and change in the composition and pH of the canal secretion that result in chronic otitis externa. This condition may be likened to eczema and is a spectrum of disease ranging from mild drying and scaling of the canal skin to complete obliteration of the canal by chronically infected hypertrophic skin. There is often intense itching, which causes the patient to scratch his or her external canal, which often causes mechanical damage to the epithelium and results in intermittent episodes of acute bacterial superinfection with acute dermatitis.

Bacteriology

More than half of the organisms recovered from an acute episode of otitis externa are Gram-negative species, and *Pseudomonas aeruginosa* accounts for 71% of the Gram-negative organisms and about 38% of the total isolates. The Gram-positive staphylococci are the second most common organisms recovered, accounting for 25% of total isolates, with *Staphylococcus epidermidis* and *Staphylococcus aureus* being most common. Other organisms include *Proteus,* streptococci, and various Gram-negative bacilli. *Aspergillus* and *Candida* are occasionally isolated from infected external ear canal, but in general they account for less than 1% of single isolates. Susceptibility profiles of the isolates reveal that *S. epidermidis* has the highest level of resistance to antibiotics such as neomycin and oxacillin and *P. aeruginosa* resistance to quinolones are rare. For the mild or uncomplicated infection, culture of the canal is ordinarily not taken, because it will usually demonstrate a mixed growth of these organisms. For recalcitrant infections, culture and susceptibility profile may assist in the choice of antibiotic therapy.

Treatment

The main principles of treatment for external otitis are local removal of debris or cerumen, drainage of the infection, reestablishment of the normal acidic environment, administration of topical antimicrobials, and prevention of recurrent infections. Debris or cerumen should be removed from the canal and drainage suctioned to increase aeration. The insertion of an ear wick is often necessary to allow penetration of a topical medication medially beyond the swollen outer canal. In the absence of systemic symptoms, necrotizing otitis externa, or significant surrounding cellulitis, topical antibiotics alone are sufficient to treat otitis externa, with adequate cleaning of the canal. Traditionally, the most common preparation is a combination of neomycin, polymixin, and hydrocortisone. Fungal infections are also treated topically after cleansing of the canal. Specific examples of antifungal agents include clotrimazole, germicidin, or tolnaftate. Acidifying solutions such as Burow's solution may also be used. The best clinical evidence demonstrates equivalent results with ear cleaning, an ear wick, and any of the choices of topical agents: acidifying agents, antibiotics, antibiotic and steroid combinations, or antifungal agents. Frequent dosing (three to four times daily) for at least 4 days is supported by the studies. Two studies demonstrated equivalent efficacy with topical ciprofloxacin or ofloxacin dosed twice daily when compared with antibiotic and steroid combination dosed four times daily. However, these agents are also more expensive than older topical antibiotics. Occasionally, a significant cellulitis or periauricular lymphadenitis requires the addition of a systemic antibiotic. Common choices of oral antibiotics are antistaphylococcal penicillins, first-generation cephalosporins, or one of the antipseudomonal fluoroquinolones such as ciprofloxacin. In addition to oral antibiotics, an oral analgesic may often be prescribed because of the significant pain and discomfort associated with the acute stage of infection.

After resolution of the acute infection, patients need to be informed of the various measures to prevent recurrent infections, such as the avoidance of any manipulation of the canal with cotton swab or any other instrument, drying of the canal after shower or swimming, and the use of a 50:50 solution of alcohol and white vinegar to displace water within the canal after exposure.

Other Forms of External Otitis

Necrotizing external otitis, also known as malignant external otitis, is a potentially life-threatening infection usually beginning in the external auditory canal and extending to the temporal bone, skull base, and adjacent structures. The disease is usually found in elderly diabetic patients or any patients with a compromised immune system. The infection is almost always caused by *Pseudomonas aeruginosa,* although other organisms have been isolated. Patients often give a history of an acute external otitis that does not resolve despite adequate local therapy. On physical examination, granulation tissue is classically found in the inferior aspect of the external canal, often obscuring the tympanic membrane. On the other hand, granulation tissue is rarely seen in routine uncomplicated otitis externa. Purulent secretion is also a common finding. Patients often describe a deeply seeded pain that travels medially. Multiple cranial nerves may be involved, especially the facial nerve. Treatment must be aggressive, both topically and parenterally. The patient is often treated with antipseudomonal therapy for an extended period of time, often for 6 weeks or more. Given the improvement in antipseudomonal antibiotics, most patients can be managed medically; currently, the role for surgery may be limited. Recent reports using antibiotics alone with local external canal cleaning and with dual-modality therapy (antibiotics and hyperbaric oxygen therapy) show improved success rate of upward of 90% to 100%.

Bullous myringitis is an acutely painful condition of the ear characterized by bullae formation on the tympanic membrane and deep portion of the ear canal. Patients often present with a characteristic history of sudden onset of very severe, usually unilateral and often "throbbing" otalgia, and may be associated with an upper respiratory tract infection. Physical examination reveals either blood-filled, serous, or serosanguinous blisters involving the tympanic membrane and/or the deep meatal wall. Because the tympanic membrane is intact, the otorrhea is usually scanty. The blisters are believed by some to occur between the richly innervated outer epithelium and middle fibrous layers of the tympanic membrane. Middle ear effusions are frequently found in bullous myringitis. On audiometric testing, the hearing loss may be conductive, sensorineural, or mixed. In most patients, hearing loss will completely recover, although in cases with severe bilateral sensorineural loss, residual high frequency deficits may persist. The etiology of the disease is currently unknown, although an association of bullous myringitis with influenza epidemics has been reported. A wide variety of organisms, both viral and bacterial, is currently implicated in this disease, including the most common agents causing otitis media. In most cases, the symptoms are self-limiting. Patients may require strong oral analgesics to relieve the pain, and close follow-up is required. Antibiotics may be used if there is any middle ear fluid, suggesting a form of otitis media, or they may be given to protect against secondary bacterial infection due to ruptured bullae.

Furuncles are not uncommon and occur in the lateral cartilaginous portion of the external canal. These are infections of the glands or hair follicles with staphylococcal organisms. A patient often presents with pain and swelling of the canal. Treatment consists of systemic antibiotics against staphylococcal organisms, topical preparations, and the placement of alcohol-soaked (70%–95%) gauze wicks until the furuncle points and bursts spontaneously. Incision and drainage are reserved for patients in severe pain with a protracted course or marked swelling.

Herpes zoster oticus or the Ramsay-Hunt syndrome typically presents with multiple characteristic herpetic vesicles around the auricle or in the external auditory canal. Patients with a history of varicella-zoster virus are susceptible to this infection during times of immunosuppression. After the vesicular eruption, patient often presents with a rapidly progressive facial paralysis. Sensorineural hearing loss and vertigo may also occur. This syndrome is responsible for 2% to 10% of all facial paralysis. The prognosis for recovery from facial paralysis is poorer than that of idiopathic Bell palsy and exhibits a more severe denervation. Steroidal and antiviral therapy may be added, particularly in the debilitated or immunosuppressed patient. In retrospective case series, acyclovir given intravenously appears to improve the outcome, whereas it is generally considered to have poor bioavailability by the oral route.

OTITIS MEDIA

Infections of the middle ear are broadly classified under the heading of otitis media. Strictly speaking, otitis media is a general term used to describe any inflammatory process involving the middle ear cleft without regard to etiology or pathogenesis. Otitis media may be further subdivided and classified according to the chronicity of the disease, presence of symptoms, appearance of the ear, or presumed etiology and pathogenesis.

Etiology

Multiple interrelated factors contribute to the development of otitis media, including infection, dysfunction of the eustachian tube (ET), allergy, and barotraumas. Eventually, irreversible damage can occur as a result of the inflammatory conditions elicited by these factors. The middle ear, connected to the nasopharynx by the ET, may be considered an extension of the nasal cavity and is lined by essentially the same upper respiratory epithelium. The ET is responsible for ventilation of the middle ear. The air within the middle ear space is slowly absorbed, resulting in a relative negative pressure. This negative pressure is relieved by opening the ET, equilibrating the pressure with that of ambient air.

Acute otitis media (AOM) often follows viral upper respiratory tract infection, and investigators have well established that the incidence of AOM is highest in winter months, when the incidence of viral upper respiratory tract infection is highest. A viral upper respiratory tract infection facilitates extension of pathogenic bacteria into the ET and middle ear cleft by causing inflammation, impairing the normal mucociliary clearance and promoting adherence of bacteria in the inflamed nasopharynx. The bacteriology of AOM is well known and varies little throughout the world. Tympanocentesis has revealed *Streptococcus pneumoniae* in 20% to 35% of patients, nontypable *Haemophilus influenzae* in 20% to 30%, *Moraxella catarrhalis* in 20%, no bacteria in 20% to 30%, and virus with or without bacteria in 17% to 44%. Normal function of the ET is vital in maintaining a healthy middle ear. Bacterial, viral, and allergic nasotubal inflammation causes not only obstructive mucosal edema but also destruction of normal mucociliary flow.

Nasopharyngeal tumors obstruct the orifice of the ET, and many patients with these tumors also present with middle ear effusion. In an adult patient without any previous history of otitis media who presents with unilateral middle ear effusion, a careful examination of the nasopharynx is mandatory to exclude the possibility of mechanical obstruction of the ET by a tumor. Radiation for these tumors also injures tubal cilia, which adds a passive dysfunction to the obstruction. Patients who have primary ciliary dyskinesia can be expected to have abnormal ciliary function of the ET and commonly have otitis media with effusion (OME) in addition to bronchiectasis and sinusitis.

Allergy has long been recognized as one of the causative factors of OME. Nasotubal mucosal congestion associated with inhalant allergy can cause obstruction of the ET. A significant association has been reported between food allergy and serous otitis media.

Barotrauma caused by changes in barometric pressure that occur during diving, flying, or therapy using hyperbaric oxygen can produce otitis media even in the presence of a normal ET. During ascent, air in the middle ear passes through the ET as it expands. In rapid descent, air in the middle ear and ET is compressed, and the ET collapses when the difference in pressure between the environment and the middle ear space becomes too great. If unequalized, the resultant high negative pressure in the middle ear causes bleeding or transudation of serum. The presence of an artificial airway and a history of dysfunction of the ET before therapy greatly increase the risk for hyperbaric oxygen-induced barotrauma and the development of serous otitis media.

Each of the causative factors just mentioned stimulates mucosa and inflammatory cells in the middle ear to release inflammatory mediators. These include histamine, prostaglandins, leukotrienes, kinins, proteases, hydrolytic enzymes, platelet-activating factor, tumor necrosis factor, γ-interferon, and nitric oxide. When produced, these inflammatory agents increase vascular permeability and secretory activity of the middle ear cavity, resulting in middle ear effusion.

Classification and Treatment

The stages of otitis media can be subdivided according to the chronicity of the disease: AOM, OME, and chronic otitis media (COM). These various forms of otitis media are dynamically interrelated regarding their cause and pathogenesis and represent the same disease process as it progresses in a continuum. For example, AOM can lead to OME with the resolution of the acute symptoms of pain and fever, and finally to COM when pathologic conditions in the middle ear have become irreversible. Patients with COM may exhibit perforations of the tympanic membrane or ossicular chain destruction with resultant hearing loss, and both are often seen when cholesteatoma or granulation tissue is present.

AOM is an acute bacterial infection of the middle ear cleft characterized by a rapid onset of otalgia and fever. In early stages, erythema and edema in mucosa of the middle ear correspond otoscopically with an erythematous tympanic membrane. As the infection progresses, purulent exudate accumulates in the middle ear, and the tympanic membrane visually appears opaque, full, or bulging. The tympanic membrane has diminished mobility on pneumatic otoscopic examination, and audiometrically there is a conductive hearing loss due to middle ear effusions.

Antimicrobial therapy is the first line of treatment in uncomplicated cases and is initially directed toward the most common pathogens. Amoxicillin has been the empiric drug of choice for treating patients with AOM, but with increased incidence of β-lactamase–producing organisms, the efficacy of amoxicillin as the best initial therapy is being questioned. Reevaluation within 24 hours is warranted for any signs of progression; otherwise, symptoms should improve significantly within 48 to 72 hours after appropriate therapy is begun. The duration of antimicrobial therapy is an issue debated and not yet resolved but is generally 7 to 10 days.

Surgical intervention is necessary when specific knowledge of the causative organism requires tympanocentesis in patients with severe otalgia, toxic appearance, and unsatisfactory response to antimicrobial therapy. Either tympanocentesis or myringotomy is effective in providing symptomatic relief by decompressing the middle ear space, but neither alone offers any advantage in resolving the infection nor in clearing the middle ear effusion over treatment with amoxicillin. In cases complicated by facial nerve paralysis, meningitis, or other intracranial extensions, however, myringotomy should be performed without delay to drain the middle ear space and to obtain material for culture.

Complications of otitis media are fortunately quite rare since the institution of routine antimicrobial therapy. However, surgical therapy is generally required in many of the intratemporal and intracranial complications that are associated with AOM such as facial paralysis, acute mastoiditis, labyrinthitis, petrous apicitis, meningitis, epidural abscess, sigmoid sinus thrombosis, and brain abscess.

OME is an inflammation of the middle ear space resulting in a collection of fluid behind an intact tympanic membrane, and the fluid may be serous or mucoid in nature. This process may be further categorized as acute, subacute, or chronic based on the duration of the disease process. In general, OME implies that severe pain and associated constitutional symptoms are lacking. Adults with previously normal hearing will find OME to be quite troublesome. They often present to the physician for evaluation of aural pressure, hearing loss, clicking, popping, or a sense of imbalance. A previous history of upper respiratory viral infection and/or AOM is common. Patients without such a history should be carefully evaluated for other potential etiologies of ET obstruction, such as adenoid hypertrophy or a nasopharyngeal tumor. Physical examination commonly reveals a poorly mobile tympanic membrane with either a yellow color (serous effusion), a gray color (mucoid effusion), or significant opacity. In case of serous effusion, air bubbles may also be visible, creating an air–liquid interface within the tympanic cavity.

For most patients with OME, the history and physical examination are usually sufficient for the diagnosis. For patients in whom the diagnosis is unclear, pneumatic otomicroscopy combined with tympanometry usually can clinch the diagnosis. Patients with unilateral persistent OME should be referred to an otolaryngologist for further management, and flexible fiberoptic nasopharyngoscopy and CT may be indicated to identify the underlying etiology. Also, patients should undergo an audiometric evaluation to assess the degree of hearing impairment, especially in patients with associated risk factors for hearing loss, such as craniofacial anomalies, neurologic and cognitive impairment, psychomotor retardation, or known syndromes associated with sensorineural hearing loss.

The natural history of OME in children has been well documented, with the best prognosis of spontaneous resolution of the effusion when it follows a recent episode of AOM. Similar data do not exist for adults with OME. In fact, most adult patients refuse protracted observation periods for spontaneous resolution of the middle ear effusion, because the constant symptoms of aural fullness, hearing loss, and imbalance are intolerable. Medical therapy for patients with OME has been directed toward its causes, such as infection, inflammation, allergy, and dysfunction of the ET. Three metaanalyses of 13 randomized clinical trials have shown that antibiotic therapy has a statistically higher clearance rate of middle ear effusion when compared with the use of placebo, but the magnitude of the efficacy is small. The use of decongestants and antihistamines has been shown to be ineffective in the treatment of patients with OME, but these should be used for concurrent sinonasal disease, if present. Studies of the efficacy of oral corticosteroids so far have failed to demonstrate a consistent beneficial effect that would justify their routine use in patients with OME.

Surgical intervention with the placement of a tympanostomy tube should be considered when observation and medical therapy fail to demonstrate timely resolution of the effusion. On the other hand, myringotomy alone proved to be no better than observation. Serous otitis media is a well-recognized complication of nasopharyngeal carcinoma and was present in 38% of patients at presentation and in 46% of patients after radiation therapy in a study of 175 patients with the disease. Treatment of the serous otitis media after radiation can be a perplexing problem. Tympanostomy tubes help to ventilate the middle ear and provide some relief of the conductive hearing loss, but long-term follow-up has found significantly more otorrhea and complications in the middle ear and a significantly greater deterioration of air conduction in tube-ventilated ears compared with ears after repeated myringotomies without tubes. Tang and others advise avoiding myringotomy altogether, with or without insertion of tubes, citing increased middle ear complication in operated ears. In a subset of patients with OME, the effusion and conductive hearing loss may persist despite reasonable medical and surgical intervention. In these situations, exploration is advocated to identify the origin of the persistent disease, and exploratory tympanotomy with or without mastoidectomy may be required.

COM is the most advanced disease state in the spectrum of otitis media, and by definition it is associated with some form of irreversible pathologic condition in the middle ear such as granulation tissue, ossicular changes, tympanosclerosis, tympanic membrane perforation, cholesterol granuloma, and cholesteatoma. Obliteration of the middle ear space may be seen as a result of severe tympanic membrane retraction, which occurs in both middle ear atelectasis and in adhesive otitis media, in which loss of mucosa results in the adherence of the tympanic membrane to the promontory and the ossicles. The diagnosis of COM can usually be made by history, otoscopy, microscopic ear examination, and appropriate audiometric assessment. Most patients have a past history of frequent AOM, intermittent foul-smelling otorrhea, hearing loss, or a combination of these. Less often, presenting complaints include tinnitus, vertigo, or otalgia. Otoscopic findings may reveal tympanic membrane perforation with or without otorrhea, tympanosclerosis, polypoid middle ear mucosa, or severe tympanic membrane retraction with or without cholesteatoma. Tuning fork examination and audiometric evaluation may reveal a mixed or conductive hearing loss. CT of the temporal bone is the radiographic study of choice in patients with uncomplicated COM.

The primary treatment modality for patients with COM is surgery, which is necessary to eradicate disease and reconstruct the hearing mechanism. Medical treatment is limited to the control of active otorrhea, which can initially be treated with frequent suction cleaning and topical antibiotics, as a powder or suspension, with or without hydrocortisone. The topical antimicrobial is selected empirically to eradicate the most commonly isolated aerobic pathogens, *P. aeruginosa* and *S. aureus*. Irrigation with 2% acetic acid solution, often made with one part white vinegar to one part distilled water or 70% alcohol, may also be effective. In adults, an oral fluoroquinolone (e.g., ciprofloxacin) may be helpful, and intravenous antibiotics are sometimes necessary.

The primary goals of surgical management of patients with COM are to identify and remove infected tissue, aerate the middle ear and mastoid, close the middle ear, reconstruct the hearing mechanism, and prevent the morbidity of future sequelae or complications. Any surgical approach should be flexible and individualized, using adaptable techniques appropriate for the pathologic conditions encountered.

LABYRINTHITIS

Labyrinthitis is a general term that refers to the inflammation of the inner ear. The inflammatory process may be a manifestation of a systemic illness or may be the specific target of an infectious agent. Although the cochlear and vestibular portions of the labyrinth communicate, the patient may not always have symptoms with both. A variety of organisms can invade the labyrinth, precipitating cochlear or vestibular infections.

Bacterial Infections

Acute bacterial infection of the inner ear is divided into serous or toxic labyrinthitis and suppurative labyrinthitis. These diseases occur in the presence of an acute or chronic bacterial otitis media, spreading from the middle ear through the round window membrane or a horizontal canal fistula.

Serous labyrinthitis is a complication of otitis media and is thought to occur when toxic mediators from otitis media reach the membranous labyrinth with an absence of bacteria in the inner ear. It is an uncommon complication, representing 1% to 3% of all intratemporal complications of otitis media. The pathogenesis of the disease is based on animal data demonstrating increased permeability of the round window membrane for the passage of macromolecules in the presence of bacterial toxic mediators and the findings of sensorineural hearing loss in humans with otitis media.

In acute suppurative labyrinthitis, whether otogenic or meningogenic, there is more severe infection of the labyrinth with direct access of the infecting organism to the bony and membranous labyrinth. The incidence of this infection is rare and currently represents only a few percent of all intratemporal complications of otitis media. The presumed route of spread for otogenic labyrinthitis is through the round window membrane, oval window, a labyrinthine fistula, or congenital abnormalities of the temporal bone. The route of inoculation for meningogenic labyrinthitis is through the internal auditory canal or the cochlear aqueduct to the membranous labyrinth. The pathology of suppurative labyrinthitis shows a wide variety of findings such as inflammation of the perilymphatic spaces of the cochlea and vestibular organs, eosinophilic staining of inner ear fluids, loss of spiral ganglion cells, and eventually the development of fibrous tissue and ossification of the membranous labyrinth over time.

The differentiation between serous labyrinthitis and suppurative labyrinthitis is based on a continuum of clinical findings, and a clear division between the two diseases is sometimes difficult to make based on clinical grounds alone. Classically, serous labyrinthitis is seen in the patient with AOM or chronic suppurative otitis media and is characterized by the sudden onset of mild to moderate hearing loss and occasionally vertigo. In most cases, the symptoms resolve with time, pointing to reversible damage thought to be due to changes in cochleovestibular ionic potential and inflammatory toxic mediators. Suppurative labyrinthitis is often presented by profound sensorineural hearing loss, otalgia, fever, nausea, emesis, and vertigo. It often coexists with AOM, chronic suppurative otitis media, cholesteatoma, or meningitis. The classic description of the disease states that the otologic changes are irreversible. The disease may progress to facial paralysis, meningitis, and other intracranial complications.

Hearing loss in meningogenic suppurative labyrinthitis is most common after infection with *Streptococcus pneumoniae,* followed by *Haemophilus influenzae* and *Neisseria meningitides*; it occurs very early in the illness. The common pathogens of AOM and chronic suppurative otitis media are thought to cause serous and suppurative labyrinthitis. The diagnostic workup of serous and suppurative labyrinthitis includes an audiogram, culture of the otogenic or meningogenic sources of the infection, and CT of the temporal bone and brain to rule out other complications.

The treatment of labyrinthitis is to prevent further progression of the damage to the inner ear organs and the resolution of the underlying infectious disease. The mainstays of therapy are culture-directed intravenous antibiotics and myringotomy with or without tube placement. Controversy exists in the literature with respect to the addition of steroid therapy to prevent hearing loss and labyrinthitis ossificans. Different randomized, prospective, placebo-controlled studies have yielded contradicting results regarding the use of steroid therapy. At present, the decision to administer steroid therapy is still controversial and should be individualized to each patient.

Viral Labyrinthitis

Based on clinicopathologic studies, a classification of neurolabyrinthitis was developed describing the labyrinthine disorders thought to be related to viruses. The classification includes acute viral labyrinthitis, acute viral neuritis, and delayed endolymphatic hydrops. Acute viral labyrinthitis describes involvement of the auditory or vestibular end organs, and acute neuritis refers to a disruption of cochlear or vestibular peripheral nerve function. With current diagnostic methods, it is not always possible to differentiate the two entities, and because therapy is not altered by the distinctions, this detail has limited practical relevance. As a result, the terms of labyrinthitis and neuritis are often used interchangeably in the literature.

Acute cochlear labyrinthitis afflicts about 5 to 20 of 100,000 persons annually in the United States, with a median age of 40 to 54 years and equal distribution between men and women. This entity is also referred to as idiopathic sudden sensorineural hearing loss (ISSNHL) and has been defined as the loss of at least 30 dB of hearing in at least three contiguous frequencies in fewer than 3 days in an otherwise healthy person. Many viruses have been implicated in ISSNHL, including influenza, parainfluenza viruses, mumps, rubeola, rubella, herpes simplex, varicella-zoster virus, cytomegalovirus, and adenovirus group. Primary infection and host–virus interaction have been hypothesized as mechanisms leading to the hearing loss. Although it is usually unilateral, it may be bilateral or sequential.

Histopathologic examination most commonly shows a loss of cochlear hair cells, most severe at the basal turn. There may be loss of supporting cells, tectorial membrane disruption, atrophy of stria vascularis, and occasionally loss of spiral ganglion neurons. Vascular etiology has also been postulated because sometimes pathology shows small vessel thrombosis and inner ear fibrosis. ISSNHL is one of the few true emergencies in otology because prompt initiation of appropriate therapy may improve or totally reverse the hearing loss. The patient usually complains of the sudden onset of hearing loss, noticed during the day or on first arising in the morning, and experiences concomitant aural fullness or tinnitus. Pain is not associated with ISSNHL. A detailed history needs to be taken to exclude the possibility of surgical, head, or pressure-induced trauma. About 50% of the patients recall a recent viral infection. The patient may complain of disequilibrium or frank vertigo. A complete physical examination should include neurologic evaluation to establish that there are no other cranial neuropathies and to detect any nystagmus.

Otologic examination should reveal normal external auditory canals and tympanic membranes bilaterally. A complete audiometric testing should be obtained as the initial step of evaluation. The audiometric configuration has significant prognostic value, with mild to moderate loss in the mid-frequency having the best rate of spontaneous recovery. Vestibular testing by electronystagmography (ENG) also has prognostic value; patients with normal ENGs have a statistically greater likelihood of hearing recovery than do those with abnormal ENGs. Magnetic resonance imaging (MRI) with gadolinium is performed to evaluate the internal auditory canal and cerebellopontine angle to exclude the possibility of a tumor. CT of the temporal bone may be used to evaluate any congenital deformity or suspected trauma. Laboratory tests may include complete blood count with differential, erythrocyte sedimentation rate, coagulation studies, glucose, lipid profile, fluorescent treponemal antibody absorption test, thyroid function, inner ear antibodies, and acute and convalescent sera for viral antibody titers.

If the patient is seen within the first 10 days after onset of the sensorineural hearing loss, steroid therapy should be initiated and tapered over the next 12 days, if there is no medical contraindication. Aspirin is contraindicated, and antacids are administered concomitantly. In a double-blind, randomized, prospective, placebo-controlled study, steroid therapy enhanced the likelihood of hearing recovery in the intermediate hearing loss range of ISSNHL. Carbogen (95% oxygen and 5% carbon dioxide) inhalational therapy is an unproven modality of treatment, as is the administration of dextran or other vasodilating agents. The prognosis for hearing recovery depends on age of the patient, audiogram type, and the presence or absence of associated vertigo. Overall, the spontaneous recovery rate to 10 dB of the opposite ear ranges from 47% to 63%. If the hearing does not recover within 1 month, if there are retrocochlear signs on audiometric testing, or if the ENG is abnormal, the possibility of a vestibular schwannoma needs to be excluded with gadolinium-enhanced MRI. Patient in whom the hearing does not recover should receive appropriate hearing aid evaluation and fitting.

Acute vestibular labyrinthitis or neuritis is a relatively common disorder. It is defined as the sudden unilateral loss of vestibular function without associated auditory or central nervous system symptoms in an otherwise healthy adult. Patients may have a single attack or multiple attacks. In contrast to ISSNHL, in which the cochlear end-organ is more commonly involved than the cochlear nerve, isolated atrophy of the vestibular nerve is the rule on histopathologic examination. The histopathologic changes seen in cases of vestibular neuritis are thought to be most compatible with a viral cause because they closely mimic the alterations seen with herpes zoster infection of the vestibular system.

Patients usually present with sudden onset of acute vertigo without any associated central nervous system or auditory symptoms. The disease often occurs with middle-aged individuals. The vertigo may be severe enough to precipitate nausea and vomiting. The acute phase generally lasts several days to a few weeks as the mechanisms of vestibular compensation adjust and complete recovery is expected within 6 months. In the acute phase, physical examination reveals a visibly ill patient. Movement tends to aggravate the dizziness and may precipitate emesis. Patients usually have spontaneous nystagmus; however, other portions of the cranial nerve examination should be unremarkable and there should be no cerebellar abnormalities except for gait unsteadiness. Audiometric evaluation is obtained to document the absence of any auditory deficit or any asymmetry. ENG testing in the acute phase may show only intense spontaneous nystagmus, but it also may document a unilateral decreased caloric response in the involved ear.

Differential diagnosis includes Ménière disease, vestibular schwannoma, and cerebellar infarction. If there is any cerebellar abnormality on neurologic examination, CT should be performed to exclude the possibility of a cerebellar infarct. MRI may be required to rule out vestibular schwannoma if there is any retrocochlear sign on audiometric testing. The attacks of Ménière disease are usually shorter in duration than those of vestibular neuritis, lasting a few hours instead of several days to a few weeks, and it is usually associated with auditory symptoms such as aural fullness, hearing loss, or tinnitus.

Treatment of vestibular neuritis is supportive in nature consisting of vestibular suppressant, hydration, and antiemetics. Commonly used vestibular suppressants include meclizine, dimenhydrinate, and diazepam. After the first few days of the acute episode, the vestibular suppressant therapy should be tapered to minimize its potential effect on the compensatory mechanisms. Early treatment with acyclovir is still experimental. Some patients may experience multiple attacks of acute vertigo with subsequent attacks being milder and briefer than the initial episode. Positional vertigo, like that of benign paroxysmal positional vertigo, may appear in the recovery phase of the acute attack. A few patients with the multiple-attack form of the disease may have sufficient symptoms to warrant vestibular section.

In the earlier classification of neurolabyrinthitis, it was also proposed that ipsilateral, contralateral, or bilateral endolymphatic hydrops is a delayed manifestation of some viral labyrinthine infections, because a subclinical viral injury to the resorptive mechanism of the endolymphatic sac eventually becomes evident clinically by fluctuating sensorineural hearing loss or episodic vertigo. An extension of the same reasoning is used in the hypothesis that Ménière disease represents a response to a subclinical viral infection. The history typically comprises an early childhood loss of cochlear or vestibular function in one or both ears, temporally related in many cases to mumps, an upper respiratory illness, or influenza. Many years later, symptoms of progressive endolymphatic hydrops appear in an apparently normal ear. Audiometric testing documents the degree of and fluctuation in the sensorineural hearing loss, and auditory brainstem response (ABR) testing is consistent with a cochlear lesion. ENG testing demonstrates a variable degree of loss of unilateral or bilateral vestibular function. Therapy is the same as for Ménière disease and is dictated according to the predominant symptoms.

BIBLIOGRAPHY

Becker W, Naumann HH, Pfaltz CR. Clinical aspects of diseases of the external ear. In: Buckingham RA, ed. *Ear, nose, and throat diseases.* New York: Thieme Medical, 1994:71.

Buchman CA, Levine JD, Balkany TJ. Infection of the ear. In: Lee KJ, ed. *Essential otolaryngology—head and neck surgery.* New Haven: McGraw-Hill, 2003:462.

Gulya AJ. Infections of the labyrinth. In: Bailey B, ed. *Head and neck surgery—otolaryngology.* Philadelphia: Lippincott-Raven, 1998:2137.

Hendley JO. Otitis media. *N Engl J Med* 2002;15:1169–1174.

Holten KB, Gick J. Management of the patient with otitis externa. *J Family Pract* 2001;50:353–360.

Jung TT, Hanson JB. Classification of otitis media and surgical principles. *Otolaryngol Clin North Am* 1999;32:369–383.

Marais J, Dale B. Bullus myringitis: a review. *Clin Otolaryngol* 1997;22:497–499.

Roland PS, Stroman DW. Microbiology of acute otitis externa. *Laryngoscope* 2002;112:1166–1177.

CHAPTER 126
Pharyngitis

Gretchen Champion

Pharyngitis is an illness frequently encountered in the primary care setting. Although the overwhelming majority of pharyngitis cases are benign and self-limiting, certain etiologies require a particular treatment or even referral. This chapter reviews the principal etiologies, treatments, and complications of pharyngitis.

Anatomically, the pharynx consists of the nasopharynx, oropharynx, and hypopharynx and includes lymphoid tissue of the tonsils and adenoids. Pharyngitis is characterized by an inflammation of some or all pharyngeal tissues. The etiology is largely infectious and reactive; however, autoimmune, congenital, or neoplastic disease may rarely play a role.

ETIOLOGY

Infectious

Viral infections cause over 35% of all cases of infectious pharyngitis. The organisms commonly seen in upper respiratory illnesses, including rhinovirus, coronavirus, parainfluenza, influenza, and Coxsackie viruses, also produce a mild to moderate pharyngitis. Adenovirus and herpes simplex virus pharyngitis are less common but produce more severe symptomatology. Epstein-Barr virus results in significant pharyngotonsillitis in patients with mononucleosis. Human immunodeficiency virus (HIV) may also manifest as pharyngitis during primary infection. Herpes simplex groups I and II may cause pharyngitis indistinguishable from bacterial entities.

Streptococcus pyogenes (group A streptococcus) is certainly the most-discussed cause of pharyngitis. This bacterium is involved in up to 15% of all cases of pharyngitis and peaks during the winter and early spring in temperate climates. Group A streptococcal pharyngitis has the potential for systemic sequelae, including acute rheumatic fever and acute glomerulonephritis.

Non–group A β-hemolytic streptococci have been associated with endemic bacterial pharyngitis in military populations and college students. Mixed anaerobic bacteria, *Staphylococcus aureus, Corynebacterium diphtheriae, Bordetella pertussis, Yersinia* sp., and *Mycoplasma pneumoniae* also cause occasional cases of pharyngitis. Organisms associated with sexually transmitted disease, including *Neisseria gonorrhoeae* and *Treponema pallidum* (syphilis), may infect the pharyngeal tissues.

Although rare, fungal infections are seen largely in immunosuppressed patients. Organisms include *Candida* sp., *Histoplasma capsulatum,* and *Blastomyces dermatitidis.*

Noninfectious

Noninfectious causes of pharyngitis include granulomatous disease, radiation, integumental disorders, and gastric reflux disease. Gastric reflux disease is prevalent in the adult population and may result in pharyngeal irritation and subsequent discomfort, mimicking infectious pharyngitis (see Chapter 61).

HISTORY AND PHYSICAL EXAMINATION

Determining the cause of a sore throat involves inquiring about the acuity, nature, and severity of disease. Symptoms in addition to "sore throat" will give clues as to the most likely etiology. Finally, the directed history should include underlying medical disease, immunodeficiency, sexual history, and prior infectious and noninfectious exposures.

Examination of the pharynx is accomplished with good lighting and should include the floor of the mouth, tongue, palate, uvula, tonsils, and posterior pharyngeal wall. The examination of the nasopharynx and hypopharynx, if indicated, can be accomplished with a mirror or nasopharyngoscope. Increased work of breathing, drooling, or stridor signals possible laryngeal obstruction and should be addressed immediately.

SPECIFIC PHARYNGEAL INFECTIONS

Viral

Pharyngeal discomfort occurs frequently during an episode of the common cold but is often not the major symptom. Symptoms such as rhinitis, malaise, low-grade fever, and cough are more characteristic of viral infections. The pharynx may appear normal or erythematous. Postnasal drip may be visualized. Tonsillar exudates are rarely seen with influenza or common cold viruses.

Epstein-Barr virus (mononucleosis) is common in young adults, and pharyngitis may be severe, exudative, and associated with generalized adenopathy. Mononucleosis is a relatively frequent cause of pharyngotonsillitis in young adults.

History suggestive of recent high-risk sexual contact should prompt investigation into HIV. Primary infection with HIV is characterized by fever, malaise, and nonexudative pharyngitis 3 to 5 weeks after inoculation. Patients with pharyngeal herpes simplex virus demonstrate small vesicles often visualized on the soft palate accompanied by severe odynophagia. Patients with adenovirus infections may have accompanying conjunctivitis.

Bacterial

Group A streptococcus pharyngitis may present acutely with odynophagia, fever, headache, abdominal pain, nausea, and tender cervical lymph nodes. Certain strains of *S. pyogenes* produce erythrogenic toxin, which results in the erythematous rash of scarlet fever. Physical examination often reveals tonsillopharyngeal erythema, exudates, soft palate petechiae, swollen uvula, and cervical lymphadenitis. Patients with acute glomerulonephritis may report hematuria.

Gonorrheal and chlamydial pharyngitis often present with mild pharyngitis and clinical suspicion based on history should dictate workup. Diphtheria is uncommon today because of wide-spread vaccination; however, cases are still reported in the United States in the unvaccinated population. The disease has a slow onset, mild pharyngeal discomfort, low-grade fever, and the characteristic dark gray membrane adherent to the tonsillopharyngeal mucosa.

Anaerobic pharyngitis, also known as Vincent angina, may present with foul breath and purulent tonsillar exudate. Lemierre disease, thrombosis of the internal jugular vein, is a condition in children and young adults caused by specific anaerobe, *Fusobacterium necrophorum,* and is associated with septic thrombophlebitis and systemic bacterial spread. Presentation is often fever, stiff neck, and dysphagia.

Peritonsillar abscesses are mixed-organism infections seen primarily in the winter. Patients present with odynophagia, drooling, fevers, and muffled voice. They often have a history of untreated pharyngitis. Physical examination reveals unilateral soft palate erythema, edema, deviated uvula, and trismus. The infection can spread to adjacent vasculature and deep neck spaces.

Epiglotitis is less common now with *H. influenzae* vaccination but still occurs. It may be associated with *S. aureus* infection in adults and may present initially as uncomplicated pharyngitis but progresses rapidly with acute airway obstruction. Patients will have severe odynophagia, stridor, and voice change. Retropharyngeal or deep space abscess can also occur and typically present with fever, trismus, severe odynophagia, or tender palpable neck abscess.

DIAGNOSIS AND TREATMENT

For most patients who present with typical infectious pharyngitis, the major clinical distinction is whether the etiology is group A streptococcus or a common viral entity. Severe signs such as fever, tonsillar exudates, rash, and adenopathy favor a group A streptococcal etiology but are by no means diagnostic. Because of the overlap in symptoms and physical examination findings, clinical evaluation is not reliable in determining the etiology. Culture of the pharynx on sheep blood agar is the standard laboratory test for group A streptococcus but takes 24 to 48 hours for results. Therefore, the rapid strep antigen test has emerged and has a specificity of 90% but sensitivity of 60%. With such a low sensitivity, persons with pharyngitis but a negative rapid strep test should have a bacterial throat culture performed.

Antibiotics prevent complications and shorten the duration of group A streptococcus pharyngitis. Simple community-acquired group A streptococcus is sensitive to a 10-day course of penicillin or amoxicillin. Erythromycin should be the medication of choice for the penicillin-allergic population. Cephalosporins and azithromycin can achieve eradication within 5 days of treatment; however, their cost generally limits their routine use. Antibiotics should generally be reserved for patients with a positive rapid strep test or positive bacterial throat culture. If given within 7 days of onset of symptoms, antibiotics are thought to prevent rheumatic heart disease. Antibiotics have not been shown to prevent acute glomerulonephritis. Antibiotics generally thought to be safe in pregnancy include penicillin, cephalosporins, erythromycin (but not erythromycin estolate), nitrofurantoin, isoniazid, and ethambutol.

Diagnosis of viral infection is usually clinical, but nasopharyngeal swab is useful for epidemics and hospital monitoring. Treatment for typical viral pharyngitis is largely supportive, including rest, analgesics, and hydration. Ibuprofen is superior to acetaminophen in relieving throat pain. The antiviral medicine amantadine is effective for type A influenza pharyngitis.

Herpes pharyngitis can be diagnosed with viral cultures of vesicular fluid. Treatment usually involves acyclovir or similar medicine. Supportive care, including analgesics, also has a role. Gonococcal pharyngitis is diagnosed by growth on Thayer-Martin media and is often treated with penicillin, tetracycline, or cephalosporins for nonresistant organisms. Syphilis is diagnosed with blood test and treated with penicillin.

Mononucleosis (Epstein-Barr virus) and HIV are diagnosed with blood tests. Diphtheria is confirmed by culture on Loeffler medium.

There are several complications of bacterial pharyngitis. Peritonsillar abscess is diagnosed on clinical examination and is treated with incision, drainage, and antibiotics. Deep neck abscesses may be life threatening due to airway and vascular involvement and require surgical evaluation. Lemierre disease is diagnosed with neck ultrasound or computed tomography and treated with antibiotics in conjunction with surgical consultation.

Any indication of airway obstruction should warrant prompt surgical evaluation. Biopsy should be performed in any patient with a persistent lesion on the tonsil or pharynx, and a high index of suspicion for pharyngeal neoplasm is important in patients with tobacco and alcohol risk factors. Gastric reflux disease, a frequent source of pharyngeal irritation, is diagnosed with esophageal pH monitoring and treated with lifestyle modifications and pharmacotherapy.

BIBLIOGRAPHY

Bisno AL. Acute pharyngitis. *N Engl J Med* 2001;344:205–211.

Bisno AL, Peter GS, Kaplan EL. Diagnosis of strep throat in adults. *CID* 2002;35:126–129.

Sheeler RD, Houston MS, Radke S, et al. Accuracy of rapid strep testing in patients who have had recent streptococcal pharyngitis. *J Am Board Fam Practice* 2002;15:261–265.

Stewart MH, Siff JE, Cydulka RK. Evaluation of the patient with sore throat, earache, and sinusitis: an evidence-based approach. *Emerg Med Clin North Am* 1999;17:153–183.

Stollerman GH. Rheumatic fever in the 21st century. *CID* 2001;33:806–814.

Thompson LDR, Wenig BM, Kornblut AD. Pharyngitis. In: Bailey B, ed. *Byron Bailey's head and neck surgery—otolaryngology,* 3rd ed. Philadelphia: Lippincott Williams & Wilkins, 2001:543–554.

CHAPTER 127
Common Oral Lesions

Wen Jiang

A multitude of different types of lesions can occur in the oral cavity and oral pharynx. The different types of lesions can be classified into one of two categories—inflammatory or neoplastic. Inflammatory lesions, generally referred to as stomatitis, may be secondary to infection, trauma, drug reactions, systemic diseases, or autoimmune disorders. Numerous neoplasms occur in the oral cavity, ranging from benign papillomas to malignancies such as squamous cell carcinoma. Neoplasms are discussed in greater detail in Chapter 128. Stomatitis is a frequent cause for a primary care visit. A simplified way of categorizing lesions is to consider them as blistering, ulcerative, red, or white lesions.

BLISTERING LESIONS

Most blistering lesions involving the oral mucosa are a result of viral infections or the oral manifestation of one of the multiple immune and nonimmune dermatologic disorders. Herpes viruses comprise the largest family of viruses that cause oral lesions. The most common type of infection is due to human herpesvirus-1 or herpes simplex virus (HSV). Clinical signs and symptoms of a primary infection usually manifest themselves within 7 days after exposure. The route of infection is by direct contact with infected fluids. Oral lesions are most prominent on the gingiva, thus the common name primary herpetic gingivostomatitis. This entity is usually seen in children between 1 and 3 years of age. The clinical presentation consists of vesicles on any mucosal surface and may be associated with moderate fever, malaise, headache, dysphagia, occasional arthralgia, and cervical lymphadenopathy. Common sites of involvement include the palate, buccal, and gingival mucosa and the vermilion borders of the lips.

In the otherwise healthy individual, the lesions resolve in 10 to 14 days without scarring. After the resolution of the primary infection, the virus migrates to regional nerve ganglia and lies dormant until reactivation. Reactivation of latent virus can be induced by various factors, the most frequently cited being exposure to ultraviolet light. Recurrent lesions, especially those on the vermilion borders of the lips, also referred to as herpes labialis, are typically associated with a distinct individualized prodrome described as a sensation of tingling, tightness, burning, or itching. Within 24 hours, the prodrome is followed by a rapid progression to vesicle formation. The vesicles then rupture and crust to form the typical "fever blister" or "cold sore." Healing usually occurs within 7 to 10 days. The frequency of reactivation is increased in immunosuppressed individuals.

The vesicles are formed by the degeneration of the epithelial cells. Histologically, the virally infected cells appear multinucleated. The nucleus is homogeneous or glassy, with nuclear material being on the perimeter of the cell. Vesicle formation is the key point for diagnosis. The diagnosis of primary herpetic gingivostomatitis is frequently made on the basis of clinical signs and symptoms with evidence of prior exposure. A fourfold rise in antibody titer to HSV-1 over a 2-week period is also confirmatory. Although viral culture is the "gold standard" for the diagnosis of HSV-1, it is not widely used because of associated costs and delay in diagnosis.

Treatment is mainly supportive, with hydration, analgesics, and antipyretics. Numerous nonprescription preparations are available; however, reports of their actual efficacy have been most often derived from anecdotal reports. Their primary value appears to be one of symptomatic relief and placebo effect rather than virucidal action. Systemic antiviral therapy (i.e., acyclovir) has been used to treat both primary and recurrent oral HSV-1 infections. Anecdotal evidence and preliminary reports indicate that early intervention with systemic acyclovir greatly attenuates the clinical signs and symptoms associated with primary herpetic gingivostomatitis. On the other hand, such treatment is ineffective when used to treat recurrent fever blisters unless it is used at the first onset of prodromal symptoms. Prophylactic use of systemic acyclovir has been reported to be effective in preventing recurrent HSV-1 infections that precipitate other conditions (e.g., erythema multiforme [EM]); however, it is of no value in preventing sunlight-induced recurrences. Topical acyclovir has been reported to greatly shorten the duration of the recurrent perioral lesions if it is applied during the prodromal period. Nevertheless, topical acyclovir is poorly absorbed through the vermillion border and perioral skin and should not be considered as a treatment of first choice. For many individuals, herpes labialis is effectively prevented by the application of lip balms and other preparations that block ultraviolet radiation to the skin.

Oral lesions of varicella-zoster virus (VZV) or human herpesvirus-3 share many similarities with those of herpes simplex. Both viruses result in primary mucocutaneous eruptions. After primary infection, VZV, like HSV-1, remains latent in nerve ganglia and can be reactivated, causing a characteristic vesicular eruption (shingles) in a dermatomal distribution. Immunosuppressive states such as malignancy, human immunodeficiency virus (HIV) infection, chemotherapy, and transplantation predispose individuals to develop shingles, although a small percentage of affected patients have a recurrent vesicular eruption without any precipitating events. Varicella-zoster is contracted by direct contact or exposure to aerosolized droplets. Clinical features of primary infection include a rash involving the trunk, head, and neck. This rash progresses to formation of vesicles that ulcerate and crust. Oral mucosal involvement is of minor significance compared with cutaneous manifestations. Oral lesions in recurrent VZV are pathognomonic and characterized by a prodrome, followed by a unilateral vesicular eruption that soon ulcerates. The most commonly involved sites are buccal mucosa, palate, and the pharynx. Recurrent VZV infection is diagnosed on the basis of clinical signs that the involved lesions are localized in an anatomic area of specific innervations and that the lesions are unilateral and do not cross the midline.

In otherwise healthy individuals, supportive care is usually sufficient for both primary and recurrent intraoral infections. Oral or intravenous acyclovir has been reported to be effective and is the drug of choice in immunosuppressed patients. Corticosteroids are contraindicated. Recurrent intraoral lesions are relatively painful; therefore, oral narcotic analgesics are often prescribed. Topical anesthetics, palliative mouth rinses, and occlusive dressings have all been used effectively as supportive measures through the ulcerative phase of the infection. Oral VZV lesions have an excellent prognosis in the immunocompetent host; however, those who are immunocompromised are at a much greater risk for extended recurrences and are relatively unresponsive to conventional therapy.

Coxsackie viruses are members of the picornavirus family and can cause two conditions that both manifest as oral blisters: hand, foot, and mouth disease and herpangina. Viral infection is normally transmitted by infected salivary droplets. Hand, foot, and mouth disease normally occurs as an epidemic primarily affecting children under the age of 5. Herpangina is an acute viral infection caused by one of several Coxsackie A viruses (A1 to 6, A8, A10, and A22).

Characteristically, the infection occurs in the summer and fall months and affects children more frequently than adults. Patients initially have a brief nonspecific prodrome of fever and malaise, followed by an erythematous pharyngitis and dysphagia. The oral vesicles are patchy, involving the soft palate, tonsillar pillars, and fauces. The vesicles rapidly rupture to form shallow ulcers covered by pseudomembrane and are surrounded by an erythematous halo, mimicking recurrent aphthous ulcers. The symptoms are normally self-limiting, and the lesions resolve within 1 week without scarring. Treatment is supportive with mouth rinses and gargles.

Many dermatologic disorders may have oral mucosal changes as part of the spectrum of disease. Often the pain and discomfort of the oral symptoms can be more significant than the cutaneous involvement. Some of the common dermatologic disorders that result in blistering of the oral mucosa include pemphigus vulgaris (PV), cicatricial pemphigoid, bullous pemphigoid, and EM.

PV is a group of acute and chronic autoimmune blistering diseases involving the skin and mucous membranes. The primary pathogenic process is the formation of antibodies against intercellular bridges between squamous cells' desmosome–tonofilament complexes that results in the loss of cell–cell adhesion and the formation of intraepithelial blisters. The disease typically affects individuals 40 to 60 years of age, with equal distribution between both sexes. In its worst form, the disease can be fatal. PV usually presents with oral erosions that can predate cutaneous lesions by weeks to months. Most patients with PV will have oral involvement at some point in the course of the disease, and more than half may have this as their presenting symptom. The diagnosis can be made with a positive Nikolsky sign with induction of a blister with minor trauma or an Asboe-Hansen sign that produces lateral extension of a blister by pressing on it. The most commonly affected sites in the oral cavity are sites with oral trauma such as gingiva, palate, and buccal mucosa. Lesions are painful vesicles that rapidly rupture, producing an ulcer with a gray membrane. To confirm the diagnosis of PV, the margin of a vesicle or bullae should be biopsied. Microscopically, lesions show intracellular edema, loss of intercellular adhesion, suprabasilar acantholysis, and a split above the basement membrane zone. Basal cells are cuboidal shaped and remain attached to the lamina propria, creating a "row of tombstones" effect. Free acantholytic squamous cells assume a spherical form called the *Tzanck cell.* On direct immunofluorescence, IgG and C3 are found deposited in the lesional and perilesional skin in the intercellular space of the keratinocytes. Indirect immunofluorescence reveals IgG autoantibodies, directed against a 130-kDa glycoprotein Desmoglein-3, a member of the cadherin superfamily. The titer of the antibody correlates with severity of disease. Treatment strategies depend on the pemphigus subtype, severity, and the rate of progression of the disease. For oral lesions, topical steroids or topical cyclosporine may be used. Systemic corticosteroids may be required to control the disease, usually continued for 1 to 3 months and then tapered. Other immunosuppressive agents such as azathioprine and methotrexate may be added to control symptoms. The disease tends to be chronic and often requires multiple agents to control new blister formation. And even with all the immunosuppressive agents available, PV has a mortality rate of 5% to 15%, often secondary to complications of therapy.

Cicatricial pemphigoid, or mucous membrane pemphigoid, is a heterogeneous, chronic, subepithelial blistering disease with various clinical and immunologic presentations. Patients present with tense vesicles that rupture easily on the cutaneous or mucosal surfaces. Most patients will have patchy oral mucosal involvement, with the most common sites being gingival, buccal, and labial mucosa. Ocular involvement is common, and the inflammation and scarring of the cornea may eventually lead to blindness. On direct immunofluorescence, a subepidermal blister is seen with a moderate mixed perivascular infiltrate. Perilesional skin usually shows a linear deposition of IgG and C3. The targeted proteins of the autoantibodies represent components of the hemidesmosomes and anchoring filaments. Topical and/or intralesional steroids can be used for localized disease, whereas systemic steroids are effective for more diffuse involvement. For chronic use, dapsone and other immunosuppressive agents such as azathioprine, cyclophosphamide, and cyclosporine may be used. The uses of topical tetracycline with niacinamide, minocycline, and topical cyclosporine have all been described in case reports.

Bullous pemphigoid is a chronic autoimmune disease affecting older adults, typically over 60 years of age. It is characterized by autoantibodies against the basement membrane zone. Cutaneous lesions often start with a prodrome of pruritus and urticaria before the eruption of tense vesicles and bullae. About 30% to 40% of patients may have oral involvement. The blisters are usually smaller than those of PV and are nonscarring. The gingiva and buccal mucosa are commonly involved. Histologically, neutrophils may predominate in an "Indian file" arrangement at the dermal epidermal junction. Neutrophils, eosinophils, and lymphocytes fill the papillary dermis. On direct immunofluorescence of perilesional skin, there is a deposit of IgG and C3 at the dermal–epidermal junction in most patients. Most patients have circulating serum IgG antibodies, but unlike PV there is no correlation between antibody titer and disease activity. There are two recognized antigens targeted by the IgG autoantibodies, bullous pemphigoid antigen-1 and -2, both encoding for proteins that are part of the intracellular hemidesmosome. Localized disease can be treated with oral antihistamine and topical steroids. Systemic prednisone with a starting dose of 1 mg/kg is the mainstay of therapy for generalized disease or severe oral or ocular involvement. Methotrexate, azathioprine in doses of 50 to 200 mg/day, or dapsone 100 to 200 mg/day can be helpful. A combination of tetracycline or erythromycin and niacinamide is often tried but has not undergone rigorous testing. A prolonged clinical remission may be seen after steroid therapy in as many as 75% of patients. Recurrences of the disease tend not be as severe as the original outbreak.

EM is a reaction pattern with characteristic erythematous bull's-eye lesions on acral skin and often dramatic involvement of the mucous membrane. The disease usually affects young healthy adults. Multiple drugs such as sulfonamides, anticonvulsants, barbiturates, and allopurinol have been implicated in the drug-induced form. However, in about 50% of the cases, the etiology of the lesions is unknown. The skin lesions consist of macules with a violaceous color that progress to true target (iris lesions) or atypical targets over several days. There are minor and major forms of EM, with minimal mucosal involvement in the minor form. The major form of EM, also referred to as *Stevens-Johnson syndrome,* is usually associated with drug reactions and often has severe and extensive mucosal involvement. In oral lesions, intact vesicles are not usually present. Instead, fibrinous membranes may be seen attached to ill-defined erosions. Anterior labial, tongue, and buccal mucosa are the common sites of involvement, with gingival lesions being less common. Ocular involvement may be severe, including keratitis and ulcerations of the cornea. The cause of EM appears to be an immune-based reaction to an antigen whether it is a drug, *Mycoplasma pneumoniae,* or the herpes antigen. The recurrent form of EM is almost universally associated with herpes simplex. Each episode of EM is usually self-limited, lasting for 2 to 4 weeks, and supportive care is required. Case-controlled studies have not shown a benefit of oral corticosteroids, although investigators have observed control of symptoms if steroids are instituted very early in the course of the disease.

ULCERATIVE LESIONS

Recurrent aphthous stomatitis (RAS) (Fig. 127.1) is a common disorder affecting 5% to 66% of examined adult patient groups.

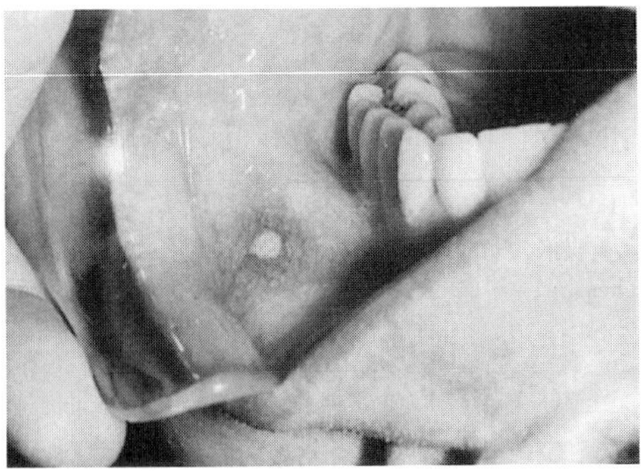

FIG. 127.1. Recurrent aphthous stomatitis. A minor aphthous ulcer with a central white ulceration is surrounded by an erythematous halo on the buccal mucosa. (From Bailey BJ, ed. *Head and neck surgery: otolaryngology.* Philadelphia: JB Lippincott, 1993, with permission.)

Patients present with recurrent bouts of one or several rounded, shallow, painful oral ulcers at intervals of a few months to a few days. There are three main presentations of RAS: minor, major, and herpetiform. The minor form is the most common, affecting 80% of the patients. The lesions are usually less than 5 mm in diameter with a gray white pseudomembrane enveloped by a thin erythematous halo. It commonly occurs in the labial or buccal mucosa and floor of the mouth. The lesions heal within 1 to 2 weeks without scarring. The major form is uncommon and severe, with oval or irregular ulcers that may exceed 1 cm in diameter. These lesions have a predilection for the lips, soft palate, and fauces; persist for up to 6 weeks; and often heal with scarring. The herpetiform is very uncommon, characterized by multiple recurrent crops of small painful ulcers that tend to fuse and produce large irregular ulcers.

A number of diseases have been associated with RAS and may suggest an etiology; however, the precise mechanism of pathogenesis has not been discovered. RAS may have a familial basis, with more than 40% of patients reporting a vague family history of oral ulceration. Nutritional factors have been suggested to be linked to RAS, such as iron, folic acid, vitamin B_{12}, and zinc deficiencies. Some studies have noted an increased prevalence of food allergies and gluten sensitivity among RAS patients. Some women with RAS have cyclical oral ulceration related to the luteal phase of the menstrual cycle.

Various infectious etiologies have also been suggested for RAS, including oral *(viridans)* streptococci and various members of the herpesvirus family. The current theory is that the most likely etiology is immunologic. Autoantibodies to oral mucosal membranes have been found. The ratio of T helper to T suppressor cells in the analysis of peripheral T lymphocytes in patients with RAS was found to be decreased, suggesting an immunologic influence. However, the precise etiology remains unknown.

If RAS is associated with systemic disease, the treatment should emphasize the correction of the underlying problem, such as the correction of vitamin deficiency or avoiding foods that may trigger an allergic reaction. All patients should be advised to use an oral hygiene procedure that is as atraumatic as possible, and all dental appliances should be checked to ensure an optimal fitting.

Various topical agents can be used, such as topical tetracycline or chlorhexidine in the forms of 0.2% w/w mouth rinse or 1% gel. Topical corticosteroids remain the mainstay of RAS treatment in most countries, although there are few well-controlled studies of their precise efficacy. Topical analgesics such as benzydamine hydrochloride mouthwash or lignocaine gel may provide some symptomatic relief of pain. Systemic immunosuppression such as prednisone and azathioprine has been suggested to be effective when there is profound pain and long-standing ulceration; however, there have been no detailed published studies on their precise clinical benefit. Treatments with colchicine, pentoxifylline, and dapsone all have been reported to give some clinical benefit. Thalidomide remains the most effective agent for the management of RAS, producing a remission in almost 50% of treated patients in one randomized controlled trial. However, it has mild adverse side effects (e.g., intolerance, loss of libido) in up to 75% of treated patients, and the risk of teratogenicity has also limited its clinical application.

Acute necrotizing ulcerative gingivitis is another example of an ulcerative lesion of the oral cavity. This disorder also is known as trench mouth or Vincent stomatitis. Its incidence has increased with the increased prevalence of acquired immunodeficiency syndrome (AIDS). Ulceration of the interdental papillae with bleeding and pseudomembrane formation occurs with a fetid odor. Systemic symptoms of fever, malaise, and lymphadenopathy also occur. Culture of these lesions reveals fusiform bacilli and spirochetes. Treatment consists of superficial debridement and antibiotics. Any patient with a persistent lesion should be referred to an otolaryngologist or oral surgeon for evaluation and biopsy.

Lupus erythematosus may have oral involvement, occurring as an erythematous plaque that develops a painful ulceration. It occurs most often in chronic discoid lupus, but any form may have oral involvement. Diagnosis requires biopsy. Histologically, degeneration of the basal cell layer is observed with lymphocytic infiltration. Immunofluorescence most often reveals IgG deposition in the basement membrane. Treatment is with nonsteroidal antiinflammatory drugs, whereas steroids are reserved for severe cases.

WHITE LESIONS

Oral lichen planus affects 1% to 2% of the general adult population and is the most common noninfectious oral mucosal disease referred to oral pathology clinics. Typical oral lesions are striations (striae of Wickham), papules, plaques, mucosal atrophy, erosions (shallow ulcers), or blisters affecting the buccal mucosa, tongue, and gingiva. Oral lichen planus is characterized histologically by a dense subepithelial lymphocytic infiltrate and epithelial basal cell destruction. Apoptotic basal keratinocytes form colloid or Civatte bodies, which appear as homogenous eosinophilic globules. Epithelial basement membrane changes are common and comprise breaks, branches, and duplications. Recent research suggests that oral lichen planus is a purely T-cell–mediated inflammatory disease, where T-cell–secreted tumor necrosis factor-α and matrix metalloproteinase-9 play critical roles in the pathogenesis of the disease. Biopsy is required to differentiate between oral lichen planus and other white or chronic ulcerative oral lesions and malignancy must also be excluded. Treatment of all patients with oral lichen planus consists of removal of all local exacerbating factors. Patients should be instructed in thorough oral hygiene. Teeth associated with oral lesions should be examined and sharp cusps or edges reduced. Superinfection with *Candida albicans* should be controlled with topical antimycotics. Patients' prescriptions should be altered if a lichenoid drug reaction is suspected. Medical treatment is generally restricted to atrophic, erosive, or symptomatic lesions. Local oral lesions can be controlled with betamethasone propionate ointment (0.05%), applied three to four times daily after meals. Generalized oral lesions are treated with a 0.25-mg dexamethasone mouth rinse twice daily after meals. Intralesional triamcinolone acetonide may be used for persistent localized erosive lesions. Finally, if lesions do not respond to topical therapy, a short course of systemic corticosteroids may be used.

Oral candidiasis is another source of white lesions in the mouth. Many *Candida* species colonize mucocutaneous surfaces in most healthy humans. They are strictly opportunistic pathogens, normally innocuous but can cause disease when the host immune system is compromised. *Candida albicans* is the most common *Candida* species isolated from the oral cavity both in health and disease, with a reported prevalence of 40% to 60% in healthy individuals. Many local and systemic factors can predispose an individual to candidiasis. Local factors include reduced salivary flow, ill-fitting dentures, epithelial changes, alteration in oral flora, or a high carbohydrate diet. Systemic factors include endocrine disorders such as diabetes, hypothyroidism, hyperparathyroidism, or adrenal suppression; dietary factors such as iron or folate deficiencies; and various immunosuppressed states due to malignancy, drug therapy, HIV and AIDS, or congenital immunodeficiency syndromes.

Oral candidiasis can be grouped into two categories, based on the distribution of the lesions. Category I consists of candidal infections confined to oral and perioral tissues (primary oral candidiasis), and category II includes disorders where oral candidiasis is a manifestation of generalized systemic mucocutaneous candidal infection (secondary oral candidiasis). The principle clinical features of category II disorders include chronic oral candidiasis, chronic cutaneous candidiasis, and chronic vulvovaginal candidiasis. Category I is further divided into acute (pseudomembranous, erythematous), chronic (pseudomembranous, erythematous, hyperplastic), and candida-associated forms (denture stomatitis, angular cheilitis, median rhomboid glossitis). Pseudomembranous candidiasis, or thrush, is the most common form, characterized by whitish or yellow creamy plaques on the surface of the oral mucosa and tongue (Fig. 127.2). The plaques may be wiped off, revealing a raw erythematous base. The plaques consist of yeast cells and hyphae, bacteria, desquamated epithelium, necrotic tissue, and inflammatory cells. The deeper parts of the epithelium show acanthosis, and the inflammatory response in the connective tissue comprises lymphocytes, plasma cells, and polymorphonuclear lymphocytes (PMNL).

Erythematous candidiasis is usually associated with the use of corticosteroids or broad-spectrum antibiotics. Clinically, it is characterized by erythematous areas generally on the dorsum of the tongue, palate, or buccal mucosa, in the absence of white plaques. Although relatively rare compared with other forms of

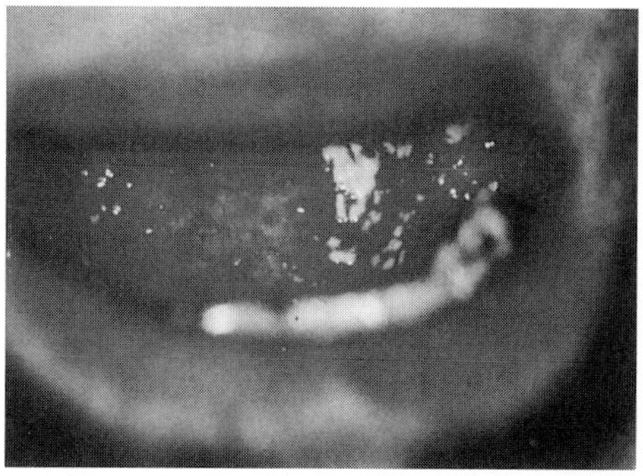

FIG. 127.2. Soft white plaques of pseudomembranous candidiasis (thrush). (Courtesy of Dr. Robert O. Greer.) (From Bailey BJ, ed. *Head and neck surgery: otolaryngology.* Philadelphia: JB Lippincott, 1993, with permission.)

oral candidiasis, up to 50% of the candidiasis associated with HIV infection may be of this form. Hyperplastic candidal lesions are chronic, discrete, raised lesions that vary from small, palpable, translucent, whitish areas to large, dense, opaque plaques. These lesions usually occur on the inside surface of the cheeks, palate, and tongue and will not rub off. Histopathologic examination of the lesions reveals parakeratosis, showing irregular separation and epithelial hyperplasia, with the yeast organism invasion restricted to the upper layers of epithelium. Classically, denture stomatitis presents as chronic erythema and edema of the denture-bearing mucosa in the elderly, especially under maxillary prostheses. Patients are usually asymptomatic or only complain of slight soreness. This entity is present in approximately 50% of complete denture wearers. Histologically, the tissues exhibit proliferative and degenerative changes with reduced keratinization and thinner epithelium. Because tissue invasion by *Candida* does not commonly occur in this form and relatively few yeasts are isolated from the mucosal surface, this entity may reflect a hypersensitivity reaction to antigens of the yeast. Angular cheilitis presents as sore, erythematous, fissured lesions affecting angles of the mouth and is commonly associated with denture stomatitis. It has also been associated with iron deficiency anemia or vitamin B_{12} deficiency. Median rhomboid glossitis is characterized by an area of papillary atrophy that is elliptical or rhomboid-like, symmetrically placed and centered at the midline of the tongue, anterior to the circumvallate papillae.

The diagnosis of oral candidiasis is made on clinical grounds with a thorough medical and dental history. Several clinical and laboratory techniques may be used to confirm a diagnosis. The presence of *Candida* hyphae can be confirmed with periodic acid–Schiff staining of a cytology smear of the pseudomembrane, thus allowing a quick and accurate diagnosis. Quantitative determination of fungal burden may be a useful marker of infection since normal carriage in 50% of the population is less than 100 colony-forming units/mL, whereas in infected individuals, counts range from 4,000 to 20,000 colony-forming unit/mL. Differentiation between different strains of *Candida* is usually not required unless in an immunocompromised host and the condition fails to resolve after appropriate antifungal treatment. In case of hyperplastic lesions, biopsy of the relevant tissue provides the most accurate diagnosis and excludes the possibility of other infectious or neoplastic process. Some 40% of patients with any type of oral candidiasis were found to have a hematologic abnormality; therefore, hematologic screening may be relevant in refractory disease. Screening is mandatory in patients with chronic mucocutaneous candidiasis, in HIV-positive individuals, and in others with systemic disease.

Medical therapy with topical applications of antifungal agents is the primary treatment modality for oral candidiasis; however, elimination of the underlying factors responsible for the development of oral candidiasis may be enough to resolve the problem. Withdrawal or substitution of broad-spectrum antibiotics can usually produce resolution of the oral fungal infection. Most commonly used topical treatment is nystatin oral suspension or nystatin pastilles four times daily for 7 to 14 days. Amphotericin suspension or lozenges used four times daily after meals may also be effective. In denture-induced candidiasis, patients must remove the denture while undertaking the topical treatment. Another option is to coat the denture-fitting surface with miconazole gel while it is being worn and repeat this three times daily for 7 to 14 days. Also, proper oral hygiene needs to be emphasized. The patient is advised to soak the denture overnight in 0.1% hypochlorite to eliminate the yeast organism. In refractory cases, oral fluconazole or itraconazole may also be used. However, underlying immunodeficiencies should always be suspected when appropriately treated pseudomembranous candidiasis fails to resolve. In patients with immunosuppression or HIV with chronic mucocutaneous candidiasis, systemic administration of ketoconazole, fluconazole, or itraconazole might be required or, rarely in the case of azole-resistant candidiasis, amphotericin. Quantitative assays of *Candida* in the oral cavity, along with cytology, can be useful in monitoring responses to antifungal therapy. Current research from several laboratories has established the importance of T lymphocytes in experimental oral candidiasis and supports clinical observations that link oral candidal infections to defects in cell-mediated immunity.

Leukoplakia is defined as white mucosal patches or plaques. This is a descriptive term rather than a disease entity. Most leukoplakic lesions are histologically benign. Some lesions, however, are cancerous or precancerous. A history of cigarette smoking, alcohol use, or both in any patient with an oral lesion should raise concern and should be a motivating factor for referral for biopsy.

RED LESIONS

Erythroplakia is a red lesion or plaque of the mucosa. This, like leukoplakia, is a description of a lesion rather than a true disease process. In contrast to leukoplakia, most erythroplakic lesions are worrisome, with 80% to 90% of lesions diagnosed as severe dysplasia or squamous cell carcinoma. These lesions often are asymptomatic, homogeneous, velvety red plaques. Biopsy is mandatory to exclude the possibility of malignancy.

Radiation mucositis is a painful inflammatory reaction of the oral mucosa to radiation therapy. The degree of injury depends on the fractionation and duration of radiation therapy, location of the lesion, and degree of oral hygiene. Radiation-induced mucositis often appears by the second week of therapy and may persist for 2 to 3 weeks after completion of radiation therapy. The lesions initially occur with diffuse erythema and swelling, followed by ulceration, which may become covered with fibrinous exudates. This condition can result in pain, decreased oral intake, systemic or local infections, and an interruption in the needed therapy. Therapy is primarily supportive. Hydrogen peroxide and water (4:1 solution) and saline and sodium bicarbonate solutions have been advocated to enhance cleansing of the oral mucosa. Patients should use a soft toothbrush to avoid any mucosal trauma. Routine oral care should be done four times a day. Numerous anesthetic or analgesic mucosal coating agents have been used to provide symptomatic relief, including Benadryl, viscous lidocaine, milk of magnesia, attapulgite (Kaopectate), Orabase, and dyclonine hydrochloride (Dyclone) or any combinations of the above.

ORAL LESIONS IN HUMAN IMMUNODEFICIENCY VIRUS INFECTION

HIV infection and AIDS pose a significant health risk in the female population. According to Centers for Disease Control and Prevention estimates, 11,082 cases of AIDS were diagnosed among women and adolescent girls in 2001 and 66% were from heterosexual transmission. It has been estimated that 20% to 50% of all patients infected with HIV will develop some oral lesions associated with the disease, and often times it is the first manifestation of infection in a previously undiagnosed patient. Most lesions are not associated with HIV infection in particular but are the result of the impaired cell-mediated immunity in HIV patients. Oral lesions can be categorized as infectious, neoplastic, and miscellaneous lesions attributable to treatment with antiviral therapy.

Oral candidiasis is the most common lesion, with 90% of patients with AIDS affected at some point during their disease course. Oral candidiasis in HIV-infected patients often portends a decline to AIDS, because the lesions are more commonly seen when CD4 counts fall below 200/mm^3. In treating oral candidiasis in HIV patients, it generally takes longer to eradicate the infection, and the relapse rate is high. Frequent or recurrent infections may necessitate treatment with systemic agents such as ketoconazole, fluconazole, or itraconazole.

Most opportunistic viral infections in HIV disease are a result of reactivation of latent herpes viruses due to decreased immune surveillance. Antibodies indicating prior exposure to herpes simplex (HSV-1) are estimated to be present in greater than 80% of the population; therefore, HSV-1 reactivation is the most common viral infection in HIV patients. Unlike immunocompetent hosts, reactivation of HSV in HIV-infected patients occur as ulcers on the nonkeratinized tissues such as labial mucosa, buccal mucosa, ventral tongue, and soft palate. Such ulcers can be extremely painful. HSV infection is typically managed well with acyclovir, with doses of 200 to 1,200 mg five times a day for 10 to 14 days. Famciclovir and valacyclovir may also be used. In the case of acyclovir-resistant strains, intravenous foscarnet may be given at dosage of 200 mg/kg.

Varicella-zoster infection is also quite common in HIV-infected population. Although the likelihood of developing herpes zoster increases dramatically when the CD4 count drops below 200/mm^3, VZV has not shown to be an independent predictor for the development of AIDS. In the orofacial region, VZV infection most commonly presents as unilateral involvement along the courses of one or more branches of the trigeminal nerve, and these may have significant complications such as meningoencephalitis and postherpetic pain. Treatment with oral or intravenous acyclovir until lesions resolve is recommended.

Epstein-Barr virus is a member of the herpes virus family, and the chief manifestation of this viral infection in the HIV-infected population is "oral hairy leukoplakia," which occurs in 24% to 33% of patients with AIDS. Usually, oral hairy leukoplakia presents as a slightly raised, painless, white, corrugated-appearing area on the lateral border of the tongue, sometimes tongue dorsum, and occasionally the buccal mucosa. Histologically, the lesions show epithelial projections in a hairlike configuration with epithelial hyperparakeratosis and hyperplasia. Little to no inflammatory infiltrate is associated with these lesions. Coinfection on the surface by *Candida* and human papillomavirus is not unusual. Oral hairy leukoplakia is nearly always asymptomatic and self-limiting and requires no treatment. Because these lesions are usually noted only when CD4 counts are less than 300/mm^3, their presence may portend a progression to full-blown AIDS within 2 years.

Kaposi sarcoma is the single most common neoplasm occurring in patients with AIDS, and there is a strong association with human herpesvirus-8. Oral Kaposi sarcoma initially presents as blue, red, or purple macules on the palate, gingival, and/or tongue that may not blanch with applied pressure. As they progress, the lesions may become raised, nodular, and extensive; there may also be ulceration, bleeding, and pain. A biopsy provides definitive diagnosis. Treatment is focused on palliation and local control, because there is no curative therapy. Those modalities such as chemotherapy, which further suppress the immune system, favor proliferation of Kaposi sarcoma. Local therapies include excision, laser ablation, radiation, or intralesional injection such as vinblastine or sodium tetradecyl sulfate.

Non-Hodgkin lymphoma is the second most prevalent intraoral neoplasm in patients with AIDS. Intraorally, the lesions present as ulcerations or soft tissue masses that are painful and enlarge rapidly, with the most common sites being the palate, retromolar trigone, tonsillar pillars, and tongue. Histologically, the lymphoma is frequently high grade, of B-cell lineage, and tends to be aggressive. Patients are treated with radiation therapy for local control and combination chemotherapy. Complete remission occurs in approximately 65% of patients, and the median survival time for individuals with AIDS-related lymphoma is between 4 and 11 months. Low CD4 counts and involvement of bone and extranodal sites are associated with poorer prognosis.

In HIV-infected patients, squamous cell carcinoma occurs in a younger population (<45 years old), often without the usual smoking and alcohol risk factor, and tends to be more aggressive. As in squamous cell carcinoma, lesions in this population may present as leukoplakia, erythroplakia, or as nonhealing ulcers or masses. Any patients with a suspected lesion should be referred to a specialist and the lesion biopsied to establish the diagnosis.

CONSIDERATIONS IN PREGNANCY

Oral lesions can be a source of difficulty during pregnancy. Patients with a history of aphthous stomatitis may have more frequent oral lesions during pregnancy. A hypothesis has been made that links the occurrence of aphthous stomatitis with hormonal changes of pregnancy or the menstrual cycle. Currently, however, no such link has been firmly established. Treatment should be similar to that in the nonpregnant state; however, steroid use should be limited and given under the supervision of the obstetrician. Tetracycline use is contraindicated because of the effects on fetal teeth and bones.

Herpes simplex stomatitis also can occur more frequently during pregnancy. Antiviral agents should be avoided in pregnancy, particularly in the first trimester, with the exception for life-threatening infections. Acyclovir has no known teratogenicity, but little is known about the extent of placental transfer of this drug. Supervision of the obstetrician is required in management of herpes simplex stomatitis during pregnancy. Both in the pregnant and nonpregnant state, any persistent lesions of unknown etiology should be referred to the otolaryngologist or oral surgeon for evaluation and possible biopsy.

BIBLIOGRAPHY

Aragon S, Jafek B, Johnson S. Stomatitis. In: Bailey B, ed. *Head and neck surgery—otolaryngology.* Philadelphia: Lippincott-Raven, 1998:627.

Bowers K. Oral blistering diseases. *Clin Dermatol* 2000;18:513–523.

Casiglia JW, Woo SB. Oral manifestation of HIV infection. *Clin Dermatol* 2000;18:541–551.

Farah CS, Ashman RB, Challacombe SJ. Oral candidosis. *Clin Dermatol* 2000;18:553–562.

Lee KW. *Color atlas of oral pathology.* Philadelphia: Lea & Febiger, 1885.

Lynch D. Oral viral infections. *Clin Dermatol* 2000;18:619–628.

Pindborg J. *Atlas of diseases of the oral mucosa.* Munksgaard, Copenhagen: WB Saunders, 1993.

Porter SR, et al. Recurrent aphthous stomatitis. *Clin Dermatol* 2000;18:569–578.

Rogers R. Common lesions of the oral mucosa. *Postgrad Med* 1992;141:53.

Rondu B, Mattingly B. Oral mucosal ulcers: diagnosis and management. *J Am Diet Assoc* 1992;123:883.

Saltsmen R, Jordan M. Viral infections. In: Burrow G, Ferris T, eds. *Medical complications during pregnancy.* Philadelphia: WB Saunders, 1988:372.

Simpson M, Gaziano E. Bacterial infections during pregnancy. In: Burrow G, Ferris T, eds. *Medical complications during pregnancy.* Philadelphia: WB Saunders, 1988:342.

Smith RM, et al. *Atlas of oral pathology.* Toronto: CV Mosby, 1981.

Sugerman PB, et al. Oral lichen planus. *Clin Dermatol* 2000;18:533–539.

Zigarreli D. Fungal infections of the oral cavity. *Otolaryngol Clin North Am* 1993;26:1069.

CHAPTER 128

Tumors of the Oral Cavity and Pharynx

Jay K. Roberts

The oral cavity and oropharynx are the sites of many different mass lesions. There are tumors that occur in one location exclusively, but most occur commonly in either location, so both regions are discussed together. Brief mention is made of tumors of the parapharyngeal space and of odontogenic tumors and fissural and odontogenic cysts. Except where specifically noted, when surgical intervention is suggested it should most often be accomplished by an otolaryngologist–head and neck surgeon.

ANATOMY

The oral cavity extends from the mucocutaneous junction of the lips anteriorly. Posteriorly, the limits are the posterior edge of the hard palate superiorly and the line of circumvallate papillae inferiorly. This space contains the lips, buccal mucosa, maxillary and mandibular alveolar ridges, retromolar trigone, floor of mouth, oral tongue (anterior two thirds), and hard palate.

The oropharynx is bound by the oral cavity anteriorly and extends to the plane of the hard palate superiorly and to the plane of the hyoid bone inferiorly. This space includes both surfaces of the entire soft palate, the tonsils, including their pillars, the tongue base from the circumvallate papillae to the base of the epiglottis, and the posterior and lateral oropharyngeal walls.

The parapharyngeal space lies lateral to the oropharynx and medial to the mandible and muscles of mastication. Structures of interest in this area include the deep lobe of the parotid, cranial nerves 9 through 12, the jugular vein, and the carotid artery.

BENIGN LESIONS OF THE ORAL CAVITY AND OROPHARYNX

Oral tori are exostoses rather than true neoplasms of the palate (torus palatinus) or mandible (torus mandibularis). They are bony hard protuberances located in the midline of the hard palate or along the lingual surface of the mandible in the region of the bicuspid. Tori occur in about 20% of the population, and the palatal location is more common. They are asymptomatic and do not require imaging. Surgery is required only rarely when they interfere with the fitting of dental prostheses.

A granular cell tumor occurs in two forms and is currently believed to be a benign proliferation of Schwann cell origin rather than a true neoplasm. Epulis of the newborn is the congenital form and occurs on the gingiva (Fig. 128.1). It is seen predominately (8:1) in females, occurs three times more commonly on the maxilla than the mandible, does not recur, and has been reported to regress spontaneously. The other form is a lesion of young adults, seen slightly more often in women and in African-Americans. The mass appears as a firm submucosal nodule most often in the tongue. Treatment of either form is conservative surgical excision.

A number of vascular lesions are seen in the oral cavity. Hereditary hemorrhagic telangiectasia (Osler-Weber-Rendu syndrome) is manifested by small bright red vascular lesions of the tongue and other oral mucous membranes. They are generally asymptomatic, but patients often require treatment due to bleeding from lesions elsewhere in the body. Varicosities of the ventral tongue and lateral tongue base are quite common in older individuals. They never require treatment. Lymphangioma and hemangioma are benign proliferations of blood and lymphatic vessels. Tongue and floor of mouth are the most common sites for these lesions in the oral cavity. They are often present at birth or shortly thereafter. Most hemangiomas regress during the first few years of life. Management of large hemangiomas is especially challenging, although a conservative approach is advocated. Temporary tracheotomy is sometimes required for airway compromise. When intervention is required, steroids or percutaneous embolization have been found to be more efficacious than cryosurgery, laser surgery,

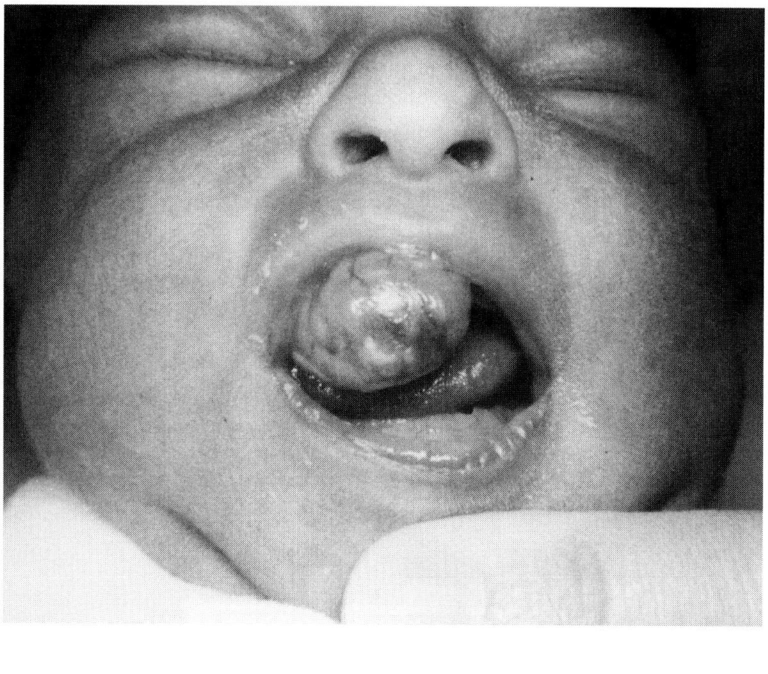

FIG. 128.1. Epulis of the newborn. Granular cell tumor of the anterior maxillary alveolus in a 1-day-old girl. The tumor was removed under local anesthesia in the nursery.

sclerotherapy, or radiation. Lymphangiomas are managed with antibiotics and steroids when infected and may be treated with surgical excision if extensive or markedly symptomatic.

Several other lingual lesions are commonly noted, including geographic tongue, median rhomboid glossitis, hairy tongue, and lingual thyroid. Geographic tongue is a condition in which certain areas of the tongue are denuded of papillae and the epithelium appears very thin. The remainder of the tongue appears normal. The surface configuration of the tongue changes over time as areas alternately desquamate and regenerate. Patients are asymptomatic, and no treatment is required. Median rhomboid glossitis is due to an embryologic abnormality. When development proceeds as expected, the tuberculum impar becomes depressed as the lateral halves of the tongue medialize. If this does not occur, the tuberculum impar is left as a surface structure. The absence of papillae in the central portion of the anterior tongue allows the underlying vessels to be very apparent, leading to the typical appearance of median rhomboid glossitis. Hairy tongue is a condition in which the filiform papillae of the dorsal surface of the tongue are markedly elongated. They are usually black or brown in color. The condition is harmless. Lingual thyroid is a condition in which the thyroid gland failed to make its descent into the neck from the foramen cecum during embryologic development. This condition becomes manifest almost exclusively in women. It is most often diagnosed in the teen years. It appears as a mass in the area of the foramen cecum, and the patient frequently complains of dysphagia, a sense of fullness, or dysphonia. The differential includes lingual tonsil, thyroglossal duct tissue, or neoplasms seen in this location such as squamous cell carcinoma, lymphoma, or minor salivary gland tumors. A thyroid scan is mandatory, because if it is a lingual thyroid, it usually is the patient's only functioning thyroid, and therefore excisional biopsy should be avoided.

A fibroma is a very common benign lesion composed of proliferating fibroblasts and is not a neoplasm. It is a fibrous overgrowth caused by chronic irritation. Some authors refer to this as fibrous hyperplasia or as fibroepithelial polyp. They occur most commonly on the tongue or buccal mucosa and appear as smooth round masses. Most often they are sessile, although they may be pedunculated. Their size ranges between several millimeters and a few centimeters, although most are less than 1 cm in size. A fibroma is not encapsulated and has a variable amount of vascularity. Conservative excision is suggested when the lesion is symptomatic, but any obvious irritating cause should also be addressed.

A number of white lesions involve the mucosa of the oral cavity and oropharynx. Lichen planus is a dermatologic disease that may manifest itself in the mouth with or without cutaneous lesions. It typically occurs in middle-aged adults, and in most series females predominate. The raised striae of reticular lichen planus seen in the buccal mucosa is characteristic, and biopsy is usually unnecessary to make the diagnosis. Erosive lichen planus is usually painful and may involve buccal mucosa, gingiva, or lateral tongue. This will sometimes be confused with discoid lupus erythematosus or squamous cell carcinoma, so biopsy is often indicated. This should be taken at the periphery of the lesion, because the central portion will often not be diagnostic. Reticular lichen planus does not require treatment; however, erosive lichen planus is best managed by steroid therapy. Focal disease may be treated topically, whereas more diffuse lesions may require topical and oral steroids.

The term *leukoplakia* is used clinically to indicate a lesion that appears white, cannot be scraped off, and which cannot be diagnosed as another lesion (Fig. 128.2). These lesions occur more commonly in elderly people and less often in women. Histologically, the majority of these show hyperkeratosis without atypia. However, approximately one fifth reveal atypia, carcinoma in situ, or invasive squamous cell carcinoma. Biopsy should be undertaken to establish a diagnosis. Further aspects of this are discussed later under Malignant Neoplasms of the Oral Cavity and Oropharynx.

A pyogenic granuloma is a benign, raised, capillary-rich lesion that, when it occurs in the oral cavity, tends to involve the gingiva. The term *pregnancy tumor* may be used for this lesion when it occurs at the gingiva of pregnant women. It is thought to be the result of overreaction to minor trauma, although hormonal changes may also be an etiologic factor. Lesions are usually sessile and friable, often between 0.5 and 2 cm in greatest dimension. They sometimes grow rapidly, suggesting malignancy. The differential diagnosis includes Kaposi sarcoma. Histologically, the pyogenic granuloma has many dilated endothelial-lined vascular spaces, budding endothelial cells, and a marked proliferation of

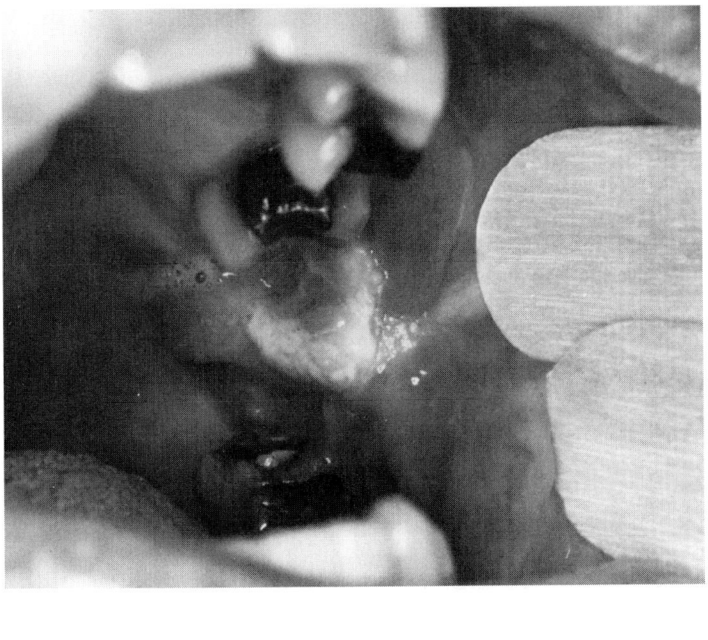

FIG. 128.2. Leukoplakia. Keratosis with marked atypia was revealed on a biopsy of this lesion appearing in the posterior aspect of the left buccal mucosa in an 84-year-old woman with no history of tobacco use.

fibroblasts. Surgical removal is the treatment of choice, although some have suggested that the pregnancy tumor not be removed until after pregnancy because of the likelihood of recurrence.

Necrotizing sialometaplasia is a benign lesion of the salivary tissue of minor salivary glands in the oral cavity occurring spontaneously or as a reaction to injury. There can be startling mucosal ulceration of the palate, which certainly could suggest squamous cell carcinoma. Because of marked squamous metaplasia of the ductal epithelium seen histopathologically, a general surgical pathologist might mistake this for squamous cell or mucoepidermoid carcinoma. Confirming the diagnosis is important to prevent unnecessary surgery. Patients heal spontaneously whether treated with biopsy, partial excision, or complete excision.

CYSTS

A mucocele is believed to occur because of traumatic injury to the duct of a minor salivary gland, allowing saliva to escape into surrounding tissues. It typically appears on the inner surface of the lower lip as a soft, compressible, slightly bluish swelling. A mucocele may also be seen on the floor of the mouth. In this location the lesion is called a ranula. The swelling generally occurs rapidly, and the lesion frequently ruptures and exudes a mucoid saliva. The lesion usually recurs quickly after each episode of spontaneous (or patient-induced) rupture. When the mucocele is recurrent or persistent, it should be excised.

Odontogenic cysts typically appear in the alveolus-gingiva, as submucosal swelling. They also may be apparent in x-rays that include dentoalveolar structures. They include the dentigerous cyst, radicular cysts, keratocysts, eruption cysts, and gingival cysts. The dentigerous cyst is most often seen in the mandible associated with the crown of an unerupted molar. It is thought to come from accumulation of fluid between the tooth crown and the reduced-enamel epithelium. A radicular cyst is asymptomatic and arises within a periodontal granuloma in the periapical area of a nonvital tooth. A keratocyst is a locally aggressive form of any of the above. The diagnosis is made on histopathology. When keratinization is seen within one of the above cysts, it is called a keratocyst. An eruption cyst is the accumulation of blood around the crown of an erupting tooth. Gingival cysts occur due to the entrapment of epithelium during palatal closure. When one discovers an asymptomatic swelling of the upper or lower jaw seen as a radiolucency on x-rays taken to include these areas, it should be evaluated by the patient's dentist or oral surgeon.

Fissural cysts occur in embryonic fusion planes and may not be apparent until young adulthood. They include the globulomaxillary cyst, which occurs in the maxilla between the canine and incisor teeth; the nasopalatine cyst, which occurs in the area of the incisive foramen and causes a mass in the midline of the hard palate anteriorly; and the nasoalveolar cyst, which may manifest as a swelling in the canine fossa beneath the base of the nostril. These may be excised surgically using an intraoral approach.

Dermoid cysts are uncommon in the oral cavity and rare in the oropharynx. They are believed to be due to entrapment of epithelial cells during embryonic development. They appear simply as a cystic swelling. Stratified squamous epithelium lines the cyst. In most instances surgical excision is recommended.

BENIGN NEOPLASMS

Squamous papilloma is a benign neoplasm seen frequently in the oral cavity and oropharynx, most commonly attached to the free edge of the soft palate or uvula. There can be multiple papillomas, usually appearing as pedunculated wartlike masses. The papilloma is rarely more than a few millimeters in greatest dimension. It is composed of finger-like projections of squamous epithelium, and it is believed to be of viral etiology. Dysplasia is distinctly unusual. The differential diagnosis includes condyloma acuminatum, focal epithelial hyperplasia, and verruciform xanthoma. If symptomatic, it may easily be excised in the office under topical or local anesthesia. Recurrence is rare.

An important category of benign neoplasms that occurs in the oral cavity and oropharynx is that of the minor salivary gland tumors. There are approximately 500 minor salivary glands in the oral cavity and oropharynx. The ratio of neoplasms of the major salivary glands (parotid, submandibular, and sublingual) to those of the minor salivary glands is 5 to 1. Over half of the minor salivary gland neoplasms occur on the palate. The distribution of minor salivary gland neoplasms parallels the distribution of the glands themselves. In the palate, minor salivary glands are not found anterior to the first molars nor are they found in the midline. Approximately 20% of minor salivary gland tumors are benign. Benign minor salivary gland tumors appear as asymptomatic masses that have been present typically for months before diagnosis. Pain is uncommon, as is ulceration. Pleomorphic and monomorphic adenoma are the most common histologic benignities. Lack of a capsule is a common histologic feature. Despite this, surgical removal is rarely followed by recurrence.

A number of other neoplasms occur rarely in the oral cavity and oropharynx, and their characteristics are similar to those that manifest elsewhere in the body. The primary symptoms are due to mass effect. Examples include lipoma, leiomyoma, rhabdomyoma, neurogenic tumors (e.g., schwannoma, neurofibroma), mesenchymoma, and plasmacytoma.

MALIGNANT NEOPLASMS OF THE ORAL CAVITY AND OROPHARYNX

Malignant tumors of the oral cavity and oropharynx account for only about 2% of all cancers occurring in women in the United States and account for only about 1% of cancer deaths in this group. The relatively low death rate is offset by the fact that successful elimination of the tumor often comes with significant functional compromise and cosmetic disability. Patients often present to the treating head and neck surgeon with advanced disease, despite the fact that the oral cavity is easy to inspect and palpate. Dentists often discover intraoral cancers before either the patient or the primary care physician becomes aware of the problem. Signs and symptoms of particular concern are otalgia, hemoptysis, voice change, dysphagia, odynophagia, ulceration or mass in the mouth that fails to resolve, or a neck mass. By far the most common histopathology is squamous cell carcinoma, which may arise anywhere in the oral cavity or oropharynx. Lymphoma is not uncommon in Waldeyer's ring (pharyngeal and lingual tonsils). Malignant minor salivary gland tumors are seen with some frequency, and mucosal melanoma is encountered rarely. Other tumors, such as sarcomas, are quite unusual.

SQUAMOUS CELL CARCINOMA

The incidence of oral carcinoma varies greatly around the world as well as in different parts of the United States. Whereas in the United States it constitutes less than 5% of the new cancers to be diagnosed each year, in certain parts of Asia it approaches 50%. This reflects different habits. As tobacco use in women has increased to approach that of men in the United States, a corresponding increase (although, of course, delayed) in the incidence of squamous cell cancer has been noted in women. In 2003, it is expected that one third of all oral and oropharyngeal carcinomas diagnosed in the United States will occur in women. This is a markedly higher proportion than noted even 10 years ago. In certain parts of the United States, the use of smokeless tobacco has been common in women for many decades. When one examines series published from these areas concerning oral cancers, one is struck by the fact that up to 93% of the tumors reported in these series occur in women.

Several etiologic factors are associated with oral cancer. The disease is most closely associated with the use of tobacco in any form. More than 90% of the patients in published series were tobacco users. Tobacco exposure causes progressive change in the exposed mucosa over time. This is demonstrated in the relatively high incidence of second synchronous or metachronous primary tumors in about 15% of the patients with squamous cell carcinoma of the upper aerodigestive tract. The extremes are a 40% to 50% incidence of second primaries in those patients who continue to smoke after presumed curative treatment of their first cancer to about 5% in those who quit tobacco use at the time of diagnosis and treatment of their first cancers. Pipe smokers have a higher incidence of cancer of the lip. It is believed that the high temperature of the pipe stem may cause irritation that leads to dysplastic change. Alcohol consumption has been shown to be correlated with oral cancers. About 75% of the patients in published series have a history of significant alcohol consumption. Tobacco and alcohol seem to work synergistically, because patients who use both seem to have a higher risk of developing oral or oropharyngeal cancer than they would with the sum of the risks of each. Solar exposure (ultraviolet light) is a risk factor for carcinoma of the lip especially. It occurs much more often in individuals who work outdoors and much more commonly in the lower lip, which is exposed more directly to sunlight.

Poor dental and oral hygiene seem also to be associated with oral cancers, but this is often compounded by the use of tobacco, alcohol, or both. Poor dentition, ill-fitting dentures, and restorative dental work in poor repair may cause irritation, leading to dysplastic changes. When two different metals come in contact, an electromotive force is set up, allowing for the flow of an electric current. This occurs, for instance, when a gold crown is placed in contact with a silver amalgam. This has been associated with recurrent dysplasia and even carcinoma in situ in the tongue on its lateral border where it contacts the interface of the two metals. Iron and riboflavin deficiencies have been associated with oral cancers. Plummer-Vinson syndrome is observed most frequently in women and is associated with achlorhydric iron deficiency, pharyngoesophageal strictures, and oral-oropharyngeal dysplasia. There are suggestions that certain occupational exposures are associated, and one sees more oral malignancy than expected in the immunocompromised, particularly those with acquired immunodeficiency syndrome, and those who have received organ transplants.

A persistent sore in the mouth is the most common symptom of oral cavity cancer. Dysphagia is the most common complaint when the primary site is in the oropharynx. Pain tends to occur rather late, and, unfortunately, many patients do not seek attention until they note pain. Often patients consult dentists because of loosening of the teeth or tooth or jaw pain. Approximately one third of the patients present with a neck mass, most often representing regional metastasis, but occasionally an ulcerated tumor will be markedly inflamed, leading to adenopathy on that basis. Weight loss is seen if the tumor has caused significant dysphagia or odynophagia. As noted earlier, most patients have a history of tobacco abuse and substantial alcohol consumption.

The physical examination is the key to diagnosing and evaluating oral cavity and oropharyngeal carcinoma. Bimanual palpation is an important part of the physical examination, because it allows one to get a better sense of the volume of tumor present. With ulcerative and endophytic tumors especially, the observable portion of the tumor may be quite unimpressive (Figs. 128.3 and 128.4). If one is examining a patient who has a heavy smoking history, it is not uncommon to see several areas of suspicious mucosa. An excellent simple aid to the diagnosis of mucosal dysplasia is the toluidine blue test. This is a painless test that allows the physician to distinguish between malignancy and other lesions that may be of concern, such as lichen planus, trauma, leukoplakia, and various benign tumors. Carcinoma in situ and invasive cancer stain bluish, whereas other lesions do not. The test helps delineate the best site for biopsy as well. False positives can occur. The procedure is as follows:

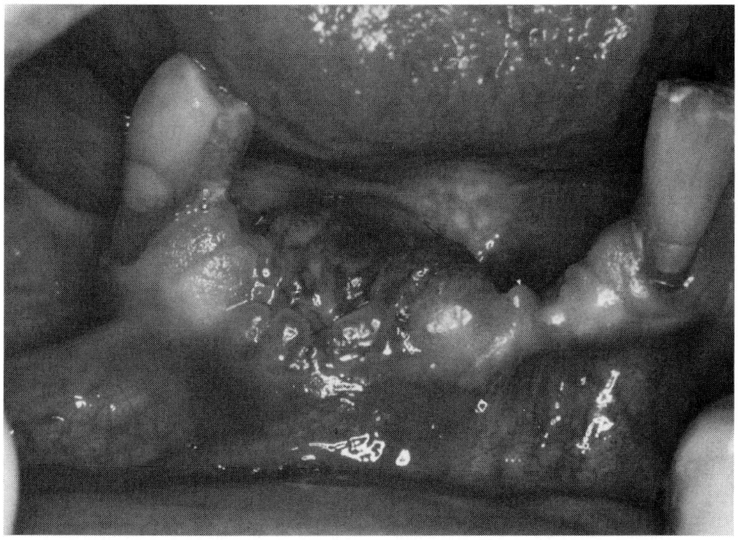

FIG. 128.3. Squamous cell carcinoma. Epidermoid carcinoma of the anterior aspect of the mandibular alveolus in an 83-year-old woman with no history of tobacco use. This was removed transorally, and the resection included a marginal mandibulectomy. The patient received excellent rehabilitation through the use of a denture.

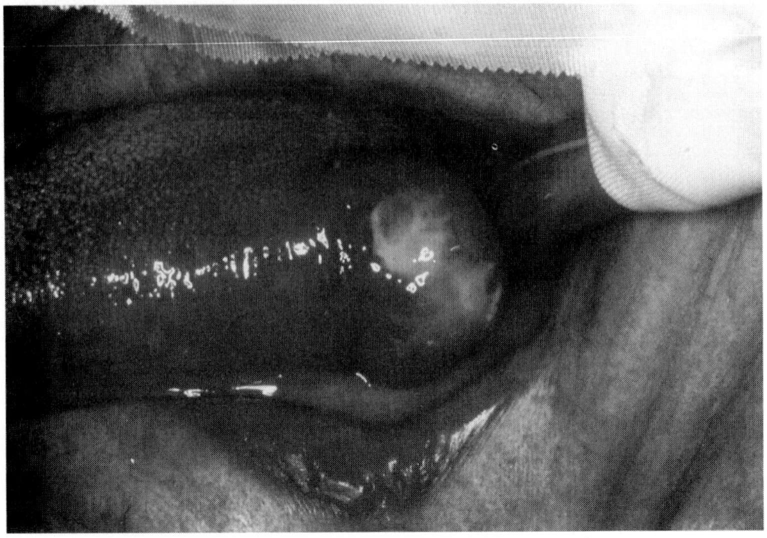

FIG. 128.4. Squamous cell carcinoma. This left lateral tongue tumor appears in a 78-year-old woman with a history of heavy tobacco and alcohol abuse. At presentation, she was staged as T1N1M0. Despite control of her local and regional disease with surgery and radiation therapy, she died of distant metastases about 18 months after treatment.

1. Rinse the mouth thoroughly with water.
2. Apply 1% acetic acid to the areas of concern with a cotton swab.
3. Remove any necrotic debris.
4. Apply 1% toluidine blue to suspicious areas.
5. Rinse the mouth with water.
6. Areas stained blue are sites for biopsy.

A careful examination of the neck is carried out to assess the patient for possible regional metastases.

Radiologic evaluation is often a useful adjunct in assessing the extent of local disease. Computed tomography is particularly helpful in assessing mandibular involvement if the tumor encroaches upon it grossly. The same is true for the bone of the hard palate and pterygoid plates. Magnetic resonance imaging can be more beneficial in assessing parapharyngeal space involvement. Other studies such as sialography, barium swallow, bone scan, and arteriography may be indicated in certain circumstances.

The most important step in evaluation of a patient with a squamous cell carcinoma of the oral cavity or oropharynx is panendoscopy with biopsy of the primary tumor, usually carried out by the otolaryngologist–head and neck surgeon. Under general anesthesia, the lesion is carefully examined and mapped, and a biopsy is obtained. Because of the significant number of patients with second primary tumors in the upper aerodigestive tract, laryngoscopy, bronchoscopy, and esophagoscopy are carried out at the same time. Any lesion found in this portion of the examination is of course mapped and biopsied as well. Some surgeons tattoo the mucosa at the margins of the tumor to assist with surgical resection should planned preoperative radiation be given or in case salvage surgery is required after failure of radiation for cure. At this point, all information is available to allow appropriate staging, which is mandatory for proper treatment planning. Staging is carried out with reference to data from the American Joint Committee on Cancer (Tables 128.1 through 128.4).

A number of modalities are used in the treatment of oral and oropharyngeal squamous cell carcinomas. Surgery, radiotherapy, chemotherapy, and combinations of these are all used with some frequency. In general, radiation and surgery are equally efficacious in stage I and II disease, and often the two are used together in stage III and IV lesions. Most would choose to use radiation for stage I and II lesions because the functional results tend to be superior with regard to speech and swallowing. Radiation, however, is likely to lead to permanent xerostomia, which patients find quite distressing. It also often leads to extraction of all dentition before treatment if the teeth are not in excellent shape.

Stage III and IV lesions, in general, benefit from treatment with both surgery and radiation. There is still some argument about whether planned preoperative irradiation followed by surgery is preferred over surgery with postoperative radiation. The advantages of planned preoperative radiation are several:

- The occasional patient has a complete response to the radiation (preoperative levels are normally about 5,500 cGy) and is taken to curative levels (usually about 7,000 cGy), thus avoiding the morbidity of surgery altogether.
- There is a theoretical advantage to irradiating tissue upon which there has been no operation. Irradiation works best in well-oxygenated tissue, and there is often significant scar tissue in the area of a major head and neck surgery. With postoperative radiation, persistent tumor is most likely to exist at the margins of resection, the area of greatest scarring, and the area of lowest oxygen tension.
- Preoperative radiation will be given. Occasionally, when postoperative radiation is planned, there is a major wound complication after the surgery, such as an orocutaneous or a pharyngocutaneous fistula, requiring many weeks of hospitalization and sometimes several reconstructive procedures. Many radiation oncologists will not irradiate an unhealed wound, and because radiation should begin within 6 weeks of operation, a postoperative wound complication sometimes means that the radiation is not given at all. In this

TABLE 128.1. Primary Tumor Classification, Oral Cavity Cancer

T1: tumor 2 cm in greatest dimension
T2: tumor >2 cm but ≤4 cm in greatest dimension
T3: tumor >4 cm in greatest dimension
T4: tumor invades bone, deep musculature of tongue, sinus, or skin

Source: Beahrs OH, Henson DE, Hutter RVP, et al., eds. *Manual for staging of cancer,* 4th ed. Philadelphia: JB Lippincott, 1992, with permission.

TABLE 128.2. Primary Tumor Classification, Oropharyngeal Cancer

T1: tumor 2 cm in greatest dimension
T2: tumor >2 cm but <4 cm in greatest dimension
T3: tumor >4 cm in greatest dimension
T4: tumor invades cortical bone, soft tissue of neck, or deep tongue musculature

Source: Beahrs OH, Henson DE, Hutter RVP, et al., eds. *Manual for staging of cancer,* 4th ed. Philadelphia: JB Lippincott, 1992, with permission.

TABLE 128.4. Stage Groupings of Oral and Oropharyngeal Cancer, TNM Classification

Stage I	T1N0M0
Stage II	T2N0M0
Stage III	T3N0M0, T1, T2, or T3N1M0
Stage IV	T4N0 or N1M0
	Any TN2 or N3M0
	Any T or NM1

Source: Beahrs OH, Henson DE, Hutter RVP, et al., eds. *Manual for staging of cancer,* 4th ed. Philadelphia: JB Lippincott, 1992, with permission.

instance one tends to observe for recurrence, and if it occurs, salvage surgery is performed with postoperative radiotherapy, assuming there is adequate wound healing.
- There is a significant reduction in recurrent disease in the cervical lymphatics when preoperative radiotherapy is given.

There are also advantages to surgery followed by radiation:

- There are fewer wound complications when surgery precedes radiation.
- Some surgeons find it easier to operate on tissue that has not been irradiated.
- In general, higher levels of radiation may be given postoperatively than preoperatively.

It is noted that when radiation is given, the ports include the cervical lymph nodes that drain the area of the primary tumor. If low cervical metastases are noted, the mediastinum is often included as well.

Surgery for squamous cell carcinoma of the oral cavity or oropharynx involves a number of considerations. Among the surgeon's concerns are whether to use a transoral, mandibulotomy, or mandibulectomy approach. Neck dissection is carried out in the presence of clinical disease, but prophylactic neck dissection is often indicated even in the apparent absence of regional disease. The reconstructive options are constantly increasing in number. Primary closure may be used for some defects, as can placement of a dermal graft. Local and regional pedicled flaps are useful in many circumstances. Consideration should be given to the use of osteomyocutaneous free vascularized flaps, particularly when there is an anterior mandibular defect. The procedure often requires several hours in the operating room. Consideration should be given to measures to prevent deep vein thrombosis. A heating blanket should be used, and blood should be available. The patient will often need to be cared for in an intensive care unit setting for the first postoperative day or two. A tracheotomy is often required for airway management postoperatively. There may be difficulties with aspiration due to postoperative swelling or the presence of an asensate regional flap or free flap placed for reconstruction. Usually, the tracheotomy tube may be removed within a week or two of surgery. The patient will most often require nasogastric feeding for 5 to 10 days after surgery. A speech pathologist is often required to provide the patient with extensive retraining with regard to speech and swallowing.

TABLE 128.3. Classification of Cervical Metastatic Disease of Oral or Oropharyngeal Cancer

N0: No clinically positive node
N1: Single ipsilateral node ≤3 cm in diameter
N2: Single ipsilateral node >3 cm but <6 cm in diameter, or multiple ipsilateral nodes ≤6 cm in diameter, or bilateral or contralateral nodes ≤6 cm
N2a: Single ipsilateral node >3 cm but <6 cm in diameter
N2b: Multiple ipsilateral nodes ≤6 cm
N2c: Bilateral or contralateral nodes ≤6 cm
N3: Nodes >6 cm

Source: Beahrs OH, Henson DE, Hutter RVP, et al., eds. *Manual for staging of cancer,* 4th ed. Philadelphia: JB Lippincott, 1992, with permission.

Chemotherapy has been used extensively in the treatment of head and neck squamous cell carcinoma. Many controlled trials have demonstrated various complete and partial response rates to numerous combinations of agents. At present, there is very little to suggest that the use of chemotherapy alone provides a significant advantage to the patient suffering from head and neck squamous cell carcinoma. Although several combinations of agents have demonstrated impressive response rates (up to 65%), none has documented an increase in survival. Adjuvant, induction, and maintenance chemotherapy have all been used, but none has yet demonstrated prolonged disease-free intervals or an increase in survival. Currently, if chemotherapy is considered in a patient with oral cavity or oropharyngeal squamous cell carcinoma, they should be enrolled in a protocol within the environment of a clinical trial.

Some organ preservation protocols, using a combination of chemotherapy and concurrent radiation, have shown survival rates similar to those achieved by radiation and surgery, but these are not yet widely accepted.

When one considers the entire population of patients currently being treated for oral cavity cancer, including all stages and all combinations of treatment modalities, one can expect a 5-year disease-free survival of about 70%. For oropharyngeal cancer, the figure is about 55%.

NONEPIDERMOID MALIGNANCIES OF THE ORAL CAVITY AND OROPHARYNX

Lymphoma in the oral cavity and oropharynx arises from the structures in Waldeyer's ring and appears as a mass in the oropharynx. Treatment depends on cell type and extent of disease. This is within the purview of the hematologist-oncologist.

Oral cavity-oropharyngeal melanoma is rare, representing only about 1% of all melanomas (Fig. 128.5). About one third of all mucosal melanomas occur in the oral cavity. This must be differentiated from the amalgam tattoo, which is a very common iatrogenic phenomenon. Mucosal melanoma most often appears as a darkly pigmented soft mass that is smooth and painless in a patient in the sixth to eighth decade of life. Amelanotic melanoma is very rare. The treatment is wide surgical

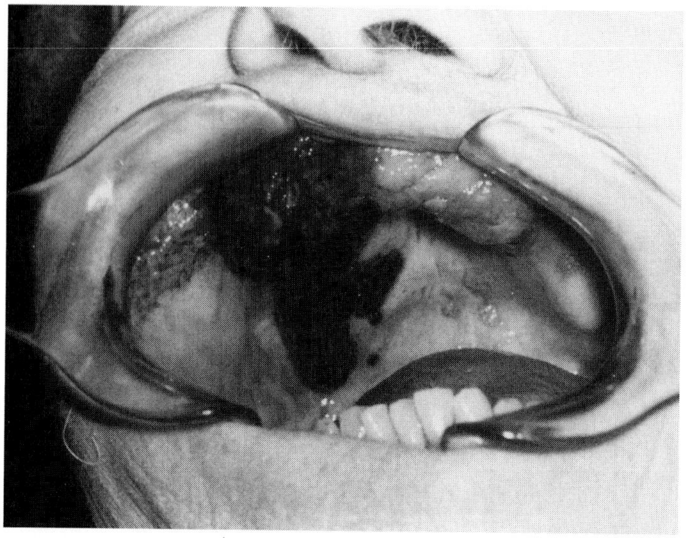

FIG. 128.5. Mucosal melanoma. This large melanoma involves the right maxillary alveolus, hard palate, and gingivobuccal sulcus in a 91-year-old woman. She also had clinical cervical adenopathy and brain metastases at the time of presentation.

excision, including neck dissection if clinical disease is apparent there. Survival is extremely poor, with most patients progressing to develop multiple metastases within a year or two. Five-year survival is only about 5% to 10%.

Minor salivary gland malignancies are seen with the same general distribution as that of the benign minor salivary gland tumors. Approximately 80% of minor salivary gland tumors are malignancies. These tumors are seen much more often in atomic bomb survivors than in other groups. There also appears to be a somewhat increased risk of salivary gland tumors of all types in women who have had breast tumors. Minor salivary gland cancers appear as painless submucosal masses that enlarge slowly over time. Imaging often reveals that these lesions have extended into the maxillary sinus, parapharyngeal space, or pterygopalatine fossa. It is uncommon for patients to present with cervical metastases. Forty percent of these malignancies are adenoid cystic carcinoma. Perineural invasion is common with this particular tumor, so local recurrence is common. There is a high incidence of distant metastasis, particularly to the lung. This distant disease may show up 20 years or more after initial diagnosis and treatment. Adenocarcinoma is the histopathology identified in about 30% of minor salivary gland malignancies. They are locally aggressive and occur in older patients. Mucoepidermoid carcinoma represents about 20% of minor salivary gland cancers. This tumor is distinctly more common in women and tends to present between ages 40 and 50. Most mucoepidermoid cancers are classified as low grade and have a very favorable prognosis. Minor salivary gland malignancies are treated with wide surgical excision and neck dissection when nodes are present clinically. Prophylactic neck dissection is not indicated because of the low incidence of cervical disease. Most would advocate radiation therapy to the primary site when dealing with a high-grade malignancy such as adenoid cystic, high grade mucoepidermoid, or adenocarcinoma. Because a relatively large percentage of minor salivary gland malignancies demonstrate recurrences at 10 or even 20 years after treatment, discussing 5-year survival does not necessarily give an accurate picture of the behavior of these tumors. Five-, 10-, and 15-year survivals are in the range of 50%, 33%, and 20%, respectively.

Sarcomas may arise from numerous tissues in the oral cavity and oropharynx, including angiosarcoma, fibrosarcoma, leiomyosarcoma, liposarcoma, osteogenic sarcoma, and rhabdomyosarcoma. The latter two occur with greater frequency than the others listed. Osteogenic sarcoma is treated most often with chemotherapy and surgery. With rhabdomyosarcoma, the most favorable results are when complete surgical excision is possible. Because significant functional compromise is usual when dealing with a patient who has had a large resection, radiation and chemotherapy after conservative surgical treatment, or even biopsy only, is the frequent mode of treatment when it occurs in the head and neck area.

PARAPHARYNGEAL SPACE

Tumors of the parapharyngeal space impinge on the oropharynx and therefore may mimic primary tumors of that area (Fig. 128.6). The structures found in this area include the deep lobe of the parotid gland, the major vessels, and several cranial nerves, as well as the cervical sympathetic chain and occasionally lymph nodes. It is not a surprise, therefore, to find that the largest numbers of tumors of this region derive from these tissues. Pleomorphic adenoma of the deep lobe of the parotid is the most common tumor found in this region, although all salivary gland histopathologies are seen here. Vascular lesions such as carotid body paragangliomas (chemodectoma) and aneurysms may be encountered. Schwannomas, ganglioneuromas, and others may arise from the neural structures in this region. Lesions occurring within the parapharyngeal space are most often benign and often asymptomatic until impressively large (Fig. 128.7). Rarely, one

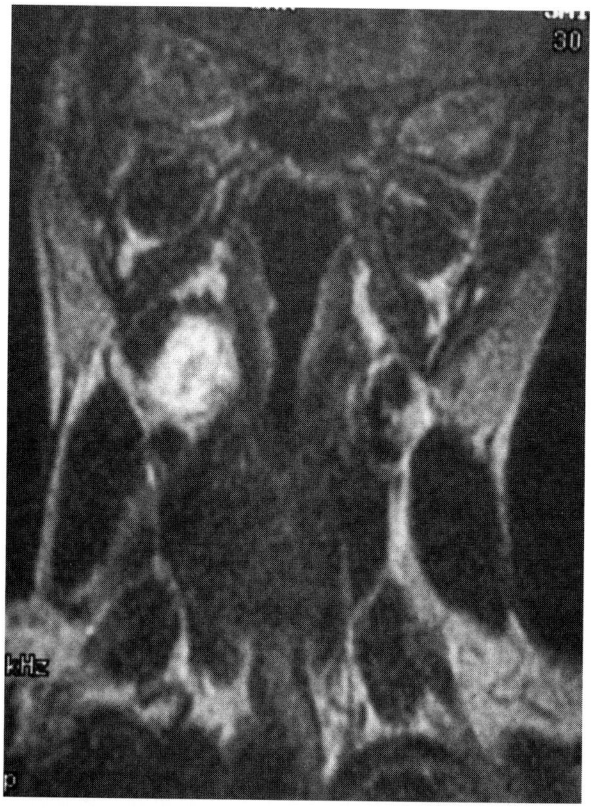

FIG. 128.6. Parapharyngeal space neoplasm. Asymptomatic ganglioneuroma of the right cervical sympathetic chain demonstrated on a magnetic resonance image of a 34-year-old woman.

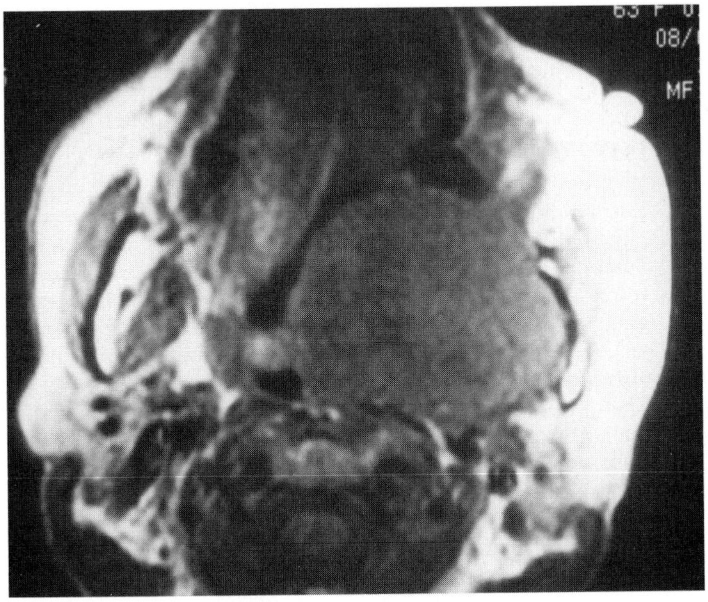

FIG. 128.7. Parapharyngeal space neoplasm. This 63-year-old woman presented with a short history of trismus. Tumor was known to have been present at least 6 years at the time of this magnetic resonance image. Resection required a lateral skull base approach. The final pathology demonstrated malignant granular cell tumor.

may find malignancy within a lymph node in this region, either a lymphoma or metastatic disease as from a squamous cell carcinoma or from a thyroid malignancy. Most are detected by the primary physician on routine physical examination of the oropharynx, where asymmetry is noted. Occasionally, the patient may present with complaints of dysphagia, voice change, sensation of a lump in the throat, or sleep apnea due to the impingement of the mass on the oropharyngeal airway at night. The best imaging of this region is obtained by magnetic resonance imaging. Depending on the size and histopathology of the tumor, it may be approached best transcervically or transorally, or a mandibular osteotomy may be required.

CONSIDERATIONS IN PREGNANCY

Most of the aforementioned lesions are benign or occur in older individuals. Nonetheless, occasionally one sees an oral or oropharyngeal lesion of concern in a pregnant woman. Fortunately, most of these lesions may be biopsied in the office under local anesthesia. Those that lie deep to the surface may be biopsied under ultrasound guidance at no risk to the developing fetus. If further imaging is required, magnetic resonance imaging may be safely accomplished during pregnancy. Once the histopathology of the lesion is known, decisions may be made as to how to manage best the pregnancy, the lesion, and the mother and fetus. Benign lesions requiring surgery may be dealt with at some point after the delivery. The difficult question comes with those pregnant patients who have a malignancy. When head and neck surgery is carried out on the mother, the major risk to the fetus is during the first trimester. Major resections have been carried out during the second and third trimesters without adverse outcome to either the fetus or the mother. If a major resection cannot be delayed until after the first trimester, consideration may be given to ending the pregnancy. Radiation therapy should also be deferred until after pregnancy.

SUMMARY

Evaluation and management of oral and oropharyngeal lesions is the life work of many otolaryngologist–head and neck surgeons, as well as some oral surgeons, general surgeons, and plastic surgeons. Because most tumors in this region are easily recognized or easily identified by appropriate biopsy, timely treatment may be effected, and most often the patient may expect a very satisfactory outcome.

BIBLIOGRAPHY

Batsakis JG. *Tumors of the head and neck.* Baltimore: Williams & Wilkins, 1979.

Cummings CW, Fredrickson JM, Harker LA, et al. *Otolaryngology-head and neck surgery.* St. Louis: CV Mosby, 1993.

Forastiere A, Koch W, Trotti A, et al. Head and neck cancer. *N Engl J Med* 2001;345: 1890–1900.

Tran LM, Mark R, Meier R, et al. Sarcomas of the head and neck. *Cancer* 1992;70: 169.

Wingo PA, Tong T, Bolden S. Cancer statistics, 1995. *CA Cancer J Clin* 1995;45:8.

Wray A, McGuirt WF. Smokeless tobacco usage associated with oral carcinoma. *Arch Otolaryngol Head Neck Surg* 1993;119:929.

CHAPTER 129
Laryngeal Neoplasms

Jay Piccirillo

The larynx is an important structure in the neck, serving as a conduit for air between the mouth and nose and the lungs. Respiration, phonation, and protection of the airway are the main functions of this structure. Disorders of the larynx can cause mild symptoms of subtle voice changes and cough to more severe complaints of dyspnea and stridor. Although most lesions in the larynx are benign, a thorough evaluation should be performed on any laryngeal neoplasm to exclude malignancy.

ANATOMY

An understanding of laryngeal tumors and the symptoms they elicit begins with an appreciation of laryngeal anatomy. The larynx is composed of rigid cartilage with a membranous back wall. At the superior aspect is the epiglottis, composed of fibroelastic cartilage. The epiglottis acts as a blockade to food, forcing ingested materials around the larynx into the piriform sinus and then the esophagus.

The vocal cords are located within the larynx. Anteriorly the right and left vocal cords come together and attach to the laryngeal cartilage by Broyle's ligament. Posteriorly the vocal cords are attached to the arytenoids, small mobile cartilages. Arytenoid movement results in abduction and adduction of the vocal cords during respiration and phonation, respectively. Fine control of the tension in these vocal ligaments allows the creation of a variety of pitches.

The vocal cords are composed of squamous epithelium, Reinke's potential space (a superficial layer of the lamina propria), the vocal ligament, and the thyroarytenoid muscle. Historically, voice production was thought to be the result of vocal fold vibration, although recent studies have demonstrated oscillation of the vocal cord mucosa responsible for vocalization. This explains why small superficial lesions can significantly alter voice.

EVALUATION

Evaluating a patient with a laryngeal neoplasm begins with a thorough history, a perceptual assessment of vocal ability, and laryngeal examination. Patients with a laryngeal neoplasm most often present with a change in voice. This is most notable and recognized earlier if the lesion occurs on the vocal cord rather than elsewhere in the larynx. Dysphasia, chronic cough, or glomus (a sensation of something in the throat) are other less common symptoms. Extensive lesions can obstruct the airway and cause respiratory difficulty or stridor.

HISTORY

A complete history must be performed on all patients with a change in voice. The onset and duration of symptoms, exacerbating factors, alleviating factors, and degree of bother should be elicited. Symptoms of short duration are often the result of an infectious or inflammatory cause, whereas persistent symptoms raise the suspicion of a malignant process. The patient should be questioned on cigarette usage and smoke exposure, which cause chronic irritation to the vocal cords and also increase the suspicion of malignancy. Occupational and recreational voice demands such as loud talking and yelling of a stockbroker or teacher and excessive singing can cause vocal trauma. Gastroesophageal reflux and postnasal drainage can cause irritation and chronic inflammation of laryngeal tissue. The patient should also be questioned about dehydration and use of drying medications because decreased lubrication of the vibratory surface of the vocal cords can restrict voice. The medical history should also be reviewed. Hypothyroidism with resultant myxedema of the vocal cords and connective tissue disorders can impair voice and mimic the symptoms of a neoplasm.

AUDITORY PERCEPTUAL ASSESSMENT

An auditory assessment of voice is an often-underused aspect of the examination. The quality of the voice is first assessed. Neoplasms often cause a hoarse or raspy character to the voice. Loss of the ability to perform high frequency low intensity vocal tasks is common in benign mucosal lesions. A breathy character to the voice or fatigue with vocalization is seen in vocal cord paralysis. Onset delays and a tremulous character of the voice are seen in spasmodic dysphonia and other neurologic disorders.

PHYSICAL EXAMINATION

Examination of the larynx is easily performed in the office in most patients. A laryngeal mirror is a quick and simple way to obtain a good view of the vocal cords. Mucosal abnormalities, color, and mobility are appreciated with this method. In patients with an exaggerated gag reflex, this may be a difficult task for both patient and physician. The mirror examination is also limited in that no permanent image is obtained. Flexible fiberoptic laryngoscopy is another effective tool to examination the larynx in the office. A scope is passed through the nose into the oropharynx. This gives good visualization of the larynx and surrounding structures. As in the mirror examination, vocal cord mobility and mucosa can be visualized. Unless the oropharynx and larynx are topically anesthetized, the subglottis and trachea are not adequately visualized.

Rigid endoscopy provides direct visualization of the larynx, subglottis, and trachea. Biopsy of suspicious lesions can be performed at the same time. A microscope can be used for enhanced visualization to detect subtle abnormalities. General anesthesia is required for this procedure.

BENIGN LARYNGEAL NEOPLASMS

Vocal Cord Nodules

Vocal cord nodules are commonly seen in patients with extensive voice demands. They occur most commonly in women and children. These lesions result from trauma to the vocal surface from excessive vibration during singing, yelling, or improper vocalization. Vascular congestion and edema occur at the area of contact of the vocal cords with resultant hyalinization of Reinke's space and thickening of the overlying epithelium. Nodules are usually bilateral and occur as white thickenings at the junction of the anterior and middle third of the true vocal cords.

Vocal cord nodules can result in loss of ability to sing high notes softly, increased breathiness, and decreased vocal endurance. Initial therapy is directed at avoiding the vocal abuse. Voice rest, refraining from loud talking, and voice therapy usually provide resolution of symptoms. Surgery is rarely necessary and not indicated unless the patient fails 6 months of voice therapy. The patient must be advised not to return to their previous voice demands after resolution of these lesions, because they can recur.

Vocal Cord Polyps

Vocal cord polyps are the most common benign lesions of the adult larynx. These lesions are usually unilateral, pedunculated, or sessile and can occur along the entire vocal cord. Generally, they occur along the anterior or middle third of the free margin of the true vocal cord and result from chronic edema. There is no sex or age predilection, although bilateral polyps are seen more commonly in women.

In contrast to vocal cord nodules, polyps require surgical excision. Microlaryngoscopy allows visualization and removal of these lesions. Postoperatively, it is important for the patient to abstain from vocal abuse and smoking. Antireflux medication can be added to prevent further irritation.

Granuloma

Vocal cord granulomas generally occur on the arytenoid. The patient often has a history of gastroesophageal reflux, although previous endotracheal intubation and trauma from chronic throat clearing are also causes. In addition to hoarseness, a sore throat and foreign body sensation are common symptoms. Any patient with a vocal cord granuloma should be evaluated for reflux unless a history of recent endotracheal intubation is reported.

Treatment involves removing the offending source of chronic irritation. Most granulomas resolve with antireflux medications and voice rest. Refractory lesions can be removed with the CO_2 laser, intralesional steroid, or Botox injection. Postoperative antireflux medications, voice rest, systemic steroids, and antibiotics aid in preventing recurrence.

Laryngeal Papillomatosis

Respiratory papilloma are exophytic lesions of the airway epithelium caused by human papillomavirus types 6 and 11. These lesions occur frequently in children and also in young adults. The childhood form is more aggressive and transmitted through the birth canal. Primigravida and vaginal delivery increase the transmission rate due to prolonged time in labor and therefore increased exposure time of the fetus to the virus. Although 1.5% to 5% of pregnant women in the United States have papilloma, routine cesarean section is not recommended because only 1 in 400 children contract the disease from actively infected mothers.

The symptoms of papilloma begin with hoarseness and progress to stridor and respiratory distress as the neoplasm enlarges. Diagnosis is made by fiberoptic laryngoscopy, demonstrating these characteristic lesions. Treatment includes surgical removal with cold instruments, the CO_2 laser, or microlaryngeal debrider. Because these lesions only involve the epithelial layer, it is important to remove only the papillary tissue and not traumatize underlying structures, such as the vocal ligament. The aggressive childhood form often requires multiple excisions due to recurrence, whereas the adult form may be treated with only one or a few surgeries. It is important to treat these lesions early so airway obstruction requiring tracheostomy is avoided. Half of patients with laryngeal papilloma will develop seeding of the tracheostoma site.

MALIGNANT NEOPLASMS

Nearly all malignant tumors of the larynx are squamous cell carcinoma. Cancer of the larynx represents 0.4% of malignant tumors in women and is more common in men. The primary risk factor for squamous cell carcinoma is cigarette smoking. Smoking combined with excessive alcohol consumption has a synergistic effect on cancer development. Lesions that arise on the vocal cords tend to produce symptoms initially and are identified at an earlier stage. Lesions elsewhere in the larynx can grow quite large before becoming symptomatic and can metastasize to regional cervical lymph nodes.

Most patients with laryngeal carcinoma present with a change in voice. Although fiberoptic laryngoscopy can identify a lesion, rigid laryngoscopy and biopsy is necessary to confirm carcinoma. Early glottic lesions can be treated with endoscopic removal or radiation therapy. More advanced lesions require more aggressive surgical treatment. Glottic and supraglottic lesions remain localized longer secondary to anatomic tissue barriers to spread, often allowing them to be treated with partial larynx-preserving surgery. In contrast, transglottic and subglottic tumors are infiltrative and invade surrounding structures, often requiring total laryngectomy.

BIBLIOGRAPHY

Bailey B. *Head and neck surgery—otolaryngology,* 3rd ed. Philadelphia: Lippincott Williams & Wilkins, 2001.

Derkay C. Recurrent respiratory papillomatosis. *Laryngoscope* 2001;111:57–69.

Silver CE, Ferlito A. *Surgery for cancer of the larynx and related structures,* 2nd ed. Philadelphia: WB Saunders, 1996.

Zeitels S, et al. Management of common voice problems: committee report. *Otolaryngol Head Neck Surg* 2002;126:333–348.

PART

15

Dermatologic Problems

CHAPTER 130

Diagnostic Techniques in Dermatology

Sophie M. Worobec

Dermatologists use several procedures to diagnose skin diseases. Those most frequently used are magnification, diascopy, skin biopsy, potassium hydroxide (KOH) preparation to demonstrate fungi or yeast, fungal culture, Wood light examination, cytodiagnosis (including Tzanck smear), testing for dermatographism, phototesting, patch and photopatch testing, and the microscopic examination of scabies preparations.

MAGNIFICATION

A magnifying lens or loupe enhances the fine details of skin lesions. The dermatoscope or skin microscope (EpiScope model 47300, Welch Allyn Inc., Skaneateles, New York) is a hand-held magnifying and illuminating instrument, similar in size to an ophthalmoscope or otoscope, that magnifies the characteristics of the skin surface 10 times. A drop of mineral oil, water, or alcohol is applied to the lesion to render the stratum corneum translucent. The dermatoscope, when gently placed against the surface of the skin, facilitates the visualization of features such as follicular plugging, Wickham striae (in lichen planus), and pigment variations within melanocytic lesions. This examination technique has been termed *epiluminescence microscopy, dermatoscopy,* or *skin surface microscopy*. The percentage of correct diagnoses of melanoma based on dermatoscopy ranges from 70% to 95%, where it is 65% to 80% based on clinical examination. If no dermatoscope is available, an otoscope can be similarly used for magnification and as a source of light in the examination of skin lesions, especially if diascopy is also performed by an experienced examiner.

DIASCOPY

In diascopy, gentle pressure is applied to skin lesions with a glass lens, two microscope slides, or a piece of firm translucent plastic to observe color changes. It is especially useful in evaluating erythematous papules or macules. Areas of erythema resulting from capillary dilatation will blanch. Purpuric lesions caused by the extravasation of red blood cells or intravascular thrombosis will not blanch, which indicates a diagnosis of vasculitis or a coagulopathy in the proper clinical context. A yellow-brown color is revealed in granulomatous lesions such as sarcoidosis, granuloma annulare, and cutaneous tuberculosis, and also in some cases of cutaneous lymphoma.

In combination with magnification and the application of a drop of mineral oil, water, or alcohol on the skin surface, diascopy reveals the dilated nail fold capillaries of scleroderma, hypertrophic coiled vessels within psoriasis plaques, and avascular areas within the Wickham striae of lichen planus.

SKIN BIOPSY

A simple procedure, skin biopsy provides relevant diagnostic information to the physician who can correctly determine what type of lesion should be sampled and when, and the appropriate size of the biopsy specimen.

Choice of Biopsy Site

The choice of biopsy site depends on the nature of the skin disease being studied. When possible, a dermatologist should evaluate the patient and make this decision. Similarly, skin biopsy material is best sent to a dermatopathologist for interpretation.

If an eruption is widespread, then an older, well-developed typical lesion (without secondary changes) at a site where a small scar will be inconspicuous is the optimal site for biopsy. However, in blistering diseases, an entire early (<24 hours old), small lesion should be removed.

When a patient has large, chronic lesions, such as patches or plaques suggestive of cutaneous T-cell lymphoma or mycosis fungoides, the most indurated lesions should be chosen, and multiple biopsy specimens often are needed. Ideally, no corticosteroids should have been used for at least 4 weeks before biopsy.

When malignant melanoma is strongly suspected, it is best to refer the patient to a physician who will be responsible for removal of the entire lesion and subsequent follow-up. If a punch or other type of incisional biopsy is chosen, it is important that it be large enough that the crucial pathology is not missed. For example, areas of regression that are white or pink clinically may reveal deeper foci of melanoma extension. A shave biopsy should be avoided when malignant melanoma is suspected because it may completely eliminate the possibility of estimating the true depth of the lesion.

Size of the Biopsy Specimen

A 3- to 4-mm punch biopsy specimen is frequently sufficient to establish the diagnosis. In certain cases of deeper tumors or lesions suspected of extending to the subcutaneous tissue, at least a 4-mm punch biopsy or an excisional biopsy should be performed. Punch biopsies are inadequate when a diagnosis of verrucous carcinoma or keratoacanthoma is being considered.

Shave biopsies may also be appropriate, especially in cases of benign epidermal tumors, such as seborrheic keratosis. The size of an excisional biopsy specimen should be determined by the area where the biopsy is to be performed and by ease of closure.

Skin Biopsy Materials

The following materials are used in skin biopsies. For anesthesia, 1% or 2% lidocaine (Xylocaine) with or without epinephrine, a 3- or 5-mL syringe, and a 27- or 30-gauge needle are used. Epinephrine should not be applied to the fingers, toes, or tip of the nose because skin sloughing may result from excessive vasoconstriction. Skin preparation solutions consist of alcohol and povidone-iodine (Betadine) or chlorhexidine gluconate (Hibiclens). Three or four sterile drapes should be available. Instruments include a No. 11 or No. 15 scalpel blade and handle, a sterile skin biopsy punch (a tubular knife), Adson forceps, suture scissors, and a needle holder. The following also are needed: nylon or Prolene suture material, five or six sterile gauze pads, a pathology specimen container, and sterile gloves. Dressing material consists of Gelfoam, Telfa pads, gauze pads, and tape or a Kerlix gauze roll.

Skin Biopsy Technique

Preparation for a biopsy includes shaving or clipping the surrounding hairs. The site is then washed gently. The area to undergo biopsy is infiltrated with a local anesthetic. In a punch biopsy, a sharp punch is firmly pressed against the skin and gently rotated until a slight give is felt. The punch is removed, and the skin plug is elevated by applying gentle pressure with an Adson forceps. The bottom of the plug is then cut with the sterile scissors. The skin tissue should not be squeezed. The specimen is placed in the pathology specimen container. The bottle should be shaken to make sure that the skin plug is immersed in the preservative solution, then immediately labeled with the patient's name, the date, and the site of the biopsy. Specimens being sent for routine pathology are placed in formalin. If tissue is being sent for an electron microscopic study, it should be placed in a special buffered glutaraldehyde solution. Tissue being sent for a direct immunofluorescence study is put in Michel transport media or snap-frozen in liquid nitrogen. Tissue for microbial culture is placed on sterile gauze in a sterile container and quickly transported to a laboratory.

Excisional biopsies are performed by using a scalpel blade to create an ellipse around the lesion in question. An edge of the ellipse is then gently elevated with a forceps, and underlying subcutaneous tissue is separated from the base with a sharp scissors. Hemostasis usually is obtained by applying gentle pressure for 1 to 2 minutes. Wound closure follows. After suturing, the wound should be covered with a dressing held in place securely with tape or gauze. It is desirable to inform the pathologist of the differential diagnosis being considered and provide a description of the skin lesion.

Complications of Skin Biopsy

Possible complications that must be included in the informed consent include allergic reaction, scarring, bleeding, infection, and pigment changes. Antibiotic prophylaxis should be provided if indicated.

POTASSIUM HYDROXIDE PREPARATION TO DEMONSTRATE FUNGI

Material from the affected area is collected on a microscope slide in the following ways. In suspected tinea corporis or candidiasis, the outer, scaly edge of a skin lesion is gently scraped with a No. 15 blade. Care must be taken to collect scale without drawing blood. Lesions of suspected pityriasis versicolor are gently rubbed with a No. 15 blade, and fine scale throughout the surface of the lesion is collected. The most scaly areas of thick, hyperkeratotic palmar and plantar lesions are scraped similarly; these may be at the center or periphery. If bullous or vesicular lesions are present, a blister roof is gently held by a forceps and removed with a curved iris scissors. Nail material can be collected with a 2-mm curette. Hairs from areas of suspected tinea capitis can be gently plucked with an Adson forceps. The collected material is placed on a glass slide for KOH examination. Similarly collected material can also be placed in a sterile container and sent for fungal cultures.

A cover slide is applied. A drop of 10% to 20% KOH or a specialized fungal stain (e.g., chlorazol black E or Swartz-Lamkin stain containing counter stains, dimethylsulfoxide, or both; available from Delasco [Dermatologic Lab and Supply], Council Bluffs, Iowa, 1-800-831-6273) is added at the side of the cover slip and allowed to percolate under the cover slip to cover the collected tissue. Excess stain is gently blotted from the slide.

The slide is briefly heated (although boiling, which can cause the KOH to crystallize, should be avoided). Heating can be omitted, but more time is then required to clarify the specimen. For thick specimens, such as nails, tops of blisters, or hairs, a 30-minute wait or longer may be necessary. Applying gentle pressure on the coverslip forces out trapped air and thins the specimen to improve visualization.

The preparation is examined microscopically in subdued light with the condenser turned to its lowest position. Fungi appear as threadlike, birefringent, branching, linear elements that cross the outlines of fading cell walls. Yeast spores vary in size, and budding is extremely useful for differentiating yeast spores from trapped air bubbles. Air bubbles have a thicker black outline and lack the birefringence of spores. A typical "spaghetti and meatballs" pattern of hyphae and spores representing *Pityrosporum orbiculare (ovale)* is seen in the lesional scrapings of pityriasis (tinea) versicolor. An experienced eye is required to differentiate artifacts such as fabric fibers and "mosaic" patterns formed by keratinocyte cell walls.

With nail material, results of KOH and fungal culture are negative in up to 65% of cases, even in the face of clinically suspected fungal disease, so that the nail material may have to be sent to a histology laboratory for microtome sectioning and periodic acid-Schiff staining to help establish the diagnosis.

KOH examination of a hair reveals arthrospores within the hair in endothrix infections, sheaths of spores surrounding the hair in ectothrix infections, and thin-walled longitudinal air spaces within the hair shaft in favic fungal hair infection.

CYTODIAGNOSIS (INCLUDING TZANCK SMEAR)

Changes induced by viruses in herpes simplex, herpes zoster, varicella, and molluscum contagiosum can be seen in cells from the base of a blister or papule. To prepare a smear, an early, unruptured blister is chosen. The roof of the blister is gently removed with a sharp scissors; the base is gently blotted with gauze, and a blunt scalpel is used to scrape the base firmly without inducing bleeding. The material on the scalpel is spread on a glass slide, and Giemsa stain or SEDI-STAIN is applied. A peculiar ballooning degeneration of the keratinocytes and the presence of multinucleated giant cells are characteristic of the lesions of herpes simplex, herpes zoster, and varicella.

The microscopic examination of material obtained with a curette from a papule of molluscum contagiosum reveals large, round, brick-shaped eosinophilic bodies (molluscum bodies).

WOOD LAMP EXAMINATION

A Wood lamp is a mercury lamp fitted with a filter that limits the emission to 360 nm; it is used to examine skin and hair in a darkened room. In disorders of depigmentation or hypopigmentation, such as vitiligo, a Wood lamp examination reveals early-developing areas that are not visible to the naked eye. The lesions of vitiligo reflect a lighter color than that of the surrounding normal skin. Hyperpigmented lesions can be seen more intensely with a Wood lamp than with visible light if the melanin pigmentation is predominantly in the epidermis. Examples of lesions accentuated with a Wood lamp are melasma, lentigo maligna melanoma, acral lentiginous melanoma, and ephelides (freckles). However, dermal hypermelanosis, as occurs in a mongolian spot, is not accentuated by Wood lamp illumination.

The urine of patients with porphyria exhibits a pinkish red fluorescence when exposed to a Wood lamp. The addition of dilute hydrochloric acid, which converts porphyrinogens to porphyrins, increases the fluorescence. However, urinary fluorescence is not always detectable, and laboratory analysis of blood, urine, and stool is necessary to establish a diagnosis of porphyria.

Erythrasma is a common bacterial infection caused by *Corynebacterium minutissimum.* It appears as brownish red patches in body folds (axillae, inframammary areas, groin) or as areas of maceration in the webs of the toes. The patches emit a coral-pink to orange-red fluorescence under the Wood lamp. In *Pseudomonas* infection, affected skin and nails exhibit a yellow-green fluorescence. Tinea (pityriasis) versicolor lesions caused by *P. orbiculare (ovale)* exhibit a yellowish fluorescence under Wood lamp illumination.

When the result is positive, a Wood lamp examination can delineate the extent of a fungal infection. Tinea corporis and tinea capitis lesions caused by *Microsporum canis, M. audouinii,* and *M. distortum* give off a brilliant green fluorescence, but not all fungal infections exhibit fluorescence. In tinea capitis caused by *Trichophyton schoenleinii* (favus), a pale green fluorescence may be seen along the entire infected hair shaft. It can be faint and particularly difficult to discern in gray hair. However, the organism currently responsible for most cases of tinea capitis, *Trichophyton tonsurans,* does not cause fluorescence, so that the result of a Wood lamp examination is negative. Sources of error include bluish or purplish fluorescence produced by ointments, skin scales, serum, crust, and salicylic acid preparations.

TESTS FOR DERMATOGRAPHISM

In a test for dermatographism, the skin is gently stroked with a blunt instrument, such as a tongue depressor or cotton-tipped applicator. The usual response is the triple response of Lewis, which consists of the appearance of a red line within 15 seconds, followed by a red flare extending laterally within 15 to 45 seconds and by a wheal in the central area of stroking within 1 to 3 minutes. In white dermatographism, a white line develops instead, and no flare or wheal is seen. The mechanism of white dermatographism is not clearly understood, but this finding confirms a diagnosis of atopic dermatitis (eczema).

PHOTOTESTING

Phototesting detects a heightened reactivity to portions (ultraviolet A, ultraviolet B, and visible light) of the sunlight spectrum and is performed to diagnose certain photosensitivity disorders. It also is used before phototherapy or photopatch testing to determine threshold sensitivities to light.

PATCH AND PHOTOPATCH TESTING

Patch testing is used to detect and document delayed hypersensitivity reactions causing allergic contact dermatitis. The indications for patch testing include a persistent eczematous dermatitis or other dermatologic disease, such as stasis dermatitis that does not heal; the test determines whether a contact hypersensitivity component is present. A screening series, the T.R.U.E. TEST, is available from GlaxoSmithKline (Research Triangle Park, North Carolina). Materials frequently used for patch testing materials include nickel, fragrances, neomycin, bacitracin, lanolin, preservatives found in personal care products, and even topical corticosteroids.

Patch testing should *never* be performed on inflamed skin. If extensive inflammation is present, false-positive reactions may occur more readily.

In photopatch testing, duplicate patch tests are applied and one set is exposed to light. Photopatch testing is indicated when a dermatitis is present in a light-related distribution and a photo allergen is suspected.

Although patch tests are simple in principle, interpreting the results and counseling patients on their relevance is complex. When the cause of a suspected contact dermatitis cannot be determined with a screening series, referral to a dermatologist with a special interest in contact dermatitis for further workup is indicated.

BIBLIOGRAPHY

Caplan RM. Medical uses of the Wood's lamp. *JAMA* 1967;202:1035.

Cram DL. Common diagnostic procedures. In: Solomon LM, Esterly NB, Loeffel ED, eds. *Adolescent dermatology.* Philadelphia: WB Saunders, 1978:39.

Fitzpatrick TB, Bernhard JD, Cropley TG. The structure of skin lesions and fundamentals of diagnosis. In: Freedberg IM, Eisen AL, Wolff K, et al., eds. *Fitzpatrick's dermatology in general medicine,* 5th ed. New York: McGraw-Hill, 1999:13.

Hoke AW. Scabies scraping. *Arch Dermatol* 1973;108:424.

Mayer J. Systemic review of the diagnostic accuracy of dermatoscopy in detecting malignant melanoma. *Med J Aust* 1997;167:206.

Patterson JW, Blaylock WK. Cutaneous diagnostic procedures for the clinician. In: *Dermatology: a concise textbook.* New York: Medical Examination Publishing (Division of Elsevier Science) 1987:35.

Storrs FJ, Rosenthal LE, Adams RM, et al. Prevalence and relevance of allergic reactions in patients patch-tested in North America, 1984–1985. *J Am Acad Dermatol* 1989;20:1038.

CHAPTER 131

Everyday Skin, Hair, and Nail Care

Sophie M. Worobec

Healthy skin requires relatively little care. The main requirements are proper cleansing, maintenance of an optimal moisture level, and protection from excessive exposure to sun, heat, cold, and wind. Physical fitness, good nutrition, and psychological well-being, even in the face of advancing age, do more for beauty than any "rejuvenating" cream.

SKIN CLEANSING

Skin cleansing removes dead skin cells, sweat, body secretions, microorganisms, and dirt. A woman's daily activities, environment, and skin characteristics determine how frequently she wishes or needs to wash. Water removes most dirt; other cleansers, such as liquid soaps, soap bars, and detergent bars, help remove lipid-soluble materials. During cold weather and with advancing age, bathing can be less frequent (sometimes only once or twice a week), and soap needs to be applied only within body folds, such as the axilla and groin. Some cleansing products incorporate moisturizers; some are labeled "fragrance-free." The list of ingredients in such products may reveal the inclusion of masking fragrances, such as rose oil. Consumers should develop the habit of carefully reading the labels of products they purchase for skin care. An example of a truly fragrance-free soap is Kiss My Face Pure Olive Oil Bar Soap. The use of sponges and loofahs is appropriate if they are not excessively abrasive. Newer plastic cleansing poufs are soft and decrease the amount of product needed to work up a lather. Astringents, fresheners, toners, and refining lotions consist of solutions of water and alcohol and can be used to remove sebum or makeup, but they may be irritating or sensitizing to some people.

BODY ODOR, FOOT ODOR, AND SWEATING

Maintaining personal cleanliness and wearing clean clothes are the most important aspects of controlling body odor. Deodorants may contain antibacterial agents and fragrances to mask body odor. Antiperspirants contain aluminum salts, which block the eccrine sweat ducts and obstruct the delivery of sweat to the skin. They can reduce axillary perspiration 20% to 40%. In some women, they may be irritating, and they should not be applied soon after shaving. Obese women may find it helpful to dust talcum powder in the axilla and groin to prevent chafing; professional bicyclists use talcum powder for the same purpose.

Heavy footwear made of synthetic materials may create a damp environment that promotes the growth of the fungi that cause athlete's foot. Dusting the feet with drying powders such as Zeasorb (or, in the presence of fungal infection, Zeasorb-AF, which contains the antifungal agent miconazole) is helpful.

MOISTURIZATION

The optimal water content for the top layer of the skin, the stratum corneum, is at least 10%. At this level, a smooth skin surface is maintained. In dry weather or during the winter in heated rooms, the ambient humidity (<60% relative humidity) is often insufficient to maintain this level of moisture in skin. Even with the use of room humidifiers, the skin begins to feel rough and may itch. The use of moisturizers is recommended to prevent and treat this common problem. Moisturizers help prevent water loss from the skin. They are best applied sparingly after bathing and patting oneself dry, but while the skin is still hydrated; any excess left on the palms is then rubbed off on a hand towel. The least expensive moisturizers are Crisco and petroleum jelly, but many people consider them too greasy, which is unfortunate, because they are fragrance-free and "do the job." Many of the moisturizers on the market contain water and glycerin (e.g., Curel lotion, Aveeno moisturizing cream). Thicker preparations include Absorbase, Aquaphor, and Eucerin. Agents such as lactic acid and urea also have water-binding properties. Lac-Hydrin lotion and cream, which are prescription products, contain 12% lactic acid and are very effective, especially when applied on ichthyotic skin and dry, cracked skin over the heels and plantar foot surfaces. Women with a tendency to acne should choose a noncomedogenic facial moisturizer, such as Neutrogena Healthy Defense Daily Moisturizer SPF 30.

PREVENTION OF SUN DAMAGE

In the past 30 years, the existence of both an intrinsic skin-aging process and an extrinsic skin-aging process that affects predominantly areas exposed to the sun (photodamage) has been increasingly recognized. The skin can be protected from the sun by minimizing midday (10 a.m.– 4 p.m.) exposure, wearing hats and protective clothing, and using sunblock skin care products. "Sunblock" products offer good protection against both ultraviolet B (UVB) and UVA wavelengths, whereas "sunscreen" products offer only UVB protection. Clothing manufactured under the trademarks of Solumbra and Coolibar is designed to protect the wearer from the sun. In general, heavy cotton denim, leather, and neoprene "wet suits" protect quite well. Rit SunGuard Laundry Treatment is a sun-blocking product that can be washed into clothing by following the manufacturer's instructions.

Sunblock products are regulated as over-the-counter drugs, and women should try different ones to see which they prefer. The development of irritation, contact dermatitis, or even photosensitivity can force a change in the use of a particular sunblock product. "Physical" sunblock products are made with zinc oxide or titanium dioxide and in general are less likely to cause adverse skin reactions. Sunblock products reduce the risk for skin cancer and photodamage only if the user does not extend the amount of time she spends in the sun. The sun protection factor (SPF) associated with these products is a laboratory-derived figure determined under strictly defined conditions. An SPF of 2 means that 50% of incipient UVB radiation is blocked. At SPF 8, 87.5% is blocked, and at SPF 16, 93.75% is blocked. However, it is not possible to calculate a person's "burn time" on a day-to-day basis with SPF figures to increase "safe" sun exposure.

Tretinoin or all-*trans*-retinoic acid products have been prescribed widely to reduce fine wrinkles, roughness, and brown spots on sun-damaged skin and to treat acne. It is prudent to minimize one's exposure to the sun or artificial UV light when using these products because studies in pigmented mice and hairless albino mice have shown that 0.05% tretinoin enhances photocarcinogenesis.

Marketing approval has been granted for the use of Renova (tretinoin emollient cream) 0.05% and Renova 0.02% as adjunctive agents in the palliation of fine wrinkles, mottled hyperpigmentation, and tactile roughness of facial skin when this cannot be achieved by a program of comprehensive skin care and sun avoidance alone. Up to 6 months of therapy may be required before improvement is seen. Renova does not eliminate wrinkles or repair sun-damaged skin, nor does it reverse photoaging or restore a more youthful skin, according to the 1998 and 2000 package inserts. It has not been established whether these products are safe and effective when used for longer than 52 weeks. Patients with visible actinic keratoses or with a history of skin cancers were excluded from Renova trials; therefore, its safety in persons with these conditions has not been established.

HAIR CARE

Shampoos remove hair oils, cellular debris, microorganisms, and other soils. The shampoo that a woman prefers will depend on her lifestyle and whether she uses other hair treatments, such as tints and permanent conditioners. Hair thickness does decline in general, even in persons in excellent health, with each decade of life past the age of 20. Women with less dense hair may wish to use a shampoo that provides "extra body." Those who swim daily may find that a "swimmer's" shampoo and conditioner will leave their hair more soft and manageable.

Free and Clear Shampoo is especially formulated for persons with contact allergies to fragrances or formalin, both of which are found in most shampoos. Additional information on shampoos is included in Chapters 136 and 139. Conditioners are added to shampoos or applied separately to facilitate combing and prevent damage from traction after washing. DHS Conditioning Rinse is also recommended for persons with a sensitive scalp. The frequency of shampooing may vary from daily to once or twice a week or less, depending on personal grooming practices and ethnic differences in hair types.

The structure of the hair and therefore preferences in hair care products differ among ethnic groups. Asian scalp hair is straight and round in cross section, with a diameter larger than that of African or Caucasian hair. Caucasian scalp hair is oval, with a "curl" to it. The scalp sebaceous glands of Africans and African-Americans are relatively inactive, and the hair shaft is oval or flat (ribbon-like), with a tendency to twist. Hair oil products are used to increase hair manageability and help style hair. The use of hair oils can result in "pomade acne" on the face, so they should be applied sparingly 1 inch back from the hairline. Some people like to wear a scarf at bedtime to prevent hair products from soiling a pillowcase and from there coming into contact with facial skin. Hair coloration changes with aging; it may darken in Caucasians with medium brown hair from the age of 20 years to middle age, after which it gradually lose pigmentation, graying then whitening. Hair coloring is becoming increasingly popular in all age groups. Paraphenylenediamine, a common ingredient of brown or black hair dyes, is a possible cause of contact dermatitis. Persons who are allergic to paraphenylenediamine can use henna dyes safely.

Permanents and, to a lesser degree, many coloring treatments weaken the hair shaft and should be carefully applied to avoid re-treating the same portion. In acquired trichorrhexis nodosa, chemical or physical agents (heat, traction, tight braiding) damage the hair shafts; hairs are short and broken, and microscopic knots or bubbles in the shafts fracture or break easily.

The amount of facial and body hair depends on the genetic background. However, an abnormal change in the facial or body hair of a woman warrants a hormonal evaluation. Hypothyroidism can be associated with course and dry hair, increased shedding of hair, loss of lateral eyebrows, and dry and rough skin. Increasing skin pallor can be a sign of systemic disease (e.g., anemia, hypopituitarism).

NAIL CARE

Fingernails vary in thickness and flexibility from person to person. As we age, the fingernails grow more slowly and become thinner, and longitudinal ridges may develop. The ingestion of gelatin or calcium does not strengthen a normal fingernail. Protecting the hands prevents nail injuries. Hands exposed to dry, cold weather or frequent washing should be protected with gloves and emollients. An intact eponychium (cuticle) prevents infection of the posterior nail fold and should not be removed. Hangnails are partially detached, dried pieces of skin at the lateral nail fold. They should be cut close to the base and covered with a bandage; they should not be picked at or torn because this may lead to secondary infection.

Carefully applied and maintained manicures are esthetically beneficial. However, the use of methacrylates as glue for wrapping nails can result in onycholysis, paronychia, and permanent damage to the nail.

Care of the toenails means wearing footwear that fits well; the most common cause of ingrown toenails is ill-fitting shoes. Toenails should be clipped straight across. Cutting them down in the corners causes the sharp ends to dig into the lateral nail folds, and granulation tissue ("proud flesh") may ultimately form. If this happens, the patient should be shown how to place a little piece of cotton between the sharp corner of the nail and the skin. The cotton should be replaced daily after a shower or bath until the nail has grown out enough that it can be trimmed properly.

"NATURAL" INGREDIENTS

"Natural" does not mean "better"; poison ivy is "all natural," yet it is the most common cause of severe contact dermatitis in North America. Skin care products may be labeled "natural" because they contain ingredients found in nature, such as α-hydroxy acids; however, these ingredients are often synthesized or manufactured for use in such products. Natural substances such as fragrances, vitamin E, lanolin, and aloe can cause contact dermatitis. In other words, "natural" materials can cause skin problems in addition to being useful.

In short, if a woman is using a skin or hair care product that pleases her, it does not make sense to switch to a more expensive product simply because it is labeled "natural."

BIBLIOGRAPHY

Bech-Thomsen N, Wulf HC, Ullman S. Xeroderma pigmentosum lesions related to ultraviolet transmittance by clothes. *J Am Acad Dermatol* 1991;24:365.

Engasser PG. Care of normal skin, hair, and nails. In: Orkin M, Maibach HI, Dahl MV, eds. *Dermatology*. Norwalk, CT: Appleton & Lange, 1991.

Jackson EM. An overview of natural cosmetic ingredient use. *Cosmetic Dermatol* 1994;7:42.

Marks R. Summer in Australia: skin cancer and the great SPF debate. *Arch Dermatol* 1995;131:462.

Renova (tretinoin emollient cream) 0.05% package insert. Raritan, NJ: Ortho Dermatological Division of Ortho-McNeil Pharmaceutical, February 1998.

Renova (tretinoin emollient cream) 0.02% package insert. Raritan, NJ: Ortho Dermatological Division of Ortho-McNeil Pharmaceutical, September 2000.

Sayre RM, Hughes SNG. Sun protective apparel: advancements in sun protection. *Skin Cancer J* 1993;8:41.

Steinem G. *Revolution from within: a book of self-esteem.* Boston: Little, Brown and Company, 1991.

Stern RS. Sunscreens for cancer protection. *Arch Dermatol* 1995;131:220.

Wolf N. *The beauty myth: how images of beauty are used against women.* New York: William Morrow, 1991.

CHAPTER 132
Rashes

Sophie M. Worobec

What is a rash? A rash is a skin eruption.

The skin diseases seen most frequently in women are acne, superficial fungal infections, seborrheic dermatitis, atopic dermatitis/eczema, warts, malignant tumors, psoriasis, herpes simplex, and vitiligo.

Dermatology is unique in that direct visual recognition often establishes the diagnosis. Many skin diseases can be identified by their unique lesions, such as the comedones of acne, the "black dots in callus" of a wart, the "iris lesions" of erythema multiforme, or the "dew drop on a rose petal" of chicken pox. The diagnosis of other conditions, such as drug rashes and contact dermatitis, may require an extensive history.

The dermatologic history includes questions about the onset (when and where the rash first appeared), course (how the rash progressed, any remissions or exacerbations), changes in appearance since the onset, systemic symptoms (e.g., fever, joint pain), local symptoms (tenderness, itching), and menstrual history; it should also be determined whether anyone close to the patient has had a skin disease. The patient's profile should include the occupational history, lifestyle and hobbies, and travel history. A review of systems helps determine whether the skin findings may be part of a disease that affects multiple systems, such as systemic lupus erythematosus (SLE), or associated with another disease, such as hepatitis or AIDS. Most patients will already have used something for their rash, and this should be ascertained. The medication history includes not only prescription medications but also over-the-counter preparations, home remedies, and personal care products.

Both SLE and syphilis have been termed the "great imitators." Fortunately, reliable serologic tests are available for both diagnoses.

Lupus erythematosus drug eruptions deserve extended mention. For example, anti-Ro (SS-A)–positive cutaneous lupus erythematosus can be induced by drugs, and causative drugs have been as diverse as terbinafine, hydrochlorothiazide, angiotensin-converting enzyme inhibitors, calcium channel blockers, interferons, and statins. Hydrochlorothiazide, procainamide, and hydralazine can cause an anti-histone antibody–positive SLE. SLE also has been reported after the long-term use of minocycline. Two new anti-tumor necrosis factor-α agents, etanercept (Enbrel) and infliximab (Remicade), have been associated with subacute lupus erythematosus. These drug-induced forms of SLE or cutaneous lupus erythematosus usually resolve after the inciting therapy has been discontinued.

Other types of drug-related cutaneous reactions vary greatly and include the following: toxic epidermal necrolysis (life-threatening); vasculitis; photosensitivity; vesicobullous, lichenoid, and acneiform reactions; alopecia; erythema multiforme; erythema nodosum; pigmentation changes; acute generalized pustulosis; and aromatic amine antiepileptic hypersensitivity syndrome. In one 5-year Finnish study of all drug reactions at one inpatient institution, the most common morphologic patterns were exanthema, urticaria or angioedema, fixed drug eruption, and erythema multiforme.

The medical history may include questions about chronic and recent illness, prior skin problems, known allergies and

TABLE 132.1. Morphology of Skin Lesions

Primary skin lesions	
Macule	Flat discoloration <1 cm in diameter (some references put no size limitation)
Patch	Flat discoloration >1 cm in diameter
Papule	Elevated lesion <1 cm in diameter
Plaque	Flat, elevated lesion >1.5 cm in diameter
Nodule	Elevated lesion >1 cm in diameter
Tumor	Rounded elevated lesion >2–3 cm in diameter (some references put no size limitation; large mass)
Vesicle	Fluid-filled elevated lesion <1 cm in diameter
Bulla	Fluid-filled elevated lesion >1 cm in diameter
Pustule	Elevated lesion filled with pus
Wheal	Elevated white to pink to red pruritic lesion; evanescent; may be yellow in the presence of severe jaundice
Secondary skin lesions	
Crust	Dried exudate attached to skin surface
Scale	Accumulation of skin "flakes"
Pustule	Elevated lesion filled with pus
Purpura	Hemorrhage into the skin; does not blanch with pressure from glass slide; small lesions are petechiae, larger ones ecchymoses
Erosion	Surface denudation limited to top layer of skin
Fissure	Linear break in the skin extending down to the dermis
Ulcer	Skin defect involving at least part of the dermis; "hole in the skin"
Excoriation	Area of erosion or ulceration produced by the patient
Atrophy	Decrease in thickness of the skin caused by partial loss of epidermis, dermis, or subcutaneous fat
Pigmentation/dyschromia	Increase of color, hyperpigmentation; decrease, hypopigmentation
Papilloma	Elevated cauliflower-like lesion
Cyst	Cavity filled with fluid or solid matter and surrounded by a sac
Lichenification	Thick plaque with accentuated skin markings
Scar	Pattern of healing in area where wound, ulceration, or disease process such as acne, herpes zoster, varicella, or porphyria cutanea tarda has occurred
Sclerosis	Circumscribed or diffuse hardening of the skin; occurs with morphea, localized or systemic scleroderma, scleroderma, chronic stasis dermatitis, chronic lymphedema, nephrogenic fibrosing dermopathy, eosinophilic fasciitis
Suggillation	Swollen "black and blue" marks, consequence of bruising

TABLE 132.2. Configurations of Skin Lesions

Type	Description	Examples
Annular	Ringlike	Tinea corporis, granuloma annulare, Lyme disease (erythema migrans)
Arciform	Incompletely formed ring, like an arc	Migratory necrolytic erythema, tertiary syphilis, mycosis fungoides
Serpiginous	Winding, like a snake	Larva migrans
Linear	In a line	Poison ivy dermatitis, linear epidermal nevi, linear scleroderma, Koebner phenomenon[a]
Guttate	Droplike individual lesions, like spots in a field	Guttate psoriasis
Dermatomal	Following a dermatomal distribution	Herpes zoster
Target-like or iris-like	Ring around a central lesion	Erythema multiforme
Reticulate	Netlike	Livedo reticularis, cutis marmorata, erythema ab igne
Grouped	Clustering of lesions in a well-demarcated area	Herpes simplex, herpes zoster

[a]The Koebner phenomenon is an isomorphic response in which lesions occur at sites of injured skin, such as a linear scratch. It is seen in, for example, psoriasis, verrucae, urticaria, and lichen planus.

what they are like, and manifestations of atopy, such as asthma, hay fever, and eczema. The family history may include questions regarding skin diseases such as psoriasis or eczema, cancer, hair or nail problems, and infectious diseases such as impetigo, scabies, varicella, herpes zoster, and herpes simplex.

The physical examination findings should be classified as primary and secondary lesions. Primary lesions are the original skin changes; secondary lesions develop with the passage of time. Pustules can be primary lesions, as in folliculitis, or secondary lesions, as when the umbilicated vesicles of herpes simplex become pustular.

The morphologic terms used to describe primary and secondary lesions are listed in Table 132.1. A rash can be further characterized by its configuration (Table 132.2) and regional distribution (Table 132.3).

In the examination of a patient with a rash, the yield of the more systematic or global examination is greater. The physician should look at more than the immediate rash that the patient points out; the patient's scalp, face, eyelids, skin behind the ears, mouth, and nails should all be assessed. The examination may reveal patterns of seborrheic dermatitis, psoriasis, eczema, or contact dermatitis. Commonly, tinea pedis helps explain a hand rash, which may itself be a tinea manus or an id reaction to the dermatophytic infection of the feet.

The spectrum of skin problems can be broadly grouped as shown in Table 132.4.

Once diagnosed, a skin problem can be treated. Individual chapters in this text address the therapy of specific diseases.

If after seeing and interviewing the patient and consulting reference books the physician cannot make a specific diagnosis, it is best to refer the patient to another physician. An experienced dermatologist can more promptly recognize a dermatosis or the need for a biopsy. Although a skin biopsy is relatively easy to perform, a dermatologist is well versed in choosing the most appropriate lesion or lesions (in the case of cutaneous T-cell lymphoma) for a biopsy. In difficult cases, a dermatopathologist can be asked to read the skin biopsy. The expertise of this specialist, gained by reading of thousands of skin slides, can help guide the patient's care. The dermatologist can help communicate the clinical findings and differential diagnosis to the dermatopathologist. Sometimes, additional laboratory work is in order (e.g., a rapid plasma reagent test and fluorescent treponemal antibody absorption test for the diagnosis of syphilis, hepatitis serology for a patient with itching, a mononucleosis test for a patient with an ampicillin rash, direct and indirect immunofluorescence for immunobullous disease, and patch testing when contact dermatitis is suspected).

Some rashes, such as a well-developed herpes zoster, are instantly recognizable; others stump even experienced and astute dermatologists. However, careful observation, a thorough history, testing, and consultation with other physicians and the literature usually narrow the diagnostic possibilities.

TABLE 132.3. Distributions of Skin Lesions

Type	Examples
Generalized	Viral eruption, drug eruption, guttate psoriasis
Photosensitive	Systemic lupus erythematosus, drug-induced lupus erythematosus photocontact allergy
Intertriginous	Intertrigo, candidiasis, inverse psoriasis, erythrasma
Symmetric	Psoriasis, atopic dermatitis, drug eruption, ichthyosis vulgaris
Asymmetric	Poison ivy dermatitis, fixed drug eruption
Along cleavage lines	Pityriasis rosea
Follicular	Acne, bacterial or yeast folliculitis, eosinophilic folliculitis, follicular eczema, keratosis pilaris, scurvy, vitamin A deficiency

TABLE 132.4. Skin Disease Groupings by Clinical Presentation

Type	Examples
Eczematous	Contact dermatitis, infestations, infections, drug reactions, atopic dermatitis, dyshidrosis, nummular eczema, stasis dermatitis, xerotic eczema
Papulosquamous	Psoriasis, seborrheic dermatitis, pityriasis rosea, secondary syphilis, tinea, lichen planus, discoid lupus, lichen simplex chronicus, cutaneous T-cell lymphoma
Vascular reactivity	Urticaria, erythema multiforme, annular erythema, toxic erythema, viral exanthems
Inflammatory	Erythema nodosum, bacterial infections, insect bites, infestations, panniculitis
Vesiculobullous	Eczematous dermatoses, viral eruptions, insect bites, scabies, bullous impetigo, Stevens-Johnson syndrome, pemphigoid, porphyria cutanea tarda, fixed drug eruption, diabetic bullae, bullae with coma, pemphigus vulgaris, dermatitis herpetiformis, epidermolysis bullosa acquisita
Pustular	Acne vulgaris, acne rosacea, folliculitis, steroid acne, gonococcemia, pustular psoriasis, candidiasis
Purpuric	Leukocytoclastic vasculitis, senile purpura, posttraumatic purpura (including suction purpura), corticosteroid excess, vascular defects, platelet disorders, clotting factor disorders
Pruritus	Various causes: xerosis; drug-induced; dermatologic disease (e.g., eczema, scabies); systemic disease (e.g., renal failure, polycythemia vera, iron deficiency anemia, hepatobiliary problems); HIV infection; psychological
Psychocutaneous	Neurotic excoriations, lip biting, hair pulling, factitial dermatitis, delusions of skin disease, dysmorphic syndrome
Life-threatening	Staphylococcal scalded skin syndrome, toxic epidermal necrolysis, toxic shock syndrome, Kawasaki disease, Rocky Mountain spotted fever

BIBLIOGRAPHY

Callan JP. "How frequently are drugs associated with the development or exacerbation of subacute cutaneous lupus?" *Arch Dermatol* 2003;139:89.

Freedberg IM, Eisen AL, Wolff K, et al., eds. *Fitzpatrick's dermatology in general medicine*, 5th ed. New York: McGraw-Hill, 1999.

Flowers FP, Krusinski PA, eds. *Dermatology in ambulatory and emergency medicine: a clinical guide with algorithms*. Chicago: Year Book, 1984.

Lynch PJ, Edwards L. *Genital dermatology*. New York: Churchill Livingstone, 1994.

Srivastava M, Rencic A, Diglio G, et al. Drug-induced Ro/SSA-positive cutaneous lupus erythematosus. *Arch Dermatol* 2003;139:45.

CHAPTER 133

Pigmentation Disorders

Sophie M. Worobec and Sheetal Mehta

Many different disorders affect skin pigmentation. This chapter focuses on the more common ones, in addition to a few rare ones, to demonstrate the spectrum of pigmentation disorders. Pigmentary disturbances can be congenital or acquired, localized or generalized. Pigmentary demarcation lines are a normal finding in up to 26% of African-Americans; they are most often seen on the dorsal and ventral surfaces of the arms, from which they extend onto the chest.

ETIOLOGY AND DIFFERENTIAL DIAGNOSIS

Skin color can be altered by disease and by exposure to heat, solar radiation, ionizing radiation, drugs, trauma, and heavy metals. Both systemic and local skin disease, in addition to therapeutic measures, can destroy melanocytes, causing temporary or permanent hypopigmentation. Hypopigmentation may follow dermabrasion, chemical peels, and destructive modalities such as cryotherapy, curettage, and electrodessication if melanocytes within the area of treatment are injured. Less intense injury leads to an inflammatory reaction, with an increased production of pigment and hyperpigmentation. Many dermatoses, even the inflamed papules and pustules of common acne, cause postinflammatory hyperpigmentation. Tanning is triggered by the activation of DNA-repair enzymes after DNA has been damaged by ultraviolet radiation. In acanthosis nigricans, increased proliferation of both keratinocytes and melanocytes produces a velvety hyperpigmentation.

Hyperpigmentation

Hyperpigmentation can be circumscribed or diffuse. Moles (nevi), freckles, and lentigines are the most common circumscribed hyperpigmented lesions. Congenital nevi, atypical nevi, lentigo maligna, and malignant melanoma are covered in Chapter 143.

Mongolian spots (dermal melanocytosis) are localized dermal aggregates of melanocytes; as a consequence of the Tyndall effect, they appear blue-gray to blue-black because of the deep location of the melanin pigment. These congenital lesions occur most often on the lumbosacral area but also occasionally on the shoulders, upper back, arms, and legs. Most mongolian spots regress by adolescence, but some persist into adulthood. These lesions are found frequently in infants of Asian, Amerindian, and African-American origin, and rarely in Caucasian infants.

Nevus of Ota is a localized hyperpigmented blue-gray or blue-brown macular lesion caused by an upper dermal nevoid aggregate of dendritic melanocytes over the distribution of the ophthalmic and maxillary divisions of the trigeminal nerve. It can extend to involve eye structures, especially the sclera; very rarely, ocular malignant melanoma has developed. It is most common in Asian, Hispanic, and African-American persons. It may be congenital but is not hereditary; more often, it appears in early childhood or during puberty and remains for life.

Melasma (chloasma, "mask of pregnancy") is a common acquired macular hyperpigmentation that appears on the face. It develops when melanin production by melanocytes is increased in response to multiple factors, including ultraviolet radiation and hormonal influences. It can be related to pregnancy or the use of oral contraceptives. Exposure to sunlight aggravates and perpetuates this condition.

Ephelides (freckles) are light brown macules, usually less than 5 mm in diameter, that occur in sun-exposed areas of fair-skinned persons. The number of melanocytes is no greater within freckles than in adjacent skin. Freckling is a marker of an increased risk for skin cancers, including melanoma.

Lentigines are circumscribed hyperpigmented brown macules in which the number of epidermal melanocytes is increased; they are slightly larger and darker than freckles. Two basic types are recognized: lentigo simplex lesions, which arise in childhood and are few in number, and actinic (solar, senile) lentigines, which arise in middle age and are numerous in sun-exposed skin. Solar lentigines (liver spots) are caused by chronic sun exposure and occur in most elderly Caucasians and in many Asians and Hispanics.

Inherited patterned lentiginosis in blacks is a benign autosomal-dominant trait characterized by the childhood onset of lentigines on the face, lips, buttocks, palms, and soles. *Multiple lentigines syndrome*, a rare but distinctive syndrome, is dominantly inherited; it is also called *LEOPARD syndrome* (lentigines, electrocardiographic abnormalities, ocular hypertelorism, pulmonary stenosis, abnormal genitalia, retarded growth and development, and deafness). Persons with this syndrome have hundreds of lentigines on the trunk, head, and extremities, including the palms and soles. Another dominantly inherited trait associated with numerous lentigines is *Peutz-Jeghers syndrome*. It is distinctive in that the lentigines occur around the mouth and eyes as well as on the lips, oral mucosa, hands, and feet in association with gastrointestinal polyps. Other rare syndromes characterized by multiple lentigines have also been described.

PUVA lentigines with melanocytic atypia have been reported in up to 4% of patients treated with psoralen and ultraviolet light of A wavelength (PUVA) for 2 years or longer.

Sun bed lentigines, also with melanocytic atypia, have been reported in persons with more than 50 exposures in UVA tanning beds.

Café au lait macules are light to dark brown, well-circumscribed macules ranging from 1 to 20 cm in size. They may be round or oval or have an irregular border. They may be present at birth or appear later in childhood. Up to 20% of all people have them, but the presence of multiple lesions suggests the possibility of an associated clinical syndrome, such as neurofibromatosis or Albright syndrome. Café au lait spots, even with associated axillary freckles, are not in themselves diagnostic of *neurofibromatosis type 1*. Lisch nodules (melanocytic hematomas of the iris) are seen in more than 97% of adult women with neurofibromatosis type 1. *Albright syndrome* consists of polyostotic fibrous dysplasia, precocious puberty in girls, endocrine dysfunction, and large café au lait spots with jagged margins resembling the coast of Maine.

Nevus spilus is a café au lait macule containing darker melanotic macules within its border. Rarely, melanomas have developed within these lesions.

Becker nevus is a pigmented hairy patch that is reported to occur in 0.5% of men, usually on the back, chest, shoulders, or neck, and in 0.1% of women. The diameter of the lesion ranges from a few centimeters to the more frequent 10 to 20 cm. A Becker nevus is not a potentially malignant lesion.

Several metabolic diseases have been associated with diffuse skin hyperpigmentation. *Addison disease* (in which vitiligo may also be a feature) is characterized by fatigue and hyperpigmentation, especially of skin crease lines and scars, as a consequence of increased pituitary secretion of melanocyte-stimulating hormone and adrenocorticotropic hormone. Other metabolic diseases associated with diffuse hyperpigmentation include *Wilson disease* (also with sky blue nail lunulae), *alkaptonuria*, *hemochromatosis*, *biliary cirrhosis*, and *porphyria cutanea tarda*.

Skin diseases in which marked postinflammatory hyperpigmentation is a feature include lichen planus and erythema dyschromicum perstans (ashy dermatosis). *Drugs* responsible for hyperpigmentation include amiodarone, busulphan, cyclophosphamide, clofazimine, doxorubicin, mechlorethamine, mephenytoin, methotrexate, paclitaxel, phenytoin, zidovudine, chlorpromazine, gold, and minocycline. Silver, bismuth, mercury, and arsenic can produce hyperpigmentation. Fixed drug eruptions, caused most often by phenolphthalein in laxatives, barbiturates, and sometimes tetracycline, can result in one or several hyperpigmented macular lesions and are often preceded by erythema and edema of the involved areas. Bleomycin can produce a linear, flagellate pattern of hyperpigmentation.

The topical use of imiquimod and fluorouracil can result in inflammation and postinflammatory hyperpigmentation. Berloque dermatitis is caused by bercapten (5-methoxypsoralen), which is present in oil of bergamot, a component of many perfumes and some hair care products. It occurs on skin to which bercapten has been applied as a phototoxic reaction and leaves a streaky, long-lasting area of hyperpigmentation.

A yellow discoloration of the skin is seen in jaundice. The sclerae are also often affected. The yellow color of carotenemia does not involve the sclerae and is accentuated on the palms and soles. Quinacrine, an antimalarial agent sometimes used to treat lupus, may also cause yellowish skin discoloration. Other drugs imparting a yellow color include canthaxanthin and phenazopyridine.

Hypopigmentation

Intrinsic hypopigmentation disorders include vitiligo, albinism, and piebaldism. *Vitiligo* affects 1% to 2% of the population in the United States. Men and women are equally affected; the predominance in women suggested by the literature is likely to reflect the willingness of women to express cosmetic concern. It can occur in persons of any age, but in 50% of cases, it begins between the ages of 10 and 30 years. Vitiligo appears to be a multifactorial disease in which multiple genetic loci interact with the surrounding environment. More than 30% of affected persons report vitiligo in a parent, sibling, or child. The lesions of vitiligo are asymptomatic and hypopigmented or completely depigmented. In early lesions, areas of perifollicular hypopigmentation may be seen; these become depigmented, extend, and coalesce, forming larger macular lesions. The lesions tend to occur over bony prominences, such as the knuckles, elbows, knees, and ankles; on the face, neck, and chest; and around orifices. Halo nevi, white patches of hair (poliosis), and prematurely gray hair are common associated problems. Vitiligo can be trichromatic, showing complete depigmentation (white), partial depigmentation (light brown), and a deeper normal brown. In vitiligo, melanocytes are locally destroyed. The cause is unknown, but associations with hyperthyroidism, hypothyroidism, pernicious anemia, diabetes mellitus, Addison disease, and very rarely internal malignancy have been noted. Most cases are idiopathic, with the formation of antibodies to melanocytes.

Oculocutaneous albinism is diffuse and may affect the eyes, hair, and skin color or the eyes alone (ocular albinism). Albinism has been classified into 10 separate phenotypes, depending on the type of defect present (i.e., absent or aberrant tyrosinase activity or altered melanin formation). In all forms, normal melanin in the skin is decreased or absent. Albinism is congenital and best initially diagnosed by comparing the patient's coloration with that of her unaffected first-degree relatives. Most cases are autosomal-recessive. Photophobia and nystagmus are frequently associated but not essential for the diagnosis.

Piebaldism is rare and occurs as an autosomal-dominant trait. It is characterized by a congenital white forelock (>90% of cases) and depigmented macules, which often contain isolated normally pigmented or hyperpigmented macules. The hyperpigmented macules are usually less than 1 cm in diameter (although larger ones have occurred) and are characteristically present both within the depigmented areas and on normal skin.

Asymptomatic hypopigmented macules that are polygonal and range from 1 mm to 2 cm in diameter are seen in *idiopathic guttate hypomelanosis*. In this common condition, lesions first appear on sun-exposed areas of the upper and lower extremities, and more rarely on the face, neck, and trunk, in early adulthood and then increase in number. They are often a cosmetic problem. The cause is unknown, although aging, exposure to the sun, and genetic background all play a role.

Skin diseases (e.g., *tinea versicolor, pityriasis alba, sarcoidosis, mycosis fungoides,* and *scleroderma*) may be associated with hypopigmentation. Hypopigmented oval to lance-ovate macules are seen in *tuberous sclerosis*. Hereditary metabolic diseases such as *phenylketonuria* can result in diffuse hypopigmentation, which is subtle and best appreciated by comparison with family members. Infectious diseases associated with hypopigmentation that should be considered if a patient has lived in an area of endemicity include *leprosy* (if sensory loss is noted within the lesions), *pinta, nonvenereal syphilis* or *bejel, yaws, onchocerciasis,* and *chronic kala-azar*.

Chemical exposure to phenolic compounds that interfere with tyrosinase activity may cause chemical leukoderma. Exposure to antioxidants (e.g., monobenzyl ether of hydroquinone) in rubber goods such as gloves or rubber pads can cause hypopigmentation. The intralesional injection or long-term topical use of corticosteroids can cause hypopigmentation.

HISTORY AND PHYSICAL EXAMINATION

A careful skin examination should be a part of the comprehensive health checkup of every patient. Pigmentary lesions should be noted. In both hyperpigmentation and hypopigmentation disorders, a careful history (date of onset, progression, general health status, medications, diet, prior or concomitant therapy, and family history of pigmentary lesions) and a careful physical examination help the clinician reach a diagnosis.

LABORATORY AND IMAGING STUDIES

A Wood light examination can help the examiner determine the true extent of hypopigmented lesions, especially in very fair-skinned persons. If tuberous sclerosis, neurofibromatosis, Albright syndrome, or one of the syndromes associated with generalized lentigines is suspected, special imaging studies and further workup may be indicated. Tyrosinase studies can be performed when albinism is a diagnostic possibility. For persons with vitiligo, a determination of the levels of vitamin B_{12}, thyroid-stimulating hormone, and antimicrosomal antibodies and a random glucose test should be considered. Thyroid abnormalities are more common in women older than 50 years of age. These and other tests should be performed as indicated by the history and physical examination findings.

If a patient has well-defined macular lesions that are hyperpigmented on sun-protected areas and hypopigmented on sun-exposed areas and that become scaly when rubbed, one of the lesions should he scraped gently with a No. 15 blade and the scales examined with potassium hydroxide (KOH) to check for hyphae and spores. A positive KOH examination result distinguishes pityriasis versicolor from pityriasis alba.

A skin biopsy is required to establish the diagnosis in cases of hypopigmentation associated with mycosis fungoides, sarcoidosis, leprosy, or other infectious diseases.

TREATMENT

Hyperpigmentation

The sine qua non of preventing or relieving melasma, freckles, and solar lentigines is protecting the skin from excessive exposure to the sun (see Chapter 131). Lesions suspected of being malignant or with the potential to become malignant should be excised (see Chapter 143).

Melasma, freckles, and solar lentigines and some cases of postinflammatory hyperpigmentation respond variably to treatment with bleaching creams and solutions containing hydroquinone (e.g., Solaquin, Eldoquin, Melanex). At bedtime, 0.025% to 0.05% tretinoin cream or gel may be added to increase bleaching. Topical corticosteroids also can lighten pigment but must be used very cautiously. Current therapy for melasma includes Tri-Luma cream (a combination of 4% hydroquinone, 0.01% fluocinolone acetonide, and 0.05% tretinoin), 20% azelaic acid cream, and chemical peels. However, all these modalities have the potential to produce untoward side effects, such as irritation and undesired hypopigmentation or hyperpigmentation. Treatment can take months and must be combined with scrupulous avoidance of excessive exposure to ultraviolet light, either from natural sunlight or a tanning parlor sunlamp.

Current therapy of solar lentigines includes laser destruction and the application of Renova (tretinoin emollient cream).

Quality-switched neodymium:yttrium-aluminum-garnet laser (QSNYL) is an alternative tool used to treat a number of benign pigmented lesions, including freckles, lentigines, nevus of Ota, and unilateral lentiginosis. Another type of laser, the alexandrite laser, has been effective in the treatment of medium brown solar lentigines. Becker nevus responds unpredictably to pigmented lesion lasers, and recurrences are common. If the lesion is part of a syndrome or a manifestation of systemic disease, the treatment should address the underlying disorder.

Hypopigmentation

Persons with vitiligo and albinism are at increased risk for the development of actinic keratoses, basal cell epitheliomas, squamous cell epitheliomas, and melanomas. Protection from sunlight with a broad-spectrum sunblock, hat, and clothing is essential (see Chapter 131).

Cosmetic cover-up with makeup (Covermark, Dermablend) or dyes (Vitadye, Dy-O-Derm) can be used over areas of vitiligo.

Efforts to treat vitiligo can be frustrating for both patients and physicians. Many approaches are used, including tacrolimus (Protopic) ointment, topical glucocorticoids, topical photochemotherapy, systemic photochemotherapy, pseudocatalase cream, multivitamin therapy, narrow-band UVB, 308-nm excimer laser, Q-switched ruby laser, and minigrafting.

The use of topical or systemic photochemotherapy with PUVA to treat vitiligo requires a large time commitment, with visits at least weekly, and burns may occur. Side effects of oral PUVA therapy include nausea and vomiting, hyperpigmentation of normally pigmented skin, itching, photoaging, increased risk for skin cancer, and increased risk for cataracts. Sunglasses and sunblock that protect against ultraviolet light must be worn for 24 hours after oral dosing. Grafting uninvolved pigmented skin into the vitiliginous area, together with PUVA therapy, has been successful in a few centers.

Another option for patients older than 12 years who have vitiligo involving 50% or more of their body surface is to undergo total depigmentation with monobenzyl ether of 20% hydroquinone cream. Side effects include irritation and contact sensitization. The resultant depigmentation is permanent, and lifetime protection against excessive exposure to the sun is necessary.

Patients with albinism should also be cared for by an ophthalmologist. In addition, a number of volunteer organizations in the United States, such as the National Organization for Albinism and Hypomelanosis (NOAH), assist patients in with dealing with vision problems and obtaining a driver's license.

Secondary hypopigmentation, as in pityriasis versicolor and even Hansen disease, abates as the underlying cause is treated.

CONSIDERATIONS IN PREGNANCY

Genetic counseling may be appropriate for women with hereditary disorders. Melasma in pregnancy is best treated by avoiding excessive exposure to the sun. Other common changes during pregnancy are darkening of the nipples, areolae, external genitalia, and sometimes the axillae and inner thighs. The linea alba becomes darkened and is then termed the *linea nigra*. Existing moles and freckles may darken. These changes partially or completely regress once pregnancy is completed. Increases in levels of estrogen, progesterone, melanocyte-stimulating hormone, and adrenocorticotropic hormone are probably responsible for the changes.

Topical formulations containing tretinoin should not be used by pregnant women. All unessential interventions should be avoided during pregnancy.

If it is uncertain whether an existing mole is undergoing a malignant change, it is best to excise it.

BIBLIOGRAPHY

Alley E, Green R, Schuchter L. Cutaneous toxicities of cancer therapy. *Curr Opin Oncol* 2002;14:212–216.

Bolognia JL, Pawelek JM. Biology of hypopigmentation. *J Am Acad Dermatol* 1988; 19:217.

Fulk CS. Primary disorders of hyperpigmentation. *J Am Acad Dermatol* 1984;10:1.

Grimes PE, Soriano T, Dytoc MT. Topical tacrolimus for repigmentation of vitiligo. *J Am Acad Dermatol* 2002;47:789–791.

Mosher DB, Fitzpatrick TB, Ortonne JP, et al. Hypomelanoses and hypermelanoses. In: Freedberg IM, Eisen AZ, Wolff K, et al., eds. *Fitzpatrick's dermatology in general medicine*. New York: McGraw-Hill, 1999:945–1018.

Pandya AG, Guevara IL. Disorders of hyperpigmentation. *Dermatol Clin* 2000; 18:91–98.

CHAPTER 134
Acne

Anita S. Pakula

Acne is the most common skin disease treated by physicians. Although it is most prevalent in adolescents, it may either persist into or initially present in adulthood. The pathogenesis of acne is multifactorial and involves hormonally induced excessive production of sebum, abnormal follicular keratinization, proliferation of *Propionibacterium acnes*, and inflammation, which is modulated by the host immune system. The clinical presentation ranges from noninflammatory comedones to inflammatory papules, pustules, nodules, and cysts that may result in permanent scarring. With as many as 30% of women in their 30s, 20% of women in their 40s, and 8% of women in their 50s having acne to some degree, the chronic nature of this disease and its psychosocial effect on the patient must not be ignored. The goals of treatment are to limit the duration and degree of disease and to prevent scarring—hence, to minimize the psychosocial consequences. Various therapeutic modalities are directed toward specific pathogenic factors. A successful treatment regimen can be devised based on an understanding of the polygenic and multifactorial nature of this disease and good communication with the patient.

PATHOGENESIS

Acne vulgaris is a disorder of the sebaceous follicles, which consist of large sebaceous glands and miniature hairs. The concentration of sebaceous follicles is highest on the face, back, and chest. The four key pathogenic factors of acne vulgaris are androgen-induced production of sebum, abnormal keratinization and desquamation of the sebaceous follicle epithelium (comedogenesis), proliferation of *P. acnes*, and inflammation.

Sebum Production

The sebaceous glands are androgen-dependent appendages of the hair follicles. They secrete lipids to lubricate the skin and hair and contain enzymes for the peripheral metabolism of androgens. The increased production of androgenic hormones during puberty appears to cause the sebaceous glands to enlarge and increase the production of sebum. The serum level of dehydroepiandrosterone sulfate (DHEA-S) rises in adrenarche and appears to be the earliest marker for the development of acne. Androgens may also decrease the concentration of linoleic acid in the sebum of persons with acne, contributing to retention hyperkeratosis and obstruction of the pilosebaceous ducts.

Comedogenesis

Abnormal keratinization of the sebaceous and follicular ducts causes the epithelial cells lining the ducts to become more cohesive and form a plug that blocks the follicular orifice. This process is referred to as *retention hyperkeratosis and comedogenesis*. The result is the formation of a microcomedo, the precursor lesion of acne.

Propionibacterium acnes Proliferation and Inflammation

The combination of excessive sebum and the anaerobic environment in the plugged follicles results in the proliferation of the anaerobic diphtheroid *P. acnes*. These bacteria trigger immune and nonimmune inflammatory reactions that further damage the follicular epithelium. *P. acnes* organisms produce lipases that hydrolyze the triglycerides of sebum into irritating free fatty acids. They also release chemotactic factors that attract neutrophils, which in turn release hydrolytic enzymes that damage the follicular wall, allowing leakage into the dermis. This process results in further inflammation and irritation.

HISTORY AND PHYSICAL EXAMINATION

A complete history should include inquiry into menstrual irregularities, medication and cosmetic use, pregnancy status, and any family history of acne and endocrine disorders. The physical examination should address the location, type, severity, and complications, such as scarring, of the acne. In addition, signs of androgen excess, such as hirsutism, androgenic alopecia, and obesity, should be noted. If an underlying androgenic disorder, such as polycystic ovarian syndrome, Cushing syndrome, or late-onset congenital adrenal hyperplasia, is suspected, then appropriate laboratory studies should be obtained.

No method for grading the severity of acne is uniformly accepted, but the classification should take into account the morphology, distribution, complications, response to therapy, and effect of the disease on the patient. Acne should be classified by the predominant type of lesion, such as comedo, papulopustule, or nodule, and then graded as mild, moderate, or severe.

TABLE 134.1. Drugs that Cause or Exacerbate Acne or an Acneiform Eruption

ACTH	Lithium
Anabolic steroids	Phenytoin
Azathioprine	Progestins (oral and implanted)
Chloral hydrate	Quinine
Corticosteroids	Rifampin
Cyclosporine	Stanozolol
Dantrolene	Testosterone
Disulfiram	Thiouracil
Halides	Thiourea
Halothane	Vitamins B_1, B_6, B_{12} (high doses)
Isoniazid	

ACTH, adrenocorticotropic hormone.

CLINICAL MANIFESTATIONS

Acne lesions can be categorized as either noninflammatory or inflammatory. Noninflammatory lesions consist of open and closed comedones. The accumulation of sebum results in the formation of a closed comedo, or whitehead. The open comedo, or blackhead, develops as a consequence of continued distention of the follicular orifice, which results in dilation and protrusion of the keratinous plug. The dark color of a blackhead is caused by melanin, not dirt. Usually, this keratinous material is sloughed without inflammation unless the lesion is traumatized.

The inflammatory lesions consist of papules, pustules, and nodules. When the follicular wall ruptures superficially, an inflamed pustule develops. Pustules have a visible central core of purulent material. Deeper rupture of the follicular wall results in a papule or nodule. Papules are inflammatory lesions measuring less than 5 mm; nodules are inflammatory lesions measuring more than 5 mm. True cysts are lined by epithelium and are the rare residua of healed pustules or nodules.

DIFFERENTIAL DIAGNOSIS

Acne rosacea is a chronic disorder of vascular hyperreactivity that more commonly affects adults between 30 and 60 years of age. A history of recurrent facial flushing is usually obtained. Comedones are usually absent, but pustules, papules, and nodules with a predilection for the nose, cheeks, and chin are common. Persistent erythema, telangiectases, and, less commonly in women, rhinophyma may result. Perioral dermatitis often occurs in younger patients and is characterized by erythema, slight scaling, and papulopustules in a perioral, perinasal, and at times periorbital distribution. Topical corticosteroids may aggravate or uncover this condition in predisposed persons. Oral antibiotics, particularly the tetracyclines and topical metronidazole (Noritate cream and MetroCream), are effective. Avoidance of stimuli that provoke flushing, such as alcohol, hot or spicy foods, and ultraviolet light, is important.

Acne cosmetica results from the frequent use of cosmetics containing lanolin, petrolatum, lauryl alcohol, butyl stearate, vegetable oils, and oleic acid. The acne is usually of the closed comedo type. Pomade acne is a form of acne cosmetica that occurs most frequently in African-Americans who use pomades or oils on their scalp and face that result in the formation of numerous comedones.

Occupational acne may occur in workers exposed to chlorinated hydrocarbons, cutting oils, coal tar derivatives, and animal and vegetable oils.

Acne mechanica occurs at sites of repeated trauma or friction. Acne lesions that develop under helmets, chin straps, bra straps, football shoulder pads, and headbands are examples.

Drug-induced acne may result from injury to the follicular epithelium; the follicular contents spill into the dermis and cause an inflammatory response. Many drugs have been reported to cause or exacerbate acne (Table 134.1). Acne may also be caused by oral contraceptives or implants containing androgenic progestins. Systemic corticosteroids may cause a folliculitis consisting of monomorphous papules on the upper trunk, arms, neck, and face.

Pyoderma faciale is an uncommon form of acne, possibly related to rosacea, that typically develops in women between the ages of 20 and 40 years; it is characterized by the rapid onset of numerous tender papules, pustules, and nodules localized to the face. Abscess formation and a reddish discoloration of the involved areas are common, as is extensive scarring.

Acne excoriée des jeunes filles is the term used to describe patients who excoriate or manipulate their acne lesions. It is most common in adolescent girls and may be a manifestation of underlying emotional stress or obsessive-compulsive disorder.

Hidradenitis suppurativa is a chronic disease in which deep inflammatory nodules, cysts, and sinus tracts develop in the axilla, groin, and perianal area. Women are more frequently affected than men.

TREATMENT

The selection of therapy should take into account the type and severity of the acne lesions. The patient must be reminded that it takes several weeks for improvement to be noted, and that maximal efficacy of the treatment may not become apparent for at least 2 to 3 months. Topical treatment should be applied to acne-prone areas, not just individual lesions. A list of the topical agents used in the treatment of acne appears in Table 134.2.

Noninflammatory Acne

Mild comedo acne may respond to over-the-counter products, which generally contain 1% to 2% salicylic acid or benzoyl peroxide in concentrations of 2.5%, 5%, or 10%. Benzoyl peroxide

TABLE 134.2. Topical Therapy for Acne

Adapalene 0.1% gel or cream (Differin)
Azelaic acid 20% (Azelex, Finevin)
Benzoyl peroxide (2.5%, 4%, 5%, 8%, 10%)
Benzoyl peroxide 5%-clindamycin 1% (BenzaClin gel, Duac gel)
Benzoyl peroxide 5%-erythromycin 3% (Benzamycin gel)
Benzoyl peroxide-sulfur (Sulfoxyl Regular and Sulfoxyl Strong lotion)
α-Hydroxy acids
Resorcinol
Resorcinol-sulfur
Salicylic acid
Sulfacetamide-sulfur (Sulfacet)
Tazarotene 0.05% and 0.1% gel (Tazorac)
Tretinoin
Topical antibiotics
Clindamycin
Erythromycin
Erythromycin-zinc (Theramycin Z)
Metronidazole (MetroGel, MetroCream, MetroLotion, Noritate)

shows bactericidal activity against *P. acnes* and is mildly comedolytic. The aqueous gels are generally better tolerated than compounds prepared in an alcohol and acetone vehicle. The gel form is usually more effective than soaps, washes, and lotions but tends to be more irritating. An irritant dermatitis manifested by erythema and peeling is common and can often be circumvented by starting treatment at a lower concentration. Contact sensitivity develops in about 1% of patients. The use of benzoyl peroxide during pregnancy has not been fully evaluated, and it is classified as a category C drug.

Moderate to severe comedo acne may benefit from the addition of the keratolytic agent tretinoin at bedtime. Tretinoin is available in a cream base at concentrations of 0.025%, 0.05%, and 0.1%. Therapy should be started with the 0.025% cream; the concentration is gradually increased as tolerated. For the patient with very oily skin, gel formulations at concentrations of 0.01% and 0.025% are available. A newer microsphere gel formulation that is available in concentrations of 0.1% and 0.04% has the advantage of being less irritating. The patient should be instructed to apply a small amount to the acne-prone areas at bedtime, 20 to 30 minutes after washing her face. Potential side effects include photosensitivity, irritation, and rarely a contact dermatitis. The patient should be warned that a transient pustular flare is common during the first few weeks of therapy. The combination of benzoyl peroxide in the morning and tretinoin at bedtime seems to have a synergistic effect; however, the potential for irritation is increased. Tretinoin may also allow topical antibiotics to penetrate more readily. Alternatively, the newer retinoids—adapalene 0.1% gel or cream and tazarotene 0.05% and 0.1% gel or cream—may be prescribed. These agents appear to be more stable in light and may be less irritating. The topical retinoids also appear to benefit inflammatory acne.

Open comedones can be easily removed with a comedo extractor. Closed comedones require puncture with a small needle or lancet first. Manipulation of inflamed lesions should be avoided.

Inflammatory Acne

Mild inflammatory papular acne benefits from the addition of a topical antibiotic. Choices include erythromycin in a solution, gel, or pad and clindamycin phosphate in a solution, lotion, gel, or pledget. A combination of benzoyl peroxide 5% and erythromycin 3% gel (Benzamycin) or benzoyl peroxide 5% and clindamycin 1% gel (BenzaClin, Duac) appears to result in less bacterial resistance than a topical antibiotic alone. Resistance should be considered if efficacy diminishes. Side effects of topical antibiotics are rare but may include local irritation and pseudomembranous colitis, which has been reported to occur with topical clindamycin.

Azelaic acid cream (Azelex, Finevin) is a newer topical agent for the treatment of mild to moderate inflammatory acne. The mechanism of action is unknown, but it appears to normalize keratinization and to have antimicrobial activity against *P. acnes*. It is applied twice daily, and although interactions with other topical agents have not been reported, it may cause irritation or allergic contact dermatitis and hypopigmentation, so that vigilance is required in patients with a dark complexion. Azelaic acid is classified as a pregnancy category B drug.

Unresponsive or moderate to severe inflammatory acne requires the addition of a systemic antibiotic. Systemic antibiotics decrease bacterial colonization and the concentration of free fatty acids in the sebum, and inflammation is decreased through the inhibition of neutrophil chemotaxis. Tetracycline, erythromycin, sulfonamides, and clindamycin are effective in the treatment of inflammatory acne, and their use is summarized in Table 134.3. Systemic antibiotics must be continued for at least 6 to 8 weeks to establish whether the patient will respond. Routine laboratory testing is generally unnecessary during long-term oral antibiotic therapy in a healthy patient. Systemic antibiotics may decrease the efficacy of oral contraceptives and cause *Candida* vaginitis.

Treatment with tetracycline or erythromycin should be initiated at a dosage of 500 mg twice daily. Tetracycline must be taken 1 hour before or 2 hours after meals. Calcium-containing foods or supplements decrease the absorption of tetracycline. Use of the estolate form of erythromycin during pregnancy has

TABLE 134.3. Summary of Systemic Antibiotic Therapy

Drug	Dosage	Advantages	Disadvantages
Tetracycline	250–1,500 mg/d	Inexpensive	Poor compliance, gastrointestinal upset, pseudotumor cerebri
Doxycycline hyclate	50–200 mg/d	Inexpensive, improved compliance	Increased photosensitivity, esophageal ulceration
Doxycycline monohydrate	50–200 mg/d	Less esophageal irritation	Relatively expensive
Minocycline	50–200 mg/d	Little resistance, little photosensitivity	Expensive, vertigo-like symptoms, rare tooth and skin discoloration, Löffler-like syndrome, drug-induced lupus
Erythromycin	500–1,000 mg/d	Inexpensive	Gastrointestinal upset, frequent resistance (30%)
Trimethoprim-sulfamethoxazole	1–2 double-strength tablets per day	Lipophilic, effective in Gram-negative folliculitis	Bone marrow suppression, drug eruptions
Clindamycin	300–450 mg/d	Effective	Limited to short-term use, pseudomembranous colitis

been associated with maternal hepatotoxicity. Tetracyclines are contraindicated during pregnancy and in children younger than 12 years of age. Doxycycline hyclate or monohydrate can be substituted in dosages of 50 to 100 mg twice daily, but these drugs are more photosensitizing. The incidence of esophageal ulceration is less with the monohydrate form. Minocycline in a dosage of 50 to 100 mg twice daily is less photosensitizing and results in less resistance but may cause ototoxicity, pigmentation of the teeth and skin, hepatotoxicity, and a drug-induced systemic lupus erythematosus-like syndrome.

Gram-negative folliculitis should be suspected in the acne patient on oral antibiotics in whom multiple pustules and nodules emanating from the nasal area develop. A bacterial culture reveals secondary colonization with *Escherichia coli, Klebsiella, Pseudomonas*, or *Proteus* species.

A patient with severe scarring or inflammatory or nodular-cystic acne that fails to respond to oral antibiotics may require referral to a dermatologist for treatment with isotretinoin. Isotretinoin is a synthetic vitamin A derivative that affects keratinization by suppressing the production of sebum and diminishing the growth of *P. acnes*. Its use is limited by the fact that it is a potent teratogen and causes numerous side effects. The usual dosage is 1 mg/kg per day taken in two divided doses. Higher dosages of up to 2 mg/kg per day can be used for patients with back and chest involvement or who have failed an initial course of isotretinoin. The duration of therapy is usually 15 to 20 weeks, with clinical improvement continuing after the medication has been stopped. Relapse is less likely to occur if a dosage of at least 1 mg/kg per day is used or a total cumulative dose of 120 mg/kg is reached. However, cumulative doses of more than 150 mg/kg appear to provide no additional benefit.

Because of the teratogenic effect of the drug, it should be prescribed only to female patients who have used two forms of contraception for at least 1 month before beginning therapy and will continue contraception for 1 month after the completion of therapy. The potential side effects should be discussed verbally with the patient and also presented to her in written form. Written forms are available in a packet supplied by the manufacturer. Baseline laboratory tests, including a complete blood cell count, liver function tests, measurement of cholesterol and triglycerides, urinalysis, and a serum or urinary pregnancy test with a sensitivity of at least 50 mIU/mL (two negative results required) should be obtained before therapy is begun. The patient should be instructed to start therapy on the second or third day of her next normal menstrual period. A transient flare of the acne is common in the first few weeks of therapy; if severe, the administration of systemic corticosteroids may be required. The laboratory tests are then repeated after 2 weeks and at monthly intervals.

The potential side effects of this drug are numerous. Cheilitis and hypertriglyceridemia are common and may be dose-dependent. Depression, photosensitivity, elevated serum liver chemistries, pyoderma, hair loss, proteinuria, hematuria, leukopenia, pseudotumor cerebri, headaches, and decreased night vision are some of the possible complications that should be monitored. Patients should be advised not to wear contact lenses during the course of therapy.

Individual papulonodular or nodular-cystic lesions can be treated with intralesional corticosteroids. The injection of 0.05 to 0.1 mL of 1.0 to 2.5 mg of triamcinolone acetonide diluted in normal saline solution is performed with a 30-gauge needle. Local atrophy and hypopigmentation are potential side effects.

Hormonal Therapy

Female patients who have acne associated with abnormal hormone studies or recalcitrant acne, and those who are not candidates for isotretinoin therapy, may respond to hormonal therapy with estrogens, glucocorticoids, or systemic antiandrogens. The patient should be evaluated for irregular menses and signs of androgen excess, such as seborrhea, hirsutism, and alopecia. Polycystic ovarian syndrome is the most common cause of female androgen excess, but adult-onset congenital adrenal hyperplasia is often overlooked.

Low doses of glucocorticoids, such as 0.125 to 0.5 mg of dexamethasone per day or 2.5 to 5 mg of prednisone per day, suppress adrenal androgen production in women with persistent acne and elevated levels of DHEA-S. Treatment is often combined with an oral contraceptive.

Estrogens, such as ethinyl estradiol or mestranol in a dose of 50 mg or more, suppress sebaceous gland activity, but the potential side effects preclude their use in most female patients. Low doses of estrogens in oral contraceptive pills may relieve acne, particularly in the newer pills, which contain fewer androgenic progestins. Ortho Tri-Cyclen, which contains norgestimate, was the first oral contraceptive to be approved by the Food and Drug Administration for the treatment of acne in women. Several newer oral contraceptives have since shown efficacy in treating acne, including those containing levonorgestrel (Alesse), desogestrel (Desogen, Ortho-Cept), and drosperinone (Yasmin). However, reports suggest an increased incidence of deep vein thrombosis with desogestrel use.

Spironolactone is an aldosterone antagonist with potent antiandrogen effects. It is effective in the treatment of acne at dosages of 50 to 200 mg/d but is not labeled for this indication. Side effects include menstrual irregularities, breast tenderness, decreased blood pressure, headaches, and hyperkalemia. Spironolactone is contraindicated in pregnancy. The problem of menstrual irregularities can be attenuated by the concomitant use of an oral contraceptive pill. Cyproterone acetate is a competitive inhibitor of the androgen receptor and is effective for acne at low doses in combination with estrogens, but it is not approved for use in the United States.

CONSIDERATIONS IN PREGNANCY

Acne may be either exacerbated or mitigated during pregnancy. It may affect the patient's self-image differently during this time, when other bodily changes are occurring. If the patient requests treatment and scarring is possible, treatment should be offered.

Topical erythromycin, clindamycin, or azelaic acid for mild acne and systemic erythromycin for severe acne are acceptable therapies during pregnancy; however, the estolate form of erythromycin must be avoided during pregnancy. Gastrointestinal upset and candidal vulvovaginitis may occur and can be especially difficult to manage during pregnancy.

Physicians treating acne in women of childbearing age, as well as during pregnancy, should be aware of the Food and Drug Administration pregnancy categories of prescribed medications.

BIBLIOGRAPHY

Bickers DR, Saurat JH. Isotretinoin: a state-of-the-art conference. *J Am Acad Dermatol* 2001;45:S125.

Bigby M, Stern RS. Adverse reactions to isotretinoin: a report from the Adverse Drug Reactions Reporting System. *J Am Acad Dermatol* 1988;18:543.

Burkman RT Jr. The role of oral contraceptives in the treatment of hyperandrogenic disorders. *Am J Med* 1995;98[Suppl IA]:130S.

Johnson BA, Nunley JR. Use of systemic agents in the treatment of acne vulgaris. *Am Fam Physician* 2000;62:1823.

Koo J. Psychosocial consequences of acne: implications and treatment options for adolescents and adults. *Cosmetic Dermatol* 1999;12:35.

Krowchuk DP. Treating acne: a practical guide. *Med Clin North Am* 2000;84:811.
Leyden J, Shalita A, Hordinsky M, et al. Efficacy of a low-dose oral contraceptive containing 20 micrograms of ethinyl estradiol and 100 micrograms of levonorgestrel for the treatment of moderate acne: a randomized, placebo-controlled trial. *J Am Acad Dermatol* 2002;47:399.
Lucky AW, Biro FM, Huster GA, et al. Acne vulgaris in premenarchal girls: an early sign of puberty associated with rising levels of dehydroepiandrosterone. *Arch Dermatol* 1994;130:308.
Nguyen QH, Kim AY, Schwartz RA. Management of acne vulgaris. *Am Fam Physician* 1994;50:89.
Pochi PE. The pathogenesis and treatment of acne. *Annu Rev Med* 1990;41:187.
Report of the Consensus of Acne Classification. *J Am Acad Dermatol* 1991;24:495.
Rothman KF, Lucky AW. Acne vulgaris. *Adv Dermatol* 1993;8:347.
Russell JJ. Topical therapy for acne. *Am Fam Physician* 2000;61:357.
Tan JKL, Vasey K, Fung KY. Beliefs and perceptions of patients with acne. *J Am Acad Dermatol* 2001;44:439.
Thiboutot DM. Acne rosacea. *Am Fam Physician* 1994;50:1691.
Thiboutot D. New treatments and therapeutic strategies for acne. *Arch Fam Med* 2000;9:179.
Usatine RP, Quan MA. Pearls in the management of acne: an advanced approach. *Primary Care Clinics in Office Practice* 2000;27:289.

CHAPTER 135
Hair Loss

Gisela Torres and Stephen K. Tyring

Hair loss can occur in any individual at any age. Hair loss is a common cause of significant anxiety for both men and women. Women, like men, experience telogen effluvium hair loss, alopecia areata, or structural changes in their hair caused by acquired abnormalities related to the use of hair cosmetics or grooming procedures. The development of hair loss or hair thinning related to poor nutrition or abnormal thyroid function is also common to both men and women. Permanent loss of hair follicles occurs in both men and women as a consequence of significant inflammation or infiltration of hair follicles with tumor cells or a granulomatous process. Changes in hair have also been reported during and after pregnancy. The most common causes of hair loss with their presentations and treatments are discussed in this chapter.

ANATOMY OF HAIR AND THE HAIR CYCLE

A hair shaft, two surrounding sheaths, and a germinative bulb form the hair follicle. The cells that proliferate to form the hair shaft are present in the hair matrix. The cells begin to differentiate at the top of the bulb, and the inner and outer root sheaths protect and mold the growing hair.

The living cells in the matrix exhibit the fastest mitotic rate of any normal human tissue. They push up into the follicular canal, undergo dehydration, and form the hair shaft, which consists of a dense, hard mass of keratinized cells covered by a sheet of platelike scales, known as the *cuticle*. A hair shaft is thus composed of three layers: An outer cuticle, a cortex, and sometimes an inner medulla. Pigment-containing melanosomes are deposited in the cortical and medullary cells, giving the hair its color. The cuticle protects and holds the cortex cells together.

The hair cycle comprises three stages: Anagen, catagen, and telogen. Anagen is the stage of active growth. Catagen is the transitional phase during which hair growth stops. The final, resting phase of the hair follicle is telogen. During this phase, the hair follicle releases the hair fiber. The shed hairs have a club-shaped appearance, and patients frequently describe them as "falling out by the roots." The duration of each stage varies with hair type and location and can be influenced by many factors. Not all the hair follicles at a particular body site are in the same stage at any one time.

The duration of anagen on the scalp is estimated to be up to 3 years. It determines hair length and is under genetic control. It is estimated that 100,000 hairs are on the scalp, and because 10% to 15% of these hairs may be in telogen at one time, an average daily loss of 100 telogen hairs can be expected.

HISTORY

When patients talk about "hair loss," they are often referring to a variety of hair disorders ranging from normal fluctuations of telogen to hair breakage or thinning to true alopecia. Damage to the structure of the hair shaft results in hair problems about which patients are often concerned. Split ends are the result of damage to the cuticle caused by brushing and mechanical or chemical cosmetic treatments. A reduced diameter of the hair shaft can be caused by systemic diseases and drugs that affect the metabolism of cortex cells in the growing hair. The presentations of various hair diseases also differ, especially between men and women. A careful history of the reported problem is therefore essential to identify and understand the underlying condition.

All patients who present with the chief complaint of hair loss should be asked routine questions to identify a genetic, medical, dietary, or physical explanation for the hair disorder and to determine whether the problem may have more than one cause. Information about the onset of the hair loss (sudden vs. gradual), its distribution, and whether it is associated with too much or too little hair elsewhere on the body may help the clinician to diagnose the hair disease. The concomitant use of medications must be carefully reviewed because many of these affect hair growth and differentiation. The patient's past and current medical history in addition to any family history of hair disease may provide useful information. Hair care procedures and products must be reviewed because they can cause or aggravate hair loss.

ALOPECIA AREATA

Alopecia areata is a nonscarring alopecia characterized by the rapid onset of total hair loss in a sharply defined area, usually round or elliptic (Fig. 135.1). No symptoms are associated, and the disease is most common in children and young adults. Approximately 1% of the population experience an episode of alopecia areata, in which hair is suddenly lost in one or several 1- to 4-cm areas of the scalp, by the age of 50 years. The eyelashes, beard, and rarely other parts of the body may be involved. The skin in these areas is smooth and hairless, or short stubs of hair may be present. The hair shaft in alopecia areata is poorly formed and breaks on reaching the surface.

Alopecia areata may progress, usually in younger persons. The loss of all scalp and facial hair is known as *alopecia totalis; alopecia universalis,* or complete loss of body hair, is the final stage of the disease. Other variants are reticular and diffuse. In the reticular variant, hair is lost in one site as hair spontaneously regrows in another site. In the diffuse variant, long anagen hairs cannot grow in involved areas.

Etiology and Diagnosis

The etiology of alopecia areata remains unknown, but the most accepted hypothesized cause is an autoimmune attack on the

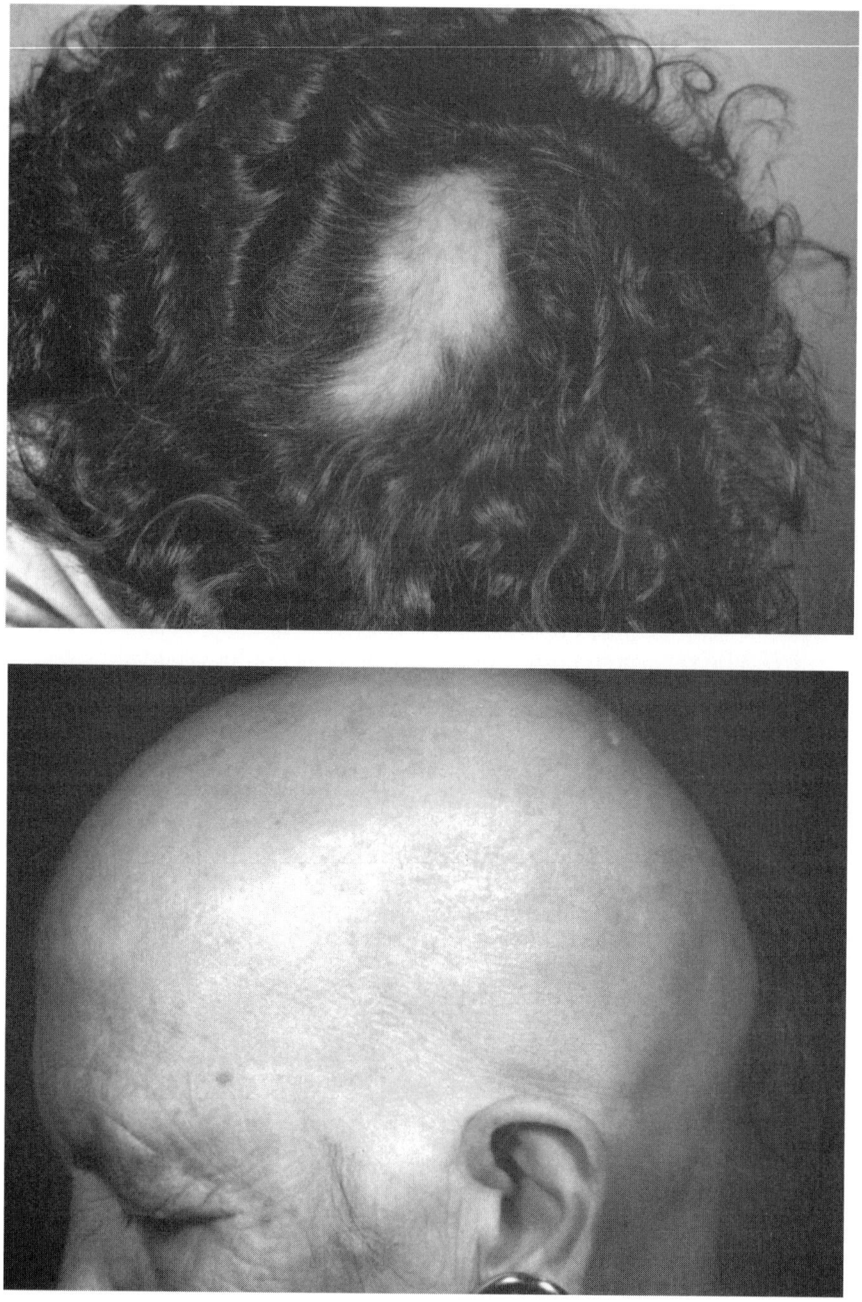

FIG. 135.1. A: Patchy alopecia areata. **B:** Extensive alopecia areata.

hair follicles mediated by T cells. In addition to the general questions asked of all patients presenting with hair loss, patients with alopecia areata should be asked about a history of other autoimmune diseases. In patients with atopy and other autoimmune conditions, such as vitiligo, diabetes, lupus, and rheumatoid arthritis, alopecia areata is generally more severe and lasts longer. Stress is frequently cited as a precipitant, but studies do not support the idea that emotional stress plays a significant role in the pathogenesis of alopecia areata. Alopecia areata appears to be partly controlled by genetic factors, although the lack of a family history does not exclude the diagnosis. Patients with early-onset alopecia areata are those most likely to have a positive family history.

In early active alopecia areata, most hair follicles convert to telogen. The light hair pull test, performed by lightly pulling on several hairs, reveals telogen hairs. Fractured hairs, which appear as black dots on the scalp, may also be seen; these are the distal segments of hairs that fractured as they exited the scalp. Patients in whom normal terminal hair does not regrow may appear totally bald, or the regrowth of short, white, vellus, or indeterminate hair may occur intermittently.

Alopecia areata is usually easy to diagnose clinically. Unusual presentations are more difficult to identify, and scalp biopsy may be needed. The diffuse variant of alopecia areata may be misdiagnosed as trichotillomania, a hair-pulling disorder. In patients with diffuse active hair loss, it may be difficult to differentiate active alopecia areata from telogen effluvium hair loss. The diffuse alopecia of secondary syphilis may also be confused with alopecia areata. Thyroid blood tests are routinely performed in patients with suspected alopecia areata, given the association with autoimmune thyroid disease and the presence of antithyroid antibodies.

Prognosis and Treatment

Regrowth usually begins spontaneously within 1 to 3 months and may be followed by loss in the same or other areas. The prognosis for total permanent regrowth of hair in cases with limited involvement is excellent. The new hair is usually of the same color and texture, although it may be fine and white. Alopecia totalis may be accompanied by cycles of growth and loss, but the prognosis for long-term regrowth is poor.

Many treatments may stimulate hair growth in alopecia areata, but at best they only suppress the underlying process. Hair growth can be stimulated in most cases with an intradermal injection of triamcinolone acetonide (Kenalog) at a concentration of 2.5 to 10 mg/mL. Injections may be repeated every 4 to 6 weeks. Atrophy, especially with the higher doses, is the major side effect. The results in most cases depend on the percentage of scalp involved, and no evidence indicates that intralesional injections of steroids alter the course of the disease. After treatment is discontinued, hair may once again be shed. This treatment should therefore be reserved for patients with a few small areas of hair loss.

When patients with recent-onset alopecia areata and baldness affecting more than 30% of the scalp were given 250 mg of methylprednisolone intravenously twice a day for 3 days successively, the course of the episode of alopecia areata was stopped in most cases. Lower doses of oral and intramuscular steroids restore hair growth, but the hair is lost when the treatment is discontinued. In one study, a 6-week taper of prednisone resulted in 25% regrowth in 30% to 47% of patients with mild to extensive alopecia areata, alopecia totalis, or alopecia universalis, with predictable and transient side effects. A combination with 2% topical minoxidil applied three times daily appeared to help limit hair loss after steroid withdrawal.

Anthralin (1%, 0.5%, 0.25%, or 0.1% Drithocreme) applied once daily in concentrations high enough to induce a visible dermatitis with erythema and mild itching has been reported to induce hair growth. The mechanism of action is unknown, but the treatment is safe and may be considered for refractory cases. Specific scalp preparations of anthralin are available and can be used in place of the cream formulations. Combination therapy with 5% minoxidil and 0.5% anthralin is more effective than treatment with either drug as a single agent.

Both topical and oral methoxsalen in combination with longwave ultraviolet light (UVA) is reported to be successful for some patients, but the relapse rate is high when treatment is stopped. A study of 102 patients concluded that psoralen with ultraviolet light of A wavelength (PUVA) is not an effective treatment for alopecia areata.

Hair growth may be stimulated by inducing a contact allergy at sites of hair loss with compounds such as diphenylcyclopropenone, dinitrochlorobenzene, and squaric acid dibutyl ester. These have been moderately effective therapeutic agents in clinical trials but are not used in routine practice. The use of dinitrochlorobenzene has been discontinued because of its potential carcinogenicity. The most frequent side effects are eczematous reactions with blistering, spreading of the induced contact eczema, and sleep disturbances.

Topical minoxidil in 2% or 5% solution (Rogaine) is approved for the treatment of male pattern baldness. The response in alopecia areata is variable. A combination with steroids and anthralin seems to be more effective. However, minoxidil does not change the course of the disease, and continual use is required to sustain growth.

Topical cyclosporine, oral cyclosporine, oral inosiplex (a synthetic immunomodulator), and topical nitrogen mustard have all been used with some success to treat alopecia areata. Hair weaves and wigs may be used by patients with alopecia totalis or universalis.

Considerations in Pregnancy

All unnecessary drugs, including those prescribed for the therapy of alopecia areata, should be discontinued during pregnancy. Exacerbation and remission of the disease may be seen during pregnancy. Patients with alopecia areata who experience postpartum thyroiditis may also have a flare of alopecia areata.

ANDROGENIC ALOPECIA

The term *androgenic alopecia* refers to the various patterns of hair loss that were originally thought to be mediated by androgen. More recent literature suggests that the mechanisms of patterned hair loss may differ in men and women. In addition, the androgen-dependent path may be only one of several paths causing similar patterned hair loss. Androgenic alopecia is variously termed *diffuse alopecia*, *female pattern alopecia*, and *male pattern baldness*, given the differences in presentation between the genders.

Androgenic Alopecia in Men (Male Pattern Baldness)

Male hair loss is the manifestation of a physiologic change induced by androgens in genetically predisposed men. It is most likely secondary to a polygenic pattern of inheritance. There are two populations of hair follicles on the scalp: androgen-sensitive follicles on the top and androgen-independent follicles on the sides and back. In genetically predisposed men, androgens cause a transformation of the terminal hair follicles and shedding of the terminal hair, which is replaced by fine, light vellus hair.

Hamilton has classified the progression and various patterns of male pattern hair loss. Type I is the triangular frontotemporal recession seen in most young men and some women after puberty. Increased frontotemporal recession accompanied by midfrontal recession is type II. Balding in a round area on the vertex follows, and the density of hair decreases over the top of the scalp (types III–VII).

TREATMENT

The desire of affected persons to undergo treatment varies, and some men opt to accept the hair loss. Medications and several surgical procedures are available for those who seek to remedy the problem. Topical minoxidil in 2% or 5% solution (Rogaine) was approved for the treatment of male pattern baldness in 1988, and the 2% solution is now available over the counter. One milliliter of minoxidil is applied to the scalp twice a day. Minoxidil may stop or retard the progression of male pattern baldness. The best results are in younger men who have been losing hair for less than 5 years and have small areas of partial hair loss on the vertex. In about one third of such men, significant hair growth will occur after 8 to 12 months of treatment. The effect of minoxidil on hair growth in the frontal and temple areas has not been specifically studied. Limited local intolerance and allergic reactions to minoxidil and the vehicle used are the most common side effects.

Finasteride (Propecia), taken daily as a 1-mg tablet, offers a promising alternative for the treatment of male pattern baldness. Finasteride is a specific inhibitor of type II 5α-reductase and decreases serum and scalp dihydrotestosterone. It acts initially to slow the miniaturization of hairs and stimulate hair growth. With continued therapy, the newly grown hairs become longer and thicker. Finasteride has proved safe and effective in men with vertex male pattern hair loss, delaying its progression and promoting hair growth. In men with hair loss in the anterior/mid area of the scalp, 1 mg of finasteride per day slowed hair loss and increased hair growth. Because finasteride is directed at correcting the underlying pathophysiology of androgenic alopecia and the hair cycle is a slow process, its initial effects increase with time. Drug-related adverse sexual experiences have been reported, which clear in men who stop taking finasteride and disappear in most men who continue taking the medication. Mild decreases in serum levels of both prostate-specific antigen and dihydrotestosterone are observed, although testosterone levels are not affected.

Hair weaves are another alternative. Strands of human hair are applied to a thin nylon filament that is anchored to the scalp with the patient's own hair.

Hair transplants have been used successfully for years to restore hair permanently. Androgen-independent hairs from the lateral and posterior areas of the scalp are used. Grafts are first implanted anteriorly to establish a frontal hairline. Subsequent grafts are placed in the affected area. In newer techniques, smaller grafts are used to produce more natural hairlines. More than 300 grafts may be necessary, and several sessions are often required, resulting in higher costs for the patient.

Surgical procedures such as excision of affected scalp can provide an instant hair effect. The procedure can be repeated every 4 weeks until hair margins converge or the scalp tissue becomes too thin. Grafts or flaps may be used later to fill any remaining void. Alternately, several types of flaps can be designed to fill voids. Surgeries and grafts are now often combined with medical treatment (minoxidil or finasteride) to produce better results.

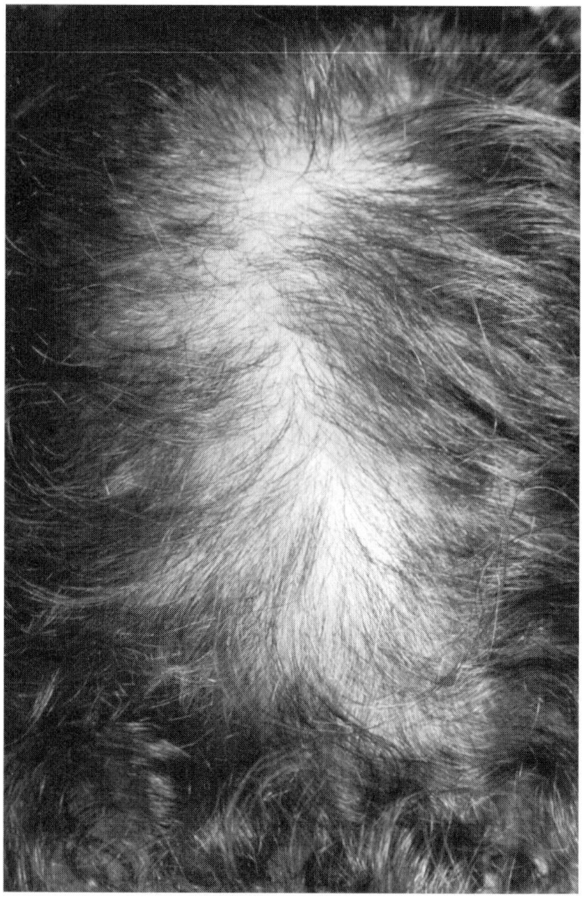

FIG. 135.2. Grade II female androgenic alopecia.

Androgenic Alopecia in Women

The hair loss typical of male pattern baldness hair occurs in women. Unlike their male counterparts, women with androgenic alopecia do not become completely bald. Beyond thinning of the hair, women may notice that their hair is finer in affected areas, and that it will not grow as long. Increased shedding may be observed. In contrast to men, women with androgenic alopecia tend to retain their frontal hairline, presumably because of increased aromatase activity. In the skin of the frontal scalp, aromatase aromatizes testosterone to estradiol, thereby decreasing the amount of dihydrotestosterone, the hormone implicated in the pathogenesis of androgenic alopecia.

Women with patterned hair loss usually complain of being able to see their scalp, and the disease makes them self-conscious. On examination, diffuse thinning over the frontal and parietal areas of the scalp with preservation of the frontal hairline is observed. This is often preceded by a telogen effluvium type of hair loss. The hairs become miniaturized and vary in diameter and length. Androgenic hair loss in women is divided into three stages, described most often by means of Ludwig's classification.

Ludwig grade I is perceptible thinning of the hair on the crown with no loss of the frontal hairline and a relatively normal part width. Ludwig grade II is pronounced thinning of the hair on the crown and an increase in the part width (Fig. 135.2). Ludwig grade III denotes obvious thinning or near-baldness on the crown with an intact hairline.

PATHOGENESIS AND DIAGNOSIS

Androgenic alopecia may develop in a woman at any time after the onset of puberty, although it most often occurs during the perimenopausal period or at times of hormonal change. Most women with patterned hair loss have normal androgen levels despite the fact that androgens may be required for the disease process. Hyperandrogenism, however, may be the cause, and therefore it is necessary to explore the patient's history of menstrual cycles, hirsutism, infertility, galactorrhea, acne, and other signs of hormonal imbalance or pituitary, adrenal, or ovarian disease. The use of specific hormones such as in birth control pills or anabolic steroids, and the use or lack of use of hormone replacement therapy in a postmenopausal woman, are also important.

The most generally accepted genetic hypothesis for this disease is autosomal dominance with incomplete penetrance and polygenic inheritance. Given the variability of this disease, it is likely that androgenic alopecia really comprises several disease entities. Most sources state that 50% of women have some type of patterned hair loss, although some studies state the prevalence to be as high as 87% in premenopausal women.

The diagnosis of androgenic alopecia is based on the history and clinical findings. It is usually considered idiopathic if the patient has no menstrual irregularities, hirsutism, severe acne, infertility, galactorrhea, or history of infertility. However, 30% to 40% of patients do have underlying endocrinologic, adrenal, or ovarian disease. If this is addressed, the hair disease may also be mitigated.

Because hair growth can be affected by thyroid function, testing for thyroid-stimulating hormone, triiodothyronine, and thyroxine should be considered. Iron and protein insufficiency can lead to hair loss and may affect a patient's response to treatment; measurement of the serum ferritin level and total iron-binding capacity and a complete blood cell count, in addition to a dietary history, may thus be warranted. If the patient does not show any signs of androgen imbalance, then sex hormone/androgen testing is irrelevant. However, if any concerning signs or symptoms are present, the levels of free and total testosterone, dehydroepiandrosterone sulfate (DHEA-S), and prolactin should be measured. Subtle abnormalities of the adrenal steroidogenic pathway may also be present; these can be detected only by adrenocorticotropic hormone (ACTH) stimulation tests. Patients with virilization and androgenic alopecia generally do have a significant abnormality of androgen metabolism, and an underlying tumor must be ruled out.

An analysis of vertical and horizontal scalp biopsy samples may be useful. Such an analysis may establish the diagnosis of androgenic alopecia and can provide information about the number of follicular units, the number of hairs in anagen and telogen, and the degree of hair differentiation, information that is helpful in predicting responsiveness to therapy. For example, a patient with significant follicular dropout will probably not respond well to therapy; instead, she may benefit more from a surgical procedure to correct the balding process.

TREATMENT

Finasteride, an inhibitor of 5α-reductase type 2, has been shown to reduce patterned hair loss in men, as previously mentioned. However, it is not as effective in women and may actually result in increased hair loss after therapy is discontinued. It should not be taken by premenopausal women, given its potential effects on fertility and teratogenicity.

Minoxidil is the only drug approved by the Food and Drug Administration for female androgenic alopecia; the topical application of 2% to 5% minoxidil promotes hair growth in women with androgenic alopecia. The recommended dosage is 1 mL twice daily. Hair growth typically peaks at 1 year. When therapy is discontinued, the hair gained is usually lost within 4 to 6 months.

Antiandrogens have been used topically, orally, and intralesionally to retard hair loss and stimulate regrowth of hair. Antiandrogens may inhibit either the conversion of testosterone to dihydrotestosterone by 5α-reductase (finasteride) or dihydrotestosterone binding to the steroid receptor. Estrogens decrease ovarian and adrenal androgen production. Spironolactone decreases testosterone production by the adrenal gland. It affects the cytochrome P-450 enzyme system, which is needed for the 17-hydroxylase and desmolase enzymes to synthesize androgens, but at the same time leads to multiple drug interactions. Spironolactone is also a mild competitive inhibitor of dihydrotestosterone binding to the androgen receptor. In some women with hirsutism, the drug decreases the growth rate and mean diameter of facial hair. Side effects include metrorrhagia, so that spironolactone is generally given with an oral contraceptive pill. Progesterone and 17α-progesterone are competitive inhibitors. However, these agents have an androgenic potential that can potentially aggravate the problem of hair loss.

Other therapies that have been tried include penetration enhancers, such as SEP-A or topical tretinoin together with topical minoxidil. The nonsteroidal drugs flutamide and cimetidine have also been tried, with limited success.

Hair dyes, permanent weaving, sprays, mousses, wigs, and other camouflage techniques can be recommended to the woman with androgenic alopecia. Hair implants and surgical removal of the involved area, as previously outlined, are more expensive alternatives, but the results are often longer-lasting and more satisfying.

CONSIDERATIONS IN PREGNANCY

Antiandrogens and finasteride can affect the fetus or fertility and therefore should not be given to premenopausal women. Antiandrogens can be associated with feminization of the male fetus. All other medications should also be discontinued during pregnancy unless the clinical circumstances indicate otherwise.

TELOGEN EFFLUVIUM

Immediate, short, and delayed anagen and immediate telogen release have been implicated in telogen effluvium hair loss. An abnormally high number of follicles enter the preshedding stage at the same time, resulting in diffuse hair loss and hair thinning (Fig. 135.3A). Patients who experience a telogen effluvium hair loss often report an association with a drug or a history of psychological or physiologic stress, such as surgery, infection, pregnancy/parturition, high fever, chronic disease, or hormonal imbalance.

Delayed anagen release is most often associated with postpartum hair loss, whereas short anagen-telogen effluvium hair loss appears to characterize patients who experience increased shedding with decreased hair length. One factor in the history that may identify delayed telogen release is an increase in hair loss after travel from an area with short hours of daylight to one with long hours of daylight; this finding suggests that in some women, light affects the hair cycle.

Etiology and Diagnosis

The diffuse hair loss seen with telogen effluvium typically affects the entire scalp, but bitemporal recession may become prominent. Typically, a normal hair cycle is resumed after the telogen effluvium process has resolved. Five types of telogen effluvium hair loss have been proposed:

1. Immediate anagen release is very common. Follicles leave anagen prematurely and enter telogen. This may be related to the use of drugs, a high fever, or another physiologic stress.
2. Delayed anagen release is associated with postpartum hair loss. The hair loss usually peaks in the second to third month after delivery.
3. Short anagen is associated with persistent hair loss. Such persons cannot grow long hair.
4. Immediate telogen release is characterized by a shortened normal telogen and initiation of anagen and is thought to be associated with drugs such as minoxidil.
5. In delayed telogen release, hair shedding follows a period of decreased shedding. In some cases, it may occur at predictable times.

The diagnosis is usually determined from the history. The physical examination findings may be relatively unremarkable. Diffuse hair loss occurs primarily on the scalp, but the pubic area and axillae may be involved. In a patient with an active telogen effluvium, the results of light hair pull tests are positive, with more than 50% of the hairs in telogen phase (Fig. 135.3B).

Laboratory Studies

The patient typically presents after the most active hair shedding has occurred. Therefore, most of the tests that are performed easily may not exclude the diagnosis of telogen effluvium because the hair disease may be resolving.

Clip and pull tests may be helpful. A clip test is performed by grasping 25 to 30 hairs between the thumb and forefinger at the scalp. The hair sample is cut with scissors, and hair 1 cm or so above the fingers is cut and discarded. The remaining sample is transferred to a glass slide, held in place with a mounting medium, and then covered with a coverslip. Hair shaft dia-

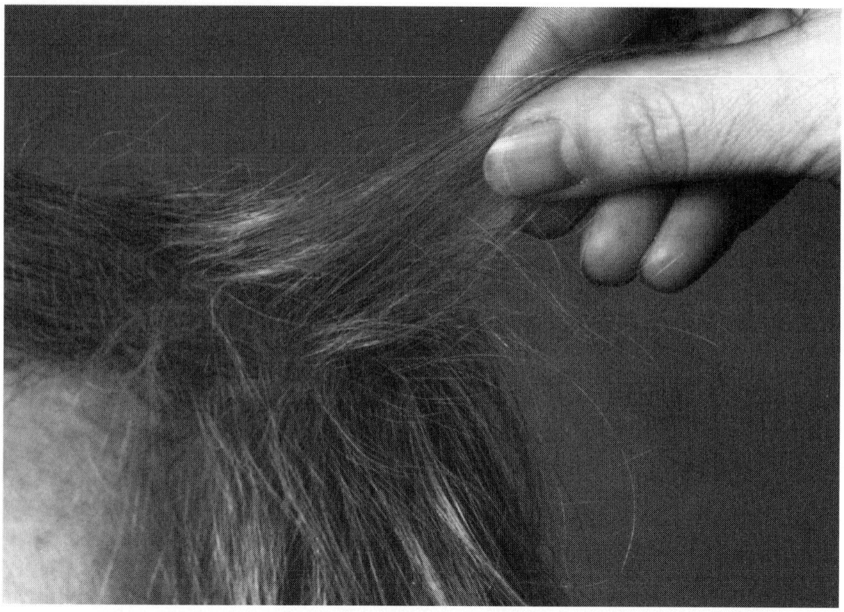

A

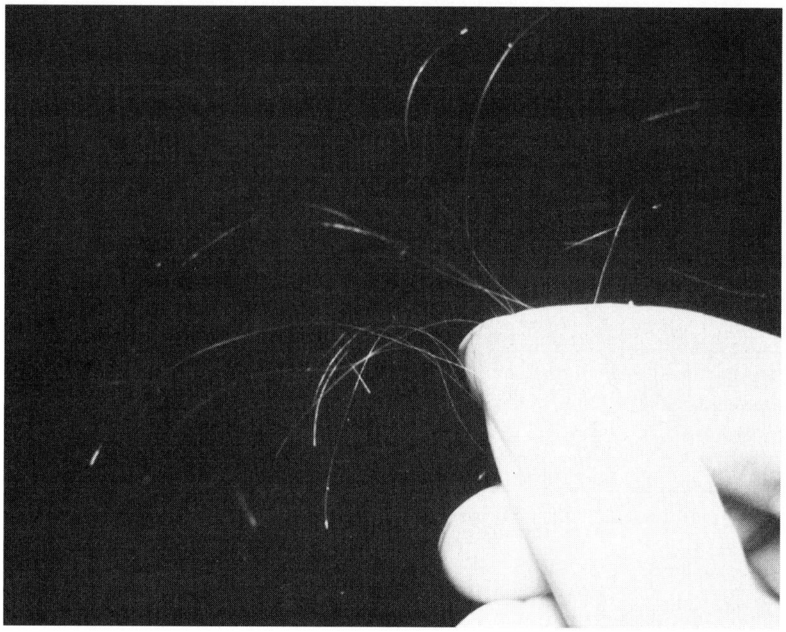

B

FIG. 135.3. A: Patient with telogen effluvium hair loss. **B:** Positive result of light hair pull test in the same patient. A similar result is seen in patients with diffuse, active alopecia areata.

meters are evaluated under the microscope. In a negative test, the hair shafts are of nearly uniform diameter; fewer than 10% of the shafts are of small diameter. In patients with a resolving telogen effluvium, typically more than 10% of the hairs are of small diameter.

Pull tests are performed by grasping 25 to 30 hairs and extracting them from the scalp with the hand or an instrument. In the normal scalp, fewer than five or six telogen hairs are detected.

If the patient presents with diffuse, active hair loss and the result of a light hair pull test is positive, a scalp biopsy (two 4-mm punch biopsy specimens for vertical and horizontal sectioning) is helpful to differentiate telogen effluvium hair loss from active alopecia areata. Establishing the correct diagnosis ensures that the patient will be properly counseled.

Women who are anemic or nutritionally deficient or who have thyroid disease may present with a telogen effluvium hair loss. Therefore, when no insult can be identified by the history, consider a serologic test for syphilis, a thyroid-stimulating hormone test, a complete blood cell count, and basic blood chemistries. The copper and zinc levels could be checked in women thought to have a poor diet.

Treatment

In general, the prognosis for most patients with telogen effluvium is good, and the hair will regrow spontaneously. Cases of seasonal telogen effluvium and immediate anagen release effluvium secondary to drugs or acute-onset physiologic events have the best prognosis. Hair growth after delayed anagen release postpartum is usually reversible, but the hair density may not return to that before pregnancy.

Once the diagnosis has been established, patients must be taught about the hair cycle and advised that hair growth will occur. Hair grows at a rate of about 0.25 mm/d, so some time will pass before the patient sees significant growth. Patients with short anagen syndrome may respond to a drug such as 2% topical minoxidil, which may prolong the anagen stage and allow hair to grow longer. Correcting an underlying abnormality such as iron deficiency may also be associated with a decrease in hair shedding and hair regrowth, but this cannot be guaranteed.

Considerations in Pregnancy

During pregnancy, many women report that their hair appears thicker. It has been suggested that estrogens prolong the anagen stage or that telogen release is delayed because of the need to conserve metabolic resources. If a pregnant woman or woman in the postpartum period notes diffuse hair loss, her iron metabolism, hematologic profile, and thyroid status should be assessed. If the patient is found to be hypothyroid or anemic, replacement therapy can be initiated; hair loss may decrease and regrowth occur.

SCARRING ALOPECIA

Scarring alopecia is caused by the destruction of hair follicles, evident clinically by the obliteration of follicular orifices and histologically by the replacement of hairs with fibrous tissue. Patients with a scarring alopecia who do not have an antecedent history of scalp symptoms, trauma, or infection may have pseudopelade. Others, such as patients with lichen planopilaris, may have an antecedent history of lichen planus. Patients should be questioned about other dermatologic and systemic diseases that may manifest on the scalp as a scarring alopecia.

Etiology and Diagnosis

A hair follicle is permanently lost if it is destroyed by inflammation, either in relation to an infectious process or to a primary skin disease of the scalp, such as lichen planopilaris or discoid lupus erythematous. Similarly, permanent scarring occurs if the hair-bearing area becomes infiltrated with a granulomatous process, such as sarcoidosis, or with tumor cells, as in metastatic disease to the scalp. The same process may occur when lesions of primary systemic amyloidosis involve hair-bearing areas. Recession of the frontal hairline in post-menopausal women, typically a nonscarring alopecia, may in some cases be associated with perifollicular erythema and a frontal fibrosing alopecia. This may be a variant of lichen planopilaris or a unique entity.

Lichen planus of the scalp presents as violaceous papules or as an area of alopecia with follicular plugging. Atrophic, circumscribed patches are associated with hyperkeratotic follicular areas and surrounding scale. In some cases, follicular spinous keratotic papules are present. If the scarring process is chronic, white areas of scalp are apparent and the follicular plugs may be lost, such that biopsy may not be diagnostic at this stage.

Pseudopelade (also known as *follicular degeneration syndrome* when seen in African-Americans or as *folliculitis decalvans* if pustular formation is present) is a central, centrifugal scarring alopecia. Its origin is unknown. Pseudopelade presents with small, glistening white patches of alopecia that resemble footprints in the snow, usually without any associated erythema or scale.

The scarring alopecia called *tufted hair folliculitis* presents with areas of scarring and tufts of hairs emerging from single openings. Patients usually have an associated superficial staphylococcal infection.

Discoid lupus, the most common cause of scarring alopecia, presents with discrete bald patches of follicular plugging with or without erythema and scaling. Eventually, the plugged follicles disappear, and the skin becomes smooth, atrophic, and scarred. Inflammation of the hair follicles leads to follicular destruction in the lesions of discoid lupus erythematosus and permanent hair loss. This scarring alopecia is one of several different forms of hair loss seen in systemic lupus, which may also cause telogen effluvium or anagen effluvium and be associated with alopecia areata. Although the lesions of discoid lupus erythematosus most often develop in patients with systemic disease, discoid lupus erythematosus also occurs in patients who do not have systemic lupus.

In women with postmenopausal frontal fibrosing alopecia of the scalp, prominent frontal and frontoparietal recession is associated with pale, smooth skin. Dermatomyositis (which can cause a diffuse and nonscarring hair loss) and scleroderma have also been reported to result in scarring alopecia.

A scarring alopecia may develop in patients with infectious processes involving the scalp if the infection is not treated. Certain infections cause scarring alopecia when they involve the scalp. Some infections in which cutaneous features are prominent include cutaneous tuberculosis, Hansen disease (leprosy), tertiary syphilis, and leishmaniasis. Eyebrow hair is often lost in leprosy.

Malignancy may also result in scarring alopecia. Infiltration of the skin by metastatic tumors or variants of mycosis fungoides (cutaneous T-cell lymphoma) can result in permanent alopecia. Both physical disruption of the follicular epithelium and the release of chemical mediators from neoplastic cells may precipitate follicular destruction.

Repeated or high doses of radiation and potent regimens of chemotherapy can permanently destroy hair follicles. Scarring alopecia is a common finding in patients with chronic graft versus host disease; the follicular epithelium may be targeted by the immune system, and perifollicular fibrosis may compress and destroy follicles.

Laboratory and Imaging Studies

Hair follicles can be destroyed in many conditions, such as infiltrative and infectious processes and primary diseases of the scalp and hair follicles. A scalp biopsy can help establish the cause of the destruction. If the entire scalp is not scarred and the disease is still active in some hair-bearing areas, it may be useful to take samples from both areas. A 4-mm specimen from a scarred area provides information about the degree of scarring. If few or no follicles are present, the patient may elect to undergo a surgical procedure to remove the scarred areas. In contrast, a specimen taken from an area of active hair loss may provide information about the diagnosis. If an immunobullous disease is suspected, another specimen can be obtained for an immunofluorescence examination. If purulent drainage is noted, the material should be cultured for bacteria and fungi.

Treatment

When *Staphylococcus aureus* is cultured from the skin of patients with inflammatory scalp diseases, antibiotic treatment may have to be continued for many weeks to eradicate the organism. Other infectious diseases associated with scarring alopecias should also be treated promptly to avoid extensive hair loss.

If the scarring alopecia is related to an infiltrative process identified by biopsy, the treatment should be directed toward the underlying process, whether a malignancy or a granulomatous condition. Similarly, if a connective tissue, autoimmune, or blistering disease is identified, the treatment should be directed toward the primary disease. If the primary cause of the scarring alopecia is physical and the result of an injury, such as a burn, the affected area can be removed surgically.

Considerations in Pregnancy

Unnecessary treatments should be avoided during pregnancy.

STRUCTURAL HAIR ABNORMALITIES AND HAIR LOSS

Structural hair abnormalities may be acquired or inherited, so it is important to ask whether the abnormality has been present from birth. A thorough review of hair care habits is recommended; in either case, some hair care practices may injure hair fibers, particularly fibers that are already abnormal. Questions about sun exposure, hair styling, frequency of shampooing, use of hair care products, and activities such as swimming may help the clinician discern the cause of a structural hair abnormality.

Etiology and Differential Diagnosis

The normal hair shaft comprises three major parts: the cortex, cuticle, and medulla (Fig. 135.4A). The four main types of structural abnormalities are fractures, irregularities, twisting, and presence of extraneous matter. Fractures may be related to a genetic disease, such as monilethrix, or physical or chemical trauma. Irregularities can be seen in both congenital and acquired hair diseases, as can coiling and twisting of the hair fiber. Extraneous matter on the hair shaft may be fungi, bacteria, or lice. A unique acquired abnormality is "bubble hair," in which bubble-like areas in the hair shaft are caused by heat, such as from a hair dryer.

Traction alopecia may result from prolonged tension created in certain hairstyles, such as braids and ponytails. Hair rollers may also cause traction alopecia. This condition is common in

A

B

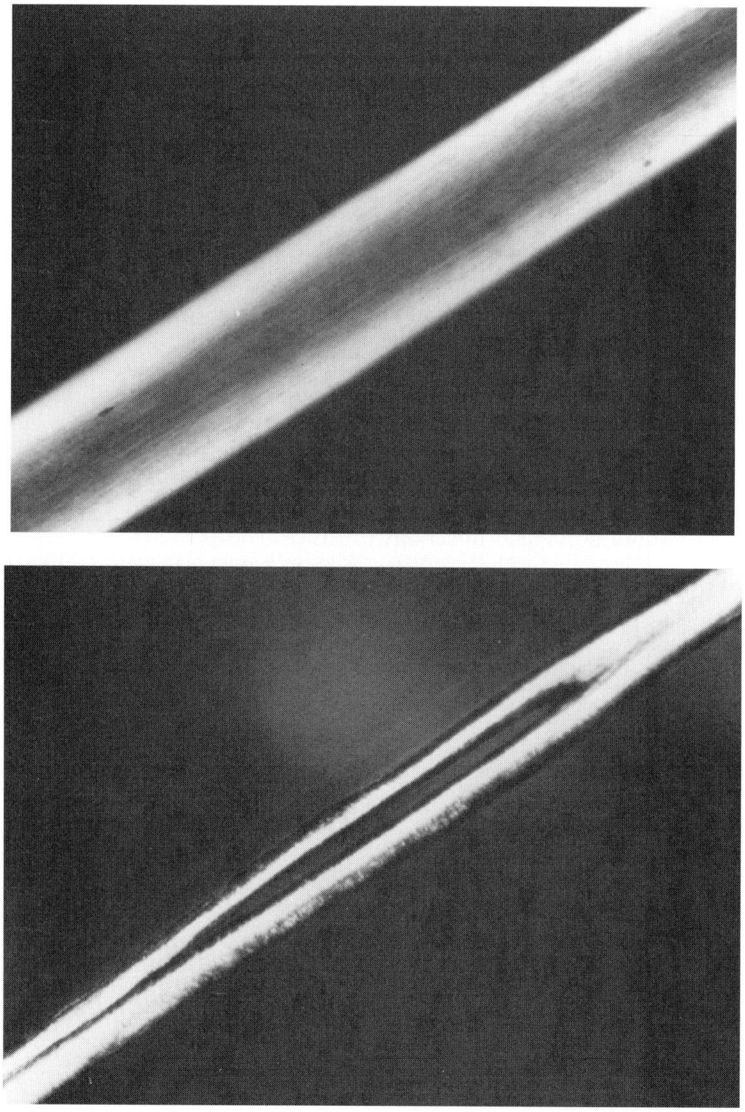

FIG. 135.4. Light microscopic examination of hair mounts from **(A)** a normal person and **(B)** a patient with uncombable hair syndrome.

African-Americans and may result in temporary or, rarely, permanent hair loss in the area exactly where the hair has been stressed. The scalp may appear normal or show evidence of inflammation or scarring.

Physical Examination

Patients may present with short hair and the chief complaint that their hair does not grow. This typically occurs in patients with structural hair abnormalities that result in fractures when the hair is manipulated, as with combing or brushing. Other patients may present with unruly hair related to knotting of the hair, longitudinal grooves, or pili bifurcati. Patients who have short, fine, brittle, dry hair from birth probably have a type of ectodermal dysplasia.

Laboratory and Imaging Studies

To be significant, hair shaft abnormalities should be seen consistently on hairs from different areas of the scalp. Hair samples should be cut at the base of the scalp and mounted in parallel on glass slides previously coated with double-faced clear tape or a mounting medium. The latter provides a permanent preparation that is free of optical distortion when examined microscopically. Scanning electron microscopy may be helpful in further identifying the structural abnormality. Polarization of mounted hairs may demonstrate alternating light and dark bands, characteristic of trichothiodystrophy.

Treatment

When a structural hair abnormality is present, the hair fiber is more prone to breakage and weathering. Therefore, simple measures such as applying conditioners and avoiding the use of hair dryers may help prevent additional damage. For patients with woolly hair or uncombable hair syndrome (Fig. 135.4B), hair-straightening methods may be tried. These can minimize the unruly appearance.

Considerations in Pregnancy

Structural hair abnormalities are usually not affected during pregnancy.

BIBLIOGRAPHY

Chartier MB, Hoss DM, Grant-Kels JM. Approach to the adult female patient with diffuse nonscarring alopecia. *J Am Acad Dermatol* 2002;47:6.

Fanti PA, Tosti A, Bardazzi F, et al. Alopecia areata: a pathologic study of nonresponder patients. *Am J Dermatol* 1994;16:167.

Headington JT. Telogen effluvium. *Arch Dermatol* 1993;129:356.

Hordinsky M. Alopecia areata. In: Olsen ED, ed. *Disorders of hair growth*. New York: McGraw-Hill, 1994:195.

Leyden J, et al. Finasteride in the treatment of men with frontal male pattern hair loss. *J Am Acad Dermatol* 1999;40:6.

Kossard S. Postmenopausal frontal fibrosing alopecia. *Arch Dermatol* 1994;130:770.

Maffei C, Fossati A, Rinaldi F, et al. Personality disorders and psychopathologic symptoms in patients with androgenic alopecia. *Arch Dermatol* 1994;130:868.

Moyes AL, Hordinsky MK, Holland E. Ectodermal dysplasias. *Diseases of the eye and skin*. New York: Lippincott Williams & Wilkins (in press).

Nayar M, Schomberg K, Dawber RPR, et al. A clinicopathological study of scarring alopecia. *Br J Dermatol* 1993;128:533.

Olsen E. Androgenic alopecia. In: Olsen ED, ed. *Disorders of hair growth*. New York: McGraw-Hill, 1994:257.

Rushton DH, Ramsay ID, James KC, et al. Biochemical and trichological characterization of diffuse alopecia in women. *Br J Dermatol* 1990;123:187.

Sawaya ME, Hordinsky MK. The antiandrogens. *Dermatol Clin* 1993;11:65.

Sawaya ME, Shapiro J. Androgenic alopecia: new approved and unapproved treatments. *Dermatol Clin* 2000;18:1.

Sperling LC. Hair and systematic disease. *Dermatol Clin* 2001;19:4.

Whiting DA. Structural abnormalities of the hair shaft. *J Am Acad Dermatol* 1987;16:1.

CHAPTER 136
Dermatitis

Christopher M. Hull and Douglas L. Powell

The term *dermatitis* is used to describe a group of inflammatory skin conditions with primary features of pruritus and cutaneous reactivity. *Dermatitis* is a descriptive term, not a specific disease, that should be reserved for describing a complex of symptoms that includes itching, burning, redness, papules, vesicles, crusting in the acute phases, and thickened plaques with accentuated skin markings (lichenification) and scaling in the chronic phases. Several diseases may be associated with dermatitic lesions, including atopic dermatitis, contact dermatitis, and seborrheic dermatitis. Therefore, dermatitis is better thought of as a reaction pattern to different stimuli and should be used to classify a group of disorders with similar clinical and histologic characteristics.

ATOPIC DERMATITIS

Atopic dermatitis (often termed *eczema*) is a chronic dermatitis characterized by pruritus and cutaneous inflammation. The prevalence of atopic dermatitis is rising, having increased several-fold during the past two decades. Atopic dermatitis is one of the most common skin disorders seen in infants and children, and although the symptoms tend to abate with age, many adults continue to have skin problems ranging from dryness, to sensitive skin, to continuing dermatitis.

Etiology

The pathogenesis of atopic dermatitis is complex and incompletely understood; it appears to be multifactorial, with contributions from genetic and environmental factors. Atopic dermatitis appears primarily in persons who demonstrate immunoglobulin E (IgE)-mediated skin reactions and in whom other allergic (atopic) conditions, such as asthma, allergies, or hay fever, tend to develop. Atopic dermatitis may have a familial basis. Epidemiologic studies demonstrate an increased risk for the development of atopic conditions in children if one or both parents are affected.

The role of allergens, especially foods, in the pathogenesis of atopic dermatitis is controversial. Approximately 10% to 20% of patients with atopic dermatitis exhibit clinically relevant hypersensitivity to food. The most common food allergens are eggs, peanuts, milk, fish, soy, and wheat. These account for two thirds of clinically relevant food allergies in atopic persons. Even if an allergen is detected with formal allergy testing, removing it from the patient's diet does not necessarily relieve the dermatitis. Therefore, routine testing for food allergies is not recommended.

Physical Examination

Atopic dermatitis evolves from the characteristic acute inflammatory dermatitis of children to a chronic lichenified dermatitis in older patients. The sites of predilection vary with age. In infants, involvement tends to be diffuse and includes the face and scalp. A predilection for the extensor surfaces (elbows, knees) is noted in children during the crawling stage. The diaper area is usually spared. In toddlers and older children, the flexor surfaces (antecubital and popliteal fossae, neck, wrists, ankles), hands, and feet tend to be involved with dermatitis. In adolescents and adults, the flexor surfaces, hands, and feet are also involved, but the lesions are generally more chronic and lichenified. The hallmark at all ages is pruritus. Several secondary changes occur in the skin, including lichenification, xerosis, excoriation, and weeping, and secondary infections develop.

Differential Diagnosis

The diagnosis of atopic dermatitis is usually straightforward, although other inflammatory skin conditions can resemble atopic dermatitis. The differential diagnosis includes seborrheic dermatitis, superficial fungal infections, contact dermatitis, tinea versicolor, stasis dermatitis, hyperimmunoglobulin E syndrome, necrolytic migratory erythema, drug eruptions, parapsoriasis, psoriasis, and early-stage mycosis fungoides. In children, rare diseases presenting with dermatitic lesions include Wiskott-Aldrich syndrome, Shwachman syndrome, histiocytosis X, and acrodermatitis enteropathica.

Laboratory Studies

The results of laboratory studies, including scratch and intradermal tests, do not correlate with exacerbation of disease. The same is true for radioallergosorbent testing (RAST). The levels of IgE and eosinophils may be elevated, but it is not necessary to test these parameters routinely for a diagnosis. If secondary infection is suspected, appropriate confirmatory tests (e.g., potassium hydroxide preparation and fungal, viral, or bacterial cultures) should be performed.

POMPHOLYX (DYSHIDROTIC DERMATITIS)

Pompholyx (dyshidrotic dermatitis) is a chronic form of vesicular dermatitis affecting the palms and soles.

Etiology

The etiology of pompholyx is unknown. Atopy may predispose patients to pompholyx because 50% of affected persons have atopic dermatitis. Emotional stress and exogenous factors, such as seasonal changes, hot or cold temperatures, humidity, exposure to nickel, and dermatophyte infections, may trigger episodes.

Physical Examination

The vesicles are deep-seated and have a tapioca-like appearance without surrounding erythema. On occasion, the vesicles may become confluent and form bullae. The blisters typically resolve without rupturing; desquamation follows. Episodes usually last 3 to 4 weeks and tend to recur.

Differential Diagnosis

The differential diagnosis of pompholyx includes contact dermatitis, pustular psoriasis, and superficial fungal infections.

NUMMULAR DERMATITIS

Nummular dermatitis is an inflammatory cutaneous eruption characterized by coin-shaped, dermatitic lesions.

Etiology

The cause of this disease is unknown. However, it is exacerbated by local factors, including excessive bathing, and irritants, such as wool and soaps. Nummular dermatitis is seen more frequently in persons with dry skin and during the winter months. It appears to be a distinct disease entity from atopic dermatitis. It is not associated with other atopic diseases, such as asthma and hay fever, and the serum IgE levels of affected persons are normal. The peak age at onset is 55 to 65 years, and a male predominance is noted.

History and Physical Examination

The lesions begin as small vesicles and papules that enlarge by peripheral extension to form erythematous, coin-shaped lesions with peripheral erosions and crusts. Central clearing may develop creating a configuration resembling that of tinea corporis. Excoriations are often present. Pruritus is variable; it can be severe and lead to significant emotional stress and difficulty sleeping.

Nummular dermatitis generally affects the extensor surfaces of the arms and legs. Involvement of the dorsal aspect of the hands and trunk is variable, and involvement of the face and scalp is unusual.

Differential Diagnosis

The differential diagnosis of nummular dermatitis includes allergic contact dermatitis, atopic dermatitis, superficial fungal infections, and psoriasis. Microscopic examination of a potassium hydroxide preparation of scale scraped from the lesion fails to reveal fungal elements in nummular dermatitis and excludes the diagnosis of tinea corporis. A contact allergen should be suspected when a patient fails to respond to appropriate therapy. Atopic dermatitis is usually associated with a personal or family history of dermatitis, allergies, hay fever, or asthma.

CONTACT DERMATITIS

Contact dermatitis is an inflammatory dermatitis caused by contact of the skin with a substance. The two forms of contact dermatitis are irritant and allergic. Irritant contact dermatitis is a nonimmunologic inflammatory reaction that occurs in nearly all persons exposed to a substance. Allergic contact dermatitis, on the other hand, is an allergic, acquired sensitivity to a substance that develops in a subset of patients previously exposed to the allergen.

Etiology

Allergic contact dermatitis is the consequence of an immunologic type IV delayed hypersensitivity response. In the initial sensitization, an antigen contacts and penetrates the skin; it is then processed by Langerhans cells and presented to T lymphocytes. The T lymphocytes bearing specific receptors for the antigen undergo clonal expansion and then enter the circulation. During the sensitization phase, no reaction develops on the skin. Subsequent exposure of the skin to the antigen leads to the elicitation phase, in which previously sensitized, clonal T lymphocytes interact with the antigen, proliferate, and release inflammatory mediators, with the development of dermatitis at the site of contact. Allergic contact dermatitis generally appears within 24 to 48 hours after exposure to the allergen.

The development of irritant contact dermatitis, on the other hand, requires no previous exposure to an irritating substance; the reaction may occur within minutes or hours after exposure. The primary factors influencing the severity of the reaction include the condition of the skin at the time of exposure, strength or concentration of the irritant, location of the contact, degree of skin moisture, and whether the irritant is occluded/trapped on the skin.

History

Many allergens can cause allergic contact dermatitis. Common ones in the United States include toxicodendron (poison ivy, oak, and sumac), nickel, fragrances, preservatives, neomycin, bacitracin, cosmetics, and rubber compounds. Allergic contact dermatitis is diagnosed based on the characteristic appearance and distribution of the eruption, the identification of potential allergens by the history, and the results of allergy patch testing. The distribution of the reaction can help distinguish allergic contact dermatitis from other forms of dermatitis in that unusual geometric shapes are frequently observed and often localized to one skin area. The distribution of allergic contact dermatitis may help identify its cause. For example, dermatitis on the face may be a reaction to foods, preservatives in cosmetics, chewing gum, hair spray, or shampoo. Dermatitis localized to the feet may result from allergy to rubber products in shoes and elastic stockings. Dermatitis in a V-shaped distribution on the neck, in the periumbilical area, or on the earlobes suggests allergy to nickel in necklaces, pants snaps, or earrings.

Common agents that cause an irritant contact dermatitis include alkalis (e.g., soaps, detergents, and bleaches), acids, antiseptics, certain foods, saliva, urine, and feces.

Physical Examination

Clinically, contact dermatitis presents as pruritic erythematous patches and plaques, with scaling usually localized to the site of contact with the allergen. Vesicles and bullae may be present acutely. On occasion, involvement is widespread, with the development of erythematous pruritic papules distant from the site of contact (auto-eczematization or id reaction). Potent allergens, such as poison ivy, oak, or sumac, cause intensely inflammatory lesions with features of erythema, induration, oozing, crusting, and occasionally blisters. Less potent allergens produce a subacute eruption marked by erythema, scaling, and thickening of the skin. Blisters are unusual in subacute reactions.

In most cases, an allergen can be identified based on the history and physical examination findings. When the allergen cannot be recognized and allergic contact dermatitis is suspected, the patient should be referred to a dermatologist for allergy patch testing. Patch testing is a safe and reliable method in which different allergens are placed on the skin and the tested area is assessed for evidence of dermatitis.

SEBORRHEIC DERMATITIS

Seborrheic dermatitis is a common skin condition, affecting 2% to 5% of the population. The clinical manifestations vary widely. Many investigators think that ordinary dandruff is the mildest expression of seborrheic dermatitis. Flares causing total-body erythroderma represent the other end of the spectrum. Most patients have relatively mild disease, however, and treatment can provide symptomatic relief and satisfactory cosmetic results.

Etiology

It is debated whether seborrheic dermatitis is primarily an inflammatory disorder or whether it is caused by a small lipophilic yeast, *Pityrosporum ovale* (also known as *Malassezia furfur*). Those who think that *P. ovale* is the primary etiologic agent point to studies in HIV-positive patients in which concentrations of *P. ovale* were higher in areas of skin affected by seborrheic dermatitis than in unaffected skin. A response to antifungal agents, particularly topical ketoconazole, favors yeast as the cause. Others question how *P. ovale* can be the primary etiologic agent when it is part of normal skin flora and does not cause disease in most people. Likewise, topical steroids, which are not fungicidal, relieve seborrheic dermatitis without having any direct effect on the yeast. Many who believe that seborrheic dermatitis is primarily an inflammatory disease argue that the proliferation of yeast exacerbates the disease by causing an increased inflammatory response to yeast antigens. Thus, either treatment of the inflammation or treatment directed against *P. ovale* results in clinical improvement.

History

Seborrheic dermatitis is a chronic condition that flares periodically. It is most prevalent in the fourth and fifth decades but can occur during puberty, and a peak of transient disease is noted in infancy. Pruritus of the scalp is common. Burning or stinging may develop in other locations, but often the lesions are asymptomatic and more of a cosmetic concern because the face is frequently involved. Seborrheic dermatitis is very common in patients with Parkinson disease and HIV infection.

Physical Examination

Greasy yellow scales with underlying erythema in well-demarcated plaques are seen on the face and scalp. Frequently affected sites include the scalp, eyebrows, nasolabial folds, and ear canals, areas where the concentration of sebaceous glands is high—hence the name of the disease. Occasionally, the central chest becomes involved, and rarely generalized erythroderma develops. Clues to the diagnosis can be obtained by asking the patient about dandruff, looking carefully in and around the ears, and observing for central facial redness.

Differential Diagnosis

Psoriasis of the scalp is often difficult to distinguish from seborrheic dermatitis; the two frequently overlap, in which case the condition is termed *sebopsoriasis*. Plaques with dry silvery scale are more typical of psoriasis. The distribution and appearance of lesions at other locations on the body provide clues to the correct diagnosis. Contact dermatitis can be another look-alike on the face but is often asymmetric. A thorough history often elicits the cause of contact dermatitis. Tinea capitis must be considered when the usual treatments fail, particularly if scaling is accompanied by hair breakage or alopecia.

Treatment

The first and most important principle of successful management is education. Parents and patients must be counseled about the chronic nature of the disease, the general principles of long-term therapy, and strategies to prevent and modulate trigger factors. The approach to the treatment of dermatitis is multimodal. Management is directed at preventing pruritus, inflammation, and secondary infection. Therapy is with antiinflammatory agents, lubrication of the skin, antipruritic agents, and antimicrobial agents when indicated. Patients must learn how to avoid trigger factors, such as skin irritants, overheating, emotional stress, and known allergens. Such education is critical in helping them to manage these chronic and often frustrating diseases.

Topical corticosteroids have been the mainstay of therapy for dermatitis because of their antiinflammatory, antipruritic, and vasoconstrictive properties. Generally, a medium- to high-potency topical steroid is required at the start of therapy to control acute inflammation except on the face and genital region, where lower-potency steroids that are not fluorinated should be used. After control has been achieved, the strength of the topical steroid can be tapered. Topical steroids should be applied twice daily. Application after bathing helps increase penetration. Ointments provide the best barrier protection and emollient action, and for a given topical steroid molecule, they are generally more potent than cream, gel, or lotion formulations. The use of ointment formulations is recommended for most patients with dermatitis, except in humid environments.

Two topical nonsteroid immunomodulators (0.03% and 0.1% tacrolimus ointment, 1% pimecrolimus cream) have been designed specifically for the treatment of atopic dermatitis and have been shown to be safe and effective nonsteroid topical alternatives. The efficacy profile of these agents is similar to that of medium-potency topical steroids, but they do not cause the adverse effects of cutaneous atrophy, steroid-induced acne, telangiectasia, and striae. They should be applied twice daily and are safe to use on the face, groin, and intertriginous areas.

The most common factor that exacerbates dermatitis is the tendency toward dry skin. Lubricants should be applied to the skin at least twice daily. Application immediately after bathing is recommended. Oil-based products (ointments and heavy creams) are better emollients than water-based ones (light creams and lotions), but the latter are more cosmetically acceptable. Products with fragrance are discouraged.

The control of pruritus is important but often difficult to achieve. Nonsedating antihistamines are commonly used and are somewhat effective. Sedating antihistamines can be useful at night to help patients sleep and control nighttime itching. Topical lotions or sprays containing pramoxine, or menthol and camphor, can also be useful adjunctive agents to help control itching.

The recognition and control of secondary infections is key to the successful management of dermatitis. Patients with dermatitis are easily colonized and infected with *Staphylococcus aureus* organisms and streptococci. Infected areas are typically excoriated, exhibiting golden crusts and at times weeping. Mupirocin cream or ointment can be used for localized secondary infections twice daily until the open areas have healed. More widespread involvement requires systemic antibiotic therapy directed at *S. aureus* and streptococci, generally for a 2-week course. Secondary infection of the skin with herpes simplex virus can complicate atopic dermatitis (eczema herpeticum) and requires systemic antiviral medications.

Systemic corticosteroids should be reserved for extensive, severe dermatitis that is refractory to other treatment measures. They have no role in the daily management of chronic disease because of their many potential side effects. Patients with severe, widespread disease that is difficult to control should be referred to a dermatologist and may require more aggressive therapy, such as ultraviolet light, methotrexate, cyclosporine, azathioprine, or mycophenolate mofetil.

The best treatment for contact dermatitis is recognition of the cause and avoidance of exposure to the specific allergen or irritant. Patients must be educated about the allergen and told about specific products that contain it. Most patch test clinics provide written educational handouts about allergens and potential sources of exposure. Otherwise, treatment is similar to that for other forms of dermatitis.

Seborrheic dermatitis responds well to both antifungal and antiinflammatory agents. The application of low-potency, nonfluorinated topical steroids twice daily works well for flares of seborrhea. Many different shampoos are effective long-term treatments when used twice a week; the suds should be rubbed over affected facial areas before rinsing. Shampoos containing a variety of medications are available, including 1% to 2% ketoconazole, 2.5% selenium sulfide, 1% zinc pyrithione, and sulfur. Patients with markedly thickened scalp scales (sebopsoriasis) can be treated with salicylic acid or coal tar shampoos to remove the scales so that other medications can penetrate more effectively. Combination treatment, such as a topical steroid cream with an antifungal shampoo, is often helpful.

If the condition does not improve with basic treatment or if the diagnosis is uncertain, the patient should be referred to a dermatologist.

CONSIDERATIONS IN PREGNANCY

Little is mentioned in the literature regarding dermatitis in pregnancy; however, because cell-mediated immunity is lessened during pregnancy and corticosteroid levels are raised, changes in the intensity of dermatitis, such as flares or resolution, would not be surprising.

Treatment should be as conservative as possible, focusing on emollients and mild soaps and cleansing agents. The use of topical corticosteroids should be kept to a minimum.

BIBLIOGRAPHY

Berbrant IM, Faergemann J. The role of *Pityrosporum ovale* in seborrheic dermatitis. *Semin Dermatol* 1990;9:262.

Egan CA, Rallis TM, Meadows KP, et al. Low-dose methotrexate treatment for recalcitrant palmoplantar pompholyx. *J Am Acad Dermatol* 1999;40:612–614.

Eichenfield LF, Lucky AW, Boguniewicz M, et al. Safety and efficacy of pimecrolimus cream 1% in the treatment of mild and moderate atopic dermatitis in children and adolescents. *J Am Acad Dermatol* 2002;46:495–504.

Faergemann J. *Pityrosporum* infections. *J Am Acad Dermatol* 1994;31(3 Pt 2):S18.

Hanifin JM, Rajka G. Diagnostic features of atopic dermatitis. *Acta Derm Venereol Suppl* 1980;92:44–47.

Hanifin JM. Atopic dermatitis in infants and children. *Pediatr Clin North Am* 1991;38:763–789.

Hanifin JM. Atopic dermatitis: new therapeutic considerations. *J Am Acad Dermatol* 1991;24:1097.

Hurwitz S. Eczematous eruptions in childhood. *Clinical pediatric dermatology*, 2nd ed. Philadelphia: WB Saunders, 1993:45.

Ive FA. An overview of experience with ketoconazole shampoo. *Br J Clin Pract* 1991;45:279.

Kemmett D, Tidman MJ. The influence of the menstrual cycle and pregnancy on atopic dermatitis. *Br J Dermatol* 1991;125:59.

Kligman AM, Leyden JJ. Seborrheic dermatitis. *Semin Dermatol* 1983;2:57.

Leung DY, Soter NA. Cellular and immunologic mechanisms in atopic dermatitis. *J Am Acad Dermatol* 2001;44:S1–S12.

Leung DY. Atopic dermatitis: new insights and opportunities for therapeutic intervention. *J Allergy Clin Immunol* 2000;105:860–876.

Leung DYM, Tharp M, Boguniewicz M. Atopic dermatitis (atopic eczema). In: Fitzpatrick TB, Freedberg IM, Eisen AZ, et al., eds. *Dermatology in general medicine*, 5th ed. New York: McGraw-Hill, 1999:1464.

Lever R. The role of food in atopic eczema. *J Am Acad Dermatol* 2001;45:S57–S60.

McGrath J, Murphy GM. The control of seborrheic dermatitis and dandruff by antipityrosporal drugs. *Drugs* 1991;41:178.

Nghiem P, Pearson G, Langley RG. Tacrolimus and pimecrolimus: from clever prokaryotes to inhibiting calcineurin and treating atopic dermatitis. *J Am Acad Dermatol* 2002;46:228–241.

Odom RB, James WD, Berger TG, eds. Atopic dermatitis, eczema, and noninfectious immunodeficiency disorders. In: *Andrew's diseases of the skin*, 9th ed. Philadelphia: WB Saunders, 2000:78–80.

Ong PY, Leung DY. Atopic dermatitis. *Clin Allergy Immunol* 2002;16:355–379.

Rietschel RL, Fowler JF, eds. *Fisher's contact dermatitis*, 5th ed. Philadelphia: Lippincott Williams & Wilkins, 2001.

Sheehan MP, Atherton DJ, Norris P, et al. Oral psoralen photochemotherapy in severe childhood atopic eczema: an update. *Br J Dermatol* 1993;129:431.
Soter NA. Nummular eczematous dermatitis. In: Fitzpatrick TB, Freedberg IM, Eisen AZ, et al., eds. *Dermatology in general medicine*, 5th ed. New York: McGraw-Hill, 1999:1480.
Stratigos JD, Antoniou C, Katsambas A, et al. Ketoconazole 2% cream vs. hydrocortisone 1% cream in the treatment of seborrheic dermatitis. *J Am Acad Dermatol* 1988;19(5 Pt 1):850.
Webster G. Seborrheic dermatitis. *Int J Dermatol* 1991;30:843.
Weston WL, Bruckner A. Allergic contact dermatitis. *Pediatr Clin North Am* 2000; 47:897–907.

CHAPTER 137
Psoriasis

Sophie M. Worobec and
Madhuri Ventrapragada

Psoriasis, a chronic skin disease, is believed to affect 0.5% to 3% of Americans, with estimates of annual treatments varying from $600 million to $3.2 billion. The disease is troublesome, causing everyday difficulties associated with itching, disfigurement, and scaliness. It can have detrimental effects on social ease, choice of clothing, and sexual relations. In the United States, some 400 people die annually of complications of psoriasis.

ETIOLOGY

The cutaneous lesions of psoriasis may consist of plaques, guttate (droplike) lesions, localized pustules, widespread pustules, and erythroderma. The disease afflicts genetically predisposed persons and is influenced by multiple genes and a wide range of trigger factors (e.g., drugs, skin injury, infection, stress). A psoriasis susceptibility allele labeled *PSOR1* has been associated with HLA-Cw6. Among monozygotic twins, if one twin is affected, the concordance for psoriasis in the second twin is 65%. Linkage to HLA-Cw6 and HLA-DR7 antigens is strong in persons with psoriasis that develops before the age of 40 years.

On histopathologic examination, psoriatic lesions have a regularly thickened epidermis with retention of epidermal cell nuclei in the stratum corneum (parakeratosis). Often, sterile subcorneal pustules containing polymorphonuclear leukocytes are present. Labeling studies have revealed that psoriatic epidermis is hyperproliferative; the normal epidermal transit time from the basal layer to the surface is reduced from 26 to 4 days.

The proinflammatory cytokine tumor necrosis factor-α (TNF-α) has been identified as an important mediator of this inflammatory and hyperproliferative skin disorder.

DIFFERENTIAL DIAGNOSIS

The differential diagnosis of psoriasis includes lichen planus, nummular eczema, lichen simplex chronicus, seborrheic dermatitis, parapsoriasis, pityriasis rubra pilaris, pityriasis rosea, drug eruptions, cutaneous lupus erythematosus, mycosis fungoides, psoriasiform tertiary syphilis, Reiter syndrome, and congenital ichthyosiform erythroderma. Localized acral pustular psoriasis resembles Bazex syndrome, in which a pustular and scaly acral eruption is an external sign of internal malignancy.

HISTORY

Psoriasis can occur at any age, from infancy until well into old age, but in most cases, the disease develops in young adults. The onset can be slow and insidious, with a few red, scaly papules coalescing into a plaque, or abrupt, with a shower of scattered scaly papules appearing on the trunk and extremities.

Therapeutic drugs associated with the new onset or exacerbation of psoriasis include beta-blockers, lithium, antimalarials, interferons, gemfibrozil, nonsteroidal antiinflammatory agents (phenylbutazone and meclofenamate), and angiotensin-converting enzyme inhibitors (captopril and lisinopril). Fluoxetine (Prozac) has been associated with the development of psoriasis after 6 and 12 months of use, a time frame similar to that observed in lithium-induced psoriasis. Both lithium and fluoxetine modulate serotoninergic function; therefore, a common mechanism may contribute to the induction of psoriatic lesions.

PHYSICAL EXAMINATION AND CLINICAL FINDINGS

Plaque psoriasis, the most common presentation, is characterized by sharply marginated erythematous plaques and papules with a tenacious silvery white scale that if picked off reveals pinpoint bleeding spots (Auspitz sign). The plaques may become confluent and cover large areas of skin. They may also appear annular or arcuate as a consequence of central clearing. The extensor surfaces of the arms and legs, especially the knees and elbows, and the lumbar area are the most common sites of involvement. The thickness of the lesions varies with location; they are usually thicker on body areas that are not folded (arms, legs, knees, elbows, back) and thinner on flexural areas (axilla and groin). Psoriasis lesions on flexural areas also tend to lack scale and are often secondarily colonized with *Candida*. The presence of scalp and nail involvement helps establish a diagnosis of inverse psoriasis. Characteristic nail changes include pitting (punctate), ridging, onycholysis, subungual hyperkeratosis, and nail plate "oil spots" or "salmon patches," which are oval to round areas of pink to reddish brown discoloration.

Guttate psoriasis is characterized by the rapid onset of multiple, small (0.5–1.5 cm), finely scaly, pink to erythematous papules over the trunk and extremities. It may be the original manifestation of psoriasis, often associated with a streptococcal throat infection, or a sign of worsening disease in patients with established plaque psoriasis.

Localized pustular psoriasis (palmoplantar psoriasis, acral pustulosis) occurs as either a sterile pustular eruption of the palms and soles or a pustular eruption of the fingers and toes with nail involvement. The nail plate may be lost, with pustules persisting in the nail bed and paronychial area. The pustules are a cloudy yellow, then turn brown and acquire a hard, keratinized surface.

Generalized pustular psoriasis (von Zumbusch type) is marked by the sudden development of sterile pustules that sometimes appear in successive waves, accompanied by fever, malaise, weakness, peripheral leukocytosis, a raised erythrocyte sedimentation rate, and sometimes hypocalcemia. The pustules may coalesce into lakes of pus or pus-laden annular lesions. Generalized pustular psoriasis may be the initial manifestation of psoriasis or develop in patients with a prior history of psoriatic lesions. A common precipitating factor for generalized pustular psoriasis is the withdrawal of systemic corticosteroid therapy. Therefore, such therapy must be avoided in the treatment of patients with known stable long-term plaque psoriasis or given with great caution to persons with disabling psoriatic arthritis.

An exfoliative or erythrodermic form of psoriasis is characterized by generalized erythema. This rare explosive form usually develops in patients who previously had plaque-type psoriasis. Associated findings may include chills, rigors, and fever secondary to poor temperature regulation; protein loss; fluid and electrolyte imbalances; sepsis; and high-output cardiac failure.

Psoriatic arthritis is more common in patients with erythrodermic, generalized pustular, intertriginous (inverse) psoriasis and in those with nail involvement. This seronegative arthritis, which is usually polyarticular and asymmetric but sometimes monoarticular, can be disabling.

LABORATORY AND IMAGING STUDIES

The history and clinical examination and a skin biopsy (in uncertain cases) establish the diagnosis of psoriasis. Additional skin tissue for direct immunofluorescence studies and serologic antibody studies should be obtained when lupus is included in the differential diagnosis. Syphilis serology may be indicated because luetic lesions are sometimes psoriasiform. A Wood light examination, potassium hydroxide preparation, fungal and bacterial cultures, and Gram stain may be appropriate to diagnose secondary yeast, fungal, or bacterial infections. Severe, explosive psoriasis can be associated with HIV infection. HIV testing should also be performed before immunosuppressive therapy is initiated for severe psoriasis. Elevated uric acid levels and albumin depletion are common in severe psoriasis. Because acral pustulosis and Bazex syndrome are clinically difficult to differentiate, a complete history should be obtained and a physical examination with age-appropriate screening for malignancy performed.

TREATMENT

All treatment approaches are directed at lessening inflammation and epidermal hyperproliferation. Patients are interested in treatments that offer long-term safety and efficacy. Topical treatments include corticosteroids, the vitamin D analogue calcipotriene (Dovonex), coal tar and its derivatives, tazarotene (Tazorac), salicylic acid, and anthralin. Gradual and careful exposure to the sun in the summertime, with care to avoid sunburn (because burns can trigger a Koebner reaction), is helpful for about 85% of psoriatic patients. However, this should not be recommended for those who are at increased risk for skin cancer or photosensitivity. In Israel, climatotherapy (2–4 weeks at the Dead Sea) is a helpful and approved therapy. In the United States, a 308-nm excimer laser has been approved for the treatment of psoriasis and is useful to manage plaques of limited size.

Avoiding skin dryness with the use of emollients and lubricants such as petroleum jelly is useful adjunctive therapy. The prompt treatment of any concurrent infections is essential because they may trigger psoriatic flares. Contact sensitization or irritating topical medications can be a cause of treatment failure, and patch testing can be used to identify this problem.

Major side effects of topical corticosteroids include cutaneous atrophy, folliculitis, and tachyphylaxis; however, they are useful in controlling localized disease. Many patients prefer a cream to an ointment base because it is less greasy and does not soil clothes. However, if thick scale is present, an ointment applied at bedtime may be more effective. Salves should be applied shortly after bathing and patting, not rubbing, the skin dry; the skin should be patted dry because percutaneous absorption is best on hydrated skin. Solutions, gels, lotions, and foams can be used for scalp treatment. The long-term use of high-potency corticosteroids on the scalp or extensive areas of the body can result in adrenal suppression and a cushingoid habitus. Therefore, every attempt should be made to wean patients from superpotent corticosteroids or decrease the frequency of use.

Tar gels and shampoos are available over the counter and help most patients; however, an irritant folliculitis that can develop into a Koebner reaction precludes their use in sensitive patients. Anthralin (Anthraderm, Drithocreme, Dritho-Scalp, Micanol) products are useful and may produce long-term remissions of plaque psoriasis, but irritation and staining of skin or clothing limit their acceptability. Salicylic acid preparations help reduce scale. Tazarotene is the first topical retinoid approved for the treatment of psoriasis and is effective when used once daily. It is available in both gel and cream formulations. Irritation is a possible side effect, and for this reason many dermatologists use it concurrently with a topical corticosteroid.

Calcipotriene ointment or cream applied twice a day is effective in reducing thick psoriatic plaques. It can be used as a first-line alternative to topical steroids or in rotation with topical steroids. Irritation develops in 10% to 17% of users, and patients should apply it sparingly for maximum benefit. The combination of calcipotriene and a topical corticosteroid is more effective than either agent alone. One approach is to use topical calcipotriene on week days and a topical steroid on weekends.

Mild to moderate disease affecting 10% or less of the total surface area can be treated by the primary care physician. Patients with more serious or refractory disease should be referred to a dermatologist. The treating physician must taken into account the patient's fertility status, desire to become pregnant, and pregnancy status when considering treatment options.

Severe psoriasis is treated with phototherapy (ultraviolet light of B [UVB] or A [UVA] wavelength), the Goeckerman regime (UVB and topical coal tar preparations), chemophototherapy with either oral or topical psoralen and UVA (PUVA), oral retinoids, and methotrexate. Broadband UVB has a long safety record and is associated with very little risk for photocarcinogenicity. Narrow band UVB is more effective than broadband UVB and in some studies as effective as PUVA. PUVA is highly effective, but long-term photocarcinogenicity is of concern.

Resistant psoriasis treated with cyclosporine has shown significant improvement. Renal toxicity is a potential side effect. Furthermore, relapse and even generalized pustular flares have occurred within several weeks after discontinuation of therapy.

Alafacept (Amevive) is the first anti–TNF-α therapy to have been granted marketing approval in the United States for the treatment of plaque psoriasis. Psoriatic skin lesions have regressed after a coexisting condition, such as Crohn disease or psoriatic arthritis, was treated with infliximab (Remicade) or etanercept (Enbrel).

Erythroderma psoriasis and generalized pustular psoriasis can be life-threatening, and many affected patients require inpatient management. Major complications include sepsis, electrolyte imbalance, and negative nitrogen balance. The retinoid acitretin (Soriatane) is highly effective in controlling generalized pustular psoriasis. Acitretin trans-esterifies into etretinate, and both of these are major teratogens. Contraception must be continued for at least 3 years after acitretin is discontinued. Etretinate was found in the plasma and subcutaneous fat of one woman (in whom sporadic alcohol intake was reported) 52 months after she had stopped acitretin therapy. Acitretin should be used only by physicians who are experienced in the use of systemic retinoids, understand the risk for teratogenicity, and have special competence in the care of severe psoriasis.

CONSIDERATIONS IN PREGNANCY

Psoriasis is twice as likely to remit than to worsen during pregnancy. In the survey of Dunna and Finlay of 65 women who had at least one pregnancy after the onset of psoriasis, the condition of most improved gradually during pregnancy but worsened again within 3 months after delivery. The same was true of psoriatic arthritis. These remissions are a consequence of higher levels of endogenous corticosteroids and endogenous interleukin-10 during pregnancy.

Many therapies are contraindicated in pregnancy (e.g., retinoids, methotrexate). Others, such as the corticosteroids, can have long-term effects that are still not fully investigated, such as the development of diabetes and hypertension in adolescence.

Generalized pustular psoriasis occurs very rarely during pregnancy and may be life-threatening. In the past, it was given the misnomer *impetigo herpetiformis*. It usually appears in the second half of pregnancy, and only one third of affected patients have a prior clinical history of psoriasis. The cutaneous eruption consists of expanding symmetric red patches that usually start in the flexures (groin, axilla, neck). Grouped pustules form at the margins; old pustules within the margin form crusts or undergo impetiginization. Erosive lesions may develop in the mucous membranes. The eruption is associated with fever, chills, asthenia, nausea, vomiting, diarrhea, low serum levels of vitamin D, and hypocalcemia. Neurologic disturbances such as confusion and convulsions were more common in the past and were probably a consequence of untreated hypocalcemia. Fetal death occurs in half of cases. The disease disappears in the postpartum period, but the risk for recurrence is increased during subsequent pregnancies.

The histopathology of the cutaneous lesions is that of pustular psoriasis. The results of direct immunofluorescence studies of skin tissue are negative. High white cell counts and sedimentation rates are common. Infection must be ruled out in the presence of fever. The intact pustules are sterile, but broken skin may become secondarily infected. The serum calcium and albumin levels should be followed, and if low, therapeutic replacement is indicated.

Prednisone in doses of up to 60 mg/d has been used to control the eruption, but it must be tapered slowly because too-sudden lowering may result in a flare-up. Placental insufficiency and stillbirth may occur even when the disease is controlled by corticosteroids. Parenteral calcium with vitamin D may be needed. Cyclosporine at doses of 4 to 5 mg/kg per day has been used successfully. It is necessary to monitor and treat any secondary cutaneous or systemic infection. Postpartum treatment with retinoids or PUVA has been reported.

BIBLIOGRAPHY

Dunna SF, Finlay AY. Psoriasis: improvement during and worsening after pregnancy. *Br J Dermatol* 1989;120:584.

Elder JT, Nair RP, Henseler T, et al. The genetics of psoriasis 2001: the odyssey continues. *Arch Dermatol* 2001;137:1447–1454.

Hemlock C, Rosenthal JS, Winston A. Fluoxetine-induced psoriasis. *Ann Pharmacother* 1992;26:211.

Javitz HS, Ward MM, Farber E, et al. The direct cost of care for psoriasis and psoriatic arthritis in the United States. *J Am Acad Dermatol* 2002;46:850–860.

Kroumpouzos G, Cohen LM. Dermatoses of pregnancy. *J Am Acad Dermatol* 2001;45:1–19.

Krueger JG. The immunologic basis for the treatment of psoriasis with new biologic agents. *J Am Acad Dermatol* 2002;46:1–23.

Lebwohl MG. Psoriasis. In: Lebwohl MG, Heymann WR, Berth-Jones J, Coulson I, eds. *Treatment of skin disease: comprehensive therapeutic strategies.* London: Mosby, 2002:533–543.

Peters BP, Weissman FG, Gill MA. Pathophysiology and treatment of psoriasis. *Am J Health Syst Pharm* 2000;57:645–662.

CHAPTER 138
Stasis Skin Changes and Disorders

Sophie M. Worobec

Chronic venous insufficiency usually occurs as a result of incompetent valvular function in the deep venous channels of the lower limbs and in the perforating veins connecting the superficial and deep venous systems. Stasis dermatitis, ulcers, and other changes are the consequences of chronic venous insufficiency. The incidence of leg and foot ulcers increases greatly with age, with venous ulceration occurring in 1% to 4% of people older than 70 years of age.

ETIOLOGY AND DIFFERENTIAL DIAGNOSIS

The venous vasculature of the lower extremities consists of the deep venous system, located within the muscular system, and the superficial system, which lies above the muscle groups. About 90% of venous return is through the deep venous system, which is subject to muscular compression. Ideally, the deep veins draw blood from the superficial system, which drains the skin venules. The contraction of calf muscles can generate a pressure of 200 to 300 mm Hg, which normally is transmitted to the deep venous system. The pressure in the superficial venous system of the lower extremities is lower than that in the deep venous system. Valves within the deep veins and perforator veins (connecting the deep and superficial venous systems) prevent the higher pressure from being transmitted to the superficial veins. In venous insufficiency, valvular dysfunction allows retrograde blood flow (up to 25% of total femoral flow) and the transmission of high pressure into the superficial veins. This pressure is then transmitted to the capillary beds of the skin and subcutaneous tissue. As a result, the endothelial pores widen, and fibrinogen molecules exude into the extracellular fluid and form fibrin complexes around the capillaries. A diffusion barrier is thus formed to oxygen and the other nutrients necessary for the healthy function of the skin and subcutaneous tissue. Decreased fibrinolytic activity and increased collagen synthesis have also been demonstrated in sclerotic areas associated with long-term stasis.

Venous insufficiency can be secondary to deep vein thrombosis (DVT), which blocks the proximal flow of blood in the deep venous system, but most patients do not have a definite clinical history of DVT or phlebitis. The incidence of venous insufficiency increases with age and the number of pregnancies. Edema of the lower legs is common. Other causes of edema include neoplastic obstruction of the pelvic veins, congenital or acquired vascular malformations of the venous or lymphatic systems, cardiac failure, and renal disease.

HISTORY

Chronic venous insufficiency is first characterized by edema of the lower legs, then by secondary changes of the skin and subcutaneous tissue. The patient may have a history of one or more episodes of phlebitis associated with pregnancy, prolonged bed rest, or trauma. Symptoms include a persistent dull ache that worsens at the end of a long period of standing or sitting with the legs in a dependent position. Stasis dermatitis manifests as pruritic eczematous changes. Leg trauma can cause bleeding of superficial varicosities.

PHYSICAL EXAMINATION AND CLINICAL FINDINGS

The earliest change of venous insufficiency, edema, is at first mild and noticeable only at the end of the day. Gradually, it worsens and is accompanied by a mild erythema, pinpoint petechiae, and the brownish pigmentation of hemosiderin deposits left by extravasated red blood cells. The skin may become thin and shiny as the edema progresses. The sites involved include the medial ankle, the dorsa of the feet (where shoe compression stops), and gradually the entire lower legs and ankles. As stasis dermatitis develops, the erythema becomes more extensive, and scaling, weeping, and crusting appear. Superficial secondary infection may occur and progress to cellulitis. Applied remedies can result in contact dermatitis of the irritant or allergic type; a new onset of vesicular lesions should alert the clinician to this possibility.

Lipodermatosclerosis is a scleroderma-like induration and fibrosis of the skin and subcutaneous tissue. It occurs in up to 30% of affected patients and often precedes venous ulceration. In the acute stage, the skin is bright red, scaly, very tender, and warm. Lipodermatosclerosis often starts above the medial malleolus. It is not preceded by trauma or illness, and the lesion is not well demarcated from adjacent normal skin. In this acute stage, lipodermatosclerosis is often misdiagnosed as morphea, cellulitis, erythema nodosum, or another panniculitis. In the chronic stage, erythema, scaling, pain, and discomfort are less pronounced, and the involved sclerotic area is sharply demarcated from the surrounding normal skin. Eventually, the entire lower third of the leg may become hard and woody, and the legs resemble inverted champagne bottles.

Venous ulcers usually develop first over the medial malleoli or anterior aspect of the leg. They usually have an irregular edematous border and a moist, granulating base. Healing often results in a thin scar that can break down with trauma. Repeated episodes of ulceration and secondary infection can result in loss of ankle mobility. Rarely, carcinoma (squamous cell or basal cell) develops in a long-standing ulcer.

LABORATORY AND IMAGING STUDIES

Doppler examination or duplex scanning can help confirm venous insufficiency. In more than 20% of patients with leg ulceration, Doppler studies reveal evidence of arterial insufficiency. Feeling the pulses may be inaccurate; arterial studies are needed to exclude arterial insufficiency in any patient before compression therapy is used.

Skin biopsy is rarely necessary. The histology of stasis dermatitis is nonspecific. Occasionally, a biopsy must be performed to rule out other diseases. The specimen should be taken from the edge of an erythematous and indurated area, which is then closed primarily after a longitudinal thin excision to prevent dehiscence and ulcer formation. A nonhealing ulcer may necessitate referral to a dermatologist for workup and biopsy to rule out a carcinoma, unusual infection, vaso-occlusive disease, or granulomatous disease. A specimen for this purpose should be large enough to include both an ulcer edge and part of the ulcer base. An exophytic component to the edge, if present, should be chosen as the biopsy site.

TREATMENT

Any coexistent arterial disease must be treated before venous disease can be treated effectively. Custom-made graded compression stockings with 30 to 40 mm Hg of pressure at the ankle are essential. These should be individualized for the patient but cannot be used by anyone with severe arterial disease. The patient should put the stockings on immediately after arising in the morning, before edema has developed, and remove them in the evening. Ace wraps can be used temporarily. Skin grafting and venous reconstruction are therapeutic options. Ligation and stripping of veins has been associated with a poorer long-term prognosis, and leg veins should be conserved because they may be needed for future use in arterial bypass surgery.

Tap water compresses can be applied to areas of weeping, crusted, or scaly dermatitis, followed by a very thin layer of a corticosteroid. This should be discontinued or tapered once the dermatitis resolves. Infections are treated as appropriate. Pentoxifylline (Trental) improves the flow of blood by decreasing its viscosity and has a labeled indication for the treatment of intermittent claudication. Off-label use has included the treatment of lipodermatosclerosis. The topical antibiotics neomycin and gentamicin should be avoided because the use of any topical agent in areas of stasis is associated with an increased incidence of allergic sensitization. If secondary allergic or irritant dermatitis is suspected, referral to a dermatologist is appropriate to help determine its cause.

Stanozolol has been used successfully to treat acute lipodermatosclerosis at a dosage of 5 mg twice a day. Fibrinolytic activity is thought to be the mechanism of its beneficial effect. The patient should be advised to take short walks, elevate the leg during the day, and avoid constricting garments.

Stasis ulcers should be monitored for signs of infection, and the infections should be treated. Deep ulcers do well with Sorbsan dressings. DuoDerm dressings with an overlying Unna boot are helpful for multiple ulcers. Large ulcers with an adequate vascular supply to support a graft may have to be grafted to heal because they may worsen without grafting.

CONSIDERATIONS IN PREGNANCY

Venous disease is more common in women with a family history of the condition. During pregnancy, several factors contribute to the formation of varicose veins: venous relaxation secondary to increased levels of hormones, expansion of blood volume, and increased venous pressure, especially in the legs, in which the iliac veins are compressed by an enlarged uterus. The relative risk for venous disease in women increases with the number of full-term pregnancies. The risk for the development of venous disease during pregnancy increases with age; it is four times higher in women older than 35 years than in women 24 years of age or younger. During pregnancy, wearing graduated compression hosiery significantly improves venous function, prevents the formation of varicose veins, and is associated with a subjective decrease in swelling, tiredness, and pain.

BIBLIOGRAPHY

Callam MJ, Harper DR, Dale JJ, et al. Arterial disease in chronic leg ulceration: an underestimated hazard? Lothian and Forth Valley Leg Ulcer Study. *Br Med J* 1987;294:929.

Coffman JD. Cutaneous changes in peripheral vascular disease. In: Freedberg IM, Eisen AL, Wolff K, et al., eds. *Fitzpatrick's dermatology in general medicine*, 5th ed. New York: McGraw-Hill, 1999:1946.

Dindelli M, Parazzini F, Basellini A, et al. Risk factors for varicose disease before and during pregnancy. *Angiology* 1993;44:361.

Goldman MP, Weiss RA, Bergan JJ. Diagnosis and treatment of varicose veins: a review. *J Am Acad Dermatol* 1994;31:393.

Kirsner RS, Pardes JB, Eglestein WH, et al. The clinical spectrum of lipodermatosclerosis. *J Am Acad Dermatol* 1993;28:623.

Korstanje MJ. Venous stasis ulcers: diagnostic and surgical considerations. *Dermatol Surg* 1995;21:635.

McCarthy WJ, Dann C, Pearce WH, et al. Management of sudden profuse bleeding from varicose veins. *Surgery* 1993;113:178.

Nilsson L, Austrell C, Norgren L. Venous function during late pregnancy: the effect of elastic compression hosiery. *Vasa* 1992;21:203.

Phillips TJ, Dover JS. Leg ulcers. *J Am Acad Dermatol* 1991;25:965.

CHAPTER 139

Superficial Fungal Infections

Boni E. Elewski

Superficial fungal infections of the skin are much less common in women than in men. The reasons for this are unclear but may be related to extrinsic differences (clothing, footwear, participation in athletic activities such as contact sports) and intrinsic differences (women perspire less profusely and have less body hair). In general, many nonfungal skin disorders are incorrectly diagnosed as being caused by fungi, whereas many true fungal infections are not correctly identified as such. The primary care physician must be familiar with the definitive methods of diagnosing cutaneous fungal infections and should also be able to prescribe cost-effective therapy. A correct diagnosis is the key to successful therapy. Cutaneous fungal infections are not usually serious, but they can be the cause of significant discomfort and a great deal of unhappiness in patients. Additionally, educating patients about ways to minimize recurrence is an important adjunct to proper therapy.

ETIOLOGY AND DIFFERENTIAL DIAGNOSIS

Fungal infections of the skin can be divided into three types: (a) superficial infections caused by the yeast *Malassezia furfur;* (b) infections of the skin, hair, and nails caused by the dermatophytes (tinea); and (c) diseases of the skin, nails, and mucous membranes caused by the yeast *Candida* (mucocutaneous candidiasis).

Tinea versicolor, which is characterized by discrete and confluent hyperpigmented or hypopigmented macules, or both, can be confused with vitiligo or postinflammatory hyperpigmentation/hypopigmentation. Dermatophyte infections of the skin (tinea corporis) can resemble psoriasis, erythema multiforme, gyrate erythemas, pityriasis rosea, and even drug-related eruptions. Psoriasis and various nail dystrophies are similar in appearance to fungal infections of the nails (onychomycosis). Hair loss caused by tinea capitis may resemble alopecia areata, trichotillomania, or bacterial pyoderma.

HISTORY

Dermatophyte fungi can be acquired from animals or soil and by person-to-person transmission. Therefore, contact or exposure to animals is important to ascertain when tinea corporis is diagnosed. Most acute infections in women are acquired from pet cats or dogs. Of course, a history of other family members with acute or chronic fungal infections is also significant. Cutaneous candidiasis is generally associated with certain key risk factors, such as diabetes mellitus, obesity, and immunosuppression. Additionally, recent dental work often precedes the onset of oral tissue *Candida* infection or perlèche. Recent antibiotic therapy may contribute to the development of vaginal candidiasis. Occupations that involve wet work contribute to *Candida* infections of the nails and web spaces. A recent manicure with forceful manipulation of the cuticle often precedes acute *Candida* paronychia.

PHYSICAL EXAMINATION AND CLINICAL FINDINGS

Tinea versicolor (pityriasis versicolor) is characterized by brown, pink, red, or white scaly patches on the trunk and proximal extremities. A common presentation during the summer is small hypopigmented areas on the trunk that fail to tan. The etiologic agent prevents the transfer of melanin from melanocytes to epidermal cells; therefore, affected patches of skin do not tan like uninfected areas. If this diagnosis is suspected, some scale should be present in addition to the color change. The presence of scale can be demonstrated by scratching one of the macular areas with a glass blade or scalpel, which will raise a small amount of fine scale. Examination of the skin with a Wood's light may reveal a weak gold or orange-brown fluorescence. Tinea versicolor is diagnosed with certainty by scraping a scaly lesion with a No. 15 scalpel blade, placing the scale obtained on a microscope slide, and adding a drop of 20% potassium hydroxide (KOH). Examination under the microscope reveals the characteristic short hyphae and yeast cells, sometimes referred to as "spaghetti and meatballs."

Dermatophytic fungi produce scaly and erythematous lesions with well-defined margins in characteristic areas of the body. Often, clearing in the center of lesions on the nonhairy skin leaves an annular, erythematous lesion with scaly borders—hence the common name of "ringworm." Dermatophyte infections are given Latin names: *tinea* ("worm") plus the area of the body affected. In tinea pedis, or fungal infection of the feet, small blisters and inflammation may develop on the edges of the soles and interdigital areas. Chronic tinea pedis is characterized by erythema, scaling, and sometimes hyperkeratosis of the soles. Tinea corporis affects other areas of the body, including the trunk, buttocks, and extremities. When the face is involved, the condition may be called tinea faciei. Tinea cruris, or dermatophyte infection of the inguinal folds, is extremely uncommon in women. Rashes in the pubic and perineal area in women are often caused by *Candida*.

Onychomycosis, or tinea unguium, is characterized by the accumulation of subungual keratin and invasion of the nail bed by fungus, resulting in a thickened, distorted, discolored, and crumbly nail. Tinea capitis, or scalp ringworm, occurs almost exclusively in children, although it is reported rarely in adults.

The confirmatory diagnosis of a dermatophyte infection requires microscopic examination of the lesion for hyphae with a KOH wet mount. The border of the lesion is scraped lightly with a No. 15 scalpel blade, and the scale obtained is placed on top of a slide. A coverslip can be used to push all of the scale into a small mound. One or at most two drops of 20% KOH solution or KOH with dimethylsulfoxide are dropped in the center of the collected scale, and a coverslip is placed over the drop. If the KOH solution does not contain dimethylsulfoxide, the slide must be heated lightly over an alcohol lamp to improve "clearing" of the epithelial cells. If the solution does contain dimethylsulfoxide, heating is not required. Under low power (×40) with reduced light, threadlike hyphae can be seen. The presence of branched, septate hyphae is confirmed under higher power (×100). This second step is necessary to make sure that artifacts are not being mistaken for hyphae. In *Candida* infections, small, thin-walled yeast cells may be noted that may be budding. Pseudohyphae, which resemble true hyphae, are pathognomonic for *Candida albicans*.

In women, *Candida* infections of the skin occur principally in intertriginous locations, such as the axillae, vulva and vagina, intergluteal fold, inframammary areas, and perianal area. Physical examination of the involved skin generally reveals bright red erythema, oozing, and superficial erosions or pustules. Patients may experience burning or itching. In another presentation, the posterior or lateral nail folds of the fingers are involved. Chronic paronychia is characterized by loss of the cuticle and retraction of the proximal or lateral nail fold with erythema. Gentle pressure on the affected area may express a small amount of yellow pus or cheesy material. This can be examined in a KOH preparation and cultured. Crusted involvement of the labial commissures (perlèche) is another presentation of candidiasis.

Onychomycosis of the fingernails, toenails, or both usually results from a dermatophyte infection of the feet. *Candida* onychomycosis of the fingernails may often progress to chronic *Candida* paronychia. The organisms then invade the nail plate itself rather than just the soft tissues of the nail fold.

LABORATORY STUDIES

Positive results of a fungal culture or KOH study should be obtained before systemic therapy is considered. It is convenient to use a dermatophyte test medium, which is an agar-containing phenolphthalein, as a color indicator. If planted scale or pus causes the medium to turn red within 7 to 14 days, the presence of a dermatophyte pathogen is confirmed. The regulations of the Clinical Laboratory Improvement Act of 1988 allow a physician to perform fungal cultures in an office laboratory so long as the findings are read as "positive" or "negative." The regulations for attempting to identify the species of an organism are more onerous. Mycology laboratories can identify the exact fungal pathogen, and such information may be useful when a systemic antifungal drug is chosen.

TREATMENT

Tinea versicolor can be treated effectively with selenium sulfide, zinc pyrithione, combinations of sulfur and salicylic acid, or one of the antifungal agents (e.g., miconazole, clotrimazole, econazole, ketoconazole, ciclopirox). Over-the-counter shampoos containing 1% selenium sulfide (Head and Shoulders Intensive Treatment) or zinc pyrithione (Zincon, Head and Shoulders) can be applied with a rough washcloth. The shampoo should be allowed to remain on the affected areas for 10 minutes and then rinsed off. Daily application for at least 1 week is recommended. Prescription shampoos such as a 2.5% suspension of selenium sulfide (Selsun), 2% ketoconazole shampoo (Nizoral), and usually ciclopirox shampoo are patient-friendly alternatives that can be used as a body wash or, in refractory cases, left on the affected areas overnight. The topical antifungal agents are much more expensive but useful in recalcitrant cases. When the condition is widespread or recalcitrant, 200 mg of systemic ketoconazole daily for 5 to 7 days, 200 mg of fluconazole daily for 3 days, or 200 mg of itraconazole daily for 5 to 7 days is an alternative. After successful treatment, the hypopigmented areas remain lighter than the rest of the skin until the patient has a chance to tan. The absence of fine scaling on the lighter areas is a good indication that no active infection is present.

Trichophyton rubrum, T. tonsurans, T. mentagrophytes, and *Microsporum canis* are the most common dermophyte pathogens. Unless systemic therapy is being considered, identifying the actual etiologic agent may be less important than firmly establishing the presence of a fungus by KOH preparation or culture. Topical antifungal agents are useful except in tinea capitis and onychomycosis, which require systemic antifungal therapy. Adjunct therapies include the application of Domeboro compresses in macerated areas and antifungal powders to absorb moisture.

Four distinct classes of topical antifungal agents currently are available. The azoles are the largest group and include the first approved imidiazoles and some variations on the basic molecule. The older agents, miconazole and clotrimazole, are available both over the counter and by prescription. The spectra of activity of all these agents against yeasts such as *Candida* and dermatophytes are similar. The following is a list of available azoles:

- Clotrimazole (Mycelex, Lotrimin AF, Lotrimin)
- Econazole (Spectazole)
- Ketoconazole (Nizoral)
- Miconazole (Micatin, Monistat)
- Oxiconazole (Oxistat)
- Sulconazole (Exelderm).

The second class is the substituted povidone and includes only ciclopirox olamine (Loprox). Like the azoles, ciclopirox is considered a broad-spectrum antifungal agent with activity against *Candida, Malassezia,* and dermatophytes.

The allylamines are the third group and include naftifine (Naftin), terbinafine (Lamisil), and Mentax, which is a benzyl amine. When used topically, they have broad-spectrum activity, but interestingly, terbinafine is not effective against *Candida* when dosed orally. The allylamines are considered fungicidal in vitro.

The fourth class includes the polyene antibiotics, amphotericin and nystatin, which have activity against *Candida* but not useful for dermatophyte infections.

Clotrimazole, miconazole (Micatin), and tolnaftate (Tinactin, Aftate) can be purchased without a prescription, so the patient may have already tried a topical antifungal agent before visiting a physician. (The patient is more likely to have tried an over-the-counter hydrocortisone preparation or topical antibiotic.) It is important that the physician determine what has previously been used so as not to be embarrassed by giving the patient a prescription version of an agent that has already been tried. When an antifungal agent is chosen in this situation, it is especially helpful to select one from a class that is available by prescription only, such as naftifine or ciclopirox.

General principles to be considered when choosing a topical antifungal are the following:

For intertriginous areas of involvement, lotions are less messy and dry more easily, and they can be applied in the morning and on return from work; a cream can be used at night but should be applied sparingly. For erythematous pruritic lesions, therapy may be initiated with an antifungal agent in combination with steroids such as clotrimazole and betamethasone (Lotrisone). Caution should be exercised because this agent contains a potent topical corticosteroid that can produce untoward side effects if used incorrectly or applied to the face and intertriginous skin. Refractory cases may respond to a combination of agents, with a topical agent from one class applied during the day and one from another class used at night.

When lesions and symptoms do not regress markedly within 1 to 2 weeks, it is probably necessary to use a systemic antifungal agent. Griseofulvin is the first choice and is usually effective for superficial dermatophyte infections; however, it has no effect on *Candida* or *Malassezia* yeast infections. A regimen for treating skin infections with ultramicrosize griseofulvin is 5 to 7 mg/kg per day for 2 to 4 weeks. An alternative is 200 mg of ketoconazole per day. If therapy is to be continued for longer than 2 weeks, it makes sense to obtain a baseline chemistry 18 panel and a complete blood cell count. Fluconazole (Diflucan) and itraconazole (Sporanox) have a much better safety profile and are also effective in mucocutaneous candidiasis.

For infections shown to be caused by the cat and dog fungus *M. canis,* itraconazole or fluconazole may be helpful.

Tinea pedis is much less prevalent in women than in men, but nonetheless some additional instruction is required. For maceration between the toes, wearing sandals may be helpful. If nylon stockings or panty hose are worn, the toes can be separated with lamb's wool, which absorbs moisture better than cotton. After bathing or showering, a hair dryer on a cool setting can be used to dry the skin between the toes. Topical antifungal agents alone often suffice, but in cases of widespread scaling with hyperkeratosis (the so-called moccasin type of tinea pedis), keratolytic agents are helpful. The concurrent nightly application of 10% to 40% urea lotion or cream (Carmol) or 12% lactic acid lotion or cream (Lac-Hydrin) may speed healing.

Onychomycosis of the toenails is extremely refractory to treatment; fingernail infections are much easier to treat. *C. albicans* is a common fingernail pathogen in women. Manicures and the use of nail cosmetics may be risk factors. Treatment options include 150 to 200 mg of fluconazole once weekly until the nail is clinically normal and 250 mg of terbinafine daily for 6 weeks in fingernail infections and 12 weeks in toenail infections. This drug is not effective in *Candida* infections, however. Itraconazole at a dosage of 400 mg daily for 1 week per month is another alternative and should be continued for 2 months (fingernails) and 4 months (toenails).

Women with onychomycosis of the fingernails or toenails can cover the nails with nail polish, which camouflages the unsightliness. Reducing the hyperkeratotic nail by filing with an emery board may also help. In those unwilling or unable to take systemic antifungal agents, 8% ciclopirox lacquer (Penlac) can be applied. Patients should be warned that cure rates are very low and that fewer than 12% of users will note an improvement.

The treatment of candidiasis requires meticulous drying of the area, adequate exposure to air, and specific anti-*Candida* therapy. Gentian violet or Castellani paint is more effective than the old-fashioned methods of drying intertriginous areas, but they have the disadvantage of coloring the skin purple. Topical antifungal creams or lotions should be used two or three times daily. Applying powder in body folds and wearing loose clothing and cotton underwear and brassieres are useful adjuncts. In highly inflamed infections, initiating therapy with a brief course of topical corticosteroid cream in combination with clotrimazole (Lotrisone), which is lightly applied to the affected areas, may be beneficial. For resistant *Candida* infections, oral fluconazole or itraconazole may be administered. Fluconazole (Diflucan) can be dosed at 150 to 200 mg/d every third day for 1 to 2 weeks; itraconazole also is effective against *Candida* infections and can be prescribed at a dosage of 200 mg daily for 1 week. The clinician should ask the patient about predisposing factors to candidiasis, such as the use of systemic corticosteroids, birth control pills, or oral antibiotics. Pregnancy, diabetes, Cushing syndrome, and AIDS may also predispose the patient to candidiasis.

Paronychial infections with *Candida* are difficult to treat. Therapy consists of avoiding exposure to water, and rubber gloves with cotton lining should be worn whenever contact is unavoidable. Systemic antifungal therapy, such as 100 to 200 mg of fluconazole once weekly for 2 to 4 weeks, can be prescribed, and topical antifungal agents can be applied to the affected area. Chronic paronychia may cause rippling or other deformity of the nails, but eventually the nails grow out normally after the paronychia has been cured.

CONSIDERATIONS IN PREGNANCY

Fluconazole should be avoided during pregnancy. It is also believed that pregnant women should not be treated with oral ketoconazole or itraconazole. Nystatin is safe to use during pregnancy because no adverse effects or complications have occurred in infants born to women treated with oral nystatin. Terbinafine is a pregnancy category B drug, but caution must be exercised in assessing the risks and benefits of treatment.

BIBLIOGRAPHY

Borelli D, Jacobs PH, Nall L. Tinea versicolor: epidemiologic, clinical and therapeutic aspects. *J Am Acad Dermatol* 1991;25:300.

Chren M-M. Costs of therapy for dermatophyte infections. *J Am Acad Dermatol* 1994;31:S103.

Cohn MS. Superficial fungal infections: topical and oral treatment of common types. *Postgrad Med* 1992;91:239, 249.

Cohen PR, Scher RK. Topical and surgical treatment of onychomycosis. *J Am Acad Dermatol* 1994;31:574.

Degreef HJ, DeDoncker PRG. Current therapy of dermatophytosis. *J Am Acad Dermatol* 1994;31:525.

Hay RJ. Antifungal therapy of yeast infections. *J Am Acad Dermatol* 1994;31:56.

Korting HC, Schafer-Korting M. Is tinea unguium still widely incurable? *Arch Dermatol* 1992;128:243.

Leyden JL. Tinea pedis pathophysiology and treatment. *J Am Acad Dermatol* 1994; 31:531.

Odds FC. Pathogenesis of *Candida* infections. *J Am Acad Dermatol* 1994;31:S2.

Roberts DT. Oral therapeutic agents in fungal nail disease. *J Am Acad Dermatol* 1994;31:578.

Sanchez JL, Torres VM. Double-blind efficacy study of selenium sulfide in tinea versicolor. *J Am Acad Dermatol* 1984;11:235.

Vidimos AT, Camisa C, Tomecki KJ. Tinea capitis in three adults. *Int J Dermatol* 1991;30:206.

CHAPTER 140

Herpes Simplex and Herpes Zoster

Gisela Torres and Stephen K. Tyring

Diseases caused by the herpesvirus family can significantly affect a woman's health, both physically and psychosocially. Rarely, these viruses are responsible for serious illness and may affect a pregnancy, causing substantial fetal harm. In this chapter, the etiology, clinical presentation, and treatment of infection with human herpesviruses 1, 2, and 3 are discussed.

HERPES SIMPLEX

Etiology

The family Herpesviridae includes a group of viruses with the following characteristics: double-stranded, linear DNA in the viral core; a 20-sided capsid containing 162 protein capsomeres assembled in the host cellular nucleus; and a lipid bilayer envelope surrounding the capsid, derived from the nuclear membrane of the infected cell. The subfamily Alphaherpesvirinae, characterized by a short reproductive cycle, rapid spread in culture, efficient destruction of infected cells, and the capacity to establish latent infection in sensory nerve ganglia, includes human herpesvirus 1 (HHV-1), HHV-2, and HHV-3 (the varicella-zoster virus).

HHV-1 is herpes simplex virus 1 (HSV-1), and HHV-2 is HSV-2. HSV-1 is best known for causing the clinical manifestations of herpes labialis, and HSV-2 for herpes genitalis. The rate of infection with HSV-1 approaches 90% in the general adult population; approximately 20% of adults are serologically positive for HSV-2 in the United States, and up to 40% worldwide. HSV-2 infection has been reported to be one of the most rapidly increasing sexually transmitted diseases. These viruses are transmitted when the mucosal surfaces or abraded skin of a susceptible person comes in contact with contaminated secretions. Virions travel from the initial site of infection to the sensory dorsal root ganglion, where latency is established. Viral replication in the ganglion with recurrent clinical outbreaks can be induced by various stimuli, such as trauma, ultraviolet radiation, extremes of temperature, stress, and hormonal fluctuations. Asymptomatic viral shedding occurs frequently and leads to transmission.

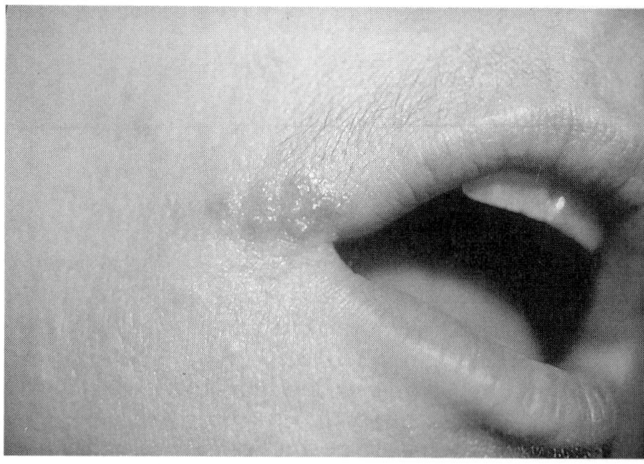

FIG. 140.1. Orolabial herpes simplex (a cold sore) demonstrating the primary lesion of herpes simplex virus 1 and 2 infection: grouped vesicles, pustules, or papules on an erythematous base.

Clinical Presentation

Primary infection with HSV is clinically more severe than recurrent outbreaks. Both HSV primary infections and recurrent episodes of viral shedding may be clinically apparent or asymptomatic.

Herpes labialis (cold sores, fever blisters) is most often associated with HSV-1 infection, although oral lesions caused by HSV-2 have been identified, usually secondary to oral-genital contact. Primary infection with HSV-1 often occurs in childhood and is usually asymptomatic; at most, 30% of infected persons experience clinically apparent outbreaks. Symptoms of primary herpes labialis may include a prodrome of fever, followed by a sore throat and mouth; submandibular or cervical lymphadenopathy may develop. In children, gingivostomatitis and odynophagia are also seen. Painful vesicles develop on the lips, gingivae, palate, tongue, or buccal mucosa, often associated with erythema and edema (Fig. 140.1). The lesions ulcerate and heal after 2 to 3 weeks. The disease remains dormant for a variable time. Pain, burning, itching, or paresthesias usually precede the recurrence of vesicular lesions, which eventually ulcerate or crust. The lesions most commonly form on the vermilion border, and symptoms of untreated recurrences last approximately 1 week.

HSV-2 is the most common cause of herpes genitalis. However, HSV-1 has been increasingly identified as the causative agent in up to 30% of primary genital herpes infections, likely as a consequence of oral-genital contact. Primary herpes genitalis develops within 2 days to 2 weeks after exposure to the virus and causes the most severe clinical manifestations. Symptoms of the primary episode last on average 2 to 3 weeks. Primary HSV-2 genital infection may be followed by bacterial superinfection and, in women, systemic complications such as urinary retention and aseptic meningitis (seen in up to 25% of women). In men, painful erythematous vesicular lesions that ulcerate form most often on the penis but may also develop in the anus and perineum. In women, primary herpes genitalis presents as vesicular/ulcerated lesions in the cervix and painful vesicles on the external genitalia, but the vagina, perineum, buttocks, and at times the distribution of the sacral nerve in the leg may also be affected. Associated symptoms include fever, malaise, edema, inguinal lymphadenopathy, dysuria, and vaginal or penile discharge. After primary infection, the virus may lie dormant for months to years until a recurrence is triggered. However, primary HSV-2 infection does not always manifest as a clinical episode, and more than half of seropositive persons do not experience clinically apparent outbreaks, although episodes of viral shedding still occur. Exposed persons with an asymptomatic primary infection may later experience an initial clinical episode of genital herpes that is not as severe as a true primary episode. Recurrent clinical outbreaks are also milder. Recurrences are often preceded by a prodrome of pain, itching, tingling, burning, or other paresthesias.

Infection with HSV can manifest clinically in other ways. Localized or disseminated eczema herpeticum (Kaposi varicelliform eruption) is a variant of HSV infection that frequently develops in patients with atopic dermatitis, burns, or other inflammatory skin conditions (Fig. 140.2). Eczema herpeticum

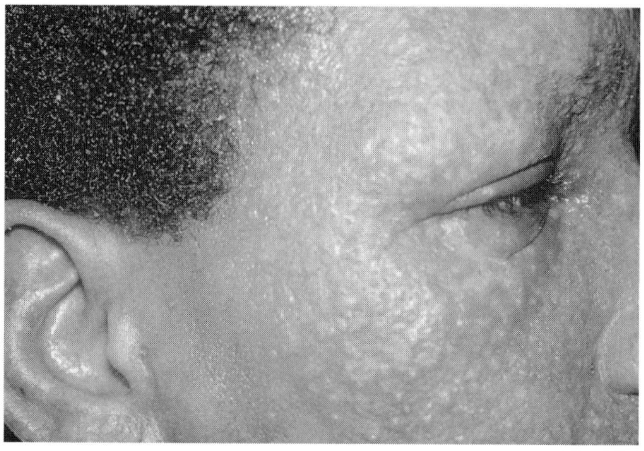

FIG. 140.2. Kaposi varicelliform eruption in a patient with atopic dermatitis. The cribriform superficial vesicles and ulcerations arose during a 2-day period. The patient had experienced two similar episodes within the preceding 18 months.

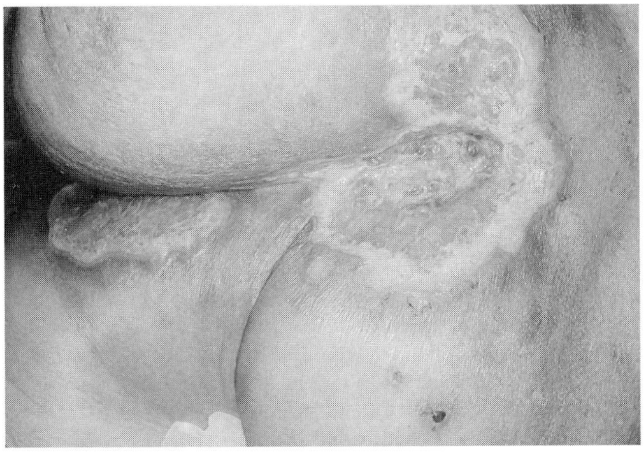

FIG. 140.3. This painful, necrotic ulceration arose during a 3-month period in a woman with AIDS. Biopsy demonstrated the cytopathologic changes of herpes infection, and culture grew herpes simplex virus 2. The lesion healed during a 5-week period while the patient was taking acyclovir.

most often affects children. Herpes whitlow, characterized by vesicular outbreaks in the hands and fingers, was formerly most often associated with HSV-1 infection and usually occurred in children who sucked their thumb and, before the widespread use of gloves, in dental and medical health care workers. However, HSV-2 herpes whitlow is increasingly recognized and is probably a consequence of digital-genital contact. Herpes gladiatorum, also caused by HSV-1, is a papular or vesicular eruption that develops on the torso of athletes who engage in sports involving close physical contact (classically wrestling). Disseminated HSV infection may occur in pregnant women and immunocompromised persons (Fig. 140.3). Patients with these forms of HSV infection may present with atypical signs and symptoms and present a diagnostic challenge.

Herpes Simplex in Pregnancy

HSV infections in pregnancy can have devastating effects on the fetus. Infections in neonates are usually caused by HSV-2; most are acquired during the peripartum period, although in utero and postpartum transmission also occurs. Factors that increase the risk for transmission from mother to infant include the presence of active primary genital infection at the time of delivery, prolonged rupture of the membranes, vaginal delivery, and the absence of transplacental antibodies. Transmission is estimated to occur once in every 3,500 to 5,000 deliveries in the United States. The clinical presentation of neonatal HSV infection ranges from localized infection of the skin, mucous membranes, or eyes to encephalitis and disseminated infection.

Laboratory Studies

In the office, Tzanck smears can be used for the rapid detection of multinucleated giant cells, although the findings are not specific for the type of herpesvirus (Fig. 140.4). HSV can be detected and typed through a viral culture of untreated lesions within 72 hours after onset. The direct fluorescence antigen assay is a frequently used diagnostic tool in hospitals; enzyme-linked immunosorbent assays and several other HSV-1 and -2 serologic assays are available to detect antibodies against these viruses. A POCkit Rapid Test for HSV-2 is now commercially available that is highly sensitive. Western blot assays are highly sensitive and specific but available only for research. HSV DNA can be detected in specific instances by the polymerase chain reaction.

Treatment and Prevention

HSV viral shedding is greatest during clinically evident outbreaks; however, transmission from seropositive persons to their seronegative partners usually occurs during periods of asymptomatic HSV shedding. Barrier methods such as condoms provide only 10% to 15% protection against the transmission of genital herpes because the virus can be transmitted to and from mucocutaneous surfaces when they are uncovered or when the integrity of the barrier is compromised. Condoms protect women more effectively than men. Various HSV vaccines have been investigated to treat and prevent herpes genitalis, but most have proved ineffective. In double-blinded randomized trials of a glycoprotein D HSV-2 vaccine, the vaccine conferred protection against the virus in women who were serologically negative for both HSV-1 and HSV-2. It did not, however, prevent HSV infection in men or in women positive for HSV-1 but negative for HSV-2. Further clinical studies of the vaccine are under way.

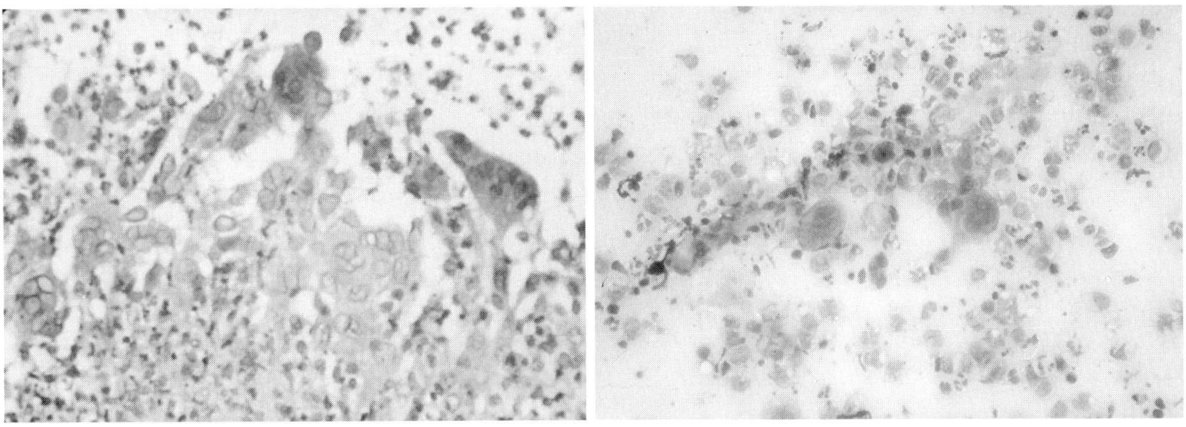

FIG. 140.4. Cytopathologic changes of herpesvirus infection. The multinucleated giant epithelial cells are diagnostic of infection with herpes simplex virus 1 or 2 or varicella-zoster virus. **Left:** Hematoxylin and eosin stain of a biopsy specimen (original magnification ×400). **Right:** Rapid Wright stain of a smear from a vesicle (original magnification ×100).

Intravenous, oral, and topical antiviral medications are available to treat HSV infection; these are most effective if administered at the onset of symptoms (Table 140.1). Oral therapy can be given episodically or for long-term suppression. Long-term suppressive therapy for genital herpes has been shown to decrease the asymptomatic shedding of HSV, and in one study, long-term valacyclovir therapy significantly decreased the transmission of HSV to the susceptible partners of HSV-2–positive persons by 50% to 77%. Indications for long-term suppressive therapy include frequent or severe outbreaks, infection in an immunocompromised person, and the gender, HSV serologic status, and reproductive capability of the patient's partner.

The treatment of both herpes labialis and herpes genitalis generally consists of episodic courses of oral acyclovir, its more bioavailable prodrug valacyclovir, or famciclovir. Commercially available topical treatments for herpes are much less efficacious than oral therapy. Resiquimod, a topical immune response modifier gel, has been shown to shorten and delay recurrent outbreaks of genital herpes in phase II clinical trials and is currently undergoing phase III clinical studies. Oral antiviral medications (acyclovir, valacyclovir, and famciclovir) may be used (off label) to treat other uncomplicated HSV conditions (e.g., herpes whitlow); the same doses that are used to treat herpes genitalis are usually recommended.

TABLE 140.1. Treatment of Herpes Simplex Virus Infections

Herpes labialis
Topical treatment for episodic outbreaks
1% Penciclovir cream (Denavir) every 2 hours for 5 days
10% Docosanol cream (Abreva) 5 times daily for 5–10 days
5% Acyclovir ointment (Zovirax topical) 5 times daily for 5 days
Oral treatment for episodic outbreaks
Acyclovir (Zovirax) 400 mg 5 times daily for 5 days
Famciclovir (Famvir) 500 mg tid for 5 days
Valacyclovir (Valtrex) 2 g every 12 hours for 24 hours (must be taken at the very first sign of symptoms/prodrome) or 500 mg bid for 5 days
Suppressive therapy
Acyclovir (Zovirax) 400 mg bid
Famciclovir (Famvir) 250 mg bid
Valacyclovir (Valtrex) 500 mg qd
Herpes genitalis
Topical treatment for episodic outbreaks
5% Acyclovir ointment/cream (Zovirax topical) 5 times daily for 5 days
Oral treatment for primary infection
Acyclovir (Zovirax) 200 mg 5 times daily for 10 days or 400 mg tid for 10 days
Famciclovir (Famvir) 250 mg tid for 10 days
Valacyclovir (Valtrex) 1,000 mg bid for 10 days
Oral treatment for episodic outbreaks
Acyclovir (Zovirax) 400 mg tid for 5 days
Famciclovir (Famvir) 125 mg bid for 5 days
Valacyclovir (Valtrex) 500 mg bid for 3 days
Long-term suppressive therapy
Acyclovir (Zovirax) 400 mg bid
Famciclovir (Famvir) 250 mg bid
Valacyclovir (Valtrex) 500 mg qd for patients with fewer that 10 outbreaks per year OR 1,000 mg qd for patients with 10 or more outbreaks per year
Complicated HSV infections
Neonatal HSV infection
Acyclovir IV 10 mg/kg every 8 hours for 10 days
Disseminated disease
Acyclovir IV 5–10 mg/kg every 8 hours for 7 days if older than 12 years OR 250 mg/m^2 every 8 hours for 7 days for children 12 years of age or younger
Acyclovir-resistant HSV infections
Foscarnet IV 40 mg/kg every 8–10 hours for 10–21 days
1% Cidofovir compounded cream/gel (not approved by FDA but recommended by CDC for localized acyclovir-resistant HSV infection)

HSV, herpes simplex virus.

Complicated HSV infections—that is, infections characterized by cutaneous or visceral dissemination and severe infections in immunocompromised hosts—should be treated promptly with intravenous acyclovir. Acyclovir-resistant HSV strains have been identified in immunocompromised patients with recurrent HSV infections, and intravenous foscarnet or cidofovir may be used in such cases. Treatment for neonatal HSV consists of intravenous acyclovir. The doses of these medications are outlined in Table 140.1.

No consensus has been reached regarding the appropriate management of expectant mothers with genital HSV infection. HSV-2–negative women should be counseled to abstain from intercourse during the third trimester with partners who may be seropositive because primary HSV infection at this time puts the fetus at high risk. The most frequently used approach in attempting to prevent vertical transmission has been to have women with clinically apparent HSV lesions during labor undergo cesarean section. However, cesarean section does not prevent all cases of neonatal infection because infection may occur in utero, and antepartum HSV cultures do not effectively predict neonatal infection. Babies born to mothers with genital HSV should be monitored closely for any signs of infection and treated promptly if signs of the disease develop. Acyclovir, valacyclovir, and famciclovir are pregnancy category B drugs. The oral administration of 400 mg of acyclovir three times daily during the third trimester of pregnancy has proved safe and effective in preventing neonatal herpes and eliminating the need for cesarean sections. Acyclovir may be administered intravenously to pregnant women with severe HSV infection because the risk that the infection poses to the infant is greater than any theoretic adverse effects of the medication. In thousands of pregnancies reported in the acyclovir registry and hundreds in the valacyclovir and famciclovir registries, these drugs have not been associated with any increase in fetal defects or difficulties during pregnancy.

VARICELLA-ZOSTER VIRUS (HUMAN HERPESVIRUS 3) INFECTION

Etiology

Primary infection with HHV-3, or varicella-zoster virus (VZV), causes chickenpox. This virus is nearly ubiquitous in the population, highly contagious, and usually acquired in early childhood. Chickenpox affects 90% of children worldwide, but it can occur in persons of any age. The virus is transmitted via contaminated secretions or respiratory droplets, or through direct contact with the skin lesions of an infected person. After exposure, an incubation period of approximately 2 weeks passes before clinical signs and symptoms develop. During this period, the virus replicates and spreads from the upper respiratory mucosa to the lymph nodes, blood, and internal organs. It then spreads from the sensory nerve endings to the dorsal root ganglion, where it remains in a latent state.

In approximately 20% of persons infected with VZV, the virus is reactivated by an unknown stimulus. Reactivation causes the clinical disease known as *herpes zoster,* or *shingles.*

Reactivation is most likely to occur in elderly and immunocompromised persons, although everyone seropositive for VZV is susceptible. In an otherwise healthy person, the chance of experiencing a second episode of shingles is less than 5%. A patient with herpes zoster is not as contagious as one with primary varicella because a susceptible person must come into direct contact with the skin lesions of the patient with shingles. In addition, a patient with shingles can transmit VZV only to a person not previously exposed to the virus or vaccine, or to a severely immunocompromised person; chickenpox, not shingles, would develop in such a case.

Clinical Presentation

After the incubation period of primary VZV infection, a prodrome of headache, fever, malaise, and gastrointestinal symptoms usually occurs. The disease is characterized by an initially pruritic erythematous macular rash that starts on the head and spreads caudally to the trunk and proximal extremities. The lesions then progress to papules and vesicles over a pink or erythematous base, often described as "dew drops on a rose petal" (Fig. 140.5). These eventually form pustules and crust after 2 to 3 weeks.

The complications of chickenpox are most common at the extremes of age. The most frequent complication is localized bacterial superinfection of the skin. Varicella pneumonia and neurologic complications such as meningoencephalitis are rare but can be fatal if not treated promptly. Reye syndrome has been described in infected children treated with aspirin. The complication rate is higher in immunocompromised persons, and primary VZV in a pregnant woman can have devastating effects on the fetus.

In the 20% of persons who acquire herpes zoster, or shingles, the virus replicates in the sensory ganglion where it previously established latency and spreads down the sensory nerve (Fig. 140.6). The inflammatory response in the nerve and ganglion often results in a prodrome of pain in the nerve distribution. The pain can be severe and is often thought to be secondary to other diseases. An erythematous vesicular rash in the dermatomal distribution of the nerve follows the prodromal neuralgia. This may be associated with malaise, fever, flulike symptoms, and ongoing pain and paresthesias. The vesicular eruption eventually crusts and resolves in approximately 2 to 4 weeks. However, the associated pain and paresthesias such as tingling, numbness, and burning usually last longer; the average time in the general population is 2 months, although the pain may persist for more than 6 months, or even years, after all signs of skin infection have resolved. This condition, known as *post-herpetic neuralgia,* is the most common and debilitating complication of herpes zoster in people older than 50 years of age. Other complications include bacterial superinfection, ocular problems, Ramsey-Hunt syndrome (facial palsy and lesions in the external and middle ear secondary to involvement of the facial or auditory nerve), nerve palsies, and visceral or central nervous system dissemination (Fig. 140.7). Dissemination and

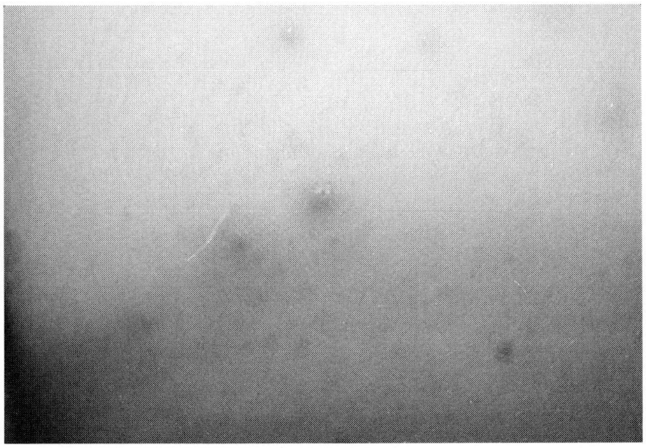

FIG. 140.5. Small (1- to 3-mm) vesicles on an erythematous macule in varicella. The vesicles undergo central umbilication, as in the lesion in the center of the figure, then crust during 3 to 7 days.

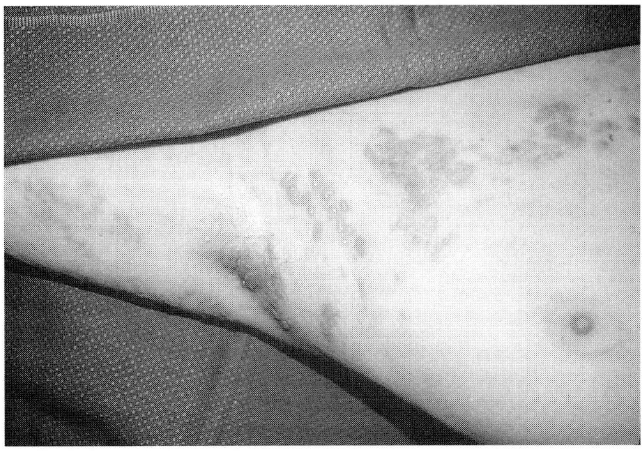

FIG. 140.6. Herpes zoster (shingles) in the left T1 dermatome. This painful eruption was preceded by 2 weeks of hyperesthesia and severe burning pain in the dermatome.

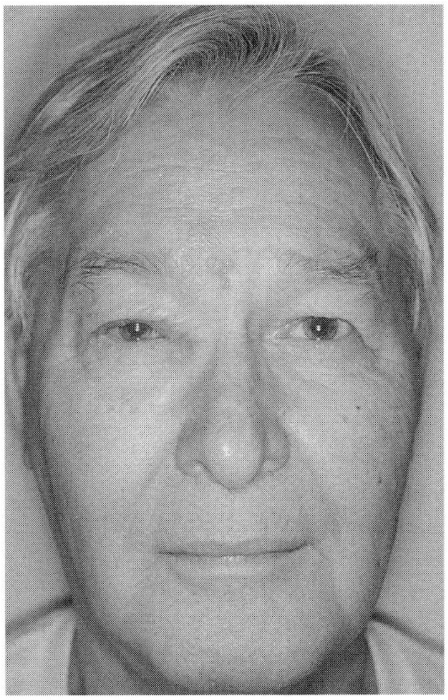

FIG. 140.7. A 36-hour-old eruption that arose after 5 days of tingling paresthesias. The patient reported tearing in the right eye and photophobia. A slit lamp examination revealed a dendritic corneal erosion. Slight erythema and a small vesicle on the tip of the nose, the area innervated by the nasociliary branch of the ophthalmic division of the trigeminal nerve, were noted.

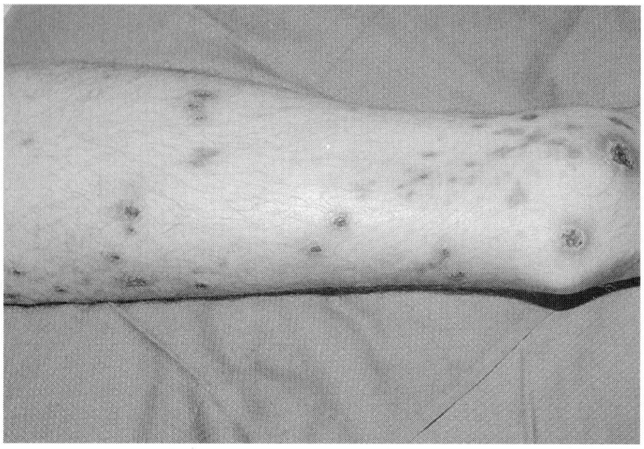

FIG. 140.8. L3 zoster had developed 3 months previously in this patient with a $CD4^+$ cell count of 64/μL. The vesicles resolved during a 3-week period, leaving the tender, 2- to 4-cm, keratotic plaques of chronic crusted herpes zoster as a residuum.

recurrence of shingles are more likely to develop in immunosuppressed persons (Fig. 140.8).

Varicella-Zoster Virus Infection in Pregnancy

The congenital varicella syndrome presents in newborns who have been exposed to VZV as limb hypoplasia, dermatomal skin scarring, and central nervous system and ocular damage. The fetuses of women exposed to VZV between weeks 13 and 20 of gestation are at the highest risk, with the syndrome developing in approximately 2%. Congenital varicella can also cause fetal demise, especially if the mother acquires varicella between 4 days before and 2 days after delivery, when the fetus/neonate is unprotected by maternal antibodies. Babies born to mothers in whom herpes zoster appeared during pregnancy do not appear to be at risk for this developmental damage.

Laboratory Studies

Both primary varicella and herpes zoster are usually diagnosed clinically. As for HSV detection, multiple laboratory tests are available. These include Tzank smears (not specific for the type of virus), serology, viral culture, polymerase chain reaction, and direct immunofluorescence assays. Serum tests for antibodies are useful in women with an unknown history of chickenpox who are planning to become pregnant because they may be candidates for vaccination.

Treatment and Prevention

Primary varicella (chickenpox) is managed both symptomatically and with systemic antiviral agents. The antiviral agents should be administered within 48 hours after the onset of rash (Table 140.2). Varicella-zoster immunoglobulin (125 U/10 kg administered intramuscularly) is available and should be given as prophylaxis to exposed pregnant women, newborns, and immunocompromised patients within 96 hours after VZV exposure. Despite the administration of varicella-zoster immunoglobulin, clinical varicella develops in more than 30% of exposed patients, but the course of the disease may be mitigated if not prevented. Pregnant women in whom chickenpox develops should be treated with oral or intravenous acyclovir, depending on the severity of the disease. The incidence of primary varicella in children has decreased dramatically since a live attenuated VZV vaccine (Oka strain) has been in use. This vaccine has been shown to be 71% to 91% effective in preventing disease altogether, and 95% to 100% in preventing severe primary disease. The vaccine is given as a single dose to recipients 12 months to 12 years of age, and as two doses 4 to 8 weeks apart to persons 13 years of age or older.

Antiviral treatment of shingles should be initiated promptly within 48 to 72 hours after the vesicular rash appears. Symptomatic treatment with analgesics and antipruritics is given along with antiviral medications (Table 140.2). Oral steroids have not been shown to add any benefit to antiviral agents in the treatment of acute shingles and are not recommended. In one study, VZV vaccine given to bone marrow transplant patients was effective in preventing shingles. Clinical trials are under way to determine whether the vaccine might also protect against herpes zoster in the general population. Post-herpetic neuralgia is difficult to treat because none of the current therapies are completely effective. Available treatments for post-herpetic neuralgia are outlined in Table 140.3. The use of gabapentin (Neurontin) plus antiviral agents during the acute phase may be neuroprotective and reduce the incidence of post-herpetic neuralgia; studies are ongoing.

TABLE 140.2. Treatment of Varicella-Zoster Virus Infections

Immunocompetent children
Acyclovir (Zovirax) 20 mg/kg po 4 times daily for 5 days
Complicated VZV infection in immunocompromised children
Acyclovir (Zovirax) 500 mg/m^2 IV every 8 hours for 7 to 10 days
Immunocompetent adults
Acyclovir (Zovirax) 800 mg po 5 times daily for 7 days
Valacyclovir (Valtrex) 1,000 mg tid for 7 days
Famciclovir (Famvir) 500 mg tid for 7 days
Complicated VZV in immunocompromised adults
Acyclovir (Zovirax) 10 mg/kg IV every 8 hours for 7 to 10 days

VZV, varicella-zoster virus.

BIBLIOGRAPHY

Brown TJ, McCrary M, Tyring SK. Antiviral agents: nonantiretroviral drugs. *J Am Acad Dermatol* 2002;47:581–599.

Corey L. Challenges in genital herpes simplex virus management. *J Infect Dis* 2002;186[Suppl 1]:S29–S33.

Fleming DT, McQuillan GM, Johnson RE, et al. Herpes simplex virus infection in the United States 1976–1994. *N Engl J Med* 1997;337:1105–1111.

TABLE 140.3. Treatment of Post-Herpetic Neuralgia

Topical treatments (skin must be healed/intact)
Topical anesthetics such as lidocaine cream, Lidoderm patch, EMLA cream, capsaicin cream
Narcotic and nonnarcotic analgesics
Anticonvulsants
Gabapentin (Neurontin) 300 mg qd with dose gradually increased to up to 1,200 mg tid as tolerated
Tricyclic antidepressants
Amitriptyline 10–25 mg qd with dose gradually increased to up to 75 mg qd
Maprotiline, desipramine
Steroids
Intrathecal methylprednisolone (only steroid treatment for post-herpetic neuralgia with significant success in trials)
Sympathetic nerve blocks
Transcutaneous electric stimulation
Acupuncture

Hata A, Asanuma H, Rinki M, et al. Use of an inactivated varicella vaccine in recipients of hematopoietic-cell transplants. *N Engl J Med* 2002;347:26–34.
Kost RG, Straus SE. Postherpetic neuralgia—pathogenesis, treatment and prevention. *N Engl J Med* 1996;335:32–42.
Rice AS, Maton S. Gabapentin in postherpetic neuralgia: a randomised, double-blind, placebo-controlled study. *Pain* 2001;94:215–224.
Rowbotham MC, Harden N, Stacey B, et al. Gabapentin for the treatment of postherpetic neuralgia: a randomized controlled trial. *JAMA* 1998;280:1837–1842.
Scott LL, Hollier LM, McIntire D, et al. Acyclovir suppression to prevent clinical recurrences at delivery after first-episode genital herpes in pregnancy: an open-label trial. *Infect Dis Obstet Gynecol* 2001;9:75–80.
Spruance SL, Tyring SK, Smith MH, et al. Application of a topical immune response modifier, resiquimod gel, to modify the recurrence rate of recurrent genital herpes: a pilot study. *J Infect Dis* 2001;184:196–200.
Stanberry LR, Spruance SL, Cunningham AL, et al. Glycoprotein D adjuvant vaccine to prevent genital herpes. *N Engl J Med* 2002;347:21;1652–1661.
Tyring S, Beutner KR, Tucker BA, et al. Antiviral therapy for herpes zoster: a randomized, controlled clinical trial of valacyclovir and famciclovir in immunocompetent subjects at least 50 years old. *Arch Fam Med* 2000;9:863–869.
Tyring SK, ed. *Mucocutaneous manifestations of viral diseases.* New York: Marcel Dekker Inc, 2002:69–144.
Wald A, Zeh J, Selke S, et al. Reactivation of genital herpes simplex virus type 2 infection in asymptomatic seropositive persons. *N Engl J Med* 2000;342:844–850.
Wald A, Langenberg AG, Link K, et al. Effect of condoms on reducing the transmission of herpes simplex virus type 2 from men to women. *JAMA* 2001;285: 3100–3106.
Whitley RJ, Weiss H, Gnann JW Jr, et al. Acyclovir with and without prednisone for the treatment of herpes zoster: a randomized, placebo-controlled trial. *Ann Intern Med* 1996;125:376–383.
Whitley RJ, Shukla S, Crooks RJ. The identification of risk factors associated with persistent pain following herpes zoster. *J Infect Dis* 1998;178[Suppl 1]:S71–S75.
Wood MJ, Johnson RW, McKendrick MW, et al. A randomized trial of acyclovir for 7 days or 21 days with and without prednisolone for treatment of acute herpes zoster. *N Engl J Med* 1994;330:896.
Wood MJ, Kay R, Dworkin RH, et al. Oral acyclovir accelerates pain resolution in herpes zoster: a meta-analysis of placebo-controlled trials. *Clin Infect Dis* 1996; 22:341–347.
Workowski KA, Levine WC. Sexually transmitted diseases treatment guidelines 2002. *MMWR Morb Mortal Wkly Rep* 2002,51:RR-6.

CHAPTER 141
Human Papillomavirus Infections (Warts)

Gisela Torres and Stephen K. Tyring

ETIOLOGY

Human papillomavirus (HPV) is a nonenveloped virus with double-stranded DNA that belongs to the Papovaviridae family. The lack of an outer envelope makes it highly stable in the environment. More than 100 different genotypes of HPV have been recognized. These are highly species-specific and specific to the tissues and anatomic areas they infect. Transmission occurs through direct contact with an infected person or with infectious virus in the environment. Autoinoculation from one area to another in the same individual is also possible. In addition, HPV infection is sexually transmitted, and some are genotypes more trophic to the anogenital mucosa.

HPV infects mucosal and skin surfaces. Epithelial cells in the basal layer of the epidermis become infected and proliferate, producing clinically apparent lesions. However, the virus may persist in the cells without inducing epithelial cell proliferation. Mucosal infection is most often associated with genotypes 6 and 11 (low-risk) and genotypes 16, 18, 30, 31, 33–35, 39, 40, 42–45, 52–59, 61, 62, 66–69, 71–74, and 82 (high-risk), which have been linked to cervical and anogenital cancers (see Chapter 28). An estimated 25% to 50% of all sexually active adults have a genital HPV infection. Other HPV genotypes cause various types of mucocutaneous lesions (Table 141.1).

TABLE 141.1. Human Papillomavirus Genotypes and Associated Diseases

HPV genotypes	Associated mucocutaneous lesions
1	Plantar warts, palmar warts
2,4,26,27,65,78	Common warts (verruca vulgaris)
3,10,27,28,49	Flat warts (verruca plana)
3,5,8,9,10,12,14,15, 17,19,20–25,36–38, 46,47,50	Epidermodysplasia verruciformis
6,11,70,83	Anogenital warts (condylomata acuminata)
6,11	Oral papillomas, recurrent laryngeal papillomatosis
6,11,16	Verrucous carcinoma
7	Butcher's warts
13,32	Oral focal epithelial hyperplasia
16,18	Laryngeal carcinoma
60	Epidermal cyst
63	Myrmecia wart

Cutaneous HPV infection is nearly ubiquitous in the adult population, although clinical manifestations usually do not develop. The susceptibility of a person infected with HPV to the development of clinically apparent warts depends on several factors. These include the quantity of virus inoculated, the immune status of the exposed person, the nature of the contact, and the degree of exposure to moisture. Although nongenital warts develop in persons of all ages, they are clearly more common in children than in adults. Persons who are immunosuppressed by medications, illness, or infection are particularly susceptible to the development of warts, which are often multiple and difficult to treat.

CLINICAL MANIFESTATIONS

Warts are the most commonly recognized clinical manifestation of cutaneous infection with HPV. They are generally classified according to their appearance (morphology) or anatomic location; for example, periungual warts are warts around the fingernail, and plantar warts are warts on the soles of the feet.

The common wart (verruca vulgaris) is generally a verrucous hyperkeratotic papule that varies greatly in size, number, and location. If the keratotic surface is removed, thrombosed capillaries that look like black dots can be seen within the wart (Fig. 141.1). The morphology of a periungual wart is similar to that of a common wart, but a periungual wart appears on the periphery of a nail, often causing pain and nail dystrophy. A verruca plana is usually a flat-topped, small, flesh-colored, minimally scaly papule that most often develops on the face and hands and also on women's legs, where it is spread by shaving. Palmar and plantar warts show a variety of clinical morphologies. If a plantar wart become hyperkeratotic, it can cause discomfort secondary to pressure. A wart can also appear as a threadlike projection on the face or neck, in which case it is called a *filiform wart* (Fig. 141.2). Butcher's warts are so called because they often appear on the fingers of people in the meat-cutting business. Epidermodysplasia verruciformis is a rare, often familial, chronic disease. It most often presents in childhood as flat warts or hypopigmented macules on the face, trunk, and extremities. The incidence of malignant conversion of the lesions of epidermodysplasia verruciformis is relatively

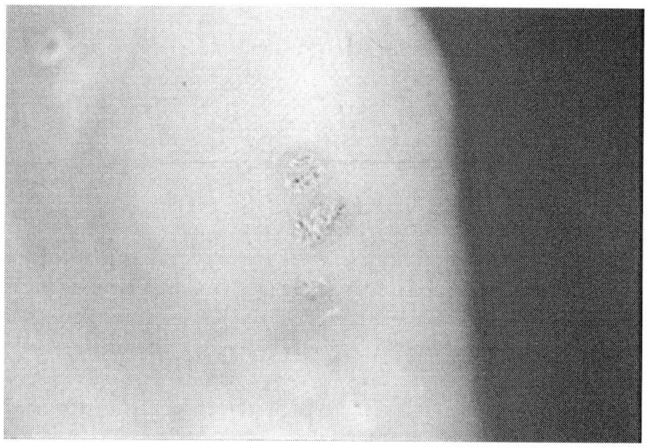

FIG. 141.1. Plantar wart (verruca vulgaris). Thrombosed capillaries are evident.

high, especially in persons infected with HPV-5 and -8, and is increased by exposure to ultraviolet light or other carcinogenic factors. Oral papillomas present as papules in the oral mucosa but may become verrucous. They can be associated with the genital serotypes of HPV secondary to oral-genital contact. Conjunctival warts and warts in other unusual areas (usually of skin trauma) have also been described. Most warts are asymptomatic unless they become irritated by trauma or pressure.

The differential diagnosis of nongenital warts includes seborrheic keratosis, nevi, keratoacanthoma, epidermolytic hyperkeratosis, Gottron papules (a manifestation of dermatomyositis), granuloma annulare, molluscum contagiosum, skin tags, lichen planus, tinea versicolor, actinic keratosis, and squamous cell carcinoma. On the feet, it is sometimes difficult to distinguish between a plantar wart and a callus or corn, an acquired digital fibrous keratoma, or a foreign body.

Warts in the anogenital area are most often condylomata acuminata. They can vary from small sessile papules, verrucous papules, and nodules to large exophytic masses and verrucous plaques. They may appear anywhere from the external genitalia to the internal genital mucosa and cervix. They are occasionally associated with mild itching or burning. Bowenoid papulosis, another manifestation of HPV infection seen on the genitalia, consists of multiple 2- to 3-mm smooth papular warts. Some of these genital lesions are caused by the high-risk HPV genotypes, and patients must therefore be closely followed for the possible development of carcinoma. The sexual partners of persons with genital warts should also be followed for any signs of malignant lesions. Squamous cell carcinoma in situ in the anogenital area, also known as *Bowen's disease*, has been associated with HPV-16 and other oncogenic types of HPV, which

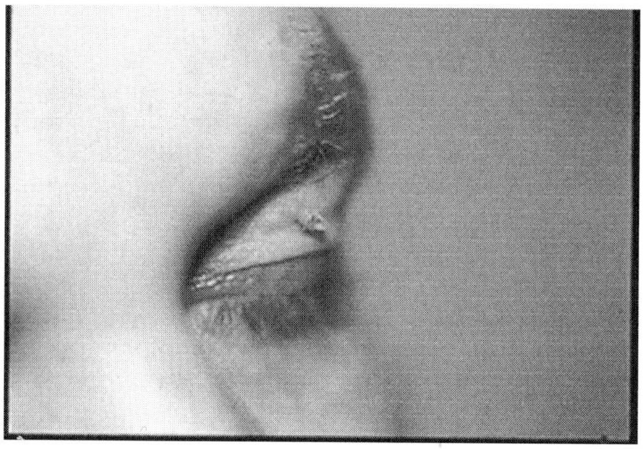

FIG. 141.2. Filiform wart.

also often cause bowenoid papulosis. A patient with these lesions should undergo a biopsy if carcinoma is suspected. It is rare for this type of squamous cell carcinoma in situ to become invasive in an immunocompetent host, but when a patient's immune system is compromised, the physician must be more cautious. Cervical dysplasia and cancer are, of course, a major concern in patients with oncogenic HPV infection; these are discussed in detail in Chapters 27 and 28.

The predominant mode of transmission of genital warts in sexually active adults is through sexual contact (Chapter 86). Nonsexual transmission may also occur. Although most genital warts in children are transmitted by other than sexual routes (e.g., vaginal delivery in women infected with HPV), sexual abuse in children must be excluded.

In the genital area, the differential diagnosis includes mainly molluscum contagiosum, squamous cell carcinoma in situ, lichen planus, seborrheic keratosis, pearly penile papules, syphilitic condylomata lata, sebaceous (Tyson) glands, and skin tags.

HUMAN PAPILLOMAVIRUS INFECTION IN PREGNANCY

HPV infection does not directly affect the course or outcome of pregnancy. However, condylomata acuminata may enlarge during pregnancy and obstruct the birth canal. Transmission of HPV to the newborn is rare but possible. Cutaneous or genital lesions may develop in children (believed to be secondary to autoinoculation). Respiratory papillomatosis in children, in which verrucae of the larynx extend into the oropharynx and bronchopulmonary airways, is often associated with the same HPV genotypes found in genital warts. This observation suggests that infection may be acquired during birth through the aspiration of contaminated maternal secretions. If the HPV type is known to be oncogenic, a small chance for the development of laryngeal cancer exists.

LABORATORY STUDIES AND DIAGNOSIS

Papanicolaou smears and colposcopy should be performed frequently in women who have any form of genital HPV infection or whose male sexual partners have genital HPV infection, given their high risk for the development of cervical cancer. Their male partners should also be screened regularly for any clinically suspect lesions, and for gay persons, some recommend anal smears. The application of a 5% acetic acid solution may aid in the diagnosis of lesions not apparent to the naked eye; the lesions turn white within minutes, but this method is not very sensitive or specific.

With warts, the diagnosis is usually based only on clinical findings. In general, if frequent treatments are failing or the patient's condition is worsening despite treatment, a biopsy should be considered. Immunohistochemical and molecular techniques can detect the presence of HPV in tissue. HPV genotyping may be helpful in determining whether a patient with apparent epidermodysplasia verruciformis is infected with an oncogenic type of HPV and can be used in conjunction with Papanicolaou smears to detect the virus.

TREATMENT AND PREVENTION

Considerable evidence suggests that a patient infected with HPV is infected for life. Therefore, the goal of treatment is to induce wart-free periods. Optimally, this should be achieved with a treatment that is no worse than the disease. Often, when patients do not respond well to treatment, increasingly aggressive treatment is attempted. Unfortunately, more aggressive therapy does not always produce a better clinical outcome.

The main reason for treating warts in parts of the body other than the genitalia is that they present a mechanical problem; they can become tender or traumatized and are often cosmetically bothersome. One option is simple observation. In healthy persons, especially children, it has been estimated that approximately two thirds of warts resolve spontaneously within 2 years. On the other hand, genital warts and bowenoid papulosis should be treated because HPV can be transmitted from the lesions to partners and because of the premalignant potential of the lesions. Treatment of the lesions will not eliminate infection because the virus is present in normal-appearing skin and mucosa adjacent to the lesions.

In the choice of a treatment, the patient's preference, anatomic location of the wart, and treatment modalities available are often the major determining factors. Patients must also be aware that recurrence is possible.

Topical therapies for warts are available over the counter, and newer prescription medications are also available. For common, flat, and palmar/plantar warts, the initial treatment usually consists of the application of acidic preparations, either alone or under occlusion. Keratolytic agents containing salicylic acid are fairly effective when applied consistently once or twice daily for several months. Patient compliance is the major limiting factor with this therapy. Physicians may elect to pare down the warts and apply 50% trichloracetic acid to the area for 2 hours; this treatment is repeated weekly. Cantharidin is another type of topical medication used in the physician's office; it induces acantholysis of the skin. After the medication is applied for 8 to 24 hours, a vesicle forms, and repeating the treatment every 1 to 2 weeks results in resolution. The two latter therapies may cause discomfort and irritation and can lead to scarring.

Topical treatments for genital warts include a variety of chemotherapeutic agents. These should be given with caution, especially to women of reproductive age and potential, because some are teratogenic or contain mutagens. Podophyllin should not be used because it contains mutagens. A 0.5% solution of podophyllotoxin (Condylox) is meant to be applied twice daily every 4 days. It can cause significant irritation, and recurrences are common. 5-Fluorouracil is another chemotherapeutic agent that has been used with some success in this setting but is teratogenic; a 5% cream is available. It is given to treat both genital and flat warts. The use of 5-fluorouracil in combination with destructive therapies has decreased recurrence. However, this treatment is associated with severe inflammation and erosions. Intralesional bleomycin has been used to treat plantar and periungual warts but must be administered with extreme caution given the potential for adverse effects.

The antiviral agent cidofovir can be compounded in a 1% to 5% cream or gel for the topical treatment of genital and widespread warts. Irritation is the most common side effect.

Interferon, one of the first drugs shown to be effective in the treatment of genital warts, is administered by injection into the dermis at the base of the wart or parenterally. Because of the side effect profile (most commonly flulike symptoms) and high cost of interferon, and because this treatment requires frequent visits, it is usually reserved for patients with large numbers of refractory genital warts, epidermodysplasia verruciformis, or laryngeal papillomatosis. Interferon is most effective if used in combination with destructive procedures, but recurrences are still possible after it is discontinued.

The immune modulator drug imiquimod (Aldara) induces interferons and is the most effective treatment for genital warts. It is also very effective in conjunction with cytodestructive methods for the treatment of other types of warts. Imiquimod is applied overnight three times per week, and in conjunction with destructive procedures, it delays and decreases the likelihood of recurrence. Mild local irritation is the most common adverse reaction.

The daily application of 0.05% retinoic acid has been used to treat flat warts. Retinoic acid is most effective when alternated with imiquimod.

Destructive procedures are used for the local removal or destruction of HPV lesions. Cryotherapy with liquid nitrogen is a frequently used modality. When applied properly, it results in a good response with minimal scarring, if any. However, warts often recur and also appear around the treated areas. Liquid nitrogen can be applied with either a spray technique, loosely wound cotton on a wooden stick, or a cryoprobe. It should be applied long enough so that the wart is completely frozen and the liquid nitrogen forms a 1- to 2-mm halo around the wart. For medium-sized to larger warts, repeated freeze-thaw cycles may improve efficacy. Surgery to excise warts usually involves curettage, electrodesiccation, and the application of hot cautery. Laser surgery has also become popular and is used for both cutaneous and mucosal warts, as in laryngeal papillomatosis. These techniques require special training and proctoring if they are to be performed effectively, and in inexperienced hands they can result in a variety of surgical complications. Recurrence is still likely, which is why treatment after these procedures with topical cidofovir, imiquimod, or interferon is increasingly accepted. Care should be taken in the treatment of plantar warts because a scar on the plantar aspect of the foot can cause a great deal of discomfort. Although treating warts removes the symptoms of infection, it is not clear whether the patient's infectivity is altered. Patients with genital warts should be educated and urged to inform their partners, both present and future, of their condition.

Papanicolaou smears and screening have had a tremendous impact on the early prevention and treatment of neoplastic cervical changes. Preventing HPV infection with vaccines is an active area of research. In one study, an HPV-16 L1 virus-like particle vaccine was effective in preventing the acquisition of this HPV viral genotype in young women. Further research is ongoing.

BIBLIOGRAPHY

Beutner KR, Reitano MV, Richwald GA, et al. External genital warts: report of the American Medical Association Consensus Conference. *Clin Infect Dis* 1998; 27:796.

Beutner KR, Becker TM, Stone KM. Epidemiology of human papillomavirus infections. *Dermatol Clin* 1991;9:211.

Koutsky LA, Ault KA, Wheeler CM, et al. A controlled trial of a human papillomavirus type 16 vaccine. *N Engl J Med* 2002;347:1645–1651.

Schiffman MH. New epidemiology of human papillomavirus infection and cervical neoplasia. *J Natl Cancer Inst* 1995;87:1345–1347.

Tyring SK, Arany I, Stanley MA, et al. A randomized, controlled, molecular study of condylomata acuminata clearance during treatment with imiquimod. *J Infect Dis* 1998;178:551–555.

Tyring SK, ed. *Mucocutaneous manifestations of viral diseases*. New York: Marcel Dekker, 2002:247–294.

CHAPTER 142
Cellulitis

Sophie M. Worobec

Cellulitis (nonnecrotizing soft tissue infection) is an acute spreading bacterial infection of the skin and subcutaneous tissue. A superficial infection of the skin is termed *impetigo*. Deeper, necrotizing soft tissue infections are characterized by necrosis of the dermis, hypodermis, fascia, and muscle.

ETIOLOGY

The causative agents of cellulitis are almost always group A β-hemolytic streptococci or *Staphylococcus aureus*. Groups G, B, and C streptococci can also be causative, especially at sites of saphenous vein harvesting for coronary artery bypass surgery. Diabetic patients are at risk for polymicrobial cellulitis, including both Gram-positive and Gram-negative bacteria and anaerobic organisms. Other agents include *Haemophilus influenzae* type b, a Gram-negative organism, especially as a cause of facial cellulitis in young children, and *Pasteurella multocida*, a Gram-negative rod, particularly after animal bites or scratches. Bacteremic bullous cellulitis may be caused by the marine bacterium *Vibrio vulnificus*. Other rare causes of cellulitis include *Pseudomonas*, *Aeromonas*, *Clostridium*, and *Legionella* species, *Helicobacter cinaedi*, and *Sphingobacterium spiritivorum*.

The foremost defense of the body against cellulitis is an intact cutaneous barrier, which can be disrupted by skin trauma or such skin diseases as severe eczema, psoriasis, stasis dermatitis, contact dermatitis, tinea pedis, and onychomycosis (especially after saphenous vein harvesting and resultant lymphatic stasis). The normal skin flora includes various aerobic and anaerobic organisms: coagulase-negative staphylococci (e.g., *Staphylococcus epidermidis*), micrococci, diphtheroids, and *Propionibacterium*. Transient colonizers of the skin include various streptococci, *S. aureus*, and Gram-negative enteric bacteria such as *Escherichia coli* and *Proteus mirabilis*. Any organism can become an opportunistic pathogen in an immunocompromised host.

Conditions commonly predisposing to cellulitis include diabetes, neoplastic disease, chronic obstructive pulmonary disease, alcoholism, malnutrition, immunosuppression, nephrotic syndrome, lymphatic or venous obstruction, atherosclerotic vascular disease, bone fractures, pressure ulcers, and drug abuse.

HISTORY AND PHYSICAL EXAMINATION

The diagnosis of cellulitis is based on the abrupt development, usually within 1 to 2 days, of a rapidly progressing area of redness, warmth, swelling, and tenderness. Lymphadenitis and lymphadenopathy, in addition to malaise, fever, chills, and other systemic symptoms of infection, may be present. Cellulitis most often develops in the lower extremities, but any part of the body may be affected. Cellulitis can be complicated by abscess formation or necrotizing soft tissue infections.

Erysipelas is a superficial type of cellulitis that affects dermal tissue; subcutaneous tissue is usually not involved. Erysipelas is characterized by an elevated, edematous, hot, bright red lesion with a sharply demarcated border. Blisters, purpura, erosions, small areas of necrosis, and scaliness may develop on affected areas.

Blistering distal dactylitis is a superficial infection of the anterior fat pad of the distal portion of the finger or toe. Most cases occur in children. Both hemolytic streptococci and hemolytic staphylococci have been isolated from these lesions. Blistering distal dactylitis is characterized by large, tense blisters on a tender erythematous base.

DIFFERENTIAL DIAGNOSIS

Impetigo is a superficial bacterial skin infection consisting of pustular or bullous skin lesions; when the lesions break, crusts develop. Ecthyma is a variant of impetigo manifested by punched-out, ulcerated, and often painful lesions that usually occur on the lower extremities.

The differential diagnosis of cellulitis includes noninfectious dermatoses such as acute contact dermatitis (lacks systemic symptoms of malaise, fever, and chills), venous thrombosis (may occur with cellulitis), recurrent breast cancer (i.e., erysipeloid carcinoma on the chest wall), and lymphatic obstruction by other tumors.

A purple, red, or violet plaque that is warm and tender on the dorsum of the hand should alert one to the diagnosis of erysipeloid, a cutaneous infection caused by *Erysipelothrix rhusiopathiae*. The organisms enter through breaks in the skin acquired during the handling of contaminated fish, shellfish, or meat.

Cellulitis should be differentiated from necrotizing soft tissue infections: necrotizing fasciitis, progressive bacterial synergistic gangrene, gangrenous cellulitis in an immunosuppressed person, and clostridial soft tissue infections. These severe, deep infections are often life-threatening and require hospitalization and a surgical and infectious disease consultation.

LABORATORY AND IMAGING STUDIES

In cellulitis, the presenting clinical picture is the basis of the diagnosis. Swabs of wounds and broken skin may be helpful, but surface swabs of unbroken skin yield little or no useful information. The results of culture of aspirates or lesional biopsy specimens are frequently negative (≥70% of cases). Blood cultures should be performed if sepsis is suspected and always in immunocompromised or debilitated patients. White blood cell counts show a leukocytosis and bandemia. Skin biopsy is usually unnecessary, but if performed, it demonstrates edema, a mixed lymphocytic and polymorphonuclear infiltrate, and sometimes bacteria with special stains. In streptococcal cellulitis of postoperative wounds, Gram staining of the discharge may reveal chains of Gram-positive cocci. In suspected cases of necrotizing fasciitis, deep incisional biopsy of the central necrotic area helps define the need for prompt surgical debridement.

Special imaging is helpful if gangrene or osteomyelitis is suspected. Rarely, bacterial skin infections may originate in a contiguous deeper focus (e.g., perforated viscus or osteomyelitis) or be caused by the hematogenous dissemination of systemic disease. Soft tissue infections of the hands should be carefully evaluated by a hand specialist to determine whether deep structures such as tendon sheaths, joints, and muscular spaces are involved. Orbital cellulitis requires urgent consultation with an ophthalmologist or a head and neck surgeon for evaluation.

TREATMENT

Most uncomplicated cases of cellulitis can be treated on an outpatient basis with a penicillinase-resistant penicillin or cefazolin. Erythromycin is a next-line agent, but careful monitoring for a response is required because resistance to this agent is increasing. Erythromycin is not indicated for erysipelas, in which the treatment of choice is oral or intravenous penicillin. Alternatives are oral amoxicillin, intravenous ampicillin, intravenous cefazolin, or vancomycin.

Because new antibiotics are constantly being introduced and patterns of resistance may change, consultation with an infectious disease service or a local microbiology laboratory may be indicated to choose the best antibiotic coverage. Hospitalization may be necessary for a compromised host at risk for sepsis, a patient who cannot reliably care for herself at home, one whose disease is progressing despite the use of oral antibiotics, or any patient who presents with a high fever, rigors, severe and rapid progression, or involvement of the face, orbit, or perineum.

Abscesses must be drained, and devitalized tissue requires debridement.

If an open wound is present and the patient has not had a tetanus toxoid booster in the last 5 years, one should be administered. If no initial tetanus series was ever received, both tetanus toxoid and tetanus immune globulin should be given.

Diabetic patients in whom Gram-negative organisms are a concern have been treated with amoxicillin-clavulanate potassium. However, this drug is expensive, and side effects include diarrhea and rash. Various quinolones are also indicated for soft tissue infections. Cefoxitin is another option. If a diabetic patient shows signs of sepsis, parenteral therapy with imipenem or a penicillinase-resistant penicillin plus an aminoglycoside antibiotic should be administered.

Parenteral antibiotic therapy of cellulitis has been given on an outpatient basis to complete treatment after hospitalization or to initiate outpatient oral therapy. A single daily parenteral dose of ceftriaxone effectively treats most cases except for some diabetic foot infections, possibly because of poor coverage of anaerobic bacteria or associated peripheral vascular disease. The pharmacokinetics of teicoplanin, a glycopeptide related to vancomycin, allow once-daily intravenous administration. However, teicoplanin cannot be used to treat infections with Gram-negative organisms; thus, a second drug is necessary when Gram-negative organisms may be involved.

Nonpharmacologic therapy should be used together with antibiotics; the affected area should be rested and moist compresses applied.

CONSIDERATIONS IN PREGNANCY

Although cellulitis is not uncommon during pregnancy, little has been written specifically about cellulitis in pregnant women.

Two severe infections caused by *Pasteurella multocida* were reported in pregnant women who had had contact with animals (licked by a dog and a cat) but no history of an animal bite. Meningitis developed in one patient, and cellulitis with a deep abscess in the other. Both were successfully treated with parenteral penicillin and cephalosporin after failing to respond to oral phenoxymethyl penicillin. The immunoglobulin G level of one patient was slightly decreased, but no other immunologic defects were detected in these women. Partial suppression of cell-mediated immunity during pregnancy may have interfered with their resistance to this infection. The risk for acquiring most infectious diseases is not increased during pregnancy, nor is the severity of infection. However, infectious diseases caused by intracellular bacterial pathogens, such as tuberculosis, viral infections, and systemic fungal, protozoal, and helminthic infections, are significantly more severe during pregnancy.

During pregnancy, higher doses of antibiotics may be needed for pharmacokinetic reasons (see Chapter 12). Renal function and the composition and amount of body fluids change as pregnancy progresses. However, little has been published about pharmacokinetics in pregnancy. Lower levels of ampicillin in serum or plasma have been documented during pregnancy, and it is suspected that levels of other antibiotics are also lower. In cases of severe infection, knowledge of the magnitude and duration of peak serum drug levels is crucial to obtain optimal levels at the site of infection, which is rarely in the bloodstream. Treatment during pregnancy may fail because peak levels of antibiotics are lower where they are needed, at the site of infection. The one exception is the treatment of lower urinary tract infection; levels of antibiotics in the urine appear to be unchanged during pregnancy.

BIBLIOGRAPHY

Bisno AL, Stevens DL. Current concepts: streptococcal infections of skin and soft tissue. *N Engl J Med* 1996;334:240–245.

Dahl PR, Perniciaro C, Holmkvist KA, et al. Fulminant group A streptococcal necrotizing fasciitis: clinical and pathological findings in 7 patients. *J Am Acad Dermatol* 2002;47:489–492.

Kahn RM, Goldstein EJ. Common bacterial skin infections: diagnostic clues and therapeutic options. *Postgrad Med* 1993;93:175.

Lindbeck G, Powers R. Cellulitis. *Hosp Prac (Off Ed)* 1993;28[Suppl 2]:10.

Marinella MA. Cellulitis and sepsis due to *Sphingobacterium*. *JAMA* 2002;288.

Philipson A. Pharmacokinetics of antibiotics in pregnancy and labour. *Clin Pharmacokinet* 1979;4:297.

Rollof J, Johansson PT, Host E. Severe *Pasteurella multocida* infections in pregnant women. *Scand J Infect Dis* 1992;24:453.

Tsao H, Swartz MN, Weinberg AN, et al. Soft tissue infections: erysipelas, cellulitis, and gangrenous cellulitis. In: Freedberg IM, Eisen AL, Wolff K, et al., eds. *Fitzpatrick's dermatology in general medicine*, 5th ed. New York: McGraw-Hill, 1999:2213–2231.

Weinberg ED. Pregnancy-associated depression of cell-mediated immunity. *Rev Infect Dis* 1984;6:814.

Zemstov A, Veitschegger M. *Staphylococcus aureus*-induced blistering distal dactylitis in an adult immunosuppressed patient. *J Am Acad Dermatol* 1992;26:784.

CHAPTER 143
Skin Cancer

Marc D. Brown

Skin cancer continues to be the most common form of cancer, with over 1 million cases per year in the United States. Fortunately, the vast majority of these skin neoplasms are easily diagnosed, can be treated by several therapeutic modalities with a high cure rate, and are usually not a cause of significant morbidity or mortality. The exceptions are melanoma and certain high-risk squamous cell carcinomas. Skin cancers do kill more than 10,000 persons annually in the United States, however, and many of these deaths may have been preventable.

The three most common types of skin cancer are basal cell carcinoma (BCC), squamous cell carcinoma (SCC), and melanoma, all with various histologic and clinical subtypes. The most common etiologic factor in skin cancer is acute or chronic exposure to ultraviolet radiation (exposure to the sun). BCC and SCC are more common in middle-aged to elderly patients; melanoma is often seen in a younger population. These skin cancers range in biologic behavior from slow-growing tumors that invade only locally to rapidly growing and metastasizing malignant carcinomas.

BASAL CELL CARCINOMA

Etiology

BCC is the most common cancer, with an estimated 1 million new cases annually in the United States. Despite its high inci-

TABLE 143.1. Etiology of Basal Cell Carcinoma

Sun exposure
Previous radiation treatment
Arsenic exposure
Trauma
Genodermatoses

dence, very few people die of BCC. This cancer typically grows slowly, and the risk for metastasis is very low. BCC affects men slightly more often than women, but the gap is narrowing as women increasingly expose their skin to the sun. The incidence of BCC increases with age; however, younger persons (in their 20s and 30s) with an initial BCC tumor are being seen more frequently.

The most common etiologic factor is exposure to ultraviolet light. BCC develops more frequently on areas exposed to the sun, such as the central face (especially the nose), ears, forehead, cheeks, neck, upper back, and chest. About 90% of all BCCs develop on the head and neck. BCC more often affects fair-skinned persons, who sunburn easily. It is also more common in those with outdoor occupations and who live in sunny climates. BCC is rare in blacks. Other predisposing factors are listed in Table 143.1.

BCCs that develop at a site of previous irradiation can grow very aggressively. The tumor appears 15 to 30 years after the x-ray treatment. Unfortunately, x-rays were used in the past to treat dermatologic conditions such as acne and tinea capitis. Exposure to arsenic is now rare, but in the past, arsenic was used in medications (Fowler solution) and fertilizer. In patients who have been exposed to arsenic, small pits in the palmar surface of the hands are an associated clinical finding.

Trauma as an etiologic factor is difficult to prove, but historically some patients note the development of BCC after trauma to the skin.

In albinism, protective melanin is lacking. In xeroderma pigmentosum, an autosomal-recessive disease, DNA repair after usual exposure to the sun is abnormal, and skin cancers develop at an early age. Ocular and neurologic abnormalities are associated with this condition. Basal cell nevus syndrome is a rare autosomal-dominant disorder characterized by the development of multiple BCCs early in life. Hundreds of tumors may form. Associated clinical findings include jaw cysts, frontal bossing, hypertelorism, bifid ribs, palmar pits, and internal neoplasms.

Clinical Findings

The several clinical types of BCC are listed in Table 143.2. The most common type is the nodular BCC, which appears as a pink to flesh-colored papule or nodule with a translucent (pearly) surface, telangiectases, and rolled borders (Fig. 143.1). Patients describe a pimple that waxes and wanes in clinical appearance but slowly enlarges. As the nodular BCC grows, central erosion or ulceration may develop; failure to heal, crusting, and bleeding typically cause the patient to seek medical attention. Pain is usually absent except in cases with perineural invasion or invasion of deeper structures, such as cartilage, which may result in tenderness. Although a BCC can be clinically recognized and diagnosed when quite small, the typical size at diagnosis is about 1 cm. If ignored or misdiagnosed, a BCC can reach an impressive size and may result in the destruction and loss of an important structure, such as an ear, nose, or eyelid.

TABLE 143.2. Types of Basal Cell Carcinoma

Nodular
Superficial
Morpheaform
Pigmented
Cystic
Basosquamous

Variants of the nodular BCC include the pigmented and cystic BCC. The pigmented BCC is brown to black as a consequence of melanin deposition in the tumor. The pigmented BCC resembles a nodular melanoma, but close inspection reveals an elevated, rolled, translucent border. The cystic BCC appears as a smooth, round lesion. If near the eyelid, it can resemble a benign hidrocystoma.

The morpheaform BCC is the most aggressive BCC. Synonyms include *sclerosing*, *infiltrative*, and *micronodular BCC*. Clinically, this BCC is poorly defined, with a scarlike appearance: it is white to yellow, flat, indurated, and firm. The infiltrative BCC has the greatest potential for deep and insidious subclinical growth and extension. A nodular BCC has a soft, mushy quality and feel that are easily distinguished, and it can be removed with a sharp curet; in contrast, the infiltrative BCC is difficult or impossible to remove with a curet. The infiltrative BCC is most likely to recur locally after treatment. The basosquamous BCC is a variant of the aggressively growing BCC and histologically shows areas of squamous differentiation within the basaloid neoplasm.

The superficial BCC appears as an ill-defined red, scaly patch or plaque, frequently on the upper back or chest but also on the face. The superficial BCC grows and spreads peripherally and rarely invades deeper subdermal structures. Because of its appearance, the superficial BCC may be misdiagnosed as a dermatitis or fungal infection and slowly enlarge for several years before a skin biopsy establishes the correct diagnosis.

Laboratory Studies

The definitive diagnosis of a BCC is made with a skin biopsy. In most cases, histologic confirmation should be obtained before treatment is begun because the histologic subtype may determine the best treatment option. A biopsy can be performed by shave or punch excision. A punch biopsy provides a deeper tissue sample and should be used for a probable morpheaform BCC. The classic histologic picture of a BCC is that of basaloid tumor islands extending from the epidermis into the dermis or subcutaneous tissue. The tumor islands stain a deep blue with hematoxylin and eosin. An orderly line of cells is seen around the periphery of dermal tumor nests (peripheral palisading), as is stromal retraction. The infiltrative BCC shows numerous small nests and finger-like tumor islands on a background fibrous stroma.

Treatment

Despite its pattern of slow growth, the BCC tumor is characterized by relentless, often extensive subclinical local invasion through soft tissue, cartilage, muscle, and even bone. Thus, treatment is imperative, although not necessarily urgent. The best treatment method for a BCC depends on several factors, including tumor size, histology, location, and previous treat-

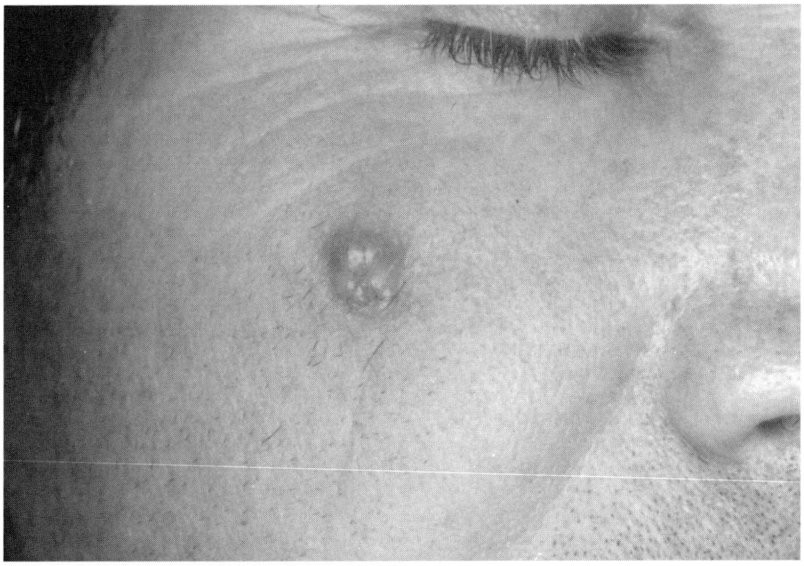

FIG. 143.1. Basal cell cancer (nodular type).

ment. These criteria help to define and distinguish low-risk from high-risk BCCs. Tumors larger than 1 cm on the face and 2 to 3 cm on the trunk are considered to be high-risk. Superficial and nodular BCCs are lower-risk than infiltrative, aggressive BCCs. Histologic evidence of perineural invasion also defines a high-risk BCC. Location is particularly important; areas that are difficult to treat include the nose and ear and the periocular, perioral, and preauricular and postauricular regions of the face. Previously treated BCCs (especially those treated with radiation) that are locally recurrent are also more difficult to treat.

A clear understanding of the indications, advantages, and disadvantages of the available modalities help the physician to adopt a uniform approach to the treatment of BCCs. Most BCCs are low-risk tumors and can be treated with a high cure rate by means of curettage, excision, cryosurgery, radiation, or laser (Table 143.3).

ELECTRODESICCATION AND CURETTAGE

Electrodesiccation and curettage is probably the method of ablation most frequently used by dermatologists for small nodular or superficial BCCs. After the tumor is removed with a sharp curet, electrodesiccation is applied to the base and periphery. This process is then repeated two times. Curettage should not be used for an infiltrative BCC, a recurrent BCC with scar tissue, or a nodular BCC that extends deeply into the subcutaneous tissue. Small tumors treated with electrodesiccation and curettage typically heal in 2 to 4 weeks with a whitish scar; treating large BCC tumors with electrodesiccation and curettage may leave a cosmetically unacceptable scar. The disadvantage of this method is a lack of clear histologic margin control.

TABLE 143.3. Skin Cancer Treatments

Electrodesiccation and curettage
Excision
Radiation
Cryosurgery
Laser
Mohs surgery

EXCISION

Excision and layered closure is best used for larger tumors and in areas where cosmesis is a concern and the skin is relatively loose, such as the neck, cheeks, and forehead. Curettage of the tumor before excision makes a clearer delineation of the margins possible. A surgical margin of 4 to 6 mm is recommended. Excision allows for permanent section margin control. Excision followed by local flap reconstruction is best performed with frozen section margin control before the flap is sutured in place.

CRYOSURGERY

Freezing with liquid nitrogen is an excellent method for premalignant lesions and superficial skin cancers. Treating deeper tumors with cryosurgery requires the use of a thermocouple to measure the depth and degree of freezing adequately. Healing may require 4 to 6 weeks.

RADIATION

Because radiation can induce skin cancers, it is best used in older patients. For patients reluctant to undergo surgery, radiation is an excellent alternative, with good cure rates and acceptable cosmesis. Disadvantages include the need for multiple treatments, possible radiation dermatitis, and lack of margin control.

LASERS

The carbon dioxide laser is destructive and can adequately remove smaller and superficial skin cancers. Wounds heal slowly. Bleeding is minimal, so this may be a good choice for patients who are taking anticoagulant medication.

The use of lasers and photosensitizing agents taken up by the tumor (photodynamic therapy) is being investigated. This method may hold promise for the nonsurgical treatment of multiple, smaller skin cancers.

MOHS SURGERY

In Mohs surgery, serial layers of skin and soft tissue are removed systematically with precise frozen section margin con-

TABLE 143.4. Prevention of Skin Cancer

Use sunscreens with SPF ≥15.
Begin sunscreen use in childhood.
Avoid most intense sun (10 a.m.–2 p.m.).
Wear protective clothing (hat, long-sleeved shirt).
Avoid tanning parlors.
Perform skin self-examination on a regular basis.

SPF, sun protection factor.

trol. Mohs surgery offers the highest cure rates and is indicated for tumors with high-risk characteristics: large size; recurrence; location on the eyelids, ears, nose, or lips; infiltrative histology; perineural invasion. Mohs surgery requires precise layered excision and tumor mapping, along with horizontal histologic frozen section and microscopic examination of all tissue removed. With this procedure, the dermatologic surgeon can track out subclinical extensions of skin cancers while removing as little normal tissue as possible. Mohs surgery is performed in an outpatient setting under local anesthesia, and the defect can be reconstructed immediately once clear margins have been ascertained.

The appropriate follow-up of patients with BCC is important because another skin cancer subsequently develops in up to 35% of patients. Most patients should be seen twice a year for a full skin examination. The use of sunscreens and avoidance of the sun should be stressed at each visit. Preventive steps are outlined in Table 143.4.

SQUAMOUS CELL CARCINOMA

Etiology

SCC is the second most common skin malignancy. More than 100,000 new cases occur in the United States each year, resulting in about 2,500 deaths. SCC originates in epidermal squamous cells and invades the dermis. If confined to the epidermis, it is referred to as *SCC in situ* or *Bowen disease*. Like BCC, SCC is most common in areas exposed to the sun because exposure to ultraviolet light is the primary etiologic factor. Frequent sites of involvement include the lower lip, ear, dorsum of the hand, and scalp. Bowen disease can be seen on the lower legs of women. SCC usually afflicts persons in their 60s or 70s.

In addition to exposure to the sun, other etiologic factors in the development of SCC include previous exposure to radiation (including radiotherapy), chronic scarring processes (e.g., burn scars, chronic skin ulcers, chronic osteomyelitis), genodermatoses, and chronic exposure to polycyclic hydrocarbons. Of interest is the association of some SCCs with human papillomavirus infection. These resemble a warty growth and can be seen on the digits or genitalia. Immunosuppressed patients are also at increased risk for SCC, especially patients with renal transplants.

Clinical Findings

SCCs that develop in skin with actinic damage typically begin as a hyperkeratotic pink to red papule, plaque, or nodule (Fig. 143.2). An SCC can grow rapidly and ulcerate centrally; when aggressive, it can double in size within weeks to months. An SCC can also metastasize, especially to the regional lymph nodes or lungs. Thus, treatment is more urgent than for the slow-growing BCC.

The common precursor lesion for SCC is actinic keratosis, which is a sun-induced premalignant lesion seen most commonly on the face, hands, arms, and scalp of fair-skinned persons. Actinic keratosis appears as a flat to slightly raised pink, scaling lesion, usually less than 1 cm in size. A hypertrophic actinic keratosis is difficult to distinguish from an early SCC, and a skin biopsy is necessary to confirm the diagnosis. Many patients with both BCC and SCC have a background of diffuse actinic keratosis. Bowen disease appears as an erythematous, scaling patch and clinically resembles a superficial BCC (Fig. 143.3).

An SCC arising in an actinic keratosis was previously thought to be unlikely to metastasize. However, more recent studies indicate that such SCCs can be very aggressive. Metastatic rates for SCC range from 2% to 40%. SCCs that develop in old scars or ulcers have a greater metastatic potential. Other risk factors for aggressive biologic behavior include size (>2 cm), deep invasion, location on the lower lip or ear, underlying immunosuppression, perineural invasion, poorly differentiated histology, and previous treatment (Table 143.5).

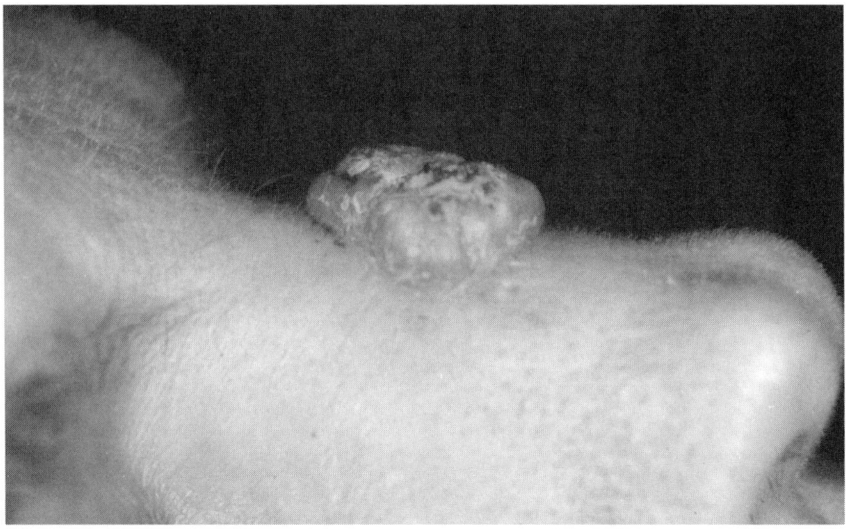

FIG. 143.2. Well-differentiated squamous cell carcinoma.

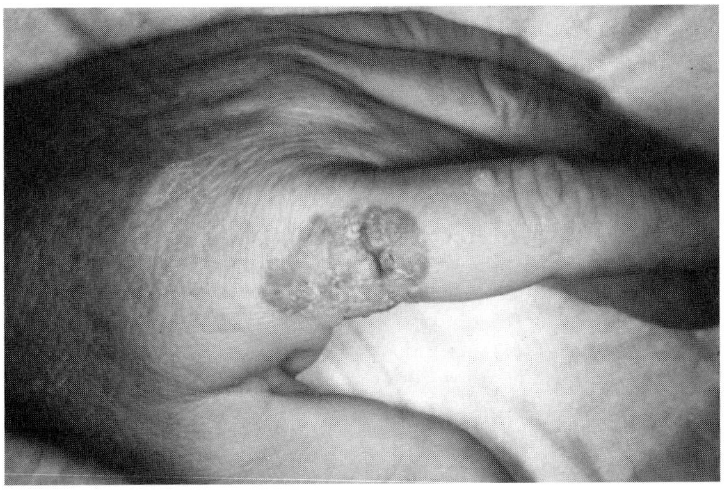

FIG. 143.3. Bowen disease (squamous cell carcinoma in situ).

Laboratory Studies

As with BCC, a skin biopsy is necessary to confirm the diagnosis of SCC. A punch biopsy is preferred to obtain a deeper specimen and so avoid missing evidence of invasion. The pathologist should report whether an invasive SCC is well differentiated, moderately differentiated, or poorly differentiated.

The classic histology of SCC is that of a neoplastic proliferation of keratinocytes arising from the epidermis and extending through the dermis and potentially into deeper subcutaneous tissue. A well-differentiated SCC shows keratin formation with horn pearls. Mitotic figures range from few with fairly normal keratinocyte architecture to frequent and atypical (poorly differentiated). Less common subtypes include lobular, acantholytic, and spindle cell variants.

Treatment

Smaller, low-risk lesions can be treated by standard methods, similar to those used for BCC, with cure rates exceeding 90%. For in situ SCC, topical 5-fluorouracil, cryosurgery, and curettage offer quick and simple treatment. For more invasive SCC, excision and margin control become more important. For high-risk SCC, Mohs surgery or wide local excision is necessary; even then, the cure rate may be only 90% to 95%. Careful palpation of the regional nodes is important, as is a screening chest roentgenogram. Sometimes, patients with a high-risk tumor on the head or neck that is deeply invasive may require elective lymph node dissection or postoperative radiation therapy. For patients with a high-risk SCC, follow-up is recommended every 3 to 4 months for the first 2 to 3 years, then every 6 months thereafter. Patients with extensive actinic keratosis may have to be seen on a regular basis.

TABLE 143.5. High-Risk Squamous Cell Carcinoma

Size >2 cm
Poorly differentiated histology
Deep invasion
Perineural invasion
Etiology (burn scar)
Location (ear, lip)

MELANOMA

Etiology

The incidence of melanoma continues to rise at a rapid and predictable rate; during the past 50 years, it has increased almost 1,000-fold. Currently, the estimated lifetime risk is about 1 in 75. More than 40,000 new cases develop annually in the United States, resulting in about 7,500 deaths. Melanoma is the most common cancer in women ages 25 and 29 and is second only to breast cancer in women ages 30 to 35. The good news is that the overall 5-year survival rate has improved, probably as a consequence of earlier detection, diagnosis, and treatment.

Ultraviolet radiation has been consistently implicated as a major etiologic factor in the development of melanoma. People at high risk are those with fair skin, a tendency to freckle, light-colored hair and eyes, and a history of severe sunburns. A family history of melanoma also increases an individual's risk. Persons with atypical moles or a large number of moles are at increased risk, as are those with large congenital nevi. Intermittent, limited but intense sun exposure appears to be the major element in the development of melanoma. Melanoma is more prevalent among persons of a higher socioeconomic class who work indoors and tend to spend weekends and vacations outdoors. Depletion of the ozone layer may also be related to the increased incidence of melanoma.

The three major precursor lesions to the development of melanoma are dysplastic nevi (atypical moles), congenital nevi, and lentigo maligna.

A dysplastic nevus is an acquired pigmented lesion of the skin. Its clinical and histologic appearance differs from that of the typical common mole. The dysplastic nevus is both a precursor and a marker lesion for the development of malignant melanoma. It is often larger than a common mole and has a variegated color, ranging from tan to dark brown. The margins are irregular and poorly defined, and the center is often raised. The exact incidence of dysplastic nevi in the general population is unknown; estimates range from 2% to 50%. Any dysplastic nevus can develop into a melanoma, although the vast majority do not. Malignant melanoma can also occur de novo on normal skin. Thus, removing all dysplastic nevi from a patient does not ensure that a melanoma will not develop. Moles that change and atypical moles should be evaluated for surgical excision.

Congenital nevi are moles that are present at birth or develop shortly thereafter. Most are small; only 1 in 20,000 newborns has a large congenital nevus. A large ("giant") congenital

TABLE 143.6. Risk Factors for Melanoma

Precursor lesions
Lentigo maligna
Congenital nevus
Dysplastic nevi
Large number of moles
Fair skin, light-colored hair, tendency to freckle
Poor tanning; history of sunburns, sun exposure
Family history of melanoma

nevus is usually defined as one larger than 10 cm. The lifetime risk that a large congenital nevus will develop into a malignant melanoma is estimated to be 6% to 8%. Excision is recommended as early as possible, although removal frequently requires extensive, multistaged surgical procedures. Small congenital nevi, which are present in 1% of newborns, are far easier to treat, but agreement has not been reached regarding the need for surgical excision. The risk for melanoma associated with a small congenital nevus is unknown; small nevi may be responsible for 3% to 15% of all melanomas, but clear data are lacking. Prompt excision is advised for a small congenital nevus that shows evidence of change other than the normal enlargement that occurs in proportion to a child's growth. A small congenital nevus may be excised prophylactically sometime around puberty, when the child can more easily tolerate excision under local anesthesia in an outpatient setting.

A lentigo maligna is a flat, macular, pigmented lesion that appears on sun-exposed areas in older persons. Sunlight is thought to have a causative role. The lentigo maligna begins as a tan, irregular, freckle-like lesion; it subsequently enlarges, and a highly irregular pigment pattern and border may develop. Growth is typically slow, but it can become quite large. A lentigo maligna is best thought of as a melanoma in situ that has the potential to evolve into an invasive melanoma. Surgical excision is the treatment of choice. Superficial treatment methods such as cryosurgery are less reliable because atypical melanocytes may extend along hair follicles and dermal appendages. Other nonexcisional treatment modalities include radiation, laser ablation, and dermabrasion, but these are associated with higher recurrence rates.

Risk factors for melanoma are outlined in Table 143.6.

Clinical Findings

The key to the successful treatment of malignant melanoma is early recognition. The characteristic clinical features of early melanoma can best be remembered as the *ABCD*s of melanoma (Table 143.7): *a*symmetry, *b*order irregularity, *c*olor variegation, and *d*iameter of more than 6 mm. Whereas most moles are round, oval, and uniform, one half of a typical melanoma is asymmetric in comparison with the other half. Margins are typically irregular. The color ranges from hues of tan and brown to black, sometimes mixed with red and pink.

TABLE 143.7. ABCDs of Melanoma Diagnosis

A—Asymmetry
B—Border irregularity
C—Color variegation
D—Diameter >6 mm

Melanoma is classically divided into four subtypes. Superficial spreading melanoma, the most common, occurs at any anatomic site but most often on the trunk and extremities. Nodular melanomas present as elevated or polypoid tumors that grow rapidly and sometimes become ulcerated with more advanced growth.

A lentigo maligna melanoma (Fig. 143.4) develops from the precursor lentigo maligna, as described previously; this is a brown to black macular lesion located on sun-exposed areas of the neck in older persons. Acral melanoma (Fig. 143.5) presents as a darkly pigmented flat to nodular lesion on the palms or soles or under the nails; this subtype is more common in African-Americans and Asians.

Any change in a preexisting mole may signal an evolving melanoma. Although most melanomas are asymptomatic, pruritus and bleeding may occur as they enlarge and become more nodular. Any mole that is symptomatic should be removed for histologic examination.

Laboratory Studies

One of the most important steps in the diagnosis and proper management of a melanoma is a timely and appropriate biopsy. The best biopsy procedure is total excisional removal of the pigmented lesion, usually with a narrow resection margin (2–3 mm). Dissection should be carried to the level of the subcutaneous tissue to obtain an accurate measurement of tumor infiltration, which is important for prognostication and the formulation of a treatment plan. Sometimes, an incisional or punch biopsy may be necessary because of the large size or location of a melanoma (e.g., a large lentigo maligna melanoma on the face). In this case, a punch biopsy specimen should be taken from the most deeply pigmented or nodular area of the suspected melanoma. No evidence indicates that a melanoma will spread from a biopsy site. Removal of a suspect pigmented lesion by shave excision or curettage is not recommended.

An important element of the histologic diagnosis is the Breslow depth, which is the vertical thickness (in millimeters) from the stratum granulosum to the deepest portion of the melanoma. The Breslow depth most accurately determines the patient's prognosis, the likelihood of metastasis, and the treatment recommendations. Other helpful information provided in the pathology report includes evidence of ulceration, regression, or angiolymphatic invasion; degree of mitotic activity; and presence or absence of precursor lesions.

Whether patients with early melanoma should undergo routine laboratory testing is controversial. No data clearly support the value of routine chest roentgenography, complete blood cell counts, and chemistry profiles. Nonetheless, many physicians think they are warranted as baseline studies. More extensive diagnostic investigations, such as computed tomography, magnetic resonance imaging, and nuclear scans, clearly are not indicated in staging asymptomatic patients with thin melanomas unless suggested by a specific finding on the physical examination. Sentinel lymph node biopsy is indicated if the Breslow depth is greater than 1 mm. If clinical palpation reveals grossly involved lymph nodes, nodal dissection without a prior biopsy is reasonable. If nodal biopsy or dissection shows metastatic melanoma, then full-body computed tomography should be performed to detect distant or visceral spread of the melanoma. More complete diagnostic radiologic studies may also be indicated for deep melanomas (>4 mm), in which the risk for metastasis is more than 50%.

A complete physical examination is important in all patients with melanoma. This begins with careful inspection and palpa-

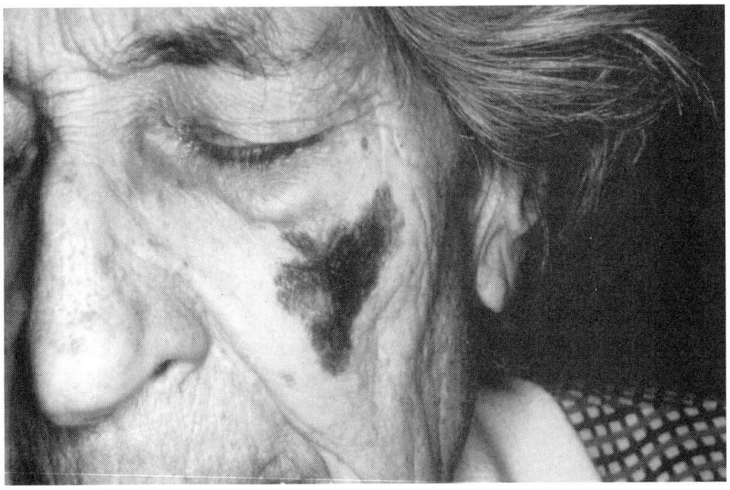

FIG. 143.4. Lentigo maligna melanoma.

tion around the area of the melanoma and a search for cutaneous metastatic lesions. Regional and distant lymph nodes are carefully palpated to detect any clinical evidence of metastatic disease. A thorough cutaneous evaluation includes examination of the scalp, conjunctivae, oral mucosa, genitalia, perianal area, nails, palms, and soles. Any liver or spleen enlargement should be noted.

Treatment

The treatment options for melanoma are based on the Breslow depth of invasion and the clinical stage. A major trend has been a decrease in the size of the margin required for reexcision after a diagnosis of melanoma. Previously, lesions of melanoma were excised with up to a 5-cm margin of normal skin. The result was often cosmetically unacceptable, and a skin-grafting procedure was required for reconstruction. More recent clinical trials indicate that thin melanomas can be excised with a much narrower margin. The optimal margin of resection is uncertain, but data suggest that resection margins of more than 2 cm do not improve survival. The dissection should be carried to the level of the deep subcutaneous tissue, but muscle fascia does not have to be removed. In most cases, the resulting defect can be closed in a side-to-side fashion or with a local flap. For melanoma in situ, without evidence of invasive disease, excision with a 5-mm border of clinically normal skin is sufficient. Theoretically, this should result in a 100% cure rate. For invasive melanomas with a Breslow thickness of less than 1 mm, a 1-cm margin of clinically normal skin is required. This results in a 5-year survival rate exceeding 95%. Thicker melanomas are associated with a higher risk for microscopic satellitosis, and therefore a wider margin of resection is required (usually 1–2 cm, depending on the Breslow depth of invasion).

Long-term follow-up is important for patients with melanoma. Late recurrences are possible, even in those whose melanomas were thin. Of greater concern is the development of a second primary melanoma. It is estimated that a second melanoma develops within 3 years in 3% of persons who have had a melanoma. A secondary primary melanoma develops in up to one third of patients with the familial atypical mole and melanoma syndrome. In addition, immunocompromised patients tend to be at high risk for the development of multiple primary melanomas. Although somewhat arbitrary, 6 months appears to be an appropriate interval between examinations for patients with thin melanomas. For patients with thicker, high-risk melanomas, return visits three or four times a year are recommended.

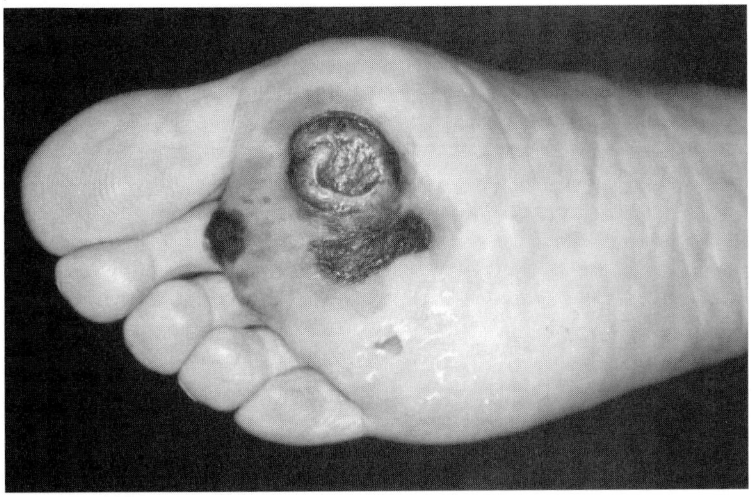

FIG. 143.5. Acral melanoma.

Considerations in Pregnancy

The issue of whether pregnancy before, during, or after a diagnosis of melanoma affects the prognosis and outcome is controversial. No data unequivocally suggest that pregnancy worsens the prognosis. However, melanoma can cross the placental barrier and affect the fetus. If a melanoma is diagnosed during pregnancy, it should be removed immediately. Some physicians advise women with melanoma to avoid pregnancy for several years after the diagnosis and thus avoid the possibility of becoming pregnant if metastatic disease develops. Obviously, this is a highly individual decision on the part of patients.

BIBLIOGRAPHY

Guidelines of care for basal cell carcinoma. *Am Acad Dermatol Bull* 1990;8[Suppl]:9.

Johnson TM, Smith JW Jr, Nelson BR, et al. Current therapy for cutaneous melanoma. *J Am Acad Dermatol* 1995;32:689.

Koh HK. Cutaneous melanoma. *N Engl J Med* 1991;325:171.

Kwa RE, Campana K, May R. Biology of cutaneous squamous cell carcinoma. *J Am Acad Dermatol* 1992;26:1.

Miller SJ. Biology of basal cell carcinoma. *J Am Acad Dermatol* 1991;24:1.

Schwartz RA. *Skin cancer: recognition and management*. New York: Springer-Verlag, 1988.

Swanson NA. Basal cell carcinoma: treatment modalities and recommendations. *Prim Care* 1983;10:443.

CHAPTER 144
Dermatoses of Pregnancy

Sophie M. Worobec and Madhuri Ventrapragada

The skin exhibits many changes during pregnancy: the nipples, areolae, and external genitalia become more darkly pigmented; a linea nigra develops on the lower abdomen; existing moles may darken; and a facial blotchy hyperpigmentation, termed *melasma*, develops in up to 70% of women. Hair growth resulting in mild to moderate hirsutism is common and resolves either in the third trimester or after delivery. In 1 to 5 months postpartum, telogen effluvium occurs; regrowth is usually seen within 1 year. Stretch marks, or striae cutis distensae, develop over the abdomen, hips, buttocks, and breasts, often with the initial presentation of itching. Skin tags may enlarge and proliferate. Hyperemia results in palmar erythema in up to two thirds of women. Both spider angiomata and cherry angiomata may appear. Existing angiomata tend to enlarge. Varicosities of the lower extremities may worsen.

Sweet syndrome, which includes a constellation of signs (fever, leukocytosis, tender red plaques, and biopsy findings of a subepidermal edema with a neutrophilic dermal infiltrate), has been reported in six patients during pregnancy. In two women, it recurred during subsequent pregnancies (Fig. 144.1).

The dermatoses of pregnancy can be divided into those that are well defined and those that are poorly defined. Among the well-defined entities are pemphigoid gestationis (PG), pruritic urticarial papules and plaques of pregnancy (PUPPP), intrahepatic cholestasis of pregnancy (ICP), and "impetigo herpetiformis," which is a form of pustular psoriasis. The first three conditions are described in this chapter, and the last in Chapter 137.

PEMPHIGOID GESTATIONIS (HERPES GESTATIONIS)

PG is an immunologically mediated bullous disease of pregnancy and the postpartum period. It is recurrent and marked by extremely pruritic urticarial papules or vesicles, which often are grouped together on an erythematous background. Urticarial plaques may be present, and bullae may evolve from the vesicles, but the mucous membranes are spared. The face, palms, and soles are rarely involved. Excoriations and crusts are common (Figs. 144.2 and 144.3).

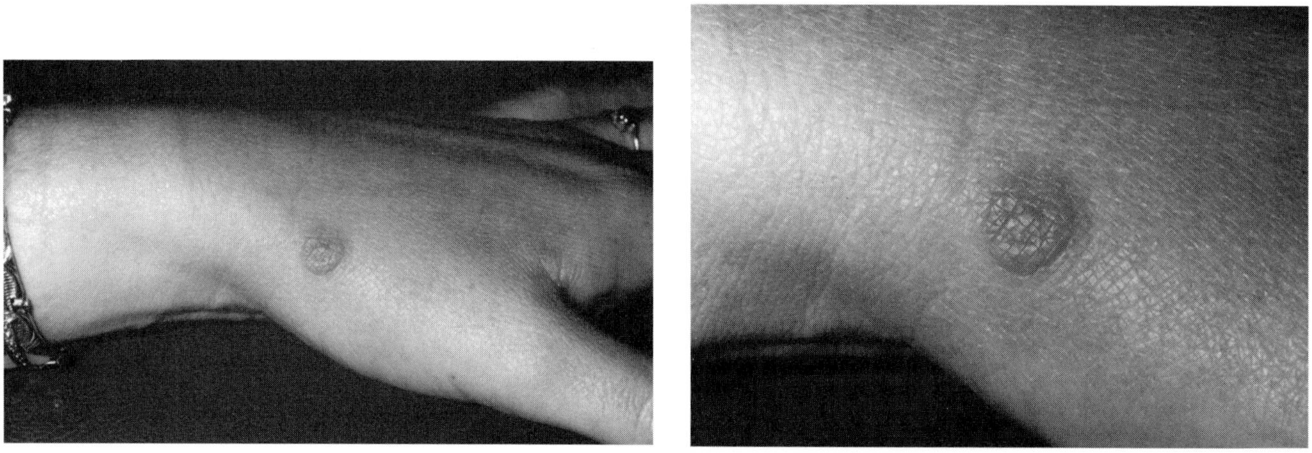

A B

FIG. 144.1. A: A pseudovesicular plaque associated with Sweet syndrome. **B:** Close-up view of the same plaque. These multiple firm, red, edematous plaques, which may recur, have an edematous feel and appear somewhat translucent, so that the term *pseudovesicular* has been used to describe them. They vary in size and duration, and after they heal, a dusky red or hyperpigmented patch is left. The diagnosis is by biopsy, which reveals a dense, neutrophilic infiltrate in the upper dermis. Sweet syndrome is associated with malignancy in approximately 30% of cases and should trigger an age-appropriate workup for malignancy. However, in six case reports, Sweet syndrome was associated with pregnancy in normal women. Pregnancy-associated Sweet syndrome may recur during subsequent pregnancies.

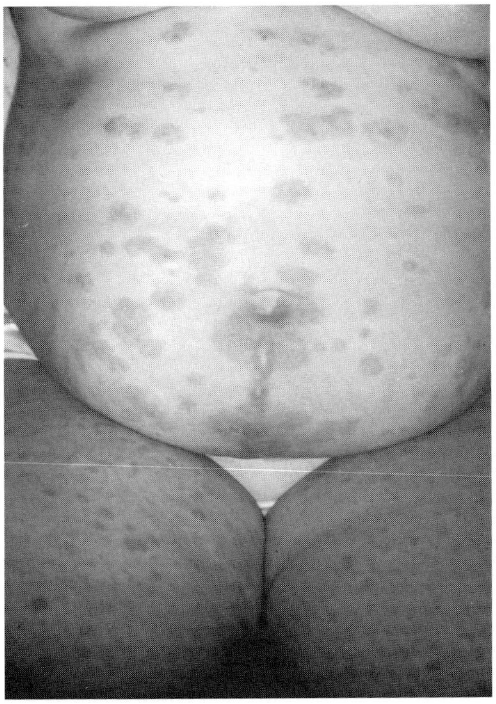

FIG. 144.2. Pemphigoid (herpes) gestationis is an immunologically mediated bullous disease of pregnancy that appears postpartum. The eruption is marked by small papulovesicles with an erythematous rim. Urticarial plaques may also be present. The lesions are in a generalized distribution. (Courtesy of Dr. Kim B. Yancey.)

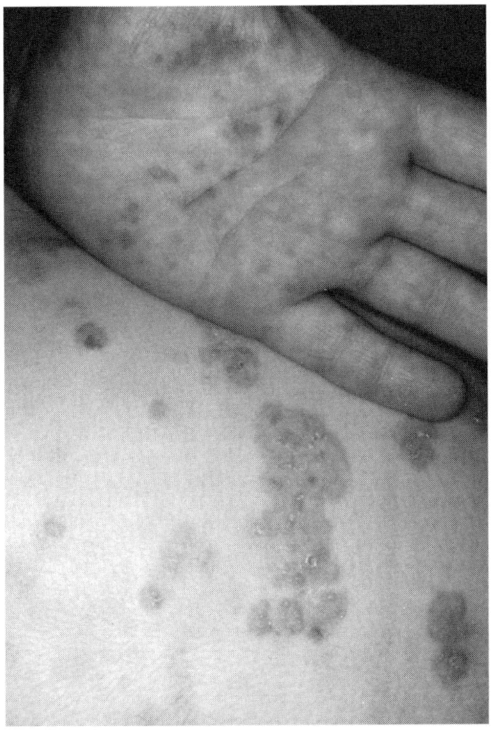

FIG. 144.3. Close-up view of the lesions of pemphigoid (herpes) gestationis. Small papulovesicles are grouped together on an erythematous background. Excoriations and crusts are common. (Courtesy of Dr. Kim B. Yancey.)

Etiology

PG has no relationship to herpes viral infection. In PG, circulating immunoglobulin G1 (IgG1) autoantibodies have been demonstrated that bind to one of two antigen sites within the epidermal basal membrane zone. One of these sites consists of a 180-kd protein, which has been identified as bullous pemphigoid antigen-2 (BPA-2); the other, BPA-1, is a 230-kd protein. These antigens are present in extracts of human placenta and amnion and also are recognized by sera from patients with bullous pemphigoid. The incidence of HLA-DR3 or HLA-DR4 or a combination of the two is increased in patients with PG. The incidence of PG has been variably estimated at 1 in 1,700 to 50,000 deliveries in the United States, 1 in 40,000 deliveries in the United Kingdom, and 1 in 60,000 deliveries in Europe.

History

The eruption most often starts in the second or third trimester, with flares common at the time of delivery or postpartum. The onset can also be in the first trimester or postpartum. Most cases resolve within a few months after delivery, with a few urticarial eruptions occurring in the first year postpartum. The eruption may recur during subsequent pregnancies and begins earlier in the subsequent pregnancy. The use of birth control pills may also cause flares. A few patients have experienced recurrences for more than 10 years postpartum. Exacerbations have been associated with hormone-producing tumors (hydatiform mole or choriocarcinoma).

One study showed an increase in fetal morbidity and mortality, but this was not confirmed in a subsequent large study. In a series of 11 cases, one intrauterine death occurred. The number of small-for-gestational-age infants born to affected mothers and the incidence of preterm delivery may be increased. Infants may rarely exhibit a transient urticarial, vesicular, or bullous eruption, which resolves after a few weeks. PG is associated with autoimmune disease, particularly Graves disease.

Physical Examination

The eruption is polymorphic and consists of papules, plaques, vesicles, and sometimes tense bullae; the lesions occur anywhere on the body but start on the abdomen in more than 50% of cases.

Differential Diagnosis

The differential diagnosis includes allergic contact dermatitis, drug eruption, and PUPPP. In rare cases, target lesions may be present, leading to a differential diagnosis of erythema multiforme or bullous pemphigoid.

Laboratory Studies

Skin biopsy shows edema of the dermal papillae and an infiltrate consisting of eosinophils, lymphocytes, and a few neutrophils. A subepidermal blister with necrosis of basal cells may be found, but routine histopathologic study alone does not distinguish PG from other blistering diseases. The diagnostic test is direct immunofluorescence of a perilesional skin biopsy specimen with demonstration of the third component of complement (C3) in a linear pattern along the basement membrane (Fig. 144.4). The deposits may persist for more than 1 year after the eruption has cleared and have also been demonstrated in the skin of infants born to affected mothers. Other immune reactants, most often IgG, have also been found along the basement membrane.

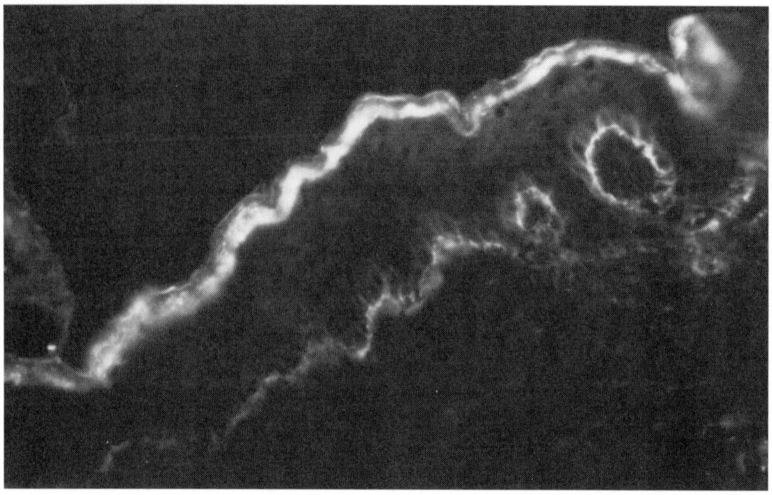

FIG. 144.4. Pemphigoid (herpes) gestationis. Direct immunofluorescence of skin close to the lesions is used to diagnose this condition. Here, the third component of complement (C3) is deposited in a linear pattern along the basement membrane. Other immune reactants, most often immunoglobulin G, may also be found along the basement membrane. (Courtesy of Dr. Kim B. Yancey.)

Treatment

The goal of treatment is to suppress the formation of blisters and relieve the intense itching. Topical corticosteroids have controlled mild cases. Systemic glucocorticoids, usually 0.5 mg of prednisone per kilogram daily (≥1 mg/kg per day), and first-generation antihistamines have been the cornerstone of treatment. The dose of prednisone can be reduced in steps if the eruption subsides, then increased at delivery as required (because the disease often flares postpartum). Plasmapheresis has been effective in severe cases, and high-dose immune globulin combined with cyclosporine has also been used. Studies do not demonstrate a difference in the number of premature or small-for-gestational-age infants with treatment, and no increase in fetal morbidity or mortality has been noted. If the mother requires treatment postpartum, breast-feeding may be difficult because antihistamines and corticosteroids pass into breast milk, and this issue should be discussed with the pediatrician. If the mother is treated with prolonged high-dose corticosteroids, infants should be monitored for adrenal insufficiency. Infants may have a transient eruption that abates spontaneously and does not require treatment.

PRURITIC URTICARIAL PAPULES AND PLAQUES OF PREGNANCY

PUPPP is a common itchy disorder that develops toward the end of the third trimester of pregnancy and rarely in the postpartum period. Red urticarial papules and plaques usually begin on the abdomen, especially within stretch marks, then spread onto the thighs and sometimes the buttocks and arms (Fig. 144.5). PUPPP affects 1 in 130 to 300 pregnancies.

Etiology

The etiology of PUPPP is unknown. Increased maternal weight gain, increased fetal weight gain, and an increased incidence of twinning in 30 patients have led to the hypothesis that abdominal distention, or a reaction to it, may be important.

History

PUPPP is much more common in primigravidas but may occur in any pregnancy. In half of the cases, lesions first develop within periumbilical striae. They usually resolve spontaneously in the postpartum period. Very rarely, a postpartum onset or exacerbation occurs. No increase in fetal loss or morbidity has been reported. PUPPP usually does not recur in subsequent pregnancies.

Physical Examination

The lesions of PUPPP are polymorphous. They consist of extremely itchy, 1- to 2-mm red urticarial papules that usually appear first on the abdomen within periumbilical stretch marks. Within days, they coalesce into plaques and spread onto the thighs, buttocks, arms, and chest but usually spare the face, palms, and soles. Microvesicular, purpuric, targetoid, or polycyclic lesions occasionally occur.

Laboratory Studies

Biopsy is usually not necessary; the diagnosis is made based on the clinical presentation. The routine histopathologic findings are nonspecific, showing upper dermal edema, a lymphohistiocytic perivascular infiltrate, and sometimes eosinophils. The results of direct immunofluorescence of the perilesional skin are negative, and this test should be performed if a diagnosis of PG is in the differential diagnosis.

Treatment

The treatment of PUPPP consists of the application of emollients and topical corticosteroids and, rarely, short courses of systemic steroids. In severe cases, some advocate the use of potent topical corticosteroids five to six times per day, or a short course of oral steroids. Successful therapy with ultraviolet light of wavelength B (UVB) has been reported.

INTRAHEPATIC CHOLESTASIS OF PREGNANCY (RECURRENT CHOLESTASIS OF PREGNANCY, PRURIGO GRAVIDARUM)

ICP is marked by severe itching that is sometimes followed by jaundice. It usually occurs in the late third trimester but is also seen earlier in pregnancy. The incidence is estimated to be 0.02% to 2.4% of pregnancies.

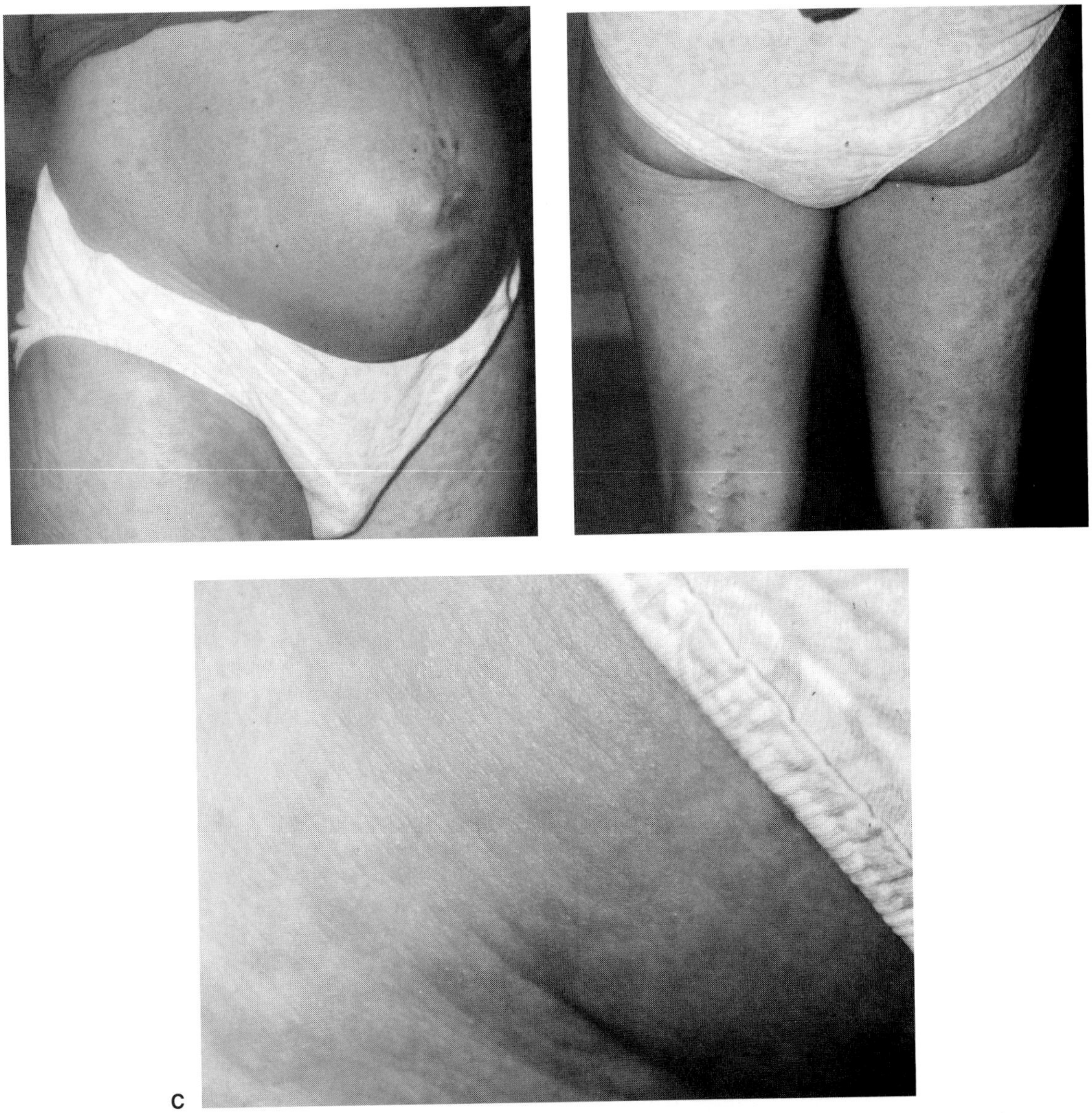

A B C

FIG. 144.5. Pruritic urticarial papules and plaques of pregnancy. This condition is characterized by red urticarial papules and urticarial plaques **(A),** which usually appear first on the abdomen and then spread to the thighs and sometimes the buttocks and arms, **(B)** seen here on the thighs. **C:** Close-up view of urticarial papules on the lower buttock.

Etiology

A genetic predisposition is suggested by reports of recurrent episodes of cholestasis of pregnancy in several members of the same family. The incidence of HLA-A31 and HLA-B8 is increased. Whether increased levels of estrogen, progesterone, or both contribute to the cholestasis is unknown.

History

Severe generalized itching that is generally worse at night and has no other cause (e.g., eczema, scabies) is the hallmark of the medical history. Fatigue, anorexia, nausea, fullness in the right quadrant, light-colored stools, dark urine, and vomiting may be present. The patient should have no history of exposure to hepatotoxic drugs or hepatitis viruses. Fat malabsorption may lead to vitamin K deficiency and weight loss in severe cases. The condition is usually not associated with risks to the mother unless she has a severe vitamin K deficiency. Fetal complications include an increased incidence of fetal distress, preterm delivery, and stillbirth. The pruritus usually resolves within a few days after delivery. The symptoms may return during subsequent pregnancies (40%–50% of patients) or with oral contraceptive use. The prevalence of gallstones in affected women is high.

Physical Examination

No primary skin lesions are present, but secondary excoriations may be widespread. Jaundice (if it occurs) may not develop until 4 weeks or later after the onset of itching. The liver may be enlarged and slightly tender. Rare uterine and intracranial hemorrhage has been reported in women with severe vitamin K deficiency.

Laboratory Studies

Mild to moderate hyperbilirubinemia, elevated serum alkaline phosphatase and acid levels, abnormal hepatic transaminase levels, and impaired sulfobromophthalein retention may be found in women with recurrent ICP. The most sensitive test is an increased postprandial total serum level of bile acid.

Impaired vitamin K absorption leads to a prolonged prothrombin time. Therefore, the prothrombin time should be monitored and vitamin K administered as necessary. Examination of the placenta often reveals nonspecific abnormalities that may cause fetal hypoxia.

Treatment

Bland emollients, topical remedies to relieve itching, antihistamines, ursodeoxycholic acid, and cholestyramine (4 g two or three times daily) have been used as treatment. In Europe, phototherapy with UVB or UVA is considered helpful. The intramuscular administration of vitamin K before delivery has been advocated by some to diminish the risk for vitamin K deficiency. Some investigators have successfully treated severe disease with oral corticosteroids.

OTHER DERMATOSES OF PREGNANCY

Four of the poorly defined dermatoses of pregnancy are discussed in the following sections.

Prurigo of Pregnancy (Prurigo Gestationis of Besnier)

Prurigo of pregnancy is described as itchy erythematous papules and nodules over the upper trunk and extensor surfaces of the extremities. It usually resolves during the postpartum period with residual hyperpigmentation. Blistering is absent, and no fetal morbidity or mortality is associated with this condition, which may be related to atopy, cholestasis, or both.

Papular Dermatitis of Pregnancy

Papular dermatitis of pregnancy is described as 3- to 5-mm red papules that quickly become crusted and excoriated, leaving a hyperpigmented scar. It is controversial whether this condition is actually a separate entity.

Pruritic Folliculitis of Pregnancy

Pruritic folliculitis of pregnancy was first described in six patients in 1981, also as 3- to 5-mm excoriated red papules. On skin biopsy, five of the six patients had sterile folliculitis. All the offspring were healthy, and the results of direct immunofluorescence were negative. The eruption resolved at delivery, within 1 month after delivery, or within 1 week after onset. Subsequent cases have been reported. The condition may be underdiagnosed. The differential diagnosis includes infectious folliculitis, eosinophilic folliculitis, PUPPP, prurigo of pregnancy, PG, steroid acne, and acne vulgaris.

Autoimmune Progesterone Dermatitis of Pregnancy

Autoimmune progesterone dermatitis is a rare cyclic skin reaction caused by sensitivity to progesterone. Skin lesions may be urticarial, papulovesicular, bullous, eczematous, or acneiform, or they may resemble those of erythema multiforme. The eruption usually appears during the luteal phase of the menstrual cycle, when progesterone levels are high.

Autoimmune progesterone dermatitis of pregnancy was reported in 1973 in a patient with a papulopustular eruption over the extremities, buttocks, and thighs during the first trimester. Some of the lesions were acneiform, and some had a psoriasiform scale. Peripheral eosinophilia, pulmonary infiltrates, and polyarteritis were associated findings. The pregnancy ended in a spontaneous abortion in the third month, as had a previous pregnancy (in the second month) in which the patient had experienced a similar dermatitis. Skin biopsy of lesional skin revealed intraepidermal eosinophilic abscesses together with lymphocytes and histiocytes, dense perivascular infiltrates, and a lobular panniculitis with eosinophilic abscesses within the subcutaneous tissue. An intradermal injection of aqueous progesterone produced a delayed hypersensitivity reaction and similar histologic findings. The dermatitis resolved after the abortion. No premenstrual flare of this patient's dermatitis was reported, although a progesterone-containing contraceptive worsened her symptoms.

IMMUNOLOGIC CHANGES OF PREGNANCY

In a report that appeared in 1995, 12% of sera from pregnant women, but only 2% of sera from women who were not pregnant, contained IgM that reacted with the epidermal proteins of 180 kd (BPA-2) and 230 to 240 kd (BPA-1) in the basement membrane zone. These women had no clinical disease; therefore, the anti-basement membrane zone antibodies can be regarded as "natural autoantibodies." The IgM antibodies exhibit a low level of affinity, in contrast to the high level of affinity of the IgG antibodies that bind to BPA-2 and BPA-1 in PG. An extension of this finding is that humoral reactivity is greater in pregnant women than in women who are not pregnant. Pregnant women produce several antibodies to both paternal and fetal antigens. The immunologic changes of pregnancy, coupled with the profound physiologic changes, are probably are responsible for the skin disorders and changes that develop during pregnancy.

BIBLIOGRAPHY

Bierman SM. Autoimmune progesterone dermatitis. *Arch Dermatol* 1973;107:896.

Borradori L, Didierjean L, Bernard P, et al. IgM autoantibodies to 180- and 230- to 240-kd human epidermal proteins in pregnancy. *Arch Dermatol* 1995;131:43.

Cohen LM, Capeless EL, Krusinski PA, et al. Pruritic urticarial papules and plaques of pregnancy and its relationship to maternal-fetal weight gain and twin pregnancy. *Arch Dermatol* 1989;125:1534.

Engineer L, Bhol K, Ahmed AR. Pemphigoid gestationis: a review. *Am J Obstet Gynecol* 2000;183:483–491.

Hirvioja ML, Tuimala R, Vuori J. The treatment of intrahepatic cholestasis of pregnancy by dexamethasone. *Br J Obstet Gynaecol* 1992;99;109.

Jurecka W. Pregnancy dermatoses. In: Lebwohl MG, Heymann WR, Berth-Jones J, et al., eds. *Treatment of skin disease: comprehensive therapeutic strategies*. London: Mosby, 2002:69.

Katz SI. Herpes gestationis (pemphigoid gestationis). In: Freedberg IM, Eisen AZ, Wolff K, et al., eds. *Fitzpatrick's dermatology in general medicine*. New York: McGraw-Hill, 1999:686.

Kroumpouzos G, Cohen LM. Dermatoses of pregnancy. *J Am Acad Dermatol* 2001;45:1–19.

Lawley TJ, Yancey KB. Skin changes and diseases in pregnancy. In: Fitzpatrick TB, Eisen AZ, Wolff K, et al., eds. *Dermatology in general medicine*. New York: McGraw-Hill, 1999:1963.

Ling TC, Coulson I. Autoimmune progesterone dermatitis. In: Lebwohl MG, Heymann WR, Berth-Jones J, et al., eds. *Treatment of skin disease: comprehensive therapeutic strategies*. London: Mosby, 2002:69.

PART

16

Psychological and Behavioral Problems

CHAPTER 145

Depression

Adrian Leibovici and Linda Chaudron

Depression, one of the most common mental disorders, is an important source of disability for both men and women. It is associated with emotional and physical distress, with dysfunction at work and in personal relations, and in extreme cases with suicide. About one fourth of all persons in the United States will experience some form of depression in their lifetime, and in about 9% of the population the symptoms will reach clinical proportions.

CLASSIFICATION AND EPIDEMIOLOGY

From a clinical viewpoint, depression can be construed as a symptom (feeling down, blue, sad, with low mood), a sign (affect depressed as observed by an objective examiner), a syndrome, or an illness.

Syndrome of Depression

Depressed mood and inability to experience pleasure (anhedonia) are the most common features of depression. They must be sustained and severe. Appetite is decreased or less frequently increased, and weight loss or gain follows in severe cases. Sleep is disturbed, in the form of insomnia or hypersomnia. Patients complain of fatigue, lack of energy, and difficulty with concentration or decision-making. Thinking is dominated by ideas of poverty, worthlessness, and guilt. Thought processes and motor function can be either slowed or sped up (psychomotor retardation or agitation). In the most extreme cases, patients exhibit delusions and suicidal thinking and behavior.

Depressive Illness

The nosology of depression is complex and evolving due to the phenomenologic and etiologic diversity of this common psychiatric condition. The official psychiatric classification of depression (*Diagnostic and Statistical Manual,* 4th edition) recognizes several broad diagnostic categories: major depressive disorder (unipolar), dysthymic disorder, bipolar disorder, cyclothymic disorder, substance-induced mood disorder, mood disorder due to a general medical condition, and adjustment reaction with depressed mood.

Major depressive disorder is characterized by a rather severe and prolonged depressive syndrome that lasts at least 2 weeks, more often several months. The natural course is usually episodic. The severity, frequency of episodes, extent of interepisodic recovery, and response to treatment vary. Women are twice as likely to develop major depression as men: lifetime prevalence in the community is 10% to 25% for women and only 5% to 12% for men. Ethnicity, education, income, and marital status do not predict depression, but the illness is 1.5 to three times more frequent in first-degree relatives of afflicted persons. A subtype of depression in which hyperphagia, hypersomnia, decreased libido, anxiety, and so-called rejection sensitivity are more prevalent in women. It is referred to as "atypical depression."

The most severe cases of depression present with extreme psychomotor retardation, nihilistic or paranoid delusions, severe weight loss, early morning awakening, and a tendency to feel worse in the morning (diurnal mood variation): This clinical picture is called melancholia.

Bipolar disorder or manic-depressive illness typically consists of alternating episodes of depression and mania. The manic state consists of elevated or irritable mood, grandiosity, decreased need for sleep, pressured speech, racing thoughts, distractibility, and increased levels of energy and goal-directed activity (sexual, professional, social). The same syndrome of somewhat lesser intensity is called hypomania. The diagnosis of bipolar disorder is made if at least one manic or hypomanic episode occurs, even in the absence of documented depressive episodes. The interval between episodes often is asymptomatic, especially early in the course of illness. Some patients tend to cycle more rapidly with aging. In severe cases, so-called mixed affective states are described: The patient experiences a mixture of depressive and manic symptoms at the same time, for instance, hyperactivity and flight of ideas on one hand and unhappiness and suicidal ideation on the other. When true mania is present, bipolar disorder 1 is diagnosed. It is equally common in both sexes and has a lifetime community prevalence of 0.4% to 1.6%. Bipolar disorder 2 is diagnosed when hypomania but not mania is present. It tends to be more common in women, and its prevalence is only 0.5%. Women with bipolar disorder tend to have more depressive and mixed episodes (i.e., dysphoric mania) than men.

Dysthymic disorder is characterized by a depressive syndrome of somewhat lesser intensity but of longer duration than major depression. The diagnostic time criterion is at least 2 years, although in most cases the illness lasts much longer. The terms chronic depression and depressive personality have also been applied. The disorder is two to three times more frequent in women. The lifetime community prevalence is 6%.

Cyclothymic disorder, referred to in the past as cyclothymic personality disorder, is a chronic condition characterized by periods of depression and periods of manic-like acceleration. The severity of symptoms and extent of disability are less than with bipolar disorder. As with dysthymia, cyclothymia lasts very long and many times defines a person's behavioral and interacting style. The lifetime community prevalence is 0.4% to 1 %, and the genders are equally affected.

These four diagnostic categories can be seen as primary, because their etiology is largely unknown. Secondary depression (Table 145.1) is also very common. It can be caused by an emotional stressor (adjustment reaction with depressed mood), by a foreign substance taken for medical or recreational reasons (substance-induced mood disorder), or by a concurrent medical condition (mood disorder due to a general medical condition). Depressive syndromes are also quite prevalent as concomitants or complications of other psychiatric conditions, such as anxiety disorders, schizophrenia, and certain personality disorders. The clinical picture of secondary depression is quite variable, ranging from brief and mild sadness to the most severe forms of melancholia. Many times the course is atypical, following that of the primary etiologic factor. Prevalence is known for certain conditions (e.g., 25%–40% of patients with Parkinson disease have depression) but less studied for others.

TABLE 145.1. Conditions Associated with Secondary Depression

Infections: Acquired immunodeficiency syndrome, influenza, mononucleosis, viral hepatitis, tuberculosis, syphilis
Collagen disease: Systematic lupus, rheumatoid arthritis, scleroderma
Malignancy: Carcinomatosis, pancreatic carcinoma
Endocrine disease: Hypothyroidism, hyperthyroidism, hypopituitarism, Cushing disease, Addison disease
Neurologic disease: Stroke, multiinfarct dementia, other dementias, brain tumor, head trauma, epilepsy (temporal lobe), Parkinson disease, multiple sclerosis
Avitaminosis: Pellagra, pernicious anemia
Iatrogenic: Antihypertensives (β-blockers, α-methyldopa), vincristine, vinblastine, cycloserine, steroidal contraceptives, cimetidine
Accidental intoxications: Thallium, mercury
Drugs of addiction: Intoxication and withdrawal (alcohol, anxiolytics, cocaine, amphetamines); intoxication (opioids, inhalants, hallucinogens, PCP)

ETIOLOGY AND PATHOGENESIS

Primary Depression

The exact cause and mechanism are unknown, but a multifactorial paradigm is generally accepted, because it accommodates facts and findings from different and sometimes competing fields. Heredity, neurochemistry and neurophysiology, gender, personality type, early emotional trauma, and life stressors have all been shown to correlate with the occurrence of depressive illness and with its natural course.

Heredity

Adoption and twin studies support the notion that both bipolar and unipolar major depression recurrent subtypes have genetic transmission, although efforts to identify a locus or depressive gene have not been successful. It is unknown if inheritance is based on a single dominant gene or a polygenic continuum or if the gene or genes are autosomal or X-linked. The phenotypic expression of genetic vulnerability is reflected in the 1.5- to 3-fold increase in prevalence in first-degree relatives of patients with major depression. First-degree relatives of persons with bipolar depression are also at increased risk of developing mood disorders.

Neurobiology

The discovery more than three decades ago that pharmacologic monoamine oxidase inhibition was associated with an antidepressant effect raised the possibility that metabolic pathways influenced by this group of enzymes could be involved in the pathogenesis of depression. Much research has been done in this area, leading to the identification of neurotransmitters, brain receptors, and specific pathways thought to be connected with mood and mood disorders. Abnormalities in serotonin and norepinephrine systems are thought to occur in mood disorders, and most antidepressants influence predominantly these two systems.

Gender

Women's greater vulnerability to depression is well documented but poorly understood. Research into gender differences has not yielded significant insights into the mechanisms of depression in general, although several theories have been advanced:

- Women have higher concentrations of monoamine oxidase, the very enzyme inhibited by one class of antidepressants.
- Women respond with mood swings to physiologic changes mediated by sexual hormones.
- Clinical and even subclinical abnormalities in thyroid hormone secretion are more common in women and have been linked to certain types of depression.
- In a male-dominated society, women are thought to display more passivity, reliance on interpersonal associations, and helplessness, which might make them vulnerable to depression when confronted with adversity and loss.

Emotional Deprivation

Animal studies in primates have shown that separation from the mother and the group in the first month of life leads to severe behavioral disturbance, consisting of withdrawal and self-aggression (anaclitic depression). Depression might be more severe and start earlier in life in persons who lose a parent in childhood; child abuse and neglect are considered important elements in the history of some patients with chronic depressive syndromes.

Stress

Adverse life events such as separation and loss (real or anticipated) are linked to depressive syndromes. They may cause depression, as in adjustment reactions, or precipitate a depressive decompensation in patients with preexisting vulnerability. Sometimes the connection between life stressors and depression is obvious, but other times it takes an astute and persistent clinician to reveal it: Many women deliberately or unconsciously conceal abandonment, painful anniversaries, sexual problems, or victimization.

Secondary Depression

Virtually any medical condition can cause depression, via some known or presumed neurochemical effect, by means of the psychological trauma of being ill (incapacity, severe prognosis, deformity), or as a combined psychobiologic reaction. For instance, severe depression associated with carcinoma of the pancreas sometimes precedes diagnosis or severe symptoms, but when the patient becomes aware of this most malignant illness, a reactive component is often superimposed.

Mood disorders are described in association with collagen diseases, infections, endocrinopathies, neoplasms, and avitaminosis. Organic processes in the brain are frequently complicated by depression. Degenerative diseases such as multiple sclerosis, Parkinson disease, or temporal lobe epilepsy can cause symptoms that are more severe than what would be expected from a psychological response to illness. Poststroke depression can pose major management problems because it interferes with the victim's effective participation in rehabilitation at a critical time. Left and anterior locations of the stroke predict a high incidence and typical clinical picture of depression; right and posterior localizations lead to less typical brain syndromes, where affect is mostly restricted and flat. Lack of energy and motivation, poor appetite and sleep, and even psychomotor retardation are characteristic to end-stage organ failure (hepatic, renal, cardiac). Depressive thought content and depressed affect and mood are sometimes present.

Steroidal contraceptives have been associated with depression, which can be severe. Other medications causing iatrogenic depression include antihypertensives (e.g., beta-blockers, α-methyldopa, reserpine), cytostatics (e.g., vincristine, vinblastine), and antipsychotic drugs.

Drugs of abuse and addiction can cause mood pathology during or after either intoxication or withdrawal. Cocaine withdrawal and alcohol intoxication, for instance, are often accompanied by intense dysphoria and suicidal tendencies, which are generally short-lived.

DIAGNOSIS

The clinical diagnosis of depression is relatively easy and should be made by any informed clinician. Several simple rules should be observed:

- The clinician should maintain a high level of suspicion in the presence of major life stressors.
- Some patients do not complain unless specific questions are asked.
- When avoided, questions about substance abuse, sexual function, and suicidality reflect the interviewer's rather than the patient's awkwardness.
- The physician's office is not always conducive to the free expression of intimate thoughts and feelings, so the clinician should try to put the patient at ease as much as possible.
- Rushing to comfort and reassure a patient who starts complaining might shut her off, and the full scope of her distress will not become apparent.
- When in doubt, the clinician should obtain psychiatric consultation.

GOALS OF TREATMENT

Symptom reduction is crucial in the acute phase of treatment: Not only is the subjective distress associated with this illness extreme (severe psychological pain), but the risks of suicide can be lowered considerably by initiating supervision and effective interventions early. Restoring function and preventing depressive relapse are the other two major objectives of treatment, becoming more relevant as the patient starts to improve.

Psychological autopsy shows that depression is a major factor in most suicides. Each time depression is diagnosed, the practitioner should assess suicide risk immediately and take appropriate action. Direct questions about the presence of death wishes, suicidal thoughts, and concrete plans to commit suicide and the availability of means to carry out such plans should be asked without hesitation. The myth that such questions might lead the patient to hurting herself is disproved by clinical reality. In fact, many times suicidal patients are reassured when unacceptable self-destructive fantasies can be shared with a sympathetic nonjudgmental professional. Certain history and clinical features are known risk factors for suicide, and their presence or absence should be determined: prior suicide attempts, family history of suicide, alcoholism in the patient or family, coexistence of severe medical illness (incurable or with intractable pain), psychotic depression, living alone, hopelessness, old age, and white race. When a significant risk of suicide is determined to be present or when in doubt, immediate evaluation by a psychiatrist should be obtained. Procrastination can be fatal: Many patients who commit suicide had seen a physician shortly before the act. This underscores the need to protect patients at risk. Mobilizing supportive family members to supervise the patient until she can be seen by a psychiatrist (suicide watch) or even calling an ambulance and forcefully transporting the patient to the hospital for evaluation is sometimes necessary.

A thorough diagnostic effort helps the clinician identify conditions that are directly causal or only contributing factors to the depressive syndrome. Specific treatment, when available, may obviate or minimize the scope of antidepressant treatment. Examples include hormone replacement in hypothyroidism; aggressive treatment of congestive heart failure; finding alternatives to offending drugs such as propranolol, oral contraceptives, and cimetidine; or addressing the patient's cocaine or alcohol addiction.

Symptomatic treatment for depression includes antidepressant medication, electroconvulsant therapy (ECT), and psychotherapy. Severity of illness, affordability, patient preference, type of depression, and previous response to treatment all play a role in the choice.

Research has been conducted in an effort to objectify the relation between the use of medication, standardized psychotherapies, or both and the outcome of treatment. It is generally accepted that mild depression, especially so-called reactive depression, can be treated with psychotherapy alone, but severe depression will not respond without antidepressant medication or ECT. In depression of moderate severity, the choice of treatment is less clear. It appears that both psychotherapy and antidepressant medication are more effective than placebo and that coadministration of medication and psychotherapy is more effective than either one alone.

ANTIDEPRESSANT MEDICATION

With the advent of newer better tolerated antidepressants, the use of medication in primary care practice and in less severe forms of depression has expanded significantly. The generalist who chooses to treat depression should maintain a certain level of familiarity with the use of different therapies. In practice, antidepressant medication is tried rather than psychotherapy, because the latter is time-consuming and requires special training and expertise.

There are several classes of antidepressant medication (Table 145.2). All antidepressants are equally effective in therapeutic doses, although a particular patient might respond to one antidepressant but not to another. The choice of antidepressant is based on the side effect profile, price, and convenience of use. The only predictors of therapeutic response for a particular drug are previous good response in the patient or in another family member. Therapeutic effect can be seen after 10 to 14 days, although in some cases it takes 6 or 8 weeks. It is important to stress with patients the lack of instant response to antidepressant medication: Along with side effects, impatience with the lack of quick symptom relief is a major source of noncompliance. Another important circumstance associated with therapeutic failure in depression is the use of antidepressant medication in insufficient dosage or for an insufficient amount of time.

The mechanism of action of antidepressants is not entirely understood, but they all seem to influence neurotransmission by enhancing noradrenergic, serotonergic, and to a lesser extend dopaminergic systems.

Selective Serotonin Reuptake Inhibitors

Selective serotonin reuptake inhibitors (SSRIs), such as fluoxetine, sertraline, paroxetine, citalopram and fluvoxamine, have become the most popular antidepressants among general practitioners. They are as effective as traditional antidepressants, at least in outpatient settings, and in most cases have a more favorable side-effect profile; specifically, they are practically devoid of side effects such as orthostatic hypotension, tachycardia, or heart block. Jitteriness, insomnia, and gastric discomfort are among the most common side effects and, with few exceptions, are tolerable. Sexual dysfunction, especially anorgasmia, can be a problem for some patients. SSRIs compete in variable degrees for the cytochrome P-450 2D6 enzyme system, which can increase levels of other medications administered concurrently (e.g., tricyclic antidepressants, some antipsychotics, coumadin, quinidine, flecainide). Fluvoxamine inhibits the 3A4 isoenzyme and may increase cardiotoxicity when coadministered with antihistaminic drugs such as terfenadine or astemizole. Overall, however, SSRIs are well tolerated and not as dangerous as other antidepressants when taken in overdose, a distinct possibility in some depressed patients. Other appealing features of this class of antidepressants are easy administration (once a day in most cases), lack of association with undesirable weight gain, and anticompulsive antianxiety properties. Sensational reports in the media linking fluoxetine (Prozac) to suicidal and homicidal ideation and behavior were based on case reports and to date have been disproved by systematic research. One major drawback of SSRIs is their high price, which should be taken into consideration with women who have limited resources.

TABLE 145.2. Commonly Used Antidepressants

Class	Generic name	Brand name	Dose range (mg/d)
Heterocyclics			
Tertiary amines	Imipramine	Tofranil	150–300
	Amitriptyline	Elavil	150–300
	Doxepine	Adapin, Sinequan	150–300
	Clomipramine	Anafranil	150–300
Secondary amines	Desipramine	Norpramin	150–300
	Nortriptyline	Aventil, Parlor	75–150
	Amoxapine	Asendin	150–450
	Protriptyline	Vivactil	15–60
	Trimipramine	Surmontil	150–300
	Maprotiline	Ludiomil	150–200
Selective serotonin reuptake inhibitors	Fluoxetine	Prozac	20–80
	Fluvoxamine	Luvox	100–300
	Sertraline	Zoloft	50–200
	Paroxetine	Paxil	20–50
	Citalopram	Celexa	20–60
Dual action	Mirtazapine	Remeron	15–45
	Venlafaxine	Effexor, Effexor XR	75–375
MAOIs (monoamine oxidase inhibitors)	Phenelzine	Nardil	45–90
	Tranylcypromine	Parnate	30–50
	Isocarboxazid	Marplan	30–50
Other	Trazodone	Desyrel	200–450
	Nefazodone	Serzone	100–500
	Bupropion	Wellbutrin, Wellbutrin SR	150–350

Dual-Action Antidepressants

A consensus is slowly emerging from clinical trials and the collective experience of many practitioners that in some cases, especially where symptoms are extremely severe, newer antidepressants affecting both serotonergic and noradrenergic transmission might be more effective. So far venlafaxine and mirtazapine can be said to belong to this new class, but others are being developed. Venlafaxine is an activating antidepressant also approved for treatment of generalized anxiety disorder. It can cause increase in supine diastolic blood pressure, especially in higher doses, and hence it is prudent to monitor blood pressure. Mirtazapine is sedating, which can be an advantage when given at bedtime to patients with insomnia. There are reports that it can lead to weight gain, which might be a limiting factor, especially in patients with hyperphagia.

Heterocyclic Antidepressants

Medications in this class used to be the first choice of antidepressant in most cases until a decade ago when they started to be slowly replaced by SSRIs. There are two subgroups of heterocyclics: tertiary amines (e.g., imipramine, amitriptyline, doxepin, clomipramine) and secondary amines (e.g., desipramine, nortriptyline, protriptyline, maprotiline). Side effects include orthostatic hypotension, tachycardia, quinidine-like delays in atrioventricular conduction, constipation, urinary retention, dry mouth, blurred vision, confusion, sedation, insomnia, and restlessness. Tertiary amines are more anticholinergic and sedative, so they are more useful in agitated depression and when insomnia is prominent. Secondary amines are "activating" and less anticholinergic: They are more suitable when psychomotor retardation is present or when it is important to avoid sedation, as in patients who work or drive. Among tricyclics, nortriptyline has become popular with psychiatrists because there seems to be a more reliable therapeutic window when blood levels are measured. Amitriptyline, once one of the most popular antidepressants, is avoided now, especially in the elderly, because it is the most anticholinergic and sedative agent. It is as effective as the other antidepressants and is the least expensive agent, which can be relevant in uninsured patients. Clomipramine, the first drug marketed in the United States specifically for obsessive-compulsive disorder, works as a potent antidepressant also.

Treatment with tricyclic antidepressants requires monitoring of physical status. A baseline electrocardiogram should be obtained, especially in at-risk patients such as the very old and the very young. Vital signs, including orthostatic changes, should be checked periodically. A typical trial in a young healthy woman might start with desipramine 50 mg at bedtime. The dose is increased gradually to 150 mg at bedtime over 1 week as tolerated. If no improvement is noted after 4 weeks, further increments in dose are attempted, up to 300 mg/d. Measuring blood levels can be useful; a steady state for any given dose is reached in about 5 days. In the elderly, the dosage needed and tolerated can be considerably lower, and increments should be more gradual—in other words, "start low, go slow."

Monoamine Oxidase Inhibitors

Phenelzine, tranylcypromine, and isocarboxazid are the only medications in this class currently in use for depression in this country. They irreversibly inhibit monoamine oxidase activity, slowing the catabolism of monoamines like norepinephrine and serotonin. They are very effective, especially when anxiety is a prominent feature, as in "rejection sensitivity depression." The most common side effects include orthostatic hypotension, mild anticholinergic toxicity, and sedation. Rarely, patients might experience a hypertensive crisis resulting from the ingestion of catecholamine precursors because the physiologic defense against such an occurrence, intestinal monoamine oxidase, is suppressed by the drug. Patients taking monoamine oxidase inhibitors must eliminate tyramine-rich foods from the diet (e.g., chocolate, coffee, wine, processed cheese, canned meats) and avoid using medications such as L-dopa or cold remedies containing sympathomimetics. Another severe complication is a serotonin syndrome (extreme, even fatal hyperpyrexia), which was associated with the coadministration of monoamine oxidase inhibitors and meperidine or other drugs like SSRIs, other analgesics, and so forth.

Other Antidepressants

Several antidepressants that do not belong to the main three classes can be very useful. Trazodone, which primarily influences the serotonin system, has a separate soporific effect that is dose related; at even low doses some patients experience relief of insomnia. High doses necessary for antidepressant effect can be prohibitively sedating. Nefazodone, which is chemically related to trazodone, is thought to present some advantage when anxiety is a prominent feature of depression. There are recent reports of liver toxicity, and liver function monitoring is advised. Bupropion is notable for its lack of negative effect on sexual function. It also has no notable cardiotoxicity, but in high doses it is associated with a higher incidence of seizures.

Drug Combinations and Antidepressant Augmentation

In psychotic depression, an antipsychotic agent is added to the antidepressant. When insomnia, agitation, or anxiety accompanying depression are severe, a benzodiazepine can be given for several weeks, until the antidepressant medication takes effect. Lithium carbonate, stimulants, and triiodothyronine are thought to enhance the action of antidepressants and are sometimes added to an established antidepressant regimen. Such associations, as well as combinations of two antidepressants, are used in refractory depression and should only be handled by a psychiatrist.

ELECTROCONVULSANT THERAPY

ECT is the most effective treatment for severe depression. It is especially indicated in patients with high suicidal risk, catatonia, agitated depression, inability to tolerate medication, lack of response to several good trials with antidepressants, and a previous response to ECT, and if it is the patient's preference. There are no absolute contraindications, and it has been given without ill effects to pregnant women. It is administered by a psychiatrist, usually in an inpatient setting, but the primary care physician should remain involved, providing support to the patient and medical consultation as needed to the psychiatrist.

TREATMENT OF BIPOLAR DISORDER

Mania and hypomania are best treated with mood stabilizers such as lithium, carbamazepine, and valproic acid. The same agents can be used when the patient is asymptomatic to prevent future episodes, but alone they are ineffective in treating depression. In acute mania, antipsychotics are necessary for sedation; in extreme cases ECT may be needed. When a patient with bipolar disorder is being treated with antidepressants, the clinician must monitor her closely for early signs of acceleration, because one of the side effects of antidepressants in this group of patients is reversal to mania.

PSYCHOTHERAPY

Mild and moderate forms of depression may respond to psychotherapy alone; in severe depression, psychotherapy can be used as an adjunct to somatic treatments. Of the more than 200 forms of psychotherapy described, several deserve to be mentioned because they are widely used, consist of better standardized techniques, and have been systematically studied against medication and against each other for efficacy.

Cognitive therapy is based on the assumption that negatively distorted thinking about oneself is crucial to the depressive syndrome and that helping the patient identify such distortions and correct them as they occur can lead to symptom reduction. Interpersonal therapy focuses on the patient's social relations, which are almost always disrupted. Whether such difficulties are causal, concomitant to, or consequences of depression, the interventions are the same, namely helping the patient resolve a grief reaction, eliminate social isolation, and negotiate new social roles. Brief dynamic psychotherapy decreases symptoms by identifying and resolving a core conflict between unacceptable wishes and social and moral constraints. Supportive psychotherapy is patient-and problem-driven rather than based on a particular theory and allows for the flexible application of many techniques, including discussion, advice, reassurance, limit setting, persuasion, confrontation, interpretation, and clarification.

In depressed women, issues such as guilt, loss, dependency, painful memories of abuse and abandonment, and low self-esteem are pertinent regardless of the treatment modality and should be investigated and addressed. Education about the nature of the depressive illness and the rationale and specifics of different treatments, including medication and ECT, can take a fair amount of time in the self-absorbed, indecisive, distraught patient. Such minimal supportive interventions can and should be attempted by all primary care providers who choose to prescribe antidepressant medication. If the practitioner is too busy for such a time commitment, it is better to refer the patient directly to a mental health professional.

SPECIAL CONSIDERATIONS IN WOMEN

Differences in prevalence notwithstanding, mood disorders have a similar clinical picture regardless of gender. In an eclectic model of illness, gender-specific social, biologic, and psychological factors are taken into account in each case, but in general, "female depression" cannot be seen as a separate illness. Nevertheless, several "vulnerable" periods occur across the life course of women and require special consideration.

For women, depression is a rather common response to gender-specific difficulties in overcoming crises and developmental milestones. The breakup of a romantic relationship, marital oppression by a dominant partner and other conflicts in which the woman feels powerless, becoming a widow, hysterectomy, and nursing home placement and living are situations in which women become extremely vulnerable to psychopathology in general and to depression in particular. The primary care provider, not the mental health professional, has the opportunity to notice the first manifestations and to take appropriate action.

Premenstrual Symptoms and Syndrome

The premenstrual period is one of physical discomforts, mood changes, and even depressive syndromes for many women. Historically, premenstrual disorders were poorly defined entities consisting of physical and psychological symptoms of variable severity with a specific temporal correlation with the menstrual cycle. The disorders have been interchangeably labeled premenstrual syndrome, late luteal dysphoric disorder, and premenstrual dysphoric disorder (PMDD).

Rigorous research has found that approximately 50% to 75% of women experience premenstrual physical changes such as abdominal pain or bloating, headaches, and breast tenderness; 30% report mood changes such as increased mood lability, irritability, or tearfulness; and 3% to 5% meet criteria for a major mood disorder, PMDD. Symptoms of PMDD must be present during most menstrual cycles in the year and include depressed mood or mood lability, anxiety, and/or anhedonia occurring 1 week before menses and disappearing within a few days of menses onset. Other symptoms include physical symptoms listed above as well as fatigue, appetite changes, feeling overwhelmed, and having difficulty concentrating. Women with PMDD may find their work, school, and relationships markedly impaired by this syndrome. Because PMDD symptoms overlap with other affective disorders, clinicians should rule out an underlying mood disorder or anxiety disorder that is exacerbated premenstrually by having women chart their symptoms for 2 consecutive months. Data indicate that SSRIs, used either continuously or intermittently, are effective in the treatment of PMDD. Intermittent dosing is recommended to begin after ovulation, during the luteal phase, and continue until 2 to 3 days after menses onset.

Considerations in Pregnant and Lactating Women

Women who are depressed during pregnancy are at higher risk for obstetric complications and for delivering low-birth-weight infants. Decisions regarding treatment should balance the goal of using as little medication as possible to minimize infant exposure and possible teratogenesis and toxicity to the infant against the risk of decompensation, with its severe consequences for both mother and child. Because of the high prevalence of depression among women of childbearing age, it is important to counsel all women regarding the implications of using psychotropics in pregnancy before starting medication.

No link between the use of heterocyclic antidepressants during pregnancy and congenital malformations could be established in several large-scale European retrospective studies of either consecutive random births or consecutive deliveries of malformed infants. Studies of SSRIs, particularly fluoxetine, sertraline, paroxetine, and citalopram, seem to indicate this class of drug is relatively safe during pregnancy. There are no reports of increased rates of major malformations in infants exposed to SSRIs. Studies of young children exposed in utero have found no differences in the behavioral and cognitive development of these children compared with unexposed children. A recent study has also found no increased rates of major malformations in infants exposed in utero to venlafaxine. Preliminary postmarketing analysis of outcomes in women treated with fluoxetine during pregnancy seems to indicate that this drug should be relatively safe as well. Other new drugs, such as bupropion and the rest of the SSRIs, are less well studied from this point of view. There is some indication that monoamine oxidase inhibitors are associated with teratogenesis in animals and humans, and they should probably be avoided in pregnancy.

The use of heterocyclics late in pregnancy has been associated with toxicity and withdrawal in the neonate. Symptoms include respiratory distress, heart failure, seizures, irritability, and anticholinergic effects such as urinary retention and tachycardia.

Although all psychotropic medications are excreted in breast milk, data indicate that most tricyclics, except doxepin, are found in very small amounts in breast milk and are most often undetectable in infant serum. Similarly, fluoxetine, sertraline, and paroxetine have been found in minimal or undetectable amounts in infant serum. The long half-life of fluoxetine may be of concern because there is one case report of an infant with therapeutic levels of its metabolite. However, in general, these medications appear to be safe to use in nursing mothers if the infant is regularly monitored by the pediatrician.

Mood stabilizers, including lithium, carbamazepine, and valproic acid, have all been shown to be teratogenic in humans. Lithium taken in the first trimester of pregnancy has been associated with a 20-fold increase in congenital malformations compared with the general population. Most frequently noted were Ebstein anomaly and other cardiovascular abnormalities. Even so, many children exposed to lithium in the first trimester have normal development. Therefore, if exposure does occur, the fetus should be monitored echocardiographically rather than automatically prescribing therapeutic abortion. Lithium equilibrates across the placenta and can be toxic to both mother and fetus, especially when given close to delivery. The newborn can present with "floppy baby syndrome" (hypotonia, lethargy, cyanosis), fetal goiter, arrhythmia, and poor sucking response. Blood levels in the mother can show dangerous increments immediately after delivery due to the sudden decrease in glomerular filtration rate. Other factors, such as edema and the use of sodium-depleting diuretics and sodium restriction for hypertension, can affect lithium levels and must be considered. The concentration of lithium in breast milk averages half of that in maternal plasma. Two cases of lithium toxicity in infants breast-fed by women taking lithium have been documented. The American Academy of Pediatrics considers lithium to be contraindicated during breast-feeding. Because of the small therapeutic window for lithium and the possibility of toxicity, if treatment with lithium is required, the infant must be closely monitored.

Carbamazepine was considered relatively safe until it was associated with craniofacial defects, nail hypoplasia, and developmental delay. There is a well-documented association between the use of valproic acid in the first trimester and spina bifida in the offspring; therefore, this medication is contraindicated in pregnancy. Both carbamazepine and valproic acid are considered compatible with breast-feeding because the concentration of these medications in breast milk averages below 10% that in maternal plasma. Cases of liver dysfunction in infants exposed to both carbamazepine and valproic acid through breast milk have been reported, so infants should be closely monitored.

Postpartum Mood Disorder

In the first 3 to 6 months postpartum about 25% of women are affected by a depressive syndrome that meets criteria for major or minor depression. Symptoms include tearfulness, mood lability, irritability, obsessive and intrusive thoughts about oneself and one's ability to be a good parent, poor appetite, difficulty falling asleep, lack of energy, and mild cognitive disturbance due to poor concentration and inattention. A small number of women develop bipolar disorder, and these women may present with a mixed picture of dysphoric and hypomanic or manic symptoms as well as psychotic symptoms. The etiology is unknown, but risk factors to consider are a personal or family history of depression and life stressors, especially a poor relationship with the child's father. Attempts to identify biologic determinants for postpartum depression, including estrogen, progesterone, thyroid hormones, or cortisone levels, have been unsuccessful. Treatment consists of a combination of pharmacotherapy (SSRIs, venlafaxine, or tricyclics in usual doses have been effective) and supportive psychotherapy (individual or group). The focus of psychotherapy is to explain the nature of symptoms and their relation to the patient's circumstances and to reassure the patient that the prognosis for full remission is quite good.

Psychotic depression, a severe form of postpartum depression, is potentially dangerous, because the patient can engage in violent behavior toward herself or her child in response to delusions or hallucinations. It responds to aggressive treatment with antidepressants and antipsychotics or with ECT and may require psychiatric hospitalization (see Chapter 147).

Postpartum depression must be distinguished from the so-called maternity blues, a period of mild depressive mood and lability starting within 3 days after delivery and lasting no more than 2 weeks. It is self-limited, but physician reassurance and support from the family are helpful. Postpartum depression usually starts after an interval of apparent well being after delivery, but in some cases what seems to have started as maternity blues progresses to a full-blown major depression.

Menopause

Historically, involutional melancholia was a depressive syndrome associated with menopause. Research to date has not supported any increased prevalence or distinct depressive syndrome during menopause. Nevertheless, women with a history of depression, particularly depression around hormonal fluctuations such as PMDD or postpartum depression, are at high risk of a depression during the perimenopausal period.

BIBLIOGRAPHY

American Psychiatric Association. *Diagnostic and statistical manual of mental disorders,* 4th ed. Washington, DC: American Psychiatric Association, 1994.

Bech P. Acute therapy of depression. *J Clin Psychiatry* 1993;54[Suppl]:18.

Burt VK, Suri R, Altshuler L, et al. The use of psychotropic medications during breastfeeding. *Am J Psychiatry* 2001;158:1001–1009.

Chaudron LH, Jefferson J. Mood stabilizers during breastfeeding: a review. *J Clin Psychiatry* 2000;61:79–90.

Elia J, Katz IR, Simpson GM. Teratogenicity of psychotherapeutic medications. *Psychopharm Bull* 1987;23:531.

Hendrick V, Fukuchi A, Altshuler L, et al. Use of sertraline, paroxetine and fluvoxamine by nursing women. *Br J Psychiatry* 2001;179:163–166.

Jensvold M, Halbreich U, Hamilton J, eds. *Psychopharmacology and women: sex, gender, and hormones.* Washington, DC: American Psychiatric Press, 1996.

Kaplan HI, Sadock BJ, eds. *Comprehensive textbook of psychiatry,* 4th ed. Baltimore: Williams & Wilkins, 1985.

Kulin NA, et al. Pregnancy outcome following maternal use of the new selective serotonin reuptake inhibitors. *JAMA* 1998;279:609–610.

Miller LJ, ed. *Postpartum mood disorders.* Washington, DC: American Psychiatric Press, 1999.

Novalis PN, Rojcewicz SJ, Peele R. *Clinical manual of supportive psychotherapy.* Washington, DC: American Psychiatric Press, 1993.

Nulman I, et al. Neurodevelopment of children exposed in utero to antidepressant drugs. *N Engl J Med* 1997;336:258–262.

Schatzberg AF, Cole JO. *Manual of clinical psychopharmacology,* 2nd ed. Washington, DC: American Psychiatric Press, 1991.

Stewart DE, Stotland NL, eds. *Psychological aspects of women's health care: the interface between psychiatry and obstetrics and gynecology.* Washington, DC: American Psychiatric Press, 2001.

Wisner KL, Zarin DA, Holmboe ES, et al. Risk-benefit decision making for treatment of depression during pregnancy. *Am J Psychiatry* 2000;157:1933–1940.

CHAPTER 146

Anxiety

Adrian Leibovici and Linda Chaudron

Anxiety disorders are the most common psychiatric problems encountered in the community. They vary in clinical presentation, etiology, prognosis, and treatment, but all have in common an excessive display of concern, fear, and worry. Proper recognition and treatment of anxiety is an important task for the primary care physician, because many cases present with physical symptoms suggestive of medical illness and many medical conditions are accompanied by anxiety. Women are particularly prone to anxiety, and overall the prevalence of anxiety is much higher than in men.

CLASSIFICATION AND PHENOMENOLOGY

Panic Disorder

Panic anxiety is characterized by discrete episodes of very intense fear with a rather sudden onset and many somatic concomitants. The object of the fear varies (e.g., death, heart attack, stroke, losing one's mind). At other times, the fear is intense but not defined. Among the most common physical symptoms are sweating, palpitations, racing heart, chest pain, shortness of breath, choking, shaking, numbness or tingling, abdominal distress, dizziness, and a fainting sensation. The frequency and intensity of attacks vary widely: Some patients have one or several each day for weeks in a row; others have symptom-free intervals of weeks and even months. Typically, patients become concerned with the meaning of symptoms ("Do I have a severe medical condition?" or "Am I going insane?") and with the possibility of additional attacks in the near future. Many times, untreated cases are complicated by avoidance of situations from which escape might be difficult in the event of a panic attack (agoraphobia). Examples include fear and avoidance of going out alone, being in a crowd, and using public transportation. Agoraphobia occurs most often as a complication of panic, but there are cases of agoraphobia without a history of panic disorder in which avoidance is caused by fear of, for instance, diarrhea or dizziness.

Generalized Anxiety Disorder

In generalized anxiety disorder, patients cannot stop worrying about upcoming events or about possible but not probable negative outcomes. This apprehensive expectation is considered excessive. Other symptoms include fatigue, feeling restless or on edge, irritability, insomnia, difficulty concentrating, and muscle tension. In general, the disorder lasts a long time, often characterizing the person's style or temperament. According to modern diagnostic criteria, symptoms must be present for at least 6 months. Similar symptoms, usually in reaction to a significant psychosocial stressor but lasting less than 6 months, are labeled adjustment reaction with anxious mood.

Obsessive-Compulsive Disorder

Obsessions are recurrent thoughts that are perceived as intrusive and inappropriate. They cause subjective distress and are time-consuming for the patient. Examples include aggressive impulses (to hurt a defenseless person or shout profanity at a funeral), fear of contamination (getting acquired immunodeficiency syndrome by shaking hands), preoccupation with remembering names of public figures, concern with having things placed in a certain order (papers on a desk or shirts in a drawer must be symmetrically arranged), and repeated doubts (wondering whether one has turned off the oven or locked the door before leaving the house). Some obsessive thoughts are abnormal only because of their repetitive nature, but other have little basis in reality; for instance, the recurrent fear that one has hit someone in traffic. Patients recognize obsessions as unreasonable and try to ignore or suppress them.

Compulsions are behaviors performed repeatedly and with a sense of urgency by patients to alleviate anxiety. Frequently, compulsive behavior alleviates the distress caused by a specific obsession. For instance, a patient concerned with cleanliness will engage in repetitive handwashing; the concern with having completed certain tasks like locking the door will trigger repetitive checking of the knob. Sometimes compulsions take a ritualistic magical form—for instance, counting up to a certain number or pacing a certain number of steps for each occurrence of an obsessive blasphemous thought. As with obsessions, compulsions are recognized as excessive and irrational by the patient. Attempts to suppress compulsive behavior cause increasing levels of urge and distress. Satisfying a compulsive need relieves the anxiety for a while, but it is not pleasurable and can make the patient feel guilty and inadequate.

Patients with obsessive-compulsive disorder either have both obsessions and compulsions or only one of the symptoms. Typically, the illness starts in childhood in men and in the third decade of life in women. The course is chronic and fluctuating, with exacerbations in response to stress. A few patients deteriorate to the point of not being able to function, even requiring institutionalization.

Specific Phobias

Patients experience severe fear in the presence or mere anticipation of a specific situation or object. Virtually anything can become the stimulus for a phobic response, but some types of exposure are more common: animals such as snakes and insects, receiving injections and seeing blood, heights, water, storms, different situations such as flying or using elevators, or being in closed spaces (claustrophobia). The fear is recognized as unreasonable and excessive by an adult patient but not by a young child. The common reaction to a phobic stimulus is avoidance, which protects the patient against experiencing anxiety. The extent of disability is proportional to the patient's circumstances in terms of the object of her phobia. A fear of heights could be inconsequential for a woman living in a flat rural region but devastating for the urban professional who must use elevators and stairs on a daily basis. When forcefully exposed to the object of her phobia, the patient experiences anxiety of panic proportions. The harder it seems to escape from such a situation, the more severe the symptoms are. In most phobia-related anxiety reactions, the patient's heart rate and breathing are accelerated, but in the blood-injection subtype most patients experience a vasovagal reaction, with hypotension and fainting.

Social Phobia

The cardinal symptom of social phobia is marked apprehension of performing in public, anticipating failure and embarrassment. The most common example is public speaking, be it a lecture, an examination, or even a friendly social gathering. Other situations include eating, drinking, or writing in public. The fear is recognized as excessive and unreasonable by adult patients. It leads to avoidance of social exposure, a more restricted life, and a fair amount of emotional suffering. Sometimes the person decides to endure the anxiety associated with exposure. The actual performance can be much better than anticipated, but not uncommonly the patient's nervousness will sabotage her efforts, leading to a poor outcome, confirmation of her fears, and a reinforcement of the phobia. The anxiety experienced by patients with social phobia ranges from anticipatory apprehension to panic. Physical symptoms such as abdominal pain, diarrhea, blushing, sweating, shaking, and palpitations are likely and tend to peak right before the feared event is scheduled to start.

Posttraumatic Stress Disorder and Acute Stress Disorder

In posttraumatic stress disorder and acute stress disorder, symptoms develop in reaction to situations in which a person is confronted with an extremely traumatic event, such as death, serious injury, assault, or credible threats of the same nature. The victim can be the person herself or others around her. The initial response is one of horror and helplessness. The traumatic event is reexperienced many times as nightmares; the imagery includes painfully realistic flashbacks. There is intense emotional distress when an unrelated memory or unintended external cue reminds the subject of the original event. There is numbing of emotional response and a deliberate effort to reject recollections associated with the trauma. For instance, patients tend to avoid people, places, or conversational subjects directly or even tangentially related. Patients have selective amnesia, a feeling of detachment, constriction of affect, and a decrease in goal-directed activities. They show increased overall arousal (insomnia, hypervigilance, irritability, exaggerated startling response, outbursts of anger).

Symptoms that develop soon after exposure and subside in no more than a month make up an acute stress disorder. When the illness lasts more than a month, a diagnosis of posttraumatic stress disorder is warranted. Traditionally, events such as war, terrorist acts, earthquakes, and other catastrophes are considered common causes of posttraumatic stress disorder. The chronic and severe abuse (physical, sexual, emotional) suffered in childhood by many patients has recently been added to the list. This is significant for women, who tend to be victimized more often (see Chapter 153).

Anxiety Disorder Due to a General Medical Condition and Substance-Induced Anxiety Disorder

Anxiety in all its forms (generalized, panic, obsessions, compulsions) can be the physiologic consequence of a medical illness or of an exogenous chemical introduced into the body, like medication, food, or recreational drugs (Table 146.1). Certain conditions associated with secondary anxiety are more common in women: hyperthyroidism, certain collagen diseases, and the use of stimulants for weight loss or of nonsteroidal antiinflammatory drugs for pain. Other common causes of anxiety include pulmonary embolism, chronic obstructive pulmonary disease and asthma, angina, arrhythmias, mitral valve prolapse, and congestive heart failure. Medications such as steroids, sympathomimetics, and coffee and caffeine-containing foods are also common offenders.

Substances of abuse such as alcohol and cocaine can cause anxiety both during intoxication and withdrawal. The diagnosis of substance or illness-induced anxiety is warranted when the onset, course, and resolution of the primary condition are correlated in time with the symptoms of anxiety.

TABLE 146.1. Secondary Anxiety

Respiratory
Chronic obstructive lung disease
Emphysema
Pneumonia
Acute respiratory failure
Cardiovascular
Pulmonary embolism
Congestive heart failure
Arrhythmias
Coronary ischemia
Endocrine/metabolic
Cushing disease and syndrome
Hypoglycemia
Hyperthyroidism
Pheochiromocytoma
Porphyria
Carcinoid
Neurologic
Encephalitis
Vestibular dysfunction
Tumors
Cerebrovascular events
Recreational drug intoxication
Alcohol, cannabis, phencyclidine, inhalants, hallucinogens, caffeine, cocaine, and amphetamine-related drugs
Recreational drug withdrawal
Alcohol, cocaine, hypnotics, sedatives
Prescription drugs
Analgesics, anesthetics, sympathomimetics, oral contraceptives and other steroids, antihypertensives, anticonvulsants, antiparkinsonians, antipsychotics, lithium, anxiolytics, antidepressants, insulin
Toxic agents
Heavy metals, paint, gasoline, pesticides, carbon monoxide, nerve gas

Anxiety can be a sign or symptom in many other psychiatric disorders, including schizophrenia, personality disorders, and depression. The relation between anxiety and depression is a close and important one but remains poorly understood. Especially in women, a syndrome characterized by anxiety attacks and severe dysphoria, meeting the criteria for both panic disorder and major depression, has been described. Both diagnoses can be made, but some advocate a separate nosologic category for mixed depression and anxiety disorder. Fortunately, somatic treatments for both depression and anxiety overlap.

A diagnosis of anxiety disorder is justified only when the extent of symptoms causes disability: Some measure of anticipatory apprehension or anxiety is a universal and normative psychophysiologic response to perceived danger. When its intensity is commensurate with the originating stimulus, anxiety has an important adaptive value, allowing the person faced with a challenging situation to mobilize her coping and fighting resources.

EPIDEMIOLOGY

Anxiety disorders are the most prevalent psychiatric illnesses noted in community studies. Women are three times more likely to have an anxiety disorder than men.

The lifetime prevalence of panic disorder in the general population ranges from 1.5% to 3.5%. Panic without agoraphobia is twice as common in women than in men; for panic with agoraphobia, the ratio is 3:1. Social phobia is more common in women than in men in community samples, but the sexes are equally represented in clinical settings. The lifetime community prevalence for this disorder is estimated to be as low as 3% and as high as 13%. Simple phobia is considerably more common in women (ratios of up to 9:1 for certain subtypes). Its lifetime community prevalence is about 12%. Obsessive-compulsive disorder is equally common in women and men and afflicts about 2.5% of the general population. The epidemiology of stress-induced anxiety disorders is less well defined.

ETIOLOGY

Biologic, psychological, and sociologic factors have been shown to play a role in generating, perpetuating, and exacerbating anxiety. A unifying theory is lacking, and, at best, one can say that the etiology of anxiety is multifactorial. A genetic factor probably exists, at least in some conditions such as generalized anxiety disorder, obsessive-compulsive disorder, and panic disorder; however, a single locus on the genome was not identified, and anxiety disorders as a group have lower heritability than other major psychiatric illnesses (e.g., schizophrenia and bipolar disorder). This opens the door to psychosocial theories, which tend to stress the connection between anxiety and fear as an instinctual response to danger. Behavioralists regard anxiety as a conditioned response to fear.

According to cognitive theory, thought distortions allow the misreading of benign stimuli as signs of real danger, which in turn leads to autonomic hyperactivity. In psychoanalytic theory, anxiety is the price we pay to keep unacceptable archaic wishes out of the realm of our awareness.

The ability to provoke attacks reliably in panic disorder patients with lactate, bicarbonate, or carbon dioxide has lent strong support to biologic theories on the etiology of all anxiety disorders. The locus ceruleus, with its high concentration of noradrenergic neurons, is implicated in the sympathetic response associated with anxiety. Other areas, such as the septohippocampal region, are thought to analyze and compare stimuli from the environment, body, and memory: Hypersensitivity of this area might explain some forms of paroxysmal anxiety. Positron emission tomography has shown hypermetabolism in the frontal lobes, especially the orbital gyri of patients with obsessive-compulsive disorder. These areas contain serotonergic neurons consistent with the efficacy of serotonin-enhancing drugs in reducing obsessions and compulsions. The neurochemical theory of anxiety revolves around the role of the γ-aminobutyric acid (GABA) receptor complex: Benzodiazepines link to it, opening calcium ion channels, and the action of GABA, the brain's main inhibitory neurotransmitter, is enhanced.

An extracranial theory for the pathogenesis of panic has been advanced. The carotid body directly stimulates a response in the brain's respiratory and circulatory centers via the 9th and 10th cranial nerves in response to subtle changes in the concentration of blood gases. According to this theory, panic is merely hypersensitivity of such a "suffocation alarm system."

COMPLICATIONS

Anxiety disorders, even when severe, may remain unrecognized and therefore untreated for long periods of time, sometimes for a lifetime. This was particularly true for women who were cast in social roles consistent with dependency, acceptability of displays of fear and weakness, and lack of pressure to overcome their symptoms. Extreme examples of women who had not left their home for decades because of agoraphobia have been documented in the literature. In general, patients with untreated anxiety disorders have a more restricted life and tend to achieve below their potential.

Many patients discover that, at least initially, drinking alcohol provides symptomatic relief. Slowly, they develop tolerance and increase their consumption. Such self-medication leads to alcoholism in many uninformed patients. Similarly, chemical alleviation of severe anxiety can lead to abuse or addiction to benzodiazepines, barbiturates, or illicit drugs.

Up to 60% of patients with panic disorder develop major depression sometime in the course of their illness. For some, this is an apparent complication of the unrelenting stress of living with intense anxiety attacks and especially with the fearful anticipation of their occurrence. Epidemiologic data suggest that extreme anxiety may represent a risk factor for suicide.

GENDER-RELATED CLINICAL ISSUES

Although the epidemiology of anxiety points to a greater vulnerability for women, the phenomenology is no different between the genders. In the absence of definitive genetic data to suggest a sex-linked transmission of anxiety disorders between generations, the psychological and sociologic literature has tried to fill in the gap by identifying the risk factors for developing anxiety that are more common in women. Modern life and the new demands and opportunities for women have received special attention: Women with underlying low self-esteem are faced with competitive careers and expectations of success, and this leads them to become apprehensive, fearful, and insecure. Phobic and panic symptoms develop as a result of new conflicts centering around such dichotomies as success versus failure, sensitive versus aggressive, feminine versus macho, and being accepted versus loss of love.

The reproductive cycle is marked by the exacerbation of preexistent anxiety or new-onset anxiety at each of its milestones (menarche, pregnancy, delivery or abortion, menopause). There is, however, a subgroup of women with preexistent anxiety who experience a decrease in symptoms during pregnancy. Many times, anxiety is self-limited and commensurate with the situation at hand. For instance, women, especially new mothers, tend to experience high levels of worry and nervousness during the first trimester of pregnancy and again close to delivery. This is in reaction to concerns about their adequacy as mothers, the well-being of the infant, and the way in which relations with their partner and family might be affected. Sympathetic listening to elicit such worries and gentle reassurance is enough in most cases. However, the practitioner must be able to recognize situations where the level of anxiety reaches clinical proportions and specific interventions are required. For instance, postpartum panic disorder and postpartum obsessive-compulsive disorder have been described. There are anecdotes of women who developed obsessional ideas about harm to the infant or compulsive rituals involving some aspect of infant care. It is hypothesized that the rapid decline of estrogen and progesterone after delivery affects serotonergic transmission in the brain, which in turn leads to anxiety symptoms. Indeed, serotonergic agents such as clomipramine or selective serotonergic reuptake inhibitors (e.g., fluoxetine, fluvoxamine) are effective in the treatment of perinatal anxiety disorders.

DIAGNOSIS

Anxiety is more difficult to diagnose than other psychiatric conditions such as depression or psychosis. Not infrequently, the clinical picture is confusing due to the vagueness of the patient's complaints, the coexistence of other emotional problems, and the tendency of the anxious patient to report numerous physical symptoms. A patient might be seen many times in the office for chest pain, shortness of breath, intolerance to cold, poor concentration, or tearfulness before mentioning more suggestive symptoms such as discrete periods of paroxysmal fear or intrusive thoughts and ritualistic behavior. The key to the successful identification of an anxiety disorder is the physician's willingness to listen to the patient's account of complaints in her own words. In the opening phase of the interview, the patient should not be interrupted—according to one study, the average primary care physician waits less than half a minute before interrupting the patient with a question that is usually meant to mold the story into preexistent nosologic category. In the second phase of the interview, if a suspicion of anxiety was generated, the physician should elicit additional information methodically, asking specific questions about the presence of other anxiety conditions (many times they coexist); the presence of medical conditions; the use of medications, drugs, alcohol, and caffeine-containing products; exposure to toxic agents implicated in the etiology of anxiety; a family history of anxiety or other psychiatric disorders; and current psychosocial stressors or past exposure to traumatic events. A thorough assessment includes a physical examination and a mental status examination. When in doubt, a formal consultation with a psychiatrist is helpful.

TREATMENT

Starting in the mid-1960s, the treatment for anxiety shifted from psychoanalytic approaches to a balanced combination between biologic and behavioral therapies. The net result is probably quite positive, with better symptom control, reduced disability, and fewer complications.

Pharmacologic Treatment

Many classes of psychotropic drugs have a role in the treatment of anxiety.

ANTIDEPRESSANTS

A major advance in the treatment of anxiety disorders was the recognition that many antidepressant medications are also effective in controlling specific conditions and symptoms such as panic, phobias, and compulsions. Such drugs are discussed in Chapter 145. In general, the same dosages are used as for depression. It is increasingly accepted that for most anxiety disorders, the preferred pharmacologic treatment is an antidepressant. Selective serotonin reuptake inhibitors (SSRIs), venlafaxine, and nefazodone have been approved for some specific anxiety disorders, but off label use is also quite common and, with the exception of bupropion, most antidepressants have been used in most forms of anxiety.

BENZODIAZEPINES

Primary care physicians write 80% of all prescriptions for antianxiety medications, psychiatrists only 20%. Of all anxiolytics prescribed, 90% are benzodiazepines. These numbers underscore the need for primary care physicians to be familiar with the proper use of benzodiazepines. Drugs in this class were first developed as muscle relaxants, but their use has extended rapidly to the treatment of insomnia, status epilepticus, and anxiety.

The first to be released was chlordiazepoxide, in 1960. About a dozen drugs in this class are approved for use in the United States. In equivalent doses, they are equally effective (Table 146.2) Benzodiazepines link to a specific receptor, part of a larger macromolecular complex that also contains receptors for the inhibitory neurotransmitter GABA. The action of this neurotransmitter is facilitated when the benzodiazepine receptors are occupied by the drug. The net result is hyperpolarization and therefore decreased firing of GABA-ergic neurons, which in turn could explain seizure and anxiety suppression.

TABLE 146.2. Benzodiazepines

Generic name	Brand name	Dosage equivalency (mg)
Clonazepam	Klonopin	0.25
Alprazolam	Xanax	0.5
Triazolam	Halcion	0.5
Lorazepam	Ativan	1.0
Diazepam	Valium	5.0
Clorazepate	Tranxene	7.5
Prazepam	Centrex	10
Oxazepam	Serax	15
Chlordiazepoxide	Librium	25
Flurazepam	Dalmane	30
Temazepam	Restoril	30

Pharmacokinetic considerations are important when choosing a particular drug in this class. For instance, the rate of onset of the therapeutic effect is very short for diazepam and flurazepam and slow for oxazepam; lorazepam and alprazolam fall somewhere in the middle. The duration of action varies with the distribution half-life when drugs are given acutely (short for diazepam, long for chlordiazepoxide, intermediate for lorazepam) and with the elimination half-life when they are given daily and a steady state is established (short with triazolam, intermediate with lorazepam, long for clonazepam). A few benzodiazepines, such as lorazepam and oxazepam, are metabolized in the liver through conjugation with glucuronic acid only, but most other drugs in this class undergo oxidative degradation. The distinction is important because effective glucuronic conjugation occurs even when liver function is restricted due to illness or age; therefore, oxazepam and lorazepam are preferable in the elderly or in the presence of advanced liver disease.

Compared with older antianxiety drugs, benzodiazepines have a favorable side-effect profile. The most common side effects are sedation, anterograde amnesia, dizziness, ataxia, and other forms of motor discoordination. They are relatively safe when taken in overdose, unlike barbiturates, the drugs they have replaced in the treatment of anxiety. Most patients treated continuously with benzodiazepines develop tolerance and a need for ever-increasing doses to sustain the therapeutic effect. Cases of addiction, iatrogenic or illicit, are not rare, and the prescribing of these drugs is highly regulated.

Dosage varies with indication and must be individualized. In generalized anxiety disorder, one starts with a diazepam equivalent of 2 mg three times a day and titrates up as needed. Most patients do not need more than the equivalent of 20 mg of diazepam daily. In panic disorder, alprazolam 0.25 mg four times a day is a good starting dose. If the patient needs more than 1 mg four times a day, a referral to a specialist should be strongly considered. Ideally, benzodiazepines should be used for limited periods only (e.g., several weeks) or on an as-needed basis to avoid habituation.

BUSPIRONE

Buspirone is a nonbenzodiazepine nonsedating anxiolytic that is relatively well tolerated and nonaddictive. It probably works by inhibiting the firing of serotonergic neurons in the raphe. Its effectiveness in generalized anxiety disorder is at best mild, but some patients find it useful. The usual dose is 5 to 10 mg three times a day, but some patients need considerably more (up to 80 mg/d).

Other Anxiolytics

Barbiturates such as amobarbital, pentobarbital, or phenobarbital were used extensively to control anxiety before the advent of benzodiazepines. They should probably be avoided because they are hepatotoxic and addictive and have no notable advantage over benzodiazepines. Meprobamate and antihistamines such as hydroxyzine have also been used for control of anxiety. Antipsychotic drugs, also called major tranquilizers, are strong anxiolytics, but their long-term use in the absence of psychotic symptoms is not indicated, given the risk of side effects like tardive dyskinesia and other movement disorders.

BETA-BLOCKERS

Drugs such as propranolol and atenolol have been advocated for use in social phobia and generalized anxiety disorder and when the peripheric consequences of anxiety (e.g., tachycardia, hyperventilation, excessive perspiration) are prominent. One starts with doses as low as 10 mg twice a day of propranolol and titrates up to 120 to 160 mg/d. Heart rate and blood pressure must be monitored for bradycardia and hypotension. Performance anxiety is a common indication.

Pharmacologic Treatment for Specific Anxiety Disorders

SSRIs are now used as first-line treatment for panic disorder. There is no indication that one SSRI is more effective than the others. Dosage is not different from treatment of depression. The first few days on an SSRI, patients might experience increased jitteriness and anxiety—this is relevant in patients already experiencing high levels of anxiety because they might give up taking medication before experiencing any benefit. This early transient effect needs to be explained in advance. Phenelzine 45 to 90 mg/d and other monoamine oxidase inhibitors (tranylcypromine, isocarboxazid) are considered by some to provide the most comprehensive pharmacologic treatment, because they seem to diminish social apprehension better than other drugs. Among tricyclic antidepressants, imipramine has been the most widely studied, but other drugs in this class (e.g., nortriptyline, doxepin) should be equally effective. The same dosage guidelines and blood levels apply as in the treatment of depression. Some studies suggest that clomipramine is a more powerful antipanic agent than imipramine. High-potency benzodiazepines such as alprazolam and clonazepam are also being used in the treatment of panic disorder. They work faster but lose their effectiveness in time due to tolerance. One strategy is to start an antidepressant and a benzodiazepine concomitantly and to taper the benzodiazepine after several weeks, when the antidepressant has become effective. Regardless of what drug is chosen, effective treatment translates into a decreased frequency and intensity of panic attacks and a better ability to confront the avoidance that is characteristic of agoraphobia.

Generalized anxiety disorder responds to judicious use of benzodiazepines. Antidepressants such as tricyclics work better than placebo but are less effective than benzodiazepines in this disorder, and beta-blocking drugs might have a role in diminishing the consequences of autonomic hyperactivity. Recently venlafaxine has been approved as an effective treatment for generalized anxiety.

Obsessive-compulsive disorder has been more resistant to therapeutic intervention than other anxiety disorders. Compulsions can be decreased by up to 60% to 80% with the use of clomipramine in usual antidepressant doses. The other tricyclics are not very effective. Sometimes a therapeutic response occurs only after 6 to 8 weeks. Obsessions are less responsive to medication than compulsions. SSRIs are somewhat useful in the treatment of this illness: In clinical practice they are used first, because of their favorable side-effect profile compared with clomipramine. Benzodiazepines and the other antianxiety drugs do not work in patients with obsessive-compulsive disorder.

Social phobia responds best to monoamine oxidase inhibitors and SSRIs. Very mild and circumscribed cases of social phobia, such as performance anxiety, respond to beta-blocking agents, but this class of drugs does not work when social avoidance is pervasive.

In acute stress disorder, the as-needed use of benzodiazepines controls the most extreme manifestations until patients regain behavioral control. Posttraumatic stress disorder has been treated with SSRIs, tricyclic antidepressants, monoamine oxidase inhibitors, lithium, antiepileptics, benzodiazepines, and beta-blocking agents.

Antianxiety Medication and Pregnancy

Some studies indicate that the use of benzodiazepines during the first trimester of pregnancy is associated with a higher incidence of cleft palate in the newborn. Most data refer specifically to diazepam, and it is not unanimous. Other benzodiazepines, such as clonazepam, are thought to have low teratogenic potential. Meprobamate is associated with an assortment of congenital defects when used during pregnancy.

Benzodiazepines cross the placenta easily due to their low molecular weight. This tendency becomes more accentuated toward the end of pregnancy. When benzodiazepines with long half-lives are used chronically, they tend to accumulate in the fetus. The neonate experiences a withdrawal syndrome consisting of hypotonia ("floppy infant"), tremor, hyperreflexia, irritability, intolerance to cold, and respiratory depression. The use of barbiturates during pregnancy can also cause withdrawal in the newborn. Nursing mothers pass benzodiazepines in milk in active form, leading to lethargy in the infant.

When weighing the risks of psychotropic medication in the pregnant or nursing woman with clinical anxiety, one must factor in the extent of her subjective distress and the relative risks to mother and child if severe symptoms are not addressed (see earlier under Complications). It is often recommended that SSRIs or tricyclic antidepressants should be used as a first choice in such situations, because they are generally better accepted for use in pregnancy.

Psychotherapy

PSYCHOEDUCATION

Much of the "talk" therapy involved in the treatment of anxiety disorders is initiated in the primary care physician's office. Regardless of the specific disorder, the primary care physician is in an excellent position to educate the patient about her illness and its treatment. In conditions such as panic disorder, psychoeducation has great therapeutic value: Telling the patient that her symptoms are due to anxiety rather than heart disease, stroke, or insanity and teaching her to relax in such circumstances can bring considerable relief. In fact, in all anxiety disorders, informing patients about the name of their condition and its prevalence has positive effects, because it gives them the needed vocabulary to refer to their illness and a sense that they are not alone experiencing it. Explaining the biologic nature of anxiety is reassuring for some patients; others do better when the role of situational factors is stressed.

Dealing with the somatic concomitants of anxiety can be challenging in patients who feel uncomfortable conceptualizing their distress in emotional terms and hope that a physical condition can be identified and treated. The physician must decide how far to go in ordering diagnostic tests and specialist consultations before exploring the psychological aspects of the problem. An "either/or" (organic versus psychogenic) approach is counterproductive, because it can lead to such iatrogenic outcomes as excessive use of diagnostic tests and consultations, overlooking legitimate coincidental medical problems, and alienating the patient by telling her that she has no medical problem but that she should see a psychiatrist. Referral for consultation or treatment, when necessary, should be discussed openly as a way of obtaining expert advice and care. The physician should reassure the patient that she is not being abandoned as a hopeless "mental case" and that the referring physician will remain involved.

The patient's lifestyle must be explored and anxiety precipitants identified and eliminated if possible. Simple measures such as proper rest and exercise, a predictable sleep/activity schedule, healthy eating, and elimination of coffee and caffeine-containing beverages can go a long way. The association between alcohol and anxiety is a very strong one: Many uninformed patients become alcoholics as they try to alleviate a preexisting anxiety disorder by drinking. The chronic drinker who tries to quit may experience various degrees of anxiety, part of a withdrawal syndrome. It is generally very difficult to treat anxiety successfully if the patient continues to drink, and patients must be forcefully confronted with this fact.

BEHAVIORAL THERAPY

The focus of behavioral therapy is to obtain symptom reduction by increasing the patient's ability to tolerate the very situations likely to make her uncomfortable. Phobias, panic, and compulsive rituals respond best to this approach. Patients are helped to identify anxiety-producing situations and list them hierarchically. A structured program of gradual exposure to these stimuli is then agreed on between therapist and patient. For instance, a woman afraid of riding the bus because that is where she had her first panic attack starts by going to the bus station to watch buses come and go. In the next stage, she gets on the bus and gets off immediately. Then she rides longer and longer distances, starting with off hours when few people are likely to ride and ending with rush hours when the bus is crowded. At each point during treatment, the patient experiences anxiety and is taught to be aware of it and to reflect on its intensity and on her ability to master it. The patient is tempted to interrupt her exposure to the anxiety-producing stimulus (for instance, by getting off the bus sooner than planned) but forces herself not to (response prevention). Gradually, tolerance to even the most dreaded situations develops and the patient becomes able to function without avoidance. The overall level of anxiety decreases, and she now uses buses without difficulty. If panic has been mitigated with medication, behavioral therapy can progress much faster and with more dramatic results.

COGNITIVE THERAPY

Initially developed for depression, cognitive therapy is now being applied in the treatment of selected anxiety conditions such as performance anxiety and social phobia. It is based on the assumption that symptoms are the result of cognitive distortions in which a negative view of oneself plays a central role. Patients are taught to consider alternative explanations to the negative assessment of situations leading to symptoms. Cognitive-behavioral therapy applies both behavioral and cognitive restructuring techniques and is emerging as a powerful and increasingly used psychotherapeutic tool.

Other therapies used in the treatment of anxiety disorders include biofeedback and relaxation, psychoanalysis or psychodynamic psychotherapy, interpersonal psychotherapy, and supportive psychotherapy. Generally, patients are referred to mental health professionals for formal psychotherapy. It is important, however, for the primary care physician to monitor progress and to be available to coordinate care with the psychotherapist as needed.

BIBLIOGRAPHY

American Psychiatric Association. *Diagnostic and statistical manual of mental disorders,* 4th ed. Washington, DC: American Psychiatric Press, 1994.

Elia J, Katz IR, Simpson GM. Teratogenicity of psychotherapeutic medications. *Psychopharmacol Bull* 1987;23:53.

Iqbal MM, Sobha T, Ryals T. Effects of commonly used benzodiazepines on the fetus, the neonate and the nursing infant. *Psych Serv* 2002;53:39–49.

Kaplan H, Sadock BJ, ed. *Comprehensive textbook of psychiatry,* 4th ed. Baltimore: Williams & Williams, 1985.

Klein D. Testing the suffocation false alarm theory of panic disorder. *Anxiety* 1994;1:t.

McGlynn T, Metcalf I-I, eds. *Diagnosis and treatment of anxiety disorders: a physician's handbook.* Washington, DC: American Psychiatric Press, 1989.

Schatzberg AF, Cole JO. *Manual of clinical psychopharmacology,* 2nd ed. Washington, DC: American Psychiatric Press, 1991.

Stewart DE, Stotland NE, eds. *Psychological aspects of women's health care: the interface between psychiatry and obstetrics and gynecology.* Washington, DC: American Psychiatric Press, 1993.

Weissman MM, Kierman GL, Markowitz IS, et al. Suicidal ideation and suicide attempts in panic disorder and attacks. *N Engl J Med* 1989;321:1209.

Zerhe IK. Anxiety disorders in women. *Bull Menninger Clin* 1995;59[Suppl A]:38.

CHAPTER 147

Psychosis

Adrian Leibovici and Linda Chaudron

None of the current definitions of psychosis has received universal acceptance. In a broad sense, psychosis refers to a psychiatric syndrome characterized by severe impairment in the ability to separate what is real from what is imagined (loss of reality testing). A more technical and narrow definition requires the presence of specific signs and symptoms, such as delusions or hallucinations.

A delusion is a false belief so rigid that it does not change, even in the face of compelling and repeated refuting evidence. The content of delusional thoughts is varied but is usually organized around several familiar themes: persecution, reference, religion, somatic symptoms, jealousy, guilt, poverty, grandiosity, and nihilism.

Hallucinations are severe perceptual distortions occurring in any sensory domain (auditory, visual, tactile, olfactory, or gustatory). Unlike illusions, where a real stimulus is perceived erroneously, hallucinations have no basis in reality whatsoever. Examples include hearing noises or voices, seeing persons or animals, feeling bugs crawling on one's skin, and being bothered by an unpleasant and otherwise unexplained smell. Other features of the psychotic syndrome include disorganization of thinking and bizarre behavior.

EPIDEMIOLOGY AND CLINICAL DESCRIPTION

Psychosis can be secondary to various physical or emotional factors or the central manifestation of a number of still idiopathic psychiatric illnesses, the most common and disabling of which is schizophrenia.

Schizophrenia

This severe usually chronic psychiatric illness is characterized by the profound disturbance of many psychological functions, although sensorium is generally preserved. The clinical picture is characterized by the presence of delusions, hallucinations, abnormal behavior and speech, and so-called negative symptoms. Patients remain oriented and generally intact cognitively. Delusions can be bizarre, such as the belief that one's internal organs have been altered by hostile forces or that one is monitored by special FBI agents with cosmic weapons. The search for pathognomonic content to schizophrenic delusions has not been fruitful, but in general ideas of reference are very suggestive of a schizophrenic process. Examples include the belief that certain events, such as radio and television broadcasts, convey special messages to the patient or that someone puts thoughts in the patient's mind (thought insertion), removes thoughts (thought withdrawal), or manipulates the patient's thinking (thought control).

Auditory hallucinations are the most prominent perceptual distortion, although virtually any sensory modality can be affected. Often patients hear voices running a distinct discourse that is perceived as separate from their thoughts. Threats, pejorative statements, or commands that the patient is more or less able to resist are common. A particular type of hallucination is almost exclusively encountered in schizophrenia: It consists of one or several voices continuously commenting on the person's thoughts or behavior.

Thought processes in schizophrenia are profoundly disturbed. This is reflected in disorganized speech, illogical associations (loose associations), answers that are only marginally connected with the question asked (tangentiality), and in severe cases, total loss of comprehensible structure or meaning (incoherence).

Deficits in volition, production of speech, and affective expression are described under the generic term "negative symptoms." Patients display difficulty initiating goal-directed activities, whether related to social interactions or work (avolition). Their speech has little spontaneous flow, and their answers are laconic (alogia). The range of emotional response in schizophrenic patients is generally restricted (blunt or flat affect), although exaggerated or incongruent affective states are also described.

The behavior of schizophrenic patients ranges from normal in certain phases of illness to profoundly disorganized in others, paralleling the extent to which thought processes are affected. For instance, a patient may go out into the cold without proper clothing or may wander dangerously in the traffic. At other times, the behavior reflects the content of delusions or hallucinations: The patient becomes hostile or even violent when confronted with a "persecutor" or when the voices tell her to defend herself. Negative symptoms also shape behavior, which explains the patient's poor ability to care for herself and the perception that she is morally weak or lazy, contributing to the social and occupational underachievement caused by this illness.

The diagnosis of schizophrenia is justified only if symptoms persist for at least 6 months. In general, the course is chronic, with onset in the late 20s for women and a few years earlier for men. Some patients have exacerbations and remissions; others remain symptomatic all the time. It is not uncommon for patients to have episodes of delusions, hallucinations, and disorganization in response to life stressors and to display only negative symptoms between episodes.

In some patients, the course toward worsening with each new decompensation leads to states of profound deficit and mental disability. Such an outcome was more common before the advent of effective treatment—hence the old term "dementia praecox," which is actually a misnomer.

There are several clinical varieties of schizophrenia. The paranoid type is characterized by the prominence of auditory hallucinations and delusions with persecutory content, although other psychological functions are somewhat better preserved. The disorganized (hebephrenic) type is dominated by disorganized speech or behavior and inappropriate affect: Sometimes patients make concrete, cheerful remarks, incongruent with circumstances. The catatonic type refers to the coexistence of a marked psychomotor disturbance during the acute phase of illness. Mutism, negativism, idiosyncratic complex movements such as immobility and plasticity (waxy flexibility), echolalia and echopraxia (repeating the interviewer's words or movements), stupor, and purposeless hyperactivity can occur in any combination or level of severity. Other types of schizophrenia are residual (predominance of negative symptoms with few if any delusions and hallucinations) and undifferentiated.

The exact prevalence and incidence of schizophrenia are not yet known because different studies have used different definitions of the illness. In general, the illness is equally prevalent throughout the world when the same diagnostic criteria are applied. The lifetime prevalence of schizophrenia is thought to range between 0.5% and 1%. The incidence is 1 per 10,000/yr. Community-based studies show no sex differences in prevalence, although hospital-based studies indicate higher rates for men. This is consistent with the assertion that women have a later onset and a better prognosis, making hospitalization less likely.

SCHIZOPHRENIFORM DISORDER

Patients presenting with signs and symptoms characteristic of schizophrenia of less than 6 months' duration receive a diagnosis of schizophreniform disorder. About two thirds of such patients progress to develop schizophrenia; the remaining third recover before the 6-month criterion for schizophrenia is met.

SCHIZOAFFECTIVE DISORDER

When major depression, mania, or a mixed affective state coexists with typical schizophrenic symptoms, a diagnosis of schizoaffective disorder is sometimes warranted, although the relation between psychosis and mood pathology is a more complex one (see Differential Diagnosis, later).

DELUSIONAL DISORDER

Another major psychotic illness is paranoia or delusional disorder. It is characterized by prominent nonbizarre delusions with better preservation of other psychological functions such as thought processes, volition, and behavior. In the persecutory subtype, patients experience delusions of persecution: one is spied on, poisoned, conspired against, and harassed. The perceived aggressor can be a work supervisor, a government agency, or a relative. The erotomanic subtype applies to patients with the delusional belief of being loved by another person, usually of a higher social status. The patient tries to contact that person through letters, telephone calls, and gifts. Stalking and even extreme aggression, including murder, can occur as patients are repeatedly rejected and their frustration increases. Although this subtype is equally prevalent in both genders, women are more often seen by clinicians; men are more likely to be handled in the legal system. The grandiose subtype is characterized by the delusion of having made a discovery or having a special relationship with a prominent public figure, such as the president or the pope. Many such persons apply for patents (e.g., perpetual motion devices). In the somatic subtype, the psychotic process revolves around one central somatic delusion, such as a foul smell emanating from the mouth or vagina or the conviction that one is contaminated with germs. Finally, in the jealous subtype, the central delusion is that the patient's spouse is unfaithful. There is no due cause, and the patient tries to intervene by following her spouse or hiring private detectives. The overall prevalence and incidence of paranoia does not differ in women and men, but men tend to be afflicted more by the jealous subtype.

ETIOLOGY AND PATHOPHYSIOLOGY

Most research into the cause and mechanisms by which psychosis develops has focused on patients with schizophrenia, although one favorite method of inquiry is looking at better-understood illnesses with psychotic symptoms and trying to extrapolate findings to schizophrenia. Many theories have been proposed, but no single model can integrate all the important correlative data accumulated. It is said that schizophrenia and related psychiatric conditions are a consequence of a complex interaction between inherited and environmental factors.

Genetic Factors

Most genetic research has been conducted in schizophrenia. The risk of schizophrenia is significantly higher in biologic relatives of affected persons than in the general population, and the relative risk increases with the degree of consanguinity, peaking in monozygotic twins. Adoption studies show that biologic but not adoptive relatives are at increased risk, apparently refuting the theories stressing upbringing as an etiologic factor. However, even in monozygotic twins there is a high degree of discordance, which leaves room for an important role to be played by environmental factors.

Current research efforts focus on genetic mapping in hopes of identifying one or several "schizophrenia genes." Another strategy is the study of genetic disorders that may present with a schizophrenic-type psychosis (e.g., homocystinuria, porphyria, Huntington chorea, and albinism). The chemical mechanisms of such illnesses might lend insights into the pathophysiology of primary psychotic illnesses, such as schizophrenia.

Congenital and Perinatal Disorders

Basic neurodevelopmental processes occurring primarily in the second trimester of pregnancy can be disrupted, resulting in psychotic symptomatology later in life. For instance, corpus callosum agenesis, arachnoid cysts, porencephaly, and other rare conditions have been shown to correlate with psychosis. Brain injury resulting from complicated pregnancy or delivery can also lead to psychotic illness in adulthood. One of the proposed pathways is brain hypoxia of whatever cause, which can disrupt proper neuronal migration in the hippocampus and results in aberrant cytologic architecture of this brain structure, thought to have an important role in cognitive-affective processes and pathology. Some of the obstetric and perinatal factors associated with psychosis later in life are listed in Table 147.1.

TABLE 147.1. Perinatal Factors Associated with Psychosis Later in Life

Viral infections during pregnancy
Maternal age >40 y
Gestational medical illnesses (e.g., diabetes, hypertension, deep vein thrombosis)
Breech presentation
Cesarean section
Forceps application or vacuum extraction
Pathology of the placenta
Hyperbilirubinemia in the newborn
Respiratory distress
Prematurity

Medical Illness

Medical and neurologic illness can cause nonschizophrenic psychosis. Probably there is more than one mechanism responsible. Here again, it is hoped that by studying the impact on the brain of such conditions, our understanding of the pathogenesis of psychotic phenomena will advance. An example is the association between epilepsy and schizophrenic-like psychosis, which occurs more frequently than would be expected by chance only. Research has shown that this is not a random association but one dependent on certain characteristics of the epileptic process. In particular, foci in the medial aspect of the temporal lobe, especially on the left side, are highly predictive of psychosis. Such observations corroborate with other data supporting notions such as localization and lateralization in schizophrenia. Some of the neurologic, medical, and toxicologic/pharmacologic factors associated with psychotic conditions are listed in Table 147.2.

TABLE 147.2. Organic Psychoses

Delirium
Uremic or hepatic encephalopathy
Hyponatremia
Collagen disease
Lupus cerebritis
Infections affecting brain tissue
Meningitis
Encephalitis
Brain abscess
Human immunodeficiency virus infection
Nutritional deficiency
Megaloblastic anemia (B_{12} or folate deficiency)
Wernicke psychosis (thiamine deficiency)
Pellagra (niacin deficiency)
Porphyria
Endocrinopathies
Hypothyroidism
Addison disease
Hypopituitarism
Cerebrovascular disease (all types of stroke can manifest with psychotic symptoms)
Cerebral tumors (primary or metastatic)
Neurodegenerative disorders
Parkinson disease
Huntington chorea
Wilson disease
Multiple sclerosis
Alzheimer disease
Epilepsy
Intoxication
Alcohol, sedatives, hypnotics, anxiolytics, cocaine, cannabis, phencyclidine, amphetamines and other stimulants
Withdrawal syndromes
Alcohol, sedatives, hypnotics, anxiolytics
Prescription medications
Analgesics, anticholinergics, antihistamines, antiparkinsonians, anticancer agents (cyclosporine), corticosteroids, muscle relaxants, antihypertensives

Structural Brain Abnormalities

Older pneumoencephalographic and newer brain computed tomography and magnetic resonance imaging studies of patients with schizophrenia and other psychotic disorders reveal the presence of subtle structural differences. Ventricles are enlarged, and the total cortical mass is reduced. Temporal horns, especially on the left side, are affected more. These changes are less prominent in women than in men. Again, the data seem to point to a special role for the temporal lobes and adjacent structures.

Functional Neuroimaging

The advent of positron emission tomography and single photon emission computed tomography have allowed in vivo studies of the intensity of some neurochemical processes in different regions of the brain. Using these techniques, researchers have shown that patients with schizophrenia have a low level of metabolic activity in the prefrontal cortex. The prefrontal cortex is an area of multimodal association linked to higher cognitive processes such as fluency of thought, volition, attention-shifting, and behavior sequencing, as well as affective expression. Symptoms such as affective blunting, avolition, and alogia are generated via hypofrontality, according to this theory.

Neurochemistry

Based on the fact that all traditional antipsychotic drugs block dopamine (D_2) receptor binding, the dopamine hypothesis of psychotic symptom formation was developed. According to this theory, functional overactivity of dopamine in temporolimbic regions leads to "positive" symptoms such as delusions and hallucinations. Dopamine blockade in these regions accounts for the antipsychotic effect of neuroleptics; dopamine blockade in the basal ganglia explains the extrapyramidal side effects of these drugs. Furthermore, based on the fact that dopaminergic fibers originating in the substantia nigra and tegmentum project onto the frontal cortex, a dysfunction of the dopamine neurotransmitter system could explain both the negative symptoms and the dulling effect of antipsychotics.

This formulation is at best simplistic. It does not account for new research identifying a variety of subtypes of dopamine receptors, the absence of D_2 receptors in frontal and temporolimbic regions, and the effectiveness of newer antipsychotics such as clozapine and risperidone, which exert potent effects on non-D_2 receptors. The role of serotonergic or D_1 receptors is being reevaluated, but to date a unifying biochemical theory of psychosis remains elusive.

Psychosocial and Cultural Factors

A complete discussion of the etiology and pathophysiology of psychosis would be incomplete without mentioning nonbiologic theories. Several decades ago such theories prevailed in this country. Severe failure of ego functioning, resulting in a subjective perception of daily tasks as overwhelming and leading to inability to adjust and function, was a common psychoanalytic interpretation of schizophrenia. Developmental failure caused by inappropriate upbringing was another favorite formulation: Attention was directed to the "schizophrenogenic" mother, described as anxious, overprotective, and enmeshed. The fact that schizophrenia is more prevalent in lower socioeconomic strata led to theories linking poverty to the etiology of this illness. Other factors, such as urbanization, industrialization, and migration, were similarly interpreted based on prevalence studies.

All these theories fail to analyze the respective connections in both directions, making unproven cause-and-effect presumptions. Does the anxious mother cause her child to develop symptoms, or is the premorbidly aloof and unresponsive child making the sensitive mother overly concerned and protective? Is poverty a cause of schizophrenia, or is schizophrenia, with its disabling functional and occupational failure, throwing the patient at the bottom of the socioeconomic ladder?

Although they do not provide convincing etiologic explanations, psychosociocultural factors are relevant in understanding the context in which psychosis develops, the dynamics of decompensation, and the success or failure of treatment. Their proper consideration allows a more complete definition of the concept of vulnerability. According to this notion, the actual occurrence of symptoms results from the cumulative and coincidental action of diverse predisposing factors, be they genetic predisposition, environmental stress, or noncompliance with treatment.

DIAGNOSIS

It is relatively easy to make a diagnosis of psychosis when the patient presents with bizarre delusions, complains of hearing voices, or displays disorganized speech and behavior. Many times, however, the clinical picture is more subtle. Paranoid patients can be so distrustful that they do not share their delusions with the physician. Indirect clues, such as a guarded attitude in the office or reports by caregivers that the patient makes frequent calls to the police and does not allow people in her house, should be properly interpreted. Depressed patients with psychosis may ruminate about lack of money and difficulty paying bills. The untrained listener may validate such complains as plausible without noticing the fact that they are unusual for that patient or that they are presented in a rigid exaggerated manner, unresponsive to reassurance. Even more difficult to identify are patients with chronic psychotic illness, presenting only with some measure of affective blunting, poor social functioning, and mild thought process disturbance, such as tangentiality and loose associations. The astute clinician takes note of such signs and obtains a thorough history. The effort could be rewarded with the finding that in the past the patient experienced more florid psychotic symptoms.

When in doubt, referral to a psychiatrist for consultation is appropriate. Rarely, projective psychological testing administered by a certified clinical psychologist can be helpful in unmasking psychotic thinking in patients who cover their thought disorder well and cannot be diagnosed clinically.

DIFFERENTIAL DIAGNOSIS

Two common errors can be made by the primary care provider once the presence of a psychotic syndrome has been established: automatic referral to a mental health professional and instituting treatment immediately, without further diagnostic inquiry. Such actions are justified only in some cases: For instance, a patient with a well-established diagnosis of schizophrenia needs psychiatric follow-up, or an acutely agitated psychotic patient needs sedation right away. In general, however, the clinician's first priority is to rule out a host of medical conditions that can present with psychotic symptoms.

Whenever possible, a thorough physical and neurologic examination should precede any other action. Along with the mental status examination (description of attention, alertness, affect, mood, thought content and processes, perception, memory, and other cognitive functions), the history and a minimum set of laboratory data (blood count and differential, chemistry profile, urinalysis) enable the physician to make a diagnostic presumption that can then be pursued and confirmed.

Delirium

The first entity to consider and rule out should be delirium, a medical emergency. Delirium is a medically induced acute confusional state that can present with high levels of behavioral and thought disorganization, as well as delusions and hallucinations. Unlike other psychotic illnesses, however, it has a rather sudden onset (hours or days). Another distinguishing feature is the fluctuation in level of alertness and orientation (waxing and waning) and the impairment in attention and concentration. Many exogenous substances and acute medical conditions can lead to this transitory insult to brain function and by definition removal of the cause is followed by resolution of mental symptoms.

The vulnerability of a person to develop delirium and the time necessary to recover from it are increased with age and the preexistence of organic brain pathology. For instance, an elderly woman with mild dementia easily develops delirium in response to moderate dehydration. Her confusion, agitation, and psychosis may linger for weeks and even months after her water and electrolyte balance is restored, much to the frustration of her physician, who might be tempted to label her as insane and in need of psychiatric hospitalization.

Dementia

Loss of memory and other cognitive functions such as speech, praxis, and visual/spatial orientation due to a progressive destruction of brain tissue defines the syndrome of dementia, which is encountered mostly in older persons. Alzheimer disease and cerebrovascular disease, alone or in combination, account for almost 80% of cases. Whatever the cause, patients develop psychopathology during the course of illness, including paranoid delusions, delusions of misidentification, disorganization of thought processes, agitation and aggression, and other psychotic symptoms. Incorrectly attributing these manifestations to a functional psychiatric illness can lead to unrealistic treatment choices and an incorrect prognosis. A history of steady and chronic memory and functional decline; a computed tomography or magnetic resonance image of the head suggestive of atrophy, small infarcts, or both; other associated features (e.g., alcoholism, repeated head trauma, hypothyroidism, vitamin B_{12} deficiency); or a family history of dementia should raise the suspicion of dementia.

Substance-Induced Psychosis

Stimulants such as methylphenidate, d-amphetamine, and certain drugs of abuse such as cocaine and phencyclidine can cause a psychotic syndrome indistinguishable from acute schizophrenia: auditory command hallucinations, ideas of reference, paranoia, assaultiveness, and intense fear. Psychosis occurs both as a result of intoxication but also of withdrawal (e.g., alcoholic hallucinosis characterized by visual and tactile hallucinations begins after alcohol levels have dropped). Many prescription drugs have been reported to cause psychotic symptoms as an untoward effect. Examples include anticholinergic agents, antiparkinsonian drugs, corticosteroids, analgesics, muscle relaxants, antihypertensives, cimetidine, and cytostatics such as cyclosporine or procarbazine.

The physician should remember the role of exogenous substances in generating psychosis and should always obtain a thorough drug history. In cases of suspected abuse, the urine or blood should be checked ("tox screens").

Medical Illness

As mentioned, psychosis can be a nonspecific manifestation of many medical conditions (Table 147.2). Proper diagnosis avoids traumatic psychiatric labeling and allows the institution of specific treatment if available. There are many anecdotes in the literature documenting patients with slow-growing brain tumors, temporal lobe epilepsy, porphyria, or degenerative neurologic conditions who had been diagnosed and treated for many years for "schizophrenia."

Primary Psychosis

In the absence of identifiable medical factors, a functional psychotic illness can be presumed. Given the accumulating evidence that illnesses such as schizophrenia and paranoia have an important biologic substrate, the term "functional" has become something of a misnomer. The term "primary psychosis" seems more appropriate, although such a category must exclude brief reactive psychosis, a nonorganic but secondary illness lasting between 1 day and 1 month that occurs in apparent response to a very stressful event.

The distinctions between schizophrenia, schizoaffective disorder, delusional disorder, and schizophreniform disorder were discussed above. There is an important overlap between affective and psychotic disorders. Sometimes schizophrenic patients experience depressive symptoms that can be an isolated or combined consequence of three factors: improvement leading to better insight into the devastating consequences of the illness (postpsychotic depression), prominent negative symptoms, and antipsychotic-induced affective blunting. On the other hand, many patients with primary affective illness become psychotic. It is notoriously difficult to distinguish between some forms of mania and florid schizophrenic decompensation.

Other psychiatric illnesses are sometimes difficult to differentiate from psychosis. Patients with panic anxiety complain of losing their mind. Their perception is genuine and very frightening, but they remain rational throughout the attack. Similarly, patients with obsessive-compulsive disorder have irrational thoughts such as having caused a car accident or being contaminated with germs or dirt. These thoughts are uncontrollably intrusive, but the patients are not psychotic because they know their fears are irrational.

Several personality disorders (borderline, paranoid, schizotypal, schizoid) can present with elements of psychotic thinking, especially when the patient is under increased stress. The diagnosis of personality disorder relies on the presence of a pervasive and stable pattern of behavior and interpersonal relationships that is maladaptive and causes subjective distress and functional disability. Personality disorders can mimic psychosis or coexist with psychotic illness. They are best diagnosed by mental health professionals based on extensive history and ongoing behavioral observations. When suspected, early referral for psychiatric consultation is advised.

TREATMENT

Secondary Psychosis

Good treatment starts with the understanding that psychosis is not an illness but a syndrome cutting across many different entities. A thorough diagnostic effort allows for specific treatment of secondary psychosis, be it correction of hypoxia, dehydration, or infection in a delirious patient; the discontinuation of an offending pharmacologic agent used for another illness; or the surgical removal of a slow-growing meningioma.

Dangerousness

The disturbed behaviors associated with psychosis can, in extreme cases, be dangerous to the patient or others. Suicide is a common complication of both psychotic depression and schizophrenia. Erratic unsafe acts such as crossing the street without paying attention to traffic or sleeping in the cold can also have life-threatening consequences. Acutely paranoid patients can be aggressive, exhibiting acts ranging from random assaultiveness to thoroughly prepared murderous plots. Caregivers have an ethical and legal duty to protect both patients and their potential victims. Early in the evaluation phase, the clinician must estimate the risks involved and decide if hospitalization, voluntary or not, should be arranged. Factors such as past behavior, command hallucinations, suicidal or homicidal thinking, and availability of social supports must be considered when making such a decision, and psychiatric consultation should be obtained as soon as possible.

Agitation

Acute psychosis is often accompanied by a fair amount of agitation. The patient is distraught and in need of subjective relief. Motor restlessness can be intense and interferes with further diagnostic examination. In such circumstances, sedation and even physical restraints are necessary. Concerns about the patient's dignity, civil rights, and proper treatment are legitimately raised only when such measures are applied too late, too early, for excessive periods of time, or without proper clinical justification. Many drugs, including antipsychotics, benzodiazepines, other nonbenzodiazepine anxiolytics, and lithium, are being used for acute sedation. A powerful and safe regimen is the combination of haloperidol 5 mg and lorazepam 2 mg, given together orally or intramuscularly, every 1 to 4 hours as needed. Antipsychotics used for acute sedation act immediately and in a nonspecific way, which is why they are also called major tranquilizers. The more specific antipsychotic effect is delayed for weeks and occurs at different, usually lower, doses.

Pharmacologic Treatment of Psychotic Symptoms

Regardless of etiology, psychotic symptoms (delusions, hallucinations, disorganization) improve with the use of specific pharmacologic and, to a lesser extent, nonpharmacologic interventions.

ANTIPSYCHOTICS

Drugs in this class are also known as neuroleptics or major tranquilizers. Until recently they all had in common the antagonism of dopamine receptors in several areas of the brain, such as the tegmentum, substantia nigra, temporolimbic structures, prefrontal lobes, and basal ganglia. The introduction of nonconventional antipsychotics such as clozapine and risperidone, with mechanisms of action involving other neurotransmitter systems, has changed the thinking on the mechanism of pharmacologic suppression of psychotic phenomena. Thus, a new class of antipsychotic drugs has emerged in the last decade: They are still called "atypical" although they have rapidly gained ground against conventional antipsychotics and are likely to replace them entirely in the not so distant future.

Conventional antipsychotics are equally effective in equivalent dosage. They differ in side effects, forming a continuum from high to low potency (Table 147.3). High-potency drugs such as haloperidol or fluphenazine cause extrapyramidal syndromes: parkinsonism, akathisia (a subjective and objective restlessness thought to be one of the major causes of noncompliance with these medications), and acute dystonia (a rather frightening, albeit benign, complication that resolves promptly with the administration of diphenhydramine 50 mg intramuscularly). Low-potency drugs such as thioridazine or chlorpromazine cause little movement disorder but are associated with orthostatic hypotension, somnolence, and anticholinergic toxicity (constipation, urinary retention, dry mouth, delirium in the elderly).

All traditional antipsychotics, when used for long periods, can cause tardive dyskinesia, a movement disorder characterized by facial tics and choreoathetoid movements of the tongue, mouth, limbs, or trunk. In some cases it improves with discontinuation of the antipsychotic; in others it is irreversible. In extreme cases it can cause swallowing or breathing problems, although its main impact is aesthetic. Tardive dyskinesia is one of the main sources of malpractice liability in psychiatry, and in some communities written informed consent before starting antipsychotic medication has become standard. Women and the elderly are thought to be at increased risk of developing tardive dyskinesia.

A very rare but potentially lethal complication of antipsychotic medications is neuroleptic malignant syndrome. It consists of hyperarousal, hyperthermia, extreme muscular rigidity, and subsequent myolysis, acute changes in mental status. Early recognition, discontinuation of antipsychotic medication, and nonspecific intensive care measures are most important, although drugs like dantrolene and even electroconvulsant therapy have been advocated in treating this condition.

Haloperidol 5 mg twice daily, or any other drug in equivalent dosage, is a usual antipsychotic dose. Higher doses are justified only when sedation is also necessary. Loading a patient with high doses of antipsychotic medication (rapid neurolepti-

TABLE 147.3. Antipsychotic Medications

Class	Generic name	Brand name	CPZ equivalent
Typical			
Low potency	Chlorpromazine	Thorazine	100
	Thioridazine	Mellaril	95
	Mesoridazine	Serentil	50
Intermediate potency	Molindone	Moban	10
	Loxapine	Loxitan	10
	Perphenazine	Trilafon	8
	Thiothixene	Navane	5
	Trifluoperazine	Stelazine	5
High potency	Fluphenazine	Prolixin	2
	Haloperidol	Haldol	2
			Usual daily dose (mg)
Atypical			
	Clozapine	Clozaril	300–900
	Risperidone	Risperidal	2–8
	Olanzapine	Zyprexa, Zydis	5–20
	Quetiapine	Seroquel	200–800
	Ziprasidone	Geodon	40–160

zation) does not achieve a faster decrease in delusions or hallucinations. The elderly and patients with coexistent liver disease might need considerably lower doses. For instance, a demented woman with paranoia and agitation might require as little as 0.25 mg of haloperidol once or twice a day. Patients who are noncompliant with oral medication benefit from depot preparations given intramuscularly, such as fluphenazine decanoate every 2 weeks or haloperidol decanoate every 4 weeks. Iatrogenic parkinsonism responds to drugs such as trihexyphenidyl, benztropine, or amantadine. Akathisia responds to small doses of propranolol (e.g., 10 mg four times a day). Although effective in decreasing delusions, hallucinations, acute disorganization, and agitation, most typical antipsychotics have little effect on negative symptoms.

With the introduction of clozapine on the market in 1991, a new class of antipsychotic drugs, "the atypicals," emerged. These drugs not only inhibit dopamine receptors, but also a subtype of serotonin receptor. It is postulated that the interplay between dopamine and serotonin receptor inhibition is responsible for some of the advantages noticed with these new compounds: decreased incidence and severity of extrapyramidal side effects, decreased tendency to cause hyperprolactinemia, and some efficacy in correcting negative symptoms like apathy and avolition.

Clozapine is considered to be the most effective antipsychotic. It does not cause tardive dyskinesia or parkinsonism and is effective in treating negative symptoms. About one third of patients with psychosis resistant to other antipsychotics do respond to and tolerate clozapine.

The high cost, cumbersome dispensing system, and association with severe side effects (e.g., agranulocytosis, seizures, tachycardia) limit its wider use. Doses range from 12.5 to 900 mg/d, with an average maintenance dose of 300 mg. Weekly white blood cell counts to prevent fatal agranulocytosis are required by the manufacturer for the first 6 months of treatment; afterward white blood cell counts can be checked every other week.

Like clozapine, risperidone is a newer antipsychotic that does not depend only on dopamine inhibition for its action. In doses of up to 3 mg twice a day it is relatively free of side effects, but at higher doses it behaves like a high-potency antipsychotic.

Olanzapine in doses up to 20 mg is also effective and, according to some, might have mild mood elevating properties. Weight gain and worsening of diabetes control have been described with its use. Quetiapine's initial dosing guidelines of about 300 mg/d have been revised upward to up to 800 mg/d, which translates into increased efficacy. Like clozapine, quetiapine is almost devoid of parkinsonian side effects, an advantage in many patients, especially those with preexistent parkinsonism.

The newest atypical antipsychotic released, ziprasidone, is now in full postmarketing testing. It can increase QTc, and electrocardiographic monitoring is recommended.

Other drugs have a more limited role in the treatment of psychosis. Benzodiazepines can be useful for acute sedation, antidepressants in psychotic depression, and lithium and other mood stabilizers in psychotic mania and as prophylaxis in bipolar disorder. Vitamin E is being advocated in the treatment of tardive dyskinesia. Electroconvulsive therapy is used for affective psychosis and in selected cases of treatment resistant schizophrenia, especially in young patients.

Nonspecific Nonpharmacologic Interventions

Interacting with a psychotic patient can be frightening, frustrating, and perplexing to the caregiver. The myth that only mental health professionals can deal with such patients can be dispelled easily by observing several simple rules. The patient must be treated with respect and the content of her delusional thoughts explored in a nonjudgmental manner. The interviewer must not try to either contradict or pretend to agree with the delusional patient but rather should focus on areas of agreement, such as the fact that the patient is upset, scared, or in need of help. Many psychotic patients calm down if their "space" is not being violated: For instance, close physical proximity or discussion of sensitive subjects is better avoided. Certain elements of the physical examination, such as the rectal and genital examination, might need to be postponed. Communication with the patient must be kept simple and direct. Too much information presented at once might be overwhelming. Patients with psychosis tend to do better with predictable routines, and become anxious and more psychotic when faced with unexpected changes. Even trivial modifications in their medication or appointments should be introduced carefully. Awareness of such basic principles allows the primary care provider to establish the therapeutic relationship necessary for the delivery of nonpsychiatric medical care, for psychiatric management in case this is provided to some extent by the primary care provider, or for successful referral to a psychiatrist. More formal interventions usually require involvement by a psychiatric provider.

Psychosocial Treatments

Several types of nonpharmacologic treatments have proven to be useful in the management of patients with subacute and chronic psychotic illness.

INDIVIDUAL PSYCHOTHERAPY

Supportive and behavioral therapies are most relevant in the treatment of psychotic patients; psychoanalytic techniques are considered by many to be of limited usefulness, if not outright detrimental. Supportive psychotherapy stresses directive interventions such as clarification, psychoeducation, explanations, encouragement, reassurance, and even advice, in contrast to analytic techniques in which the therapist remains more neutral and detached and the main intervention is interpretation.

Severely regressed patients respond to behavioral techniques such as modeling, reinforcement of desirable behaviors by contingency application of rewards, extinction of psychotic or undesirable behavior, and so forth. Some of the goals of psychotherapy include improving coping ability and social skills, increasing understanding of the illness and its proper treatment, decreasing psychotic thinking and inappropriate behavior, decreasing subjective distress, and avoiding noncompliance and relapse.

FAMILY

Family involvement in the care of psychotic patients is crucial. Family therapy with or without patient participation, multifamily therapeutic groups, and self-help and advocacy groups are all useful modalities. They can achieve important goals such as education about the illness, emotional support, practical tips about dealing with sick relatives, and information about community resources.

ENVIRONMENTAL MANIPULATION

The social management of patients with psychosis centers on creating a protective environment in which exposure to different life stressors is controlled. Group homes, social clubs, day programs, occupational therapy, vocational training, and sheltered workshops are components of such an environment. The goal is to help the patient return to the highest level of socialization tolerable.

CONSIDERATIONS IN PREGNANCY AND POSTPARTUM

Puerperal Psychosis

Between 1 and 2 per 1,000 deliveries are complicated by a psychotic syndrome. The exact definition of puerperal psychosis is controversial. Many believe that most cases reflect either a better accepted category of postpartum affective disorder or a psychotic episode in an already affected woman who decompensates in response to the psychological stress of pregnancy and delivery. The clinical picture is variable, but there is always a symptom-free interval between delivery and onset of at least 2 to 3 days. Sleep disorder, rapidly changing course, irritability, and mood lability are almost always present. Nihilistic delusions about the infant or pregnancy include the belief that the child is dead or defective or denial of having an infant altogether. Command hallucinations to harm the infant are of particular concern. In some cases schizophrenic-type symptoms predominate: thought disorganization, bizarre delusions, and hallucinations. The most common presentation is affective psychosis. Symptoms include delusions of guilt and worthlessness, crying, death wishes, and suicidal and infanticidal ideas. In most patients these thoughts are intrusive and ruminative. Manic and mixed affective states are also described. An infrequent variety of puerperal psychosis is the pseudoorganic type: Patients are confused and show memory and other cognitive deficits.

The illness can have an early onset, in which case affective symptoms tend to predominate. Late-onset cases (more than 3 weeks after delivery) present with the schizophreniform syndrome and tend to occur in older women with preexistent psychopathology.

The cause of puerperal psychosis is unknown. In some patients, some form of psychopathology precedes the pregnancy or becomes evident during gestation. Many patients with recurrent psychotic affective illness, particularly bipolar, experience their first episode of illness postpartum. Attempts at finding a correlation between postpartum psychosis and endocrine markers such as progesterone, estrogen, follicle-stimulating hormone, prolactin, and thyroxin have been unsuccessful.

Treatment includes pharmacotherapy aimed at the most prominent symptoms. Antipsychotics and antidepressants are used in combination for the psychotically depressed patient. Risperdal up to 3 mg twice daily and venlafaxine up to 225 mg once a day exemplifies such a regimen. Lithium and other mood stabilizers can be used alone or in combination with antipsychotics for manic symptoms. Antipsychotics alone are appropriate for the nonaffective varieties. In all cases, lack of response to medication raises the need for electroconvulsive therapy, which is quite effective.

In the acute phase, the safety of the mother and the infant must be thoroughly evaluated. Suicide, infanticide, and child neglect or abuse are common complications. Puerperal psychosis is a psychiatric emergency, and the woman should be referred for psychiatric evaluation. Hospitalization is almost always necessary; some advocate hospitalizing both patient and child if possible. As the patient improves, she can benefit from supportive psychotherapy. Therapies concentrate on issues such as her relationships with her child, her partner, and her mother. Individual, marital, or group settings can all be useful, and enlisting the support of family, friends, and social services is appropriate. The prognosis for resolution of acute symptoms is good.

Preexistent Psychotic Illness and Pregnancy

Women with already diagnosed psychotic conditions such as schizophrenia pose special management problems when they become pregnant. Even before conception, the practitioner might be faced with the need to provide the would-be mother and her partner with genetic counseling: The offspring of a schizophrenic mother has a 10-fold higher risk of developing schizophrenia. The risk of decompensation to the mother during and after pregnancy, her parenting skills, and her suitability to overcome the many challenges of motherhood must be discussed so that an informed decision can be reached. After conception, the mother's mental status should be followed closely and the pregnancy considered high risk. Once the infant has been delivered, social services are always called on to provide support and to assess the safety of the mother and the child.

Use of Somatic Treatments and Pregnancy

Antipsychotic drugs are crucial in the treatment of psychotic illness regardless of etiology, and their use or avoidance during and immediately after pregnancy is associated with several potential problems and risks. When making a prescribing decision, the clinician must consider the risks of structural teratogenicity, behavioral teratogenicity, and maternal and newborn toxicity on the one hand and danger to the fetus and mother if the untreated patient decompensates on the other.

The few large retrospective and prospective studies of possible correlations between structural congenital malformations and the use of neuroleptics during pregnancy showed conflicting results. There may be a slight increase in malformations, especially if the drugs were used between the 4th and 10th weeks of pregnancy. This preliminary conclusion is derived primarily from the California Child Health and Development Project, in a study of 19,000 births between 1959 and 1966 that originally showed no significant differences between women who had used antipsychotics and women who did not. A reanalysis of the data in 1984 by Edlund and Craig showed that mothers who used neuroleptics between the 4th and 10th weeks had a 5.4% chance of giving birth to malformed children, as opposed to 3.2% for the rest of the sample. Another large study conducted in France by Rumeau-Rouquette and coworkers found that use of neuroleptics in the first trimester was associated with a 3.5% risk of malformations in the infant, higher than the 1.6% risk for the rest of the sample (chromosomal abnormalities were excluded). On the other hand, a large prospective study of over 50,000 births found no correlation between the use of antipsychotics during pregnancy and congenital malformations. Teratogenicity is somewhat higher in case reports and small retrospective studies. Interpreting the existing data on teratogenicity is made difficult by a number of confounding variables: Children of untreated psychotic women may have a higher risk of malformations; many of the women included in the analysis took small doses of phenothiazines as antiemetics only; and no consideration was given to concurrent use of other drugs, diagnosis, age, number of pregnancies, dose, or length of exposure.

Even less is known about the behavioral teratogenicity of antipsychotics. Learning delays, hyperactivity, and other disturbances of motor activity have been blamed on virtually any central nervous system active medication used by the mother during pregnancy. A critical review of the literature reveals a still undeveloped methodology and a paucity of long enough follow-up studies. Presently, there is very little in the scientific literature regarding the consequences of using atypical antipsychotics during pregnancy. None of the antipsychotics available can therefore be considered safe in this regard.

The use of neuroleptics during the third trimester of pregnancy may cause an extrapyramidal syndrome in the neonate that lasts up to several months. Symptoms include hypertonia, psychomotor agitation, hyperreflexia, and initial delay in learning tasks. The effect might be dose related. Exaggerated neonatal jaundice and a syndrome characterized by cyanosis and respiratory distress have been described, especially with the use of high doses of chlorpromazine.

All antipsychotics are excreted in breast milk. Several studies showed that except for mild drowsiness, there are no major negative consequences to infants breast-fed by mothers taking antipsychotics. However, no studies have evaluated the excretion of the newer atypical antipsychotics and the effects on the nursing infant.

In practice, antipsychotics can be used during and immediately after pregnancy if necessary. Delirium, severe acute psychosis, and the likelihood of psychotic decompensation if medication is withheld are acceptable indications. Treatment of nausea with phenothiazines or the use of antipsychotics for anxiety or nonspecific tranquilization should be avoided. In patients who are well compensated on antipsychotics and want to become pregnant, an attempt to discontinue the medication in the first trimester or in the weeks preceding delivery can be made. During such an effort, the patient must be monitored closely for early signs of decompensation. Some advocate the use of high-potency drugs such as haloperidol during pregnancy, but there are few solid data to support a particular drug over others.

BIBLIOGRAPHY

American Psychiatric Association. *Diagnostic and statistical manual of mental disorders*, 4th ed. Washington, DC: American Psychiatric Press, 1994.

Burt VK, Hendrick VC. *Postpartum psychiatric disorders: concise guide to women's mental health.* Washington, DC: American Psychiatric Press, 1997:63–77.

Cohen L, Rosenbaum J. Psychotropic drug use during pregnancy: weighing the risks. *J Clin Psych* 1998:59[Suppl 2]:18–28.

Elia J, Katz IR, Simpson GM. Teratogenicity of psychotherapeutic medications. *Psychopharmacol Bull* 1987;23:531.

Novalis PN, Rojcewicz SJ, Peele R. *Clinical manual of supportive psychotherapy.* Washington, DC: American Psychiatric Press, 1993.

Schatzberg AF, Cole JO. *Manual of clinical psychopharmacology,* 2nd ed. Washington, DC: American Psychiatric Press, 1991.

Stewart D, Stotland NL, eds. *Psychological aspects of women's health care: the interface between psychiatry and obstetrics and gynecology.* Washington, DC: American Psychiatric Press, 1993.

Yoshida K, Smith B, Graggs M, et al. Neuroleptic drugs in breast-milk: a study of pharmacokinetics and of possible adverse effects in breast-fed infants. *Psychol Med* 1998;28:81–91.

CHAPTER 148

Addictive Disorders and Substance Abuse

Deborah Martina Smith

ILLICIT DRUG USE

Descriptive Epidemiology

An estimated 14.0 million Americans are illicit drug users (use within the month before interview) according to the 2000 National Household Survey on Drug Abuse (NHSDA). Marijuana is the most commonly used illicit drug. One half of the users of drugs other than marijuana (3.8 million) were using psychotherapeutics nonmedically. The rate of past month illicit drug use among both adults and youths was higher among those that were currently using cigarettes or alcohol compared with those not using either substance. In 2000, the rate of past month illicit drug use was 42.7% among youths 12 to 17 years who used cigarettes. The rate of illicit drug use was 65.5% among youth heavy drinkers. Overall, approximately half (49%) of current illicit drug users were under age 26.

There are gender differences in the prevalence of substance abuse and drug dependence disorders. Men were reported to have a higher rate of current illicit drug use than women (7.7% vs. 5.0%) in 2000. However, among youths aged 12 to 17, the rate of current illicit drug use was similar for boys (9.8%) and girls (9.5%). The rates of nonmedical use of psychotherapeutic drugs (pain relievers, tranquilizers, stimulants, and sedatives) were similar for males (1.8%) and females (1.7%). This is the class of abused drugs with the next highest prevalence after marijuana. Although associated with intense public commentary and individual and societal repercussions, cocaine and heroin use are much lower in overall prevalence (≤1%).

An emerging trend in substances of abuse is the use of the "club drugs" among teens and young adults. 3,4-methylenedioxymethamphetamine (MDMA), flunitrazepam (trade name Rophynol), γ-hydroxybutyrate (GHB), and ketamine are among the drugs used in nightclubs, bars, and raves. In high doses these drugs cause a variety of adverse effects, including malignant hyperthermia. MDMA is a synthetic psychoactive drug with both stimulant and hallucinogenic properties. Street names for MDMA are "ecstasy," "Adam," "hug," "beans," and "love bug." MDMA is usually ingested in pill form, but some users snort it, inject it, or use it in suppository form. Recent research links MDMA use to long-term damage to those parts of the brain critical to thought, memory, and pleasure. There has been some preliminary evidence that this damage is more severe in women.

GHB, flunitrazepam, and ketamine are predominantly central nervous system depressants. Because they are generally colorless, tasteless, and odorless, they can be added to beverages and ingested unknowingly. With these characteristics, these drugs emerged as "date-rape" drugs. This phenomenon is also known as "drug-facilitated" rape.

Since 1990, GHB has been abused in the United States for its euphoric, sedative, and anabolic effects. Street names include "liquid ecstasy" and "Georgia home boy." Coma and seizures can occur after abuse of GHB, and when combined with methamphetamine there appears to be an increased risk of seizure. Combining use with alcohol potentiates the effects. GHB and two prodrugs, γ-butyrolactone and 1,4-butandiol, have been involved in overdoses and deaths in addition to date rapes. The latter two drugs are industrial solvents, and all three are available in gyms, raves, health food stores, and are sold over the Internet.

Flunitrazepam (Rophynol) has been identified as being of particular concern as a cause of drug-facilitated rape. It is a benzodiazepine that is not legally approved for marketing in the United States. Street names for the drug include "rophies," "roofies," "roach," and "rope." Flunitrazepam incapacitates victims and prevents them from resisting sexual assault. It produces anterograde amnesia such that individuals will not remember events while under the influence of the drug. If mixed with alcohol, the drug can be lethal.

Ketamine is an anesthetic that has been approved for use in humans and animals. Currently, most ketamine legally sold is for veterinary use. It can be injected or snorted. Street names include "special K" or "vitamin K." At certain doses ketamine can cause dreamlike states and hallucinations. At high does, the drug causes delirium and respiratory depression.

Addictive disorders include a range of disorders related to the use of a substance. These substances are both legal and illegal drugs. There are 11 classes of psychoactive drugs. In addition to alcohol, caffeine, and nicotine, the list includes amphetamines and related drugs, cannabis (marijuana), cocaine, hallucinogens, inhalants, opioids, phencyclidine, and the class of sedative hypnotics and anxiolytics.

The term *substance-induced disorders* refers to a group of disorders caused by a substance (i.e., substance intoxication or withdrawal). Substance dependence describes a disorder characterized by cognitive, behavioral, and physiological symptoms related to the repeated use of a substance in addition to significant substance-related problems. Substance abuse describes a pattern manifested by recurrent and significant adverse consequences related to repeated use of a substance. Unlike substance dependence, it does not include a pattern of tolerance, withdrawal, or compulsive use.

Etiology and Social Context

The biologic basis for addiction disorders has not yet been completely elucidated. There is evidence of a genetic predisposition for substance abuse disorders other than alcoholism. However, there are many environmental variables. The multifaceted social context in which women develop substance abuse disorders must be appreciated if appropriate evaluation and treatment support is to be provided.

Women are highly stigmatized for substance abuse and dependence. Women experience more family disruption than men as a result of their substance abuse. Increasingly, as women's roles have changed, there is more visibility to their impairment in the occupational setting. There is also a greater likelihood than in the past that substance-abusing women will have had contact with the criminal justice system.

Sex, sexuality, and sex roles play a part in the initiation, continuation, and consequences of substance abuse in women. Women are often initiated into drug use by a man, particularly an intimate partner. This is commonly the case with injection drug use. Prior childhood as well as adult sexual assault is a significant risk factor for the development of substance abuse in women. Sexual assault, along with other types of interpersonal violence, increase the risk of posttraumatic stress disorder. Posttraumatic stress disorder has been identified in at least 50% of treatment-seeking substance-abusing women.

Screening and Diagnosis of Substance Abuse

Primary care physicians should have a systematic approach to screening for substance abuse, because few patients spontaneously volunteer this information. Although all patients should be asked about substance use, those with a previous history of substance abuse or a family history of such abuse may be at higher risk. The CAGE and T-ACE screening questionnaires designed for alcohol abuse screening are presented later in the chapter. In primary care practice these brief instruments can serve as a template for screening for other substances. Additional information is obtained by careful physical examination and toxicology screening.

The review of systems, physical, and mental status examinations are conducted to disclose evidence of recent or current drug use, intoxication, withdrawal syndromes, and medical consequences. The following are examples of medical problems correlated with drug use that may be observed through physical assessment and ancillary testing:

- Adverse pregnancy outcomes
- Anemia
- Anxiety disorders
- Cancers of the liver, esophagus, oropharynx, and stomach
- Cardiovascular disease (e.g., phlebitis, cardiomyopathy)
- Cellulitis related to injection drug use
- Cirrhosis
- Dental disorders
- Depression
- Eating disorders and malnutrition
- Hepatitis B and C
- Menstrual cycle disorders and other gynecologic conditions
- Secondary effects of traumatic injuries
- Sexual dysfunction
- Sexually transmitted infections, including human immunodeficiency virus infection
- Tuberculosis
- Upper respiratory tract infections.

Other medical issues include lack of preventive screening such as regular Pap smear testing and mammography.

Urine Testing

Urine testing may be useful in verifying substance abuse suspected by clinical indicators in the history and physical examination. Such testing also is useful in monitoring the progress of drug rehabilitation and in screening for relapse. Obtaining a toxicology screen requires informed consent and the ability to discuss the results in a nonjudgmental manner. Drugs that can be identified in a urine screen include marijuana, cocaine, amphetamines, opiates, phencyclidine, lysergic acid diethylamide, methaqualone, barbiturates, benzodiazepines, and steroids. However, the urine toxicology test detects only recent use.

Frequent users are more likely to be detected by urine screening than occasional users. Results of urine tests remain positive after the last use of amphetamines for 24 to 72 hours, cocaine for 24 to 72 hours, opiates for 2 to 4 days, marijuana for 7 to 30 days, alcohol for 8 to 16 hours, lysergic acid diethylamide for 2 to 3 days, phencyclidine for 7 days, and benzodiazepines for several weeks. Once the patient has been screened for substance use, the next step is to assess the extent of this use and the associated adverse effects to determine what treatment, if any, is indicated.

Treatment

The treatment of substance abuse or dependence is aimed at reversing the health and social problems associated with the substance of use. The first step in treatment is for the individual to accept that substance abuse or dependence is a treatable disease. The principles of effective drug abuse treatment as outlined by the National Institute on Drug Abuse are discussed below and illustrated in Fig. 148.1.

- *No single treatment is appropriate for all individuals.* Matching treatment settings, interventions, and services to each individual's particular problems and needs is critical to her ultimate success in returning to productive functioning in the family, workplace, and society.
- Drug-free counseling covers a variety of approaches that have in common only the absence of provision of any medication. Outpatient drug-free treatment emphasizes intensive and long-term treatment and involves psychotherapy. This therapy is reserved for individuals who are highly motivated and have better-than-average verbal skills.

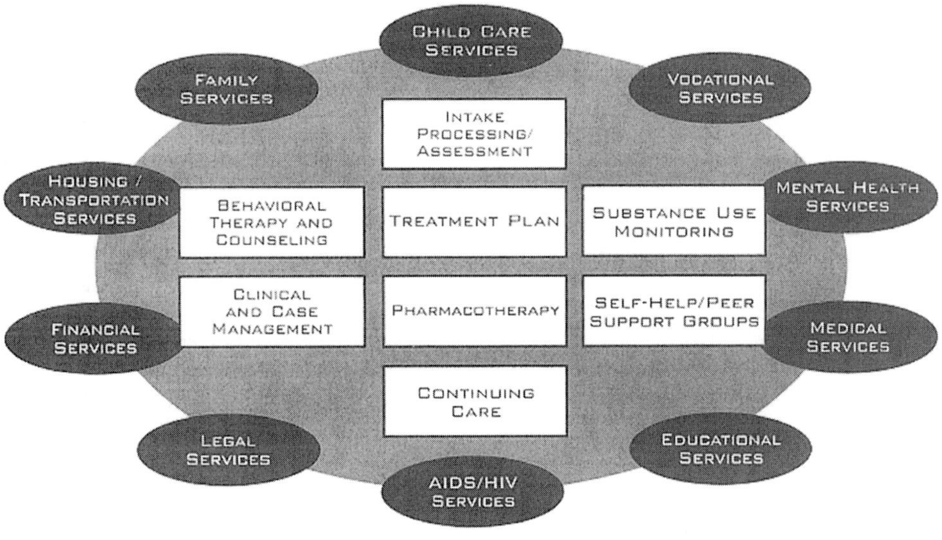

FIG. 148.1. Components of comprehensive drug abuse treatment. The best treatment programs provide a combination of therapies and other services to meet the needs of the individual patient.

- Self-help groups (i.e., Alcoholics Anonymous) involve a series of meetings in which individuals discuss the experience and problems in a forum. The meetings follow a format and are cost-free, there is no waiting list, no records of the meeting are taken, and a traditional 12-step progression to abstinence and a change in lifestyle is followed. Women-only groups should be an option.
- Inpatient drug-free treatment programs are residential rehabilitation programs that follow the philosophy of personal growth by involvement in a community of individuals who share similar difficulties. Many of these centers admit individuals under court orders who were given the choice of compulsory treatment or a return to incarceration. Women face barriers to using inpatient and residential treatment because of child care and family responsibilities.
- *Treatment needs to be readily available.* Because individuals who are addicted to drugs may be uncertain about entering treatment, taking advantage of opportunities when they are ready for treatment is crucial. The provider must have a working knowledge of the treatment resources in the community.
- *Effective treatment attends to multiple needs of the individual, not just her drug use.* To be effective, treatment must address the individual's drug use and any associated medical, psychological, social, vocational, and legal problems.
- One specific medical issue encountered in primary care practice is pain management. Although providers may have well-founded concerns about potential drug-seeking behavior, these concerns may interfere with clinical judgment about the appropriateness of using narcotic analgesics. Like other clients, substance abusers often are undertreated for acute pain. Medication for pain control, including narcotics, should never be withheld merely because a client has a history of substance abuse.
- When developing a pain treatment plan, distinctions must be made among patients who are actively using illicit opioids and receiving treatment for pain, former drug abusers who no longer use drugs, and clients in methadone maintenance. Clients actively abusing heroin or prescription opioids and those on methadone maintenance should be assumed to have some degree of drug tolerance, which necessitates higher starting doses and more frequent dosing intervals of pain medication than in the nonaddicted client. Patients who are actively abusing drugs often manifest psychological disorders that influence pain perception (depression, anxiety), requiring concomitant treatment. Chronic pain management in substance abuse disorder clients is most effective if there is close primary care follow-up and coordination of a treatment plan with substance abuse treatment professionals. Pain management specialists should be consulted as needed to examine alternative management strategies.
- *An individual's treatment and services plan must be assessed continually and modified as necessary.* This ensures that the plan meets the person's changing needs. A patient may require varying combinations of services and treatment components during the course of treatment and recovery. In addition to counseling or psychotherapy, a patient at times may require medication, other medical services, family therapy, parenting instruction, vocational rehabilitation, and social and legal services. It is critical that the treatment approach is appropriate to the individual's gender, ethnicity, and culture. There is an increasing emphasis on providing gender specific treatment or standard treatment in women only groups or settings.
- *Remaining in treatment for an adequate period of time is critical for treatment effectiveness.* The appropriate duration for an individual depends on her problems and needs. Research indicates that for most patients, the threshold of significant improvement is reached at about 3 months in treatment. After this threshold is reached, additional treatment can produce further progress toward recovery. Because people often leave treatment prematurely, programs should include strategies to engage and keep patients in treatment. Primary care physicians are often involved with patients after they have completed intensive outpatient or inpatient treatment. Continuing motivational support to assist patients in staying with treatment is important.
- *Counseling (individual and/or group) and other behavioral therapies are critical components of effective treatment for addiction.* In therapy, patients address issues of motivation, build skills to resist drug use, replace drug-using activities with construc-

tive and rewarding nondrug-using activities, and improve problem-solving abilities. Behavioral therapy also facilitates interpersonal relationships and the individual's ability to function in the family and community. Brief interventions in the primary care setting can reinforce these skills that contribute to maintaining treatment.

- *Medications are an important element of treatment for many patients, especially when combined with counseling and other behavioral therapies.* The U.S. Food and Drug Administration (FDA) has approved three pharmacotherapies for illicit opiate addiction: methadone, *l*-alpha-acetyl-methadol (LAAM), and naltrexone. Methadone and LAAM are very effective in helping individuals addicted to heroin or other opiates stabilize their lives and reduce their illicit drug use.
- Methadone is a synthetic potent opioid agonist that is cross-tolerant with heroin. Methadone is well absorbed orally and has a half-life in plasma of 16 to 48 hours. A single daily dose achieves satisfactory plasma concentrations with only a twofold variation in peak-to-trough concentrations. Like morphine and heroin, methadone acts mainly on the receptors, which are believed to be important for analgesia, euphoria, respiratory depression, tolerance, and dependence. Methadone can be used both for detoxification of the opioid addict and as maintenance treatment to substitute for heroin and other opioids that are typically injected. The rationale for use of methadone depends on the fact that it can be administered orally and has a long half-life, which prevents withdrawal symptoms from occurring (heroin has a half-life of only 3 to 4 hours).
- At high doses, usually above 60 mg/dL, methadone attenuates the effects of heroin and may decrease the frequency of heroin injection. Doses need to be individually adjusted: most patients can be managed satisfactorily with methadone doses between 60 and 100 mg/dL, but some patients require higher dosages, and a few do well on less. Methadone treatment is one of the treatment options for opiate users but it is often not available in rural areas. It reduces the risk of HIV infection because it decreases the frequency of injection as well as high-risk sex behaviors. Methadone treatment also retains a higher proportion of illicit drug users on treatment than any other modality.
- LAAM is an opiate agonist. It has a half-life of 72 to 92 hours, which is a longer half-life than methadone, but otherwise has similar properties to methadone. LAAM is given orally three times per week.
- Naltrexone is an opioid antagonist with no intrinsic agonist properties. It blocks the opiate receptors, thereby preventing the euphoric high produced by opiates. It is well absorbed orally and has a half-life of approximately 72 hours. It is given orally three times per week. Naltrexone is also an effective medication for some opiate addicts with co-occurring alcohol dependence.
- Clonidine is a centrally acting antihypertensive agent that is helpful in managing opiate withdrawal in outpatient settings. It works by suppressing the autonomically mediated signs and symptoms of withdrawal. It is not approved by the FDA for this purpose.
- Antidepressants have been used both for cocaine detoxification and maintaining abstinence. The rationale for antidepressant treatment in patients with cocaine abuse comes from the clinical observation that depression may precede or follow cocaine use. Antidepressant treatment seems to be most effective for patients with diagnosed cocaine abuse who have antecedent or consequent symptoms of severe depression.
- *Addicted or drug-abusing individuals with coexisting mental disorders should have both disorders treated in an integrated way.* Because addictive disorders and mental disorders often occur in the same individual, patients presenting for either condition should be assessed and treated for the co-occurrence of the other type of disorder. Collaborative management with mental health specialists and addiction medicine specialists will likely be the most productive primary care clinical practice.
- *Medical detoxification is only the first stage of addiction treatment and by itself does little to change long-term drug use.* Medical detoxification safely manages the acute physical symptoms of withdrawal associated with stopping drug use. Although detoxification alone is rarely sufficient to help addicts achieve long-term abstinence, for some individuals it is a strongly indicated precursor to effective drug addiction treatment.
- *Treatment does not need to be voluntary to be effective.* Strong motivation can facilitate the treatment process. Sanctions or enticements in the family, employment setting, or criminal justice system can increase significantly both treatment entry and retention rates and the success of drug treatment interventions. There are controversies regarding the criminalization of drug use behaviors in women, particularly those who have victimization histories. Many women face child custody issues as a result of their drug abuse. The risk of losing involvement with their children can be a strong motivating force for many women to seek drug treatment. However, it can also represent a fear factor that keeps women from presenting for care. This is particularly a problem among pregnant substance abusing women.
- *Possible drug use during treatment must be monitored continuously.* Lapses to drug use can be anticipated during treatment. The objective monitoring of a patient's drug and alcohol use during treatment, such as through urinalysis or other tests, can help the patient withstand urges to use drugs. Such monitoring also can provide early evidence of drug use so that the individual's treatment plan can be adjusted. Feedback to patients who test positive for illicit drug use is an important element of monitoring.
- *Treatment programs should provide assessment for HIV and acquired immunodeficiency syndrome, hepatitis B and C, tuberculosis, and other infectious diseases.* Counseling to help patients modify or change behaviors that place themselves or others at risk of infection is a part of a comprehensive approach to infectious disease prevention. This includes counseling to reduce high-risk sex behaviors and injection practices. Counseling also can help people who are already infected manage their illness and prevent further complications. Primary care physicians should provide hepatitis A and B and tetanus toxoid immunizations to appropriate candidates.
- *Recovery from drug addiction can be a long-term process and frequently requires multiple episodes of treatment.* As with other chronic illnesses, relapses to drug use can occur during or after successful treatment episodes. Addicted individuals may require prolonged treatment and multiple episodes of treatment to achieve long-term abstinence and fully restored functioning. Participation in self-help support programs during and after treatment often is helpful in maintaining abstinence.

Substance Use and Abuse during Pregnancy

Substance abuse by the pregnant woman is a major problem because of the associated perinatal complications. These include an increased incidence of stillbirths, intrauterine growth retardation, meconium-stained amniotic fluid, premature rupture of the membranes, maternal hemorrhage (placental abruption or placenta previa), and fetal distress. Prenatally drug-exposed infants have variable development consequences. Other than neonatal abstinence or withdrawal syndromes, it is difficult to pinpoint drug-specific effects. Polysubstance abuse is common so that a fetus may have had in utero exposure to alcohol, cigarette smoking, and illicit drug use.

In the combined 1999 and 2000 NHSDA samples, 3.3% of pregnant women aged 15 to 44 years reported using illicit drugs in the month before interview. This rate is significantly less than the rate among nonpregnant women aged 15 to 44 years (7.7%). However, young women merit specific attention. Among pregnant women aged 15 to 17 years, the rate of use was 12.9%, nearly equal to the rate for nonpregnant women of the same age (13.5%).

Identification of substance abuse in pregnant women is more difficult than obtaining epidemiologic data. Maternal report of the substance abuse often is inaccurate because of the fear of medical or social consequences. Affected women may have cognitive impairments while intoxicated or as long-term sequelae or they may be uncooperative and nonadherent, creating a difficult clinical care situation. The obstetric management of the pregnant patient should involve a multidisciplinary team. This team includes nurses, social workers, mental health providers, and substance abuse providers. At the initial visit, a history and physical examination should elicit information relative to substance abuse or dependence. It is often easier for the clinician to conduct screening for smoking and for the patient to respond. A positive history of smoking has been demonstrated to be a good preliminary screen for risk of substance abuse in pregnancy.

Although cocaine and heroin use are relatively low in prevalence among pregnant women, a history of such use, especially injection drug use, should prompt a complete screen for bloodborne infectious diseases. Injection drug use is a well-established risk for acquisition and transmission of HIV infection and hepatitis B and C. Women who use crack cocaine as well as other substances often have histories of exchanging sex for drugs or money with multiple partners and are also at risk of sexually transmitted infections. Screening for tuberculosis is also recommended.

Obstetric care is otherwise as indicated by the course of the pregnancy and complications that may arise. Delayed onset of prenatal care often results in limited opportunities for certain types of screening and surveillance that are gestational age specific. Ultrasound for dating and monitoring of fetal growth are generally required, as are late third trimester fetal well-being studies. Primary care clinicians should be collaborating with perinatal and addiction specialists if they are providing care during pregnancy. Understanding of the intensity of prenatal care required is necessary if the primary care clinician is responsible for preapproval or preauthorization procedures.

Drug use may be monitored by urine toxicology screening at intervals during prenatal care. The prenatal care provider must carefully consider the consequences of routine mandatory screening, realizing that in certain situations flexibility is important. Providing ongoing prenatal care is essential, even if it means that certain pregnant women do not have a urine toxicology screen at every visit. Social alienation, stigmatization, fear of losing custody of other children, and fear of prosecution prevent many women from adhering to prenatal visits. Punitive responses when toxicology confirms relapse to drug use are counterproductive.

The treatment of opiate abuse during pregnancy, detoxification, and provision of maintenance therapy can be safely undertaken. Typically, the detoxification period is the first step in treating opiate abuse and may take from 3 to 7 days. Opiate agonist therapy, including the use of methadone, is used. Detoxification should take place in a medically monitored setting with care by provided by knowledgeable clinicians. Fetal monitoring is commensurate with the gestational age. Women can be maintained on methadone for the duration of pregnancy. Increases in dose requirements due to the metabolic and physiological changes of pregnancy are not uncommon. If necessary, split dosing can be used to avoid untoward side effects and withdrawal symptomatology.

The postpartum period and continuing care in the year after pregnancy provide important opportunities for women to receive treatment for substance abuse. The completion of evaluation and treatment for medical complications of substance abuse is an essential component of a comprehensive approach to care. Interconceptional care to include education to reduce high-risk sex behaviors and the provision of contraception is a key step in ensuring treatment success. For many women breast-feeding is appropriate and should be encouraged with instructions for infant care.

Pregnancy and childbirth are times when women can be motivated to change unhealthy behaviors. Health care providers should use this motivating force with counseling and education, realizing that the potential is great for success when childbearing women are enrolled in a comprehensive multidisciplinary treatment program.

Summary

In a national survey of primary care physicians and psychiatrists, 32% of physicians indicated that they do not inquire routinely about illicit drug abuse. Psychiatrists and obstetrician-gynecologists were most likely to screen for drug abuse. Obstetrician-gynecologists were least likely to intervene. Details of whether this behavior differed with pregnant women were not studied. Only 55% of physicians reported that they routinely recommend formal addiction treatment to drug abusing patients, and a not insignificant minority (15%) did not offer any intervention. Psychiatrists were most likely to intervene but were more likely to refer patients to a 12-step program.

Primary care clinicians should be optimistic about the ultimate effectiveness of screening, diagnosis, evaluation, and treatment of substance abuse disorders and their role in providing elements of care. Substance abuse disorders are chronic illnesses not unlike many others that are encountered in clinical practice.

SMOKING AND ALCOHOL USE AND ABUSE

Concurrent use of tobacco and alcohol are frequent, and the two substances represent the only two legally produced and marketed mood-altering drugs available for self-prescription. Cigarette smokers are more likely to be alcohol users than nonsmokers, and heavy alcohol users are more likely to smoke than nondrinkers. The medical consequences of co-occurring use of tobacco and alcohol are often encountered in clinical practice, and primary care clinicians provide counseling and treatment to support change in patterns of use.

Descriptive Epidemiology

Since 1971, the NHSDA has been the primary source of information on the prevalence and incidence of illicit drug, alcohol, and tobacco use in the civilian population aged 12 years and older. The 2000 NHSDA report listed important findings regarding tobacco and alcohol use in the population as a whole and in women and girls. These findings are described.

NATIONAL OVERVIEW

In 2000, an estimated 65.5 million Americans reported current use of a tobacco product, a prevalence rate of 29.3% among persons aged 12 and older. Cigarette smoking accounted for 85% of the tobacco use.

An estimated 104 million Americans reported current use of alcohol, a prevalence rate of 46.6% among persons aged 12 years and older. Of these drinkers, one fifth (46 million people) participated in binge drinking. Binge drinking is defined as five or more drinks on the same occasion at least once in the last 30 days.

AGE

In 2000, current cigarette smoking rates increased steadily by year of age, reaching a high of 41.4% at age 20. Overall, 13.4% of youths aged 12 to 17 were current cigarette users (smoking all or part of a cigarette in the past month). The smoking rate for adults aged 26 and older remained fairly constant at 24% to 25%.

The age of peak prevalence for current alcohol use, binge drinking, and heavy alcohol use is 21. Binge and heavy alcohol use rates decrease with increasing age. While half of the population aged 45 to 49 are current drinkers, only 1 in 5 persons is a binge drinker and less than 1 in 20 is a heavy drinker.

GENDER

In 2000, males aged 12 and older were more likely than their female counterparts to report past month use of any tobacco product. Approximately 35.2% of males were current users compared with 23.9% of females. However, for youths aged 12 to 17, the rate was higher for females (14.1%) than males (12.8%). Data combined for 1999 and 2000 revealed that 18.6% of pregnant women aged 15 to 44 smoked cigarettes as compared with 29.8% of nonpregnant women in the same age range.

Males were more likely to report current alcohol use than females, except among the youth aged 12 to 17 when rates were comparable. Among pregnant women aged 15 to 44 years in 1999 and 2000 combined, 12.4% used alcohol and 3.9% reported binge drinking.

RACE AND ETHNICITY

In 2000, current cigarette smoking rates were 42.3% among American Indians and Alaska Natives, 32.3% among persons reporting more than one race, 25.9% among whites, 23.3% among blacks, 20.7% among Hispanics, and 6.5% among Asians. There are differences in smoking rates within Hispanic and Asian subpopulations. For youth aged 12 to 17, black females had lower rates of lifetime, past year, or past month use of cigarettes than their white or Hispanic counterparts.

Whites were more likely than any other racial or ethnic group to report current alcohol use (50.7%). The lowest current drinking rates were reported for Asians (28.0%). For youth aged 12 to 17, black girls were also considerably less likely to report any alcohol use, binge drinking, or heavy use when compared with white or Hispanic girls.

ASSOCIATION WITH ILLICIT DRUG USE

Cigarette smokers are more likely to use illicit drugs than nonsmokers; 15.6% of smokers reported current illicit drugs compared with 3.2% of nonsmokers. The level of alcohol use was strongly associated with illicit drug use in 2000. Among heavy drinkers aged 12 and older, 30% were current illicit drug users.

Etiology

Family and peer influences, demographics, advertising, economics, and alcohol and tobacco availability have all been identified as social determinants of the initiation of tobacco and alcohol use among adolescents. Habitual smoking and alcohol dependence are also both behaviors that are partly determined by genetic influences. Twin studies and family studies have been used to explore the genetic predisposition to dependence. Twin and adoption studies provide evidence for a genetic contribution to risk for either alcohol or nicotine dependence that is estimated to account for 40% to 60% of risk in people of European descent.

Behavioral mechanisms are also important in the initiation of smoking and drinking. Although nicotine and alcohol have different target sites in the central nervous system, they share certain acute pharmacologic effects such as relief of anxiety and stress. Therefore, self-medication, sensation seeking, and impulsivity may be involved in the initial use of both nicotine and alcohol. There may also be some synergistic effects between nicotine and alcohol that promote the development of tolerance and dependence of one or both substances. Certain behavioral phenomenon associated with alcohol or cigarette smoking also result in conditioned responses for the use of the substances. Such sensory cues may play a greater role in determining smoking behavior in women. Examples of cues are being near an area where smoking is permitted or passing in the vicinity of a liquor store. There are differences between substances that need further elucidation. In general, initial alcohol use results in mostly social drinking, with some persons developing alcohol dependence, whereas most smokers develop nicotine dependence.

Medical Consequences: Smoking

The medical consequences of cigarette smoking are devastating, affect virtually every organ system, and are completely preventable. Cigarette smoking is the largest single risk factor for premature morbidity and mortality in women living in the developed world. Less than 100 years ago tobacco use by women was limited. Public display of smoking became a declaration of independence by women and was equated with fashion and glamour. The gender gap in smoking prevalence narrowed by the mid-1980s, and women now risk losing their life expectancy advantage over men based on tobacco usage alone. Women also experience unique reproductive health and pregnancy-related consequences as a result of cigarette smoking. Table 148.1 represents a compilation of medical consequences of smoking in women. Reproductive health and pregnancy-related consequences are treated separately. In the few circumstances in which there is evidence of a reduced risk of a disease or condition, it should be emphasized that this effect does not recommend smoking. These risk reductions are caused by estrogen-deficiency effects of smoking.

Identification and Assessment of Tobacco Use in Primary Care Practice

At least 70% of current smokers say they want to and intend to quit. The most common reason for quitting cited by both men and women is for health-related reasons. Almost 70% of current smokers have at least one visit to a physician in a given year, yet only about half of all smokers receive advice from their physician to stop smoking. The single most important step in addressing tobacco use and dependence is screening for use. It is recommended that the query regarding tobacco use should be treated as an additional vital sign and should be asked at every visit. If the patient responds in the affirmative, then the readiness of the patient to make an attempt to quit smoking must be ascertained. The time line that the patient and clinician should have in mind is within the next 30 days. Women have lower smoking cessation rates, but studies have reported no major or

TABLE 148.1. Medical Consequences of Smoking in Women

Effect	Strong evidence	Suggestive evidence
Cardiovascular and pulmonary systems	Major cause of coronary heart disease with increased risk in oral contraceptive users Increased risk of ischemic stroke and subarachnoid hemorrhage 90% of mortality from chronic obstructive pulmonary disease in women Reduced rates of lung growth in adolescent girls	
Endocrine and immune systems		Increased risk for Graves ophthalmopathy Increased risk for human immunodeficiency virus infection
Musculoskeleton and skin	Decreased bone density and increased risk of hip fractures in postmenopausal current smokers Decreased wound healing Increased risk for onset of psoriasis	Increased facial wrinkling Elevated risk of rheumatoid arthritis Reduced risk of osteoarthritis of knee Increased risk of cholecystitis and cholelithiasis
Gastrointestinal tract	Former smokers at increased risk for ulcerative colitis Increased risk for Crohn disease Increased risk for peptic ulcer disease	
Neurologic and ophthalmologic disorders	Increased risk for cataracts and age-related macular degeneration Decreased risk for Parkinson disease	
Psychiatric disorders	Smokers are more likely to be depressed High smoking prevalence in schizophrenia, anxiety disorders, attention deficit disorder, and alcoholism	
Risk for neoplasia	90% of all lung cancer deaths in women Increased risk for cervical and vulvar cancers Increased risk for cancers of oropharynx, pancreas, kidney and bladder, liver and colon-rectum	Increase in cancer of larynx and esophagus
Drug interactions	Pharmacokinetic interactions Alcohol-delayed gastric emptying Increased clearance Caffeine (56%) Clozapine Olanzapine (98%) Propanolol—oral (77%) Decreased half-life Heparin Theophylline (63%) Pharmacodynamic interactions Benzodiazepines—decreased sedation Beta-blockers—less effective blood pressure and heart rate reduction Opioids—decreased analgesic effect	Decreased serum concentration Chlorpromazine (24%) Haloperidol (70%) Insulin-decreased subcutaneous absorption Possible higher dose requirement
Preventive health	Women with ≥1 pack per day cigarette use: lower rates of mammography and Pap tests	
Public health	Exposure to environmental tobacco smoke is a cause of lung cancer in nonsmoking women	

Source: Women and smoking: a report of the Surgeon General—2001; Wolf R. Use and abuse of tobacco, alcohol and drugs; Zevin S, Benowitz NL. Drug interactions with tobacco and smoking: an update; Rakowski W, Clark MA, Ehrich B. Smoking and cancer screening in women for ages 42–75: associations in the 1990–1994 National Health Interview Surveys, *Prev Med* 1999;29:487–495,with permission.

consistent differences among women's and men's motivation for wanting to stop smoking, readiness to stop smoking, or general awareness of the harmful health effects of smoking. Yet more women than men identify future health, present health, and the effect that their smoking has on others as important motivating factors for smoking cessation. Additional research suggests that women are not as well informed of the gender-specific health consequences of smoking and are less likely to recognize that there are health benefits to smoking cessation.

Smoking Cessation and Nicotine Treatment Methods

The National Cancer Institute (NCI) reports the following key findings in guidelines for clinician practice:

- Tobacco dependence is a chronic condition that often requires repeated intervention.
- Effective treatments do exist that can produce long-term and permanent abstinence from smoking.
- Patients who are willing to attempt to quit should be provided with treatment options that have been identified as effective.
- Patients who are unwilling to make a quit attempt should be provided with a brief intervention that is designed to increase their motivation to quit.

Strategies for office-based assistance to patients for smoking cessation based on NCI guidelines are summarized in Table 148.2.

Numerous first-line pharmacotherapies now exist and have been assessed for effectiveness in increasing long-term smoking abstinence. First-line therapies include five FDA-approved products: bupropion SR, nicotine gum, nicotine inhaler, nicotine nasal spray, and the nicotine patch. If pharmacotherapy is used in light smokers, consideration should be given to reduc-

TABLE 148.2. Strategies for Treating Tobacco Use and Dependence

"A"	Action	Strategy for implementation
"Ask"	Implement an office-wide system that ensures that the tobacco use status of every patient is queried and documented at each visit.	Expand the vital signs to include tobacco use or include an identification system such as a chart sticker.
"Advise"	In a clear, strong, and personalized manner, urge every tobacco user to quit.	Personalize the advice, for example, by tying tobacco use to current health or illness, social issues, impact of smoking on others.
"Assess"	Determine the willingness to quit within the next 30 days.	Encourage participation in an intensive treatment, provide a motivational intervention to persons not yet willing to quit, provide additional information to special populations such as adolescents.
"Assist"	Help patient to develop a quit plan that includes setting a quit date.	Provide problem-solving, social support, recommendations for pharmacotherapy and supplementary educational materials.
"Arrange"	Schedule follow-up contact, either in person or telephone. Evaluate how other office personnel can be involved.	Timing is important and contact should preferably occur within 1 week of the quit date, a second contact in 1 month. Reinforce success, identify any problems encountered, and anticipate challenge ahead. Assess pharmacotherapy use and consider more intensive treatment.

Source: *Treating tobacco use and dependence.* Quick Reference Guide for Clinicians, with permission.

ing the dose of the nicotine replacement products. Full prescribing information is available in the package insert, and sources that can be accessed via the Internet. Second-line pharmacotherapies for which there are clinical guidelines but no labeled indication for smoking cessation are clonidine and nortriptyline. Clonidine therapy has been evaluated and been found to have some effectiveness but has a significant side-effect profile. These second-line agents can be considered for patients unable to use primary therapies or who were unsuccessful using them.

Many patients are unwilling to make an attempt at smoking cessation or have previously attempted and failed. About one third of smokers attempt to quit each year, and approximately 10% to 15% of individuals are successful in quitting with each attempt. Therefore, multiple attempts at quitting and multiple clinical interventions are to be anticipated. The cessation process can be viewed as a cycle with short-term and long-term successes. One aspect of practice-based smoking interventions is to move a smoker along the continuum of change. This change process involves the stages of change: precontemplation or preparation, contemplation, and action. Individuals who are not yet thinking about quitting or are contemplating quitting should receive interventions designed to increase their motivation to move to the next stage of change.

The recommended practice is to provide counseling using the "5 R's" as outlined in the NCI guide for clinicians. The "5 R's"—*Relevance, Risks, Rewards, Roadblocks, and Repetition*—are designed to motivate smokers who are unwilling to immediately quit. Smokers may be unwilling to quit due to misinformation, concern about the effects of quitting, or demoralization because of previous unsuccessful quit attempts.

Relevance: Encourage the patient to indicate why quitting is personally relevant, being as specific as possible. Motivational information has the greatest impact if it is relevant to a patient's disease status or risk, family or social situation (e.g., having children in the home), health concerns, age, gender, and other important patient characteristics (e.g., prior quitting experience, personal barriers to cessation).

Risks: The clinician should ask the patient to identify potential negative consequences of tobacco use and highlight those that seem most relevant. The clinician should emphasize that smoking low-tar/low-nicotine cigarettes will not eliminate these risks. The risks include acute risks such as respiratory difficulties, long-term risks such as lung cancer, and environmental risks such as higher rates of smoking in children of smokers.

Rewards: The clinician should ask the patient to identify potential benefits of stopping tobacco use and highlight those that seem most relevant to the patient. Examples of rewards include that home, car, clothing, and breath will smell better or being a good example for children.

Roadblocks: The clinician should ask the patient to identify barriers or impediments to quitting and note elements of treatment (problem-solving, pharmacotherapy) that could address barriers. Typical barriers might include withdrawal symptoms, fear of failure, weight gain, lack of support, depression, and enjoyment of tobacco.

Repetition: The motivational intervention should be repeated every time a patient in the precontemplative or contemplative stage presents for care. Tobacco users who have failed in previous quit attempts should be told that most people make repeated quit attempts before they are successful.

Several factors are of special significance to women as they attempt to quit smoking. There is some evidence that women experience more severe withdrawal symptomatology if their quit date and first week of smoking cessation coincides with the luteal phase as compared with the follicular phase of the menstrual cycle. It seems reasonable to explore the menstrual cycle timing of smoking cessation with some women to optimize their motivation and potential success.

Weight gain after smoking cessation is reported as a concern by women more often than by men. Smoking is related to body mass index, and both male and female smokers have a lower body mass index than nonsmokers. Nicotine is believed to be the component of cigarette smoke that is responsible for the effects on weight, although the impact on food intake and metabolic rate is limited. Physical activity and other factors mediate this effect.

There may be differences among women as to how concerns about weight change are identified and reported. Different aspects of body image, fitness, clothing size, or other ways of representing body habitus change may be important. African-American women report a preferred body weight that is significantly higher than white women and are more likely to be satisfied with their body shape. Adolescents are particularly likely to equate smoking with weight concerns and to report they are smoking expressly for the purpose of maintaining their weight.

The average weight gain in the year after quitting is 6 to 11 pounds. Weight control programs as adjunctive treatment in smoking cessation have not been found to improve long-term smoking cessation or reduce relapse. In fact, there is evidence for an inverse relationship between food restriction and smoking cessation. Animal and human research have demonstrated that food restriction increases drug use. Addition of an exercise program to smoking cessation may have a positive impact, but it is not known whether there are differences between men and women. Women may overestimate postcessation weight gain, and although gain is expected, many women indicate an unwillingness to tolerate weight change. Therefore, cognitive-behavioral treatment for smoking cessation has been proposed as a useful approach to address dysfunctional attitudes about weight gain, body image, and overall health. Elements of cognitive-behavioral treatment such as problem solving can be incorporated into primary care practice or the patient can be referred for more intensive participation in an external program. Bupropion SR and nicotine replacement products, in particular nicotine gum, have been shown to delay, but not prevent, weight gain.

Another factor of special significance to women during smoking cessation is depression. Depressive mood, anxiety, nervousness, and irritability are common symptoms to appear with nicotine abstinence. Most of these symptoms appear to peak within the first 1 to 2 weeks after smoking cessation and then return to baseline. Among participants in smoking cessation programs, more women than men report a history of depression. The stimulant effects of cigarette smoking reduce negative affect in individuals with depression or propensity for depression. Most studies of antidepressant treatment in smoking cessation have not addressed gender. Bupropion and nortriptyline appear to be effective in individuals with a history of depression. Selective serotonin reuptake inhibitors are under study for their role in adjunctive therapy for smoking cessation. Fluoxetine has demonstrated some effectiveness in individuals with higher depression scores, a diagnosis of depression, or a history of alcoholism. Behavioral interventions that address mood have been also been demonstrated to be helpful, but there are no gender-specific results.

Many aspects of social relationships and roles appear to influence smoking behavior in women. The identification of support from family, friends, and newly developed relationships such as a discussion group is an important part of the quit plan. There appears to be a short-term advantage for women in achieving smoking cessation with increased social support. Consistency and permanence of support may be factors related to long-term outcomes, but this area requires further investigation.

Medical Consequences: Alcohol

Alcohol dependence is characterized by tolerance to the intoxicating effects of alcohol, uncontrolled drinking behaviors, social and medical consequences, and alcohol withdrawal. Most individuals do not meet the criteria for alcohol dependence, but many drink alcohol to levels that are associated with health consequences.

The role of primary care in the management of alcohol related health consequences includes the following:

- Primary prevention of inappropriate alcohol use
- Screening to identify women who are problem drinkers
- Secondary prevention of the complications of harmful alcohol use
- Clinical care of alcohol withdrawal and other medical consequences
- Providing various modalities of treatment for alcohol abuse and dependence or arranging for that treatment.

One standard drink is defined as 12 fluid ounces (oz.) of beer, 5 fluid oz. of wine, or 1.5 fluid oz. of distilled spirits. These amounts equate to approximately 12 to 15 g of ethanol. Ethanol is oxidized to acetaldehyde by alcohol dehydrogenase in the liver, accounting for approximately 90% of metabolism. Acetaldehyde in turn is converted to acetate by aldehyde dehydrogenase. When alcohol intake is heavy, the liver microsomal ethanol-oxidizing system is induced to augment metabolic capacity. Women have lower alcohol dehydrogenase activity and therefore have higher blood alcohol concentrations than men after consuming similar amounts of alcohol per kilogram of body weight. A general guide is that one drink per hour can be metabolized and that two to three standard drinks will result in blood alcohol concentrations in the range of the legal limits. Approximately 50% of Japanese and other Asian populations have aldehyde dehydrogenase isoenzymes with reduced enzymatic activity. Under these circumstances alcohol intake results in a characteristic flushing reaction associated with nausea, vomiting, sweating, and palpitations. As a result, alcohol use and abuse in these populations is decreased. The drug disulfiram is an inhibitor of aldehyde dehydrogenase and the production of the flushing reaction in the presence of alcohol is the basis for its use as aversive therapy. Similarly, this adverse reaction occurs with metronidazole use and alcohol and is the rationale for the drug interaction warning. Metronidazole is the primary therapy indicated for trichomoniasis and bacterial vaginosis.

The health consequences of alcohol intake can be mapped along a U-shaped curve. Light to moderate drinking (essentially one to two standard drinks per day) has been studied extensively, and there is good evidence for a cardioprotective effect. This effect is thought to be mediated via high-density lipoprotein, changes in platelet function, stimulation of clot dissolution, and cellular signaling processes. The "French Paradox" is the term used to describe the experience of Europeans who drink considerably more alcohol on a daily and lifetime basis than Americans and have greater dietary intake of saturated fats yet have lower rates of coronary artery disease. The effects of alcohol are presumed to be interacting with multiple other factors.

Table 148.3 is a summary of medical consequences of alcohol in women. Reproductive and pregnancy-related consequences are treated separately.

Identification and Assessment of Alcohol Use in Primary Care Practice

Screening by questionnaires is a better way of detecting excessive alcohol use than laboratory testing. The social stigma of alcohol abuse or alcoholism is greater for women than men, and women are less likely to be intoxicated when presenting for medical evaluation other than in the emergency room setting. Therefore, the approach to screening should be direct, routine, but nonjudgmental. In the event of denial, when signs or symptoms point to the contrary, the interview process should always close in an open-ended fashion that allows the patient the opportunity to modify her responses in the future.

If the response to an initial question about any use of alcohol is positive, then the *CAGE* screening test is recommended to ascertain problem drinking. The *CAGE* screen consists of four questions:

- "Have you ever felt that you ought to **C**ut down on your drinking?"
- "Have people **A**nnoyed you by criticizing your drinking?"'
- "Have you ever felt **G**uilty about your drinking?"

TABLE 148.3. Medical Consequences of Alcohol Abuse and Dependence in Women

System	Strong evidence	Suggestive evidence
Cardiovascular and renal	Heavy drinking: cardiomyopathy, arrhythmias, hypertension, stroke Impaired acid-base, fluid and electrolyte balance	
Endocrine and immune	Increased susceptibility to bacterial infection: pneumococcal pneumonia and *M. tuberculosis* Pseudo-Cushing syndrome Insulin resistance Hypoglycemia, hyperuricemia, and hypertriglyceridemia	Exacerbating of human immunodeficiency virus–induced and trauma-induced immunosuppression Adolescent growth hormone suppression
Musculoskeletal and skin	Osteoporosis and osteomalacia	
Gastrointestinal tract	Esophageal and gastric motility disorders, gastritis, esophagitis, malabsorption, primary and secondary nutritional disorders Acute and chronic pancreatitis Fatty liver, hepatitis and cirrhosis Accelerated hepatitis C damage	
Neurologic and ophthalmologic	Direct toxic effects: temperature dysregulation, sleep disturbances, disorders of coordination, and mood Withdrawal syndrome Encephalopathies Posttraumatic abnormalities	Hemorrhagic stroke
Hematologic	Hemachromatosis Sideroblastic, megaloblastic, and hemolytic anemia Impaired platelet production and function	
Psychiatric disorders	Substance-independent comorbid depression, anxiety disorders Substance-induced syndromes	
Risk for neoplasia	Cancer of tongue, larynx, pharynx, and esophagus	Colorectal cancer Breast cancer
Drug interactions	Potentiation of depressant effects of narcotics and sedative drugs Alterations in drugs metabolized by cytochrome P-450 systems	
Preventive health Social health	Accidental falls, motor vehicle accidents (DWI/DUI), domestic violence, sexual assault, parenting and child custody concerns, homelessness, high-risk sexual behavior	

Source: Alcohol's effect on organ function; Diamond I, Jay CA. Alcoholism and alcohol abuse, with permission.

- "Have you ever had a drink first thing in the morning to steady your nerves or get rid of a hangover (an *E*ye-opener)?"

Each positive response is assigned one point. Scores of two or more should prompt further evaluation of the patterns of alcohol use with special attention to binge drinking and complete clinical evaluation. Ascertainment of other consequences of harmful alcohol use such as adverse social (change in child custody), legal (driving while intoxicated), or occupational (excessive sick leave warning) events is essential to the evaluation process. With the consent of the patient, family members or significant others may be interviewed to be a source of information on the degree to which harmful use of alcohol is taking place. These interviews also afford the clinician an opportunity to assess barriers and facilitators of external support to the patient.

Treatment Modalities for Harmful Alcohol Use

As with smoking cessation, once a problem has been identified the next step on the part of the clinician is assessing patient readiness to change. Denial of harmful drinking behavior is representative of the precontemplative stage. Acknowledgment and consideration of change is contemplation. The patient who has decided to quit drinking but not yet begun treatment is in the determination stage. The initiation of treatment and achieving abstinence is the action stage of change. Once in recovery, the maintenance stage begins and relapse prevention interventions are important. Relapse is also a stage of change in that it is to be anticipated when recovering from a complex illness. Primary care clinicians are likely to be caring for patients who are attempting to try treatment again as well as for the first time.

Many studies support the effectiveness of brief interventions in reducing harmful drinking. All types of practice settings have been evaluated and found to be conducive to intervention by the dedicated clinician. However, brief counseling and motivational interventions require a different perspective. Many clinicians, especially physicians, are trained to provide very specific prescriptions or proscriptions. This type of counseling may make clinicians feel uncomfortable with the elements of negotiation that are involved. To date there is no single script for providing brief counseling and motivational interventions, but important elements that serve as a template to foster an immediate or ongoing relationship between provider and patient have been suggested.

The *FRAMES* concept is one such approach. *FRAMES* is a mnemonic that stands for Feedback, Responsibility, Advice, Menu of options, Empathy, and Self-efficacy:

- Feedback is provided about specific behaviors. This may be related to the chief complaint or presenting clinical situation.
- Responsibility for making change is understood to belong to the patient. The clinician is able to make a definitive statement in this regard while subsequently rendering support and assistance.
- Advice on what to do next that is related to a specific harmful drinking behavior and the need to change use.
- Menu of options are provided and is based on the severity of the problem.
- Empathy is expressed for the challenges of treatment.

- Self-efficacy is promoted by reinforcing any positive action demonstrated by the patient.

There is little research on gender-specific aspects of this approach to providing counseling. There are clinical practice approaches to women's health issues that may either enhance or diminish effective intervention for alcohol abuse and dependence. Informed decision-making and nondirective options counseling have been the standard in a variety of areas of reproductive health such as prenatal genetic diagnosis or contraceptive choice. Past experience with this type of counseling may improve the effectiveness of the clinician in providing substance use and abuse interventions. However, women with substance use problems are often highly stigmatized, particularly when pregnant or parenting, and are subjected to judgmental, alienating, and sometimes coercive treatment. These approaches are counterproductive.

Some patients have far more severe degrees of impairment than can be managed in the office setting. The need for management of withdrawal symptoms, the presence of serious comorbid psychiatric and medical conditions, other substance abuse disorders, and eating disorders may require that the primary care clinician refer the patient to an addiction medicine specialist. Other treatment settings include outpatient care with varying levels of patient contact in a dedicated alcohol treatment program, medically monitored inpatient or residential treatment, or intensive medical treatment in a hospital setting. Self-help or 12-step programs are often used alone or in conjunction with other treatment modalities, especially as part of aftercare. Clinicians with addiction training and expertise best manage acute withdrawal syndromes and detoxification. There is no consensus on the need for pharmacotherapy during mild withdrawal other than the use of thiamine/B-complex vitamins. Long-acting benzodiazepines have been recommended for use to increase patient comfort. Oxazepam may be preferred in the presence of liver damage. Beta-blocker therapy is being used in some settings. Primary care clinicians may also participate in the management of patients who are on relapse prevention medications. Disulfiram and naltrexone, an opioid antagonist, are the two FDA-approved medications for reducing the risk of alcohol use relapse. There is no reliable information on gender-specific effects.

Several factors are of special significance to women as they attempt to change harmful drinking patterns. The context and meaning of alcohol and other drug use in women's lives are important in the treatment process and treatment outcomes. Relationships, including with children, are often highly dysfunctional among women with alcohol and other substance use and abuse problems. The substance use may have proceeded the dysfunction or been part of a response to it. A history of interpersonal violence, including sexual assault, is prevalent among women with problem drinking behaviors. Group counseling for women only, education on healthy sex and sexuality, parenting skills workshops, and individual therapy are all examples of the types of interventions that may be of specific value to women. Unmet child care needs are barriers to adherence to intensive outpatient programs and to participation in residential treatment.

Alcohol dependence in women frequently presents with comorbid depression and other psychiatric disorders, such as posttraumatic stress disorders. The depression and anxiety disorders may be substance independent (primary) or substance induced (secondary). There is a developing clinical care literature on the use of selective serotonin reuptake inhibitor therapy for both types of disorders. Patients with preexisting depression should be treated with these agents as indicated. There is evidence that patients may be treated with both an selective serotonin reuptake inhibitor and naltrexone as well. This is an additional area where consultation or referral may be of value in the primary care setting.

Complementary and Alternative Medicine

There is widespread interest in the use of complementary and alternative medicine and practices for all types of health conditions. The use of various modalities has been asserted for the treatment of tobacco and nicotine dependence, but systematic research has been limited. Acupuncture is the stimulation of points considered to be channels or pathways for the body's energy or chi. There is no direct correlation with anatomic structures used in allopathic medicine. Investigations of the role of acupuncture, acupressure, and electroacupuncture in tobacco and alcohol dependence treatment have yielded mixed results on the outcomes of abstinence and relapse prevention.

Explorations in other treatments such as autogenic relaxation training facilitated by biofeedback, homeopathy, intercessory prayer, and hypnotherapy have been reported but do not withstand evidence-based review. There are no entries for substance abuse in the German Commission E Monographs, which is a therapeutic guide for herbal medicines. The herb kudzu root is used in traditional Chinese medicine to treat alcohol intoxication and abuse. Limited study of the proposed active moiety, an isoflavone, has been undertaken. A single small human clinical trial showed no difference compared with placebo for effects on sobriety.

Reproductive Health and Tobacco and Alcohol Use

Tobacco use and harmful drinking are associated with adverse impact on all aspects of reproductive health and pregnancy. There is strong evidence for increases in primary and secondary infertility and younger age of menopause among cigarette smokers. There is suggestive evidence for increased risk of dysmenorrhea, secondary amenorrhea, menstrual irregularity, and ectopic pregnancy and spontaneous abortion. Alcohol abuse is similarly associated with luteal phase changes, hyperprolactinemia, sexual dysfunction, and possibly premature ovarian failure.

Although there is a great deal of emphasis placed on illicit drug use during pregnancy, tobacco and alcohol use rates in pregnancy are two- to fourfold higher. Cigarette smoking in pregnancy is associated with an increased risk of preterm premature rupture of membranes, placental abruption, placenta previa, low-birth-weight and small for gestational age infants, and a general increased risk for perinatal mortality, fetal death, and sudden infant death syndrome. Cigarette smoke has hundreds of compounds in it, and other products of combustion are considered to be causative in these adverse effects, chiefly carbon monoxide and free radicals.

The most important effect of prenatal alcohol exposure is the fetal alcohol syndrome and its variants. The Institute of Medicine recommended criteria for fetal alcohol syndrome and alcohol-related effects to include circumstances in which characteristics of the facial anomalies and neurodevelopmental, behavioral, and cognitive abnormalities can be accounted for even if maternal alcohol exposure cannot be confirmed.

Women who smoke are less likely to breast-feed their infants, and prenatally alcohol-exposed infants may have poor suckling and impaired breast-feeding. There are controversies as to whether or not any safe level for alcohol ingestion exists during pregnancy and lactation. Clearly, there are exposed infants who do not have any adverse effects. Women who inadvertently had a glass of wine before recognizing their pregnancy should not be unduly alarmed. However, evidence does exist for the significance of binge drinking during pregnancy. Among pregnant women, binge drinking has been found to be independently associated with younger age (≤30 years) and current smoking.

Screening for tobacco use in pregnancy should follow the same practice guidelines as for nonpregnant smokers. Behavioral interventions are also similar, although the need to foster change in a short period suggests that referral to a targeted smoking cessation program may of greater benefit. Self-help educational materials should be directed toward pregnant women as opposed to the general population. In some sectors the use of nicotine replacement therapy in pregnancy remains controversial, but there appears to an emerging consensus that the risk of unmitigated cigarette smoking is greater than the use of pharmacotherapy. Generally, nicotine replacement therapy is reasonably indicated for use as an adjunct for pregnant women who are unable to quit with behavioral therapy alone. Intermittent use formulations are recommended because they deliver a lower total daily dose of nicotine. Similarly, the gum, spray, or inhaler could be used while breast-feeding, making it possible to monitor timing of nicotine replacement therapy dosing and breast-feeding.

The CAGE questionnaire for screening for harmful alcohol use has been reported to lack sufficient sensitivity for screening during pregnancy. A recommended variation on this rapid screen is *T-ACE:*

- *T*olerance: "How many drinks does it take to make you feel high?"
- "Have people *A*nnoyed you by criticizing your drinking?"
- "Have you ever felt that you should *C*ut down on your drinking?"
- "Have you ever had a drink first thing in the morning to steady your nerves or get rid of a hangover (an *E*ye-opener)?"

Brief counseling interventions and motivational interviewing remain the mainstay of clinical support for reduction in problem drinking during pregnancy. Once again, structural factors such as transportation and child care as well as the impact of interpersonal violence cannot be underestimated as to their significance in the outcome of alcohol treatment.

Many women stop smoking or using alcohol during pregnancy for the health of the infant and act in the face of strong social pressures. These factors may lessen in intensity in the postpartum period, and women are prone to relapse. If women have unresolved issues underlying their substance use or have new stressors, then relapse is even more likely. There is a void in the services to women beyond the immediate postpartum period, and it is important for primary care clinicians to provide continuity of care.

Prevention

The primary care clinician has an important role in the prevention of morbidity and mortality associated with tobacco use and harmful drinking. Primary prevention involves clear presentation of risk and health consequences to nonusers to preempt initiation of use. When use and abuse do occur, secondary prevention involves recognizing problems for women such as trauma or eating disorders that are associated with high risk for substance use. Providing interventions to treat these conditions and others can prevent initiation or escalation of substance use. Tertiary prevention involves screening, diagnosis, and treatment of the medical and psychological consequences of substance use.

BIBLIOGRAPHY

Abbot NC, Stead LF, White AR, et al. Hypnotherapy for smoking cessation (Cochrane Review). *The Cochrane Library* 2002; Issue 1.

Archie CL, Anderson MM, Gruber EL. Positive smoking history as a preliminary screening device for substance use in pregnant adolescents. *J Pediatr Adolesc Gynecol* 1997;10:13–17.

Blumenthal M, ed. *The complete German Commission E Monographs: therapeutic guide to herbal medicines.* Boston: Integrative Medicine Communications, American Botanical Council, 1998.

Bobo JK, Hosten C. Sociocultural influences on smoking and drinking. *Alcohol Tobacco* 2001;24:225–232.

Brady KI, Randall CL. Gender differences in substance use disorders. *Psych Clin North Am* 1999;22:241–252.

Centers for Disease Control and Prevention. National Center for Chronic Disease and Prevention and Health Promotion. *Women and smoking: a report of the Surgeon General, 2001.*

Chasnoff IJ, Neuman K, Thornton C, et al. Screening for substance use in pregnancy: a practical approach for the primary care physician. *Am J Obstet Gynecol* 2001;184:752–758.

Dempsey DA, Benowitz NL. Risks and benefits of nicotine to aid smoking cessation in pregnancy. *Drug Safety* 2001;24:277–322.

Ebrahim SH, Diekman ST, Floyd RL, et al. Comparison of binge drinking among pregnant and nonpregnant women, United States, 1991–1995. *Am J Obstet Gynecol* 1999;180:1–7.

Fiore MC, Bailey WC, Cohen SJ, et al. *Treating tobacco use and dependence.* Quick reference guide for clinicians. Rockville, MD: U.S. Department of Health and Human Services. Public Health Service. October 2000.

Friedman PD, McCullough D, Saitz R. Screening and intervention for illicit drug abuse: a national survey of primary care physicians and psychiatrists. *Arch Intern Med* 2001;161:248–251.

Little HJ. Behavioral mechanisms underlying the link between smoking and drinking. *Alcohol Tobacco* 2001;24:215–224.

National Institute on Drug Abuse. *Principles of drug addiction treatment: a research-based guide.* NIH Publication No. 99-4180, October, 1999.

Perkins KA, Levine M, Marcus M, et al. Tobacco withdrawal in women and menstrual cycle phase. *J Consult Clin Psychol* 2000;68:176–180.

Rigotti NA. Treatment of tobacco use and dependence. *N Engl J Med* 2002;346: 506–512.

Samet JH, Rollnick S, Barnes H. Beyond CAGE: a brief clinical approach after detection of substance abuse. *Arch Intern Med* 1996;156:2287–2293.

Sokol RJ, Martier SS, Ager JW. The T-ACE questions: practical prenatal detection of risk-drinking. *Am J Obstet Gynecol* 1989;160:863–868.

Stratton K, Howe C, Battaglia F, eds. Institute of Medicine. *Fetal alcohol syndrome: diagnosis, epidemiology, prevention, and treatment.* Washington, DC: National Academy Press, 1996.

Substance Abuse and Mental Health Services Administration. Center for Substance Abuse Treatment. *Practical approaches in the treatment of women who abuse alcohol and other drugs.* DHHS Publication No. (SMA) 94-3006. Rockville, MD: 1994.

Substance Abuse and Mental Health Services Administration. *Summary of findings from the 2000 National Household Survey on Drug Abuse.* Office of Applied Studies, NHSDA Series H-13 DHHS Publication No. (SMA) 01-3549. Rockville, MD: 2001.

Substance Abuse and Mental Health Services Administration. Center for Substance Abuse Treatment. Treatment Improvement Protocol Series (TIPS), TIP10, TIP15, TIP 20.

Svikis D, Henningfield J, Gazaway P, et al. Tobacco use for identifying pregnant women at risk of substance abuse. *J Reprod Med* 1991;42:299–302.

White AR, Rampes H, Ernst E. Acupuncture for smoking cessation (Cochrane Review). *The Cochrane Library* 2002; Issue 1.

Wolf R. Use and abuse of tobacco, alcohol, and drugs. In: Parish LC, Brenner S, Ramos-e-Silva M, eds. *Women's dermatology: from infancy to maturity.* Pearl River, NY: The Parthenon Publishing Group, 2001:491–509.

Zevin S, Benowitz NL. Drug interactions with tobacco smoking: an update. *Clin Pharmacokinet* 1999;36:425–438.

CHAPTER 149
Eating Disorders

Michelle P. Warren and Jennifer E. Dominguez

The term "eating disorders" usually refers to the conditions anorexia nervosa and bulimia nervosa, which are diagnosed clinically based on criteria set forth by the American Psychiatric Association in the *Diagnostic and Statistical Manual of Mental Disorders,* 4th edition (DSM-IV). These disorders typically begin during adolescence or young adulthood, and more than 90% of those afflicted are female. Women are much more likely than men to base their perceptions of self-worth on physical appearance. A cultural preoccupation with youth and slimness has resulted in a considerable increase in these disorders over the past several decades. Although these disorders represent extreme cases of nutritional restriction, recent studies have linked hypothalamic amenorrhea with subclinical dieting and high intensity exercise. These conditions present a serious health risk for a large number of otherwise healthy women. Despite this, obesity remains the most common nutritional disorder in the developed world. Ironically, although we have become a nation obsessed with dieting, the percentage of obese women has increased in all age groups and ethnicities.

Obesity does not appear as a clinical diagnosis in the DSM-IV because it has not been established that it is consistently associated with any psychological or behavioral syndrome. It has become apparent that some obese people engage in bingeing behaviors but without the compensatory behaviors to maintain weight within a normal range. This new binge eating disorder appears for the first time, as a set of research study criteria, in the appendix of DSM-IV.

Anorexia nervosa, bulimia nervosa, weight-loss and exercise-associated amenorrhea, obesity, and binge eating disorder all have in common an incompletely understood multifactorial etiology with resulting multiple treatments that are less than efficacious.

ANOREXIA NERVOSA

Anorexia nervosa is a disorder in which previously healthy persons lose weight to the point of emaciation while continuing to view themselves as fat. Described by Hilde Bruch as the "relentless pursuit of thinness," the starvation, at least in the initial stages, is self-imposed. The disorder occurs primarily in females (90%) with a mean onset at age 14 or, alternatively, a bimodal onset at ages 14 and 18. Onset after the third decade is rare. The initial stereotypic patient was a white, intelligent, perfectionistic, upper- or upper-middle-class adolescent, often from an intact professional family. About 1 in every 100 middle-class adolescent girls suffers from anorexia nervosa. The disease is much more prevalent among professional ballet dancers and female athletes in sports with rigid standards for thinness, such as figure skating and gymnastics. However, this view is simplistic: The disorder occurs, although less frequently, in males (especially among athletes in sports with rigid weight standards), the elderly, all ethnic backgrounds, and persons in all industrialized countries.

Etiology and Diagnosis

The exact etiology of anorexia nervosa is unknown. It is thought to be a combination of sociocultural, psychological, and organic factors. Although the illness has been traced back as far as the 13th century and described in the medical literature since the 17th century, its incidence and prevalence have increased markedly during the past several decades. Some argue that this increase is due to the current cultural ideal of an extremely thin female body, others attribute it to a glamorized presentation of anorexia nervosa in the mass media, and still others attribute it to the stress on women to succeed as wife, mother, and career professional simultaneously without adequate preparation. The woman who develops this disorder has usually felt helpless and ineffectual for a long time, with her actions always being in response to others. She fears being incompetent and a "nothing," but others have perceived her as being self-assured. She develops a rigid discipline over eating and weight loss, often after experiencing a lifestyle change, to have a feeling of power and control over one aspect of her life. The anorectic person behaves at this point in a way similar to animals and humans starved for other reasons, with a preoccupation with food, high consumption of chewing gum and caffeine-containing beverages, hoarding behavior, and sleep disturbance. One exception is that although most food-deprived persons tend to slow down activity to conserve energy and are aware of their emaciated condition, persons with anorexia nervosa have a high almost driven energy level and a distorted body image. The family interaction style of many of these patients is one of conflict avoidance.

There appears to be a genetic predisposition that makes some persons susceptible to the disorder after they begin to lose weight. There continues to be controversy over the possible genetic relation between anorexia nervosa and other eating disorders and affective disorders.

The diagnosis of anorexia nervosa is based on clinical criteria developed by the American Psychiatric Association and published in DSM-IV (Table 149.1). They include weight loss or failure to gain weight, leading to a body weight less than 85% of expected; intense fear of fatness; disturbance in body image (not just a feeling of fatness but an actual exaggeration of their own body measurements but not those of other persons); and amenorrhea of at least 3 months or failure to menstruate without hormone administration. The new diagnostic criteria divide both anorexia nervosa and bulimia nervosa into purging and nonpurging types. This has eliminated the need to give about 50% of eating disorder patients both diagnoses, simultaneously or sequentially. Women who have an eating disorder and yet do not fulfill the full criteria for anorexia nervosa or bulimia nervosa or binge eating may be diagnosed as "Eating Disorders Not Otherwise Specified" as described in the DSM-IV.

TABLE 149.1. DSM-IV Diagnostic Criterion 307.1: Anorexia Nervosa

A. Refusal to maintain body weight at or above a minimally normal weight for age and height (e.g., weight loss leading to maintenance of body weight less than 85% of that expected; or failure to make expected weight gain during period of growth, leading to body weight less than 85% of that expected).
B. Intense fear of gaining weight or becoming fat, even though underweight.
C. Disturbance in the way in which one's body weight or shape is experienced, undue influence of body weight or shape on self-evaluation, or denial of the seriousness of the current low body weight.
D. In postmenarcheal females, amenorrhea (i.e., the absence of at least three consecutive menstrual cycles). A woman is considered to have amenorrhea if her periods occur only after hormone (e.g., estrogen) administration.

Specify type

Restricting type: During the current episode of anorexia nervosa, the person has not regularly engaged in binge eating or purging behavior (i.e., self-induced vomiting or the misuse of laxatives, diuretics, or enemas).

Binge eating/purging type: During the current episode of anorexia nervosa, the person has regularly engaged in binge eating or purging behavior (i.e., self-induced vomiting or the misuse of laxative, diuretics, or enemas).

Source: American Psychiatric Association. *Diagnostic and statistical manual of mental disorders,* 4th ed. Washington, DC: American Psychiatric Association, 1994, with permission.

History

The patient with anorexia nervosa may present with a medical complaint such as fatigue, dizziness, weakness, constipation, abdominal pain, or bloating. Because of primary or secondary amenorrhea, often patients will present to a gynecologist. Alternatively, she may be brought to a physician by concerned parents, teachers, colleagues, or a spouse because of significant weight loss, while she denies any adverse symptomatology and points out her high energy level. Adult patients in therapy may be referred by a therapist and often have not been seen by a physician for years. The patient should be questioned about all the above symptoms.

It is important to get an accurate history of previous weights, both high and low, as well as the degree of weight loss over time. The physician should assess why the patient decided to go on a diet, how she feels about her current appearance, and what weight goal she wishes to attain, if any. Some patients, although not actively suicidal, would like to "shrink away to nothing." As patients have become more sophisticated, most report that they realize their weight is too low. If asked, however, how they feel about their thighs, most readily admit to feeling fat.

It is also important to take a detailed dietary history. The patient with anorexia nervosa does not, at least initially, have a loss of appetite or a decrease in craving for any nutrient. Snacks containing concentrated sweets and any foods with identifiable fats (e.g., butter, margarine, salad dressing) are eliminated first. As the disease progresses, intakes frequently reach 300 to 800 calories a day. The patient prefers to eat alone, because the eating process is usually lengthy and highly ritualized, with the food arranged in a specific pattern and eaten in a particular order. Many patients automatically count calories but overestimate the amount of calories they consume. The patient should be questioned about her knowledge of eating disorders, including which television programs or magazine articles and books she has read. This knowledge may prove useful in discussing the patient's diagnosis.

If the patient admits she has anorexia nervosa, it is important to find out when the diagnosis was made (in contrast to when the patient believes the problem began); past symptoms, especially in comparison with current complaints; and previous treatments, including psychotherapy, pharmacotherapy, and hospitalization.

Physical Examination and Clinical Findings

The most notable finding on physical examination is the degree of loss of subcutaneous fat, which may or may not be accompanied by a degree of muscle wasting. It is crucial to examine these patients without clothing. Because patients with this disorder tend to be cold, they often dress in multiple layers of clothing, which are not perceptible. It is important to measure both height and weight. In the younger teen, there may not be a history of weight loss but rather failure to gain weight when expected to or, even more serious, growth failure and delayed puberty. Other physical findings are those of any cachectic patient: lower core body temperature, acrocyanosis of extremities, low or low-normal blood pressure, and bradycardia. Indications of extreme starvation requiring emergency intervention include the development of lanugo hair, leg edema, orthostatic hypotension, and a weight loss greater than 40%.

Laboratory and Imaging Studies

Patients may be at considerable medical risk and yet have completely normal laboratory findings. The degree of weight loss, the symptomatology, and the duration of illness do not necessarily correlate with the degree of laboratory abnormalities. The changes that occur in the hypothalamic-pituitary-adrenal axis in patients with anorexia nervosa are closely related to the extent of weight loss and in most instances are consistent with those occurring in other forms of starvation. Routine tests to confirm hypothalamic amenorrhea should be performed, including follicle-stimulating hormone (FSH), luteinizing hormone (LH) estradiol, and prolactin. If a careful history reveals anovulation with signs of androgen excess, dehydroepiandrosterone sulfate and testosterone may be performed. This will eliminate syndromes of androgen excess, prolactin-secreting adenomas, and other pituitary abnormalities. Routine tests, including complete blood count, chemistries, and liver profile, are sufficient to note stability. Abnormalities related to starvation may include lowered white blood cell count with neutropenia, lowered total red blood cell count, macrocytic anemia, elevated or very low cholesterol, elevated liver function tests, reduced creatinine clearance, and an abnormal creatinine kinase level. A serum creatinine level in the high-normal range should be seen as abnormal, because with reduced muscle mass the value should be low. A computed tomography may show cortical atrophy. An electrocardiogram should be obtained. A prolonged QT interval is an ominous sign. The echocardiogram of the severely anorexic patient reveals small heart size with mitral valve prolapse. Anorexia nervosa may also result in bone mineral depletion and eventually osteopenia, osteoporosis, and stress fractures; these finding may not be reversible. Therefore, evaluation of bone density with dual-energy x-ray absorptiometry is recommended.

Treatment

There is no entirely satisfactory treatment approach for anorexia nervosa, and the disorder is associated with a mortality rate of 5% to 18%. Treatment must be individualized and multifaceted. The severity of the illness may determine whether inpatient or outpatient treatment is appropriate. The treatment team, in either setting, should include at a minimum a physician to monitor weight status and medical condition and a therapist to address the underlying psychological issues. If the physician is not dealing with nutritional education and concerns about the eating process, a nutritionist with expertise in eating disorders should be included, as well as additional therapists for group or family therapy. All members of the team must be in close communication to ensure the patient gets a consistent message. A contract signed by the patient and all her providers is recommended.

Initial treatment is directed toward reestablishing a weight compatible with survival and may necessitate an inpatient setting. Extreme caution should be taken when refeeding severely malnourished patients, because rapid refeeding can result in hypophosphatemia, cardiac arrest, and delirium. Behavior modification techniques are also often used during the early stage of treatment. Nutritional supplements may be administered by mouth, by nasogastric or nasoduodenal tube, or rarely by peripheral or central hyperalimentation. The achievement of an appropriate weight and normalized eating habits is a long-term goal. Individual psychotherapy is often augmented by group or family therapy.

Numerous pharmacologic agents, including chlorpromazine, fluoxetine, lithium, and tricyclic antidepressants, have been used in the treatment of anorexia nervosa but with variable success. Because severe cachexia results in a flat affect resembling depression, many clinicians reserve the use of antidepressants for patients who meet criteria for depression after the refeeding process. An agent used with some success is the serotonin antagonist cyproheptadine, which in high doses (32 mg/d) may result in appetite increase and mood elevation.

Appropriate treatment of the bone loss seen in anorectic patients is unclear and warrants further study. To date, the most effective means of treatment is through weight gain and resumption of normal menstrual periods. Although it was previously thought that the lack of periods and loss of estrogen secretion were responsible for the bone loss, recent studies suggest that other mechanisms may be involved. Although many anorectics are treated with oral contraceptives, no evidence suggests that this is beneficial. Furthermore, it may prevent evaluation of improvement and resumption of menstrual cycles. The same is true of hormone replacement therapy. Supplementation with calcium or vitamin D may be advisable, but more aggressive forms of therapy, such as bisphosphonates and nasal calcitonin, are not recommended for use in premenopausal women.

Considerations in Pregnancy

Many patients develop secondary amenorrhea before significant weight loss has occurred or have persistent amenorrhea after weight has been regained. This may reflect psychogenic factors operating on the hypothalamus or some deficit in carbohydrate intake. Starvation ultimately results in prepubertal patterns of LH secretion, but resumption of weight does not necessarily reverse this pattern. Patients meeting full diagnostic criteria for anorexia nervosa have primary or secondary amenorrhea and could not become pregnant under normal circumstances, but there have been anorectic women who have conceived using a fertility agent. However, there is a high miscarriage rate of 25% to 30% in this population, as well as a high frequency of low-birth-weight infants born to women who are underweight. There is no evidence that a past history of anorexia nervosa, regardless of length or severity, precludes later normal childbearing if weight has returned to normal and cycles resumed.

BULIMIA NERVOSA

Bulimia, from the Greek for "ox-hunger," refers to an eating pattern in which a large quantity of food is consumed over a brief period of time. In bulimia nervosa, patients maintain their weight despite eating binges by engaging in purging behaviors (e.g., self-induced vomiting, use of laxatives, diuretics, or diet pills) or periods of starvation or excessive exercise. Although practiced by the ancient Greeks and Romans, bulimia nervosa became a clinical diagnostic entity for the first time in 1980, with the publication of the DSM, 3rd edition. It affects primarily women (90%) and has its onset most often during mid- to late adolescence. The diagnosis reflects a spectrum of behavior that in its mildest form does not impinge on functioning in aspects of life not connected with food and may be self-limited. At the other end of the spectrum is an extremely severe disorder in which all waking hours are spent eating and purging with significant dysphoric mood, suicide attempts, stealing, and abuse of alcohol and other drugs; the prognosis for this severe form is guarded despite treatment. Because this syndrome is often secretive, it is difficult to diagnose. In a separate condition known as bulimia nervosa, the bulimic behavior accompanies severe weight loss, as anorexia nervosa.

Etiology and Differential Diagnosis

The etiology of bulimia nervosa is unknown with biologic, psychological, and societal factors all implicated, as with anorexia nervosa. It is hypothesized that patients with bulimia nervosa have a dysregulation of serotonin that results in a loss of normal serotonergic inhibition of carbohydrate intake. Another hypothesis is that bulimic patients may be responding to heightened levels of pancreatic polypeptide Y when they initiate a binge. The endogenous peptide neuropeptide Y has also been implicated, because it stimulates feeding when administered in various hypothalamic areas.

Bulimic persons seem to be at increased genetic risk for the development of affective disorders and alcoholism, because there is often a history of depression or alcoholism in first-degree relatives. Persons with bulimia usually feel a lack of self-control and manifest poor self-esteem. They are often compulsive, depressed, and anxious and feel a lack of control over their lives. Bulimics often have a history of other impulsive behavior, such as drug or alcohol abuse. Stealing, shoplifting, and sexual promiscuity may be part of the syndrome. Family interactions are often problematic; the problems vary from parental absence to enmeshment. Despite controversy in the literature, it appears that the incidence, severity, or duration of physical or sexual abuse is not greater among bulimic patients than in the female population as a whole. Such a history, however, may have a negative impact on therapy and perhaps on prognosis. The psychological literature views the binge-and-purge cycle as a mechanism for regulating tension states that may be the result of sexual urges, impulsivity, boredom, anxiety, or aggression. It has been postulated that the bingeing behavior is maintained because these persons attempt to maintain a weight lower than what is constitutionally comfortable for them by habitually fasting and feeling hungry during parts of the day. Patients usually report dissatisfaction with their body and a societal pressure to be thin. Obesity may exist in other family members. The patient may also be overweight to some degree, and the disorder begins after a period of dietary restriction.

TABLE 149.2. DSM-IV Diagnostic Criterion 307.51: Bulimia Nervosa

A. Recurrent episodes of binge eating. An episode of binge eating is characterized by both of the following:
   (1) Eating, in a discrete period of time (e.g., within any 2-h period), an amount of food that is definitely larger than most people would eat during a similar period of time and under similar circumstances.
   (2) A sense of lack of control over eating during the episode (e.g., a feeling that one cannot stop eating or control what or how much one is eating).

B. Recurrent inappropriate compensatory behavior in order to prevent weight gain, such as self-induced vomiting; misuse of laxatives, diuretics, enemas, or other medications; fasting; or excessive exercise.

C. The binge eating and inappropriate compensatory behaviors both occur, on average, at least twice a week for 3 months.

D. Self-evaluation is unduly influenced by body shape and weight.

E. The disturbance does not occur exclusively during episodes of anorexia nervosa.

Specify type

Purging type: During the current episode of bulimia nervosa, the person has regularly engaged in self-induced vomiting or the misuse of laxatives, diuretics, or enemas.

Nonpurging type: During the current episode of bulimia nervosa, the person has used other inappropriate compensatory behaviors, such as fasting or excessive exercise, but has not regularly engaged in self-induced vomiting or the misuse of laxatives, diuretics, or enemas.

Source: American Psychiatric Association. *Diagnostic and statistical manual of mental disorders,* 4th ed. Washington, DC: American Psychiatric Association, 1994, with permission.

The diagnosis of bulimia nervosa is a clinical one. The current diagnostic criteria from the DSM-IV (Table 149.2) include recurrent episodes of rapid consumption of a large amount of food in a discrete period of time (bingeing), a feeling of lack of control over eating during this bingeing period, regular engagement in behaviors to prevent weight gain due to the bingeing, and a fear of being overweight. In addition, patients must engage in an average of at least two binge eating episodes a week for at least 3 months to meet the criteria.

History

The primary care physician is in a position to make an early diagnosis of an eating disorder. This rarely happens, however, because the patient appears healthy, and it is rare that a teenager or adult voluntarily admits to bingeing or purging episodes. For this reason, it is recommended that a dietary history aimed at detecting an eating disorder be obtained from all girls, adolescents, and adult women. Psychological treatment is usually not sought for a number of years. Many adult bulimic patients seek medical attention only because it is a prerequisite for their eating disorder treatment program.

The woman with frequent episodes of bingeing followed by self-induced vomiting often complains of sore throat and hoarseness. Other complaints may include weakness, dizziness, constipation, headache, chest pain, abdominal pain, bloating, muscle cramps, and a general sense of not feeling well. Many patients have episodes of secondary amenorrhea despite appropriate weight for height. The patient should be questioned about the occurrence of any of these symptoms.

In contrast to adult patients who are self-referred, many teenagers are brought to treatment after being discovered by their parents. They view purging as a weight-control technique and have no desire to change. Unlike the solitary bingeing of the adult, teenagers may binge and vomit in groups.

Physical Examination and Clinical Findings

The physical examination is usually entirely normal. Benign painless swelling of the parotid or submandibular glands has been reported and is reversible when the binge-and-purge cycles end. There may also be characteristic superficial ulcerations, hyperpigmented calluses, or scars on the dorsum of the hands of patients who use their fingers to induce vomiting. With repeated emesis, the acid vomitus causes a loss of tooth enamel that affects the palatal side of the upper teeth, beginning with the molars and moving centrally. This ultimately results in dental caries and significant abnormalities of bite.

Other medical complications include reflux esophagitis, esophageal tears, and aspiration pneumonia. Life-threatening complications, such as ventricular fibrillation due to hypokalemia, renal failure, gastric rupture, toxic megacolon after prolonged laxative abuse, seizures, and tetany, have also been reported. The use of syrup of ipecac to induce vomiting has been associated with death in bulimic patients due to cardiotoxic effects.

Laboratory Studies

Laboratory studies are often entirely normal. Many patients are careful not to purge for a day or two before a physician visit. The physician should determine when the last purging episode occurred. The physician must explain the potential medical complications of purging behavior, reminding the patient that normal laboratory studies do not imply that her health may not be placed in danger immediately after purging. The most common electrolyte abnormality is an elevated serum bicarbonate level, indicative of a metabolic alkalosis. Other abnormalities include hypochloremia, hypokalemia, and hypomagnesemia. Occasional patients require oral potassium supplementation on a daily basis. Patients may also have an elevated serum amylase level, which in many cases is a result of an elevation of the salivary (not pancreatic) isoenzyme. Analysis of the reproductive hormones may reveal an anovulatory profile with normal estrogen secretion or hypothalamic amenorrhea with low to normal gonadotropins.

Treatment

Treatment of bulimia remains a major therapeutic challenge, because many of the associated behavioral abnormalities appear resistant to treatment. Most patients are treated in an outpatient setting. An inpatient or day hospital setting, using a therapeutic approach similar to that used for patients with anorexia nervosa, is occasionally indicated. Treatment of bulimia nervosa with psychotherapy alone is not sufficient. The symptom of bingeing and purging must be addressed directly through behavioral approaches such as aversion therapy, behavior modification, and most recently cognitive-behavioral restructuring. Several controlled outpatient psychotherapy trials have been conducted on bulimic adults with generally good short-term results. Although the details of the programs vary—some use individual therapy, others group therapy or a combination of individual and group therapy—they had several elements in common. Most treatment programs emphasize nutrition counseling; some even prescribe specific dietary intake for patients. There is also a strong emphasis on eliminating binge eating and vomiting, as well as on establishing normal eating patterns. Several programs include assertiveness training or relaxation training. Almost all programs place an emphasis on self-monitoring. Many programs emphasize specific behavioral paradigms, such as stimulus control, response delay, and problem-solving technique.

Pharmacotherapy plays an important adjunctive role in the treatment of bulimia nervosa. Evidence linking bulimia to major affective disorders has led to the hypothesis that antidepressant medications might be an effective treatment. Controlled, double-blind, placebo trials have been carried out using tricyclic antidepressants with success. A patient who initially has a good response to imipramine may later develop tachyphylaxis and respond well to a different tricyclic.

The mood disturbance of some bulimic patients has been noted to be similar to that of patients with atypical depression. This term is used to describe patients who, when depressed, retain reactivity to environmental events and experience two or more of the following: increased appetite or weight gain, oversleeping, severe fatigue, and extreme sensitivity to personal rejection. Studies suggest that patients with atypical depression respond better to monoamine oxidase inhibitors than to tricyclic antidepressants. The use of monoamine oxidase inhibitors requires strict adherence to a tyramine-free diet and thus calls for careful patient selection and close monitoring.

There has also been interest in and success with use of the specific serotonin agonists, especially fluoxetine. This medication is an antidepressant and also produces a decrease in appetite, particularly for carbohydrates, as a side effect. This drug has a safer and better-tolerated side-effect profile (no dry mouth or constipation and little if any cardiotoxicity). Narcotic antagonists, such as naltrexone, have been reported to reduce the frequency of bingeing and purging under both double-blind and open-label conditions. Such agents remain confined to the research setting. Because some bulimic women seem to have seasonal fluctuations of bingeing consistent with seasonal affective disorder, light therapy has been tried with some success.

Considerations in Pregnancy

Obstetricians should take an initial history designed to detect the presence or history of eating disorders in their pregnant patients. The pregnant bulimic patient physically appears normal but represents a high-risk pregnancy. She may be able to eat an adequately balanced diet with vitamin supplementation during the pregnancy and yet continue to binge and purge on a daily basis. Medications such as fluoxetine that may have controlled symptoms in the nonpregnant state are contraindicated. As with other chronic illnesses, the pregnancy should be planned with the patient in remission and off all medications. Normal full-term infants have been born to actively bulimic women who have received high-risk care throughout their pregnancy. Anecdotally, these women are at higher risk for postpartum depression.

WEIGHT LOSS, DIETING, AND EXERCISE

Anorexia nervosa and bulimia are extreme examples of nutritional aberrations. However, there is considerable evidence of subclinical eating disorders in weight-stable nonathletic women diagnosed with functional hypothalamic amenorrhea. Studies suggest a pattern of depressed metabolic rate and reproductive dysfunction due to an energy deficit qualitatively similar to that seen in anorexic patients. The prevalence of amenorrhea among female athletes is also thought to be related to a negative energy balance produced when energy expenditure exceeds caloric intake. The consequences of the amenorrheic condition, particularly for young women, are not confined to the reproductive system and can result in severe bone deficiencies.

Etiology, Diagnosis, and History

The physiologic basis for hypothalamic amenorrhea is disruption of the hypothalamus pulsatile secretion of gonadotropin-releasing hormone (GnRH). The pulse generator seems to be very sensitive to stress and metabolic factors and is highly sensitive to environmental insults, particularly weight loss. GnRH secretion also seems to be sensitive to decreased energy intake, particularly when expenditure of exercise exceeds dietary intake. Inhibition of GnRH results in depressed secretion of LH and FSH from the anterior pituitary and in turn little or no ovarian stimulation and estradiol production.

Patients with weight-loss–associated amenorrhea generally weigh 10% to 12% less than ideal body weight and have a history of dieting and severe restriction of dietary fat. Menstrual irregularities can range from prolongation of the follicular phase or shortening of the luteal phase to prolonged amenorrhea. Patients are generally healthy, without distorted body image. Although amenorrhea is often the presenting symptom, a history of weight loss may not be volunteered. However, seeking information about recent dieting and weight loss is an important adjunct to the history. If amenorrhea has occurred over a lengthy time, or at a young age, a history of fracture, particularly stress fractures, should be obtained.

Women with exercise-associated amenorrhea generally range from normal to underweight, with those who are 10% to 12% below their ideal weight at the greatest risk. Diagnosis of exercise-associated menstrual dysfunction is made by eliciting a history of exercise, generally of an endurance type such as long-distance running. Nevertheless, aerobics or any intense training regime may be associated with this problem. It may be helpful to ask specifics about daily activity or miles run to quantify the exercise. This condition is most common among athletes in sports in which low body weight is desirable, such as long-distance running, ballet, gymnastics, or figure skating. As above, a detailed dieting and fracture history should be elicited.

Physical Examination, Clinical Findings, and Laboratory Studies

Because these patients are generally healthy and of normal or slightly less than normal weight, physical examination should reveal little. Pulse rate and blood pressure may be low. However, other causes of amenorrhea should be ruled out, including syndromes of androgen excess, prolactin-secreting adenomas, other pituitary abnormalities, thyroid condition, pregnancy, or a chronic medical condition.

The endocrine profile for both of these conditions is similar. LH secretion is lowered, when examined in detail, and there may be a reversal to a 24-hour pubertal secretory pattern. As seen in anorexia nervosa, LH secretion may occur in spurts during sleep. Although prolactin levels are normal, the LH/FSH ratio is generally decreased. Response to GnRH is variable, but estrogen levels are generally low. Occasionally, patients may become anovulatory with a positive response to a progesterone challenge, which is a good prognostic sign. Women with exercise-associated amenorrhea also often have low metabolic rates and triiodothyronine levels.

If medical history reveals a significant history of fracture or of extended amenorrhea, especially in young women, a dual-energy x-ray absorptiometry scan to measure bone density is recommended. Although under normal circumstances weight-bearing exercise is associated with increased bone density, studies of amenorrheic athletes have shown consistently lower bone mass than their normally cycling counterparts. It is thought that this mechanical load does not compensate for poor nutrition and may in fact put these athletes at an increased risk of injury.

Treatment

For women with weight-loss associated amenorrhea, a return to normal weight or an adjustment of dietary habits should reverse the condition. This can often be accomplished through nutritional counseling. Exercise-induced amenorrhea is easily reversible and often corresponds with a decrease in exercise. However, for elite athletes this may not be possible, and nutritional intervention may be necessary.

As in the case of anorexia nervosa, clinical studies have not consistently supported the efficacy of oral contraceptives and estrogen therapy in treating hypothalamic amenorrhea. These may, in fact, mask the underlying dysfunction and do not improve bone mass. The same is true of hormone replacement therapy. Treatment for osteopenia should include normalization of weight and body composition and supplemental calcium and vitamin D. Other more aggressive forms of therapy, such as bisphosphonates and nasal calcitonin, are not recommended for use in premenopausal women.

Complications in Pregnancy

There is a high rate of spontaneous abortion (25%–35%) among underweight women, as well as a high risk of giving birth to infants who are small for their gestational age.

OBESITY

Obesity may be defined as a maladaptive increase in the amount of energy stored as fat. There is no method to determine accurately the optimal amount of body fat stores or the ideal body weight for a given person. Published weight tables, such as those of the Metropolitan Life Insurance Company, are generally used to determine ideal body weight, although they reflect the actual weight of insured adults. A better measure is a body mass index (BMI), which takes into account the relation between height and weight. The most frequently used BMI is the Quetelet index (weight in kilograms divided by height in meters squared [kg/m^2]). The most accurate office measure of body fat is the direct measurement of subcutaneous fat mass at various anatomic sites, usually the triceps and subscapular, using skinfold calipers. Other methods for measuring body fat include hydrostatic weighing, bioelectrical impedance analysis (four-electrode plethysmography used to determine total body water), total body potassium, and total body dual-photon densitometry.

Etiology

Obesity is a heterogeneous group of disorders that can result from various pathophysiologic mechanisms. The familial nature of obesity has been noted for generations. When both parents are obese, about 70% of their children will be obese. Studies comparing heights and weights of adult adoptees with those of their adoptive and biologic parents, studies of monozygotic twins reared together and apart, and studies of pairs of monozygotic twins deliberately overfed have indicated a larger role for genetics than previously thought. Although these studies indicate the importance of genetics, they do not tell us what precisely is inherited.

A person may have hypertrophic obesity due to an increase in fat cell size, hyperplastic obesity due to an increase in cell number, or a combination of both. In certain persons, new fat cells may develop during any period of weight gain throughout life. This is probably genetically determined. It is hypothesized that weight reduction does not decrease the number of fat cells and that once individual fat cells reach a normal size, weight reduction stops.

Human studies have lent support to the "set point" theory, which states that each person has a genetically determined biologic weight (the set point). The organism defends its body weight (much like a thermostat) against pressure to change, even if the weight is far above the culture's ideal. Historically, investigators believed there was a discrete hunger center in the lateral hypothalamus and a satiety center in the ventromedial hypothalamus. It is now recognized that the process of feeding is considerably more complex and that these "centers" are more like "systems" that regulate feeding behavior via an interplay of central and peripheral pathways, including other brain areas, neurotransmitters, circulating metabolites, and hormones. These include neuropeptide Y, dopamine, norepinephrine and epinephrine, and serotonin.

The high prevalence of obesity in the United States may be due, at least in part, to unlimited access to palatable foods. Sweetness (sugar content) is a weaker determinant of overeating than both fat content and variety. It is thought that some overweight persons may be more prone to eat in response to visual or olfactory cues, regardless of hunger. Fewer than 1% of obese patients have endogenous obesity as a result of endocrine or hypothalamic abnormalities or defined genetic syndromes. These few patients are usually readily identified in childhood because of growth failure.

Many epidemiologic studies, prospective, cross-sectional, and retrospective, have shown that the risk of developing certain health problems and a shortened life span is higher among overweight persons than among those who are not overweight of the same sex, race, age, and socioeconomic status. The risks increase with the degree of obesity.

There are two patterns of fat distribution. The upper segment obesity pattern (abdominal, apple, or android) is associated with a higher risk of developing physiologic complications than the lower segment pattern (femoral-gluteal, gynoid) pattern. The pattern of fat distribution can be determined visually or by measuring the circumferences of waist and hip. A waist-to-hip ratio of 0.8 or higher in females is high enough to provide that risk. The body's content of visceral fat, as determined by computed tomography or magnetic resonance imaging, may be a better predictor of risk than the waist-to-hip ratio.

Physiologic complications include hyperinsulinism, insulin resistance, acanthosis nigricans, non–insulin-dependent diabetes mellitus, cholesterol gallstones, hypertension, atherogenic lipid profile, coronary vascular disease, stroke, gout, exacerbation of arthritis, obstructive sleep apnea, menstrual abnormalities, and complications of anesthesia, surgery, and pregnancy. The types of cancer associated with obesity in women include gallbladder and biliary passages, breast, cervix, endometrium, and ovary. Complications such as acanthosis nigricans, hyperinsulinism, hypertension, atherogenic lipid profile, and obstructive sleep apnea can begin before puberty if the child is sufficiently overweight.

History

The history should include information about the age at onset of excessive weight gain, maximum weight attained, and any identifiable precipitating events or circumstances. Note should be made of the presence of chronic or earlier serious health problems, previous starvation, abdominal surgery, or prolonged bed rest, all of which have been associated with the onset of excessive weight gain. A detailed menstrual history, including any fertility problems or pregnancies, should be elicited. Most obese girls have an early menarche, often by age 10. Soon after, they may develop secondary amenorrhea or dysfunctional uterine bleeding. The clinician should also inquire about the use of pharmacologic agents known to result in obesity (e.g., steroids, antipsychotic, and antidepressant medications). Because obesity is associated with polycystic ovarian syndrome, in about 30% of cases this condition should be considered, especially if patients present with an irregular menstrual cycle or infertility. In addition to enlarged sclerocystic ovaries, serious comorbid conditions associated with polycystic ovarian syndrome include diabetes, heart disease, dyslipidemia, and hypertension. It is also associated with hirsutism, acne, alopecia, as well as acanthosis nigricans, which is linked to insulin resistance (see Chapters 36 and 37).

The family pattern of weight gain and history of obesity-related conditions such as diabetes, high blood pressure, heart disease, and cancer should be elicited. The clinician should obtain any history of similar disorders in the patient. Further information about the family's attitude toward obesity and any perceived relation between eating and various moods and life stresses is important in gaining a perspective on which therapeutic strategies have the best probabilities for success. It is important to assess why the patient is seeking medical attention at this time and her motivation to lose weight. Patterns of eating should be investigated, including the number of meals and snacks per day, the rate of eating, food preferences, the degree of hunger and satiety, and the occurrence of bingeing and nocturnal eating. The patient should be asked, in detail, about previous efforts at weight loss.

The impact of obesity on social functioning, including peer relationships, leisure activities, and school or work performance, should be assessed. In today's culture, with its emphasis on slimness, the child, adolescent, or adult who is obese may have difficulty with self-image and peer relationships. Several studies have shown that children and adolescents, when offered a choice of friends, prefer a person with a physical handicap rather than one with obesity. Other studies have found a striking similarity between the psychological traits of obese adolescent girls and those of racial minorities who have been victims of prejudice. Discrimination against the obese in education and employment has been well documented. Although most obese adults do not have a poor self-image, a pathologically poor self-image is found in persons who become or remain obese during adolescence. Such persons view themselves as disgusting and avoid their own reflection. They divide the world into fat people, who are bad, and thin people, who are good. These severe body image disturbances seem to develop during a critical period of adolescence, when negative views of peers and significant adults are incorporated into the teenager's developing self-concept. Such body image disturbances persist with remarkably little change over long periods of time, even after weight reduction.

Physical Examination and Clinical Findings

The physical examination should include careful measurement of height, weight, and circumferences of waist and hip, with calculation of the BMI and waist-to-hip ratio. Blood pressure measurements should be made with an appropriately sized cuff, using a thigh cuff if necessary. Insulin resistance may result in acanthosis nigricans (a velvety darkening of the skin due to melanocyte deposition in the dermis; it is found at the neck and often in the axillary and inguinal regions) and hyperandrogenism, which is manifested as hirsutism. The clinician should note the distribution of body fat, acne, and the color of striae if present. Special attention should be paid to the thyroid gland, the back, and weight-bearing joints. It is often difficult to detect organomegaly or masses on the abdominal examination or to palpate the ovaries on the pelvic examination.

Laboratory Studies

The insulin response to oral glucose is greatly elevated in the obese person, and fasting levels of both glucose and insulin should be obtained. A normal fasting insulin is not sufficient, however, to rule out hyperinsulinism or insulin resistance. Obese females tend to have higher levels of triglycerides, very-low-density lipoprotein, low-density lipoprotein, and total cholesterol and lower levels of high-density lipoprotein than their lean counterparts. A complete 12-hour fasting lipid profile must be obtained to calculate the ratio of total cholesterol to high-density lipoprotein. A low high-density lipoprotein level responds to weight reduction and exercise.

Obesity may cause infertility due to ovarian dysfunction in the absence of grossly abnormal menses, as may occur in luteal phase insufficiency. Obese females may also develop oligomenorrhea or secondary amenorrhea. The most common cause is polycystic ovarian syndrome. The extent to which obesity plays a causative role has not been determined. Diagnostic studies include measurement of serum LH, FSH, estrone, dehydroepiandrosterone, androstenedione, and testosterone. Imaging studies of the ovary, such as pelvic ultrasound, are needed to assess ovarian size and function.

Morbidly obese females are at risk for obstructive sleep apnea, which may develop into hypersomnia and the pickwickian syndrome. Observers may report that the patient snores loudly and sometimes seems to stop breathing. Such patients warrant polysomnography and may benefit from continuous positive airway pressure as an alternative to tonsillectomy, adenoidectomy, and uvulectomy or tracheostomy while losing weight.

Treatment

The basis for the treatment of obesity is to lower energy intake below that of energy expenditure. This might be easier and more effective if we had a classification of human obesity based on etiology and pathogenesis. However, the classification used to determine the type of obesity treatment is that of mild, moderate, and severe or morbid obesity. Mild obesity is characterized as a weight 20% to 40% over ideal body weight, as defined by standard tables of height and weight, or a BMI of 27 to 30 (25 for women); moderate obesity as a weight 41% to 100% over ideal body weight or a BMI of 30.1 to 35; and severe obesity as more than 100% above ideal body weight, with a BMI above 35.

Ninety percent of all obese persons have mild obesity and may not have any physiologic problems for which weight loss would be indicated. Some degree of weight loss may be important for women with upper segment obesity. Mild obesity should be treated with conservative methods, if at all.

Patients with moderate (9.5%) and severe obesity (0.5%) usually require treatment. The amount of weight required to reverse physiologic problems may be in the range of 5% to 10% rather than achieving ideal body weight. Patients who cycle between weight loss and gain might actually be doing themselves more harm than if they just remained obese, but this is not true for the moderately and extremely obese. If conservative treatments fail, these women may be treated with very-low-calorie diets (VLCDs), pharmacotherapy, or surgery.

CONSERVATIVE APPROACHES

Most weight-loss programs include a diet, nutrition education, behavior modification, and exercise. Diets are most likely to succeed if they are highly individualized, based on current eating patterns, degree of motivation, intellect, amount of family support, and monetary considerations. Such a diet plan should aim for a loss of 1% of body weight per week. Dozens of weight-loss books are on the market; many make untrue and sometimes dangerous claims. A physician should be consulted before instituting any new diet. The distribution of protein, fat, and carbohydrate is important to lose the maximum amount of adipose tissue with a minimum loss of nitrogen. This is provided by the American Heart Association's step I diet: 20% of calories from protein, 30% of calories from fat (less than one third from saturated, more than one third from monounsaturated, and one third from polyunsaturated), and 50% of calories from carbohydrates, preferably complex carbohydrates that are high in fiber. Vitamin and mineral supplements should be used with diets providing fewer than 1,200 calories a day.

Before the diet program begins, the woman must have a realistic expectation about the rate of weight loss. It takes an energy deficit of 3,500 to 3,600 kcal to lose 1 pound. Compliance with new dietary habits for a prolonged period to attain and maintain weight loss is a major difficulty. Weigh-in and counseling sessions on a weekly or biweekly basis are essential initially, with biweekly or monthly reassessment required for many during both weight loss and maintenance.

Behavioral programs focus on how to eat, on the assumption that eating habits must change to maintain weight loss. Women are asked to keep a food diary and the circumstances surrounding its consumption (time, place, activity, mood). This identifies specific behaviors to be targeted for change. Programs may focus on changing the ways and conditions under which foods are eaten. Studies on the effectiveness of behavioral treatment indicate that its advantage is not in the amount of weight lost but rather in the maintenance of weight once loss has occurred.

Although the role of physical activity in the development of obesity is unclear, an exercise program should be a part of every weight-reduction plan. It is important to recommend an exercise program that does not require elaborate expensive facilities, such as walking or climbing stairs. As with behavioral change strategies, exercise is more important for weight maintenance than for weight loss. Compliance with exercise programs, however, is poor: studies report a 25% to 75% dropout rate.

Treatment programs for the mildly obese, with their emphasis on lifestyle changes, are conducted primarily within self-help groups and commercial programs. Self-help groups include Overeaters Anonymous and Take Off Pounds Sensibly. The success of such groups parallels that of groups such as Alcoholics Anonymous in the treatment of alcoholism. Commercial diet programs, of which Weight Watchers International is the prototype (the oldest and the largest, claiming a yearly membership of 3 million), include diet, behavior modification, and exercise. Commercial diet programs tend not to collect or release data on attrition and success rates. A recent study of a commercial weight-reduction program in the United States, however, found an attrition rate of 50% at 6 weeks and 70% at 12 weeks. Similar high attrition rates were reported in five other programs on three continents.

VERY-LOW-CALORIE DIETS

There is no universally accepted definition of a VLCD. Most commonly, it provides 400 to 800 calories a day (protein-sparing modified fasts) but is formulated to provide all essential nutrients and to result in a positive nitrogen balance. VLCDs should not be confused with the liquid protein diets of the 1970s, which contained poor-quality protein and resulted in over 60 deaths related to cardiac atrophy. Current diets provide protein from meat, fish, or fowl (served as food) or from egg and milk sources. In the latter case, the protein is powdered, mixed with vitamins and minerals, and hydrated (by the patient) into liquid form. The amount of carbohydrate to be included, if any, is controversial.

These diets should be restricted to persons at least 30% overweight. Contraindications include a recent myocardial infarction; a cardiac conduction disorder; a history of cerebrovascular, renal, or hepatic disease; cancer; type I diabetes; and pregnancy. Attrition rates vary from 15% to 68%. Treatment by VLCD is often delivered by a multidisciplinary team that includes a physician, a behavioral psychologist, a dietitian, and perhaps an exercise specialist. No studies have been conducted, however, to compare the results of team treatment with those of treatment by a single physician.

Usually, treatment by VLCD involves four phases. During the 1- to 4-week introductory phase, the patient is placed on a traditional 1,200- to 1,500-calorie diet with increased exercise. The VLCD itself follows for 8 to 16 weeks. Then, conventional foods are gradually reintroduced during a 4- to 8-week refeeding period, a time of high anxiety for the patient. The program generally ends with a maintenance phase, during which the patient is instructed in methods of maintaining weight loss. Less than a third of patients participate in formal weight-maintenance programs.

Patients should be examined by a physician once a week during the VLCD phase and should have blood studies biweekly. Complications associated with VLCD include gallstones, elevated uric acid level, and anemia. Symptoms are usually confined to the first few days and include fatigue, dizziness, muscle cramping, headache, gastrointestinal distress, cold intolerance, dry skin, and hair loss. Most patients do not report hunger, probably because of ketosis. Although the resting metabolic rate is depressed during the dieting process, it rises to a level appropriate for the patient's new body weight.

The average weight loss on a VLCD for 12 to 16 weeks is 20 kg. The weight loss is usually less for women, especially those who are very short, because they have lower caloric needs. Patients tend to regain most of their weight within 1 to 5 years; it is unknown whether participation in a formal weight-maintenance program would improve these findings. Patients may retain some of the health benefits despite regaining much of the weight.

PHARMACOTHERAPY

Many short-term trials of 4 to 12 weeks have shown that appetite suppressant drugs produce weight losses two to four times that of placebo. These drugs include dexfenfluramine, fluoxetine, sibutramine, and phenylpropanolamine. Dexfenfluramine has been studied most extensively, including a 1-year trial known as INDEX (International Dexfenfluramine Study) that involved 822 patients from 24 centers in nine countries. Results from this randomized double-blind trial of dexfenfluramine 15 mg twice daily or placebo indicate that such a drug might aid in extended weight loss over time or would be an aid in maintenance of weight loss after VLCD. Several recent studies have reported positive findings on the efficacy of metformin, an antihyperglycemic agent, along with a low-calorie diet in treating obesity in diabetic patients.

According to licensing regulations, the pharmacologic treatment of obesity is limited to short periods, usually 12 to 16 weeks. This is based on a belief that obesity can be treated as a short-term disorder, similar to pneumonia, rather than as a chronic disease, such as diabetes. The question of longer term, even lifelong, administration of drugs for the management of obesity has been raised. This is based on the facts that obesity is a major health problem, that the management of severe physiologic and psychological disorders depends on weight loss, that only sustained weight loss results in sustained medical benefits, and that current therapy too often ends in failure. Pharmaceutical companies are expanding their efforts to develop new drugs to be used in the long-term treatment of extreme obesity.

SURGERY

Surgery is indicated for highly selected patients who are more than 100 pounds above ideal body weight and who have a serious illness responsive to weight loss for which no previous treatment has been successful. A woman selected must understand the surgery and the requirement for lifelong postoperative care. She must be emotionally stable, without any tendency toward self-destructive behavior. Perioperative mortality in severely obese patients having a primary operation to control obesity is below 1% in centers specializing in this type of surgery.

Two surgical techniques are reasonably safe and effective: gastric restriction and gastrointestinal bypass. In the former, patients decrease their food intake to avoid the intense discomfort and vomiting that occur when small additional amounts of food are eaten. The greatest flaw with the procedure is that liquids and semisolids of high caloric density can pass through the pouch in excess (e.g., potato chips, chocolate) and that overdistention can cause the pouch to distend. Gastric restriction procedures have a higher dropout rate, indicating that conscious modification of eating behavior is more difficult to achieve.

Gastrointestinal bypass surgery may result in diarrhea or the dumping syndrome and requires the patient to take vitamin and mineral supplements. These patients also report a change in eating patterns, consuming fewer fats, sweets, and milk and milk products. Studies have shown less depression, anxiety, irritability, and preoccupation with food during weight loss subsequent to the gastric bypass procedure than had occurred during previous nonsurgical attempts at weight reduction. About 50% of severely obese persons maintain a weight loss of greater than 50% of excess weight 5 years after surgery; this exceeds the success of any other treatment.

Considerations during Pregnancy

Among pregnant women, 20% are more than 120% over ideal weight for height and 5% are over 150% of ideal weight for height. Complications of pregnancy such as hypertension, diabetes mellitus, and urinary tract infection, but not anemia, are increased in the obese woman, and the greater the obesity, the higher the risk. The risk of developing gestational diabetes in the severely obese woman is four or more times greater than in the nonobese woman, and the risk of developing all forms of diabetes in pregnancy is more than six times greater. Obese pregnant patients are more likely to have subnormal weight gain, a primary cesarean section, macrosomic infants, and higher morbidity with premature infants. Maternal obesity had no major effect on neonatal death rates. However, obese mothers with antenatal complications had a neonatal mortality rate three times that of nonobese mothers with antenatal complications. The offspring of obese mothers are more likely to be obese; this has been related to decreased total energy expenditure, not to increased food consumption.

BINGE EATING DISORDER

Estimates of the prevalence of "moderate" binge eating range from 23% to 87%. Some of these obese bingers may be carbohydrate cravers who display a high demand for carbohydrate because of its ultimate action on brain neurotransmitter metabolism. Such persons are described as having more rigid and extreme dieting attitudes and substantial psychological distress. Several studies conducted before the development of the new DSM-IV research criteria indicated that obese bingers had less psychopathology and dietary restraint than did patients with bulimia nervosa. Obese binge eaters, as compared with obese nonbingers, had greater lifetime rates of affective disorder and more often had histrionic, borderline, or avoidant personality disorders. This is an active research area.

BIBLIOGRAPHY

Al-Othman FN, Warren MP. Exercise, the menstrual cycle, and reproduction. *Infertil Reprod Med Clin North Am* 1998;9:667.

American Psychiatric Association. *Diagnostic and statistical manual of mental disorders,* 4th ed. Washington, DC: American Psychiatric Association, 1994:539.

Bachrach LK, Guido D, Katzman D, et al. Decreased bone density in adolescent girls with anorexia nervosa. *Pediatrics* 1990;86:440.

Bjorntorp P, Brodoff BN, eds. *Obesity*. New York: JB Lippincott, 1992.

Brownell KD, Foreyt JP, eds. *Handbook of eating disorders: physiology, psychology, and treatment of obesity, anorexia, and bulimia*. New York: Basic Books, 1986.

Brownell KD, Rodin J. Medical, metabolic, and psychological effects of weight cycling. *Arch Intern Med* 1994;154:1325.

Garbaciak JA, Richter M, Miller S. Maternal weight and pregnancy complications. *Am J Obstet Gynecol* 1985;152:238.

Garrow JS. Drugs for the treatment of obesity: what do we need? *Pharmac Med* 1990;4:213.

Guy-Grand B, Apfelbaum M, Crepaldi G, et al. International trial of long-term dexfenfluramine in obesity. *Lancet* 1989;2:1142.

Hatsukami DK, Mitchell JE, Eckert ED. Eating disorders: a variant of mood disorders? *Psychiatr Clin North Am* 1984;7:349.

Hudson JL, Pope HG, Jonas JM. Treatment of bulimia with antidepressants: theoretical considerations and clinical findings. In: Stunkard AJ, Stellar E, eds. *Eating and its disorders*. Research Publications: Association for Research in Nervous and Mental Disease. Vol. 62. New York: Raven Press, 1984:259.

Marcus MD, Wing RR, Ewing L, et al. Psychiatric disorders among obese binge eaters. *Int J Eating Disord* 1990;9:69.

Mehler PS. Diagnosis and care of patients with anorexia nervosa in primary care settings. *Ann Intern Med* 2001;134:1048.

Newman MM, Halmi KA. The endocrinology of anorexia nervosa and bulimia nervosa. *Endocrinol Metab Clin North Am* 1988;17:195.

Schneider LH, Cooper SJ, Halmi KA, eds. The psychobiology of human eating disorders: preclinical and clinical perspectives. *Ann N Y Acad Sci* 1989;575.

VanItallie TB, Lew EA. Overweight and underweight. In: Lew EA, GaJewski J, eds. *Medical risks: trends in mortality by age and time elapsed*. New York: Praeger, 1990.

Warren MP. Anorexia, bulimia, and exercise-induced amenorrhea: medical approach. In: Bardin CW, ed. *Current therapy in endocrinology and metabolism*. Philadelphia: BC Becker, 1991.

Warren MP, Fried JL. Hypothalamic amenorrhea: the effects of environmental stresses on the reproductive system—a central effect of the central nervous system. *Endocrinol Metab Clin North Am* 2001;30:611.

Warren MP, Locke RJ. Anorexia nervosa and bulimia. In: Sciarra JJ, ed. *Gynecology and obstetrics*. Philadelphia: Lippincott Williams & Wilkins, 2000.

CHAPTER 150
Intimate Partner Violence

Elizabeth deLahunta Edwardsen

Intrafamily violence is becoming acknowledged as a significant widespread health problem. Family violence can be divided into child abuse, elder abuse, sexual abuse or rape, and spouse or intimate partner violence. Although lagging behind child abuse, intimate partner violence is gaining recognition by the medical community. Multiple medical societies are giving a medical perspective to health-related issues resulting from abusive relationships.

Intimate partner violence occurs between two persons involved in an intimate relationship (dating, cohabitating, or marriage), either heterosexual or homosexual. The violence may be actual or threatened. There is a repetitive pattern of coercive behavior in which one partner's basic rights are unacknowledged. This behavior may include physical, sexual, verbal, or emotional abuse.

HISTORICAL PERSPECTIVE

Children and wives have been regarded as property in many cultures since the beginning of recorded time (Table 150.1). Beatings were condoned as corrective discipline; this abuse was

TABLE 150.1. Cultural Sayings

China: A bride received into the home is like a horse that you have just bought: You break her in by constantly mounting her and continually beating her.
Great Britain: A woman, an ass, and a walnut tree, bring the more fruit, the more beaten they be.
Italy: As both a good horse and a bad horse heed the spur, so both a good woman and a bad woman need the stick.
Nigeria: A woman is like a horse: He who can drive her is her master.
Poland: He who loves much beats hard.
Russia: A wife is not a pot; she will not break so easily.
United States (Benjamin Franklin): Love well, whip well.

TABLE 150.2. Timeline: Sanctions of Abuse

2000 BC	Babylon, Laws of Hammurabi sanction wife abuse
1000 BC	Egyptian evidence, fracture incidence of female mummies greater than male mummies
15th century	Rules of Marriage
1768	British common law, "Rule of Thumb"
1871	Rule of thumb denounced by Massachusetts Supreme Court
1874	Qualifier in North Carolina Supreme Court, "permanent injury..."
1920	Laws sanctioning spouse abuse are repealed in United States
1960s	First modern reports of wife abuse
1970	Kitty Genovese incident
1971	First shelter for abused women, London

perceived as a necessary form of physical chastisement to maintain family order, as deemed appropriate by the man of the house. The Laws of Hammurabi, written in Babylon in 2000 BC, include the first recorded sanctioning of wife abuse (Table 150.2). Egyptian evidence from paleopathologists revealed that female mummies had more fractures than male mummies, despite the fact that men were the warriors of that society. These fractures of female mummies, primarily skull fractures, are presumed to have been inflicted during domestic disputes. A medieval scholar in the 15th century stated that it was better to damage the body and save the soul than vice versa, thereby condoning intimate partner violence. British common law placed some limitation on spouse abuse with the "rule of thumb," which allowed a man to beat his wife with a rod no bigger than his thumb. As recently as 1970 in Queens, New York, a woman named Kitty Genovese was murdered by her partner in full view of several neighbors; they failed to intervene on her behalf because they saw the incident as a private matter, not a crime. Until recently, the legal system enforced a "stitch rule" that recognized a complaint as valid only if a woman suffered serious or permanent injury and only if the abuse was witnessed.

MAGNITUDE OF THE PROBLEM

In the United States, approximately 12 million women have been physically abused at least once by a male partner. Battering has been declared the most common source of injury to women, more common than auto accidents, muggings, and rapes by a stranger combined. Approximately one fourth of all female homicides are committed by a present or former intimate partner. The vast majority of violence against women, including wife battering and sexual assault, is perpetrated by people known to the victim. Intimate partner violence costs billions of dollars each year. Medical costs include hospitalizations and emergency department and office visits; many of these encounters do not address the underlying abuse, perpetuating the violence. Other costs include absenteeism from work, police responses to incidents, legal interventions, social work involvement, damaged property, and relocation expenses.

ELEMENTS OF INTIMATE PARTNER VIOLENCE

The theme of all violent acts is the desire to obtain or retain power and control over another person. Many methods are used by the perpetrator, often without the awareness of anyone but the partner (Fig. 150.1). Psychological torture is often the most injurious over time. Isolation is effective because it alters the victim's perception of reality. With total control over what a woman can do, whom she sees and talks to, and where she goes, the victim soon begins to believe the reality that her partner projects.

Emotional abuse lowers a woman's self-esteem. By putting her down or making her feel bad about herself, calling her names, making her believe she is crazy or playing mind games, a man can erode a woman's sense of worth. She is taught repeatedly by her partner that she is incompetent, immoral, unattractive, and unintelligent. She begins to believe that no one else could love her and that she needs her partner to navigate her life.

Economic abuse includes making her ask for money, giving her an allowance, taking her money, making her accountable for every penny spent, not permitting her to have a bank account or credit cards, not permitting her to be employed, and forcing her to sign joint tax returns without reviewing them.

Sexual abuse may involve making her perform sexual acts against her will, physically attacking the sexual parts of her body, treating her like a sex object, not permitting infection-control measures or birth control, and either not permitting her or forcing her to have an abortion.

Children are also used as an avenue to maintain power. A man may make a woman feel guilty about the children, use the children to give messages, or use visitation as a way to harass her. He may also abuse the children.

Threats psychologically immobilize many women. Often a man makes or carries out threats to hurt a woman, her family, or her possessions: Threats to take the children or harm them, to murder or harm the partner, to commit suicide, or to report her to welfare or immigration services are common.

Traditional thinking about male privilege within the home routinely exists. The woman may be treated like a servant, removed from any major decisions, and expected to act as if her partner is the "master of the castle." In the setting of loss of all other means of control and the resulting low self-esteem and fear, intimidation has a large foothold. Looks, actions, gestures, a loud voice, smashing things, and destroying her property readily convey to a woman that she must act as demanded by her partner or deal with the consequences. The threat of physical violence is always present and can lead to severe injury or death.

SOCIOPSYCHOLOGICAL INDICATORS

The prototype of an abusive relationship includes previous exposure of both partners to violence in their childhood homes, forced social isolation of the female partner, greater perceived stress (e.g., financial concerns, pregnancy), and substance abuse. Traditional views of marriage, family unity, and a commitment for life are common. Religious leaders and family members often support preservation of the relationship despite the violence. Societal portrayal of a woman as a nurturer and caretaker with ultimate responsibility for the well-being of the family, even to the sacrifice of herself, is upheld. Marriage is recognized by the couple and their friends and family as the preferred social status for all women. In the event of separation, children are perceived as disadvantaged without both parents, despite previous disharmony within the home and long-term ill effects of exposure to violence.

Characteristics of Battered Women

Battered women cross all racial, religious, socioeconomic, age, and educational boundaries. A battered woman, as a child, was

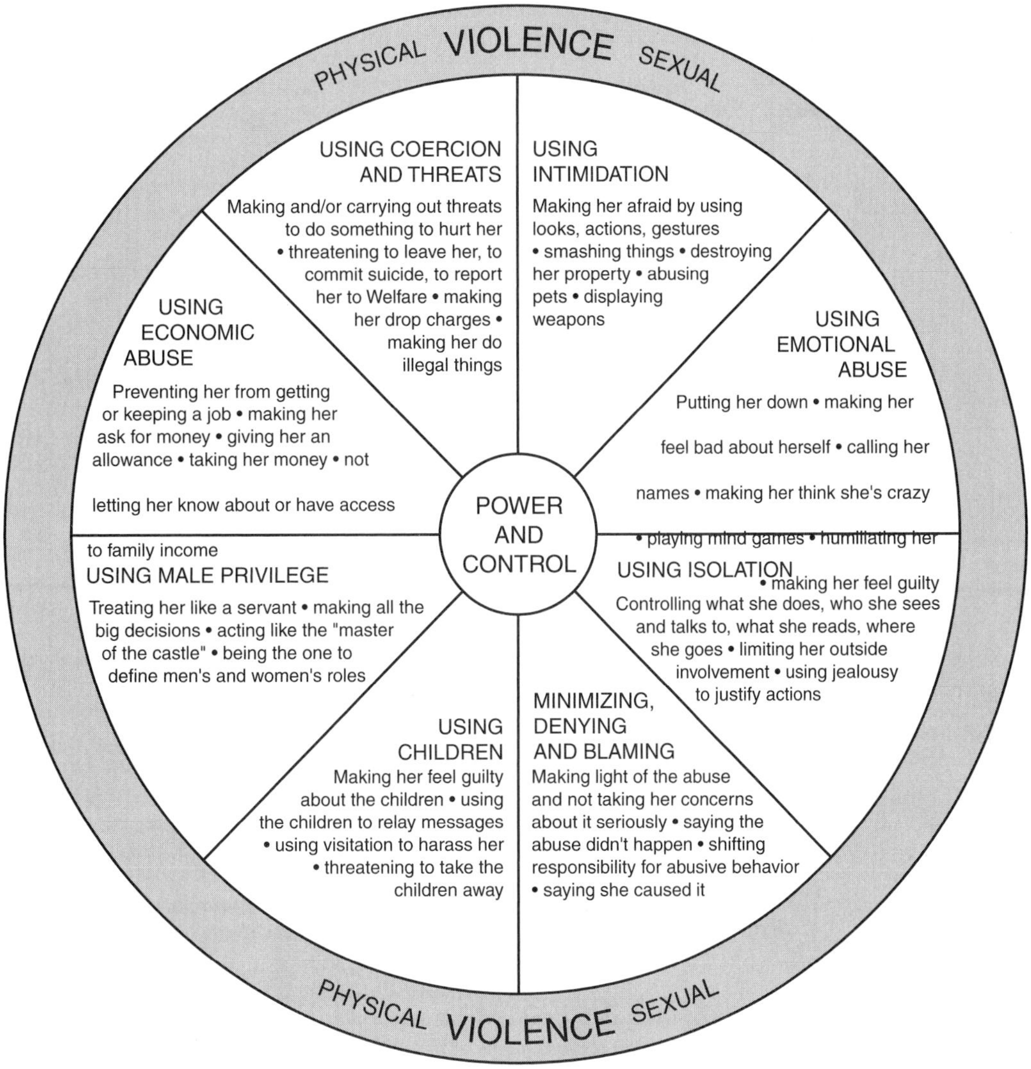

FIG. 150.1. Power and control wheel delineates the forms of abuse that may be encountered in an abusive relationship. The central issue is the need for one partner to attain or maintain power and control in the relationship. The rim of the wheel portrays the presence of physical violence or the threat of physical violence as an ever-present element in an abusive relationship. Physicians may use this wheel to help their patients identify abusive aspects of personal relationships.

frequently portrayed as "Daddy's little girl." The woman often has limited life experience and few job skills, lacks self-esteem, and subscribes to the feminine sex role stereotype. Sex is a means to establish intimacy. She is financially dependent and fearful of rejection by her friends and family. She accepts personal responsibility for the batterer's actions, believing that her inadequacies create conflict. She believes that no one can help her resolve her predicament except herself. She suffers from guilt and may deny the terror and anger she feels. She appears passive to the world but has learned to manipulate her environment so she does not get killed. Severe stress reactions with psychophysiologic complaints develop over time. Unfortunate myths imply that battered women must be masochistic, asking for or provoking repeated batterings, or they would seek outside help and leave the relationship.

Characteristics of Batterers

Like battered women, batterers come from all racial, religious, socioeconomic, and educational backgrounds. They often have been victims of child abuse. Most are violent only with their partners and may be perceived as congenial in all other aspects of life ("Dr. Jekyll and Mr. Hyde"). The batterer does not necessarily suffer from mental illness. He seeks ultimate control over all components of his family life. The abuser is often an underachiever for his level of education, lacks self-confidence, and has difficulty with intimacy. He uses sex as an act of aggression. He believes in male supremacy and the stereotypic masculine role in the family. He is pathologically jealous without justification and may interrogate his partner until she admits imagined infidelity. He does not accept responsibility for his actions and blames his partner for contrived faults that incite his "justified" response. The batterer poorly controls his aggression. He has severe stress reactions, during which he may use alcohol and other substances along with partner beating to cope. He does not believe he should suffer negative consequences for his actions and minimizes the extent of the violence. He continues to batter because he has learned that violence, or the threat of violence, maintains his power. Until recently, society has made little effort to end the cycle of violence and has condoned it with silence.

A typical abusive episode occurs in the home, often in the kitchen, during periods of greatest interpersonal interaction.

Dinnertime, evenings, weekends, and holidays are common. Persons outside the family rarely witness these episodes.

BARRIERS TO IDENTIFICATION

There are significant barriers to the identification of intimate partner violence. Physicians may distance themselves from the problem to make themselves and their families appear less vulnerable. Some physicians still perceive intimate partner violence as a private matter in which medical personnel should not meddle. Sadly, some physicians advocate corporal punishment and cannot see intimate partner violence as a crime. Frustration may be high with a seemingly unchangeable problem and may create a false impression that medical efforts are too time consuming and ultimately futile. There may be fear of entanglement in legal processes. Psychosocial problems appear complicated, and some physicians may feel powerless outside their area of expertise. Identifying intimate partner violence can be like opening Pandora's box: numerous often unforeseen issues arise. To improve the identification of intimate partner violence, physicians must become knowledgeable about historical, physical, and circumstantial clues that lead to the recognition of a potentially abusive relationship.

PATIENT ASSESSMENT

The role of health care providers who evaluate women is primarily one of identification and acknowledgment of potential abuse. A high level of suspicion is essential. Women should be questioned directly about the potential for intimate partner violence in their lives as part of any routine or emergency visit. A history must be conducted in a safe environment with a supportive attitude from all health care providers. Confidentiality is paramount.

Table 150.3 lists several misconceptions about intimate partner violence. One is that an injury is accidental unless proven otherwise. On the contrary, intimate partner violence must be addressed and excluded to avoid possibly grave consequences if not identified. Other misconceptions include the belief that injuries from abuse are always life-threatening; that alcohol, drugs, depression, or psychological problems cause intimate partner violence rather than result from intimate partner violence; and that victims are reluctant to accept help. Unfortunately, lack of acknowledgment of a battered woman's experience can lead to further battering and pathology. If not validated, the victim feels greater isolation and is less likely to pursue efforts to leave the batterer. Psychopathology, including chronic anxiety, and phobias may evolve. Substance abuse, low self-esteem, a sense of hopelessness, and posttraumatic stress disorder often emerge as a consequence (not a precipitant) of intimate partner violence. Also, the cycle of intimate partner violence is usually perpetuated and escalates if not interrupted. Therefore, medical providers should *universally screen* all women about the existence of intimate partner violence in their relationships.

In a medical setting, clues to intimate partner violence can be found in a structured interview. Interviewing should start with general questions that become more direct as needed to allow the patient to reveal her circumstances in a comfortable fashion (Table 150.4). When directly asked, many female trauma patients, across all socioeconomic classes, report intimate partner violence as the cause of their injuries. The interview must be conducted in a safe, confidential, caring, and nonjudgmental fashion. Victims of intimate partner violence expect health care providers to initiate discussions surrounding the abuse. A woman's partner and family should not be present when screening for abuse. Creative ideas may need to be used to separate a possessive partner or overly protective family member. Discussions may be held privately during excursions to provide a urine specimen or obtain a radiograph.

Signs and symptoms of the battering syndrome are as varied as the victims themselves. Indicators can be learned to improve the identification of abuse (Table 150.5). A woman who is fearful, nervous, jumpy, hesitant, embarrassed, or self-destructive should raise the index of suspicion for intimate partner violence. An overly attentive partner who wishes to be present for the entire encounter is a red flag. He may answer all questions for the patient (including personal data such as the timing of her last menses). A delay in presentation, inconsistency between the injury pattern and the explanation provided, and injuries indicative of trauma are clues to abusive relationships, similar to child abuse and elder abuse. Multiple current medications often include sedatives. Repeated presentations to the health care system, sometimes only discovered by a review of substantive medical records, often include recurrent injuries, depression, anxiety, psychosomatic complaints, chronic pain syndromes, and substance abuse.

Constant fear and low self-esteem lead to anxiety and depression. Many women become overwhelmed by helpless-

TABLE 150.3. Misconceptions Regarding Intimate Partner Violence

Injuries are accidental unless proven otherwise.
Abusive injuries are typically life threatening.
Alcoholism, drug abuse, depression, and other psychosocial problems are the cause of battering.
Abuse victims are reluctant to accept help.
Abuse is a problem of poor, minority, and unemployable people.
Abuse is a family problem that can be prevented when women learn to cope or parent more effectively.

TABLE 150.4. Interviewing Questions and Statements

1. Abuse and violence are epidemics in our society; therefore, we are asking all women about the possibility for abuse in their lives in addition to other health problems.
2. Please be assured that whatever you say will be kept confidential; if you are or have been abused, we would like to give you a chance to talk about it. I will not push you to do anything you do not want to do.
3. Are you (have you ever been) in a relationship with someone who has ever physically hurt or threatened you?
4. We all fight/disagree sometimes with the people we live with. When you disagree at home, are you ever afraid of what your partner might do to you, your children, or your possessions?
5. Has your partner threatened to kill you?
6. Does your partner ever try to control what you do, where you go, your money, or relationships with your family and friends?
7. Does your partner ever force you to engage in unwanted sex or sex that makes you feel uncomfortable?
8. Your injuries concern me. Injuries such as these are often caused by abuse. Could this be happening to you?
9. If you ever are abused, please come back.
10. We see many women who have been abused. Remember, help is available.

TABLE 150.5. High-Risk History for Intimate Partner Violence

Incident
- Mechanism described by patient does not fit injury
- Delay in seeking care

Past medical history
- "Accident-prone" patient
- Frequent health care visits (review past medical history)
- Drug/alcoholism (partner or patient)

Family circumstances
- History of children being abused
- High stress in family (e.g., financial concerns, pregnancy)
- Marital problems

Patient affect
- Patient evasive/guarded, embarrassed, depressed
- Patient denies abuse too strongly
- Patient minimizes injury or demonstrates inappropriate responses (cries, laughs)

Interaction with partner
- Patient has hypervigilant behavior with partner
- Patient defers to partner
- Partner hovers

TABLE 150.6. Typical Findings of Abuse

Central injuries
- Black eyes
- Front teeth injuries
- Midface injury
- Neck injury
- Breast/abdomen (particularly during pregnancy)
- Miscarriage/vague gynecologic complaints (e.g., pelvic pain)

Hidden injuries
- Injuries to hidden sites (covered by clothes)
- Internal injuries

Defensive injuries
- Midarm injuries

Inconsistent injuries
- Injuries to areas not prone to injury by falls
- Symmetric injuries
- Old as well as new injuries
- Injuries to multiple sites

Abusive mechanism of injury
- Weapon injuries or marks
- Strangulation marks
- Bites/burns (scald, cigarette)

ness and hopelessness and become psychologically immobilized. Repressed rage may evolve into suicidal and homicidal ideation. Hypervigilance and startle responses may develop with stimuli as common as closing a door or someone entering the room. Sleep disturbances, nightmares, eating disturbances, fatigue on awakening, thought disorganization, and mood swings can be presentations of depression and posttraumatic stress disorder. Psychosomatic presentations include phobias, choking sensations, heart palpitations, numbness or tingling of the extremities, dizziness, and nervousness. Complaints of asthma exacerbations and allergies increase. Chronic pain syndromes most often involve headaches, gastrointestinal symptoms, and chest, pelvic, or back pain. A battered woman may complain of abuse directly; however, abusive episodes are sometimes disguised as falls or assaults by a stranger.

PHYSICAL EXAMINATION AND CLINICAL FINDINGS

The physical examination should be conducted with the patient privately. A high suspicion for abuse must exist in the mind of the examiner to avoid missing characteristic signs of abuse (Table 150.6). The pattern of injury may point to intimate partner violence. The victim may have injuries consistent with using a defensive posture, such as arms raised above the head. Central injuries to the face, head, neck, breasts, abdomen, and genitals are prevalent in intimate partner violence; accidental injuries, in contrast, normally affect the extremities. Victims of intimate partner violence are 13 times more likely to sustain injuries to the chest, breast, or abdomen compared with victims of accidents.

Most violence-related injuries are minor, although life-threatening injuries may result after escalating violence. The mechanisms of injury include punching, kicking, slapping, biting, choking, rape or sexual assault, smothering, attempted drowning, scalding, and using weapons. Some women report threatening actions and injuries by their partners driving motor vehicles. A pattern of multiple injuries (e.g., contusions, lacerations, black eyes, concussions, joint dislocations, fractures, miscarriages) in varying stages of healing is highly suspicious.

LABORATORY AND IMAGING STUDIES

On initial presentation, further assessment of physical injuries should be pursued as with any similar injury from nonabusive circumstances. However, if abuse is identified, evaluation of psychosomatic complaints may be shortened in lieu of psychiatric evaluation and other interventions, as appropriate.

TREATMENT

Treatment must include both physical and emotional care. Referral to subspecialists may be indicated, based on the extent of physical injuries or the degree of psychopathology. However, all primary care physicians or physicians who see women with initial presentations need a basic level of knowledge and understanding of intimate partner violence to coordinate care, to advise of potential future treatment courses, and to counsel. Unfortunately, the current pattern of medical response often contributes to the battering syndrome. Nonetheless, battered women are most amenable to interventions in the medical setting, especially if they have presented with problems related to abuse. The mnemonic "SCRAPED" can assist health care providers to remember key elements of intimate partner violence for identification and treatment (Table 150.7).

TABLE 150.7. Mnemonic to Identify and Treat Intimate Partner Violence

Identification	Treatment
S Screen	**S** Safety
C Central injuries	**C** Crime
R Repetitive injuries	**R** Referral
A Abuse (physical + psychological)	**A** Acknowledge abuse
P Possessive partner	**P** Protocols
E Explanation inconsistent	**E** Evidence collection
D Direct questions	**D** Documentation

A team approach is ideal in addressing and intervening in the problem of intimate partner violence. Prehospital personnel, physicians, nurses, social workers, mental health personnel, clergy, advocacy groups, law enforcement groups, and the legal profession can all contribute. However, uninformed health care providers or advocates may increase the danger to patients. *Safety planning* is one of the most important interventions. Patients need to have a safe disposition and information about potential future risks to their life and health. It is helpful if some essential items (clothes, money, keys, legal documents, a few sentimental possessions, and children's needs) can be stored in a safe easily accessible location. Patients need to have a plan for where they might go if the violence escalates.

Mandatory reporting of intimate partner violence exists in many states. However, as an autonomous and competent adult, a woman can decide if she wishes to file a report with the police or seek legal action. A physician may educate and encourage a particular action but should respect and support the patient's decision. Reporting should be done only with the knowledge of the battered woman and in accordance with state law. Discussion of restraining orders and how to obtain them would be helpful. The woman is generally acutely aware of her situation and what action will maintain her safety and future options. Patient confidentiality must be observed in all instances.

When intimate partner violence is suspected, the victim's emotional status must be assessed. A battered woman may experience many sequelae of chronic victimization (e.g., substance abuse, hopelessness, posttraumatic stress disorder). She may sense imminent doom and have constant apprehension. The clinician should determine what efforts she has made to cope with the violence and whether she can function at home or work.

The clinician must also assess the future risk to the victim and any children in the home. Without proper identification and intervention, the natural course for intimate partner violence is chronic battering with escalation over time. At the time of presentation, a woman may be at the greatest risk for serious physical impairment or even death, especially if separation from the partner is pursued. Safety issues must be addressed: 30% of women who were murdered in 1990 were killed by their husbands or boyfriends. Children in the home may also be at risk. Assessing the safety of a woman's environment and her need for alternate lodging is critical to prevent further injuries. Emergency shelters are available across the nation. Factors associated with potential lethality are listed in Table 150.8.

The need for legal assistance, referrals, and follow-up must be determined. Legal assistance and appropriate follow-up should be arranged. The victim may wish to pursue criminal or civil court procedures. A contact person should be identified and a phone number provided. Shelters and other resources should be explained, even if these services are not used.

The physician must avoid blaming the victim and focusing on the woman and her presumed psychopathology. The physician must also avoid the frustration of expecting a single encounter to reverse years of victimization and learned helplessness. Simply recognizing and acknowledging the abuse moves a battered woman immeasurably forward. Options must be presented, but the physician must accept the woman's choice nonjudgmentally. Such acceptance may start to reverse years of low self-esteem and help her make her own informed decisions.

Medical conditions should be diagnosed and managed in the usual fashion. Medications, particularly tranquilizers, are discouraged, because they can erode the woman's ability to solve problems, serve as her own advocate, and seek help. Efforts to assist the woman to make substantive changes in her social situation and avoiding blame are integral parts of the health care plan.

Treatment plans that include couple or family counseling are usually unsuccessful and are extremely risky for the woman. Intimate partner violence is an issue of power and control, not a communication flaw. Ultimate responsibility for the violence belongs to the perpetrator and not the victim.

Documentation of findings in the medical record establishes the credibility of a battered woman if she seeks legal aid (most commonly for divorce proceedings or child custody settlements). Repetitive trauma and frequent health-related visits are the usual pattern. Stating the history in the patient's words and using a body map to document injuries are helpful (Fig. 150.2). Photographs should be obtained, when indicated, as

TABLE 150.8. Risk for Lethality

Escalation of violence
Children in the home
Batterer threatens to kill spouse
Presence of a weapon
Use of drugs and alcohol

Source: McLeer S. The role of the emergency physician in the prevention of domestic violence. *Ann Emerg Med* 1987;16:1155, with permission.

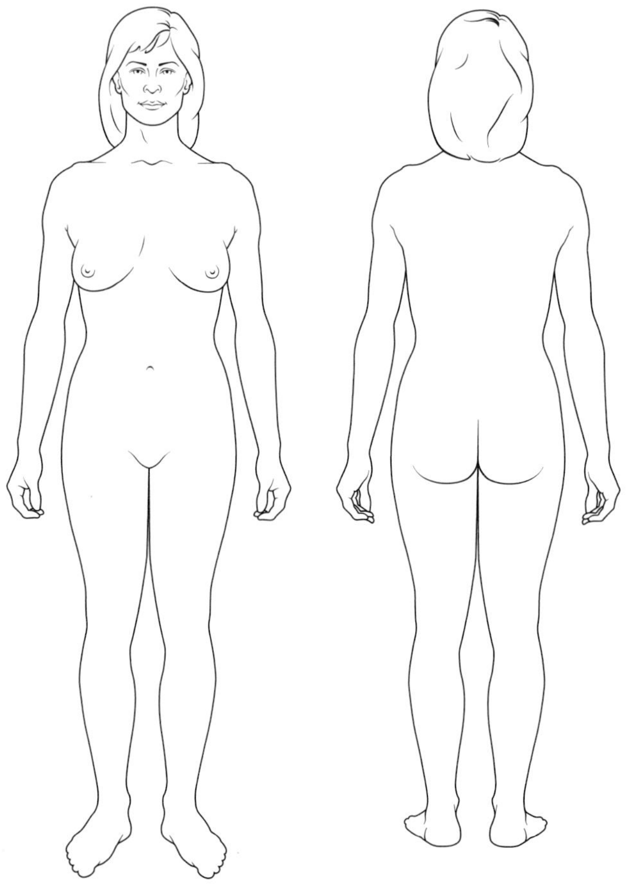

FIG. 150.2. Body map. (McFarlane J, Parker B. *Abuse during pregnancy: a protocol for prevention and intervention.* White Plains, NY: March of Dimes Birth Defects Foundation, 1994, with permission.)

part of evidence collection. An objective opinion of any inconsistencies identified during the evaluation should be charted. Concern has been raised regarding discrimination against women involved in violent relationships who seek health or life insurance. Advocacy groups are actively pursuing this matter.

BATTERING CYCLE

The cycle of intimate partner violence includes three phases (Fig. 150.3). The first is a tension-building phase in which small incidents are portrayed as monumental inadequacies of the woman. The male partner becomes more volatile, but the woman accepts this behavior to avoid a more severe outburst. High anxiety in anticipation of imminent abuse causes the woman to "walk on eggshells." The second phase is an acute battering, which may cause serious injury or extreme fear. The third phase involves reconciliation. This "honeymoon" period is filled with remorse and apologies from the batterer and renewed hopefulness on the part of the victim that the abuse will cease. Nurturing attention by the batterer reaffirms the belief that the relationship is stable and enduring.

Why Women Stay

Women stay in abusive relationships for various reasons. There is an ever-present threat of escalating physical violence to herself and her children. The resulting fear is well substantiated by statistics showing that a woman's greatest risk is at the moment she attempts to leave an abusive relationship. There is no guarantee that the battering will cease. Any attempt by the woman to assume control over the relationship or life circumstances usually leads to escalation of the violence. She may see no alternative to her circumstances, because she may be without financial resources, alternate housing, or employment. Her dismal situation may still be preferable to the unknown. Immobilization, both physical and psychological, can be a reality. Having learned helplessness, many women cannot avail themselves of new possibilities, even when there are alternatives. Cultural, family, and religious values remind her that she has a duty to her partner and maintaining family unity. Previous experiences with law enforcement agencies may have reinforced the belief that only she can help herself. She accepts partial or complete responsibility for the difficulties in her household. An emotional attachment to the batterer may linger.

Psychological Evolution

A battered woman goes through several psychological stages as she attempts to understand her home situation. Initially, she denies the abuse and refuses to admit that she has been beaten or that there is a problem in the relationship. She offers excuses for her partner's violence and refers to the injuries as accidents. She believes that the violence will never happen again. She feels guilty and accepts the problem as her responsibility. She believes she deserves to be beaten due to flaws in her character that incite her partner's violent actions. In time, a woman becomes enlightened that she no longer needs to assume responsibility for the battering. She recognizes that no one deserves to be beaten. However, she is still committed to the relationship and hopeful that things will work out. A traumatic bond may have formed in the setting of a power imbalance and the periodic nature of the abuse and nurturing. (Similar bonding has been described between hostages and their captors.) Many women overestimate the benefit of keeping the family unit intact.

Ultimately, the woman realizes and accepts that she cannot stop his violent behavior. She decides that she will no longer submit to his violence and that she can change her attitude about herself and start a new life. This process has a different time frame for every woman. Most women return to the relationship and the batterer several times before successfully severing all ties. Often an impetus to leave is recognizing the ill effects the violence is having on the children (child abuse, poor coping and interpersonal skills, educational difficulties, poor anger control, eating disorders, anxiety, depression, early sexual activity, substance abuse) or a recent escalation in the violence. At these moments, the reasons to leave become clearer. A woman sees the potential for safety from mental and physical abuse for herself and her children. She develops increased feelings of control over her life and independence. She can feel self-respect, self-confidence, and a sense of identity. Also, increased peace of mind ensues. Future relationships, ideally, are founded in equality (Fig. 150.4).

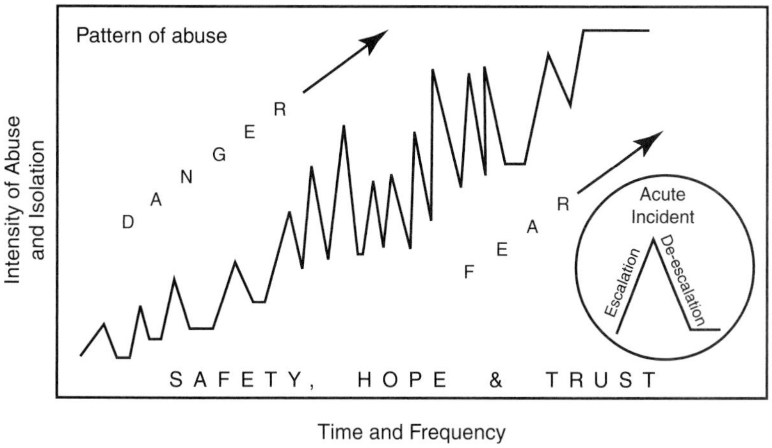

FIG. 150.3. Graph illustrating the pattern of abuse.

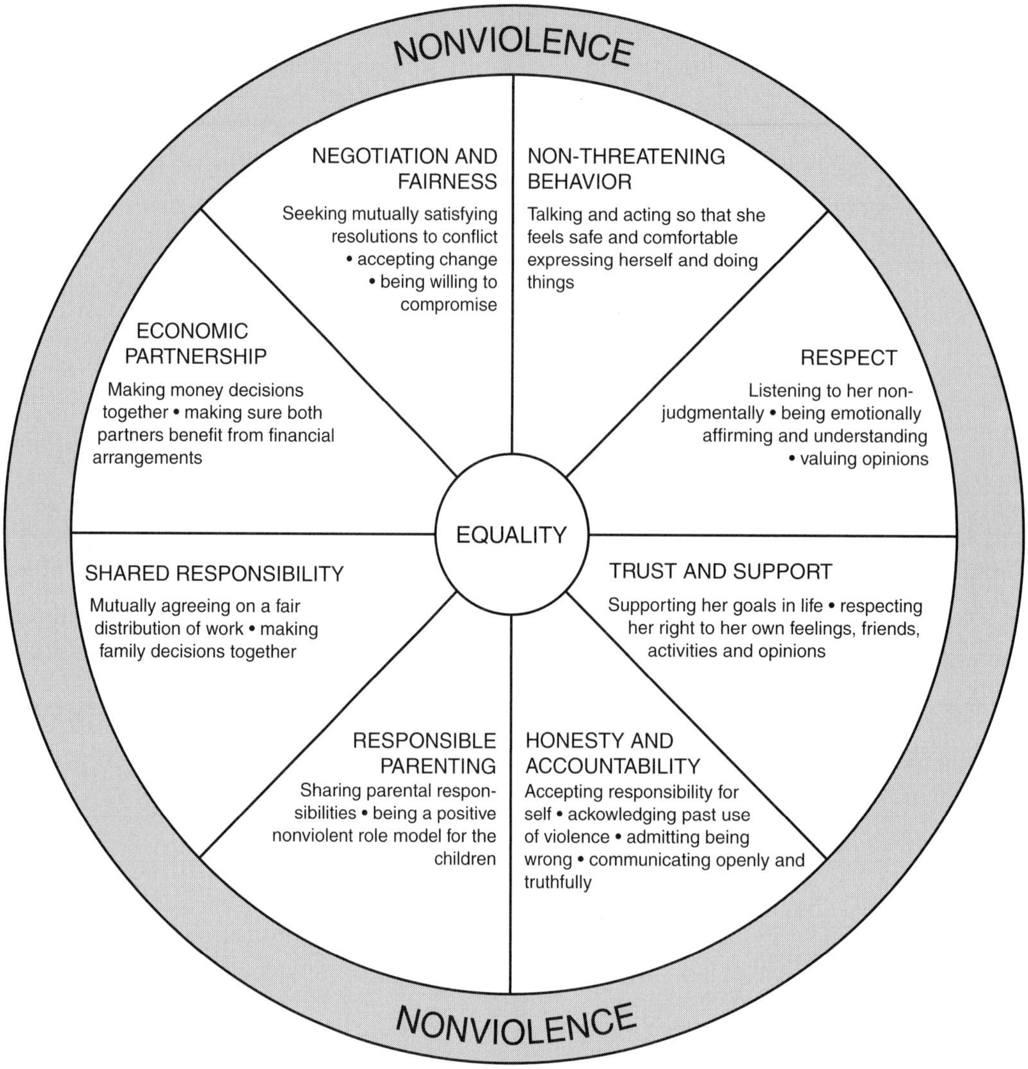

FIG. 150.4. The equality wheel shows elements of a mutually supportive relationship. Nonviolent means of interrelating are incorporated into all aspects of the relationship. Physicians may use this wheel to educate their patients about more egalitarian interaction styles.

CONSIDERATIONS IN PREGNANCY

Intimate partner violence may occur for the first time or escalate during pregnancy. Physical abuse occurs in 37% of obstetric patients across all class, race, and educational boundaries. In the first 4 months and the last 5 months of pregnancy, respectively, 154 per 1,000 and 170 per 1,000 pregnant women are assaulted by their partners. Morbidity and mortality during pregnancy caused by intimate partner violence include placental separation; antepartum hemorrhage; fetal fractures; rupture of the uterus, liver, or spleen; preterm labor and miscarriage; and low birth weight.

CONCLUSION

Intimate partner violence is an epidemic that cannot be ignored. Efforts must be made toward increasing identification of these victims and improving documentation on their behalf. All women must be assessed for possible victimization secondary to intimate partner violence. A standard approach is listed in Table 150.9. With continuing education, proper identification and intervention can interrupt the cycle of violence and convey the following to all victims of intimate partner violence:

- The medical profession cares. We want you to be safe.
- No person deserves to be beaten.
- This is not your fault.

TABLE 150.9. Approach to Patients who are Victims of Abuse

Screen all women
Identify abuse
Validate experience
Safety planning
Maintain confidentiality
Report only with patient's knowledge
Document objectively
Empower the woman to make her own informed decisions

- Battering is a crime.
- Intimate partner violence is common for all types of women.
- Abuse is usually a repetitive event.
- Help is available.

The most important contribution physicians can make to ending abuse and protecting the health of victims is to identify and acknowledge the abuse. Health care professionals at all levels of training must be taught about identification, assessment, and intervention for survivors of intimate partner violence.

BIBLIOGRAPHY

American Medical Association. *Violence: a compendium from JAMA, American Medical News, and the specialty journals of the American Medical Association.* Chicago: AMA, 1992.
Ferrato D. *Living with the enemy.* New York: Aperture Foundation, 1991.
Hoff L. *Battered women as survivors.* New York: Routledge, 1990.
Kilgore N. *Sourcebook for working with battered women.* Volcano, CA: Volcano Press, 1992.
Martin D. *Battered wives.* Volcano, CA: Volcano Press, 1981.
Salber PR, Taliaferro E. *The physician's guide to domestic violence.* Volcano, CA: Volcano Press, 1995.
Sonkin DJ, Durphy M. *Learning to live without violence: a handbook for men.* Volcano, CA: Volcano Press, 1989.
Stark E, Flitcraft A. Spouse abuse. In: Rosenberg M, Fenley M, eds. *Violence in America: a public health approach.* New York: Oxford University Press, 1991.
Walker LE. *The battered woman.* New York: Harper & Row, 1979.

CHAPTER 151

Childhood Physical Abuse

Ann M. Lenane

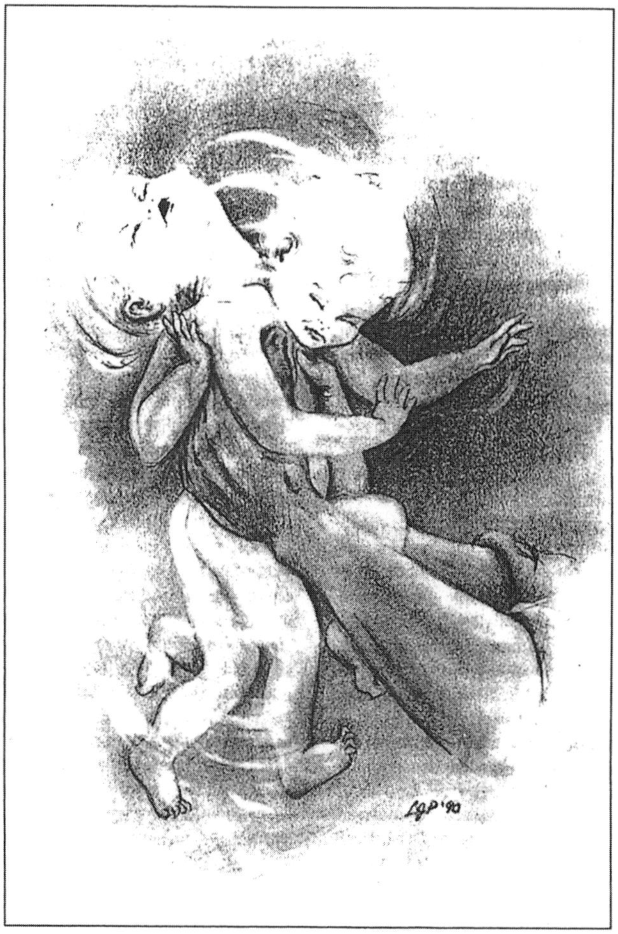

FIG. 151.1. The shaken infant. (From Kleinman PK. *Diagnostic imaging in child abuse,* 2nd ed. St. Louis: Mosby, 1998, with permission.)

In 1946, Caffey first described fractures in the long bones of infants with subdural hematomas, now known as shaken baby syndrome (SBS) (Fig. 151.1). Currently, we know a great deal about the medical and social aspects of child abuse, but we still face more of the unknown in this complex problem.

In 1999, the most recent year with compiled data, there were an estimated 2,974,000 referrals received by United States child protective agencies, 60% of which were accepted and investigated. Of these, 29% were determined to be child abuse or neglect. These data indicate that the rate of victimization is 11.8 per 1,000 children, with the highest risk in the 0- to 3-year-old age group. Of these cases, 58% were child neglect, 21% were physical abuse, and 11% were sexual abuse. A child with a history of abuse had a threefold risk of future abuse, compared with a child with no such history. It is estimated that 1,100 children died from abuse or neglect in 1999.

For every abused child, there are multiple victims: the child, the parents, extended family, and the child's entire community. As we strive to learn more about child abuse, we continue to hope we can someday prevent it. This chapter is an overview, and not a comprehensive guide, to the evaluation of child physical abuse.

Types of child physical abuse include fractures, bruises, burns, and abusive head trauma, often known as SBS. Each is described separately, although more than one may occur in the same child.

TAKING THE HISTORY

Children do not present to a health care provider with a chief complaint of child abuse. More often, a child presents with an injury or with a variety of symptoms, and it is the job of the medical provider to recognize the possibility of abuse. Because most abused children have a history of injuries, the medical providers who care for children must be familiar with the following warning signs of child abuse:

- Does the injury fit the history?
- Does the history fit the age/developmental stage of the child?
- Is the injury a burn or human bite?
- Are there any inconsistencies in the story?
- Was care sought promptly and appropriately?
- Is hygiene appropriate for the circumstances?
- Is there evidence of substance abuse?
- Is there evidence of domestic abuse?

If these questions raise any suspicion of child abuse, a complete evaluation should be done, including a review of past medical records and psychosocial history, taken by a social worker, if one is available. The medical provider should also keep in mind that certain vulnerable children are susceptible to being abused (Table 151.1).

TABLE 151.1. Child Abuse Risk Factors

Caretaker risk factors	Child risk factors
Young parents	Premature infant
Single parents	Fussy, colicky infant
Economic stress	Developmental delay
Poor impulse control	Physical disability
Past abuse as a child	Chronic medical condition
Substance abuse	Autism
Mental health problems	Attention deficit hyperactivity disorder
Domestic violence	
Lack of social/emotional support	
Low socioeconomic status	

PHYSICAL EXAMINATION

If any risk factors are identified, the medical provider should perform a complete physical examination of the child, looking for a medical explanation for the physical findings and avoiding initial accusations of child abuse. However, the provider must be aware of the difference between accidental and abusive injury patterns. If the injuries seem to be nonaccidental, the case must be reported to the appropriate child protection agency. Further, the child may not be discharged until that agency provides for safe disposition of the child. The following sections summarize the types of injuries that may indicate abuse.

Bruises

Bruises are the most common skin manifestations of child abuse; however, they are also frequently seen in accidental trauma. If the medical provider sees bruises suspicious for child abuse, he or she should document the size, shape, and color of each bruise, photographing it, if possible.

Accidental injuries tend to be over bony prominences, such as the orbit, nose, forehead, chin, the spinous processes along the back, the knees, elbows, and hipbones. Bruises from abuse are usually found behind the ears, on the cheeks, neck, chest, abdomen, back, buttocks, genitalia, and inner surfaces of the extremities. Bruises reflecting a pattern of an object should also be suspected for possible abuse. Most professionals with childcare responsibilities are trained to recognize the outlines left by familiar objects of abuse, such as electrical cords and belts.

Policies regarding corporal punishment vary, but in most states, a spanking that leaves bruises or scars is considered child maltreatment. Certain cultural healing practices, such as coining and cupping, often leave a pattern or mark on affected children, but these are traditional healing techniques, and not considered child abuse. Other medical causes of bruises include illnesses, such as meningococcemia and leukemia, and coagulopathies, such as idiopathic thrombopenic purpura (ITP). These can be identified by their clinical presentation and laboratory studies and thus should not be misdiagnosed as child abuse. Although Mongolian spots and hemangiomas are occasionally confused with bruises, an experienced medical provider can usually differentiate them.

Burns

Burns are another skin manifestation of child abuse. Unlike familiar childhood bruises, burns in young children are unusual enough that a complete social history and physical examination should be done for any child presenting with a burn. Most burns are caused by scalding liquids or hot objects. The key to determining the possibility of abuse is comparing the medical history with the physical findings.

In situations of hot liquid burns, the pattern, temperature of the liquid, and exposure time are important factors in classifying the burn as accidental or abusive. Often, an unintentional liquid burn leaves the shape of an inverted pyramid. The most severely burned skin is at the point of impact, surrounded by a more superficially burned area, often with splash marks. But deliberately scalded skin has a sharp line of demarcation between the burned and unburned areas. When an infant has been dipped into hot water, the gluteal and inguinal creases may be spared. The hands/arms of the perpetrator may be mildly burned. In cases of extremity burns, there is often a "stocking/glove" distribution, reflecting the way the arm or leg was dipped into the hot liquid.

In cases of hot object burns, accidental injuries tend to be on the palms or the fingers or the edge of an iron may burn an exposed body part. But abusive burns are often full thickness and reflect the pattern of the heated object, such an iron, steam radiator, curling iron, or a cigarette. The temperature of the object and the exposure time are major factors in identifying the burn as being abusive. Some medical conditions may mimic burns. These include severe diaper dermatitis, epidermolysis bullosa, impetigo, cellulitis, staphylococcal scalded skin syndrome, and erysipelas.

Fractures

Fractures are common in accidental childhood injuries, but certain fractures are more suggestive of being nonaccidental. Kleinman grouped pediatric fractures as being highly, moderately, or minimally suspicious for abuse. High-risk fractures include classic metaphyseal lesions, also called bucket handle or corner fractures, and rib fractures. Low risk fractures include long bone fractures and clavicle fractures.

Other fractures of concern are transverse or oblique/spiral fractures of the humerus, femur, or tibia in a young child, skull fractures with a history of a low velocity or short distance fall, any fracture in a nonambulatory child, and femur fractures in infants less than 1 year of age. Multiple fractures at different stages of healing are also highly suggestive of abuse.

The history of the injury should be consistent with the physical findings, if the injury was accidental. Thus, fractures that are considered high risk for abuse could be explained by a high-speed motor vehicle crash. Consultation with a pediatric orthopedic surgeon is invaluable in determining whether the fracture fits the history. Also, a radiologist skilled in pediatric radiology should evaluate the films to identify fractures and other bony abnormalities. In cases of a suspicious fracture or suspected child abuse in a child under 2 years of age, a skeletal survey should be done to determine the medical cause for "brittle" bones and occult fractures. In children over 2 years of age, the yield of this set of radiographs is lower and should only be done as clinically indicated.

Abdominal and Thoracic Injury

Thoracic, abdominal, and pelvic injuries are relatively rare in young children. In the absence of a history of major trauma, such as a high velocity fall or a motor vehicle crash, these injuries should be suspect for abuse. The usual mechanisms of these injuries (with the exception of rib fractures in infants, see earlier) may be one's punching, throwing, or kicking the child.

The damages sustained include esophageal tears, pharyngeal injury, pulmonary contusion, pneumothorax, hemothorax, duodenal hematoma, liver laceration, splenic laceration, pancreatic injury, mesenteric tears, renal injury, and retroperitoneal hematomas.

Often, thoracic trauma may present with difficulty in breathing or rapid respiratory rate, whereas abdominal trauma often presents with abdominal pain, lethargy, and vomiting. The physical examination may reveal thoracic or abdominal tenderness, and there may not be visible bruising. With no history of trauma, only when the evaluation shows no medical etiology to explain the symptoms would the diagnosis of child abuse be suspected. The medical evaluation, including laboratory and radiographic studies, would be similar to that for any pediatric trauma patient. A surgeon with expertise in pediatric trauma should be consulted.

Thoracic and abdominal injuries are unusual manifestations of child abuse. Nonetheless, medical providers must be aware of the medical evaluation of these injuries and the need to report them to the appropriate child protection agency.

Oral Injuries and Bites

Oral injuries are rare in child abuse, but it is critical to be aware that injuries to the inside of an infant's mouth can be highly indicative of abuse. Further, it is essential to thoroughly examine the mouth of any child where there is probable abuse. Such injuries include cuts to the inside the mouth in a child with no teeth, cuts or injury to the frenulum or uvula, and any bruising inside the mouth. Accidental oral injuries are usually accompanied by trauma to the lips, nose, or chin. In the absence of these, any injury inside the mouth should raise suspicion.

Bites are fairly commonplace injuries among young children. They are rarely accidental, in the true sense; however, one child inflicting a bite upon another is not considered child abuse. In cases of a child with a witnessed bite by another child, with no risk factors for child abuse, further evaluation for abuse would not be necessary. If the lesion is questionable, or there are other risk factors, efforts should be made to determine whether the perpetrator was an adult or child.

If a dentist is unavailable to evaluate the bite, photographs should be taken, with a measuring device included in the photograph. Thus, a dentist or forensic odontologist can view the photograph and make a determination. Additionally, a psychosocial assessment should be done to decide the safe disposition of the child while the dental evaluation is pending.

Abusive Head Trauma and Shaken Baby Syndrome

SBS has become well known. Child abuse experts often substitute the term "abusive head trauma" to reflect both the violent nature of the event and the possibility of other types of head trauma, such as impact. The phrase depicts the constellation of symptoms that appear when a child, usually an infant, is violently shaken by a caretaker. Such an infant presents for medical evaluation with symptoms such as fussiness, lethargy, seizure activity, fever, vomiting, poor feeding, and apnea. A bump may be noted on the infant's head if an impact blow was part of the event. SBS is estimated to be fatal in 25% of cases. The survivors have morbidity that is dependent on the degree of injury. In one study, 54% of shaken infants had deficits in motor tone and coordination, and 85% had deficits in attention.

Many of these infants present in extremis and initially undergo infant resuscitation. Once the infant is stable, a more detailed assessment may reveal laboratory or radiographic evidence of a traumatic event. If SBS is suspected, the evaluation consists of a complete physical examination, laboratory studies, such as complete blood count, coagulation screen, electrolytes, hepatic and pancreatic injury panels, urinalysis, toxicology screen, and blood type screen.

In addition, a head computed tomography and a skeletal survey are performed. The head computed tomography in SBS may show subdural hematoma, subarachnoid hemorrhage, parenchyma hemorrhage, cerebral edema, hypoxic ischemic changes, and skull fractures. In the skeletal survey, possible injuries include classic metaphyseal lesions of abuse and rib fractures. The rib fractures are caused by manual pressure on the ribs as the infant is held; the metaphyseal fractures are caused by the flailing of the arms and legs as the infant is shaken (Fig. 151.1). An experienced ophthalmologist should do the retinal examination, searching for retinal hemorrhages, which are seen in up to 80% of shaken infants, but rare in accidental head injury.

Usually, infants with abusive head trauma require hospital admission, often to a pediatric intensive care unit. The appropriate child protection agency should be notified to assist with discharge planning and determine whether there are other children in the home who may be at risk.

Munchausen Syndrome by Proxy

A recently recognized area of child abuse, Munchausen syndrome by proxy (MSBP), also called pediatric condition falsification (PCF), is an extremely complex situation involving a child who presents with a factitious condition caused by the caretaker. The categories of symptoms due to MSBP/PCF include perceived illness, enforced invalidism, and fabricated illness. The children's symptoms include acute life-threatening events; apnea; seizures; blood in the urine, stool, emesis, or sputum; rashes; fevers; sepsis; and metabolic abnormalities. To reach the diagnosis requires an astute medical team and a detailed medical/investigative effort.

Several interesting features suggest MSBP/PCF. Initially, the father may be unaware of the true nature of the problem and is often minimally involved. The biologic mother is the most frequent perpetrator (75%–98%). She herself may have factitious illnesses, along with mental health problems, including depression or personality disorders. She may have a medical background (30% in one study). Feeling at ease in the medical setting, the mother is often friendly with the medical staff. She typically hovers around the child, apparently very devoted to his or her care, and is content to have her child remain in the hospital. She is eager to have the child undergo extensive testing, while the medical team struggles for an explanation. Once MSBP/PCF is suspected, complex toxicology screening or covert video surveillance is frequently necessary to prove the diagnosis.

Management consists of referral to the appropriate protective agency, often a trial removal of the child from the home (resulting in resolution of the symptoms if the diagnosis is correct), and addressing other critical mental health issues. MSBP/PCF is a dangerous form of child abuse. Follow-up studies have found that 10% of victims of die from their "injuries." Most survivors suffer long-term medical and psychosocial morbidity.

SUMMARY

Child abuse is a common problem with potentially devastating outcomes for children, families, and society. Those who care for children must have an understanding and ability to recognize this complex problem and be aware of the necessary steps required to protect children.

BIBLIOGRPAHY

Belfer RA, Klein BL, Orr L. Use of the skeletal survey in the evaluation of child maltreatment. *Am J Emerg Med* 2001;19:122–124.

Brill PW, Winchester P, Kleinman MD. Differential diagnosis. I. Diseases simulating abuse. In: Kleinman PK, ed. *Diagnostic imaging of child abuse,* 2nd ed. St. Louis: Mosby, 1998.

Caffey J. Multiple fractures in the long bones of infants suffering from chronic subdural hematoma. *AJR Am J Roentgenol* 1946;56:163–173.

Conway EE. Nonaccidental head injury in infants: the shaken baby syndrome revisited. *Pediatr Ann* 1998;27;10:677–690.

Ewing-Cobbs L, Prasad M, Kramer L, et al. Inflicted traumatic brain injury: relationship of developmental outcome to severity of injury. *Pediatr Neurosurg* 1999;31:251–258.

Jenny C, Taylor RJ, Cooper M. *Diagnostic imaging and child abuse: technologies, practices, and guidelines.* Washington, DC: Medical Technology and Practice Patterns Institute, 1996.

Lenane AM. Child abuse. In: Garfunkel LC, Kaczorowski J, Christy C, eds. *Mosby's pediatric clinical advisor instant diagnosis and treatment.* St. Louis: Mosby, 2002: 226–228.

Monteleone JA. Munchausen syndrome by proxy. In: Monteleone JA, Brodeur AE, eds. *Child maltreatment: a clinical guide and reference,* 2nd ed. St. Louis: GW Medical Publishing, 1998.

Nimkin K, Kleinman PK. Imaging of child abuse. *Radiol Clin North Am* 2001;139: 843–864.

Reece RM. *Child abuse: medical diagnosis and management.* Philadelphia: Lea & Febiger, 1994.

Reece RM, Ludwig S, eds. *Child abuse: medical diagnosis and management,* 2nd ed. Philadelphia: Lippincott Williams & Wilkins, 2001.

Wagner GN. Bitemark identification in child abuse cases. *Pediatr Dentist* 1986;8: 96–100.

www.acf.dhhs.gov/programs/cb/publications/cm99/high/htm. Highlights of the 1999 National Child Abuse and Neglect Reporting System.

CHAPTER 152
Sexual Assault

Joseph Kozlowski and Phyllis C. Leppert

Sexual assault is a medical emergency. Eighteen percent to 43% of women responded to national surveys that they have been sexually assaulted at some time in their lives.

The major motive for sexual assault is aggression. Sexual assault is defined as any sexual act performed by one person on another without that person's consent. Rape is defined by the U.S. Justice Department as "carnal knowledge" through the use of force or threat of force. Consent is total agreement and is based on choice. Having sex as a result of being tricked or lied to is not consent.

When a victim is sexually assaulted, she loses control over her life for that period of time. She not only feels fear and pain but can suffer emotionally. This can affect her sexual, physical, and social functioning. It may take years before a victim can put the experience behind her and function on a somewhat normal level. Victims hesitate to report assault because of humiliation, feelings of guilt, fear of retribution, and disillusionment with the criminal justice system.

There are many mistaken beliefs about sexual assault. Some of these include the notion that women are asking for sex by smiling at a man or by the way they dress or dance. Other beliefs are that in the absence of physical resistance or injury, sexual assault has not occurred, or that sex is a man's right if he spends money on a date. A similar belief is that if a woman knows a man and invites him into her home or is on a date with him, unwanted sex is not rape. The truth is that being on a date or being alone with someone is not an invitation to have sex. Forced sexual intimacy is a form of violence, not an act of manhood.

Common myths concerning rape stem from society's historical attitudes toward women. Rape is not the result of a spontaneous sexual urge. Rape is much more, because it represents a violent assault, rather than a sexual assault, on a woman's body and psyche that often results in physical injury. Acts of mental brutality, threats, and intimidation are common. Death is a common fear of a woman during rape, and in about 1% of rapes homicide does occur.

MANAGEMENT OF SEXUAL ASSAULT VICTIMS

An estimated 80,000 victims are treated each year, including infants and the elderly. The staff of each medical facility must determine whether it is prepared to meet the needs of a sexual assault victim. A useful approach is to train a team that can work well together. This limits the number of personnel who come in contact with the victim and provides better security in gathering and storing legal evidence. The team can be composed of nurses, physicians, physician assistants, and nurse practitioners, all of whom should be trained in evaluating a sexual assault victim.

In addition to the team, a well-trained counselor who is available 24 hours a day can counsel victims concerning medical, legal, or social problems. Immediate contact with a counselor may be a way to prevent victims from suppressing memory of the assault. The counselor can also offer emotional support during legal proceedings if the victim wishes to prosecute.

Team members should know state and local laws regarding sexual assault. Informed consent must be obtained before collection of evidence and forensic examination of the victim. Obtaining consent allows the victim to regain a sense of control over the examination. The victim should be placed in a private secure room where a history can be taken and a physical examination performed. The examiner is responsible for treating injuries and performing appropriate laboratory tests to detect, prevent, and treat sexually transmitted infections. Other tests should be performed to detect pregnancy and to prevent it if the victim desires. The victim should meet a support person, such as a rape crisis counselor, preferably before the examiner sees her. The support person can stay with the victim through the examination.

PHYSICAL EXAMINATION

An initial assessment for unstable vital signs, altered consciousness, peritoneal injury, and pain alerts the examining provider to serious injuries. Rape victims can sustain major nongenital physical injuries, and such injuries should be tended to first. If a weapon such as a knife or gun was involved, treatment should follow appropriate resuscitation maneuvers and diagnostic studies.

A few rape victims have moderate to severe genital injuries. Most of these include upper vaginal lacerations, although intraperitoneal extension of such lacerations is rare. Injuries to the anal canal cause mucosal lacerations. The use of photoscopy to evaluate these injuries is justified. Most mucosal injuries need no intervention, because most minor mucosal bleeding resolves without intervention. For some victims, the impending pelvic and rectal examinations may be their first, and these victims need reassurance. All procedures should be explained, and the victims should be involved immediately in all decisions regarding the examination and consent forms. This is done to help restore a victim's feeling of self-respect and dignity. Nothing during the examination should suggest force.

After assessing the acute injuries, a nonjudgmental history should be taken. To spare the victim the distress of having to repeat the narration of the assault unnecessarily, only one member of the team should obtain the history. Basic details about the assault are necessary to ensure that all injuries are detected and to guide the medicolegal examination. The victim's general appearance and demeanor should be noted. Some victims remain calm; others are hysterical or even withdrawn. Most victims feel frightened, humiliated, degraded, and angry. A concise history, not excessively detailed, written in a legible fashion works best. Unnecessary frivolous information may result in discrepancies with the police report that can adversely affect future criminal proceedings: Minute details taken at a time of acute emotional crisis may appear inconsistent or contradictory in court.

The history should include the date, time, and location of the assault; the race, identity, and number of assailants; the nature of the physical contacts; and the use of weapons, restraints, foreign bodies, drugs, and alcohol. The body orifices involved (oral, vaginal, or rectal) should be reported. If digital penetration occurred or if foreign bodies were used, this should also be reported. Questions should be asked about whether the attacker ejaculated and where this occurred. If ejaculation occurred, the examiner should ask whether it occurred on clothing or on the victim's body. Contraceptive devices, such as condoms, may have been used by the attacker or by the victim. The victim may have bathed, douched, showered, urinated or defecated, washed her mouth, brushed her teeth, used a tampon, or changed her clothing. These activities could alter evidence after the assault and should be documented.

Gynecologic medical history should be recorded, including past infections, contraceptive use, last menstrual period, and last consensual intercourse. Also noted should be the victim's gravidity and parity, whether she is pregnant, and the date of her last Pap smear. The medical history should include allergies, any medications the victim is taking, and tetanus immunization status.

Marks of violence should be documented, including scratches, bruises, rope imprints, bite marks, lacerations, points of tenderness, abrasions, ecchymoses, and linear abrasions. Nongenital injuries occur in 20% to 50% of sexual assaults.

Documentation with photographs is indicated if physical trauma is evident. Police agencies can send a qualified forensic photographer to take the photographs. Documentation on a traumagram or body diagram creates a visual depiction of injuries.

EVIDENCE GATHERING

Saliva

The first step in gathering evidence involves oral swabs and smears. Saliva samples should be obtained and the swabs streaked over clean glass slides and placed in slide folders. The swabs are then air dried before they are placed in sealed paper box containers marked "oral swabs." An additional saliva sample is obtained on a filter paper the victim places in her mouth. Only the victim may handle the filter paper with bare hands. The filter paper is thoroughly saturated, air dried, and inserted into the envelope marked "saliva sample."

Trace Evidence

To minimize the loss of evidence, the victim should disrobe over a large piece of examination table paper or a clean sheet. Clothes and the paper or sheet are then placed in a paper (not plastic) bag for forensic testing. Wet or damp clothing should be air dried before packaging; if wet clothing is wrapped, mold and mildew can damage evidence. The victim's underwear should be collected and placed in the paper bag provided. A Wood's lamp can be used to locate semen stains. Care should be taken not to shake the clothing, because microscopic evidence may be lost. If the victim has changed clothes after the assault, the examiner should ask her to bring the clothing in for the police so evidence may be collected.

Debris Collection

Debris (e.g., leaves, fibers, glass, dirt, or hair) is sometimes found on the victim's body. To collect this evidence, the victim is placed on a paper sheet and she brushes off the debris. Any foreign material found on her body is collected, and the folded sheet is placed in the appropriate envelope.

Dried Secretions

Dried secretions from bites or ejaculation deposits are sampled by taking a swab moistened with one or two drops of water or saline. The area of the stain or suspected dry secretion is swabbed carefully, and the swab is allowed to air dry. These swabs are placed in an envelope marked "dried secretions."

Fingernail Scrapings

Many times women scratch their attackers, although some victims may not realize this. To collect evidence, a paper sheet with a wooden or plastic scraper is provided for each of the victim's hands. Each hand in turn is held over the paper sheet when scraping all fingernails so that any debris falls on the paper. After all the fingers have been scraped, the scraper is placed in the center of the paper, and the paper is folded and placed in an envelope. Each paper is marked "left" or "right" for the respective hands.

Pulled Head Hairs

Pulling hair strands for evidence collection is considered by many to be traumatic to victims of sexual assault. Examiners must use their judgment, based on the victim's physical and emotional well-being and her decision. If the victim agrees to the gathering of head hair, the examiner should use the thumb and forefinger, not forceps or scissors, to pull five hairs from each of five scalp locations for a total of 25 hairs. These hairs are placed in an envelope.

Pubic Hair Combings

A sterile comb and paper sheet should be provided for collecting pubic hair combings. The paper sheet is removed and placed under the victim's genital area. Using the comb provided, pubic hair is combed in downward strokes so that any loose hair or debris falls on the paper sheet. To reduce embarrassment and increase a sense of control for the victim, she may prefer to do the combing. The sheet is carefully removed. The comb is placed in the center of the sheet and the sheet is folded and returned to the envelope marked "pubic hair combings."

Pulled Pubic Hairs

Pulling pubic hair for evidence is another traumatic experience for sexual assault victims. Again, professional judgment regarding whether to complete this step should be based on the victim's physical and emotional well-being and preference. She may feel more comfortable pulling these hairs herself. The thumb and forefingers, not forceps, are used to pull 15 full-length hairs from various locations of the pubic area for sampling. The hairs are placed in the envelope designated "pulled pubic hairs."

PELVIC EXAMINATION

Genital trauma may be a result of sexual assault. The inner thighs, vulva, and vagina are assessed for signs of trauma such as bruises, lacerations, and erythema. Injuries to the genitalia should be characterized and photographs taken. Small abrasions of the fourchette and distal vagina may be evaluated with the aid of a colposcope, if available. Injuries to the labia and clitoris, with evidence of erythema and engorgement, may last for several hours after intercourse. The examination should evaluate the status of the pelvic reproductive organs and should document possible infections. It is generally unnecessary to use a speculum.

When evaluating injuries and collecting specimens in prepubescent or adolescent females, an adult-sized speculum should never be used; even a pediatric speculum may cause further trauma. Specimens for culture and forensic analysis may be obtained by using a glass eyedropper or a cotton-tipped applicator. For prepubescent children, a vaginal, not cervical, specimen is indicated for a culture to test for sexually transmitted disease. If extensive injury or the presence of foreign bodies cannot be ruled out, the examination might cause further trauma to the child. If the child is too distressed to cooperate, an examination under anesthesia is appropriate.

In adults, appropriate specimens include cervical, gonorrhea, and chlamydia cultures. Using two swabs simultaneously, the vaginal vault is carefully swabbed. Both swabs are allowed to air dry and are placed in boxes marked "vaginal DNA." Using two additional swabs, the same swabbing procedure is repeated and two smears are prepared on slides. These are allowed to air dry. When the slides are dry, they are placed in slide folders marked "vaginal smears."

ANAL SWABS AND SMEARS

The anal region is examined if anal penetration has occurred. Many victims do not admit that anal penetration has occurred due to embarrassment, so an anal examination should be performed on every victim. Signs of trauma may include laceration, abrasion, or edema. Swabs of the anal region should be moistened with saline or distilled water before the collection process. The anus is carefully swabbed with two swabs, and two smears are prepared on slides. The swabs and smears are allowed to air dry. Cultures can be taken at this time if appropriate. The swabs and smears are placed in boxes marked "anal."

KNOWN BLOOD SAMPLES

Using the blood tubes provided for collecting serum and plasma and following normal phlebotomy techniques, blood samples are drawn. The tubes are filled to maximum volume and returned to tube holders. If the victim received a blood transfusion before the examination, "transfusion" should be written on a piece of paper and taped to the blood tubes.

Blood tests to be performed include those for pregnancy, hepatitis B, and human immunodeficiency virus (HIV), as well as rapid plasma reagin tests and the Venereal Disease Research Laboratory test. Basic information about the risk of HIV infection, methods of testing, and confidentiality should be reviewed with the victim. Counseling should also be provided. The patient should be told of the need for HIV retesting in 12 weeks, 6 months, and 1 year. Rapid plasma reagin tests should also be repeated in 12 weeks.

SEXUALLY TRANSMITTED DISEASES

Gonorrhea, syphilis, and *Chlamydia trachomatis* are the three most common sexually transmitted diseases transmitted during a sexual assault. Other infections, such as *Trichomonas vaginalis*, genital herpes, genital warts, HIV, and hepatitis B, also can be transmitted. Prophylactic antibiotic therapy is routinely prescribed. If the victim is known to be pregnant at the time of the assault, 250 mg erythromycin every 6 hours is given orally for 10 days to prevent chlamydia infection. If the victim is not pregnant, 100 mg doxycycline twice a day is given orally for 10 days. For gonorrhea, one dose of 125 mg ceftriaxone should be given intramuscularly. For trichomonas infection, one dose of 2 g metronidazole is given orally (see Chapter 86). Hepatitis B vaccine can be offered after confirmation of positive antibody status. Treatment is 0.06 mL/kg hepatitis B immune globulin intramuscularly, to be repeated in 1 month if the victim's serology is negative. Tetanus prophylaxis is appropriate for victims with trauma who are not current with their immunizations.

PREGNANCY PREVENTION

Patients who wish pregnancy prevention can be given two oral contraceptive tablets, each containing 50 mg ethinyl estradiol, taken 12 hours apart, or three contraceptive tablets, each containing 35 mg ethinyl estradiol, taken 12 hours apart. This treatment should be offered regardless of the time of the last menstrual period. An antiemetic (e.g., one promethazine [Phenergan] rectal suppository, 25 mg) can prevent nausea and vomiting caused by the oral contraceptives. Statistically, the risk of pregnancy is small: 2% to 4% of women not using contraceptives at the time of assault become pregnant. Hormonal therapy is effective if given within 72 hours of the assault. If pregnancy is diagnosed as a consequence of an assault, the victim can be counseled on her options, including pregnancy termination.

FOLLOW-UP CARE AND REFERRAL

Many sexual assault victims are lost to follow-up care. They also have limited recall about retesting, treatment, and referral. They should receive a sheet that outlines a list of follow-up appointments and treatments received during the evaluation. The outline should list a schedule of follow-up laboratory testing with dates. These tests include sexually transmitted disease cultures after antibiotic therapy and repeat blood tests for syphilis and HIV at 3- and 6-month intervals. Information about referral agencies, such as rape crisis groups and names and telephone numbers of staff members at various medical facilities, should also be given.

Some communities have rape crisis centers that provide counseling and support for the victim. Some victims may hesitate to request help because they want to forget the experience. It is desirable to make a referral at the initial visit. Support may include resources for housing, money, child care, notification of significant others, and counseling about future litigation. Talking about the event is helpful. The initial impact of an assault is shock, disorganization, disbelief, and disorientation. Victims do not feel safe even in their own homes. There may be a long period of adjustment. Friends and family may believe that the victim has adjusted to the event, but the victim may be denying the experience and making unrealistic attempts to resume everyday life. Family members may experience the same reactions as the victim. Initially, feelings of hopelessness, disbelief, and shock are common. Victims can experience somatic symptoms, such as headaches, abdominal pain, sleep disturbances, nightmares, eating disorders, nervousness, and irritability. These complaints may actually be signs of posttraumatic stress disorder. Some victims, when exposed to certain stimuli, can undergo flashbacks in which they reexperience the assault. These symptoms can persist for weeks, months, or years.

Recovery is influenced by the victim's personality and by the characteristics of the assault. Date rape victims may believe they can no longer trust anyone close to them. Victims assaulted by strangers may believe there is no way to prevent an attack and no environment in which they are completely safe. In the last stages of integration, the victim accepts the reality of the assault and the validity of her emotional response.

Primary care physicians and obstetrician-gynecologists often provide ongoing care for sexual assault victims. Understanding the psychological changes that occur after an assault is paramount in being able to treat these patients. Most victims report fearing death and feeling unsafe. A sense of shame, guilt, helplessness, and lowered self-esteem can affect relationships with boyfriends, spouses, and family. Depression is a common consequence of an assault.

Various sexual dysfunctions can occur, including orgasmic failure. Some victims prefer a prolonged abstinence from sexual activity or experience altered sexual response. Some permanently decrease their sexual activity. The spouse or significant other typically reacts in an overprotective fashion. This may make the victim believe she cannot take care of herself, so such overprotectiveness should be discouraged. Allowing the victim to express herself, particularly with feelings of anger, provides an important step in regaining self-control. Spouses and significant others of sexual assault victims often feel helpless and vulnerable and may also suffer from depression.

VULNERABLE INDIVIDUALS

Children, the elderly, handicapped, and mentally ill persons are especially vulnerable to sexual assault. One study reported that 26% of women who were treated for sexual assault in an urban emergency room were those with a diagnosis of a major psychiatric illness. Children who are victims of sexual abuse may present initially to rape crisis centers. Sexual abuse in children and adolescents is defined as any sexual activity they do not understand and to which they cannot give informed consent. Therefore, sexual abuse in the pediatric age group includes sexual intercourse, genital fondling, and exposing children to pornography and sexual exploitation. The parent or another adult may become concerned about the child's behavior or by symptoms of vaginal discharge or a genital or anal abnormality. A child may make a statement to an adult that suggests she may be sexually abused. The primary care provider must be aware that other physical conditions such as a streptococcal vaginal or anorectal infection or lichen sclerosis may be mistaken for signs of sexual abuse in a child. Suspected childhood sexual abuse is an emergency. The primary care provider should not attempt to diagnosis childhood sexual abuse and should immediately refer the child and family to a medical team that is experienced in the diagnosis and treatment of this problem. Childhood sexual abuse has serious long-term consequences for those who have been subjected to it. Adults who have been sexually abused in childhood are at risk for depression, eating disorders, and posttraumatic stress disorders. These same adults may have trouble in forming intimate relationships and are at risk for promiscuous behavior.

SUMMARY

Sexual assault is one of the fastest growing violent crimes in the United States. Victims of sexual assault sustain both physical and emotional trauma. Health care professionals caring for these women have a duty to provide sensitive compassionate treatment. Professional objectivity, in compliance with state statutory requirements, in evaluating sexual assault victims is paramount. This can help ensure that vital information is accessible for criminal proceedings. Follow-up and sustained psychological support are essential to help the victim make the transition from victim to survivor and allow healthy daily activities to resume. Childhood sexual abuse also has long-term sequelae. Children and adolescents suspected of being sexually abused must be referred for expert care.

BIBLIOGRAPHY

American Academy of Pediatrics. Guidelines for the evaluation of sexual abuse in the prepubertal child. *Pediatrics* 1999;103:186–191.

Beebe DK. Emergency management of the adult female rape victim. *Am Fam Phys* 1991;43:2041.

Dupre AR, Hampton HL, Morrison H, et al. Sexual assault. *Obstet Gynecol Surv* 1993;48:640.

Dwyer JD. Examination and treatment of the sexual assault victim. *Phys Assist* 1987;11:100.

Eckert LO, Sugar N, Fine D. Characteristics of sexual assault in women with major psychiatric diagnosis. *Am J Obstet Gynecol* 2002;186:1284–1291.

Hampton HL. Care of the woman who has been raped. *N Engl J Med* 1995;332:234.

Hick DJ, Minkin MJ, Solola A. Examining the rape victim. *Patient Care* 1986;20:98.

Joffe MD, Rubin D. Sexual abuse and rape. In: Burg FD, Ingelfinger JR, Polin RA, et al., eds. *Gellis and Kagan's current pediatric therapy.* Philadelphia: WB Saunders, 2002:395–398.

Kirkland K, Mason RE. Victims of crime: the internist's role in treatment. *South Med J* 1992;85:965.

Silverman D, McCombie SL. Counseling mates and families of rape victims. In: McCombie SL, ed. *The rape crisis intervention handbook: a guide to victim care.* New York: Plenum Press, 1980:173.

Young WW, Bracken AC, Goddard MA, et al. Sexual assault: review of a national model protocol for forensic and medical evaluation. New Hampshire Sexual Assault Medical Examination Protocol Project Committee. *Obstet Gynecol* 1992;80:878.

CHAPTER 153
Posttraumatic Stress Disorder

Phyllis C. Leppert

In the 19th century, physicians identified a cluster of symptoms associated with trauma and developed treatment methods for this disorder. However, the symptoms of this stress-induced emotional disorder have been known since antiquity. They were well described by Homer and Cicero. What is now known as posttraumatic stress disorder (PTSD) was originally recognized in soldiers exposed to the death and carnage of battle. Pepys described the syndrome in his diary of the Great London Fire of

1666, and physicians described it in the American Civil War. In World War I it was known as "shell shock." In World War II the symptoms were correctly identified as both physiologic and psychological. Modern examples of events that caused post-traumatic stress disorder in individuals are the Oklahoma City bombing in 1995 and the events of September 11, 2001. According to the National Institute of Mental Health, 5.2 million U.S. adults have PTSD each year.

DESCRIPTION AND ETIOLOGY

The cluster is a triad of symptoms that includes an intrusive reexperienced event, avoidance responses to evidence of the event and generalized emotional numbing and isolation, and physiologic systemic arousal that does not predate the trauma. Persons experiencing PTSD have witnessed or been confronted with events that involve actual or threatened death, serious injury, or a threat to the physical integrity of others or self. They are persons who are overwhelmed by a particular stressful experience. The emotional response in adults is one of intense fear, helplessness, or horror. Children become disorganized or agitated. The trauma is relived by recurrent and intrusive distressing recollections, including images. In children, this may occur in play. Recurrent dreams occur as well. There is usually a sense that the traumatic event is actually recurring. This is felt as reliving the trauma, with illusions, hallucinations, and dissociative episodes. There is then intense psychological distress from the cues that come to symbolize the trauma. The physiologic symptoms are activated by these internal and external cues, and the victim comes to avoid these disturbing stimuli. The traumatized person avoids thoughts, feelings, or discussions associated with the event, as well as people identified with the trauma. The victim feels detached and estranged, is unable to have loving feelings, and is disinterested in participating in social activities. There is often a sense of guilt if others have died and the victim has lived.

To a person with PTSD, the future seems short: "I'll never marry," "I'll die young." Physiologic symptoms include trouble falling asleep or waking up early, outbursts of anger, exaggerated startle, and difficulty in concentration. Many persons affected are hypervigilant. By definition, the symptoms must be of at least 1 month's duration and produce clinically significant distress or social impairment. PTSD is acute if the duration of symptoms is less than 3 months and chronic if it has lasted more than 3 months. In delayed-onset PTSD, the symptoms occur 6 months or more after the stressful event.

The concept of PTSD has been broadened and is used to include symptoms that follow combat trauma, rape, torture, natural disasters, and acute and chronic medical disorders, as well as other categories. The current criteria for acute PTSD require that symptoms must follow the trauma, not precede it, and cannot be due to the effect of drug abuse or medication. The symptoms must last at least 2 days and occur within 4 weeks of the event.

Severe trauma, such as torture, rape, or combat, produces PTSD in many persons. The prevalence of PTSD for combat veterans is about 30%; it is over 90% in prisoners of war or victims of torture.

Research studies in animals and humans have demonstrated the specific brain areas and neurologic circuits involved in the emotions of fear and anxiety. Fear is a protective emotion that has evolved to assist an individual in dealing with real danger. The fear response is coordinated by the amygdala and is an automatic and rapid protective response that occurs in multiple physiologic systems in the body. There are neurologic changes that result from the activation of the autonomic nervous system as well as hormonal responses activated by the hypothalamic-pituitary adrenal system. These physiologic responses control and stimulate the output of cortisol, norepinephrine and epinephrine, resulting in increased energy for fighting or running away from danger. Recent research has shown that some anxiety disorders may be associated with an abnormal activation of the amygdala.

Brain imaging studies show that the hippocampus appears to be different in individuals with PTSD compared with those without this disorder. These differences in the hippocampus are thought to be responsible for intrusive memories and flashbacks. Persons with PTSD have lower cortisol levels but higher epinephrine and norepinephrine levels that those without PTSD. In addition, individuals with PTSD continue to produce high levels of natural opiates even after a dangerous event has passed.

The natural history of PTSD is not always clear, but it seems to be severe for several years and then gradually diminishes. Sleep difficulties and intrusive thoughts persist. Persons so affected carefully avoid anything reminding them of the trauma. Persons who have experienced PTSD usually have a marked decrease in tolerance for serious trauma of any type. However, victims can let go of the memories and the event and lead successful lives. Over time, those who have persistent symptoms have chronic depression and generalized anxiety. The incidence of PTSD after rape or assault in women may exceed 50% during the first months after the occurrence. In several months and up to 1 year it is 25% to 30%, and after several years it is 5% to 10%.

DIFFERENTIAL DIAGNOSIS

The differential diagnosis of PTSD must include other disorders with similar symptoms. Other illnesses, such as schizophrenia, could be considered. Depression, anxiety, and substance abuse should also be considered as potential diagnoses. Extreme trauma, such as occurs in concentration camp victims, hostages, or battered women, produces a form of PTSD in which a wide range of symptoms and personality changes occur. In childhood, chronic sexual or physical abuse may lead to a substance abuse disorder, eating disorders, antisocial personality, borderline personality disorder, chronic pain disorder, or hypochondria. The primary care clinician must be aware, however, that the diagnosis of PTSD is often missed.

The clinician must be sensitive and allow a person with PTSD to have psychological space. Comments such as "That must have been very painful" may appear glib. The clinician will have personal emotional reactions to the description of severe trauma as well. The history should be taken gently. The person may be asked "Have you ever been in a war? A disaster? A severe accident?" "Have you ever been attacked or assaulted?" The clinician could say "We have learned that physical and sexual abuse is more common than we thought." This statement could be followed by gentle further inquiry. These questions should not be asked initially in the history taking.

PTSD does not involve the normal traumatic stress recovery process: It is more intense and the symptoms are more diverse and more numerous. The primary care provider should be alert to the possibility of PTSD and should refer women to experts for therapy. The appropriate therapy for a particular type of trauma is currently under study. Therapy consists of pharmacotherapy, cognitive-behavioral therapy, and exposure therapy. Exposure therapy allows the patient to gradually and repeatedly relive the traumatic experience under controlled conditions to help work through the fear.

TABLE 153.1. Acute Stress Reaction

Physical signs and symptoms: chest pain, chills, thirst, fatigue, nausea, dizziness, headaches, rapid pulse, elevated blood pressure, difficulty breathing, sweating.
Cognitive signs: confusion, nightmares, hypervigilance, poor problem solving, disorientation, altered alertness, impaired abstract thinking, disorientation.
Behavioral signs: withdrawal, inability to rest, pacing and erratic movement, changes in social activity, loss of appetite, changes in speech patterns.
Emotional signs: excess fear, guilt, or grief; panic; denial; anxiety; agitation; anger; depression.

EMOTIONAL FIRST AID

After a traumatic event such as episodes of war, a hurricane, tornado, fire, or airplane or car crash, individuals will experience an acute stress reaction. Individuals who have been raped, sexually or physically abused, or a victim of a violent crime will also express and acute stress reaction (Table 153.1).

Primary providers, when caring for persons who have sustained acute trauma, can take steps to prevent PTSD. Victims of rape should be offered crisis intervention and counseling. The information given must be honest, adequate, unambiguous, and timely. Victims of a disaster or trauma such as rape need to feel secure. Psychological support, defusing, debriefing, and sometimes psychopharmacologic treatment are needed. Customs and rituals are important in all cultures and assist in the grief and mourning process. They may promote a feeling of safety. Rituals are also carried out within the community, and this helps in expressing feelings and providing a sense of relief. Studies have demonstrated that when people are given the opportunity to talk about their experiences as soon as possible after a catastrophic event, the symptoms of PTSD may be reduced.

Emotional first aid is simple treatment that occurs immediately and in close proximity to the place where the emotional breakdown occurred. The patient is expected to recover quickly. It includes acceptance of feelings and symptoms, identification of resources and activities, realization of the psychologically painful situation and acceptance of reality, optimism, not blaming others, acceptance of help and support, and the resumption of daily life. The way an individual responds to stress depends on their genetic makeup, physical activity, and the normalcy of their sleep–wake cycle.

Persons at high risk for stress-related psychological disorders include survivors with psychiatric problems; close relatives of suddenly or traumatically deceased persons; children, especially if separated from parents; the elderly, mentally retarded, and handicapped; traumatized survivors; and body handlers. For instance, in New York City after September 11, 2001, PTSD was more frequent among those who survived the collapse of the twin towers and who thought they might have done more to help others. Health care professionals and other professionals who waited in vain for the predicted thousands who would be hospitalized also suffered from PTSD.

Although primary physicians are not involved in the ongoing therapy of persons with definite PTSD or with the total psychological therapy of persons at risk of developing it, primary physicians should be alert to the existence of PTSD and dedicated to preventing it.

BIBLIOGRAPHY

Allen SN, Bloom SL. Group and family treatment of post-traumatic stress disorder. *Psychiatr Clin North Am* 1994;17:425.

American College of Obstetrics and Gynecology. *ACOG Today* 2001;45:10:1.

Blank AS Jr. Clinical detection, diagnosis, and differential diagnosis of posttraumatic stress disorder. *Psychiatr Clin North Am* 1994;17:351.

Harvard Mahoney Neuroscience Institute Letter. *Stress and the Brain* 8:3:1–3. Fall 2001/Winter 2002.

Lundin T. The treatment of acute trauma: post-traumatic stress disorder prevention. *Psychiatr Clin North Am* 1994;17:385.

McFarlane AC. Individual psychotherapy for post-traumatic stress disorder. *Psychiatr Clin North Am* 1994;17:393.

National Institute of Mental Health. Facts about Post-Traumatic Stress Disorder. www.nimh.nih.gov/anxiety/ptsdfacts.cfm. Accessed January 12, 2003.

Sutherland SM, Davidson, JRT. Pharmacotherapy for post-traumatic stress disorder. *Psychiatr Clin North Am* 1994;17:409.

Tomb DA. The phenomenology of post-traumatic stress disorder. *Psychiatr Clin North Am* 1994;17:237.

Subject Index

Page numbers followed by f indicate figures; those followed by t indicate tabular material.

X

Y

Z